Introducing CourseCare from Cengage Learning

Available exclusively to Cengage Learning, **CourseCare** is a revolutionary program designed to provide you and your students with an unparalleled user experience with your Cengage Learning Digital Solution.

Digital solutions experts provide you with one-on-one service every step of the way—from finding the right solution for your course to training to ongoing support—helping you to drive student engagement.

Over 12,000 instructors have experienced CourseCare. Here is what they are saying...

- **100%** agree that the trainer was knowledgeable.
- **96%** agree the training was relevant.
- **95%** agree they would recommend the **CourseCare** training to a colleague
- **93%** agree that because of **CourseCare** they are more likely to suggest their colleagues use a Cengage Learning digital solution.

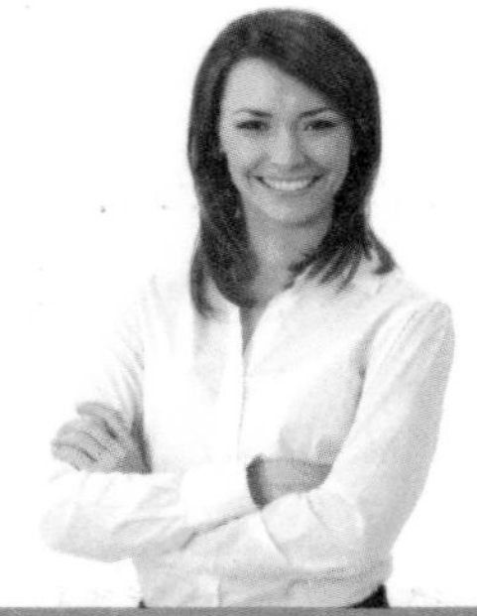

Digital Solutions Managers & Sales Representatives

Your Digital Solutions Manager and Sales Representative partner with you to understand your unique needs and provide you with the right digital solution to meet your goals. They continue to work with you, ensuring that your Cengage Learning Digital Solution keeps pace as your course evolves.

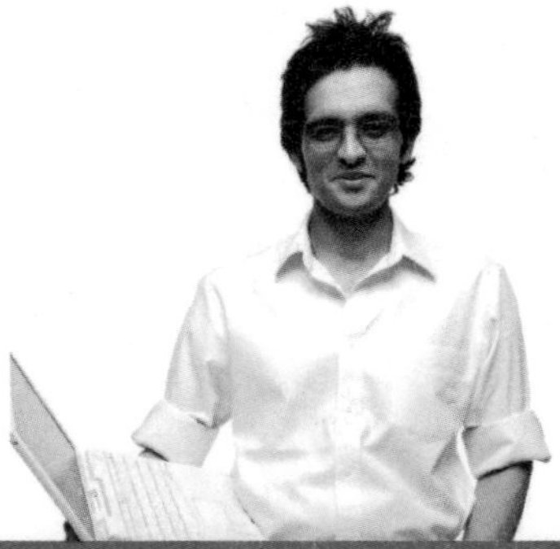

Service & Training Consultants

Your Service and Training Consultant provides professional training on your digital solution that is flexible to meet the demands of your busy schedule. Online or face-to-face, we can work with you to deliver a highly customized training program designed to meet your specific needs and requirements.

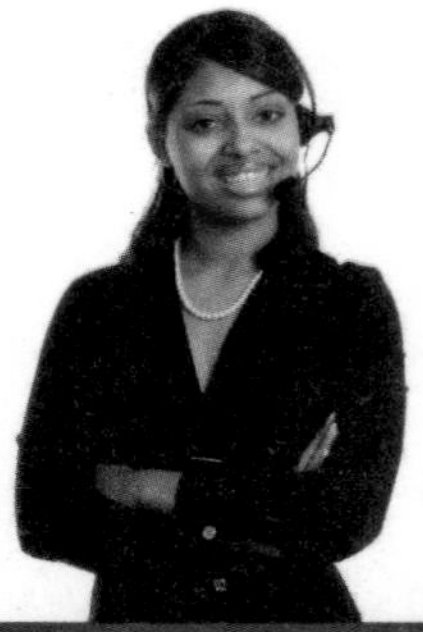

Digital Solutions Coordinators

Your Digital Solutions Coordinator is your dedicated resource, assuring that your course has a smooth start and stays on target to meet your goals. From set-up to student activation and usage reports, your Digital Solutions Coordinator ensures that you and your students are getting the full benefit of your Cengage Learning Digital Solution.

Explore your Medical Assisting options at: **www.cengage.com/coursecare**
or contact your Cengage Learning representative for more information.

www.cengage.com/coursecare

source code: 12M-HC0133

EDITION 7

Medical Assisting

Administrative and Clinical Competencies

Michelle Blesi, MA, BA, CMA(AAMA)
Program Director, Medical Assisting
Century College – East Campus
White Bear Lake, MN

Barbara A. Wise, RN, BSN, MA (Ed)

Cathy Kelley-Arney, BSHS, MLT-C

DELMAR
CENGAGE Learning™

Australia • Brazil • Japan • Korea • Mexico • Singapore • Spain • United Kingdom • United States

DELMAR
CENGAGE Learning

Medical Assisting: Administrative and Clinical Competencies, Seventh Edition
Michelle Blesi, Barbara A. Wise, Cathy Kelley-Arney

Vice President, Editorial: Dave Garza
Director of Learning Solutions: Matthew Kane
Executive Editor: Rhonda Dearborn
Managing Editor: Marah Bellegarde
Senior Product Manager: Sarah Prime
Editorial Assistant: Lauren Whalen
Vice President, Marketing: Jennifer Baker
Marketing Director: Wendy E. Mapstone
Senior Marketing Manager: Nancy Bradshaw
Senior Production Director: Wendy A. Troeger
Production Manager: Andrew Crouth
Content Project Manager: Thomas Heffernan
Senior Art Director: Jack Pendleton
Senior Technology Product Manager: Mary Colleen Liburdi

Library of Congress Control Number: 2011926859

ISBN-13: 978-1-111-13512-6

ISBN-10: 1-111-13512-6

Delmar
Executive Woods
5 Maxwell Drive
Clifton Park, NY 12065
USA

Cengage Learning is a leading provider of customized learning solutions with office locations around the globe, including Singapore, the United Kingdom, Australia, Mexico, Brazil, and Japan. Locate your local office at **www.cengage.com/global**

Cengage Learning products are represented in Canada by Nelson Education, Ltd.

To learn more about Delmar, visit **www.cengage.com/delmar**

Purchase any of our products at your local bookstore or at our preferred online store **www.cengagebrain.com**

Printed in the United States of America
5 6 7 17 16 15

THIS EDITION IS DEDICATED TO BARBARA A. WISE

Barb was a wonderful colleague, mentor, and friend. She had a real passion for helping others and loved to see those less fortunate prosper. I met her through Connie Krebs (one of the original coauthors of this text), who mentored me until her death. After, Barb graciously stepped in and continued to provide me with guidance and support.

Barb's love for education was the driving force in creating this quality textbook. She was a wonderful writer who enjoyed sharing her knowledge. She always challenged me to take my writing to a higher level and to never settle for mediocrity. And, her marvelous wit kept us all smiling!

She is gone, but will never be forgotten. Her words will live on for many years to come!

Michelle Heller,
Colleague and Contributor to the Seventh Edition

I feel lucky to have worked with Barb on two editions of this book.

Professionally, I knew her as someone who always did her research, submitted thorough manuscripts, listened to (almost) everything I suggested, and never missed a deadline. Personally, she became a dear friend. I knew her to be tireless in every aspect of her life, generous and devoted to her family and friends.

She started writing the first edition of this book in 1983 with two colleagues, and has been the driving force behind all seven editions. She was meticulous and diligent—she took every reviewer comment to heart and hired accuracy checkers for every chapter she wrote. She wanted the book to be as appealing as possible, in content, format, and graphics.

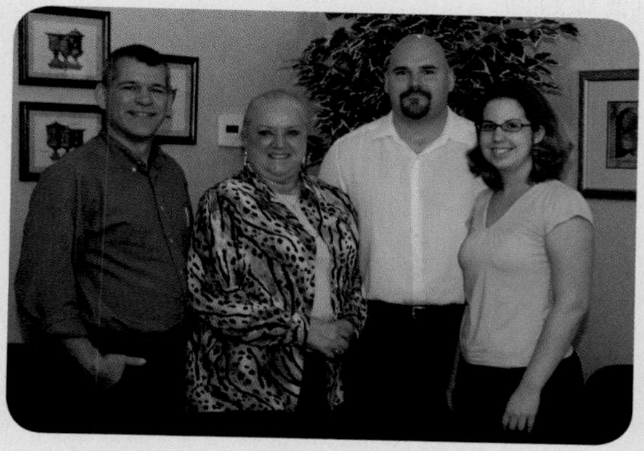

Posing for a picture during the photo shoot for the sixth edition. Left to right: Tom Stock (photographer), Barbara Wise, Jack Pendleton (Senior Art Director), Sarah Prime. *Delmar/Cengage Learning.*

Barb often told me that she was surprised at the success of the book; I always replied that I wasn't. I'll miss her style and humor, and will never forget her spirit and passion.

Sarah Prime,
Senior Product Manager

As the Editor for Medical Assisting, I feel privileged to have worked, laughed and learned from Barb. She has shared her drive for knowledge with several generations of Medical Assisting students and educators. She had a passion for life and for learning. Her imprint on Medical Assisting education will be felt for generations to come.

Rhonda Dearborn,
Executive Acquisitions Editor

Brief Contents

Contents

Procedures

How to Use the Text:

A Guided Walkthrough

Certification Connection

	Ch. 3	Ch. 4
CMA (AAMA)		
Word building and definitions	X	X
Uses of terminology		X
RMA (AMT)		
Word parts	X	X
Definitions	X	X
Common abbreviations		X
Spelling	X	
CMAS (AMT)		
Use and spell basic medical terms appropriately	X	X
Identify root words, prefixes, and suffixes	X	X
Define basic medical terms	X	X

Certification Connection. At the beginning of each unit, this element draws a link from text content to certification exams from the American Association of Medical Assistants (AAMA) and American Medical Technologists (AMT).

Chapter 37

The Medical History and Patient Screening

CHAPTER OBJECTIVES

In this chapter, you will learn the following:

KB KNOWLEDGE BASE

1. Spell and define, using the glossary at the back of this text, all the Words to Know in this chapter.
2. Explain the purpose of screening in today's medical office.
3. Describe the process for screening and determining the urgency of a patient's condition.
4. Identify the skills necessary to conduct a patient interview.
5. List the characteristics of the patient's chief complaint and the present illness.
6. Explain the purpose of ob
7. Identify the components and their documentation.
8. Compare and contrast the and social and occupational
9. Discuss the genogram and explain why it is useful.
10. Explain how the review of systems is obtained and documented.

Chapter Objectives. Chapter objectives are presented at the beginning of each chapter and are categorized according to Knowledge Base, Skills, and Behaviors curriculum standards.

S SKILLS

1. Perform in-person screening.
2. Obtain and record a patient health history.

B BEHAVIORS

1. Demonstrate professionalism by being courteous and diplomatic; showing respect, empathy, and cultural sensitivity; maintaining privacy and confidentiality; and adapting to change.
2. Apply critical thinking skills in performing patient assessment and care.
3. Use language and verbal skills that enable patients' understanding and appropriate, congruent body language and other nonverbal skills.
4. Apply active listening skills.
5. Demonstrate awareness of the territorial boundaries of the person with whom communicating.
6. Demonstrate recognition of the patient's level of understanding in communications.
7. Analyze communications in providing appropriate responses and feedback.
8. Recognize and protect personal boundaries in communicating with others.
9. Demonstrate sensitivity to patient rights
10. Use time management

WORDS TO KNOW

allergies
biases
chief complaint (CC)
clinical diagnosis
emergent
familial
genogram
interview
objective
over-the-counter (OTC)
patronizing
prioritizing
remedies

Words to Know. Key terms and ideas are presented in a list at the beginning of each chapter and are highlighted the first time they appear. A glossary are included at the end of the text.

- **Essential Coverage of Anatomy and Physiology.** In Chapters 23–35, the structure and function of each body system is followed by a discussion of the common diagnostic examinations and diseases and disorders of that system. To facilitate learning, an expanded outline format organizes the description, signs and symptoms, etiology, and treatment for each disease. New features in this section include *Body System Interrelationships* and *Age-Related Body System Characteristics.*

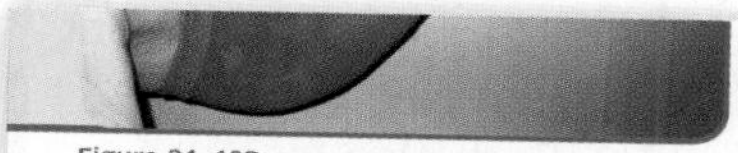

Figure 31–10B: Compression sleeve and glove. *Courtesy of Barbara A. Wise.*

Rheumatoid Arthritis (Room′-a-toyd Ar-thri′-tis)

Description—This chronic systemic inflammatory autoimmune disease affects the joints and surrounding muscles, tendons, ligaments, and blood vessels. It affects women three times more often than men. It occurs primarily between the ages of 20 and 60, with a peak onset period between 35 to 45.

Signs and symptoms—The symptoms develop insidiously, then become localized in joints, usually bilaterally. Following inactivity, the affected joints stiffen, swell, and

AGE-RELATED BODY CHARACTERISTICS

The immune system decreases in effectiveness as we age. When born, passive immunity is transmitted from the mother to the infant. This is increased even more by the passing antibodies through breast milk. By 18 months this immunity has waned. Routine immunizations given to infants and children provide immunity to the usual childhood diseases as well as previous life threatening diseases. People with compromised immune systems, chronic diseases, or certain risk factors, as well as the aged, are routinely given a flu vaccine as a means of providing a short term resistance to influenza. The elderly and other people with chronic conditions are given a pneumonia vaccine to provide resistance to that disease. As we have just read, some new vaccines may influence the immune system to prevent us from initially developing certain cancers or many prohibit recurrence.

- **Example** boxes appear throughout the book but, especially, in application chapters such as those that contain medical terminology and dosage calculations.

EXAMPLE

Practice defining and building medical terms associated with the special senses.

A. Define ***ophthalmologist***.

Step 1: Start with the suffix, *-logist*, meaning "one who studies."
Step 2: Identify the prefix. There is no prefix.
Step 3: Identify the combining form, *ophthalm/o*, meaning "eyes."

Putting it all together, the definition is "one who studies or specializes in the eyes" (a term given to a medical doctor for this field).

B. Build a medical term that means "***a condition of tiny or small ear***."

Step 1: Start with the suffix, *-ia*, "condition (of)."
Step 2: Identify the prefix, *micro-*, "tiny or small."
Step 3: Identify the combining form, *ot/o*, "ear."

Putting it all together, *micro-* + *ot/o* + *-ia* becomes "microtia."

Without these changes, the resulting word would have been "microotoia."

Table 4–9 lists and defines the combining forms, prefixes, and suffixes related to the special senses.

THE REPRODUCTIVE SYSTEM

There are separate reproductive systems for the male and female. Each system has its own associated terms.

The reproductive system is responsible for enabling the human race to reproduce and perpetuate the species through new birth. Thus, this section introduces terms not just specific to the reproductive system but also to human development from fertilization through birth.

The primary structure associated with the female reproductive tract is the ovary (of which there are two); the remaining structures are accessory organs. Included in these accessory organs are the uterus, the fallopian or uterine tubes, the vagina, and external accessory organs such as the female breasts. Combining forms associated with this system are deeply rooted in Greek and Latin terms, making it more difficult to remember and memorize the terms.

The primary structure in the male reproductive system is the testis (of which there are two); the remaining

communicate in the most efficient and effective manner for each individual. Patients may be shy or embarrassed by their problems or questions and may not ask and answer direct questions. Therefore, excellent listening skills are vital to understanding what the patient is trying to convey. Be familiar with information about the patient before proceeding with an explanation. This will help determine how to communicate best with each individual.

CLINICAL PEARL

Never assume that a patient already knows the information you are conveying. Sometimes a patient will state that he or she understands something to keep from being embarrassed. If you sense that this is the situation, you should briefly repeat the information to ensure that you are receiving the information accurately.

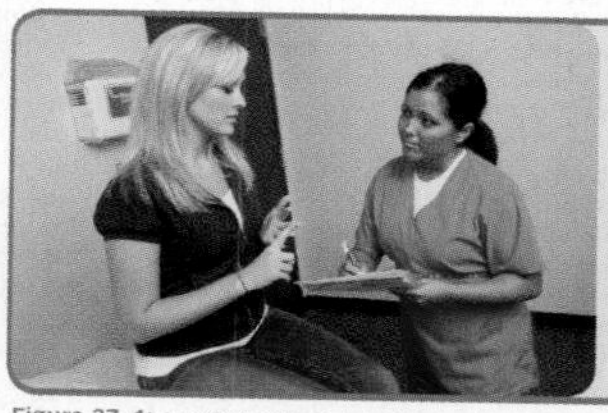

Figure 37–1: A medical assistant and patient are in a private area discussing symptoms and assessing the patient's condition. This is called in-person screening. *Delmar/Cengage Learning*

- **Clinical Pearls** are short, straightforward pieces of advice based on experience or observation. These boxes bridge the gap between text material and the real world, highlighting key practical activities that must be performed on the job.

- **Media Links** connect procedures and text to corresponding video or animation content on the Premium Website.

versatile allied health occupations in today's health care environment. American Medical Technologists (AMT)—a certifying organization for medical assistants—describes the medical assistant as "an integral member of the health care delivery team, qualified by education and experience to work in the administrative office, the examining room and the physician office laboratory. The medical assistant is also a liaison between the doctor and the patient and is of vital importance to the success of the medical practice."

To become a successful medical assistant, you

MEDIA LINK

View the video, "Qualities of a Successful Medical Assistant," for this chapter on the Premium website

Skills and Responsibilities of the Medical Assistant

As health care progresses, so do the skills and responsibilities of the medical assistant. The field of medical

- **Patient Education** boxes present important issues to discuss with patients before and during tests and examinations.

PATIENT EDUCATION

The medical assistant is often involved in patient education, which can include supplying information about diseases and disorders, explaining diagnostic tests, and providing instruction in health care procedures. Recording the patient's health history may identify areas in which educational materials can be helpful. Your office policy may make it appropriate for you to mention these resources. To instruct a patient properly, the medical assistant must know the material. Be prepared to answer any questions from the patient. If you cannot answer one of the patient's questions, tell the patient that you do not know the answer but will ask the physician. Never try to answer a question that you are not prepared to discuss. You could give incorrect information that could harm the patient's well-being. Never give information that is beyond your scope of practice. In teaching a patient about health care and all that is involved in medical well-being, the primary goal of the medical assistant should be good communication. Refer to Chapter 8 for more on patient education and detailed information about instructing patients according to their needs.

PROCEDURE 54–6 Administer an Intramuscular Injection

MEDIA LINK: View the animation, "Intramuscular Injection Animation," on the Premium Website for this chapter

PURPOSE: To inject large amounts of medication, 0.5 mL to 3.0 mL, and oil-based substances or irritating solutions that are more easily tolerated in the muscle tissue

EQUIPMENT: Medication (sterile water for injection in vial or ampule), cotton balls, alcohol prep, adhesive bandage or hypoallergenic tape, sterile needle (usually 1 to 3 inches, 18G to 23G), medication tray, patient's chart, pen, gloves

S SKILL: Prepare, verify, and administer proper doses of medications for intramuscular injections.

S SKILL: Demonstrate appropriate aseptic technique as it applies to medication administration.

S SKILL: Demonstrate proper disposal of used syringes and needles.

Procedure Steps	Detailed Instructions and/or *Rationales*
1. Wash and glove hands.	
B 2. Prepare the syringe with the ordered amount of medication, ***verifying all ordered doses or dosages prior to administration.***	Read the label of the medication and compare it with the order.
B 3. Identify the patient and explain the procedure, ***using language the patient understands.*** Ask patient to remove clothes, if necessary.	Identify the patient by using two identifiers. Compare the medication order (again) with the patient's chart.
B 4. Allow the patient to ask questions ***and show awareness of any patient concerns regarding the procedure.*** Respond to the patient as appropriate.	
5. Select and prepare the injection site with an alcohol prep. Allow the alcohol to air dry.	Do not blow on the area to dry the alcohol. *The area may be contaminated by microorganisms in the exhaled air.*
6. Secure a large area of skin (to accommodate the large amount of medication) between the thumb and finger of one hand and, with the other hand, hold the syringe securely. Insert the needle at a 90-degree angle with a steady penetration. Let go of the skin.	
7. With one hand, hold the barrel of the syringe while pulling back on the plunger slightly with the other hand to make sure a blood vessel has not been penetrated. If no blood appears in the syringe, proceed by slowly pushing down on the plunger to expel medication into the muscle.	If blood appears in the syringe, pull the needle out carefully at the angle of entry. *Blood in the needle indicates the possibility of the needle placement being within a blood vessel. Medication injected directly into the bloodstream caus[...] undesirable as well a[...]* medication, syringe, [...] syringe and medicatio[...]
8. Remove the needle quickly by the same angle of injection and wipe the site with a cotton ball. Gently massage the area.	*Massaging helps distr[...] tissues.*

Step-by-Step Procedures. Each procedure starts with Purpose, Equipment and Supplies, Skill reference, and Media Link (if applicable). Each also includes step-by-step instructions in one column with additional detail and rationales next to each step. Affective (behavior) steps are called out with special icons and color. Documentation examples follow procedures where appropriate.

Chapter Summaries. Now in bulleted format, these summaries recall the main knowledge base objectives within the chapter.

CHAPTER SUMMARY

- The field of medical assisting is one of the most versatile allied health occupations in today's health care environment. The majority of medical assistants work in ambulatory care settings or outpatient health care facilities.
- Medical assistants may work with physicians in a sole proprietorship (solo practice), in a partnership (two or more physicians), or in a multi-provider clinic (group practices with three or more physicians). Other health care environments include urgent care centers and the patient-centered medical home model.
- The three main areas of medical assisting are general, administrative, and clinical. *General skills* include communication skills, legal matters, instruction, and operational functions. *Administrative skills* include scheduling appointments, working with medical records, insurance and coding, billing and collections, and bookkeeping. *Clinical skills* include aseptic technique, minor surgery, collecting, pro-

on the phone (except in emergencies), insurance forms should be filed in chronological order, record requests for next-day surgeries should be sent to the surgery center ASAP, and deposits must be made every day.

- Priority level for working the floor should be as follows: (1) assisting the provider with emergencies and other procedures, (2) rooming patients, (3) performing procedures, and (4) working on pending tasks.
- American Association of Medical Assistants (AAMA) offers the CMA (AAMA) credential, continuing education opportunities, the publication *CMA Today*, and other services. Members must recertify every five years.
- American Medical Technologists (AMT) offers the RMA (AMT) credential and the CMAS (AMT) credential, continuing education opportunities, and the publications *AMT Events* and *CE Journal of CE Topics and Issues*. The organization offers certifica-

Study Tools. At the end of each chapter, reinforce your understanding of the concepts covered through activities in the Workbook, Premium Website, Learning Lab, CourseMate, and Web Tutor. Use this element as a study plan and checklist to get the most out of the entire learning package.

STUDY TOOLS

Workbook	Activities for Chapter 1
Premium Website	
MEDIA LINK	View this **Media Link** for Chapter 1: • Qualities of a Successful Medical Assistant
StudyWARE	**StudyWARE™ Software** with quizzes and activities for Chapter 1
	Audio Library of medical terms
	Online access to **Critical Thinking Challenge 2.0**
CourseMate	Activities and Quizzes for Chapter 1
WebTutor	Activities and Quizzes for Chapter 1

Check Your Knowledge Review. Solidify your understanding of the chapter through certification-style review questions.

CHECK YOUR KNOWLEDGE

1. To be successful as an MA, you must learn a specific:
   a. Knowledge base
   b. Set of skills
   c. Behaviors
   d. All the above
2. All of the following are clinical skills EXCEPT:
   a. Filing patient records
   b. Phlebotomy
   c. Administering medications
   d. Wrapping instruments
3. Medical assistants who perform both clinical and administrative skills are referred to as:
   a. Survivalists
   b. Capitalists

7. Which of the following would take priority over all other floor tasks?
   a. Rooming patients
   b. Performing procedures
   c. Tasking
   d. Assisting the provider with a procedure
8. Which of the following organizations provides the RMA credential?
   a. AAMA
   b. AMT
   c. AAPC
   d. NHA
9. Which of the following organizations' focus is primarily on certifying medical billers and coders?

Preface

Medical Assisting: Administrative and Clinical Competencies, Seventh Edition is a proven, competency-based learning system with a 25-year history of success. It is written in an interesting, easy-to-understand format and covers the knowledge, skills, behaviors, and values necessary to prepare you to become a thriving, multi-skilled medical assistant. It can be used in a variety of settings:

- For a structured classroom setting, with the expertise of a qualified instructor
- For individualized instruction of learning in programs of diversified training because much of the content and format are appropriate for self-study
- For on-the-job training in a provider's office, where the learning package serves as a supplement to employee instruction and as a resource manual
- For review by medical assistants who wish to prepare for the certification exam

Information is presented in five major sections: foundational knowledge, front office tasks, anatomy and physiology, back office tasks, and preparing for employment. These sections are further divided into 20 units with 59 chapters.

RENEWED, REFRESHED, AND REINVENTED

The entire learning system—which includes a variety of print and digital components for all learner types—is designed to be an interactive guide as you embark on a career in medical assisting. The Seventh Edition has been renewed, refreshed, and reinvented to make it even more accessible and innovative for today's dynamic health care environment:

- *Chapters and Content:* Major reorganization of units and chapters to streamline material; new chapters on the Physician's Office Laboratory (Chapter 44) and Dosage Calculations (Chapter 52)
- *New Feature Elements:* Media Links, Clinical Pearls, Examples, Study Tools
- *Skills and Procedures:* More than 25 new procedures
- *Today's Topics and Trends:* Some of the new topics include scope of practice, emergency preparedness and safety, ICD-10, and basic math and dosage calculations. (A complete list of new topics follows in the next section.)
- *Procedure Layout:* Easily identify affective (behavior) curriculum standards through special icons; also includes procedure steps with side-by-side rationales, detailed instructions, and documentation examples
- *Chapter Objectives and Summaries:* Objectives are presented in categories of Knowledge Base, Skills, and Behavior; summaries now in bulleted formatting
- *Curriculum Correlations:* To meet the latest curriculum standards for medical assisting programmatic accreditation, mapping tools are included in text Procedures, Workbook Competency Checklists, and the Instructor's Manual.
- *Innovative Technology:* Premium Website content, Learning Labs, CourseMate, and Web Tutor ancillaries provide engaging and useful learning experiences. Read more about these digital solutions in the Comprehensive Learning System section.

NEW TOPICS IN THE SEVENTH EDITION

Unit 1

- Professionalism, time management skills, and personal appearance
- New Procedure: Display Professionalism
- Professional organizations: National Center for Competency Testing
- Alternatives to the traditional medical model and related medical therapies

Unit 2

- New placement of medical terminology chapters to come earlier in the text
- More focus on medical terminology word building, with numerous examples

Unit 3

- Sources of law
- Medical assistant scope of practice
- Patient Self-Determination Act
- American Medical Technologists' Standards of Practice
- Differentiating legal, ethical, and moral issues
- Personal, professional, and organization ethics
- Personal ethics and professional performance
- Reporting illegal and unsafe behavior

Unit 4

- New Procedure: Respond to Nonverbal Communication
- Fundamentals of psychology, including Maslow's hierarchy of needs and Kübler-Ross's five stages of grief
- Adaptive and nonadaptive coping skills
- Self-awareness
- Critical thinking skills
- Communicating with diverse patient populations
- New Procedure: Instruct Patients According to Their Needs
- New Procedure: Advocate on Behalf of Patients

Unit 5

- New Procedure: Perform a Telephone Screening
- New Procedure: Call a Patient with Test Results
- Community resources
- New Procedure: Create a List of Resources for Patient Health Care Needs
- New Procedure: Create a List of Resources for Emergency Preparedness
- Ergonomics and computer use
- Practice management software
- Electronic health records software
- Guidelines for evaluating Internet resources

Unit 6

- New Procedure: Receive Patients
- New Procedure: Explain Office Policies
- Electronic health records
- CHEDDAR chart note format

Unit 7

- New Procedure: Verify Insurance Coverage
- New Procedure: Obtain a Managed Care Referral and Precertification
- Diagnostic-related groups
- CPT coding rules
- ICD-10-CM and ICD-10-PCS
- Electronic coding

Unit 8

- Single-entry and double-entry bookkeeping
- Computerized bookkeeping
- Filing paper claims
- Clearinghouses
- Posting insurance payments
- Explanation of benefits and remittance advice
- New Procedure: Apply Insurance Payments and Adjustments to Patient Accounts
- Billing secondary insurance
- Computerized billing
- Posting patient payments
- New Procedure: Post an NSF Check
- Credit balances and refunds
- Collections laws

Unit 9

- Direct deposit for bank deposits
- Basic accounting formulae (A/R ratio, collections ratio, cost ratio)
- Cost analysis
- Financial records

Unit 10

- New Procedure: Open the Office and Evaluate for Safety
- Safety signs, symbols, and labels
- Material safety data sheets
- New Procedure: Clean a Spill
- Personal safety
- New Procedure: Fire Preparedness
- Emergency preparedness and evacuation
- New Procedure: Develop a Safety Plan for Emergency Preparedness
- New Procedure: Prepare Employee Payroll

Unit 11

- Body structure and function across the life span, for each body system
- Interrelationships of body systems table
- Age-related characteristics boxed elements

Unit 12

- New Procedure: Sanitize an Instrument
- New Procedure: Disinfect an Instrument
- New Procedure: Patient Positioning

Unit 13

- Respiratory examinations
- New Procedure: Pulse Oximetry
- New Procedure: Plot Data on a Growth Chart

Unit 14

- Chapter 43 combines all blood collection material into one chapter
- Order of draw
- New Chapter 44 with CLIA and categories of testing, safety in the POL, and POL guidelines
- New Procedure: Perform Hemoglobin A1C Screening
- Wound cultures

Unit 15

- Chapter 48 combines all radiology material into one chapter

Unit 16

- Chapter 49 focuses on preparing for surgery (previously two units)
- Surgical asepsis
- New Procedure: Surgical Scrub
- Positioning the patient for surgery
- Draping

Unit 17

- Additional drug references besides the PDR
- Handling medications in the medical office
- Systems of measurement
- New Chapter 52, a review of basic math and dosage calculations
- Chapter 52 is reorganized to group all oral and non-injectable medication
- New Procedure: Call in a Complete and Accurate Prescription to a Pharmacy
- The Seven Rights of medication administration
- New Procedure: Record a Medication Entry in the Patient's Chart
- Chapter 54 is reorganized to focus on injections and immunizations only
- Documenting injections
- Patient preparation and documentation of immunizations

Unit 18

- Chapter 55 combines several units from the previous edition to refocus chapter on medical emergencies
- Office policy manual and documentation
- Responding to an emergency
- Documenting emergencies
- CPR
- Documenting CPR and AED procedures

Unit 19

- Body mechanics and ergonomics
- 2010 Dietary Guidelines for Americans
- 2011 MyPlate program

Unit 20

- Practicum content refocused to discuss how the student should act, dress, and behave
- Starting your job search
- Interviewing and interview follow-up
- New Procedure: Write a Thank-You Letter Following an Interview

COMPLETE LEARNING SYSTEM: STUDENT SUPPLEMENTS

Workbook

(ISBN 978-1-1111-3514-0)

Explore the text content through Words to Know Challenges, Review Questions, and Application Activities for each chapter. The Workbook has been fully revised to align with the content in the seventh edition. Use the Competency Checklist section to evaluate performance of the text procedures and map to specific ABHES and CAAHEP curriculum standards.

The Competency Checklists have been completely reformatted to match the text procedures exactly and provide instruction to download the specific material needed to complete the procedure. New Procedure Forms can be downloaded from the Premium Website, and Scenario Information for procedures can be found in the Instructor's Manual.

Competency Checklist
Procedure 36–1: Complete an Incident Exposure Report

ABHES Curriculum

MA.A.1.4.e	Perform risk management procedures
MA.A.1.4.f	Comply with federal, state, and local health laws and regulations

CAAHEP Core Curriculum

IX.P.6	Complete an incident report
IX.P.8	Apply local, state, and federal health care legislation and regulation appropriate to the medical assisting practice setting

Task:	To provide documentation required by OSHA in the event an employee becomes injured or is exposed to blood or body fluids. A post-exposure plan must be followed and an incident report must be filled out.
Supplies & Conditions:	OSHA Form 301 (Injury and Illness Incident Report), pen.
Standards:	A maximum of three attempts may be used to complete the task. The time limit for each attempt is 15 minutes, with a minimum score of 70%. **Scoring:** Determine student's score by dividing points awarded by total points possible and multiplying results by 100.
Forms:	Procedure 36–1 Scenario with Procedure 36–1 Form. Procedure forms can be downloaded from the Premium Website; procedure scenarios are included in the Instructor's Manual.

Premium Website

(www.cengagebrain.com)

This robust, password-protected website is designed to maximize learning in providing a multimedia approach to learning the concepts presented in this text. Follow the directions on the printed access card to log on at www.cengagebrain.com. In the student resources:

- Use the **Media Link** library to view the videos and animations referenced in the text.
- Download the **Procedure Forms** needed to complete the Competency Checklists. The forms can be completed electronically and saved or printed and completed manually.
- Practice chapter concepts with the **StudyWARE™ Software** (described later in this section).
- Practice your pronunciation and recognition of medical terms by using the **Audio Library**; you may search for terms by word or body system.
- Use **Mobile Downloads** of Spanish or English glossary terms for practice.

- Complete the popular **Critical Thinking Challenge 2.0** and **Competency Challenge 2.0** programs (described later in this section).

StudyWARE™ Software

StudyWARE™ is interactive software included with many of Delmar Cengage Learning's products and lets you have fun while increasing knowledge. Learning activities and quizzes correlating to each chapter of the text helps you study key concepts and test your comprehension with immediate feedback.

- Activities include Championship, Maze, and Flash Cards
- Anatomy & Physiology image labeling and spelling bee games
- Surgical Instruments flash cards
- Dosage Calculation & Basic Math tutorials

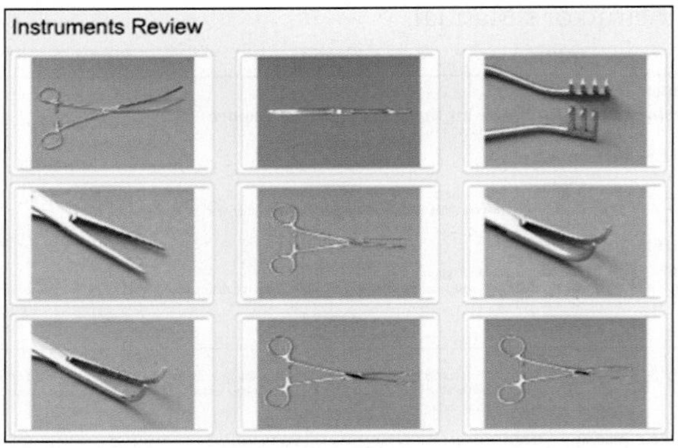

Critical Thinking Challenge 2.0

In the Critical Thinking Challenge 2.0, you are working in a medical office during your practicum. You will be confronted with a series of situations in which you must use your critical thinking skills to choose the most appropriate action in response to the situation. Your decisions will be evaluated in three categories: how they affect the practice, the patient, and your career. The 2.0 version includes 10 video-based scenarios with more branching options. After successfully completing the program, print out a Certification of Completion.

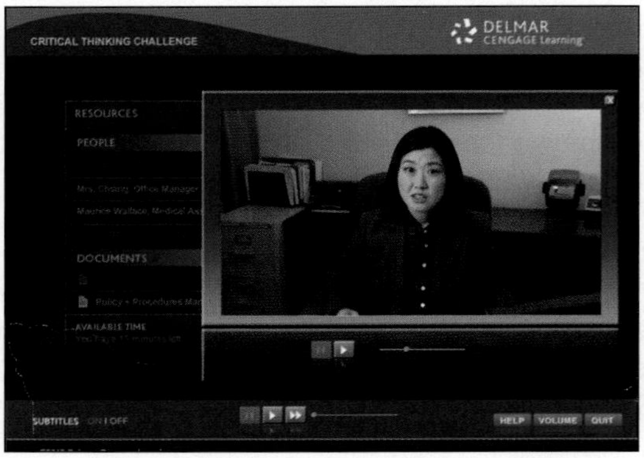

Competency Challenge 2.0

Simulating a "Week in the Life" of a medical assistant, Competency Challenge 2.0 includes video-based case studies that provide an opportunity to test your knowledge and understanding of the educational competencies for the medical assistant. The 2.0 version features interactive activities, better assessment, and printable quiz scores and competency checklist. Monday through Thursday focuses on 26 video-based case studies with interactive exercises; Friday is a capstone event that applies the competencies practice to a realistic patient case study.

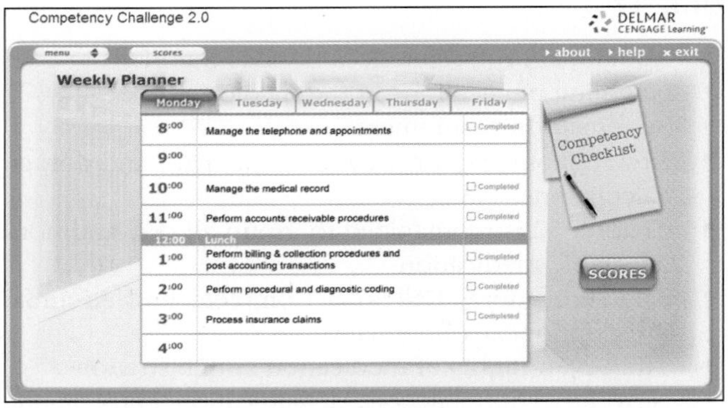

Learning Lab

(ISBN 978-1-1331-2736-9 or 978-1-1331-2735-2)

Learning Lab maps to learning objectives and includes interactive activities and case scenarios to build students' critical thinking skills and help retain the more difficult concepts. This simulated, immersive environment engages users with its real-life approach. Each Learning Lab has a pre-assessment, three to five learning activities, and post-assessment organized around the units in this text. The post-assessment scores can be posted to the instructor grade book in any learning management system. The amount of time the student spends within the Learning Lab can also be tracked.

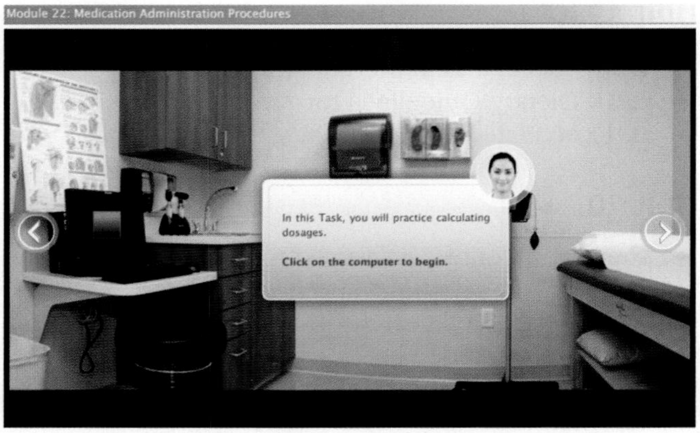

CourseMate

(ISBN 978-1-133-28264-8 or 978-1-133-28263-1)

CourseMate helps you make the grade with several components: (1) an interactive eBook, with highlighting, note taking, and search capabilities; (2) interactive learning tools, including quizzes, flashcards, videos, games, and presentations; and (3) Engagement Tracker, a first-of-its-kind tool that monitors student engagement in the course. Go to www.cengagebrain.com to access these resources and look for this icon CourseMate, which denotes a resource available within CourseMate.

COMPLETE LEARNING SYSTEM: INSTRUCTOR SUPPLEMENTS

Instructor's Manual

(ISBN 978-1-1111-3513-3)

The Instructor's Manual provides mapping to ABHES and CAAHEP curriculum, lesson outlines, suggestions for classroom activities, answer keys for the text and Workbook, and Procedure Scenario information to complete the Competency Checklists. Additionally, find information about using the Critical Thinking Challenge 2.0 and the Competency Challenge 2.0 in your course.

Instructor Resources

(ISBN 978-1-1111-3516-4)

Spend less time planning and more time teaching with Delmar Cengage Learning's Instructor Resources. As an instructor, you'll find this CD-ROM offers invaluable assistance by giving you access to all your resources anywhere at any time. Features of the Instructor Resources CD-ROM include:

- A Computerized Test Bank in ExamView with more than 2,600 questions. Each question contains a reference to the text page number and ABHES and CAAHEP curriculum standard.
- Instructor presentation slides created in Microsoft® PowerPoint for each chapter.
- An Image Library of more than 500 images from the text.
- Customizable Instructor's Manual files.

Instructor Companion Site

(Access at www.cengage.com/login)

Log on to the Instructor Companion Site to gain access to CourseForward Curriculum (described in more detail later in this section). In addition, access all the resources found on the Instructor Resources CD-ROM (presentation slides, Test Bank, Image Library, and Instructor's Manual) and all content on the student Premium Website. Access at www.cengage.com/login with your Cengage instructor account. If you are a first-time user, click Create a New Faculty Account and follow the prompts.

CourseForward Curriculum

CourseForward is a modular curriculum solution that breaks down content into topics for ease of learning and serves as a roadmap for course material. CourseForward is designed for instructors to spend less time planning and more time teaching. Some of the features of CourseForward include equipment lists, homework assignments, in-class discussion topics and suggested responses, individual and group activities, and chapter content mapped to activities and assignments.

WebTutor™ Course Cartridge

(Blackboard ISBN 978-1-1111-3523-2)
(Angel ISBN 978-1-1111-3518-8)
(WebCT ISBN 978-1-1116-4005-7)

WebTutor™ is an Internet-based course management and delivery system designed to accompany this text. Its content is available for use in Blackboard, Angel, and WebCT. Available to supplement on-campus course delivery or as the course management platform for an online course, features of the WebTutor™ include:

- Online quizzes for each chapter
- Online glossary
- Slide presentations in Microsoft® PowerPoint
- Communication tools, including a course calendar, chat, email, and threaded discussions

Contributors

Yvonne Burbrink, BS, RMA(AMT)
Curriculum Manager
Medical Assistant Program
Corinthian Colleges
Santa Ana, CA
Unit 20: Workplace Readiness

Virginia Busey Ferrari, BA, MHA
Adjunct Professor
Business, Computer Science and Career Technical Education
Solano Community College
Fairfield, CA
Unit 4: Professional Communications
Unit 5: Business Communications
Unit 10: Managing the Medical Office Environment

Cecile R. Favreau, MBA, CPC
Professional Relations Specialist
UMass Memorial Medical Group
Adjunct Faculty Member at Salter College
West Boylston, MA
Unit 7: Medical Insurance and Coding

Michelle Heller, CMA(AAMA), RMA(AMT)
Adjunct Faculty Member
Columbus State Community College
Columbus, OH
Unit 1: Health Care Roles and Responsibilities

Brina Hollis, PhD
Director Healthcare Programs–Cleveland Market
Bryant & Stratton College
Parma, OH
Unit 16: Minor Surgery Procedures

Sherri Mason, RN, BSN, LNCC
Unit 6: Beginning the Patient's Record
Unit 17: Medication Administration Procedures

Michael R. Meacham, JD, MPH
Associate Professor
Department of Health Leadership and Management
Medical University of South Carolina
Charleston, SC
Unit 3: Medical Law and Ethics

Sandra Marmolejo Romero, BSN, RN, CPHQ
Adjunct Associate Professor
Bilingual Medical Assistant Program
Southwestern Community College District
San Diego, CA
Unit 2: Medical Terminology
Unit 8: Billing and Payment for Medical Services
Unit 9: Banking and Accounting Procedures

Lynn A. Skafte, BA, CMA(AAMA)
National Medical Assisting Program Coordinator
School of Health Sciences
Rasmussen College
Bloomington, MN
Unit 15: Laboratory Procedures

Acknowledgments

A textbook of this nature requires the input and assistance of many friends, professional colleagues and acquaintances, subject matter experts, and the publishing team. The authors are particularly grateful to the reviewers, listed on the next pages, who continue to be a valuable resource. Their insights, comments, suggestions, and attention to detail are very important in guiding this book as it evolves. Special acknowledgment to Helen Houser, RN, MSHA, at Phoenix College; and Lori Malone, CMA(AAMA), at Century College, East Campus, for their detailed suggestions and feedback, which helped shape the development of this edition.

ANATOMY AND PHYSIOLOGY CHAPTERS 23–35

The invaluable contributions to Chapters 23–35 from physicians, nurse practitioners, nurse specialists, and educators are above and beyond recognition. These professionals have invested many hours in reviewing content and identifying material to be deleted, updated, or added. Words alone are not adequate to express our appreciation for their unselfish gift of time and professional expertise to ensure the accuracy and currency of this text.

A very special acknowledgment goes to Cheryl Baxter, RN, MS, who is a pediatric nurse practitioner and an educator for Ohio's Child Care Program. She is an Advanced Cardiac Life Support Instructor and lectures on child abuse. She also serves as Medical Director for the Medical Assistant Program at Columbus State Community College. Cheryl contributed many hours of her time to review all 13 chapters of Anatomy and Physiology, making suggestions relating to pediatrics. In addition, she spent many hours brainstorming with this author the age-related changes occurring in the body and the interaction of the body systems in disease conditions that is incorporated in this edition. Her assistance and expertise are immeasurable.

With great appreciation, we acknowledge the following professionals who contributed knowledge, expertise, and feedback to the seventh and previous editions:

Chapter 23 Anatomic Descriptors and Fundamental Body Structure

Stephen D'Ambrosio, PhD, Professor of Radiobiology and Pharmacology, Ohio State University, College of Medicine (fourth, fifth, and seventh editions)

Carmen Carpenter, RN, MS, CMA(AAMA), Chair, Allied Health Science and Medical Assisting, South University, West Palm Beach, FL (sixth edition)

Chapter 24 The Nervous System

Claire V. Wolfe, MD, Physical Medicine and Rehabilitation (sixth and seventh editions)

Chapter 25 The Senses

Todd E. Whitaker, MD, ophthalmologist (seventh edition)

Janet McOwen, RN, ophthalmology (sixth edition)

Lawrence Koegel, MD, otorhinolaryngologist (sixth and seventh editions)

Chapter 26 The Integumentary System

Julio C. Cruz, MD, dermatologist (seventh edition)

Kelly Zyniewicz, MD, dermatologist (fifth and sixth editions)

Chapter 27 The Skeletal System

John S. Wolfe, MD, orthopedic surgeon

Chapter 28 The Muscular System

John S. Wolfe, MD, orthopedic surgeon

Chapter 29 The Respiratory System

Paul R. Beery II, MD, MS, FACS, Intensivist, Assistant Professor of Clinical Surgery, Ohio State University Hospitals (seventh edition)

Karen Bishop, RN, MS, CNP, nurse practitioner, pulmonary practice (sixth edition)

Phil Diaz, MD, pulmonologist and researcher for Ohio State University (fourth and fifth editions)

Chapter 30 The Circulatory System

N. Howard Kander, MD, FACC, interventional cardiologist (sixth and seventh editions)

Chapter 31 The Immune System

Peter J. Kourlas, MD, hematologist/oncologist (sixth and seventh editions)

Lisa Smith, RN, MS, AOCN, oncology clinical nurse specialist (fifth edition)

Elaine Glass, RN, MS, OCN, oncology clinical nurse specialist (fourth edition)

Chapter 32 The Digestive System
Thomas Ransbottom, MD, gastroenterologist (sixth edition)

Chapter 33 The Urinary System
Ashay Patel DO, urologist (seventh edition)
Henry Wise, MD, urologist (fifth edition)
Michelle Steed, RN, BSN, clinical nurse manager, Urology Services and Dialysis, Riverside Methodist Hospital (fifth edition)

Chapter 34 The Endocrine System
Manuel Tzagournis, MD, endocrinologist and professor emeritus, Internal Medicine, Division of Endocrinology, Diabetes, and Metabolism, Ohio State University Hospitals (sixth and seventh editions)

Chapter 35 The Reproductive System
R. Dennis Blose, MD, obstetrician/gynecologist (seventh edition)
Christine Dombroski, RNC, NP, nurse practitioner, OB/GYN and women's health (fifth and sixth editions)
Ashay Patel, DO, urologist (seventh edition)

Reviewers

Theresa Addison, NCMA
Former Medical Department Chair
Formerly with Remington College
Shreveport, LA

Cheryl H. Bordwine, BHA, MBA, RMA (AMT)
Director/Professor
Medical Assisting Program
College of the Mainland
Texas City, TX

Estelle Coffino, MPA, RRT, CPFT, CCMA
Director, Allied Health Programs
The College of Westchester
White Plains, NY

Sue Coleman, LPN, AS
Director of Healthcare Education
National College
Lynchburg, VA

Kelly Collins, MA, CPT
Instructor, Allied Health
Tulare Adult School
Tulare, CA

Rita Cordova, CMA(AAMA), RN, MSN
Director of Medical Assisting
Herzing University
Madison, WI

Cherika deJesus, BS, CMA(AAMA)
Minnesota School of Business
Brooklyn Center, MN

Laurie Dennis, CBCS
HIBC Instructor
Florida Career College
Clearwater, FL

Esther Diaz, CCMA-AC
Health Academy Instructor
Sweetwater High School
National City, CA

Jane W. Dumas, MSN, CCMA, CHI (NHA)
Allied Health Department Chair
Remington College – Cleveland West Campus
North Olmsted, OH

Kathryn Emery, CMA(AAMA)
Instructor
AAMA
Lake Elsinore, CA

Teresa England-Lewis, RN, MSN
Health Occupations Instructor
North Montco Technical Career Center
Lansdale, PA

Ellen Halibozek, MS, CPC
Curriculum Manager
Corinthian Colleges
Santa Ana, CA

Theresa Henderson, CCMA-AC, CMA(AAMA), CPT 1
Medical Instructor
Fontana Unified School District
Fontana, CA

Claudia N. Hewlett, AS
Medical Assisting Senior Lead Instructor
Remington College
Memphis, TN

Stephanie Hollan, BSM
Department Chair
Houston, TX

Helen Houser, RN, MSHA MA
Program Director
Phoenix College
Phoenix, AZ

Rosemary C. Johnson, MSPA, FHFMA
Adjunct Professor
Capital Community College
Hartford, CT

Beth Laurenz, MBA, BS, AAS, LPN, CMA(AAMA)
Director of Healthcare Education
National College
Columbus, OH

Penny Lee, CMA(AAMA), CAHI
Program Director of Medical Assisting
MedTech College
Greenwood, IN

Marta Lopez, MD, RMA(AAMA)
Program/Clinical Coordinator and Assistant Professor
Medical Assisting Program
Miami Dade College-Medical Center Campus
Miami, FL

Alice Macomber, RN, RMA (AMT), RPT, AHI, CPI, BXO
MA Program Director
Keiser University
Port St. Lucie, FL

Wilsetta McClain, RMA (AMT), NCPT, EMT-B, ABC
Department Chair
Baker College of Auburn Hills
Auburn Hills, MI

Pat Moody, RN
Medical Assisting Clinical Instructor
Athens Technical College
Athens, GA

Mickey Obermire, CLT
Teacher
Clovis Adult Education
Clovis, CA

Donna Otis, LPN
Medical Instructor
Metro Business School
Rolla, MO

Aaron Paschall
Curriculum Coordinator
Heritage Education
Denver, CO

June M. Petillo, MBA, RMC, NCP
Director of EHR
Adjunct Instructor
Capital Community College
Hartford, CT

Agnes Pucillo, BSN, LPN
Allied Health Instructor
Prism Career Institute
Cherry Hill, NJ

Machelle Rougely, BSM, RMA (AMT)
Program Director
Westwood College
Dallas, TX

Cathy D. Soto, PhD, MBA, CMA(AAMA)
Program Director
Medical Assisting Technology Program
El Paso Community College
El Paso, TX

Traci L. SuSong, MBA/HCM, CMA(AAMA), CMRS
Program Director
Bryant and Stratton College
Parma, OH

Wanda D. Strayhan, MS, CCMA, CBCS
Program Chair, Allied Health
Florida Career College
Clearwater, FL

Georgia Turner, BBA, CHI, CBCS
Instructor
Jefferson State College
Birmingham, AL

Lisa Zepeda, MS
Instructor
San Joaquin Valley College
Visalia, CA

Section

1

Medical Assisting Foundations

Unit

1

Health Care Roles and Responsibilities

The health care industry is one of the oldest and most respected professions in the world. The field of medicine has been around for thousands of years, dating as far back as 3000 BC. Some scientists even suspect that medicinal properties were used far before the first documented findings.

Medical pioneers paved the way for today's engineers to create innovative technology and medications that cure and treat some of the most complex of diseases. Because of these innovations, our quality of life is much better, and the average life span has increased by several years.

The evolution and specialization of medicine has encouraged many health care specialties and subspecialties to emerge, even creating several tiers of practitioners to work in each area. Medical assisting is not only one of the fastest growing health care occupations today but also among the most versatile careers.

Chapter 1 explores the skills and responsibilities of the medical assistant, examines behaviors necessary to be successful in the health care industry, and discusses various credentialing opportunities.

Chapter 2 looks at medical historians, who set the wheels in motion for the technology and pharmaceuticals we have today. It also discusses the physicians, midlevel practitioners, and allied health professionals that comprise the health care team and investigates the various types of medical establishments in which these professionals work.

Certification Connection

	Ch. 1	Ch. 2
CMA (AAMA)		
Displaying professional attitude	X	
Working as a team member to achieve goals	X	X
Professional communication and behavior	X	
Consent	X	
Patient written authorization		
Time management	X	
Revocation/suspension of license		X
Performing within ethical boundaries	X	
Responsibility and rights: (1) Patient (2) Physician (3) Medical assistant	X	X
RMA (AMT)		
Identify and employ professional conduct in all aspects of patient care	X	
Employ appropriate interpersonal skills with (1) employer/administration; (2) coworkers; (3) vendors; (4) business associates	X	X
Employ active listening skills	X	
Identify and understand laws, regulations, and acts pertaining to the practice of medicine		X
Understand credentialing requirements of medical professionals	X	
Recognize the importance of professional development through continuing education	X	
Inform patients of test results per physician instruction		
CMAS (AMT)		
Employ human relations skills appropriate to the health care setting	X	
Display behaviors of a professional medical administrative specialist	X	
Participate in appropriate continuing education	X	
Observe and maintain confidentiality of records, charts, and test results	X	

Chapter 1 The Medical Assistant

OBJECTIVES

In this chapter, you will learn the following:

KB KNOWLEDGE BASE

1. Spell and define, using the glossary at the back of the text, all the Words to Know in this chapter.
2. Describe the role of the medical assistant.
3. List seven questions individuals should ask themselves before becoming a medical assistant.
4. Identify typical skills and job responsibilities of the medical assistant.
5. List the types of establishment in which medical assistants work.
6. Describe the outlook for medical assistants over the next several years.
7. Define professionalism and describe behaviors that are necessary when working in a professional capacity.
8. Describe the ideal appearance of a medical assistant and factors that influence appearance.
9. List four basic goals of time management.
10. Describe items or situations that take priority when working in an administrative or clinical capacity.
11. List and describe professional organizations that certify or credential medical assistants.
12. Discuss the importance of becoming credentialed and the steps necessary for becoming credentialed through the organizations discussed in this chapter.

S SKILLS

1. Demonstrate professionalism.

B BEHAVIOR

1. Apply active listening skills.
2. Demonstrate awareness of the territorial boundaries of the person with whom communicating.
3. Demonstrate sensitivity to the message being delivered.
4. Demonstrate awareness of how an individual's appearance affects anticipated responses.
5. Demonstrate dependability, punctuality, and a positive work ethic.
6. Exhibit a positive attitude and a sense of responsibility.
7. Maintain confidentiality at all times.
8. Be cognizant of ethical boundaries.
9. Exhibit initiative.
10. Adapt to change.
11. Express a responsible attitude.
12. Be courteous and diplomatic.
13. Conduct work within the scope of education, training, and ability.

WORDS TO KNOW

accreditation
Accrediting Bureau of Health Education Schools (ABHES)
administrative skills
advocate
altruism
American Academy of Professional Coders (AAPC)
American Association of Medical Assistants (AAMA)
American Medical Technologists (AMT)
appearance
behaviors
Certified Clinical Medical Assistant (CCMA)
Certified Medical Administrative Assistant (CMAA)
Certified Medical Assistant, CMA (AAMA)
clinical skills
Commission on Accreditation of Allied Health Education Programs (CAAHEP)
confidential
empathic
general skills
generalist
innate
knowledge base
medical assistant
multi-provider clinic
National Center for Competency Testing (NCCT)
National Certified Medical Assistant (NCMA)
National Certified Medical Office Assistant (NCMOA)
National Healthcareer Association (NHA)
partnership
Patient-Centered Medical Home (PCMH)
provider
Registered Medical Assistant, RMA (AMT)
skills
solo practice
tactful
time management
urgent care center

THE ROLE OF THE MEDICAL ASSISTANT

The field of medical assisting is one of the most versatile allied health occupations in today's health care environment. **American Medical Technologists (AMT)**—a certifying organization for medical assistants—describes the **medical assistant** as "an integral member of the health care delivery team, qualified by education and experience to work in the administrative office, the examining room and the physician office laboratory. The medical assistant is also a liaison between the doctor and the patient and is of vital importance to the success of the medical practice."

To become a successful medical assistant, you must acquire a specific **knowledge base** (theory) and **skills** (procedures) while also demonstrating specific **behaviors** (professional characteristics or attitudes). You will see these three bolded terms in the Objectives section at the beginnings of most of these chapters.

Is Medical Assisting Right for You?

How do you know whether medical assisting is right for you? According to the **American Association of Medical Assistants (AAMA)**—a professional organization for medical assistants—if you can answer yes to the following questions, medical assisting is probably for you:

- Are you looking for a meaningful job?
- Do you like helping others (Figure 1–1)?
- Do you have an interest in health and medicine?
- Are you a "people person"?
- Are you good at multitasking, easily switching tasks throughout the day?
- Do you like variety in your job?
- Would you like to enter a career in an expanding field?

The following sections describe some of the specific responsibilities of medical assistants.

MEDIA LINK

View the video, "Qualities of a Successful Medical Assistant," for this chapter on the Premium Website.

Skills and Responsibilities of the Medical Assistant

As health care progresses, so do the skills and responsibilities of the medical assistant. The field of medical assisting is continuously evolving. In an effort to keep up with the changes, the AAMA routinely completes an occupational analysis, which identifies three broad areas of practice for certified medical assistants.

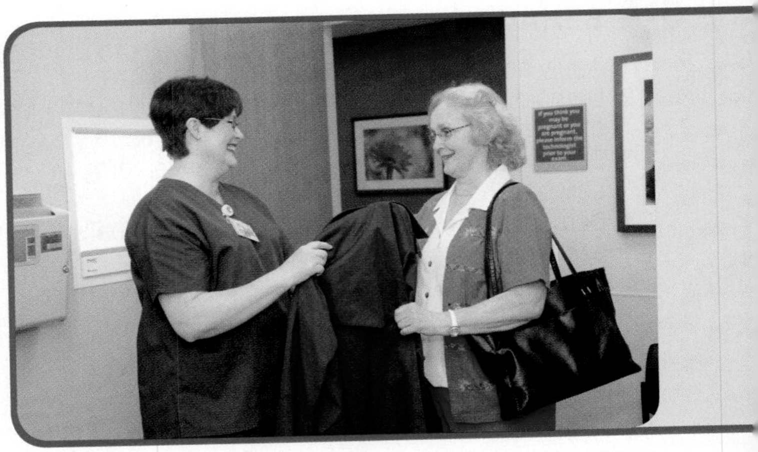

Figure 1–1: The medical assistant assists the patient by taking her coat to hang it up for her. *Delmar/Cengage Learning.*

Although this analysis is performed specifically for members of the AAMA, the skills listed are applicable to all medical assistants across the spectrum. The areas are identified as **general**, **administrative**, and **clinical**. Mastery of these skills prepares medical assisting students to be integral members of today's health care team.

General Skills

Medical assistants must have wonderful communication skills and the ability to think critically and analyze information. The general skills of the medical assistant can be divided into four major categories:

- *Communication:* The medical assistant should take on the role of a communication liaison when working with patients. This skill is necessary to promote important exchanges of information between the **provider** (physician, nurse practitioner, or physician assistant) and the patient. Good communication skills also promote positive interaction with coworkers, supervisors, and external associates that conduct business with the practice.
- *Legal and ethical concepts:* These are concepts concerned with legal, ethical, moral, and professional conduct in the execution of medical assisting duties. These skills help prevent unnecessary litigation and keep the medical assistant practicing within his or her scope of practice.
- *Instruction:* Today's medical assistant is taking on a larger role in patient education. Patient education topics include disease prevention and management, medication management, and overall health maintenance. Another very important role of the medical assistant is to be an **advocate** for the patient because it is important for patients to know that they have someone looking out for them.
- *Operational functions:* These are functions that are necessary to keep the equipment and facility running effectively.

PATIENT EDUCATION

Today's medical assistants are becoming more active in patient education by taking on the role of a health coach (Figure 1–2). Topics frequently covered with patients include disease prevention, health maintenance, and medication management. To be at the top of your game, always check with the provider before conducting these sessions to determine essential goals for the session. Start each session by allowing the patient or patient's family members to identify their goals as well for the session. Researching this information prior to the session enhances the learning process and aids in overall patient compliance.

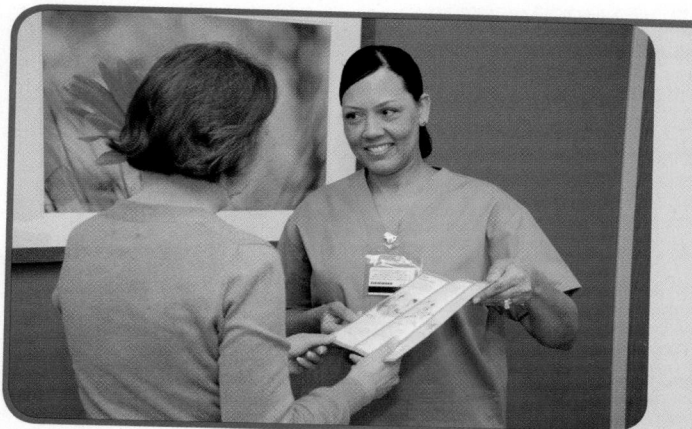

Figure 1–2: The medical assistant acts as a health coach as she reviews important information within the patient brochure. *Delmar/Cengage Learning.*

Administrative Skills

Performing administrative skills helps manage the business affairs of the practice and includes two categories—administrative procedures and practice finances. The following skills are listed under this category:

- Scheduling appointments
- Performing inpatient and outpatient admissions and procedures
- Creating and maintaining the patient's medical record
- Filing medical records and other documents
- Performing procedural and diagnostic coding for reimbursement
- Performing billing and collection procedures
- Performing bookkeeping and financial procedures
- Preparing submittal ("clean") insurance forms.

Clinical Skills

Performing clinical skills is an extension of the provider's role of assessment, examination, diagnosis, and treatment. These are divided into three categories, which include fundamental practices, diagnostic procedures, and patient care on the occupational analysis chart. Some skills from this category include:

- Identification of the roles and responsibilities of the medical assistant in the clinical setting as well as of other team members in the medical office.
- Application of principles of aseptic technique and infection control
- Performance of vital signs
- Performance of sterilization and minor surgery procedures
- Collection and processing of specimens
- Performance of lab tests (Figure 1–3)
- Performance of electrocardiograms (ECGs or EKGs)
- Administration of medications
- Performance of phlebotomy procedures

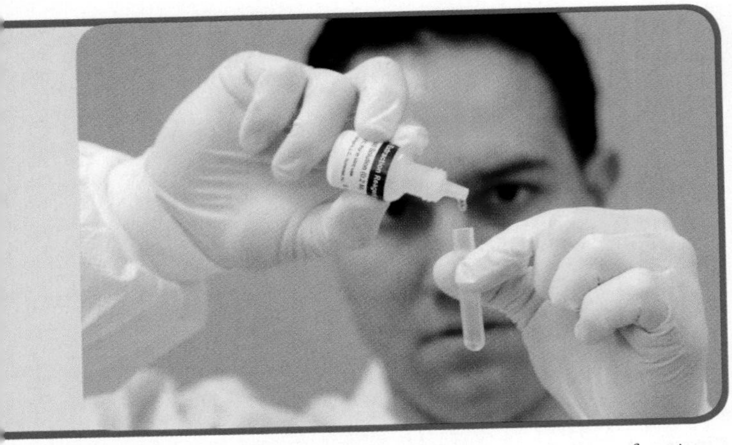

Figure 1–3: In this figure, the medical assistant is performing one of the many lab tests medical assistants routinely perform. *Delmar/Cengage Learning.*

- Performance of patient screenings
- Preparation of patients for examinations, procedures, and treatments
- Response to emergencies

Many medical assistants work as **generalists**, meaning that they perform both clinical and administrative duties in addition to general responsibilities. Other medical assistants specialize in administrative procedures whereas others prefer working in clinical positions exclusively.

Boundaries of Medical Assistants

Medical assistants must know the boundaries, or scope of practice, of the profession (Figure 1–4). In general, medical assistants cannot examine, diagnose, or prescribe treatment, but can perform duties mentioned earlier in the chapter. Each state has its own medical practice acts that may dictate what types of medications medical assistants can administer and whether additional credentialing is required to take X-rays. Chapter 5 expands on the medical assistant's scope of practice.

Medical Assistant Work Environment

Medical assistants work in a variety of settings, although the majority of them work in ambulatory care environments. Some of the types of practices in which medical assistants work include doctor offices, specialty practices, urgent care centers, clinics, hospitals, labs, insurance companies, billing companies, and government agencies. The actual business of practicing medicine in these organizations can be conducted in several ways.

Solo Practices

Some physicians prefer to have a **solo practice**, also called a sole proprietorship, meaning that the individual physician alone makes all decisions regarding the practice. Being employed as a medical assistant in this type of office requires you to have both administrative and clinical skills essential for the smooth operation of that practice, especially if you are the only employee. This type of businesses is rare today because of the expenses involved in running a business.

Partnerships

In a **partnership**, two or more physicians have a legal agreement to share in the total business operation of the practice. In this case, usually two to several medical assistants (or other members of the health care team) are employed to care for patients and conduct business.

Multi-Provider Clinics

Multi-provider clinics are group practices, which consist of three or more providers who share a facility for the purpose of practicing medicine. In this model, the providers share expenses, income, equipment, records, and personnel. Many times, these practices are owned by hospitals, management groups, or insurance companies. Usually, several professionals make up the health care team in this setting. Medical assistants, lab technicians, radiology technicians, nurses, physician assistants, and the physician work together in providing health care.

Urgent Care Centers

Urgent care centers are ambulatory care centers that take care of patients with acute illness or injury and those with minor emergencies. These centers originated in the 1970s and have grown in popularity over the past couple of decades. Urgent care facilities are usually open seven days a week and are especially busy during times when other clinics and offices are closed. Patients are normally seen in the order of arrival except in emergencies. Many of these centers are started by emergency room physicians and are equipped with radiographic equipment, lab equipment, splinting supplies, and emergency equipment. Medical assistants with X-ray certification are often desirable because of their versatility.

Patient-Centered Medical Homes

The American Academy of Providers (AAP) describes the **Patient-Centered Medical Home (PCMH)** as:

> A team-based model of care led by a personal physician who provides continuous and coordinated care throughout a patient's lifetime to maximize health outcomes. The PCMH practice is responsible for providing for all of a patient's health care needs or appropriately arranging care with other qualified professionals. This includes the provision of preventive services, treatment of acute and chronic illness, and assistance with end-of-life issues. It is a model of practice in which a team of health professionals,

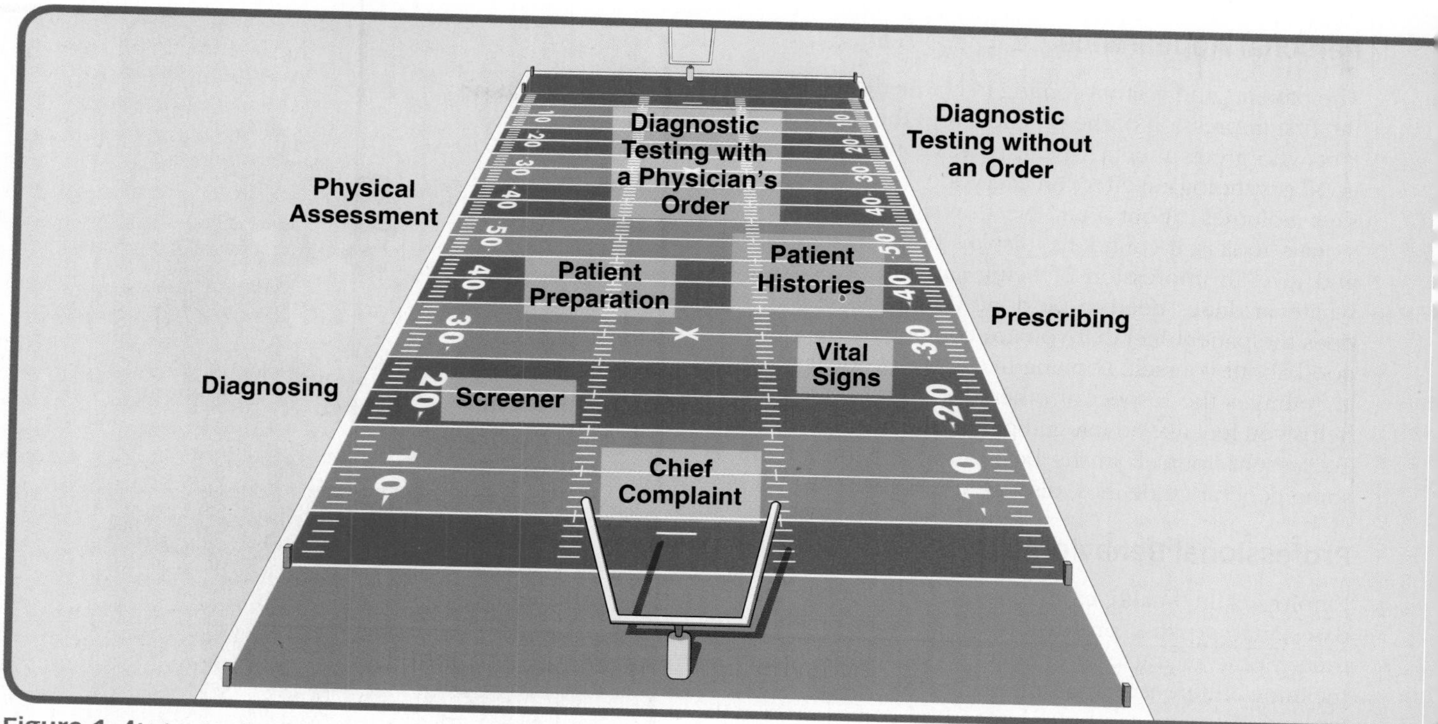

Figure 1–4: This football field illustrates boundary lines for what a medical assistant can do. The out-of-bound markers illustrate what the medical assistant cannot do. *Delmar/Cengage Learning.*

coordinated by a personal physician, works collaboratively to provide high levels of care, access and communication, care coordination and integration, and care quality and safety.

The PCMH is more of a partnership between the PCMH team and patient. The provider oversees all of the patient's care and focuses on the patient's total health rather than on a specific condition. Electronic medical records are a big part of the PCMH model, and patients have continuous access to their records in this model. Early findings have shown that patients thrive in this model, which helps reduce health care expenses. Medical assistants are very good for this model due to their flexibility and affordability. For more information about this model, visit the Website from the American College of Providers (ACP) and Patient-Centered Primary Care Collaborative groups at www.emmisolutions.com/medicalhome/acp/.

Job Outlook for Medical Assistants

The job outlook for medical assistants looks very promising. This is due to the versatility of medical assistants as well as to our aging population. The following excerpt is from the United States Department of Labor, Bureau of Labor Statistics:

> Employment of medical assistants is expected to grow 34 percent from 2008 to 2018, much faster than the average for all occupations. As the healthcare industry expands because of technological advances in medicine and the growth and aging of the population, there will be an increased need for all healthcare workers. The increasing prevalence of certain conditions, such as obesity and diabetes, also will increase demand for healthcare services and medical assistants. Increasing use of medical assistants to allow doctors to care for more patients will further stimulate job growth.

DEMONSTRATING PROFESSIONALISM

Being a part of the health care team requires the medical assistant to demonstrate professionalism and professional behavior on an array of levels. Evolving into a professional is not something that just happens; it is a process that develops throughout one's career. Webster defines professionalism as, "the conduct, aims, or qualities that characterize or mark a professional or a professional person." One of the most important traits of a medical professional is **altruism** or selflessness—an unselfish concern for the welfare of others. As a health care professional, you should display professionalism not only to patients but also to supervisors, coworkers, vendors, and outside business associates. The following section describes desirable characteristics and behaviors of a professional medical assistant.

Personal Appearance

The patients and visitors coming into a medical office gain the first impression of the practice from the medical assistant who greets them. A neat, professional person has a good psychological effect on everyone. Your **appearance** says volumes about you. Neat, well-groomed professionals look self-confident, display pride in themselves, and give an impression of being capable of performing whatever duties need to be done (Figure 1–5). Not only does the patient feel that you are competent, but you feel good about yourself. Looking like a professional not only encourages the respect of others for your profession but helps you feel like an integral part of the health care team. To present yourself in the best possible light, adhere to some general guidelines, discussed in Table 1–1.

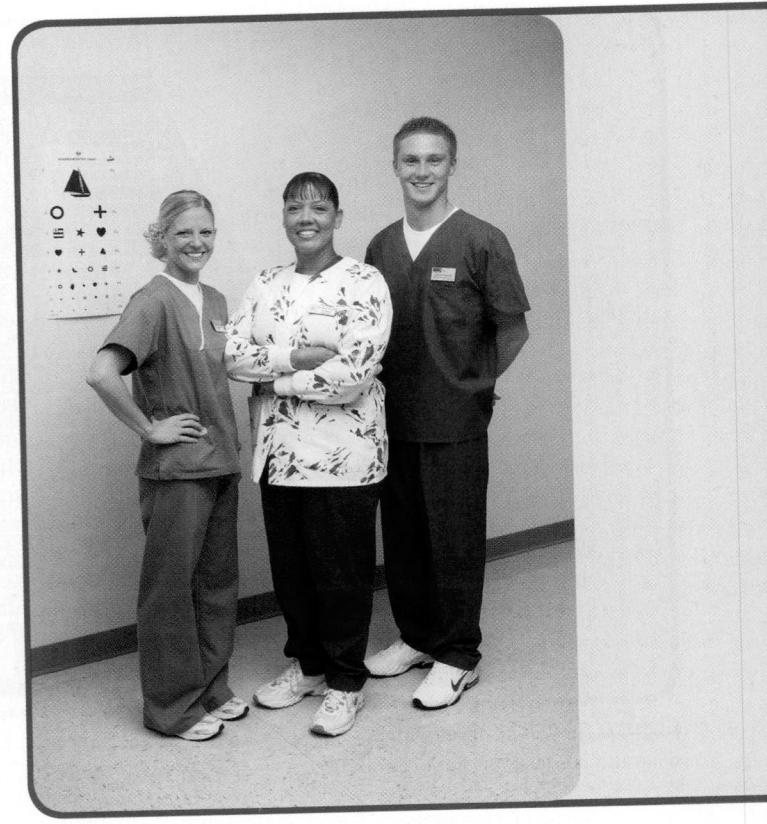

Figure 1–5: Medical assistants should always look very professional. Uniforms should always be crisp and clean. *Delmar/Cengage Learning.*

Professional Behaviors

Employers in health care settings often pursue candidates that possess professional behaviors or character traits. Some characteristics seem to be almost **innate**—meaning inherent or natural—whereas others must be learned. All traits can be enhanced by consciously making an effort to improve them. Your ability to work well with your employer, supervisors, and coworkers and your effectiveness in dealing with patients is greatly influenced by your personal characteristics. Table 1–2 is a list of professional characteristics that are necessary to possess when working as a health care worker.

TABLE 1–1 How to Project a Professional Appearance

Cleanliness	This is the first essential for good grooming. Take a daily bath or shower and use a deodorant or antiperspirant. Shampoo your hair often. Brush and floss your teeth at least twice a day. Use mouthwash or breath mints when necessary.
Posture	The ease with which you move around reflects your poise and confidence. Posture affects not only your appearance but also the amount of fatigue you experience.
Hand care	Keep your fingernails manicured and cut well below the fingertips. Start each day with an aseptic hand wash, paying close attention to nails. Keep hand cream or lotion in convenient places to use after washing your hands. Follow institutional guidelines in relation to polishes. (Most facilities prohibit nail polish and art.)
Hair	Keep your hair clean and away from your face. Long hair should be worn up or fastened back.
Proper attire	Attire may vary with medical specialty. When uniforms are required, they should be clean and free of wrinkles and fit well. Uniform shoes should be kept clean and have clean shoestrings; hose must not have runs. Pay attention to the undergarments you wear beneath the uniform so that they do not show through the fabric of your uniform and that t-shirts or other long-sleeved shirts look professional.
Jewelry	Do not wear jewelry except for a watch or wedding ring. A single small earring may be worn in each ear. Not only does jewelry look out of place, it is a great collector of microorganisms. Novelty piercings, such as nose rings and tongue studs, are not appropriate for professional grooming.
Fragrances	Perfumes, colognes, and aftershave lotions can be offensive to some patients, especially if they have allergies or are suffering from nausea. If you feel it is necessary to wear something, use one with a light, clean-smelling fragrance.
Cosmetics	Cosmetics should be tasteful and skillfully applied.

TABLE 1–2 Professional Traits

Accurate	Be detailed and make certain that information is correct. Accuracy is vital: Not being accurate in the medical field can cost a patient his or her life.
Adaptable	The ability to adjust or make fit. Your willingness to be flexible and to cooperate will be noticed by your employer or supervisor and coworkers and reciprocated as a result of your actions.
Courteous	Be polite and well mannered. In a professional environment, courtesy is not optional, and manners really do matter.
Confidential	Be prudent and conscious—especially in your speech. Never give out any information regarding a patient without the patient's written permission. To do so is a violation of privacy laws and can result in termination, expensive fines, and possible jail time.
Dependable	Be reliable and responsible. Supervisors and coworkers need to be able to trust you to show up for work and to follow through with what you say you are going to do.
Empathic	Put yourself in another person's shoes; think about what is best for the patient.
Honest	Be trustworthy and truthful. Dishonesty can result in harm or even death to the patient. Being dishonest also causes others to feel you have no integrity. Once integrity is lost, it is very hard to regain.
Initiative	Show ambition; do things that need to be done without being told—as long as it is within your scope of practice.
Patient	Act calm when things don't necessarily go as planned or as quickly as planned.
Punctual	Be in exact agreement with time; showing up for work before you are scheduled to be there and returning from breaks on time.
Respectful	Show regard for others even if you disagree with their message; be respectful of others' property, culture, position, or opinion. Respect is a two-way street. To gain respect—you have to give it!
Tactful	Be able to perceive a situation and know the right thing to say or do. Tact is especially difficult and important when dealing with ill people.

CLINICAL PEARL

At times, your personal life can spill over into your professional life. Social networking sites such as Facebook have caused some employers to reconsider hiring particular individuals due to disreputable postings or distasteful photographs. Think about what the information or photographs you share say about you before you post them.

Personal Qualities

In addition to character traits, other personality qualities affect the way character traits are perceived. An individual might demonstrate initiative, dependability, honesty, and other traits, but if he or she is not likable, that individual will struggle in bonding or getting along with others. These qualities can be more difficult to acquire because they seem to be connected to one's personality. Let's look at some of these qualities in Table 1–3 and in Procedure 1–1, which follows the table.

TABLE 1–3 Positive Personal Qualities

Friendly attitude	A real, concerned, caring viewpoint; your attitude can be your greatest asset or your biggest stumbling block. A good attitude has to be cultivated and nourished. Having a good outlook on life carries over into every area and promotes a general well-being.
Genuine smile	A genuine smile conveys that you acknowledge others and are interested in being of service.
Perception as a professional	To look your best, you must be in good health. This means that you practice what you preach: Have a well-balanced diet, get plenty of rest, and avoid smoking.

PROCEDURE 1–1 Displaying Professionalism

PURPOSE: To display professional qualities in all aspects of your position and thus to be respected as a reputable medical assistant.

EQUIPMENT: Because this is more of a mindset than a procedure, the scenarios selected by your instructor will dictate conditions and supplies with which to practice this procedure. In general, you must exhibit a professional appearance and professional characteristics as you play out the scenarios selected by your instructor to measure each step. Some steps can be in the fashion of questions and answers rather than as an actual scenario.

S **SKILL:** Displaying Professionalism

	Procedure Steps	Detailed Instructions and/or *Rationales*
B	1. ***Exhibit dependability and punctuality by being on time and following through with what you say you are going to do.***	*Supervisors, peers, and patients need to know they can count on you. If you are constantly running late or not following through with prearranged commitments, others feel they can't trust you.*
B	2. ***Display a professional appearance.***	Your uniform should be clean, free of wrinkles, and include appropriate under-attire. Hair should be clean and tied back (if applicable), and jewelry should be kept to a minimum. Hands should be freshly washed between each patient, and nails should be clean and short. *The patient will be much more accepting of your role as a health care professional if you look the part. (If you fail to cover tattoos and wear facial and tongue piercings, it could cause the patient to feel uncomfortable and ask for someone other than you to care for him or her.)*
B	3. ***Engage in active listening skills during all encounters.***	*Good listening skills improve the communication process.*
B	4. ***Be aware of territorial and professional boundaries in the workplace.***	*Knowing and abiding by the territorial boundaries you are assigned assists in positive relationships with supervisors and colleagues. Being aware of professional boundaries also helps prevent medical litigation.*
B	5. ***Exhibit a positive work ethic.***	*A positive work ethic tells both patients and coworkers that you enjoy your line of work and helps build respect for you as a professional.*
B	6. ***Display sensitivity when working with colleagues and patients.***	*Patients and coworkers feel you really care about them when you are sensitive toward their feelings, and you conduct yourself in a positive manner.*
B	7. ***Demonstrate courtesy to patients and coworkers.***	Never interrupt someone when they are speaking and be alert to things you can do for patients and coworkers that will assist them in times of need. *This also helps others have respect for you.*
B	8. ***Display tact and diplomacy in dealing with patients and others.***	*Being tactful and diplomatic assists others in receiving messages that might otherwise be awkward.*
B	9. ***Adapt to changes when necessary.***	*Unexpected changes are common in health care. Being flexible assists you in being a good team player.*
B	10. ***Remain confidential at all times.***	*Divulging confidential information can lead to distrust, loss of respect, and possible fines concerning patient confidentiality*

TIME MANAGEMENT

Time management refers to an assortment of skills, tools, and practices that manage time during daily activities and when accomplishing specific projects. To be an efficient professional, you must take control of your time rather than allowing time to take control of you Figure 1–6. Time management specialists focus on a principle referred to as Pareto's Principle, or the 80-20 rule, which states that as little as 20 percent of your labors result in 80 percent of your results. To be efficient with your time, focus on the 20 percent of your work that yields the greatest results.

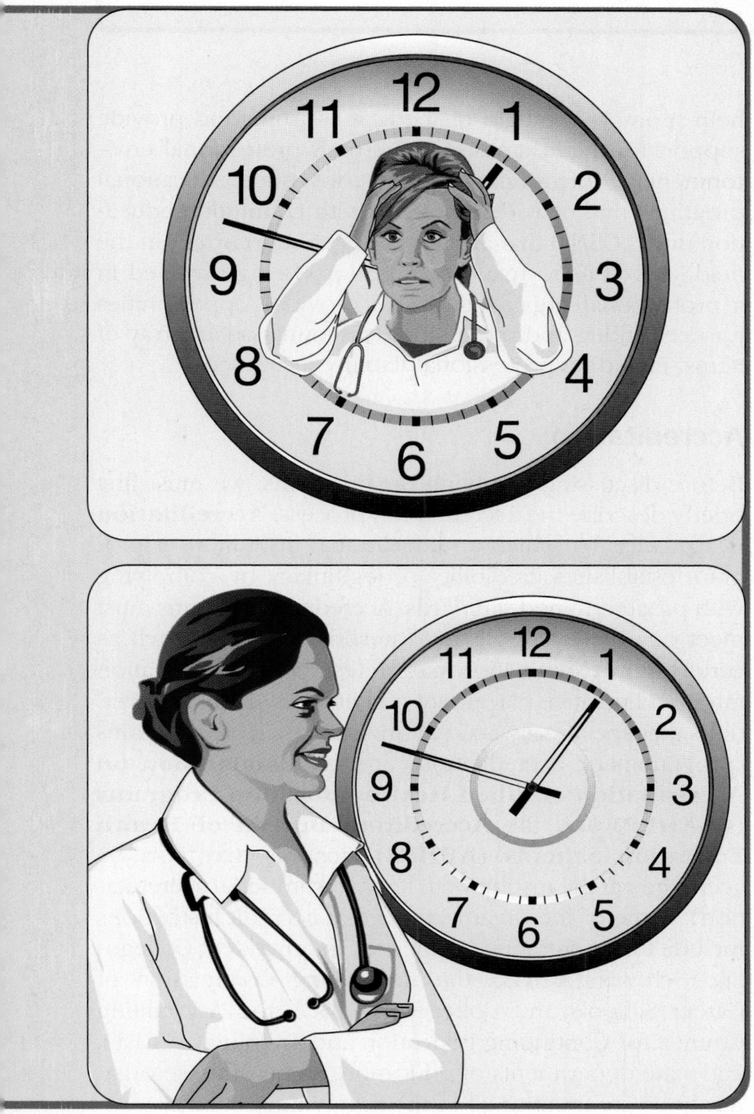

Figure 1–6: Time can take control of you, or you can take control of time by staying organized and managing your schedule in an efficient manner. *Delmar/Cengage Learning.*

The following list is a set of goals that assist you in being more efficient with your time:

- *Make a daily list of tasks and projects that must be completed.* Prioritize the list so that if you are unable to complete all tasks, the ones that are most important will be completed. When you are just beginning your career, you might need an experienced individual such as a supervisor to help identify tasks that have priority.
- *Learn to say no to low-priority requests—especially those that are optional.* Supervisors might ask whether you are able to take on some new responsibilities in addition to your old responsibilities. If your plate is already full, thank the supervisor for considering you for the task, but politely state that your schedule is already very full and that you don't want to run the risk of performing poorly because you have taken on too much.
- *Don't be a perfectionist for tasks that don't require your best effort.* Some tasks, such as accounting tasks and patient procedures, require great precision and accuracy, but others do not. For example, if you find that you spend a great deal of time composing email messages, it might be more timely just to call the individual rather than trying to find the perfect words to put in a written message.
- *Stay away from bad habits that rob you of your time such as surfing the Internet or using the phone for extended lengths of time.* Additionally, Internet surfing and texting to personal friends and family members are usually not tolerated in the workplace.

When working in an administrative capacity, patients in the office usually take priority over patients calling in to the office except in emergency situations. Filing insurance claims usually have time limits; claims should be filed by date so that you never miss a deadline. Other timely tasks such as record requests for patients who have next-day surgeries and depositing patient and insurance payments take priority over tasks that can wait until the next day.

The clinical side of medical assisting has a natural progression as well. Table 1–4 sums up what takes priority when working in a clinical capacity.

Staying organized also assists in time management. Keep your desk area and patient rooms clean and organized. Figure 1–7 illustrates both a disorganized desk and a nicely organized desk. You can act more efficiently if your desk is neat and clean. All patient rooms should be set up in the same manner. This helps in retrieving items quickly and provides you with more time to work on other tasks.

TABLE 1–4 Floor Management Priority Table

First Priority	**Assisting the provider with emergencies and procedures.** Learning to anticipate when a patient might need a special procedure performed is a good skill to cultivate. The medical assistant can save time by preparing items necessary for the procedure ahead of time, but do not open any supplies until a direct order is given to perform the procedure.
Second Priority	**Rooming patients.** When a room becomes vacant, clean and prepare it for the next patient. Retrieve the patient from the reception area, document the patient's chief complaint, and perform vital signs. Try to stay one to two rooms ahead of the provider; the provider should never have to wait for the medical assistant to room a patient.
Third Priority	**Performing procedures and dismissing patients.**
Fourth Priority	**Working on pending files that have tasks** (calling back patients with test results, calling in prescriptions per the physician's order, and so on).

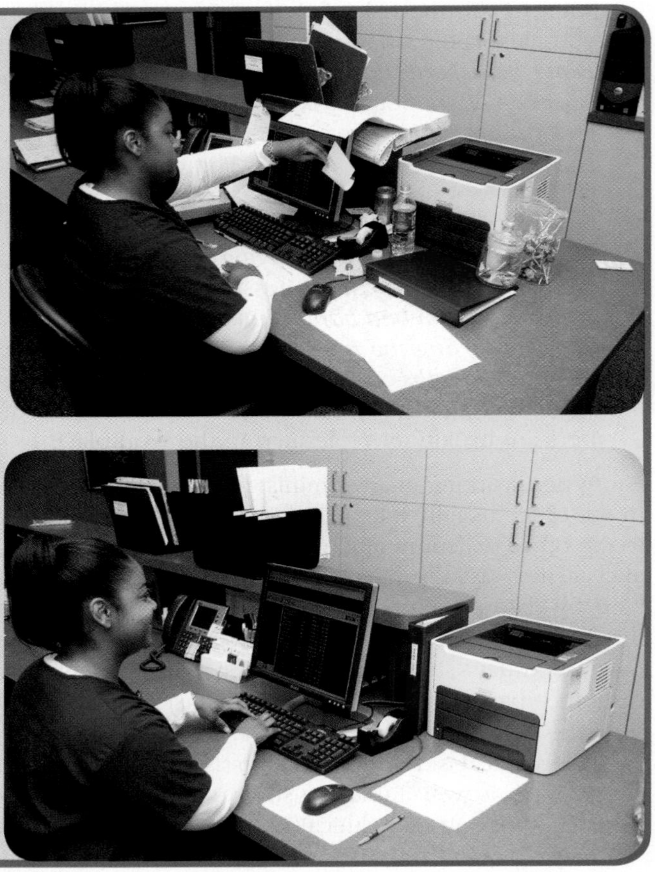

Figure 1–7: A cluttered, disorderly desk makes it difficult to stay organized (top photo), whereas a clean, orderly desk enables you to be much more efficient with your time (bottom photo). *Delmar/Cengage Learning.*

PROFESSIONAL ORGANIZATIONS FOR MEDICAL ASSISTANTS

A variety of organizations provide professional services for medical assistants, including credentialing and continuing education opportunities. These organizations help promote the field of medical assisting and provide support for medical assistants in their professional environments. Professional organizations offer educational programs that provide members with continuing education units (CEUs) that are necessary to stay current in the field as well as to retain certification. Being involved in a professional organization also provides opportunities for networking and professional discounts on an array of items, including professional liability insurance.

Accreditation

Before discussing certifying organizations, we must first briefly describe the accreditation process. **Accreditation** is a process by which an educational institution or program establishes credibility or legitimacy by complying with predetermined standards. Accredited programs must meet or exceed established thresholds in areas such as certification examination pass rates, student graduation rates, and positive placement percentages. Two organizations that specifically accredit medical assisting programs (programmatic accreditation) are the **Commission on Accreditation of Allied Health Education Programs (CAAHEP)** and the **Accrediting Bureau of Health Education Schools (ABHES)**. Schools may also be accredited at the institutional level (institutional accreditation). Some of the organizations that accredit institutions include the Accrediting Council for Independent Colleges and Schools (ACICS), the Accrediting Commission of Career Schools and Colleges (ACCSC), the Accrediting Council for Continuing Education and Training (ACCET), and state departments of education. Some of these organizations are mentioned in the following sections.

American Association of Medical Assistants

The American Association of Medical Assistants (AAMA) (Figure 1–8) traces its roots to 1955. At that time, the primary purpose of the AAMA was to raise the standards

AFFILIATE OF THE AMERICAN ASSOCIATION OF MEDICAL ASSISTANTS

CERTIFIED MEDICAL ASSISTANTS: HEALTHCARE'S MOST VERSATILE PROFESSIONALS

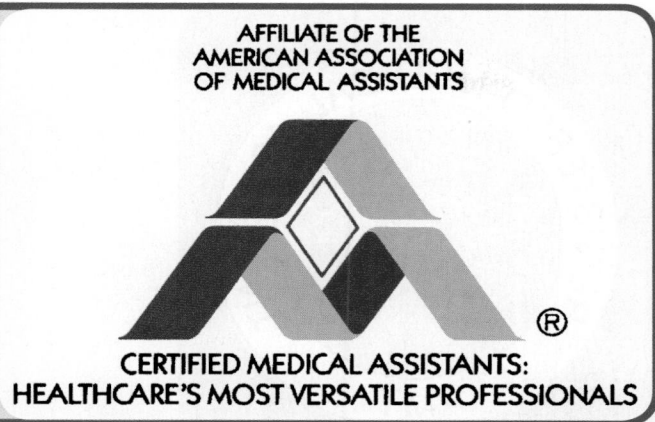

Figure 1–8: AAMA Logo. *Courtesy of the American Association of Medical Assistants.*

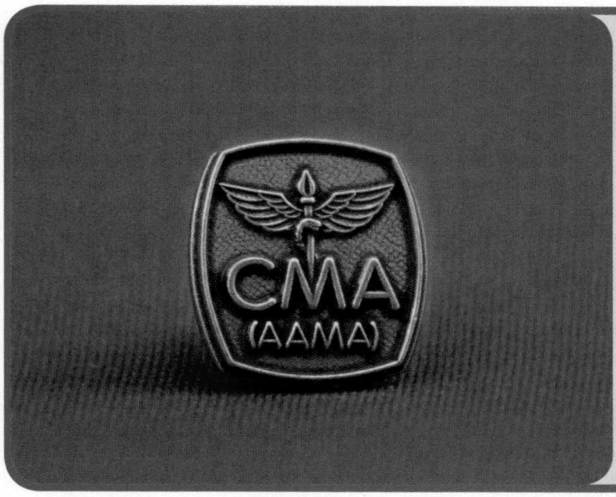

Figure 1–9: Certified Medical Assistant (CMA) (AAMA) pin. *Courtesy of the American Association of Medical Assistants.*

of the medical assistant to a professional level. (Medical assisting wasn't a recognized career at that point.) Physicians realized then, as they do now, that health care professionals were needed to assist them in a multitude of office duties for which nurses had not been trained. They also needed help in the physician-patient relationship. Today, medical assisting is formally recognized as an allied health profession, and educational programs are eligible for federal funding by the Bureau of Health Manpower. AAMA members receive a bimonthly magazine, *CMA Today*, which is devoted to educational articles written by experts in allied health and related fields. Legislation issues that affect the medical assistant's right to practice are often featured in this magazine.

Certification Examination

The AAMA offers certification testing for medical assisting graduates that meet specific prerequisites. The credential, **Certified Medical Assistant, CMA (AAMA)** (shown in Figure 1–9), is awarded to participants who successfully pass the AAMA's national certification exam. The credential was changed to include the (AAMA) addendum starting on January 1, 2008, to help differentiate the credential from similar health care certifications.

Graduates of medical assisting programs accredited by CAAHEP or ABHES are eligible to take the CMA (AAMA) certification exam. Tests are given throughout the year at various Prometric testing centers around the country. Each candidate is allowed a 90-day period in which to take the exam; applications are due at least 90 days in advance of the first of the month in which the candidate wants to test. Areas of knowledge and topics covered in the exam are listed in the *CMA (AAMA) Certification/Recertification Examination Content Outline*, which can be found on the AAMA Website at www.aama-ntl.org.

As of January 1, 2010, all newly certified and recertifying CMAs (AAMA) are considered current for 60 months following the end of the calendar month of his or her initial certification or most recent recertification. (So, those taking their test on March 15, 2013, are considered current through March 31, 2018.)

Recertification reinforces the validity of the CMA credentials and helps maintain continued acceptance by providers, patients, and other health care professionals. This requirement may be met in one of two ways:

1. By earning 60 continuing education units or hours or academic or other formal credit. The category breakdown of points must be as follows: 10 administrative, 10 clinical, 10 general, plus 30 from any combination of the categories.
2. By retaking the certification examination.

American Medical Technologists

The American Medical Technologists (AMT) organization (Figure 1–10) was founded in 1939 and is a certification and membership society for several allied health professionals, including medical assistants, medical laboratory technologists and technicians, phlebotomists, medical lab assistants, medical administrative specialists, and others. A national board of directors is elected to conduct the business of the organization such as educational programs, legal concerns, certification, and other national issues. Members receive professional publications, *AMT Events* and *CE Journal of CE Topics and Issues*, which provide timely information and educational articles of interest to medical assistants.

AMT
American Medical Technologists
Certifying Excellence in Allied Health

Figure 1–10: AMT Logo. *Courtesy of the American Medical Technologists.*

Certification Examination

In 1972, the American Medical Technologists (AMT) association initiated a nationally recognized certification process to address the needs of medical assistants and award the title of **Registered Medical Assistant, RMA (AMT)**, following the successful completion of a program accredited by a recognized accrediting body and after passing the national certification examination (Figure 1–11). The RMA (AMT) exam is designed to evaluate the competence of the entry-level medical assistant. The AMT also offers a certification for individuals specializing in front-office procedures, the Certified Medical Administrative Specialist, CMAS (AMT).

The format and questions on the exam are developed by the Examinations, Qualifications, and Standards Committee of the AMT. After applicants receive their Authorization to Test letter, they can schedule their examination at any PearsonVUE testing center. To view the content outline of this examination, go to the AMT Website at www.amt1.com, click the tab for Certification, and then click the link for Medical Assistants or Medical Administrative Specialists. Successful examinees must recertify every three years by obtaining the required number of CEUs.

Additional criteria for certification through the AMT include graduating from a formal medical services training program of the United States Armed Forces or having been employed in the medical field for a minimum of five years. Those who desire to become certified through the AMT must send a completed application form to the AMT headquarters office with the application fee and any other pertinent documentation.

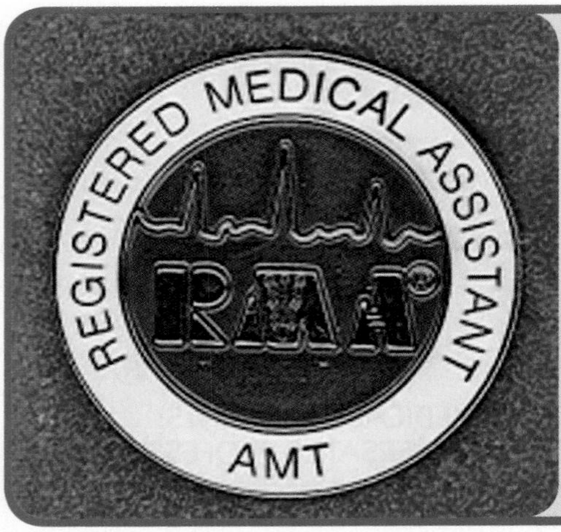

Figure 1–11: Registered Medical Assistant (RMA) pin. *Courtesy of the American Medical Technologists.*

National Center for Competency Testing

The **National Center for Competency Testing (NCCT)** (Figure 1–12) is a national certification organization that has been in existence since 1989. The organization certifies medical assistants as well as other health care professionals, including phlebotomists, patient care technicians, medical office assistants, insurance and coding specialists, ECG technicians, and other health care specialists.

The mission of the NCCT is to enhance the professional stature and employability of its members through credentialing and continuing education. The organization offers a free-of-charge benefit for individuals that maintain active certification status, referred to as My Professional Center (MPC), a Website that offers professional growth, career development, and professional and personal networking opportunities.

National Center for Competency Testing

Figure 1–12: NCCT Logo. *Courtesy of the National Center for Competency Testing.*

Certification Examination

For medical assistants, the NCCT offers certification examinations for **National Certified Medical Assistant (NCMA)** (Figure 1–13) and **National Certified Medical Office Assistant (NCMOA)**. Certification requirements include high school graduation (or equivalent) and graduation from an NCCT-approved medical assisting program or two years of qualifying full-time employment in addition to an application fee. The NCCT must receive the candidate's application within two weeks of the requested test date. Examination centers are scattered throughout the country. Candidate certification is valid for a period of five years from the date of certification indicated on each candidate's certificate. NCCT-certified individuals must participate in the renewal process by accruing 14 clock hours of continuing education annually through completion of courses provided or preapproved by NCCT. To learn more about the NCCT, go to its Website at www.ncctinc.com.

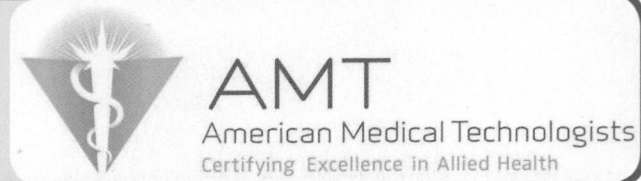

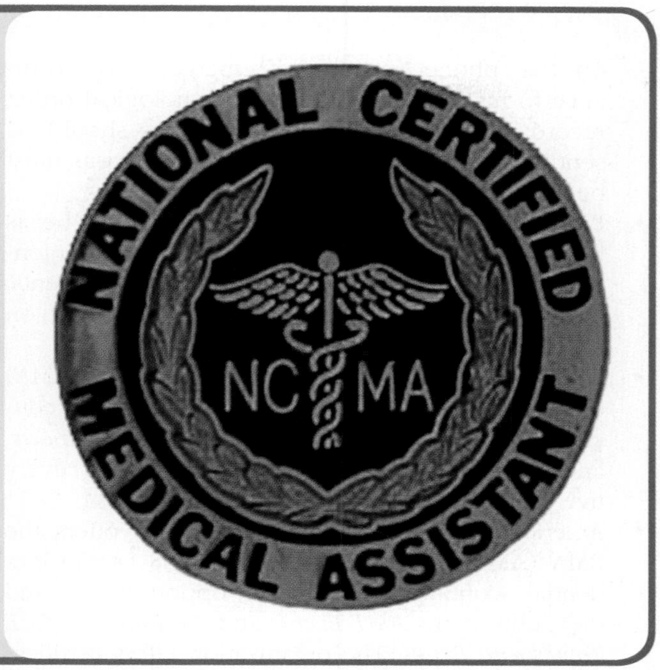

Figure 1–13: National Certified Medical Assistant (NCMA) pin. *Courtesy of the National Center for Competency Testing*

National Healthcareer Association

The **National Healthcareer Association (NHA)** (Figure 1–14) was established in 1989 as a certification agency. Today, the NHA provides products and services to health care professionals, including continuing education, program development, career and networking services, and 10 certification exams for several allied health care areas, including **Certified Clinical Medical Assistant (CCMA)** and **Certified Medical Administrative Assistant (CMAA)**.

Certification Examinations

To qualify to sit for a certification exam, you must be a graduate of an NHA-approved health care training program or have one or more years of full-time job experience and a high school diploma or GED. Exams are given at NHA-approved testing sites across the country and may be administered online or in traditional paper-and-pencil testing format. For more information, visit the NHA's Website at www.nhanow.com. To recertify, candidates either retake the exam or obtain ten CEUs every two years.

American Academy of Professional Coders

Medical assistants working in an administrative capacity might want to obtain certification as a medical coder.

NHA National Healthcareer Association
National Healthcareer Association
"The Benchmark in Allied Healthcare Certification"

Figure 1–14: Logo of the NHA. *Courtesy of the National Healthcare Association.*

The **American Academy of Professional Coders (AAPC)** was founded in 1988 to promote professionalism and encourage and support education, networking, and certification in the medical billing and coding areas. The AAPC offers training (both distance learning and traditional classroom options) through its Independent Study Program and the Professional Medical Coding Curriculum. The AAPC also offers continuing education through its annual national conference, workshops, webinars, and several publications, including *Coding Edge Magazine*, *EdgeBlast e-Newsletter*, *Billing Insider e-Newsletter*, and *ICD-10 Connect e-Newsletter*. For more information, visit the AAPC's Website at www.aapc.com.

Certification Examinations

According to the AAPC, "AAPC certifications allow medical coders, billers, and other health care professionals to:

- Validate superior knowledge and expertise in various medical coding environments
- Earn 20% more than non-credentialed coders (according to a 2009 AAPC Salary Survey)
- Show credentials nationally recognized by employers, provider societies and government organizations
- Have confidence in their ability to capture lost revenue for their practice, diminish post-payment risk and protect their practice from unfavorable audit results." (Source: www.aapc.com/certification)

AAPC offers several types of certifications, including:

- CPC® (Provider Practice)
- CPC-H® (Outpatient Hospital/Facility)
- CPC-P® (Payer)

Other certifications are available as well. To remain in good standing, credentialed members are required to renew membership annually and submit 36 hours of continuing education units every two years for verification and authentication of expertise.

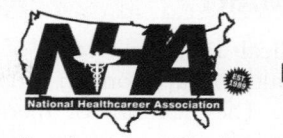

CHAPTER SUMMARY

- The field of medical assisting is one of the most versatile allied health occupations in today's health care environment. The majority of medical assistants work in ambulatory care settings or outpatient health care facilities.
- Medical assistants may work with physicians in a sole proprietorship (solo practice), in a partnership (two or more physicians), or in a multi-provider clinic (group practices with three or more physicians). Other health care environments include urgent care centers and the patient-centered medical home model.
- The three main areas of medical assisting are general, administrative, and clinical. *General skills* include communication skills, legal matters, instruction, and operational functions. *Administrative skills* include scheduling appointments, working with medical records, insurance and coding, billing and collections, and bookkeeping. *Clinical skills* include aseptic technique, minor surgery, collecting, processing and testing specimens, performing ECGs, administering medication, screening patients, assisting with procedures and treatments, and responding to emergencies.
- The job outlook for medical assistants is very good. The field of medical assisting is expected to grow 34 percent through 2018.
- A professional appearance includes looking neat, well-groomed, and self-confident. Looking like a professional provides patients with a good first impression of you and the practice.
- Professional behaviors include being accurate, adaptable, courteous, confident, dependable, empathic, honest, initiative-taking, patient, punctual, respectful, and tactful.
- Personal qualities of a medical assistant include a friendly attitude, genuine smile, and good health.
- Time management refers to an assortment of skills, tools, and practices to manage time during daily activities and when accomplishing specific projects. Goals that assist with time management include making a daily prioritization list, learning to say no, not being a perfectionist when it is not necessary, and avoiding unproductive habits.
- When working in an administrative capacity, patients in the office take priority over patients on the phone (except in emergencies), insurance forms should be filed in chronological order, record requests for next-day surgeries should be sent to the surgery center ASAP, and deposits must be made every day.
- Priority level for working the floor should be as follows: (1) assisting the provider with emergencies and other procedures, (2) rooming patients, (3) performing procedures, and (4) working on pending tasks.
- American Association of Medical Assistants (AAMA) offers the CMA (AAMA) credential, continuing education opportunities, the publication *CMA Today*, and other services. Members must recertify every five years.
- American Medical Technologists (AMT) offers the RMA (AMT) credential and the CMAS (AMT) credential, continuing education opportunities, and the publications *AMT Events* and *CE Journal of CE Topics and Issues*. The organization offers certification testing for other allied health professions as well. Members must renew their certification every three years.
- The National Center for Competency Testing (NCCT) offers the NCMA credential and the NCMOA credential, continuing education opportunities, and the "My Professional Center" Website that offers professional growth, career development, and professional and personal networking opportunities. The organization offers certification testing for other allied health professions as well. Members must renew their certification every five years.
- The National Healthcareer Association (NHA) offers the CCMA and CMAA credentials as well as continuing education, program development, and career and networking services. The organization offers certification testing for other allied health professions as well. Certified individuals must renew their certification every two years.
- Administrative MAs might want to obtain certification as a medical coder. The American Academy of Professional Coders (AAPC) offers several certifications, including CPC, CPC-H, and CPC-P, among others. It also provides education, networking opportunities, and several publications for members.

STUDY TOOLS

Workbook	Activities for Chapter 1
Premium Website	
MEDIA LINK	View this **Media Link** for Chapter 1: • Qualities of a Successful Medical Assistant
StudyWARE	Activities and Quizzes on the **StudyWARE™ Software** for Chapter 1
	Audio Library of medical terms
	Online access to **Critical Thinking Challenge 2.0**
CourseMate	Activities and Quizzes for Chapter 1
WebTutor	Activities and Quizzes for Chapter 1

CHECK YOUR KNOWLEDGE

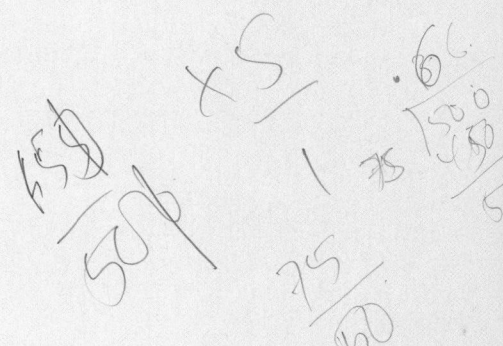

1. To be successful as an MA, you must learn a specific:
   a. Knowledge base
   b. Set of skills
   c. Behaviors
   d. All of the above
2. All of the following are clinical skills EXCEPT:
   a. Filing patient records
   b. Phlebotomy
   c. Administering medications
   d. Wrapping instruments
3. Medical assistants who perform both clinical and administrative skills are referred to as:
   a. Survivalists
   b. Capitalists
   c. Generalists
   d. Commonists
4. Employment opportunities for medical assistants are expected to grow by what percentage through 2018?
   a. 32%
   b. 34%
   c. 36%
   d. 38%
5. A term that means selflessness is:
   a. Altruism
   b. Apathy
   c. Empathy
   d. Egocentric
6. Putting yourself in another person's shoes is:
   a. Sympathy
   b. Apathy
   c. Empathy
   d. None of the above
7. Which of the following would take priority over all other floor tasks?
   a. Rooming patients
   b. Performing procedures
   c. Tasking
   d. Assisting the provider with a procedure
8. Which of the following organizations provides the RMA credential?
   a. AAMA
   b. AMT
   c. AAPC
   d. NHA
9. Which of the following organizations' focus is primarily on certifying medical billers and coders?
   a. NCCT
   b. AMT
   c. AAPC
   d. NHA
10. Which of the following certifying organizations offers a personal Website titled "My Professional Center" that offers professional growth, career development, and professional and personal networking opportunities?
    a. NCCT
    b. AAPC
    c. AMT
    d. AAMA

WEB LINKS

American Association of Medical Assistants: www.aama-ntl.org/

American Medical Technologists: www.amt1.com

National Center for Competency Testing: www.ncctinc.com

National Healthcare Association: www.nhanow.com

American Academy of Professional Coders: www.aapc.com

RESOURCES

Heller, M., and Veach, L. (2009). *Clinical Medical Assisting: A Professional, Field Smart Approach to the Workplace*. Clifton Park, NY: Delmar Cengage Learning.

Lindh, W., Pooler, M., Tamparo, C., and Dahl, B. (2010). *Delmar's Comprehensive Medical Assisting Administrative and Clinical Competencies* (4th ed.). Clifton Park, NY: Delmar Cengage Learning.

Morris, M. J. (2005). *The First Time Manager: The First Steps to a Brilliant Management Career*. London: Kogan Page.

Chapter 2

The Health Care Team and the Medical Environment, Past and Present

OBJECTIVES

In this chapter, you will learn the following:

KB KNOWLEDGE BASE

1. Spell and define, using the glossary at the back of the text, all the Words to Know in this chapter.
2. Discuss licensure and certification as it applies to health care providers.
3. List and describe different types of physicians and non-physician specialties.
4. Describe the role of the midlevel practitioner and list three examples of this type of provider.
5. List and describe four types of nurses.
6. Discuss the role of other allied health professionals and state how they fit into the medical environment.
7. Describe why Hippocrates is known as the father of medicine.
8. Identify the contributions of early and modern medical pioneers.
9. Describe the role of the government legislation and organizations in health care.
10. Compare and contrast the terms *complementary* and *alternative* therapies.
11. List and describe fifteen types of alternative therapies.

WORDS TO KNOW

acupuncture
alternative therapy
apprenticeship
apothecaries
ayurvedic medicine
biofeedback
caduceus
complementary therapy
doctor of medicine (MD)
doctor of osteopathic medicine (DO)
doctorate
epidemic
guilds
Hippocratic oath
homeopathy
hospitalist
magnet therapy
medical biller
medical coder
medical office manager
midlevel practitioner
naturopathy
nurse anesthetist
nurse midwife
nurse practitioner
Patient Protection and Affordable Care Act
phlebotomist
placebo effect
plague
provider
physician assistant
Pythagoras
reciprocity
revocation

HEALTH CARE PROVIDERS

Medical assistants are agents or representatives of the health care provider. A health care **provider** is an individual licensed to examine, diagnose, and prescribe treatment to patients seeking assistance. An organization such as a hospital or clinic can also be referred to as a health care provider. Oftentimes, when you think of health care providers, you think of physicians, but an array of health care professionals are considered health care providers. The following sections explore each type.

Physicians

Physicians invest many years in learning how to practice medicine, which is the art and science of the diagnosis, treatment, and prevention of disease and the maintenance of good health. Their training, education, and practical experience include a four-year undergraduate degree, four years in medical school, and three to eight years of internship and residency.

Licensure

Physicians must now pass all sections of the United States Medical Licensing Examination (USMLE) prior to receiving a medical license. "The USMLE® provides medical licensing authorities with a common evaluation system for applicants for initial medical licensure. Designed to be taken at different points during medical education and training, the USMLE assesses a physician's ability to apply knowledge, concepts and principles, and to demonstrate fundamental patient centered skills" (AMA).

Licensure requirements will vary by state but in general physicians applying for licensure must:

- Be of legal age.
- Be of good moral character.
- Have graduated from an approved medical school.
- Have completed an approved residency program or its equivalent.
- Be a resident of the state in which the physician is practicing.
- Submit proof of successful completion of all three steps of the United States Medical Licensing Examination (USMLE).

Physicians must continue their education following licensing by completing continuing medical education (CME) units. The number of CME units will vary by state.

Reciprocity

In the past, physicians meeting all necessary requirements for licensure had an opportunity to be licensed by another state through a process referred to as **reciprocity**. This is where one state recognizes the licensing requirements of another state as being similar or more stringent than their own. This process is looked down upon today due to the ease of attaining fraudulent licenses in multiple states. As a result, many states do not license physicians through reciprocity.

Revocation

Each state's Board of Medical Examiners provides procedures for **revocation** or suspension of licensure. In some states, the board has the power to revoke a license, and in other states, a special review committee has this authority.

A physician may lose the license to practice medicine if convicted of a crime such as murder, rape, violation of narcotic laws, or income tax evasion. A medical license may also be revoked for unprofessional conduct. The most usual offenses in this category are betrayal of patient-physician confidence, illegal use of drugs and alcohol, and inappropriate sexual conduct with patients.

A license may be revoked because of proven fraud in the application for a license. In some cases, fraudulent diplomas are used. Fraud in the filing of claims for services that were not rendered and fraud in the use of unproven treatments are also grounds for revocation of a license.

Physicians who are found to be incompetent to practice because of mental incapacity also may have their license revoked.

Doctor of Medicine and Doctor of Osteopathic Medicine

One of the areas of greatest confusion is the differentiation between **doctors of medicine (MDs)** and **doctors of osteopathic medicine (DOs)**. Holders of either degree have similar educational requirements, are licensed physicians, and may use all accepted methods of treatment; the difference in the degrees originates from somewhat different schools of thought. DOs place specific emphasis on the body's musculoskeletal and nervous systems, preventive medicine, holistic patient care, and patient education.

In the United States, medical licensing boards permit DOs to perform the same duties as MDs. Additionally, physicians of both schools, MDs and DOs, must satisfactorily complete board examinations and be licensed in the state in which they wish to practice medicine. Whether you find employment working for either a DO or an MD, you will be able to apply the same administrative and clinical knowledge and skills.

General or Family Practice

A physician in general or family practice sees all kinds of patients with all kinds of problems. If, however, the symptoms of a case suggest a serious or perhaps unknown cause, the physician might refer the patient to a specialist for further diagnosis or treatment. When the patient's specific need or problem has been remedied or the recovery plan has been established, the patient returns to the family doctor for continued care.

Physician Specialties

The advances in modern medicine have made it impossible for physicians to study every aspect of medicine. Because of this, some have become medical specialists, focusing on a specific kind of medicine. To help you become familiar with these specialties, Table 2–1 contains basic information concerning each area.

Specialty areas require additional years of study in the particular area of choice, usually requiring a minimum of two or as much as six years of additional study. After satisfactorily accomplishing all requirements, the physician is awarded a certificate of competency in the specialty area and is recognized as a diplomat or fellow of that specialty.

TABLE 2–1 Physician Specialists

Specialty	Title of Practitioner	Area of Specialization	Types of Patients Seen
Allergy	Allergist	Diagnosing and treating conditions of altered immunologic reactivity (allergic reactions)	Adults of all ages, children, both sexes
Anesthesiology	Anesthesiologist	Administering anesthetic agents before and during surgery	Adults of all ages, children, both sexes
Cardiology	Cardiologist	Diagnosing and treating abnormalities, diseases, and disorders of the heart	Adults of all ages, children, both sexes
Dermatology	Dermatologist	Diagnosing and treating disorders of the skin	Adults of all ages, children, both sexes
Endocrinology	Endocrinologist	Diagnosing and treating diseases and malfunctions of the glands of internal secretion (hormones)	Adults of all ages, children, both sexes
Family practice	Family practitioner	Similar to general practice in nature, but centering on the family unit	Adults of all ages, infants and children of all ages, both sexes
Gastroenterology	Gastroenterologist	Diagnosing and treating diseases and disorders of the stomach and intestines	Adults of all ages, children, both sexes
Geriatrics	Gerontologist or geriatrician	Diagnosing and treating diseases, disorders, and problems associated with aging	Older adults, both sexes
Gynecology	Gynecologist	Diagnosing and treating diseases and disorders of the female reproductive tract; strong emphasis on preventive measures	Female adolescents and adults
Hematology	Hematologist	Diagnosing and treating diseases and disorders of the blood and blood-forming tissues	Adults of all ages, infants and children, both sexes
Hospital	**Hospitalist**	Work with patients admitted to the hospital. They work in many departments and reduce the load of hospital visits for the primary care provider and specialist.	Adults of all ages, children, both sexes
Infertility	Infertility specialist	Diagnosing and treating problems in conceiving and maintaining pregnancy	Couples who desire to have children but cannot

(continues)

TABLE 2–1 *(Continued)*

Specialty	Title of Practitioner	Area of Specialization	Types of Patients Seen
Internal medicine	Internist	Diagnosing and treating diseases and disorders of the internal organs	Adults of all ages, both sexes. Do not typically treat children.
Nephrology	Nephrologist	Diagnosing and treating diseases and disorders of the kidney	Adults, children, both sexes
Neurology	Neurologist	Diagnosing and treating diseases and disorders of the nervous system	Adults, children, both sexes
Nuclear medicine	Nuclear medicine specialist	Diagnosing and treating diseases with the use of radionuclides	Adults, children, both sexes
Obstetrics	Obstetrician	Providing direct care to women during pregnancy and childbirth and immediately thereafter	Pregnant patients
Occupational medicine	Occupational medicine specialist	Diagnosing and treating diseases or conditions arising from occupational circumstances (e.g., disorders caused by chemicals, dust, or gases)	Adults of all ages, both sexes
Oncology	Oncologist	Diagnosing and treating tumors and cancer	Adults of all ages, children, both sexes
Ophthalmology	Ophthalmologist	Diagnosing and treating diseases and disorders of the eye	Adults of all ages, children, both sexes
Orthopedics	Orthopedist	Diagnosing and treating disorders and diseases of the bones, muscles, ligaments, and tendons and fractures of the bones	Adults of all ages, children, both sexes
Otorhinolaryngology	Otorhinolaryngologist, commonly referred to as an ENT (ear, nose, and throat) specialist	Diagnosing and treating disorders and diseases of the ear, nose, and throat	Adults of all ages, children, both sexes
Pathology	Pathologist	Performing analysis of tissue samples to confirm diagnosis	Usually has no direct contact with patients
Pediatrics	Pediatrician	Diagnosing and treating diseases and disorders of children; strong emphasis on preventive measures	Infants, children, and adolescents
Physical medicine	Physical medicine specialist	Diagnosing and treating diseases and disorders with physical agents (physical therapy)	Adults, children, both sexes
Plastic surgery	Plastic surgeon	Evaluates and improves appearance of scars, deformities, and birth defects; also provides elective procedures that patients desire for aesthetic purposes	Adults of all ages, children, both sexes
Psychiatry	Psychiatrist	Diagnosing and treating pronounced manifestations of emotional problems or mental illness that might have an organic cause	Adults of all ages, children, both sexes. (*Note*: Child psychiatry is a further specialized field dealing exclusively with children and adolescents.)

Specialty	Title of Practitioner	Area of Specialization	Types of Patients Seen
Pulmonary specialties	Pulmonary, thoracic, or cardiovascular specialist	Diagnosing and treating diseases and disorders of the chest, lungs, heart, and blood vessels	Adults, both sexes
Radiology	Radiologist	Diagnosing and treating diseases and disorders with Roentgen rays (X-rays) and other forms of radiant energy	Adults of all ages, children, both sexes
Sports medicine	Sports medicine specialist	Diagnosing and treating injuries sustained in athletic events	Adults, especially young adults (athletes), both sexes
Surgery	Surgeon	Diagnosing and treating diseases, injuries, and deformities by manual or operative methods	Adults of all ages, infants, children, both sexes
Trauma medicine	Emergency provider (commonly referred to as ER or trauma provider because most work in hospital emergency rooms)	Diagnosing and treating acute illnesses and traumatic injuries	Adults of all ages, infants, children, both sexes
Urology	Urologist	Diagnosing and treating diseases and disorders of the urinary system of females and genitourinary system of males	Adults of all ages, infants, children, both sexes

In addition to specialty areas, some physicians have a particular interest that is not a specialty but is an area they believe worthy of their time and effort to help their patients toward better health. These areas are viewed as subspecialties or areas of special interest.

Non-Physician Specialties

Many other health care professionals with the title of doctor are not physicians but provide services to patients. Table 2–2 lists the ones with whom you are most likely to have contact.

CLINICAL PEARL

A basic understanding of the term *doctor* might be helpful. It comes from Latin and means "to teach." Persons who hold doctoral degrees (**doctorates**) are entitled to be addressed as "Doctor" and to write the initials that stand for their doctorate after their name; for example, PhD or MD. Doctorates are attainable in most disciplines, such as nursing, mathematics, education, chemistry, philosophy, and so on. In the medical field, the "Dr." abbreviation denotes the person's qualification to practice medicine. In other fields, it means the person has achieved the highest academic degree awarded by a college in the particular discipline.

Midlevel Practitioners

Health care providers such as **nurse practitioners (NPs)** and **physician assistants (PAs)** are sometimes referred to as **midlevel practitioners**. They are able to examine patients, order diagnostic tests, and prescribe certain types of medications. Activities for midlevel practitioners are usually directed or dictated by a supervising physician, although in some states, nurse practitioners have more autonomy and can work independently of a physician. Midlevel practitioners are gaining acceptance by patients all over the country. Some patients feel more comfortable with these practitioners because they are often able to spend more time with patients than physicians can. The medical assistant should be familiar with state delegation laws and whether an NP or PA can delegate particular responsibilities to medical assistants.

Nurses

The American Nurses Association (ANA) describes nursing as the following:

> *Nursing is the protection, promotion, and optimization of health and abilities, prevention of illness and injury,*

TABLE 2–2 Non-Physician Specialties

Specialty	Title of Practitioner	Degree	Area of Specialization	Types of Patients Seen
Chiropractic	Chiropractor	DC, or doctor of chiropractic	Manipulative treatment of disorders originating from misalignment of the spinal vertebrae	Adults of all ages, children, both sexes
Dentistry	Dentist	DDS, or doctor of dental surgery, DMD, or doctor of dental medicine	Diagnosing and treating diseases and disorders of the teeth and gums	Adults of all ages, children, both sexes
Optometry	Optometrist	OD, or doctor of optometry	Measuring the accuracy of vision to determine whether corrective lenses are needed	Adults of all ages, children, both sexes
Podiatry	Podiatrist	DPM, or doctor of podiatric medicine	Diagnosing and treating diseases and disorders of the feet	Adults of all ages, children, both sexes
Psychology	Psychologist	PhD, or doctor of philosophy	Evaluating and treating emotional problems; these professionals give counseling to individuals, families, and groups	Adults of all ages, children, both sexes

alleviation of suffering through the diagnosis and treatment of human response, and advocacy in the care of individuals, families, communities, and populations.

There are several types of nurses. The role of the nurse practitioner has already been discussed. The following descriptions apply to other nursing categories.

Registered Nurse

In the United States, a registered nurse (RN) is defined as a professional nurse who has completed a course of study at a state-approved school of nursing and passed the National Council Licensure Examination (NCLEX-RN). RNs are licensed to practice by individual states. Employment settings for RNs include hospitals, convalescent facilities, clinics, and home health care, to name a few. (A registered nurse is not considered a provider but is mentioned in this section because this section discusses other types of nurses. This is a starting point for nurses who become providers.)

Nurse Anesthetist

A **nurse anesthetist** is an RN who is certified to administer anesthesia. The initials CRNA stands for certified registered nurse anesthetist and means that the RN has completed an anesthesia training program and passed the certification test to administer anesthesia. CRNAs normally work in hospitals and ambulatory surgical centers as well as in a host of other surgical environments.

Nurse Midwife

A **nurse midwife** is a professional RN who has had extensive training and experience in labor and delivery. Most states require a certification in addition to the state nurse license. The midwife assists the birthing mother throughout her pregnancy, the delivery of her infant at home or in a medical facility, and the postpartum period. Nurse midwives manage normal pregnancies and deliveries that potentially have no risks of developing complications.

Licensed Practical Nurse

Sometimes referred to as licensed vocational nurses (LVNs), licensed practical nurses (LPNs) are trained in basic nursing techniques and direct patient care. They practice under the direct supervision of an RN or a provider and are employed in hospitals, convalescent centers, nursing homes, and home health care. (LPNs are not considered providers.)

HEALTH CARE TEAM MEMBERS

Many other health professionals provide specific care to patients (Figure 2–1). They work in a variety of settings such as hospitals, laboratories, municipal safety divisions, provider offices, pharmacies, convalescent and extended care facilities, and for home health care agencies. It is important for you to have some understanding of the specific duties for which they have been trained and their role in total patient care. Unless you work for

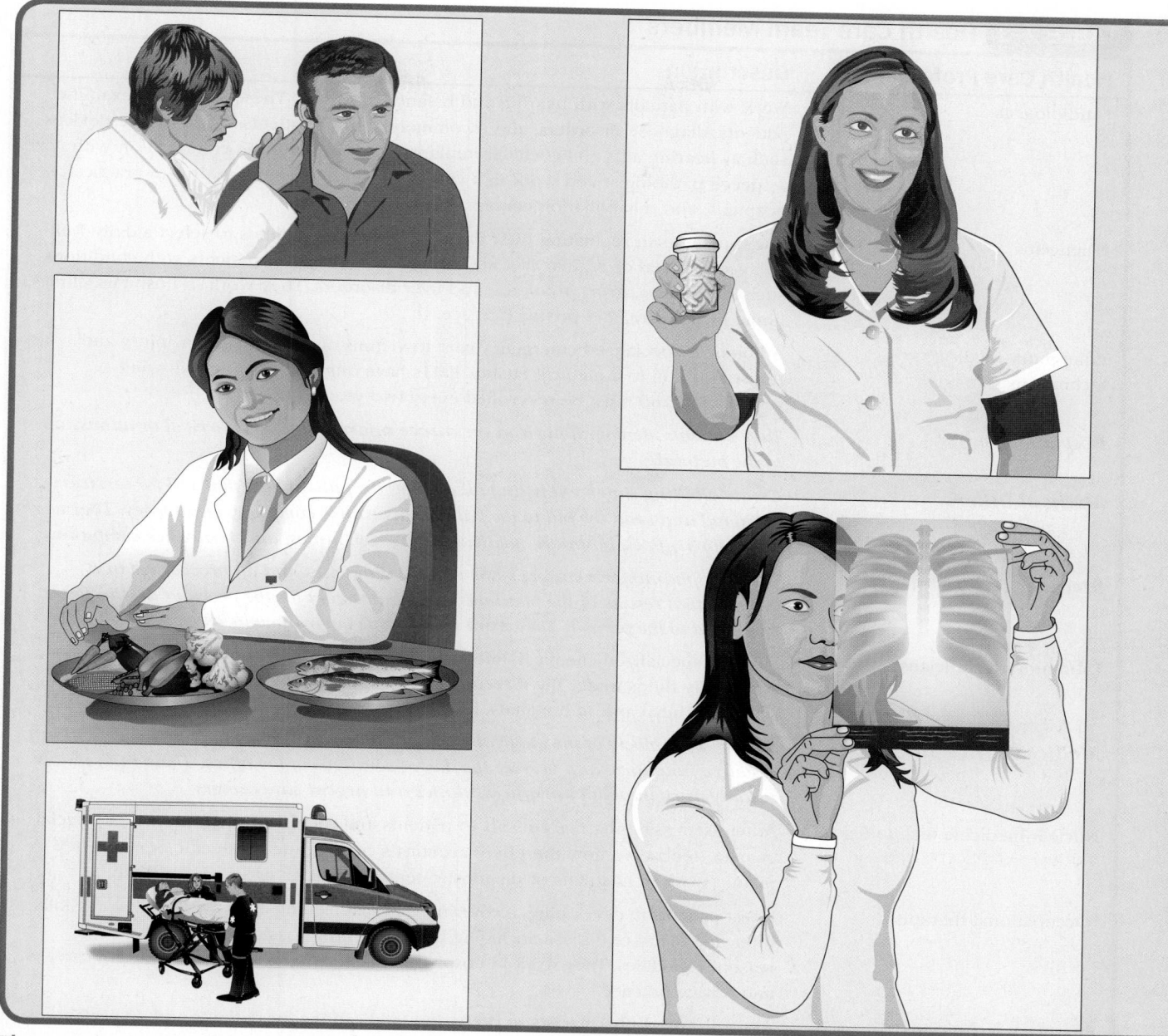

Figure 2–1: Allied health professionals; clockwise from top: Audiologist, pharmacy technician, radiology technician, emergency medical technician, and nutritionist. *Delmar/Cengage Learning.*

a hospital, or in a group practice or clinic, you probably will not work directly with most of these team members, but you might have contact with them by telephone or by written communication. Often, patients can have several health problems at the same time, and cooperation with other members of the health care team to accommodate the patient is vital. Knowing the role each professional plays in the total health care of patients enables you to speak more intelligently with others in the medical field and become more efficient in your role as the medical assistant. You might even be able to take on some of these roles as a medical assistant with additional experience and training. Specialized roles for medical assistants will be italicized in Table 2–3.

Table 2–3 provides a listing of health care professionals and their descriptions.

A BRIEF HISTORY OF MEDICINE

To understand fully the high technical level of current health care and the responsibilities of those who provide it, we must look back at its history and learn how it

TABLE 2–3 Health Care Team Members

Health Care Professional	Description
*Audiologists	Work with patients with hearing and balance disorders. These specialists examine patients, diagnose disorders, and recommend and fit patients with assistive devices such as hearing aids and cochlear implants. They can work in combination with a speech pathologist and work in a variety of settings including private practice, hospitals, and rehabilitation centers.
*Dieticians	Assist patients in regulating their diets. They instruct patients to select a daily well-balanced special or regular diet and design meal plans for patients with conditions such as diabetes, heart problems, and liver disorders. They work in hospitals, clinics, home health care, and private practice.
Emergency medical technicians (EMTs)	Administer specialized emergency care to victims of acute illness or injury and transport them to a medical facility. EMTs have ongoing training following certification and must be recertified every two years.
Hospital registrars	*Take patients' demographic and insurance information upon arrival or admission to the hospital.*
Medical billers	*Create a billing statement listing all charges the patient has incurred for services rendered and send the bill to the patient, insurance company, or attorney. They work in doctor's offices, hospitals, medical billing companies, and insurance companies.*
Medical coders	*Use an alphanumeric coding system for all diagnoses and all procedures in a manner that results in the maximum reimbursement for the provider and in fewer fees billed to the patient. They work in the same environments as medical billers.*
Laboratory technicians	Perform specialized chemical, microscopic, and bacteriologic tests of blood, tissue, and bodily fluids under the direction of a pathologist, other provider, or medical scientist. They work in hospitals, laboratories, and clinics.
Medical Office Manager	*Supervise members of the medical office staff, coordinate schedules, perform human resource functions, and oversee the daily operations of the office. These individuals usually work in physician offices, clinics and urgent care centers.*
Nuclear medicine technologists	Administer radiopharmaceuticals to patients and then scan the body with a special camera to observe how the pharmaceuticals concentrate in specific organs. They mainly work in hospitals or diagnostic centers.
*Occupational therapists	Assist patients in developing, recovering, and maintaining daily living and work skills following injury or disease, including helping improve basic motor functions and reasoning abilities. They work in hospitals, rehabilitation centers, home health care, and private practice.
Pharmacy technicians	Assist licensed pharmacists in preparing medications for patients and, in certain cases, administering the medicine. They also assist in clerical duties such as telephone communication, typing, and filing and, often, in patient education regarding medicines. (Requirements and duties can vary in different states.) Professional certification can be obtained through individual state pharmacy boards. They often work in hospitals and store chain pharmacies.
Phlebotomist	*A phlebotomist is a healthcare worker whose primary responsibility is to obtain blood samples. Other duties include the transportation, handling, and processing of blood specimens for analysis. Phlebotomists work in a variety of settings including doctor's offices, outpatient laboratories, skilled nursing facilities, and hospitals.*
*Physical therapists	Evaluate, diagnose, and treat movement disorders in patients with musculoskeletal injuries and illness. Treatments can include therapeutic exercise, functional training, manual therapy techniques, assistive and adaptive devices and equipment, and physical agents and electrotherapeutic modalities. They usually work in hospitals, rehabilitation centers, home health care, and private practice.

Health Care Professional	Description
Radiology technicians *General X-ray machine operators*	Take X-rays and CAT scans and, sometimes, administer non-radioactive chemicals to help illuminate structures on the X-ray. They work in hospitals, diagnostic centers, and clinics. *Some medical assistants are able to obtain a limited permit to take x-rays in an ambulatory health care setting. (This will vary by state.) The permit is often referred to as a general x-ray machine operator's (GXMO) license. A GXMO usually performs x-rays of the chest, extremities, spine, and sinuses in ambulatory settings.*
Respiratory therapists	Perform procedures of treatment that maintain or improve the ventilatory function of the respiratory tract in patients. They work in hospitals, nursing homes, and home health care.
Sonographers	Create images of structures within the body by using sound waves instead of X-rays. Although people think of the sonography associated with OB/GYN practices, sonography aids in the diagnosis of many other conditions as well. Sonographers work in hospitals, diagnostic centers, and specialty offices such as cardiovascular and OB/GYN practices.
Surgical technologists	Assist the surgeon and surgical team before, during, and after a procedure. They set up the operating room and instruments before surgery and help in the cleanup following surgery. They work in hospital OR departments and ambulatory surgical centers.

*Indicates those that professionals that might also work in private practice.

has developed. Ancient times were filled with infectious disease and **epidemics** (affecting large numbers of individuals in a population) as well as illnesses and injuries caused by dietary deficiencies and unhealthy or hostile environments. Eighty percent of primitive human beings died by the age of 30 as a result of hunting accidents or violence. Primitive individuals lived primarily alone, so there was little risk of widespread diseases or **plagues** (potentially infectious life-threatening diseases, usually transmitted by bites of rodent fleas to humans). However, when they began settling in communities, farming, and domesticating animals, epidemic diseases resulted from overcrowding, filth, and the natural presence of microorganisms. Initially, tuberculosis, tetanus, malaria, smallpox, typhus, typhoid, and, later, leprosy ravaged early civilizations.

Ancient Civilizations

Because people in ancient times did not understand the concept of microorganisms or the function of the human body, the presence of disease was credited to evil spirits and demons brought on as punishment for disobedience to the gods. Therefore, medical practice became the role of priests or medicine men. Treatments involved rituals to drive out demons.

Egypt

Evidence found in Egyptian tombs and on papyri indicates the people of the area around the Nile River had developed a level of medical practice as early as 3000 BCE. Egyptian providers were priests who studied medicine and surgery in the temple medical schools. They tried to drive out evil spirits with spells and concocted potions. In addition to magic, they also used about one third of the medicinal plants still used in pharmacies today.

Egyptians believed that blood in the body flowed through canals like those constructed along the Nile for irrigation. When it was thought that the body's canals were clogged, they were opened by bloodletting or the application of leeches. The leech not only removed blood and disease toxins but also produced hirudin in the process, which prevented coagulation. The use of leeches continued until the nineteenth century and is now being reintroduced following some surgical procedures and in specific traumas where a large amount of blood is present within the tissues.

India

The Hindus in India had the world's first nurses and hospitals. They employed extensive use of drugs, including those for anesthesia that undoubtedly assisted with the main Hindu contribution to the art of healing: surgery. Their knowledge of anatomy was limited, but their surgeons performed a fairly technical form of cataract and plastic surgery. Early writings reveal that they used approximately 120 surgical instruments in a variety of procedures.

China

The Chinese, India's neighbors, had a highly developed center of early medical learning. Their belief in evil spirits as the cause of illness gradually changed; they began searching for medical reasons for illness. About 3000 BCE, the emperor, who was known as the father of Chinese medicine, followed a document called *Great Herbal* (a translation), which contained more than a thousand drugs; some are still in use today. The art of acupuncture was originally used as a means to drive out demons. Today, the ancient procedure has become a respected alternative form of treatment.

Greece

The Greeks also played a large role in the development of medicine. Beginning about 2000 BCE, they invaded many lands and established a remarkable civilization. They acquired knowledge from those they conquered but still practiced religious and healing rituals. They believed Apollo, the sun god, taught the art of medicine to a centaur who in turn taught others, including Asklepios, the Greek god of healing, who lived around 1250 BCE. The priests in the temples of Asklepios (also called Aesculapius) used massage, bathing, and exercise in treating patients. They also depended on the magical power of large, yellow, nonpoisonous snakes. After patients purified themselves by bathing and made offerings to the god, they were given tablets to read that described cures of former patients. Then they were put into a drug-induced sleep in the temple. During the night, the snakes licked the wounds and Asklepios applied salves. The god was usually depicted holding a staff with a serpent coiled around its shaft. This is probably the origin of the medical symbol known as a **caduceus** (Figure 2–2), even though it shows two instead of one coiled serpent, as did the staff of Aesculapius.

Hippocrates, the founder of scientific medicine, was a Greek physician born in about 460 BCE on the Island of Cos. During his 99 years of life, he took medicine out of the realm of priests and philosophers and produced an organized method of gaining knowledge through the means of observation. He taught that illness was the result of natural causes and not punishment for sin. He advocated examining a patient's environment, home, and place of work. He stressed the importance of diet and cleanliness. He felt medical knowledge could be acquired only through accurate clinical observation of the sick. He discovered that the course of certain diseases could be traced by listening to the chest of a patient. More than 2,000 years passed before a French physician named Laennec invented the stethoscope to improve this method of observation.

Hippocrates studied with the most distinguished teachers of the day. He practiced in many parts of the Greek world and was admired for his cures. He wrote many detailed studies, among which are ones on prognostics, fractures, and surgery. He is best known for his code of behavior, known as the **Hippocratic oath**, however, some scholars believe that the oath was written by **Pythagoras.** Physicians often repeat a modernized version of the oath sometime around graduation from medical school (Figure 2–3). For all his accomplishments, Hippocrates became known as the father of medicine.

The Roman Empire

Except for the teachings of Claudius Galen (featured in Table 2–4), the Romans made almost no contribution to medicine but established superior methods of sanitation and water supply. They realized disease was connected to filth and overcrowding. They drained the marshes to reduce the incidence of malaria and instituted laws to maintain public health and clean streets. They built an extensive underground sewer system and pure water aqueducts capable of bringing an estimated 300 million gallons of drinking water a day into the city. Medical officers and surgeons served in the army. A private hospital system was also developed, first for the wealthy and slaves, then for the campaign armies. Later, public hospitals were founded, and the hospital movement expanded with the growth of Christianity and its tradition of caring for the sick.

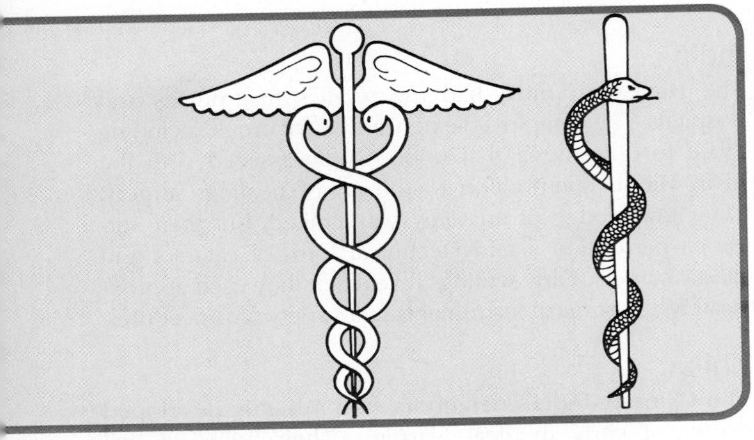

Figure 2–2: A caduceus (left) and the staff of Aesculapius (right). *Delmar/Cengage Learning.*

Medieval History

The great Roman Empire was overrun by barbarians; Europe was controlled by Teutonic tribal groups whose people were agricultural, and established health standards vanished. The centers of learning and medicine decayed. From the fifth to the sixteenth centuries, little progress was made in medical knowledge or practice.

Eventually, medicine passed into the hands of the Christian church and Arab scholars. The church did not foster medical science. It recommended prayer and fasting because it believed that illness was a punishment for sin. Christianity forbade human dissection, so anatomy and physiology died except for the erroneous pages of Galen. Priests again became healers, using exorcism and holy relics to cure the sick.

OATH OF HIPPOCRATES

I swear by Apollo, the physician, and Aesculapius and health and all-heal and all the Gods and Goddesses that, according to my ability and judgment, I will keep this oath and stipulation:

TO RECKON him who taught me this art equally dear to me as my parents, to share my substance with him and relieve his necessities if required; to regard his offspring as on the same footing with my own brothers, and to teach them this art if they should wish to learn it, without fee or stipulation, and that by precept, lecture, and every other mode of instruction, I will impart a knowledge of the art to my own sons and to those of my teachers, and to disciples bound by a stipulation and oath, according to the law of medicine, but to none others.

I WILL FOLLOW that method of treatment which, according to my ability and judgment, I consider for the benefit of my patients, and abstain from whatever is deleterious and mischievous. I will give no deadly medicine to anyone if asked, nor suggest any such counsel; furthermore, I will not give to a woman an instrument to produce abortion.

WITH PURITY AND WITH HOLINESS I will pass my life and practice my art. I will not cut a person who is suffering from a stone, but will leave this to be done by practitioners of this work. Into whatever houses I enter I will go into them for the benefit of the sick and will abstain from every voluntary act of mischief and corruption; and further from the seduction of females or males, bond or free.

WHATEVER, in connection with my professional practice, or not in connection with it, I may see or hear in the lives of men which ought not to be spoken abroad I will not divulge, as reckoning that all such should be kept secret.

WHILE I CONTINUE to keep this oath unviolated may it be granted to me to enjoy life and the practice of the art, respected by all men at all times but should I trespass and violate this oath, may the reverse be my lot.

Figure 2–3: The Hippocratic oath. *Adapted from the Hippocratic oath.*

The Arab Empire

A second storehouse of medical knowledge was in the Moslem Arab Empire, which, by 1000 CE, extended from Spain to India. The Arabs were eager for knowledge, and the classical learning was translated into Arabic. Medicine began a revival. Arab physicians learned much about epidemics, but their great knowledge of chemistry resulted in their major medical contribution in pharmacology. They also continued the Roman system of hospitals, including at least four major teaching centers. One had specialized wards for specific conditions. All patients were admitted regardless of race, creed, or social status. Upon departure, patients were given sufficient money to cover their convalescence.

Medical Schools

The union of medical knowledge from both the East and the West produced an outstanding medical school at Salerno, Italy, around 850 CE. It was believed to be founded by a Jew, a Roman, a Greek, and an Arab and was open to both men and women of all nationalities. Because it was not a church school, it could teach medicine using a sound basis and became the convalescent center for wounded Crusaders. By the twelfth century, it had a highly organized curriculum upon which students were examined and issued degrees to become the first true doctors. Both anatomy and surgery were taught, but it was still based upon animal dissection. Other medical centers followed, including ones in Paris, Oxford, and Cambridge. Despite earlier progress, however, religious and scholarly factions prohibited advancement. Medical teaching was predominately oral because books were scarce. (For example, the medical school in Paris had only 12 books at the end of the fourteenth century.) Dissection was rare. One university did secure the right to dissect one executed criminal every three years, but it allowed only a superficial examination of the chest and abdomen.

Barber Surgeons

Medieval European surgeons' practice was limited to nobility, the high clergy, and wealthy merchants. Other patients and minor surgeries were treated by ignorant barber surgeons. They cut hair, practiced bloodletting, opened abscesses, and occasionally did amputations—all with the same razor. Their trademark became the white poles around which they wrapped their blood-stained bandages. The red and white pole is still seen today outside of barbershops.

The Great Diseases

Two of the greatest medieval diseases were leprosy and the bubonic plague. Leprosy was present in the early centuries, brought perhaps by the Roman soldiers. It was

TABLE 2–4 Medical Pioneers through the Eighteenth Century

Name and Date	Country of Residence	Contribution
Alcmaeon 500 BCE	Greece	Dissected animals to study sight and hearing.
Hippocrates 460 BCE–379 BCE	Greece	Known as the father of medicine. See chapter reference.
Aristotle 384 BCE–322 BCE	Greece	A contemporary of Hippocrates, was a philosopher and scientific genius and became the tutor of Alexander the Great. He brought together medicine, biology, botany, and anatomy. His findings were based upon animal dissection because human dissection was illegal.
Claudius Galen CE 121–CE 199	Turkey and Rome	Physician, surgeon, and anatomist. He wrote more than 500 anatomy books, but his theories were flawed because he studied the anatomy of pigs, dogs, and Barbary apes. He believed that the body was composed of and regulated by four humors (fluids) of life—blood, phlegm, black bile, and yellow bile—and that an imbalance of these resulted in illness. His viewpoints were accepted until the sixteenth century.
Rhazes CE 860–CE 932	Arab Empire	Produced about 150 books, including a medical encyclopedia weighing 22 pounds. He based his diagnosis upon observation of disease, and his major contribution was distinguishing smallpox from measles. He is also credited with the use of animal gut sutures to sew wounds.
Trotula Platearius Sometime between 1100 and 1200	Italy	Earliest known female physician. She specialized in obstetrics and gynecology and wrote a textbook, *Diseases of Women*, which was used for 700 years.
Ambroise Paré 1510–1590	France	A French surgeon; he discovered it was possible and much more successful to tie bleeding vessels with a ligature than to burn them with a cautery. He invented special forceps to grasp arteries and developed new techniques for treating fractures and dislocations.
Andreas Versalius 1514–1564		An anatomist who did his own dissections on corpses that he took from the gallows or bought from grave robbers. He determined that the structures he dissected were not as Galen had described. From his studies he wrote one of the most influential anatomy books of its time.
William Harvey 1578–1657	England	Observed that blood in the arteries always flowed away from the heart while blood in the veins flowed toward it, with valves that prevented it from changing direction.
Antony Van Leuwenhoek 1632–1732	Netherlands	Built more than 200 microscopes (some of which magnified up to 270 times), allowing him to see, for the first time, red blood cells.
Gabriel Fahrenheit 1688–1736	Germany	A physicist who introduced the thermometric scale and developed the mercury thermometer.
Edward Jenner 1749–1823	England	Gave the first vaccination to an 8-year-old boy, using the exudate from a cowpox lesion of a dairymaid. He injected the boy with smallpox two months later, but it did not develop.
Rene Laennec 1781–1826	France	Invented the stethoscope because he could not hear the heart and lungs of an obese patient with his ear. It was originally a rolled-up piece of paper but became a wooden tube.

Note: BCE and CE are abbreviations for "Before the Common Era" and "Common Era."

one of the few diseases recognized as being contagious but was believed to be a result of sins against God. The afflicted were herded into leper houses outside the towns, forbidden to marry, proclaimed dead citizens, and ordered to wear a black cloak with white patches. In 1313, King Philip the Fair wanted to burn them all but was forbidden by the church. Incidences of leprosy decreased with the coming of the Black Death (the bubonic plague), which killed many lepers. *Black death* described the dark, mottled appearance of the corpse due to hemorrhages beneath the skin. (In 1905, it was determined that this disease was caused by a bacillus that grew in fleas of infected black rats.) The disease was devastating. Symptoms included sudden shivering, headache, vomiting, and pains in the abdomen and limbs, followed by delirium. Large, painful boils appeared at the body joints, and, unless treated, it proved fatal in five days. Other variations included the pneumonic plague, which affected the lungs and caused death in three days, and the septicemic plague, caused by direct bacillus injection into the blood by the flea, which caused death within 24 hours.

The Renaissance

Beginning in Italy in the fourteenth century, there was a revival of culture and concern for life. Gradually, people began to escape the limitations of the church and adopted a new attitude toward the human body. The classical artists, Michelangelo, Dürer, and da Vinci, began to practice dissection to depict the human body—especially the bones, muscles, and internal organs—accurately.

The Guilds

The practice of medicine in the beginning of the seventeenth century was divided among the members of three **guilds** (an association of persons engaged in a common trade or calling for mutual advantage and protection): the physicians, the surgeons, and the **apothecaries** (pharmacists). The physicians were the most prestigious because they usually possessed a university degree. They preferred studying, teaching, and debating the theories of disease to actually dealing directly with the sick. They limited their practice to the upper classes. The surgeons were considered inferior to the physicians. They were divided into two classifications: Surgeons of the Long Robe and the more humble barber surgeons. Only a few surgeons held university degrees. They were trained largely in hospitals or through **apprenticeships** (a period of time during which one is bound by agreement to learn some trade or craft). Barber surgeons used their razors for opening veins as well as for barbering. The apothecaries were tradesmen and were permitted to treat people with the drugs they made, prescribed, and sold. They were the general practitioners for the masses and learned through apprenticeships.

Many pioneers made contributions to medicine throughout the early ages. Table 2–4 provides a listing of these individuals and describes their contributions.

Modern Medicine

Humans had been "practicing" medicine for thousands of years, but only since the development of the microscope and the discovery of microbes has it progressed. With the emphasis on scientific inquiry, medicine changed rapidly. Tables 2–5 and 2–6 list many of the medical pioneers who made contributions since the 1800s. These pioneers provided us not only with technology but with practices that have improved overall morbidity and mortality rates. Women are among the contributors in this era and, today, are some of the most respected medical scientists and physicians in the world.

The Impact of Government on Health Care

The federal government has provided much impetus and influence in the growth of medicine through funding, grants, and regulations.

Table 2–7 lists organizations and legislation that have affected the delivery of health care. A review of the information will give you some insight about why certain policies and procedures are followed in the medical office.

ALTERNATIVES TO THE TRADITIONAL MEDICAL MODEL

A great deal of interest has also arisen in methods of health care other than the traditional medical model. Some authorities make a distinction between the various types of related therapies. One type is called **complementary therapies**. These are treatments that are considered to supplement or add to the conventional form of medicine. Some examples are the use of massage, acupressure, **acupuncture** (Figure 2–4), and hypnosis. Another type of therapy is called **alternative therapy**. This is interpreted by some as meaning a method used instead of conventional medicine. Often, alternative therapies are not validated by research, and no scientific evidence exists that they are or can be therapeutic. Some people have claimed cures from these and other remedies, but without scientific study, the placebo effect or spontaneous healing cannot be ruled out. (A **placebo effect** refers to the fact that some people respond favorably to a known ineffective treatment because they believe it is working. This occurs in about 30% to 40% of patients.) In this chapter, the word *related* will be

TABLE 2–5 Medical Pioneers in the Nineteenth Century

Name and Date	Country of Residence	Contribution
W. T. G. Morton 1819–1868	United States	Introduced the use of ether to make his patients more comfortable during surgery.
Florence Nightingale 1820–1910	England (primarily)	Founder of modern nursing. She was sent with 38 nurses to care for Crimean War casualties. She established a formal school of nursing at St. Thomas Hospital in London in 1860.
Clara Barton 1821–1912	United States	A Civil War nurse; recognized the need for support services for soldiers. She established the American Red Cross in 1881 and served as its first president.
Elizabeth Blackwell 1821–1910	United States	First woman physician in the United States. She was rejected by 17 schools before being accepted. In 1853, she and two woman physicians opened a medical college for women in New York and, in 1857, a hospital exclusively for women.
Louis Pasteur 1822–1895	France	A chemist who discovered microorganisms could be destroyed by heating. The treatment of milk with heat to destroy organisms carries his name, pasteurization. He also discovered a vaccine to prevent and treat rabies.
Joseph Lister 1827–1912	England	A surgeon who realized microbes in the air caused infections after surgery. He used diluted carbolic acid to disinfect the skin, his hands, and instruments and developed a pump to spray the air. This was the foundation for medical asepsis.
Wilhelm von Roentgen 1845–1923	Germany	Discovered X-rays, which were later called Roentgen rays in his honor. This gave physicians the ability to see inside the body without surgery.
Elias Metchnikoff 1845–1916	Russia	Worked at Pasteur's Institute and became director after Pasteur died. He discovered how white blood cells protect the body from disease.
Walter Reed 1851–1902	United States	An army major serving in Cuba; he discovered the cause of yellow fever was a virus carried by a mosquito. By preventing bites, the disease was curtailed, and the Panama Canal was built.

TABLE 2–6 Medical Pioneers in the Twentieth and Twenty-First Centuries

Name and Date	Country of Residence	Contribution
Marie Curie 1867–1934	Poland	First world-famous woman scientist. She discovered radium, and her work led to the use of radium in the treatment of cancer.
Alexis Carrel 1873–1944	France	Came to the United States and discovered severed arteries could be joined and again be functional. Also did animal research transplanting bones, blood vessels, and organs.
Elise Strang L'Esperance 1878–1959	United States	Graduated from medical school established by Elizabeth Blackwell. She had a concern for early cancer detection and established the Strang Clinic.

Name and Date	Country of Residence	Contribution
Sir Alexander Fleming 1881–1964	Scotland	While experimenting with bacteria, a mold accidentally drifted onto a culture and prevented the bacteria from growing. Later, this mold was studied and became the beginnings of penicillin.
George Papanicolaou 1883–1962	United States	Worked at the Strang Clinic diagnosing cervical cancer. His discovery, the Pap test, has become routine and has saved the lives of thousands of women.
Sir Frederick Banting 1891–1941	Canada	Discovered and isolated insulin in 1921, giving diabetics a more normal life.
Gerhard Domagk 1895–1964	Germany	A bacteriologist experimenting with mice, he discovered a red dye called prontosil killed coccus-family organisms. This led to the development of sulfa drugs that cure 90% of coccal infections.
Jonas Salk 1914–1995	United States	With a team of researchers, he successfully isolated the polio virus and developed the first vaccine for polio.
A. B. Sabin 1906–1993	United States	Developed an attenuated oral vaccine for polio.
Michael DeBakey 1908–2008	United States	The first to use an external heart pump successfully in a patient. He also pioneered the use of Dacron grafts to replace or repair blood vessels.
Willem J. Kolff 1911–2009	Netherlands	A Dutch physician who invented the first artificial kidney and went on to build all sorts of artificial organs, including the first artificial heart.
Charles Hufnagel 1916–1989	United States	Replaced a heart valve with the first artificial one in 1953.
C. Walton Lillehei 1918–1999	United States	Pioneered open-heart surgery. With two electronic engineers, perfected a pacemaker with silver-plated wires going through the chest and attaching to the surface of the heart.
Ake Senning 1915–2000	Sweden	The first to implant a pacemaker.
Frank B. Colton 1923–2003	Poland/United States	Developed the first oral contraceptive (Enovid) in 1960.
Peter Safar 1924–2003	United States	Wrote *ABC of Resuscitation* in 1957. The American Heart Association adopted his A-B-C system of CPR in 1977.
Patrick Steptoe 1913–1988, and Dr. Robert Edwards 1925–	England	Credited with the world's first successful in vitro fertilization on November 10, 1977, and the birth of the first test-tube baby on July 25, 1978.
Dr. Robert Jarvik 1946–	United States	Designed the first permanently implantable artificial heart, known as the Jarvik-7. First surgery with the Jarvik-7 took place in 1982. Today's version is known as the SynCardia temporary CardioWest and is approved as a temporary bridge for those awaiting heart transplants.
Ray W. Fuller 1935–1996	United States	Fuller with some help from other researchers at Eli Lilly and Co. is credited with the development of Prozac (leading anti-depressant with low side effects). Developed in 1972 and marketed in 1987.

(continues)

TABLE 2–6 *(Continued)*

Name and Date	Country of Residence	Contribution
Stanley Cohen 1935– and Herbert Boyer 1936–	United States	Credited with cloning genetically engineered molecules (1973). Their contributions have led to the development of synthetic insulin, a clot-dissolving agent for heart attack victims, and a growth hormone for underdeveloped children.
Nicholas Terrett and Peter Ellis (Pfizer) 1998	England/United States	Discovered sildenafil citrate (Prozac). Originally developed as a heart medication but became known for its side effects of penile erection. Synthesized in 1996 and marketed in 1998.
AbioCor company 2001	United States	Developed the first totally implantable artificial heart, implanted in a patient in 2001. Unlike the Jarvik-7, this device has no external wires, which helps reduce infection in the recipients receiving these devices.

TABLE 2–7 **Organizations and Legislation Affecting Health Care**

Date	Organization/Legislation	Description
1930	Food and Drug Administration	Legislation that gave status to Public Health Service and the Food and Drug Administration. In 1953, the two became part of the Department of Health, Education, and Welfare, which has since become the Department of Health and Human Services.
1930	National Institutes of Health (NIH)	Had its beginnings in 1887 as a laboratory, researching the causes of cholera and tuberculosis. There was no treatment for either disease. In 1930, the NIH was established under the U.S. Department of Health and Human Services (DHHS). There are 13 research institutes (e.g., the National Cancer Institute) that work to improve health and provide information to health care professionals. They support biomedical research in the cause and prevention of disease at the institutes and at universities and hospitals.
1946	Hill–Burton Act	Provided for the improvement and construction of hospitals. Big cities renovated existing buildings and established ICU units, trauma centers, and outpatient services. Small towns and rural areas were provided with regional health centers.
1948	World Health Organization (WHO)	A specialized agency of the United Nations that cooperates to control and eradicate disease worldwide. It shares information and technology and delivers medical supplies and drugs where needed.
1965	Medicaid	A title under the Social Security amendments that provides government funding to the states help pay for the medical care of indigents. States establish criteria for qualification and set fee schedules to reimburse providers who perform services.
1966	Medicare	National health insurance for persons over 65 or those who are blind, disabled, or have certain kidney conditions. It is administered by the Centers for Medicare and Medicaid Services (CMS) through the DHHS. Medicare has Part A, which covers hospitalization, and Part B, which covers physicians and other medical providers.
1967	Clinical Laboratory Improvement Amendments (CLIA)	Established guidelines for operating laboratories. A congressional investigation into physicians' office labs (POL) resulted in the 1988 amendments. The labs were found deficient in both quality of service and results, mainly due to lack of accredited technologists. The new law set standards for laboratories and listed tests that were exempt from CLIA that could be performed in a POL with a certificate of waiver.

Date	Organization/Legislation	Description
1968	Uniform Anatomical Gift Act	Allows living individuals to indicate their desire for their body or organs to be gifted to research, transplant services, or a tissue and organ bank at the time of their death.
1970	Occupational Safety and Health Administration (OSHA)	Originally an act to reduce the incidence of injury, illness, and deaths in the workplace. It is under the U.S. Department of Labor. Since the end of the 1980s has been extended to the health care industry. The threat of HIV and AIDS brought about guidelines to protect workers from blood-borne organisms by requiring compliance to standards covering body fluids, needles, sharps, spills, personal protective equipment, and other hazards.
1970	Controlled Substances Act	The Drug Enforcement Administration (DEA), which is part of the U.S. Department of Justice, works with all levels of government to address the serious use and abuse of drugs. Providers must apply for registration and receive a DEA number to administer, prescribe, or dispense drugs. The act also specifies the proper storage or disposal of controlled drugs.
1996	Health Insurance Portability and Accountability Act (HIPAA)	HIPAA legislation is intended to limit health administration costs, provide for patient information privacy, and prevent fraud and abuse. The regulations deal with many areas, such as electronic transmission of data, release of personal information, security of records, establishing individuals as HIPAA officers, and so on.
2006	Medicare D	Everyone who receives Medicare is eligible to join a prescription drug plan to assist in payment of medication costs. Multiple insurance companies provide plans from which to choose coverage based on drugs covered, drug costs, monthly premiums, copayments, and deductible costs.
2010	**Patient Protection and Affordable Care Act**	Intended to expand access to health insurance, provide additional consumer protections, and reduce costs of health care. See Chapter 5 for more detail.

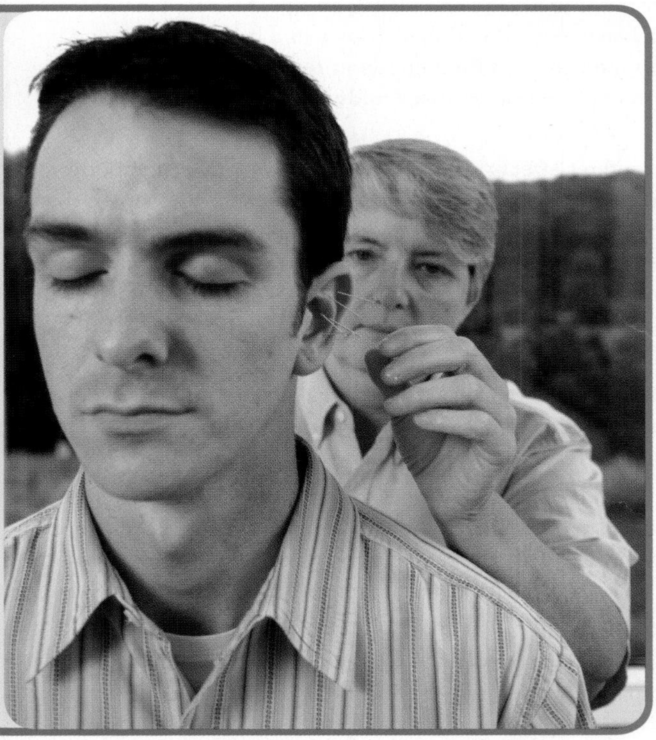

Figure 2–4: A patient receives acupuncture on his ear. © Bob Stockfield, *Courtesy of National Center for Complementary and Alternative Medicine.*

used to mean any treatment, either complementary or alternative, because the therapies might not be labeled by their practitioners, and to our knowledge, no authority has developed a classification standard.

The National Center for Complementary and Alternative Medicine defines these therapies as "medical practices that are not commonly used, accepted, or available in conventional medicine." In the *Alternative Medicine* booklet by Harvard Medical School, another definition states, "those interventions not taught widely in U.S. medical schools nor generally available in U.S. hospitals." Currently, an effort is being made by medical science to become more knowledgeable about therapies from other cultures and those of previous generations in this country. It is trying to distinguish which ones are safe and effective, which are effective but can carry health risks, which are ineffective, and which are both ineffective and unsafe. Some medical schools are introducing courses on alternative therapies to provide physicians with a knowledge of unconventional choices for their own evaluation and to be able to provide care and advice to patients who might select adjunct (added to) treatments.

Table 2–8 is a brief look at several therapies that promote some form of medical intervention or treatment.

TABLE 2–8 Different Types of Complementary or Alternative Therapies

Type of Therapy	Description
Acupuncture	A form of traditional Chinese medicine that is also practiced by the Japanese, Koreans, and French. It consists of using extremely thin, sterilized needles, sometimes electrified with low voltage, that are inserted on points along the network of 12 body meridians (channels) to connect the levels from the organs to the skin. It is used as an anesthetic or to treat pain.
Aromatherapy	A treatment that uses essential oils extracted from plants for a therapeutic effect. Different oils are used for specific conditions, such as lavender for first aid of burns, neroli for anxiety, and tea tree for antibacterial and antifungal action. These can be diffused through the air, inhaled, or absorbed through the skin with massage. Oils can also be used as a compress, in wound care, or as a mouth rinse.
Ayurvedic medicine	The traditional healing system of India and perhaps the oldest formal medical system in the world. It addresses mental and spiritual well-being and physical health. Ayurveda identifies three types of energies that are present in all things: vata, pitta, and kapha. The practitioner tries to assess the proportion of the energies and customize a health program to bring them into a health balance. Sickness results from the energies being out of balance.
Biofeedback	A method that enables a person, usually with the help of electronic equipment, to learn to control otherwise involuntary bodily functions. Therapeutic uses can be helpful with asthma, cardiovascular disorders, headaches, incontinence, insomnia, irritable bowel syndrome, controlling stress, and neuromuscular problems.
Faith	Numerous clinical studies have concluded that patients who receive prayer, in addition to treatment, respond more favorably than those who don't. As a result of these studies, more medical schools now include spirituality training within their curricula. Even though some physicians and health care providers do not accept the power of faith and prayer, many do recognize something or someone else was responsible for a patient's unexpected recovery.
Homeopathy	Homeopathy is a 200-year-old system of medicine based on the Law of Similars: If a dose of a substance can cause a symptom, that same substance in minuscule amounts can cure the symptom. It is a highly controversial form of medicine and lacks any scientific explanation of why it might work. The dose of a substance is diluted many times in a base of water and alcohol, sometimes to the point that no molecules of the ingredient remain. Holistic healers, such as naturopaths, herbalists, chiropractors, acupuncturists, midwives, and even some medical doctors also use the drugs.
Humor	The physical response to humor and laughter affects most of the major systems of the body, increasing heart rate and blood pressure and improving muscle tone. Research has shown that humor can play a part in reducing anxiety. More research is needed to understand the role of humor in recovery or coping with illness. It is known that laughter increases NK cell activity, lymphocyte proliferation, monocyte migration, and the production of IL-2 and IgA, which are positive effects in the immune system.
Hypnosis	Hypnotherapy provided by a therapist is actually supported by more scientific research than many other complementary therapies. Clinically, hypnotherapy has been used in childbirth; to provide acute or chronic pain relief; for stress management; to control certain phobias; for postamputation phantom limb pain, nausea, and hypertension; in irritable bowel syndrome; and for other conditions.
Magnet therapy	Magnet therapy is based on the theory that each cell possesses an electromagnetic field and that disease occurs as a result of an electromagnetic imbalance. Therapy involves placing small magnets close to the skin to correct the imbalance. The magnets are especially popular for pain relief, but some magnet manufacturers also state that the therapy aids in reducing constipation, inflammatory processes, and depression.
Massage	Therapeutic massage is the second most popular related therapy in the United States and can be covered by insurance. It encompasses a wide range of approaches, using hands to manipulate muscles and soft tissue. It is a powerful means to treat stress-related conditions, such as insomnia, headaches, and irritable bowel syndrome, and health conditions such as sciatica and depression. There are many other variations of massage.

Type of Therapy	Description
Hand reflexology	This practice claims there is a map on the hands that matches a corresponding body part. Stimulating these points on the hand sends impulses to help the muscles in the corresponding body part relax and blood vessels open to increase circulation, therefore allowing more oxygen and nutrients to enter and promote healing.
Naturopathy	This is a multidisciplinary approach to health care based on the belief that the body has power to heal itself. Treatment is based on assessment of the correct diet, rest, relaxation, exercise, fresh air, clean water, and sunlight the patient is receiving. Herbal products, detoxification procedures, massage, hydrotherapy, counseling, and advice on lifestyle might be used. It can also use homeopathy and acupuncture.
Tai Chi	This is a Chinese movement discipline that improves strength, flexibility, and sense of balance. It can help reduce frailty and falls in elderly patients. It involves a series of fluid movements performed while relaxed but maintaining focus on a pattern of movements. Proper breathing with the exercises helps integrate the body and mind and enhance the flow of qi and overall health.
Visualization and guided imagery	Visualization refers to what you see in your mind's eye, whereas imagery involves all the senses. The therapy works when patients visualize some activity affecting their problem. An example might be a patient with cancer visualizing immune cells attacking the malignant cells and destroying them. The more senses used, the more real it will seem to the brain. There is evidence that it reduces nausea with chemotherapy, reduces postoperative pain, shortens hospital stays, and reduces anxiety.
Yoga	This is a discipline of breath control, meditation, and stretching and strengthening exercises that is thought to promote mental, physical, and spiritual well-being. It has been practiced for thousands of years. There are many types of yoga. It places great emphasis on mental and physical fitness. It increases strength; balance; flexibility; and, some claim, energy and calmness. It consists of breathing exercises, assuming a number of positions, and meditation.

CHAPTER SUMMARY

- A health care provider is an individual licensed to examine, diagnose, and prescribe treatment to patients seeking assistance. An organization such as a hospital or clinic may also be referred to as a health care provider.
- Physician training includes a four-year undergraduate degree, four years in medical school, and three to eight years of internship and residency. The physician must successfully complete all sections of the United States Medical Licensing Exam (USMLE) prior to becoming fully licensed to practice medicine. Licensure requirements are established by each state. Physicians can lose their license to practice medicine if convicted of a crime or for unprofessional conduct.
- Previously, physicians moving to another state were able to be licensed in the new state through reciprocity. Reciprocity, is a practice in which one state recognizes the licensing requirements of another state as being similar or more stringent than their own.
- A physician in general or family practice sees all kinds of patients with all kinds of problems. The advances in modern medicine have made it impossible for physicians to study every aspect of medicine. Because of this, some have become medical specialists, focusing on a specific kind of medicine. Table 2–1 contains basic information concerning each area.
- There are many other health care professionals with the title of doctor who are not physicians but provide services to patients. Table 2–2 lists the ones with whom you are most likely to have contact.
- Health care providers such as nurse practitioners (NP) and physician assistants (PA) are sometimes referred to as midlevel practitioners. They are able to examine patients, order diagnostic tests, and prescribe certain types of medications.
- A registered nurse (RN) is defined as a professional nurse who has completed a course of study at a state-approved school of nursing and passed the NCLEX-RN exam. A nurse anesthetist is an RN who is certified to administer anesthesia. A nurse midwife

is a professional RN who has had extensive training and experience in labor and delivery. Licensed practical nurses (LPNs) are trained in basic nursing techniques and direct patient care.

- Table 2–3 provides a listing of other health care professionals and their descriptions.
- Many medical pioneers made contributions throughout the early ages. Table 2–4 provides a listing of these individuals and describes their contributions.
- Hippocrates was a Greek physician and is considered the father of medicine. He is best known for his code of behavior known as the Hippocratic oath, a modernized version of the oath sometime around graduation from medical school. physicians repeat as they enter practice.
- Tables 2–5 and 2–6 list many of the modern medical pioneers who have made contributions since the 1800s. These pioneers provided us not only with technology but with practices that have improved overall morbidity and mortality rates.
- The federal government has provided much impetus and influence in the growth of medicine through funding, grants, and regulations. Table 2–7 lists organizations or legislation that has affected the delivery of health care.
- One type of related therapy is complementary therapies, which are treatments that supplement or add to the conventional form of medicine. Another type of therapy is alternative therapy, meaning a method that is used instead of conventional medicine. Table 2–8 is a brief look at several therapies that promote some form of medical intervention or treatment.

STUDY TOOLS

Workbook	Activities for Chapter 2
Premium Website StudyWARE	Activities and Quizzes on the **StudyWARE™ Software** for Chapter 2
	Audio Library of medical terms
	Online access to the **Critical Thinking Challenge 2.0**
learninglab	Module 1: Health Care Roles and Responsibilities
CourseMate	Activities and Quizzes for Chapter 2
WebTutor	Activities and Quizzes for Chapter 2

CHECK YOUR KNOWLEDGE

1. Which of the following would *not* be an example of a health care provider?
   a. Medical assistant
   b. Physician
   c. Nurse practitioner
   d. Chiropractor
2. When one state's medical board recognizes the licensing requirements of another state's medical board as being similar to or more stringent than its own.
   a. Endorsement
   b. Revocation
   c. Reciprocity
   d. None of the above
3. This physician specialist looks after patients admitted to the hospital.
   a. Physician partner
   b. Hospitalist
   c. Physiatrist
   d. Hospital physician
4. Which of the following specialists would be considered a midlevel practitioner?
   a. Podiatrist
   b. Psychologist
   c. Nurse practitioner
   d. None of the above

5. This health care professional administers radiopharmaceuticals to patients and then scans the body with a special camera to observe how the pharmaceuticals concentrate in specific organs.
   a. Radiological technician
   b. Radiologist
   c. Ultrasound technician
   d. Nuclear medicine technologist
6. Which of the following is considered one of the humors described by Galen?
   a. Phlegm
   b. Tears
   c. Mucus
   d. Nasal drippings
7. The legislation that was designed to make health care more accessible to those who wouldn't otherwise be able to afford health care benefits.
   a. HIPAA
   b. Health Care Reform Act
   c. PPACA
   d. OSHA
8. These treatments are considered to supplement or add to the conventional form of medicine.
   a. Alternative therapies
   b. Supplemental therapies
   c. Addendum therapies
   d. Complementary therapies
9. This type of medicine identifies three types of energies that are present in all things.
   a. Ayurvedic medicine
   b. Biofeedback
   c. Acupuncture
   d. Homeopathy

WEB LINKS

American Board of Medical Specialties: www.abms.org

American Medical Association: www.ama-assn.org

American Osteopathic Association: www.aoa-net.org

National Institutes of Health: www.nih.gov

Biography Base: www.biographybase.com/biography/Galen.html

RESOURCES

Abiomed. *Heart Replacement. www.abiomed.com/products/heart_replacement.cfm.* (Retrieved 15 Dec. 2010)

American Medical Association. *Health Professions Education Directory.* Web. (Retrieved 12/15/2010) *www.ama-assn.org/ama/pub/education-careers/careers-health-care.page.*

Clayman, C. B. (1989). *The American Medical Association Encyclopedia of Medicine.* New York: Random House.

"FSMB Licensure Examinations USMLE Step 3 Welcome." *FSMB Welcome to Federation of State Medical Boards.* Web. 22 Mar. 2011. *www.fsmb.org/m_usmlestep3.html.*

Health Care HealthCare.gov. Understand the Affordable Care Act Healthcare.gov. Web. 22 Mar. 2011. *www.healthcare.gov/law/introduction/index.html.*

Lindh, W., Pooler, M., Tamparo, C., and Dahl, B. (2010). *Delmar's Comprehensive Medical Assisting Administrative and Clinical Competencies* (4th ed.). Clifton Park, NY: Delmar Cengage Learning.

Louderback, J. (2003). *Medical Miracles.* McClean, VA: Gannet Satellite Information Network.

Marks, G., and Beatty, W. K. (1973). *The Story of Medicine in America.* New York: Charles Scribner.

"Medical Licensure." *American Medical Association - Physicians, Medical Students & Patients (AMA).* Web. 22 Mar. 2011. *www.ama-assn.org/ama/pub/education-careers/becoming-physician/medical-licensure.page.*

Unit

2

Medical Terminology

Working in the medical field, whether in an administrative or clinical role, demands that you have a strong working knowledge of medical terminology, the language used in the health care setting. As a medical assistant, you must be able to define and build medical terms, spell terminology correctly, and use proper application of medical terms when working with patients and fellow health care professionals. Specifically, you apply these skills to explain medical terminology so the patient understands the meaning and can interpret physician orders. For the success of your career, it is essential for you to develop a working relationship with this language of medical terminology.

Certification Connection

	Ch. 3	Ch. 4
CMA (AAMA)		
Word-building and definitions	X	X
Uses of terminology	X	X
RMA (AMT)		
Word parts	X	X
Definitions	X	X
Common abbreviations		X
Spelling	X	
CMAS (AMT)		
Use and spell basic medical terms appropriately	X	X
Identify root words, prefixes, and suffixes	X	X
Define basic medical terms	X	X

Chapter

3 Introduction to Medical Terminology

OBJECTIVES

In this chapter, you will learn the following:

KB KNOWLEDGE BASE

1. Spell and define, using the glossary at the back of the text, all the Words to Know in this chapter.
2. Receive an introduction to Greek and Latin origins of medical terms.
3. Understand how prefixes alter the meaning of a medical term and be able to use prefixes appropriately with combining forms.
4. Understand how suffixes change a medical term and how to use suffixes appropriately with combining forms.
5. Define the difference between a word root and combining form.
6. Gain an understanding of how to break medical terms apart properly to aid in defining their meaning.
7. Demonstrate a basic knowledge in building medical terms.
8. Determine whether a term is singular or plural and demonstrate knowledge of converting medical terms from singular to plural and vice versa.

WORDS TO KNOW

combining forms	prefix	suffix
plural	singular	word root

ORIGIN OF MEDICAL TERMINOLOGY

Many medical assisting students find it exciting to learn this new language of medical terminology. Initially, medical terminology can seem foreign to you; however, with study and practice, you will learn to speak and write this unique language with confidence and ease.

It is important to know that most medical terms derive from Greek or Latin origins. The Romans of ancient times recorded their teachings in Latin; the Romans were one of the first people to develop medical procedures, diagnoses, and treatments. At about the same time, Greek physicians were also developing medical studies and recording their findings in the Greek language. Thus, you will find that a great majority of the medical terms you encounter today have either Latin or Greek foundations.

For example, the Romans believed that a woman's uterus was what caused her to be moody and unpredictable; with this belief, they used the combining form of *hyster/o* to denote that part of a woman's anatomy. They weren't that far off the mark if you consider their findings carefully—think about moods and emotions associated with the menstrual cycle (premenstrual syndrome or PMS) as well as with menopause.

In addition to Greek and Latin origins, some terms are associated with a physician or person who discovered a particular part of the anatomy or a disease. For instance, the Fallopian tubes are named after Fallopius, the physician who discovered them and named them after himself. The surgical term designated for delivering a baby by other than a natural method (referred to as a cesarean section) is supposedly the manner in which Julius Caesar was delivered into this world.

Other cultures have influenced medical terminology as well but, by and large, the Greek and Latin languages have had the greatest impact on the language of health care. Through memorization and constant review of the **prefixes, suffixes, word roots**, and **combining forms**, which you will be introduced to in this chapter, you can learn this new language!

As you read and study this chapter, you will find that there are distinct differences in the various components of medical terms:

- The prefix is the component that goes at the *beginning* of a word and modifies its meaning.
- The suffix is the component found at the *end* of a word and completes the medical term. A suffix can change a word from a noun to an adjective when added to either the word root or the combining form.
- Word roots and combining forms are the foundations of the word that identifies the structure or anatomy being described and to which a suffix or a prefix is added. The difference between the word root and the combining form is that a vowel is added to the word root when necessary to make the terms easier to pronounce and more logical.

One of the best tools to help learn medical terminology is to make flash cards and refer to them often. Can you recall being in elementary school and using flash cards for the multiplication tables? Although it might seem very basic at the postsecondary level, using this type of review has proven effective in imprinting medical terminology on memory. Concentrate on the prefixes, suffixes, and word roots that give you the most problems. Another tool to help you learn medical terminology is your StudyWARE™ software on the Premium Website. On it, you will find electronic flash cards and audio pronunciations for many of these terms as well as animations to help illustrate some of the concepts in this chapter.

This chapter provides an introduction to the world of medical terminology, meant to give you a foundation on which to build your knowledge. Accept the challenge of learning this new language and talking the talk of health care!

PREFIXES

A prefix is a word part found at the beginning of a medical term. A prefix actually changes or modifies the word root in the medical term. Often, prefixes indicate a location, presence or absence, quantity, size, frequency, or position. When a prefix is separated from the term, most often the prefix is followed by a hyphen.

To see how a prefix can change the meaning of a term, let's look at the medical term *gastric*, which means "pertaining to the stomach." If the prefix *hypo-* (meaning "below or underneath") is added, it becomes *hypogastric*, which now has a different meaning: "pertaining to below the stomach." This is quite different than the original term with which we started. In this particular case, the prefix *hypo-* is indicating location. Common prefixes are listed in Table 3–1.

Exceptions

Usually, prefixes are not altered when added to a combining form or word root; however, there are a few are exceptions to this. A basic rule is that if the combining form or word root begins with a vowel, you would select the most appropriate prefix that is applicable that ends in a consonant.

Look at the following example for a better understanding. Let's build a medical term that means "a condition of no urine." The medical term *uria* means a condition of urine, and, referring to Table 3–1, there are two choices for a prefix that relate to "no/without": *a-* and *an-*. According to the basic guideline, the best selection for the prefix would be *an-*. When applied to the word root, the resulting term is *anuria*. If the prefix

TABLE 3–1 Common Prefixes

Prefix	Meaning	Example
a-, an-	Without	*Arrhythmia* is without a rhythm; *anuria* is a condition without urine.
ante-, pre-, pro-	Before	*Antenatal* or *prenatal* vitamins are vitamins taken before the baby is born. *Prophylactic* medications are used before a disease might occur.
anti-, contra–	Against	*Anticoagulants* are chemicals that work against the blood's clotting ability. Many medications are *contraindicated* when using other medications, meaning that they are against being used together.
bi-, diplo-	Two	*Bilateral* means "pertaining to two sides"; *diplococci* are bacteria appearing in pairs (twos).
brady-	Slow	*Bradycardia* is a condition of a slow heart (rate).
circum-	Around	*Circumference* is the measurement around an object.
de-	Away from	*Dehydration* is the process of taking water away from the body.
dia-, trans-	Through	*Diathermy* is a treatment modality of passing heat through the skin to the underlying tissues. *Transcutaneous* medications are absorbed through the skin.
dys-	Abnormal, painful, difficult	*Dysuria* is a condition of painful urination.
ecto-	Outside	*Ectopic* pregnancies occur when the ovum becomes fertilized outside of the uterus.
endo-	Within	*Endoscopies* are procedures in which an instrument is placed within the body for viewing structures.
epi-	Upon, over	The *epidermis* is the outermost layer of skin over the dermis.
eu-	Normal, good	*Euthyroid* indicates that thyroid function is normal.
ex-, exo-, extra-	Out of, away from, outside	*Exophthalmos* is an abnormal condition of the eyeballs in which they appear to be out of the sockets, *exoskeleton* is a skeleton on the outside of the body, and *extracurricular* refers to activities outside of the classroom.
hemi-, semi-	Half	*Hemiplegia* is paralysis occurring on one side of the body; *semiconscious* is being half conscious and half unconscious.
hyper-, poly-	Above normal, excessive	*Hyperthermia* is an abnormal body temperature above normal; *polyuria* is a condition of excessive urination, often occurring in diabetic patients.
hypo-, sub-	Below normal, below, underneath, inferior	*Hypodermic* injections are administered below the dermis of the skin. *Substernal* chest pain would be underneath the breastbone of the rib cage.
inter-	Between	*Intercostal* spaces are located between the ribs.
intra-	Within	*Intracellular* fluid is the fluid found within the cells.
iso-	Same	*Isotonic* saline has the same pH as blood.
mal-	Bad, not adequate	*Malabsorption* occurs when the body has bad or inadequate absorption through the gastrointestinal tract.
megalo-, mega-, macro-	Large, big	*Megalocytes* are large cells.
micro-	Small, tiny	A *microscope* is an instrument used for viewing tiny things.
mono-	One	A *monocyte* is a cell that contains only one nucleus.

Prefix	Meaning	Example
multi-, pluri-	Many	*Multipara* indicates that a woman has had more than one pregnancy (many pregnancies).
oligo-	Few, scanty, sparse	*Oliguria* is a condition in which scanty urine is produced.
pan-	All	*Pancytopenia* is an abnormal decrease in the number of all cells
peri-	Around	*Perianal* pertains to the area around the anus.
post-	After, following	*Postmortem* is after death.
quadra-, quadri-	Four	*Quadrants* are imaginary divisions of four sections; *quadriplegia* is the paralysis of all four extremities.
re-	Again, backward	*Reproduce* is to produce again.
super-, supra-	Above, superior, more	*Superman* has powers above the normal mortal man; *suprapubic* is the area immediately above the pubis.
tachy-	Fast, abnormally fast	*Tachycardia* is a condition of an abnormally fast heartbeat.
ultra-	Beyond	An *ultrasound* is a radiological procedure that goes beyond the speed of sound.
uni-	One, single	*Unilateral* pertains to one side only.

of *a-* had been selected, the resulting term would have been *auria*—doesn't that look strange?

Another exception to note is changing the prefix to make the medical term easier to pronounce. For example, look at the term *antacid*, meaning "against acid." It's doubtful that you have ever seen or will see the term *antiacid*, although according to the rules of prefixes, that is really the way the term should be written. Learning the prefixes and their meanings is the most effective way to apply your knowledge for building medical terms.

SUFFIXES

A suffix is a word part added to the end of a word and completes a medical term. When suffixes are written as separate components, they begin with a hyphen followed by the suffix. Suffixes usually indicate a procedure, condition, disorder, or disease. Some suffixes are actually stand-alone nouns that can be added to combining forms for more specificity of a particular term. Suffixes can change a medical term to an adjective as well.

To see an example of these situations, let's look at a word you are probably familiar with, *pyromaniac*, which means "pertaining to an obsession with fire." This term is created when the combining form *pyr/o* ("fire") is added to *mania* (a stand-alone term that can also be used as a suffix, meaning "an unusual preoccupation or obsession"), followed by the suffix *-ac* ("pertaining to"), which completes the word and changes the term to an noun.

Dissecting a term is a good exercise to show how suffixes make a medical term complete. To take a medical term apart to define it, you should (1) start with the suffix, then (2) identify the prefix (if there is one), and, finally, (3) determine the word root(s) or combining form(s). As you go through this chapter, these steps will be further discussed and reinforced, so you will become more comfortable with the process. As you learn the meanings of combining forms, breaking medical terms apart to define them will become more logical for you. Now, let's take a term and dissect it to see how this process works (see Figure 3–1).

EXAMPLE

Define *hydrophobic* (hydr/o + phob/o + -ic)

Step 1: Start with the suffix. The suffix *-ic* means "pertaining to."

Step 2: Identify the prefix. There is no prefix in this term.

Step 3: Determine the combining form. There are two combining forms: *phob/o* means "abnormal fear," and *hydr/o* means "water."

Definition: "Pertaining to an abnormal fear of water"

Hydrophobia, "an abnormal fear of water," is another term for rabies. Animals infected with rabies avoid water because they cannot swallow—the rabies paralyzes the throat muscles, which is also why affected animals froth at the mouth and drool.

A list of common suffixes and their meanings can be found in Table 3–2.

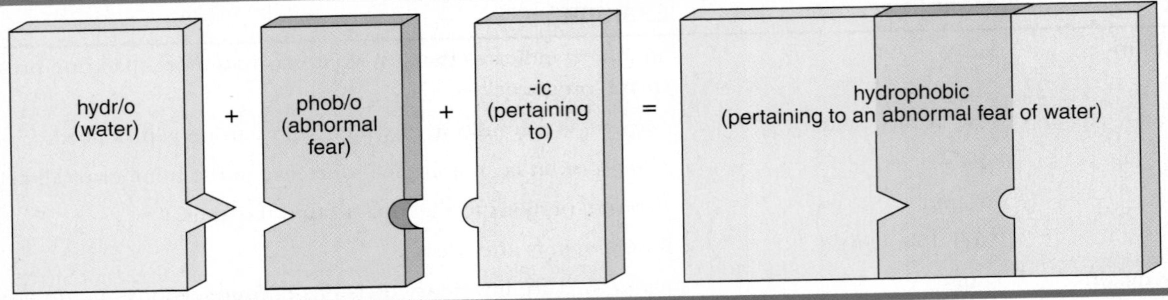

Figure 3–1: *Hydrophobic* means "pertaining to an abnormal fear of water." *Delmar/Cengage Learning.*

TABLE 3–2 Common Suffixes

Suffix	Meaning	Example
-ac, -al, -ar, -ary, -eal, -ia, -ic, -ory, -ous -tic	Pertaining to, condition (of)	*Ventricular* pertains to the ventricles.
-ad	Toward	*Caudad* is toward the tail.
-algia, -dynia	Pain	*Arthralgia* is pain in the joint(s). *Cephalodynia* is pain in the head or a headache.
-ase	Enzyme	*Amylase* is an enzyme that breaks down starches.
-asthenia	Weakness	*Myasthenia gravis* is great muscle weakness.
-blast	Baby, immature	*Erythroblasts* are immature red blood cells most often found in the bone marrow.
-cele	Hernia, abnormal protrusion	A *rectocele* is an abnormal protrusion from the rectum.
-cide, -cidal	Killing, destroying	*Bacteriocidal* solutions kill bacteria.
-crine	To secrete	The *endocrine* system secretes hormones.
-cyte	Cell	A *leukocyte* is a white blood cell.
-derma	Skin	*Scleroderma* is "hard" skin.
-ectasia, -ectasis	Stretching, dilating	*Bronchiectasis* is a lung condition in which the bronchioles are stretched out permanently.
-ectomy	Surgical removal	A *hysterectomy* is the removal of the uterus.
-edema	Swelling, fluid accumulation	*Lymphedema* is fluid accumulation and swelling when the lymph nodes cannot circulate lymph back through the vascular system, usually due to an obstruction.
-ema, -iasis, -ism, -lepsy, -osis	Condition, abnormal condition	*Erythema* is a condition with redness; *hyperthyroidism* is a condition of above-normal thyroid function; *candidiasis* is a condition of a yeast infection; *hidrosis* is a condition of abnormal sweating. *Narcolepsy* is an abnormal condition of sleep.
-emesis	Vomiting	*Hyperemesis* is excessive vomiting.
-emia	Blood	*Anemia* is a condition of low (no) blood.
-esthesia	Sensation, feeling	*Anesthesia* produces a lack of feeling or sensation.
-gen, -genesis, -genic	Producing, production, production of, formation	A *carcinogen* is something that produces cancer, *carcinogenesis* is the formation of cancer, and *carcinogenic* is a substance capable of producing cancer.

Suffix	Meaning	Example
-globin, -globulin	Protein	*Hemoglobin* is the protein in red blood cells that transports oxygen; an *immunoglobin* is a protein that helps protect us against infections.
-gram	Recording	An *electrocardiogram* is a recording of the heart.
-graph	Instrument used to record	An *electrocardiograph* is the instrument used to make an electrocardiogram.
-graphy	Process of recording	*Electrocardiography* is the process of recording the heart's beat.
-itis	Inflammation	*Gastritis* is inflammation of the stomach.
-kinesia, -kinesis	Movement	*Dyskinesia* is painful movement of the body.
-logist	One who studies	A *cardiologist* is one who studies the heart.
-logy	The study of	*Cardiology* is the study of the heart.
-lysis, -lytic	Destruction	*Hemolysis* occurs when red blood cells are destroyed.
-malacia	Softening	*Nephromalacia* is a condition occurring when the kidney(s) soften.
-mania, -manic	Abnormal preoccupation or obsession	*Pyromania* is an abnormal obsession with fire, and a *pyromaniac* is a person with this preoccupation.
-megaly	Enlargement	*Acromegaly* is enlargement of the extremities.
-meter, -metry	Measuring device, process of measuring	A *spirometer* measures the amount of air inhaled and exhaled through the respiratory system. *Pelvimetry* is the process of measuring a pregnant woman's pelvis.
-oid	Resembling	*Osteoid* is resembling bone.
-oma	Tumor	A *lipoma* is a fatty tumor.
-opia	Vision	*Diplopia* is double vision.
-ose	Sugar	*Lactose* is the sugar found in milk.
-ostomy	Formation of a new opening	A *gastrostomy* is a new opening in the stomach to provide nutrients to patients who are unable to swallow.
-para, -parous	Bearing, producing child	*Unipara* refers to a woman who has given birth to one child.
-pathy	Disease	*Lymphadenopathy* is a disease of the lymph glands.
-penia	Deficiency	*Thrombocytopenia* is a deficiency of clotting cells (platelets).
-pepsia	Digestion	*Eupepsia* is normal digestion.
-pexy	Surgical fixation	*Mastopexy* is surgical fixation of the breasts.
-phage, -phagy, -phagia	To eat or digest	*Macrophages* are large cells that ingest foreign matter. *Dysphagia* is difficult or painful digestion.
-phasia	Speaking	*Dysphasia* is difficult speaking, as in laryngitis.
-phil, -philia	To love	An *eosinophil* loves the red dye found in Wright's and Giemsa's stains.
-phobia	Abnormal fear	*Necrophobia* is an abnormal fear of death.
-phonia	Sound	*Aphonia* is the lack of sound (or not being able to hear sound).
-phrenia, -phrenic	Mind, diaphragm	*Schizophrenia* is a split personality; the *phrenic* nerve stimulates the diaphragm.
-plasty	Surgical repair	*Rhinoplasty* is surgical repair of one's nose.
-plegia, -plegic	Paralysis	*Quadriplegia* is paralysis of four limbs; a *quadriplegic* is a person who has this condition.

(continues)

TABLE 3–2 (*Continued*)

Suffix	Meaning	Example
-pnea	Breath or breathing	*Dyspnea* is difficult breathing.
-poiesis	Formation	*Hematopoiesis* is the formation of blood.
-ptosis	Sagging or drooping	*Blepharoptosis* is a drooping eyelid.
-rrhage, -rrhagia	Heavy discharge	*Hemorrhage* is a heavy discharge of blood.
-rrhaphy	Suturing	*Cardiorrhaphy* is a suturing of the heart.
-rrhea	Discharge, flowing	*Diarrhea* is flowing of feces through the anus.
-rrhexis	Rupture	*Cardiorrhexis* is a rupture of the heart.
-scope, -scopy	Instrument, process of using the instrument	*Microscopes* are instruments used to view tiny objects; *microscopy* is the process of examining the tiny objects.
-somnia	Sleep	*Polysomnia* is much sleep.
-stasis	Stopping	*Homeostasis* is the process of stopping processes in the body to maintain an equilibrium.
-stenosis	Narrowing	*Esophagostenosis* is the narrowing of the esophagus.
-stomy	Opening	*Gastrostomy* is making a new opening into the stomach.
-tome	Instrument used for cutting	A *gastrotome* is an instrument used for cutting into the stomach.
-tomy	The process of cutting	*Nephrotomy* is the process of cutting into a kidney.
-trophic, -trophy	Nutrition	*Atrophic* pertains to a lack of nutrition, commonly found in limbs that have been bound by casts.
-uria	Urine	*Dysuria* is painful or difficult urination.
-version	Turning	*Cardioversion* is turning or converting the heart to a normal rhythm.

WORD ROOTS AND COMBINING FORMS

Word roots are the foundation of a medical term and usually describe part of the body. Sometimes, word roots indicate color. A combining form is simply a word root that has a vowel added to the end of the word root. This makes it easier to combine with suffixes or other word roots. Usually, the combining form vowel is not used if the suffix begins with a vowel. Earlier in this chapter, you learned that hydrophobic means "pertaining to a fear of water." In that example, both a combining form (hydr/o) and a word root (phob) are joined to create the term. It made sense to use the combining form hydr/o to facilitate pronunciation while using the word root phob because the suffix (-ic) started with a vowel.

Most often, the combining form vowel is an *o*, but other vowels may be used, depending on the word root; the other two most common vowels seen in combining forms are *a* and *i*. Some examples of combining forms and word roots are listed in Table 3–3.

TABLE 3–3 Common Combining Forms and Word Roots

Combining Form	Word Root	Meaning
cardi/o	cardi	heart
cyan/o	cyan	blue
muscul/o, my/o, myos/o	muscul, my, myos	muscle
neur/o, neur/i	neur	nerve
ren/o, nephr/o	ren, nephr	kidney
gastr/o	gastr	stomach
ur/o	ur	urine
oss/e, oste/o	oss, oste	bone
leuk/o	leuk	white
colon/o	colon	colon
colp/o	colp	vagina

In Chapter 4, you will learn many more combining forms and word roots as they pertain to individual body systems.

Remember, the difference between combining forms and word roots is simply that a combining form has a vowel added to the word root to help in connecting suffixes or other word roots and combining forms. The combining form vowels make the medical term easier to pronounce and more sensible. Keep in mind that different books identify combining forms in various manners, so you might come across a different way of identifying combining forms; however, the principle is the same regardless of the designation.

BREAKING A MEDICAL TERM APART

Earlier in this chapter, we dissected the term *hydrophobic* to learn about its meaning. During that process of breaking a medical term apart in an attempt to define it, we followed these steps:

1. ***Start with the suffix***. A suffix usually indicates a procedure, condition, disorder, or disease and always goes to the right (back of the word). It is denoted with a hyphen to the left. (*Example: -ectomy, surgical removal of.*)
2. ***Next, identify the prefix***. A prefix often indicates a location, presence or absence, quantity, size, frequency, or position and always goes to the left (front of the word). It is denoted with a hyphen to the right. (*Example: hyster-, referring to the uterus.*) One important point to note is that not every medical term contains a prefix.
3. ***Identify the word roots and combining forms***. The word root or combining form is the part of the word that defines a part of the anatomy (or sometimes a color), and there can be more than one of these in a medical term.

When you put all the word components together, you have a very basic definition of the medical term. Now, let's apply these rules to break down and define a simple term (see Figure 3–2).

EXAMPLE

Define *hypogastric*
(*hypo-* + *gastr/o* + *-ic*)

Step 1: Start with the suffix, *–ic*, which means "pertaining to."
Step 2: Identify the prefix, *hypo-*, meaning "below" or "underneath."
Step 3: The word root is *gastr* (the combining form would be *gastr/o*), which means stomach.

Definition: "pertaining to below the stomach"

MEDIA LINK

To view this process visually, you can go to the Premium Website and play the "Word Parts Working Together" animation.

See how easy that was? It is just a process of learning the components and remembering the rules. Now, let's take another example.

EXAMPLE

Define *endocarditis*
(*endo-* + *cardi/o* + *-itis*)

Step 1: Start with the suffix, *–itis*, meaning "inflammation."
Step 2: Identify the prefix, *endo-*, meaning "within."
Step 3: Identify the combining form. The term contains one combining form, *cardi/o*, which refers to the heart.

Definition: "inflammation within the heart"

Remember that there are several prefixes that mean the same thing, several suffixes that mean the same, and root words and combining forms that are alike. Learning the most appropriate application of each takes time and practice.

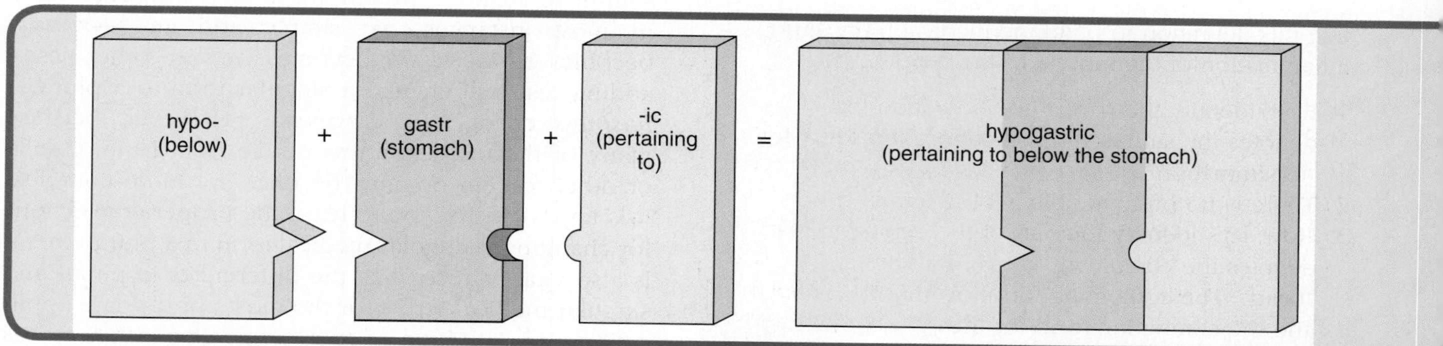

Figure 3–2: A medical term may be taken apart to determine its meaning. *Hypogastric* means "pertaining to below the stomach." *Delmar/Cengage Learning.*

BUILDING A MEDICAL TERM

Now that we have dissected some medical terms, you are ready to try building a medical term on your own, starting with a definition. At this point, we know you have not memorized the various prefixes, suffixes, and combining forms; however, you can refer to Tables 3–1, 3–2, and 3–3 to find the definitions for the word parts in these examples. The earlier you are exposed to this process, the easier it will be for you. Remember the rules:

1. Start with the suffix and identify its meaning.
2. Next, see whether there is a prefix; if there is one, determine its meaning.
3. Finally, determine the word roots or combining forms and define them.

EXAMPLE

Use the following definition to build a medical term, remembering the rules: "A condition of painful urine."

1. First, identify the part of the definition that denotes the suffix: "A condition of." The suffix for "condition" is *–ia*.
2. Next, identify the part of the definition that denotes the prefix because it modifies the medical term: "painful." The prefix for "painful" is *dys-*.
3. The final step is to identify the word root or combining form: "urine." The word root for "urine" is *ur*. (Because the suffix [-ia] begins with a vowel, we'll choose the word root.)

Here is what happens when all the various components are combined:

Dys- + ur + -ia = dysuria

Now, let's build a term that uses multiple combining forms instead of just one word root; note the difference in how the terms are constructed.

EXAMPLE

Use this definition to build the medical term: "An inflammation of the muscle of the heart."

1. First, identify the part of the definition that denotes the suffix: "inflammation." The suffix for "inflammation" is *-itis*.
2. There is no prefix modifying the terms.
3. Now, let's identify the part of the definition that denotes the combining forms: "muscle" and "heart." The combining form for "muscle" is *my/o*, and the combining form for "heart" is *cardi/o*.

Looking at the combining forms for muscle and heart, it makes sense to use the combining form *my/o* when putting them together (my**o**cardio). However, if the combining form (cardi/o) is used when adding the suffix (-itis), it appears illogical and hard to pronounce because the suffix also begins with a vowel. Look at each possibility; you can see how strange one of the terms seems as opposed to the other:

my/o + cardi/o + -itis = myocardioitis ***(incorrect)***

or

my/o + cardi + -itis = myocarditis ***(correct)***

MEDIA LINK

Go to the Premium Website and play the "Combining Word Roots" animation to see how another term is constructed with more than one word root.

SPELLING MEDICAL TERMINOLOGY

Spelling is *very* important when writing medical terminology; misspelling a term can mean the difference in a diagnosis or treatment. Some medical terms are pronounced the same, so you need to know the application of the medical term in each of those instances to spell it properly in a patient's medical record. For example, *ilium* and *ileum* are pronounced identically, although they are entirely different structures. If a health care provider asks you to obtain pre-authorization for a patient to have a portion of the small intestine removed and you type the term *iliectomy*, you would be requesting pre-authorization for the patient to have a portion of a hip bone removed! So, be very careful and attentive to your spelling.

FORMING PLURALS FROM SINGULARS

In our everyday English language, it is relatively simple to make a **plural** form of a **singular** term. In most instances, we simply add an *s—runner* becomes *runners*, *car* becomes *cars*. In other cases, adding "es" will change a singular term to a plural—*business* changes to *businesses*. However, because many of the medical terms derive from Latin, Greek, or other foreign origins, the rules are more complex. It is important for you to learn the proper conversions for changing a singular medical term to a plural one. It is also vital to recognize the differences in plural and singular medical terms for the most appropriate application and definition of such terms. For instance, it is not uncommon to hear lay people say "appendixes" rather than "appendices"—the correct plural form for the singular form *appendix*. This example shows the rule for singular words ending with the letter *x*: drop the *x* and add *ces* instead. Practice makes perfect, so when you are unsure about the proper conversion from singular to plural and vice versa, consult a reference rather than make an error.

Table 3–4 lists the basic rules for changing singular medical terms to plurals and applications of each.

TABLE 3–4 Singular to Plural

Singular Ending	Plural Ending	Example
-a	-ae	*Vertebra* (singular) becomes *vertebrae* (plural).
-ex, -ix	-ices	*Apex* (singular) changes to *apices* (plural); *appendix* (singular) becomes *appendices* (plural).
-is	-es	*Diagnosis* (singular) becomes *diagnoses* (plural).
-nx	-nges	*Phalanx* (singular) with one digit such as finger or toe, when counting more than one, changes to *phalanges* (plural).
-um	-a	*Atrium* (singular) changes to *atria* (plural).
-us	-i	*Bacillus* (singular) becomes *bacilli* (plural).

CHAPTER SUMMARY

- Most medical terms derive from Greek or Latin origins. Some terms are associated with a physician or person who discovered a particular part of the anatomy or a disease.
- A prefix is a word part always found at the beginning of a medical term that changes or modifies the word root in the medical term. Prefixes often indicate a location, presence or absence, quantity, size, frequency, or position.
- A suffix is a word part added to the end of a word to complete that term, usually indicating a procedure, condition, disorder, or disease. Some suffixes are actually stand-alone nouns that can be added to combining forms for more specificity of a particular term. Suffixes can change a medical term to an adjective as well.
- A word root most often describes part of the body and sometimes denotes color.
- Combining forms are word roots that have a vowel added to the end of the word root, which makes it easier to combine with suffixes or other word roots. Most often, the combining form vowel is an *o*; the other two most common vowels seen in combining forms are *a* and *i*.
- To take a medical term apart to define it, you should (1) start with the suffix, then (2) identify the prefix (if there is one), and, finally, (3) determine the word root(s) or combining form(s).

STUDY TOOLS

Workbook	Activities for Chapter 3
Premium Website	
MEDIA LINK	View these **Media Links** for Chapter 3: • Word Parts Working Together • Combining Word Roots
StudyWARE	Activities and Quizzes on the **StudyWARE™ Software** for Chapter 3
	Audio Library of medical terms
	Online access to the **Critical Thinking Challenge 2.0**
CourseMate	Activities and Quizzes for Chapter 3
WebTutor	Activities and Quizzes for Chapter 3

CHECK YOUR KNOWLEDGE

1. In the term "tachycardia," what part of the word is the prefix?
   a. ta-
   b. tach-
   c. tachy-
   d. There is no prefix in this word.
2. In the term *pyromania*, what part of the word is the suffix?
   a. pyro-
   b. mani/o
   c. –mania
   d. –ania
   e. –ia
3. The suffix in the term *rhinitis* is ___________, and it means ___________.
   a. –is, abnormal condition
   b. –is, inflammation
   c. –itis, abnormal condition
   d. –itis, inflammation
4. Which of the following terms is in its singular form?
   a. Bacillus
   b. Bacteria
   c. Scapulae
   d. Veins
5. If a health care provider determines that more than one condition is causing a patient's illness, which of the following would be correct?
   a. Diagnosis
   b. Diagnosises
   c. Diagnoses
   d. Diagnoseses

WEB LINKS

MedTerms Medical Dictionary: www.medterms.com

Chapter

4

Understanding and Building Medical Terms of Body Systems

OBJECTIVES

In this chapter, you will learn the following:

KB KNOWLEDGE BASE

1. Spell and define, using the glossary at the back of the text, all the Words to Know in this chapter.
2. Demonstrate the ability to select and define combining forms for each body system.
3. Demonstrate the ability to add prefixes appropriately to combining forms for each body system.
4. Demonstrate the ability to add suffixes appropriately to combining forms for each body system.
5. Be able to break medical terms apart to define their meanings.
6. Appropriately use medical terms in applications.

WORDS TO KNOW

acne vulgaris
alimentary canal
alopecia
ascites
atria
atrium
bicuspid
bolus
cell
cervicitis
cholecystolithiasis
chyme
cryptorchidism
cusp
dermatology
dialysis
diaphragm
digestive
erythrocyte
external
feces
femoral
femur
gastrointestinal (GI)
histologist
human organism
hyperglycemia
inferior vena cava
integumentary system
internal
jaundice
leukocyte
medial
micturition
mitral
myocardium
nephron
neuron
ophthalmologist
pneumonitis
polyneuralgia
pyelonephritis
septum
superior
superior vena cava
thorax
tissue
tricuspid
ventricle
viscera

STRUCTURE OF THE HUMAN BODY

A comprehensive discussion of the anatomy and physiology of the body appears in Unit 11, but a brief introduction to help you understand the organization of the body is essential in this chapter.

The basic unit of the human body is the **cell**, which is composed of many smaller units. The combining form for cell is *cyt*/o, and the suffix for the same word is *-cyte*. In subsequent parts of the chapter, you will see more references to cells that are specific to tissues and organs. For instance, **erythrocytes** are red blood cells that will be discussed in the circulatory system; **leukocytes** are white blood cells that are essential to our immune systems in that they help protect us from infections in various ways. Cells organize to become **tissue**, and tissues become organized to form *organs*. The combining form for tissue is *hist*/o, so when you come across the word **histologist**, you will be able to identify that this is someone who studies or specializes in tissues. Organs work together to be organized into *organ systems*, which ultimately are organized into the **human organism**, a very highly structured living being. The organ systems that comprise the living human body will be referenced in this chapter as related to medical terminology.

THE INTEGUMENTARY SYSTEM

The skin, or the **integumentary system**, is the most external and visualized as well as the largest organ of the human body. The skin is our first line of defense against foreign invaders, so protecting the skin is of utmost importance in remaining healthy. The study of the skin is called **dermatology** and is less commonly referred to as the integumentary system. Most people do not fully realize or appreciate the complexity of the skin and its structures, nor the important role the skin plays in keeping us healthy and protected from external dangers. Technically, the skin is composed of three layers: the outermost or the *epidermis*; the "true" skin or *dermis*; and the anchoring layer, which is actually below the skin, the *hypodermis*. Several layers make up the epidermis; they are discussed in Unit 11. The integumentary system includes not only the skin but the nails of the hands and feet, hair on various areas of the body, sweat glands, oil glands, the specialized glands of the ear that produce wax, and the associated structures for each of these.

Some terms related to the integumentary system must be memorized because they will not break down into components. An example of one of these terms is **alopecia**, the medical term meaning baldness. Another example is **acne vulgaris**, an unfortunately common affliction with teenagers; *vulgaris* literally means "ordinary, common." As you are reading through Unit 11, acquaint yourself with these various diseases and disorders to be proficient in problems associated with the skin as well as with diagnosis and treatments for such problems.

The skin is the most **external** or superficial organ we have. Injuries that occur beneath this structure would be considered **internal** or deep injuries.

Table 4–1 lists and defines the most common combining forms related to the integumentary system.

TABLE 4–1 Integumentary System

Combining Form	Definition	Example
adip/o, lip/o	Fat	*Adipose* tissue is the layer just below the skin, consisting primarily of fat cells. A *lipoma* is a benign, fatty tumor.
albin/o, leuk/o	White, without color	*Albinism* is a condition in which there are no melanocytes to provide color to the skin, giving the person a white appearance. *Leukoderma* is abnormal patches of white skin.
cutane/o, derm/o, dermat/o, integument/o	Skin	A *subcutaneous* injection is given beneath the skin's layers; a *dermatologist* is one who specializes in disorders of the skin.
cyan/o	Blue	*Cyanosis* of the nail beds or lips is a bluish tint due to the lack of oxygen.
erythem/o	Red	*Systemic lupus erythematosus* is an autoimmune disease often characterized by a red butterfly rash on the face.

Combining Form	Definition	Example
melan/o	Black	*Malignant melanoma* is a black tumor of the skin.
onych/o	Nail	*Onychomycosis* is an abnormal fungal infection of the nails.
scler/o	Hard, hardening	*Scleroderma* is a condition of hardened skin.
xanth/o, icter/o	Yellow	*Xanthoderma* is yellowish-appearing skin. A patient described as being *icteric* has a yellow discoloration of the skin from a liver disorder. Sometimes the word *jaundice* is used for the same condition.
xer/o	Dry	*Xeroderma* is a condition of extremely dry skin.

THE MUSCULOSKELETAL SYSTEM

Beneath the integumentary system, the musculoskeletal system forms the structural support that enables us to stand upright. Within this system are the bones of the skeletal system as well as the muscles that move the bones. There are 206 bones in the human body; by learning the name of each of the bones, you will have a good basis for knowing the combining forms for each of them. Additionally, when you learn the combining forms for the names of the bones, it will be easier to identify other structures. For instance, the combining form for **femur** (the thighbone) is *femor/o*. Although that might not seem significant now, later, when you hear a reference to the **femoral** artery, based on your working knowledge of the bones of the body, you will know that this artery is located in the upper leg (thigh). The human body also has 646 muscles, but you won't need to know as many of those for combining forms as you will for bones. Classifications of the muscle types, such as smooth muscle or striated muscle, and terms pertaining to the membrane separating the muscles and attaching the muscles will be your most common usage. One of the most common combining forms for muscle is *my/o*; this fact should help you in defining terms you encounter with other body systems.

EXAMPLE

Practice defining medical terms associated with the musculoskeletal system. An example of a term that uses the *my/o* combining form is ***polymyositis***. Try breaking this term apart to define it.

Step 1: Start with the suffix, *-itis*, meaning "inflammation (of)."
Step 2: Identify the prefix, *poly-*, meaning "many."
Step 3: Identify the combining form, *my/o*, meaning "muscles."

Putting it all together, the definition is "inflammation of many muscles."

Polymyositis is a muscle disease characterized by the simultaneous inflammation and weakening of voluntary muscles in many parts of the body.

Table 4–2 identifies and defines the most common combining forms for the musculoskeletal system.

THE CARDIOVASCULAR SYSTEM

The cardiovascular system, also known as the circulatory system, is composed of the heart and its associated structures. These are vessels that carry blood rich in oxygen and nutrients throughout our bodies all the way to the cellular level, and there are vessels that transport the used by-products for disposal by the body.

The heart is composed of three layers of muscle and divided into right and left sections with two chambers in each of these sections. The left side of the heart is responsible for pumping the oxygen and nutrient-rich blood out through the aorta and ultimately to the cellular level. The right side of the heart receives the oxygen-poor, waste-rich blood, which is pumped back through

TABLE 4–2 The Musculoskeletal System

Combining Form	Definition	Example
ankylos/o	Stiffening	*Ankylosing spondylitis* is an abnormal stiffening of the spine that results in a lack of mobility.
arthr/o	Joint	*Arthritis* is inflammation of a joint.
carp/o	Wrist (bones)	*Carpal tunnel syndrome* affects the nerves in the wrist.
cervic/o	Neck	The *cervical* spine is the group of vertebrae that compose the neck.
chondr/o	Cartilage	*Costochondritis* is an inflammation of the cartilage around the ribs that often mimics the pain of a heart attack.
cost/o	Ribs	When performing an electrocardiogram, the medical assistant must locate the *intercostal* spaces for proper electrode placement.
crani/o	Skull, head	The *cranial* cavity is located within the skull.
dactyl/o	Digit	*Dactylography* is the process of taking someone's fingerprints.
femor/o	Femur (thighbone)	The *femoral* artery is located near the femur in the upper part of the leg.
fibul/o	Fibula (smaller bone in the calf)	A *fibular* fracture would be a break of the fibula.
humer/o	Humerus (upper bone in the arm)	When one hits the *humeral* nerve, it is often described as hitting the funny bone.
ili/o	Ilium (pelvic bones)	The *iliac* crest of the pelvis is used as a landmark for administering intramuscular injections.
lamin/o	Lamina of a vertebra	A *laminectomy*, removing a portion of the vertebra, may be performed by a surgeon to relieve back pain.
mandibul/o	Mandible (lower jaw, the only movable bone in the skull)	*Temporomandibular joint* (TMJ) pain occurs when the bone of the mandible does not align correctly with the temporal bone to which it is attached.
maxill/o	Maxilla (upper jaw)	*Maxillary* sinuses are located just above the maxilla of the face.
muscul/o, my/o	Muscle	*Muscular* pertains to muscles; the **myocardium** is the muscular portion of the heart.
orth/o	Straight, straighten	An *orthopedist* is one that specializes in straightening bones.
oste/o	Bone	*Osteitis* is inflammation of a bone.
patell/o	Patella (knee cap)	The *patellar* reflex is solicited when striking a patient's leg just below the knee cap.
pelv/i	Pelvis	The *pelvic* cavity is housed within the bony structure of the pelvis.
phalang/o	Fingers or toes	*Phalangitis* is inflammation of a finger or a toe.
rachi/o, spondyl/o, vertebr/o	Vertebra(e), spine	*Rachitis* and *spondylitis* are both inflammation of the vertebrae or spine. The *vertebral* column is composed of the bones of the spine.
stern/o	Sternum (breastbone)	*Substernal* chest pain is pain described as being just below the breastbone, often indicating a heart attack.
ten/o, tend/o, tendin/o	Tendon	*Tendonitis* is inflammation of a tendon.
tibi/o	Tibia (shin)	A *tibial* contusion, caused by striking the shin, is quite painful.

the lungs for reoxygenation. The heart is usually described as being **medial**, or located mostly in the middle of the chest or **thorax**. The venous structures that return oxygen-poor blood to the lungs include the **superior vena cava**, which is the large vein that collects blood from the upper (superior) structures such as the head and neck. The **inferior vena cava** is the corresponding large vein that collects blood from the lower (inferior) structures such as the legs, abdomen, and pelvic regions.

The heart is also divided into right and left sections by tissue called the **septum**. As mentioned, the left side of the heart is responsible for routing the oxygen-rich blood through the aorta, arteries, and arterioles to supply the cells with necessary oxygen and nutrients. The right side of the heart receives the oxygen-poor blood from the cells for routing to the lungs for an exchange of carbon dioxide and oxygen. The heart is further divided into four chambers: The two **superior** structures are called the **atria** (plural for **atrium** because there is a right and a left), and the two inferior structures are called the **ventricles** (plural for ventricle). Aiding the proper flow of blood through the heart are valves that prevent regurgitation of the blood back into chambers of the heart. By learning the prefixes for numbers, you can identify the structure of the valves more easily. The **bicuspid** or **mitral** valve is located between the left atrium and left ventricle. The prefix of *bi-* refers to the number two, so you would know the valve has two sections or **cusps**. The reference to mitral goes back to Roman times and the mitral (or head covering) that priests wore for Roman Catholic services. These large hats were composed of two pieces of material, thus the reference to two. The valve that maintains proper blood flow through the right side of the heart between the atrium and ventricle is the **tricuspid** valve—of course, the prefix of *tri-* refers to the number three.

The aorta, arteries, and arterioles are the vessels that transport the oxygen-rich blood throughout the body. The exchange between the oxygen and carbon dioxide (this is the blood that has waste products) occurs at the capillary level, and the blood is then routed through the venules, veins, and vena cavae before being returned to the right side of the heart. The vessels transporting the blood from the left side of the heart are more muscular and thicker-walled than the vessels returning the blood to the right side of the heart because they are under great pressure. Unit 11 provides a more in-depth discussion of the structural differences in arteries and veins and the reasons for these differences.

Also included with the cardiovascular system are the blood system, lymphatic system, and immune system. The vascular part of the system that routes the blood cells throughout the body helps protect the body by providing immunity and responses to pathogenic invaders and transports lymph fluid.

EXAMPLE

Practice defining and building medical terms associated with the cardiovascular system.

A. Define ***phlebotomist***.

Step 1: Start with the suffix, *-ist*, meaning "one who."
Step 2: Identify the prefix. There is no prefix.
Step 3: Identify the word root or combining form(s). There are two: *phleb/o* (meaning "vein") and *tom* (meaning "[surgical] incision").

Putting it all together, the definition is "one who [makes a surgical] incision into a vein."

This is exactly what a phlebotomist does when taking your blood. Those trained in phlebotomy use needles to make a small incision into a superficial vein to aspirate blood for diagnostic testing.

B. Now, let's build a word for "***pertaining to the atrium and ventricle***."

Step 1: Start with the suffix. The suffix for "pertaining to" is *-ar*.
Step 2: Identify the prefix. In this case, there is no prefix.
Step 3: Identify the word root(s) or combining form(s). There are two: "atrium" (which is *atri/o*) and "ventricle" (which is *ventricul-*).

Putting it all together, *atri/o* + *ventricul-* + *-ar* becomes "atrioventricular."

Note the use of the combining-form vowel for ventricle and absence of the one for atrium. Remember your basic rules: if you are adding combining forms, and the second word component begins with a consonant, the combining-form vowel is used with the first. However, if adding a component that begins with a vowel, the combining form vowel is usually dropped, as it was in *ventricul/o*.

It is important for you to be familiar with the combining forms relating to the cardiovascular system, identified and defined in Table 4–3.

THE RESPIRATORY SYSTEM

When you think of breathing, you likely think only of the lungs; however, there is much more to the respiratory system than the lungs. One must envision the pathway of air into the body to realize all the structures that comprise the respiratory system. Air first enters the body through the mouth or the nose, moves down through the throat (*pharynx*), the voice box (*larynx*), the airway (*trachea*), the bronchi, the bronchioles, and ends at the *alveoli*, the microscopic air sacs that exchange oxygen and carbon dioxide through the processes of inspiration (breathing in) and expiration (breathing out).

TABLE 4–3 The Cardiovascular System

Combining Form	Definition	Example
aden/o	Gland	*Lymphadenopathy* is often found with viral illnesses such as infectious mononucleosis.
angi/o, vas/o	Vessel	*Angioplasty* may be performed to repair or remove a blockage found in a blood vessel.
aort/o	Aorta	An *aortic* aneurysm is a ballooning out of this major vessel and is frequently life-threatening.
arteri/o	Artery	*Temporal arteritis* is an inflammation of the temporal artery.
ather/o	Yellow, fatty plaque	*Atherosclerosis* is hardening of the arteries due to deposits of yellow, fatty plaque.
atri/o	Atrium (atria), upper chambers of the heart	The *atrioventricular* node is located between the atrium and ventricle of the heart and provides stimulation for the heart's beat.
cardi/o	Heart	*Cardiac* surgery pertains to surgery on the heart.
erythr/o	Red	*Erythrocytes* are the red blood cells, which are responsible for transporting oxygen.
hem/o, hemat/o	Blood	*Hemodialysis* is cleansing of the blood by a machine; a *hematologist* is one who specializes in blood disorders.
leuc/o, leuk/o	White	*Leukocytes* are the white cells that help protect the body from infections.
lymph/o	Lymph	*Lymphoma* is a tumor found in the lymph system.
phleb/o, ven/o	Vein	A *phlebotomist* or *venipuncturist* is a person who draws a patient's blood for diagnostic testing.
splen/o	Spleen	When a person's spleen becomes overactive and removes too many blood cells, a *splenectomy*, removal of the spleen, might have to be performed.
thromb/o	Clot	*Thrombophlebitis* is an inflammation of a vein due to a blood clot.
ventricul/o	Ventricle, lower chambers of the heart	*Ventricular bigeminy* is an abnormal heart rhythm involving the ventricles of the heart.

The lungs are located superior to the abdominal organs, positioned just above the **diaphragm**, which is the muscle that literally divides the body's thoracic cavity from the abdominal cavity. You may find it surprising that the right and left lungs are not identical to one another as is the case with the kidneys. Both lungs are composed of lobes. The right lung has 3 lobes (superior, inferior, and middle) while the left lung has 2 lobes (superior and inferior), but the right lung is shorter than the left lung to provide enough room for the liver to be positioned beneath the diaphragm. The left lung is narrower to provide room for the heart. Therefore, having a lobectomy is different from having a pneumonectomy. Remember that the suffix *-ectomy* means "surgical removal," so the difference in these two operations is that the lobectomy is the removal of only a lobe of the lung, whereas the pneumonectomy is the removal of an entire lung. Another important set of terms in relation to the respiratory system includes those that refer to air or oxygen, which keeps our organs, tissues, and cells healthy. Probably one of the more common combining forms you already know is *aer/o*; think about the terms *aerobic* and *aerodynamic*. Another common combining form for air or oxygen is *ox/o*; an example is pulse oximeter, a device usually clipped to a finger to measure the oxygen content in the blood without actually taking any blood from the patient.

EXAMPLE

Practice defining and building medical terms associated with the respiratory system.

A. Define ***pneumonitis***.

Step 1: Start with the suffix, *-itis*, meaning "inflammation (of)."
Step 2: Identify the prefix. There is no prefix.
Step 3: Identify the word root, *pneumon*, meaning "lung(s)."

Putting it all together, the definition is "an inflammation of the lungs."

B. Build a word that means "***pertaining to difficult (painful) voice or speaking***."

Step 1: Start with the suffix, *-ia*, "pertaining to."
Step 2: Identify the prefix, *dys-*, "painful."
Step 3: Identify the word root or combining form, *phon/o*, "voice/speaking."

Putting it all together, *dys-* + *phon/o* + *-ia* becomes "dysphonia."

CLINICAL PEARL

Remember that if the suffix begins with a vowel, the combining form vowel is dropped.

You must learn the terms associated with the structures of the respiratory system as well as those pertaining to the process of breathing. A listing and definitions of the combining forms and suffixes related to the respiratory system are provided in Table 4–4.

THE GASTROINTESTINAL SYSTEM

Often when one thinks about the **gastrointestinal (GI) system**, the stomach is what comes to mind. Just as with the respiratory system, many structures comprise the gastrointestinal or **digestive** system, as well as accessory structures that assist with the digestion of nutrients that are taken into the body.

When nutrients are taken into the body, the first place the food enters is through the mouth. Within the mouth are several digestive structures such as the tongue, teeth, and salivary glands. As food is chewed, the tongue and teeth help break it into smaller parts; the tongue mixes saliva with the smaller parts and pushes the food back to the throat as a **bolus**. This bolus makes its way through the pharynx to the esophagus and is deposited in the stomach. The stomach secretes enzymes and gastric juices to liquefy the bolus further. The bolus is then transformed into **chyme** and moved into the first portion of the small intestine, the duodenum. The small intestine is divided into three sections: the duodenum, the jejunum, and the ileum. Most of digestion occurs within the small intestine.

The next structure in the journey is the large intestine, which is also divided into parts. The first part of the large intestine is the cecum, the part of the large intestine from which the appendix projects; this is followed by

TABLE 4–4 Common Combining Forms and Suffixes Related to the Respiratory System

Combining Form	Definition	Example
aer/o	Air	*Anaerobic* microorganisms prefer a lack of air for growth.
atel/o	Imperfect	*Atelectasis*, when taking the literal definition, means imperfect stretching. In premature infants, atelectasis indicates that the lungs cannot expand fully.
bronch/o, bronchi/o	Bronchus (bronchi)	*Bronchitis* is an inflammation of the bronchi found in upper respiratory tract infections; *bronchiectasis* is an abnormal stretching of the bronchi.
bronchiol/o	Bronchioles (little bronchi)	Toddlers are often diagnosed with *bronchiolitis*, an inflammation of the bronchioles.
laryng/o	Larynx (voice box)	A *laryngectomy* is the surgical removal of the larynx, usually due to cancer.
lob/o	Lobes	*Lobar* pneumonia indicates an infection in only one lobe of a lung. A *lobectomy* is the surgical removal of a lobe of a lung.

(continues)

TABLE 4–4 *(Continued)*

Combining Form	Definition	Example
muc/o	Mucus	The *mucous* membranes are responsible for secreting mucus in the respiratory tract.
nas/o, rhin/o	Nose	*Nasal* sprays are used in the nose to alleviate symptoms of *rhinitis*, an inflammation of the nose and nasal passages.
ox/o	Oxygen	*Hypoxia* is a condition of below-normal oxygen levels.
pharyng/o	Pharynx (throat)	The *pharyngeal* tonsils are the lymph glands found in the back of the throat.
pleur/o	Pleura (membrane surrounding each lung)	*Pleurisy* is an inflammation of the pleura around one of the lungs.
pneum/o, pnemon/o	Lung, air	A *pneumothorax* is a collapsed lung from air rushing in; *pneumonitis* is an inflammation of a lung, more commonly known as *pneumonia*.
pulmon/o	Lung	Chronic obstructive *pulmonary* disease (COPD) is a disease that affects the lungs and the oxygen levels.
sinus/o	Sinus(es)	*Sinusitis* is an inflammation of the sinuses, often from an allergic reaction.
spir/o	To breathe	A *spirometer* is a device that measures the amount of air a patient breathes in and out. *Respiratory* literally means "pertaining to repeat(ed) breathing."
tonsill/o	Tonsil(s)	In repeated cases of strep throat, a *tonsillectomy*, surgical removal of the tonsils, may be performed.
trache/o	Trachea (windpipe)	A *tracheotomy* is performed when a person is unable to breathe through the mouth or nose; this involves creating a new opening for air to pass.
Suffix	**Definition**	**Example**
-ptysis	To spit	*Hemoptysis* is spitting up blood.

the *ascending* colon (ascending refers to going up), the *transverse* colon (transverse means across), the *descending* colon (going down), the *sigmoid* colon (sigmoid means "resembling an *s*"), and then the *rectum* and the *anus*. The large intestine's responsibility is primarily to reabsorb water and package the waste for disposal as **feces**. Thus, the digestive system, or **alimentary canal**, begins at the mouth and terminates at the anus, making it quite a complex system indeed. (*Aliment/o* is the combining form for "nutrition," and the suffix *-ary* refers to "pertaining to"; that is certainly the function of the alimentary canal.) Within the digestive system are accessory organs that assist in the processing of nutrients; these include the teeth, tongue, liver, pancreas, and gallbladder. The proper medical term for the appendix is *vermiform appendix*; the word *vermiform* loosely means "shaped or appearing like a worm" (*verm/i*). Refer to Unit 11 for figures illustrating the digestive system—the appendix does look a lot like a worm!

Some terms are not constructed like other medical terms in this chapter, and you need to memorize these. For instance, **viscera** is a collective term that means the internal organs, and **ascites** is an abnormal fluid accumulation in the abdominal cavity. The abdominal cavity is lined and protected by a membrane known as the peritoneum (you might identify the suffix *-eum*, which means membrane). Look at the term *cirrhosis*. Literally defined, this word means "a condition of yellow," but that does not make much sense medically. However, if you know anything about this disease, the patient many times will present with a yellow discoloration of the skin (**jaundice**) because the liver is no longer functioning normally. The problem with this generality is that not all patients with cirrhosis have a yellowish skin color. When the condition was first diagnosed in Greek medicine, because physicians at that time did not have the medical technologies we have, the patient was diagnosed based on the yellowish color caused by the failing liver; hence, the term as we know it. The term *jaundice* is derived from the French term for yellow; once again, it is probably easier if you memorize the term as meaning "a yellowish discoloration of the skin."

EXAMPLE

Practice defining and building medical terms associated with the gastrointestinal system.

A. Define ***cholecystolithiasis***.

Step 1: Start with the suffix, *-iais*, meaning "abnormal condition."
Step 2: Identify the prefix. There is no prefix.
Step 3: Identify the combining forms, *cholecyst/o* (meaning "gallbladder") and *lith/o* (meaning "stones").

Putting it all together, the definition is "an abnormal condition of gallbladder stones," or, more commonly, gallstones.

B. Build a term that means "***surgical removal of half of the stomach***."

Step 1: Start with the suffix, *-ectomy*, "surgical removal."
Step 2: Identify the prefix meaning "half." Of the two prefixes that mean this, we will use *hemi-*.
Step 3: Identify the combining form, *gastr/o*, "stomach."

Putting it all together, *hemi-* + *gastr/o* + *-ectomy* becomes "hemigastrectomy."

CLINICAL PEARL

When you combine the word components to make the medical term, review to see whether a combining-form vowel needs to be dropped to make the correct medical term. The combining-form vowel is not used when combining with the suffix because the suffix begins with a vowel.

Table 4–5 identifies and defines the most common combining forms and suffixes associated with the gastrointestinal system.

THE URINARY SYSTEM

The urinary system is instrumental in ridding the human body of waste products that build up in the bloodstream and excreting that waste in the form of urine. The urinary system is composed of two kidneys, two ureters, one bladder, and one urethra. The body filters the blood in the **nephrons** of the kidneys; the nephrons are the microscopic functional cells of the kidney. Think about the specialist you would be referred to if you were having problems with your kidneys—a nephrologist, not a kidneyologist. Ultimately, the process of secreting urine for transport out of the body begins in the nephrons of the kidney; after the blood has been filtered and waste products removed, the urine is sent through the ureters to the bladder. The filtration process that occurs within the nephron and its complicated microscopic structure is a highly complex procedure that is explained in detail in Unit 11. The bladder is responsible for housing the urine until there is a sufficient quantity to be transported out of the body by voiding, or **micturition**. Many medical terms relate to the urinary system, so an introduction to the terminology is necessary here.

The most common combining form on which many of the urinary system medical terms are based is *ur/o*, so learning this word component will help you interpret many of the terms associated with this system. *Ur/o* refers to the urine. A urologist is a specialist who is consulted when a patient is having problems with micturition (voiding). One common problem associated with the urinary system is formation of kidney stones, which are commonly referenced in that manner; however, the terms *renal calculi* and *nephrolithiasis* are also appropriate for this abnormal condition. When the kidneys fail to function properly, the waste products that would normally be transported out of the body in the urine build up in the bloodstream. Patients experiencing this condition often must have their blood artificially cleansed by **dialysis**. Otherwise, a condition known as *uremia* will occur, a term that literally means "urine in the blood."

TABLE 4–5 Common Combining Forms and Suffixes Related to the Gastrointestinal System

Combining Form	Definition	Example
abdomin/o	Abdomen	*Abdominal* pain is pain felt in the abdomen.
aden/o	Gland	*Sialadenitis* is inflammation of the salivary glands.
aliment/o	Nourishment, food	*Hyperalimentation* is the process of providing more or additional nourishment.
amyl/o	Starch	*Amylase* is an enzyme secreted by the pancreas that breaks down starches into simple sugars.

(continues)

TABLE 4–5 *(Continued)*

Combining Form	Definition	Example
an/o	Anus	An *anal* fissure is a tear in the anus, the terminal portion of the digestive (GI) tract.
append/o, appendic/o	Appendix	An *appendectomy* is the surgical removal of the appendix, a small projection off the cecum; *appendicitis* is the condition that most frequently leads to this operation.
bucc/o	Cheek	Dentists frequently administer local anesthetic into the *buccal* (cheek) area.
cec/o	Cecum (first segment of the large intestine)	The ileocecal junction is where the small intestine merges with the large intestine.
cheil/o	Lip(s)	*Cheilitis* is an inflammation of the lip.
cholecyst/o	Gallbladder	*Cholecystolithiasis* is the condition most commonly referred to as gallstones.
choled/o	Common bile duct	*Choledolithotomy* is the process of removing stones from the common bile duct.
col/o, colon/o	(Large) intestine, colon	A *colostomy* is the formation of a new opening into the colon; a *colonoscopy* is the process of using a lighted instrument to visualize the colon.
dent/i, dent/o odont/o	Tooth (teeth)	A *dentist* is a tooth specialist.
duoden/o	Duodenum (first section of the small intestine)	*Duodenal* ulcers develop as a result of too much stomach acid passing from the stomach into the duodenum.
enter/o	(Small) intestine	*Enteral* stasis is a condition that occurs when digestion fails to take place in the small intestine.
epiglott/o	Epiglottis	*Epiglottitis* is an inflammation of the epiglottis, the structure that closes over the trachea to prevent food from passing into the respiratory system.
esophag/o	Esophagus (food tube)	*Esophageal* ulcers can occur when a patient has gastroesophageal reflux disease (GERD) and acid backs up into the esophagus.
gastr/o	Stomach	A *gastrectomy* is partial surgical removal of the stomach.
gloss/o, lingu/o	Tongue	*Ankyloglossia* is a condition of being “tongue tied.”
hepat/o	Liver	*Hepatitis* is a viral inflammation of the liver; at least five viruses cause hepatitis.
ile/o	Ileum (last section of the small intestine)	The *ileocecal* junction is where the ileum joins with the first section of the large intestine, the cecum.
intestin/o	Intestine	*Gastrointestinal* pertains to the stomach and intestines.
jejun/o	Jejunum (second section of the small intestine)	A *jejunectomy* is the surgical removal of the jejunum.
lith/o	Stone, calculus	*Sialolithectomy* is the surgical removal of salivary stones.
or/o, stomat/o	Mouth	*Oral* means pertaining to the mouth.
pancreat/o	Pancreas	*Pancreatitis* is an inflammation of the pancreas that causes the patient a good deal of pain; *pancreatic* secretions include amylase, lipase, and insulin.

Combining Form	Definition	Example
periton/o	Peritoneum	The *peritoneal* cavity is lined by the peritoneum and houses the viscera.
pharyng/o	Pharynx (throat)	*Oropharyngeal* means "pertaining to the mouth and the throat."
proct/o, rect/o	Rectum	A *rectal* examination involves digital examination of the rectum; a *proctologist* is a specialist in rectal diseases.
sial/o	Saliva	*Sialolithiasis* is a condition of having stones in a salivary (gland).
sigmoid/o	Sigmoid colon	A *sigmoidectomy* is the surgical removal of the sigmoid colon, part of the large intestine.
Suffix	**Meaning**	**Example**
-ase	Enzyme	*Amylase, protease,* and *lipase* are all enzymes that break down food products for assimilation into the body.

EXAMPLE

Practice defining and building medical terms associated with the urinary system.

A. Define ***pyelonephritis.***

Step 1: Start with the suffix, *-itis*, meaning "inflammation (of)."
Step 2: Identify the prefix. There is no prefix.
Step 3: Identify the combining forms, *pyel/o* (meaning "renal pelvis") and *nephr/o* (meaning "kidney").

Putting it all together, the definition is "inflammation of the renal pelvis and kidney."

In this particular term, kidney is a bit redundant because the combining form *pyel/o* refers to the renal pelvis, which is contained within the kidney.

B. Build a medical term that means "***the process of viewing the bladder with a lighted instrument***."

Step 1: Start with the suffix, *-scopy*, "process of using a lighted instrument."
Step 2: Identify the prefix. There is no prefix.
Step 3: Identify the combining form, *cyst/o*, "bladder."

Putting it all together, *cyst/o* + *-scopy* becomes "cystoscopy."

Remember that the process of viewing is different from the instrument used for the examination. A "scope" is the instrument, but "scopy" is the process of using that scope.

TABLE 4–6 Common Combining Forms Related to the Urinary System

Combining Form	Definition	Example
bacteri/o	Bacteria	*Bacteriuria* indicates the presence of bacteria in the urine, usually from a urinary tract infection (UTI).
cyst/o	Bladder, sac	A *cystoscopy* is viewing the interior of the bladder with a lighted instrument.
glomerul/o	Glomerulus, filtering unit of a nephron	*Glomerulonephritis* is an inflammation of the glomerulus of the nephrons.
hemat/o	Blood	In some cases of nephrolithiasis, *hematuria*, or blood in the urine, is present.
lith/o	Stone, calculus	*Nephrolithiasis* is a condition of having kidney stones.
nephr/o, ren/o	Nephron, functional cell of the kidney, kidney	A *nephrectomy* is the removal of a kidney; the *renal* artery supplies blood to the kidney.
noct/o	Night	Older patients frequently complain of *nocturia*, a condition of having to get up during the night to void.
py/o	Pus	*Pyuria* is the presence of pus in the urine.

(continues)

TABLE 4–6 *(Continued)*

Combining Form	Definition	Example
pyel/o	Renal pelvis	*Pyelolithotomy* is the surgical removal of kidney stones from the renal pelvis.
ur/o, urin/o	Urine	*Pyuria* is an abnormal condition of pus in the urine; a *urinometer* is an antiquated device that was used to measure the specific gravity of urine.
ureter/o	Ureter	An *ureteroscopy* is the procedure of viewing the ureter(s) with a scope.
urethr/o	Urethra	A voiding *cystourethrogram* is an examination that is done while a patient is voiding, which allows visualization of the bladder and the urethra.

Table 4–6 lists and defines the most common combining forms associated with the urinary system.

THE NERVOUS SYSTEM

There are two major divisions to the nervous system: the central nervous system, consisting of the brain and spinal cord, and the peripheral nervous system, the portion that allows for awareness of surroundings through various receptors and communications with the brain. The brain is protected by the bony covering of the skull or cranium, whereas the fragile and delicate spinal cord is protected by the vertebrae of the spinal column. Without proper functioning of the nerve impulse centers in the brain as well as an intact spinal cord, voluntary movement of the extremities would be difficult if not impossible. The functional cells of the nervous system are **neurons**, so many of the medical terms related to the nervous system are based on this term. There are also various parts of the brain and its protective covering, known collectively as the meninges.

EXAMPLE

Practice defining and building medical terms associated with the nervous system.

A. Define ***polyneuralgia***.

Step 1: Start with the suffix, *-algia*, meaning "pain."
Step 2: Identify the prefix, *poly-*, meaning "many."
Step 3: Identify the combining form, *neur/o*, meaning "nerve."

Putting it all together, the definition is "pain in many nerves."

B. Build a medical term that means "***pertaining to the nerves and muscles***."

Step 1: Start with the suffix, *-ar*, "pertaining to."
Step 2: Identify the prefix. There is no prefix.
Step 3: Identify the combining forms, "nerves" (*neur/o*) and "muscles" (*muscul/o*).

Putting it all together, *neur/o* + *muscul/o* + *-ar* becomes "neuromuscular."

CLINICAL PEARL

Look carefully at how the term *polyneuralgia* was constructed: The second combining form began with a consonant, so the combining form vowel was maintained, but the suffix began with a vowel, so the combining form vowel was dropped.

For this system of the body, it is essential to learn the combining forms associated with the parts of the brain and the membranes lining the brain for protection as well as some of the pathologic conditions that affect the nervous system. Table 4–7 lists and defines the common combining forms associated with the nervous system.

THE ENDOCRINE SYSTEM

The endocrine system is a unique system within the human body. The word *endocrine*, when broken down into its components (*endo-* and *crin/o*), literally means to "secrete within." Although each gland produces a secretion, it is not visible externally because the product—a hormone—is released directly into the bloodstream—hence, to secrete within. Laboratory tests can measure the level of hormones in the bloodstream to determine whether they are adequate. These are quite common blood tests drawn in health care providers' offices.

The organs of the endocrine system also are very specific in the way they operate; each hormone secreted by an endocrine organ targets a specific organ. The same hormone will not affect any other organ within the body.

For instance, when the pituitary gland releases thyroid stimulating hormone (TSH), the hormone travels straight to the thyroid gland to stimulate it to produce more hormones for increasing the metabolism. But if your body needed more insulin, TSH would have absolutely no effect on your blood sugar. (Insulin's job is to lower blood sugar levels.) Often, the endocrine system and its secretion of hormones is likened to a lock and key; only one key will fit a lock, and only one hormone affects a particular organ.

The terms you will encounter related to this system most often refer to specific endocrine glands.

EXAMPLE

Practice defining and building medical terms associated with the endocrine system.

A. Define ***hyperglycemia***.

Step 1: Start with the suffix, *-emia*, meaning "blood."
Step 2: Identify the prefix, *hyper-*, meaning "above normal, excessive."
Step 3: Identify the combining form, *glyc/o*, meaning "sugar or glucose."

Putting it all together, the definition is "above normal blood sugar (or glucose)."

B. Build a medical term that means "***an abnormal condition of below-normal parathyroid (function)***."

Step 1: Start with the suffix, *-ism*, "abnormal condition of."
Step 2: Identify the prefix, *hypo-*, "below normal."
Step 3: Identify the combining form, *parathyroid/o*, "parathyroid."

Putting it all together, *hypo-* + *parathyroid/o* + *-ism* becomes "hypoparathyroidism."

CLINICAL PEARL

Another prefix that means "below normal" is *sub-*, but this prefix is less common than *hypo-*. With practice, you will learn which term creates a particular medical term.

Table 4–8 lists and defines the endocrine glands' combining forms and suffixes.

THE SPECIAL SENSES

The special senses include the organs that provide vision, hearing, balance and upright stature, smell, and taste. Also included are the receptors of the skin that enable the sense of touch, pain, and temperature (although there are few medical terms specifically associated with these senses). Most of the word components you must learn are associated with the various organs in the special senses. The organs associated with the senses include the *eye*, *ear*, *tongue*, and receptors embedded in the skin. The receptors in the skin associated with the sense of touch are varied in that some receptors differentiate between heat and cold *(thermoreceptors)*, whereas others help in the sensation of pain *(nociceptors)*. In some cases, more than one combining form is associated with an organ, so learning the most appropriate word component is essential to success with this section. For instance, both *ophthalm/o* and *opt/i* are combining forms for the eye, and *ot/o* and *aur/o* are combining forms for the ears. *Gloss/o* and *lingu/o* both refer to the tongue. Follow the examples to define and build medical terms.

TABLE 4–7 Common Combining Forms Related to the Nervous System

Combining Form	Definition	Example
cerebell/o	Cerebellum	If there is an interruption in *cerebellar* nerve impulses, voluntary movements of the body become difficult.
electr/o	Electricity	An *electroencephalogram* (*EEG*) is a recording of the electrical impulses transmitted by the brain.
encephal/o, cerebr/o	Brain, cerebrum	Viral *encephalitis* is an inflammation of the brain by a virus; the *cerebral* part of the brain is what gives each individual unique personalities and thought processes.
mening/o	Meninges	*Meningococcal encephalitis* is an infection of the meninges resulting in inflammation of the brain.
neur/o	Nerve	*Neuralgia* is a generalized term meaning pain in a nerve.
phas/o	Speech	Occasionally when a patient has a stroke, *aphasia*, or inability to speak, can occur.

TABLE 4–8 Common Combining Forms and Suffixes Related to the Endocrine System

Combining Form	Definition	Example
gluc/o, glyc/o	Sugar, sweet	*Glucosuria* and *glycosuria* both mean "sugar in the urine."
parathyroid/o	Parathyroid glands	*Hyperparathyroidism* is a condition of excessive parathyroid activity.
thym/o	Thymus gland	*Thymosin* is a hormone secreted by the thymus gland.
thyr/o	Thyroid gland, shield	*Thyrotoxicosis* is a serious condition of the thyroid being "poisoned."
toxic/o	Poison, toxin	See previous example.
Suffix	**Definition**	**Example**
-oid	Resembling	*Thyroid* means "resembling a shield."
-ose	Sugar	*Sucrose* and *lactose* are different types of sugars than *glucose*.

EXAMPLE

Practice defining and building medical terms associated with the special senses.

A. Define ***ophthalmologist***.

Step 1: Start with the suffix, *-logist*, meaning "one who studies."
Step 2: Identify the prefix. There is no prefix.
Step 3: Identify the combining form, *ophthalm/o*, meaning "eyes."

Putting it all together, the definition is "one who studies or specializes in the eyes" (a term given to a medical doctor for this field).

B. Build a medical term that means "***a condition of tiny or small ear***."

Step 1: Start with the suffix, *-ia*, "condition (of)."
Step 2: Identify the prefix, *micro-*, "tiny or small."
Step 3: Identify the combining form, *ot/o*, "ear."

Putting it all together, *micro-* + *ot/o* + *-ia* becomes "microtia."

Let's review how "microtia" was constructed because it is slightly different from some of the other examples presented in this chapter. First, an exception was made when the prefix was added in that the *o* at the end of *micro-* was dropped because the combining form begins with a vowel. Remember that this is unusual, and it is not common practice to change prefixes in such a manner. Also, because the suffix begins with a vowel, the combining form vowel was dropped. Without these changes, the resulting word would have been "microotoia."

Table 4–9 lists and defines the combining forms, prefixes, and suffixes related to the special senses.

THE REPRODUCTIVE SYSTEM

There are separate reproductive systems for the male and female. Each system has its own associated terms.

The reproductive system is responsible for enabling the human race to reproduce and perpetuate the species through new birth. Thus, this section introduces terms not just specific to the reproductive system but also to human development from fertilization through birth.

The primary structure associated with the female reproductive tract is the ovary (of which there are two); the remaining structures are accessory organs. Included in these accessory organs are the uterus, the fallopian or uterine tubes, the vagina, and external accessory organs such as the female breasts. Combining forms associated with this system are deeply rooted in Greek and Latin terms, making it more difficult to remember and memorize the terms.

The primary structure in the male reproductive system is the testis (of which there are two); the remaining structures are accessory organs and include the internal structures such as the epididymis, the vas deferens, the seminal vesicle, the prostate gland, and the bulbourethral or Cowper's glands. The remaining structures are categorized as external reproductive organs.

The cycle of development of an embryo until it becomes a neonate or infant is also pertinent. At fertilization, the result of the combination of the sperm and the ovum is termed a zygote; the zygote will not implant itself into the uterine wall for about three days. After the zygote implants, it is called an embryo until the

TABLE 4–9 Common Combining Forms Related to the Special Senses

Combining Form	Definition	Example
audi/o	Sound, hearing	An *audiogram* is a record of how well a patient is able to hear various pitches of sound.
aur/o, ot/o	Ear	*Aural* and *otic* drops are used in the ear to soften ear wax. *Microtia* is a condition of very small ears.
blephar/o	Eyelid	*Blepharoptosis* is a sagging (drooping) eyelid.
conjunctiv/o	Conjunctiva(e)	*Conjunctivitis* is an inflammation of the mucous membrane lining of the eye, commonly referred to as pink-eye.
corne/o	Cornea	A *corneal* abrasion is a scratch on the cornea of the eye.
myring/o, tympan/o	Ear drum	A *myringotomy* is often performed on children to relieve pressure on the ear drum; *a tympanic* thermometer is one inserted into the ear canal to measure temperature.
ocul/o, ophthalm/o	Eye	*Ocular* implants are placed in the eye; an *ophthalmologist* is a specialist in the eye and associated diseases.
olfact/o	Smell	The *olfactory* nerve endings in the nose provide the sense of smell.
retin/o	Retina	*Retinal* surgery would be performed to repair a detached retina.
Prefix	**Definition**	**Example**
presby-	Aging, elderly	*Presbyopia* and *presbycusis* are medical terms given to diminished vision and hearing associated with the aging process.
Suffix	**Definition**	**Example**
-cusis	Hearing	*Presbycusis* is the medical term given to hearing loss that occurs as a result of the aging process.
-ptosis	Sagging or drooping	*Blepharoptosis* is a sagging (drooping) eyelid.

end of the eighth week of development, after which it is called a fetus. While the embryo or fetus is developing and growing, it is enclosed in a protective sac known as the placenta or amniotic sac. After the fetus has been delivered outside of the mother's body, it is referred to as a neonate or newborn until the fourth week of life, at which time it is called an infant. This term applies until the child is a year old.

EXAMPLE

Practice defining and building medical terms for the female reproductive system.

A. Define ***cervicitis***.

Step 1: Start with the suffix, *-itis*, meaning "inflammation (of)."
Step 2: Identify the prefix. There is no prefix.
Step 3: Identify the combining form, *cervic/o*, meaning "neck" (of the cervix, in this case).

Putting it all together, the definition is "inflammation of the neck (of the uterus)."

B. Build a medical term that means "***surgical removal of an ovary, fallopian tube, and uterus***."

Step 1: Start with the suffix, *-ectomy*, "surgical removal (of)."
Step 2: Identify the prefix. There is no prefix.
Step 3: Identify the combining forms, "ovary" (*oophor/o*), "fallopian tube" (*salping/o*), and "uterus" (*hyster/o*).

Putting it all together, *oophor/o* + *salping/o* + *hyster/o* + *-ectomy* becomes "oophorosalpingohysterectomy."

In "oophorosalpingohysterectomy," the first combining form vowel was retained because the next combining form begins with a consonant. The same is true when the third combining form is added; however, the combining form vowel for uterus was dropped because the suffix begins with a vowel.

EXAMPLE

Practice defining and building medical terms for the male reproductive system.

A. Define ***cryptorchidism***.

Step 1: Start with the suffix, *-ism*, meaning "condition (of)."
Step 2: Identify the prefix. There is no prefix.
Step 3: Identify the combining forms, *crypt/o* (meaning "hidden") and *orchid/o* (meaning "testes").

Putting it all together, the definition is "a condition of hidden testes."

When one of the testes fails to descend as it should, it remains in the abdominal cavity rather than in the scrotum, and, thus, the testis is hidden. Hence, the description, "a condition of an *undescended* testis," might be more appropriate.

B. Build a medical term that means "***the process of producing or originating sperm cells***."

Step 1: Start with the suffix, *-genesis*, "originating or beginning."
Step 2: Identify the prefix. There is no prefix.
Step 3: Identify the combining form, *spermat/o*, "sperm."

Putting it all together, *spermat/o* + *-genesis* becomes "spermatogenesis."

After you learn more about the anatomy of the reproductive systems for both the male and female, come back to this chapter and refresh your knowledge of the medical terms. Table 4–10 lists and defines the combining forms associated with the reproductive system and human development through birth.

COMMON ABBREVIATIONS

In addition to the many medical terms, abbreviations are also common references to the various body systems. Table 4–11 offers a brief introduction to some of these; you will learn more as you progress through the book.

TABLE 4–10 Common Combining Forms Related to the Reproductive System

Combining Form	Definition	Example
amni/o	Amnion	*Amniocentesis* is a surgical puncture of the amnion (amniotic sac) for diagnostic testing for birth defects.
cervic/o	Neck, cervix (neck) of the uterus	*Cervical* cancer may be revealed with the use of a Pap smear.
colp/o, vagin/o	Vagina	A *colposcopy* is examination of the vagina with a lighted instrument; *vaginitis* is inflammation of the vagina, usually bacterial or fungal.
embry/o	Embryo	*Embryology* is the study of human development through the eighth week after conception.
gravida	Pregnancy	The terms *nulli gravida* indicates a woman has never been pregnant.
gyn/o, gynec/o	Female, woman	A *gynecologist* is a specialist in the anatomy of the female reproductive system.
hyster/o, metr/o, uter/o	Uterus	A *hysterectomy* is the surgical removal of the uterus; a *uteroscopy* might be performed prior to the surgery. *Metrorrhagia* is uterine bleeding at a time other than the monthly cycle.
lact/o	Milk	*Prolactin* is a hormone secreted by the pituitary gland so a mother can nurse her baby by producing milk.
mamm/o, mast/o	Breast	A *mammogram* is a common radiologic test for detection of breast cancer; a *mastopexy* may be done to correct sagging breasts.
men/o	Month, menstruation	*Menopause* is when a woman no longer has monthly periods.

Combining Form	Definition	Example
nat/o	Birth	A *neonate* is a newborn; the *prenatal* period pertains to the months prior to the baby's birth.
oophor/o, ovari/o	Ovary	An *oophorectomy*, surgical removal of an ovary, may be performed in the case of an *ovarian* cyst.
orch/o, orchi/o, orchid/o, test/o	Testes	*Cryptorchidism* is a condition in which one or both testes (testicles) have not descended in the male and can require an *orchiopexy* to correct. *Testosterone* is the hormone produced by the testes in the male.
ov/o	Egg	Ov/o means "pertaining to an egg"; an oval is shaped like an egg.
prostat/o	Prostate	A *prostatectomy* is the surgical removal of the prostate.
salping/o	Tube (fallopian)	*Salpingitis* is an inflammation of the fallopian tube that can impede pregnancy.
sperm/o, spermat/o	Sperm	A *spermaticide* kills sperm and prevent pregnancy.

TABLE 4–11 Common Medical Abbreviations

Abbreviation	Meaning
Abd, Abdo	Abdomen
AF	Atrial fibrillation
ASHD	Arteriosclerotic heart disease
BP	Blood pressure
CA, ca	Cancer, carcinoma
CAD	Coronary artery disease
COPD	Chronic obstructive pulmonary disease
CSF	Cerebrospinal fluid
CVA	Cerebrovascular accident (stroke)
DM	Diabetes mellitus
ECG, EKG	Electrocardiogram
EEG	Electroencephalogram
EGD	Esophagogastroduodenoscopy
FBS	Fasting blood sugar
Fx	Fracture
GERD	Gastroesophageal reflux disease
GI	Gastrointestinal
GU	Genitourinary
GYN	Gynecology
HPV	Human papilloma virus
IV	Intravenous
MI	Myocardial infarction
OA	Osteoarthritis
OD	Right eye
OP	Osteoporosis
OS	Left eye

(continues)

TABLE 4–11 *(Continued)*

Abbreviation	Meaning
OU	Each eye or both eyes
PVD	Peripheral vascular disease
THR	Total hip replacement
TKR	Total knee replacement
TMJ	Temporomandibular joint
UA	Urinalysis
UGI	Upper GI (series)
URI	Upper respiratory infection
UTI	Urinary tract infection
VF	Ventricular fibrillation

CHAPTER SUMMARY

- The steps for breaking a medical term apart to define it or to build a medical term, you should (1) start with the suffix, (2) identify the prefix (if there is one), and (3) determine the word root(s) or combining form(s).
- The basic unit of the human body is the cell (combining form *cyt*/o). Cells organize to become tissue (combining form *hist*/o), and tissues become organized to form *organs*. Organs work together to be organized into *organ systems*, which ultimately are organized into the human organism.
- The skin (*cutane*/o, *derm*/o, *dermat*/o, *integument*/o), or the integumentary system, is the most external and visualized organ in the human body and is the largest organ of the human body. The study of the skin is called dermatology.
- Within the musculoskeletal system are the bones (*oste*/o) of the skeletal system as well as the muscles (*muscul*/o, *my*/o) that move the bones. One of the most common combining forms for muscle is *my*/o. There are 206 bones in the human body; by learning the name of each of the bones, you will have a good basis for knowing the combining forms for each of them.
- The cardiovascular system is composed of the heart (*cardi*/o) and its associated structures. The aorta (*aort*/o), arteries (*ateri*/o), and arterioles are the vessels that transport oxygen-rich blood (*hemo*/, *hemat*/o) throughout the body. The blood is then returned to the heart through the venules, veins (*phleb*/o, *ven*/o), and vena cavae.
- In the respiratory system, air (*aer*/o) first enters the body through the mouth or the nose (*nas*/o, *rhin*/o), moves down through the throat (*pharynx*, *pharyng*/o), the voice box (*larynx*, *laryng*/o), the airway (*trachea*, *trache*/o), and into the lungs (*pulmon*/o) to the bronchi, the bronchioles (*bronchiol*/o), and, at the end, the alveoli, the microscopic air sacs that exchange oxygen (*ox*/o) and carbon dioxide through the processes of inspiration (breathing in) and expiration (breathing out).
- Many structures comprise the gastrointestinal or digestive system, as well as accessory structures that assist with the digestion of nutrients taken into the body. The GI system begins at the mouth (*or*/o) and terminates at the anus (*an*/o), making it quite a complex system.
- The urinary system is instrumental in ridding the human body of waste products that build up in the bloodstream and excreting that waste in the form of urine (*ur*/o, *urin*/o). The urinary system is composed of two kidneys (*ren*/o), two ureters (*ureter*/o), one bladder (*cyst*/o), and one urethra (*urethr*/o).
- There are two major divisions to the nervous (*neur*/o) system: the central nervous system, consisting of the brain (*encephal*/o) and spinal cord, and the peripheral nervous system, the portion that enables awareness of surroundings through various receptors and communications with the brain.
- The terms you encounter related to the endocrine system most often refer to specific endocrine glands such as the thyroid (*thyr*/o), the parathyroid (*parathyroid*/o), and the thymus (*thym*/o).
- The special senses include the organs that provide vision (eye, *ocul*/o and *ophthalm*/o), hearing (ear, *aur*/o and *ot*/o; hearing, *audi*/o), balance and upright stature, smell (*olfact*/o), and taste. Also included are the receptors of the skin that enable the sense of touch, pain, and temperature.

- There are separate reproductive systems for the male and female. Each system has its own associated terms. The primary structure associated with the female reproductive tract is the ovary (*oophor*/o, *ovari*/o); the remaining structures are accessory organs. The primary structure in the male reproductive system is the testis (*orch*/o, *orchi*/o, *orchid*/o, *test*/o).

STUDY TOOLS

Workbook	Activities for Chapter 4
Premium Website	
StudyWARE	Activities and Quizzes on the **StudyWARE™ Software** for Chapter 4
	Audio Library of medical terms
	Online access to the **Critical Thinking Challenge 2.0**
learning**lab**	Module 2: Medical Terminology
CourseMate	Activities and Quizzes for Chapter 4
WebTutor	Activities and Quizzes for Chapter 4

CHECK YOUR KNOWLEDGE

1. Which of the following is the correct medical term for dry skin?
   a. Xanthoderma
   b. Xeroderma
   c. Scleroderma
   d. Erythemaderma
2. The term *epigastric* means:
   a. pertaining to upon the stomach.
   b. pertaining to below the stomach.
   c. pertaining to above the stomach.
   d. pertaining to near the stomach.
3. The combining forms *ili*/o, *lamin*/o, *mandibul*/o, and *maxill*/o pertain to which body system?
   a. Lymphatic
   b. Musculoskeletal
   c. Cardiovascular
   d. Integumentary
4. Aphonia means:
   a. a condition of no speech.
   b. a condition of no recording.
   c. a condition of painful speech.
   d. a condition of no voice.
5. The combining form in "stomatitis" means:
   a. body.
   b. inflammation.
   c. mouth.
   d. stomach.
6. Billie hadn't been feeling very well, so she decided to visit Dr. Burress, a ________, a specialist in the study of the blood. Dr. Burress examined Billie and ordered some blood tests; he asked the ________ to draw the specimens.
   a. hematologist, phlebotomist
   b. hematologist, cardiologist
   c. cardiologist, phlebotomist
   d. cardiologist, venipuncturist
7. The combining form in "colposcopy" relates to the ________ system.
   a. gastrointestinal
   b. endocrine
   c. reproductive
   d. nervous

WEB LINKS

MedTerms Medical Dictionary: www.medterms.com

RESOURCES

Ehrlich, A. (2009). *Medical Terminology for Health Professions* (6th ed.). Clifton Park, NY: Delmar Cengage Learning.

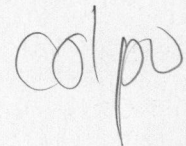

Unit

3

Medical Law and Ethics

Chapter 5
Legal Issues

Chapter 6
Ethical Issues

Legal and ethical issues arise so frequently in the everyday life of a medical assistant. How do we balance the requirements of patient confidentiality against the public's right to be aware of a dangerous situation? The law provides the tools and framework for crafting an answer. Likewise, how do we judge the performance of our providers? Again, the law provides an answer.

Granted, sometimes we might not like or agree with the answer. That is not the point. We are obligated to live within the rules we have, as a society, determined to be in the best interest of either the individual or the public. You are not, as a medical assistant, expected to know all the nooks and crannies of the law. You are, however, expected to be aware that law exists to address many of the situations you will encounter in your practice and to be aware of what the law requires of you in those circumstances.

Certification Connection

	Ch. 5	Ch. 6
CMA (AAMA)		
Legislation	X	
Drug Enforcement Administration (DEA)	X	
Medical records	X	
Releasing medical information	X	
Provider–patient relationship	X	
Maintaining confidentiality	X	
Performing within ethical boundaries		X
RMA (AMT)		
Medical law	X	
Understand the application of the Clinical Laboratory Improvement Amendments of 1988 (CLIA '88)	X	
Medical law: Terminology	X	
Principles of medical ethics and ethical conduct		X
CMAS (AMT)		
Apply principles of medical law and ethics to the health care setting	X	X
Recognize legal responsibilities of, and know scope of practice for, the medical administrative specialist	X	
Know basic laws pertaining to medical practice	X	
Know and observe disclosure laws (patient privacy, minors, confidentiality)	X	X
Know the principles of medical ethics established by the AMA		X
Recognize unethical practices and identify ethical responses for situations in the medical office		X

Chapter 5 Legal Issues

OBJECTIVES

In this chapter, you will learn the following:

KB KNOWLEDGE BASE

1. Spell and define, using the glossary at the back of the text, all the Words to Know in this chapter.
2. Define "law" and describe the sources of law.
3. Compare and contrast criminal and civil law.
4. Describe tort law.
5. Explain the difference between intentional and unintentional torts and provide examples of each.
6. List and describe the elements of negligence and medical malpractice.
7. Compare and contrast provider and medical assistant roles in terms of standard of care.
8. Describe the doctor–patient relationship, discussing the concepts of a contract and consent.
9. Identify and describe the types of advance directives presented in this chapter.
10. Explore issue of confidentiality as it applies to the medical assistant.
11. Describe the governmental agencies that regulate matters in health care; examine specific statutes that affect the medical office.
12. Explain the federal laws discussed in this chapter that affect the provider office.

WORDS TO KNOW

acceptance
advance directives
agent
beyond a reasonable doubt
capacity
common law
compensatory damages
consent
consideration
defendant
federal law
felony
Good Samaritan Act
guardian
gross negligence
Health Insurance Portability and Accountability Act (HIPAA)
informed consent
jurisdiction
legislating
libel
living will
medical malpractice
misdemeanor
negligence
offer
plaintiff
power of attorney
preponderance of the evidence
privileged communication
property right
prosecution
punitive damages
respondeat superior
slander
standard of care
standard of proof
state law
statute
statute of limitations
statutory law
supremacy clause
vicariously liable
wrongful death

WHAT IS "LAW" AND WHO MAKES IT?

The common definition of law is, in the broadest sense, a system of rules, usually enforced through a collection of institutions commonly recognized as having the authority to do so (Hart, 1961). An anonymous legal proverb refers to the law as "a seamless web," referring to the fact that pieces of law frequently interact with one another. For example, the successful **plaintiff** in a **medical malpractice** case receiving a large jury award can suddenly find he or she has a problem involving tax law. And sometimes someone who intentionally causes a grievous injury to another won't be adjudged guilty of criminal conduct but can still be held liable under civil law.

EXAMPLE

This was the infamous O.J. Simpson case. A civil court found that Simpson killed his ex-wife and her boyfriend after the criminal trial had found him not guilty.

Law is derived from several sources, predominately legislative bodies and courts, and law is developed at multiple levels in the United States. The United States Congress, of course, makes **federal law** when it passes legislation. The Patient Protection and Affordable Care Act (health care reform) that was passed in 2010 is a good example. Because of the **supremacy clause** in the United States Constitution, laws created by Congress apply to everyone in the United States. The federalist system of the United States, however, is complex because in addition to the Congress making federal law, state legislatures make **state law** that applies to everyone within the state but not to those who don't live or work there. Requirements for provider licensing, for example, can be different in Connecticut than they are in Pennsylvania. The final layer in this structure consists of local governments. Counties, cities, townships, and other units of government can pass resolutions or ordinances that govern conduct within those **jurisdictions**. Setting a speed limit on a residential street is a good example. The process by which any of these entities develops law is called **legislating,** and the outcome—the final product of the process—is called a **statute**. Thus we are governed by **statutory law** as handed down by the Congress, the state legislature, or the local government.

It is also true to say that the United States Supreme Court also "makes" law by interpreting the constitution. In *Roe v. Wade*, for example, the Supreme Court found that a woman had a constitutional right to privacy under the Fourth Amendment but that her privacy rights had to be balanced against the state's interest in protecting life and protecting the mother's health. In that case, the court noted that the state's legitimate interest in protecting life increased during the pregnancy. The court then resolved the apparent conflict by increasing the ability of the state to restrict abortion by trimester. The court found the state's interests were strongest in the third trimester of the pregnancy, thereby permitting the state to restrict or prohibit abortion (except in cases to preserve the life or health of the mother). In the first trimester, the state's interests are the weakest, so the court determined the state could not interfere with the woman's right to privacy—in this case, the right to an abortion—in any way (*Roe v. Wade*, 1973).

The other kind of law that courts truly do make is the **common law**, also known as *case law* or the law of *precedent*. The term has its origins in ancient England and is based on customs of the day that came to be recognized by the courts in the forms of judgments. Basically, ancient courts would look to societal customs and compare those with the conduct of the **defendant**. This process was referred to as "finding the law." If the defendant's conduct did not fit the norm, the court would enter a decree in favor of the **plaintiff**. This form of law came about because of the need to address situations not covered by statute. English courts thus sat as a court of law (dealing with interpretation and application of statues) and as a court of equity (dealing with community expectations and customs). Common law arose from this concept of equity. The concept of **negligence** arises from the common law. Discussion of that concept in detail follows.

As a medical assistant, you must know how to comply with state and federal law especially and, sometimes, local government requirements. In most cases, the kinds of law with which you will come in contact are statutory, although, as we shall see, that is not always the case. You must understand the common law and know the difference between criminal law and civil law as well. As you can see from Figure 5–1, both state and federal statutes and state and federal court decisions affect the health care provider.

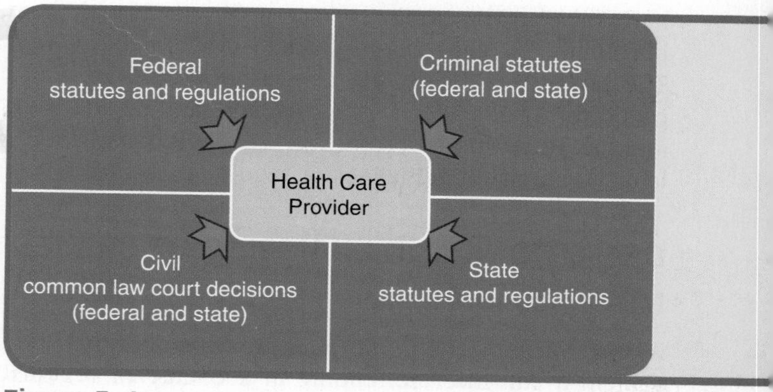

Figure 5–1: Sources of law affecting health care providers.
Delmar/Cengage Learning.

CRIMINAL VS. CIVIL LAW

An ocean's worth of difference stands between these two sub-branches of the law. Criminal law is (1) exclusively statutory and (2) deals with one who has performed an act prohibited by law or failed to perform an act required by law. In either instance, the person on trial is the defendant; the unit of government bringing the charges is the plaintiff, frequently referred to as the **prosecution**. Civil law is a collection of rules that govern the conduct and affairs of people—their rights—the infractions of which are not crimes.

In criminal law, there are two kinds of crimes: **misdemeanors**, punishable by imprisonment in a jail for less than one year, assessment of a fine, or both; **felonies**, which are punishable by imprisonment in a state prison for more than one year (and sometimes punishable by death). Determining what crime belongs in each category is a job for the state legislature.

The other distinction between criminal and civil law is the **standard of proof** required to impose a penalty on the defendant. In a criminal case, the standard of proof is very difficult: **beyond a reasonable doubt**. Simply put, when the defendant is on trial for a crime, the prosecution must prove that the defendant committed the act beyond a reasonable doubt as determined by a jury of the defendant's peers. In other words, 12 people must absolutely agree that the act was committed and that the defendant committed it. In the famous O.J. Simpson case, there was in the mind of the jury a reasonable doubt about whether Simpson killed Ron Goldman and Nicole Brown Simpson; thus, Simpson was found not guilty. After that verdict, however, the Goldman and Brown families brought a **wrongful death** action in civil court and were able to demonstrate by a **preponderance of the evidence** (the standard of proof required in civil court) that Simpson did indeed commit the murders and should be held to account in money damages paid to the families (Bugliosi, 1997).

Seldom, however, is involvement with the law so dramatic. The nature of criminal law is to protect a person and his or her property from those who would do harm or steal. The criminal justice system deals with them in roughly the same fashion you see on *Law and Order*. The police investigate; the district attorney (sometimes called the state's attorney) prosecutes; the jury decides, and the judge imposes sentence, usually following legislatively mandated guidelines or requirements.

DEFINITIONS AND EXAMPLES OF CRIMES

Misdemeanors

A misdemeanor is a crime punishable by less than one year in a jail, most commonly in a county or regional jail, not a state prison. Sometimes the punishment can include a fine, or a fine might be imposed instead of sending the defendant to jail.

EXAMPLE

BISMARCK, N.D. (AP)—November 9, 2010

It's green.

It was offered as payment.

But it's not money.

A North Dakota man has been sentenced to six days in the slammer, after offering pot for payment in a bar. Richard Hanley Junior has pleaded guilty to misdemeanor marijuana possession and disorderly conduct. Authorities say he bumped into a server at a Bismarck bar. Drinks were spilled and another employee demanded payment. Prosecutors say Hanley offered to make good on the booze with a baggie of pot (Associated Press, 2010).

You just can't make this stuff up! Misdemeanors are offenses that can often be avoided by using some commonsense judgment. The preceding Example box presents an extreme situation; other examples might be someone who breaks into the vending machine to steal money; an irate neighbor who destroys a shrub growing on a contested property line, and so forth.

Felony

This category of crime is much more serious. These are crimes committed by people who intend to do significant harm to another, either through depriving him or her of property or injuring him or her personally. For our purposes, we'll divide felonious acts into four categories: murder, manslaughter, robbery, and burglary.

Murder

The traditional definition of murder is the "unlawful killing of another with malice aforethought" (Blackstone, 1765). This concept is still good, although legislatures have defined a number of degrees of murder based on the level of premeditation by the defendant or the status of the victim.

EXAMPLE

A particularly gruesome example is the home invasion of Dr. William Petit, Jr., of Cheshire, CT. On the evening of July 23, 2007, two men broke into the home, beat Dr. Petit and bound him, and ransacked the house in search of valuables. After forcing

Mrs. Petit to go to a bank for cash, the conspirators raped, tortured, and killed Mrs. Petit and her two daughters, ages 11 and 17. They then set the house on fire and escaped. Somehow, Dr. Petit survived. One of the perpetrators was convicted; the other will face trial in the future (Griffin and Kovner, 2010).

Clearly, in this example, this was a case of first-degree murder. The perpetrators planned the attack in advance and carried it out, inflicting brutal harm to the family.

Manslaughter

Manslaughter is the unlawful killing of a human being without malice. It is of two kinds:

- *Voluntary*—Upon a sudden quarrel or heat of passion.
- *Involuntary*—In the commission of an unlawful act . . . or without due caution and circumspection, of a lawful act which might produce death. (U.S. Code, n.d.)

Voluntary manslaughter involves a violent act by one person on another. The following case is a good example.

EXAMPLE

James Peters and Thomas Minton had been drinking in Peters' apartment on the evening of May 1, 2009. Minton got into an argument with Mrs. Peters, whereupon Mr. Peters stood up from the wheelchair that he used occasionally and told Minton to leave. Instead of leaving, Minton lunged toward Peters. Peters retaliated by stabbing Minton nine times. The initial charge was murder, but the presiding judge at the preliminary hearing reduced the charge to manslaughter because there was no evidence Peters' actions were intentional or premeditated (Pope, 2009).

Involuntary manslaughter most commonly involves a death arising from a motor vehicle accident. Frequently, the driver is under the influence of alcohol or drugs.

EXAMPLE

Jessica Lynn Shekell, a 23-year-old woman, pleaded guilty to killing two sisters and injuring two minors while driving drunk on the wrong side of the freeway in Anaheim. Shekell had been drinking with her friends at a couple of bars in Placentia when she was driving on the wrong side of the freeway and collided with Sally Miguel's vehicle.

Sally Miguel and her sister, Patricia, were killed in the crash. Their nieces and Sara Miguel survived the crash but suffered serious injuries.

Shekell has pleaded guilty to two felony counts of gross vehicular manslaughter with gross negligence while intoxicated: a felony count of driving under the influence of alcohol, causing bodily injury; and a felony count of driving with a blood-alcohol level of more than .08 percent, causing bodily injury. She also received sentencing enhancements for causing great bodily injury. Shekell faces up to 19 years and eight months in prison (Guisti, 2010).

Robbery

Robbery is the unlawful taking of money or goods of another from his or her person or in immediate presence by force or intimidation, such as in the following case.

EXAMPLE

Iniguez and McIntosh went to a West Leola Street home in Pasco in May 2005 and showed a shotgun. After forcing their way in and tying up the occupants, the intruders took the occupants' jewelry and wallets (*TriCity Herald*, 2009).

Burglary

Burglary is similar to robbery: It involves the taking of money or property belonging to another. The difference is that burglary does not involve the presence of the victim. This is literally the case of someone breaking into a home to steal jewelry while the family is out of town.

A medical assistant should seldom be exposed to criminal law. There are, however, times and places when this knowledge will be helpful to you. The provider who knowingly bills Medicare for tests and procedures not actually performed on patients is committing a crime. The medical assistant who has knowledge of what the provider is doing and participates in the scheme can also be guilty of criminal conduct.

THE LAW OF TORTS

The concept of a *tort* arose from the ancient English tradition discussed earlier. This is a branch of common law. The term comes from the Latin *tortum*, which means "wrong," and some good examples of torts include automobile accidents, product liability, slander and libel, and, of course, medical malpractice. The person who is harmed by the conduct of another may use tort law to sue the person who caused the harm and receive both **compensatory damages** and **punitive damages**.

Torts can be both unintentional and intentional. Automobile accidents, a baseball through the window, or a rock flying from the lawnmower are all accidents; they are all unintentional. Acts referred to as *intentional torts*, such as **libel** and **slander**, trespass, and intentional infliction of emotional distress, are those incidents in which the defendant could reasonably foresee that harm would result to the plaintiff.

Libel and slander are two forms of the same thing: defamation of character. Thus, if one says, "Dr. Jones is an awful provider; he's killed at least a dozen of his patients," the person doing the talking may be held liable for damages if Dr. Jones can show (a) that the statement was untrue and (b) that he was damaged as a result. This would be a case of slander because it is a spoken defamation. Libel is a written defamation; thus, if one makes a similar entry on his or her Facebook page or blog, Dr. Jones's action would be for libel.

Negligence

Although the category of intentional torts is interesting and has lots of examples of bad behavior, it is the unintentional acts that most often concern medical office professionals. "Simple" negligence can—and often does—rear its ugly head without warning or notice. That is the central point of it: that it happens by mistake or accident. Unlike intentional torts, negligence is not planned or contrived in advance in any way. The underlying principle that establishes whether the plaintiff can collect for damages in the case of the negligence is the **standard of care** the defendant owed to the plaintiff.

EXAMPLE

Richard and Jim go on a hunting trip. Richard turns and fires his shotgun at what he thinks is a flock of pheasants. He misses, however, and some of the buckshot hits and injures Jim. Jim can sue Richard and collect an amount of money to pay for the care resulting from his injuries (compensatory damages). Jim might also be able to recover money if Richard was wantonly reckless in the way he handled the gun (punitive damages).

In the example, the questions are these: Did Richard owe Jim a duty regarding how he pointed, aimed, and shot his gun? Did Richard live up to that duty? If he did, there is no suit. If he did not meet the standard imposed by the duty, there would be liability on Richard's part—meaning he would have to pay for Jim's care. And if the jury found that Richard's conduct was unreasonably reckless, it could also award punitive damages. This is a case of negligence.

The legal foundation for the concept of negligence is this: Everyone owes everyone else the duty to behave "reasonably" (Blackstone, 1765). If you don't behave reasonably and someone is injured as a result of your conduct, you will be liable for damages. Most of the time, this duty to behave reasonably is in the negative: that is, a duty to avoid doing something like pointing a gun at a hunting companion. When two people have a particular relationship to one another—for example, doctor and patient—the concept of an *affirmative duty* arises. In cases like this, the provider possesses an affirmative duty to, for example, treat the defendant's disease if the provider knows the patient is ill. Likewise, the provider has an affirmative duty to examine the patient to diagnose illness as well.

Several factors can point to negligence—or not—by the defendant:

1. A *duty* of care must be owed by the defendant to the plaintiff.
2. The defendant must have committed a *breach* of that duty.
3. The plaintiff must have suffered harm (*injury*).
4. And that harm must be a result of the defendant's breach of duty (*causation*).

Thus, in our hunting accident:

1. Richard owed Jim the duty of not pointing and discharging a gun in Jim's direction.
2. Richard pointed and discharged the gun at Jim.
3. Jim was injured.
4. Richard's firing the weapon caused Jim's injury.

Now, what happens if we change the facts? Richard still makes the same move with his gun and fires it in Jim's direction. But none of the buckshot hits Jim. *No liability results because Jim wasn't injured.* And if we look at it slightly differently once again: Richard makes the same move, but this time doesn't fire: *No liability results because Richard didn't violate the duty of care he owed Jim.* Likewise, if, later in the trip, Jim is checking his weapon, it discharges and some of the buckshot injures himself, *no liability results because Jim's injury is not a result of anything Richard did.*

Although there are some statutory considerations in addition to common law negligence, the concept can be applied to the medical assistant.

EXAMPLE

An elderly patient presents at the provider's office for a routine physical exam. You record the history and the vital signs accurately. The examination goes well and, because of the patient's age, the provider orders a pneumonia vaccination. You prepare the injection and administer it. But because it is flu season and you weren't paying full attention, you mistakenly inject the patient with flu vaccine. The patient has a known allergy to eggs, and she becomes violently ill and requires hospitalization.

In this example:

1. You owed a duty of care to the patient that included injecting the correct vaccine.
2. You injected the patient with the wrong vaccine.
3. The patient became ill and required hospitalization.
4. Her illness was a result of your injection.

Thus, in this case, the medical assistant was negligent in the care of the patient. Now, let's think of the medical assistant who provides administrative support for the office and handles records.

EXAMPLE

The provider has completed the exam of the patient, has noted the presence of a swelling around the lymph nodes in the throat and has determined that watchful waiting is the best course for this patient at this time. He orders her to return in four weeks for a follow-up exam. You are handling checkout for the patient and misread the order as four months and schedule the patient accordingly. The patient returns for her exam after four months. It turns out that she has a rapidly growing cancer that has now metastasized beyond her throat. Her surgery, radiation, and chemotherapy will be long, costly, and painful. She will be fortunate to survive. What result?

In this example:

1. You owed a duty of care to the patient to correctly interpret the provider's orders on check-out.
2. You mistakenly scheduled the follow-up exam for 4 months from the date rather than 4 weeks.
3. You permitted the patient's cancer to advance beyond its early stage, causing severe injury through the trauma of care for advanced cancer to the patient.
4. This result occurred because the patient was not being seen on follow up in a timely manner, a result of the error in reading the order.

Again, the conduct of the medical assistant was negligent resulting in injury to the plaintiff. And in both cases, the medical assistant would be held solely liable for the damages, except for one very important concept: ***respondeat superior***, which comes from the Latin, "let the master answer." This doctrine of law holds that the employer is **vicariously liable** for the acts of the employee (Flight, 2011). In this case, the notion of "let the master answer" is clear because the medical assistant was performing duties on behalf of the provider—doing something clearly within the scope of his employment (U.S. Bureau of Labor Statistics, 2009). This concept does not mean the medical assistant is absolved of responsibility. The medical assistant may be sued, in addition to the provider, because each person is responsible for his or her own actions.

We see in these examples how the concept of negligence begins to touch the provider's office as well as the medical assistant. And with that in mind, we turn to a very special subspecies of negligence: medical malpractice.

Medical Malpractice

Remember when we discussed "standard of care"? This concept is central to the idea of medical malpractice. Simply put, did the doctor render treatment—or fail to provide treatment—consistent with the standard of care expected of people with his or her training and experience in similar circumstances? The provider has a special relationship with the patient (we'll discuss the nature of the relationship in a bit) and thus has an affirmative duty of care toward the patient. If the provider fails to exercise the responsibility associated with that duty, whether affirmative or not, then he or she would be held liable for the damages caused.

A medical assistant owes the duty of *reasonable* care. He or she must take appropriate steps to check the type and dosage of medication before administering it to the patient and must take appropriate steps to ensure that the paperwork regarding charts and follow-up appointments is completed accurately (Cowdrey and Drew, 1995).

It is because of that special relationship between the provider and the patient that the elements of negligence change a bit from what was discussed earlier. Here are two additional elements, highlighted, not a part of the standard negligence lawsuit:

1. There is a *relationship* between the provider and the patient.
2. That *relationship created a duty* of the provider toward the patient.
3. The duty was of the nature of a professional *standard of care*.
4. The provider *breached* the duty to the patient.
5. The patient had a resulting *injury*.
6. The patient would not have sustained the injury but for the provider's breach of duty (*causation*) (Flight, 2011).

Following are descriptions of each of these elements:

- *Relationship*: The relationship of the provider to the patient is created by the offer of care by the provider and an acceptance by the patient. This is fundamental contract law (covered at more length in following sections of this chapter).
- *Duty:* The nature of the duty the provider owes the patient has several dimensions. First, if the provider knows of an abnormal test result or observation on examination, he or she has a duty to tell the patient. The provider has a duty to diagnose medical conditions and, finally, a duty to treat known medical conditions (*Glidden v. Maglio*, 2000).
- *Standard of care:* The provider must use the same standard of care in rendering diagnosis or treatment as would be used by a competent practitioner in the same class as the defendant in similar circumstances (*Mitchell v. Hadl*, 1991).
- *Breach of duty:* The provider must have failed to act upon the duty he owed the plaintiff. This includes failing to undertake and affirmative duty to act (*Noble v. Sartori*, 1990).
- *Injury:* The plaintiff must have suffered an injury (*Redder v. Hanson*, 1964).
- *Causation:* The failure of the provider to act according to duty, or a failure to act in a manner consistent with providers in similar circumstances, must be the cause of the injury. This can be a direct cause, or it can be referred to as something that would not have occurred "but for" the provider's failure to act (*Holtzclaw v. Ochsner Clinic*, 2002).

Although all of this might seem simple enough and pretty straightforward, the nature of medical malpractice litigation is that it is, in fact, intensive. That is to say, literally thousands of facts can go into an alleged incident of medical malpractice, and the defendant can raise key concepts to protect himself from liability. Plausible defenses to medical malpractice allegations are:

- *Statute of limitations:* Most states have a **statute of limitations** law. This tells all who would file a lawsuit that they have a limited period of time in which to bring their claim. In the case of medical malpractice claims, an injured patient generally has two years from the date the injury is discovered in which to file his or her lawsuit. The theory is that two years should be sufficient time to discover whether one has been injured at the hands of his or her provider or other medical provider. If one does not bring suit within the statutory time period, the case will be dismissed (*Crawford v. McDonald*, 1972).
- *Contributory negligence:* This term describes an action by the plaintiff that has contributed to the injury he or she has suffered. When the plaintiff does something that has in fact contributed to his injury the provider cannot be blamed. So the family of a person who lied to a provider about the drugs he or she had consumed and subsequently died of from a drug overdose will not be able to bring a successful malpractice action because the provider unknowingly administered more of the drug on which the patient was already intoxicated. The patient has a duty to be truthful with the provider (*Rochester v. Katalan*, 1974).
- *Emergency:* Generally speaking, both Good Samaritan statutes and common law will protect a medical provider when he or she responds to an emergency situation. This is true for both the provider and the medical assistant. There is a key question to consider as a threshold. First, is there a relationship between the provider and the victim in an accident? If the medical assistant bypasses the accident, no relationship is established; the six-factor medical malpractice analysis does not apply, and no liability will attach to the medical assistant. If the medical assistant stops to render aid, a relationship is established, and the medical malpractice analysis applies. After that relationship is established, the medical assistant owes a victim a duty of care and will not be held liable for further injury to the accident victim unless he or she commits **gross negligence** in providing care.

Medical malpractice is a source of considerable controversy among policy makers. Some states have imposed statutory caps on punitive damages, meaning that the plaintiff can recover only actual damages and up to the cap, or limit, on punitive damages, which are imposed to "punish" the defendant. Many states have not enacted a cap, and there is no federal legislation on the issue. Providers and other medical services providers argue that many of the malpractice judgments are excessive and contribute to higher insurance premiums. In addition, they argue, the possibility of being sued and subject to those excessive verdicts causes them to practice defensive medicine, ordering additional tests that serve only a marginal clinical purpose but will protect the provider in the event of a malpractice allegation.

Conversely, plaintiffs and their attorneys argue that punitive damages work to deter future malpractice and call attention to the plight of the injured patient in a way that is undeniable to the medical services community. This issue was not addressed in the health care reform legislation passed in 2010, and it is likely to resurface from time to time in the future; however, there is a special relationship between doctor and patient that sets the stage for potential medical malpractice litigation.

THE DOCTOR–PATIENT CONTRACT

The relationship between doctor and patient is in the nature of a contract. The provider, by holding himself out to provide medical services, is making an **offer** to care for the patient. When the patient makes an appointment, she is indicating **acceptance** of the offer. And when she assures the medical assistant taking the appointment that she has insurance and will pay the co-pay, **consideration** has changed hands, forming a valid contract for care between the patient and the provider. This is all that is required to form a contract: offer, acceptance, and consideration. From that point on, the provider has an affirmative duty to care for the patient to the professional standards associated with a doctor of similar training and experience (Flight, 2011).

A contract can be *express* or *implied*. The scene in the following paragraph is an "express contract," meaning the parties clearly expressed their respective intentions. Often, a contract can be implied from the facts.

EXAMPLE

Consider the patient suffering chest pain, difficulty breathing, and perspiration who goes to an urgent care center operated by a local hospital. A nurse staffing the center consults with a provider by phone who inquires about the patient's symptoms, medical history, and related matters. The provider then advises the patient to return home and call his medical group, an affiliate of the hospital, in the morning. The patient does so, gets in bed, and never wakes up because he died from a heart attack in his sleep. Is this a contract? Yes; when the provider inquired about the patient's symptoms and history, he or she established enough of a relationship to be the patient's provider, especially since he or she should have known from the symptoms that the patient needed immediate care (*O'Neill v. Montefiore Hospital*, 1960).

However, to form a contract, both parties must have the **capacity** to enter into a contract. This means the person must be (a) the age of majority as determined by the state in which the contract is formed, or (b) an emancipated minor, meaning a person under the age of majority but who is completely self-supporting, and (c) not the victim of a legal disability, meaning either a person who is mentally incompetent or is under the influence of drugs that alter the mental state (Flight, 2011; Cowdrey and Drew, 1995).

The matter of capacity is important for another reason. In our example, the **consent** of the patient clearly existed: he went to an urgent care center. But the question is, "Who can give consent?" And what if they can't give it?

A parent or **guardian** can give consent for a minor child; a person who is the age of majority or who is an emancipated minor can give consent for him- or herself, provided that person is not under any legal disability. And, as one might suspect, there is always an exception for emergencies, for example, the minor child who arrives at the hospital with severe and multiple traumas as a result of a car accident, whose life is in jeopardy if untreated, and the parents cannot be located. The providers and the hospital will not be held liable for providing care. The result is different, however, if the injury or condition is not life threatening. In those cases, courts have ruled that the provider cannot proceed to treat without parental consent (Cowdrey and Drew, 1995).

Rights of the Parties to the Contract

Like any other contract, the people who make a contract have certain rights. In business, many of these rights will be spelled out in the contract document. In most cases involving health care providers, however, the contracts are oral agreements and thus subject to both statutory and common law interpretations. As a medical assistant, you will be required to understand the provider's obligations to the patient (remember, you are the doctor's "**agent**") as well as the provider's rights in the doctor–patient relationship. As these are mutual rights and responsibilities, often in conflict, we can examine them as a series of questions that might be raised from both sides of the relationship.

Is It Abandonment of the Patient or a Proper Refusal of Care?

We discussed previously how a contract may be formed, thereby imposing a duty of care on the provider. But when can the provider be relieved of that duty? There are only a few circumstances in which a provider can end the duty of care after it has been established. The provider has that duty until the relationship is terminated by:

1. mutual consent of the patient and the doctor.
2. patient dismissing the doctor.
3. the changed circumstance under which care is no longer needed.
4. provider withdrawal from the relationship by providing the patient with written notice with reasonable time to find a new provider (*Miller v. Greater Southeast Community Hospital*, 1986).

As in the O'Neill case in the preceding example, it doesn't really take much to establish the provider's duty of care. And when in that situation, the provider cannot on a whim disregard the patient. Providers are compelled to provide care:

- when the patient is disabled with HIV (*Bragdon v. Abbot*, 1988).
- when the patient has sued the provider group for malpractice and there has not been enough time to notify the patient to seek a new doctor (*Tierney v. University of Michigan Regents*, 2003).

- when the relationship with the patient has not been continuous (*Haidak v. Corso*, 2004); when the abandonment could constitute a criminal act (*Mack v. Soung*, 2000).

In other words, when there are ethical considerations (*Haidak*) or an antidiscrimination law such as the Americans with Disabilities Act (*Bragdon*), or the need for emergency treatment (*Tierney*), a provider can be held liable for breach of contract and perhaps for medical malpractice if the patient is harmed by the abandonment.

Is the Patient Entitled to Privacy or Is the Doctor Required to Report?

The patient has a right to expect his or her communications with his or her provider to be kept confidential. That is the nature of the privileged communications in the relationship. The privilege, however, is not without some exceptions. The provider is required by statutes in most states to report child abuse and elder abuse. Indeed, even when test results are inconclusive as to child sexual abuse, the provider will be held harmless for reporting such suspicions (*Johnfroe v. Children's Hospital*, 2008). When there is a requirement to report abuse, the privilege is no excuse for failure to report; thus, courts will protect the provider for abiding by the law. Although the advent of HIPAA (discussion follows) provides an additional layer of assurance for the patient regarding his or her personal health information, it also is not an absolute guarantee when the public interest demands disclosure. For example, HIPAA permits disclosure of information to a family member unless the patient objects; when subpoenaed as part of litigation; when the provider has a legal duty to report, as in cases of abuse or contagious diseases; and when needed for public health activities, law enforcement purposes, or similar needs (Miller, 2006).

The proper outlook on this matter is that the patient is entitled to privileged communications and privacy of his or her personal health information unless a clear exception is determined by the office administrator in consultation with legal counsel.

Who Decides What Care to Provide or Accept: The Doctor or the Patient?

This question really turns on the issue of **informed consent**. Before a doctor can treat the patient, the patient must provide informed consent. At least that is the way it works most of the time. There are, as there in all things, exceptions to the rule.

The first concern in this question refers again to the capacity-to-contract issue mentioned previously. To provide consent, one must be competent. The secondary matter is whether the patient consented or refused care. See Figure 5–2 for a brief look at the question.

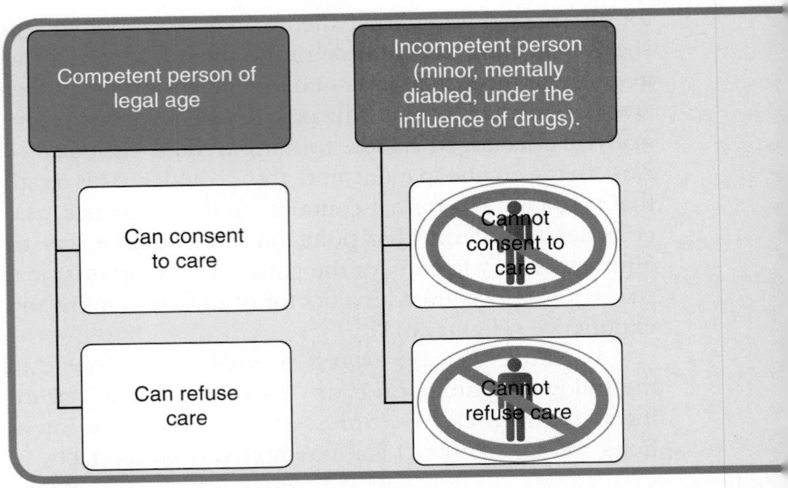

Figure 5–2: Competency and consent. *Delmar/Cengage Learning.*

A competent person can refuse care, even if terminally ill (*Cruzan v. Director, Missouri Dept. of Health*, 1990). This means he or she can decline a ventilator, hydration, nutrition, blood transfusion, and any other life-saving or life-prolonging treatment. There are some very limiting exceptions regarding the protection of a third party and prevention of suicide, but, otherwise, a person has a liberty interest in refusing care (*Cruzan v. Director, Missouri Dept. of Health*, 1990). However, a person who is not competent by reason of age, disability, or impairment resulting from drugs or alcohol cannot give informed consent, nor can he or she refuse care. Indeed, the provider will be found negligent for accepting and abiding by an impaired person's refusal of care.

Special circumstances do exist, however. A parent or legal guardian can consent to care on behalf of a minor child. Even the divorced parent who has visitation rights, when in custody of the minor, has authority to consent (Morrissey, Hoffman, and Thorpe, 1986), but a parent cannot refuse care for the minor if the illness is life threatening (The Sullivan Group, 2010).

Patient Self-Determination Act

The Patient Self-Determination Act (PSDA) represents a milestone in establishing patient rights with respect to a health care provider (42 U.S.C. 1395 cc (a), 1990). In the most basic terms, the PSDA requires any health care provider accepting Medicare or Medicaid to inform the patient (1) of his or her right to accept or refuse treatment, (2) of his or her rights regarding advance directives under state law, and (3) of any hospital or provider policies regarding withholding or withdrawing life-sustaining equipment (Ulrich, 1999). Further, the Act requires the provider to ask the patient about any **advance directives**. As you can conclude from the second requirement, informing the patient about his or her rights under state law, there are some variations from state to state regarding the use of **powers of attorney** and **living wills**. As a medical assistant, it might become your responsibility to provide this notice to the patient and inquire about any advance directives he or she might have made. The durable power of attorney or health care **power of attorney** is an instruction from the patient to all who might need to know that the patient has empowered a representative to make health care decisions and the discontinuation of life support. In a broad sense, the power of attorney authorizes the person named by the patient to consent, refuse consent, or withdraw consent regarding any medical service or procedure (Kansas Bar Association, 2010). A living will is a document prepared by the patient as a statement of his or her medical wishes. It is distinguished from the power of attorney by the fact that a living will does not designate anyone else to make decisions but, rather, outlines what the patient wants or doesn't want regarding life-saving or life-sustaining measures. It is a document that speaks for the patient when he or she cannot speak for him- or herself (Alexander, 1991).

Medical Records

A medical record is a collection of information about a patient. There are a number of reasons careful maintenance of this record is critically important. The first is medical: If the patient needs additional treatment or is referred to another provider, that caregiver can make note of prior conditions and events that might be relevant in the current circumstance. In addition, licensing authorities require copious records to be kept. Finally, the record becomes a document by which the standard of care is substantiated in the event of future litigation. It is, in short, a summary of the patient's maladies and what was done to treat them. An adequate record includes:

1. Documentation of each patient encounter, including the reason for it, relevant history, exam findings, and prior test results; it should also include a clinical impression or diagnosis, a plan for care, and the date and legible identity of the provider.
2. Past and present diagnoses.
3. Rationale for results of diagnostic and ancillary services.
4. Patient's progress, including response to treatment or noncompliance.
5. Notation of risk factors.
6. Written plan for care, including prescriptions, referrals, consultations, and follow-up instructions (Texas Medical Liability Trust, 2010).

Hospitals own the records they make; so do providers. This gives those providers a **property right** to the record, and they can restrict its availability. Although ownership usually confers the right to do with the property whatever the owner wants, that is *not* the case with medical records. Although the provider or the hospital might own the paper on which the information is written and the file folder in which it is kept, there are a number of stakeholders in the record. Providers are ethically obligated to forward the record to another provider who assumes responsibility for care of the patient. A court can order the records to be produced in a wide variety of circumstances. The patient or the duly appointed patient's representative has a right to view the record. All these factors underscore the necessity for extraordinary care in maintaining the record.

Electronic Medical Records

From a legal perspective, these are the same as a written record; however, they present novel situations posing an increased threat to privacy. The primary advantage of using computer databases for medical records is the ease of transferring the data from one provider to the next. If a provider and a hospital have medical record systems that can communicate to one another, it is easy for the provider to access information on his or her patient that was gathered by the hospital, such as lab results and imaging data. The primary disadvantage is the vulnerability of these records to invasion of the patient's privacy. The federal government has provided substantial financial incentives for providers and hospitals to migrate records to an electronic format (Lewis, 2010). The use of electronic medical records facilitates comprehensive, safe care for the patient, and their use will expand dramatically in the years ahead (Bates, 2003).

The electronic medical record facilitates access to information of importance to the providers. For example, a patient sees his or her primary care provider and reports his or her medications; as a follow-up, the provider orders a standard lab set. The next week, the patient goes to a cardiologist as a routine follow-up to his coronary history. When he sees her, she has immediate access to the patient's medications so she can avoid overdosing or prescribing a contraindicated drug. Likewise, she won't need to order additional lab tests because she has the results on the computer screen in her exam room. In this way, the patient's care is better coordinated and safer and reduces costs.

Changing Medical Records

Don't! A medical record should not be altered or amended in any way unless it is necessary to make the record more accurate or more complete. If a change is appropriate, the time and date of the change should be noted along with language specifically pointing out the change (Texas Medical Liability Trust, 2010).

Confidentiality and Release of the Medical Record

The provider and the hospital have the right to restrict the record to their premises. The patient has a right to expect the provider to keep all aspects of the record confidential. This right extends back to Hippocrates and is now enshrined in law. The Supreme Court said that "the entire health care system is built upon the willingness of individuals to share the most intimate details of their lives with the health care providers. . . . [And] the need for privacy has long been recognized as *critical* to the delivery of needed medical care (*Citizens for Health v. Levitt*, 2006).

Not only is the ethical obligation to safeguard the record reinforced by court decisions, but there is statutory law on the subject: the **Heath Insurance Portability and Accountability Act**, also known as **HIPAA**. In 1996, Congress passed HIPAA to, among other things, ensure that an employee leaving his or her job could take at least some insurance coverage with him or her. At the same time, Congress addressed the growing concern about the erosion of patient privacy (Freudenheim, 1991). The notion of patient privacy is where law meets ethics, and more of the latter is discussed in the next chapter.

There are two reasons the question of confidentiality of records is so important: First, sometimes there is a legitimate public interest in having records released, perhaps even over the patient's objection. The second purpose is to protect the individual's interest in making an informed, independent decision regarding his or her care and not being forced to accept a predetermined course of action. Although the burdens imposed on providers to comply with HIPAA can seem burdensome, the act does provide some guidance on these questions.

> The HIPAA Privacy Rule provides federal protections for personal health information held by covered entities and gives patients an array of rights with respect to that information. At the same time, the Privacy Rule is balanced so that it permits the disclosure of personal health information needed for patient care and other important purposes. (Department of Health and Human Services, 2010)

For the medical assistant, HIPAA means understanding that the material in the medical record is part of a **privileged communication** between the provider and the patient. In a phrase, do not discuss any patient or his or her condition outside the office.

EXAMPLE

A woman who was employed by a caterer had a condition that raised false positives on the test for syphilis. The woman was *not* afflicted. A nurse in the office was at a social affair that happened to be catered by the patient's employer. In casual conversation, the nurse mentioned to the hostess that the patient was being treated for syphilis. The information affected the patient's employment and the employer's business. The court found there was good cause for slander against the nurse (*Schlesser v. Keck*, 1954; Flight, 2011).

This is clearly an example of an unauthorized disclosure of protected health information. As a medical assistant, you should avoid at all times this type of discussion with friends, family, and acquaintances.

Mandatory Release of the Record

Occasionally, the medical office or hospital can be compelled to provide an individual's medical record. In the case of all infectious diseases, such as measles and sexually transmitted diseases (STDs) such as herpes, HIV, syphilis, and so on, a provider is *required* to report the findings to the local health department. This is a case when the public interest in preventing the spread of this type of disease to serve the public's safety, outweighs the privacy interest of the patient. As a follow-up to receiving notice of an STD, the department will attempt to locate the sexual partners of the patient to inform them so they may seek treatment. The department might also attempt to locate the sexual partners of *those* individuals to prevent the further spread of disease. The factor that weighs most heavily here is that a person could be infected without his or her knowledge or consent; therefore, the government steps in to identify sources of this disease and attempts to limit further infection. Likewise, in the case of infectious diseases such as measles, providers are required to report that diagnosis to the local health department. The same reasoning applies: The public's interest in preventing the spread of a disease to which people have been exposed without their prior knowledge outweighs the patient interest in confidentiality. This type of reporting to a local health agency is statutory law in all states.

Providers and hospitals can also be required to report certain crimes that fall into the same category. A rape victim loses the privacy of her status when she goes to the hospital or sees a doctor and shares her condition. Rape is a reportable offense, along with domestic abuse, elder abuse, and child abuse. If the health care professional knows of, or reasonably suspects, the existence of one of these conditions, he or she is required to report it to law enforcement authorities.

In addition to these mandated reporting requirements, a health care provider can be ordered by a court to release medical records when the health status of either defendant or plaintiff is at issue in the trial. Typically, this is a malpractice case in which legal counsel for the defense seeks all of the plaintiff's medical records. Part of the defense might be a preexisting condition that would be found on examination of the medical record. Likewise, in motor vehicle accidents, one who was injured might seek the medical record of the driver to demonstrate that his or her vision was below minimum standards or that he or she had some other medical impairment that made him or her unfit to drive. Or the driver-defendant in such a case might want the plaintiff's medical record to demonstrate a preexisting condition. For example, if a plaintiff brought suit alleging whiplash, the relative status of the plaintiff's neck becomes an issue. If the medical record revealed that the patient had previously been treated for a bulging spinal disk in the neck area, the defense would have a good argument that the car accident did not cause the injury alleged by the plaintiff.

Thus, the contract between the doctor and the patient places important responsibilities on both sides. After there is a contract between the two, assuming capacity and competency of the patient to provide informed consent to the provider's care, a substantial burden rests on the provider's office to care for the patient and protect the privilege of communication between the parties and the privacy of the record that tracks the medical history of the patient. The privilege of the communication between doctor and patient is nearly inviolate; the medical community is not accorded quite the same degree of protection from discovery. Although access to it is very limited, there are instances when the patient's interest in privacy gives way to the public's interest in ensuring the safety of the citizens at large.

GOVERNMENTAL REGULATION OF THE PROVIDER OFFICE

It is common to hear people refer to the "alphabet soup" of governmental agencies. Each agency has a distinctive and different mission. Government regulation is part—a substantial part—of the landscape when it comes to the practice of medicine. The next several pages review briefly which agencies regulate matters in health care and examine specific statutes that affect the medical office.

Occupational Safety and Health Administration (OSHA)

The Occupational Safety and Health Administration (OSHA) is a product of the legislative act by the same name, the Occupational Safety and Health Act (U.S. Code, 2010b). The goal of both the legislation and the agency is to ensure that employers have safe work environments for employees, which do not have hazards such as extreme cold or heat, toxins, danger from mechanical devices, or noise that would damage a person's hearing. The law is administered by OSHA, which is an agency within the U.S. Department of Labor. The statute permits it to set health and safety standards by regulation.

The Act applies to hospitals and provider offices; indeed, it applies to "any person engaged in a business affecting commerce who has employees" not including governmental agencies (U.S. Code, 2010b). Under the terms of the law, employers are to maintain safe working conditions and use methods that are appropriate to protect workers. Employers also have a duty to be familiar and comply with the appropriate standards of safety applicable to them and to provide protective equipment for employees.

The primary interest regarding OSHA to medical office personnel is in the area of exposure to bloodborne pathogens. The health concern in this case includes the transmission of hepatitis B, hepatitis C, and HIV/AIDS, among others. OSHA has adopted a comprehensive plan to address the issue of needlesticks, the most common accident that can transmit these diseases (OSHA, 2010).

Clinical Laboratory Improvement Amendments of 1988

Historically, providers have done a clinical examination and an interview without additional testing to form a hypothesis regarding a diagnosis. And if additional lab tests were needed, they were sent out to a laboratory for analysis. In more recent times, however, most provider offices maintain a "CLIA lab." Provider office labs may do such things as fungal cultures, urine dipsticks, and wet mounts of vaginal secretions. Many do minor blood testing; specialists such as nephrologists and hematologists rely on their ability to examine blood or urine specimens. Today, a provider office lab is critically important, as central to the provider function as his or her stethoscope.

In 1988, Congress adopted legislation regulating all laboratories, including the relatively small ones found in provider practices (U.S. Code, 2010c). It requires a provider or a mid-level practitioner to obtain the sample, thus a medical assistant will never find himself or herself in this situation. Nonetheless, being generally aware of both the law and the CDC regulations adopted in enforcement of the law is helpful.

Because, in the operation of any laboratory, there may be exposure to infectious disease, and to ensure that tests performed follow appropriate protocols, labs must be accredited. Obviously, care is required in the operation of a lab. Thus, certain procedures are mandated by regulation; qualifications for director of the lab are specified in regulation; and, of course, any lab seeking to be paid under Medicare or Medicaid must meet the specifications defined in the law and its accompanying regulations (Code of Federal Regulations, 2004).

Food and Drug Administration (FDA)

The Food and Drug Administration's mission has three parts: to protect the public's health by ensuring that safe pharmaceutical products and diagnostic devices make it to the market in a timely fashion, to ensure ongoing effectiveness and safety of those products by monitoring their use in the market, and to help the public get appropriate and accurate information that is based on scientific evidence (Helm, 2007). And although the direct regulatory reach into the provider's office is minimal, the extensive regulation of the pharmaceutical and medical device industries makes awareness of the FDA role important. Because the provider's office relies on prescription drugs to help patients, by regulating drug products, the FDA has significant influence on the decisions a clinician may make. And paramount, of course, is ensuring that the provider office has accurate information about the drugs it prescribes.

There are, however, several areas in which provider offices are directly touched by the FDA. The first, and perhaps most important, is the required reporting of adverse effects of prescription drugs. This is part of the FDA's post-marketing analysis referred to as a Phase 4 clinical trial. Recall that the second part of the FDA's mission is to assure the public of the safety and effectiveness of prescription drugs already on the market. To this end, the FDA requires all health care providers to report adverse events (Food and Drug Administration, 2010b).

Second, providers are to report adverse events resulting from the use of any medical device. Although this does not apply to all provider offices, it applies to hospitals, nursing homes, and ambulatory surgery centers and to any provider office where ambulatory surgery is being conducted. The initiative regarding the reporting of all adverse events arising from either drugs or devices is called MedWatch. The FDA recommends all professionals within user-facilities to be familiar with their organization's reporting process (Food and Drug Administration, 2010c).

From a practical perspective, it is important for the medical assistant to ensure that the prescription pad is stored in a safe place. It should not at any time be accessible to any unauthorized personnel such as patients or clerical staff in the office.

The Drug Enforcement Administration (DEA)

The Drug Enforcement Administration is critically important to the provider practice and others who have the responsibility of dealing with pharmaceuticals, particularly controlled substances. This agency has broad enforcement power over the distribution of narcotics and other drugs, both legal and illicit. Established by Executive Order of President Nixon in 1970, the DEA serves as a "single unified command to combat 'an all-out global war on the drug menace'" (Drug Enforcement Administration, 2010a). Simply put, it has authority over providers prescribing certain pain killers as well as authority to conduct search and seizure operations of international smugglers dealing in heroin.

Within DEA is the Office of Diversion Control. It is this part of the agency with which providers most often interact. Specifically, this is where a provider applies for the DEA registration that permits them to handle, dispense, and prescribe various controlled substances. (This registration also applies to pharmacies and hospitals.) Upon finding that the provider is licensed in the state where he or she is practicing and making an otherwise suitable application that includes specifying the schedule of drugs he or she wants authority to prescribe, the agency will issue a registration number. Registrations are valid for three years. If the provider relocates his or her office or changes his or her name, he or she must contact the DEA and apply for an amended registration (Drug Enforcement Administration, 2010b). Unit 17 discusses the DEA further.

FEDERAL LAWS AFFECTING THE PROVIDER OFFICE

Patient Protection and Affordable Care Act

In 2010, Congress passed and the President signed into law the most sweeping piece of health care legislation in decades, the Patient Protection and Affordable Care Act (PPACA), also known as health care reform. This legislation might have a dramatic impact on the delivery of health care services because it will change the way health care providers are paid. Emphasis will be on payment for performance and adherence to quality measures instead of fee for service. Likewise, there might be better reimbursements for the providers who use practice extenders for those patients whose illnesses are so minor that they really don't require the attention of a provider.

The other significant change resulting from this law will be a dramatic increase in the number of Americans who will have health insurance, and, after they have it, many will be more likely to seek care in a provider's office instead of in the hospital emergency room. Thus, patient volumes might increase substantially in providers' offices, especially for those who provide primary care.

Although the major parts of the legislation deal with health insurance and expanding coverage, there will no doubt be significant changes in the way medical services are delivered as a result. Medical assistants should remain aware of public policy issues like this one that could well affect how they do their job.

Health Insurance Portability and Accountability Act (HIPAA)

Before the enactment of the Patient Protection and Affordable Care Act, the most significant health care–related legislation in decades was unquestionably the Health Insurance

Portability and Accountability Act (HIPAA). Passed in 1996, this far-reaching legislation has had a profound effect on the practice of medicine in every provider setting.

Title I of the legislation ensures the continuation of health insurance coverage for workers and their families when they change or lose their jobs. Title II requires the creation of national health identification for providers, health insurance plans, and employers while at the same time establishing national standards for health care data exchange. This section was intended to simplify the administrative functions of health care to improve efficiency and encourage the use of electronic data interchange among providers, insurers, and employers. Because of the vastness of the effort and the relative ease and speed of transmitting data electronically, the privacy rights of patients became a critically important issue. In partial compliance with Title II, the U.S. Department of Health and Human Services has developed and issued the Privacy Rule. It is this aspect of HIPAA that is most important to medical assistants.

> A major goal of the Privacy Rule is to ensure that individuals' health information is properly protected while allowing the flow of health information needed to provide and promote high quality health care and to protect the public's health and well-being. The Rule strikes a balance that permits important uses of information while protecting the privacy of people who seek care and healing (DHHS, 2010).

Application of the Privacy Rule: What Are Covered Entities?

- *Health insurance plans:* The rule applies to almost every kind of health insurance plan. An exception is made for employer-sponsored plans that have fewer than 50 employees and for certain government programs such as food stamps.
- *Providers:* Any provider who uses electronic transmission of data as part of a standard transaction (such as submitting a claim to be paid) is covered by the rule.
- *Business associates:* Any person or organization performing work for a covered entity in which they might receive personal health information is also covered. This could be consultants who work on claims processing, billing, and utilization review. And when a business associate is involved, a written agreement must exist between the covered entity and the business associate in which the associate recognizes the application of HIPAA to his or her work (DHHS, 2010).

Application of the Privacy Rule: What Is Protected?

All protected health information (PHI) is protected from unauthorized disclosure. This means that any information related to (1) the patient's physical or mental health, past and present; (2) any information related to payment for services associated with any past or present physical or mental health condition; and (3) any information related to the treatment or care of that patient is protected. In addition, this protection specifically applies to any information that would identify the individual patient such as name, address, social security number, certain demographic information, and other material that might reasonably identify the patient receiving the care. All of this is considered personal health information, and the unauthorized disclosure of it is banned under the Privacy Rule.

The rule goes on to specify that a covered entity can disclose the information only to the patient, to an insurance plan for payment, and to the Department of Health and Human Services when it is conducting a review of utilization patterns. PHI can also be used internally for analysis of quality or health care operations. In addition, disclosure is authorized when required by a law or court order, to protect the public health (such as in reporting certain infectious diseases), to protect domestic abuse victims, for certain judicial and administrative proceedings, for certain law enforcement purposes, to aid funeral directors, and in some cases for research (DHHS, 2010).

The rule also specifies that any information that is disclosed or released must disclose only the minimum necessary to serve the intended purpose of the disclosure. Further, the covered entity must have policies in place limiting internal access to those who have good reason to have the information and must have policies spelling out the routine disclosure of information as part of a standard operating procedure such as billing an insurance carrier. A covered entity must also have a policy addressing the disclosure of its privacy policy to patients and must provide notice of this policy to the patient (DHHS, 2010).

To emphasize the importance of compliance, the Department of Health and Human Services has developed a range of fines that can be imposed for violations occurring after February 18, 2009. Each violation is punishable by fines ranging from $100 to $50,000 with an annual cap of $1.5 million. In certain cases, there will be no fine, but the enforcement of the regulation is intended to deter deliberate unauthorized disclosures as well as to minimize the mistaken, incidental disclosure. In extreme cases, criminal penalties are appropriate and will be prosecuted (DHHS, 2010).

EXAMPLE

Temptation is sometimes overwhelming. Our curiosity about others, celebrities in particular, can sometimes cloud our judgment. In 2008, the *Los Angeles Times* reported that as many as 25 staff members, including six providers, could be disciplined for unauthorized access and disclosure of records pertaining to Britney Spears while she was a patient at the UCLA Medical Center. As many as 13 employees were fired and six suspended, and another six providers would be otherwise disciplined. Although the electronic nature of medical records threatens patient privacy, the use of passwords to detect who accessed which records and when can determine accurately the identity of those who are not authorized (Ornstein, 2008).

The Good Samaritan Act

All states have adopted some form of a **Good Samaritan Act**. As the name implies, it speaks of who would act as the good Samaritan in providing assistance to one in need. The nature of these laws is to protect individuals who decide to provide help and serve those who are injured. The underlying policy is that the law wants to avoid punishing those who engage in helping others. This is a form of legal immunity; if the volunteer responding to a crisis makes an error in treatment, he or she will not be held liable for the mistake. Usually, two conditions apply: First, the aid must be provided at the scene of the emergency, and, second, the law will not apply if the volunteer is seeking a reward or fee. The following is a good example of a Good Samaritan Act from the State of Hawaii.

EXAMPLE

Any person who in good faith renders emergency care, without remuneration or expectation of remuneration, at the scene of an accident or emergency to the victim of the accident or emergency shall not be liable for any civil damages resulting from the person's acts or omission, except for such damages as may result from the person's gross negligence or wanton acts or omissions (Hawaii Revised Statutes, 2010).

There are a couple of important considerations before we leave this topic. First, this law applies to everyone. It is not solely for doctors. In other words, if you, the medical assistant, come upon a person at an accident scene and render aid, you will be held harmless for any mistakes you might make unless you show a wanton disregard of danger to the victim. If you continue past the accident, you have no duty. When you stop to provide assistance, however, you must remain until someone with comparable or better training arrives. So long as you, or the doctor, or the citizen on the street (a) have no prior clinical relationship with the victim, (b) stop and render aid that is reasonable, (c) and have no expectation of being paid for the service, the volunteer who steps up to provide help will be protected from any mistakes he or she might make.

Americans with Disabilities Act (ADA)

The Americans with Disabilities Act of 1990 is referred to as civil rights legislation designed to prohibit discrimination against individuals based on disability. "Disability" is defined as "a physical or mental impairment that substantially limits a major life activity" (42 U.S.C. sec. 12112, 1990). It applies to employment, public transportation, public entities, commercial facilities, public accommodations, and telecommunications. For example, hotels are required to make accommodations for guests who might be disabled; buses, trains and airplanes must make similar accommodations. This can mean having wider doorways, showers that are accessible without a bathtub, personal assistance in boarding and disembarking, ramps in commercial buildings for those who use a wheelchair, and so forth. Likewise, in the employment setting, the employer must be prepared to make similar accommodations to those qualified to do the job who might not, for example, be able to walk without assistance. Employment interviews must be focused on the job components and the applicant's ability to perform them. So, for example, although it would be inappropriate to consider one who uses a wheelchair as a baggage handler in an airport, the person who is a research assistant would not be required to lift heavy objects and, thus, could not be kept from the job because he or she uses a wheelchair.

Like all civil rights legislation, the ADA is not without controversy. Although many labor and civil rights groups banded together to advocate for its passage, business and religious groups opposed it as either too costly or an unwarranted intrusion of the federal government into charitable or state affairs.

As a medical assistant, you might come in contact with the ADA as part of the provider team that certifies a patient to be disabled. Like all matters in your work, you must take great care to ensure the accuracy of the documentation. This is an area in which the patient's right of privacy is limited by his or her claim to be disabled to have the protection of the act. Be aware that because the patient needs the certification, there can be some inclination to provide information that is otherwise confidential or privileged. Do not, for example, provide information over the phone to a prospective employer. When you receive a form from an employer requesting information related to the disability, make certain the patient has consented to the release of the information and that conclusions in any such form are appropriately documented in the patient's chart (EEOC, 2008).

Uniform Anatomical Gift Act

As part of its responsibilities, the National Conference of Commissioners on Uniform State Laws has developed the Uniform Anatomical Gift Act. This means that the versions of legislation governing organ donations are substantially the same from state to state. It is basically a template for public policy.

The UAGA governs organ donations for (1) organ transplantation and (2) the transfer of anatomical gifts of one's deceased body for use in the study of medicine. The UAGA was first written in 1968 and has been revised twice since. In 2007, 20 states had adopted the UAGA.

The act prohibits the trafficking of human organs and profiteering from donations for transplant or therapy. The UAGA prescribes the form by which organ donations can be made and provides that if there is no such document, a surviving spouse can make the gift. Likewise, the act lists other relatives, in a specific order, who can make the gift if there is no surviving spouse. Finally, the act limits the liability of health care providers who act in good faith on representation of a deceased patient's wishes.

CHAPTER SUMMARY

- In the broadest sense, law is a system of rules enforced through a collection of institutions that have the authority to do so.
- Congress makes federal law; these laws apply to everyone in country. In addition, state legislatures make state law that applies to everyone within that particular state. Finally, local government entities can pass resolutions or ordinances that govern conduct within those jurisdictions.
- Laws are also derived from the court system; these become common law, also known as case law or the law of precedent.
- Criminal law (1) is exclusively statutory and (2) deals with one who has performed an act prohibited by law or failed to perform an act required by law.
- Civil law is a collection of rules that govern the conduct and affairs of people and their rights, infractions of which are not crimes.
- The term *tort* comes from the Latin *tortum*, which means "wrong"; tort law is a branch of common law. Torts can be unintentional (accidental, such as negligence) or intentional (such as slander, libel, and medical malpractice).
- Four elements must be present for negligence to apply: (1) a *duty* of care owed by the defendant to the plaintiff, (2) a *breach* of that duty by the defendant, (3) harm (*injury*) suffered by the plaintiff, (4) and that harm a result of the defendant's breach of duty (*causation*).
- Six elements must be present for medical malpractice to apply: (1) a current *relationship* between the provider and the patient, (2) that *relationship created a duty* of the provider toward the patient, (3) the nature of that duty required a professional *standard of care*, (4) the provider *breached* the duty to the patient, (5) the patient had a resulting *injury*, and (6) the patient would not have sustained the injury but for the provider's breach of duty (*causation*).
- The relationship between doctor and patient is in the nature of a contract. From that point on, the provider has an affirmative duty to care for the patient to the professional standards associated with a doctor of similar training and experience (an expected standard of care).
- Contracts can be *express* (meaning the parties clearly expressed their respective intentions) or *implied* (meaning the parties agreed by nonverbal actions or conduct). Before a doctor can treat a patient, the patient must provide consent.
- Durable power of attorney authorizes the person named by the patient to consent, refuse consent, or withdraw consent regarding any medical service or procedure. A living will is a document prepared by the patient as a statement of his or her medical wishes but does not designate anyone else to make decisions.
- Some of the federal agencies that regulate matters in health care and affect the medical office include the Occupational Safety and Health Administration (OSHA), the Clinical Laboratory Improvement Amendments of 1988 (CLIA), the Food and Drug Administration (FDA), and the Drug Enforcement Administration (DEA).
- In addition, many laws govern medical offices, including the Patient Protection and Affordable Care Act (PPACA), the Health Insurance Portability and Accountability Act (HIPAA), the Good Samaritan Act, the Americans with Disabilities Act of 1990 (ADA), and the Uniform Anatomical Gift Act.
- Although medical assistants cannot be expected to know all the particulars of the law, they should be aware that many of the actions in a provider's office do have legal consequences and conduct themselves accordingly.

STUDY TOOLS

Workbook	Activities for Chapter 5
Premium Website StudyWARE™	Activities and Quizzes on the **StudyWARE™ Software** for Chapter 5
	Audio Library of medical terms
	Online access to the **Critical Thinking Challenge 2.0**
CourseMate	Activities and Quizzes for Chapter 5
WebTutor	Activities and Quizzes for Chapter 5

CHECK YOUR KNOWLEDGE

1. In the United States, law is predominantly derived from:
   a. legislative bodies.
   b. executive orders.
   c. voter referendums.
   d. international courts.
2. What is the Latin phrase that means "let the master answer"?
   a. *Respondeat superior*
   b. *Res ipsa loquitur*
   c. *Subpoena duces tucem*
   d. *Ex post facto*
3. Which of the following defines a contract?
   a. Offer, consent, acceptance
   b. Offer, acceptance, consideration
   c. Offer, consideration, consent
   d. Consent, consideration, acceptance
4. What is the Act that protects a provider from liability for any civil damages when he or she gives emergency care?
   a. Health Insurance Portability and Accountability Act
   b. Americans with Disabilities Act
   c. Good Samaritan Act
   d. Occupational Health and Safety Act
5. Which of the following is NOT considered personal health information protected from unauthorized disclosure under HIPAA?
   a. Information included in a study that cannot be used to identify the patient
   b. Information related to a patient's past mental health
   c. Information related to a patient's present physical health
   d. Information related to the treatment or care of a patient
6. It is the goal of which government agency to ensure that employers provide safe work environments for employees?
   a. DEA
   b. FDA
   c. OSHA
   d. ADA

WEB LINKS

U.S. Department of Health and Human Services, HIPAA Information: www.hhs.gov/ocr/privacy/

Americans with Disabilities Act: www.ada.gov/

Occupational Health and Safety Administration: www.osha.gov/

Drug Enforcement Administration: www.justice.gov/dea/index.htm

U.S. Food and Drug Administration: www.fda.gov/

Clinical Laboratory Improvement Amendments: www.cms.gov/clia/

REFERENCES

Alexander, G. "Time for a New Law on Health Care Advance Directives." *Hastings Center Law Journal*, 42, no. 3 (1991):755–778.

American Bar Association. (2010). *Division for Public Education: Law for Older Americans*, from American Bar Association: Defending Liberty,

Pursuing Justice: www.abanet.org/publiced/practical/patient_self_determination_act.html. (Retrieved December 28, 2010)

Americans with Disabilities Act. (1990). 42 U.S.C. sec. 12112. *U.S. Code*. Washington, DC: United States Congress.

Associated Press (b). Nebraska.TV: www.nebraska.tv/Global/story.asp?S=13470138. (Retrieved November 9, 2010)

Associated Press. ABC 6 Action News (WPVI, Philadelphia, PA). abclocal.go.com/wpvi/story?section=news/bizarre&id=7773146. (Retrieved November 9, 2010)

Bates, D. W., M. E. "A Proposal for Electronic Medical Records in U.S. Primary Care." *Journal of the American Medical Infomatics Association* (2003):1–10.

Blackstone, W. (1765). *Commentaries on the Laws of England*. London: Clarendon Press.

Bragdon v. Abbot, 524 U.S. 624 (U.S. Supreme Court 1988).

Bugliosi, V. (1997). *5 Reasons Why O.J. Simpson Got Away with Murder*. Seattle: Island Books.

Centers for Disease Control and Prevention. (2010). *Current CLIA Regulations*. wwwn.cdc.gov/clia/regs/toc.aspx. (Retrieved October 12, 2010)

Code of Federal Regulations, Part 493 Laboratory Requirements. (2004) Washington, DC: U.S. Government.

Citizens for Health v. Levitt, 549 U.S. 941 (U.S. Supreme Court 2006).

Cowdrey, M., and Drew, M. (1995). *Basic Law for the Allied Health Professions*. Sudbury, MA: Jones and Bartlett.

Crawford v. McDonald, 187 S.E. 2d 542 (Georgia Supreme Court 1972).

Cruzan v. Director, Missouri Dept. of Health, 497 U.S. 261 (U.S. Supreme Court 1990).

Department of Health and Human Services. (2010). *Health Information Privacy*. www.hhs.gov/ocr/privacy/hipaa/understanding/index.html. (Retrieved October 12, 2010)

Department of Health and Human Services. (2010). *Health Information Privacy*. www.hhs.gov/ocr/privacy/hipaa/understanding/summary/index.html. (Retrieved December 28, 2010)

Drug Enforcement Administration. (2010a). *DEA History*. www.justice.gov/dea/history.htm. (Retrieved October 18, 2010)

Drug Enforcement Administration. (2010b). *Office of Diversion Control*. www.deadiversion.usdoj.gov/drugreg/faq.htm#top. (Retrieved October 18, 2010)

Drug Enforcement Administration. (2010c). "Cases Against Doctors." Office of Diversion Control: www.deadiversion.usdoj.gov/crim_admin_actions/admin_2007.htm. (Retrieved October 18, 2010)

eMedExpert. (October 26, 2010). *Bupropin (Wellbutrin) Medical Facts*. www.emedexpert.com/facts/bupropion-facts.shtml. (Retrieved October 30, 2010)

FamilyDoctor.org. (September 2010). *Advance Directives and Do Not Resusicate Orders*. familydoctor.org/online/famdocen/home/pat-advocacy/endoflife/003.html. (Retrieved December 28, 2010)

Flight, M. (2011). *Law, Liability, and Ethics for Medical Office Professionals*. Clifton Park, NY: Delmar Cengage Learning.

Food and Drug Administration. (2010b). *FDA Basics*. www.fda.gov/AboutFDA/Transparency/Basics/default.htm. (Retrieved October 30, 2010)

Food and Drug Administration. (2010c). *MedWatch*. www.fda.gov/Safety/MedWatch/HowToReport/ucm085568.htm. (Retrieved October 18, 2010)

Food and Drug Administration. (2010d). *Radiation-Emitting Products*. www.fda.gov/Radiation-EmittingProducts/default.htm. (Retrieved October 18, 2010)

Food and Drug Administration. (March 2, 2005). *FDA Provides Updated Patient and Healthcare Provider Information Regarding Crestor*. www.fda.gov/NewsEvents/Newsroom/PressAnnouncements/2005/ucm108414.htm. (Retrieved October 18, 2010)

Freudenheim, M. (1991). "Guarding Medical Confidentiality." *New York Times*, January 1, p. 1.

Glidden v. Maglio, 722 N.E.2d 814 (Massachusetts Supreme Court 2000).

Griffin, A., and Kovner, J. (2010). "Jury Finds Steven Hayes Guilty." *Hartford Courant*, October 6, p. A-1.

Guisti, M. L. (November 2, 2010). "Woman Convicted of Felony Vehicular Manslaughter Involving DUI Crash." Orange County Criminal Lawyer Blog: www.orangecountycriminallawyerblog.com/2010/11/woman-convicted-of-felony-vehi.html. (Retrieved November 8, 2010)

Haidak v. Corso, D.C. App LEXIS 34 (District of Columbia 2004).

Hart, H. (1961). *The Concept of Law*. New York City: Oxford University Press.

Hawaii State Legislature. (2010). *Hawaii Revised Statutes Section 663-1.5*. www.capitol.hawaii.gov/site1/hrs/default.asp. (Retrieved October 18, 2010)

Helm, K. A. "Protecting the Public from Outside the Provider's Office: A Century of FDA Regulation from Drug Safety Labeling to Off-Label Promotion." *Fordham Intellectual Property, Media and Enterprise Law Journal*, 18 (2007):117–186.

Holtzclaw v. Ochsner Clinic, 831 So. Wnd 495 (Lousiana Court of Appeals 2002).

Johnfroe v. Children's Hospital, 537 So. 2d 383 (LA Court of Appeals 2008).

Kansas Bar Association. (2011). "Living Wills and the Durable Power of Attorney for Health Care." www.ksbar.org/public/public_resources/pamphlets/living_wills.shtml (Retrieved April 25, 2011)

Legal Information Institute, Cornell University Law School. United States Constitution (1791). topics.law.cornell.edu/constitution/billofrights. (Retrieved October 15, 2010)

Lewis, N. (March 11, 2010). "Feds Add $162 Million to EMR Funding." *InformationWeek Healthcare*: www.informationweek.com/news/healthcare/EMR/showArticle.jhtml?articleID=223900079. (Retrieved October 15, 2010)

Mack v. Soung, 95 Cal. Rptr. 2d 830 (CA Court of Appeals; 3rd District 2000).

Miller v. Greater Southeast Community Hospital, 508 A. 2d 927 (District of Columbia 1986).

Miller, R. D. (2006). *Problems in Health Care Law* (9th ed.). Sudbury, MA: Jones and Bartlett.

Mitchell v. Hadl, 816 S.W.2d 183 (Kentucky Supreme Court 1991).

Morrissey, J., Hoffman, A., and Thorpe, J. (1986). *Consent and Confidentiality in the Health Care of Children: A Legal Guide*. New York: Free Press, Macmillan.

Noble v. Sartori, 799 S.W. 2d 8 (Kentucky Supreme Court 1990).

O'Neill v. Montefiore Hospital, 202 N.Y.S. 2d 436 (New York Supreme Court 1960).

Ornstein, C. (March 15, 2008). "Prying in Britney Spears' Medical Records May Cost Employees' Jobs." *Los Angeles Times*: articles.latimes.com/2008/mar/ 15/local/me-britney15. (Retrieved December 28, 2010)

Occupational Health and Safety Administration. (2010). "Bloodborn Pathogens and Needlestick Prevention." www.osha.gov/SLTC/bloodbornepathogens/index.html/. (Retrieved October 12, 2010)

Patient Self-Determination Act. (1990). 42 U.S.C. 1395 cc (a). Washington, D.C.: U.S. Government.

Pope, J. (2009). "Man Pleads No Contest in Voluntary Manslaughter Case." *Las Vegas Sun*, August 2, p. 1-B.

Pozgar, G. (2007). *Legal Aspects of Health Care Administration* (10th ed.). San Francisco: Jones and Barlett.

Pozgar, G. D. (2007). *Legal Aspects of Health Care Administraton* (10th ed.). Sudbury, MA: Jones and Bartlett.

Redder v. Hanson, 338 F.2d. 244 (US Courtr of Appeals 1964).

Rochester v. Katalan, 320 A. 2d 704 (Delaware Supreme Court 1974).

Roe v. Wade, 410 U.S. 113 (U.S. Supreme Court 1973).

Schlesser v. Keck, 271 P. 2d 588 (California Supreme Court 1954).

Texas Medical Liability Trust. (2010). *Risk Managment: Guide for Provider Practices*. Austin, TX: Texas Medical Liability Trust.

Tierney v. University of Michigan Regents, 669 N.W. 2d 575 (Michigan Court of Appeals 2003).

TriCity Herald. (October 9, 2009). "Justices Reaffirm Pasco Man's Robbery Conviction." www.tri-cityherald.com/2009/10/09/748069_justices-reaffirm-pasco-mans-robbery.html. (Retrieved October 12, 2010)

The Sullivan Group. (2010). "Provider Law Review: Refusal of Care." www.thesullivangroup.com/risk_resources/refusal/refusal_2_refusal.asp. (Retrieved October 15, 2010)

Ulrich, L. P. (1999). *The Patient Self-Determination Act*. Washington, DC: Georgetown University Press.

United States Department of Labor: Bureau of Labor Statistics. (December 17, 2009). *Occupational Outlook Handbook*, 2010–2011 Edition. www.bls.gov/oco/ocos164.htm. (Retrieved October 12, 2010)

U.S. Code. (n.d.). Manslaughter, Title 18, Chapter 51, section 1112. *United States Code*. Washington, D.C.: U.S. Government.

U.S. Code. (1970). Title 29, chapter 15. Occupational Safety and Health Act. U.S. Congress.

U.S. Code. (2010b). Title 29, chapter 15. Occupational Health and Safety Act . *United States Code*. Washington, DC: United States Government.

U.S. Code. (2010c). Title 42, Chapter 6A, sec. 201. Clinical Laboratory Improvement Amendments. *United States Code*. Washington, DC: United States Goverment.

U.S. Equal Employment Opportunity Commission. (September 9, 2008). *Facts about Americans with Disabilities Act*. www.eeoc.gov/facts/fs-ada.html. (Retrieved December 28, 2010)

Whitaker, W. (1880). "The Law of Slander as Applicable to Providers." *The American Law Register*, 465–470.

Chapter

6 Ethical Issues

OBJECTIVES

In this chapter, you will learn the following:

KB KNOWLEDGE BASE

1. Spell and define, using the glossary at the back of the text, all the Words to Know in this chapter.
2. Discuss the concepts of autonomy, beneficence, and distributive justice and how they apply to ethical issues in health care.
3. List and describe at least six ethical issues in health care.
4. Differentiate between legal, ethical, and moral issues affecting health care.
5. Compare personal, professional, and organizational ethics.
6. Identify where to report illegal and unsafe activities and behaviors that affect the health, safety, and welfare of others.
7. Discuss the role of cultural, social, and ethnic diversity in ethical performance of medical assisting practice.
8. Identify the effect personal ethics can have on professional performance.

WORDS TO KNOW

autonomy
beneficence
distributive justice
ethics
extrinsic
intrinsic
morals
organizational ethics
professional ethics
values

WHAT IS ETHICS?

Ethics is one of those intangible elements of life we deal with on a daily basis. Being aware of what is and is not ethical is essential for a successful career as a medical assistant. An ethical dilemma becomes apparent when there does not appear to be any justice through the legal system. This is also the case when there is no clear-cut right or wrong on any matter. It might also be true when the right behavior leads to the wrong outcome.

ETHICAL ISSUES IN HEALTH CARE

In health care, the term *bioethics* is commonly used, emphasizing the principles of **autonomy**, **beneficence**, and **distributive justice** (Slee, Slee, and Schmidt, 2008). The term finds its origins in the implications of scientific research as well as in medical practice. Generally, when we discuss bioethics, we are discussing ethical issues with significant, often literally life-or-death, ramifications for the patient.

When we speak of autonomy for the patient, we are recognizing that the patient has a right to make determinations for him- or herself. In the context of health care, when we recognize the autonomy of the patient, we are recognizing that it is the patient who has the right to make decisions about his or her life, death, and health.

The concept of beneficence requires people to do what is in the best interests of others. Thus, there are times when the concept of beneficence is at odds with the concept of autonomy.

Finally, distributive justice is the principle by which we as a society (or the health care community) decide to allocate resources that are in scarce supply. Because health care costs continue to rise, not everyone will have the same access to care. Likewise, there can be physical or geographic constraints to a person's access to care. There are a variety of approaches to this particularly complex issue, including:

- *An egalitarian approach:* Everyone gets equal share.
- *An earned approach:* Those who deserve get more.
- *A libertarian approach:* Each gets what he or she can legitimately get.
- *A social justice approach:* Allocation should be made to maximize the number of people helped.

EXAMPLE

The issue of distributive justice is especially timely today. In the health care market, in which people cannot afford a flu vaccination, should one be made available to them for free? What about a high-cost MRI study to evaluate a potential back injury? Should the cost make a difference in the outcome of the decision?

These are, of course, questions that have no definitive right (or wrong) answer. Regardless of which approach you believe is correct, someone else will believe his or her approach is just as right as yours. Table 6–1 presents descriptions of ethical issues relating to health care, some of which you will read in the following examples.

Ethical Issue: Abortion

Consider the issue of abortion from these three perspectives—autonomy, beneficence, and distributive justice. Why? One who perceives the issue as one of patient *autonomy* is likely to believe that the woman has a right to self-determination over what happens to her body. In this line of thought, the patient is the mother and she has a right to determine the state of her own health and what happens to her body. However, those who see this as an issue of *beneficence* might take the position that, because the fetus cannot speak for itself, those of us who can should act in the best interests of the fetus—that is, to provide it an opportunity to live. Much of this line of reasoning depends on one's values and faith with regard to the beginning of life. If one believes life begins at the moment of conception, the person acting with beneficence would take steps to protect the life of the unborn. Finally, in the third perspective, *distributive justice*, one would believe that if this procedure is legally available, it should be available to all. In this case, this person would advocate that Medicaid should fund abortions so they are available to the poor as well as to the insured and those able to pay.

At times, as we all know, these perspectives can boil over into the political and legal arenas. In *Roe v. Wade*, the Supreme Court attempted to fashion an uneasy balance between these principles. Using a trimester test, the Court basically said a woman's right to autonomy diminishes the further along in the pregnancy she is, whereas the fetus's right to life becomes more pronounced during the same time period. The court was not asked to, nor did it, address the issue from a distributive justice perspective.

Ethical Issue: Cryonics

Similarly, the issue of cryonics can be considered through all three principles. Simply put, one who sees the patient as autonomous might find that a person has a right to decide whether he or she wants to be frozen in time in the hope of coming back to life in the future; the person who is acting beneficently might find that such an act is not in the best interest of the patient, and one concerned with distributive justice might not have an objection to the procedure, as such, but would argue that it shouldn't be done until such time as it is available to everyone.

TABLE 6–1 Ethical Issues in Health Care

Field	Description of Ethical Issue
Abortion	Artificial termination of pregnancy
Artificial insemination	Introduction of semen into the oviduct or uterus by artificial means
Assisted suicide	Helping a terminally ill person to commit suicide
Contraception	Birth control by using various contraceptive measures
Cryonics	A process whereby the body of a seriously ill or a deceased individual is frozen to stop the decomposition of tissues
Eugenics	Improving genetic qualities by means of selective breeding
Euthanasia	Killing an individual (or animal) without making him or her suffer from pain
Gene therapy	The process of replacing defective genes with normal or genetically altered genes.
Genetically modified food	Consumption of food derived from genetically modified organisms
Human cloning	Creating a genetically identical copy of a human
Human enhancement	Overcoming the limitations of the body by artificial means
Life extension	Attempts either to slow down or reverse the processes of aging to maximize life span
Life support	Resorting to medical equipment to keep an individual alive
Organ transplantation	Unfair donation of any part of the body on the basis of race, class, and so on
Psychosurgery	Brain surgery carried out to ease the complications associated with mental or behavioral problems
Sex reassignment therapy	Medical procedures pertaining to sex reassignment of both transgendered and intersexual individuals
Suicide	The act of killing oneself
Surrogacy	A process whereby a woman agrees to carry and deliver a child for a contracted party
Vaccination	A dispute over the morality, ethics, effectiveness, and safety of the vaccination process
Xenotransplantation	Surgical procedure in which tissue or whole organ is transferred from one species to another.

Ethical Issue: DRGs and Capitated Payments

The matter of diagnostic-related groups (DRGs) and capitated payments raises special concerns. The DRG limits the amount a hospital can be paid based on the diagnosis, irrespective of any complications that might develop. Likewise, a capitated payment to a provider (a set number of dollars per patient per month) limits the payment to a provider to a set amount each month, despite how ill the patient might be. The questions here are, does the provider have an incentive to release the patient from the hospital too early to save the hospital money? Similarly, does the provider have an incentive to limit care to minimize patient care expense and maximize revenue from the capitated payments?

The answer to each is yes. That's the point of paying providers using DRGs and capitated rate—to hold down *unnecessary* costs. That's the operative word: *unnecessary*. Providers have, of course, an obligation to first do no harm and to render his or her best efforts to provide care. The provider's sense of professional ethics is what stands between adequate care and substandard care motivated by the payment structure. To this end, the provider should always consider the patient's best interests—act with beneficence—in light of all other circumstances.

CLINICAL PEARL

Critical Thinking Exercise: Review the list of ethical issues in Table 6–1. Think carefully about each one and consider it from all three of the central paradigms of ethics, autonomy, beneficence, and distributive justice. Can you see how you can view these issues from each of the three perspectives? How does that shape your view of each of these concerns?

Ethics and Diversity

We live in a multicultural world, and the world is becoming more diverse each day. As medical professionals, you have a responsibility to care for all people equally without regard to race, creed, or color. Although it is relatively easy to tell ourselves that we harbor no ill will toward those who do not look like us, it can be difficult to meet them on their own terms. What this means is that to be fully respectful of all patients, you must recognize—and respond appropriately to—ideas and elements from other ethnic and cultural backgrounds that might be different from your own.

Some elements with which you should be familiar, or at least be aware of, include manner of dress, communication style, consciousness of time, values and beliefs, and so on. In short, to render care with full respect toward each individual, the medical assistant must be sensitive to the fact that people of different cultures have different ways of seeing things. As much as we might be tempted to believe our view of the world is correct and others must be mistaken, perspectives regarding the ideas previously listed vary, and there is no right or wrong about them. Thus, patients wearing a burka or a dashiki should be accorded the same care as those wearing a dress or a polo shirt. Further, one should be aware that those who dress in such fashion may well have ideas and beliefs that clash with Western ideas of health care and those views must be treated with respect.

DISTINGUISHING LEGAL, ETHICAL, AND MORAL JUDGMENTS

There often are no clear-cut lines separating law, ethics, and **morals**—three types of categorizing principles. That which is legal might not be ethical in certain situations. What seems morally correct might not be legal. Sometimes, these are distinctions without differences; more often, they are joined seamlessly by contours that are not immediately recognizable. Whatever the case, a medical assistant must be able to distinguish among the three.

The discussion of legal issues in Chapter 5 should be helpful here. If you know of statutes or court decisions, those are matters of law and should be treated as such, which is to say the dictates should be followed.

EXAMPLE

We know that HIPAA requires particular measures to ensure the privacy rights of patients. However, we also know that, occasionally, confidential information should be disclosed to a law enforcement authority. Your job is to understand, in this example, that patient information remains private until you (or your employer) are ordered by a court of law to disclose that information as part of the evidence-gathering function in a legal case.

Ethics Check Questions

Ethical matters, however, are seldom so clear, and that should be one point of distinction. If there is no legal guidance, the question is not one of law but one of ethical conduct. Thus, when you see an ethical issue that causes you to ask, "What's the right thing to do?" look to three questions:

- What promotes the right of the patient's determinations about his or her own health?
- What is in the best health interests of the patient?
- Is performing (or not performing) the act in question fair to others?

So what is the difference among legal, ethical, and moral issues? As noted in Chapter 5, legal issues are those that arise from societal norms that have been either found as part of common law or enacted into statute. These usually involve the allocation of rights and responsibilities between human beings. Moral issues stem from a belief system in which one makes judgments about right and wrong. Ethical issues, especially in the professional context, are those that arise from "a set of standards and rules promulgated by various professions and enforced against its members" (Slee, Slee, and Schmidt, 2008).

EXAMPLE

Consider this scenario: In a state where early termination of a pregnancy is *legal* because it has not been outlawed by the state legislature, a married woman successfully obtains an abortion from her OB/GYN provider. She has not told her husband for reasons known only to her. The medical assistant in the office believes not only that abortion is *morally* wrong, but that the marriage is an institution kept sacred only if husband and wife share everything between them. She is acquainted with both the husband and wife because they all go to the same church. Can the medical assistant inform the husband of the wife's actions?

In this example, the medical assistant may not inform the husband for two reasons: (1) the medical assistant has an *ethical* obligation to keep patient information confidential, and (2) sharing such information would also be a *legal* violation because it is covered by HIPAA.

EXAMPLE

Two medical assistants are employed in a primary care provider's office. The provider, like many doctors, routinely accepts sample drugs from pharmaceutical companies and gives them to patients, at no charge, to get them started right away on a prescription or to let them try the drug to see whether they get relief from their symptoms. There are usually plenty of samples in the cabinet. One medical assistant has found that she can take some of the samples with no one noticing. Indeed, she then sells the medicine to friends and neighbors regardless of the appropriateness of the medication. One evening, you, one of the medical assistants, see her from down the hall. She is clearly taking drugs and putting them in a purse the size of a beach bag. Office protocol does not allow for this procedure. You are unaware of any authority she might have received from someone else in the office to remove the drugs. She might have permission because the doctor routinely supports the community's free clinic. What do you do?

In this example, it is entirely possible that the medical assistant has permission to remove the drugs and is doing so at the request of the provider. It is equally possible, however, that the medical assistant is committing a crime. This is a *legal* wrong and, for many people, also *morally* incorrect. Because you don't know whether this is a crime in progress, you have no obligation to call the police. On the other hand, because this action clearly violates office policy, some kind of intervention is appropriate. Your *ethical* obligation is to report what you saw to your supervisor as soon as possible because, at the very least, this action is unsafe and could be illegal.

What to Report, to Whom, and When

In this example, you could not conclude a crime was in progress, given the office history of supporting the free clinic. So responding ethically by raising the matter with the superior was appropriate. However, by changing the facts slightly—perhaps the provider in the office did *not* support the free clinic, it was after hours, and the behavior of the person removing the drugs was fidgety and nervous—you could reasonably conclude a crime was being committed and, thus, should notify the police immediately.

Although not everything can be quite as clear as witnessing a crime in progress, there are some rules and guidelines:

- *Criminal conduct*: On those rare occasions when you might witness a crime in progress, it is appropriate to notify the local police.
- *Patient information:* You will never go wrong by NOT discussing this sort of information with anyone other than the patient or the attending provider. The only exception to this would be when served with a court order directing you to comply. (It would most likely be the provider who would be so served; however, this could happen to you.)
- *Provider misconduct:* This one is a bit more complicated, assuming you work for the provider in question. If, for example, you are aware that a provider in the office where you work is showing up for work under the influence of alcohol, you do have an ethical obligation to act on that information. After all, the well-being of the patient is your *first* concern. The question is where you turn to act? In most cases, there will be a practice administrator or office manager or even another provider in the office. Your ethical obligation is to act in accordance with the best interests of the patient. Following this path relieves you of whatever duty you might think you owe in terms of telling a patient directly, which should NOT be done. You also have an obligation to your employer and, if you can address the situation from within, follow that course.
- *Office staff misconduct:* Consider the medical assistant who is aware that a nurse is disclosing information about a celebrity patient to a blogger. Again, putting the patient's interest at the forefront makes the answer a bit easier. This person's activity needs to be disclosed to the practice administrator or office manager.

PROFESSIONAL ETHICS

Codes of ethics prescribe behavior for professionals, **professional ethics**, in many industries, associations, and fields. The American Medical Association (AMA) has a comprehensive *Code of Medical Ethics* that speaks to a wide range of matters arising in the professional conduct of a doctor (American Medical Association, 2011). The AMA Code is comprehensive, addressing the provider's conduct in interprofessional relations, hospital relations, confidentiality, fees, records, and professional rights, among others. In addition, the AMA publishes opinions arising out of controversies in each of the 10 categories of the code. You can find the AMA's Code of Medical Ethics on the AMA Website, www.ama-assn.org.

As a medical assistant, you, too, are subject to a code of professional conduct when joining organizations such as the American Association of Medical Assistants (AAMA) or the American Medical Technologists (AMT). Figure 6–1 shows the AAMA's Code of Ethics; Figure 6–2 presents the AMT's Standards of Practice. The AAMA also has a creed (Figure 6–3), a brief set of fundamental

CODE OF ETHICS
of the American Association of Medical Assistants

The Code of Ethics of AAMA shall set forth principles of ethical and moral conduct as they relate to the medical profession and the particular practice of medical assisting.

Members of AAMA dedicated to the conscientious pursuit of their profession, and thus desiring to merit the high regard of the entire medical profession and the respect of the general public which they do serve, do pledge themselves to strive always to:

A. render service with full respect for the dignity of humanity;
B. respect confidential information obtained through employment unless legally authorized or required by responsible performance of duty to divulge such information;
C. uphold the honor and high principles of the profession and accept its disciplines;
D. seek to continually improve the knowledge and skills of medical assistants for the benefit of patients and professional colleagues;
E. participate in additional service activities aimed toward improving the health and well-being of the community.

Figure 6–1: AAMA Code of Ethics. *Courtesy of the American Association of Medical Assistants, Inc. Revised October 1996.*

beliefs, that provides guiding principles by which to practice medical assisting.

As you can see, the various codes of ethics and standards of practice set forth a general standard of behavior. They do not, and cannot be expected to, provide guidance for every specific question that can arise. Thus, the medical assistant must use his or her best judgment regarding the application of ethical considerations to any given situation.

EXAMPLE

As a medical assistant, you are not legally bound to obtain continuing education to maintain a license, for example. However, the AMT's Standards of Practice requires members to "strive to increase technical knowledge"; similarly, the AAMA's Code of Ethics requires members to "seek to continually improve knowledge and skills."

ORGANIZATIONAL ETHICS

Organizational ethics represent the **values** by which the organization conducts its business. Organizations frequently include a values statement as part of their mission and vision statements.

AMT STANDARDS OF PRACTICE

AMT seeks to encourage, establish, and maintain the highest standards, traditions and principles of the practices which constitute the profession of the Registry. Members of the AMT Registry must recognize their responsibilities, not only to their patients, but also to society, to other health care professionals, and to themselves. The following standards of practice are principles adopted by the AMT Board of Directors, which define the essence of honorable and ethical behavior for a health care professional:

1. While engaged in the Arts and Sciences, which constitute the practice of their profession, AMT professionals shall be dedicated to the provision of competent service.
2. The AMT professional shall place the welfare of the patient above all else.
3. The AMT professional understands the importance of thoroughness in the performance of duty, compassion with patients, and the importance of the tasks, which may be performed.
4. The AMT professional shall always seek to respect the rights of patients and of health care providers, and shall safeguard patient confidences.
5. The AMT professional will strive to increase his/her technical knowledge, shall continue to study, and apply scientific advanced in his/her specialty.
6. The AMT professional shall respect the law and will pledge to avoid dishonest, unethical or illegal practices.
7. The AMT professional understands that he/she is not to make or offer a diagnosis or interpretation unless he/she is a duly licensed physician/dentist or unless asked by the attending physician/dentist.
8. The AMT professional shall protect and value the judgment of the attending physician or dentist, providing this does not conflict with the behavior necessary to carry out Standard Number 2 above.
9. The AMT professional recognizes that any personal wrongdoing is his/her responsibility. It is also the professional health care provider's obligation to report to the proper authorities any knowledge of professional abuse.
10. The AMT professional pledges personal honor and integrity to cooperate in the advancement and expansion, by every lawful means, of American Medical Technologists.

Figure 6–2: AMT Standards of Practice. *Courtesy of the American Medical Technologists.*

MEDICAL ASSISTANT'S CREED

The creed of the American Association of Medical Assistants reads as follows:

I believe in the principles and purposes of the profession of medical assisting.
I endeavor to be more effective.
I aspire to render greater service.
I protect the confidence entrusted to me.
I am dedicated to the care and well-being of all people.
I am loyal to my employer.
I am true to the ethics of my profession.
I am strengthened by compassion, courage, and faith.

Figure 6–3: Medical Assistant's Creed. *Courtesy of the American Association of Medical Assistants, Inc. Revised October 1996.*

EXAMPLE

Go online and read the mission, vision, and values statements of two outstanding health care organizations:

- Cleveland Clinic: http://my.clevelandclinic.org/about/overview/mission_history.aspx
- Geisinger Health System: www.geisinger.org/about/mission.html

You might note some significant similarities even though the statements are worded very differently. Both are committed to excellence, compassion, teamwork or collaboration, and integrity, among many other similarities. These are significant statements, not merely a collection of nice-sounding words on paper. These values statements reflect organizational cultures that value their employees as well as their patients. These are examples of organizations that will go above and beyond for both patients and employees.

Ethical organizations support and empower their employees. Employees are encouraged to learn more and develop skills and knowledge to improve the patients' experiences. And employees are rewarded accordingly by both **intrinsic** and **extrinsic** means. Employees are encouraged to adhere to high ethical standards. What this means, in part, is that when an employee spots unethical behavior, he or she should call the Compliance Hotline or some similar reporting mechanism. The employee should be proud of the fact that he or she is part of the better angels of the organization. That is an intrinsic reward, pride in knowing one is upholding the high standards of the organization. Likewise, the employee who is given an end-of-year bonus as part of a unit that had the highest patient satisfaction scores is receiving an extrinsic reward.

There is an overall framework for an organization to facilitate ethical behavior. Although leadership is an important element that will be discussed in following sections, generally, four characteristics in the *organization* (not in the *leader)* encourage ethical behavior:

1. A written code of standards
2. Training for officers, managers and employees in the subject of ethics
3. Availability of advice for employees confronting ethical issues
4. A system (or systems) for confidential reporting (McDaniel, 2004)

The chief mechanism for development of an ethical culture within an organization, however, rests with the organization's leadership. Values statements, training, and reporting mechanisms are all hollow without the active engagement and support of the organization's leaders. This is why we say leaders must "walk the talk." In several studies undertaken during a 20-year period, employees consistently ranked honesty as the single most admired characteristic in a leader by, margins of 80 percent and higher (Kouzes and Posner, 2003). In a nutshell, good leaders are honest and try to create an improved and more ethical organization. This element is critical because it provides a set of standards for improving individual and, thus, organizational behavior.

PERSONAL ETHICS AND PROFESSIONAL PERFORMANCE

What does all this mean to you, the medical assistant? These ethical considerations are intended to enhance your professional performance. If you are inclined to be very social, you will need to be very aware of this tendency when dealing with the private health information *of a patient.* Or if you believe that after you have completed this course of study and pass your certification exam that you will never again crack a book or attend an educational session, perhaps this line of work is not for you.

Whatever your personal perspective might be regarding ethical matters, you must adapt your personal views to be in complete alignment with the ethical standards of your profession and the organization in which you are employed.

CHAPTER SUMMARY

- An ethical dilemma becomes apparent when there is no clear-cut right or wrong answer, when right behavior leads to a wrong outcome, or when there does not appear to be any justice through the legal system. Moral issues stem from a belief system in which one makes judgments about right and wrong.
- The concepts of autonomy, beneficence, and distributive justice can be helpful in viewing ethical issues in health care. The concept of autonomy means that the patient has a right to make determinations for him- or herself. The concept of beneficence requires people to do what is in the best interests of others. Distributive justice is the principle by which we as a society (or the health care community) decide to allocate resources that are in scarce supply.
- There are many ethical issues in health care; some of the issues are discussed in Table 6–1 and include abortion, artificial insemination, euthanasia, life support, organ transplantation, surrogacy, and vaccination.
- As a medical professional, you have a responsibility to care for all people equally, without regard to race, creed, or color. To render care with full respect toward each individual, you must be sensitive to the fact that people of different cultures have different ways of seeing things.
- There often are no clear-cut lines separating law, ethics, and morals. What is legal might not be ethical in certain situations. What seems morally correct might not be legal. The medical assistant must use his or her best judgment regarding the application of ethical considerations to any given situation.
- Whatever your personal perspective might be with regard to ethical matters, you must adapt your personal views to be in complete alignment with the ethical standards of your profession and the organization in which you are employed.
- Professional organizations often include various codes of ethics and standards of practice that speak to member conduct and behavior. Providers are expected to uphold the AMA's Code of Medical Ethics. As a medical assistant, you will be subject to a code of professional conduct when joining organizations such as the AAMA or the AMT.
- Organizational ethics represent the values by which the organization conducts its business.

STUDY TOOLS

Workbook	Activities for Chapter 6
Premium Website	
StudyWARE	Activities and Quizzes on the **StudyWARE™ Software** for Chapter 6
	Complete the following **Competency Challenge 2.0** activity: • Thursday, 1 PM: Respond to Legal and Ethical Issues
	Audio Library of medical terms
	Online access to the **Critical Thinking Challenge 2.0**
learninglab	Module 3: Legal and Ethical Issues
CourseMate	Activities and Quizzes for Chapter 6
WebTutor	Activities and Quizzes for Chapter 6

Chapter 7

Verbal and Nonverbal Communications

OBJECTIVES

In this chapter, you will learn the following:

KB KNOWLEDGE BASE

1. Spell and define, using the glossary at the back of the text, all the Words to Know in this chapter.
2. Recognize the elements of oral communication, using a sender–receiver process.
3. Identify the components of the standard communication model.
4. Identify styles of verbal communication.
5. Recognize communication barriers and identify techniques for overcoming them.
6. Give examples of nonverbal communication.
7. Explain *perception* and state its importance in communication.
8. Describe Maslow's Hierarchy of Needs and Dr. Kübler-Ross's Stages of Grief.
9. List commonly used behavioral defense mechanisms and give an example of each.
10. Describe and list coping skills for dealing with stress.
11. Identify the role of self boundaries in the health care environment.

S SKILLS

1. Respond to nonverbal communication.

B BEHAVIORS

1. Be attentive and apply active listening skills.
2. Demonstrate respect for individual diversity.
3. Demonstrate empathy in communicating with patients.
4. Use appropriate body language and other nonverbal skills in communicating with patients and their families.
5. Demonstrate awareness of territorial boundaries of the person with whom communicating.

WORDS TO KNOW

active listening
articulate
communication
compensation
conceptualize
contradict
convey
denial
displacement
distort
empirically
incongruous
intellectualization
interpret
intuition
malinger
perception
projection
rationalization
reference points
regression
repression
stress
sublimation
suppression

THE COMMUNICATION PROCESS

According to Webster's New Dictionary, **communication** can be defined as "the exchange of thoughts, messages, or information, as by speech, signals, writing, or behavior." To become effective in the art of communication, it can help to **conceptualize** the communication process, as shown in Figure 7–1. The message originates with the sender. The encoded message takes form based upon the sender's **reference** points. The message is picked up by the intended receiver, who immediately begins to decode it based on reference points. In responding (or providing feedback), the whole process is reversed: the original receiver becomes the sender, and the original sender becomes the receiver. In receiving this feedback, the original sender (now the receiver) can assess and evaluate how well the original message was received and **interpreted** and make any necessary adjustments or clarification.

The communication process is further clarified by the use of the standard communication model, which has six components: the sender, an encoder, a medium, a decoder, a receiver, and a message. To understand communication, think of communicating with another person by using the Internet, as illustrated in Figure 7–2 and explained in Table 7–1.

When communicating verbally, the spoken word must be delivered in an **articulate**, clear manner if the intended message is to be received. Correct pronunciation and proper grammar help convey meaning. You must also be aware of the rate of the spoken word—that is, how fast you are speaking. Patients need to be spoken to in a pleasant and unrushed manner so that the information has a chance to register, and questions can be asked. Eye contact is an important tool in body language and conveying your message (Figure 7–3). However, you must be aware of cultural sensitivities regarding eye contact and personal touch.

Communication Styles

To be an effective communicator, you must be able to identify and adapt to the communication styles of others. You must watch and listen carefully to your patient and

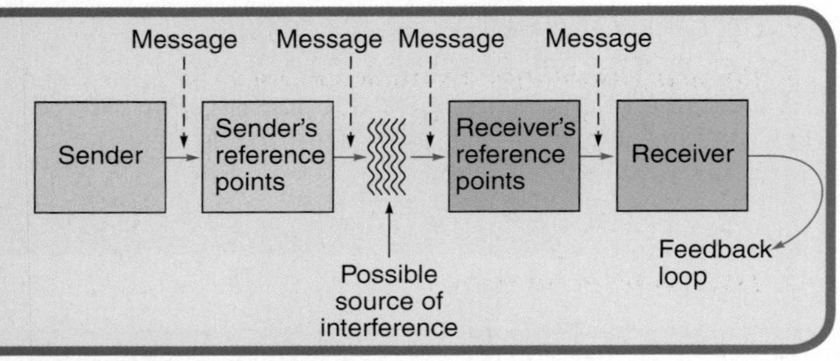

Figure 7–1: The communication process. *Delmar/Cengage Learning.*

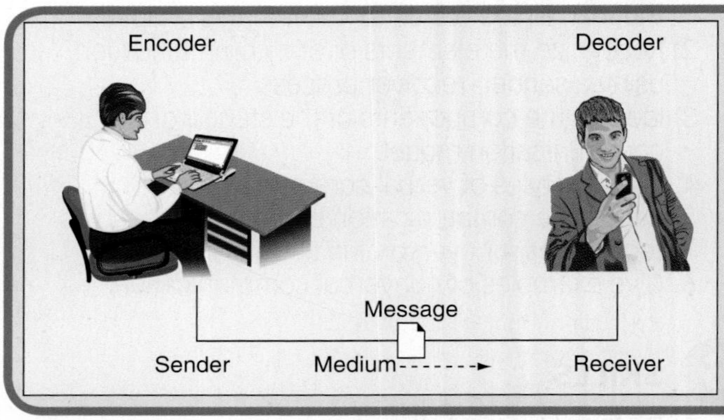

Figure 7–2: The standard communication model. *Delmar/Cengage Learning.*

TABLE 7–1 The Components of the Standard Communication Model and Their Definitions

Sender	The sender is what or who is trying to send a message to the receiver.
Encoder	In the general case, messages cannot be directly inserted onto the communications medium. An example is words spoken on the telephone, actually converted into electrical impulses, which then can be transmitted by wires.
Message	Using this mode, we have an encoded message that is transmitted by the medium.
Medium	The medium is the method that transmits or sends the message. The medium can be the phone system, the Internet, and many other electronic systems using wires. Even television and radio can use electromagnetic radiation as well as other nontraditional mediums, such as bongo drums.
Decoder	The decoder then takes the encoded message and converts it to a form the receiver understands, such as by a phone system with voice or Internet (electronic) message. A human cannot understand electronic impulses; therefore, the decoding provides the form for the user to understand in actual words.
Receiver	The receiver is the intended target (or user) of the message.

Adapted from: Jeremy Bowers (2003), *The Ethics of Modern Communication*. http://www.jerf.org/writings/communicationEthics/node1.html. Retrieved 11/16/2010.

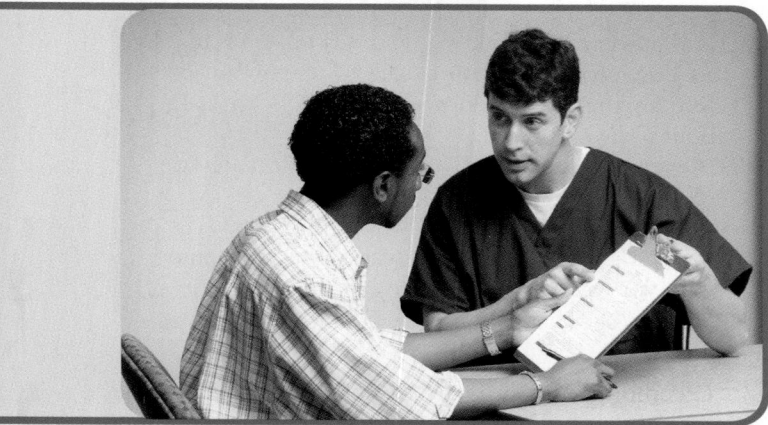

Figure 7–3: Make eye contact with patients when communicating verbal messages. *Delmar/Cengage Learning.*

identify his or her style and then carefully adjust your communication to be most effective.

People process and communicate information in three basic ways:

1. *Visual.* Visual people need to see pictures or see it in writing. Visual learners make up about 65 percent of the population and relate most effectively to written information, notes, diagrams, and pictures. A visual learner will most likely take notes, even if written information is presented.
2. *Auditory.* Auditory people learn by hearing. An auditory learner tends to listen to a lecture and then take notes afterward or rely on printed notes; these learners make up about 30 percent of the population.
3. *Kinesthetic.* Kinesthetic people think in terms of sensations or feeling, often move their hands when talking, and respond physically as well as verbally. Kinesthetic learners learn effectively through touch and movement and space and learn skills by imitation and practice; these learners make up only 5 percent of the population.

If you first identity the other person's communication style and then make adjustments to your communication style based on it, you are much more likely to receive a positive response. When you recognize your patient's learning style, examples of adjustments include:

- *Visual:* Provide written material and be sure there is opportunity for the patient to make notes.
- *Auditory:* Provide clear instructions and information and provide an opportunity for the patient to ask questions to reinforce information. Also, provide time for note-taking after the session.
- *Kinesthetic:* Make adjustments for space, therapeutic touch, and reflective (mirror) feedback.

Communication Barriers

The whole communication process seems simple enough, and generally it works well. However, many things can happen to affect the quality of the message or even **distort** it. You must be aware of these potential problems.

Foremost is the issue of reference points. For example, the spoken message might include terminology familiar to you but unknown to the patient. From your studies, you would be familiar with the term *epistaxis*, but a patient has likely not taken a medical terminology course; thus, using *nosebleed* would be more appropriate when talking with a patient. If you used the term *epistaxis*, even though the patient can hear you say the word, your message might not be understood. Talking to patients on a level they can easily understand is a skill requiring quick judgment. You have to adapt to a vast number of personalities when **conveying** information.

There are other barriers to communication, and you must work through them to provide quality patient care. A communication barrier is defined as anything that gets in the way of interpreting a message correctly. Three common barriers include:

1. *Physical disabilities.* Examples include deafness, loss of sight, or other physical problems.
   - *Overcome this barrier by adjusting your volume of speech, using an interpreter, offering Braille or large-print materials, and so on.*
2. *Psychological attitudes and prejudice.* This refers to personal opinions formed, for example, about alternative lifestyle individuals or certain ethnic or religious groups.
   - *Overcome this barrier by avoiding touching or eye contact if a cultural or religious barrier; always have a family member with patient in exam room.*
3. *Cultural diversity.* Not all patients speak, read, write, or understand English.
   - *Overcome this barrier by using interpreter services for the patient and family member; have printed materials available in multiple languages.*

Patients with special needs require extra understanding. Often a family member, friend, or caregiver will accompany the patient, thereby helping with your task of transmitting necessary information for correct interpretation. It is important, however, for you to speak to all patients directly, to be an active listener, and to repeat information as necessary. Having the patient repeat back what you said can also help ensure correct decoding of information. Be sure to include the patient in his or her health care discussions and do not converse only with another person. Chapter 8 further discusses patient communications and cultural sensitivity.

There can be many sources of interference or distractions such as others talking and phones ringing as well as phone conversations, coworkers, and interruptions. Therefore, it is best to speak one on one with the patient in an area where there is not likely to be any distractions or interference.

Active Listening

Listening involves giving attention to persons trying to communicate with you and taking an active interest in what they are saying. **Active listening** is the participation in a conversation with another by means of repeating words and phrases or giving approving or disapproving nods. This signals to the message sender that you are hearing and following what is being said. This method of conversation is highly recommended between health care providers and patients in communicating needs because it requires both parties to interact. The listener must make an effort to pay attention and follow the speaker. Taking a patient into an exam room or to a quiet space is the most appropriate way to communicate important information.

It takes time to build skills and confidence in communicating. Always greet your patients by name, listen carefully, and master the art of the open-ended question. The following is an example of a conversation in which the medical assistant is using active listening skills while taking the patient's chief complaint:

EXAMPLE

Medical assistant: "Good morning Mrs. Owen. Can you tell me what problems you have been having?"

Mrs. Owen: "Well, I've been having a lot of indigestion lately, about a month or so, and I take antacids for it, but it isn't going away. It bothers me a lot in the evening."

Medical assistant: "I'm sorry to hear that Mrs. Owen. When you say that you've been having what you think might be indigestion for approximately a month, and it seems worse at night, and you take antacids for this problem, does it help?"

Mrs. Owen: "It seems to a little, but this indigestion never goes away completely."

Medical assistant: "Could you please tell me what other kinds of medication you are taking?"

Mrs. Owen: "I only take aspirin sometimes for arthritis pain."

Medical assistant: "How much and how often are you taking the aspirin?"

Mrs. Owen: "Come to think of it, I have been taking aspirin about three or four times a day for the past two months."

Medical assistant: "Thank you Mrs. Owen. I wrote all this down for the doctor to talk to you about. Is there anything else you need to see Doctor Lang about today?"

Mrs. Owen: "No, thanks. I just want my stomach to feel better."

Medical assistant: "The doctor will be with you shortly. Can I get you some water or a magazine while you wait?"

Common courtesy is an art and skill proven to be an asset in the medical field while communicating. In a professional setting, it is essential to be polite. *Please*, *thank you*, *excuse me*, and *May I help you?* should be words in frequent use. In this way, the entire health care staff will show respect for others and a sense of caring.

Perception

Perception in the context of communication may be considered as being aware of one's own feelings and the feelings of others. The feelings you have about other people's moods and the way they act are perceptual, unspoken communication between you. **Intuition** is another term for perception in this sense. Although they cannot be measured **empirically**, these feelings can be strong indeed. Therefore, they must be recognized and reckoned with.

Being perceptive is a skill acquired with experience and practice. Being attentive to the needs of others and your surroundings will improve your perception skills. Anticipating the needs of others (patients, providers, coworkers) is a part of perception that enhances your effectiveness.

intuition — gut feeling

NONVERBAL COMMUNICATION

How often have you heard the saying, "It's not always what you say but how you say it"? Nonverbal communication can be defined best as the procedure of communicating with a person or party without using any form of speech to grab the audience's attention or to exploit a message. This type of communication is not written or spoken, but it conveys a message just the same.

Nonverbal communication helps express a thought and can make your message more easily understood. However, it can also oppose or **contradict** a verbal message. In *The Power of Nonverbal Communication*, Henry H. Calero said, ". . . it is the congruent or **incongruent** silent messages that greatly influence the message a person receives" (p. 2). Thus, to be properly understood, it is critical for your nonverbal communication to match the message of your verbal communication.

EXAMPLE

Some examples of incongruent verbal and nonverbal communication:

- Viktor says, "No," while nodding his head yes.
- Sally says "I agree," while rolling her eyes.

When communicating with patients, your tone of voice should be happy and sincere, indicating a positive attitude. Always display positive body language, giving warm facial expressions, using appropriate gestures, and maintaining eye contact; these are all nonverbal communication skills and cues that help reinforce the words you are speaking. Nonverbal communication is displayed in a number of ways, described in detail in the following sections.

CLINICAL PEARL

Be ready to respond to some of these nonverbal messages and cues you might receive from patients:

- "I don't understand" or "I don't fully understand." This could be displayed by subtle changes in the expressive lines around the eyes and mouth and perhaps the entire head leaning slightly to one side.
- "What you are communicating is upsetting me." This can be indicated by the subtle way the shoulders have hunched up, a look in the eyes, and a rise in voice pitch.

MEDIA LINK

View the video on "Communicating with Patients" for this chapter on the Premium Website.

Body language is a complex communication process. It involves unconscious use of posture, gestures, and other forms of nonverbal communication. It is important to be aware of body language because a positive verbal message can be misinterpreted or contradicted by negative body language. For example, a patient might say, "I'm OK," while grimacing with pain, indicating a conflicting message.

Appearance

The image you project is of utmost importance—the one chance to make a first impression. Image includes your overall appearance, expression of confidence and skills, and empathy. Appropriate dress, uniform, or business-like attire should be worn. Your professional appearance sends a nonverbal message that you have authority, confidence, and knowledge.

Facial Expression

Part of perception is being aware of how others think you feel or see you. You create this impression partly by your facial expression. You wear your expression like a billboard, so you will want to convey relaxed and pleasant facial expressions. The most common example of a positive, happy facial expression is a smile (Figure 7–4). This nonverbal signal conveys a positive attitude. It is especially important to be pleasant and friendly to those seeking medical attention because worries concerning their condition are already on their minds. A positive attitude and a receptive awareness show in your facial expression.

Eye Contact

Eye contact is one of the most powerful body language skills. It tells the patient that you are interested in giving and receiving messages of mutual concern and interest. Use of eye contact while engaging in conversation permits an open, honest transmission of thoughts and ideas. Looking away while people are talking to you makes them feel that what they are saying is not important. Interest and attention soon disappear and the intent of your message can be distorted or lost.

CLINICAL PEARL

You must always be sensitive to individual needs when communicating with patients. In certain cultures, making continuous eye contact with a person during a conversation can be interpreted as rude.

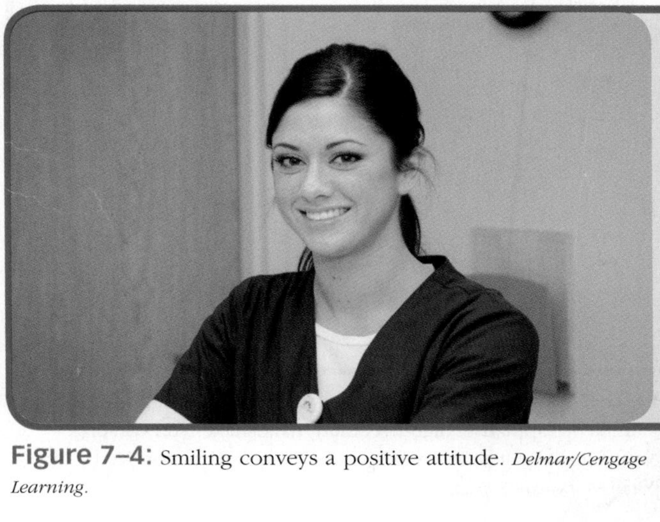

Figure 7–4: Smiling conveys a positive attitude. *Delmar/Cengage Learning.*

Gestures

Another way of transmitting nonverbal messages is by gesturing. Gestures are body movements that enhance what is being said. You might know people who talk with their hands. Using hand and body gestures to accentuate a point can help the receiver understand your meaning. To emphasize the subject matter in conversation, gestures help convey the message.

In the medical field, you will encounter many people who are from different cultures, countries, and social backgrounds. Some gestures, facial expressions, or remarks might be offensive to them. Use caution when you are not sure of a remark or gesture because the meaning might be interpreted differently than your intent.

We use many gestures daily that have become such a part of our personalities that we do not even realize we do them. Some positive and popular gestures are thumbs up, okay, high-five, applause, winking, and a handshake (Figure 7–5). In our society, these are all ways of showing signs of acceptance, encouragement, appreciation, and friendliness. When using these gestures, your intended message is understood without saying anything at all. Some of the ways of telling whether a person is upset or not interested (negative body language) are crossed arms, looking at one's watch, rolling of the eyes, tapping of the foot or fingers, sighing, and talking under one's breath. There are still other gestures that are rude and socially unacceptable. If a patient displays this type of behavior, it might be necessary to call for assistance from a supervisor or coworker.

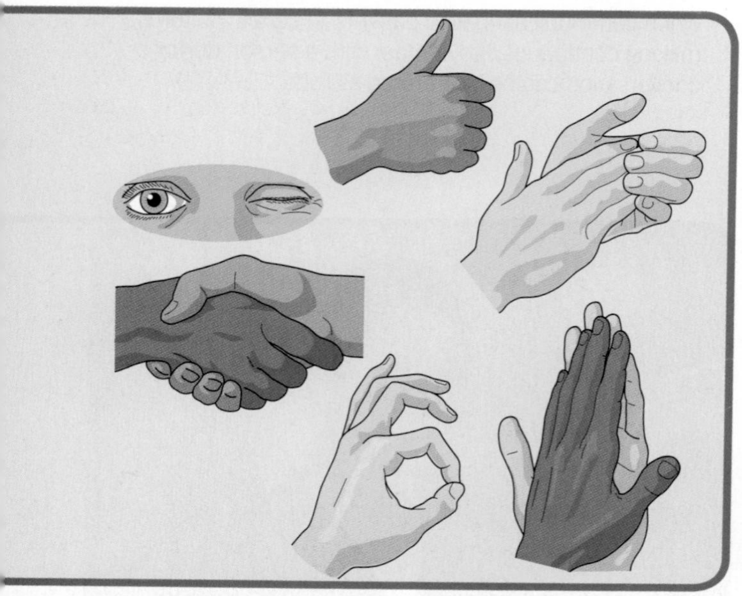

Figure 7–5: Common positive gestures (clockwise, from top): thumbs up, applause, high-five, okay, handshake, and winking. Note that some gestures might not be perceived as positive by all patients. *Delmar/Cengage Learning.*

Distance

There is also a proper distance you should maintain when speaking to others. If you are engaged in a personal conversation, the generally acceptable space between two people is from 1.5 to 4 feet. For social conversation among people, the distance between people is from 4 to 12 feet, which is about the distance at which you and your patients will be communicating. In a public setting, the space can be 12 to 25 feet. Keep in mind that touch, gestures, and language barriers are important considerations when communicating with patients. Generally, if someone is moving away from you while you are speaking, he or she may be doing so to create more space or because you are too close for comfort.

Silence

Another powerful nonverbal communication tool is silence. This method can be frustrating for the person to whom it is directed. When a patient exhibits this nonverbal way of communicating, you might need to ask supervisor, a physician, or another staff member for assistance (Figure 7–6).

Therapeutic Touch and Relationships

A comforting touch helps patients feel that you care and gives them a sense of security and acceptance:

- A handshake is a sign of friendship.
- A hug conveys feelings of warmth and affection (but only if you are certain of the acceptable boundaries expressed by the patient or by office protocol; it is appropriate to ask the patient's permission).
- Patting someone on the back and saying "Good for you" provides positive reinforcement. You

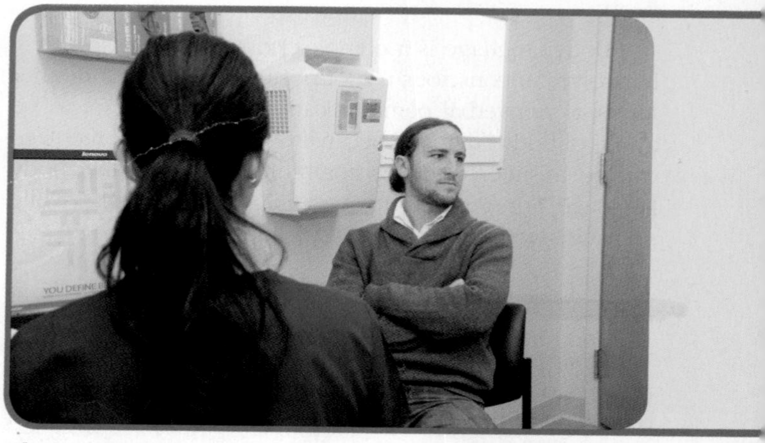

Figure 7–6: The patient is silent and avoiding eye contact with the medical assistant. When a patient is silent and avoids eye contact, such as this patient, it is helpful to solicit help from another individual more experienced in these situations. *Delmar/Cengage Learning.*

might do that in praise of a patient who followed the prescribed treatment of the physician, lost 10 pounds, and needs positive recognition of these achievements to encourage continued compliance.

Studies have shown that patients who have been touched, by a hand on the shoulder or a hand held, respond significantly better in treatment than those not touched (Figure 7–7). You always want to be sensitive to the patient's reaction when touching is involved. The least threatening place to touch someone is on the arm between the elbow and the wrist.

There are, however, patients who might be offended by your touching them or whose religious beliefs, culture, or ethnic origin do not allow this. When touching patients in the office to offer comfort or praise, it would be best to do so in the presence of other professionals for your protection against possible misunderstandings. This safeguards you from being unfairly accused of touching someone inappropriately.

Therapeutic relationships include your use of empathy, impartial behavior, and understanding of emotional behavior in working with patients.

COMMUNICATING EMOTIONAL STATES

As you've learned, communication is a complex process, and you must be aware of all its facets so that complete information exchange can occur. The perceptive medical assistant should be able to determine what questions to ask a patient to determine whether the look on the patient's face matches the patient's emotional demeanor.

You may use the following questions to find out the emotional states of the patients during in-person screening. After greeting the patient with a kind "hello" and calling him or her by name, you might want to ask a variation of "What seems to be the problem today?" ("What brings you here to see the doctor today?" or "Can you tell me about the problem you seem to be having?" or "Can we talk about what has been giving you concern that brings you in to see the doctor?" are some other examples.) The patient's response to this question indicates the chief complaint or purpose of the visit. Adding the following question is a technique especially helpful in extracting additional information from patients to assist in attaining the proper diagnosis: "And what are you dealing with every day?"

When a patient presents for a follow-up visit, ask, "Are you feeling any better since you last saw the doctor?" or "You don't seem to be feeling too well; do you feel any better?" or "Can you tell me how you've been doing since you were here last?" Avoid asking questions such as "How are we feeling?" and never use so-called pet names such as honey or sweetie, which can be interpreted as disrespectful or rude. A helpful tool in eliciting information from patients is use of an intake questionnaire. This encourages the patient to focus on what health issues bring him or her in to the office, prompts him or her for recent consultations you will need to have available for the doctor, and obtains a current list of medications. Patient screening and intake questionnaires are discussed further in Chapter 37.

Hearing patients' answers can provide a general idea of how they feel emotionally. Of course, you can accomplish this only by taking time to find out. That means giving the patients your undivided attention when you are present with them. You need communication skills and genuine concern to establish this rapport. Repeating back to the patient what you heard for clarity and accuracy can help bridge any potential gap in communication. Remember that the manner in which you speak, your tone of voice, and your body language convey your attitude to others. Make sure that your professionalism and compassion show when you serve your patients.

You can be instrumental in pointing out factors that can interfere with a particular treatment approach planned by the physician. Some of these factors are presented in Table 7–2. Patients will likely respond to

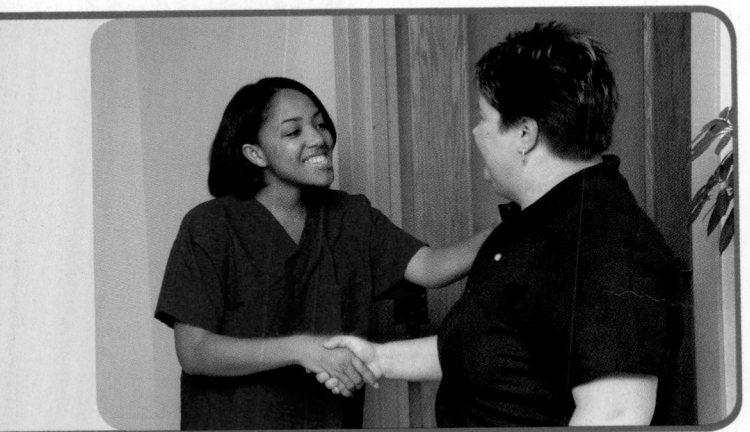

Figure 7–7: The medical assistant is reinforcing a positive message through therapeutic touch. *Delmar/Cengage Learning.*

TABLE 7–2 Factors That Can Interfere with Patient Compliance in Treatment Plans

Travel (business or pleasure)
Work schedule (irregular hours)
Relocating/moving
Lifestyle/cultural influences
Economic concerns
Comprehension of physician's orders
Disability/mental incompetence
Being unclear about the directions or the importance of the treatment plan

and comply with the physician's orders more readily if you convey a genuine concern for their well-being with each contact. If a patient seems quieter than usual, you might discover in the course of your interaction that the patient is preoccupied by a problem that he or she will reveal if you show interest and take time to listen.

Often, a statement that begins with "I" can open up a conversation. For instance, you may say to a patient, "I noticed as you were walking in today that you don't seem to be as lively as usual. Is anything in particular bothering you?" This gives patients a positive impression that you care about how they are and that you are showing it. This can make the patient feel more at ease and might increase compliance with the physician's orders. You play an important role in assisting both physician and patient in providing quality health care.

Using the statements that begin with "I" can be helpful when communicating with anyone, not only patients. You could use an "I" statement with a coworker, such as, "I noticed the filing is getting piled up; can I help you?" This way of offering help is a nonconfrontational approach that makes it easy to elicit a positive response. When you converse with your coworkers, it is important to speak sincerely and communicate your feelings in a professional and positive tone, just as you do with patients. This can help promote the spirit of teamwork among coworkers.

PROCEDURE 7–1 Respond to Nonverbal Communication

PURPOSE: Recognize and respond to nonverbal communication while taking a patient's chief complaint

EQUIPMENT: Patient's chart, pen (if paper chart), computer (if EHR). You need to elicit information about the patient's chief complaint for the physician. Additionally, you notice in the chart that today is the patient's birthday.

S SKILL: Recognize and respond to nonverbal communication.

Procedure Steps	Detailed Instructions and/or *Rationales*
1. Ask the patient the reason for today's office visit. The patient does not respond to your question and looks away.	
B 2. ***Demonstrating perception of nonverbal cues and the patient's level of comprehension,*** ask the question again.	*It is important to communicate on the patient's level of comprehension. Nonverbal cues can help you adapt to individual patient needs.*
3. Ask open-ended questions and use other techniques discussed in this chapter to start a conversation and avoid silence.	The questions and techniques you use should be tailored to individual patient needs. For example because today is the patient's birthday, you might wish the patient a happy birthday.
B 4. ***During entire contact with patient, use appropriate and effective verbal and nonverbal communication skills.***	This includes: • Demonstrating empathy in communicating with patients, family, and staff. • Applying active listening skills. • Using body language and other nonverbal skills in communicating with patients, family, and staff. • Demonstrating respect for individual diversity.
B 5. ***During entire contact with patient, maintain appropriate distance from patient.***	*This demonstrates awareness of territorial boundaries of the person with whom communicating.*
6. When you have obtained the chief complaint and documented it in the patient's chart, thank the patient and say that the physician will be in shortly.	

FUNDAMENTALS OF PSYCHOLOGY

Understanding some fundamentals of psychology is an important element in your job as a medical assistant. It will help you become an effective communicator and understand needs and grief. Abraham Maslow's Hierarchy of Needs and Dr. Elisabeth Kübler-Ross's Five Stages of Grief are often studied.

Maslow's model consists of five stages of needs, as shown in Figure 7–8. The first four are grouped together as "deficit needs," meaning if something is missing in any of the first four categories, you experience that as a need. These four stages are:

1. *Physiological:* Basic survival needs (food, water, air, sleep)
2. *Safety:* Stability (protection, health, order)
3. *Belongingness and Love:* Being with someone or a group (friendship, family, meaningful employment)
4. *Esteem:* Respect, self-respect, confidence, and independence

The fifth and highest level is:

5. *Self-Actualization:* At this stage, you tend to be a problem solver and place a great deal of emphasis on family and long-term relationships.

When Dr. Elisabeth Kübler-Ross, author of *Death and the Dying Patient*, researched death and dying, she found that most people went through a process of five stages when dealing with grief, especially over terminal illness and death. The five stages are: denial, depression, bribery, anger, and resolution. Dr. Kübler-Ross also found that some people, individuals with a sense of purpose in their lives, didn't go through first four stages, but immediately went to the fifth stage, resolution.

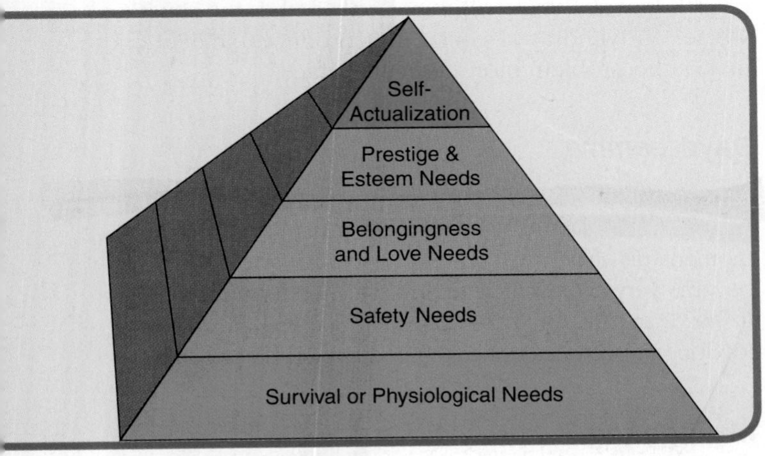

Figure 7–8: Maslow's hierarchy of needs. *Adaptation based on Maslow's Hierarchy of Needs.*

In your practice as a health care professional, you need know how and why Maslow's hierarchy and Kübler-Ross's research are important in relation to working with patients.

- Kübler-Ross's grief model was developed initially as a model for helping dying patients cope with death and bereavement; however, it has been expanded to include the concept and provide insight and guidance for coming to terms with personal trauma and change and for helping others make emotional adjustments and cope, whatever the cause.
- Everyone is motivated by needs. Maslow's Hierarchy of Needs helps explain how these needs motivate us all.
- Both Kübler-Ross's and Maslow's theories are helpful to understand and to use with patient interaction in difficult times. Implementing coping skills helps communication and promotes empathy with a patient and his or her family's needs.
- Examples of organizations that can assist patients and family members struggling with illness include:
    - Local chapter of hospice
    - American Cancer Society
    - Compassion and choices
    - Children's hospice international
    - Center to advance palliative care
    - Your local hospital resources

DEFENSE MECHANISMS

Defense mechanisms are largely unconscious acts we use to help us deal with unpleasant and socially unacceptable circumstances or behaviors and to make an emotional adjustment in everyday situations. We all use various defense mechanisms from time to time. However, habitual use of these mechanisms can result in negative feelings or outcomes. A method to resolve unpleasant circumstances is to look for creative solutions rather than to dwell on the problem. This not only helps resolve the dilemma but increases your quality and effectiveness.

Repression

The most commonly used defense mechanism is **repression**, which means holding feelings inside or forcing unacceptable or painful ideas, feelings, and impulses into the unconscious mind. Feelings of hostility, jealousy, or intense anger do not vanish and can surface in dreams or subtle behaviors. Repression, like all the defense mechanisms, tends to protect us from unwanted messages about ourselves that make us feel bad.

Suppression

Suppression describes a condition in which the person becomes purposely involved in a project, hobby, or work so that a painful situation can be avoided. Rather than face a difficult problem within a relationship, for instance, some throw themselves into their work so much that there is little or no time for the relationship. This is a way to avoid communication because the legitimate work has to be done. However, this does nothing to relieve the root cause of the **stress**. Stress can be defined as a physical, mental, or emotional response to events that cause bodily or mental tension.

Displacement

Displacement is the transfer of emotions about one person or situation to another. A typical example of displacement when working as a medical assistant might be as follows: In the course of the day, you have many duties to perform for others, and one patient in particular becomes overly demanding or difficult. You hold back the strong feelings that arise and deal with the situation professionally. Later in the evening at home, you allow the pent-up anger to surface and direct it at a family member.

Projection

In **projection**, you might unconsciously blame another person for your own inadequacies. An extreme form of projection can lead to hostile, even aggressive behavior if you perceive another person to be the cause of the painful feelings. For example, an obese patient who has gained a few pounds might blame you, arguing that the scales were set up or read incorrectly.

Rationalization

With **rationalization**, you justify behavior with socially acceptable reasons and tend to ignore the real reasons underlying the behavior. This self-disciplined, unconscious act might seem harmless, but habitual use can become nonproductive or even destructive because it distorts reality. A typical rationalization might be, "I dieted strictly all day; therefore, it's okay to eat a couple of candy bars later in the evening after supper."

Intellectualization

Intellectualization is still another means of denying socially unacceptable feelings or strong feelings that cannot be easily expressed. With this mechanism, you use reasoning to avoid confronting emotional conflicts and stressful situations. For example, you might discuss all the facts and provide endless information about how to begin caring for an elderly relative, elaborating on special diets and home health care to avoid dealing with the true feelings of sadness that can accompany the person's illness.

Sublimation

Sublimation is used unconsciously to express socially unacceptable instinctive drives or impulses in approved and acceptable ways. An example of sublimation might be a 30-year-old father who is a frustrated athlete forcing his child to excel in a sport or an artist unconsciously directing sexual impulses in the form of constructive writing, sculpture, painting, or photography.

Compensation

Compensation is somewhat similar to sublimation. When you use this defense mechanism, you use a talent or an attribute to the fullest to compensate for a realized personal shortcoming. For example, a person who can no longer participate in sports because of illness or injury might find satisfaction in writing about the game, helping with coaching, or becoming an ardent fan of a well-known team.

Temporary Withdrawal

Temporary withdrawal is a retreat from facing a painful or difficult situation. This avoidance of something unpleasant is another way of protecting ourselves from disagreeable feelings. Watching TV or reading excessively to avoid dealing with an issue are common types of withdrawal. Putting off issues only makes the situation worse. As withdrawal goes on, it produces anxiety and makes the problem more difficult to face.

Daydreaming

A healthy type of temporary withdrawal that all of us do from time to time is daydreaming. This is a way to escape momentarily from reality and relax. At times, you can become very creative and return refreshed from daydreams. If, however, this form of escape is done too often and for too long, it becomes unhealthy and should be of concern.

Malingering

Another common defense mechanism is **malingering**. When you malinger, you deliberately pretend to be sick to avoid dealing with situations that are unpleasant or cause anxiety. A malingering individual might stay home sick on a day when he or she was to give a presentation when, in fact, that person is not sick and is actually enjoying the time at home.

Denial

Denial seems to be a commonly used defense mechanism. It is the refusal to admit or acknowledge something so that you do not have to deal with a problem or situation. When you are not accepting the phases of life that might produce anxiety, you sometimes use denial as an emotional defense. When one who has been given the diagnosis of a terminal illness does not accept the reality of it and believes that a recovery is certain, that person is going through the denial stage.

Regression

Regression is behaving in ways that are characteristic of an earlier developmental level. This usually happens in times of high stress. For example, a college student consoles herself during final exam week with eating hot fudge sundaes as she did as a child with her mother whenever problems at school piled up. Occasionally, someone might regress to sucking his or her thumb or twirling hair when stressed or very tired.

Procrastination

This defense mechanism is a threat to efficiency. It robs us of time and energy if we let it become a habit. An example of procrastination would be "always putting off until tomorrow what you can do today." There is nothing wrong with doing as much as you can within reason and ability in a day and leaving some things to do the next day as long as you prioritize and make sure that time-sensitive work is completed. The problem with procrastination is that, over time, it becomes easier to put off more tasks. This creates stress on the job for you and coworkers because there is so much to do the next day, and catching up is difficult. To have a cohesive team, you want to complete your work on time and offer to assist others if they need help.

COPING SKILLS

Coping skills, like defense mechanisms, can be positive or negative. We use our coping skills to get through situations nearly every day. Coping skills offset disadvantages in day-to-day life, a tool for adapting to the circumstances at hand. Positive coping helps you through situations at nearly the same level of effectiveness as those who do not have the disadvantage. Use of negative coping skills can provide short-term relief or distraction but can ultimately worsen the circumstance. A common example of negative coping skill is abuse of alcohol or drugs. You also use adaptive and nonadaptive coping skills. Refer to Tables 7–3 (adaptive) and 7–4 (nonadaptive) to understand how you would apply these skills to your personal and professional life.

Self-Awareness and Personal Boundaries

The importance of valuing self and being self-aware comes with an understanding of personal boundaries. Your personal boundary can be defined by the amount of physical and emotional space you allow between yourself and others. In an article titled, "Boundaries: The Importance of Valuing Yourself," Cindy Ricardo proposes that there are two main types of boundaries: physical and emotional.

Physical boundaries include your body, your sense of personal space, sexual orientation, privacy, money, home, and safety. In the example of personal space, when someone gets too close to you, your reaction is to take a step back to maintain a boundary that you have established. When you move back, you send a nonverbal message to the other person that he or she is invading your personal space.

Ricardo says that emotional and intellectual boundaries are just as important in protecting your sense of self-esteem and your ability to separate your feelings from the feelings of others. Sometimes it's not as obvious when these boundaries are invaded, for example:

- Blaming others for problems
- Telling others what to think or how to act
- Allowing another person's mood to dictate your mood

Medical assistants, in both administrative and clinical capacities, have many opportunities daily to observe patients' mental and emotional states. These observations have a direct influence on your behaviors, which in turn directly influence your overall health. Keep in mind that all medical personnel are patients too. Therefore, all the information we learn about patients applies to us as well. A true understanding of oneself is the primary key to understanding others. Use adaptive coping skills as a reference tool for self-awareness and handling stress.

Learning about yourself requires you to take a good hard look at who and what you really are. When assessing your "self," your individual presence might come to mind first. This presence comprises both your physical self (your body) and your self-image (how you view yourself). Another aspect of self, as termed by psychologists, is the self-as-process. This refers to the ongoing process inside each of us that deals with constant changes or adjustments in our lives. Your response to others is dealt with by your social self. You identify strongly with many

TABLE 7–3 Adaptive Coping Skills

Deep breathing	Breathe in through the nose and out through the mouth. Breathe in for five seconds and out for 10 seconds.
Diet and exercise	Reduce salt and sugar intake. Take walks.
Stretching	Stretch in the morning and at night.
Talking	Talk with friends, counselors, or pastors.
Journaling	Keep a diary and record your thoughts and feelings.
Planning	Create to-do lists and mark items off when they are complete. Stay organized.
Sleeping	Make your bedroom an inviting place to be. Establish a regular sleep schedule, even on weekends. Don't consume caffeinated beverages in the evening. Don't drink alcohol two to three hours before going to bed. Eat light meals in the evening. Don't smoke in the evening (or at all).
Change thoughts	Replace negative thoughts with positive thoughts.
Music	Listen to relaxation tapes.
Positive affirmations	Use statements such as. "I can trust myself through and through," "I am beautiful," and "Every day in every way I am better."
Create boundaries	Sometimes more distance is needed in relationships. Surround yourself with people who build you up rather than those who tear you down.
Spirituality	Use meditation or prayer. Seek meaning and purpose in human existence.
Humor	When we laugh, endorphins that reduce stress are released.
Communication skills	When speaking with others, use statements such as, "When you ____, I feel ____." Use effective communication techniques such as paraphrasing, asking open-ended questions, and reflection.

TABLE 7–4 Nonadaptive Coping Skills

Drinking	Isolation
Drug Use	Obsessions
Gambling	Shopping over credit
Sex addiction	Over- or under-eating
Road rage	Avoiding responsibilities
Hanging onto anger	"Yes, but …"
Inappropriate boundaries	

roles. Finally, you have an ideal self. This is what you picture yourself to be—the perfect model you have of yourself.

We are, indeed, complex beings, capable of doing just about anything we choose and achieving the goals we set for ourselves. A good way to begin a basic assessment of yourself is by making a list of all the strengths you have as well as of all your weaknesses. This technique can help point out your abilities and qualities and identify areas that need to be changed or improved. Keeping a journal or a diary, even if only temporarily, is another way to vent feelings, look at problems, and realize and assess your behavior patterns to know your true self better.

An ideal time to reevaluate yourself and renew your goals and aspirations is annually on your birthday. Many people prefer the traditional New Year's resolution. Knowing yourself helps you become a more complete person and helps you relate to others more effectively.

CHAPTER SUMMARY

- The standard communication model has six components: the sender, an encoder, a medium, a decoder, a receiver, and a message. The message originates with the sender. The encoded message takes form based upon the sender's reference points. The message is picked up by the intended receiver, who immediately begins to decode it based on reference points. In responding (or providing feedback), the whole process is reversed: The original receiver becomes the sender, and the original sender becomes the receiver.
- People often fall under one of three communication styles: visual, auditory, or kinesthetic.
- Nonverbal communication includes body language, facial expression, eye contact, gestures, distance, silence, and therapeutic touch.
- Perception means to be aware of one's own feelings and the feelings of others. Anticipating the needs of others (patients, providers, coworkers) is a part of perception that enhances your effectiveness.
- Abraham Maslow developed a Hierarchy of Needs that is often studied. The needs include: Physiological, Safety, Belongingness and Love, Self-Esteem, Self-Actualization.
- Dr. Elisabeth Kübler-Ross's five stages of grief are denial, depression, bribery, anger, and resolution.
- Common defense mechanisms include repression, suppression, displacement, projection, rationalization, intellectualization, sublimation, compensation, temporary withdrawal, daydreaming, malingering, denial, regression, and procrastination.
- We all use some—perhaps many—of these defense mechanisms from time to time. If they are used without conscious awareness, they can be relatively harmless. However, habitual use of defense mechanisms can veil reality and interfere with facing personal issues and crises as well as hinder open and honest communication with others.
- Coping skills offset disadvantages in day-to-day life and are tools for adapting to the circumstances at hand; they can be adaptive (such as deep breathing, diet and exercise, or journaling) or nonadaptive (such as avoiding responsibilities or drug use).

STUDY TOOLS

Workbook	Activities for Chapter 7
Premium Website	
MEDIA LINK	View these **Media Links** for Chapter 7: • Communication • The Importance of Appearance
StudyWARE	Activities and Quizzes on the **StudyWARE™ Software** for Chapter 7
	Audio Library of medical terms
	Online access to **Critical Thinking Challenge 2.0**
CourseMate	Activities and Quizzes for Chapter 7
WebTutor	Activities and Quizzes for Chapter 7

CHECK YOUR KNOWLEDGE

1. A patient who is grimacing and wincing would be communicating:
   a. nonverbally.
   b. verbally.
   c. affectively.
   d. intellectually.
2. Which of the following terms describes being aware of one's own feelings and the feelings of others?
   a. Body language
   b. Gestures
   c. Empathy
   d. Perception

3. All the following are examples of body language except:
   a. appearance.
   b. facial expressions.
   c. tone of voice.
   d. gestures.
4. Which of the following would convey a positive attitude?
   a. Frown
   b. Smile
   c. Clenched teeth
   d. Fist
5. Which of the following would be part of active listening?
   a. Handshake
   b. Eye contact
   c. Repeating information given by the patient
   d. Both b and c
6. Which of the following describes an unconscious act that helps one deal with an unpleasant situation?
   a. Coping skills
   b. Defense mechanism
   c. Excuse
   d. Problem solving
7. The ongoing method inside each of us that deals with changes and adjustments in our lives is our:
   a. ideal self.
   b. social self.
   c. self-as-process.
   d. self-image.

WEB LINKS

Educational Psychology Interactive: www.edpsycinteractive.org

Mental Help Net: *www.mentalhelp.net*

REFERENCES

Bowers, Jeremy. (2003). *The Ethics of Modern Communication*. www.jerf.org/writings/communicationEthics/node1.html. (Retrieved 11/16/2010)

Calero, Henry H. (2005). *The Power of Nonverbal Communication*. Aberdeen, WA: Silver Lake Publishing.

Ricardo, Cindy. "Boundaries: The Importance of Valuing Yourself." Self-Growth.com. www.selfgrowth.com/articles/Boundaries_the_importance.html. (Retrieved 11/16/2010)

Chapter 8 Applying Communication Skills

OBJECTIVES

In this chapter, you will learn the following:

KB KNOWLEDGE BASE

1. Spell and define, using the glossary at the back of the text, all the Words to Know in this chapter.
2. Define critical thinking and list the steps in applying critical thinking skills to a problem.
3. Identify resources and adaptations that are required based on individual needs, including culturally diverse, pediatric, geriatric, difficult, or uncooperative patients.
4. Identify different patient education formats and describe the steps to follow when providing patient education.
5. Recognize the role of patient advocacy in the practice of medical assisting.
6. Discuss the role of assertiveness in effective professional communication.
7. Describe relationships among the medical assistant, the employer, and coworkers and how to resolve conflict.
8. Explain methods of communicating information in the medical office.
9. Describe the purpose of staff meetings and employee evaluations.

S SKILLS

1. Instruct patients according to their needs.
2. Document patient education.
3. Advocate on behalf of patient.
4. Use the Internet to access information related to the medical office.

B BEHAVIORS

1. Demonstrate empathy and respect for individual diversity in communicating with patients.
2. Apply active listening skills.
3. Communicate on the patient's level of comprehension and demonstrate recognition of the patient's level of understanding.

WORDS TO KNOW

advocacy
analytical
assertive
Confidential Communication Preference (CCP) form
critical thinking
empathy
evaluation
job description
patient education
petty
reflective communication

CRITICAL THINKING SKILLS

As discussed in Chapter 7, we use many coping skills and defense mechanisms to deal with difficult or stressful situations in our complex daily lives. Another approach to handling interpersonal problems and concerns is to use **critical thinking** (or problem-solving) skills.

Most definitions of critical thinking are based on cognitive developmental theories such as those of Piaget, King and Kitchener, and Bloom and Kohlberg and involve a process of:

1. "Deciding what you think and why you think it;
2. Seeking other views and evidence (developing arguments using supportive evidence); and
3. Deciding which view is most reasonable." (Ruggiero, 1989)

Taking a step-by-step approach helps you look realistically and logically at a problem. This method encourages **analytical** thinking and confident decision making. Use these basic steps of critical thinking when problem solving:

1. Determine just what the problem is and write it down. Ask whether there is a contributing problem chain or series of events.
2. Gather facts and ideas to help you decide what to do about it.
3. List possible decisions and what you think each outcome will be. Use analytical and creative thinking.
4. Prioritize your decisions and begin testing them one by one until results are satisfactory to you and others concerned.

If results are not satisfying, begin again with step one. Often, step one alone triggers an answer to a problem. Sitting down and writing out the problem is often most therapeutic. When you begin using this skill to think logically about major problems, such as changing employment, relocating geographically, or locating a suitable day care facility, you will think more logically in all matters. Making a habit of this skill will increase your peace of mind and reduce stress because you will deal with problems more efficiently and spend less time and energy worrying about what to do. This skill can be a great stride toward eliminating procrastination.

MEDIA LINK

View the "Attributes of a Critical Thinker" video for this chapter on the Premium Website.

COMMUNICATING WITH PATIENTS

Your ability to be an effective communicator with patients and providers will set you apart from others. There are numerous situations encountered in the medical office that require the application and use of excellent communication skills. Table 8–1 lists communication tips you will find useful. These skills take time to develop. You want to start small and become more comfortable at each step to increase your confidence. Hone your skills by practicing these tips with family and coworkers.

Communicating with Special Needs Patients

Patients with special needs require unique and individually tailored methods to communicate instructions. As a medical assistant, you must learn to communicate with patients with disabilities such as a hearing or visual impairment. One method, known as reflective (or mirrored) communication, can be especially helpful for any patient requiring special attention. **Reflective communication** means to afford the opportunity to examine behaviors and interactions, act as a verbal "mirror," and restate what the patient has said for clarification by all parties.

TABLE 8–1 Communication Dos and Don'ts

Dos	Don'ts
Maintain eye contact and use a warm and friendly greeting such as: "Good morning, Mrs. Jones, it's nice to see you today."	Don't forget to use common courtesy and don't look away while others are speaking.
Listen and take an active interest in what the patient is saying.	Don't talk too much about yourself. Let patients talk about themselves.
Ask open-ended questions.	Avoid questions that require only a yes or no answer.
Comment on something the patient is wearing or a common interest or current event.	Avoid political or religious discussions.
Be friendly, open, confident, and caring.	Don't hang back or be aloof in the conversation.
Be confident.	Don't be overconfident or off-putting.

Interpreter services are available for language assistance with hearing impaired and visually impaired patients. You must be aware of these services and the method to contact an interpreter. It is best to have these services arranged in advance of the patient appointment so there are no delays. Be sure you review the patient schedule and work together with the scheduling coordinator to be notified in advance of a scheduled patient with special needs. Most often, special needs patients are accompanied by a family member or caregiver. If so authorized by the patient, you may also share the instructions (verbal and written) with the family member or caregiver. Be sure to let both the patient and caregiver know to contact you immediately for any questions regarding the care instructions.

MEDIA LINK

View the "Patient Education Session with a Deaf Patient" video for this chapter on the Premium Website.

Communicating with Culturally Diverse Patients

To provide the best health care to all patients, it is important to be sensitive to the diverse cultural backgrounds of patients. The U.S. Department of Health and Human Services has sponsored research for recommendations to provide culturally and linguistically appropriate services (CLAS) to patients to improve access to care, quality of care, and, ultimately, health outcomes.

It is important for health care organizations, doctors, and medical staff to understand and respond with sensitivity to the needs and preferences of these patients during their health encounter. The American Institutes for Research has defined cultural competencies as "the social groups influencing a person's culture and self-identity [which] include not only race, ethnicity, and religion, but also gender, sexual orientation, age, disability, and socioeconomic status."

It is critical to incorporate cultural diversity awareness into your routine when performing your medical assistant duties. Use role playing and critical thinking skills to envision your current perceptions of patients and how you might treat patients differently with an understanding of diversity. Table 8–2 provides a quick reference guide to cultural concepts, skills, and knowledge.

Communicating with Pediatric Patients

There is also a different approach to communicating with pediatric patients. Remember that children are not just small adults, and they and their families require a much different approach than with adult patients. Dr. John M. Purvis suggests using four Es (*encouragement, **empathy**, enlistment, and education)* to engage the child in health care matters. The language you use is important because you want to avoid intimidating the young patient. Refer to examples in Table 8–3.

MEDIA LINK

View the "Working with Pediatric Patients" video for this chapter on the Premium Website.

Communicating with Geriatric Patients

The already complex communication processes can be further complicated by age, which can require additional patience and skill. A number of factors affect geriatric patients in their ability to communicate effectively with

TABLE 8–2 Cultural Concepts, Skills, and Knowledge

Concepts	Skills	Knowledge
Culture forms an important part of a patient's identity.	Have a basic understanding of the patient's language.	Knowledge of common foods of different cultures
The meaning of various nonverbal and verbal communications can be different in different cultures.	Be able to interpret patient verbal and nonverbal behaviors in a culturally relevant manner.	Knowledge of the significance of common verbal and nonverbal communications of different cultures
Communication of cultural understanding and respect is critical to build a relationship with a patient.	Be able to communicate an understanding of a patient's culture as a means of strengthening the patient relationship.	Knowledge of family structure and the roles of family members of different cultures

Adapted from: Laura Kristal, Patrick W. Pennock, Sandra McLaren Foote, and Carl W. Trygstad, "Cross-Cultural Family Medicine Residency Training," *Journal of Family Practice*, 17, no. 4 (1983):683–687. Division of Family Medicine, University of California, San Diego School of Medicine.

TABLE 8–3 Words and Phrases to Use When Working with Pediatric Patients

Instead of Saying...	Say this Instead...
Deformity	Appearance
Worry	Wonder
Perform an X-ray	Take a picture
Problem	Finding

Source: John M.Purvis, M.D., "The Challenge of Communicating with Pediatric Patients," *American Academy of Orthopaedic Surgeons*, (February 2009). http://www.aaos.org/news/aaosnow/feb09/clinical5.asp. Retrieved 11/17/2010.

TABLE 8–4 Working with Older Patients

Greet them warmly and by Mr., Mrs., or by first name. Avoid using euphemisms such as "Honey" or "Dear."
Introduce yourself, stating your name and position.
Seat patients in a quiet, comfortable, well-lit area.
Provide assistance in reading or filling out forms.
Physically assist the patient as needed.
If patients are in the examination room for long periods of time, check on them and keep them updated on how long the wait might be.
Use therapeutic touching, with the patient's permission, and office protocol. Lightly touching the patient's shoulder, arm, or hand might help the patient relax.
Say goodbye at the conclusion of the visit.

Adapted from: Thomas E. Robinson, George L. White, and John C. Houchins, "Improving Communication with Older Patients: Tips from the Literature," *Fam Pract Management*, 13, no. 8 (2006 Sep):73–78. www.aafp.org/fpm/2006/0900/p73.html. (Retrieved 11/17/2010)

health care providers and willingness to comply with medical regimens. The normal aging process, involving sensory loss, decline in hearing or memory, retirement from work, and separation from family and friends, affects communication functionality. Table 8–4 presents some tips to smooth patient visits and communication. Additionally, providing older patients with a written visit summary is a good tool to communicate and help them remember the key points of their visit (see Figure 8–1).

Communicating with Families

You must be careful to respect the patient's privacy when discussing health care issues with family members because of the legal aspect of complying with patient's

Key items we discussed today:

Your blood pressure is 140/90. Your goal is less than 130/85.

New medications:

Benazepril (Lotensin) 10 mg – one tablet per day

Instructions:

Take your pill when you get up in the morning. Go for a short walk every morning and again in the afternoon. Cut back on salt and alcohol. Your next visit is in 2 weeks.

Call our office if you have any question, or your symptoms become worse.

Figure 8–1: An example of a Patient Visit Summary.
Delmar/Cengage Learning.

communication wishes, which should be documented on the patient's **Confidential Communication Preference (CCP) form**. Confirm with the patient in private whether he or she wishes the health matter to be discussed during this visit. Do not relay information to the patient or family that the provider has not directed you to do so. Many times, the provider will discuss abnormal results or serious health conditions directly with the patient and family, and this responsibility will not fall on you. If a patient or family member presses you for information, be polite and tell the patient you will relay his or her questions or concerns to the provider and make sure he or she receives a response. Read the dialogue in the following Example box, which provides an example of effective communication and customer service skills for this type of situation.

EXAMPLE

Patient/Family says, "Does my test result show cancer?"
Medical Assistant says, "I was able to get a copy of the report and have given it to Dr. Long. He will be able to discuss it with you."
Patient/Family says, "Can you just tell us yes or no?"
Medical Assistant says, "I'm sorry, but I am not trained to interpret test and lab results. It is best to discuss it with Dr. Long, and I will make sure he is aware of your concerns."

Prior to the patient's departure, you can score customer service points by following up with the patient (and family member[s]) to see that their questions or concerns have been answered. This is a good opportunity for them to let you know whether they have any additional questions you can relay to the physician.

Communicating with Difficult or Uncooperative Patients

As a medical assistant, you will encounter difficult or uncooperative patients who make unreasonable demands or refuse to cooperate. The best approach is to hold off any negative judgments and try your best to accommodate the requests. By taking steps to defuse difficult patients, the doctor can now spend quality patient care time without unnecessary interruption.

Follow these steps to defuse and resolve the matter:

1. Let the patient vent.
2. Express empathy to the patient. The tone of your voice goes a long way. Use a genuinely warm and caring tone to enhance the meaning of empathic phrases.
3. Begin problem solving. Ask the patient questions to help clarify the situation and cause of the problem and double-check the facts.
4. Mutually agree on the solution. Be careful to not make a promise you cannot keep.
5. Follow up. You will score big points by following up with your patient to see whether the problem has been resolved. This is sometimes referred to as service recovery.

PATIENT EDUCATION

Often, the provider will ask you to provide **patient education**. This can include verbal instructions, printed materials, or electronic formats. Larger organizations can have an education department with materials readily available, or offices might contract with a company, such as Krames Patient Education, that makes the educational materials accessible by print or electronic means. Patient education in the ambulatory setting keeps patients healthier and medical conditions from worsening and can reduce the need for hospitalization. Patients can be taught the importance of prevention, early treatment, and overall health maintenance.

You must first assess the patient's ability to comprehend the instructions. Use reflective communication skills, repeating the clear, concise instructions to patient. It is often best to provide a written copy of the educational materials for the patient to take with him or her. These materials should be available in languages other than English, so be sure to determine the primary language of the patient. You must instruct the patient according to his or her individual needs. Examples of common patient education topics are listed in Table 8–5.

TABLE 8–5 Patient Education Topics

Managing Your Cholesterol
Living Well with Diabetes
Quitting Smoking
Understanding Cardiac Catheterization
Low-Fat Eating
All about Arthritis
Understanding Breast Biopsy

You should document patient education sessions in the patient's chart, referencing the provider's order and information provided, including follow-up instructions for the patient (Figure 8–2). It is important to be attentive to how patient education is administered and documented. Patient education is more than just teaching facts and demonstrating skills. It is an essential component of good patient care. Why document? Documenting patient education promotes continuity and consistency in care, improves efficiency, and minimizes professional liability. Document the following:

- The date, time, topic, and purpose of the patient education session.
- The provider who ordered the education session.
- Who was present at the session (interpreters, family, and so on).
- The patient's comprehension and responses to the session. Patient education includes what the patient learns. In addition to a brief description of the topics covered, documentation should include a note about the interaction and response of the learner (for example, "Patient asked …"). Also include information about the patient's reactions and feelings as well as responses to your open-ended questions.
- Describe written materials given to the patient or include copies of educational materials in the chart. Detailed information about the educational materials helps with the continuity of care, avoids unnecessary repetition, and helps build on lessons already learned.
- Describe any verbal information that wasn't included in the written materials.
- Your signature

Procedure 8–1 shows the steps involved in instructing patients.

07-12-20XX 4:30 p.m.	Blood glucose procedure demo per Dr. Rao. Interpreter Sharon Jones was present. Pt was able to successfully demonstrate entire procedure. Gave pt glucose unit, controls, strips, and home care instructions. Pt to f/u in 1 month for FBS per Dr. Rao. J. Andrews, CMA(AAMA)

Figure 8–2: Example of documentation of a patient education session. *Delmar/Cengage Learning.*

PROCEDURE 8–1 Instruct Patients According to Their Needs

PURPOSE: Complete the patient intake and instruct patient and family according to the patient's needs as directed by the provider.

EQUIPMENT: Patient's chart, pen (if paper chart), computer (if EHR), patient education materials.

S **SKILL:** Instruct patients according to their needs.

S **SKILL:** Document patient education.

Procedure Steps	Detailed Instructions and/or *Rationales*
1. Greet the patient and any other person present in the room by name.	
B 2. Provide a written copy of the instructions and review them one by one verbally with the patient, ***using language the patient can understand.***	
3. Ask the patient to repeat the instructions (act as a verbal mirror) and restate what is said for clarification by all parties.	*Ensures that the patient understands what you have said.*
B 4. ***During entire contact with patient, use appropriate and effective verbal and nonverbal communication skills.***	This includes: • Demonstrating empathy in communicating with patients, family, and staff. • Applying active listening skills. • Using body language and other nonverbal skills in communicating with patients, family, and staff. • Demonstrating respect for individual diversity.
B 5. ***During entire contact with patient, maintain appropriate distance from patient.***	*This demonstrates awareness of territorial boundaries of the person with whom communicating.*
6. Provide your name and office phone number if there are additional questions.	
7. Document in the patient's chart what information and instructions were given concerning the procedure.	

PATIENT ADVOCACY

Patient **advocacy** can be defined in many ways. Advocates promote and protect the rights of patients, frequently through a legal process. Patients are also represented in response to health care, insurance matters, prescription drug coverage, the Department of Motor Vehicles (DMV), and matters with large health care institutions. Counseling and information is also provided to patients about their rights as well as intervention with health care providers as needed. Patient advocates intervene, assist, manage, and fight for their patients or to promote issues. Patient advocates take the burdens of dealing with physician, insurance companies, or medical or other issues during their illnesses. They represent their clients, for instance, when there are disputes with medical bills.

A medical assistant can help patients with matters affecting their health, legal, or financial status such as medical bills and job discrimination related to the patient's medical condition within their scope of practice and responsibilities. Other examples of patient advocacy include:

- Living will: Provide the forms and explanation of the process.
- Billing questions: Verify proper procedure and diagnosis code, deductible, and appeal process if required.
- Pharmacy questions and coverage: Verify insurance coverage and generic versus name-brand prescriptions.
- DMV: Complete forms or provide the information required by the DMV for the patient to obtain a disabled-person placard.

PROCEDURE 8–2 Patient Advocacy

PURPOSE: Advocate on behalf of the patient to be considered as a candidate for the pharmaceutical company's free drug program, as directed by the provider.

EQUIPMENT: Paper, pen, computer, release of information, letterhead, envelopes.

S SKILL: Advocate on behalf of patients.

S SKILL: Use the Internet to access information related to the medical office.

Procedure Steps	Detailed Instructions and/or *Rationales*
1. Using the Internet, obtain the drug manufacturer's name and address and protocol for requesting free drug program candidacy. Follow instructions from the manufacturer to assist the patient with the process.	One Website resource is RxAssist (www.rxassist.org).
2. Download and complete the appropriate form or prepare a letter to the drug manufacturer with all relevant information regarding patient and financial status.	Procedure Form 8–2 (mock application form) can be used to complete this activity.
3. Print the form (or letter) and give it to the provider for prescription information and signature (if required).	Some applications might require a letter from the provider in addition to, or in place of, the application form. In a medical office, you would print the letter on office letterhead.
4. Make three copies of signed form (or letter). Prepare one copy to be mailed to the pharmaceutical company, one copy to be mailed to the patient, and one copy to be filed in the patient's chart (or scanned and uploaded to the patient's chart if electronic).	
5. Document in the patient's chart when the form (or letter) was sent and create a reminder for follow-up.	
6. Notify patient of the outcome of the request.	

Patients' perspectives are sometimes different when they think of what a patient advocate is. The following is often considered advocacy:

- Compassion
- Behavior
  - Being shown concern for their questions and worries
  - Being treated with dignity
  - Being kept informed
  - Having attention paid to their special needs
  - Respecting their cultural, racial, and religious needs

See Procedure 8–2.

COMMUNICATING WITH THE HEALTH CARE TEAM

Communicating with the health care team will occur in a variety of methods: verbal, written, and electronic. It is imperative for all communications to be respectful and professional. Any communications regarding a patient become part of the patient's legal medical record. Therefore, you must always take special care to document accurately and protect the integrity of the communication, regardless of the medium used.

You are part of a team, which includes the office staff, physician(s), office manager, and patients. It is essential for you to commit yourself to the common goal of quality patient care. Communicating effectively with all members of the team is fundamental to your job performance. Authors Karen Leland and Keith Bailey discuss "Four Essential Truths of Human Interaction" in their book, *Customer Service for Dummies*:

1. Different people have different working styles. Your working style may be very different from your coworker's style. Use self-awareness to identify these differences and adapt.
2. Be aware of your coworker's sensitivity and tailor your communication to be appropriate for each person with whom you interact.
3. You prefer some people over others. While you will personally get along with certain people over others, it is important to be able maintain a working relationship with all of your coworkers.
4. You can't judge a book by its cover. Avoid forming opinions about other people without getting to know them first.

Effective Professional Communication

Effective professional communication within the office is an essential component of your responsibilities within the medical practice. You will be responsible for taking the initiative and being **assertive** (but not aggressive) in communicating with others. As defined by Carl Benedict, licensed clinical professional counselor, "assertive communication is a style in which individuals clearly state their opinions and feelings, and firmly advocate for their rights and needs without violating the rights of others. Assertive communication is born of high self-esteem. These individuals value themselves, their time, and their emotional, spiritual, and physical needs and are strong advocates for themselves [and others], while being very respectful." On the other hand, "aggressive communication is a style in which individuals express their feelings and opinions and advocate for their needs in a way that violates the rights of others. Thus, aggressive communicators are verbally and/or physically abusive."

Professional communication relies on a certain set of expectations. As a professional in your area of expertise, the expectation is that patient safety, patient care, patient privacy, and provider proficiency are met within the time frame and schedules given. Expectation implies a high degree of certainty and usually involves the concept of preparing or envisioning. Figure 8–3 is one example of a comprehensive list of expectations for a medical assistant in a particular facility.

Roles and Responsibilities in the Medical Office

For a medical office to run efficiently, you will also be required to know and understand the roles and responsibilities of others in addition to your own expectations. One method that defines the roles and boundaries is the organizational chart (see Figure 8–4), which spells out the reporting structure and roles and is updated at any time there are personnel changes. The organizational chart should be prominently posted with other human resource and office policy postings. In a typical medical office, there are providers and staff. In a larger medical group, there is usually one provider who holds the role of managing provider, assuming the management role for all the providers in the group. The office manager (sometimes referred to as practice manager) usually reports to the managing provider. In the large medical group with a corporate office, there are likely to be additional layers of practice management and directors.

Many providers in both private and group practices find it necessary to employ several medical assistants. To thrive as a team, a great deal of cooperation and respect for one another is necessary for a harmonious relationship to be maintained. You will most likely be given a specific **job description** at the onset of your employment. This is to set clear expectations, encourage each employee in a particular area, and promote efficiency. Be cautious of overstepping boundaries because this can cause friction and misunderstandings. At the same time, all staff members must be willing to pitch in when help is needed, *provided it is within your scope of practice*.

The ideal medical office is where patients and medical staff are going about the business at hand in a pleasant, efficient manner. Coordinating a medical office requires great skill. There are multiple layers of policy, regulation, and personalities that affect the day-to-day operations. Harmony, smooth schedules, up-to-date filing, and referrals would reflect a model practice. However, there are often numerous interruptions, emergencies, and staffing schedule changes that affect the operation. Each member of the staff has a unique set of values, principles, and standards to offer. Mutual respect and trust enhance the teamwork and efficiency.

The number of employees varies in each type of medical practice. Some providers in private practice employ only one medical assistant to perform both administrative and clinical duties. This is a tremendous responsibility and requires a highly motivated and mature personality. A good rapport with your employer is necessary to accomplish the objectives of quality patient care. Usually, a good friendship and respect develops between the provider and medical assistant over time, and working together is an enjoyable learning experience for both. Interest in each patient is easy to cultivate because individual contact is made at each office visit. You can get to know patients quite well because of frequent interaction and phone conversations with patients. You will soon become the provider's eyes and ears by supplying important patient information obtained in this manner.

Communication lines must remain open with this one-to-one relationship, as in all employer–employee

MA Task/Check List

1. Patient Prep—Completed one to two days in advance of the patient visit.
   a. Reviews physician's daily schedule
   b. Pull or review EHR patients chart for visit
   c. Abstract patient problem list, medications, and allergies in to EHR.
   d. Reviews last visit notes for any pending results. If results are not in EHR either scanned or on flow sheet, print a copy from patient portal
   e. One month in advance—reviews physician's schedules and sends appropriate orders (lab, mammogram, etc.) for CPE to patient in advance of appointment.

2. Patient Intake
   a. Informs patients if physician is behind schedule and offers to sit in waiting room or exam room (if exam room space is available).
   b. Documents patient information timely and accurately in patient's medical record/EHR.
   c. Observes patient's symptoms and conditions and is alert for the very ill patient who may need emergency care and immediately notifies the physician.
   d. Documents accurate vital signs in chart. Include chief complaint, pain scale if complaint of pain. Last Menstrual Period if between ages 13-60 years. (This includes, height [without shoes], weight, BP, pulse, temperature.)
   e. Review the current allergy list with the patient and make needed updates to the allergy profile.
   f. Review the current medications with patient and update any changes by history.
   g. Complete smoking ad hoc form in the AEMR.
   h. Ask patient if he or she has an Advance Directive (Document Patient Response on the Advance Directive form in the EHR. If not ask patient if he or she would like to have some information. (Give patient the information.) Record in the EHR that information was provided and the date that it occurred. If patient has Advance Directive, make sure it is scanned in to the EHR (including from paper chart).
   i. Complete any point of care tests per physician's protocols. (Example: Complete a Blood Glucose on all diabetic patients.) Order test in EHR and document results in the EHR form.
   j. Prepare patient for type of exam by setting up patient and room (Example: Pap Test), have required instruments, lab slides, and materials ready for the physician, paper requisitions completed on Micro and Pathology specimens.
   k. Documents that will require physician signatures need to be completed with the patient's demographic information prior to physician review.
   l. Follow up instructions, test instructions and directions should be given to the patient. Utilize handout materials from the various departments.
   m. Schedule needed diagnostic tests and treatments.
   n. Document no-show appointments, canceled appointments in medical record/EHR and Schedule. Reports to physician for follow-up requirements.
   o. Ensures that the physician does not wait between patients (his or her next patient should be ready when the physician completes their prior exam).

3. In Office Tasks and Procedures
   a. Complete any ordered injections, ear lavages, EKGs, etc. per physician's verbal or written orders.
   b. Document completed procedure orders on task list of EHR.
   c. Complete administration forms attached to the task list. Including the documentation of Manufacturers and Lot # in EHR (document the NDC number on forms per protocol for each injection, and also document on billing form).
   d. Document TB results following physician review and document in patient's medical record.
   e. Assist physician with any required procedures including setting up equipment.
   f. Instruct patients on proper handling of specimens.
   g. Place printed lab reports in physicians required location. Alerts physician on any critical results.
   h. All lab reports to be scanned into EHR until further notice when integration success rate is deemed acceptable.
   i. Completes all call-backs to patients as directed by provider.

4. Office Orders
   a. Complete orders per physician requests for charges.
   b. Void orders as needed per physician request.
   c. Direct Referral—complete the order entry fields in the EHR, and then print a requisition for the patient. Fax referral to the referring office as notification.
   d. Authorizations—complete the order by entering data in the order entry fields, print requisitions, and send to the appropriate insurance carrier.
   e. Outpatient Testing—place orders in the EHR and print requisitions for patients. Some paper written requisitions are still required such as Mammograms and Pathology.

5. Results and Consults
   a. Pull patient's charts for results, consults and other patient information. Attach results to paper chart.
   b. Review and pull any critical type results for physician to see immediately.
   c. Place in physicians designated area for results review.

Figure 8–3: Sample medical assistant expectations for a particular facility. *Delmar/Cengage Learning. (continues)*

6. Forms
   a. Complete form information such as demographic information prior to physician review (all demographic, CCP, NOPP, and Insurance information to be scanned into EHR prior to physician seeing patient). Other forms requests—complete the information and attach for physician to review.
   b. Pull and attach chart with form (only) if needed.

7. Messaging
   a. Receive incoming calls from patient and ensure that messages are taken accurately reflecting patients questions and concerns.
   b. Utilize message templates to ensure that the needed information is obtained for the physician.
   c. Document the message response into the EHR.
   d. Contact patients with physician's instructions.
   e. If patient has an urgent message, MA will contact the physician or managing physician immediately.
   f. Complete all call backs to patients as directed by provider.

8. Refilling Medications
   a. Medication refills may be placed in the EHR per physician's written protocols. All refills should be approved by physician prior to the medication order entry. MA's must be accurate when entering medication orders due to the auto faxing to pharmacy. Physicians will cosign all medication orders. Narcotics refills must be approved by physician prior to entering the medication in EHR. All narcotics will be on hold from auto faxing until the physician signs the order.
   b. If physician does not allow MA to enter the refills for auto fax, then he or she will complete the medication order entry by document. Don't print and fax the refills directly to the pharmacy.
   c. Notify patient that prescription has been sent to pharmacy.

9. HIPAA
   a. Maintain patient confidentially at all times and assure the security of patient data.
   b. Do not allow anyone to document using his or her log in.
   c. When selecting patients for EHR documentation, they search patient properly and ensure that they are documenting on correct patient's medical record/EHR.

10. Scanning and Abstracting into EHR
   a. Scan documents into EHR by selecting correct patient and note type (indexing).
   b. Use document map to subject the note type correctly which improves the physicians required time to search for documents.
   c. Notify site manager when scanning is not completed each day.
   d. Obtain site manager approval when a document needs to be in-errored in the EHR system.

11. Other Office Tasks
   a. Assist with maintenance of equipment and supplies.
   b. Clean and stock exam rooms for needed supplies.
   c. Assist and train other Medical Assistants as required.
   d. Place supply or medication orders as directed.
   e. Understand the business office operations/procedures and current accepted insurance plans.
   f. Complete referrals and prior authorizations for patients
   g. Provide back–up coverage for receptionists by answering and documenting messages, schedules appointments in the registration system, updates accurate patient demographic data, and obtains required registration forms.
   h. Provide back–up coverage for check in/check out and the required duties of the position(s).
   i. Maintain physician's filing and/or scanning into the EHR.
   j. Scan to EHR any additional documents flagged by providers from paper charts.
   k. Maintain consults on file per protocol, shred other documents after scanning that can be retrieved (such as from Patient Portal).
   l. File back paper charts.
   m. Maintain medication logs and temperature logs.
   n. Sort mail, faxes, and lab reports and distribute to providers.

12. Computer Skills
   a. Log on and off daily to the computer.
   b. Keep tablet on docking station or charged on power cord during non use.
   c. Secure the tablet in locked secure storage area prior to leaving office.
   d. Check to ensure that the printers have paper for the printing of requisitions.
   e. Notify support center with any system errors while using the EHR.
   f. Maintain proficiency and accuracy in the required applications: EHR, Scheduling, Patient Portals, Windows, and Microsoft Office programs (Word, Excel, Outlook/email).
   g. Notify site manager immediately if employee becomes aware of any computer issue that affects his or her position such as security violation, proficiency, or training needed.

Note: These duties or work flows will change or evolve as office policies and EHR becomes fully implemented and upgraded.

Figure 8–3: *(continued)*

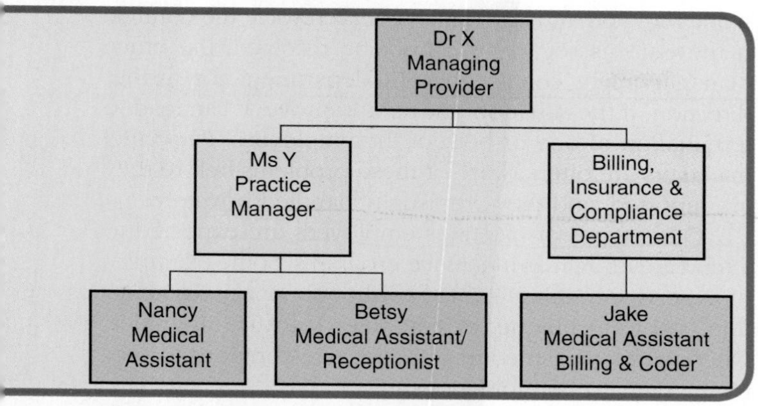

Figure 8–4: A basic organizational chart. *Delmar/Cengage Learning.*

relationships. If misunderstandings occur, they must be rectified as soon as possible. Table 8–6 presents techniques for communicating with coworkers in the event of a misunderstanding. Small problems can mushroom into more complex problems if misunderstandings are not cleared up in a timely manner. Solutions to these problems must be worked out together. You must be competent and assertive in decisions concerning administrative, clinical, and personal employment matters.

The provider usually delegates responsibility for office management to one employee, a position often referred to as practice manager. This frees the provider to attend to patients and relieves the provider of personnel management. This is a major area of importance, especially in large clinics with many employees. In large medical groups, the office might be also be supported by a human resources (HR) department for personnel management and payroll.

Working closely with others can be rewarding and challenging. In a large medical practice or clinic, where there are many employees, a certain amount of give and take must prevail. Completing assigned tasks is expected so that the work is shared equitably. **Petty** differences, defined as trivial or of little importance, should be settled with tact. An example of a petty difference would be differences in choice of clothing, uniform, hair style, and so on, something that has little if any effect on the practice. Always remain professional, and if you have a personal conflict you are unable to resolve, it is best to take the matter to your office manager for a private discussion and resolution. Sometimes a petty difference can in fact escalate and need to be addressed directly by the office manager. An example might be a disagreement on personal appearance choices, but if the clothing or hygiene becomes objectionable to patients or violates office policies, the matter may be better addressed by the office manager.

TABLE 8–6 Phrases That Help Resolve Conflict

That would upset me as well.
I understand what you're saying.
I can see why you'd feel that way.
I know this is really frustrating for you.
I'm sorry.

CLINICAL PEARL

In certain situations, it is almost always best to take the issue to the office manager. Examples include:

- Medication error: If you or another medical assistant has made a medication error, go directly to the office manager so that proper office procedures are followed, and the provider and patient are notified accordingly.
- Coworker tardiness (and effect on patients, providers, and practice): If habitual tardiness is affecting the practice, providers, patients, and coworkers, the manager should be notified so that corrective action is taken.
- Falsifying (or errors on) time card: There can be serious consequences for errors or falsifying time cards, which are legal documents. If you become aware of such a situation, immediately notify your office manager so that corrective action can be taken.
- Patient complaints: Depending on the nature of the complaint, it is wise always to let the manager know. If the complaint is of long wait times, you can be proactive and keep patients informed to defuse any adverse affect. If there is a trend regarding a specific type of complaint, your manager will certainly want to know so the cause can be identified and corrected. Always display empathy and understanding with the patient in resolving complaints.

Sharing enlightening experiences and significant events with other employees is a natural inclination but should be done during non-patient hours to protect the professional office setting. Self-discipline and self-control is necessary and expected in a professional setting.

Methods of Communication in the Medical Office

There are a variety of methods to communicate important information to staff members. An intra-office memo is one means, especially between regularly scheduled staff meetings. Most communications are now sent electronically (email or instant messaging). Become familiar with your office policy on intra-office communication, including restrictions and privacy expectations on electronic communication. You must be proficient in computer technology and software applications. There are times a written document (often a memo) is provided, requiring each employee to read and sign it, indicating that the information has been received, and then passed on to the other employees for signature as well. This helps ensure that all employees are informed and is especially useful in a notification of a new or change in office policy. Word of mouth is not a reliable way to relay an important announcement because it might not reach everyone or might be misinterpreted or changed as it passes from one person to another.

Some offices and clinics use a bulletin board as a means of intra-office communication. Notices of educational programs, seminars, or meetings are posted for all members of the staff to read, in an area such as the staff room or eating area.

Participating in Staff Meetings or In-Services

Most medical offices hold regular staff meetings that all employees are expected to attend. They are usually set and chaired by the office manager or the provider. The meetings are usually held in the medical office either before or after patient care hours and are announced far enough in advance so that arrangements can be made for staff to attend. Many staff meetings are scheduled at regular times (e.g., the second Friday of each month, a meet-and-eat meeting at noon every other Wednesday). At these meetings, decisions concerning office policy changes are reached and problems are discussed (Figure 8–5). This is a time for new ideas to be expressed and exchanged and for all members of the staff to get more acquainted with each other. If you are part of a large medical practice, oftentimes, ice breakers are used as a group exercise to help people get to know themselves, one another, and the nature of their group. This often will spur teamwork, creative thinking, and problem solving.

In some situations, conflict arises between employees that can be impossible to resolve. This type of situation should not be brought up in a staff meeting. You must try to work out your differences with your colleague directly at first. If this is not successful, take the matter to your office manager. Your office manager will work with you and your colleague to resolve the conflict. If the issue is severe or cannot be resolved, the office manager might contact the HR department for further direction. If the situation does not improve, it can lead to termination of one or both of the employees. Personnel managers are often aware of these problems before they are reported, and they are usually handled privately.

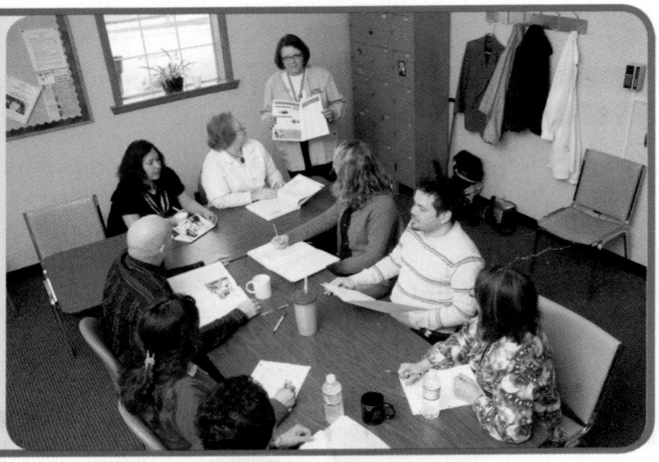

Figure 8–5: Providers or office managers hold regular meetings in the office to communicate important information to the members of the staff. *Delmar/Cengage Learning.*

Other types of meetings employees are expected to attend are known as in-service programs. Some examples of in-service training include cardiopulmonary resuscitation, sterile technique, or computer software upgrades. Often, employers encourage holiday celebrations to promote better working relationships.

Performance Reviews as an Avenue for Communication

In most employment situations, an **evaluation** of work performance is made on an annual basis and filed in your permanent employment record. The initial employment review is usually held after a probationary period of 30, 60, or 90 days. In this meeting, you and your employer (most likely your immediate supervisor, such as office manager) will discuss your job performance. Evaluation forms outline the most important qualities and abilities needed for the job and include a section for strengths and weaknesses to be listed. (Employee evaluation forms are discussed further in Chapter 22, "Managing the Office.")

Employers are always aware of an employee's behavior. Little goes unnoticed when you share a daily routine. Your attitude shows at all times. Even if the word *attitude* is not part of the evaluation, the other categories cover it comprehensively. Consider setting performance goals so that you accomplish your duties and objectives and attain a high level of job performance (see Table 8–7).

Initiative is an important factor. Demonstrating resourcefulness will help you advance in your career. Following office policy is also important. Being on time and dependable on the job are always pleasing to employers. Absences and tardiness are difficult to tolerate from employees who make it a habit. Another area of extreme importance to employers is the quality and quantity of your work. Performing assigned tasks in a reasonable amount of time, without needing to be reminded, is a valuable trait.

The employee evaluation need not be a threat to the conscientious medical assistant. It is a time when questions about advancement and salary may be openly

TABLE 8–7 Personal Performance Goals

Open and honest communication
Working as a team
Developing creative solutions
Soliciting suggestions
Planning effectively
Having a vision and goals

discussed. If you have lived up to the standards of the job, your performance should receive a favorable review.

Some employers find that annual evaluations motivate employees and keep communication lines open. It is important to set up performance goals, with managers conducting 30-day or quarterly reviews prior to annual performance evaluations so there are no surprises for the employee or manager. Using effective and open communication, you will have the opportunity to review goals and objectives with feedback, determine whether there are barriers, and decide whether you would want or need to make any changes. By creating performance goals, you take ownership of your aspirations, achievements, and objectives and establish a clearer path to any necessary changes for personal and organizational improvement.

Some offices and employers choose not to have official evaluations but wish employees to discuss whatever is on their mind at any time. For some office personnel, this works quite well. For the private practice provider with one or two medical assistants, this is usually the case.

CHAPTER SUMMARY

- Critical thinking is an approach (one of many coping skills) to handle interpersonal problems and concerns, using a step-by-step approach to problem solving.
- Communicating with culturally diverse, pediatric, geriatric, and difficult or uncooperative patients involves the use of resources and adaptations based on individual needs.
- Patient education can include verbal instructions, printed materials, or electronic formats. Using reflective communication skills, provide information to patients as requested by the provider.
- Patient advocacy is a critical role of the medical assistant to advocate, promote, and protect the rights of patients. Advocacy includes issues affecting patients such as prescription drug benefits, DMV disability placard, a living will (advanced directive), and billing matters.
- The medical assistant must be assertive, but not aggressive, in communications. Assertive people value themselves; their time; and their emotional, spiritual, and physical needs and are strong advocates for themselves and others while being very respectful.
- Relationships among the medical assistant, the employer, and coworkers should be defined with an organizational chart, outlining the roles and boundaries of each. A job description and expectation list further defines roles and responsibilities. Effective communication and conflict resolution skills are paramount in resolving petty differences and real or perceived conflict.
- There are a number of methods of communicating information in the medical office, including an interoffice memo, electronic message (email, instant message, or EMR transmission), and personal or staff meetings. You must be familiar with the policy, expectations, and restrictions concerning office communications.
- Staff meetings and employee evaluations are necessary to communicate information or initiate discussion concerning office policies, problems, and organizational change. Evaluations are part of assessing your work performance. Performance goals set forth what you wish to accomplish prior to your next evaluation (goals and objectives).

STUDY TOOLS

Workbook	Activities for Chapter 8
Premium Website	
MEDIA LINK	View these **Media Links** for Chapter 8: • Attributes of a Critical Thinker • Patient Education Session with a Deaf Patient • Working with Pediatric Patients
StudyWARE	Activities and Quizzes on the **StudyWARE™ Software** for Chapter 8
	Complete the following **Competency Challenge 2.0** activity: • Thursday, 3 PM: Provide Patient Instruction
	Audio Library of medical terms
	Online access to the **Critical Thinking Challenge 2.0**
learninglab	Module 4: Professional Communications

CourseMate	Activities and Quizzes for Chapter 8
WebTutor	Activities and Quizzes for Chapter 8

CHECK YOUR KNOWLEDGE

1. All the following are steps to problem solving except:
   a. determining what the problem is and writing it down.
   b. using creative thinking.
   c. gathering facts and ideas to help you decide what to do.
   d. putting off dealing with the problem until you are able to solve it.
2. Which of the following is key to patient compliance when providing patient education?
   a. Information
   b. Motivation
   c. Criticism
   d. Nonchalance
3. The medical assistant must learn to relate to which of the following people?
   a. Patient
   b. Provider
   c. Coworkers
   d. a and b only
   e. All of the above
4. All the following are necessary for an enjoyable work atmosphere except:
   a. cooperation.
   b. respect.
   c. liking your coworkers.
   d. honesty.
5. All the following are qualities of an efficient medical assistant except:
   a. versatility.
   b. beauty.
   c. initiative.
   d. self-starting.
6. Which of the following could be part of a staff meeting?
   a. In-service program
   b. Policy changes
   c. Discussing a personality conflict
   d. None of the above
   e. Both a and b
7. Which of the following can be used as a means of intra-office communication?
   a. Bulletin board
   b. Email
   c. Intra-office memo
   d. All of the above

WEB LINKS

Krames patient education materials: www.krames.com

REFERENCES

Kristal, L., Pennock, P. W., McLaren Foote, S., Trygstad, C. W. "Cross-Cultural Family Medicine Residency Training." *Journal of Family Practice*. 17, no. 4 (1983):683–687. Division of Family Medicine, University of California, San Diego School of Medicine.

Leland, K., and Bailey, K. (2006). *Customer Service for Dummies*. Hoboken, NJ: Wiley Publishing.

Osborne, H. *In Other Words … Making Sure It Works … Documenting Patient Education*. (January 2000). *Boston Globe On Call* magazine. www.healthliteracy.com/article.asp?PageID=3819. (Retrieved 11/17/2010)

Purvis, J. M. "Engaging with Younger Patients." (May 2009). www.aaos.org/news/aaosnow/may09/clinical2.asp. (Retrieved 11/17/2010)

Robinson, T. E., White, G. L., and Houchins, J. C. "Improving Communication with Older Patients: Tips from the Literature." *Fam Pract Manag*. 13, no. 8 (2006 Sep):73–78. www.aafp.org/fpm/2006/0900/p73.html. (Retrieved 11/17/2010)

Section

2

The Front Office

Unit

5

Business Communications

The medical assistant must be prepared to deal efficiently with the unending variety of telephone calls and electronic messages received daily. A pleasant voice, good listening skills, clear communication skills, and excellent customer service techniques are essential. You must practice patience, demonstrate compassion, and exercise good judgment to those in need of such attention. You must be proficient in computer skills, spell accurately, and write legibly. You will have an opportunity to demonstrate your knowledge of anatomy, medical terminology, spelling, grammar, and punctuation when you answer the office phone or respond to email as you complete messages and charting. These are fundamental skills of verbal and written correspondence. Processing incoming and outgoing mail might also be one of your responsibilities. Written communication skills must be as flawless as possible to reflect a professional environment.

Office communications today can be made in a variety of modes: electronic, wireless, paper, or a combination (known as hybrid). There are electronic medical records (EMR). Also in use are patient portals, through which patients can create their own electronic health records, known as personal health records (PHR); communicate with their doctor electronically; request lab results, referrals, and appointments; and, in some instances, communicate with doctors by email. Transmitting medical information can create some privacy challenges that you as a medical assistant must make your highest priority.

Certification Connection

CMA (AAMA)	Ch. 9	Ch. 10	Ch. 11
Adapting communication to an individual's needs	X		
Computer concepts (components, applications, Internet services)			X
Equipment operation, maintenance, and repair			X
Fundamental writing skills		X	
Patient interviewing techniques	X		
Prioritizing incoming and outgoing data (e.g., importance, urgency, recipient availability)	X	X	
Professional communication and behavior	X		
Receiving, organizing, prioritizing, and transmitting information	X	X	
Recognizing and responding to verbal and nonverbal communication	X		
Telephone techniques	X		
Understand the modalities for incoming and outgoing data (e.g., mail, fax, telephone, computer)		X	

(continues)

Certification Connection

	Ch. 9	Ch. 10	Ch. 11
RMA (AMT)			
Computer applications		X	X
Employ active listening skills	X		
Employ appropriate telephone etiquette	X		
Employ effective written and oral communication	X	X	
Employ email applications			X
Form business documents and correspondence appropriately		X	
Inform patient of test results per provider's instructions	X		
Instruct patient by telephone	X		
Perform appropriate telephone screenings	X		
Process incoming and outgoing mail		X	
Receive, process, and document results received from outside provider		X	
Transcription and dictation			X
CMAS (AMT)			
Communications	X	X	
Employ effective written and oral communication	X	X	
Employ email applications			X
Form business documents and correspondence appropriately		X	
Fundamentals of computing			X
Medical office computer applications		X	X
Process incoming and outgoing mail		X	

Chapter 9

Telephone Communication

OBJECTIVES

In this chapter, you will learn the following:

KB KNOWLEDGE BASE

1. Spell and define, using the glossary at the back of the text, all the Words to Know in this chapter.
2. Explain the proper protocol for answering the telephone in the medical office.
3. Describe methods of screening and routing incoming calls.
4. List the information that should be documented in all telephone messages.
5. Describe the different types of telephone calls a medical assistant might have to answer in the medical office and explain how each should be handled.
6. Describe the types of community resources for patients' health care needs and emergency services and how to research current information.

S SKILLS

1. Perform a telephone screening.
2. Obtain a telephone message from a recording device or outside answering service.
3. Telephone a patient with test results, observing HIPAA regulations and following the instructions of the provider.
4. Create a list of resources for patient health care needs.
5. Create a list of community resources for emergency preparedness.

B BEHAVIORS

1. Demonstrate empathy in communicating with patients, family, and staff.
2. Apply active listening skills.
3. Demonstrate sensitivity appropriate to the message being delivered.
4. Analyze communications in providing appropriate responses and feedback.
5. Implement time management principles to maintain effective office function.

- inc cover letter
- Hipaa

WORDS TO KNOW

anticipate
Confidential Communication Preference (CCP)
confirmed
empathy
etiquette
express
fax
patient portal
personality
screening
teleconferencing
triage

THE DIRECTOR OF FIRST IMPRESSIONS

The telephone is the center of all activity in the medical office just as it is with any business. The professional attitude conveyed to the caller is critical to the success of the business of practicing medicine. Consider the following:

- On average, it takes a person about 10 seconds to pick up on your attitude from listening to the tone of your voice.
- Developing excellent telephone customer service (in both tone and words) is one of the *most valuable* business skills you can acquire.

As such, you are the *Director of First Impressions* for the medical office. Because the phone call is often the first contact a patient has with the office, your manner of speaking and the **empathy** you convey are part of establishing an appropriate image of the practice. Your voice is part of your **personality**, but over the phone, your voice *is* you. Does your telephone personality reveal a confident, courteous, friendly, and efficient medical assistant? Inflection in your voice can be heard in the manner of your speaking. See Table 9–1.

You must **anticipate** the needs of the patient and provider by asking the proper questions to route accurate information to the appropriate person with the level of urgency required. You must be courteous, articulate, and a careful and active listener to establish successful communication.

ANSWERING THE TELEPHONE

Answering each call as soon as possible, no matter what the nature of the call, is most efficient and promotes a positive atmosphere. Nearly all medical facilities have telephones with multiple lines, and many offices have an automated system that directs the caller and then places the call in queue. While on hold, the automated system often will provide information such as the provider's profiles, prescription refill policies, office hours, emergency contact information, and hold times. When the phone rings into the office, someone should answer each line as soon as possible, at least by the third ring.

The following is an excellent example of how to answer a call with a smile on your face. Answer the phone, "Good morning, Central Medical Center, Ellen speaking, how may I help you?" This will most often prompt the caller to give his or her name and the reason for the call. Make sure you get all the information needed, repeating back the information to the caller to make sure you have recorded his or her request accurately. Let the caller know when he or she may expect a response (make sure you give a reasonable time frame and one you can keep). If you do not have a response within the original time frame quoted, call the patient back and let him or her know you are still waiting and will call back as soon as you have the information. Good customer service does not keep callers waiting without a reply. Patients can become very anxious when waiting for medical results, so frequent updates are often appreciated.

When you are finished with the conversation, it is best to allow the caller to hang up first. If you hang up first, you might miss something the patient wanted to add. When you finish the call, say "Goodbye" or "Goodbye, Mrs. Jones." Keep all calls as brief as possible while being pleasant and professional. Limit personal calls to a minimum during working hours.

MEDIA LINK

On the Premium Website, view the "Telephone Personality" video for this chapter.

Handling Multiple Ringing Lines

Sometimes all lines ring continually. When you have more than one line coming in to the office, place your first call on hold properly, find out who is on the second line, and determine whether it is an emergency (or a hospital or doctor calling). Then you can put the second caller through if an emergency, or on hold if not, while you finish the first call.

TABLE 9–1 Phone Tone and Etiquette

If Your Phone Tone is ...	It Translates as ...
Monotone (a flat voice)	"I'm bored and have absolutely no interest in what you're talking about."
Slow speed and low pitch	"I'm depressed and want to be left alone."
A high-pitched and empathic voice	"I'm enthusiastic about this subject!"
An abrupt speed and loud tone	"I'm angry and not open to input."
High pitch combined with drawn-out speed	"I don't believe what I'm hearing."

Basic guidelines for handling several ringing lines include:

- Excusing yourself and asking the patient you are speaking with whether you may place him or her on hold.
- Answering the second call, determining the nature of the call (be sure it is not an emergency), and asking whether he or she can hold. (Another exception is that a doctor or hospital calling to speak with the provider in your office should be put through immediately and not placed on hold.)
- Return to the first call and thank him or her for holding.
- Resolve the first call and return to the second call.

TELEPHONE SCREENING

An established phone **screening** manual (sometimes called a **triage** manual) should be kept near each phone for reference so that each person who answers the phone will ask standard questions and give the standard response as has been pre-authorized by the provider (see Figure 9–1).

You should learn how to proceed logically through a set of questions that will reveal the caller's condition and help determine, if necessary, how soon the patient should be seen by a provider. This process is called telephone screening. If you do not know how to handle a patient, or if the questions have not been addressed in the manual, referring the problem to one who is more experienced is necessary and appropriate. Never guess in response to a patient's questions and do not treat any question lightly. Document, in detail, all the information obtained from the patient and relay or attach a message for the doctor to review. Telephone screening is a perfect example of anticipating needs. In this case, anticipate what the doctor will need, such as relevant patient information and symptoms, lab results, consult results, last appointment, next appointment, blood pressure, and temperature and mark the message urgent if determined so or advised by patient.

If there is a serious telephone emergency that cannot be handled in the facility, it is best to refer the patient to an emergency medical service and explain that it will send someone as soon as possible to help. It might be best to direct the person to an emergency room of the nearest hospital. It is important to have all emergency phone numbers listed by each phone in the office. In stressful times, this will be helpful in giving the patient phone numbers he or she might need quickly or in calling an emergency service for the patient (see Procedure 9–1 later in this chapter). Medical assistants must ask questions of coworkers and supervisors as they learn how best to deal with problems.

If you are speaking to a patient face to face at the office and you must answer the phone, say to the patient, "Excuse me for a moment, please," answer the phone call, and then continue with what you were doing. All emergency calls must be handled immediately.

Routing Calls in the Medical Office

Table 9–2 lists examples of calls received in the medical office and where they should be routed. Knowing where to send a call when it comes in can save time, avoid frustration, and score service points.

You will find that patients will frequently ask to speak with the provider. Never say, "The doctor is busy," because this can give the impression that the doctor does not want to be bothered by the caller. Be aware of the statements you make in reporting why the provider cannot speak on the telephone. It would be much better to state, "The doctor is with a patient now. May I take a

UPPER RESPIRATORY INFECTION (URI)

Temperature / Fever?

SHORTNESS OF BREATH?

Chest Tightness?

Chest Discomfort or PAIN?

Wheezing?

Duration of Symptoms? (e.g., 1 day or 2 weeks)

What have they done about it so far? (e.g., ASA, Tylenol, OTC cough meds or decongestant)

Be SPECIFIC when DESCRIBING the COUGH: Productive or Nonproductive, and Color

Any history of pneumonia or asthma?

Ask patient if he or she thinks he or she needs to be seen, and HOW URGENT?

Figure 9–1: Example of a page in a phone screening manual. *Delmar/Cengage Learning.*

TABLE 9–2 Routing Calls in the Medical Office

Type of Call	Immediately Routed to Provider	Record Message for the Provider	Routed to Clinical Medical Assistant	Routed to Administrative Medical Assistant
Any situation deemed to be an emergency by the provider	X			
Critical lab results	X	X (route to the provider immediately after recording the results)		
Patient requesting test results (attach results to message)	X (abnormal results)		X (if results are normal and protocol approved by provider)	
Billing or insurance calls				X
Prescription refills			X (or provider)	
Referrals			X	
Scheduling appointment				X
Another provider	X			
Hospital calling for orders	X			
Patient complaints		X (and to supervisor and quality department)		
Patient requesting medical advice	X (usually set up patient appointment)			
Third-party request for information about a patient (if not billing or provider referral–related, check CCP for authorization to release)	X			X (check CCP)

message and we will return the call as soon as possible?" The caller will usually respect the right of others to have the full attention of the provider and will not expect to interrupt the doctor except for an emergency.

Non-Emergency Calls

If the person on the phone needs additional information or if the call is going to take a while, excuse yourself from the phone call by saying, "May I put you on hold for a moment?" However, if it will be more than one minute, the caller should not be put on hold; in this case, say, "May I call you back with that information?" Be sure to check the patient's phone number before hanging up because it might have changed since the patient's last appointment. Find out a good time to call back, including later times in case the provider wants to talk with the patient. When a caller is on hold, be mindful of the length of the hold time. It can be helpful to have recorded information for the caller while on hold (such as immunization and procedure updates); however, be aware of leaving callers on hold too long because they will let you know how many times they have heard the recording.

Transferring Telephone Calls

If you need to transfer a patient's call to another department or office, first give the caller the phone number, the extension, and the person's name to whom you are transferring him or her in case a disconnection occurs. You should signal (or page) the person and, when the person answers, explain who is waiting to speak to him or her and give a brief summary of the issue. Pull the chart for the provider if the patient is calling for information and have the pertinent data readily available (e.g., labs, test result, consult, chart notes). If using a public address system, be very careful with confidentiality, stating only the person's name and that he or she has a call on a particular line. After the person picks up the line, you may give additional information as needed. All messages should be recorded in the patient's chart. If using a paper chart, be sure to record on paper per office protocol. If using EMR, document the message in the message journal of the patient's chart and route to the appropriate person.

Refer to Procedure 9–1 for the steps to follow when performing telephone screening.

PROCEDURE 9–1 Perform a Telephone Screening

PURPOSE: Answer the telephone promptly and professionally, by the third ring, identifying yourself and the office

EQUIPMENT: Telephone, paper, pen, computer—if available

S SKILL: Perform a telephone screening.

Procedure Steps	Detailed Instructions and/or *Rationales*
1. Answer the phone promptly (by the third ring) in a polite and pleasant manner. Identify the office and yourself by name.	Your voice must be clear and distinct. Speak at a moderate rate, expressing consideration for the needs of the caller.
B 2. ***Apply active listening skills*** and correctly record the name and phone number of the caller, the reason for the call, and the date and time of the call.	Be sure to obtain the correct spelling, DOB, M/F, and pronunciation of the caller's name.
B 3. Before placing a caller on hold, determine whether the call is an emergency situation and, if so, process the call immediately, using the screening (triage) manual, ***demonstrating sensitivity appropriate to the message being delivered.***	
B 4. Use the telephone screening (triage) manual to ask the appropriate questions and document the patient's responses. (***Analyze communications in providing appropriate responses and feedback.***)	
B 5. If a caller must be placed on hold, try to check with him or her periodically to let him or her know you haven't forgotten about him or her, ***demonstrating empathy in communication with patients, family, and staff.***	
6. Accurately document the information in a message (paper or electronic) and route to provider with appropriate level of urgency.	
7. After screening and routing the call, sign off on message (paper or electronic) with final action taken.	
B 8. Complete all calls on hold in a timely manner. Screen and complete as many calls as possible before adding names to the provider's call-back list, ***implementing time management principles to maintain effective office function.***	

Interpreter Services

There are unique challenges for providers and health care facilities across the nation in meeting the cultural and language needs of their patient populations. Many health care facilities have systems to address patients' language needs (often referred to as interpreter services), such as noted in Figure 9–2, but often, systems to address patients' cultural needs are less defined. This might be attributable to a lack of resources; however, in some cases when resources are available, they are not being used or processes are not being followed. This is one reason accurate patient demographic data collection

USE OF INTERPRETERS: QUICK REFERENCE GUIDE

For the following situations a qualified employee interpreter (QEI), Tele-Interpreters, Interpreters Unlimited, or Interpreter Consulting Services, Inc. (CSI, sign language) must be used:

1. All informed consents*
2. Do Not Resuscitate process
3. Organ donation process
4. History and physicals
5. Explanation of diagnosis, plan for medical treatment, procedures for surgery
6. Family conferences
7. Discharge instructions
8. Extensive social worker interventions
9. Patient complaints
10. Patient requests requiring medical intervention
11. Medication instructions and possible side effects.
12. Legal issues (advance directives, guardianship, etc.)
13. Document restricting patient rights or benefits, e.g., Medicare denial letters.

*For orally translated forms, must use Tele-Interpreters, Interpreters Unlimited, or Interpreting and Consulting Services, Inc. (ICS, sign language), **NOT** a QEI.

Tele-Interpreters (Phone Service)

- Call 800-XXX-XXXX
- Give Access Code
- Give Tele-Interpreters operator campus/location and cost center where interpretation is being done. This is for trending use over time.

Interpreters Unlimited

- Call 800-XXX-XXXX to schedule.
- Provide campus, department, location, and your name for invoicing purposes.
- Complete Agency Interpreter Evaluation, Orientation Checklist and Confidentiality forms. Send completed forms to your Quality Management Department.
- An invoice is sent to department using the on-site interpreter.
- Department manager signs the invoice to verify use; adds the cost center where interpretation was done.
- Department manager sends the invoice to the Community Health Alliance for approval and payment.

Interpreting and Consulting Services, Inc. (ICS) – (American Sign Language)

- Call 800-XXX-XXX to schedule, ask for Interpreting Services. An answering service may take your name and an interpreter will call you back to schedule. You can also schedule on the website: www.[website].com.
- Provide campus, department, location, and your name for invoicing purposes.
- Complete Agency Interpreter Evaluation, orientation checklist and confidentiality forms. Send completed forms to your Quality Management Department.
- An invoice is sent to department using the on-site interpreter.
- Department manager signs the invoice to verify use; adds the cost center where interpretation was done.
- Department manger sends the invoice to the Community Health Alliance for approval and payment.

Qualified Employee Interpreters (QEI)

- Check to see if your medical practice has internal Qualified Employee Interpreters (QEI).
- Call the department director/supervisor to see if the employee (QEI) can be released.
- Employee uses the code for interpretation time on his or her time card.
- Requesting staff completes the Interpreter Evaluation form and sends to Human Resources Department.

Physicians: Physicians who are bilingual in the patient's preferred language may interpret for their patients and should document that they spoke to their patient in the patient's preferred language. Physicians are to use a Qualified Employee Interpreter, Tele-Interpreters, Interpreters Unlimited, or Interpreting and Consulting Services, Inc. (ICS) if they are not bilingual.

Figure 9–2: Use of Interpreters: Quick Reference Guide (example). *Delmar/Cengage Learning.* *(continues)*

Documentation Required: Whenever Interpreters are used, documentation shall be placed in the patient's medical record indicating:

a. The full name of the person who acted as the Interpreter and ID number if from an agency
b. The Interpreter's position, if an employee or physician
c. The Interpreter's agency, if appropriate
d. If the Interpreter is a family member, the relationship of the Interpreter to the patient and the reason why a QEI or agency interpreter did not interpret for the patient.

If the patient or patient's legal representative's preferred language is not one for which a vital document has been translated, the phone interpretation service shall be called to orally translate all the forms, e.g., consent forms for the patient/patient's legal representative. The staff member will include the document in the medical record and will record the following:

I have accurately and completely read the (document) to (Tele-Interpreter's ID# or name), a professional interpreter with Tele-Interpreters Inc. To the best of my knowledge the document was accurately translated into (identify language), the patient's or legal representative's primary language, that he/she understood the terms and conditions and acknowledged his/her agreement by signing the English document. (signed by nurse/physician)

Check with your manager to determine what Interpreter services your office or department has available. Your manager will be able to determine what forms need to be translated and in to which languages (different requirements for different states).

Figure 9–2: *(continued)*

is a priority as a tool to improve services to a diverse population.

Hospitals and providers should have policies in place regarding the provision of language services and should not rely on patients' friends, family, or other ad hoc interpreters. It is your responsibility to become familiar with your office policies regarding interpreter services: how to access language services, and how to work with an interpreter.

DOCUMENTING TELEPHONE CALLS

Documenting telephone messages is of vital importance and should be treated likewise. It is critical to record the date, time, name, date of birth, M/F, phone number(s), and detailed and accurate message along with your name or initials. All calls should be documented in the same manner; see Table 9–3 for items that must be documented and Figure 9–3 for an example. Urgent messages should be marked urgent and given to the doctor immediately. Be sure to pull the chart and have all relevant information to the call attached to the message (e.g., lab reports, test results, consults, prescription requests, and so on). If you are in an office using electronic messaging with EHR, attach the relevant information to the message to expedite care (Figure 9–4). All messages must be signed off (both paper and electronic) to confirm that final action has been taken. This usually entails that the last person to contact the patient shall sign off and file or save to chart and notify patient of action.

A telephone message pad (Figure 9–5) and pen should be placed by each office telephone. You cannot rely on memory in a busy office. Record the message using office protocol for office messaging (electronic or paper). Offices may choose to customize message templates to suit their individual needs best. Loose papers are not advised in patient charts. A date stamp may be used.

An electronic message template example might look like the one shown in Figure 9–6, with options for medication renewal, save to chart, subject (message type), patient name, caller name, phone number, and body for message. Electronic messages also often allow you to select a priority level, depending on the time sensitivity of the message.

TABLE 9–3 Key Elements When Recording a Phone Message to the Patient's Chart

- Caller's full name, spelled correctly, date of birth, M/F
- A detailed and accurate message indicating nature of the call
- If requesting prescription, include name and phone number of pharmacy, drug name, dosage, last refill date
- If requesting lab or test information (results), attach report to message
- Action required (attach to message or chart if available; if not available, state so)
- Date, time of call, initials of person receiving call
- Phone number of caller—including the area code if appropriate—and if OK to leave message (verify with CCP)

Date/time
Mr. Silvers called to let Dr. Lang know that his dentist, Dr. Edwin Blair, gave him an antibiotic, penicillin 500 mg, #32, 4x da, for 8 days, for an abscessed tooth.

Figure 9–3: Example of documenting a phone message in the patient's chart. *Delmar/Cengage Learning.*

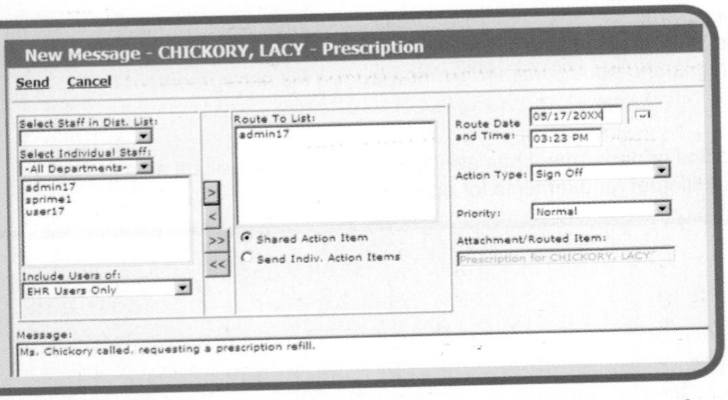

Figure 9–4: In an office with EHR, you can link relevant information to the patient's message to expedite care. *Courtesy of TriMed Technologies, Corp.*

Table 9–4 summarizes the basic guidelines for handling the telephone in the medical office.

Confidentiality and Returning Patient Messages

When returning patient messages, confidentiality in accordance with regulations established by Health Insurance Portability and Accountability Act of 1996 (HIPAA) is of primary concern. Data regarding patients may not be given out over the telephone to anyone unless the patient has give written permission for the release of specific information with a signature. This authorization is often given with a **signature. This authorization is often given with a Confidential Communication Preference (CCP)** (see Figure 9–7).

Recording Messages from Messaging Devices

Email, voice mail, pagers, and other answering devices make communications much more accessible than ever before. Internal EHR messaging, lab portals, and prescription refills can be available to doctors day and night, although replies to patients are not to be expected outside normal business hours.

Answering machines are useful for short periods such as during lunch time; however, answering services are more likely used outside office hours. The answering service can relay a message to the office by email, fax, or phone or contact the doctor by cell phone or pager if the

MESSAGE FROM								
For Dr	Name of Caller	Rel to Pt	Patient	Pt Age	Pt Temp	Message Date / /	Message Time AM PM	Urgent ❑ Yes ❑ No
Message:							Allergies	

Respond to Phone #	Best time to Call AM PM	Pharmacy Name / #	Patient's Chart Attached ❑ Yes ❑ No	Patient's Chart #	Initials
DOCTOR – STAFF RESPONSE					
Doctor's / Staff Orders / Follow-Up Action					

	Call Back ❑ Yes ❑ No	Chart Message ❑ Yes ❑ No	Follow–Up Date / /	Follow–Up Completed Date/Time / / AM/PM	Response by

Figure 9–5: A telephone message form. *Delmar/Cengage Learning.*

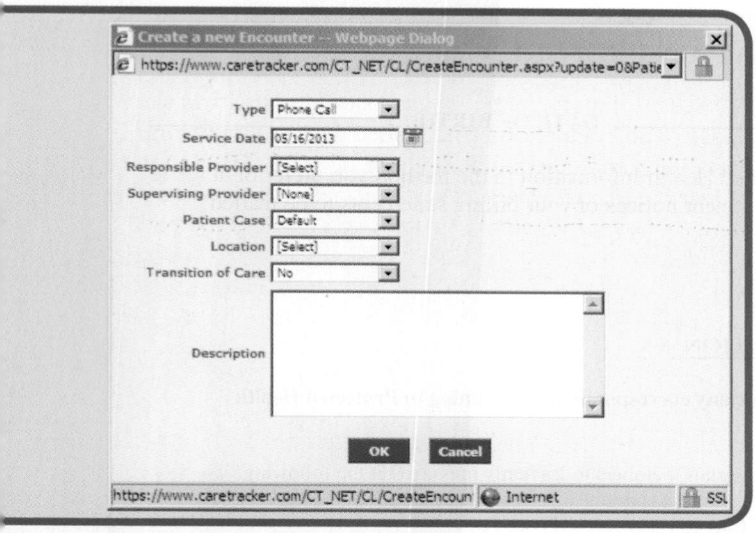

Figure 9–6: An electronic message template. *Courtesy of Ingenix CareTracker.*

call is determined to be an emergency or the doctor is on call. A method of informing the patient of how to reach the doctor must be available 365 days a year, which is why an answering service is often employed. Messages from the answering service need to be returned in the order of importance within an appropriate and reasonable time period. Remember to check the **fax** machine and **patient portal** for other patient-related messages. Refer to Procedure 9–2 for the steps to follow when obtaining telephone messages from a phone recording device or answering service. If available, use a headset and take your messages hands-free from the phone. This is a much more efficient way to take messages and ergonomically friendly to your neck and shoulders. You can then write or use your keyboard to take your messages as you talk with patients. Be sure to position your phone or headset properly to reduce noise and maximize clarity, as shown in Figure 9–8.

Phones, private branch exchange (PBX) systems, and EHR applications vary widely, so you should be honest about your knowledge and experience. Ask to have the features explained and demonstrated so you use the proper technique. Proper training will ensure that you are a valuable team member providing reliable, efficient customer service in a professional manner. Remember that the entries you make in a patient's chart are now part of a legal medical record.

TABLE 9–4 Guidelines for Handling the Provider's Telephone

1. Answer the telephone as promptly as possible, with a smile.
2. Keep a pad and pen next to the telephone at all times.
3. Verify the caller's name and correct spelling. If an adult calls about a child, make sure you have the correct last name and date of birth. Do not assume the child's last name is the same as the caller's name.
4. Determine the reason for the call.
5. Handle as many telephone calls as you possibly can without disturbing the provider. Provide message and documentation, including attaching the backup and chart when needed by the provider for review.
6. If the provider prefers to speak to a patient, call the provider to the telephone after asking who is calling. Pull the patient's chart and give it to the provider.
7. Whenever possible, if you cannot handle the call alone, take a message for the provider. The provider will tell you what to do or call the patient back as time allows.
8. Make a memorandum for the provider of every telephone call. Use printed telephone memorandum pads that show the date, time of call, name of caller, telephone number, date of birth, and sex and send the message (or electronic message in the EMR) to the provider.
9. Always know where to reach the provider. If the message is urgent and the provider is not in the office, page or telephone at once and relay the message.
10. If the provider cannot be reached, have the message by your phone. When your employer checks in, you may relay the message.
11. Learn how much medical information the provider wishes you to give over the telephone. Patients frequently call the office because they have forgotten the provider's instructions about treatments or medications. If these instructions are clearly stated in the chart, or in a preapproved triage manual, it might be possible for the assistant to repeat them to the patient.
12. When answering a second line, determine whether it is an emergency or another provider before placing the caller on hold and returning to finish the first call.
13. Allow the caller to say goodbye and to hang up first.

CONFIDENTIAL COMMUNICATION PREFERENCE

PLEASE PRINT

PATIENT NAME: ______________________________ **DATE OF BIRTH:** ____/____/____

You may request to receive confidential communications of Protected Health Information in the method you prefer or at an alternative address. For example, you may not want your appointment notices or your billing statements to be mailed to your home where it might be seen by others.

Please select all that applies. Sign and date below.

PROTECTED HEALTH INFORMATION

I. Laboratory, X-ray, test results, billing statements, and/or any correspondence pertaining to Protected Health Information (PHI).

I authorize Dr. / NP ______________________ or the staff members to leave my messages at the following:

☐ DO NOT LEAVE A MESSAGE OTHER THAN TO RETURN CALL.

☐ **Y** ☐ **N** Leave results on answering machine or voice mail

☐ **Y** ☐ **N** Home Phone ( ) ______________________

☐ **Y** ☐ **N** Work Phone ( ) ______________________

☐ **Y** ☐ **N** Cell Phone ( ) ______________________

☐ **Y** ☐ **N** Other Phone ( ) ______________________

☐ **Y** ☐ **N** Please mail my results to: ______________________

____

☐ **Y** ☐ **N** Other Person(s) authorized:

Name	**Phone #**	**Relationship**
	( )	
	( )	

II. Billing Statements and Correspondence:

Any correspondence related to your health information will be automatically mailed to your home address, unless indicated otherwise. Do you agree to this ☐ **Yes** ☐ **No** If No, please provide alternate address:

ADDRESS	CITY	STATE	ZIP CODE

III. Automated Reminder Calls:

We are currently utilizing a reminder service that places automated reminder calls. Disclosure of selected demographic information and date/time of your scheduled appointment are provided, in order to contact you as a reminder that you have an appointment for treatment or medical care at the listed entity. You have the right to request not to be contacted or change your request at any time to terminate this service.

☐ **YES** I wish to be reminded of my upcoming appointments using this automated reminder service.
☐ **NO** I do not wish to be reminded of my upcoming appointments using this automated reminder service.

Thank you for assisting us to serve you more effectively.

______________________ ____/____/____

Patient Signature (or Legal Representative) **Date**

FOR STAFF USE ONLY: ITS Notified Date ____/____/____ Staff Initials: ________

Figure 9–7: Confidential Communication Preference. *Delmar/Cengage Learning.*

PROCEDURE 9–2 Obtain a Telephone Message from a Phone Recording Device

PURPOSE: To obtain accurate message(s) from a recording device or answering service, obtaining all necessary information from the caller to process requests correctly.

EQUIPMENT: Telephone message device; pen; paper, phone message log, or computer; appropriate patients' charts

S SKILL: Obtain a telephone message from a recording device or outside answering service.

Procedure Steps	Detailed Instructions and/or *Rationales*
1. Assemble all necessary items in an area away from noise and distractions.	
B 2. Check the recording device or call the answering service and, ***using active listening skills***, write out each message accurately.	You might have to listen to the recording more than once to obtain complete information because some voices can be difficult to understand. It is a good practice to ask another staff member to listen if you have difficulty.
3. Check fax machine and office email for additional messages. Clarify any discrepancies in emails or faxes with the service.	*Sometimes answering services will send you an email message or a fax, which provides you with a hard copy that can be filed in or scanned to the patient's chart.*
4. Sign your initials after the message and ensure that you have written the date and time of the message.	
5. List all patients who leave messages so you can pull their charts.	
B 6. ***Prioritize messages according to the nature of their seriousness and distribute to the appropriate staff member, provider, or department to be processed.***	

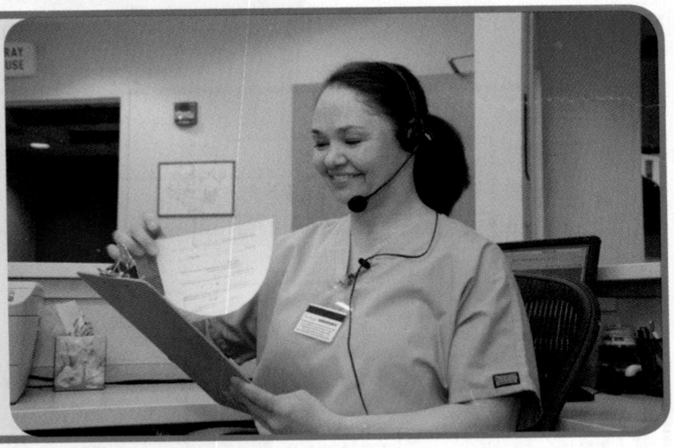

Figure 9–8: The medical assistant is using a headset to answer calls to free her hands to multitask by using the keyboard, taking messages, opening mail, and performing other office duties. *Delmar/Cengage Learning.*

If you have not seen by doc for 3 years, it becomes a new pat.

COMMON TYPES OF PHONE CALLS

Working in the medical office requires you to be aware of the most frequent types of phone calls received in the medical office. They are:

- Patients who are calling for appointments, prescriptions, or the results of tests
- Referrals
- Emergency calls
- Other providers, hospitals, or laboratories
- Personal calls and general business calls

Appointments

When scheduling appointments, positively identify the patient and confirm the last appointment date. Be sure to use at least two identifiers of the patient, including date of birth as well as last and first names. If you are working for a doctor with a closed practice (no longer accepting new patients), it is important to confirm that you are booking only current patients. Be sure you check with the doctor or office manager if there is a change in status or if the doctor will accept new patient referrals.

You must also assess the type of appointment needed and note in the schedule (e.g., Comprehensive Physical Exam [CPE], follow-up, immunization, new patient, and so on) because each type of appointment can carry a different billing code, require a different amount of time for the visit, and have different eligibility for insurance reimbursement. For example, a typical CPE will not be reimbursed by insurance if the appointment is less than one calendar year from the previous CPE appointment. Appointment schedule templates most often have time slots held for same-day or urgent visits (Figure 9-9). Use these appointments to book first from your phone calls of the day for patients requiring more immediate attention. Use your screening methods to determine which patients need to be seen in the same-day and urgent time slots. You will also want to book any open appointments slots in order during the day. (For instance, if you have three morning and two afternoon appointments open at the beginning of the day, fill your morning appointments first.)

Patients who phone for appointments should be given a choice of two appointment times. Usually, one of the two times will be satisfactory, and this will eliminate the patient's asking for multiple dates and times that are available. The appointment should be **confirmed** by reading the scheduled time back to the patient after it has been recorded in the appointment book or scheduling system. Frequently, medical offices place reminder calls to patients 24 to 48 hours in advance of appointments. See Table 9–5 for some helpful telephone scheduling tips. Scheduling is discussed further in Chapter 12.

Prescription Refills

Each office has its own rules for prescription refills. It is important for you to learn the rules of the office in which you work and follow them without exception. The general rule is that a medical assistant does not give out information or call in a prescription without the **express** direction of the provider. Write a message for the request for prescriptions in legible handwriting with detailed accuracy or document in the EMR. If a patient requests a prescription refill, you need to know the name and phone number of the pharmacy as well as the name of the medication, strength, and prescription number and when the prescription was last filled. Record the telephone number at which the patient can be reached in case the provider needs to talk with the patient before prescribing the medication. The provider might need to examine the patient first, in which case you would need to call and schedule an appointment.

Many prescription refill requests are now sent to the office by electronic messaging, known as easyscripts or surescripts (often referred to as e-scripts), directly from the pharmacy. In addition, patients may also request prescription refills through patient portals. EHR applications such as CareTracker from Ingenix (www.ingenix.com) or RelayHealth (www.relayhealth.com) offer patient portal capabilities.

It might be the office policy for prescription refill requests to be faxed (or sent electronically) from the pharmacy versus a request from the patient. It is important for you to be aware of and adhere to the office policies regarding prescription refill requests. Be certain to enter all the information accurately on the prescription refill, including the name of the medication, strength, number of refills, and dosage. Be sure all information is accurately entered into the patient's chart (whether paper or EMR) and that you have followed the express direction from the provider (see Figure 9–10). Upon completion, notify the patient that the prescription has been sent to the pharmacy so that the patient may pick up the medication.

TABLE 9–5 Telephone Scheduling Dos and Don'ts

Instead of saying ...	Say this ...
"When would you like to come in?"	"Do you prefer mornings or afternoons?"
"Are you a patient here?"	"When did we last see you?"
"What is the problem?"	"What is the reason for the visit?"

Test Results

Patients will call the office on a daily basis to request test results. Always observe your office policy for releasing results. Most providers will want to speak with the patient personally if the test results are abnormal, although some

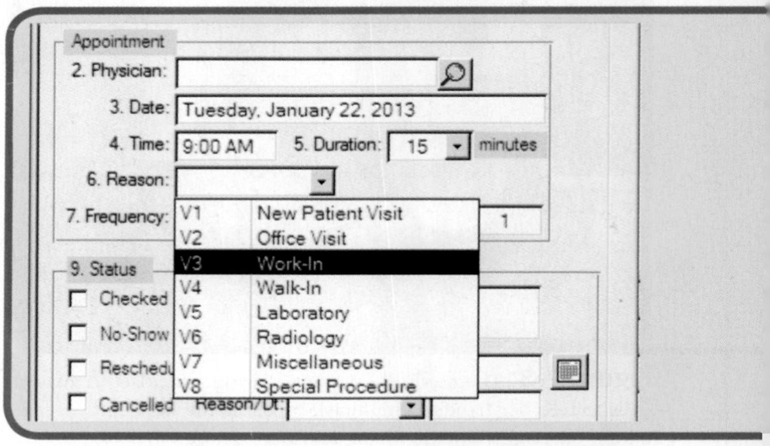

Figure 9–9: A patient appointment form template that allows Work-in and Walk-in appointment options. *Delmar/Cengage Learning.*

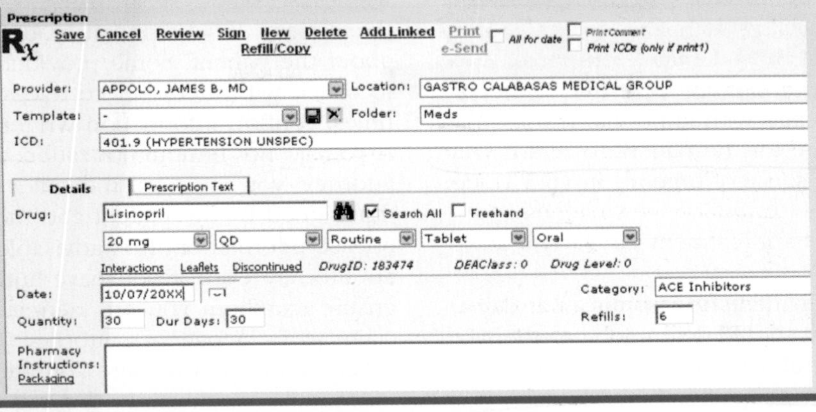

Figure 9–10: Prescription refill request in an EHR application. *Courtesy of TriMed Technologies, Corp.*

providers allow the medical assistant to give normal results over the telephone (see Procedure 9–3). Be sure to attach the results of the test, lab result, or consult report for the provider to review along with the message for the provider to call the patient. To ensure quality care, all lab reports, tests, consult reports, and outside testing received should go first to the provider for review and signoff, known as validation, prior to being filed

PROCEDURE 9–3 Telephone a Patient with Test Results

PURPOSE: Using the necessary equipment, follow all the steps in the procedure and inform the patient about laboratory or other test results. Protect PHI (protected health information) according to HIPAA and document the call.

EQUIPMENT: Patient's chart (paper chart or EMR), telephone, lab results, pen

S **SKILL:** Telephone a patient with test results, observing HIPAA regulations and following the instructions of the provider.

Procedure Steps	Detailed Instructions and/or *Rationales*
1. Obtain patient's chart, with test results attached, from the provider (with instructions on message to patients).	*The provider must review all test results before they can be released to the patient. Do not release any results that have not been initialed (validated) by the provider.*
2. Check the patient's chart for the signed privacy notice (CCP) to determine who may receive the information.	Be sure to check the signed notice to determine whether it is permissible to leave information on an answering machine.
3. Telephone the patient, identifying yourself and the office.	
4. Identify the person you are speaking to.	Information can be given only to the patient or to persons authorized by the patient to receive PHI.
B 5. Inform the patient about test results and any instructions from the provider. ***Demonstrate empathy in communication with patients, family, and staff.***	
B 6. Ask the patient to repeat the results to be sure he or she has the correct information, ***demonstrating recognition of the patient's level of understanding.*** Instruct the patient to call the office with any questions.	
7. Allow the patient to hang up first.	*Allowing the patient to hang up first eliminates the possibility of missing a question or statement from the patient.*
8. Document the call in the patient's chart.	

or scanned into the patient's chart. Always review the patient's CCP prior to calling with any results to confirm which number to call and authorization to leave messages or speak with other parties. It is generally best not to leave a message with abnormal results. You should leave the message for the patient to return your call, without revealing a sense of urgency in your voice.

Follow-up Calls

Often, providers advise patients to call the next day to report their progress. You should determine whether you are to take the call and relay the message to the doctor (always record the patient's report in his or her chart) or if the provider wishes to speak directly to the patient. It is also a good practice to check with the provider to see whether you should contact the patient if you do not receive the follow-up call from the patient by a predetermined time. Make sure you have the current home, cell phone, pager, or work number(s) before the patient leaves your office so that you will be able to call back if necessary. It is also a good practice to make sure that the patient's chart has a current phone number of a relative or friend if the the patient cannot be contacted.

Professional Calls

When a doctor telephones to speak to your provider, politely ask the caller for his or her name and inform the provider. Professional **etiquette** dictates that the provider will not keep a colleague waiting unless the provider is involved with an emergency or surgical procedure. Be sure to ask whether the call is regarding a patient and whether you should pull the chart. This is an example of anticipating the needs of your provider. It is also wise to obtain the name and phone number of the caller in case the call is disconnected.

Calls received in your office regarding X-ray or laboratory results need to be recorded with precise accuracy. Always record the name of the person giving the report and the phone number in case your doctor wants to call back for further information. It is best to read back everything you have written down to be sure it is correct and complete before allowing the caller to leave the line. Attach the message along with the patient's chart for review by your doctor.

Business, Personal, and Legal Calls

Your provider should let you know how to handle calls from family members, business associates, and salespeople. Calls from attorneys requesting information about a patient must be handled with great caution. Attorneys know that patients must give written permission to divulge information to anyone regarding their health, yet attorneys will call and ask for information. Pull the patient chart and look for authorization listing the name of the attorney and the signature of the patient. If you find it, you may answer questions about the patient. Some providers might still want you to check with them before releasing information. At all times, confirm information written on the patient's CCP. If you do not find authorization listing the name of the attorney, you must tell the caller to send an authorization signed by the patient and then you will be able to release information. It is advisable to return a call from an attorney even if you have authorization so you can ensure to whom you are talking. Anyone can call and claim to be a patient's attorney. Unless you know the caller, you cannot be sure you are talking to the correct individual. You must also be aware of office policy and your provider's preference. Most providers prefer to be advised of requests from attorneys. In addition, a quality department review might be required prior to release of patient information.

Only information that has been authorized by the patient in writing, with the patient signature, may be given to another party. Otherwise, the patient record is considered confidential information, and you can be liable for your actions. Follow the office and organizational quality department protocols. Be sure to record the call and information released by telephone or copied for attorneys or other parties from patient charts. Patients have the right to know who has accessed their medical information, and their charts should reflect each and every release of information.

Common practice is for medical assistants to refer business or legal calls to the office manager. Check with your provider or employer regarding the policy.

Long-Distance Calls

You might need to place long-distance calls. If you are calling an area outside of your time zone, you should consult the telephone directory for the map of time zones (Figure 9–11) so you can establish the appropriate time to call. Take into consideration when it is lunch break in a different time zone so that you do not waste time trying to phone an office when the staff is not available to take your call. Be sure you know the code needed to dial for your long-distance service in addition to the telephone numbers of the persons you need to call. A record book should be kept on all long-distance calls.

DIFFICULT CALLERS

As a medical assistant, there are times you encounter difficult callers. When patients make demands by asking for something that is unreasonable and difficult to provide, your first reaction can be annoyance. The best approach is to hold off any negative judgments and try your best to accommodate the requests.

If the caller is cursing, give the caller the benefit of the doubt and politely say "I really want to help you,

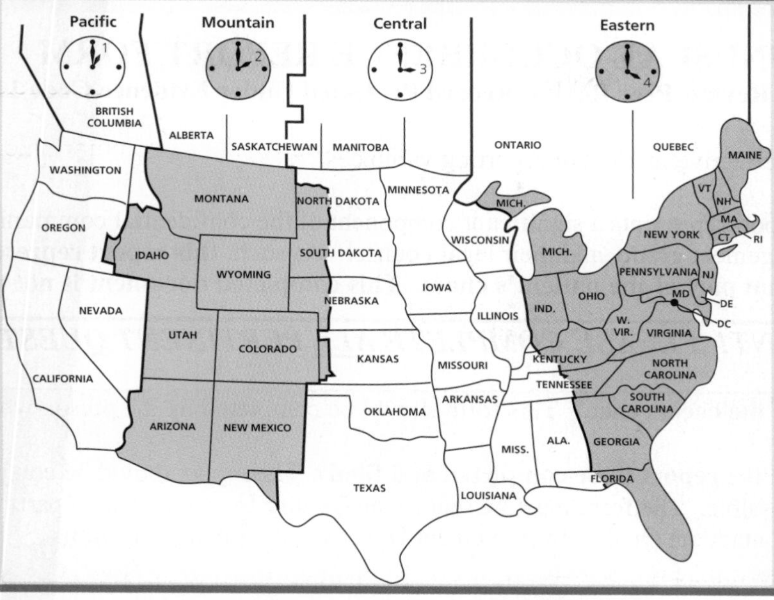

Figure 9–11: Refer to a time zone map when placing long distance calls. *Delmar/Cengage Learning.*

but I'm having trouble with the kind of language you are using. Can you please refrain from using that kind of language?" Give the caller a second chance and another warning if the language persists. If this does not work, let the caller know that you are no longer the person who can help and inform your supervisor of the problem. If a caller makes are any threats, document the identity of the caller, the nature of the threat, advise you are no longer the person who can help, and inform your supervisor. End the call in a professional manner.

If a caller makes any threats, you must document the details of the call, notify your supervisor or provider, and, if deemed appropriate, contact the police department. Most medical offices will have you (or your supervisor) complete a document called an Unusual Occurrence Report (UOR, see Figure 9–12) which is then forwarded to the quality department for review or action. Careful and accurate documentation is required in circumstances surrounding a threat or complaint.

TELEPHONE SERVICES

Phone Menus

Most business phone systems have a menu for the caller to be connected to the proper person or department. By pushing the correct number as directed by the recorded message (e.g., "Press one to reach the billing department, press two to speak to the scheduling department, press three for prescription refills"), the caller can be connected to the desired party. The system is designed to be more efficient, route to the proper person or department, prevent the caller from being disconnected, or be kept on hold too long. The caller should be instructed at the beginning of the recording to immediately hang up and call 911 or EMS (as applicable to caller's geographical area) if there is a medical emergency.

Conference Calls

The telephone can be used to simultaneously conduct conversations with several people in various locations at the same time. This allows business to be conducted, meetings to occur, and professional or personal communication to be carried out. Conference calling saves time, travel, and money—all important in managing practice expenses. If your phone system is not equipped to allow multiple connections, conference calls may be arranged with your local phone service provider.

Teleconferencing

Teleconferencing is a means of exchanging information much like a conference call, except everyone can see and hear each other at the same time. All are linked by way of telecommunications equipment. There are cameras, speaker phones, connection devices, and television or computer monitors in each location. The phone company for the meeting originator will contact all other sites and network the phones. With the aid of the phone, camera, and monitors, participants can see and talk to each other. A teleconference can involve several people in many locations. Ideas can be presented, concerns expressed, and new techniques shown; teleconferencing is the next best thing to actually being together in a meeting, yet it conserves travel time and expense.

UNUSUAL OCCURRENCE REPORT FORM

Quality Review/Peer Review Record Protected Under Evidence Code 1157

Purpose: To provide an effective method of reporting variances.

Confidentiality: This report represents a significant component of the confidential communication between physicians, nurses, management group, and their legal counsel. As such, **this report represents privileged communication and is not part of the patient's chart. This completed document is not to be photocopied**.

IMPORTANT! PLEASE COMPLETE ALL PERTINENT QUESTIONS!

- **Who should report the occurrence?** This form should be completed by the person who has knowledge of the occurrence.
- **When and where is the report to be completed and filed?** The report should be completed as soon after the occurrence as possible. The form must be sent to the Quality Improvement Department within 24 hours after occurrence. Contact the Quality Improvement Department with any questions.

- **Name and Position of Staff member involved**__________
- **Date and time of event:**__________

1. **Patient's Name:** __________ (M) (F)
   Address:__________
   Diagnosis:__________ DOB:__________
   Attending physician:__________ PCP:__________
   HMO: ☐ Yes ☐ No
   Health Plan:__________ ID#:__________

2. **Location of event:**
   ☐ Office (Name of practice)__________
   ☐ Hospital (Name of hospital)__________
   ☐ Other__________

3. **Patient factors prior to event:**

☐ alert	☐ intoxicated	☐ uncooperative	☐ developmentally disabled
☐ confused	☐ medications	☐ suicidal	☐ depressed
☐ agitated	☐ sedated	☐ unconscious	☐ anesthetized

4. **Categories of event:**

☐ **Falls**:	☐ ambulating	☐ from bed/table	☐ other	
☐ **Medications**:	☐ missing	☐ given	☐ omitted	☐ extra dose
	☐ time variance	☐ wrong route	☐ wrong dose	☐ wrong Rx
	☐ wrong patient	☐ Rx filled incorrectly	☐ other	

Figure 9–12: Unusual Occurrence Report. *Delmar/Cengage Learning.*

☐ **Procedure/Treatment:** ☐ wrong patient ☐ lost specimen ☐ procedure omitted ☐ procedure delayed ☐ other ☐ orders not carried out ☐ no consent signed ☐ radiation exposure ☐ technique ☐ NPO violated

☐ **Equipment:** ☐ shock ☐ not available ☐ improper use ☐ mechanical prob. ☐ other
Equipment name:________________
Manufacturer:________________ Serial #:________________

☐ **Safety/Security:** ☐ damage to property ☐ HIPAA/Privacy ☐ lost/stolen property ☐ unauthorized presence ☐ wet floor ☐ drug count variance ☐ drug tampering ☐ drug key variance ☐ fire ☐ other

5. Written description of the event: (attach additional sheet if necessary)
____
____

6. Additional persons involved: Patient/Staff/Visitor
Name: ________________ Name: ________________
Address: ________________ Address: ________________
Phone #: ________________ Phone #: ________________

7. Review:
1. Does medical record adequately reflect event? ☐ Yes ☐ No
2. Patient's status
   a. Pre-event: ________________ b. Post-event: ________________
3. Effect/Outcome: ☐unknown ☐deficit
   (comment)________________
   ☐ increased LOS ☐ death ☐ additional tx required (comment)________________

8. Action taken: ☐ Refer for medical review ☐ Administrative review ☐ Notify carrier

9. Corrective action taken: (Attach policy and procedure affected)
____
____

10. Procedures followed:
☐ MD/Attending notified Time notified: ________ By whom: ________
☐ Medical records secured ☐ Original x-rays secured ☐ Lab/path. Secured

11. Family/Patient attitude after event:
☐ unaware ☐ angry ☐ understanding ☐ cooperative ☐ belligerent ☐ threaten law suit

Additional information:________________
Prepared by: ________________ Title: ________________
Signature: ________________ Date: ________________
Site Manager/Supervisor: ________________ Date: ________________

Figure 9–12: *(continued)*

COMMUNITY RESOURCES

It is a good idea to keep an up-to-date index of your most frequently called numbers by the telephone, as well as resources for patients and emergency preparedness (see Figure 9–13 and Procedures 9–4 and 9–5). Review Table 9–6 for a list of some of the frequently called numbers in a medical office. You will be able to locate these resources through such means as office

COMMUNITY RESOURCE	SERVICES PROVIDED	CONTACT INFORMATION
CDC	Vaccine Information; Travel advisories; Current health related information.	(xxx) xxx-xxxx
Child Protective Services	Services, information, and reporting protection for minors.	(xxx) xxx-xxxx
Home Health	Patient services in home setting such as postoperative, diabetes care.	(xxx) xxx-xxxx
Senior Services	Patient services to seniors, including diabetes education and monitoring, blood pressure screening.	(xxx) xxx-xxxx

Figure 9–13A: Community resources for patient health care needs (examples). *Delmar/Cengage Learning.*

COMMUNITY RESOURCE	CONTACT INFORMATION
Centers for Disease Control and Prevention (CDC)	**www.cdc.gov** Centers for Disease Control and Prevention, 1600 Clifton Rd, Atlanta, GA 30333, U.S.A. 800-CDC-INFO (800-232-4636) TTY: (888) 232-6348, 24 Hours/Every Day cdcinfo@cdc.gov
Medical Reserve Corps	**Office of the Civilian Volunteer Medical Reserve Corps** Office of the Surgeon General U.S. Department of Health and Human Services 5600 Fishers Lane, Room 18C-14 Rockville, MD 20857 Telephone: (301) 443-4951 Fax: (301) 480-1163 **www.medicalreservecorps.gov**
Police Department	Call 911 for emergency Call (xxx) xxx-xxxx (local number) for non-emergency business

Figure 9–13B: Community resources for emergency preparedness (examples). *Delmar/Cengage Learning.*

PROCEDURE 9–4 Create a List of Resources for Patient Health Care Needs

PURPOSE: Use research tools and techniques to create a list of community resources related to patients' health care needs

EQUIPMENT: Computer with Internet access, telephone directory, and local hospital directory

S SKILL: Create a list of resources for patient health care needs.

Procedure Steps	Detailed Instructions and/or *Rationales*
1. Assemble required items (telephone, telephone book, pen, paper, computer with Internet access).	
2. Using the telephone book and Internet, research the community resources available in your area, create a list of available health care resources, and identify the services provided by each.	You might have to use more than one search engine and verify resources for accuracy.
3. Verify the information with a follow-up telephone call to the community resource for most current information to be documented.	*Information might be outdated;, you want to include the most current information available and update periodically.*

Procedure Steps	Detailed Instructions and/or *Rationales*
4. Create a list in a spreadsheet format (using Microsoft Excel or Word, for instance). In the spreadsheet, identify the communication resource(s), services provided, and contact information.	
5. Print the resource document.	Refer to Figure 9–13A as an example.

PROCEDURE 9–5 Create a List of Resources for Emergency Preparedness

PURPOSE: Use research tools and techniques to create a list of community resources for emergency preparedness

EQUIPMENT: Computer with Internet access, telephone directory, and local hospital directory

S SKILL: Create a list of community resources for emergency preparedness.

Procedure Steps	Detailed Instructions and/or *Rationales*
1. Assemble required items (telephone, telephone book, pen, paper, computer with Internet access).	
2. Using the telephone book and Internet, research community resources available in your area; create a list of community resources for emergency preparedness.	You might have to use more than one search engine and verify resources for accuracy.
3. Verify the information with a follow-up telephone call to the resource.	*Contact information (telephone numbers, Websites, etc.) might be outdated; you need to have the most current resource information available.*
4. Create the list in a spreadsheet format (Microsoft Excel or Word). In the spreadsheet, identify the community resource for emergency preparedness, services provided, and contact information (Website address, physical address, telephone and fax numbers).	
5. Print the resource document.	Refer to Figure 9–13B as an example.

TABLE 9–6 Frequently Called Numbers (Partial List)

911	Insurance companies	Answering services
Local hospital(s)	Referrals and authorizations department	Office manager
Ambulance/Patient transport systems	Provider specialists	Pager/cell phone for provider
Lab services	Home health	Quality department; HR department
IT department	Senior services	Office extensions
Pharmacies		

materials and directories, the Internet, intranet, and telephone book. Use Internet portals for access to telephone numbers and addresses to research available additional community resources, for both patient health services and emergency preparedness. (See Table 9–7 and Table 9–8 for sample lists. Please note that these are just a sampling of numbers that might be helpful, not a complete list.) This can be a good tool for researching not only local resources but also state and federal resources such as the CDC, Medicare, and Department of Motor Vehicles (DMV). You may also use such sources as the Yellow Pages (www.yellowpages.com) and MapQuest (www.mapquest.com). Using these search engines can often cut down on your research time and give you options if looking for multiple sites and locations. Be sure always to have a copy of the most current telephone book, as well as the current directory for the local emergency clinics, hospitals, providers (in network), and specialists, on hand in the office, and be sure to verify the current information.

TABLE 9–7 Community Resources for Patient Health Care Needs (Partial List)

Senior services	Osteoporosis centers	Child Protective Services
Home health services	Research department	Emergency Medical Services
Lab services and locations	DMV	Education and training services
Diabetes programs	CDC (including vaccine information, travel advisories, etc.)	Public health services
Women's health centers		

TABLE 9–8 Community Resources for Emergency Preparedness (Partial List)

Medical Reserve Corps	CDC	Ambulance/patient transport companies
American Medical Association (AMA)	Fire department	Local hospital directory of contact information
OSHA	Police department	

CHAPTER SUMMARY

- Answer the phone with a greeting and then state the medical office name and your name; for example, "Good morning, Central Medical Center, Ellen speaking, how may I help you?" Answer calls as soon as possible, at least by the third ring, and with a smile on your face.
- Sometimes referred to as "triage," telephone screening is a method to determine the nature of the call, accurately describe patient symptoms, and determine level of urgency, using standard questions and standard responses in a template form that has been pre-authorized by the provider. The medical assistant is responsible for routing incoming calls, which is the act of transferring the call or routing the message to the appropriate person, with the required level of urgency, following patient privacy (HIPAA) guidelines and office procedure.
- Document the following information in each telephone message: date, time, patient (caller) name (verify spelling), DOB, M/F, call-back phone number(s), information requested or to be relayed (including symptoms from screening template), and your name (or initials).
- Typical calls the MA receives or places in the medical office include patients calling for appointments, prescriptions, or test results; referrals; emergency calls; other providers, hospitals, or laboratories; and personal calls and general business calls.
- Keep an up-to-date index of your most frequently called numbers, as well as resources for patient health care needs and emergency preparedness, by the telephone.

STUDY TOOLS

Workbook	Activities for Chapter 9
Premium Website MEDIA LINK StudyWARE	View this **Media Link** for Chapter 9: • Telephone Personality
	Activities and Quizzes on the **StudyWARE™ Software** for Chapter 9
	Audio Library of medical terms
	Online access to the **Critical Thinking Challenge 2.0**
CourseMate	Activities and Quizzes for Chapter 9
WebTutor	Activities and Quizzes for Chapter 9

CHECK YOUR KNOWLEDGE

1. Which of the following is NOT considered a guideline (protocol) for answering the telephone in the medical office?
   a. Answer the telephone as promptly as possible, with a smile.
   b. Put the caller on hold as quickly as possible.
   c. Handle as many telephone calls as you possibly can without disturbing the provider. Provide message and documentation, including attaching the call-back number and chart when needed by the provider for review.
   d. Document only the important calls.
   e. None of the above
   f. b and d
2. Identify methods of screening and routing incoming calls.
   a. Determine nature of call.
   b. Accurately describe patient symptoms.
   c. Determine level of urgency.
   d. Use standard questions and respond in a template form pre-authorized by the provider.
   e. All of the above
   f. b and c only
3. Which of the following is incorrect when documenting a telephone message?
   a. Record nature of call only if urgent message
   b. Caller's full name
   c. Date of birth
   d. M/F (sex)
   e. Date and time of call
4. Which types of telephone calls will a medical assistant have to answer in the medical office?
   a. Appointments
   b. Prescription refills
   c. Follow-up calls
   d. Difficult calls
   e. All of the above
   f. a, b, and d
5. Which of the following describe the types of community resources for patients' health care needs?
   a. Senior services
   b. Lab services and locations
   c. Occupational Health and Safety Administration
   d. Police department
   e. All of the above
   f. a and b only

WEB LINKS

Centers for Disease Control and Prevention: www.cdc.gov

Joint Commission: www.jointcommission.org

MapQuest: www.mapquest.com

Medical Reserve Corps: www.medicalreservecorp.gov

Ingenix: www.ingenix.com

Relay Health: www.relayhealth.com

United States Postal Service: www.usps.com

Confidentiality Education Group (CEG): www.cc.nih.gov/ccc/ceg/info.html

Webopedia: www.webopedia.com

Yellow Pages: www.yellowpages.com

Chapter

10 Written Communication

OBJECTIVES

In this chapter, you will learn the following:

KB KNOWLEDGE BASE

1. Spell and define, using the glossary at the back of the text, all the Words to Know in this chapter.
2. List seven types of correspondence used in the medical office and identify when each is used.
3. Name instances when form letters and templates may be indicated.
4. Explain the purpose of information sheets.
5. List the pros and cons of using email.
6. List three precautions to take to avoid acquiring a virus through email.
7. Explain how HIPAA affects correspondence.
8. Recognize elements of fundamental writing skills, including spelling, parts of speech, sentence structure, punctuation, capitalization, and treatment of numbers.
9. Name and describe the 12 components of a business letter.
10. Identify three letter styles.
11. Explain how to sort, open, and annotate incoming mail.
12. List six classifications of mail.
13. Explain the purpose of the following: certificate of mailing, certified mail, restricted delivery, return receipt.

S SKILLS

1. Compose a business letter and prepare it for mailing.

WORDS TO KNOW

adjective	conjunction	etiquette	punctuation
adverb	context	hyphen	stationery
annotate	contraction	master	template
apostrophe	correspondence	noun	verb
clause	domestic	postscript	watermark
compose	ellipsis	proofread	word processor

CORRESPONDENCE IN THE MEDICAL OFFICE

Communication as previously defined is "the exchange of thoughts, messages, or information by speech, signals, writing, or behavior" (*Webster's New Dictionary*). In its broader sense, correspondence can be thought of as any exchange of information between persons. There are many forms of communication, such as talking, gesturing, or writing. Written communication is often called **correspondence**. Correspondence or written communication in the medical office can include sending notes; interoffice communications (IOCs); email; information recorded to the patient's chart; form letters; information sheets; and business, professional, and personal letters. In a physician's office, written communication is used:

- To inform the staff officially of a policy or decision.
- To inform patients or customers of a policy or decision.
- To contact professional colleagues.
- To correspond with professional associations.
- To respond to or request a medical consultation.
- To engage in business communications with medical suppliers, financial consultants, attorneys, and insurance companies.
- To send a message regarding a patient (by written message, EHR, patient portal, or email).
- To send personal messages.

Interoffice Communication

IOC is an informal, memo-style communication that is usually specific to one concern. It is an effective way of being certain that everyone is aware of some event, policy, concern, and other internal communication, circulated electronically (email) or by copy of a memo.

Informal Notes

Informal notes would be indicated for times when thanks, congratulations, or similar expressions are desired. Usually, these are personal and informal in nature. Often, they are written on a first-name basis.

Personal Letters

The physician might ask for assistance with personal correspondence. It is common for medical assistants to correspond with travel agencies, mail order catalogs, uniform or clothing suppliers, and specialty shops. You should be able to **compose** (write) the necessary letter after receiving the specific information desired so all the provider has to do is provide a signature.

Professional Letters

Providers might need to write to their professional associations, licensing boards, and other physicians regarding some issue or concern affecting personal medical activities or their professional practice. Perhaps your employer holds an office in a medical society that requires communicating with the members or issuing the group's opinion on a particular subject to the community or media. Some providers hold office on a hospital medical board, which might necessitate issuing written communication. Providers who participate in research do a great deal of professional correspondence regarding the experimental studies being conducted. Some providers enjoy writing professional journal articles about a unique patient or explaining a procedure they have developed. Obviously, these specific writings require detailed dictation and perfect transcription.

Some professional letters might not be very detailed. Suppose your employer wrote a medical journal article about a new method of treatment he has developed that has proved very successful. The medical association planning committee is scheduling presenters for its next convention. Your employer has received a request to make a presentation about his new treatment at the convention and asks you to write a response for his signature. In preparation for this task, you and the provider refer to the office calendar and his personal schedule. He discovers that he and his family have scheduled a vacation to begin the day after the conference closes, but he could make the presentation at the beginning of the meeting. You confer with the office scheduler to block off the additional days. Refer to Procedure 10–1 for guidelines to compose a response to a communication.

Form Letters and Templates

The greatest amount of correspondence, aside from documenting in a patient's chart, is of the business type required to manage the affairs of the practice. This would include referrals, consultations, annual examination reminders, collection letters, school and work releases, suppliers of equipment and materials, and other correspondence necessary to the office operation. These types of correspondence can be individually composed, or prewritten form letters and **templates** may be used.

Form letters are especially well suited for:

- Return-to-work or school approvals (following surgery or illness).
- Annual diagnostic examination reminders (CPEs, eye examinations, Pap tests, mammograms, sigmoidoscopies).
- Delinquent account reminders, usually in about three increasing levels of request intensity.

- Noncompliance, missed appointments, and dismissal from practice.
- Office visit verifications (for work or school absence).
- Athletic participation approvals.
- Information to referred patients such as appointment confirmation, office location, information needed, and examination preparation.

Prewritten form letters can be developed and stored electronically on computers. When needed, the letter is pulled up; the appropriate date, name, address, amount due if a collection letter, and relevant information is added. It is then printed without the need to prepare the total letter. The **master** of each hardcopy form letter is stored electronically and in a file folder. Copies are made as needed. Specific information appropriate to the recipient is entered in the blank areas. Be sure to check the patient's chart for a signed form to release information and be certain there are no restrictions about where or to whom information can be sent.

A template is an electronic file (or preprinted document) with a predesigned, customized format. Examples of templates are fax cover sheets or patient information letters, ready to be filled in. Your **word processing** program (such as Microsoft Word) has numerous built-in templates. Explore these to create documents you will use frequently. In addition, you can use the mail merge feature to send the same letter to multiple recipients.

Information Sheets

Information sheets provide specific written instructions regarding the examinations and diagnostic tests performed in your office. They help reinforce what you have explained and serve as a reminder after the patient leaves the office. Cast care and fever control are examples of types of information sheets that can be provided. They also typically explain to patients how to prepare themselves for a particular test or what to expect when the test is performed. Usually, there is a place on the form to enter the date and time the examination is scheduled. Information sheets can be prepared and stored in the files to be used as needed and are an excellent example of patient education material.

Email

Email allows for the almost instant exchange of information. In addition, the advantage of transmitting written material makes it appropriate for transferring reports, documents, correspondence, and most forms of written communication. Not only can material from one computer be sent to another, but material can also be scanned from other sources and sent over the Internet.

When you receive communication, you can open your email and read the information. If you wish to save it, it can be printed out or saved electronically. Be cautious of emails that might contain viruses. To comply with patient privacy and Health Insurance Portability and Accountability Act (HIPAA) guidelines, all electronic communications, including email, must provide security measures such as restricted user access, encryption, and passwords.

The instantaneous nature of email makes it a popular method of communicating in business settings. With the advantages come some disadvantages, including some challenges regarding privacy issues. Some pros and cons of using email need to be addressed:

- *Pros:* Email is a powerful tool, enabling us to communicate at times without picking up the phone or, worse, getting on a plane. It provides round-the-clock convenience and service, reducing costs and increasing productivity at work.
- *Cons:* Email communications are far more likely to be misinterpreted than if you were to have those same communications face to face.

Review Table 10–1 for more pros and cons.

TABLE 10–1 Pros and Cons of Using Email

Pros	Cons
It enables communication with many people by sending the same email to multiple recipients simultaneously.	It isn't the best medium for communicating certain emotional or highly charged issues.
It leaves a trail, so the history of a conversation can be traced.	It is often overused as a substitute for phone and in-person communication.
It provides an easy reference to past communications.	It isn't as secure, private, and confidential as people think.
It doesn't require customers (patients) to be available to send them a message.	It can be used in a court of law as evidence and increases company liability risk.
It saves time when you need to communicate but don't have time for small talk.	It can be problematic when dealing with time-sensitive issues that require immediate responses.
It enables you to attach pertinent files without the delay of other mail delivery systems.	

As with other forms of communication, the content of email messages reflects on their author. Therefore, you must send articulate, accurate messages. It requires an established **etiquette** that helps ensure that good manners are the rule rather than the exception in cyberspace:

- Emoticons are icons that express emotions, such as ☺ or ☹, but should not be used in the professional setting.
- Abbreviations such as FYI, FAQ, and BTW are popular in email, but should be used sparingly in the professional setting (avoid text message–style writing).
- Don't overuse cc.
- Always review your email before sending!

Show consideration for other people by asking "How would I feel if I received this message?" Respect readers' time by keeping messages clear and concise, but be sure to provide enough information for readers to understand what is being said or requested. Good emails are to the point but not so short that they create the impression of being rudely curt. Most people lean toward being one or the other—being an over-communicator or an under-communicator. Other considerations:

- *Ownership and intellectual property:* Whose email is it? The Electronic Communications Privacy Act ruled that internal emails are the property of the company that pays for the email system, thereby giving the company the right to search your mailbox. EXAMPLE: Do not copy or forward company policy, procedural files, or information owned by the organization.
- *Privacy:* Emails can be sent or forwarded by accident or without knowledge or permission. EXAMPLE: Do not copy or forward information owned by the organization; especially be mindful of never emailing a patient's information without the express written consent of the party and verification of the recipient.
- *Legal considerations:* E-mails can be recovered (even deleted ones) and used for evidence in civil and criminal court cases. EXAMPLE: Simply deleting an email that has negative connotations does not protect you (or the organization) from its being recovered and used in a legal proceeding. Be very cautious about the nature of the email because it creates a permanent record of the matter.
- *Freedom of speech:* Carefully consider what you say in email to avoid later regrets and possibly having to defend yourself. EXAMPLE: Avoid sending an email when you are upset; once sent, you cannot retrieve those thoughts. You might have the right to say what is on your mind, but there can be repercussions from your actions.

Email and Computer Viruses

With the increased use and dependence on the Internet for communication and information gathering, you need to be aware of the very real threat that computer viruses pose. A virus is information sent electronically to interfere with or destroy your electronic files. You must be especially careful with the use of email. The following rules can help keep your computer virus-free:

1. Before opening an email, look at the subject and who sent it. If you receive an email from an unfamiliar source or with a suspicious subject (e.g., the subject is out of character with what you would expect to receive from the sender), do not open it! Delete and purge the suspicious email immediately.
2. Never open an executable or script file (files with .exe or .vbs suffixes) unless you are expecting to receive such a file from the sender. Opening these types of files is particularly dangerous because they can cause any number of actions, ranging from sending an email to everyone in your address book to completely erasing the contents of your hard drive.
3. Use antivirus software to scan emails before opening them (either through your email server or from your local mail application). Keep in mind that this is not entirely effective because new viruses are being created and deployed continuously and might not be detectable even if you have the most up-to-date virus database.

More information about protecting your computer from viruses is discussed in Chapter 11.

COMMUNICATION AND HIPAA REGULATIONS

Communications that include personal information about patients require specific handling. You must employ effective written communication skills adhering to ethics and laws of confidentiality. With the enactment of HIPAA, rules about the security of patients' personal health information (PHI) as contained in medical records were identified. Care must be taken to protect the integrity of the information and prevent disclosure to entities that are not directly involved with the provision of health care. Most physicians have developed specific release of information forms that follow HIPAA guidelines. Patients are requested to sign these forms giving permission for providers to communicate personal information. Some instances would be:

- Patient personal use.
- Life insurance questionnaire.
- Disability insurance questionnaire.

A release form is not required when releasing information pertaining to the patients' care. Some examples of instances would be:

- To request a consultation from a specialist.
- To provide results to the referring physician from a specialist.
- To provide information to a hospital or nursing care facility.
- To an insurance company for payment of services.

The patient is provided with a written statement from the provider's practice that explains its adherence to the HIPAA regulations regarding his or her personal information. Patients are asked to sign a form indicating that they have received a copy of this document. This is often referred to as a Notice of Privacy Practices (NOPP).

Procedures must be in place to comply with HIPAA and protect the privacy of patient information with electronic applications (email and EHR). Security measures must include encryption, firewall software and hardware, personnel passwords, access restrictions, and activity logs.

Access to the patient's record can be limited within an office to only those people who have a need to view the chart. Therefore, preparing written (or electronic) communication can be limited to those approved individuals. Others would be prohibited from access to patient information by the security officer as directed by the HIPAA regulations.

WRITING GUIDELINES

Any communication you prepare should be written using proper grammar and punctuation and have no misspelled words. It also must be spaced on the page properly and be neat and clean. Try not to use the same major word twice in the same or even consecutive sentence. Resources for writing are available from many sources: books, word processing programs, and Web resources (see Table 10–2). The following sections will assist you in producing attractive, error-free communications.

Spelling

You must check any word whose accuracy you are not sure of. When using a word processing program, use of the spell-check feature can be of great assistance. However, do not rely solely on this feature because it is possible for the word to be spelled correctly but also to be a word out of **context**. Examples of this are using "their" for "there," "cite" for "sight," "rite" for "right," "your" for "you're," and others. In addition, medical terminology can be marked by spell check as incorrect because these words are not in the spell check's dictionary.

There are 14 rules about spelling that are very helpful when you understand how to use them, shown in Figure 10–1. Here are some ideas that might help you become a more accurate speller:

- If you cannot seem to spell certain words correctly, try making an alphabetical list of them to use as a quick reference.
- Make a mental picture of the word correctly spelled.
- Pronounce the word correctly several times.
- Write the word, dividing it into syllables and inserting accent marks.
- Write or type the word several times.
- Learn to use general and medical dictionaries when you are in doubt.

Parts of Speech

To compose effective, well-written communications, you must be aware of the eight parts of speech and how they are used. Review Table 10–3. After you have the spelling and the parts of speech under control, it is time to put the words together in sentences.

TABLE 10–2 Resources for Writing

Book Resources	Word Processing Resources	Web Resources
Thesaurus	Spelling/grammar check	Writer's resources
Dictionary	Reference books	Dictionary
Medical dictionary	Thesaurus	Thesaurus
Grammar handbook		Encyclopedia
Style book (*The Chicago Manual of Style*; *CBE Style Manual*; *AMA Manual of Style*)		

RULE 1. *I* before *E*, except after C. Write *ie* when the sound is "*ee*," as in: *Achieve, Field, Grief, Yield*

- **EXCEPT after *C*, as in: Conceive, Deceive, Perceive, Receive**
- **Other EXCEPTIONS: Leisure**

RULE 2. Write *ei* when the sound is not long *e*, as in: *Height, Weight, Vein, Sleigh*

- **EXCEPTIONS: Friend, Mischief**

RULE 3. The prefixes *mis-, il-, in-, im-,* and *dis-* do not change the spelling of the root word.
Mis + spell = misspell
Il + legal = illegal
In + audible = inaudible
Im + mature = immature
Dis + appear = disappear

RULE 4. Only one English word ends in *sede* (*supersede*). Only three words end in *ceed (exceed, proceed,* and *succeed)*. All other words end in *cede: concede, recede, precede.*

RULE 5. The suffixes *–ly* and *–ness* do not change the spelling of the root word.
Sudden + ly = suddenly
Truthful + ness = truthfulness

- **EXCEPTIONS: Words ending in *y*. Change *y* to *I* before any suffix not beginning with *i*:**

Happy + ly = happily
Kindly + ness = kindliness

RULE 6. Drop the *e* from the end of a word before adding the suffixes *–al, -ed, -ing,* and *–able.*
complete – completed – completing
observe – observable
spine – spinal

- **EXCEPTIONS: Words ending in ce and ge usually keep the silent e when the suffix begins with *a* or *o* in order to preserve the soft sound of the final consonant.**

Notice + able = noticeable
Change + able = changeable

RULE 7. Keep the final *e* before a suffix beginning with a consonant.
Large + ly = largely
Care + ful = careful
Care + less = careless

- **EXCEPTIONS: Argument (argue + ment), Truly (true + ly)**

RULE 8. With words of one syllable ending in a single consonant preceded by a single vowel, double the consonant before adding *–ing, -ed,* or *–er.*
Sit + ing = sitting
Dip + ed = dipped
Run + er = runner

RULE 9. If a one-syllable word ends in a single consonant not preceded by a single vowel, do not double the consonant before adding *–ing, -ed,* or *–er.*
Reap + ed = reaped
Heat + ing = heating

RULE 10. To make a word ending in *y* plural, check the letter before the *y*. If it is a vowel, just add *s*. If it is any other letter, change the *y* to *I* and add *es*.
Birthday – birthdays
Toy – toys
City – cities
Fly – flies

RULE 11. Most nouns (names of people, places, things, ideas) become plural by adding *s.*
Boy – boys
Dog – dogs

Figure 10–1: Spelling rules. *Delmar/Cengage Learning.* (*continues*)

RULE 12. The plural of nouns ending in *s, x, z, ch,* or *sh* is formed by adding *es.*

Wax – waxes
Dish – dishes
Waltz – waltzes

RULE 13. The plural of most nouns ending in *f* is formed by adding *s*. The plural of some nouns ending in *fo* or *fe* is formed by changing the *f* to *v* and adding *s* or *es*.

Gulf – gulfs
Belief – beliefs
Knife – knives
Life – lives

RULE 14. The plural of nouns ending in *o* preceded by a vowel is formed by adding *s*. The plural of nouns ending in *o* preceded by a consonant is formed by adding *es.*

Patio – patios
Ratio – ratios
Tornado – tornadoes
Hero – heroes

- **EXCEPTIONS: Eskimos, Silos**

Figure 10–1: *(continued)*

TABLE 10–3 The Eight Parts of Speech

Speech Part	Description	Word Examples	Example of Use
Noun	The name of anything, such as a person, a place, an object, an occurrence, or a state	assistant, office, attention, laboratory, Texas, computer	The *assistant* draws *blood* and takes it to the *laboratory*.
Pronoun	A substitute for a noun	she, her, he, him, his, which, some, everyone, it, their, they, nobody	*He* called *her* to see whether *she* knew whether *anyone* else was going to the in-service program.
Verb	A word or word group that expresses action or a state of being	write, perform, cut, assist, attend, run, jump, enter am, is, are, will be, have been, feel, seem, appear	The assistant *measured* the patient's blood pressure and *entered* the findings on the chart.
Adjective	Describes, limits, or restricts a noun or pronoun	efficient, dedicated, tall, thin, dependable, irregular	Joyce is an *efficient* and *dependable* medical assistant.
Adverb	Modifies a verb, adjective, or another adverb. Adverbs commonly end in -ly and answer questions.	How? What? When? Where? How often?	*Frequently*, Jane arrives *early* for work and often stays *late*.
Preposition	Shows the relationship of an object to some other word in the sentence	of, with, without, for, above, below, on, from, between	*Between* you and me, Dr. Morrison's handwriting is, *without* a doubt, the most difficult to read.
Conjunction	Connects words, phrases, and clauses	and, but, or, for, because, if, so, yet, while	We can work Jane in *if* she can be here by 1:00 *but* not at 3:00 as she requested.
Interjection	Used to express strong feeling or emotion. These words are usually followed by an exclamation point or a comma.	oh, hurray, ouch, wow	*Hurray*! We received the research grant.

Sentence Structure

When writing letters, write in complete thoughts. A *simple sentence* consists of only one complete thought, that is, one independent clause with a subject and a verb.

EXAMPLE

- Physicians examine patients.
- Physicians prescribe medication.
- The receptionist scheduled appointments.

A *compound sentence* contains two or more independent clauses, separated by a comma.

EXAMPLE

- The physician dictates letters, and the medical assistant transcribes them.
- Administrative medical assistants perform clerical duties, and clinical medical assistants perform clinical duties.
- Laboratory technicians analyze specimens, and medical assistants assist with physical examinations.

A *complex sentence* contains one independent clause and one or more dependent **clauses**. A dependent clause cannot stand alone as a sentence.

EXAMPLE

- The doctor, who is off on Thursdays, sees allergy patients in the morning. (An adjective clause)
- Patients are sometimes quite apprehensive when they come to the office for diagnostic examination. (An adverb clause)
- Physicians require patients to receive proper instructions for diagnostic procedures. (Noun clause)

A *compound-complex sentence* contains two or more independent clauses plus one or more dependent clauses.

EXAMPLE

- Medical assistants should seek continuing education because of the evolution of new technology and new procedures in the medical field.

Written material should be composed of sentences of differing lengths and complexity to match appropriately the written matter being prepared. Patient referral or business letters require concise material, whereas personal correspondence or medical articles can contain more variety. In any correspondence, be careful not to make run-on sentences or any sentence containing too many clauses.

Punctuation

To make sentences easier to read and to tell a reader when you come to the end of a thought, a variety of marks called **punctuation** are used. Review Table 10–4.

Capitalization

Capitalize names of persons and places, the first word in a sentence, names of holidays, principal words in titles of major works, and any product or title that might be trademarked. Many medical terms begin with a capital letter because they are names of the physicians who named them. Medications are usually trademarked. Be especially careful to check every word in a heading or title for correct spelling. Use your medical dictionary or a good general dictionary. Always have these reference books in the office.

Numbers

The use of numbers must be consistent. If you use a specific reference style book (such as *The Chicago Manual of Style*), follow its instructions for using numerals or spelling out the numbers. Also, follow the rules your employer wishes to be used for your office.

In the absence of other references and if the physician's preference is unknown, usually any number under 10 is spelled out, whereas those above are expressed in numeric form. A partially contradicting general rule says to spell out the number if it can be done in one or two words. A number at the beginning of a sentence must be spelled out. A person's age and the time of day are usually written in figures. Dates, street numbers, and page numbers are written in figures. When several numbers are mentioned within a short space, figures should be used for all of them.

Proofreading

All written communication must be **proofread** before it is sent. This is a process of carefully reading printed material and marking errors for correction. Although spell check and immediate feedback of composition errors from word processing software will identify most common errors, it will still miss the correctly spelled wrong word and out-of-context words.

TABLE 10–4 Punctuation Marks

Punctuation	Mark	Usage and Examples
Apostrophe	’	Used in **contractions** to signify that one or more letters have been left out ***Who’s*, meaning *who is*, should not be confused with *whose*; *there’s*, meaning *there is*, is not to be confused with *theirs*.** Used to signify possession in a noun **The medical assistant’s stethoscope hangs in the examination room.**
Colon	:	Used to formally introduce a word, a list, a statement or question, a series of statements, or a long quotation. It is used after the salutation of a business letter and between numbers denoting time.
Comma	,	If something or someone is sufficiently identified, the description following is considered nonessential and should be surrounded by commas **The medical assistant, who is part of the medical team, needs to be especially careful in attending to details.** To separate words and word groups with a series of three or more To separate two adjectives when the word can be inserted between them To separate two sentences if it would help avoid confusion To surround degrees or titles used with names To surround words such as *therefore* and *however* when they are used as interrupters When beginning sentences with introductory words such as *well*, *now*, or *yes* To separate two strong clauses joined by a coordinating conjunction: *and*, *or*, *but*, *for*, *nor* To separate a statement from a question
Ellipsis	. . .	When omitting a word, phrase, line, paragraph, or more from a quoted passage. To create ellipsis marks with a PC, type the period three times and the spacing will be automatically set, or press Ctrl + Alt and the period once. **The regulation states, “All agencies must document overtime . . .”**
Exclamation mark	!	Used after words, expressions, or sentences to show strong feeling
Parenthesis	( )	Used to enclose matter apart from the main thought. Even though it may contain a complete sentence, it does not have to start with a capital or end with a period; however, if it is an interrogative statement (question), it ends with a question mark.
Period	.	Placed at the end of a sentence
Semicolon	;	Used between two independent clauses of a compound sentence when they are not joined by a conjunction, unless they are very short and are used informally. Can also be used for clarity.
Question mark	?	Question marks are placed after every direct question.
Quotation marks	“ ”	Used to enclose a direct quote A comma, question mark, or exclamation mark is placed inside the quotation marks *if it is a part of the quotation* and outside if it applies to the main clause.

Watch for certain things that seem to be problems, such as:

- Words ending in "s"
- Combinations of punctuation
- Capital letters
- Numbers
- Apostrophes, hyphens, and dashes
- Periods and commas
- Two-letter words
- Double letters in words.

Proofreading requires concentration and attention to details in a step-by-step process. Career proofreaders use at least a three-read system. First, they read through the material to make sure it makes sense and to check for errors in composition such as a misaligned margin, paragraph indents, spacing on the page, and so on. Then they read for content, to make certain correct words, punctuation, and grammar is used. Last, they do a check of spelling. Going through these steps should ensure an error-free communication. Good transcription, composing skills, and the ability to produce error-free communications are very desirable traits and an asset to the physician's practice.

PREPARING BUSINESS LETTERS

A business letter has several distinct components. The word processing software default formatting is usually appropriate for composing letters. The following identifies and provides a description of each part of a business letter. Refer to the sample letters in Figure 10–2.

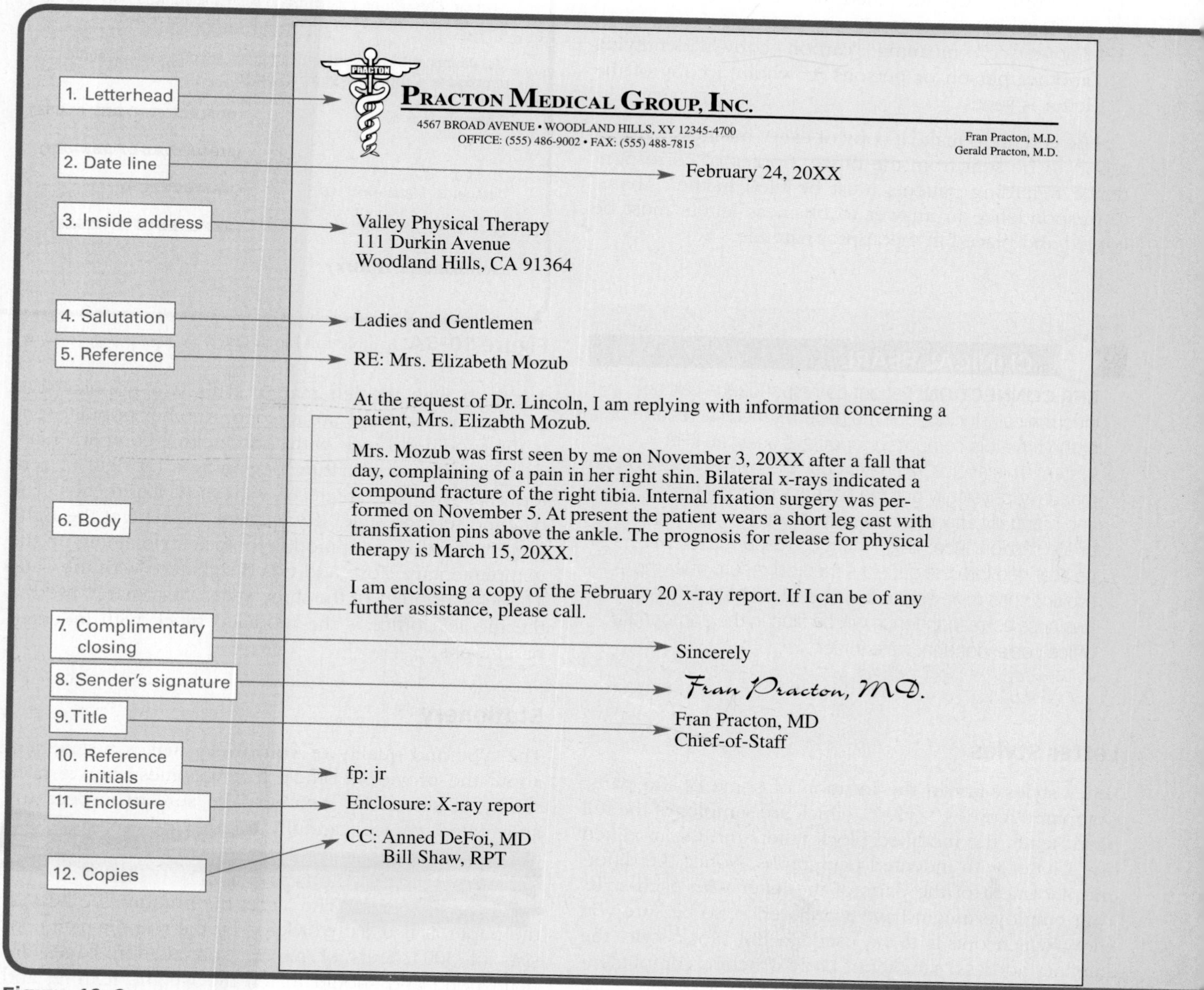

Figure 10–2: Components of a business letter. *Delmar/Cengage Learning.*

1. *The letterhead:* Preprinted name, complete address, and phone number (optional)
2. *Date line:* Date letter is dictated—or composed if not dictated
3. *Inside address:* Address of person to whom the letter is being sent
4. *Salutation:* The greeting to the recipient
5. *Reference:* To identify what or about whom the letter is concerning
6. *Body:* The content of the letter
7. *Complimentary closing:* Expressing the closing of the letter
8. *Sender's signature:* Signature of the writer
9. *Title:* Writer's title if appropriate (e.g., Vice President, Director)
10. *Reference initials:* Initials of the letter typist
11. *Enclosures:* Any identified materials to be sent with the letter
12. *Copies:* "cc," meaning "carbon copy," identifying another person or persons to whom a copy of the letter is sent.

Be certain to make a copy of every business letter or report to be sent from the office. Copies of correspondence regarding patients must be filed in their charts. Correspondence in answer to business letters must be copied and placed in the appropriate file.

Samuel E. Matthews, MD
100 East Main Street-Suite 120
Yourtown, US 98765-4321

August 15, 20-- **(DATELINE)**

Robert Smith, M.D.
50 North Broad Street
Mytown, US 43200 **(INSIDE ADDRESS)**

Dear Dr. Smith: **(SALUTATION)**

RE: Amy D. James **(REFERENCE)**

I am referring Amy James to your office for an eye examination. She is complaining of some difficulty with reading. She will be returning to school soon, and her parents wish to ensure that her vision is properly corrected.

Ms. James will call your office for an appointment. I would appreciate a report of your findings.

Sincerely yours, **(COMPLIMENTARY CLOSE)**

(SIGNATURE OF SENDER)

Samuel E. Matthews, MD **(NAME TYPED)**

lk **(REFERENCE INITIALS)**

(ENCLOSURE, IF ANY)

Figure 10–3A: Sample full block letter. *Delmar/Cengage Learning.*

CLINICAL PEARL

EHR CONNECTION: Patient correspondence can be electronically included in the patient's medical record at the time it is composed for offices using an EHR system. This avoids having to copy the correspondence manually, physically pull the patient's medical record, and manually affix the correspondence in the appropriate section. Incoming patient correspondence will be scanned into the patient's medical record after the provider has reviewed and marked it with validation. Business correspondence will be filed in the appropriate office correspondence file folder.

Letter Styles

Letter styles vary in the location of some of the parts. Compare Figures 10–3 A–C, which are samples of the full block letter, the modified block letter, and the modified block letter with indented paragraphs. Notice the different placement of the parts of the letter with each style. Your employer might have a preference, so be sure you know which one is to be used. In full block style, the dateline, address, salutation, body of letter, complimentary close, typed signature, and the initials of the typist are flush with the left margin. This is a popular style because no tab stops are needed. Another popular style is the modified block with the dateline, complimentary close, and typed signature beginning a bit right of center. This style is compatible with most letterheads. The dateline sets the style. If you place the date at the right, you must follow with modified block style, lining up the complimentary close and typed signature with the date. The least popular of the three styles customarily used in the medical office is the modified block with indented paragraphs.

Stationery

The type and quality of **stationery** makes a statement about the provider's office. If it becomes your responsibility to select the stationery, be sure to inspect any anticipated choice carefully. The letterhead style and content is usually the choice of the provider. Letterhead stationery and matching envelopes are usually 16-, 20-, or 24-pound weight. The larger the number, the heavier the paper. It is usually ordered by the ream, which consists of 500 sheets of paper. Continuation pages are plain bond and should match the weight, texture, and

Samuel E. Matthews, MD
100 East Main Street-Suite 120
Yourtown, US 98765-4321

August 15, 20-- **(DATELINE)**

Robert Smith, M.D.
50 North Broad Street
Mytown, US 43200 **(INSIDE ADDRESS)**

RE: Amy D. James **(REFERENCE)**

Dear Dr. Smith: **(SALUTATION)**

I am referring Amy James to your office for an eye examination. She is complaining of some difficulty with reading. She will be returning to school soon, and her parents wish to ensure that her vision is properly corrected.

Ms. James will call your office for an appointment. I would appreciate a report of your findings.

(COMPLIMENTARY CLOSE) Sincerely yours,
(SIGNATURE OF SENDER)

(NAME TYPED) Samuel E. Matthews, MD
(TITLE IF NEEDED)

lk **(REFERENCE INITIALS)**
(ENCLOSURE, IF ANY)

Figure 10–3B: Sample modified block letter. *Delmar/Cengage Learning.*

Samuel E. Matthews, MD
100 East Main Street, Suite 120
Yourtown, US 98765-4321

August 15, 20-- **(DATELINE)**

Robert Smith, M.D.
50 North Broad Street
Mytown, US 43200 **(INSIDE ADDRESS)**

RE: Amy D. James **(REFERENCE)**

Dear Dr. Smith: **(SALUTATION)**

I am referring Amy James to your office for an eye examination. She is complaining of some difficulty with reading. She will be returning to school soon, and her parents wish to ensure that her vision is properly corrected.

Ms. James will call your office for an appointment. I would appreciate a report of your findings.

(COMPLIMENTARY CLOSE) Sincerely yours,
(SIGNATURE OF SENDER)

(NAME TYPED) Samuel E. Matthews, MD
(TITLE IF NEEDED)

lk **(REFERENCE INITIALS)**
(ENCLOSURE, IF ANY)

Figure 10–3C: Sample modified block letter with indented paragraphs. *Delmar/Cengage Learning.*

brightness of the letterhead. A **watermark** appears on bond paper and should read across the paper in the same direction as the typing. You can determine the correct watermark side by holding the paper to the light.

Composing the Letter

Steps in the process to produce a final copy without errors are to:

- Determine what information must be included (a) to answer a letter, (b) to respond to a verbal request, (c) to request information, and (d) to obtain a specific response.
- Determine the style for the letter and set margins for appropriate placement on the page.
- Select the typeface and font size.
- Compose a rough draft, using concise, easy-to-understand sentences. Use the words *I* and *we* as infrequently as possible, especially to begin sentences. Remember that it is awkward to use the same word twice in one sentence or even in consecutive sentences. Use a thesaurus to increase the variation of words to make the content more interesting.
- Proofread the draft and edit the content. Eliminate redundant (extra, unnecessary) phrases.
- Compose the final copy and prepare the envelope.
- Sign it or give it to the sender to sign.

You can prepare a letter from dictated notes or from a dictation machine tape, or you can compose it at the keyboard. Certain formatting standards must be considered when preparing a letter. The following are points to remember as you perform Procedure 10–1:

- The date typed indicates when the content of the letter was dictated.
- The month is spelled out in full. (Traditional style is month/day/year; military style is day/month/year.)
- The inside address should be copied exactly from the correspondence to be answered or as printed in the phone book or medical society directory.
- A courtesy title is used. (Use Mr., Mrs., Miss, or Ms. or, if gender unknown, use Mr.)
- Do not use Dr. before the physician's name if MD follows.
- If a street address and box number are given, use the box number.

- The words *North*, *South*, *East*, and *West* preceding street names and *Road*, *Street*, *Avenue*, and *Boulevard* are *not* abbreviated.
- The words *Apartment* and *Suite* are typed on the same line as the address and are separated by a comma. *Apartment* may be abbreviated if the line is long.
- The name of the city is spelled out and is separated from the state by a comma.
- The state name can be spelled out or abbreviated and is separated from the ZIP code by one space; there is no punctuation between the state and the ZIP code.
- A proper salutation is "Dear," followed by the title and the person's last name. If the correspondence is to a colleague or friend, a first name is appropriate. (Ask the physician.) When writing to a business, use "Dear Sir" or "Dear Madam."
- To use a reference line, type "RE:" and then the person's full name and date of birth. (*The reason for including the date of birth is to be sure the report is attached to the correct patient chart when received by the referring provider.*) This line goes two spaces *below* the salutation, flush with the left margin in block style. It may be lined up with the date and follow the address in the modified block style. It is a common error to type the reference line prior to the salutation because that is where most physicians who dictate correspondence name the person.
- Always double space between paragraphs, flush left with block style and indented five spaces with modified block.
- If a second page will be necessary, stop the first page at the end of a paragraph, if possible. If not, include at least two lines from the broken paragraph on the bottom of the first page.
- The bottom margin must measure at least one inch.
- The last word on a page cannot be divided.
- Capitalize only the first word of a complimentary closing; follow it with a comma.
- The formality of the letter determines the closing: "Cordially," or "Sincerely," is considered informal, whereas "Very truly yours," is more formal.
- The sender's name is entered four spaces below the closing, exactly as on the letterhead; an official title follows on the same line, separated by a comma, or it can be typed on the next line with no comma.
- The typist's initials, in lower case, are placed two spaces below the sender's name. When the sender will not be signing the letter, both the dictator's (in upper case) and typist's initials are used. Typists do not use their reference initials on letters they sign.
- When items will be enclosed with the letter, enter "Enclosure" or "Encl." one or two lines below reference initials; number and identify if more than one enclosure is included.
- If copies are sent to others, enter "cc" (for carbon copy) and the other receiver's name one or two spaces below the initials or last notation. When more than one individual is carbon copied, list their names alphabetically or by rank. When a copy is sent to another person without the knowledge of the recipient, it is known as a *blind carbon copy* (bcc). No notation is placed on the recipient's letter, but *bcc* is placed on the file copy to indicate it was sent.
- A **postscript** (PS) is entered two spaces below the last notation.
- When using a second page, a heading of the patient's name, page number, and date is entered either vertically or horizontally, one inch from the top. If the letter does not concern a patient, the receiver is listed.
- The letter continues on the third line after the heading; the page should contain at least two lines of a paragraph.
- Print a draft copy and proof it. Proofing on screen is difficult because you cannot view the entire letter at one time. Correct and save the copy. Print the letter on a letterhead.
- Prepare an envelope and give with letter to the writer for a signature.

PROCEDURE 10–1 Compose a Business Letter

PURPOSE: Draft a letter (or response to communication received).

EQUIPMENT: Computer, paper (letterhead), received correspondence

S SKILL: Compose a business letter and prepare it for mailing.

Procedure Steps	Detailed Instructions and/or *Rationales*
1. Assemble equipment and supplies; bring up the word processing screen. Select your letter style.	

Procedure Steps	Detailed Instructions and/or *Rationales*
2. Correctly type the date, inside address, appropriate salutation, and reference line.	• Position the cursor down at least three lines below the letterhead. • Select letter style and type and enter the date. Be sure the location is appropriate for the chosen style. • Move cursor to the fifth line (or appropriate number of spaces) below the date. • Enter the inside address. Be sure the address is in the appropriate location for the style of letter. Use the appropriate courtesy title and enter the name exactly as printed on the received letterhead or as is in the phone or medical society directory. • Double space after the last line of the address. • Enter the appropriate salutation followed by a colon. • Double space. • Enter the reference line in the location appropriate for letter style (i.e., type RE:; enter the name of the patient or person and date of birth about whom the letter is written). • Double space.
3. Correctly type or enter the body (content) of the letter.	• Be sure the paragraph style is appropriate to the style of the letter. • Always double space between paragraphs. • If a second page is needed, end the first page at the end of a paragraph. If this is not possible, place at least two lines of the paragraph on the first page. Do not divide the last word on the first page. • When a second page is necessary, enter the second page heading in vertical or horizontal format; include the name, page number, and date. • Double space.
4. Correctly enter the closing elements: a complimentary closing, sender's name and official title, typist's initials, enclosures, cc or bcc recipients, and postscript.	• Go down four lines. • Enter the sender's (provider's) name in letter style format exactly as printed on letterhead. An official title follows the name on the same line, separated by a comma, or it is placed directly below with no comma required.
	• Double space. • Enter typist's initials. • Single or double space if enclosing materials. • Enter the preferred style enclosure. Number and identify if there is more than one enclosure. • Single or double space if copies will be sent. • Enter cc and the recipient(s) name(s). Enter bcc on the file copy if sending a blind copy. • Double space. • Enter PS for postscript, if desired.
5. Print a draft copy and proofread the letter, making any necessary corrections.	

(continues)

(continued)

Procedure Steps	Detailed Instructions and/or *Rationales*
6. Print the letter on letterhead and prepare an envelope.	
7. Present the letter with envelope to the person (provider) for signature.	
8. Make a copy and file a copy in the chart (or scan in EHR), if it concerns a patient, or in the appropriate business folder.	

Consultation Letters

In a specialist's office, one of the most common letters received is a request from another provider for a consultation with a patient (Figure 10–4). You will often find it necessary to correspond with the patient if you need to send any special instructions, directions to your office, and other information. Be certain the material has ample time to arrive at the patient's home before the date of the examination. The content of the correspondence usually covers:

- The reason for the appointment.
- The date and time of the appointment. (It should request notification if the appointment cannot be kept and advise the patient of any policy regarding missed or late cancelled appointments and associated charges.)
- A statement saying that if the patient has any questions to please feel free to call your office. Be sure to include your office's phone number.
- *Note: If a prior authorization is required by the patient's insurance company, it should be so stated in an appointment or referral correspondence.*
- The observation that the office visit will require a follow-up letter from the specialist to the referring provider, identifying the findings, diagnosis, and recommended course of treatment.

Samuel E. Matthews, MD
100 East Main Street, Suite 120
Yourtown, US 98765-4321

October 7, 20--

ENC: Blue Cross Insurance
cc: Patient Chart

Robert Smith, M.D.
50 North Broad Street
Mytown, US 43200

Dear Dr. Smith:

I am referring Susan B. James (6/19/19XX) to your office for evaluation of severe headaches of approximately six months duration. She was treated initially at a pain clinic in Yourtown. Susan will be calling your office for an appointment. I am sure you will find her to be a most cooperative patient.

I would appreciate a report of your diagnosis and recommended course of treatment.

Sincerely,

Samuel E. Matthews, M.D.
lk

Figure 10–4: Sample referral letter. *Delmar/Cengage Learning.*

HANDLING INCOMING MAIL

The amount of mail coming into a medical office depends on the number of providers. Many types of mail come into a physician's office. Office policy determines whether it is sorted and placed on the provider's desk or the office manager's desk or whether a combination of both occurs in relation to the type of mail received. The actual processing of the mail may be done by the manager, receptionist, administrative medical assistant, or mail clerk. Your employer might want to review all the mail personally and request that you open only the envelopes and arrange everything neatly on the desk. Some providers allow the mail to be opened and sorted, referring only to professional or personal material that requires their response; anything pertaining to the practice operation is handled by the office manager.

The office policy manual should give instructions regarding the handling of mail. If no manual is available, the office manager or the provider should be consulted. Following are some generally accepted practices.

Sorting Mail

Incoming mail should first be sorted; Table 10–5 presents examples of mail a medical office receives. Any mail marked *personal* should be placed on the provider's or office manager's desk unopened. Special delivery

TABLE 10–5 Mail Received in the Medical Office

Special delivery mail
Special messenger mail
Correspondence from patients
Payments from patients
Payments from insurance companies
Requests for information from insurance companies
Referral letters or reports from providers
Laboratory reports
Hospital reports
Professional organization mail
Professional journals
Magazines
Newspapers
Advertisements
Promotional literature and samples from pharmaceutical companies

mail or special messenger mail should be opened immediately. Mail may be sorted into categories, such as mail from patients, physicians, insurance companies, and miscellaneous sources. Other classes of mail, such as magazines, professional journals, and newspapers, should be separated from drug samples and advertisements.

Opening Mail

When opening mail, you need a letter opener, paper clips, a stapler, and a date stamp. It is more efficient to stack all envelopes so that they are facing in the same direction. A quick tap on the desk will move contents away from the flap side of the envelope. Open each letter along the flap edge, being careful to remove all contents from each envelope. As the mail is removed, be sure the contents contain the same name and return address shown on the envelope. Some offices want you to keep the envelope with the mail received, and certainly you should if it is needed to help identify the contents. Otherwise, you may discard the envelopes.

Date-stamp the correspondence and attach any enclosures. If an enclosure is indicated on the letter but is missing, it is necessary to write "None" after the "Encl." notation and circle it to indicate the need for follow-up.

Always be cautious opening mail. If you are suspicious of a letter or package, take appropriate precautions and contact the United States Postal Service (USPS). The USPS has suggested that certain things would make a letter seem suspicious:

- It is unexpected or from someone you do not know.
- It is addressed to someone no longer at your address.
- It is handwritten and has no return address or bears one that you cannot confirm is legitimate.
- It is lopsided or lumpy in appearance.
- It is sealed with an excessive amount of tape.
- It is marked with restrictive endorsements such as *Personal* or *Confidential*.
- It has excessive postage.
- It is wrapped with string (against postal regulations, indicating it could have been delivered by other means).
- Sound is coming from a package.

If such a letter or package should arrive, what should you do? ***Never handle a letter or package that you suspect is contaminated***; additionally:

- Don't shake it, bump it, or sniff it.
- Wash your hands thoroughly with soap and water.
- Notify local law enforcement authorities.

Processing Incoming Mail

Follow office policy and provider preference when processing incoming mail, including routine office expense bills, insurance forms, and checks for deposit. Be sure to endorse stamp immediately any checks with the practice's stamp. If cash is received in the mail, you should always seek a witness to verify the amount of money and have that person sign a receipt along with you to be sent to the patient. This helps avoid the possibility of the patient saying that more was sent than was actually found in the envelope. This can happen quite innocently by human error.

Unless you are specifically directed otherwise, you should always make sure all patient-related hospital summaries; dictated operative notes; referring physician reports; and other hospital, laboratory, or special examination reports are seen by the provider and initialed before they are filed (or scanned if using EHR). Requests regarding patients or other office matters should be placed in a designated area for the physician to see and respond to each day.

You can perform a valuable, timesaving service for the physician by **annotating** the incoming mail or identifying important points to be noticed. If any correspondence or a patient's chart will be needed to answer mail, it should be pulled and placed with the mail to facilitate the response.

Notifications of meetings should be made available to the provider daily. Miscellaneous correspondence and professional journals are often placed under the stack of mail. Some providers want to see all supply catalogs and pharmaceutical company descriptions of products. In other offices, many of these items are disposed of immediately, especially if they concern areas of practice the office does not provide. Items that may be needed for future reference should be placed in a designated file. Be sure to verify the current policy with your provider and office manager.

Drug samples that may be used should be logged on an inventory sheet and placed in a designated, secure area for future use. Samples that will not be used should never be placed in the trash because they could cause harm to individuals taking them without medical evaluation and advice. Often, community clinics and service organizations can make good, safe use of donated samples. The office should have a secure box to collect samples for this purpose. Once again, be sure to follow office policy regarding drug samples.

Mail Received during Vacations

When the provider is away from the office for professional meetings or on vacation, you might be asked to read all mail carefully and decide how each piece will be handled. You should discuss what to do with urgent mail before the provider leaves. The provider might want you to call to discuss or, in some cases, to copy and forward the mail. If the provider is a member of a group practice, he or she might want you to consult with a partner or on-call provider to review mail and messages. This is especially critical for urgent medical matters. Never send an original document by mail; send only copies and comply with HIPAA regulations. If the provider will be away for a long time, you might need to send mail more than once. If so, be sure to number the envelopes consecutively and keep track of what you send so that you can be sure all the mail is received. When responding to the person who sent urgent mail, you might wish to send a brief note explaining the reason for the delay in answering.

If the office will be closed temporarily or permanently, be sure to go to the post office and complete a form to have mail held or forwarded to another address. Never send the form by mail because it can be delayed. The USPS cannot take verbal orders for this purpose. Allowing mail to accumulate invites theft. You can also request "Hold Mail Service" from the USPS Website (currently limited to certain ZIP codes, so check online if you qualify), which will allow your mail to be held safely at the post office. Mail can be held from 3 to 30 days with this feature.

PREPARING MAILINGS

The USPS uses some of the most advanced, innovative technologies for reading and sorting mail. Some of these technologies are presented in Table 10–6. These advanced technologies read the address on the envelopes you mail, so you must address the envelopes properly to aid in accurate reading and efficient delivery.

TABLE 10–6 USPS Mail Technology

The postal service uses more than 10,000 pieces of automated processing equipment to sort nearly half the world's mail volume.
Intelligent Mail® services increase the value of mail for the postal service and its customers. Intelligent Mail barcodes uniquely identify pieces of mail as well as trays, sacks, and containers of mail and track them through the mail processing system.
The flats sequencing system is the postal service's latest piece of equipment. It sorts large envelopes and magazines, known as "flats," at 37,000 pieces per hour in carrier walk sequence.
The delivery input/output subsystem machine reads and verifies the address on a piece of mail, sprays a barcode, and sorts the mail at 39,000 pieces per hour.
The postal automated redirection system automatically forwards nearly 3 billion pieces of mail every year. In 2008, 46 million postal customers submitted address changes.
The USPS is the world leader in optical character recognition technology; its machines read 93 percent of all hand-addressed letter mail.
The advanced facer canceller system positions letter mail and cancels stamps at 36,000 pieces per hour.
The delivery barcode sorter reads the barcode on letter mail and sorts pieces at 36,000 pieces per hour.
The automated flat sorting machine sorts flat mail at 17,000 pieces per hour.
The automated package processing system processes packages and bundles of mail at more than 9,500 pieces per hour.

Source: United States Post Office, www.USPS.com.

Addressing the Envelope

Addresses can now be read by computers using optical character readers (OCRs) if handwritten or typed. Refer to the USPS bulk mail–rate products and services, and you will find that you might qualify for a discount on postage, but the address must be typed or machine printed to be eligible. Use a standard type font because script or executive-type letters run together. It is best to check with the local post office or USPS Website on an annual basis for the most current rates and terms for bulk mailing.

For **domestic** mail, the post office city, state, and ZIP code or ZIP + 4 should appear, in that order, on the bottom line of the address. However, if all three elements will not fit on that line, the ZIP code or ZIP + 4 may be placed on the line immediately below the post office and state, aligned with the left edge of the address block. The standard two-letter state abbreviations should also be used (see Figure 10–5). The ZIP + 4 codes should always be printed as five digits, a **hyphen**, and four digits. The hyphen should be treated as any other character as far as spacing and stroke width are concerned. Figure 10-6 shows a properly addressed envelope with all components in the correct format and location. This address can be read easily by the OCR equipment.

Mail addressed to foreign countries should include the country name printed in capital letters (no abbreviations) as the only information on the bottom line.

Alabama	AL	Montana	MT
Alaska	AK	Nebraska	NE
Arizona	AZ	Nevada	NV
Arkansas	AR	New Hampshire	NH
California	CA	New Jersey	NJ
Canal Zone	CZ	New Mexico	NM
Colorado	CO	New York	NY
Connecticut	CT	North Carolina	NC
Delaware	DE	North Dakota	ND
District of Columbia	DC	Ohio	OH
Florida	FL	Oklahoma	OK
Georgia	GA	Oregon	OR
Guam	GU	Pennsylvania	PA
Hawaii	HI	Puerto Rico	PR
Idaho	ID	Rhode Island	RI
Illinois	IL	South Carolina	SC
Indiana	IN	South Dakota	SD
Iowa	IA	Tennessee	TN
Kansas	KS	Texas	TX
Kentucky	KY	Utah	UT
Louisiana	LA	Vermont	VT
Maine	ME	Virginia	VA
Maryland	MD	Virgin Islands	VI
Massachusetts	MA	Washington	WA
Michigan	MI	West Virginia	WV
Minnesota	MN	Wisconsin	WI
Mississippi	MS	Wyoming	WY
Missouri	MO		

Figure 10–5: Two-letter state abbreviations. *Adapted from the United States Postal Service, www.usps.com.*

EXAMPLE

MR THOMAS CLARK
117 RUSSELL DRIVE
LONDON WIP6HQ
ENGLAND

Mail addressed to Canada may use either of the following formats when the postal delivery zone number is included in the address.

EXAMPLE

MRS HELEN SAUNDERS	MRS HELEN SAUNDERS
1010 CLEAR STREET	1010 CLEAR STREET
OTTAWA ON K1AOB1	OTTAWA ON CANADA
CANADA	K1AOB1

The post office will furnish additional information on mailing to foreign countries if assistance is needed.

Preparing the Envelope

When the mail has been signed, fold it and place it in the envelope (see Figure 10–7 A–C).

Ensure that the envelope is a proper size. Envelopes smaller than $3\frac{1}{2} \times 5$ inches do not meet standards. Envelopes larger than $6\frac{1}{8} \times 11\frac{1}{2}$ inches are acceptable but must be processed by hand and will require additional postage (see Table 10–7).

Stamp or Meter Mail

The expenditure of sending mail should be evaluated to determine the most cost-effective method to use. Your local post office and the USPS Website can furnish you with current information, postage rates, categories, and regulations. The USPS now offers postage and shipping discounts when you use the Website. Look for specials and promotions to reduce costs of postage and handling.

Mail may be either stamped or metered. Stamps may be purchased at a post office or purchased online and printed. If you have a large volume of mail, it is preferable to use a postage meter. Meters offer features such as a moistener to seal the envelopes (usually at a fixed cost to purchase). This allows you to enter a number of envelopes for mailing (such as monthly comprehensive

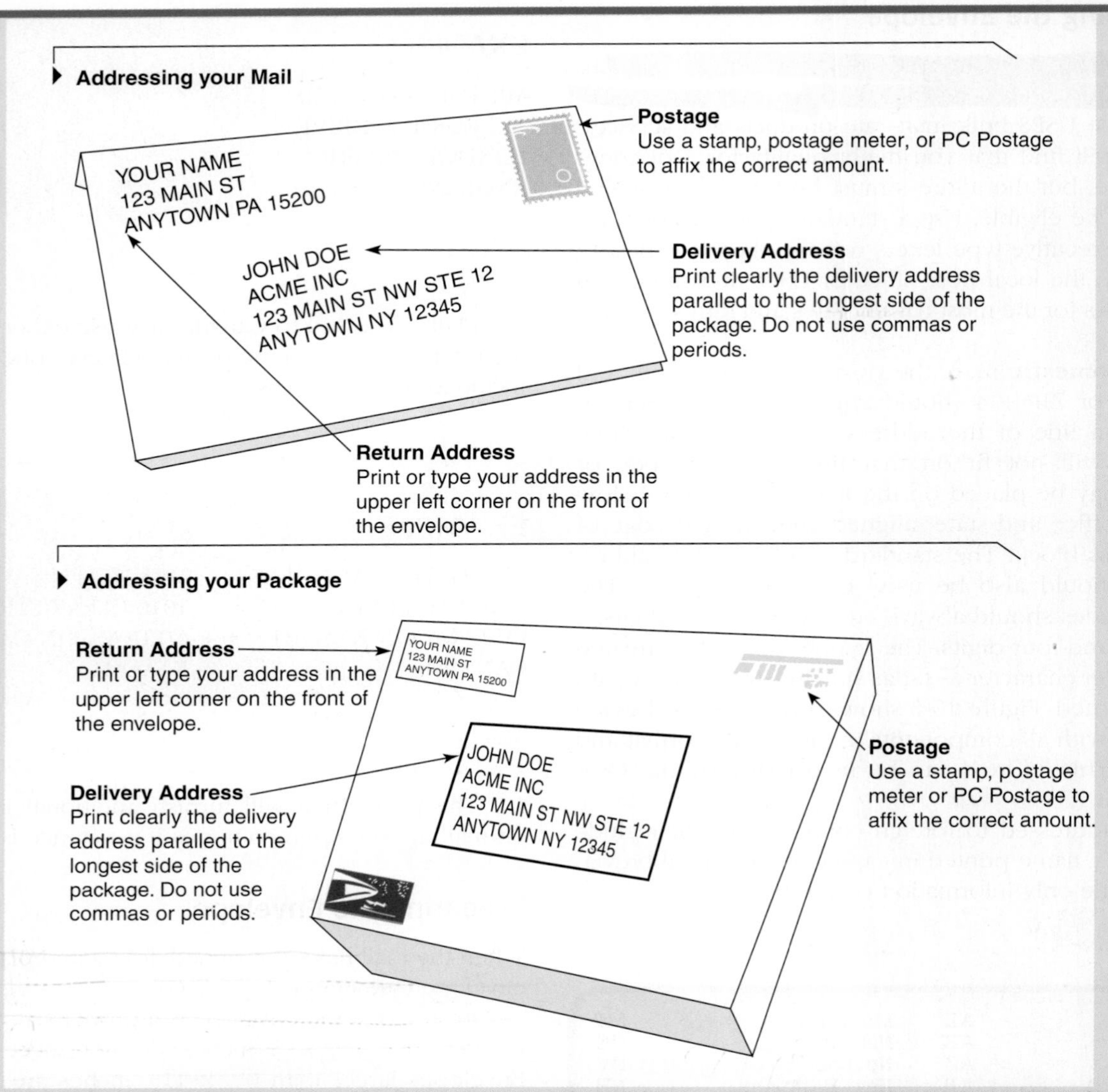
Addressing your Mail
YOUR NAME
123 MAIN ST
ANYTOWN PA 15200
JOHN DOE
ACME INC
123 MAIN ST NW STE 12
ANYTOWN NY 12345
Postage
Use a stamp, postage meter, or PC Postage to affix the correct amount.
Delivery Address
Print clearly the delivery address paralled to the longest side of the package. Do not use commas or periods.
Return Address
Print or type your address in the upper left corner on the front of the envelope.
Addressing your Package
Return Address
Print or type your address in the upper left corner on the front of the envelope.
YOUR NAME
123 MAIN ST
ANYTOWN PA 15200
JOHN DOE
ACME INC
123 MAIN ST NW STE 12
ANYTOWN NY 12345
Delivery Address
Print clearly the delivery address paralled to the longest side of the package. Do not use commas or periods.
Postage
Use a stamp, postage meter or PC Postage to affix the correct amount.

Figure 10–6: Addressing your mail. *Adapted from the United States Postal Service, www.usps.com.*

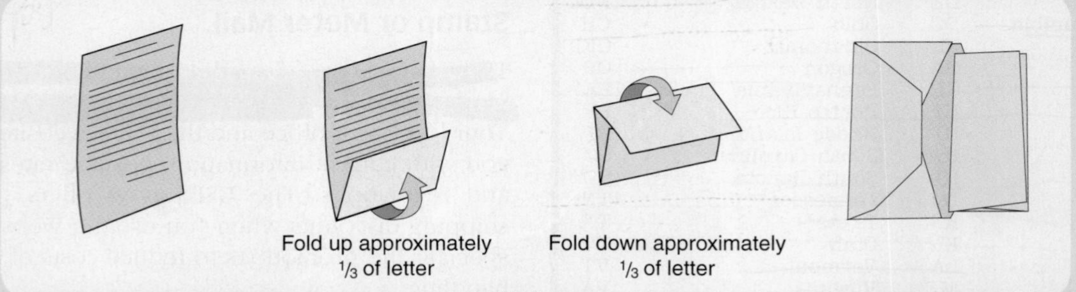
Fold up approximately 1/3 of letter
Fold down approximately 1/3 of letter

Figure 10–7A: Folding of a letter for a standard size business envelope. *Delmar/Cengage Learning.*

physical exam reminders) at a bulk rate. You also save time by not having to go to the local post office.

To expedite the processing of metered mail, remember to (1) check and change the date on the meter daily, (2) apply the correct amount of postage by weighing the mail before affixing postage, (3) check the imprint to be sure it is clear and readable, and (4) use fluorescent ink in the meter.

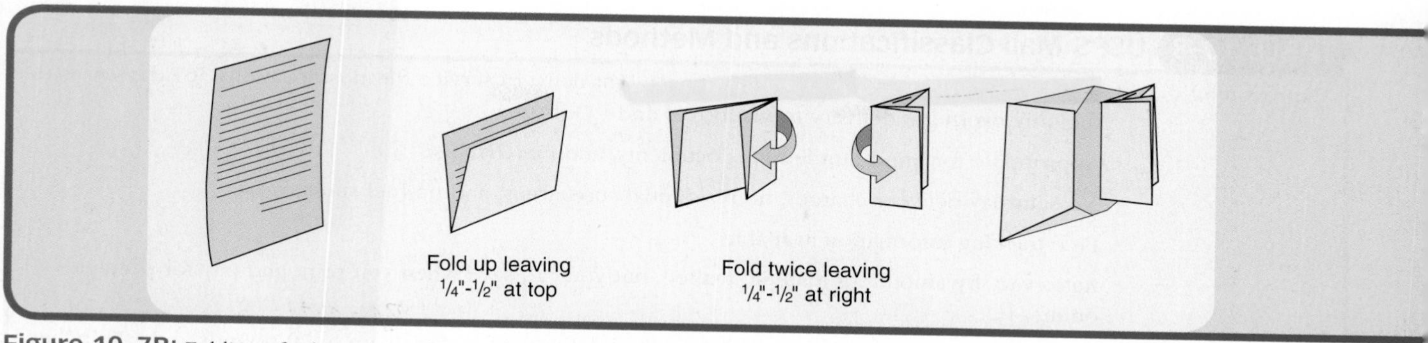

Figure 10–7B: Folding of a letter for a 6¾" envelope. *Delmar/Cengage Learning.*

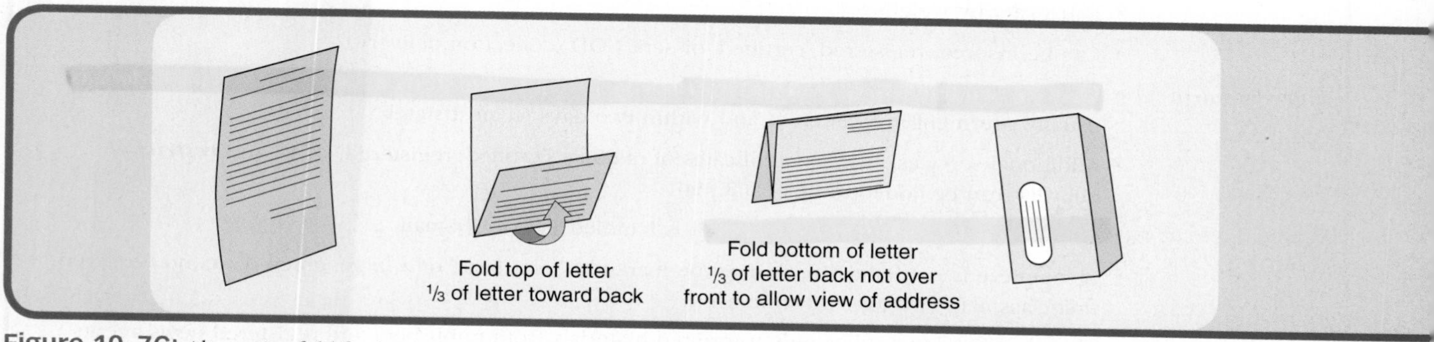

Figure 10–7C: Alternative fold for business envelope. *Delmar/Cengage Learning.*

TABLE 10–7 Mail Pieces and Dimensions

Mail Piece		Description	Length	Height
Postcard	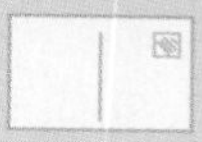	Rectangular cardstock mail piece not contained in envelope	5-inch minimum, 6-inch maximum	3.5 inch minimum, 4.25-inch maximum
Letter (up to 3.5 ounces)	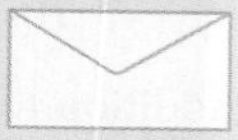	Small, rectangular mail piece no thicker than $\frac{1}{4}$ inch	5-inch minimum, 11.5-inch maximum	3.5-inch minimum, $6\frac{1}{8}$-inch maximum
Large Envelope	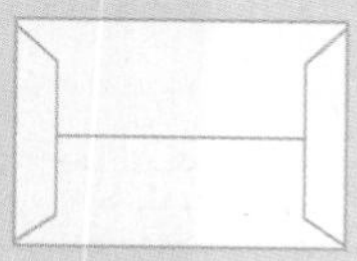	Flat, rectangular mail piece no thicker than $\frac{3}{4}$ inch	11.5-inch minimum, 15-inch maximum	$6\frac{1}{8}$-inch minimum, 12-inch maximum
Package	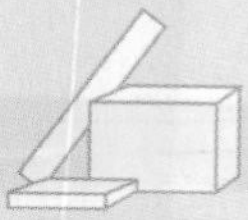	A three-dimensional mail piece contained in a box, thick envelope, or tube, weighing up to 70 pounds	Length + girth (distance around the thickest part of the package) cannot exceed 108 inches. (Parcel post cannot exceed 130 inches.)	

Adapted from United States Postal Service, www.usps.com.

Mail Classifications

The USPS has many informative bulletins and booklets regarding the classifications, mailing standards, special mailing services, and other customer services they offer. These are available at your local post office and through the USPS Website. Most mail from the provider's office will probably be first class, but a brief discussion of the classifications with their variations and additional methods of mailing is included for your information in Table 10–8. If

TABLE 10–8 USPS Mail Classifications and Methods

Express mail	• The fastest service and is guaranteed overnight delivery service for most locations 365 days a year; the only overnight delivery to mailboxes and P.O. boxes • Appropriate for important letters, documents, and merchandise • No Saturday delivery charges, no residential surcharges, and no fuel surcharges • Free tracking information available • Rates vary by amount of material mailed, but you can save when you print and pay for postage online
Priority mail	• Provides preferential handling and expedited delivery of materials up to 70 pounds and 108 inches in combined length and width • Priority Mail stickers, labels, envelopes, and boxes provided at no charge • Rates vary by weight • Can be insured, registered, certified, or sent COD (collect on delivery)
First-class mail	• Used for sending letters, postcards, stamped cards, greeting cards, checks, and money orders; is usually overnight in local cities and within two days to most states • Additional services, such as certificates of mailing, certified, registered, COD, and ***restricted*** delivery, can be added to first-class mail • If a piece is heavier than 13 ounces, it is handled as priority mail • If the piece is not letter size, it must be marked "First Class," or a large, green-diamond-bordered first-class mail envelope must be used
Periodicals	• This classification applies only to printed materials from publishers and registered news agents approved for Periodical privileges • Magazines or newspapers mailed by others will use first-class or standard mail (A) rates
Standard mail (A)	• A classification used by retailers, catalogers, and other advertisers to promote products and services. This classification also permits anyone to mail a parcel weighing less than one pound • Eligible nonprofit organizations can take advantage of the special rates when mailing in excess of 200 pieces, each weighing less than 16 ounces, or for sending more than 50 pounds per mailing
Standard mail (B)	• For parcels weighing one pound or more, up to 70 pounds • The delivery time can take up to nine days • If a first-class mail piece is attached or enclosed, you will pay for it in addition to the standard mail (B) parcel charge • Insurance to cover the value of articles mailed can be purchased • There are special rates for books or catalogs

Source: United States Postal Service.

you have special mailing needs, it would be advisable to consult with your local post office for advice and up-to-date regulations because they tend to change periodically.

Special Mailing Services

There are other special mailing services you might want to use when mailing personal or confidential patient information, presented in Table 10–9. These are in addition to the various classifications already discussed.

If you have mail returned because the patient has moved and left no forwarding address, refer to the patient's chart and demographic form. Try contacting the patient's alternative phone numbers for current information, but be careful to follow HIPAA guidelines and patient CCP. When a letter is returned after an attempt has been made to deliver it, you must prepare a new envelope and put on new postage before re-mailing it. A letter is sometimes returned if you have made an error, such as transposing numbers in an address.

Other services are available is there is a need for them. FedEx and UPS offer other delivery alternatives. Access their Websites for information, rates, services, shipping labels, and pickup.

TABLE 10–9 Special Mailing Services

Certificate of mailing	• This is a receipt showing evidence that the piece was mailed. It is helpful when you want to prove that something was mailed or a deadline was met. • It is purchased at the time of mailing. • There is no proof of delivery, and no insurance against loss is provided with the certificate.
Certified mail	• This provides proof of mailing and delivery of the mail. The sender receives a mailing receipt when the item is mailed, and a receipt of delivery is kept at the recipient's post office. A proof-of-delivery return slip can be purchased. • Appropriate to use if the provider is terminating services to a patient for some reason; a signed return receipt should be purchased to provide evidence to be placed in the discharged patient's chart. • This service is available only for first-class or priority mail and does not carry insurance protection.
Collect on delivery (COD)	• Use this when you wish to collect payment for merchandise or postage when the item is delivered. The receiver must have ordered the material. • It can be used with first-class, registered, express, priority, or standard mail. • Fees include insurance coverage limited to $1000.
Insurance	• Insurance can be purchased for up to $5000 for regular standard mail and for mail sent at priority or first-class mail rates and automatically includes delivery confirmation. • A restricted delivery, return receipt, or special handling service can be purchased for items insured over $200.
Registered mail	• Registered mail is the most secure option offered, providing protection for valuables and important mail. • Registered articles are placed under tight security from the point of mailing to the point of delivery. First-class mail or priority mail postage is required. • Return receipt and restricted delivery is available. • Insurance up to $25,000 can be purchased for items sent by registered mail.
Restricted delivery	• Restricted delivery means that the mail is delivered only to a specific addressee or someone authorized to receive mail for the addressee. • This can be used to be certain that only the patient receives specific communication such as lab reports, a copy of a consultant examination, or any other personal material.
Return receipt	• Return receipt is the sender's proof of delivery. • It can be purchased at the time of mailing for mail sent COD; express mail insured for more than $50; or registered, certified, or restricted mail. The receipt shows who signed for the item and the date it was delivered.

Source: United States Postal Service.

CLINICAL PEARL

The restricted delivery method of sending correspondence works well to maintain compliance with HIPAA rules. It is always advisable to check the patient's chart to see whether there are restrictions for sending sensitive personal information. With restricted delivery, you would be certain only the patient receives the correspondence. For example, a wife could be assured that her husband would not open a lab report that has an abnormal finding before she had a chance to read it. Or, if mail is sent to a place of business, a secretary would not open and read personal communication.

CHAPTER SUMMARY

- Seven types of written correspondence are used in the medical office: sending of notes; interoffice communications (IOC); email; information recorded in the patient's chart; form letters; information sheets; and business, professional, and personal letters.
- Form letters and templates are usually indicated to manage the affairs of the practice. This includes referrals, consultations, annual physical reminders, collection letters, school and work releases, and other correspondence necessary to the practice operation.
- An information sheet provides specific written instruction regarding the examination and diagnostic test(s) performed in your office, helping serve as a reminder to the patient after he or she leaves the office. Cast care and fever control are examples that can be provided on an information sheet.
- There are pros and cons of using email. Email is a powerful tool, enabling instant communication and greater productivity, round-the-clock convenience, cost reduction, and easy reference to past communications by referencing sent emails. It doesn't require the customer (patient) to be available to send a message, and files can be attached to the message. However, it is far more likely to be misinterpreted by the receiver than would face-to-face communications, isn't as secure or private as people think, and can be problematic in legal or time-sensitive issues.
- You must take precautions to avoid acquiring a virus through email. A general rule is to look at the subject and sender before opening the message. If it is from an unfamiliar source or displays a suspicious subject, do not open it. Never open an executable or script file (files with .exe or .vbs suffixes) unless you are expecting to receive such a file from the sender. Use antivirus software to scan emails before opening them.
- Communications that include personal information about patients require specific handling and compliance with HIPAA rules. Care must be taken to protect the integrity of the information and prevent disclosure to entities that are not directly involved with the provision of health care.
- Any communication you prepare should be written using proper grammar and punctuation and have no misspelled words. Components of fundamental writing skills include spelling, parts of speech, sentence structure, punctuation, capitalization, and treatment of numbers.
- A business letter has 12 distinct components. These include:
  - The letterhead: Preprinted name, complete address, and phone number (optional)
  - Date line: Date letter is dictated—or composed if not dictated
  - Inside address: Address of person to whom the letter is being sent
  - Salutation: The greeting to the recipient
  - Reference: To identify what or about whom the letter is concerning
  - Body: The content of the letter
  - Complimentary closing: Expressing the closing of the letter
  - Sender's signature: Signature of the writer
  - Title: Writer's title if appropriate (e.g., Vice President, Director)
  - Reference initials: Initials of the letter typist
  - Enclosures: Any identified materials to be sent with the letter
  - Copies: "cc," meaning "carbon copy," identifies another person or persons to whom a copy of the letter is sent
- There are three letter styles, the full block letter, the modified block letter, and the modified block letter with indented paragraphs.
- Many types of mail come into a provider's office. You must know how to sort, open, and annotate incoming mail. Sort the mail into categories; mail marked personal should be placed on the provider's or manager's desk unopened. Sorting categories include mail from patients, providers, insurance companies, and miscellaneous sources. When opening mail, use a letter opener, paper clips, stapler, and date stamp. Use caution with suspicious letters or packages. Annotate the mail by identifying important points to be noticed.
- The USPS has many informative bulletins and booklets regarding the classifications of mail. They include express mail, priority mail, first-class mail, periodicals, standard mail (A), and standard mail (B). You should be familiar with the classifications and methods.
- Use special mailing services when you want to mail personal or confidential information. These services include certificate of mailing, certified mail, collect on delivery, insured, registered mail, return receipt, and restricted delivery.

STUDY TOOLS

Workbook	Activities for Chapter 10
Premium Website StudyWARE	Activities and Quizzes on the **StudyWARE™ Software** for Chapter 10
	Complete the following **Competency Challenge 2.0** activity: • Thursday, 9 AM: Respond to Written Communication
	Audio Library of medical terms
	Online access to the **Critical Thinking Challenge 2.0**
CourseMate	Activities and Quizzes for Chapter 10
WebTutor	Activities and Quizzes for Chapter 10

CHECK YOUR KNOWLEDGE

1. Of the following items, which are advantages of using email?
   a. Can be used in a court of law as evidence
   b. Provides easy reference to past communications
   c. Saves time and paper
   d. a and c
   e. b and c
2. Identify which is NOT a type of form letter or information sheet.
   a. Reply to AMA regarding provider speaking engagement
   b. Work status note
   c. Athletic participation approvals
   d. Annual diagnostic test or examination notice
3. Which of the following are parts of speech?
   a. Noun
   b. Verb
   c. Adjective
   d. Pronoun
   e. All of the above
   f. a and d
4. Describe how mail received during vacation might be handled.
   a. Hold all mail until the provider returns.
   b. Read all mail and decide how each piece will be handled.
   c. Call the physician to discuss daily mail.
   d. Call the physician to discuss urgent mail.
   e. b and d
   f. a and c
5. Which is not a classification of mail?
   a. Certified
   b. Internet address
   c. Registered
   d. Express

WEB LINKS

Centers for Disease Control and Prevention: *www.cdc.gov*

Confidentiality Education Group (CEG): *www.cc.nih.gov/ccc/ceg/info.html*

Ingenix CareTracker: *www.ingenix.com/ehr/caretracker*

Joint Commission: *www.jointcommission.org*

Medical Reserve Corps: *www.medicalreservecorp.gov*

United States Postal Service: *www.usps.com*

Webopedia: *www.webopedia.com*

Chapter 11 Operating Computers and Office Equipment

OBJECTIVES

Upon completion of this unit, you will learn the following:

KB KNOWLEDGE BASE

1. Spell and define, using the glossary at the back of the text, all the Words to Know in this chapter.
2. Define the computer terms listed in this chapter.
3. Differentiate between computer hardware and software and be able to give examples of each.
4. Define application software and application suites and be able to give an example.
5. Explain the capabilities of practice management software, electronic health records software, and encoder software.
6. Explain why caution should be taken when gathering information from the Internet and describe four guidelines for finding credible information on the Internet.
7. Explain the computer term *downtime* and describe when this would be used.
8. List five machines, other than the computer, that are commonly found in medical offices and describe what they do.

S SKILLS

1. Operate and maintain a copy machine.
2. Operate a transcriber to produce a printed copy from recorded material.
3. Perform maintenance activities to ensure the operability of administrative and clinical equipment.

WORDS TO KNOW

continuity of care
dictation
electronic health record (EHR)
encoder
ergonomic
facsimile (fax)
hardware
HL7 Protocol
interface
peripheral
software
transcription

THE COMPUTER

In *Computer Fundamentals for an Information Age,* authors Shelly and Cashman define a "computer [as] an electronic device, operating under the control of instructions stored in its own memory unit, which can accept and store data, perform mathematical and logical operations on that data without human intervention, and produce output from the processing."

Computers come in a variety of makes, styles, sizes, capacities, and price ranges. Some can be carried like a small notebook; others are large, designated primary network machines. Many can convey sound, and some are capable of responding to voice commands. Most offer wireless connectivity and feature a mouse and keyboard.

The computer has changed the way information is processed and stored, and you must be proficient with computer skills in today's medical office. With technology constantly changing, it is necessary to update and learn new applications almost continuously. It would be wise to take every opportunity possible to acquire additional skills.

Providers are aware of the advantages of using computers in the office. The computer can facilitate claims processing; the necessary information is entered on the office computer and sent directly to insurance clearinghouses and insurance companies. This eliminates paperwork, and the speed of reimbursement is enhanced considerably. Some providers find the computer essential if they are engaged in research and need to identify quickly all patients with a specific diagnosis. It is also valuable in the quick identification of patients taking a particular drug if the manufacturer should issue a warning about side effects.

Written communication is more efficient with the use of computer software. Practice management software can help eliminate human error in totaling charges and receipts while quickly providing financial status figures. Electronic medical records allow offices to enter all patient information and office visit progress notes instead of writing on charts. Information once contained in numerous file cabinets can be stored on networks and can be called up with a few keystrokes. The computer is useful for inventory control of office supplies, personalizing form-letter mailings for collections, rescheduling annual checkups, and gathering research data. Maintaining the privacy of personal information stored in computers is critical and is addressed by Health Information Portability and Accountability Act (HIPAA) regulations.

Computer Terms

With the development of the computer came a whole new vocabulary of technical terms as well as new meanings for old words. To communicate with is important to understand and use comp Table 11–1 lists some of the most commor relating to the computer and its componer

CLINICAL PEARL

A system must be established to limit access computer information in relation to the requir of the job. Employees with computer access s have a password to safeguard the information. the display on a monitor from being viewed by Reposition a flat screen monitor or use a scree

TABLE 11–1 Computer Terms

Term	Meaning
Attachment	A file such as a letter or document that you send along with an email message.
Back up	Duplicate of data files made to protect information. Records should be backed up daily. Some experts recommend twice daily.
Boot	To start up a computer.
CD-ROM	**C**ompact **D**isk-**R**ead **O**nly **M**emory; a type of optical disk capable of storing large amounts of data, typically 650–700 megabytes (MB). Reads only CDs.
CPU	**C**entral **P**rocessing **U**nit, or the brain of the system. The memory is made up of **bits**. A bit is a single **BI**nary digi**T**. *Binary* refers to a situation in which only two choices are possible: for example, yes/no, on/off, pass/fail. *Digit* refers to a single number. A bit is either 0 or 1. A **byte** is the fundamental group of bits a computer will treat as a word. A byte consists of 8 bits. A 16-bit processor is twice as fast as an 8-bit processor. One **K** (kilobyte) is equal to 1,024 bytes. A 64-K computer can handle 65,536 bytes. The greater the number of bytes, the greater the memory.
Disk	A round plate on which data can be encoded. There are two basic types of disks: *magnetic disks* and *optical disks*.

(continues)

TABLE 11–1 *(Continued)*

Term	Meaning
Disk drive	The device used to get information on and off a disk.
Domain	A group of computers and devices on a network, which are administered as a unit with common rules or procedures. On the Internet, domains are defined by IP addresses. All devices sharing a common part of the IP address are said to be in the same domain.
DVD-ROM	Digital Versatile Disc or Digital Video Disc. Optical disc storage format commonly used for video or data storage. Holds a large amount of data compared to the CD-ROM. DVD-ROM holds 4.3 GB of data. Reads both CDs and DVDs.
File	A single, stored unit of information that is given a file name by which it can be accessed from storage.
Hardware	The electronic, magnetic, and electromechanical equipment of a computer system (such as keyboard, disk drive, monitor, CPU, and printer).
Input	Data or commands entered on the computer.
Interface	The hardware and software that enable individual computers and components to interact.
Memory	Internal storage areas on the computer.
Microprocessor	A silicon chip that contains a CPU.
Modem	**MO**dulator/**DEM**odulator—a device or program that enables a computer to transmit data over telephone or cable lines.
Output	What the computer produces after recorded information is processed, revised, and printed out.
Peripheral	Anything you plug into a computer—for example, a printer, USB flash drive, monitor, or scanner.
Prompt	Messages issued to a user, requesting information necessary to continue processing.
RAM	**R**andom **A**ccess **M**emory—a temporary, or volatile, memory. RAM is synonymous with main memory, the memory available for programs to use. When you turn off the computer, this memory is gone unless it is saved.
ROM	**R**ead **O**nly **M**emory—the permanent special memory that stores programs to boot the computer or store diagnostics.
Server	A computer or device on a network that manages network resources; examples would be file servers (storage devices), print servers (to manage one or more printers), network servers (to manage network traffic), database servers (to process database queries), and Web servers (serve up Web pages).
Software	Computer programs necessary to direct the hardware of a computer system to perform specific tasks.
Terminal	In networking, a terminal is a personal computer or workstation connected to a mainframe. The personal computer usually runs terminal emulation software that makes the mainframe think it is like any other mainframe terminal.

Hardware and Software

When discussing computers, reference is made to hardware and software. **Hardware** refers to the hard disk drive, the CPU, the monitor, and the keyboard (Figure 11–1). **Software** refers to the application programs containing instructions to the computer that enable it to perform tasks. A computer, by itself, cannot do anything without software for accessing and inputting data. You interact with the software programs to produce correspondence, maintain records, calculate financial statements, and perform many other tasks. Software is commonly available on CD-ROM (Figure 11–2) or DVD-ROM or downloadable from the Internet to be installed on the computer's hard drive. When you input data with a software program, the data resides in the computer's main memory until it is saved in a file on the hard drive or other storage device.

The main storage component for a computer is its hard drive, which stores enormous amounts of information that can be retrieved almost immediately. Various types and capacities of storage devices are available to supplement internal hard drive storage capacity. Table 11–2 list some examples.

Personal computers (PCs) store their software programs as well as input data on their hard drive. In offices with several workstations, the individual computers or terminals can be networked to a server or mainframe computer. The server or mainframe computer can contain databases, applications, and stored files to be shared in the office. This arrangement frees up hard drive space on

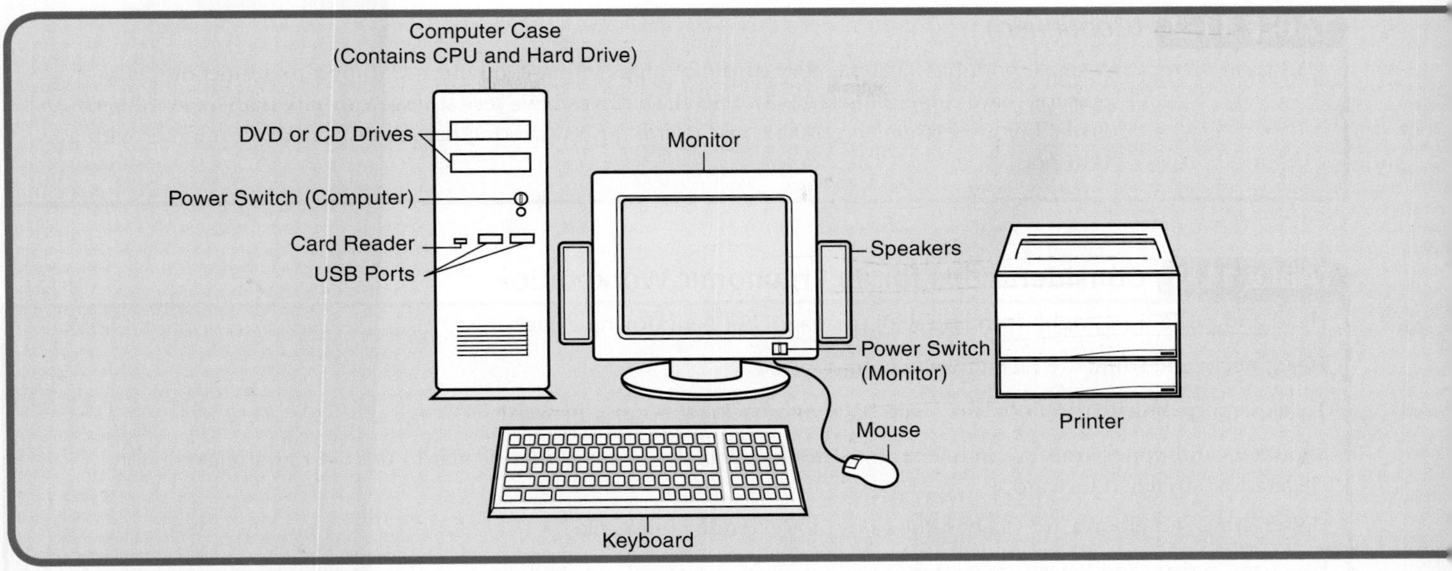

Figure 11–1: Computer hardware. *Delmar/Cengage Learning.*

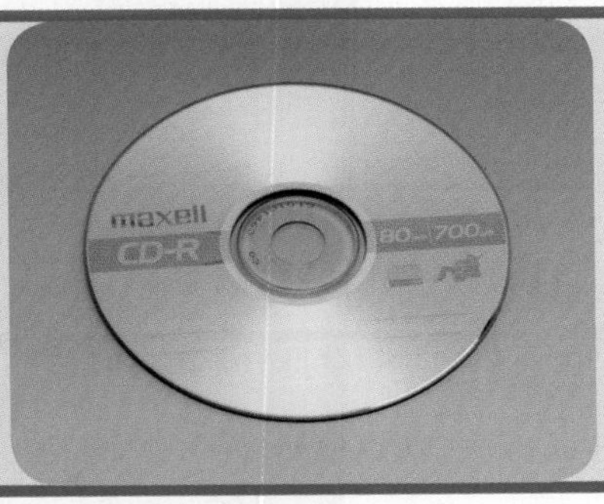

Figure 11–2: CD-ROM. *Delmar/Cengage Learning.*

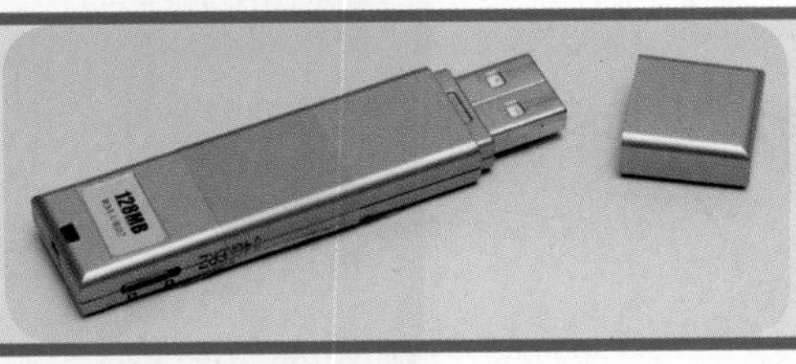

Figure 11–3: USB flash drive. *Delmar/Cengage Learning.*

the individual workstations and provides a centralized location from which client applications such as email can be accessed. A properly networked system permits input and record updates from all stations and allows the information to be accessed from all stations.

ERGONOMICS AND COMPUTER USE

When using the computer, evaluate the workstation for health and safety considerations by performing an ergonomic assessment. **Ergonomics** programs provide a work environment that promotes wellness, and minimizes musculoskeletal disorders. Improper setup of workstations or repeated use of computer equipment can result in injury. Be sure to request an evaluation and appropriate equipment necessary to avoid alignment or repetitive injuries. Proper lighting, height, keyboard, mouse, and headset are items that should be addressed. Table 11–3 is a checklist to set up a proper ergonomic workstation. Figure 11–4 represents good posture and ergonomics while using a computer.

TABLE 11–2 Types and Capacities of Storage Devices

CD-R	**CD-R**ecordable. Data can be saved (burned) onto this disk by using a computer with a CD burner. After the CD is burned, data can be retrieved, but no additional data can be added to it. Can typically store 650–700 MB.
CD-RW	**CD-ReW**ritable disk. This type of disk enables you to write onto it in multiple sessions. Storage capacity is the same as CD-R.
DVD+R and DVD-R	**DVD-R**ecordable disk. A DVD-R disk can record data only once, and then the data becomes permanent on the disc.
External hard drive	A peripheral (external) hard drive that can be connected to a computer through a USB port or Firewire (IEEE 1394). External hard drives are useful for backing up or storing large amounts of data beyond the capacity of the computer's internal hard drive.

(continues)

TABLE 11–2 *(Continued)*

USB flash drive	A small, portable flash memory card that plugs into a computer's USB port and functions as a portable hard drive (Figure 11–3). USB flash drives have less storage capacity than external hard drives but are extremely portable and useful for transferring data to or from any computer with a USB port.

TABLE 11–3 **Considerations for an Ergonomic Workstation**

Head and neck are upright or in line with the torso, not bent down or back.
Head, neck, and trunk are faced forward, not twisted.
Trunk is perpendicular to floor; may lean back into backrest but not forward.
Shoulders and upper arms are in line with the torso, generally about perpendicular to the floor and relaxed, not elevated or stretched forward.
Upper arms and elbows are close to the body, not extended outward.
Forearms, wrists, and hands are straight and in line, forearm at about 90 degrees to the upper arm.
Wrists and hands are straight, not bent up or down or sideways toward the little finger.
Thighs are parallel to the floor, and the lower legs are perpendicular to floor. Thighs may be slightly elevated above knees.
Feet rest flat on the floor or are supported by a stable footrest.

Source: U.S. Department of Labor, Occupational Safety and Health Administration. www.osha.gov

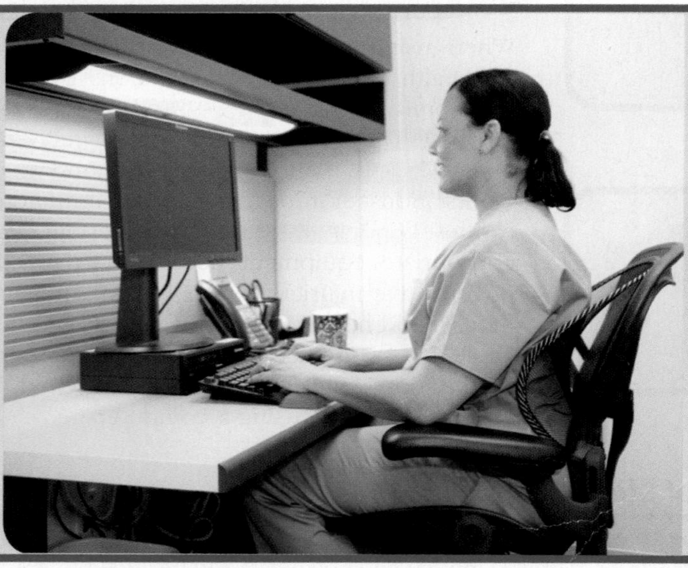

Top of monitor at or just below eye level

Head and neck balanced and in-line with torso

Shoulders relaxed

Elbows close to body and supported

Lower back supported

Wrists and hands in-line with forearms

Adequate room for keyboard and mouse

Feet flat on the floor

Figure 11–4: Good posture and ergonomics at a workstation. *Delmar/Cengage Learning.*

CLINICAL PEARL

The Occupational Safety and Health Administration provides eTools for ergonomic computer workstation setups, at www.osha.gov/SLTC/etools/computerworkstations/components.html.

MEDIA LINK

View the "Ergonomics" video for this chapter on the Premium Website.

COMPUTER APPLICATION SOFTWARE

Computer application software capabilities are virtually limitless. Application software allows users to interact with the computer to perform specific tasks such as word processing, database management, spreadsheet preparation, and music or video playing. These programs enable users to produce text documents, perform bookkeeping, create graphic designs, manage medical office operations, and many other activities. An application suite includes multiple applications programs bundled together, often with related functions. Such suites usually include, at minimum, a word processing program, spreadsheet program, and presentation software. Popular suites include Microsoft® Office (which includes Word®, Excel®, PowerPoint®, and OneNote® programs) or Apple iworks® (which includes Pages®, Numbers®, and Keynote® programs).

Word processing software is available for all computers; some examples of software programs are Microsoft® Word®, Apple® Pages®, or Corel® WordPerfect®. These programs provide almost limitless composition of written and graphic materials. You can select from a number of print font styles and sizes, which can be bolded, italicized, underlined, superscripted or subscripted, printed with shadows, and more. You can vary line spacing and margins and set columns, borders, bullets, and tabs. You can rearrange content by highlighting, cutting, and then pasting it in the new location. It is possible to insert page breaks, use auto shapes that allow you to add text boxes, draw lines, input clip art or content from files, draw and insert tables, and much more. With practice, you not only can create quality standard correspondence but also outstanding reports, articles, and presentations for your employer.

Medical offices might use educational software programs, another type of applications software, for patient education. The medical assistant can load the programs into the computer, discuss with patients what they will see, and ask whether patients have further concerns after they complete the viewing. Informational programs have been developed for diabetes, cancer, pregnancy, health hazards of smoking, and many other subjects.

Practice Management Software

Practice management software is a type of application software that manages the operations of a medical practice and is available from a variety of companies. The functionality of practice management software varies, depending on the program, but typically allows a medical office to schedule appointments, record patient demographics and insurance information, process claims, perform insurance and billing routines, and generate financial reports. Many programs enable users to look up patient treatment or payment history easily, print patient mailing labels, find phone listings, or set up a recall and reminder system.

The patient demographics screen provides for the entry of account information for each patient (Figure 11–5). All the data needed to bill the account properly is included. It provides information needed for billing such as primary and secondary insurance.

The transactions entry screen, or procedure posting screen, allows users to apply procedure charges to patient accounts and then generate completed insurance forms. This is where all charge entries are done, including the entries for payments made at the time of service. During charge entry, a running total of the account is displayed at all times. When you have finished making entries for the patient, the account updates immediately. Procedure and diagnosis codes are built into the program and can be searched by number or by description (Figure 11–6). Many programs can send insurance forms electronically directly to insurance clearinghouses, or claims can be printed. Accurate submission of claims means a higher percentage of payment and less rejection of claims.

Financial reports can be prepared with a minimum of effort when data is regularly entered on the computer. Accounts receivable may be printed by date or age or in alphabetical order and broken down between insurance company and patient. A detailed summary of income between two given dates can be easily prepared. The report of charges between any two dates can be accessed in detail or summary. A day sheet can be easily prepared. Providers might find a need for a statistical report of diagnosis and procedure code usage, which can be retrieved from the stored data. Reports can also be sorted and output by individual patient, provider, or insurance company.

The utility menu screen, or file maintenance screen, in a practice management application gives you access to all the functions you need to set up and maintain the custom files to be used by the system, establish the format for your custom forms, and do the maintenance work to keep your system running efficiently. After these files are established, the data in them is a keystroke away when the system is in use.

It is important to note that these illustrations of computer screens and descriptions of functionality are only a sampling of the many office procedures possible with computers.

Electronic Health Records Software

An **electronic health record (EHR)** captures all patient health information harvested from one or more encounters in any health care delivery system (such as a medical office, hospital, urgent care center, and so on). The information captured includes demographics, progress notes, vital signs, current medications, allergies, immunizations,

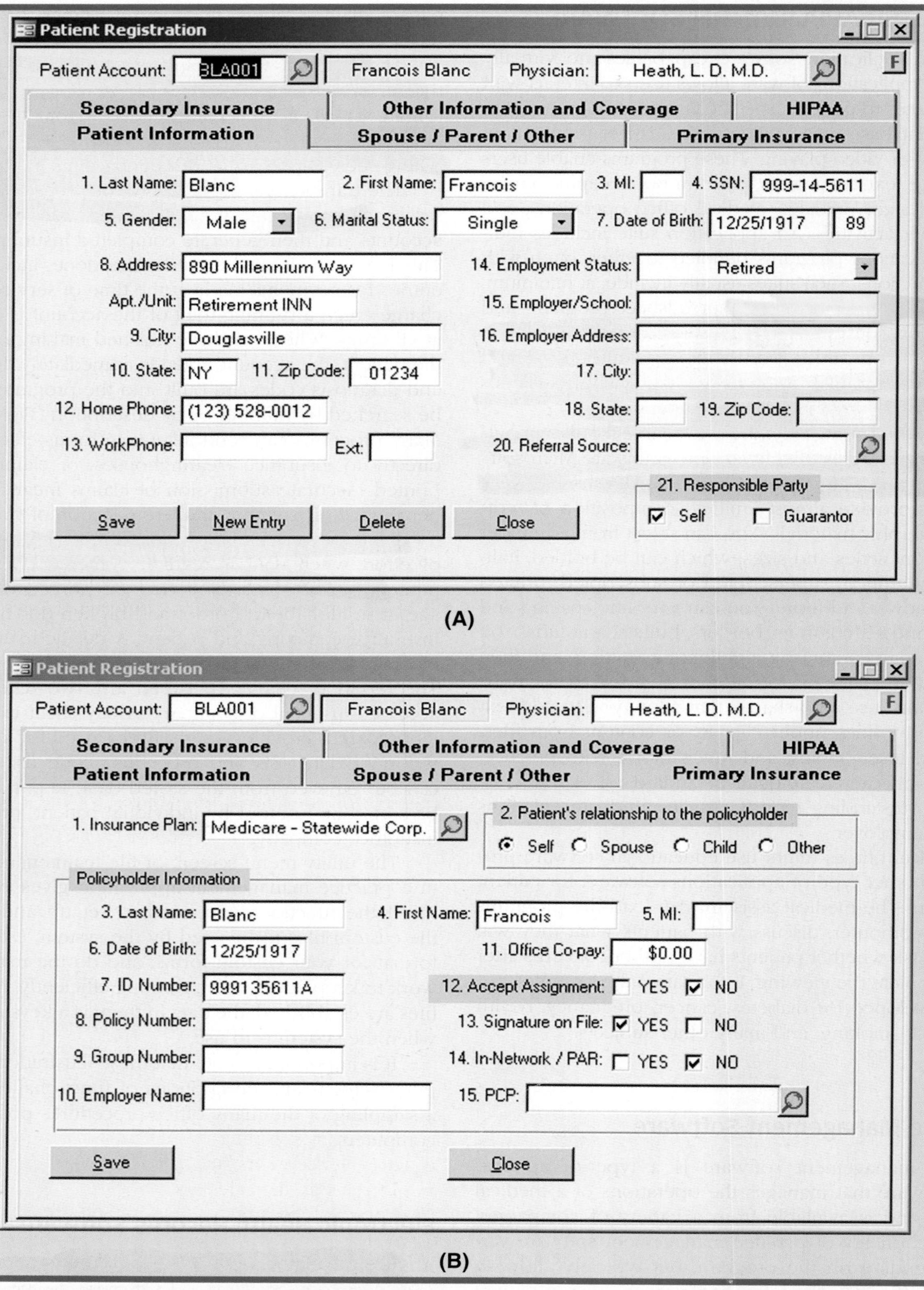

Figure 11–5: The patient information screen contains areas to input (A) demographic information and (B) insurance information.
Delmar/Cengage Learning.

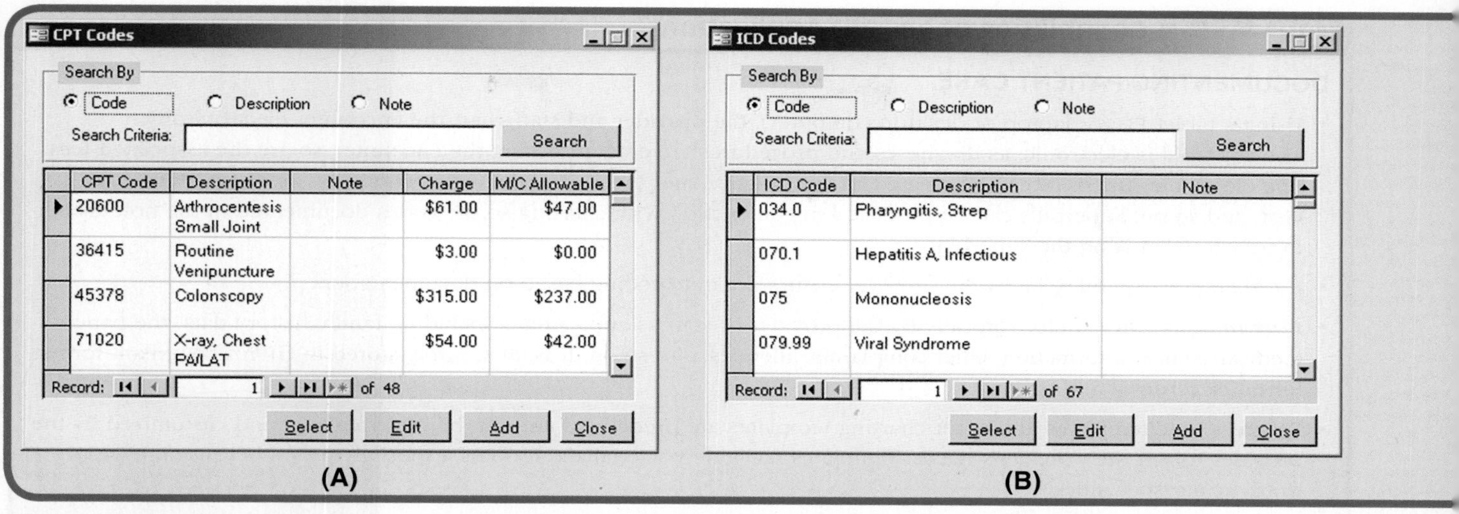

Figure 11–6: Screens showing (A) CPT procedure codes and (B) ICD-9-CM diagnosis codes. *Delmar/Cengage Learning.*

lab orders, and more. EHR software enables providers to document all care received by the patient—tests performed, treatments prescribed, patient education given, and so on. Figure 11–7 shows a sample screen in EHR software.

Use of EHR software significantly enhances efficiency in the medical office in many ways, improving workflows, reducing paper usage, and shrinking costs. EHR systems are *inclusive* of features such as appointment scheduling, collections, and reports, resulting in the highest level of care. As you document in an EHR, it is your responsibility to ensure data integrity; you must always be certain you are documenting in the correct patient's chart and entering accurate information in a professional manner.

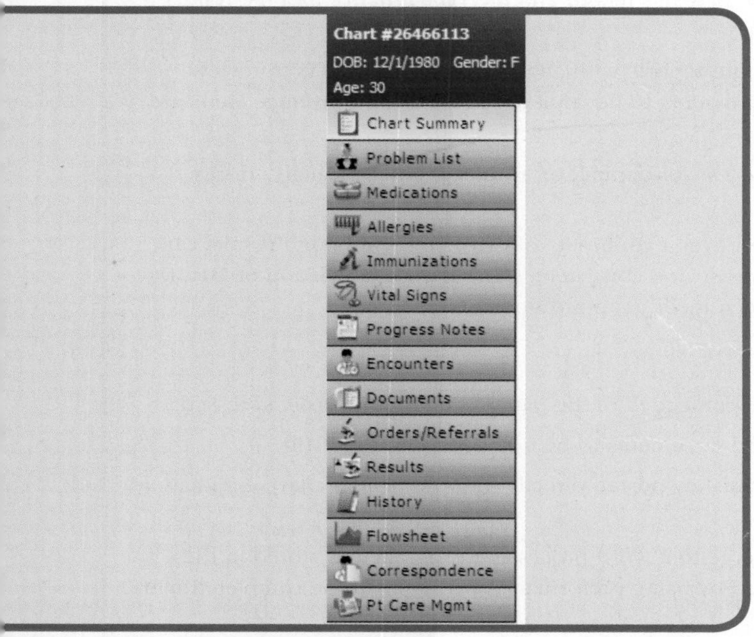

Figure 11–7: Electronic chart tabs within EHR software. *Courtesy of Ingenix CareTracker.*

Review Table 11–4, which provides a listing of some of the functionality EHR software can provide. Note that not all EHR software might have all the features listed; the features listed in the following table provide examples of what EHR software is capable of doing.

EHR software often integrates with practice management software to combine the patient's care with the tracking, billing, and reporting aspects associated with that care.

EHR Software and Downtime

Inevitably, the practice will experience times when the computer systems are not operating. This is referred to as downtime. Preparations must be made to convert to paper, using manual scheduling and messaging, billing, and a downtime form for the patient encounter (see Figure 11–8).

Encoder Software

Encoder software is available as a powerful application for all CPT®, HCPCS, ICD-9, and ICD-10 code sets, and Medicare coding guidelines. This software will improve coding accuracy and billing performance and reduce rejected claims. With optional functionality features, other advantages to using encoder software include:

- Compliance editing
- Robust code checking
- Increase in the rules set
- Improved compliance and accuracy for accelerated claims payments
- Fee calculator
- Color code edits
- Modifier crosswalk
- Cross-coder relationships
- Medicare CCI edits
- LMPR/LCD and NCD policies

TABLE 11–4 Capabilities of an EHR Application

DOCUMENTING PATIENT CARE

- Using a tablet PC (or laptop or desktop computer), the provider and staff chart the encounter electronically. The superbill is electronic; as diagnoses and procedures are entered during the encounter, so are the associated fees. The electronic superbills can be created by the practice, and there can be many versions: by provider, by type of visit, and so on. Superbills can be produced in conjunction with charting so the codes documented in the note match exactly to what is on the superbill.
- E / M coding capability helps the provider ensure accurate coding based on documentation.
- *Everything* is entered electronically by the provider or staff as appropriate, including family history data, the patient's medical/clinical information, chief complaints, allergies, and so on. It is all securely stored in HIPAA-compliant format for quick retrieval and review.
- Progress note templates and other charting templates are predefined and can be easily created and customized by the provider to suit the provider's needs. Templates facilitate personalized formats, especially useful because they apply to particular specialties.
- Using voice and handwriting recognition, providers can dictate or make notes directly into the patient's electronic record for quick input of notes and encounter information.

PRESCRIBING MEDICATIONS

- Prescription management capabilities include providing information and alerts on dosages, allergies, and possible interactions with other medications.
- A drug formulary allows the provider to make selections based on the patient's insurance coverage, and the provider's favorites list can be developed.
- Prescriptions can be submitted electronically, directly to the patient's pharmacy. In addition, EHR software can support prescription printing and faxing.
- Ineffective and discontinued drugs and negative reactions to a specific drug(s) are tracked. Even samples and prescriptions issued by other providers can be tracked easily.

LAB ORDERS AND RESULTS

- With interfacing to and from several major labs, the provider can order lab tests directly through the patient's record. When results are ready, they automatically post back into the patient's record and *alert the practice that the results are in, with highlights on any abnormalities.*
- Other points of interest regarding labs—The provider can route reports with attached notes for others to review, review diagnoses from previous encounters, select outside providers to be copied on results, and produce Medicare waivers for tests that might not be covered.
- Protocols can be established to automate the notification process for panic-level results, whereby a high-priority message is sent to the provider, notifying of the problem.
- All results can also flow through to flow sheets for evaluation over a continuity of care. All the inbound results can be received through standard **HL7 protocols**, making setup easy and consistent. (**HL7** is an abbreviation of **Health Level Seven**, the standard for exchanging information between medical applications.)

DOCUMENT MANAGEMENT

- Images (patient photos, insurance cards, other scans) can be embedded in the patient's chart and easily accessed.
- Document management enables all types of files and scanned documents to be uploaded into the EHR.
- Faxes can be automatically routed to an email inbox and ultimately posted directly into the patient chart, eliminating the need to gather paper faxes and scan them.
- Letters (consult, attorney, and so on) can be generated to merge to a word processing program and stored in the patient's record for reference. These can be quickly generated by using preformatted text and can be completed with voice recognition.

- **Provider's Home Page** acts as a virtual inbox for the provider, providing a snapshot view of daily schedules, health maintenance items requiring immediate attention, items requiring signature approvals, and an intra-office messaging system that tracks and documents all office communications and patient care.
- An inbox/outbox view of action items is available to streamline messaging.
- Doctor's Home Page eliminates stacks of charts, sticky notes, and reports on the provider's desk and places them in an easily viewable electronic format, using no paper.

HEALTH REMINDERS

- EHR software can assist the practice and provider to ensure that **continuity of care** protocols are followed and that patients who need to be seen based upon their medical condition are alerted as such to the practice and provider when follow-ups are due.
- EHR software can include plans, guidelines, and protocols for the management of specific conditions based on factors such as age, sex, diagnosis, and lab result values.
- The system can generate alerts for appointment recall, prescription refills, and laboratory orders.
- When a patient's record is accessed, a screen can alert the provider about any due or overdue health maintenance tasks as well as any suggested protocols for that patient.

PATIENT PORTALS

- Patient portals allow patients to communicate with the practice and providers, using a secure username and password.
- Patients may be given rights (as set by office policy) to input or update demographic information, request appointments and prescription refills, check lab test results, or review billing statements.

Ingenix® and 3M™ are popular suppliers of encoder software. Chapter 15 contains more information about using encoder software.

The Internet

The Internet is a system of interconnected computer networks by which to access information from all over the world. To access the Internet, you need a computer, a modem, and a Web browser (application software that enables you to access the Internet). Using your Web browser, you can type in a specific Web address to go to a specific topic page. To search for a topic without a specific Web address, you can enter appropriate keywords into a search engine such as Yahoo, Google, or Bing. In return, you receive a listing from which you can select a more specific entry.

The Internet can be a great source of data from health organizations such as the American Cancer Society and the Centers for Disease Control and Prevention (CDC). Through the Internet, you can schedule airline, hotel, and other services directly without going through various agents; research community resources; and look up ZIP codes and phone numbers. It is possible to enter, obtain, and exchange information as well as conduct business transactions such as banking, all electronically. You can look at books, museums, associations' publications, the world's encyclopedias, and so much more.

However, be cautious. The Internet contains a wealth of information, but not all of it is good information. Anyone can create a Web page, so serious problems can be associated with some online sources. Carefully evaluate content posted online and be savvy in recognizing trusted sources.

> **CLINICAL PEARL**
>
> Patients should be warned especially about going online to seek medical advice or purchase medications. Self-medication could cause serious problems from drug interactions with the prescribed medications ordered by the provider.

Take certain precautions when reading and evaluating websites. Remember, no official agency reviews or evaluates the information posted on the Internet. You

Appt Date/Time: ______________ **Co-Pay:** ________

Patient Last Name: ______________________ **First Name:** ______________________

DOB __________ **Age** ______ **Visit Date** (Encounter Date) ______________

MD ______________ **Practice Location** ______________________

MA Adult Intake: (Ad Hoc Charting) B/P ________ Ht ______ Wt ______ BMI ______ LMP ______

T ______ P ______ R ______ 02 ______

Allergies: (Allergy Profile)

____

____

____

Medications: (Medication Profile)

____

____

____

____

____

____

____

____

____

____

____

____

Chief Complaint: ______________________ **Onset of Symptoms** ______________

Pain Scale: 1 2 3 4 5 6 7 8 9 10

New Problem (Problem List)

____

ORDERS (Super bill) (POC test, Lab, Imaging, Referrals/Authorizations and Misc. Orders)

E & M ______________________ **Dx** ______________

______________________ **Dx** ______________

______________________ **Dx** ______________

______________________ **Dx** ______________

______________________ **Dx** ______________

Dx Codes ______, ______, ______, ______ **CPT Codes** ______, ______, ______, ______

RX(Easy Script) ______________________ Dose ______

Route ______________ Frequency ______________ Duration ______________

Instructions ______________________________________

RX(Easy Script) ______________________ Dose ______

Route ______________ Frequency ______________ Duration ______________

Instructions ______________________________________

RX(Easy Script) ______________________ Dose ______

Route ______________ Frequency ______________ Duration ______________

Instructions ______________________________________

Figure 11–8: EHR downtime form. *Delmar/Cengage Learning.*

Physicians Visit Notes__________

S – from patient
O – measured
A – diagnosis
P – plan

Assessment/Plan/Instructions __________

Follow up Visit:__________

Figure 11–8: *(continued)*

might want to follow some simple website guidelines such as:

1. Check the source. Are there links to professional affiliations or are there professional credentials?
2. Be cautious about personal testimonies from users; they often are receiving monetary compensation for making statements.
3. Watch for dates of the information; the information can be very old and no longer valid.
4. Use your analytic and critical thinking skills to interpret *scientific* studies or reports. Who did the research? How many people were included in the study? Is the amount of time spent appropriate to arrive at the stated conclusions? Is there more than one study on the subject to give its results credibility?

As you become more familiar with technical reading and practice analyzing information, you will be able to make good decisions. Technology has made great changes in the way we access and exchange information, and it is important for you to learn to use new technologies.

COMPUTER SECURITY

Regardless of whether your office has practice management software or EHR software you must employ best practices for safe computer use. There are a number of considerations for security:

1. Physical access (computers, screens, printers, fax, copier): You must take action to protect patient information from being viewed by unauthorized users. Use screen privacy shields and automatic screen savers; place equipment out of high traffic and visual sight areas.
2. Use passwords for each computer and software application and set applications to log off automatically if inactive for a specified period of time.
3. Catalog all information system components:
   a. Hardware: computer workstation and tablets, printers, PDAs, scanners, modems
   b. Software: Operating system, billing software, practice management, email, EHR, database
   c. Network: Routers, hubs, phone and cable lines, wireless, firewall software and hardware
4. Back up data to ensure integrity from loss, disaster, human error, hard drive error, virus, or equipment damage. Use the appropriate level of secure backup for the practice:
   a. Tapes
   b. CDs
   c. Offsite
5. Keep network and communication safeguards intact: To defend against attacks and viruses, install firewalls (hardware and software devices that protect an organization's network from intruders). A firewall denies access to unauthorized users and applications and creates audit trails or logs that identify who accessed the network and when. Firewalls also issue alarms if repeated unsuccessful attempts or abnormal activities occur.
6. Keep antivirus software up to date: Viruses attach themselves to emails, program files, and data files. Be vigilant in keeping antivirus software current. Operating systems and the services and programs they run can be inherently open to attack.
7. Understand encryption: HIPAA security standards require you to assess whether unencrypted transmissions of health information are at risk of being accessed by unauthorized entities. If they are, some form of encryption should be considered. Examples are:
   a. Patient billing and information exchanged with payers and health plans
   b. Usage and case management; authorization and referrals
   c. Patient health information gathered from or displayed on a website or portal
   d. Lab and other clinical data electronically sent to and received from outside labs
   e. Word processing files used in transcription and transferred electronically
   f. Emails between providers and patients or between attending and referring providers and their offices
8. Vendor and business relationships chain of trust: Demand that all vendors and business partners fully understand the HIPAA security standards.
9. Access and security levels to EHR should be monitored and tracked (see Figure 11–9).

Electrical surges and power outages can destroy information currently being used by the computer if it has not yet been saved by the operator or automatically by the program. Loss of data due to electrical surges and power outages can be prevented by the installation of a protective device known as an uninterrupted power supply (UPS), which contains a battery backup system. A UPS is capable of sensing a surge or outage and automatically switches to a backup battery to preserve the data. The size of the battery determines the length of time the electronic equipment can be sustained. The primary purpose is to allow you time to save your document, exit the program, and shut down your system until the power is again stable.

It is very important to establish a backup policy to make copies of office programs and data. Often, this is performed each night. Computer hard drives can crash, causing the loss of all programs and stored data. Programs and extensive data can be copied by a peripheral tape backup device, thereby providing a

"Peer review" – newsletter

Staff Security Request Form								
Name of Practice Site								
Site Manager Name								
Select only one security position for each staff member								
Staff Name	Employee Number	Current Position	Site Manager/ Office Coordinator	Front	MA	MA-Orders	Batcher Insurance Biller	Medical Records
Physician Signatures								
Physician Name								
Physician Name								
Physician Name								
Approval								

Figure 11–9: Staff security request form. *Delmar/Cengage Learning.*

durable copy of information. All central computer data should be backed up on tape daily. Some offices even contract to have materials backed up to an offsite facility to protect against loss of files from fire or natural disaster.

OFFICE EQUIPMENT

In addition to computers, a variety of machines and equipment are required to manage the business operation of a medical office. Large multi-provider offices and clinics have more patients and employees and therefore require a greater number of machines and larger-capacity equipment. Smaller offices and single-provider practices might have less-specialized equipment. The following section discusses the types of common office management equipment found in a medical practice.

Copy Machine

The copy machine is extremely important to the efficiency of the office (Figure 11–10). A photocopy of correspondence, an insurance form or patient's insurance card, a patient's record, laboratory reports, or account information is often needed. Frequently, prepared literature, information sheets, and initial information forms require copying. Some offices might use the copier for monthly billing. The accounting record is copied, folded, and inserted into an envelope and mailed, thereby eliminating preparation of a separate statement.

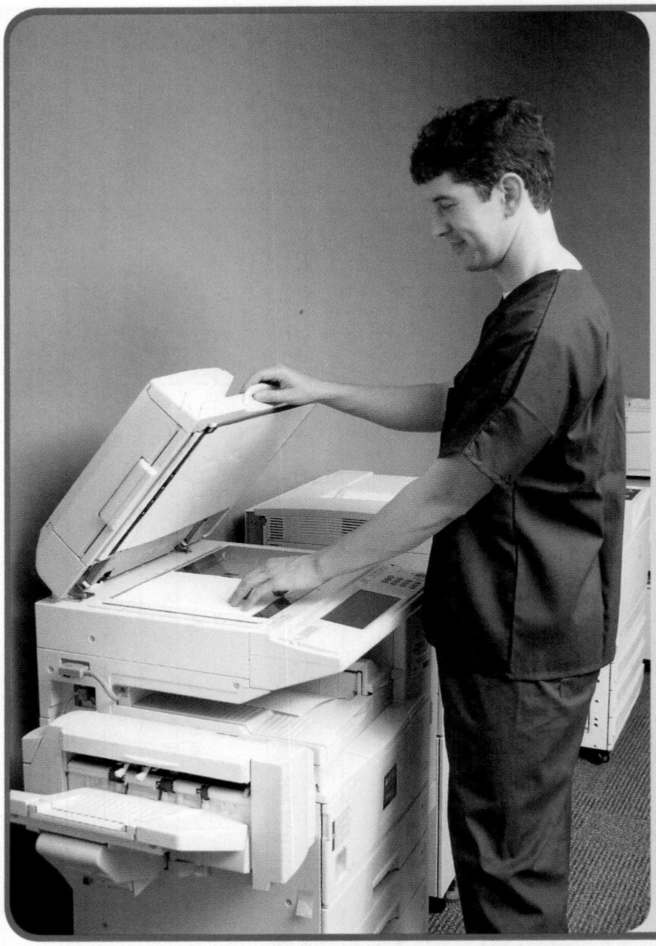

Figure 11–10: The medical assistant using a copy machine. *Delmar/Cengage Learning.*

CLINICAL PEARL

Care should be taken to avoid copying material that carries a copyright protection because this is considered illegal unless permission to copy is obtained from the writer or publisher.

Routine maintenance will improve the quality of copies. Offices should have service arrangements with suppliers of equipment and copy materials. Service representatives can demonstrate how to clean the glass, feed rollers, and surfaces and how to maintain the toner. Large copiers can be programmed to perform several functions such as enlarging or reducing copy size, stapling, sorting, off-set stacking, one- or two-sided copying, and insertion of cover sheets. You should ask for additional instruction before attempting to perform these functions. If there is a paper jam or the copier is in some way inoperable, it might be necessary to call the technician for service.

You might be assigned to provide routine cleaning and maintenance of the copier. Usually, each morning, the glass and rollers should be cleaned and the exterior wiped of dust or smudges. Pick up any discarded paper clips or staples that might get into the copier. The paper supply should be filled and the toner checked and replaced as needed. Depending on the model, some toner cartridges can be refilled by a service provider at reduced costs. Be sure to have at least one replacement cartridge in reserve, depending upon the amount of copying done in your office.

Newer models of office copy machines are capable of serving as printers and scanners, in addition to simply making copies, and can be connected directly to the office computer network. Instead of a document being sent to a printer and then using a copier to make copies, the printer is built into the copier, thereby eliminating one paper copy and one peripheral piece of equipment. A copy machine can produce copies at a much lower cost than a printer, and the features of speed, collating, off-set stacking, and others can be very time saving. The all-in-one printer, fax, scanner, and copy machine is attached to the computer and replaces four individual pieces of equipment.

PROCEDURE 11–1 Operate and Maintain a Copy Machine

PURPOSE: Accurately prepare settings on a copy machine to produce a duplicate of the original in the size, number, and order desired

EQUIPMENT: Copy machine, paper, and material to be copied

S SKILL: Operate and maintain a copy machine.

Procedure Steps	Detailed Instructions and/or *Rationales*
1. Assemble the material to be copied and prepare the copy machine for use. Turn on the copy machine; check the paper supply.	Some offices leave the machine on all day because it requires a warm-up period before it can be used. If this is not your office policy, turn the machine off when finished. Ensure adequate paper supply. *Some machines can jam when supply becomes too low.* Also, check the paper in the appropriate size supply tray. *The last person using the copier may have used colored paper, a different size, or letterhead paper.*
2. Determine the number of copies needed.	• You usually make one file copy of every letter you send. If copies are to be sent with the letter, you need additional copies. • Two copies of most medical legal reports are needed. • If you are making copies of instruction sheets for patients, copy enough for a month's use at one time.
3. Correctly operate the copy machine. a. Adjust the settings for what you want to copy (size, orientation, and so on) and for the number of copies needed. b. Raise the lid and place the material to be copied, one sheet at a time, place in the feed tray or face down on the glass. c. Close the lid. d. Press the button or key pad to activate the copier.	Settings: Legal- or letter-size paper; regular copy, lighter, darker (can be adjusted as needed to produce acceptable copy); regular, reduced, or enlarged copy; number of copies
4. When finished copying, prepare the copy machine for the next job. a. Remove the original(s) and copies. b. Return the machine to standard settings if you changed them. c. Clean any fingerprints or other smudges appropriately. d. Restock paper supply if necessary. e. Turn off machine (if office policy dictates).	

Fax Machine

Facsimile (fax) machines (Figure 11–11) can be used by hospitals, providers' offices, and clinics to send and receive information regarding patients over telephone lines. The machine makes it possible to send and receive letters, medical reports, laboratory reports, and insurance claims. Providers can use the fax machine to receive and send prescription orders to pharmacies, and the office can also use it for ordering office or medical supplies.

Learn the specific procedure for operating the fax machine you will be using. Following are general rules that are important for the use of any fax machine:

1. Always remove paper clips and staples from material to be scanned so you will not damage the fax machine.
2. Make a test copy if the document has color. Dark colors may block copy and can slow transmission.
3. Do not use correction tape or fluid on documents to be transmitted.
4. Do consider using typed words for numbers to avoid problems with interpretation.
5. If the material you are faxing is confidential, before sending it, call to alert the recipient to be watching for the material.
6. The first sheet of any transmission is called the fax cover page (Figure 11–12). It includes the date, name of recipient, recipient's address and fax number, and the number of pages being sent (including the fax page). The name and fax number of the sender will also be included. Any special information required for routing instructions should be added. The fax page (or cover sheet) should also include a *confidentiality notice.*
7. Be familiar with error messages the fax machine might display and learn how to correct these problems. The machine might be equipped with built-in service diagnostic codes that can be automatically transmitted over telephone lines to a service provider. Most service calls can be resolved by telephone, therefore reducing costly equipment downtime and labor costs.
8. You might need to resend a message if noise or interference on the telephone line resulted in an unclear transmission or the transmission's not going through.
9. Check to be sure the transmission is completed. The display will indicate that the message was sent, identifying the date and time of transmission. Remove the original from the machine.

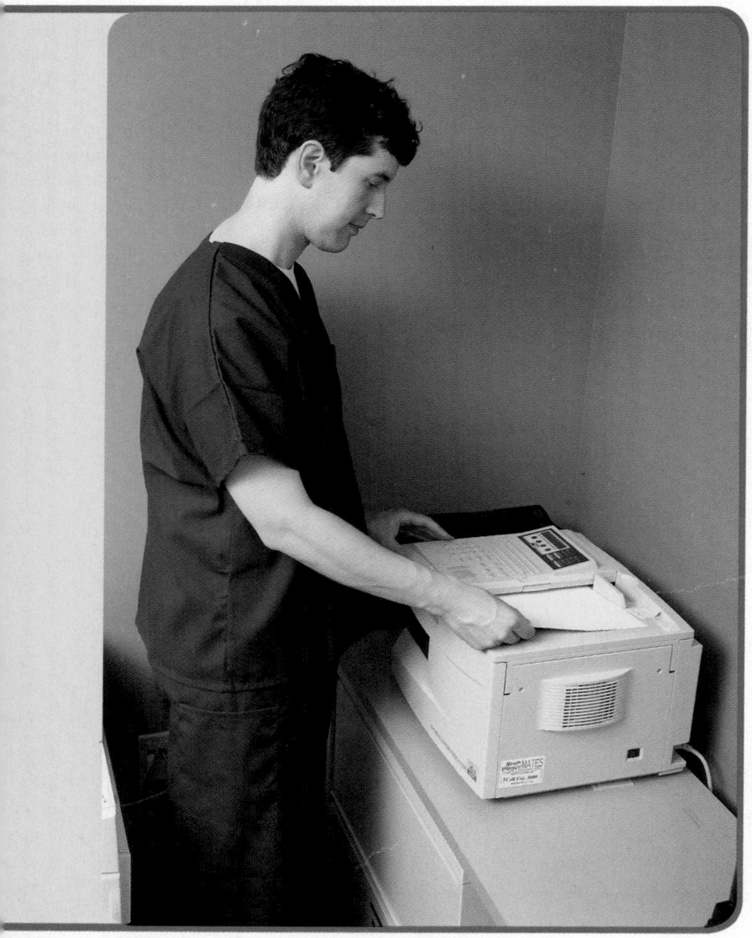

Figure 11–11: The medical assistant using a fax machine.
Delmar/Cengage Learning.

Dictation-Transcription Machine

The most common forms of dictation-transcription equipment used in the provider's office are the desktop machines (Figure 11–13). Several kinds of machines are available: a unit for **dictation** only, a unit for **transcription** only, or a combination unit that can be used for both purposes. Many providers use portable dictation equipment. The provider might use it in the office, in the car, at home, or while attending meetings. Some providers dictate their notes following each patient's appointment. When office hours are over, they will give you the tape so their observations, comments, and findings can be entered on the respective patient's EHR or paper chart.

The technology for dictation and digital voice recording is constantly improving and changing. You must keep up to date with the changes in technology for efficiency in dictation and transcription and the integration and interoperability with other software programs. Some offices outsource dictation or have specific transcribers in the office.

The dictation equipment must be kept in operating order at all times. Check to be certain it is ready for use, replace the batteries as needed, and maintain current supplies.

Community Practice
123 Main Street
Yourtown, US 12121
Phone (555) 555-1212
Fax (555) 555-1234
www.communitypractice.exa

PRACTICE NAME

Fax Cover Sheet

To:	From:
Fax:	Pages:
Phone:	Date:
Re:	cc:

❑ Urgent ❑ For Review ❑ Please Comment ❑ Please Reply ❑ Please Recycle

CONFIDENTIALITY NOTICE: This fax transmission, together with any attachments, contains confidential information that is prohibited from disclosure. This information is intended only for the use of the individual(s) or entity to whom it is intended, even if addressed incorrectly. If you have received this e-mail in error, please immediately notify the sender by fax or phone at the address shown. Please delete it from your files if you are not the intended recipient. You are hereby notified that any dissemination or copying of this message or any attachment is strictly prohibited. Thank you for your compliance.

MESSAGE:

Figure 11–12: A fax cover sheet example. *Delmar/Cengage Learning.*

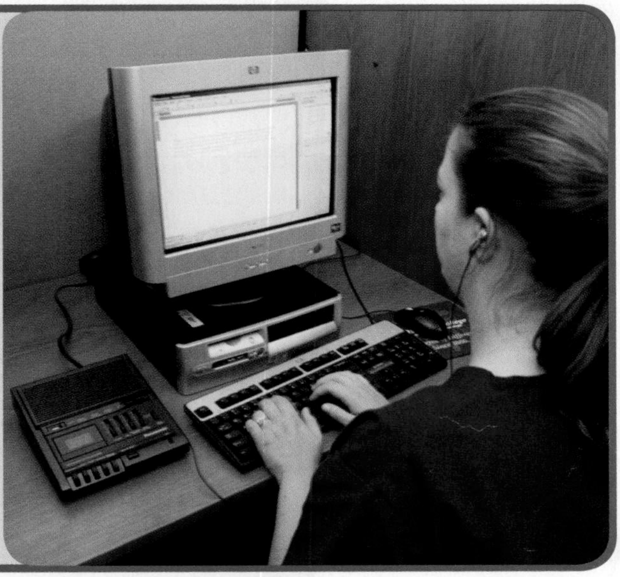

Figure 11–13: Dictation-transcription machine. *Delmar/Cengage Learning.*

When preparing to do transcription, keep in mind some helpful guidelines. If you know a certain transcription is a priority, do it first. It is also best to do the oldest dictation first so you can get caught up to date. Try to work where it is quiet and you won't be interrupted. After you select the tape, insert it in the machine, and you are ready to begin. Refer to Procedure 11–2 to transcribe a dictated document.

Many medical offices and providers are now using speech recognition software. One popular application is Dragon Naturally Speaking® (such as Dragon Medical 10.1), which allows the user to create transcription-free medical records, email, and correspondence up to three times faster than most people type, with up to 99% accuracy. Dragon Naturally Speaking offers seamless compatibility with Microsoft Office and networks and works in EHR programs. Use of voice recognition software has been found to reduce cost and turnaround time compared with traditional transcription methods. As with any transcription or voice recognition program, there can be difficulties setting up the profiles and accuracy. Be certain to carefully proofread to eliminate any errors.

PROCEDURE 11–2 Operate a Transcriber

PURPOSE: Operate the transcriber, to complete an accurate transcription within a specified time period

EQUIPMENT: Transcriber, dictation tape, headset, foot control, computer, and paper

S SKILL: Operate a transcriber to produce a printed copy from recorded material.

Procedure Steps	Detailed Instructions and/or *Rationales*
1. Assemble equipment and supplies. Turn on the transcriber; verify that a headset with earphones and the foot control are attached to the unit. Adjust the headset with earphones.	Earphones should not be shared to *prevent the spread of organisms.*
2. Insert the tape and prepare to perform the transcription, following the provider's instructions. a. Press the play tab or the pedal to listen for the beginning of the dictation. b. Listen for the provider's instructions. c. Adjust the volume, tone, and speed controls for clearest communication reception.	
3. Bring up the word processing screen and enter the recorded information. a. Set margins and tabulator stops as needed. b. Alternately press and release the foot pedal to listen to and transcribe the recorded material.	Consult a dictionary if a word is unfamiliar. If you are unable to understand a word or words, leave a blank note in the place on the tape and ask someone else to listen. If necessary, ask the dictating provider for assistance so you can complete the work.
4. Turn off the machine and place accessory items in their proper storage space. Save the dictation tape.	*Save the tape in case questions arise before the provider will approve the report or sign the document.*
5. Erase the tape following approval of the material or provider's signature on the document so the tape can be used again.	

Printers

To produce hard copies from computer files, you must have a printer. Two types of printers are appropriate for a medical office: inkjet or laser. An inkjet printer can print in different modes. In draft mode, less ink is used and the page can be printed faster. For a professional-looking finish, letter quality mode is used and, therefore, the printing process is slower. The purpose of the draft setting is to conserve printer toner or ink when printing a large number of pages of a document that is not in its final stages. Inkjet printers cost less than laser printers, but their ink cartridges are more expensive, meaning that the ink cost per printed page is higher. Inkjet printers can be more economical in offices with a lower volume of printing. Laser printers are usually preferred in an office environment with higher printing volume. Additionally, the print quality is much better.

Smart Phones and Pagers

Providers use smart phones or pagers so they can be contacted regardless of where they are or what they are involved in. A smart phone is a cell phone that also has features similar to a personal digital assistant (PDA) or computer, such as the ability to send and receive email and access the Internet or other software programs. In 2009, the Manhattan Research Taking the Pulse research reported that 64% of providers owned a smart phone and projected that the number would increase to 81% by 2012. A pager is a small electronic device that can receive (and sometimes transmit) signals and short messages. If the provider uses this technology, you would dial the pager number and enter the phone number from which you are calling. This transmits the number to the pager, and the phone number of the caller and the message will be displayed.

EQUIPMENT MAINTENANCE

The medical assistant might be asked to keep track of equipment maintenance because a number of office and clinical equipment pieces must remain operational (Figure 11–14). Most machines come with a manual for routine maintenance. Daily maintenance includes cleaning various parts (with appropriate materials), checking and resetting consumables, replacing parts, and troubleshooting. For example, refer to Figure 11–15 for scanner maintenance. Refer to Procedure 11–3 to perform routine equipment maintenance.

Equipment Maintenance Checklist

Date: 4/10/20XX Taken by: S. White, MA

	Item	Perform maintenance	Inspected	Repairs needed
1.	Copier	Clean glass, rollers, check toner	✓	—
2.	Printer	Clean, check cartridge/toner	✓	Noisy, call service
3.	Computer	Clean glass, check power cord, cables	✓	—
4.	Exam table 1	Clean, check cover	✓	Cover worn
5.	Electric exam table 2	Clean, check cover, power cord, operable	✓	—
6.	Sphygmomanometer 1	Check cuff, tubing, valve, bulb	✓	Bulb soft
7.	Sphygmomanometer 2	Check cuff, tubing, valve, bulb	✓	—
8.	Ophthalmoscope 1	Power supply, cord, bulb	✓	—
9.	Ophthalmoscope 2	Power supply, cord, bulb	✓	Replaced bulb
10.	Exam light 1	Clean, power cord, bulb	✓	—

Figure 11–14: An example of a completed equipment maintenance checklist. *Delmar/Cengage Learning.*

DAILY CARE

❑ Cleaning Materials
Soft, dry cloth
Cleaner F1 [Part # CA99501-0013 (or isopropyl alcohol)]

❑ Recommended Cleaning Cycle

Location	Standard Cleaning Cycle
Pad ASSY	Clean every 1,000 scanned sheets The scanner may need to be cleaned more frequently depending on the type of documents being scanned
Pick Roller	
Feed Roller	
Plastic Roller	
Glass	

❑ Cleaning the ADF
Open the Automatic Document Feeder (ADF)
Push the ADF button
Pull ADF cover toward front of scanner
Clean with a soft, dry cloth moistened with Cleaner F1

Pad ASSY	Clean the rubber surface downward using caution not to bend the pick springs
Pick Roller	Lightly clean the Pick roller using caution not to scratch the surface or Mylar
Feed Rollers	Hold both the "**Send to**" and "**Scan**" buttons on the **Operator Panel** and lightly hold the moistened cloth against the rollers
Plastic Rollers	Lightly clean the rollers using caution not to damage the adjacent sponges
Glass	Clean lightly

Close the ADF until the ADF button locks

(A)

TROUBLESHOOTING

❑ Removing Jammed Documents
Remove any documents from the ADF Paper Chute
Open the ADF
Push the ADF button
Pull ADF cover toward front of scanner
Remove the jammed document
Close the ADF until the ADF button locks

❑ Remedying Typical Troubles
Is the AC adapter properly connected?
Is the Power button on?
Is the ADF closed completely?
Are documents loaded in the ADF Paper Chute correctly?
Are fewer than 50 sheets of paper loaded?
Are the documents free of staples, paper clips, etc.?
Does the scanner need cleaning?
Do the consumables need to be replaced?
Are the consumables installed correctly?

❑ Items to Check Before Calling for Help
Model number
Serial number
*These numbers can be found on the sticker located on the back of the scanner

(B)

Figure 11–15: Example of equipment maintenance instructions for a scanner. (A) Daily care instructions and (B) Troubleshooting instructions. *Delmar/Cengage Learning.*

PROCEDURE 11–3 Perform Routine Maintenance of Administrative and Clinical Equipment

PURPOSE: Inspect each item for cleanliness and safe condition and ensure operability. Provide routine maintenance. Note and report any equipment requiring repair.

EQUIPMENT: Equipment list, clipboard, pen, and access to any necessary maintenance supplies

S SKILL: Perform maintenance activities to ensure the operability of administrative and clinical equipment.

Procedure Steps	Detailed Instructions and/or *Rationales*
1. Assemble equipment and supplies.	
2. Inspect each item on the list for cleanliness and record findings. If not clean, clean the item appropriately.	

Procedure Steps	Detailed Instructions and/or *Rationales*
3. Check the equipment for safety factors: a. Electric cord and plugs b. Loose screws or bolts	
4. Check for operability: a. Test any light source; replace burned-out bulbs. b. Inspect items for wear; order replacement parts. c. Briefly operate seldom-used equipment.	*Operate seldom-used equipment to ensure that it is in working condition if needed.*
5. Check required operational standards: a. Freezer temperature b. Refrigerator temperature c. Autoclave test strip	
6. Correctly fill out the equipment maintenance checklist, sign it, and submit it to the appropriate person for action. a. Write the date on the maintenance checklist. b. Note and report equipment that requires repairs.	

CHAPTER SUMMARY

- With the numerous computer applications and software used in the medical office today, it is important to understand and use computer language.
- Computer hardware refers to the hard disk drive, the CPU, the monitor, and the keyboard. Software refers to the application programs containing instructions that enable it to perform tasks such as word processing, scheduling, and recording EHRs.
- Application software allows users to interact with the computer to perform specific tasks such as word processing, managing databases, preparing spreadsheets, and playing music or videos. An application suite usually includes, at a minimum, a word processing program, spreadsheet program, and presentation software (such as Microsoft Office® or Apple iWorks®).
- Practice management software manages the operations of a medical practice and is available from a variety of companies. Functionalities can vary but typically allow a medical office to schedule appointments, record patient demographics and insurance information, process claims, perform insurance and billing routines, and generate financial reports.
- No official agency reviews or evaluates the information posted on the Internet; therefore, take precautions when reading and evaluating websites. Follow these four guidelines when using the Internet:
  1. Check the source. Are there links to professional affiliations or are there professional credentials?
  2. Be cautious about personal testimonies from users; they often are receiving monetary compensation for making statements.
  3. Watch for dates of the information; the information might be very old and no longer valid.
  4. Use your analytic and critical thinking skills to interpret *scientific* studies or reports. Who did the research? How many people were included in the study? Is the amount of time spent appropriate to arrive at the stated conclusions? Is there more than one study on the subject to give its results credibility?
- *Downtime* is a term describing when the computer systems are not operating. The office must have downtime forms and procedures in place for this occurrence. Downtime forms and procedures are

used when there is a power outage or connectivity issue (wireless connection is unavailable, telephone lines are out, and so on).

- A number of machines are used in a medical office in addition to the computer. Examples include:

1. Copy machine: photocopies correspondence, insurance forms, laboratory reports, and so on.
2. Fax machine; sends and receives information regarding patients over telephone lines.
3. Dictation-transcription machine: available as desktop or portable equipment, enabling providers to dictate their notes and for others to transcribe them.
4. Printer: produces hard copies from computer files.
5. Pagers: Providers commonly wear pagers so they can be contacted regardless of where they are. Today, cell phones with data features are commonly used in lieu of or in addition to pagers.

STUDY TOOLS

Workbook	Activities for Chapter 11
Premium Website MEDIA LINK	View this **Media Link** for Chapter 11: • Ergonomics
StudyWARE	Activities and Quizzes on the **StudyWARE™ Software** for Chapter 11
	Audio Library of medical terms
	Online access to **Critical Thinking Challenge 2.0**
learninglab	Module 5: Business Communications
CourseMate	Activities and Quizzes for Chapter 11
WebTutor	Activities and Quizzes for Chapter 11

CHECK YOUR KNOWLEDGE

1. Which types of material are often photocopied?
   a. Patients' insurance card(s)
   b. Patients' drivers license
   c. Patients' Social Security card
   d. Lab reports
   e. a, b, and c
   f. a and d
2. Identify when dictation is NOT used.
   a. Patient notes
   b. Patient appointment time
   c. Patient observations
   d. Patient findings
3. Which is NOT a computer term?
   a. IOC
   b. Virus
   c. Attachment
   d. Interface
4. All of these are computer programs, except:
   a. digital voice recorder.
   b. medical practice management software.
   c. electronic health records software.
   d. encoder software.
5. Which is NOT referred to as computer hardware?
   a. PDA
   b. Router
   c. Printer
   d. Scanner
   e. Modem
6. Explain why backing up computer data is necessary.
   a. Deletes unwanted information
   b. Human error
   c. Virus
   d. Hard drive error
   e. All of the above
   f. b, c, and d

WEB LINKS

Relay Health: www.relayhealth.com

Ingenix: www.ingenix.com

REFERENCES

"Provider Smartphone Adoption Rate to Reach 81% in 2012." *Providers in 2012: The Outlook for On Demand, Mobile, and Social Digital Media*. www.manhattanresearch.com/newsroom/Press_Releases/provider-smartphones-2012.aspx (Retrieved 12/28/2010)

Unit

6

Beginning the Patient's Record

Chapter 12
Scheduling Appointments and Receiving Patients

Chapter 13
The Medical Record, Documentation, and Filing

Maintaining organization and a regular flow of activity in the medical office not only ensures that the schedule remains on course, but it directly influences the perception of professionalism patients, vendors, and visiting providers develop when in the office. A professional, relaxed, and orderly appearance reassures patients that their examinations and assessments will be thorough and accurate. The patient's first impression will likely remain with him or her, influencing several factors. It can determine his or her willingness to continue with the practice but can also alter how well that patient will trust that the instructions provided should be followed. A terse, disorganized appearance will give an impression of less than competent practice, whereas a relaxed, well-prepared demeanor will inspire confidence and compliance with provider instructions and recommendations.

The most professional attitudes, competent practice, and exceptional customer service will be of little benefit if accurate documentation of patient visits, examinations, findings, and reports are not maintained meticulously and filed in a timely fashion. A loss of a single report can have a dire impact on a patient's outcome. A missed laboratory value that could have been easily corrected or a pathologic diagnosis of cancer being filed incorrectly that results in treatment is not being instituted may put the entire practice at risk—and everyone's jobs. By having predictability in the schedule, staff members experience decreased stress, achieve goals, and interact positively with one another, providing a much more pleasant and productive work environment. From a business and legal perspective, an orderly flow to the workday ensures that results, reports, and financial documents are maintained and filed accurately, protecting both the patient and the medical personnel from loss or missed information.

Certification Connection

	Ch. 12	Ch. 13
CMA (AAMA)		
Records management		X
Scheduling and monitoring appointments	X	
RMA (AMT)		
Medical receptionist/secretary/clerical: Terminology	X	X
Reception	X	
Scheduling	X	
Records and chart management		X
CMAS (AMT)		
Appointment scheduling	X	
Reception	X	
Medical records management		X

Chapter

12 Scheduling Appointments and Receiving Patients

OBJECTIVES

In this chapter, you will learn the following:

KB KNOWLEDGE BASE

1. Spell and define, using the glossary at the back of the text, all the Words to Know in this chapter.
2. List and explain the various methods of scheduling and the advantages and disadvantages of each method.
3. Describe scheduling guidelines.
4. Recognize office policies and protocols for handling appointments.
5. Identify critical information required for scheduling patient admissions and procedures.
6. Describe how the administrative medical assistant should greet and receive patients.
7. List the information that should be obtained for every new patient.
8. Explain the importance of discussing general office policies to patients.

S SKILLS

1. Schedule appointments for new and established patients, using established priorities.
2. Schedule a referral appointment for a patient.
3. Schedule an inpatient admission for a patient.
4. Apply HIPAA rules regarding privacy and release of information.
5. Gather complete patient information and verify insurance coverage.
6. Explain general office policies.

B BEHAVIORS

1. Use language and verbal skills that enable patients' understanding.
2. Demonstrate sensitivity to patient rights.
3. Incorporate the Patient's Bill of Rights into personal practice and medical office policies and procedures.

WORDS TO KNOW

audit trail
charge slip
clustering
double-booking
encounter form
flex time
matrix
modified wave
obliterate
open hours
no show
referral
single-booking
streaming
unstructured
utilization
wave

PREPARING THE APPOINTMENT SCHEDULE

Among the most primary and vital functions of medical office management is in scheduling appointments. Proper scheduling keeps the patient flow at a satisfactory pace for the provider and all office personnel and promotes a good professional working relationship. Office hours can be scheduled with appointments made during specific times or left as an open, **unstructured** block of time.

Establishing a Matrix

Weekly schedules for the provider(s) and other licensed practitioners in the facility should be accessible to everyone in the office to keep an organized routine and to know where to locate them in case of emergency. Regular office hours should be posted at the entrance of the medical facility, on appointment cards, and on other printed materials. More discussion about an office policy manual is provided in Chapter 22.

Several styles of appointment books are available that allow for scheduling as far out as a year or more. A standard appointment book printed with daily hours ranging from 8:00 AM to 5:00 PM, is shown in Figure 12–1. Custom appointment books can be ordered for offices with special needs. Computerized scheduling is most helpful for keeping track of schedules for multiple practitioners in an office.

Computerized appointment scheduling has been increasingly replacing paper appointment books and most likely will be one component of a medical practice management software system (see Figure 12–2). Such a system is most effective when multiple terminals are used throughout the office working through a single server. A paper report can be printed each morning or the evening prior to the workday in case of downtime due to computer failures. Daily backups to a secondary external drive or an offsite data management service are highly recommended.

A computerized appointment system offers the capability of locating the next available time or a specific date and time, showing appointments already scheduled, and printing copies of the daily schedule. In addition to helping with daily organization, printed copies of the schedule may be filed with accounting records of each day to serve as supporting legal documents in the event of financial audits or legal proceedings or maintained for a specified time period for retrieval on demand at a later date.

The appointment book or computer schedule should be formatted with a fixed **matrix**. A matrix refers to blocking off time slots in a paper schedule with an X or having specified time periods automatically blocked out in the computer's schedule screen, as shown in Figure 12–3. Spaces blocked by an X indicate that the provider or other health care professional will not be available during those times to treat patients. For example, nothing should be scheduled between the hours of 8:00 AM and noon on Thursdays, and nothing scheduled before 9:00 AM and after 4:45 PM on Fridays. Either the provider(s) will not be available to see patients or that segment of time is being reserved for urgent conditions or same-day appointments.

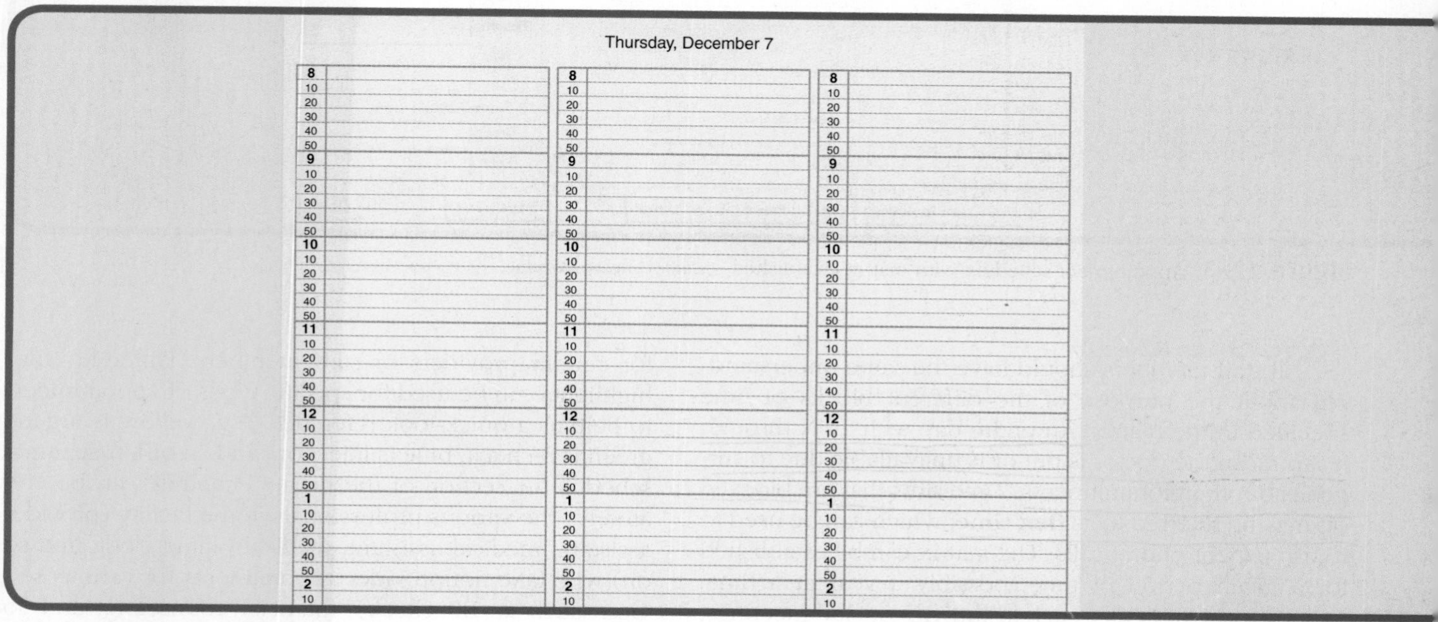

Figure 12–1: Paper appointment book page. *Delmar/Cengage Learning.*

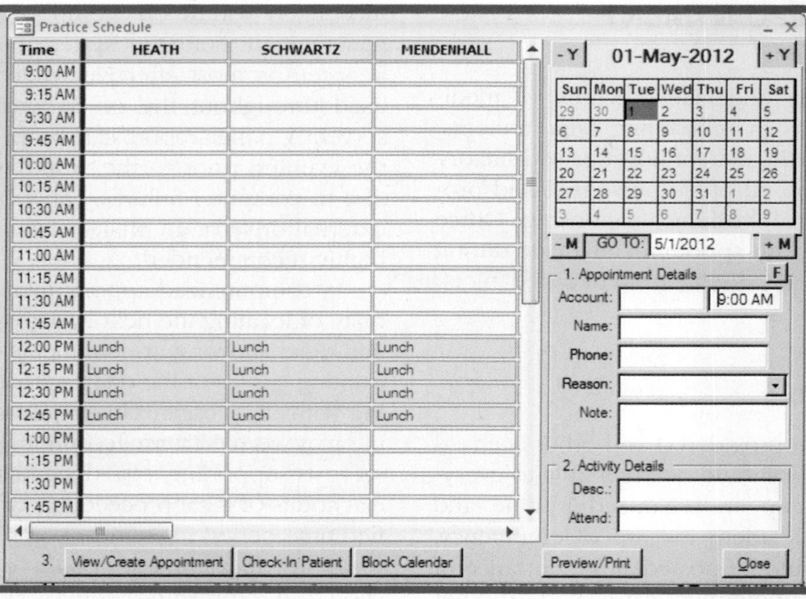

Figure 12–2: Computerized appointment schedule for multiple providers. *Delmar/Cengage Learning.*

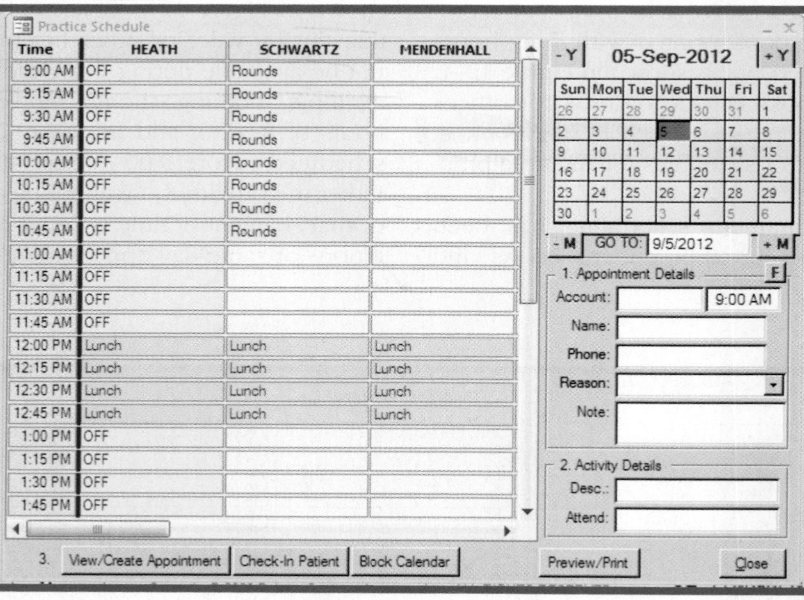

Figure 12–3: Appointment schedule with matrix established. *Delmar/Cengage Learning.*

All staff members should have the same understanding about the purpose of the different blocks of time specified in the matrix. An entire day with an X through it can mean the doctor is out or is unavailable due to surgeries or other commitments. Time slots that are blocked off may be referred to as **flex time**, which can be used to return patient phone calls. The matrix can be established for a given period of time, possibly a year at a time. Include known breaks, such as lunches or staff meetings, and regular hospital days, surgery days, or fixed days off for certain providers or staff members. Different color highlights can be used for specific types of appointments to help as a quick-look reference (e.g., yellow is urgent, green is recheck, blue is injection, and so on). A separate schedule or section of the master schedule can be created for the various professionals in the facility (provider assistant, medical assistant, medical billing clerk, and so on) who take nonprovider appointments for various services such as BP checks, financial counseling, and so on. The amount of time set aside for different types of appointments and different times of days for specific appointment categories should also be considered when constructing the matrix. Concise and consistent scheduling will prevent many conflicts and make the daily office routine much more efficient.

Methods of Scheduling

After the matrix has been established, the preferred style of scheduling is adopted based upon the particular medical practice, the provider's preference, and availability of the staff. Scheduling appointments can be done through any of the following methods, either alone or in combination: **clustering, double-booking, open hours, single-booking, streaming, wave**, and **modified wave**. Table 12–1 lists these methods of scheduling with a description of the purpose of each.

CLINICAL PEARL

Working patients into the schedule is likely a practice providers prefer to avoid but can be used in the event of an urgent need. Often, a patient's appointment does not take as long as scheduled, or a patient will fail to show for a scheduled appointment, opening time in the schedule. Before offering to work in a patient, make sure the patient's provider feels that it will be possible to examine and treat the patient in the amount of time estimated to be available. Clearly explain to the patient that this is not a routine practice, and it should not be expected in the future. Also, let the patient know that being worked in might require a significant wait. It is essential for all parties to understand clearly what is to occur for this exception in scheduling to be successful.

TABLE 12–1 Methods of Scheduling

Scheduling Method	Description	Pros	Cons
Clustering	Scheduling patients for specific type of visits or procedures at specific times; e.g., Monday mornings can be reserved for new patients, Wednesday afternoons for immunizations and school physicals.	Streamlines evaluations of patients with similar complaints. Visit paperwork can be prepared in batches ahead of time. Unnecessary personnel can focus on other tasks during cluster visits.	If one visit gets off track or requires more time than anticipated, it can throw the appointment flow off track. Focusing on categorized complaints might not leave opportunities to individualize evaluations.
Double-booking	The same appointment time is given to two or more patients.	Processing two patients at the same time may be more time efficient, enabling the provider to see one patient while waiting for a result on the other.	If a problem arises with one patient, it can delay the evaluation of the other, causing the rest of the schedule to get behind.
Walk in/Open hours	No scheduled appointment. Patients sign in upon arrival and are seen by the provider in that order.	Offers patients an opportunity to present for complaints that have an unexpected onset.	If a patient's complaint is more complex, or several patients succumb to the same problem, it can overwhelm available personnel and resources.
Single-booking	Used when an appointment for a patient will take a longer period of time. Single-booking means a single patient is booked for a specific amount of time.	Enables the provider to focus on one patient and thoroughly assess complaints.	When patients' problems are straightforward and easily addressed, this method might leave gaps in the schedule that could otherwise be used more efficiently to see other patients or perform needed ancillary tasks.

(continues)

TABLE 12–1 *(Continued)*

Scheduling Method	Description	Pros	Cons
Streaming	Appointments are scheduled for a particular amount of time based on patient need. This type of scheduling is designed to keep a continuous flow of patients coming through the office.	When used well, may keep a steady flow of patients with the most effective use of time slots.	When an unexpected problem presents and sufficient time has not been allotted, subsequent visits may be delayed.
Wave	Patients are scheduled during the first 30 minutes of each hour, leaving the last 30 minutes for same-day appointments.	Provides ample time for unexpected visits and staff to keep up with charting, filing and other tasks and preparing for the next visit in the second half hour. Most effective use might be seasonal, as in flu season or periods where large special events are taking place in the area.	Excessive downtime when the last half hour is not needed and patients do not present. A lag in the schedule can adversely affect the flow of the office by altering workflow tempo.
Modified wave	Scheduled the same as wave but with the exception of scheduling patients in the last 30 minutes at 10–20 minute intervals.	Same benefit as a wave with the added benefit of seeing more patients in the same allotted time period.	Same as the wave; however, scheduling more patients in a given period can contribute to a backup when patients are late, providers delayed, or other unexpected events arise.

Appointment Documentation

As with all medical documents, appointment entries should never be erased or **obliterated** with correction fluid. Appointment schedules are legal documents and should be kept for a period determined by individual state laws, usually about three years. A valid record of all appointments should be kept, regardless of whether the appointment was actually kept. In fact, a history of **no shows** and cancelled appointments can be helpful in defending claims against an office or provider.

Use a consistent procedure when altering the schedule for an acceptable purpose. In a paper scheduling system, one common practice is to use a large letter C at the beginning of the person's name to indicate a cancellation, or C&C to indicate that the patient did Call to tell you why the appointment had to be Canceled. Draw a single line through the original entry with the date and insert your initials and the correction made underneath it to avoid the appearance of attempting to conceal information or making a fraudulent entry after the fact. All entries must be legible. A stamp might be used to record the missed appointment or, in the case of electronic records, the changes made will be automatically stored as an **audit trail**. Figure 12–4 provides a suggested list of some commonly used abbreviations that may be used in the appointment schedule. More important, whatever abbreviations are used should be clear and consistent within a particular practice. A more extensive list of abbreviations appears in the appendix of this text.

Time Management Analysis

Over the course of a month or more, a periodic evaluation of scheduling procedures can be undertaken to determine how to manage time in the office best. Data reflecting the number of work-ins, cancellations, and no shows as well as the time spent with specific exams and complaints of patients will help determine the best way to revise scheduling techniques. Appointments can then be adjusted into short, medium, long, and extended time slots for various procedures, exams, and consultations. Often, a patient might require multiple procedures to be scheduled or must arrange to see more than one doctor

BP✓	blood pressure check
C&C	called and canceled
C	canceled
Cons	consultation
CP	chest pain
CPE (CPX)	complete physical examination
ECG	electrocardiogram
FU	follow-up examination
Inj	injection
Lab	laboratory studies
NP	new patient
NS	no show
P&P	pap and pelvic
PT	physical therapy
Re✓	recheck
Ref	referral
RS	reschedule
Sig	sigmoidoscopy
S/R	suture removal
Surg	surgery

Figure 12–4: The entire staff must know abbreviations specific to the practice and their meanings and use them consistently. Here is a sample list. *Delmar/Cengage Learning.*

in an office or a medical center in a given period of time. When possible, coordinating all these appointments for the patient on the same day will decrease the number of trips or days the patient must take off from work, and this extra effort and expression of concern can help inspire confidence in the office medical staff. The medical assistant should be prepared to offer brief explanations and general instructions for commonly ordered procedures, exams, or treatments. (However, it is the ultimate responsibility for the ordering specialist, not the medical assistant, to ensure the patient's understanding and obtain informed consent for various procedures.) Printed instructions may be sent with an appointment card as a reminder prior to the scheduled appointment, which will help the patient prepare for the exam and reduce anxiety. Further discussion and helpful information about diagnostic examinations is provided in Units 14 and 15.

Although the optimal situation is that patients are seen in the time allotted and on time, situations arise when schedules are interrupted and adjustments must be made. This can create disappointment and tension with patients, providers, and staff members. It is important to maintain composure and a professional demeanor at all times, understanding again that the frustration is likely not directed at any one person but at the undesirable situation or chain of events. Surveys have shown that patients usually tolerate up to a half-hour wait well, but longer waits can increase dissatisfaction. Recognizing that the patient's time is just as valuable as the provider's time will help in handling delays professionally. The patient should be notified tactfully and as soon as possible when a scheduling issue is recognized. One resolution might be to offer the patient a choice to continue waiting (even if it will be longer than expected) or to reschedule the appointment for another time altogether. Giving the patient a choice is generally appreciated and might be all that's necessary to alleviate the tension created by unforeseen delays.

CREATING PATIENT APPOINTMENTS

Patients who request appointments over the phone or in person deserve the same courtesy. Arrive at a mutually agreeable appointment day and time and confirm it by repeating it to the person prior entering it in the appointment book or computer. When making the appointment entry, be sure to include the name of the patient, the parent's name when appropriate, reason for visit, provider to be seen, date, time, and current phone number. The current phone number is critical for appointment confirmation and ready access if an appointment needs to be altered. In the case of a new patient, be sure to obtain complete information so that a chart may be prepared ahead of the initial appointment time, and the patient can be notified before the scheduled appointment if needed.

Certain times of the year can bring conditions that schedule conflicts, such as colds and flu in the winter months, injuries during winter and spring breaks from school, and rashes and other ailments related to summer, incur. Take these into account when preparing the daily schedule, especially those specific to a particular geographic area of practice specialty. Figure 12–5 offers a list of some helpful points to keep in mind when scheduling appointments. The saying, "Time Is Money," is a good thought to consider. It should remind us to use time well and for the purpose intended. Efficient use of the provider's time and of the entire staff in treating patients is the main purpose of a schedule.

A new patient must provide you with complete information not only so that you can prepare a chart for the initial appointment but also in case it becomes necessary to reach the patient before the scheduled appointment.

Appointment Scheduling over the Phone

Excellent communication skills, a solid knowledge of the signs and symptoms of diseases and disorders, and an understanding of medical terminology and anatomy enable the medical assistant to perform telephone screening proficiently and prepare an efficient schedule. A precise assessment of a patient's condition and actively listening to the patient's report of his or her symptoms is referred to as telephone screening. When the patient phones in with a request to see the doctor, determine the caller's identity, including the correct spelling of the caller's name, and whether that person is a new or existing patient to the practice.

Proficiency in assessing problems over the phone will come with experience. A preapproved telephone screening manual or a medical office handbook

1. Is the patient's name spelled correctly?
2. Is an appointment available in the next hour?
3. Are the date and time understood?
4. Is there enough time for this type of appointment to be completed?
5. Is there another patient in this same time slot?
6. Does the patient prefer morning or afternoon?
7. Can the same day and time be used for a series of appointments for this patient to help with remembering the appointments?
8. What is the alternate time that can be offered if this appointment is refused?
9. Has the appointment been entered in the book or computer?
10. Was an appointment card given to the patient?

Figure 12–5: Questions to be answered when making appointments. *Delmar/Cengage Learning.*

reinforces continuity among staff members and helps avoid omissions. All employees who answer such calls should use the same format and ask the same questions every time of each patient who reports similar symptoms. Following set screening guidelines previously approved by the provider helps stratify patients based on severity and urgency. Record what the patient says rather than paraphrasing his or her comments. Ask the patient precise questions and wait for the response. Ask the caller what has been tried to relieve the problem and whether it has been successful. Record exactly how much and how often which medications, home remedies, or other treatments have been used. Do not omit any information the patient says even if it seems trivial or unimportant. The information provided should be able to guide the type, urgency, and length of appointment to be scheduled.

Health insurance providers often influence which providers the patient seeks treatment from. In the case of health maintenance organizations (HMOs), providers who contract with a specific company are designated as being in network. Many times, a patient is calling to schedule an appointment because the provider is on a list of in-network providers. If the provider is unable to accept new patients, it is courteous to suggest one or two other providers who might currently be accepting new patients.

Follow-Up Appointments

The medical assistant assists patients by receiving payments and arranging necessary follow-up or referral appointments. The provider will indicate the need for a follow-up visit on the charge slip, or he or she might instruct the patient to arrange an appointment. It is always best to make the follow-up appointment prior to the patient's leaving the office. Write the time and date on an appointment card or provide him or her with a printout, giving the patient an opportunity to review the information prior to leaving. Figure 12–6 shows an example of an appointment card given to the patient. Also provide the patient with any appropriate printed instructions or educational materials regarding his or her condition, further treatment, or scheduled studies at the same time.

Appointment cards or forms provided to patients should include the full name of the provider, complete address, phone number, and type of practice printed clearly on them. In the case of a new practice or changed location, consider offering the patient a small map or printed directions to the office. For multiple office locations listed on a single form, circle the correct location to avoid future confusion. Many appointment cards for professional services state that the patient must give the staff a 24-hour notice if a change in the scheduled appointment must be made; a verbal reminder helps reinforce this policy and can be helpful in maintaining a smooth schedule, as does a telephone reminder of the appointment provided the day before.

Regular follow-up appointments can be made by sending recall notices in the mail, rather than trying to schedule annual appointments a year in advance, to remind the patient it is time to schedule an appointment. An example is a reminder for an annual Pap test. Many offices send reminder notices of appointments that were made in advance. The patient may be asked to complete the card before leaving the office to ensure that the contact information is correct.

Procedure 12–1 lists the steps in appointment scheduling.

Appointment for *Linda Parker*

On *Thurs. 4/5* at *9:30* AM/PM

With Dr. Catherine Lang—Baldwin Family Practice Center

712 Central Parkway

Central City, XX Zip Code

Telephone # 000/555-5000 Fax # 000/555-5001

If unable to keep this appointment, please give 24-hours notice or a charge will be made for the reserved time.

Figure 12–6: An example of a typical appointment card to give the patient; it has the date (and day) and time of the next scheduled appointment. *Delmar/Cengage Learning.*

PROCEDURE 12–1 Schedule Patient Appointments

PURPOSE: In a simulated situation, schedule an appointment for a patient by either appointment book or computer, remembering to follow HIPAA guidelines for safeguarding protected health information (PHI)

EQUIPMENT: Appointment book, appointment cards, or computer with scheduling program

S SKILL: Schedule patient appointments.

Procedure Steps	Detailed Instructions and/or *Rationales*
1. Determine which method will be used for scheduling: appointment book or computer entry. a. If using a paper scheduling system, mark off the hours when the provider will be unable to see patients. b. If using an electronic scheduling system, open the appointment scheduler and navigate to the correct date.	Include daily hospital rounds, lunch hour, meetings, and vacation.
2. Schedule appointments for new and existing patients, using established priorities. Write patients' names in the schedule book or enter them in the appropriate spaces on the appointment screen.	Record patients' names and phone numbers for easy access in case they need to be contacted. *New patients*: Choose a specified day or block out sufficient time for a new-patient appointment. Collect all necessary contact information and personal information to verify appointment. *Existing patients*: Offer to schedule the patient's next appointment prior to the patient's leaving the office. Ask the patient whether he or she has a preference for a particular day and morning or afternoon. As appropriate, offer the first available day that either fits with the provider's request for the next appointment or the patient's preference.
3. Complete an appointment card and give it to the patient or print out an appointment reminder slip, using the scheduling software.	Be sure to record the appointment first in the appointment book and then on the appointment card.

Referral Appointments

Patients often need to be referred to other facilities for diagnostic testing and to specialists outside the expertise of the practice's provider. For the patient's insurance company to pay for these visits, the referring provider, or the primary care provider in the case of HMOs, must submit a **referral** to the hospital, specialist, or other provider. The referring provider will direct the patient to a participating provider listed on the patient's insurance plan. To facilitate this process, keep a list of names, addresses, and phone numbers of providers to which the employer wishes to refer patients in different specialty areas (see Procedure 12–2).

Often, explaining this to the patient is one of the most important duties of the medical assistant. In some states, the law requires the insurance company to warn patients if using a nonparticipating provider will cause them to incur significant medical expenses. The patient is ultimately responsible for payment of all services received regardless of the referral source. The medical assistant can help patients avoid excess charges by verifying that a provider is contracted to accept the patient's insurance plan and ensuring that preauthorization has been obtained.

Scheduling Inpatient Admissions

When calling to have a patient admitted to the hospital, be prepared to provide all necessary information. When scheduling a hospital admission, identify the attending provider for the admission, the service the patient is to be admitted to (i.e., whether medical, surgical, or obstetric), the admission date requested, and the type of reservation (inpatient, ambulatory surgery, or outpatient). Additional information that might be required:

1. Full name of the patient (include birth names of married women or children)
2. Age and date of birth
3. Gender
4. Marital status
5. Social Security number
6. Address (including ZIP code)
7. Telephone numbers (home, pager or cell phone, and work)
8. Designated contact person or closest relative
9. Primary insurance and Social Security number of guarantor (person who will be responsible for the hospital charges)
10. Employer and work telephone number of guarantor
11. Hospital insurance coverage, with verification of preauthorization
12. Name, address, and phone number of referring provider
13. Provider's diagnosis and plan of care for the **utilization** committee review (do not guess!)
14. For scheduled surgery, provide the expected date of surgery, name, and length of procedure, type of planned anesthesia, estimated blood units to be held or used, and radiology services needed.
15. For preadmission testing, offer the date, time, and names of lab tests, X-rays, ECG, and type of patient preparation required.

Certain medical conditions justify inpatient hospital care for what would otherwise be an outpatient procedure based on severity of the illness or intensity of services. The provider will indicate what condition warrants such a condition of admission.

PROCEDURE 12–2 Arrange Referral Appointments

PURPOSE: In a professional manner, schedule appointments for an outpatient procedure and an inpatient admission

EQUIPMENT: Patient's chart with referral request, phone directory, phone, pen, and paper

S SKILL: Schedule an outpatient procedure.

S SKILL: Schedule an inpatient admission.

Procedure Steps	Detailed Instructions and/or *Rationales*
1. Obtain patient's chart with request for referral to other facility. Determine whether pre-authorization is required.	If the patient has an HMO, wait for preauthorization before continuing.
2. Locate and record correct phone number and address of referral's office.	
3. Place the call to the referral office and provide the administrative medical assistant with all appropriate information.	Information includes: • Your name, provider's name, practice address, and phone number. • Patient's name, address, insurance information, and reason for the appointment. Include the name of the contact person making the appointment or one who will be available if questions arise prior to the appointment date. • Indicate whether a referral request confirmation will be mailed or faxed. • For future reference, record in the chart the name of the person who is taking the information.

Procedure Steps	Detailed Instructions and/or *Rationales*
4. Prepare a copy of all information pertinent to the appointment to give to the patient, including the time, day, date, name, address, and directions to the facility if needed. If the patient is not present when the appointment is made, phone the patient to provide the necessary information.	If the patient is present at the time of the referral appointment call, confirm the date before finalizing the conversation, when possible.
5. Fax or mail a confirmation letter.	*This establishes a written record for both the referring office and the office receiving the referral to facilitate follow-up on both sides.*
6. Send a follow-up letter to the patient with printed instruction, referral's contact information, directions, and appointment time.	*The letter provides the patient with written information that can be referenced at a later time.*
7. Record all actions in the patient's chart and initial the patient's chart with date and time, signifying that the request was completed.	*Documentation of actions taken provide verification at a later time.*

Charting Examples

Outpatient note: Dr. Agrawal indicated Mrs. Kelly should be referred for a surgical consult. Verified that Dr. Johnson is listed in patient's insurance plan as participating provider. Signed HIPAA release faxed with visit notes to Dr. Brad Johnson's office [general surgeon] at 555-123-4567. Also spoke with receptionist, Jennifer Smith, regarding referral. Appointment date for Mrs. Kelly 1/27/2011 at 9:30 am. Appointment card given to Mrs. Kelly with address of office and Jennifer's name for additional contact if needed.	Inpatient note: Dr. Patel (surgeon) wants Mr. Garcia to be admitted for laparoscopy and possible open cholecystectomy. Admission coordinator, Jane Andrews at St. Joseph's Hospital, verified that she received admission orders. Mr. Garcia has been advised to go to hospital the day before admission to have labs performed. Orders for labs faxed to hospital. Date and time and preadmission patient instructions were given to patient. He was also advised that admitting department will have paperwork for him to sign prior to admission. Dr. Benson is patient's primary care provider and copies of all information along with date and time of planned procedure faxed to his office. He will see patient in hospital as attending provider.

MAINTAINING THE SCHEDULE

To maintain a reasonable work flow in the office, scheduling appointments must be done in time slots that are realistic for not only presenting complaints of the patients but also with the abilities of both provider providers and staff members in mind. The best means of doing this is to develop a standard within the practice of how much time is allotted for each type of visit. A blood pressure check might require only 10-minute intervals, whereas a new patient examination requires 45 minutes to an hour. Over time, these amounts may be adjusted either longer or shorter but should be continually assessed according to what is appropriate for the individual practice environment.

Another aspect of maintaining a realistic schedule is to help the provider and other practitioners stay on schedule. When it appears the schedule is getting behind and catching up is nearly impossible, the medical assistant might be asked to call patients and delay their arrival time or offer to reschedule them for another day. Explain tactfully to any patients who are waiting that the schedule is running behind by a given amount of time but they will be seen as soon as possible. Make a notation in the patient's chart regarding the reason the appointment needed to be rescheduled and how long the patient waited before leaving or being rescheduled along with his or her response to the change in schedule.

Walk-In Patients

Although unusual, a patient who has not made an appointment might arrive in the office. A sign posted near the reception window can indicate the office hours and that patients are seen by appointment *only*. When a patient arrives who has no appointment, explain that an appointment is necessary. If an appointment slot is available, it might be offered with the express understanding that it is an exception and not the usual practice. If no time slot is available, politely offer to schedule the soonest appointment that is available and appropriate for the patient's complaint. Patients who are persistent can be referred to the office manager or provider for further discussion. In the case of an emergency, notify the provider, offer emergency assistance as needed, and have another staff member notify 911.

Late Patients

Habitually late patients present yet another challenge to maintaining a reasonable schedule. An established office policy regarding repeated late arrivals should be part of new-patient packets. Document patterns of late arrival or missed appointments in the chart and request that the provider or office manager discuss the office policy with the patient. When there are extenuating circumstances, such as transportation, child care, or work-associated problems, an exception should be made and a solution sought to prevent future problems. For example, in some practices, late arrivals are rescheduled when the patients arrive 10 to 15 minutes past the scheduled appointment. The length of time should be part of the written policy and acknowledged and adhered to by all staff.

Canceled or Missed Appointments (No Shows)

When a patient cancels or does not show for a scheduled appointment, note this in the person's chart and offer the appointment time to another patient when possible. Notify the provider of the schedule change and whether the patient called to cancel or was a no show. The provider will advise whether further action is warranted based on the patient's previous appointment history and medical condition. For example, a missed follow-up for a muscle strain might not be cause for concern, but a diabetic patient missing an appointment for wound care and dressing changes is at an increased risk for serious infection, and attempts at rescheduling are usually indicated. Record the appointment as canceled or as a no show in the schedule and in the patient's chart. Telephone the patient to remind him or her of the missed appointment and offer to reschedule. If the patient cannot be reached by phone, mail a letter regarding the missed appointment, offering to arrange another appointment. If the patient's condition warrants, a second letter with a certified return receipt may be sent to determine the patient's status and to demonstrate that all efforts were made to contact him or her.

Business Appointments

In addition to medical appointments and unexpected schedule disruptions, other professionals can arrive in the practice unannounced or call for an appointment to present the provider with new information regarding medications, office equipment, medical supplies, or other business opportunities. The most efficient use of time and to avoid having the visit interfere with the regular office schedule is to offer a regular appointment slot. A reserved appointment slot will allow the provider adequate time to acquire desired information on products with ample time for questions and answers. On occasion, representatives might offer to bring complimentary items, including lunch and other treats for the office staff. There are federal laws regarding what is an acceptable amount, so always be sure to obtain approval from the provider or office manager. Sample medications left must be handled appropriately and will be addressed in the pharmacology section of this text. Be sure to obtain the provider's approval prior to distributing any products left to patients or to staff members. Determine what length of time slot the provider would like reserved for such visits; some might not wish to see representatives themselves and ask instead that they talk to the office manager or medical assistant or mail information. Politely interrupt to let the provider know when a colleague or family member drops in for a visit. Based on the number of patients present, consider offering a polite reminder of the number of patients still waiting before the meeting begins.

GREETING AND RECEIVING PATIENTS

The administrative medical assistant working at the front desk is often the first person a patient encounters in the office. This is a very significant role. It is extremely important for the patient's initial experience to be very positive; to ensure this, the administrative medical assistant should:

- Greet patients promptly and courteously (Figure 12–7).
- Maintain eye contact when talking to patients.
- Call patients by their full names.
- Actively listen to patient remarks and show that you care about their concerns.
- Explain patient instructions thoroughly.
- Do not question or discuss personal matters with patients in the reception room.
- Respect the patient's right to confidentiality.

The administrative medical assistant should be positioned within the office to have a clear view of the reception room. If the space is behind a wall with a glass window partition, the reception room may not be seen easily. A dividing window offers the advantage of privacy

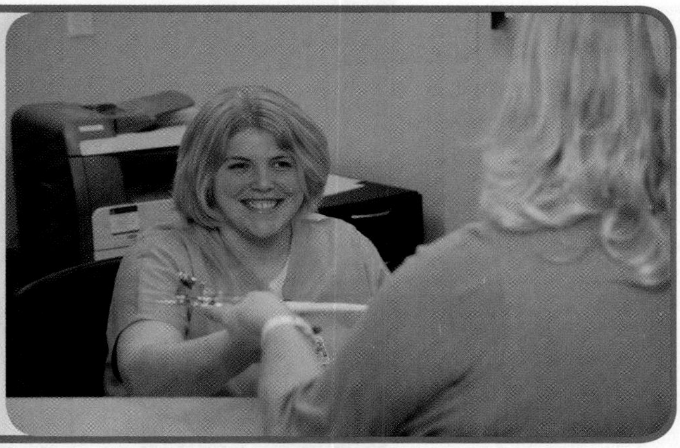

Figure 12–7: The administrative medical assistant should greet each patient with a warm and friendly smile.
Delmar/Cengage Learning.

for telephone conversations, talking with patients, or performing other duties but can interfere with noticing the new arrivals who might not report to the window when they come in. A very ill patient should not be required to or allowed to sit in a reception room. As soon as possible, assist the patient into an examination room where the patient can be made comfortable until the provider can see him or her. Remember to ensure the patient's safety. Warn the patient (and advise any companions) to be careful while lying on the narrow examination table.

Monitoring the social climate of the reception area can reveal behaviors that could cause an unfavorable impression of the office or have an adverse effect on others, such as the use of offensive or obscene language or unauthorized soliciting in the office. Addressing any situations professionally and as politely as possible early on can prevent escalation and additional problems. It might be necessary to have the provider or office manager intervene and, in very rare circumstances, law enforcement might be required if the person becomes aggressive.

Patient Sign-In

Even when appointment times have been assigned to patients, having patients sign in when they arrive is a good policy (Figure 12–8). Sign-in sheets help identify new patients who might need to complete forms and help track arrival times and waiting times. The sign-in sheet should not request any personal information because it will be out where others can read it. Consider just asking for a first name, time of arrival and general reason for appointment (i.e., new patient, follow-up, blood pressure check, and so on), or whoever receives patients might complete the sign-in instead of patients.

New Patients

The administrative medical assistant or receptionist might be charged with the responsibility of ensuring that new-patient information forms are completed. If this is done through an interview, be sure that others cannot overhear the questioning process (Figure 12–9). Another common method for acquiring new-patient information is to have the patient or parent fill out the forms. It is important to give clear instructions and ask whether there are any questions. If a patient appears reluctant to complete the form or exhibits difficulties that indicate a reading problem, quietly offer to assist in completing the forms in a closed room where confidentiality can be maintained. Check to be sure this form is complete and signed by the responsible party. Procedure 12–3 discusses the steps in obtaining new-patient information.

The following information should always be obtained:

- Patient's full name (if obtained by interview, verify the spelling)
- Date of birth (DOB)
- Social Security number (SSN)
- Marital status
- Current address and length of time at that address
- Telephone numbers at home and at work or pager, cell phone, email, and fax numbers
- Name and relationship of person legally responsible for charges. Under normal circumstances, parents are considered responsible for the charges of their children. Oral agreements are not necessarily binding, and the individual who will pay the bill needs to sign a simple statement before care is given. This statement may be a form prepared by the provider or office manager or a handwritten statement (Figure 12–10). Additionally, a child or mentally disabled person might be a ward of the state, and the state will be responsible for charges.
- Patient's occupation, including the name, address, and phone number of employer. Also record the spouse's work information if available.
- Health insurance information. Ask to see the patient's identification cards for all plans that provide coverage for the patient and make a copy of both sides of the card(s) as documentation that coverage is in force at the time of the visit. A signed release of information separate from the one printed on insurance forms might be required in some states and should be completed at the time of the first visit (Figure 12–11).
- A copy of the patient's driver's license or the driver's license number and expiration date. This information is helpful in verifying the patient's identify and in locating him or her later if needed.
- If referred, write down the referral source. This information might helpful if there is trouble locating the patient or he or she moves without leaving a forwarding address.

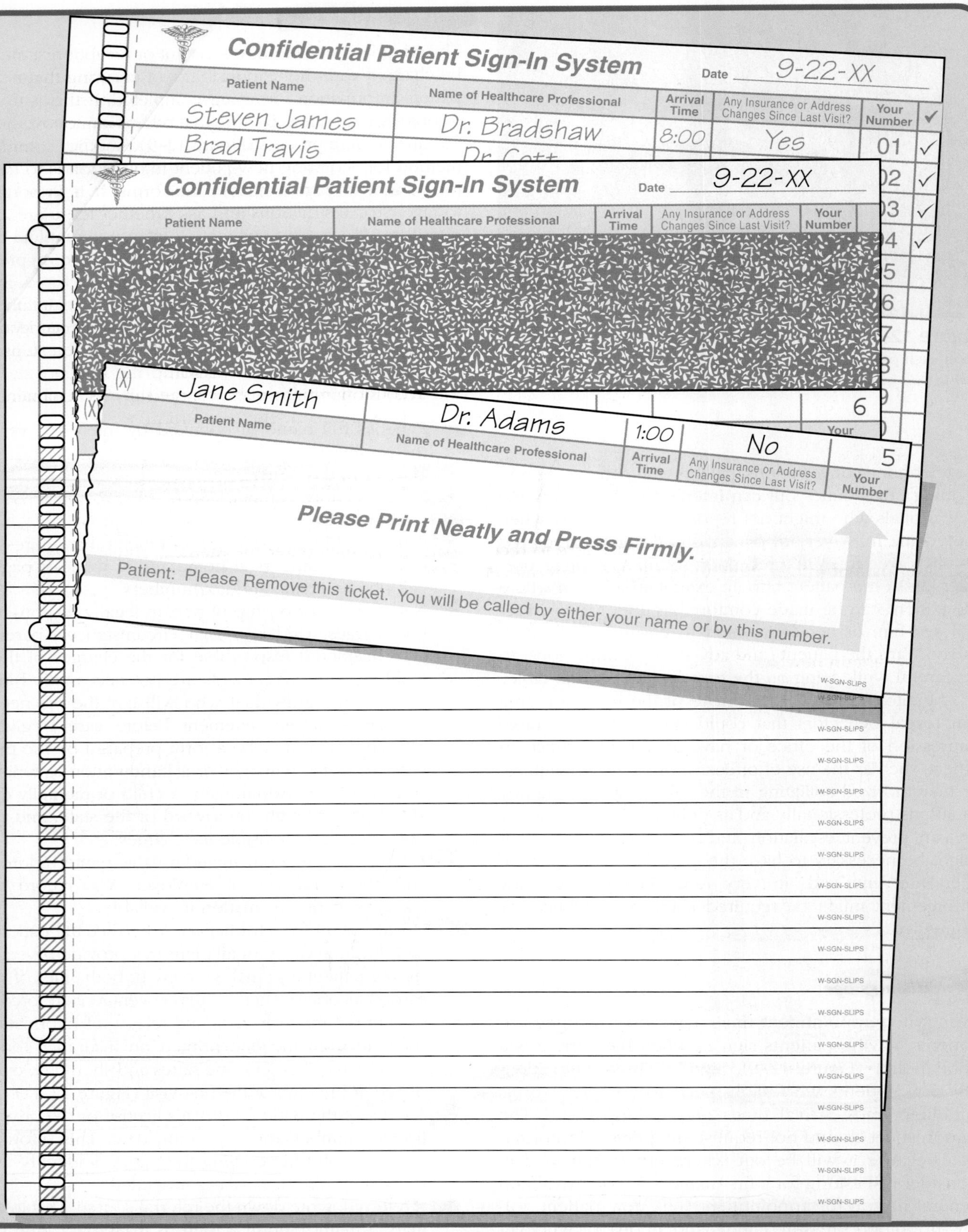

Confidential Patient Sign-In System
Date 9-22-XX
Patient Name
Name of Healthcare Professional
Arrival Time
Any Insurance or Address Changes Since Last Visit?
Your Number
Steven James
Dr. Bradshaw
8:00
Yes
01
Brad Travis
Confidential Patient Sign-In System
Date 9-22-XX
Patient Name
Name of Healthcare Professional
Arrival Time
Any Insurance or Address Changes Since Last Visit?
Your Number
Jane Smith
Dr. Adams
1:00
No
5
Please Print Neatly and Press Firmly.
Patient: Please Remove this ticket. You will be called by either your name or by this number.
W-SGN-SLIPS

Figure 12–8: Patients should sign in upon arrival at the medical office. *Delmar/Cengage Learning.*

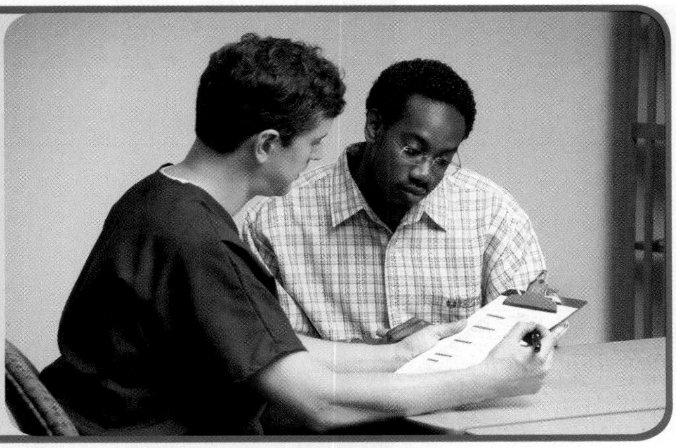

Figure 12–9: A medical assistant and patient are in a private area discussing the patient's completed information form. *Delmar/Cengage Learning.*

Verifying Insurance and Preparing Charge Slips

Verify the patient's insurance coverage by phoning the insurance company or electronic verification with the company. Place a copy of the verification or scan of the card and completed insurance forms in the patient's financial file with any other referral materials.

In an office without electronic health records, the administrative medical assistant has the responsibility for preparing **encounter forms** (also known as **charge slips**) that accompany the patient charts. The encounter form lists the procedures, with the respective codes, that are appropriate or most frequently performed in the office. It also includes a space for the patient's name and date and any additional information requested. Clinics may prepare charge cards to stamp the patient's name and account number on the charge slip. See Chapter 14 for an example of an encounter form.

PROCEDURE 12–3 Receive a New Patient and Create a New Patient Chart

PURPOSE: Complete the steps in the procedure to receive patients as they enter the medical office, including obtaining patient information and verifying insurance eligibility

MATERIALS: New patient form, patient's insurance card, encounter form, chart folder, tabs, and computer

S **SKILL:** Obtain new patient information.

S **SKILL:** Verify insurance information.

S **SKILL:** Apply HIPAA rules concerning privacy and release of information.

Procedure Steps	Detailed Instructions and/or *Rationales*
1. Greet the patient promptly and courteously, calling the patient by full name. Maintain eye contact when talking to the patient.	
B 2. Ask the new patient to complete a new-patient information form; or, in a private area, ask preliminary questions. ***Do not question or discuss personal matters with patients in the reception room. Offer to assist the patient if it appears he or she is having difficulty.***	*A medical history is part of the medical and legal records and should be checked for accuracy.*
3. Prepare a new patient chart: a. If using EHR, create a new patient chart, using the information provided on the information form. b. If using paper charts, prepare a patient folder with the patient's name and pertinent information. Include any new information in the patient's chart. Transfer information from the form to the chart sheet. Insert the chart, sheets, and information form in the folder.	

(continues)

(continued)

Procedure Steps	Detailed Instructions and/or *Rationales*
4. Ask the patient for the insurance card: a. If using EHR, scan the insurance card and attach it to the patient's chart. b. If using paper charts, copy the insurance card (both sides). Place the copy in the patient's folder.	
5. Verify insurance by phoning the insurance company or by submission through the EHR program.	*Person-to-person contact may be necessary for less than fully automated systems and should be followed up with receipt of a fax verification of eligibility from the insurance company.* For either partially or fully automated systems, a fax or emailed verification may be received from the insurance company to verify coverage. Either the electronic or paper verification should be entered in the patient's chart.
6. Prepare an encounter form and attach it to the chart. Place the folder in the area reserved for charts of patients to be seen.	

Jason E. Jackson, MD
8247 Central Avenue
Stockdale, NY 23456-7890
345-678-9100

Date: 6-17-XX Patient: Julia Renee Price
Party Responsible for Payment: Martina J. Burnette

I, Martina J. Burnette, agree to pay for all examinations and treatments for Julia Renee Price.

Margo Little 6-17-XX
Witness Date

Figure 12–10: Example of a third-party liability statement. *Delmar/Cengage Learning.*

MEDICAL RECORDS RELEASE Date ____________

I, Kendra Leigh Forest, 4406 Slate Run Drive, Bluestone MI, request that all of my medical records be released from:

Catherine R. Lang, MD
431 S. Water Street
Bluestone, MI 12345-6789
123/789-0123

To: Jason E. Jackson, MD
8247 Central Avenue
Stockdale NY 23456-7890
345/678-7890

Sonia D Philips 3-7-xx Kendra Leigh Forest 3-7-xx
Witness Date Patient Date

Figure 12–11: Records release form. *Delmar/Cengage Learning.*

Before the patient is seen, the encounter form is completed and attached to the chart, and the chart is placed in a designated area until the patient is taken to the examination room. As the provider completes the examination or treatment, the charge slip is available for the appropriate entries to be made on the slip.

EXPLAINING OFFICE POLICIES

In the course of medical treatment, patients tend to feel anxious about all the new and unfamiliar experiences of interviews, tests, examinations, and financial issues they encounter. One way to ease fears and maintain good rapport with patients is to communicate clearly what is expected of patients in the practice as well as what patients can expect from the office staff.

Patient's Bill of Rights

Posting a Patient's Bill of Rights is one way to communicate the legal rights patients have while under the care of a practitioner or facility but also what rights they have *ethically*. Such a bill of rights, unlike that of the U.S. Constitution, is not part of law but rather an outline of legal and ethical guidelines observed by the practice and the patient. Some of the components of a patient's bill of rights would include:

- Patients should be and should expect to be treated professionally with respect and courtesy at all times and, most important, when they are feeling most vulnerable, such as when receiving unpleasant news.
- Patients should have a clear understanding of what they can expect regarding how their privacy will be protected and how their personal information will be used.
- Patients have a right to participate actively in the decisions made in providing their health care and procedures and to undergo only those procedures for which they provide informed consent.
- Patients should be advised of what means of communications will be used to contact them regarding medical information, how insurance billing will be handled, any safety procedures they are expected to observe while in the office, and what they can expect from the practice's employees in general.

Office policies should be outlined briefly at the initial visit with an offer to answer specific questions and more in-depth explanations provided as needed throughout the patient's subsequent episodes of care. Office policies pertaining to patients are developed and derived from both the legal and ethical responsibilities of the practice to its patients. Although it is not necessary always to spell out which is which, the well-informed medical assistant will be able to clarify the difference when patients request more information.

Explain office policies by using a tone of voice and body language that conveys a business-like demeanor. Do not be apologetic, implying that the policies might be inconvenient or unimportant. Do not appear judgmental, suggesting that the patient will not or is not really expected to comply with the stated policies and that they are just being stated because it was demanded by the supervisor. Look at the person directly, speak clearly, and look for signs that further explanation or clarification is needed. Some persons might be reluctant to ask for additional information. When the policies have been discussed, offer an opportunity for the patient to ask questions. Answer questions as completely and as clearly as possible in the time allotted. Refer any questions or concerns outside of the medical assistant's realm or ability to address to the officer manager, provider, or other staff member as appropriate.

HIPAA Privacy Notice

To maintain legal requirements regarding patient privacy under the Health Insurance Portability and Accountability Act (HIPAA), patients new to the practice should be asked to read and sign a HIPAA Privacy Notice outlining when and how their personal health information can be disclosed to another party and when it will not be. (See Figure 12–12.)

If the reason for the visit includes a planned admission, an explanation of how the patient's medical information will be shared with the hospital is appropriate. Releasing a patient's personal and medical information to an attorney also requires a signed consent form under HIPAA. Genetic testing, mental health and therapy records, and substance abuse records require special consents for their specific release and should not be included as part of a general release of information. An exception to this requirement for signed consent is in the case of a public health risk or emergency situation as identified by appropriate authorities, in which case, the patient must be informed that the information was released.

Informed Consent

An international declaration as well as U.S. federal law requires patients to be informed in advance and provide written informed consent before their information can be used in research unless personal identifiers are removed. Personal information is sometimes retrieved through a database search to offer patients the opportunity to participate in research protocols. This activity first requires approval by a panel of medical and community experts, usually referred to as an ethical review board or institutional review board, to ensure that patient safety and confidentiality is being protected. This type of information should not just be retrieved and compiled arbitrarily without first making sure that appropriate steps have been taken to protect patients' information. Failure to do so is both a legal and an ethical violation that could result in fines and revocation of certification or licensure.

Patients should never be expected to undergo invasive procedures or surgeries or participate in research activities without providing informed consent. Informed consent is not just the act of having a patient sign a consent form but is a process of providing all relevant information to the patient regarding the potential risks and benefits needed to make an informed decision regarding whether they feel they should proceed. (Refer to Chapter 5 for a more in-depth discussion on informed consent.)

CLINICAL PEARL

Although the *consent form* may be offered for signature and witnessed by the medical assistant, the actual consent for the procedure must be obtained through explanation and discussion by the practitioner who orders or performs the procedure. For instance, the medical assistant may witness the patient signing a consent form for surgery but only after the surgeon has explained all the risks and benefits of the surgery to the patient's satisfaction and answered all the patient's questions. If any element of the consent process is missing, the consent has not been legally obtained.

Your Practice Name Here

Authorization for Disclosure of Health Information

Patient Name:____________________

Date of Birth:____________________ Phone:____________________

Address:____________________

City:____________________ State:____________________ Zip:____________________

1. *I authorize the use or disclosure of the above named individual's health information as described below.*
2. *The following individual or organization is authorized to make the disclosure:*

Name:____________________

Address:____________________

City:____________________ State:____________________ Zip:____________________

3. The type and amount of information to be used or disclosed is as follows: (include dates where appropriate)

_____ Complete health records

_____ Physical exam

_____ Immunization record

_____ Other (please specify):____________________

_____ Lab results/X-ray reports

_____ Consultation reports

4. I understand that the information in my health record may include information relating to sexually transmitted disease, acquired immunodeficiency syndrome (AIDS), or human immunodeficiency virus (HIV). It may also include information about behavioral or mental health services and treatment for alcohol and drug abuse.

5. *This information may be disclosed to and used by the following individual or organization.*

Name:____________________

Address:____________________

City:____________________ State:____________________ Zip:____________________

*For the purpose of*____________________

6. I understand that I have a right to revoke this authorization at any time. I understand that if I revoke this authorization I must do so in writing and present my written revocation to the health information management department. I understand that the revocation will not apply to my insurance company when the law provides my insurer with the right to contest a claim under my policy. Unless otherwise revoked, this authorization will expire on the following date, event, or condition: ____________________.

7. If I fail to specify an expiration date, event, or condition, this authorization will expire in sixty days. I understand that authorizing the disclosure of this health information is voluntary. I can refuse to sign this authorization. I need not sign this form in order to ensure treatment. I understand that I may inspect or copy the information to be used or disclosed, as provided in CFR 164.524. I understand that any disclosure of information carries with it the potential for an unauthorized redisclosure and the information may not be protected by federal confidentiality rules. If I have questions about disclosure of my health information, I can contact:

____________________,

Privacy Officer for____________________.

____________________ ____________________

Signature of patient or legal representative Signature of witness

Date:____________________ Date:____________________

PLEASE NOTE: This information has been disclosed to you from confidential records protected from disclosure by state and federal law. No further disclosure of this information should be done without specific, written, and informed release of the individual to whom it pertains or as permitted by state law and federal law 42 CFR, part II.

Figure 12–12: Example of a new patient information form, including HIPAA disclosure(s). *Delmar/Cengage Learning.*

Insurance Billing

Most general and specialty practices perform insurance billing as a courtesy to their patients. It is not a legal requirement for them to do so. Filing insurance claims can be confusing, so having the practice perform this task increases payment and decreases time to payment. One of the consent forms usually signed by a new patient gives assignment of benefits to the provider, which means that the patient gives permission for the provider to bill the patient's insurance directly for payment rather than the patient submitting his own insurance forms for repayment. A practice may not have the personnel resources to perform secondary billing in addition to billing the primary insurance, so the patient should have this explained at the time of service to avoid any confusion. For an elective or cosmetic procedure, payment in full can be required prior to the procedure being performed. Emergency or urgent procedures might not allow time for preauthorization and could possibly result in decreased or only partial payment from the insurance company. The patient should be advised that he or she might be responsible for the remainder that exceeds the authorized amount and any co-pays that apply. Explaining payment options and billing procedures in advance can help avoid most misunderstandings regarding financial matters.

Patient Responsibility

Although it is important to recognize the patient's rights when providing care, the patient should be advised of his or her responsibilities to the provider, the practice, and the staff. The patient has a responsibility to be honest and report all symptoms, injuries, and any medications, drugs, or herbal remedies he or she is currently using. Without complete information, good medical decisions cannot be made, and treatments might be prescribed that are actually harmful. When contracting with the provider for medical care, the patient agrees to make payment for services rendered. The provider has the right to expect the patient to keep his or her account in good standing to maintain the business and pay expenses related to the building and staff payrolls. The patient also has an obligation to treat the staff with courtesy and respect. Keep in mind that not all people are brought up with the same understanding of what is respectful. Different cultures define respect and disrespect based on very different behaviors. Reserve judgment and do not jump to conclusions. Maintain a professional and polite demeanor regardless of the behavior. If a patient uses profane language or clearly inappropriate behavior, have a witness come into the room and calmly inform the patient that his or her behavior is inappropriate for the situation and should cease immediately. Medical staff members are

PROCEDURE 12–4 Explain General Office Policies

PURPOSE: Explain both the practice's expectations for patients as well as what legal and ethical rights the patient can expect

EQUIPMENT: Quiet room free from distraction, printed patient education materials

S **SKILL:** Explain general office policies to a new patient.

S **SKILL:** Apply HIPAA rules regarding privacy and release of information.

S **SKILL:** Incorporate the Patient's Bill of Rights into personal practice and medical office policies and procedures.

Procedure Steps	Detailed Instructions and/or *Rationales*
1. Identify patient.	
B 2. Invite the patient into a room free of distractions and ***close the door to maintain and protect the patient's privacy.***	*Provide an environment in which the patient can engage in an active discussion.*

(continues)

(continued)

Procedure Steps	Detailed Instructions and/or *Rationales*
B 3. Introduce yourself, identify your role in the practice, and tell the patient what to expect from the conversation, ***using language the patient can understand and making the patient feel at ease.***	Example: "Good morning, I'm Janet, the medical assistant for Dr. Jones. I would like to give you an explanation of our office policies for new patients. It will help familiarize you with the way our office runs and what you can expect." *Doing this offers the patient a better understanding of what kinds of questions you are prepared to answer.*
4. Provide preprinted information and policies, preferably in the patient's native language (or with verification through a translator followed by documentation of patient's response to explanations).	*Visual reinforcement of printed policies helps the patient understand better and remember key points.*
B 5. ***Individualize the conversation and discussion based on the patient's needs and reason for visit. Analyze communications in providing appropriate responses and feedback.***	
6. Provide the patient with an opportunity to ask questions.	*Ensures that the patient fully understands what has been explained.*
7. Refer questions to appropriate others for further explanation or clarification.	*Make sure the patient has all needed information.*
8. Document time, date, patient response, and any materials provided in the patient record.	*Create a record of the conversation for later reference.*

Charting Example

12/1/XX 9:30 am	Office policies discussed with Mr. Davidson, particularly policy regarding smoking as patient is a known smoker. Stressed importance of compliance with office policies and procedures, especially since compressed oxygen cylinders are used and maintained in office. Patient acknowledges and agrees. Copy of printed policy provided to patient. T. Gutierrez, RMA(AMT)

not expected to tolerate physical or verbal acts of abuse or sexual harassment. If any of these are experienced, notify the supervisor or provider at once. Based on the situation, the patient can be asked to leave or even be subject to legal actions.

Payment Planning

The medical assistant can help patients who are going to have a baby, elective surgery, or extensive therapy by helping them understand in advance what costs will be outside of what insurance will pay. Reviewing insurance coverage with the patient can help him or her develop a payment plan that can help alleviate additional stress following the event. Some providers use a cost estimate sheet to give the patient an idea of the costs associated with surgery or long-term treatment (Figure 12–13). The estimate might include the approximate cost of the anesthetist, any consultants, special equipment, and hospital charges. It is important for the patient to understand that the anticipated costs provided on the estimate are just that—an estimate. In the event of unforeseen complications or additional problems, expenses are likely to be higher than the estimate. Covering this topic thoroughly prior to providing care helps prepare the patient better and decreases financial losses to both the patient and the practice.

If the patient will need to pay a substantial sum out of pocket, it might be necessary to discuss in advance how payments will be made. The insurance company

SURGERY COST ESTIMATE

Catherine R. Lang

123-789-0123

Patient ______________________ Date __________

Scheduled surgery time: __________

At ______________________ Hospital/Medical Center

On the day of your scheduled surgery you should arrive at ______ AM/PM and go to the ______ floor.

Check with your insurance company for the cost that you are expected to pay (your co-pay) unless your insurance covers the total cost. Plan for budgeting payments or coinsurance for this service.

For your information, in addition to the hospital costs for your surgery without complications, you will be charged for the following:

- Operating Surgeon __________ $______ to $______
- Assisting Surgeon __________ $______ to $______
- Anesthetist __________ $______ to $______

The total cost of the surgery and related charges are based on the length of time for the procedure. Your costs also will vary with the procedure's complexity and length of time of your hospital stay. For the surgical procedure that you are having, the average length of stay in the hospital is ____ days. The hospital room charges depend on your preference of a semi-private or private room. Be sure to bring your insurance information with you the day of your surgery. You will be telephoned ahead of time by a hospital admissions clerk to discuss specific information and to give you a confirmed time for your surgery. This person may also ask you to come to the hospital a few days or a week before your surgery to do a series of blood tests and a preadmission exam.

If you have any questions or concerns, please call us at the number at the top of this estimate.

Figure 12–13: Surgery cost estimate and information sheet. *Delmar/Cengage Learning.*

Catherine R. Lang, MD
431 S. Water Street
Bluestone, MI 12345-6789
123-789-0123

FEDERAL TRUTH IN LENDING STATEMENT

For Professional Services Provided

Patient ______________________ Date __________

Address ______________________________

—

____

—

Parent/Guardian ______________________________

1. Fee for Service $__________
2. Down Payment $__________
3. Unpaid Balance $__________
4. Amount Financed $__________
5. Finance Charge $__________
6. Annual Percentage Rate of Finance Charge
7. Total Amount of Payments (#s 4 + 5) $__________
8. Deferred Payment Price (#s 1 + 5) $__________

Total payment due (#7) is payable to Dr. Catherine R. Lang at the above address in monthly payments of $________, the first of which is payable on __________, 20XX. Each subsequent payment is due on the 15th of each month until paid in full.

__________ ______________________________

Date Signature of Patient/Parent/Guardian

Figure 12–14: A federal Truth in Lending form. *Delmar/Cengage Learning.*

might deny payment for a portion of the charges. Costs can often accumulate over a long period of treatment, as with physical therapy or rehabilitation. The Truth in Lending Act, which is enforced by the Federal Trade Commission, specifies that when an agreement is made between the provider and a patient for payment in more than four installments, the provider is required to provide a detailed description of finance charges (Figure 12–14). The patient should sign the disclosure or description in the presence of a witness and the signed form kept on file for two years or longer if required by local law. If the provider makes no specific arrangement for more than four payments for the full amount, rather than more installment amounts, the signed statement may not be necessary.

Credit Card Usage

Credit and debit cards are used in almost every facet of personal business, including paying co-pays, deductibles, and coinsurances. Flexible and medical spending accounts are established by employers to set aside a portion of an employee's pre-taxable income for use during the calendar year to pay for projected medical expenses or prescription medications. The office should display a sign indicating which methods of payment are accepted. The bank at which the practice keeps accounts might be able to provide a sign to post that shows the logos of the different types of cards accepted.

CHAPTER SUMMARY

- Scheduling appointments can be done effectively using matrixes in either computer-based systems or handwritten scheduling books.
- The schedule can be not only an organizational tool but also a time management tool by using it to analyze the time efficiency of the office.
- Different types of appointments might require various approaches and the collection of different types of information.
- Whether done in person or by phone, scheduling all types of patient appointments requires consideration for the patient's schedule and should always include collection of complete and accurate contact information.
- The well-prepared medical assistant will be able to explain both the practice's expectations for patients as well as the legal and ethical rights the patient can expect.
- By understanding and being prepared to discuss payment methods and arrangements, the medical assistant can help patients to plan ahead and alleviate stressors related to prospective expenses.

STUDY TOOLS

Workbook	Activities for Chapter 12
Premium Website StudyWARE	Activities and Quizzes on the **StudyWARE™ Software** for Chapter 12
	Complete the following **Competency Challenge 2.0** activity: • Monday, 8:00 AM, Manage the Telephone and Make Appointments
	Audio Library of medical terms
	Online access to the **Critical Thinking Challenge 2.0**
CourseMate	Activities and Quizzes for Chapter 12
WebTutor	Activities and Quizzes for Chapter 12

CHECK YOUR KNOWLEDGE

1. A *matrix* refers to what?
   a. Establishing blocks of time in a schedule for different types of appointments and scheduled breaks
   b. The material that holds printed or copied material together
   c. A method to connect different computers in the office
   d. Tangle of ethical and legal dilemmas faced by an office practice
2. Which type of scheduling might be most helpful to streamline evaluations of patients with similar complaints?
   a. Double-booking
   b. Wave
   c. Streaming
   d. Cluster
3. When explaining office policies to patients, all the following should be included EXCEPT:
   a. What the patient can expect from the office staff
   b. How the provider allocates the earnings made through the business management of the practice
   c. What types of confidentiality protections are in place
   d. How the patient is expected to behave while receiving services from the office
4. Which of the following types of information will not be required when prearranging a hospital admission?
   a. Insurance numbers
   b. Patient's demographic data
   c. Types of services expected during the admission
   d. Diagnosis chosen by the medical assistant

5. Which is the most appropriate action for greeting patients when they arrive in the office?
   a. They should be taken immediately to an exam room to protect their confidentiality.
   b. Have them sign in on the sign-in sheet with their full name, specific reason for visit, and social security number to avoid confusing them with other patients who might have similar names.
   c. Greet the patient by his or her full name and make eye contact.
   d. None of these is appropriate.

WEB LINKS

Patient Protection and Affordable Care Act, Patient Bill of Rights: *www.healthreform.gov/newsroom/new_patients_bill_of_rights.html*

American Hospital Association Patient Bill of Rights: *www.patienttalk.info/AHA-Patient_Bill_of_Rights.htm*

Chapter 13

The Medical Record, Documentation, and Filing

OBJECTIVES

In this chapter, you will learn the following:

KB KNOWLEDGE BASE

1. Spell and define, using the glossary at the back of the text, all the Words to Know in this chapter.
2. Discuss principles of using electronic medical records.
3. Identify types of records common to the health care setting.
4. Describe various types of content maintained in a patient's medical record.
5. Differentiate between subjective and objective information.
6. Identify systems for organizing medical records.
7. Identify both equipment and supplies needed for filing medical records.
8. Describe indexing rules.
9. Discuss pros and cons of various filing methods.

S SKILLS

1. Describe and demonstrate the process of making a correction to a progress note entry.
2. File medical records.
3. Maintain organization by filing.

B BEHAVIORS

1. Consider staff needs and limitations in establishment of a filing system.

WORDS TO KNOW

audit
charting
chief complaint
Chief complaint, History, Examination, Details, Drugs/Dosages, Assessment, and Return Visit (CHEDDAR)
chronologic
documentation
ethnicity
history physical impression plan (HPIP)
indexing
meaningful use
objective
privacy officer
problem-oriented medical record (POMR)
progress notes
purge
subjective
subjective objective assessment plan (SOAP)
tickler file

THE PURPOSE OF RECORDS

A complete and accurate medical record is a combination of the patient's personal information, personal medical history, known family history, social habits, medications, occupational exposures, and different types of testing performed. When any one of these is absent, the provider is without all the data needed to make an accurate diagnosis and plan further care. The medical assistant plays a pivotal role in compiling and maintaining all the elements of a complete medical record to facilitate the provider's evaluation and manage the patient's course of treatment.

The patient's personal information contains demographic information that includes gender, **ethnicity**, religion, age, marital status, living arrangements, children, occupation, and insurance information. Gender is relevant to certain types of disease processes and treatments, as is ethnicity. Persons from different ethnic groups might share a genetic propensity toward certain diseases or disorders. Some ethnic and religious groups have dietary practices that can prevent them from accepting specific types of medical care, and some practices can even interfere with prescribed drugs and treatments. Age is important when evaluating diseases of childhood, adolescence, childbearing years, and the older adult. Marital status, children, and living arrangements provide information regarding potential stressors as well as support systems. Occupation and insurance information can indicate exposures to environmental hazards or toxins and whether the person has financial support for treatment.

The medical record serves as a way to maintain and document the course of medical evaluations, treatments, and changes in condition. **Charting** progress lays out a chronological account of the patient reports, provider's evaluation, prescribed treatment, and responses to treatment as well as the need for further follow-up. Recording communications that occur between provider and other health care professionals further enforces continuity in the patient's care and helps eliminate incompatible therapies or duplication of efforts that can lead to unnecessary expense or even overdoses of medications. Copies of all reports from various providers, tests, diagnostic procedures, or interventions should be carefully maintained and shared among providers.

In addition to maintaining optimal patient care, a complete and accurate record provides legal protection for both the patient and the provider. To support a patient's accounts of injury, the provider would need to refer to the medical record. The provider would also require a complete medical record if he or she needed to defend him- or herself against legal action brought by a patient. No matter the reason for the requested records, a patient must provide a signed authorization before any information may be released (Figure 13–1). The authorization must specifically indicate who should receive the information and for what purpose it will be used. In the case of mental health records, substance abuse treatment, or genetic testing, additional authorization is required in addition to a general release of information.

The medical record may also be used for insurance purposes. Patient records help verify that claims filed for payment are based on accurate and appropriate treatments as approved through the contract between the company and the provider and meet federal laws that address reimbursement. Insurance companies may send a representative to perform periodic chart **audits** (inspections) of patients insured by the company. Medical offices receive an overall grade that reflects the thoroughness and quality of their recordkeeping. Offices that consistently score low jeopardize future contracts with those insurance companies.

Records can also be helpful in conducting research. A searchable database of patient records can help identify patients who might benefit from inclusion in clinical research protocols. Clinical trials can offer the advantage of a treatment otherwise unavailable to the patient and additional care he or she might not have otherwise received.

HIPAA AND THE MEDICAL RECORD

The Health Insurance Portability and Accountability Act of 1996, or HIPAA as it is commonly called, required many changes for health providers as well as for health insurance carriers. Although the act has a larger scope than just privacy of health records, privacy is the specific focus of information discussed in this unit. The areas that pertain primarily to records management include:

1. Maintaining the privacy of health information.
2. Establishing standards for any electronic transmission of health information and related claims.
3. Ensuring the security of all electronic health information.

The HIPAA Privacy Rule for all medical data became effective in April 2003 to provide standards for patients' confidential, personal information. Medical facilities realized that they needed to limit what information was released and to whom it was released. HIPAA is more lenient than most realize, and the Privacy Rule allows each organization to do what it feels is reasonable within the mandated guidelines, although it does not dictate the manner in which organizations will comply with the rule. All health care providers have specific policies and procedures in place to document the organization's compliance. It is essential for every employee to comply with the policies that apply to any health information released. Most institutions employ a designated HIPAA officer whose responsibility it is to

AUTHORIZATION FOR RELEASE OF INFORMATION

Section A: Must be completed for all authorizations.

I hereby authorize the use or disclosure of my individually identifiable health information as described below.
I understand that this authorization is voluntary. I understand that if the organization authorized to receive the information is not a health plan or health care provider, the released information may no longer be protected by federal privacy regulations.

Patient name: Hilda F. Goodman **ID Number:** 4309

Identity of person/organization disclosing protected health information

Persons/organizations providing information:
Practon Medical Group, Inc
4567 Broad Avenue
Woodland Hills, XY 12345-4700

Persons/organizations receiving information:
Jennifer P. Lee, MD
400 North M Street
Anytown, XY 54098-1235

Identity of those authorized to use protected health information

Specific description of information [including from and to date(s)]:
Complete medical records from 4-22-XX to 9-15-XX

Specific description of information to be used or disclosed with dates

Section B: Must be completed only if a health plan or a heath care provider has requested the authorization.

Purpose for disclosure

1. The health plan or health care provider must complete the following:
   a. What is the purpose of the use or disclosure? Patient relocating to another city
   b. Will the health plan or health care provider requesting the authorization receive financial or in-kind compensation in exchange for using or disclosing the health information described above? Yes__ No X
2. The patient or the patient's representative must read and initial the following statements:
   a. I understand that my health care and the payment for my health care will not be affected if I do not sign this form.
   Initials: hfg
   b. I understand that I may see and copy the information described on this form if I ask for it, and that I get a copy of this form after I sign it.
   Initials: hfg

Section C: Must be completed for all authorizations.

The patient or the patient's representative must read and initial the following statements:

Expiration date

1. I understand that this authorization will expire on 12 / 31 / 20XX (DD/MM/YR).
Initials: hfg

Individual's right to revoke this authorization in writing

2. I understand that I may revoke this authorization at any time by notifying the providing organization in writing, but if I do not it will not have any effect on any actions they took before they received the revocation.
Initials: hfg

Redisclosure conditions

3. I understand that any disclosure of information carries with it the potential for an unauthorized redisclosure and the information may not be protected by federal confidentiality rules.
Initials: hfg

Individual's signature

Hilda F. Goodman
Signature of patient or patient's representative
(Form MUST be completed before signing)

September 15, 20XX
Date

Date of signature

Printed name of patient's representative:__________

Relationship to the patient:__________

YOU MAY REFUSE TO SIGN THIS AUTHORIZATION
You may not use this form to release information for treatment or payment except when the information to be released is psychotherapy notes or certain research information.

Figure 13–1: Authorization for release of information. *Delmar/Cengage Learning.*

understand the rulings, train the staff in aspects of the ruling, and keep abreast of all changes with respect to HIPAA regulations and recommendations. A designated **privacy officer** must keep track of who has access to protected health information within a facility.

With the trend to replace paper records with **electronic health records (EHR)**, additional considerations pertain to records management and HIPAA compliance. A Security Rule within HIPAA mandates that not only the privacy of medical records but also the security of the records must be guaranteed. The focus of the Security Rule applies to paper records but is primarily concerned with electronic information and methods to protect it from invasion, accidental disclosure, or loss. Within the

Security Rule, providers must demonstrate compliance in four core areas:

1. Ensure confidentiality, integrity, and availability of all electronic protected health information (PHI) the providers compose, receive, maintain, or send out.
2. Have policies and procedures in place to protect against use or disclosures of the electronic information that is not required or permitted under the Privacy Ruling.
3. Have policies and procedures in place to protect against threats or hazards to the protected health information records.
4. Demonstrate compliance with the Security Ruling within the workplace.

There are varying detailed categories within the rule to show compliance. In the event of an audit, the Centers for Medicare and Medicaid Services (CMS) will ask for **documentation** to evaluate how that office is complying with requirements of the Security Rule. Categories reviewed during an audit include:

- Administrative safeguards
- Physical safeguards
- Technical safeguards
- Organizational requirements
- Documentation

Office new-employee orientation and periodic updates should include training in maintaining records security. Understanding the rationales that pertain to health care record security helps ensure that office personnel maintain the requirements necessary for compliance.

ELECTRONIC HEALTH RECORDS

The National Alliance for Health Information Technology (NAHIT) has established definitions for electronic medical records (EMR), electronic health records (EHR), and personal health records (PHR). The NAHIT defines EMR as the electronic record of health-related information for an individual that is created, gathered, managed, and consulted by licensed clinicians and staff that is maintained through a single organization involved in the individual's health and care. EHR differs from EMR in that it is the aggregate electronic record of health-related information on an individual that is created and gathered cumulatively across more than one health care organization and is managed and consulted by licensed clinicians and staff involved in the individual's health and care. An EMR can be more useful from a specialist's perspective because it focuses more directly on a particular diagnosis, whereas the EHR, being of more benefit from an insurance company or health maintenance organization perspective, will include different types of encounters for multiple problems. PHR or personal health records are simply the collection of medical records compiled and maintained by the individual.

The National Institutes of Health (NIH) uses the Health Information Management Systems Society's (HIMSS) definition of EHRs:

> The Electronic Health Record (EHR) is a longitudinal electronic record of patient health information generated by one or more encounters in any care delivery setting. Included in this information are patient demographics, progress notes, problems, medications, vital signs, past medical history, immunizations, laboratory data, and radiology reports. The EHR automates and streamlines the clinician's workflow. The EHR has the ability to generate a complete record of a clinical patient encounter, as well as supporting other care-related activities directly or indirectly via interface—including evidence-based decision support, quality management, and outcomes reporting (retrieved 7/24/2010 from www.ncrr.nih.gov/publications/informatics/ehr.pdf).

EHRs provide improved management of patient records and facilitate more efficient billing for services. They also enable providers within an institution or system to use interactive flow sheets and develop customized order sets that can be great time savers. Over the long term, the hope for EHRs is to streamline medicine not only within facilities or systems but to provide continuity and emergency access to patient information when the patient is in a locale away from regular providers, as on vacations or business trips. Such a nationalized system can also facilitate the harvesting of broader sets of data used to evaluate public health problems over a population and subdivide the results into various smaller sets. This can be applicable to environmental exposures such as air and water pollution, dietary influences of different regions, propensities for cancers across a region or population, and many other factors.

When President George W. Bush addressed the American Association of Community Colleges' annual convention in 2004, he commented that the United States was behind the times regarding patients' records. He remarked that the current health care system still used paper files and still dealt with the multitude of associated problems associated with paper, including the resulting threats to security of the information contained in personal health records. Since that time, the federal government has provided incentives for medical practices to convert to electronic health records through approving projects that encourage the implementation of such technology in medical practices.

To qualify for these incentives, providers must satisfy **meaningful use** performance measures that indicate the practice is using the electronic record rather than just having a system in place to benefit from the incentive program. Among these are transmitting more than 40 percent of their prescriptions electronically, providing patients copies of their electronic health information within three days more than 50 percent of the time, and obtaining patient demographic data a minimum of 50 percent of the time. These are only examples. The 2010 update can be found at www.ofr.gov/OFRUpload/OFRData/2010-17207_PI.pdf [retrieved 7/23/2010].

Advantages of EHRs include:

- Availability of a searchable database that records patients' demographics, allergies, lab results, and improved accessibility of the record to health care providers.
- Radiology and laboratory departments that can transmit results directly to the provider, reducing the time to treatment and notification of critical values.
- Electronically entered prescriptions that minimize errors related to illegible handwriting and reduce the time for prescriptions to be available to the patient. Software screens medications for interactions and allergies, decreasing the chance of an adverse reaction.
- Aiding in reminding the health care provider when routine testing should occur, such as mammography, vaccinations, and cardiovascular procedures.
- In a multi-specialty facility or practice, facilitating coordination of care among providers and eliminating duplicate or incompatible testing and treatment.
- Chart notes that can be available immediately when a patient needs a referral or consultation with another provider.
- Voice recognition software that improves availability of printed records and decreases costs by eliminating the need for transcribing dictated notes.
- Assigning CPT and ICD codes at the time of the visit, streamlining the process of filing insurance claims.
- A photograph of the patient, which can be included in some software applications to ensure that the correct patient's record has been selected.
- Trending that might also help identify problems that might not be identified as early as when using traditional paper records.

Although EHR does not completely eliminate the necessity for paper records, it does decrease it. The use of EHR can streamline efficiency of health care, billing, and personal information security. Electronic records can also improve the health of an entire population by providing an accessible platform for deriving information that can help identify trends such as childhood obesity or flu epidemics. The provider and staff of a practice must, however, take all necessary precautions to ensure the security of electronic information and guard against its unauthorized access or use.

PARTS OF THE MEDICAL RECORD

The medical record is divided into the following sections:

- Administrative data
- Financial and insurance information
- Correspondence
- Referral
- Past medical records
- Clinical data
- Progress notes
- Diagnostic information
- Lab information
- Medications

Patient files are generally arranged in an orderly fashion in sections as follows (with the chart opened flat): progress notes are on the right with physical exam form under them; imaging reports and lab reports are shingled on the inside (right) back cover of the chart; and on the inside cover (left) are immunization records, medication list, and patient data. This is one way to organize a chart. Follow the existing office policy. When filing additional documents in a patient's chart, place them in order of dates with the most current date on top. See Procedure 13–1.

Subjective vs. Objective Information

The information in the medical record is classified as subjective or objective. The **subjective** information is supplied by the patient and includes routine information about the patient, past personal and medical history, family history, and chief complaint. The provider and various members of the health care team provide **objective** information (e.g., vital signs, exam findings, diagnostic tests, and so on). The objective information includes examination, laboratory results, special procedure findings, X-ray reports, diagnoses, prescribed treatments, and progress notes. Table 13–1 provides examples of subjective and objective information.

TABLE 13–1 Subjective and Objective Statements and Information

Subjective	Objective
I have a headache.	The patient's temperature is 37.9°C/100.2°F.
I'm feeling palpitations.	Your heart rate is elevated at 120 beats per minute.
You don't look well.	The patient's skin is pale and diaphoretic, and he is grimacing.
My baby is fussy.	The child has not stopped crying for 12 hours and will not take fluids.
Mrs. Jones has flushed skin and says her mouth feels dry.	Mrs. Jones is a diabetic with a sugar of 325 mg/dl by fingerstick testing.

Administrative, Financial, and Insurance Information

Prioritize matters in order of importance and complete each task one at a time to help reduce stress and improve efficiency. At the first visit, every patient should be asked to provide the necessary demographic information on the patient data form as completely as possible. This includes such data as full name, Social Security number (SS#), birthdate, spouse's name, address, work and home phone numbers, insurance information, emergency contact information, and so on. Demographic and insurance information should be verified at every visit and any changes updated on both the patient's chart and in the computer (Figure 13–2). A very important item for a new patient is the HIPAA privacy statement that should be completed with the first encounter and checked for accuracy at every visit. A sign posted in the reception area and at the checkout window might be a simple question to patients such as, "Do we have your current address and phone number?" or "Please let us know if there are any changes in your personal information." Some offices post a sign or notice on the back of the exam room door so that a patient can read the reminder while waiting to be seen and let the medical assistant know of any changes.

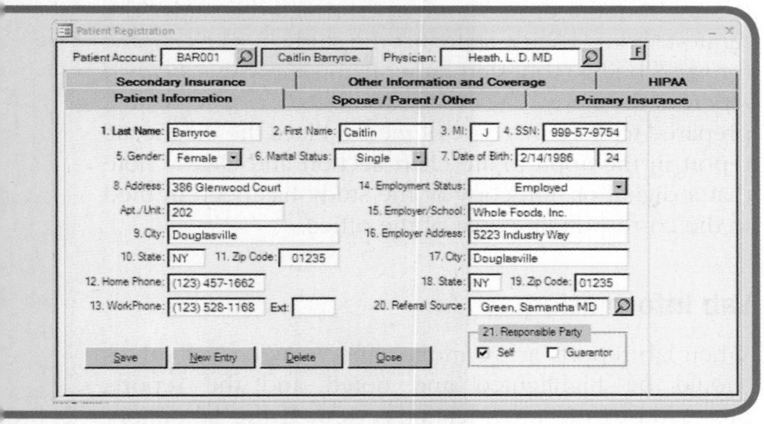

Figure 13–2 A: Confirm the patient's demographic information and update the record with any changes. *Delmar/Cengage Learning.*

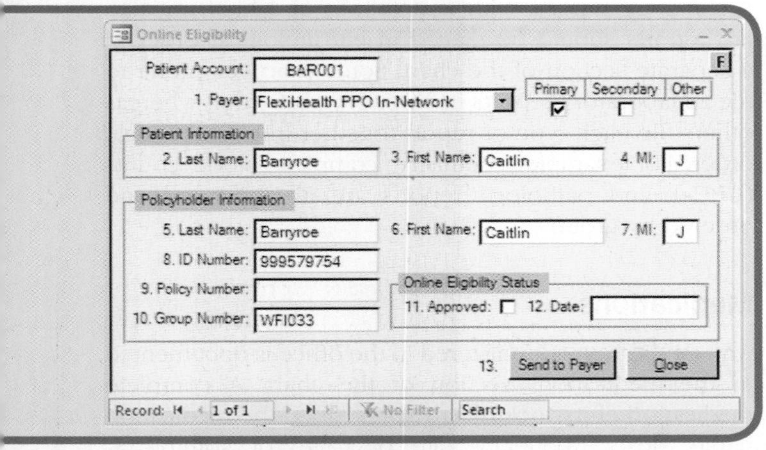

Figure 13–2 B: Verify insurance information at each visit. EHR software typically has an online eligibility feature by which to verify coverage. *Delmar/Cengage Learning.*

Financial and insurance information should be guarded carefully. This includes insurance policy numbers, credit card information, and any legal documents that might be required when the patient is seen as part of a workers' compensation claim, disability evaluations, or as part of accident or injury evaluations and treatments. It is important for this information to be protected and maintained accurately and clearly to protect the patient's financial well-being as well as to ensure that claims are processed correctly and appropriately. For instance, a patient may be seen by a practice for both regular medical visits that are billed to the patient's private insurance as well as for other instances, when the visit is charged through an attorney for personal injury or workers' compensation as part of a workplace-related injury or illness. Maintaining accurate documentation of each is important to avoid confusion and to be sure that visits are billed correctly.

Correspondence and Referrals

All correspondence received, whether medical or financial, concerning the patient should be maintained in the record. Referral or follow-up letters from specialists, informational or request-for-information letters from insurance companies, and any correspondence from the patient should be filed in the patient's chart as soon as possible after it is received. In an EHR, correspondence is scanned and uploaded into the patient's chart for easy retrieval.

Past Medical Records

A routine activity in admitting new patients to a practice is to request medical records from prior providers for continuity of care and to provide a basis of comparison for new events. By having a baseline from which to work, the provider can avoid duplicating unnecessary evaluations, tests, and treatments that have previously failed. Not only does this improve the level of care and efficiency by decreasing the time required to arrive at an accurate diagnosis, but it also prevents subjecting the patient to unnecessary discomfort and expense while keeping insurance costs down.

Even though patients have a legal right to their medical information, the chart belongs to the provider or the practice. A patient should never leave the office with a chart. Some patients might have information in the medical chart that could be damaging to them if they read it. For example, mental health notes or diagnoses that the patient does not have the capacity or educational ability to understand can cause emotional harm. A provider's order is required before any information in the chart can be released. The provider will indicate which reports and comments are authorized to be copied for release to the patient. Copies or written summaries of a patient's health records are usually the format chosen to send to another provider or health care facility.

Progress Notes

Progress notes, as the name implies, document the progress of each patient. Progress notes are entered in the chart chronologically and encompass many types of encounters and communications with the patient, mostly those that occur within the practice but also to record information about the patient from *outside* the practice (Figure 13–3). By maintaining a record of visits, prescription refills, all calls that pertain to the patient, and all calls that the patient has had with any member of the health care team, a more comprehensive assessment of the patient's presenting problems can be completed. All interactions that take place between the patient and the medical office should be recorded in the patient's progress notes. Progress notes should be arranged in chronological order, with the most recent date on top and each entry timed, dated, and initialed or signed. If several notes are recorded on a page, the last note on the page should be the most recent. A note is entered for each no show, cancellation, telephone call, or prescription.

The provider or licensed practitioner will likely indicate a preferred format for all notes, which should be adhered to for consistency. One recommended format for progress notes is to label the initial visit for any condition as a specific **chief complaint** (preferably in the patient's own words) and subsequent visits for the same problem titled as "follow up for (complaint) initially seen on (date)." The chief complaint or presenting problem is a brief description of the reason for the patient's visit. A history of the present illness and any remedies taken by the patient are included with any prescription and over-the-counter (OTC) medications currently used. The patient's medication and drug allergies should be recorded and updated during each subsequent visit. Use abbreviations that are standard and recognizable to the staff and specialty when charting information. Record complaints, as well as any pertinent negatives or signs and symptoms the patient denies, which are also useful pieces of information in making the final diagnosis. Pain levels must be assessed and recorded on the chart by using the standard scale of 1 to 10, with 10 being the worst or children's pain scales such as Wong-Baker faces or the Oucher! scales. The provider will complete the progress notes by listing all objective finding, assessment, and plan for further treatment and by signing the chart after the patient's examination is completed. Refer to Chapter 37 for more information on the medical history and patient screening.

Diagnostic Imaging Information

Imaging used to refer only to roentgen films (X-rays), but the digital age has brought about the ability to view and transmit all types of imaging, including both still and real-time images and at a much higher quality of resolution (Figure 13–4). X-rays are still valuable diagnostic tools and particularly older images can be copied by an X-ray department and maintained for baseline comparisons to be made with more recent films. However, cardiac catheterizations, echocardiography, fetal ultrasound, cerebral angiograms, gastrointestinal studies with contrast, magnetic resonance imaging (MRIs), and many other types of examinations may be stored and copied on digital systems and can be either transmitted electronically to provider practices, providing they have the proper hardware and software to receive and view the studies, or copies can be made and sent by CD or DVD media. (Usually, the CD/DVD will contain sufficient software to run on various types of computer systems.) Patients may hand-carry these copies to the practice from other practices, or the medical assistant might be asked to request a copy from the provider who performed the study. The request should clearly state that the study in its electronic format is being requested rather than simply the *dictated report* of the study. The office should have a specific area prepared to store this type of media. Place the diagnostic report in the appropriate chart section and clearly note that a digital or film copy of the study has been in filed in the corresponding area of the office.

Lab Information

When lab reports arrive in the office, any critical values should be highlighted and noted and the reports presented to the provider for review. If the laboratory technician phoned regarding the results prior to receiving the final copy, a note should be entered in the progress notes along with any action taken at that time. Any preliminary reports with annotations and final initialed lab reports should be placed in chronological order in a separate section of the chart. Some practices prefer to file all laboratory reports in chronological order, whereas others file each type of report together in chronological order. For example, chemistry, complete blood counts (CBCs), and pathology reports are all separated and ordered by groups.

Medications

Any medication administered in the office is documented in the medications section of the chart. A complete medication entry includes the prescriber, the medication name, dose, frequency, site or route of administration, special preparation if applicable, time given, and any observation period following administration and

Progress Note

Michael Adams, MD

Patient: Mary James

Date of birth: 3/21/1954

March 17, 2010 9:38 AM: Ms. James called to request a copy of her records sent to cardiovascular surgeon, Dr. Kelly. HIPAA form and release of information forms signed and verified. Dr. Adams okayed transfer of records. Faxed to Dr. Kelly's office, Jenny Powell, CMA(AAMA) ______________________________

March 17, 2010 1:15 PM: Verified with Jamie at Dr. Kelly's office that faxed records were received and complete. Jenny Powell, CMA(AAMA) ______________

March 29, 2010 10:13 AM: Received phone call from Dr. Kelly's Office that Ms. James is scheduled for aortic valve replacement on April 14th, first case at Memorial Hospital. Dr. Kelly's office will send consultant and operative notes. Melissa Johnson, MA ____________

April 17, 2010 11:17 AM: Received operative notes, consultant records and copies of intraoperative imaging related to surgery. Dr. Adams has reviewed and intialled; reports filed in patient record. Amy Smith, RMA(AMT) ______________________

April 20, 2010 11:30 AM: Received request from coagulation clinic for patient's last visit notes. Notified that patient will be started on Coumadin. Updated patient's medication record, sent requested information after verifiying release of information form signed. Jenny Powell, CMA(AAMA) ______________________

Figure 13–3: Progress note in a paper medical record. *Delmar/Cengage Learning.*

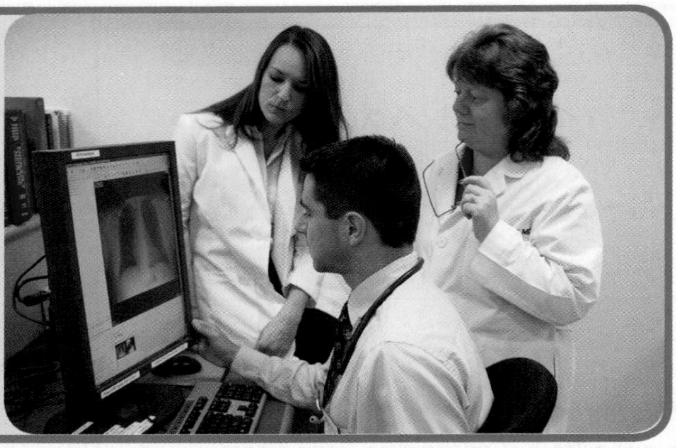

Figure 13–4: Three providers view an X-ray within an EHR system. *Delmar/Cengage Learning.*

patient's response to the treatment (Figure 13–5). In the case of vaccines, which are covered in Chapter 53, lot numbers, manufacturer name, and expiration date are also required information to be included in the record.

Copies of prescriptions are also be included as part of the chart. Whether provided as a hand-carried prescription, mailed to the patient, called or faxed to a pharmacy, or sent electronically, a record of all prescriptions given to the patient is essential to maintaining a complete patient record. Some practices prefer to keep a running log of prescriptions and when they are refilled or discontinued, which should also be maintained in this section. It should always be clear how the prescription was provided for other office personnel who review the chart to verify information, for instance, if a pharmacy calls with questions or a patient loses a paper prescription and requests a duplicate.

Progress Note

John Campbell, MD

Patient: Joshua Lawrence
Date of birth: 5/14/2005
Today's weight: 44 lbs = 20 kg

September 19, 2010 1:12 PM Ms. Lawrence bring Joshua in this morning after complaints of 3 days of fever and sore throat. Dr. Campbell has seen. Rapid strep positive, culture prepared for send out. Order for PenVK received. Kelly Anderson, MA. ———

1: 40 PM Administered first dose of PenVK 50 mg/hg = 1000 mg po. Prescription given, instructions provided. Kelly Anderson, MA ———

2:00 PM Patient still in office with mother, awaiting paperwork. Noticed rash developing on arms and trunk. Child denies difficulty breathing. Dr. Campbell notified. Order for Benadryl elixir received. Gave Benadryl 25 mg orally per Dr. Campbell's order. Child took without problems. Asked mother to remain in waiting room for observation. Kelly Anderson, MA ———

2:30 PM Child drowsy but no further symptoms. New prescription provided to mother with instructions. Allergy to penicillin documented in chart, sticker placed on front of record and in computer. Kelly Anderson, MA ———

Figure 13–5: A complete medication entry within the patient's progress notes. *Delmar/Cengage Learning.*

PROCEDURE 13–1 Organize a Patient Chart

PURPOSE: Prepare an accurate and complete patient chart to submit to the provider for final review

EQUIPMENT: Chart or folder, patient records, privacy forms, tabs

S SKILL: Organize a patient's medical record.

Procedure Steps	Detailed Instructions and/or *Rationales*
1. Prepare chart or folder for patient. Verify accurate spelling of name. Include demographics, insurance information, privacy forms, and emergency contact information.	
2. Retrieve and compile available reports and information. Verify that all records are for the correct patient before including in the record.	*Misfiled and misidentified records are very difficult to locate later.*
3. Sort and organize records by type: operative notes, progress notes from various providers, laboratory reports, radiology, medication flow sheets, immunization records, and so on.	Organize and tab appropriate sections of the chart. Look for gaps in records where additional information might need to be requested or clarified. Follow the same organizational format for all patients to help avoid omitting important information.
4. Verify accuracy and completeness and submit to provider for final review.	Provides an opportunity for any desired information to be requested.

CHARTING IN THE PATIENT RECORD

Each office has its own method of charting patient information during visits. In some practices, the medical assistant might record the findings of a physical examination as it is being completed and, in others, the provider might write or type all physical findings and progress notes during or immediately following the visit. If dictation is still used rather than EHR or voice recognition software, the medical assistant must transcribe the tape as soon as possible into the desired format with the time and date, placing the completed report in the patient's chart with a notation indicating that the report was transcribed and for whom—for example, "As dictated by Dr. H. G. Brown." Most dictated reports also bear a disclaimer stating that the report has or has not been reviewed for accuracy following dictation.

In the early 1970s, Lawrence L. Weed, M.D., a professor of medicine at the University of Vermont's College of Medicine, originated a system of recordkeeping for patients that he named the **problem-oriented medical record (POMR)**. Progress notes are organized and entered based on the source from which they come whether from a provider, laboratory, or other source. The POMR record begins with the standard database information, including patient profile, chief complaint, review of systems, physical examination, and laboratory reports. Another page lists chronic problems with dates of service for each problem. Finally, another section contains information such as medication lists, preventive care lists, and education information that has been provided to the patient (Figure 13–6). This enables the provider to review at a glance the patient's past history without having to read through each individual entry of the progress notes. When using paper records, the provider can make an overall assessment of the patient's health status to date. It works especially well in group practice settings because it promotes the continuity of patient care among the group members. This same information is incorporated into the platform of EHR systems.

MEDIA LINK

Media Link: View the "Problem-Oriented Medical Record" video for this chapter on the Premium Website.

Problem and Medication List

Patient Name: **DOB:**
Allergies: **Pharmacy #**

Date	Dx #	Chronic Problems	Dx #	Chronic Medications	Date	Refills					
					Start	Date					
					Stop	Initials					
					Start	Date					
					Stop	Initials					
					Start	Date					
					Stop	Initials					
					Start	Date					
					Stop	Initials					
					Start	Date					
					Stop	Initials					
					Start	Date					
					Stop	Initials					
					Start	Date					
					Stop	Initials					
					Start	Date					
					Stop	Initials					
					Start	Date					
					Stop	Initials					

Preventive	Date	Date	Date	Date	Date	Date
History Update Every 2 Years						
Breast Exam (plus Self-Exam)						
Mammogram						
DEXA						
Diabetic Blood Sugar Monitoring						
Diabetic Foot Care						
Diabetic HbA1c						
Diabetic LDL						
Diabetic Retinal Exam						
Diabetic Proteinuria						
Fasting Glucose						
Lipid Panel						
Pap/Pelvic						
Prostate Exam, PSA						
Rectal Exam						
Sigmoid/Colonos						
Stool for Occult Blood						
Testicular Exam (plus Self-Exam)						

Immunizations

Vaccination	Schedule	Date	Date	Date	Date
Hepatitis	As appropriate				
Influenza	At risk—q1y				
Pneumovax	At risk X 1				
Td Booster	PRN—q10y				

Education

	Date	Date	Date	Date
Advanced Directives/ Power of Attorney				
Alcohol/Drug Use				
Birth Control/Menopause				
Diabetes				
Diet				
Exercise				
Smoking				
Stress				

Figure 13–6: A sample patient problem and medication list that also provides space for dates and details of preventive actions, patient education, and immunizations as well as for the patient's pharmacy phone number. *Delmar/Cengage Learning.*

SOAP and HPIP

One of the most frequently used data collection methods for patient visits is the **SOAP** note or **Subjective Objective Assessment Plan** (Figure 13–7).

SOAP stands for:

S—Subjective impressions
O—Objective clinical evidence
A—Assessment or diagnosis
P—Plans for further studies, treatment, or management

This process makes the chart easier to review and helps in follow-up of all problems the patient might have. A similar system of recording medical information about patients is the **History Physical Impression Plan (HPIP)** method:

H—History (subjective findings)
P—Physical exam (objective findings)
I—Impression (assessment/diagnosis)
P—Plan (treatment)

Figures 13–8 A and B show these two methods of charting patients' medical information. Notice how similar they are. Following these formats in recording findings of patients yields better point-of-care service because there is a logical sequence to follow. There is less chance of overlooking a problem or a plan to treat patients.

OUTLINE FORMAT PROGRESS NOTES

Patient Name Yvette Garcia

Page 4

Prob. No. or Letter	DATE	S Subjective O Objective A Assess P Plans
5	9/6/XX	Patient complains of two days of severe high epigastric pain and burning,
		radiating through the back. Pain accentuated after eating.
		On examination there is extreme guarding
		and tenderness, high epigastric region
		no rebound. Bowel sounds normal. BP 110/70
		R/O gastric ulcer, pylorospasm
		To have upper gastrointestinal series.
		Start on Cimetidine 300 mg daily
		Eliminate coffee, alcohol & aspirin
		Return two days.

Figure 13–7: Example of SOAP progress note page. *Delmar/Cengage Learning.*

Ms. Sabrina Katherine Lake *DOB 12/23/1977*
01/29/XX

Subjective	*Pt states, "I've been feeling very tired and weak for the past month," LMP 01-15-XX very heavy flow. Exam: 6 # Wt loss since last visit 12/19/XX.*
Objective	*BP 112/70, Hb 10.4, Hct 31%. Decrease in muscle strength, pale.*
Assessment	*R/O anemia.*
Plan	*CBC with diff sent to lab, return in 1 week.*

Figure 13–8A: An example of the SOAP method of charting. *Delmar/Cengage Learning.*

Mr. Dennis J. Roberts *DOB 8/25/XX*
3/4/XX

(H) Hx	*C/O severe H/A Rt side of his head lasting several hours to up to 3 days; has had 4 in the past 6 wks, pain is increasing each time; takes ASA for pain.*
(P) PX	*Neurologic exam shows slight tremor in both hands.*
(I) Impression	*R/O encephaloma.*
(P) Plan	*CAT scan of cranium. Refer to Clearbrook Neurological Associates.*

Figure 13–8B: An example of the HPIP method of charting. *Delmar/Cengage Learning.*

CHEDDAR

CHEDDAR is the acronym for **Chief complaint, History, Examination, Details, Drugs/Dosages, Assessment, and Return Visit**. It is another method for charting that encourages providers to include greater detail of the information obtained during the interview and examination (Figure 13–9).

- *Chief complaint:* This is the presenting problem and should be recorded in the patient's words. Any unusual descriptions should be placed in quotation marks. A report of "just not feeling well" should be qualified further. Whether a complaint of illness or injury, as much subjective information should be obtained as possible to include location of the pain; radiation to any areas; quality: sharp, dull, throbbing, aching; severity assessed using a pain scale of 1–10 or, for children, a Wong-Baker faces scale; associated symptoms; aggravating factors; alleviating factors; and the time and onset of the symptoms.
- *History:* A list of the patient's prior medical history, including systemic problems; injuries; surgeries; allergies to food, environmental triggers or medications; social habits such as smoking and alcohol use; safety measures observed such as bicycle helmet and seatbelt use; exercise habits; and any other health maintenance. This is also an area in which to include any relevant family history.
- *Examination:* This section is for objective findings of the examiner. Include responses to moving the patient or the patient's inability to perform a given task due to a cognitive or physical disability and whether these deficits are baseline for the patient, depending on prior history.
- *Details of problems and complaints:* Results of additional testing may be placed here in a separate section.
- *Drugs and dosages:* A comprehensive list of ALL medications, both prescription and over-the-counter drugs, as well as any herbal remedies or illicit substances

Progress note

Amanda Patel, DO
123 Parkridge Circle
Cincinnati OH
555 444 1212

Patient: Andrew Cunningham
Date of birth: 7/2/1984
Today's weight: 185 lbs

11/2/2010. [*Chief complaint*] Mr. Cunningham arrives in the exam room with complaints of pain in his left knee that began while playing basketball. He went up for a jump shot and collided with another player on the way to the floor, causing him to invert the knee after foot made contact with the floor. He describes an immediate burning sensation and difficulty bearing weight.

[*History*] Two prior surgeries for ACL repair on right knee and MCL repair on left knee, all while playing high school varsity sports. No serious medical problems. NKDA.

[*Examination*] Mild swelling noted at the joint but there is no warmth or erythema noted. Positive drawer sign. 2+ popliteal, dorsalis pedis and posterior tibialis pulses. Slight antalgic gait.

[*Details*] Will send for X-ray and MRI. Requesting old films of prior injuries for comparison.

[*Drugs*] Using Advil 400 mg 3 times daily for pain with adequate relief. Former smoker, quit 5 years, prior 10 pack year history. Alcohol: 2 beers twice a week. Denies illicit drugs. Smoked marijuana once in high school but none since.

[*Assessment*] Advised Andrew that it's possible this is a severe sprain but suspect torn ligament. Withhold diagnosis until imaging studies have been completed. Advised to wear DonJoy neoprene brace he still has from prior injuries and avoid weight bearing as much as possible. No basketball for now. Ice as needed.

[*Return Visit*] Schedule for return in two weeks after imaging studies.

Amanda Patel, DO

Figure 13–9: An example of the CHEDDAR method of charting. *Delmar/Cengage Learning.*

used. Patients might not be forthcoming or volunteer information regarding non-prescribed use of substances but will often provide details when asked for further information. Assure them that the information is confidential. However, all information is obtainable in the event of legal proceedings so if information is provided, it should be recorded accurately.

- *Assessment:* After obtaining all relevant data, a diagnosis or assessment can be made and appropriate testing and treatment can be prescribed.
- *Return visit:* Indicate when and if a return visit is required for follow-up or for routine health maintenance.

Dating, Correcting, and Maintaining the Chart

When documenting the patient's chief complaint or any other information in progress notes, the date and time the note is taken, as well as any dates and times the patient provides regarding the complaint, are important and should be recorded accurately. Indicate AM or PM when noting the time unless using military time. Whenever a patient is given a prescription or reported or relayed provider advice over the phone, the date and time of the encounter should be recorded. Failed appointments by either cancellation or no show are noted with date and time as well. In an electronic chart, the EHR software automatically attaches a date and time to each entry. When starting a new page in a paper medical record, record the patient's name and birth date at the top of each page. Anyone who enters notes in the chart must date and sign his or her own entries.

In making a correction on handwritten progress notes, the incorrect entry should have a single line drawn through it and the correction written above it or following it and be completed with the time and date. *Never* use correction fluid or erase the error because it can appear as a fraudulent entry. Begin the note with "correction" or "late entry" when appropriate or indicate the reason for the correction. Write or print neatly and make sure to spell the patient's name correctly. In the case of a difficult name to pronounce, ask the person to provide a phonetic spelling with accent symbols to show the correct pronunciation.

Charting is part of the permanent medical *and* legal record. Using black ink makes much better photocopies of the record. When you are finished with a patient's chart, straighten and tidy the forms before filing it, being sure that no pages are hanging over the edge and that papers in the chart are not crumpled. Over time, creases in paper can cause them to rip or become unreadable, damaging the integrity and completeness of the record. After filing additional information in a patient's chart, file it appropriately as soon as possible. Patient charts should be filed when not in use to decrease clutter and minimize the chance of misplacing them.

The common practice for transcription is that dictated notes are transcribed as soon as possible following the visit. The transcriptionist prepares the notes and proofreads for errors before printing. However, if an error is found in the progress or chart note at a later time, a single line should be drawn through the error with a correction made, followed by the date, time, and initials of the person making the correction.

Each medical specialty has unique terms and phrases that are most frequently used. Most medical offices have software applications that perform spelling checks of anatomical terms, surgical terms, and medications as the text is typed within the program. Spell checker options for word processing packages usually include a feature that enables the user to customize it by adding specific words into the spell checker's dictionary. Many providers also use abbreviations in handwritten notes and dictation specific to their respective specialties. A working knowledge of such words helps identify hard-to-read handwritten entries. However, if in doubt, always ask the author for clarification. See Figure 13–10 for steps to follow in managing records.

Tracking Medical Records

Every office, whether using paper charts or electronic medical records, has a system to track outstanding work that must be completed before releasing the chart to be filed. In offices with paper charts, the office might separate the charts at the provider's station or desk into specific stacks. The provider might work through stacks of paper charts, from most urgent to least, throughout the day or save them all for the end of the day. Divisions can include:

- Charts to be filed
- Prescription refills
- Lab results

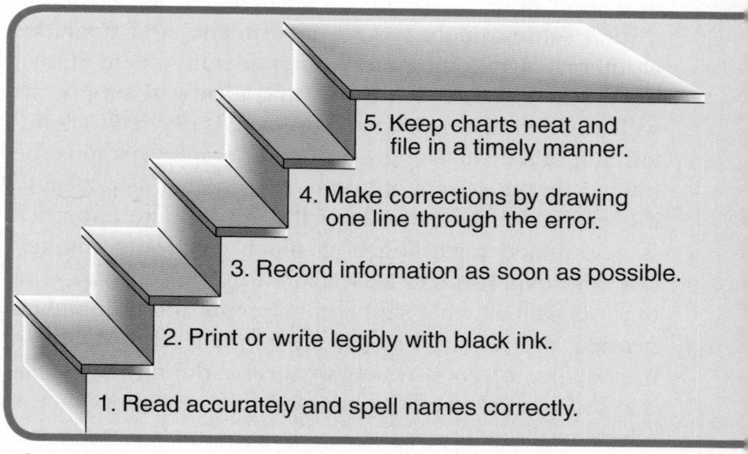

5. Keep charts neat and file in a timely manner.
4. Make corrections by drawing one line through the error.
3. Record information as soon as possible.
2. Print or write legibly with black ink.
1. Read accurately and spell names correctly.

Figure 13–10: Follow these steps for proper records management. *Delmar/Cengage Learning.*

- Coding and financial corrections
- Charts awaiting dictation
- Referrals

EHRs might have a prompt set up to prioritize which records are waiting for review to help facilitate this process when records are kept electronically. The medical assistant should keep track of and complete any assigned work such as logging prescription call-ins, phoning patients with lab results, and sending completed paper charts to the central filing area. Time management is essential when working on these tasks. The style and method of addressing assigned tasks depends upon the habits of the providers in the practice. Working on the items that are available throughout the day helps decrease the workload at the end of the day and makes the workflow more efficient.

FILING MEDICAL RECORDS

Although computers are rapidly replacing paper filing systems, an understanding of the mechanics of a traditional, noncomputerized system will provide a better understanding of the organizational steps required in filing. There can still be providers who have not yet fully automated their offices and are still using paper charts. There are still others who feel that their practice is small enough that full computerization is not necessary for that particular practice. Hence, any combination of automation and paper record systems can be found in a given practice. It is most advantageous for the medical assistant to understand and be prepared to assist with either type of system.

To adequately prepare and maintain a productive and organized filing system, the most important first step is to include staff needs and limitations in determining how to establish and implement a particular filing system. In a larger practice, the necessary financial commitment required to automate the filing fully will be repaid in a short time. In contrast, a smaller practice or one in a rural setting might require investments and upgrades at intervals when the practice can tolerate the additional expenses. Software, hardware, and technical support as well as whether a dedicated employee is needed to maintain the office versus which existing employees must be trained on the system are other considerations critical to the successful outcome. After the appropriate approach is determined regarding how much electronic automation and expense can be tolerated in a given period of time, as well as what staff commitments and training are needed, the required steps can be planned to maintain the balance of good customer service during the transition along with an efficient system that best supports the efforts of the entire staff.

Assembling and filing the patient's medical record are necessary to good patient care. Records must be filed systematically; accuracy in assembling and filing the patient's medical record is essential. Carelessly filed records result in chaos in the office. Reports that are lost or filed in the wrong chart or hidden in stacks of unfiled material result in many hours of unproductive time spent searching for them. An efficient office requires accurate filing daily. Not only does this maintain efficiency, it also reduces the chance of accidental loss of correspondence and reports.

Every office that requires paper records to be filed has storage units for this purpose. Files come in many styles, shapes, and sizes. There are vertical or lateral file cabinets, card index files, open shelf files, and tub files (Figure 13–11). To save space, many offices use movable shelving systems. Automated shelving units not only save space but provide extra security for the medical records. The carriers rotate automatically to bring the requested files in reach to avoid reaching, bending, or wasting steps that can result in workplace injuries. The work surface area is adjustable to a standing or sitting position, providing an ergonomically correct work height for all workers.

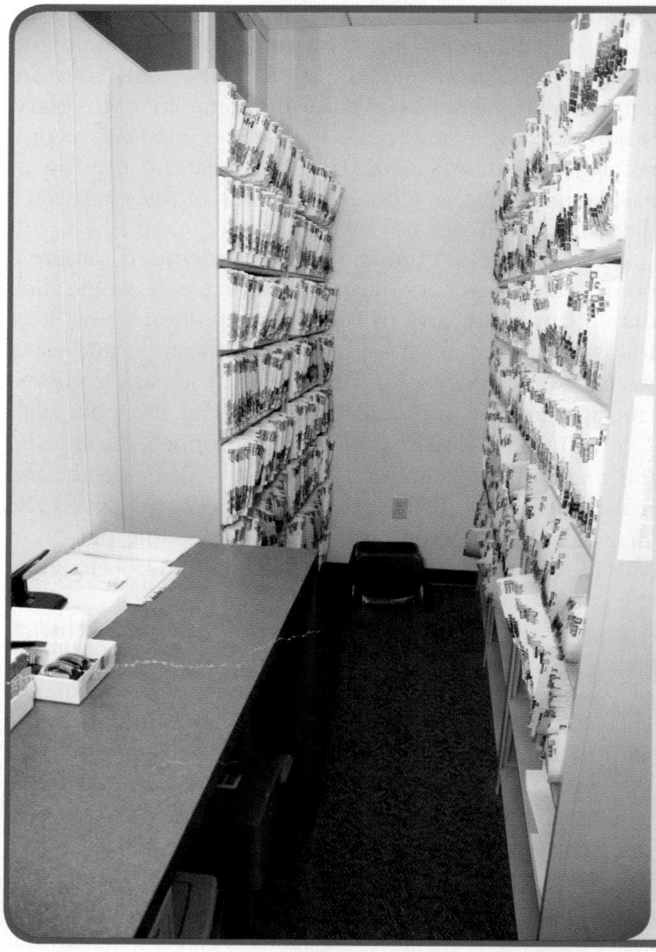

Figure 13–11: Charts in open shelf files. *Delmar/Cengage Learning.*

Safety is an important consideration when working with file cabinets. Leaving a file drawer open at floor level can create a fall hazard. Pulling out more than one file drawer at a time in a vertical file cabinet can cause it to tip over. Always be careful when pulling a file drawer out to reach material in the back because some drawers do not have a stop to keep the entire drawer from falling out.

CLINICAL PEARL

Caution: Some file cabinets can tip over and fall if the entire top drawer is pulled out completely and there is not have enough weight in the bottom drawer(s). This can be a problem especially with new file drawers as they are being filled with charts. To prevent this, begin by placing files in the bottom drawers first to avoid the possibility of injury. Keep all drawers, cabinet doors, step stools, or any other source of a possible accident closed or out of the path of others.

Steps in Filing

Folders or cards are easily filed alphabetically or numerically, but the procedure for filing reports and letters requires several steps (Figure 13–12).

Step One: Inspecting

Generally, the medical assistant is the first to *inspect* reports. The reports are divided into negative/normal and positive/abnormal for the provider to read. Some providers might have the medical assistant send reports or phone patients about diagnostic reports if the reports are normal or negative. The provider should review all reports regardless of the findings. After the provider reads a report, a check mark in the right upper corner of the document or a circle around the abnormal finding is made in red, and a notation is made about the follow-up (e.g., "Repeat mammography in 3 months," "Schedule an appointment for consultation," "Needs chest X-ray," and so on). See Figure 13–13. A letter might be dictated, or a referral might be necessary.

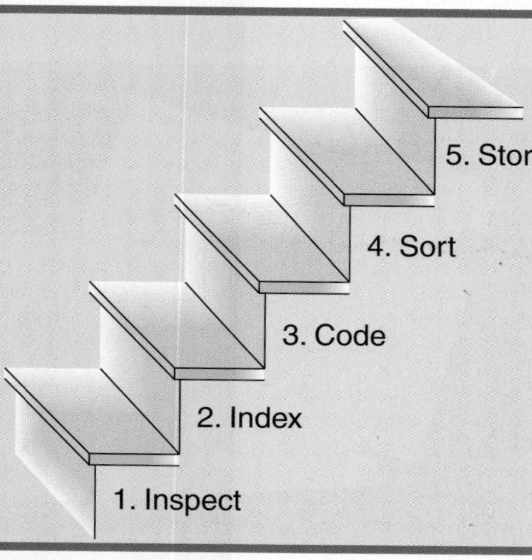

Figure 13–12: Follow these steps when filing medical records. *Delmar/Cengage Learning.*

Patient: Carol Sue Lamp ✓

City Hospital
Troy, Ohio

ROENTGEN FINDINGS

Examination of the pelvis. AP supine including the upper third of the femora bilaterally visualizes advanced degenerative arthritis of the right hip with narrowing almost to obliteration of the hip joint space and with degenerative changes and cystic formation affecting the articulating surfaces of the head of the femur as well as the acetabulum. The remaining pelvis and left hip appears essentially normal.

Impression: Advanced degenerative arthritis right hip, otherwise normal pelvis and left hip.

Figure 13–13: The check mark in the upper right-hand corner of this report shows that the provider has read the report and notified the patient, and it is ready to be released to file in the patient's chart. *Delmar/Cengage Learning.*

Step Two: Indexing

The second step is **indexing**. This requires you to make a decision about the name, subject, or other identifier under which you file the material. Materials for patients should be filed under the patient name. Research papers can be filed under illness, procedure, treatment, medication, or author. A cross-reference can be helpful in finding things later (Figure 13–14). For example, a research paper might be filed under the title, "Diabetes," and a cross-reference to the article placed under the author's name, "Allen, John."

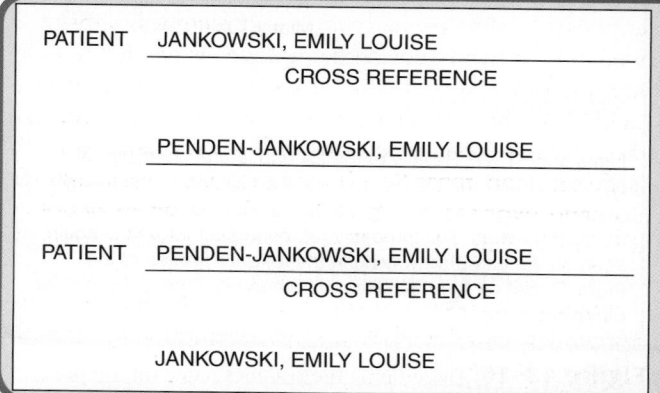

PATIENT JANKOWSKI, EMILY LOUISE

CROSS REFERENCE

PENDEN-JANKOWSKI, EMILY LOUISE

PATIENT PENDEN-JANKOWSKI, EMILY LOUISE

CROSS REFERENCE

JANKOWSKI, EMILY LOUISE

Figure 13–14: Example of a cross-reference card for effective and efficient filing. *Delmar/Cengage Learning.*

Step Three: Coding

Coding is the third step and is done by marking the index identifier on the papers to be filed. If the name, subject, or a number appears on the paper, underline or circle it, preferably with a colored pencil or a color highlighter (Figure 13–15). (The employer might have a preference about the color to be used for the coding process.) If the name, subject, or other caption does not appear on the material to be filed, write the caption in the upper right-hand corner. The person reviewing the chart or report should sign off on it to signify that the patient has been contacted. The provider should review all charts and indicate that he or she is aware that the orders were carried out. As soon as all tasks have been completed and the patient has been informed, the chart is ready to be filed.

Step Four: Sorting

The fourth step is to *sort* the material. A desk sorter can be used to put papers in alphabetic order after they have been coded. This sorter or an expanding alphabetic file for sorting reports, mail, and other items can provide a temporary file of these records until they can be placed in the patient's permanent chart. On days when it is especially hectic and all the filing has not yet been completed, this means of sorting can help you locate a particular report quickly. This can be a practical answer to more efficient filing because each letter of the alphabet is in groups and, thus, filing goes much more quickly. Also, there are times when the patient's chart is in another department, and mail, for example, can be placed in this temporary file for ease in obtaining information to answer a phone call without having to take time out to get the entire chart.

Step Five: Storing

The final step is *storing*. Locate the file drawer or shelf with the appropriate caption. Next, find the folder in which the reports are stored. Lift the folder and place it on a flat surface before adding any material. This procedure makes it easier for to ensure that the caption on the folder agrees with the caption on the paper to be filed. Place the papers with the heading to the left and the most recent material on top. Some offices attach laboratory reports to the folder in a shingle fashion. The first is attached at the bottom of the page, and each subsequent report partially overlaps the previous ones, folding the bottom of the page to a size that prevents it from hanging out of the folder and being damaged when filed.

Patient: Marsha Leonard

Tri-County Hospital
Miami, Ohio

ROENTGEN FINDINGS

Films of 8/31/XX. Review of the PA and lateral chest film of 8/31/XX shows the traches to be shifted slightly to the left by a soft tissue mass in the right thoracic inlet in the superior mediastinal area. This probably represents tumor and is again seen on the lateral view lying in the anterior portion of the thoracic inlet on the right. Heart is otherwise normal. Lungs are otherwise clear.

Figure 13–15: Underlining the patient's name on a report, usually in colored ink or a highlighter, is one way of signifying that the patient has been notified and that the report has been released to be filed in the patient's chart. *Delmar/Cengage Learning.*

Filing Supplies

Filing supplies include guides, OUTguides or OUTfolders, folders, vertical pockets, index tabs, and various colored self-stick number and letter labels as well as the standard office equipment such as stapler, staple remover, tape, and so on. (Figures 13–16 and 13–17). A properly organized filing system has many dividers or guides that identify sections within the file.

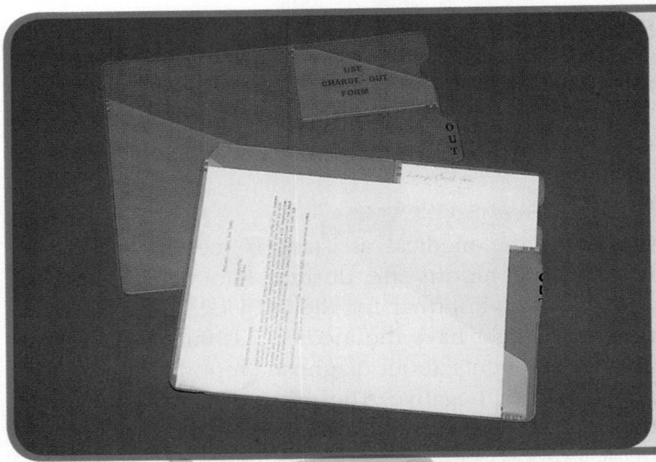

Figure 13–16: Examples of OUTguide folders. *Delmar/Cengage Learning.*

Figure 13–17: Examples of top-cut and end-cut file folders. *Delmar/Cengage Learning.*

The guides should be constructed of heavy material to stand up under continual wear. They reduce the area to be searched and enable you to locate a folder more quickly. The number of guides used is a matter of personal preference determined by each office.

An OUTguide or folder temporarily replaces a folder that has been removed. It is thick and can be of a distinctive size and color for easier detection. The use of OUTguides makes refiling much easier and alerts the medical assistant to missing files. The OUTguide can also have lines for recording information such as where the missing folder might be located, or it can have a plastic pocket for inserting an information card. In a large office with several providers and employees, it is essential to know who has the folder when it is out of the file. Occasionally, a record can be sent to another provider or treatment facility, and it is extremely important for this information to be recorded. The OUTfolder is also useful in providing a place to file material until the original folder is returned.

A color coding system can expedite both filing and finding folders. Ordinary manila folders can be coded with colored strips or dots along the edge of the folder. The coding can identify portions of the alphabet or patients of different providers within an office. Color coding is also useful in identifying different types of insured patients. Everyone should have a key to the color coding through use of a procedure manual or posted chart.

A more sophisticated and efficient way of creating color-coded labels can be achieved by using a printer. Software programs are now available that can create color-coded indexing, text, bar codes, graphics, and full color images directly onto label paper or printable folders by using your desktop color printer.

Offices that bar code their files can eliminate the need for OUTguides by scanning files prior to leaving the file area. The file clerk not only scans records when they leave the file area but also scans records in each department at least once or twice a day. This provides a great tracking system when the file leaves one area and is moved to another area. When the clerk inserts the file name into the computer, the file name pops up and identifies in chronologic order each department that has had the file since its initial removal. This system not only reduces the search time but also greatly decreases the number of lost files.

Storage units that house alternate types of media are established as drawers, open shelves, or racks. Shelves or drawers can store CDs or DVDs containing imaging studies. Racks can be most suitable for filing copies of X-ray films.

When working with a computerized or paperless filing system, additional orientation is needed about how to use the special filing equipment on the job. Storage of a vast array of information regarding patient records, employee information and payroll, scheduling, statistics regarding medical conditions, office management, taxes, inventory, and a host of other records can be filed and stored using practice management software with easy retrieval whenever necessary. This eliminates clutter and the need for filing space.

FILING SYSTEMS

Most filing systems are based directly or indirectly on an alphabetic arrangement. In alphabetic filing, the names of persons, firms, or organizations are arranged as in the telephone directory. This is the simplest and most commonly used method of filing.

In numeric filing, the material is arranged in numeric order in the main file. The main file is supplemented by an alphabetically arranged card index. The number under which a given item is to be filed can be determined by referring to the alphabetic card index file.

A subject file is based on an outline or classification of the subject matter to which the material refers. In a provider's office, it is customary to maintain files of reference materials accumulated by subject matter.

In geographic filing, material is arranged alphabetically by political or geographic subdivisions such as country, state, city, and even street, and each subdivision is alphabetized.

Chronologic filing refers to filing according to date. Arranging documents with the most current date on top is recommended.

Files can be arranged by color-coding them in either alphabetic or numeric order or by category. Each category (e.g., allergy patients, workers' compensation, charts of patients who are delinquent in payments, and so on) is assigned a different color to expedite patient care and process payment of services. This type of indexing also helps reduce the time that it takes to file and retrieve patient charts. Misfiles are quickly spotted with this system. Also, the colors of the charts are very bright and attractive. The office manager is generally the one who makes the decision about filing systems.

Table 13–2 discusses the pros and cons of each filing system.

Filing Alphabetically

The most common method of filing is alphabetic. Patient charts are filed in alphabetic order. They are also labeled with colorful numeric codes (Figure 13–18). Procedure 13–2 explains the steps necessary in filing alphabetically.

The rules for filing material alphabetically must be learned. They are as follows.

Rule 1. In filing the names of persons, the surname or last name is considered first, the first name or initial second, and the middle name or initial third.

EXAMPLE

John E. Brown is filed as Brown, John E.

TABLE 13–2 Filing Systems

	Pros	Cons
Alphabetic	Easily understood and followed	Unusual name spellings can create confusion. Requires independent recall of the last name of patients often referred to by first names, as in pediatric practices. Some letter prefixes will have many files, others few, so volumes will be unevenly distributed.
Numeric	Distributes files evenly over given spaces	Requires cross reference of names with assigned values to retrieve files by patient name.
Geographic	Useful in community health environments	Requires a degree of familiarity of a certain area. Successful use limited to frequent updates.
Subject	Helpful in epidemiology or research or for maintaining business records including insurance	Can create difficulty in retrieving files on a particular person or subject quickly without first matching cross-references for author or company.
Chronologic	Useful for setting up callbacks of patients for follow-up visits at specified intervals	Limited to only special tasks; not helpful for regular maintenance of the entire record.

Figure 13–18: A patient chart in an alphabetic filing system.
Delmar/Cengage Learning.

Rule 2. Names are filed alphabetically in an A-to-Z sequence from the first to the last letter, considering each letter in the name separately and each unit separately.

- When the surnames of two persons are spelled differently, the first and middle names or initials are not considered. See the first two names in the preceding list. The order of these two names is determined by the fourth letter in the surname.
- When a shorter surname is identical with the first part of a longer surname, the shorter name is listed first. The rule is sometimes stated as "nothing before something." See the fifth and sixth names in the preceding list.
- When the surnames are alike, the order in filing is determined by the first names or initials. When the surname and first names or initials are alike, the filing order is determined by the middle names or initials. See the fourth and fifth names in the preceding list.
- An initial is listed before a name beginning with the same letter. See the second and third names in the preceding list. This again is the example of "nothing before something."
- An abbreviated first or middle name is treated as if it were spelled out in full. See the fourth and fifth names in the preceding list.

EXAMPLE

The following names are listed in correct filing order:
Allard, Wm.
Allen, E. S.
Allen, Edna
Allen, Wm. A.
Allen, William C.
Allens, M. R.

Rule 3. A prefix, such as Mc, Mac, De, Le, and von, is considered as part of the surname.

EXAMPLE

MacAdams, Bruce
McAdams, Helen

Rule 4. Most firm names are filed as they are written. The apostrophe is disregarded in filing.

EXAMPLE

Herb's Auto Service
Walters Printing Company

Rule 5. Firm names that include the full name of an individual are filed with the name of the individual transposed.

EXAMPLE

Edward Wenger Company is filed as Wenger, Edward Company.

Rule 6. When the article *the* is part of a title, it is placed in parentheses and disregarded in filing.

EXAMPLE

Sam the Barber is filed as Sam (the) Barber
The Family Steak House is filed as Family Steak House (The).

Rule 7. *And*, *for*, *of*, and so on are disregarded in filing but are not omitted.

EXAMPLE

Adams & Smith Pharmacy is filed as Adams (&) Smith Pharmacy.

Rule 8. Abbreviations such as *Co.*, *Inc.*, or *Ltd* in a firm name are indexed as though spelled out.

EXAMPLE

Frank Smith Co. is filed as Smith, Frank Company.

Rule 9. Hyphenated surnames and hyphenated firm names are indexed as one unit.

EXAMPLE

Dunning-Lathrop & Assoc. Inc. is filed as Dunning-Lathrop (&) Associates, Incorporated
Lester Smith-Mayes is filed as Smith-Mayes, Lester.

Rule 10. Numbers are usually filed as though spelled out.

EXAMPLE

5th Avenue Store is filed as Fifth Avenue Store.

Rule 11. Professional or honorary titles are not considered in filing but should be written in parentheses at the end of the name for identification purposes.

EXAMPLE

Dr. Anne Lewis is filed as Lewis, Anne (Dr.)
President John Kennedy is filed as Kennedy, John (President)
Prof. William S. Smith is filed as Smith, William S. (Prof.).

Titles are filed as written when they are part of a firm name. Foreign or religious titles followed by one name are also filed as they are written.

EXAMPLE

Dr. Scholl's Foot Powder
Prince Phillip

Rule 12. Terms of seniority, such as *Junior*, *Senior*, *Second*, or *Third*, are not considered in filing. If two names are otherwise identical, the address is used to make the filing decision in the order: state, city, street.

EXAMPLE

Willard Keir, Sr., is filed as Keir, Willard, Sr. (Cleveland, Ohio)
Willard Keir, Jr., is filed as Keir, Willard, Jr. (Columbus, Ohio)

Rule 13. File the names of federal, state, or local government departments first by political division and then by name of department.

EXAMPLE

Drug Enforcement Administration, Cincinnati, Ohio, is filed as Cincinnati, City, Drug Enforcement Administration, Cincinnati, Ohio.

PROCEDURE 13–2 Use an Alphabetic Filing System

PURPOSE: Within an alphabetic filing system, accurately file and store a new file and then prepare an OUTguide and pull an existing file.

S SKILL: Items to be filed, cabinet for files, name of patient file to be pulled, OUTguide (card)

S SKILL: Maintain organization by filing.

Procedure Steps	Detailed Instructions and/or *Rationales*
File a New Item	
1. Use the rules for filing items alphabetically.	Double-check the spelling of the name for accuracy when using the cross-reference file.
2. Determine the appropriate storage file.	
3. When filing new material, scan the guides for the area nearest the letters of the name on the items you have to file.	When filing items such as lab reports or letters, be extremely careful to place them in the correct chart. Remove the chart, open it, and place the item in the chart with the top of the item toward the top of the inside of the chart on the appropriate left or right side. Be sure to place dated items in chronologic order with the most recent date on top.
4. Place the folder in the correct alphabetic order between two files.	Be sure to insert the new file *between* two other folders and not *within* another folder, where it could be lost.
Pull an Item from Existing Files	
5. Find the name of the patient in the alphabetic file. Double-check the spelling of the name for accuracy.	
6. Complete the OUTguide with the date and your name or with the name of the person requesting the chart.	
7. Pull the file needed and replace with the OUTguide.	

Filing Numerically

The second filing method used, especially in very large clinics, is the numerical system (Procedure 13–3). This system provides the most patient privacy because all that is visible on the folder is the patient number (Figure 13–19). As mentioned before, a cross-index or cross-reference is required in the form of an alphabetic card file, and a number is assigned to each patient. First locate the alphabetic card to determine the patient's number and then locate the numbered file.

Most offices use the same number of digits for each number assigned, and the numbers are always filed in order from smallest to largest. If the zero (0) falls before another number, it is disregarded when filing. A system

Figure 13–19: A patient chart in a numeric filing system. *Delmar/Cengage Learning.*

using six digits would begin 000001, 000002, 000003, and so on.

Some systems use the same terminal digit or digits to designate shelves or drawers. The patients are assigned numbers, which are separated into twos (2s) or threes (3s). The numbers are then read from the right-side group of numbers to the left-side group. After the last two or three digits are grouped and sorted in numeric order, sort by the middle digits. Finally, sort by the first group of digits.

EXAMPLE

The numbers of charts in one series might end in 25 and another series might end in 35. Charts labeled 10-07-25 and 02-17-25 would then be filed separately from charts labeled 08-17-35 and 12-25-35.

The order of the preceding numbered charts would be:
02-17-25
10-07-25
08-17-35
12-25-35

PROCEDURE 13–3 Use a Numeric Filing System

PURPOSE: Within a numeric filing system, accurately file and store a new file and then prepare an OUTguide and pull an existing file

EQUIPMENT: Items to be filed, cabinet for files, name of patient file to be pulled, OUTguide (card)

S SKILL: File medical records.

S SKILL: Maintain organization by filing.

Procedure Steps	Detailed Instructions and/or *Rationales*
File a New Item	
1. Use the rules for numerical filing.	Double-check spellings for accuracy when using the cross-reference file.
2. Determine the appropriate storage file.	
3. Match the first two or three numbers with those already in the file. If using terminal digits, match the last two numbers.	
4. Match the remaining numbers with those in the file.	
Pull an Item from Existing Files	
5. Find the name of the patient in the card file to obtain the account number. Double-check the spelling of the name for accuracy.	
6. Complete the OUTguide with the date, name of person pulling file, or name of requestor.	
7. Locate the file.	
8. Pull the requested file and replace with the prepared OUTguide.	

Filing by Subject

In a medical office, it is necessary to have files for business information. You must file financial records, copies of inventory, copies of orders, and records of supplies and equipment received. You should have a file for tax records, insurance policies, and canceled checks. The subject headings of these files would be relatively easy to determine, but it is more difficult to determine where to file some general correspondence or reprints of medical research publications.

Very often, reprints are filed with a cross-index, one file for the subject and one for the author with a listing of available reprint subjects. The miscellaneous folder is an important subject file. When you have one letter on a subject, it should go into the miscellaneous file indexed by subject or names. The material in each subject file is filed in chronologic order with the most recent entry on top. When five papers are assembled in the miscellaneous file on one subject or person, a separate folder should be prepared and the material removed from the miscellaneous file.

Tickler Files

A chronologic file is commonly called a **tickler file** and is used as a follow-up method for a particular date (Figure 13–20). The file may be an expanding file, a card file, or even a portion of a file drawer. It consists of dividers with the names of all the months and dividers numbered from 1 to 31 for the days of the month.

Some offices have patients fill out a card to be sent as a reminder to return for examination, testing, or injections. The patient addresses the card, and the office retains it in the tickler file to be mailed at the appropriate time. Place the month card in the front of the file each month and check each day to see whether anything needs to be done.

Reminders for equipment servicing, carpet cleaning, completing monthly orders, making an appointment for a patient to have elective surgery, sending a reminder to a patient who needs to be seen for follow-up, and scheduling a speaker for an in-service are among the many types of reminders that can be included in this file. These cards should have the party's name and phone number, the date and reason for the reminder, the referral facility phone number, and so on. There should also be a line for the person who completes the task to sign and date that it was completed.

The tickler file should be the responsibility of the administrative medical assistant, who is generally the person who handles the reception of and checkout duties for patients. This file should be checked every day at the same time. After the reminder is sent, the card should be kept for a period of weeks, months, or however long your employer or office manager requires. This is a smart practice because it serves as a reference in case of a misunderstanding or a question about how the patient or a referral was notified, when it was made, and who was responsible.

Many software companies now manufacture programs that serve as electronic tickler files that can be installed on office computers. The programs are automated to pop up on the screen to remind an individual of the task due to be completed.

Desktop Files

A convenient desktop file such as the one shown in Figure 13–21 makes it easy to flip to the phone number or address you need quickly. Other helpful materials that will fit neatly on the desktop are a list of frequently called referral facilities, pharmacies, labs, and hospitals. Using supplies that make your job easier is most practi-

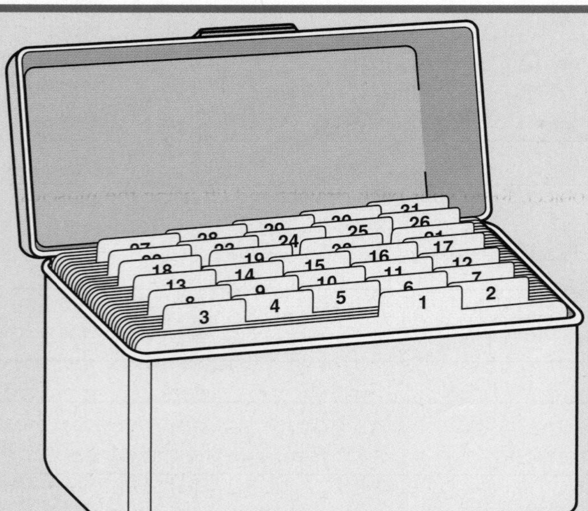

Figure 13–20: Using a tickler file such as this helps plan and keep track of important dates, events, and responsibilities.
Delmar/Cengage Learning.

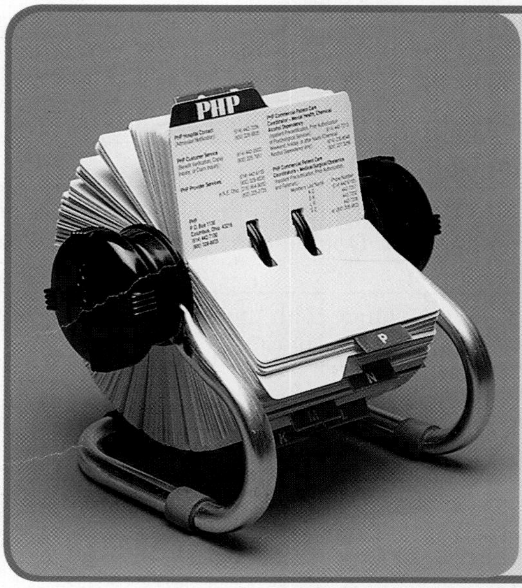

Figure 13–21: This desktop Rolodex file takes up little space but still provides fingertip access to important phone numbers.
Delmar/Cengage Learning.

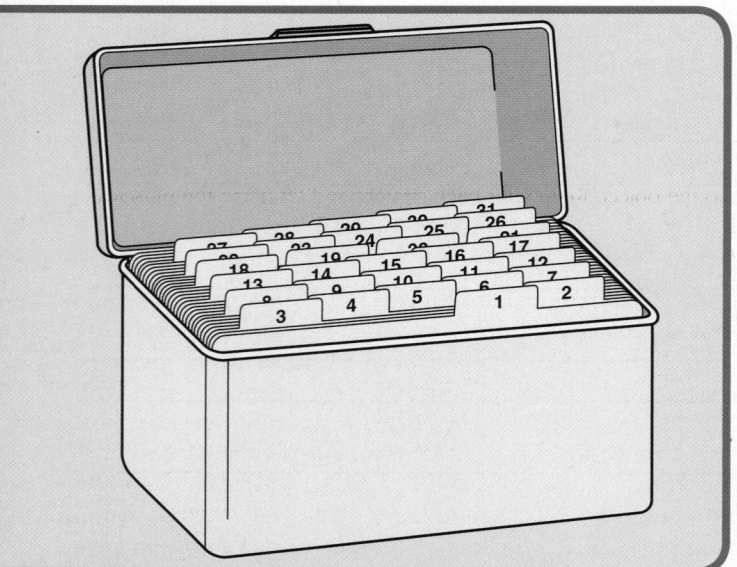

cal. Being efficient in recordkeeping is a key factor in helping the workday go smoothly.

Finding a Missing Chart

There are times when a chart seems nowhere to be found. There are a few steps to consider in locating the missing chart. First, go to the files where the chart you need should be and look through several of the charts in front of and after this location. The chart might have been accidentally placed within one of the other charts near where it belongs. Second, check the name of the chart you need and see whether the chart was filed alphabetically by the person's first name. Next, check the day's schedule and see whether the chart is out for the patient to be seen. If you know the person was seen earlier in the day or week and you cannot locate the chart, look on the day's schedule when the patient was last seen and check in several of the charts of those seen before and after the patient. It could have been placed within one of those charts by mistake. If you still cannot find the chart, the other logical places to look are on the desk of the provider, in the insurance or billing department, with the lab technician or office manager, or on the cart of the charts being pulled for the day or charts to be filed.

STORING AND PURGING FILES

In all medical practices, the shelves holding the files become full at some point, and there is no room for any more charts. Periodically you must purge files of those patients who are no longer being seen by the provider(s). **Purge** means to clean out. Thinning out the inactive charts can be done to make room on the file shelves or in drawers for new and active patients. Inactive files must be maintained for a period of time but may be stored in an offsite area when needed. Purging files might be based on when the shelves become too full or on an established schedule. Using color-coded year tab stickers can make it easier to identify the files that are next to be purged. To be most efficient, purging should be approached systematically. When files are boxed, make sure they are labeled accurately.

Use good body mechanics when moving volumes of files and charts to prevent back strain and other injuries. Figure 13–22 shows correct movement when lifting to prevent injury. Using correct technique and proper equipment, large numbers of files can be easily transported safely and efficiently.

HIPAA requires all medical records, signed consent forms, authorization forms and any other HIPAA-related documents to be retained for six years. Records of deceased patients must be maintained for two years. State laws can have additional requirements for records retention but cannot be less than federal regulations. Refer to the American Health Information Management Association's (AHIMA) Website for state-specific requirements (www.ahima.org). Some practices may choose to maintain files indefinitely, so transferring inactive files to disk significantly decreases the costs of storage space. Security is necessary in keeping this stored information regarding patients confidential. Files should be secured at all times. This includes appointment books, laboratory logs, telephone message books, the facility's triage manual, and any other records that contain identifying information or that pertains to care provided by the practice. Professional liability insurance policies, life insurance policies, canceled checks, wills, licenses, deeds, stocks, and bonds should be kept in a safe or in a fireproof box. Keep receipts for business and medical equipment and any warranties in fireproof storage until the equipment is no longer in use.

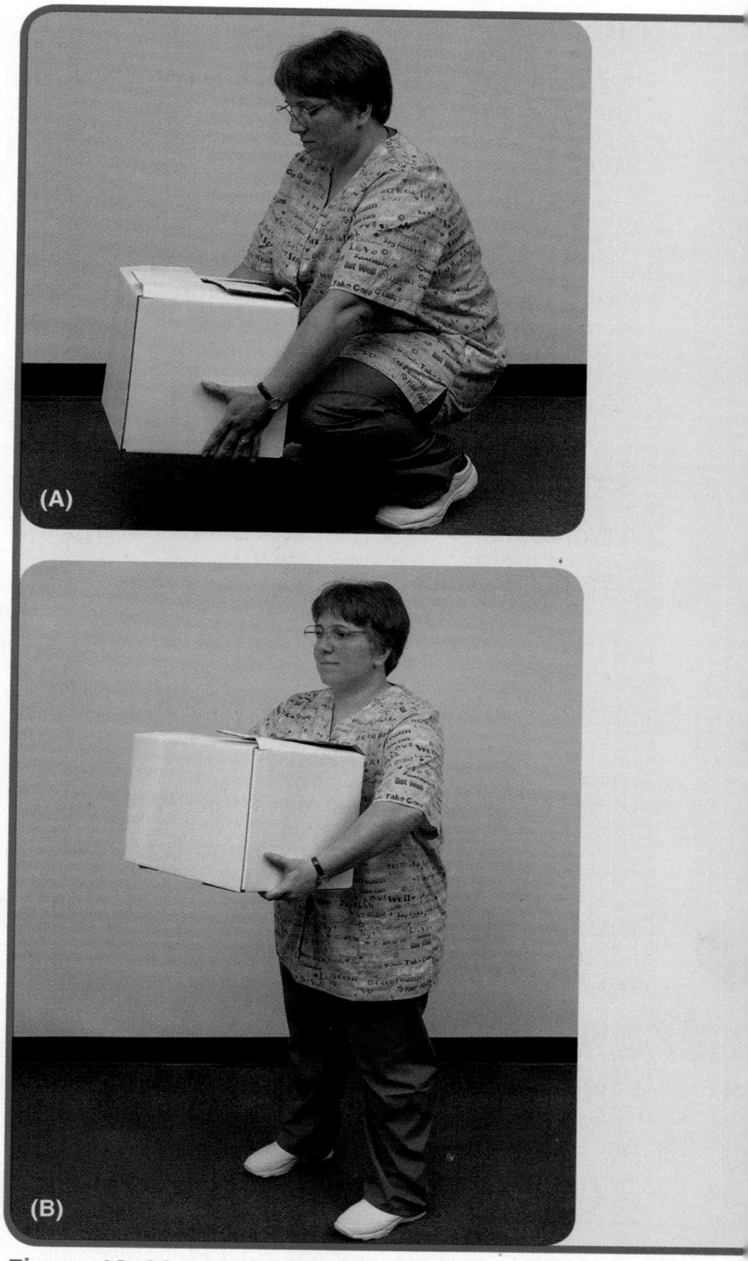

Figure 13–22: (A) Bend at the knees and hips and stand close to the object. Keep your back straight and lift using the muscles in your arms and legs, not your back. (B) Once lifted, keep the object close to your body. *Delmar/Cengage Learning.*

CHAPTER SUMMARY

- Medical records serve multiple purposes. They facilitate continuity of medical care between providers; serve as documentation to verify necessity of procedures for insurance reimbursement, and provide a chronological record of events to build subsequent care upon.
- HIPAA protections in place are designed to maintain the security of patient information while enabling providers to share critical information about patients.
- Understanding the parts of the medical record offers a basis by which to manage and maintain patient information better.
- Even though the trend is toward electronic health records (EHRs), many practices are still at different stages in the transition. Understanding the mechanics of filing and pulling records as well as how to organize the contents provides a better foundation for the medical assistant who works in a practice in transition and helps him or her learn how to manage EHRs.

STUDY TOOLS

Workbook	Activities for Chapter 13
Premium Website	
MEDIA LINK	View this following **Media Link** for Chapter 13: • Problem-Oriented Medical Record
StudyWARE	Activities and Quizzes on the **StudyWARE™ Software** for Chapter 13
	Complete the following **Competency Challenge 2.0** activities: • Monday, 10 AM, Manage the Medical Record
	Audio Library of medical terms
	Online access to the **Critical Thinking Challenge 2.0**
learninglab	Module 6: Beginning the Patient's Record
CourseMate	Activities and Quizzes for Chapter 13
WebTutor	Activities and Quizzes for Chapter 13

CHECK YOUR KNOWLEDGE

1. Which of the following items are NOT part of a patient's demographic information?
   a. Gender
   b. Ethnicity
   c. Religion
   d. Lab values
   e. Marital status
2. The medical record:
   a. documents patient progress.
   b. verifies necessity of services to insurance billing.
   c. serves as a means of communication between providers.
   d. all of the above.
3. The S in SOAP stands for:
   a. Subjective.
   b. Subordinate.
   c. Symptomatic.
   d. Standard.
4. CHEDDAR is an acronym used for:
   a. determining which accounting method is used in the practice.
   b. conducting a patient encounter.
   c. retrieving patient billing information.
   d. evaluating laboratory results.

5. "Meaningful use" refers to:
   a. how a prescription is taken.
   b. what type of labs are ordered.
   c. billing practices.
   d. the manner in which electronic health records are used.
6. Advantages of electronic health records include:
   a. eliminating the need for transcription.
   b. decreasing or eliminating errors related to poor or illegible handwriting.
   c. abolishing the need to secure patient files.
   d. providing a means for patients to diagnose themselves and decrease medical costs.
   e. a and b only.
   f. all of the above.
7. Regarding storing medical records, which is TRUE?
   a. Patient records must stored indefinitely.
   b. Records must be maintained for 15 years.
   c. Records may be purged on a regular basis to make room for new charts.
   d. Records of deceased patients may be destroyed after a death certificate is received.

WEB LINK

American Health Information Management Association: www.ahima.org

REFERENCES

"Practice Brief—Retention of Health Information (updated)." American Health Information Management Association: library.ahima.org/xpedio/groups/public/documents/ahima/bok1_012547.pdf. (Retrieved 1/10/2011)

Unit

7

Medical Insurance and Coding

Health insurance has evolved over approximately the past 150 years and has done so more rapidly in the past 30 years or so to provide more affordable coverage to subscribers and their dependents. The introduction of insurance has resulted in a need for the development of a uniform mechanism for the providers to use to report the services they provide to their patients: the Healthcare Common Procedure Coding System (HCPCS). Also, to substantiate the medical necessity for the services provided, the International Classification of Diseases, 9th Edition, Clinical Modification (ICD-9-CM) system was developed to report the diagnoses associated with those services. The chapters in this unit explore the concept of health insurance as well as the coding systems by which providers are reimbursed for the care they provide.

Certification Connection

	Ch. 14	Ch. 15
CMA (AAMA)		
Documentation/reporting: workers' compensation	X	
Coding systems		X
Third-party billing	X	
RMA (AMT)		
Insurance: Terminology	X	X
Plans	X	
Claims	X	X
Coding		X
Insurance finance applications	X	
CMAS (AMT)		
Insurance processing	X	
Coding		X

Chapter 14

Health Insurance

OBJECTIVES

In this chapter, you will learn the following:

KB KNOWLEDGE BASE

1. Spell and define, using the glossary in the back of the text, all the Words to Know in this chapter.
2. Identify and define the different types of insurance.
3. Identify and define the different models of managed care.
4. Discuss referral procedures for patients in a managed care program.
5. Describe procedures for implementing both managed care and insurance plans.
6. Discuss utilization review principles.
7. Discuss workers' compensation as it applies to patients.
8. Discuss types of provider fee schedules.
9. Describe the concept of RBRVS.
10. Define Diagnostic-Related Groups (DRGs).

S SKILLS

1. Obtain a managed care referral and precertification, including documentation.
2. Obtain a preauthorization, including documentation.
3. Verify eligibility for managed care services.

B BEHAVIORS

1. Demonstrate assertive communication with managed care and insurance providers.
2. Demonstrate sensitivity in communicating with both providers and patients.
3. Communicate in language the patient can understand regarding managed care and insurance plans.

WORDS TO KNOW

advance beneficiary notice (ABN)
allowed amount
assignment of benefits
accept assignment
birthday rule
capitation
carrier
coinsurance
conversion factor
coordination of benefits
copayment
deductible
dependent
diagnosis-related group (DRG)
fee-for-service
fee schedule
flexible spending account (FSA)
gatekeeper
geographic practice cost index (GPCI)
health maintenance organization (HMO)
health reimbursement account (HRA)

- health savings account (HSA)
- indemnity
- independent practice association (IPA)
- Medicare
- Medicaid
- Medigap
- preauthorization
- precertification
- preferred provider organization (PPO)
- primary
- seconday
- subscriber
- utilization review
- waiver

THE PURPOSE OF HEALTH INSURANCE

Health insurance was introduced as a mechanism for consumers to prepay for coverage of health care benefits so that they would not have to pay for the care when they received it. Since its development, insurance has evolved from coverage that pays for catastrophic illnesses and injuries only to coverage that encourages preventive care and services. Consumer-directed health plans have been the most recent addition to health insurance coverage and provide patients with more control over the decisions they make for the care they seek.

The debate continues regarding just how much of our medical expenses insurance should cover. One belief is that if patients are kept involved in paying for portions of their health care, they will make wiser spending choices than they would if insurance paid 100% of all health care expenses.

The traditional type of insurance that once covered the cost of medical care is fast becoming extinct. Even though traditional private insurance is fading, there are still individuals who choose to pay high premiums so that they have the flexibility to seek medical care from health care professionals of their choice. This is known as **fee-for-service** care. Fee-for-service care is still very attractive to many individuals who want the freedom to seek care from any provider and not worry about whether they are remaining in their network.

Terms Used in Health Insurance

A number of terms are unique to health insurance, some of which are presented in Table 14–1. They are discussed throughout the chapter in context and are included here to help you gain familiarity with them.

TABLE 14–1 Terms Used in Health Insurance

Advance beneficiary notice (ABN)	Required by Medicare when a service is provided to a beneficiary that is either not covered or the provider is unsure of coverage.
Allowed amount	The maximum amount an insurer will pay for any given service.
Assignment of benefits	The authorization, by signature of the patient, for payment to be made directly by the patient's insurance to the provider for services.
Authorization to release medical information (release of medical information form)	A form that must be signed by the patient before any information may be given to an insurance company or any other third party.
Beneficiary	Person entitled to benefits of an insurance policy. This term is most widely used by Medicare.
Capitation	The health care provider is paid a fixed amount per member per month for each patient who is a member of a particular insurance organization regardless of whether services were provided.
Carrier	Term used to refer to insurance companies that reimburse for health care services.
Catastrophic Plans	Individual and family health insurance plans that emphasizes coverage for hospitalization or serious illnesses (may also be referred to as hospital-only or short term plans).
Civilian Health and Medical Program of the Veterans' Administration (CHAMPVA)	Established in 1973 for the spouses and dependent children of veterans who have total, permanent, service-connected disabilities.
CMS-1500	The standard claim form designed by the Centers for Medicare and Medicaid Services to submit provider services for third-party (insurance companies) payment.

(continues)

TABLE 14–1 *(Continued)*

Coinsurance	The percentage owed by the patient for services rendered after a deductible has been met and a copayment has been paid.
Coordination of benefits (COB)	Procedures insurers use to avoid duplication of payment on claims when the patient has more than one policy. One insurer becomes the primary payer, and no more than 100 percent of the costs are covered.
Copayment	A specified amount the insured must pay toward the charge for professional services rendered at the time of service.
Deductible	A predetermined amount the insured must pay each year before the insurance company will pay for an accident or illness.
Diagnosis-related group (DRG)	A prospective payment system developed by Yale University and used by Medicare and other insurers to classify illnesses according to diagnosis and treatment. DRGs group all charges for hospital inpatient services into a single bundle for payment purposes.
Effective date	The date when the insurance policy goes into effect.
Explanation of benefits	A printed description of the benefits provided by the insurer to the beneficiary.
Fee disclosure	The action of health care providers informing patients of charges before the services are performed.
Fee schedule	A list of predetermined payment amounts for professional services provided to patients.
Gatekeeper	A term given to primary care providers because they are responsible for coordinating the patient's care to specialists, hospital admissions, and so on.
Group insurance	Insurance offered to all employees by an employer.
Health maintenance organization	Group insurance that entitles members to services provided by participating hospitals, clinics, and providers.
Indemnity plan	A commercial plan in which the company (insurance) or group reimburses providers or beneficiaries for services; allows subscribers more flexibility in obtaining services.
Independent practice association (IPA)	A type of HMO in which contracted services are provided by providers who maintain their own offices.
Individual insurance	Insurance purchased by an individual or family who does not have access to group health insurance. Applicants for coverage can be denied based on preexisting conditions or subjected to higher premiums. This is scheduled to be eliminated in 2014 as part of the Patient Protection and Affordable Care Act passed in 2010.
Limiting charge	The maximum amount a nonparticipating provider can collect for services provided to a Medicare patient.
Loss-of-income benefits	Payments made to an insured person to help replace income lost through inability to work because of an insured disability.
Managed care	A health care delivery system that combines the delivery of health care and payment of the services.
Medicaid	A joint funding program by federal and state governments (excluding Arizona) for the medical care of low-income patients on public assistance.
Medicare	A federal program for providing health care coverage for individuals over the age of 65 or those who are disabled.
Medicare fee schedule	A list of approved professional services Medicare will pay for with the maximum fee it pays for each service.

Medigap (Medifill)	Private insurance to supplement Medicare benefits for payment of the deductible, copayment, and coinsurance.
Member provider	A provider who has contracted to participate with an insurance company to be reimbursed for services according to the company's plan.
National Committee for Quality Assurance (NCQA)	A nonprofit organization created to improve patient care quality and health plan performance in partnership with managed care plans, purchasers, consumers, and the public sector.
Nonparticipating provider	A provider who is not contracted with an insurer and can collect total charges for services provided. Exception: Provider can collect only 115 percent of the Medicare Provider Fee Schedule allowed amount for Medicare beneficiaries.
Out-of-area	The term used to identify services HMO members receive outside of their specified geographical area.
Participating provider	A provider who has contracted with an insurer and accepts whatever the insurance pays as payment in full.
Patient status	Refers to a patient's eligibility for benefits; the basis upon which benefits are being provided (i.e., inpatient, outpatient, ER, office, and so on).
Point-of-service (POS) plan	An open-ended HMO, which delivers health care services using both a managed care network and traditional indemnity coverage. Care sought outside the managed care network results in higher out-of-pocket costs for the member.
Precertification	Approval obtained before the patient is admitted to the hospital or receives specified outpatient or in-office procedures.
Preexisting condition	A condition that existed before the insured's policy was issued.
Preferred provider organization (PPO)	A network of providers and hospitals that are joined together to contract with insurance companies, employers, or other organizations to provide health care to subscribers and their families for a discounted fee.
Premium	Monies paid for an insurance contract.
Relative Value Units	Numeric values assigned to payment components of the Resource-Based Relative Value Scale (RBRVS).
Resource-based relative value scale (RBRVS)	Fee schedule based on relative value units assigned for resources providers use to provide services for patients: provider work, practice expense, malpractice expense.
Service area	The geographic area served by an insurance carrier.
Subscriber	The person who has been insured; an insurance policy holder.
Third-party payer	An insurance carrier who is not the doctor or patient but who intervenes to pay the hospital or medical bills per contract with one of the first two parties.
TRICARE (Civilian Health and Medical Program of the Uniformed Services, CHAMPUS)	Established to aid dependents of active service personnel, retired service personnel and their dependents, and dependents of service personnel who died on active duty, with a supplement for medical care in military or public health service facilities.
Usual, customary, and reasonable (UCR) fee	The amount commonly charged for a particular medical service by providers in a specific geographical area; amounts are used to develop allowed amounts.
Utilization management (review)	A method of controlling health care costs by reviewing services to be provided to members of a plan to determine the appropriateness and medical necessity of the care prior to the delivery of the care.

(continues)

TABLE 14–1 *(Continued)*

Waiver	A document outlining services that will not be covered by a patient's insurance carrier and the cost associated with those services. Patient signature indicates that he or she understands that these services will not be covered and that he or she agrees to pay for the service out of pocket.
Workers' compensation	Government program that provides insurance coverage for those who are injured on the job or who have developed work-related disorders, disabilities, or illnesses.

MANAGED CARE DELIVERY SYSTEMS

Managed care is a system of health care that integrates the delivery and payment of health care for covered persons (patients, or subscribers) by contracting with selected providers for comprehensive health care services at a reduced cost. Managed care delivery systems have specific standards for providers and programs for quality assurance and utilization review.

A main goal of managed care is to provide health care with an emphasis on prevention. The theory is that by helping patients obtain care sooner rather than later, providers are able to identify problems at an early stage and improve the patient's quality of life while controlling the costs associated with an illness. For example, during an annual physical (covered by the patient's managed care plan), an individual is found to have a suspicious lump under his or her arm. Through early detection and treatment, the patient's life might be saved or at least his or her quality of life is improved. However, if the patient had traditional insurance or no insurance, there might be a delay in finding the lump and, when the patient discovers the lump him- or herself and decides to seek care, he or she has to pay more out of pocket, and the resulting delay in treatment could have life-threatening consequences.

As a mechanism to assess the quality of care provided by managed care plans, The National Commission on Quality Assurance (NCQA) was established. NCQA is an independent organization that sponsors The Health Plan Employer Data and Information Set (HEDIS), which consists of performance measures to evaluate managed care plans. Report cards for each plan are developed using this data so that employers can then make informed decisions about the plans they offer to their employees. Quality reviews by NCQA are not required but provide further evidence of a plan's commitment to providing quality care and accountability if it is willing to subject itself to this type of scrutiny.

Managed care plans employ a large staff of provider and professional relations representatives. These representatives periodically call on providers' offices personally to provide new information, distribute new policy manuals, offer assistance in navigating through their Websites, and answer questions the staff or providers might have regarding that particular company. Also, monthly newsletters are either mailed or available on the company's Website to providers' offices to keep them apprised of changes between representative's visits. Some managed care plans also offer periodic seminars on their policies and claim-filing procedures.

Today, managed care delivery systems continue to gain prominence in the types of plans employers are offering employees (see Figure 14–1).

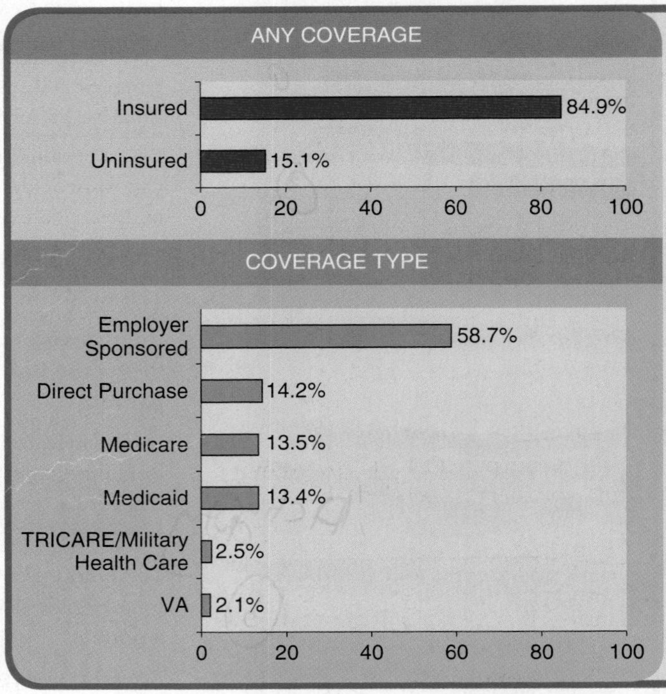

Figure 14–1: Comparison of health insurance coverage by survey, 2008. Adapted from "Table 5. Health Insurance Coverage by Survey: 2009." *Health Insurance Coverage Working Paper: 2009 American Community Survey.* U.S. Census Bureau, 2009, American Community Survey.

TYPES OF INSURANCE PLANS

Commercial Health Insurance Plans

A large segment of the population is covered by commercial insurance plans, which are owned and run by private companies. These private companies control the price of premiums paid and specify the benefits they will provide. Blue Cross and Blue Shield health insurance plans are generally well-known examples of commercial health insurance plans. Originally, Blue Cross was set up to pay for hospital expenses (but now covers outpatient services as well); Blue Shield was originally used to pay for providers' services. In the early years, Blue Cross and Blue Shield was an indemnity-type plan with an annual **deductible** and **coinsurance**. They have changed with today's health care demands and, with the increase in popularity of managed care plans, they now offer a variety of plans—HMO, PPO, point of service (POS), HSA, and HRA as well as indemnity-type.

Indemnity-Type Insurance

Indemnity-type insurance has the least amount of structural guidelines for patients to follow. Patients are able to see the provider of their choice without having to deal with listings of participating providers and other managed care guidelines. The patients are also able to see specialists without having to obtain referrals from another provider. However, this freedom of choice comes at a higher cost to the patient. Premiums are generally higher, and the plan has an annual deductible that must be satisfied before the insurance company will cover any of the patient's expenses. Traditional indemnity coverage is sometimes referred to as an 80/20 plan. This means that the carrier will pay 80 percent of the expenses, and the insured will pay the other 20 percent after the deductible has been satisfied. When a patient is covered by an indemnity-type plan, most practices will file the claim with the insurance company on the patient's behalf.

Health Maintenance Organizations (HMOs)

Health maintenance organizations (HMOs) require their members to choose a primary care provider (PCP) to oversee their medical care. The PCP is responsible for referring the patient to a specialist and approving additional services if needed; for that reason, the PCP is referred to as a **gatekeeper**. The PCP is encouraged to use the specialists listed with the HMO panel of providers. Sometimes, a referral is necessary outside the panel because the specialty might not be part of the panel. Even though there have been a number of evolutions of the standard HMO model, many of these newly developed models also require patients to have a referral to seek care from a specialist, which requires the patient to have a PCP.

HMOs are plans set up to provide comprehensive health care with an emphasis on wellness and preventive medicine. HMOs encourage annual physicals and PAP tests, breast self-exams, testicular self-exams, mammographies, and, in general, request people to see their provider as soon as any problems are noticed because preventive measures help reduce medical care costs. Well-child care is also promoted, including periodic visits for screenings of height, weight, vision, and hearing; neurologic exams; immunizations at appropriate intervals; and tuberculosis (TB) Mantoux tests. Other services include counseling about nutrition, exercise programs, stress management, weight control, low-fat diet, smoking cessation, drug rehabilitation, and the like. All these services are provided in an effort to keep people well and thereby cut the costs of medical care.

HMO contracts offer people affordable health care plans because they are provided through an individual's place of employment at a reasonable cost. The employer pays a large amount of the cost for the plan. The employee's cost is a reasonable group premium rate for health insurance coverage (part of their employee benefits) that requires only a copayment at the time of the medical service, usually $10 to $25, and can vary, depending on whether the patient is seeing his or her PCP or a specialist. When a patient is covered by an HMO, the provider's office files the claim with the insurance company on the patient's behalf.

Today, managed care is an organized system of medical team members and groups who provide quality and cost-effective care that encompasses both the delivery of health care and the payment of these services. In addition to providers, the HMO also contracts with hospitals, laboratories, and other ancillary services such as pharmacies.

Staff-Model HMOs

Staff-model HMOs are plans in which the providers are employed by the HMO, and all services (physical therapy, radiology, and so on) are provided by the practice. The PCP is responsible for routine care and referrals. True emergency (life-threatening) care does not require preauthorization. If the patient is traveling outside the HMO geographic service area, he or she must call and obtain preauthorization of any nonemergency care. Failure to do so will result in the HMO's refusing payment of the services.

Group-Model HMOs

Group models are multispecialty practices contracted to provide health care services to members. The providers may be reimbursed on a capitated basis. **Capitation** means that providers are paid a set fee per patient on their patient listing each month, whether the patient is seen one or more times or not at all. However, over the past 10 to 15 years, this method of reimbursement between HMOs and provider groups has become rarer because many have converted to a fee-for-service type of reimbursement.

Preferred Provider Organization (PPO)

A preferred provider organization (PPO) is another type of HMO and has gained in popularity. The organization consists of a network of providers and hospitals that contract to provide an insurance company or an employer with services for their members or employees at a discount rate. This benefits the insurance company by reducing the cost of care, which in turn should reduce the cost of the insurance for the employer. The providers benefit by gaining a group of patients for whom they can receive payments. The patient must select a primary care provider and receive referrals for care outside the network. If patients choose to obtain care outside the network, their out-of-pocket costs (copayments, coinsurance, and deductibles) will be higher. Premiums, deductibles, and copayments tend to be higher in PPOs than in traditional HMOs but less than traditional fee-for-service plans.

Point-of-Service (POS) Plans

Point-of-service (POS) plans allow members greater freedom in their choice of care. They do not have to select a PCP and can self-refer to specialists. If they choose to use a non-panel provider, the benefit is more like an indemnity plan with a deductible and coinsurance. If they choose a panel provider, they receive the HMO benefit of only paying a copayment with no deductible or coinsurance responsibility.

Independent Practice Associations (IPA)

Independent practice associations (IPA), also known as individual practice associations, consist of providers who practice in their own individual offices and retain their own office staff and operations. The association provides more equitable leverage in establishing contracts with HMOs and other insurance organizations.

CONSUMER-DRIVEN HEALTH PLANS (CDHP)

not taxed

Insurance companies and employers like to see consumers making informed choices regarding use of their health care dollars. The federal government created consumer-driven health plans (CDHPs)—specifically health savings accounts (HSA)—in 2003. Insurance companies have also responded to the demands for additional options beyond HMOs, PPOs, and traditional coverage by developing CDHPs. The plans typically have high deductibles and lower monthly premiums. One belief is that health care services are overused because consumers think, "I do not know what my doctor charges, I just know I pay a co-pay." When patients have CDHP-type coverage, they no longer think of going to the provider's office and just paying a co-pay; instead, they want to know how much the service is going to cost before it is provided because a set amount of money is available to pay for their health care through the high-deductible plans described in the following sections. Several plans are now available that offer different options to meet the needs of the public.

Health Savings Account (HSA)

A **health savings account (HSA)** is a tax-sheltered savings account that can be used to pay for medical expenses; it is similar in concept to an individual retirement account (IRA), but for health care. Any amount not used in a given year remains in the account and continues to gain interest. An HSA has a high deductible and must be paired with a qualified health plan. Preventive care is not subject to the deductible. Contributions to the plan can be made by the employee or employer. The maximum contributions for 2010 are $3,050 for an individual and $6,150 for a family. Small medical expenses can be paid for through the HSA, up to the deductible amount, as long as they are considered a qualified medical expense. Some examples of qualified medical expenses are ambulance service, braces, home improvements to assist a disabled person, and telephone or TV equipment to assist the hearing and visually impaired. Examples of nonqualified expenses include babysitting and child care for a healthy individual, funeral expenses, and diaper service. Usually, PPO-type coverage kicks in to pay for medical expenses after the deductible is met.

Health Reimbursement Account (HRA)

Like an HSA, a **health reimbursement account (HRA)** pays for medical expenses. It can be paired with a standard or high-deductible health plan. An employer can contribute to an HRA, but an employee cannot. In 2010, there are no restrictions to the amount of money that can be deposited into an HRA. The employer owns the money in this account, and it might not be portable when the employee leaves the company. However, the amount can be rolled over from one year to the next, and the account can be used in conjunction with a flexible spending account (FSA).

Flexible Spending Account (FSA)

A **flexible spending account (FSA)** is referred to as a cafeteria plan. There are three components to the plan:

- Health insurance premiums
- Qualified medical expenses
- Dependent care expenses

The plan is usually funded by the employee with pretax dollars. In some instances, an employer might contribute small amounts. This is a "use it or lose it" type plan. The money belongs to the employee; however, any unused amounts at the end of the year are returned to the employer. An employee should give careful consideration

4

to how much money he or she wants to put in the plan, knowing that if he or she does not use it, it will be lost. Qualified medical expenses are the same as for the HSA, HRA, and FSA. Employees are not required to pay any federal, Social Security, or state (in most cases) taxes on contributions.

GOVERNMENT HEALTH PLANS

Medicare

Medicare (as well as Medicaid, discussed later) was enacted originally in 1965 as part of the Social Security Act and was part of the Social Security Administration. In 1977, it was transferred to the Department of Health and Human Services and to the Health Care Financing Administration (HCFA). This name was later changed to Centers for Medicare and Medicaid Services (CMS) in 2001.

Medicare is a program of health insurance administered under the Social Security Administration for people over the age of 65 who meet the eligibility requirements and have filed for coverage. In addition, people who are disabled, receiving Social Security benefits, or in end-stage renal disease, regardless of age, are also eligible. Patients are issued a membership card to verify their coverage (Figure 14–2). Most patients now carry additional coverage to supplement their Medicare coverage to help offset the expenses of the annual deductible and coinsurance due after Medicare has paid its portion. The term *Medigap* is sometimes used to describe this type of supplemental insurance. It is important for patients to understand that most supplemental plans only cover the deductible and coinsurance after Medicare has paid for services. These plans do not cover the cost of services that Medicare does not cover at all.

Part A of Medicare is for hospital coverage, and any person who is receiving monthly Social Security benefits is automatically enrolled. Along with health care costs in general, the annual deductible increases each year.

Part B of Medicare is for payment of other medical expenses, including office visits, X-ray and laboratory services, and the services of a provider in or out of the hospital. The premiums are automatically deducted for those who wish the coverage and are on Social Security, railroad retirement, or civil service annuity. Other eligible individuals pay premiums directly to the Social Security Administration.

A benefit that was introduced for Part B beneficiaries as of January 1, 2005, was the Initial Preventive Physical Exam, otherwise known as the Welcome to Medicare visit. Traditional Medicare does not cover a preventive exam; however, this benefit was introduced to provide the opportunity for newly enrolled Medicare beneficiaries to gain access to covered screenings and shots. This is a "once in a lifetime" benefit that is available only during the first 12 months of Medicare coverage, and beneficiaries are responsible only for the 20 percent coinsurance.

To be noted is that as a result of the Patient Protection and Affordable Care Act of 2010, all Medicare beneficiaries will become eligible for an annual wellness visit with no cost sharing.

Part C of Medicare

Also known as Medicare Advantage, Part C is the segment of Medicare that enables beneficiaries to select a managed care plan as their primary coverage. This type of coverage is provided by private insurance companies approved by Medicare to provide this type of coverage. Medicare Advantage plans are in operation in many

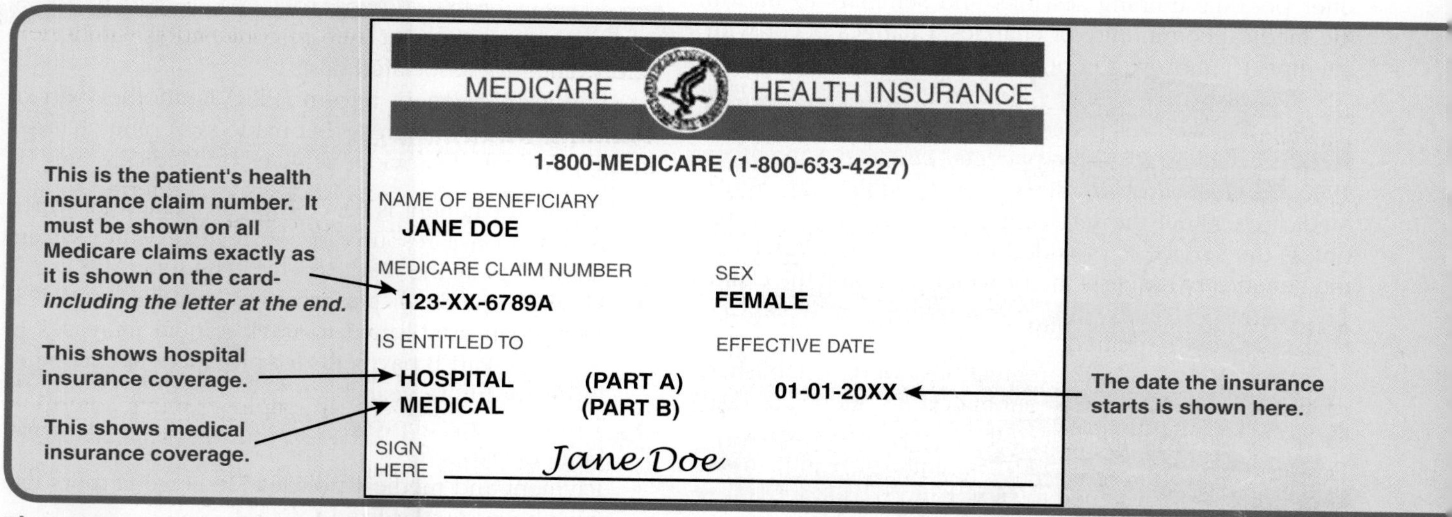

Figure 14–2: Medicare identification card. *Delmar/Cengage Learning.*

states. The plans usually offer the patient additional services outside of what traditional Medicare covers. Patients can be insured with a Medicare Advantage plan, and their Medicare coverage becomes secondary to the Advantage plan. If a patient chooses, he or she may also carry supplemental insurance. Benefits vary from plan to plan. You must keep abreast of the plans offered in your area. It is not uncommon for patients to ask questions about their coverage while they are in the office. It is helpful if you are able to offer them telephone numbers of the Advantage plans so the patient can address the details of their coverage and related questions.

Part D of Medicare

With the increasing cost of prescription medications to the Medicare population and the lack of coverage through standard Medicare, Part D was created to provide coverage for both generic and brand-name drugs. Coverage is provided through either a specific Medicare Part D plan or a Medicare Advantage plan. Beneficiaries are responsible for paying a monthly premium in addition to standard cost-sharing of a copayment and/or coinsurance.

Medicare uses Social Security numbers along with an alpha character to define the beneficiary's health insurance claim (HIC) number. This number identifies the patient when submitting claims. A Social Security number followed by the letter *A* indicates that the Social Security number belongs to the cardholder. If the number is followed by the letter *B*, it indicates that the Social Security number belongs to the cardholder's spouse.

Medicare Administration and Claims Processing

Physician providers and medical assistants must keep current with the regulations governing health care and processing of claims. Professional organizations, in-service education providers, and insurance companies offer periodic training sessions and seminars to inform the medical community of changes. Changes occur with attempts to improve the health care delivery system.

The Omnibus Budget Reconciliation Act (OBRA) of 1989 required all providers and suppliers to submit Medicare claims for their patients, effective September 1990. Providers and suppliers are not required to file the Medicare claim if the service is not covered by Medicare unless the service is provided on an assigned basis and the beneficiary requests the provider to submit the claim. Claims must be filed within a year of the time the service is received by the patient.

After May 1, 1992, regulations were established requiring that all claims submitted to Medicare had to be on an original CMS-1500 claim form (shown in Figure 14–3). The CMS-1500 is a uniform health insurance claim form designed to standardize requested information and the method in which it is submitted.

To be HIPAA compliant, providers are required to submit all Medicare claims electronically, effective October 2005. This requirement applies whether Medicare is the primary or secondary coverage for the patient. The only practitioners currently who can bill Medicare with the hardcopy CMS-1500 forms are businesses with fewer than 10 full-time employees, including providers.

In some cases, the Medicare insurance carrier automatically sends the amount not covered on to a private secondary insurance carrier, which may pay the deductible and the 20 percent not covered, eliminating the need to fill out additional forms.

Providers who sign a contract with Medicare to be a participating provider receive payment directly from Medicare for services rendered. Providers who choose not to be a participating provider can charge only 10 percent above the Medicare participating provider fee schedule amount for the service rendered. They cannot balance bill the patient for the difference between the limiting charge and their total charges.

Patients insured with Medicare Part B have an annual deductible to satisfy (pay) before any portion of their medical expenses are paid by Medicare; Table 14–2 shows recent deductible amounts. The deductible is paid to the provider of services.

The deductible is expected to continue to rise due to the continued increase in costs associated with medical care. Medicare pays 80 percent of the approved amount after the deductible is satisfied. The remaining 20 percent is paid by either the patient's supplemental insurance, after that deductible is satisfied, or by the patient. For example, a patient is seen in the provider's office for follow-up of medical conditions and the provider bills Medicare for an office visit. According to the provider's Medicare fee schedule, the allowed amount for the visit is $100; Medicare will reimburse the provider $80 and the patient or the supplemental plan will be responsible for payment of the additional $20. Medically necessary lab services are paid at 100 percent and the patient is never billed for associated costs.

Physician payment reform (PPR) is another part of OBRA passed by Congress that made sweeping changes in the payment of provider services by Medicare Part B.

- The PPR payment is based on a fee schedule, which is based on a resource-based relative value system referred to as the Medicare fee schedule (MFS).
- Medicare volume performance standards (MVPS) have been established to track annual increases in Medicare Part B payments for providers' services and levels for future years.
- Various financial protections for the beneficiary have been developed.
- Payment and medical policies Medicare carriers use have been standardized.

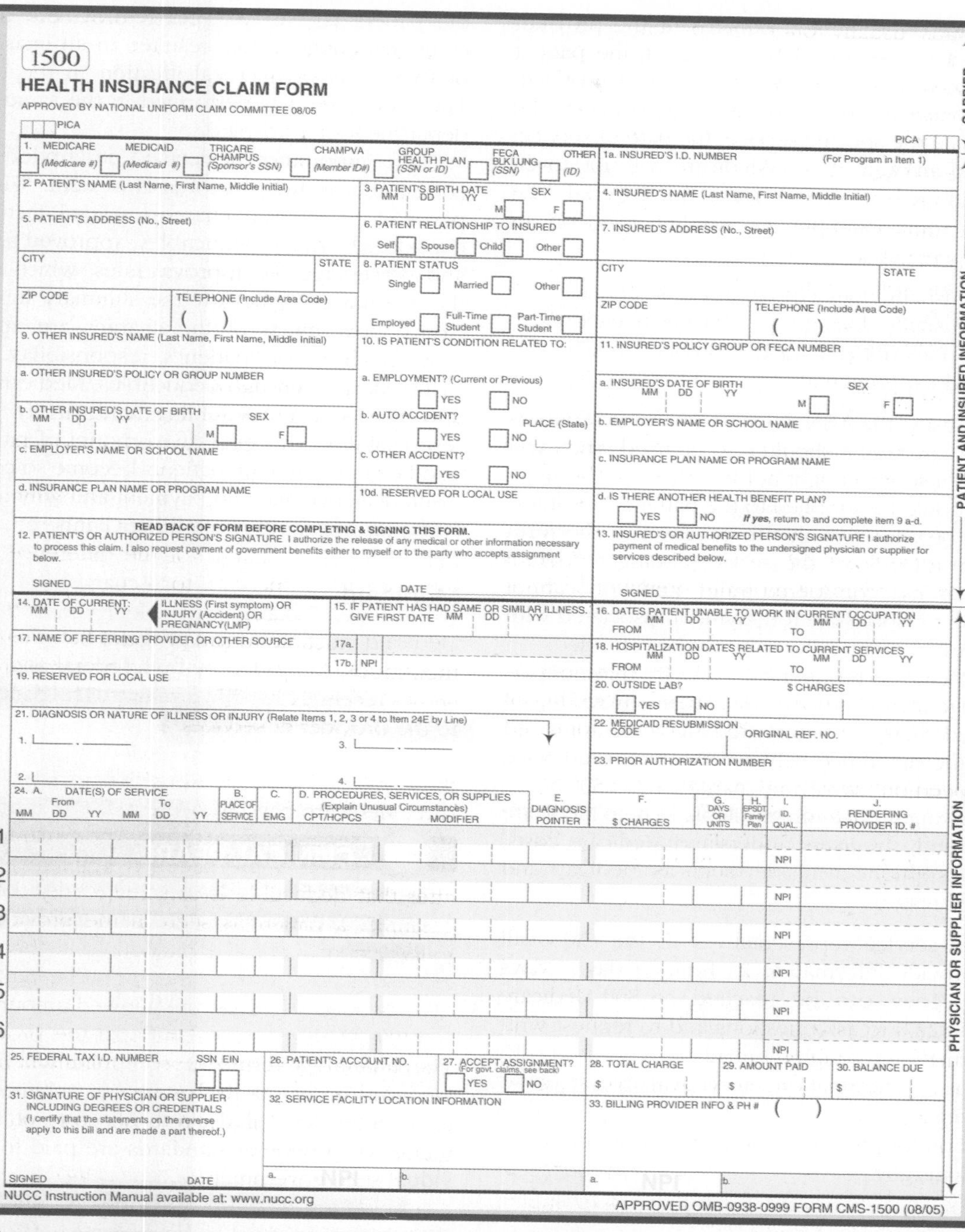

1500

HEALTH INSURANCE CLAIM FORM

APPROVED BY NATIONAL UNIFORM CLAIM COMMITTEE 08/05

PICA

CARRIER

PICA

1. MEDICARE (Medicare #) MEDICAID (Medicaid #) TRICARE CHAMPUS (Sponsor's SSN) CHAMPVA (Member ID#) GROUP HEALTH PLAN (SSN or ID) FECA BLK LUNG (SSN) OTHER (ID)

1a. INSURED'S I.D. NUMBER (For Program in Item 1)

2. PATIENT'S NAME (Last Name, First Name, Middle Initial)

3. PATIENT'S BIRTH DATE MM DD YY SEX M F

4. INSURED'S NAME (Last Name, First Name, Middle Initial)

5. PATIENT'S ADDRESS (No., Street)

6. PATIENT RELATIONSHIP TO INSURED Self Spouse Child Other

7. INSURED'S ADDRESS (No., Street)

CITY STATE

8. PATIENT STATUS Single Married Other

CITY STATE

ZIP CODE TELEPHONE (Include Area Code) ( )

Employed Full-Time Student Part-Time Student

ZIP CODE TELEPHONE (Include Area Code) ( )

9. OTHER INSURED'S NAME (Last Name, First Name, Middle Initial)

10. IS PATIENT'S CONDITION RELATED TO:

11. INSURED'S POLICY GROUP OR FECA NUMBER

a. OTHER INSURED'S POLICY OR GROUP NUMBER

a. EMPLOYMENT? (Current or Previous) YES NO

a. INSURED'S DATE OF BIRTH MM DD YY SEX M F

b. OTHER INSURED'S DATE OF BIRTH MM DD YY SEX M F

b. AUTO ACCIDENT? YES NO PLACE (State)

b. EMPLOYER'S NAME OR SCHOOL NAME

c. EMPLOYER'S NAME OR SCHOOL NAME

c. OTHER ACCIDENT? YES NO

c. INSURANCE PLAN NAME OR PROGRAM NAME

d. INSURANCE PLAN NAME OR PROGRAM NAME

10d. RESERVED FOR LOCAL USE

d. IS THERE ANOTHER HEALTH BENEFIT PLAN? YES NO *If yes,* return to and complete item 9 a-d.

READ BACK OF FORM BEFORE COMPLETING & SIGNING THIS FORM.

12. PATIENT'S OR AUTHORIZED PERSON'S SIGNATURE I authorize the release of any medical or other information necessary to process this claim. I also request payment of government benefits either to myself or to the party who accepts assignment below.

SIGNED DATE

13. INSURED'S OR AUTHORIZED PERSON'S SIGNATURE I authorize payment of medical benefits to the undersigned physician or supplier for services described below.

SIGNED

PATIENT AND INSURED INFORMATION

14. DATE OF CURRENT: MM DD YY ILLNESS (First symptom) OR INJURY (Accident) OR PREGNANCY(LMP)

15. IF PATIENT HAS HAD SAME OR SIMILAR ILLNESS. GIVE FIRST DATE MM DD YY

16. DATES PATIENT UNABLE TO WORK IN CURRENT OCCUPATION FROM MM DD YY TO MM DD YY

17. NAME OF REFERRING PROVIDER OR OTHER SOURCE 17a. 17b. NPI

18. HOSPITALIZATION DATES RELATED TO CURRENT SERVICES FROM MM DD YY TO MM DD YY

19. RESERVED FOR LOCAL USE

20. OUTSIDE LAB? YES NO $ CHARGES

21. DIAGNOSIS OR NATURE OF ILLNESS OR INJURY (Relate Items 1, 2, 3 or 4 to Item 24E by Line)

1. 2. 3. 4.

22. MEDICAID RESUBMISSION CODE ORIGINAL REF. NO.

23. PRIOR AUTHORIZATION NUMBER

24. A. DATE(S) OF SERVICE From MM DD YY To MM DD YY B. PLACE OF SERVICE C. EMG D. PROCEDURES, SERVICES, OR SUPPLIES (Explain Unusual Circumstances) CPT/HCPCS MODIFIER E. DIAGNOSIS POINTER F. $ CHARGES G. DAYS OR UNITS H. EPSDT Family Plan I. ID. QUAL. J. RENDERING PROVIDER ID. #

1 NPI
2 NPI
3 NPI
4 NPI
5 NPI
6 NPI

PHYSICIAN OR SUPPLIER INFORMATION

25. FEDERAL TAX I.D. NUMBER SSN EIN

26. PATIENT'S ACCOUNT NO.

27. ACCEPT ASSIGNMENT? (For govt. claims, see back) YES NO

28. TOTAL CHARGE $

29. AMOUNT PAID $

30. BALANCE DUE $

31. SIGNATURE OF PHYSICIAN OR SUPPLIER INCLUDING DEGREES OR CREDENTIALS (I certify that the statements on the reverse apply to this bill and are made a part thereof.)

SIGNED DATE

32. SERVICE FACILITY LOCATION INFORMATION a. NPI b.

33. BILLING PROVIDER INFO & PH # ( ) a. NPI b.

NUCC Instruction Manual available at: www.nucc.org

APPROVED OMB-0938-0999 FORM CMS-1500 (08/05)

Figure 14–3: CMS-1500 claim form. *Courtesy of the Centers for Medicare and Medicaid Services. Reprinted according to www.cms.gov website content reuse policy.*

TABLE 14–2 Medicare Deductible for 2008–2011

2008	$135
2009	$135
2010	$155
2011	$162

Medical Necessity and Services Not Covered

Medicare is permitted to pay only for services or supplies that are considered medically reasonable and necessary for the diagnosis given. Medicare will not pay for cosmetic surgery or experimental, unproven, or investigational services. Beginning in 2005, *new* Medicare beneficiaries were provided coverage for one routine physical exam. There are other preventive screenings and tests for which Medicare offers limited benefits. If the provider does provide a service that is not covered, the patient must be informed in advance, and the patient must sign an advance beneficiary notice (ABN) (Figure 14–4). The notice must state the specific service, the date of service, the anticipated amount of cost Medicare will not cover, and the specific reason the service is not covered. The following are some examples of wording used on an ABN:

- Medicare usually does not pay for this service.
- Medicare usually does not pay for this injection.
- Medicare does not pay for this service because it is considered experimental.

In addition to using the ABN when you know a service is statutorily not covered, it should also be used when you anticipate that a service might not be covered. The same information should be supplied to the patient. This information must be shared with the patient and the form completed in advance of the services being rendered; otherwise, it is not considered valid, and you cannot hold the patient responsible for payment associated with the service. Any money collected must be refunded.

Current Medicare requirements specify that nonparticipating surgeons must notify all patients in writing of their estimated charge, the estimated Medicare-approved charge, and the difference between the two in advance of elective operations involving charges over $500.

The following services are available to help Medicare beneficiaries and caregivers understand Medicare costs, coverage, and options available (such as Medigap and Medicare Advantage):

- Customer service representatives at the CMS call center provide information 24 hours a day, 7 days a week. They can be reached at 800-Medicare (800-633-4227) to ask questions and to request written information through the mail.
- A Web-based information site is available at www.medicare.gov.
- Information for providers and their staff is accessible at www.cms.gov.

Medicare Reimbursement

Remember that Medicare reimburses the approved fee at the rate of 80 percent after the patient has paid his or her annual deductible amount. Secondary payment is then sought to cover the 20 percent not covered. Many secondary carriers likewise will pay 80 percent (of the 20 percent not covered of the approved amount, after the deductible is met). The remaining small percentage and the initial annual deductible is the responsibility of the patient. Figure 14–5 shows a summary of the Medicare and secondary insurance explanation of benefits reports resulting from an actual minor medical situation in the approximate order they were received. In this example, the patient is a 65-year-old female who had a suspicious mammogram that resulted in an incisional biopsy of two areas of microcalcification in the same breast. The procedure was performed in the same-day surgery department of a hospital.

The importance of detailed descriptions, procedure codes, and accurate records is evident. With insurance payment of medical charges, several factors must be considered: annual deductibles, approved fee schedules, and percentages of approval rates, which all influence the amount paid. Review the summary in Figure 14–5. Notice how much of the charges are approved and how much is the patient's responsibility. Follow the initial charges through deductibles, Medicare, secondary coverage, sometimes refiling, and, finally, the patient's responsibility. This excessive amount of paperwork is a good example of why patients become so confused with insurance coverage and payment and why medical assistants seem never to finish filing claims.

Medicaid

Medicaid is a government program that was implemented in 1965 and is funded by both federal and state governments. Medicaid is health care coverage for individuals of limited or low income.

CLINICAL PEARL

Medicaid patients should be treated medically, personally, and professionally in the same manner as any other patient.

The federal government sets minimum standards for Medicaid coverage. Each state can enhance the benefits to a higher level if desired. All costs of any enhancements to the federal standards are paid for by the individual state government.

There are different categories of eligible recipients, including pregnant women and aged, blind, or disabled individuals, to name a few. Eligibility requirements can differ from state to state. Medicaid cards are issued to recipients on a monthly basis. Always verify current coverage before rendering services to ensure that your provider will be paid. There are time limits for filing claims for reimbursement.

Patients covered by Medicaid must seek care from a participating provider; not all providers are Medicaid providers. Providers are not required to accept Medicaid patients, nor are they required to apply to participate with Medicaid. A provider must be participating to receive reimbursement for services provided. If a provider does

(A) **Notifier(s):**
(B) **Patient Name:** *(C)* **Identification Number:**

ADVANCE BENEFICIARY NOTICE OF NONCOVERAGE (ABN)

NOTE: If Medicare doesn't pay for *(D)*_____________ below, you may have to pay.

Medicare does not pay for everything, even some care that you or your health care provider have good reason to think you need. We expect Medicare may not pay for the *(D)*____________ below.

*(D)*_______________	*(E)* Reason Medicare May Not Pay:	*(F)* Estimated Cost:

WHAT YOU NEED TO DO NOW:

- Read this notice, so you can make an informed decision about your care.
- Ask us any questions that you may have after you finish reading.
- Choose an option below about whether to receive the *(D)*____________ listed above.

Note: If you choose Option 1 or 2, we may help you to use any other insurance that you might have, but Medicare cannot require us to do this.

***(G)* OPTIONS:** **Check only one box. We cannot choose a box for you.**

☐ **OPTION 1.** I want the *(D)*__________ listed above. You may ask to be paid now, but I also want Medicare billed for an official decision on payment, which is sent to me on a Medicare Summary Notice (MSN). I understand that if Medicare doesn't pay, I am responsible for payment, but **I can appeal to Medicare** by following the directions on the MSN. If Medicare does pay, you will refund any payments I made to you, less co-pays or deductibles.

☐ **OPTION 2.** I want the *(D)*__________ listed above, but do not bill Medicare. You may ask to be paid now as I am responsible for payment. **I cannot appeal if Medicare is not billed.**

☐ **OPTION 3.** I don't want the *(D)*__________ listed above. I understand with this choice I am **not** responsible for payment, and **I cannot appeal to see if Medicare would pay.**

***(H)* Additional Information:**

This notice gives our opinion, not an official Medicare decision. If you have other questions on this notice or Medicare billing, call **1-800-MEDICARE** (1-800-633-4227/**TTY**: 1-877-486-2048).

Signing below means that you have received and understand this notice. You also receive a copy.

(I) **Signature:**	*(J)* **Date:**

According to the Paperwork Reduction Act of 1995, no persons are required to respond to a collection of information unless it displays a valid OMB control number. The valid OMB control number for this information collection is 0938-0566. The time required to complete this information collection is estimated to average 7 minutes per response, including the time to review instructions, search existing data resources, gather the data needed, and complete and review the information collection. If you have comments concerning the accuracy of the time estimate or suggestions for improving this form, please write to: CMS, 7500 Security Boulevard, Attn: PRA Reports Clearance Officer, Baltimore, Maryland 21244-1850.

Form CMS-R-131 (03/08) Form Approved OMB No. 0938-0566

Figure 14–4: Advance Beneficiary Notice. *Courtesy of the Centers for Medicare and Medicaid Services. Reprinted according to www.cms.gov website content reuse policy.*

DATE OF FORM	DATE OF SERVICE	SOURCE OF FORM	PROVIDER OF SERVICE	SERVICE PROVIDED—CODE	CHARGE	MEDICARE APPROVED	MEDICARE PAID	SECONDARY INSURANCE PAID	PATIENT RESPONSIBILITY	COMMENTS
2005										
10/9	9/27	Medicare	Radiologist #1	Mammogram—7609L XA Both Breasts	$135.00	$65.91	-0-	-0-	$65.91	$65.91 applied to '05 deductible
11/2	10/3	Medicare	Surgeon	Office Consult—99242	$105.00	$89.56	$36.38	-0-	$53.18	$44.09 applied to '05 deductible
11/10	10/11	Medicare	Primary physician	Office Consult—99243 ECG—93000 Chest x-ray—71020-XA Blood draw—36415	$130.00 54.00 69.00 7.00 $260.00	$119.40 25.68 34.71 3.00 $182.79	$95.52 20.55 27.77 2.40 $146.24	-0- -0- -0- -0-		$36.55 to be billed to insurance
11/30	10/17	Medicare	Radiologist #2	Place needlewire—19290 X-ray needlewire placement in breast—76096-26 X-ray specimen—76098-26	$275.00 140.00 22.00 $437.00	$152.40 28.73 8.21 $189.34	$121.92 22.99 6.57 $151.48	-0- -0- -0-	$30.48 $5.74 $1.64 $37.86	
11/30	10/17	Medicare	Surgeon	Excision breast lesion—19125	$800.00	$428.42	$342.74	-0-		$85.68 to be billed to insurance
11/20	10/17	Medicare	Anesthesia #1	4.3 Anesthesia—00400 Chest skin surgery QKQS	$350.40	-0-	-0-	-0-	-0-	Requested information had not been received.
11/20	10/17	Medicare	Pathologist	1 Tissue exam—88305-26 1 Tissue exam—88307-26 1 Consult in surgery—88329	$165.00 230.00 70.00 $465.00	$41.26 86.65 49.61 $177.52	$41.26 86.65 49.61 $177.52	-0- -0- -0-	-0- -0- -0-	Lab services are paid at 100% of the Medicare allowable. Patient does not owe any copay or coinsureace on lab work.
11/20	10/17	Medicare	Anesthesia #2	4.3 Anesthesia—00400 Chest skin surgery QKQS	$111.25	-0-	-0-	-0-	$111.25	Charges denied, other insurance may pay.
11/20	10/17	Insurance	Surgeon	Procedure—excision				$68.55	$17.13	Insurance paid 80% of $68.55
12/2	10/11	Insurance	Prmy Phys	Medical x-ray, testing	$260.00			$29.24	$7.31	Insurance paid 80% of $36.55
12/14	10/3	Insurance	Surgeon	Medical	$105.00	$89.56	$36.38	$42.55	$10.63	Insurance paid 80% of $53.18
12/15	10/17	Medicare	Hospital	Laboratory Radiology Pharmacy Surgical service	$155.00 399.00 182.88 2,317.92 $3,054.80	$1,527.40	$916.44	-0-	$610.96	Deductible met.
2006										
1/5	10/3 and 10/17	Statement	Surgeon	Balance after insurance payments		—	—		$24.44	Pt bal after Medicare and insur.
1/16	10/11	Statement	Prmy Phys	Balance after insurance payments					$7.31	Pt bal after Medicare and insur.
1/27	10/17	Insurance	Hospital	Surgical services	$3,054.80	$1,527.40	$916.44	$610.96	-0-	Paid in full by insurance.
1/26	10/17	Insurance	Radiologist #2	X-ray services balance after insurance payments	$437.00	$189.34	$151.48	$30.29	$7.57	
2/12	10/17	Statement	Radiologist #2	X-ray services balance after insurance payments	$437.00	$189.34	$151.48		$7.57	Remaining balance due.

Figure 14–5: Summary of insurance explanation of benefits form and medical statements received in connection with one routine breast incisional biopsy procedure. *Delmar/Cengage Learning.*

not participate and provides treatment to a Medicaid patient, it is very unlikely that he or she will receive any payment from Medicaid.

Medicaid HMO plans are offered within some states' programs. Participation in traditional Medicaid does not mean a provider is automatically participating in the HMO; typically, a separate contract must be signed.

Workers' Compensation

Employees in the United States have the benefit of being covered by workers' compensation laws. For many years, the name of the coverage was known as workman's compensation, but it was changed to avoid connotations of gender bias. Every state has these laws to cover employees who are injured while working or become ill as a result of their work. In addition to state statutes, federal statutes cover federal employees injured on the job—United States Longshoremen and Harbor Workers' Compensation, Federal Coal Mine Health and Safety Compensation, and special benefits for workers in the District of Columbia. The state compensation laws cover those workers not protected by federal statutes. The employer pays the premium for workers' compensation insurance, with the premium based on the risk involved in performance of the job as well as on the company's loss history.

Providers who treat patients under workers' compensation plans are usually required to register with the state Workers' Compensation Board on an annual basis. The code assigned to each provider limits care to a particular medical specialty.

There are four principal types of state benefits: (1) the patient may have medical treatment in or out of a hospital; (2) if a temporary disability is present, the patient may receive weekly cash benefits in addition to medical care; (3) when a percentage of permanent disability is found, the patient is given weekly or monthly benefits, and in some cases a lump-sum settlement; or (4) payments are made to dependents of employees who are fatally injured. Benefits also include comprehensive vocational rehabilitation for severely disabled employees.

In most states, the report of an industrial injury is initiated by the employer and sent to the provider, who reports to the insurance company responsible for paying the claims (Figure 14–6). A few states have their own state fund for workers' compensation, and in these states the forms must be forwarded to the state office responsible. Time requirements for filing a claim vary. When the provider receives the form, it is considered authorization for treatment.

A patient who has an industrial injury should have a separate file set up for that injury and a separate account card. If the patient's record is required in a court case for settlement of the claim, there is no chance of violating the patient's confidentiality if other medical records are in a separate file. The patient is never billed in these cases unless treatment was given without authorization or was considered excessive by the Workers' Compensation Commission, in which case you may bill the patient's private insurance and then the patient for the portion denied by the commission. Patients who have a continuing partial or permanent disability are reevaluated at intervals, and the provider must furnish a supplemental report.

The medical assistant must keep current files of procedures and forms because these are frequently changed. The public affairs section or office services section of your state workers' compensation carrier will furnish any needed information. Visiting the Website of the Bureau of Workers' Compensation for your state on a frequent basis is also a good way of staying abreast of updates and changes.

The complete and accurate preparation of forms ensures prompt payment of services. The following details are necessary for reimbursement:

- An accurate claim number appears on all forms and bills.
- The patient's complete name, the date, and the nature of the treatments are included.
- The payee name, address, and number are listed on the form.
- Fees for laboratory or X-ray examinations with interpretations are attached.
- If a surgical billing, a copy of the operative report is attached.
- Fee totals are accurate.
- Forms and bills must be legible.
- The form is signed by the provider.

A bill can be disallowed if it is not filed within the statutory time limit. If the claim is rejected for late filing and your records prove your original billing was filed within the statutory time limit, that information should be submitted for reconsideration of the claim. Always retain a copy of your billing. A code number should identify each patient.

TRICARE and CHAMPVA

As part of the United States Department of Defense, the Civilian Health and Medical Program of the Uniformed Services TRICARE (CHAMPUS) was established to aid active service personnel and their dependents, retired service personnel and their dependents, and dependents of service personnel who died in active duty, with a supplement for medical care in military or Public Health Service facilities. The word **dependent** refers to spouses and dependent children. All members of TRICARE (CHAMPUS) over the age of 10 are issued an identification card. A patient who lives within 40 miles of a

Ohio | Bureau of Workers' Compensation

First Report of an Injury, Occupational Disease or Death

By signing this form, I:
- **Elect to only receive compensation and/or benefits that are provided for in this claim under Ohio workers' compensation laws;**
- **Waive and release my right to receive compensation and benefits under the workers' compensation laws of another state for the injury or occupational disease, or death resulting from an injury or occupational disease, for which I am filing this claim;**
- **Agree that I have not and will not file a claim in another state for the injury or occupational disease or death resulting from an injury or occupational disease for which I am filing this claim;**
- **Confirm that I have not received compensation and/or benefits under the workers' compensation laws of another state for this claim, and that I will notify BWC immediately upon receiving any compensation or benefits from any source for this claim.**

WARNING:
Any person who obtains compensation from BWC or self-insuring employers by knowingly misrepresenting or concealing facts, making false statements or accepting compensation to which he or she is not entitled, is subject to felony criminal prosecution for fraud.
(R.C. 2913.48)

Tear off this sheet and return the completed form to your employer's managed care organization (MCO) or to your local BWC custo mer service office.

Injured worker and injury/disease/death info.

Last name, first name, middle initial | Social Security number | Marital status ☐ Single ☐ Married ☐ Divorced ☐ Separated ☐ Widowed | Date of birth

Home mailing address | Sex ☐ Male ☐ Female | Number of dependents

City | State | 9-digit ZIP code | Country if different from USA | Department name

Wage rate $ ______ Per: ☐ Hour ☐ Month ☐ Week ☐ Year ☐ Other | What days of the week do you usually work? ☐ Sun ☐ Mon ☐ Tues ☐ Wed ☐ Thur ☐ Fri ☐ Sat | Regular work hours From ______ To ______

Have you been offered or do you expect to receive payment or wages for this claim from anyone other than the Ohio Bureau of Workers' Compensation? ☐Yes ☐No If yes, please explain. | Occupation or job title

Employer name

Mailing address (number and street, city or town, state, ZIP code and county)

Location, if different from mailing address

Was the place of accident or exposure on employer's premises? ☐ Yes ☐ No
(If no, give accident location, street address, city, state and ZIP code)

Date of injury/disease | Time of injury ______ ☐ AM ☐ PM | If fatal, give date of death | Time employee began work ______ ☐ a.m. ☐ p.m. | Date last worked | Date returned to work

Date hired | State where hired | Date employer notified | State where supervised

Description of accident (Describe the sequence of events that directly injured the employee, or caused the disease or death.) | Type of injury/disease and part(s) of body affected (For example: sprain of lower left back)

Benefit application release of information – I am applying for a claim under the Ohio Bureau of Workers' Compensation Act for work-related injuries that I did not inflict. I affirm that I elect to receive compensation and benefits under the Ohio workers' compensation laws for my claim, and I waive and release my right to file for and receive compensation and benefits under the laws of any other state for this claim. I request payment for compensation and/or medical benefits as allowable, and authorize direct payment to my medical providers. I permit and authorize any provider who attends, treats or examines me, and the Ohio Rehabilitation Services Commission (where relevant) to release medical, psychological, psychiatric, vocational or social information that is casually or historically related to my physical or mental injuries relevant to issues necessary for the administration of my claim to BWC, the Industrial Commission of Ohio, the employer in this claim, the employer's BWC managed care organization and any authorized representatives. My previous or future BWC claims may affect decisions made in this claim. Proper administration of the present claim may require BWC to share claims information with the employers of record (or their authorized representatives) and/or my authorized representative for any and all such previous or future claims. The released claims information may include any record maintained in my claim files.

Injured worker signature | Date | E-mail address | Telephone number | Work number ( )

Treatment info.

Health-care provider name | Telephone number ( ) | Fax number ( ) | Initial treatment date

Street address | City | State | 9-digit ZIP code

Diagnosis(es): Include ICD code(s)

Will the incident cause the injured worker to miss eight or more days of work? ☐ Yes ☐ No | Is the injury causally related to the industrial incident? ☐ Yes ☐ No

E code | 11-digit BWC provider number | Date

Health-care provider signature

Employer info.

Employer policy number | **Check if** ☐ Employer is self-insuring ☐ Injured worker is owner/partner/member of firm

Telephone number ( ) | Fax number ( ) | E-mail address | Federal ID number | Manual number

Was employee treated in an emergency room? ☐ Yes ☐ No | Was employee hospitalized overnight as an inpatient? ☐ Yes ☐ No

If treatment was given away from work site, provide the facility name, street address, city, state and ZIP code

☐ **Certification** - The employer certifies that the facts in this application are correct and valid.

☐ **Rejection** - The employer rejects the validity of this claim for the reason(s) listed below:

For self-insuring employers only
☐ **Clarification** - The employer clarifies and allows the claim for the condition(s) below:
☐ **Medical only** ☐ **Lost time**

Employer signature and title | Date | OSHA case number

BWC-1101 (Rev. 1/31/2011)
FROI-1 (Combines C-1, C-2, C-3, C-6, C-50, OD-1, OD-1-22)

This form meets OSHA 301 requirements

Figure 14–6: First report form for workers' compensation. *Courtesy of Ohio Bureau of Workers' Compensation.*

uniformed-services hospital needs a nonavailability statement to be cared for in a civilian provider's office. This simply means that the necessary services are not available at the service hospital or that for medical reasons it would be better to continue care under the civilian provider who has been treating the patient. Authorization is not necessary if the patient lives more than 40 miles from a military medical facility that could furnish the necessary care.

The Civilian Health and Medical Program of the Veterans' Administration (CHAMPVA) was established in 1973 for the spouses and dependent children of veterans who have total, permanent, service-connected disabilities. This service is also available for the surviving spouses and dependent children of veterans who have died as a result of service-connected disabilities. The local VA hospital determines eligibility and then issues identification cards. The insured members can then choose their own private providers. There are deductibles and cost-sharing requirements your office needs to be aware of.

If your office needs additional information on military benefits programs, you can contact your local health benefits advisor (HBA) at the nearest military hospital or clinic or the office of TRICARE (CHAMPUS) in Aurora, Colorado. Check out TRICARE's Website at www.tricare.osd.mil for contact information by the Web or telephone.

PATIENTS WITH NO INSURANCE

The most current numbers published by the U.S. Census Bureau indicate that 50.7 million people in the United States did not have health insurance in 2009. With that number of people without insurance, it is inevitable that a provider office will encounter patients who do not have health insurance but need medical care. When patients without health insurance are seen in the provider office, they are classified as self-pay patients. In other words, they are expected to pay for the services rendered out of their own pocket and usually at the time the service is rendered. In these situations, it is advisable to require payment at the time of service to avoid any delay in reimbursement and to avoid lengthy and costly collection processes.

PRIMARY AND SECONDARY INSURANCE COVERAGE

Keeping up to date with patients' current insurance coverage can be a challenge. Patients can have more than one insurance plan. Often, families have coverage from each spouse's place of work. Many insurance companies include a non-duplication of benefits or **coordination of benefits** clause in the policy. If a child is covered by both parents' insurance, it will be necessary to determine who is considered the **primary** carrier (responsible for payment first) and who is the **secondary** carrier (responsible for payment after primary coverage). The charges are filed first with the primary carrier. After the claim has been processed and an explanation of benefits is received, the balance is submitted to the secondary carrier for payment. The charges are usually covered, or nearly so, with both plans. Responsibility for primary coverage is based upon the language contained in the policies. For example, one spouse might have a good plan as a fringe benefit; the other might decide to refuse the option to contribute to a plan and instead participate in a supplemental coverage that will become the secondary coverage. There can be many variables.

Covering dependent children is another variable. The primary coverage is usually responsible, but if both parents have equal coverage, another variable might be the determining factor. In this situation, the **birthday rule** applies. This rule states that:

- The plan of the parent whose birthday occurs first in the calendar year is primary, and the other parent's plan is secondary.
- If both parents have the same birthdate, the plan in effect the longest is primary.
- If the parents divorce and retain their plans, the parent with custody is primary.
- If a court order exists that dictates which parent is responsible for medical expenses, the court order supersedes the birthday rule.

Medicare and Supplemental Insurance

Most Medicare patients have some form of supplemental or Medigap insurance to cover the deductible and the 20 percent coinsurance. Remember to ask for their current information and insurance card because changes can occur from one visit to another.

CLINICAL PEARL

Make a copy of both sides of the Medicare and supplemental insurance cards for your records if the office is still using a paper-based medical record system. However, if the office is using an electronic medical record system, scan the patient's identification card into the record.

Medigap is health insurance offered by private companies to persons eligible for Medicare benefits and is specifically designed to supplement Medicare benefits. Medicare generally forwards the claim information directly to the Medigap carrier, thus saving the office staff time. It is important to ask the patient about any supplemental insurance at the time of service. If the patient does not have a commercial supplemental insurance and is unable to pay the deductible or coinsurance, the patient might be eligible for Medicaid. In this case, Medicare would be the primary insurance, and Medicaid would be secondary and the coverage billed for the balance, deductible, and coinsurance.

Another variable with primary and secondary coverage occurs when a person qualifies for Medicare by virtue of age but remains employed. If the employee continues to work and is employed by a company with 20 or more employees, the group plan is billed as primary and Medicare is billed as secondary. Health insurance coverage provided through employment group plans terminates when the employee retires, and Medicare becomes the primary coverage. Supplemental coverage is often available through the company's retirement plan. However, if a Medicare beneficiary is retired but has a working spouse with health insurance, and the beneficiary is an eligible dependent on the spouse's policy, then the spouse's plan becomes primary and Medicare is secondary. Medicare is also secondary when patients are receiving Veterans Administration benefits.

Additionally, keep in mind that Medicare patients tend to continue to carry their traditional red-white-and-blue insurance card even if they have opted into a Medicare HMO. A patient may present a traditional Medicare card when actually insured by one of the HMOs. It is important to verify with the patients whether they have coverage only through Medicare or through a Medicare Advantage plan. The Medicare Advantage plan will be their primary insurer, but they must maintain their coverage through Medicare Parts A and B to continue to be eligible for the Advantage plan. This means the patient must continue to pay his or her Part B premium and can also be responsible for paying a premium to the Advantage plan as well. Posting a sign that says, "Please give your insurance card to the receptionist when you arrive—thank you" (Figure 14–7) helps with obtaining current information from all patients. Current insurance information is imperative to bill correctly for services.

Please present your insurance card to
the receptionist when you arrive for
your appointment.
Thank you!

Figure 14–7: Signs such as this are often posted in the reception area. *Delmar/Cengage Learning.*

VERIFYING INSURANCE COVERAGE

When greeting the patient in the office upon arrival for an appointment, ask the patient for a current insurance card (or for all current ones). Make a copy of both sides of the card; the copy is needed to complete forms or to request information regarding that patient and his or her coverage. It is a good idea to write the date at the bottom of each card copy when the copy is made. The date alerts the medical assistant of the last time a copy of the card was obtained. If the document is scanned into an electronic medical record (EMR), the date it is scanned indicates the most current card. Also, in conjunction with an EMR, offices use an electronic patient registration system that should be updated with the current insurance information.

It is imperative for a patient's insurance coverage to be verified each time he or she is seen in the office to ensure that the correct insurer is billed and the provider receives timely reimbursement. You can verify a patient's coverage in a number of ways. Some insurers have a dedicated phone line you can call to verify the patient's coverage. With current technology, however, it is often more cost-effective and efficient to use one of the other available online technologies to obtain the information. Some offices have a point-of-service device, which looks similar to a credit card machine. This device can be used either to swipe the patient's identification card or to enter the patient identification number manually and obtain coverage information. Some offices use an online tool on the insurer's Website to obtain the information. The point-of service device and Website tools are preferred to the phone call because they are less time consuming, and you are then able to print out the results. Procedure 14–1 lists the steps in verifying insurance coverage.

If, after providing services to the patient and submitting a claim, the service is denied for lack of coverage, the office can then supply proof that it provided the service in good faith because it checked eligibility and it was active at the time the service was rendered. Many payers reimburse providers under these circumstances upon appeal. This usually results from retroactive adjustments made to patient's coverage possibly due to a job change or nonpayment of premiums, for example.

Good communication skills and capacity to understand the different types of insurance coverage, managed care or otherwise, are imperative to provide explanations to patients and providers when problems arise with insurance eligibility, coverage for services or procedures, and claims payment or rejection issues. The many types of coverage and the rules that go with them are often very confusing to providers and patients alike. Even though patients have a particular type of insurance coverage, there is no guarantee that they fully understand their benefits or the coverage type they have. Patients and providers expect the office staff to understand the coverage and be able to explain it to them in a manner in which they can comprehend.

PROCEDURE 14–1 Verify Insurance Coverage

PURPOSE: Verify the patient's insurance coverage prior to rendering service to prevent claim rejection due to patient ineligibility for coverage

EQUIPMENT: Computer, patient identification card, insurance Website address, individual password for access on Website

S **SKILL:** Accurately perform insurance coverage verification.

Procedure Steps	Detailed Instructions and/or *Rationales*
1. Access Website for patient's insurance carrier.	Enter insurance company Website address in the Web address field. *Going directly to the insurer's site allows for up-to-date eligibility information.*
2. Locate the section of the Website for Provider Information.	On the insurance company homepage, click Providers. *This displays options that relate to provider-specific functionality.*
3. Enter protected area of Website.	Enter user ID and password and then click Enter. (The individual steps might vary, depending on the Website.) *These areas are password protected to prevent inappropriate access to member information.*
4. Access area of Website for verifying eligibility.	Click Check Patient Eligibility. *This brings you to the location in which to enter patient eligibility information.*
5. Complete all required fields on the screen.	Enter patient information in all required fields, including patient name, ID number, date of birth, and so on. *This identifies the member for whom you are requesting eligibility information.*
6. Verify on screen that you have the correct patient information and that the patient is eligible for coverage.	Review patient information that is presented on screen and identify whether the patient has active coverage. *This prevents rejections for services that were provided when patient was not covered by insurance and allows the office to obtain corrected information about coverage from the patient prior to services being rendered.*
7. Print results for inclusion in the patient's record either on paper or scanned into EMR.	Select the print function on the screen. *Documentation that eligibility was verified at the time of service allows the office to dispute rejections for eligibility when a patient is retroactively terminated.*
B 8. Notify the patient if the insurer indicates that he or she is not eligible for services. ***Ensure that you communicate in language the patient can understand, while demonstrating sensitivity to the patient's situation.***	Let the patient know that the insurance company information indicates that he or she has no insurance coverage for the date of service and, if the service is provided, he or she will be responsible for payment of the service. *This allows the patient to contact his or her insurance company to find out why he or she is not covered and provides him or her with advance notice that he or she will be responsible for payment.*

UTILIZATION REVIEW

Managed care plans perform utilization review/management as a method of assessing the quality and appropriateness of the care provided to its members. These reviews are performed prior to the service being rendered (prospectively) or after the care has been provided (retrospectively). Methods for utilization management include: preauthorization, precertification, predetermination, concurrent review, and discharge planning.

Preauthorization and Precertification

The terms *precertification*, *preauthorization*, and *predetermination* refer to obtaining plan approval for services prior to the patient receiving them. Many times, these terms are used interchangeably, but there are technical differences.

- **Precertification** refers to seeking approval for a treatment (surgery, hospitalization, diagnostic test) under the patient's insurance contract. See Procedure 14–2 for steps in obtaining a managed care referral for treatment.
- **Preauthorization** relates not only to whether the services are covered but also whether the proposed treatment is medically necessary. See Procedure 14–3 for steps in obtaining preauthorization for a procedure.
- **Predetermination** refers to the discovery of the maximum amount of money the carrier will pay for primary surgery, consultation service, postoperative care, and so on.

Although these conditions are all similar because they affect the patient's ability to receive services, they are also specific and different in their application and effect on the patient's coverage.

PROCEDURE 14–2 Obtain a Managed Care Referral and Precertification

PURPOSE: Establish a referral for specialty care to prevent claims rejections for services rendered by the specialist

EQUIPMENT: Computer, patient identification card, specialist name, specialist NPI, number of visits requested, insurance Website address, individual password for access on Website

S SKILL: Accurately obtain a managed care referral.

Procedure Steps	Detailed Instructions and/or *Rationales*
1. Access Website for patient's insurance carrier or use other technology the office offers for electronic administration.	Enter insurance company or technology provider Website address in the Web address field. *Allows for immediate response to referral request.*
2. Enter protected area of Website.	Enter your user name and password. *This allows access to the secure segment of the Website where patient information is stored.*
3. Access area of Website for requesting a referral.	Click Request Referral section of the Website. *Brings up the template for completion of the referral request.*
4. Complete all required fields on the screen.	Enter the required patient information, usually designated by an asterisk (*). Also be sure to indicate the requesting provider name and NPI as well as the name and NPI of the provider the patient is being referred to and the number of visits requested. *Providing this information allows the payer to assess the request and approve it.*
5. Verify on screen that you have the correct patient information.	Review all data entry before submitting the request. *Avoids unnecessary refusals due to incorrect information.*
6. Note referral number.	Either print a copy of the approval screen or, at minimum, document the referral number for future reference. *Allows a point of reference in case the provider to whom the patient was referred has any problems being paid for the service he or she provides.*

PROCEDURE 14–3 Obtain a Preauthorization for a Procedure

PURPOSE: Obtain preauthorization for a procedure to avoid claim rejection

EQUIPMENT: Access to computer and Internet, preauthorization form for patient's insurance carrier, and patient information for completion of form

S SKILL: Complete the process for obtaining a preauthorization.

Procedure Steps	Detailed Instructions and/or *Rationales*
1. Research procedure to determine whether preauthorization is required.	Open your Web browser and type www.bcbsma.com. On the site, click Providers and then click Medical Policies. On the medical policy page, select View Alphabetic Listing and click O. Click Obesity Surgery 379. Scroll through the policy until you reach the Authorization Information section. *This information indicates that the procedure will require prior authorization.*
2. Locate the prior authorization form.	Use the Preauthorization Request for Surgical Management of Obesity form supplied at the end of this chapter.
3. Complete prior authorization form correctly.	Patient name: Albert Jefferson BCBSMA ID #: XXH987654321 Date of surgery: Use date one month after current date Date of birth: 08/16/1975 BP: 125/80 Height/Weight: 5'10"/346 lbs. Current BMI: 50 Facility name: Boston General Hospital MD name: Dr. Steven Papodopoulos Dx: 278.01, 250.00 Procedure: 43846 Provider indicates patient is well-motivated, enrolled in a pre and post program, has a strong desire to lose weight, and has been unsuccessful with other weight-loss approaches. *Proper completion of form expedites the process and aids in obtaining authorization.*
4. Fax the form to the patient's insurance organization.	

Concurrent Review and Discharge Planning

While a patient is hospitalized, all treatments, tests, and procedures are reviewed before they are provided to assure their medical necessity. Once a patient is ready to leave the hospital, discharge planning is used to assure that the patient is being discharged to the most appropriate setting and with the services or supplies that they require.

ACCEPTING ASSIGNMENT AND FEE SCHEDULES

As discussed earlier in the chapter, Medicare and other insurance carriers enlist physicians and other providers to sign up as approved or preferred providers in their network. This means that the provider agrees to treat subscribers enrolled in the network for an agreed upon, discounted, rate for services. This rate is referred to as a **fee schedule**. In return for being willing to participate and accept a reduction in charges, the provider is ensured a supply of patients (the subscribers enrolled in the network). Providers often contract with many carriers to be able to provide services for a large group of current as well as future patients.

The contracted provider agrees to accept the **allowed amount** as his or her fee; this agreement is known as **accepting assignment**. The difference between the amount charged and the payment received is written off by the provider as a provider adjustment. The physician, or any other provider, can charge the patient only for the part of the deductible that has not been met and any coinsurance or copayment that is due. The amount to be collected from the patient appears as a patient responsibility amount on the provider payment advice or remittance advice received from the payer. The provider can also charge for any service *not* covered by the patient's insurance. If the provider is charging for a noncovered service, be certain the patient understands that the charges will be his or her responsibility. Many payers either recommend or require the provider to obtain a statement signed by the patient. This statement should indicate that the fee is *not* covered so that the patient cannot later refuse to pay and claim noncoverage was unknown. These statements are known as **waivers** (for commercial insurance) or advanced beneficiary notice (for Medicare patients, discussed earlier in this chapter).

All providers, whether they choose to participate or not, must abide by Medicare laws. When the provider does *not* accept assignment, the patient is responsible for the entire bill (even if it is higher than the Medicare-approved amount) and pays the provider directly. However, even in this situation, when a provider does not accept assignment, the most that can be charged is 115 percent of the Medicare-approved non-participating provider amount. Providers who exceed limits can be fined.

Usual, Customary, and Reasonable (UCR)

Some insurance companies use the usual, customary, and reasonable (UCR) basis of payment to calculate the allowed amount for contracted providers. This amount is calculated based on the amount usually charged for a particular service by providers within a particular geographical region. Although some payers still use this methodology for calculating fee schedules, many are now using the Medicare provider fee schedule as a basis for their fee schedules.

Resource-Based Relative Value Scale (RBRVS)

The resource-based relative value scale, or RBRVS, is the methodology Medicare uses to create the Medicare provider fee schedule (MPFS). The MPFS is developed by using relative value units (RVUs) assigned to each service. The payment components consist of:

- *Physician work*, which accounts for the level of skill and amount of time required by the provider to perform the service or procedure (judgment, skill, effort).
- *Practice expense*, which reflects the overall cost to the provider for performing the service or procedure (rent, utilities, equipment expense, salaries).
- *Malpractice expense*, which accounts for the cost of liability insurance. Surgeon / obstetrician

Each of these components is then adjusted for geographical cost differences by multiplying each by a **geographic cost practice index**. This results in different payment amounts, depending on the location of the provider's practice, and amounts can vary from state to state and even within the same state, depending on whether the location is considered urban or suburban. The **conversion factor** is the dollar amount that converts the RVUs into a fee (see Figure 14–8).

Diagnostic-Related Groups (DRGs)

Diagnosis related groups (DRGs) were developed by Medicare as a basis for the Inpatient Prospective Payment system and adopted by other insurance carriers as a method for reimbursing inpatient care at hospitals. Each discharge is categorized into a DRG based on a patient's principal and secondary diagnoses, including comorbidities and complications. DRG groups are organized into mutually exclusive categories called major diagnostic categories (MDCs), based loosely on the body systems (i.e., musculoskeletal system, cardiovascular system, and so on). Each DRG is assigned a payment weight based on the average resources required to treat a Medicare patient in that grouping.

This system was designed to encourage hospitals to operate more efficiently by finding better ways to provide safe and effective care to their patients. The length of stay for a patient does not have an impact on the amount of reimbursement under this methodology unless the patient is transferred. The expectation is that some patients will stay longer and some will have reduced stays and that both provide a balance in the cost of providing patient care.

MAINTAINING CURRENCY

Staying informed and up to date with Medicare, other insurance carriers, and health care insurance regulations is a never-ending process. Ideally, in each medical office, someone is designated the claims filer and is expected to maintain currency. This can be done in various ways. Medicare updates are discussed in bulletins available monthly to the practice in addition to weekly notifications from the local Medicare carrier. Many prac-

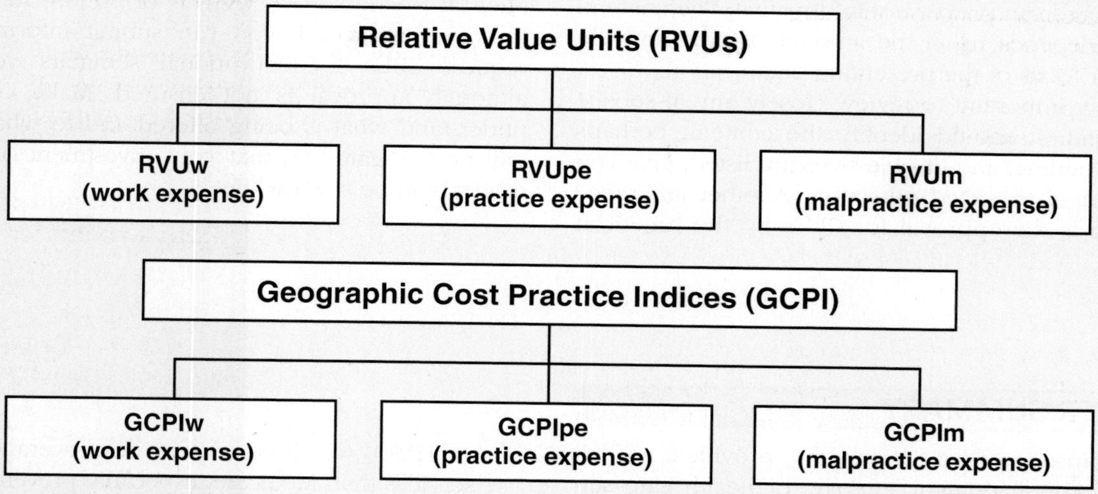

Medicare Physician Fee Schedule (MPFS) Formula

[(RVUw x GCPIw) + (RVUpe x GCPIpe) + (RVUm x GCPI)] x CF = Payment

EXAMPLE: Using the sample data below, the MPFS payment for a Level IV office visit in Buffalo, New York is calculated as $133.09.

[(2.00 x 1.000) + (1.51 x 0.944) + (0.12 x 0.720)] x $37.8975
[2.00 + 1.42544 + 0.0864] x $37.8975
3.51184 x $37.8975 = $133.09

Conversion Factor = $37.8975

CPT Code	Description	RVUw	RVUpe	RVUm
99201	Office/Other Outpatient Visit, New Patient, Level 1	0.45	0.50	0.02
99202	Office/Other Outpatient Visit, New Patient, Level 2	0.88	0.79	0.06
99203	Office/Other Outpatient Visit, New Patient, Level 3	1.34	1.13	0.10
99204	Office/Other Outpatient Visit, New Patient, Level 4	2.00	1.51	0.12
99205	Office/Other Outpatient Visit, New Patient, Level 5	2.67	1.80	0.14

Contractor No.	Locality No.	Locality Name	GCPIw	GCPIpe	GCPIm
00803	01	Manhattan, NY	1.094	1.351	1.586
00803	02	NYC Suburbs & Long Island	1.068	1.251	1.869
00803	03	Poughkeepsie/N NYC Suburbs, NY	1.011	1.075	1.221
14430	04	Queens, NY	1.058	1.228	1.791
56521	05	Rest of New York State (e.g., Buffalo)	1.000	0.944	0.720

Figure 14–8: Formula for determining provider fee schedule payments. *Delmar/Cengage Learning. (2010 Current Procedural Terminology, ©2009 American Medical Association. All rights reserved.)*

tice specialty organizations have newsletters, specific to their needs, to keep members informed. Other insurance carriers send newsletters to their participating providers, describing any changes in their coverage or processing. Oftentimes, these newsletters are made available on insurance plan Websites, and you can sign up to be notified when they are available.

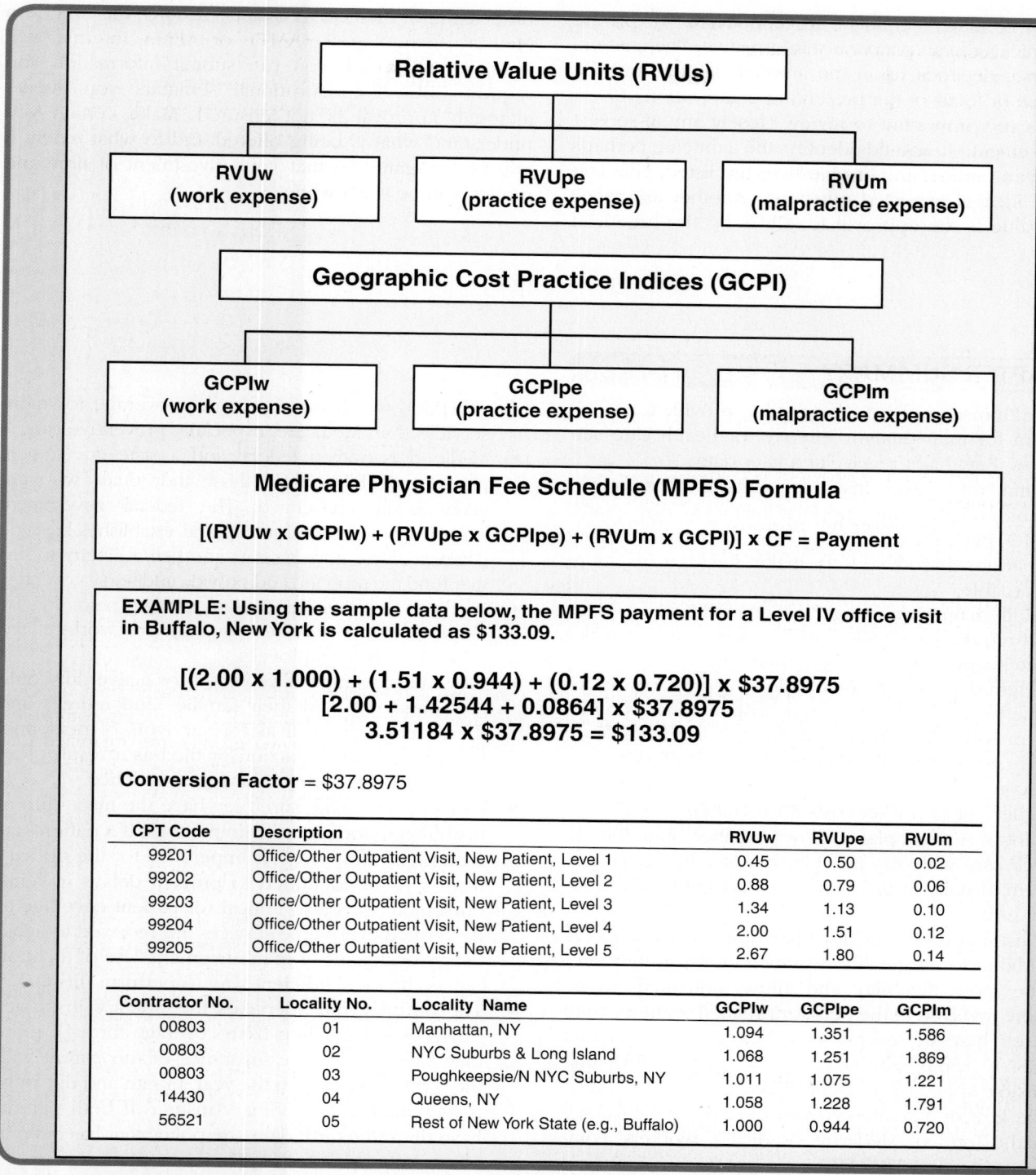

Seminars are conducted frequently. The annual major update seminar sponsored by your state medical association is practically a requirement for any practice to survive. Other seminars are conducted by private companies and can prove very informative. The content, of course, depends upon the amount of time and the expertise or focus of the presenting organization.

It is very important to review closely any in-service advertisement. It should identify the content, perhaps include an outline, and, if objectives are listed, give you a good idea of expected outcomes. Another assurance of its value is the approval for CEUs by the American Association of Medical Assistants (AAMA), the American Medical Technologists (AMT), or ARMA International. If not preapproved, you can submit information and request CEUs for educational seminars you attend, although approval is not ensured. Make certain you understand what is being offered and to what extent it will be presented so that your investment of time and money will be worthwhile.

CHAPTER SUMMARY

- Health insurance was designed to provide a mechanism for individuals to prepay for health care services they might receive at a later date.
- Commercial health insurance consists of indemnity plans and the more popular managed care plans: HMO, PPO, POS, and IPA. These models have many variations introduced to make health care more affordable.
- Health maintenance organizations (HMOs) are plans that require patients to have a primary care provider (gatekeeper) who manages their care.
- Preferred provider organizations (PPOs) consist of a network of providers and hospitals that contract to provide an insurance company or an employer with services for their members or employees at a discount rate. Going out of the network results in higher out-of-pocket costs for members.
- Point-of-service plans allow members freedom to seek care with any provider but at a higher cost to them, usually in the form of a deductible and coinsurance.
- Consumer-driven health plans are the most recent addition to the health insurance industry; they provide more flexibility and allow individuals to be more involved in the decisions related to their health care. There are several types: health savings account (HSA), health reimbursement account (HRA), and flexible spending account (FSA).
- The government also provides health care coverage in the form of Medicare, Medicaid, workers' compensation, and TRICARE.
- Medicare provides coverage to individuals who are 65 years old or older, individuals who are disabled, and those who have end-stage renal disease. Medicare Part A covers inpatient hospital care, skilled nursing facility care, rehabilitation services, hospice care, and some home health services. Part B covers provider visits, outpatient hospital care, and some services Part A does not cover. Some Medicare eligible individuals elect to have their coverage through an HMO, which often provides coverage for more services than Medicare, especially preventive care.
- Medicaid is both a federal and a state government program established for those individuals who are economically challenged. The federal government supplies some of the funding and establishes baseline coverage. State governments are then at liberty to further fund the program and provide additional coverage.
- Workers' compensation is coverage paid for by employers and provides coverage for work-related injuries to their employees.
- TRICARE coverage is provided for active-duty military personnel and their families and retirees and their families as well as for survivors of personnel who were killed in action or died as a result of an injury suffered during their time of service.
- Offices must make sure they have the most current insurance information from patients. If a patient has multiple insurances, it is imperative for the primary insurer to be identified to prevent delays in reimbursement. It is also critical for patient coverage to be verified every time services are received to avoid delays or denials of reimbursement. Use of technology is the most efficient way to perform this task.
- The birthday rule identifies the primary insurance carrier when children have coverage through more than one parent. The insurance of the parent with the birthday earliest in the year, month and day only, is identified as the primary insurer. If both parents have the same birth date, the policy that has been in effect the longest is the primary carrier.
- Preauthorization and precertification must be obtained when necessary to avoid payment denials.
- When a provider contracts with an insurer, he or she agrees to accept assignment, which means that he or she will be paid directly for his or her services and will accept the insurer's allowed amount as payment in full for services provided.
- Fee schedules are created by payers to identify the amount they will pay for services they will cover.

Usual, customary, and reasonable methodology uses the typical amount charged by providers for a particular service in that geographical area.

- RBRVS is the most common methodology used in calculating fee schedules, using relative value units assigned to work experience, practice expense, and malpractice expense, and adjusting them based on the region of the country. A conversion factor is then applied to convert the resulting RVUs into dollars.

STUDY TOOLS

Workbook	Activities for Chapter 14
Premium Website StudyWARE	Activities and Quizzes on the **StudyWARE™ Software** for Chapter 14
	Audio Library of medical terms
	Online access to the **Critical Thinking Challenge 2.0**
CourseMate	Activities and Quizzes for Chapter 14
WebTutor	Activities and Quizzes for Chapter 14

CHECK YOUR KNOWLEDGE

1. If a Medicare patient is being provided with a service that might not be covered, the office should:
   a. not provide the service.
   b. have the patient sign a waiver.
   c. have the patient call Medicare.
   d. have the patient sign an ABN.
2. The components used to calculate the Medicare physician fee schedule are:
   a. practice expense, malpractice expense and physician work.
   b. year's provider has been practicing medicine.
   c. rent, utilities, and staff salaries.
   d. none of the above.
3. A consumer-driven health plan in which only the employer contributes and the money is not lost at the end of the year is called a:
   a. health savings account.
   b. flexible savings account.
   c. health reimbursement account.
   d. medical savings account.
4. The government health plan that covers individuals who have a limited or low income is:
   a. Medicare.
   b. TRICARE.
   c. Medicaid.
   d. Social Security.
5. The percentage a patient pays for services after the deductible has been met is called:
   a. copayment.
   b. deductible.
   c. fee for service.
   d. coinsurance.
6. Insurance that provides coverage only for catastrophic illnesses and injuries is sometimes referred to as:
   a. self-pay.
   b. workers' compensation.
   c. hospital-only.
   d. managed care.
7. Methods used to verify patient coverage include:
   a. telephone.
   b. point-of-service device.
   c. plan Website.
   d. all of the above.
8. The maximum amount a nonparticipating provider can charge for a Medicare patient service is called the:
   a. limiting charge.
   b. maximum reimbursement.
   c. fee schedule.
   d. capitation.

9. What do managed-care delivery systems emphasize to help control costs?
   a. Quality assurance
   b. Preventive care
   c. Utilization review
   d. a and b
   e. a and c

10. The amount a patient must pay before his or her insurance will begin to pay is known as:
    a. coinsurance.
    b. copayment.
    c. deductible.
    d. fee for service.

WEB LINKS

Centers for Medicare and Medicaid Services: www.cms.gov

Council for Affordable Health Insurance: www.cahi.org

TRICARE: www.tricare.mil

Workers' compensation: www.workerscompensation.com

Chapter 15

Procedural and Diagnostic Coding

OBJECTIVES

In this chapter, you will learn the following:

KB KNOWLEDGE BASE

1. Spell and define, using the glossary at the back of the text, all the Words to Know in this chapter.
2. Name the two main classifications of codes and explain their basic difference.
3. Describe how to use the HCPCS coding system.
4. Describe how to use the CPT coding system and list eight general CPT coding rules.
5. Identify the symbols in the CPT manual and their meaning.
6. Identify the key components of an E/M service.
7. List circumstances under which modifiers should be used.
8. Explain the meanings of both the reason rule and sequencing.
9. Describe how to use the ICD-9 coding system and list four general ICD-9-CM coding rules.
10. Describe the impact the conversion to ICD-10-CM will have on the delivery of health care.
11. Define four types of insurance fraud and why they should be avoided.

S SKILLS

1. Accurately locate and apply CPT code(s).
2. Accurately locate and apply ICD-9-CM code(s).

B BEHAVIORS

1. Work with the provider (if appropriate) to achieve the maximum reimbursement.

WORDS TO KNOW

bundled
carrier
comorbidity
contributory factors
Current Procedural Terminology (CPT)
downcoding
encounter form
general equivalence mappings (GEMs)
Healthcare Common Procedure Coding System (HCPCS)
International Classification of Diseases (ICD)
key components
modifier
primary diagnosis
reason rule
reimbursement
sequenced
specificity
unbundled
upcoding

INTRODUCTION TO CODING

Coding is, in reality, the conversion of written descriptions of disease or injury, procedures, and services into numeric or alphanumeric designations to achieve uniform data that can be entered easily into electronic processing and storage systems. Accurate and precise coding not only helps optimize reimbursement, it is essential for carrier acceptance. The provider's **reimbursement** is based upon the codes that are submitted. Mistakes not only cost the provider, but patients are also affected when services are not covered.

The coding systems established a way to communicate numerically with carriers and at the same time provided a means to collect numeric data for national and international purposes. It is a complex system, but with experience, it becomes more manageable.

THE HISTORY OF CODING

While medical care was evolving into a highly technical service, another need was surfacing: some method of collecting health data so that providers, scientists, and government agencies could assess the incidences and treatments of diseases. As early as the 1890s, a provider developed a classification of causes of death. From this beginning, the American Public Health Association recommended that this classification system be adopted by those responsible for recording deaths in Canada, Mexico, and the United States. It was decided that the classification should be revised every 10 years. In 1938, the fifth revision had evolved into the **International Classification of Diseases (ICD)**. A few years later, hospitals began trying to classify diseases, and their medical records departments used a modified ICD version to code and index records.

The initial reason for classifying deaths was to provide a means of statistically assessing the prevalence of certain diseases or disorders or the incidences of fatal injuries. Later, codes were used to retrieve medical records by diagnosis or surgical procedure to be useful in medical research and education. As other applications became evident, the system provided a method of identifying the incidence of diseases and disorders being treated throughout the world. Reported prevalence provides statistics for assessing the status of people within and among various countries. As the need for greater **specificity** of medical conditions became desirable, the codes were revised, expanded, and refined.

By 1978, the World Health Organization published the ninth version of the ICD (ICD-9) and in the United States the *International Classification of Diseases, 9th Revision, Clinical Modification (ICD-9-CM)* was issued. ICD-9-CM codes became useful for reporting all medical care on claim forms for Medicare, Medicaid, and other third-party payers of medical services. Later, the impact of the Catastrophic Coverage Act of 1988 on the provider's office changed the way providers manage their practices, and ICD-9-CM coding has been required on all Medicare and other government health care claims since April 1, 1989. ICD-9-CM will remain in use until the 10th revision is adopted for use in the United States on October 1, 2013.

The American Medical Association (AMA) first published **Current Procedural Terminology (CPT)** in 1966, and subsequent editions expanded the code set and descriptions. Five-digit codes were introduced in 1970, and in 1983, CPT was adopted as part of the **Healthcare Common Procedure Coding System (HCPCS)**; its use was mandated in reporting Medicare Part B services. In 1986, HCPCS codes were required for reporting to Medicaid agencies, and in July 1987, the Omnibus Budget Reconciliation Act (OBRA) mandated the use of CPT codes for reporting outpatient hospital surgical procedures. As a result of the Medicare Modernization Act of 2004, new, revised, and deleted codes must be implemented every January 1.

HEALTHCARE COMMON PROCEDURE CODING SYSTEM (HCPCS)

The Healthcare Common Procedure Coding System (HCPCS) is comprised of two levels:

- *Level I:* Current Procedural Terminology (CPT) codes
- *Level II:* National codes

This section focuses on the Level II National codes (discussion of CPT codes follows in the next section). The National codes are approved and maintained jointly by the Centers for Medicare and Medicaid Services (CMS), the Health Insurance Association of America, and the Blue Cross Blue Shield Association. Health care professionals such as dentists, orthodontists, and some technical support services such as ambulance services cannot report their services with CPT codes because there are no codes in that coding system that properly report them. Thus, HCPCS Level II codes were developed to identify products and supplies for which there are no CPT codes.

HCPCS Level II codes are composed of one alpha and four numeric characters. *J* codes identify injectables that are provided to patients in an office or outpatient setting. *G* codes are temporary codes for procedures, services, and supplies. Codes beginning with K, Q, and S also represent temporary codes until a definitive decision is made about an appropriate CPT code assignment.

The HPCPS Level II manual has two sections, the Index and the Tabular List of codes. The search for the correct HCPCS code begins in the Index, which has services and supplies listed in alphabetic order. Some editions also have a drug table to make finding the codes for drugs administered in the office easier. When the description is found, the code or codes should be verified by looking in the Tabular List.

When appropriate, the correct HCPCS modifier should be appended to provide additional information about the circumstances surrounding the service. It is also possible to report both CPT codes and HCPCS Level II codes on the same claim. An example would be a patient who comes in for a therapeutic injection; a CPT code would be assigned for the administration of the drug, and a HCPCS Level II code would be assigned to the drug supply if the provider's office purchased the drug that was administered.

HCPCS codes are published annually. Not all insurance companies recognize HCPCS codes, so it is advisable to verify company policies before sending claims with HCPCS Level II codes on them. It is also advisable to check with an insurance carrier when both a CPT code and Level II HCPCS code are available to report. Most commercial insurance companies require the CPT code; however, Medicare requires the HCPCS code when a CPT code description is general.

CURRENT PROCEDURAL TERMINOLOGY (CPT) CODING

As discussed, Current Procedural Terminology (CPT) is also known as Level I of the Healthcare Common Procedure Coding System (HCPCS). The Current Procedural Terminology (CPT) manual has a systematic listing and coding of procedures and services performed by providers. Each procedure or service is identified with a five-digit code, which is used to report services. The main body of the material is listed in six sections; see Table 15–1.

Within each section are subsections with anatomic, procedure, condition, or descriptor subheadings. The procedures and services with their identifying codes are presented in numeric order with one exception: The entire Evaluation and Management section is placed at the beginning of the listed procedures. Most providers use these codes in reporting a significant portion of their services. At the end of the CPT manual are the appendices and the index.

TABLE 15–1 Six Sections of the CPT Manual

1.	Evaluation and Management (E/M)	99201–99499
2.	Anesthesiology	00100–01999, 99100–99140
3.	Surgery	10021–69990
4.	Radiology	70010–79999
5.	Pathology and Laboratory	80047–89398
6.	Medicine	90281–99199, 99500–99607

Using the CPT Manual

The introduction in the CPT manual gives excellent instructions on the use of CPT terminology and coding. The book is divided into specialty sections, but codes from any section may be used to give an adequate description of a treatment or procedure rendered by a qualified provider. The introduction offers guidelines at the beginning of each section to define items that are necessary to interpret and report the procedures and services found in that section.

In some instances, a specific procedure or service might need to be slightly altered, and if this is the case, instructions and Appendix A explain the use of **modifiers**. Modifiers inform third-party payers that circumstances for that particular code have been altered. Some examples of when modifiers would be used are if unusual events occurred, if a service was performed by more than one provider, or if only the professional or technical component of a radiologic procedure is being billed.

If you cannot find a code listed for a procedure or service the provider has performed, a provision has been made for the use of specific code numbers for reporting unlisted procedures. When an unlisted code is reported, a copy of the operative note must also be sent so that the payer can determine what was performed and then determine the appropriate reimbursement.

CPT manuals are updated annually. When the new CPT manual is issued each year, it is important to check the codes you are using to be sure they have not changed. Appendix B in the CPT manual provides a complete list of the codes deleted, revised, and added to the book. The **encounter form** (also called a superbill) should be checked to ensure that all codes remain accurate and valid. Encounter forms can be preprinted with the most frequently used CPT and ICD-9-CM codes in a specific medical office. If changes have occurred, the encounter form must be revised and reprinted. Finally, codes should be checked and updated in the office's practice management software.

The AMA also offers versions of the CPT manual in CD format, and the CPT manual's contents can be downloaded to a computer. Other coding publications are available for immediate download as well. You can view these publications by visiting the Website at www.ama-assn.org.

CPT Symbols

The 2010 CPT manual uses symbols to indicate specific information about code numbers (Figure 15–1). Review Figure 15–2, a sample of breast incision and excision

Current Procedural Terminology Codebook Symbols

New code

● 64650 Chemodenervation of eccrine glands; both axillae

Revised code (altered procedure descriptor)

▲ 44310 Ileostomy or jejunostomy, non-tube

New or revised text (other than the procedure descriptors)

▶◀ 90760 Intravenous infusion, hydration; initial, up to 1 hr
▶(Do not report 90760 if performed as a concurrent infusion service)◀

Add–on code

+11732 Avulsion of nail plate, each additional nail plate (list separately in addition to code for primary procedure)

Modifier –51 exempt

⊘ 17004 Destruction (e.g., laser surgery) of 15 or more lesions

Conscious Sedation

⊙ 33233 Removal of permanent pacemaker pulse generator

Product Pending FDA Approval

⁄⁄ 90736 Zoster (Shingles) vaccine, live, for subcutaneous injection

Reference to *CPT Assistant*, Clinical Examples in Radiology and *CPT* Changes book

47000 Biopsy of liver, needle: percutaneous
➔ *CPT Assistant* Fall 93:12

Figure 15–1: Symbols in the CPT manual. *Delmar/Cengage Learning (2010 Current Procedural Terminology © 2009 American Medical Association. All rights reserved.)*

BREAST
Incision

19000	Puncture aspiration of cyst of breast
+19001	each additional cyst (List separately in addition to code for primary procedure) (Use 19001 in conjunction with 19000) (If imaging guidance is performed, see 76095, 76096, 76393, 76942)
19020	Mastotomy with exploration or drainage of abscess, deep
19030	Injection procedure only for mammary ductogram or galactogram (For radiological supervision and interpretation, see 76086, 76088) (For catheter lavage of mammary ducts for collection of cytology specimens, use Category III codes 0046T, 0047T)

Figure 15–2: Sample CPT codes showing procedures and symbols to denote new, revised, add-on, and surgical procedures only. *Delmar/Cengage Learning (2010 Current Procedural Terminology © 2009 American Medical Association. All rights reserved.)*

codes, and note the + symbol, indicating an add-on code. In addition, notice the descriptive language and symbols that explain the specificity of the procedure.

Evaluation and Management Services Guidelines

The Evaluation and Management (E/M) section codes are divided into 17 categories of provider services, beginning with "Office and Other Outpatient Services" and ending with "Other Procedures." The E/M codes are related to medical services as opposed to surgical services. Figure 15–3 illustrates two of the five codes used for a new-patient office visit. Each code description identifies

NEW PATIENT

99201 **Office or other outpatient visit** for the evaluation and management of a new patient, which requires these three key components:

- **a problem-focused history;**
- **a problem-focused examination;**
- **straightforward medical decision making.**

Counseling and/or coordination of care with other providers or agencies are provided consistent with the nature of the lproblem(s) and the patient's and/or family's needs. Usually, the presenting problem(s) are self limited or minor. Physicians typically spend 10 minutes face-to-face with the patient and/or family.

99202 **Office or other outpatient visit** for the evaluation and management of a new patient, which requires these three key components:

- **an expanded problem-focused history;**
- **an expanded problem-focused examination;**
- **straightforward medical decision making.**

Counseling and/or coordination of care with other providers or agencies are provided consistent with the nature of the problem(s) and the patient's and/or family's needs. Usually, the presenting problem(s) are of low to moderate severity. Physicians typically spend 20 minutes face-to-face with the patient and/or family.

Figure 15–3: Sample E/M codes for new-patient office or other outpatient services. *Delmar/Cengage Learning (2010 Current Procedural Terminology © 2009 American Medical Association. All rights reserved.)*

TABLE 15–2 Key Components and Contributory Factors in E/M Code Descriptions

Key Components	Contributory Factors
• Level of history obtained	• Amount of time the provider spent
• Level of examination performed	• Counseling
• Degree of decision making involved	• Coordination of care
• Nature of the presenting problem	

the **key components** as well as **contributory factors** that must be met to report that code; Table 15–2 lists these key components and contributory factors. Another factor that affects some of these code descriptions is whether the patient is new or established.

The actual performance of any diagnostic test or study requires separate and specific coding in *addition* to the appropriate E/M code. Several other items unique to the section are described in the E/M guidelines, which are fairly easy to read and understand. If you refer to the first page of the E/M section of the CPT manual, you will see codes for a new patient that show four levels of history and examination. Selecting the appropriate E/M and CPT codes is a complex clinical decision that is ultimately the responsibility of the provider. Completion of Procedure 15–1 provides you with practice in locating and applying CPT codes.

CPT Coding Rules

To determine a CPT code, select the name of the procedure or service that most accurately identifies the service performed. This could be a diagnostic procedure, radiologic examination, or surgery. Additional procedures or pertinent services may be listed, including any modifying or extenuating circumstances.

Generally, services performed in the office are marked on the patient's encounter form by the provider (Figure 15–4). Care must be taken not to miss items such as injections, urinalysis, blood samples, or the need to use a modifier. If you must code from operative reports, you must review the description the surgeon dictated to be certain all pertinent codes have been identified.

Any service or procedure that is coded *must be* adequately documented in the medical record. If clarification is needed because the documentation is unclear about what procedure or service was performed, seek assistance from the provider. Remember, if a service is not documented, it should not be coded; payers regard undocumented services as never having been performed. Another important factor to remember is that the codes have to be **sequenced** in relation to the intensity and level of service provided. This means listing the primary reason for the office visit first and other reasons next in order of their importance.

General rules for assigning CPT codes are as follows:

1. Analyze the provider's statement or description for the service provided and isolate the main term. If anything is not clear (due to poor handwriting, and so on), check with the provider.
2. Identify the main term in the index.
3. Check for any relevant sub-terms under the main term. Verify the meaning of any unfamiliar terms or abbreviations.
4. Note the code(s) found in the index for the main term or sub-term(s).
5. After locating the term and the code in the index, verify each code in the respective section of the manual to be sure the description matches the procedure or service performed.
6. Never code directly from the index. Always cross-reference the code or codes found in the index with the actual code descriptions.

PROCEDURE 15–1 Perform Procedural Coding

PURPOSE: Accurately locate and assign the correct CPT code from information indicated on a patient encounter form

EQUIPMENT: Patient encounter form and current CPT manual

S **SKILL:** Accurately locate and apply CPT code(s), working with the provider (if appropriate) to achieve maximum reimbursement.

Procedure Steps	Detailed Instructions and/or *Rationales*
B 1. Review the encounter form; ***check with provider regarding any uncertain items, working to achieve maximum reimbursement.***	Look over the entire encounter form to make sure that all procedures and services performed are identified. *All services should be identified and reported as appropriate. If anything is not clear (such as poor handwriting), check with the provider.*
2. Identify the procedure indicated on the encounter form. Determine the main term for the procedure performed. Read the description of the procedure and isolate the main term.	*This helps you locate the code. The isolated main term is what you look up in the CPT index.*
3. Turn to the alphabetic index in the CPT manual. Turn to the letter the main term begins with and then locate the main term.	*Locating the main term in the index narrows the search for the code.*
4. Search through any sub-terms listed under the main term. Look for the sub-term that further narrows the code options; research each code listed.	*The sub-term provides either one code or several codes that must be verified.* Write down each code listed for the appropriate sub-term and review the descriptions in the main part of the manual. ***Never ever code directly from the index!*** *Always verify each code description, even if there is only one, to be sure you are selecting the correct code.*
5. Indicate the correct code on the encounter form next to the narrative for the procedure.	*This makes it easier for the staff member of the billing department to enter the code from the encounter form.*

7. Many times, one specific code is provided; the description should be reviewed and compared to the procedure or service provided. In other cases, there will be multiple codes or code ranges, all of which will need to be reviewed to locate the correct code. Verify the descriptions to select the correct code.
8. In all cases, it is necessary to review all descriptions of codes listed for main terms and sub-terms to be sure the correct code is selected.

ICD-9-CM CODING

International Classification of Diseases, 9th Revision, Clinical Modification (ICD-9-CM) is required on all claims to report morbidity and mortality of the patient. ICD-9-CM codes describe the *disease* or *condition* presented by the patient. Use of ICD-9-CM codes establishes the medical necessity for the services and procedures provided to the patient. The diagnosis reported on a claim indicates why the patient sought care, and the CPT and HCPCS codes establish what was done for the problem. The diagnosis must justify the service or procedure(s) performed. Without medical necessity, the claim will be denied. The ICD-9-CM code selected by the provider must be as specific to the patient's diagnosed condition as possible. These codes must be appropriate for the procedure or service performed for the patient and reported with CPT codes, or payment will not be approved by the **carrier**.

PLEASE RETURN THIS FORM TO RECEPTIONIST

NAME ______________________

Receipt No: ______________________

PLACE OF SERVICE: ( ) OFFICE ( ) NEW YORK COUNTY HOSPITAL ( ) COMMUNITY GENERAL HOSPITAL ( ) RETIREMENT INN NURSING HOME ( ) ______________________ DATE OF SERVICE ____________

A. OFFICE VISITS - New Patient

Code	History	Exam	Dec.	Time	
____99201	Prob. Foc.	Prob. Foc.	Straight	10 min.	______
____99202	Ex. Prob. Foc.	Ex. Prob. Foc.	Straight	20 min.	______
____99203	Detail	Detail	Low	30 min.	______
____99204	Comp.	Comp.	Mod.	45 min.	______
____99205	Comp.	Comp.	High	60 min.	______

B. OFFICE VISIT - Established Patient

Code	History	Exam	Dec.	Time	
____99211	Minimal	Minimal	Minimal	5 min.	______
____99212	Prob. Foc.	Prob. Foc.	Straight	10min.	______
____99213	Ex. Prob. Foc.	Ex. Prob. Foc.	Low	15 min.	______
____99214	Detail	Detail	Mod.	25 min.	______
____99215	Comp.	Comp.	High	40 min.	______

C. HOSPITAL CARE

	Dx	Units	Code	
1. Initial Hospital Care (30 min)	____	____	99221	______
2. Subsequent Care	____	____	99231	______
3. Critical Care (30-74 min)	____	____	99291	______
4. each additional 30 min.			99292	______
5. Discharge Services			99238	______
6. Emergency Room	____	____	99282	______

D. NURSING HOME CARE

	Dx	Units	Code	
Initial Care - New Pt.				
1. Expanded	____	____	99322	______
2. Detailed	____	____	99323	______
Subsequent Care - Estab. Pt.				
3. Problem Focused	____	____	99307	______
4. Expanded	____	____	99308	______
5. Detailed	____	____	99309	______
5. Comprehensive	____	____	99310	______

E. PROCEDURES

	Dx	Code	
1. Arthrocentesis, Small Jt.	____	20600	______
2. Colonoscopy	____	45378	______
3. EKG w/interpretation	____	93000	______
4. X-Ray Chest, PA/LAT	____	71020	______

F. LAB

	Dx	Code	
1. Blood Sugar	____	82947	______
2. CBC w/differential	____	85031	______
3. Cholesterol	____	82465	______
4. Comprehensive Metabolic Panel	____	80053	______
5. ESR	____	85651	______
6. Hematocrit	____	85014	______
7. Mono Screen	____	86308	______
8. Pap Smear	____	88150	______
9. Potassium	____	84132	______
10. Preg. Test, Quantitative	____	84702	______
11. Routine Venipuncture	____	36415	______

F. Cont'd

	Dx	Units	
12. Strep Screen	____	87081	______
13. UA, Routine w/Micro	____	81000	______
14. UA, Routine w/o Micro	____	81002	______
15. Uric Acid	____	84550	______
16. VDRL	____	86592	______
17. Wet Prep	____	82710	______
18. ____________	____	____	______

G. INJECTIONS

	Dx	Code	
1. Influenza Virus Vaccine	____	90658	______
2. Pneumoccocal Vaccine	____	90772	______
3. Tetanus Toxoids	____	90703	______
4. Therapeutic Subcut/IM	____	90732	______
5. Vaccine Administration	____	90471	______
6. Vaccine - each additional	____	90472	______

H. MISCELLANEOUS

1. ____________ ____ ______
2. ____________ ____ ______

AMOUNT PAID $ ____________

Mark diagnosis with (1=Primary, 2=Secondary, 3=Tertiary)

DIAGNOSIS NOT LISTED BELOW ______________________________

DIAGNOSIS	ICD-9-CM	1, 2, 3
Abdominal Pain	789.0	______
Allergic Rhinitis, Unspec.	477.9	______
Angina Pectoris, Unspec.	413.9	______
Anemia, Iron Deficiency, Unspec.	280.9	______
Anemia, NOS	285.9	______
Anemia, Pernicious	281.0	______
Asthma w/ Exacerbation	493.92	______
Asthmatic Bronchitis, Unspec.	493.90	______
Atrial Fibrillation	427.31	______
Atypical Chest Pain, Unspec.	786.59	______
Bronchiolitis, due to RSV	466.11	______
Bronchitis, Acute	466.0	______
Bronchitis, NOS	490	______
Cardiac Arrest	427.5	______
Cardiopulmonary Disease, Chronic, Unspec.	416.9	______
Cellulitis, NOS	682.9	______
Congestive Heart Failure, Unspec.	428.0	______
Contact Dermatitis NOS	692.9	______
COPD NOS	496	______
CVA, Acute, NOS	434.91	______
CVA, Old or Healed	438.9	______
Degenerative Arthritis (Specify Site) ____________	715.9	______
Dehydration	276.51	______
Depression, NOS	311	______
Diabetes Mellitus, Type II Controlled	250.00	______
Diabetes Mellitus, Type II Controlled	250.02	______
Drug Reaction, NOS	995.29	______
Dysuria	788.1	______
Eczema, NOS	692.2	______
Edema	782.3	______
Fever, Unknown Origin	780.6	______
Gastritis, Acute w/o Hemorrhage	535.00	______
Gastroenteritis, NOS	558.9	______
Gastroesophageal Reflux	530.81	______
Hepatitis A, Infectious	070.1	______
Hypercholesterolemia, Pure	272.0	______
Hypertension, Unspec.	401.9	______
Hypoglycemia NOS	251.2	______
Hypokalemia	276.8	______
Impetigo	684	______
Lymphadenitis, Unspec.	289.3	______
Mononucleosis	075	______
Myocardial Infarction, Acute, NOS	410.9	______
Organic Brain Syndrome	310.9	______
Otitis Externa, Acute NOS	380.10	______
Otitis Media, Acute NOS	382.9	______
Peptic Ulcer Disease	536.9	______
Peripheral Vascular Disease NOS	443.9	______
Pharyngitis, Acute	462	______
Pneumonia, Organism Unspec.	486	______
Prostatitis, NOS	601.9	______
PVC	427.69	______
Rash, Non Specific	782.1	______
Seizure Disorder NOS	780.39	______
Serous Otitis Media, Chronic, Unspec.	381.10	______
Sinusitis, Acute NOS	461.9	______
Tonsillitis, Acute	463.	______
Upper Respiratory Infection, Acute NOS	465.9	______
Urinary Tract Infection, Unspec.	599.0	______
Urticaria, Unspec.	708.9	______
Vertigo, NOS	780.4	______
Viral Infection NOS	079.99	______
Weakness, Generalized	780.79	______
Weight Loss, Abnormal	783.21	______

ABN: I UNDERSTAND THAT MEDICARE PROBABLY WILL NOT COVER THE SERVICES LISTED BELOW

A. ____________ B. ____________ C. ____________

Date ____________ Patient Signature ____________

Doctor's Signature ______________________

RETURN: ____________ Days ____________ Weeks ____________ Months

DOUGLASVILLE MEDICINE ASSOCIATES
5076 BRAND BLVD., SUITE 401
DOUGLASVILLE, NY 01234
PHONE No. (123) 456-7890
EIN# 00-1234560

❑ L.D. HEATH, M.D. NPI# 9995010111
❑ D.J. SCHWARTZ, M.D. NPI# 9995020212
❑ SARA O. MENDENHALL, M.D. NPI #9995030313

Figure 15–4: Patient encounter form. *Delmar/Cengage Learning.*

Using the ICD-9-CM Manual

The ICD9-CM manual is organized into three volumes.

1. Volume I is a tabular list, organized into 17 chapters, with conditions listed by body systems in one chapter and by conditions according to their causes in another chapter. Other information in Volume I includes supplementary classifications such as V-codes (factors influencing health status and contact with health service) and E-codes (external causes of injury and poisoning). Volume I also contains appendices of:
   - M-codes—Morphology of Neoplasms
   - Classification of Drugs by the American Hospital Formulary
   - Classification of Industrial Accidents According to Agency
   - List of Three-Digit Categories
2. Volume II is an alphabetic index organized into three main sections:
   - Section 1—Alphabetic Index to Diseases and Injuries
   - Section 2—Table of Drugs and Chemicals
   - Section 3—Index to External Causes of Injuries and Poisonings (for assigning E-codes)
3. Hospital coders use Volume III to code procedures. (Providers' offices use the CPT coding for their procedures, so this section or volume is *not* used for coding in the medical office.) Some references include this content as Section 4—Index to Procedures within Volume II, not as a separate volume.

In addition, many manuals have enhancement variations. Some are loose-leafed, and some highlight codes to be avoided or codes that require additional information. Some carry additional explanations of diseases or disorders, whereas others are color coded to identify cautions, signs, symptoms, external causes, and so on.

One example of an ICD-9-CM manual is published by Ingenix. Most provider offices use the manual that has only Volumes I and II. The tabular section with disease classifications and increasingly specific codes is arranged numerically from 001 (Infectious and Parasitic Diseases) to 999.9 (Other and unspecified complications of medical care, not elsewhere classified). Review the partial page shown in Figure 15–5 and note the following features that help ensure accurate coding:

- Boxes preceding the ICD-9-CM code indicate that a fourth and/or fifth digit are required for greater specificity.
- Code descriptions have colored backgrounds to indicate the type of code and bring attention to unspecified or other specified codes.
- At the bottom of each page, a key indicates what the different symbols represent.
- The diagnosis with a proper code is easily recognized. Note the description of the conditions in 240.0 and 240.9.
- In addition to the codes, notice the black boxed *excludes* feature that indicates other code numbers used for these conditions.
- New lines of information are identified with a solid black diamond, whereas a revised line is an outlined black diamond.
- This particular code book also includes anatomic illustrations of various body structures to aid in selecting codes (not shown).

ICD-9-CM Coding Rules

The general ICD-9-CM coding rules are:

1. Code correctly and completely any diagnosis or procedure that affects the care, influences the health status, or is a reason for treatment on that visit.
2. Code the minimum number of diagnoses that fully describe the patient's care received on that visit. The diagnosis must reflect the patient's need for treatment, X-rays, diagnostic procedures, or medications.
3. Code each problem to the highest level of specificity (third, fourth, or fifth digit) available in the classification (see Figure 15–5). Sequence codes correctly so that it is possible to understand the chronology of events (e.g., the reason for the visit and care).
4. The *main rule* to remember is the **reason rule**, which says that the reason for the patient visit (encounter) is coded *first*. This is the **primary diagnosis**; any other issues the patient presents with (**comorbidities**) are coded next, in order of importance. This includes chronic conditions that must be considered or will be affected by the treatment for the primary diagnosis.

There is one exception when the main rule does not apply: if, after the patient has been examined, another condition is discovered that differs from the condition for which the patient had originally sought treatment. In this situation, the diagnosis that required the greatest amount of effort would be coded first.

ICD-10-CM AND ICD-10-PCS

The Centers for Medicare and Medicaid Services (CMS) have published a final rule in the *Federal Register*, indicating that the implementation and use of *International Classification of Diseases, 10th Revision, Clinical Modification* (ICD-10-CM) and *International Classification of Diseases, 10th Revision, Procedure Coding System* (ICD-10-PCS) must take place on October 1, 2013. The ICD-10-CM coding system has been in existence since 1990 and used by most other industrialized countries in the world. The United States is the last such country to implement this system. It has been known for quite some time that the existing ICD-9-CM system

Chapter heading

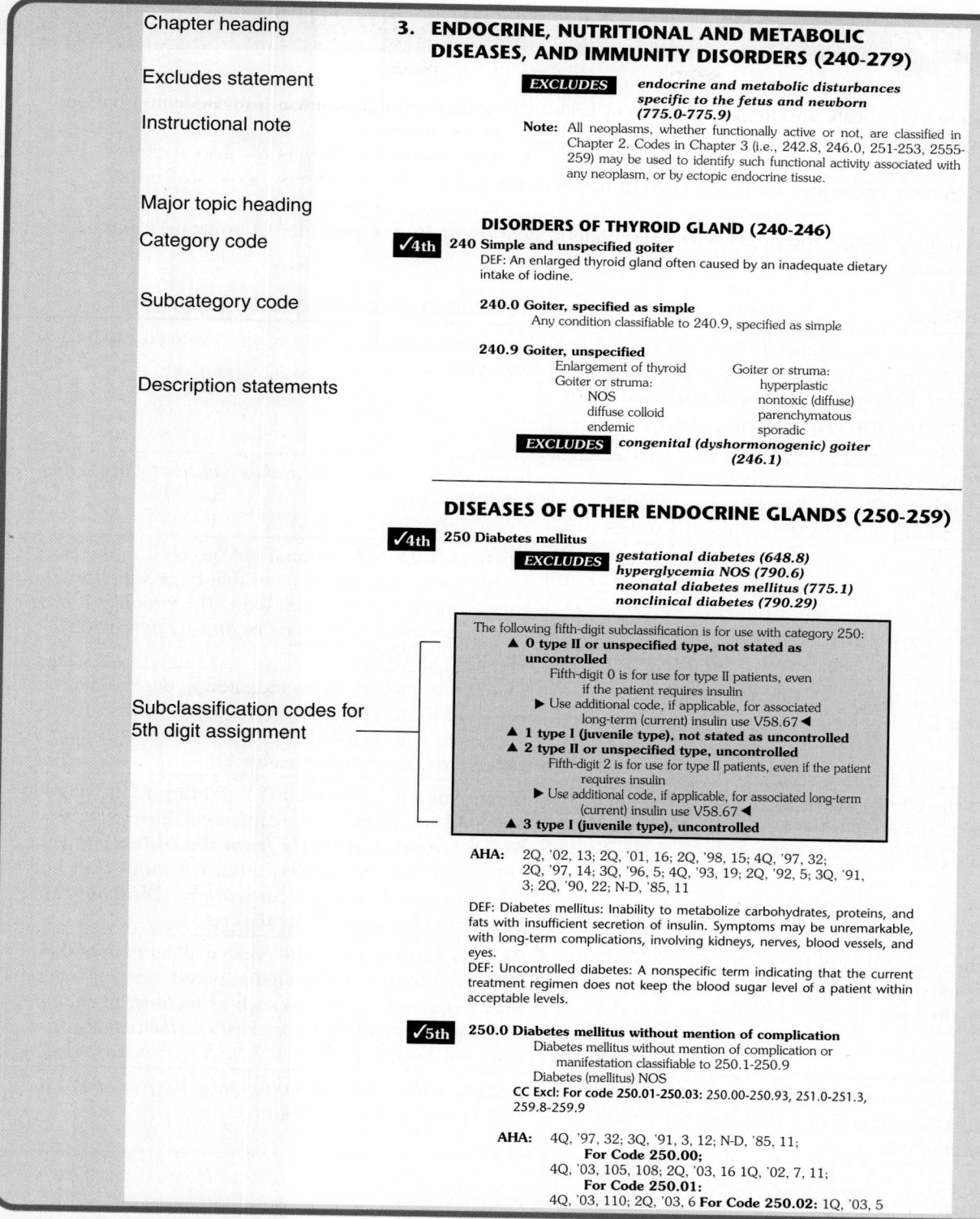

3. ENDOCRINE, NUTRITIONAL AND METABOLIC DISEASES, AND IMMUNITY DISORDERS (240-279)

Excludes statement

EXCLUDES ***endocrine and metabolic disturbances specific to the fetus and newborn (775.0-775.9)***

Instructional note

Note: All neoplasms, whether functionally active or not, are classified in Chapter 2. Codes in Chapter 3 (i.e., 242.8, 246.0, 251-253, 2555-259) may be used to identify such functional activity associated with any neoplasm, or by ectopic endocrine tissue.

Major topic heading

DISORDERS OF THYROID GLAND (240-246)

Category code

✓4th **240 Simple and unspecified goiter**

DEF: An enlarged thyroid gland often caused by an inadequate dietary intake of iodine.

Subcategory code

240.0 Goiter, specified as simple

Any condition classifiable to 240.9, specified as simple

240.9 Goiter, unspecified

Description statements

Enlargement of thyroid
Goiter or struma:
- NOS
- diffuse colloid
- endemic

Goiter or struma:
- hyperplastic
- nontoxic (diffuse)
- parenchymatous
- sporadic

EXCLUDES ***congenital (dyshormonogenic) goiter (246.1)***

DISEASES OF OTHER ENDOCRINE GLANDS (250-259)

✓4th **250 Diabetes mellitus**

EXCLUDES ***gestational diabetes (648.8)***
hyperglycemia NOS (790.6)
neonatal diabetes mellitus (775.1)
nonclinical diabetes (790.29)

Subclassification codes for 5th digit assignment

The following fifth-digit subclassification is for use with category 250:

▲ **0 type II or unspecified type, not stated as uncontrolled**
Fifth-digit 0 is for use for type II patients, even if the patient requires insulin
► Use additional code, if applicable, for associated long-term (current) insulin use V58.67 ◄

▲ **1 type I (juvenile type), not stated as uncontrolled**

▲ **2 type II or unspecified type, uncontrolled**
Fifth-digit 2 is for use for type II patients, even if the patient requires insulin
► Use additional code, if applicable, for associated long-term (current) insulin use V58.67 ◄

▲ **3 type I (juvenile type), uncontrolled**

AHA: 2Q, '02, 13; 2Q, '01, 16; 2Q, '98, 15; 4Q, '97, 32; 2Q, '97, 14; 3Q, '96, 5; 4Q, '93, 19; 2Q, '92, 5; 3Q, '91, 3; 2Q, '90, 22; N-D, '85, 11

DEF: Diabetes mellitus: Inability to metabolize carbohydrates, proteins, and fats with insufficient secretion of insulin. Symptoms may be unremarkable, with long-term complications, involving kidneys, nerves, blood vessels, and eyes.

DEF: Uncontrolled diabetes: A nonspecific term indicating that the current treatment regimen does not keep the blood sugar level of a patient within acceptable levels.

✓5th **250.0 Diabetes mellitus without mention of complication**

Diabetes mellitus without mention of complication or manifestation classifiable to 250.1-250.9
Diabetes (mellitus) NOS

CC Excl: For code 250.01-250.03: 250.00-250.93, 251.0-251.3, 259.8-259.9

AHA: 4Q, '97, 32; 3Q, '91, 3, 12; N-D, '85, 11;
For Code 250.00:
4Q, '03, 105, 108; 2Q, '03, 16 1Q, '02, 7, 11;
For Code 250.01:
4Q, '03, 110; 2Q, '03, 6 **For Code 250.02:** 1Q, '03, 5

Figure 15–5: Partial page from ICD-9-CM diseases tabular list. *From ICD-9-CM for Hospitals—Volumes 1, 2, and 3, 2005 Professional. Reprinted with permission.*

PROCEDURE 15–2 Perform Diagnostic Coding

PURPOSE: Accurately locate and assign the correct ICD-9-CM code from information indicated on a patient encounter form

EQUIPMENT: Patient encounter form and current ICD-9-CM manual

S **SKILL:** Accurately locate and apply ICD-9-CM code(s), working with the provider (if appropriate) for maximum reimbursement.

Procedure Steps	Detailed Instructions and/or *Rationales*
B 1. Review the narrative diagnostic finding(s) indicated on the encounter form and either underline or highlight them; ***check with provider regarding any uncertain items, working to achieve maximum reimbursement.***	*This isolates the diagnosis(es) for which you should be searching.*
2. Identify the main terms in the diagnostic statement(s). Read each diagnosis and identify the correct term to be looking up in the index.	*Isolating the main terms makes it easier to locate the possible codes.*
3. Locate the alphabetic index of the ICD-9-CM manual and the correct main term.	Open the ICD-9-CM manual to Volume II in the front of the book. Turn to the letter that begins the term you have identified as the main term. *This provides a starting point from which to proceed in finding the correct diagnosis code(s).*
4. After locating the main term, review any sub-terms listed.	Search through the terms indented under the main term and locate the appropriate term. A three- to five-digit code will be listed after it. *This narrows down the code(s) that need to be reviewed.*
5. Turn to the tabular list of the ICD-9-CM manual and locate the code listed beside the sub-term in the index.	Locate Volume I – Tabular List and turn to the page for the code you found in the alphabetic index. ***Never ever code directly from the index!*** *Always cross-reference the code(s) found. The index does not have any notes or coding conventions that should be considered before selecting the code.*
6. Read the description of the code and any coding conventions related to the code. Continue the process until you have found the correct code.	Read the description of the code, making note of the need for a fourth or fifth digit as noted. Also pay attention to any coding conventions such as *includes* or *excludes*. *Reading the notations helps clarify further whether the code you are selecting is truly the correct code to assign.*
7. On the encounter form, write down the code you have determined best describes the condition that is reported.	*Assigning the code and noting it on the form helps the billing staff code the encounter.*

is inadequate to report morbidity in the twenty-first century. Specifically, ICD-9-CM:

- Lacks sufficient specificity and detail.
- Is running out of capacity, and the code structure doesn't allow for medical advances in technology and a growing need for quality data.
- Is obsolete and no longer reflects current knowledge of disease processes, medical terminology, or the modern practice of medicine.
- Does not allow for the comparison of costs and outcomes of different medical technologies.
- Will not support the U.S. transition to health data exchange between providers in the United States.

TABLE 15–3 Crosswalk for ICD-9-CM to ICD-10-CM

ICD-9-CM	ICD-10-CM
372.05 – Acute atopic conjunctivitis	H10.10 Acute atopic conjunctivitis, unspecified eye
	H10.11 Acute atopic conjunctivitis, right eye
	H10.12 Acute atopic conjunctivitis, left eye
	H10.13 Acute atopic conjunctivitis, bilateral

ICD-10-CM consists of more than 68,000 codes—and is a significant increase from the existing 13,000 ICD-9-CM codes. The codes allow for greater specificity in reporting diagnoses, facilitating better tracking of quality of care and assessment of treatment outcomes (see Table 15–3). The value of ICD-10-CM is realized in:

- Greater coding accuracy and specificity.
- Higher-quality information for assessing quality, safety, and efficiency.
- Improved efficiency of care, resulting in lower costs.
- Reduced coding errors.
- Ability to recognize the advances in medicine and technology.
- That the United States will now be using the same coding system as the rest of the world.
- Improvement in tracking and responding to international public health threats.
- Enhanced ability to meet HIPAA electronic transaction and code set requirements.
- Accommodating future expansion of the codes.

The impact of changing to this coding system is very significant. All coders, providers, hospitals, and insurance companies must become proficient in the coding system because it is very different from the current system; Table 15–4 shows a comparison of the two systems. There will now be 21 chapters, and the supplementary classifications will be found within each chapter; no more E and V codes as we know them today.

In conjunction with the implementation of ICD-10-CM, the inpatient hospital procedural coding system will also be updated to the ICD-10-PCS system. (Note that providers' offices will continue to report their services with CPT and HCPCS National codes.) Just as with the diagnoses, the procedure codes needed to be updated to allow for reporting the more advanced procedures in modern medical technologies. The number of codes will increase from 3,768 to more than 89,916.

TABLE 15–4 Comparison of ICD-9-CM and ICD-10-CM Formats

ICD-9-CM	ICD-10-CM
3–5 characters	3–7 characters
First character is numeric or alpha (E or V)	First character is alpha
Characters 2–5 are numeric	Characters 2–7 are alpha or numeric
Always at least 3 characters	Always at least 3 characters
Use of decimal after 3 characters	Use of decimal after 3 characters

TABLE 15–5 Comparison of ICD-9-PCS and ICD-10-PCS Formats

ICD-9-PCS	ICD-10-PCS
3–4 characters (always at least 3)	7 characters
All characters are numeric	Each character can be alpha or numeric (alpha characters are not case-sensitive)
Use of decimal after 2 characters	No decimal

Four major objectives guided the development of ICD-10-PCS:

1. *Completeness* There is a unique code for all substantially different procedures. The ICD-9-PCS codes are so restrictive that the same code is often used regardless of whether the approach or body part is different.
2. *Expandability* The structure of this new system allows for expansion of the codes as new procedures are introduced and performed.
3. *Multiaxial* Each character within a code should have the same meaning within the same procedure section and across other procedure sections.
4. *Standardized Terminology* Meanings of terms within ICD-10-PCS should be the same regardless of whether they have multiple meanings in everyday usage.

Just as with the ICD-10-CM coding system, the PCS codes will be very different from the current ICD-9-CM; see Table 15–5 for a comparison.

To make the transition to ICD-10-CM/PCS somewhat smoother, the National Center for Health Statistics has created crosswalks, referred to as **general equivalence mappings (GEMs)**, as tools to help convert an ICD-9-CM/PCS code to an ICD-10-CM/PCS code and vice versa.

The conversion to the ICD-10-CM/PCS codes enables comparison of mortality and morbidity data as well as providing better data for:

- Assessing the quality of care provided to patients.
- Developing and redesigning payment systems.
- Claims processing.
- Clinical decision making.
- Tracking public health.
- Identifying fraud and abuse.
- Conducting research.

ELECTRONIC CODING

As the need for accuracy and optimization of reimbursement grows, even more pressure is put upon coders to make sure the codes they are reporting are accurate and properly convey the diagnoses and services that are provided. One way to assist coders in their efforts is to use software that converts medical documentation of diagnoses, services, and procedures into codes (Figure 15–6). Use of these products helps coders report codes accurately, thus reducing the primary reason for claim denials. The software also has decision support screens that help the coder determine which code is most appropriate for the patient's problem and the service or procedure performed.

A number of these programs are on the market, and some are even available for free. Exercise caution when selecting and using these programs to be sure that they are updated on a regular basis and that the sources are reputable. There are software vendors who will provide these products either as Web-based programs or as a software package that is loaded onto a computer. Before purchasing or using any of these products, it is advisable to research the sponsoring organization to be sure it is reputable. Some available products are Encoder Pro from Ingenix, Codefinder from 3M, SpeedECoder, and Code Ryte.

CODING ACCURACY

It is imperative for any codes submitted for reimbursement to be accurate. **Unbundling** codes, reporting multiple procedure codes for services when only one code is appropriate, is considered fraudulent billing and could result in stiff penalties and fines if found to have been done intentionally.

When a facility coder assigns ICD-9-CM diagnosis codes that do not match patient documentation, with the intention of increasing reimbursement to the facility through the DRG system, serious penalties and fines will be levied against the facility for submitting fraudulent claims. This practice is known as **upcoding**.

Another concern related to coding accuracy is the arbitrary practice of some insurance carriers to **bundle** codes, by which they either ignore additional codes reported on a claim and reimburse one of the lesser codes, or they ignore modifiers through secret edits built into their claims processing system.

Downcoding is another payer practice in which a reported Evaluation and Management service is reduced to a lower level based strictly on the ICD-9-CM code reported. For instance, a provider bills 99214 based on the documentation in the patient record, but the insurer, upon receipt of the claim, arbitrarily reduces the code to 99213 based on the reported diagnosis. It is the responsibility of the provider's staff to be aware of these practices and take proper action in the form of appeals to be certain that the provider is being paid appropriately based on the documentation in the patient's record.

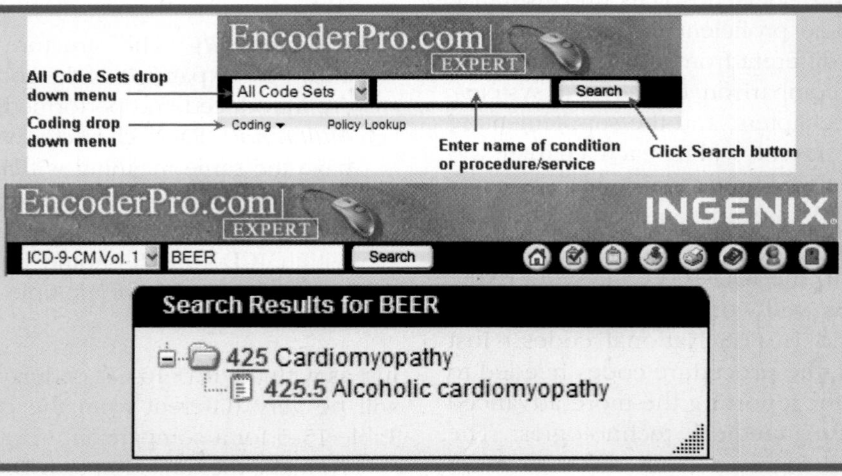

Figure 15–6: Using encoder software to look up codes. *Courtesy of Ingenix EncoderPro.*

As a result of HIPAA and, more recently, the Patient Protection and Affordable Care Act that was passed in 2010, more stringent programs are being implemented by the government and other third-party payers to audit records to ascertain whether there are any cases for which they can retract payments or deny payments due to fraud and waste. Along with tighter controls on prevention, the penalties for committing fraud are being increased, and providers will be required to adopt compliance programs that meet specific requirements.

Incorrect coding can result in suspicion of fraud or waste. An individual's diligence in providing accurate coding will help the practice avoid disruption if it is the target of an investigation. Implementing a compliance program within each individual practice ensures that all guidelines, rules, and regulations are being adhered to and can prevent the practice from being targeted. Those responsible for the coding within a practice must remain current in their knowledge of the coding guidelines and the government and payer guidelines, rules, and regulations. It is their professional responsibility to do so to protect their employer as well as themselves from undue suspicion and investigation.

Medicare Audit

The importance of complete records and documentation is never as critical as when the office is involved in a Medicare audit. Audits may be conducted if there is any question about the amount of service rendered in exchange for the claims paid. Records are essential to provide evidence that diagnoses and treatments were appropriate and that the services paid for were actually provided. The level of service must also be documented. Failure to document the level of service adequately could cause downcoding by Medicare and result in a charge of fraud. Anyone knowingly submitting a false claim or creating a false record or statement to receive payment from the federal government will be fined a civil penalty of not less than $5,500 and not more than $11,000. Documentation is essential. Remember: When records are reviewed by third-party payers, "If it is not documented, it was never done." Office staff should monitor providers' records and inform them of what is needed if necessary. Not only does it ensure adequate documentation but it also ensures that the provider receives the maximum reimbursement due. Documentation for each patient encounter must include the following:

- Reason for the encounter
- All relevant history
- Physical examination findings
- Orders for diagnostic tests and ancillary services
- Prior diagnostic test results
- Assessment, clinical impression, or diagnosis
- Plan for care

All entries must be legible, complete, dated, timed, and authenticated.

CHAPTER SUMMARY

- Providers use two coding systems to report their services in order to be paid by commercial and government payers: Healthcare Common Procedure Coding System (HCPCS), consisting of Level I Current Procedural Coding System (CPT), and Level II National codes. The second system is known as the *International Classification of Diseases 9th Revision, Clinical Modification* (ICD-9-CM).
- Coding is the conversion of written descriptions of diseases, injuries, procedures, and services into numeric or alphanumeric characters.
- Current Procedural Terminology (CPT) consists of six sections. Level II National codes are used to report supplies and services for which there are no current CPT codes.
- Modifiers are used with HCPCS codes to indicate something different about the way the service or procedure was performed.
- Guidelines are provided for the use of CPT codes to help coders determine correct use and reporting.
- Symbols within the CPT manual either call attention to a code or provide additional information for the coder so that he or she accurately assigns the code.
- Most providers use Evaluation and Management services; they are listed at the front of the manual even though the code set is at the highest range.
- The key components of an E/M service are history, examination, and medical decision making. Other contributory factors are nature of presenting problem, counseling, coordination of patient care, and time spent with the patient.
- Specific CPT coding rules have been developed to help with the assignment of codes. Understanding these rules helps the coder perform the job more effectively and efficiently.
- Providers use encounter forms in their practices to record the services provided to patients in their offices or clinics or on an inpatient basis. These forms contain the most commonly used codes and must be updated when the codes change annually.

- International Classification of Diseases, 9th Revision, Clinical Modification (ICD-9-CM) is required on all claims to report morbidity and mortality of the patient. Use of ICD-9-CM codes establishes the medical necessity for the services and procedures provided to the patient.
- The ICD-9-CM manual is divided into three volumes: Volume 1–Tabular List of Diseases; Volume 2–Index to Diseases; Volume 3–Alphabetic Index and Tabular List of Procedures.
- Just as with CPT, coding rules must be reviewed and followed to avoid errors in assignment and reporting diseases.
- Sequencing of diagnoses is important. The primary reason the patient is being seen should be listed as the primary diagnosis. Any additional diseases or injuries treated at the same encounter should also be reported as well as those that are not necessarily treated but medically managed.
- ICD-10-CM/PCS will be implemented on October 1, 2013, in the United States. This is a major revision of the current ICD-9-CM coding system and allows for more specificity in reporting conditions as well as for more growth in the coding system.

STUDY TOOLS

Workbook	Activities for Chapter 15
Premium Website	
StudyWARE	Activities and Quizzes on the **StudyWARE™ Software** for Chapter 15
	Complete the following **Competency Challenge 2.0** activity: • Perform Procedural and Diagnostic Coding
	Audio Library of medical terms
	Online access to the **Critical Thinking Challenge 2.0**
learning**lab**	Module 7: Medical Insurance and Coding
CourseMate	Activities and Quizzes for Chapter 15
WebTutor	Activities and Quizzes for Chapter 15

CHECK YOUR KNOWLEDGE

1. There are _____ coding systems for providers to use in reporting their services for reimbursement.
   a. 2
   b. 3
   c. 6
   d. 4
2. HCPCS stands for __________.
   a. Health Codes and Procedure Coding System
   b. Healthcare Common Procedure Coding System
   c. Health & Common Procedure Caring System
   d. Healthcare Current Procedural Coding System
3. How many sections can be found in the CPT manual?
   a. 4
   b. 6
   c. 5
   d. 7
4. Which section of CPT is used by almost every provider specialty?
   a. Surgery
   b. Anesthesia
   c. Radiology
   d. Evaluation & Management
5. Which form do providers use to indicate services they have provided?
   a. Superbill
   b. Invoice
   c. Encounter form
   d. a and b
   e. a and c

6. Which key components must be considered when a provider is selecting a visit level?
   a. History, exam, patient condition
   b. Exam, medical decision making, number of tests performed
   c. History, exam, medical decision making
   d. Medical decision making, number of diagnoses, time spent
7. ICD-10-CM/PCS will be implemented in the United States on __________.
   a. October 31, 2011
   b. January 1, 2012
   c. January 1, 2013
   d. October 1, 2013
8. What can a coder use to ensure correct coding?
   a. CPT manual
   b. Coding guidelines
   c. Provider directives
   d. State government regulations
9. Using ICD-9-CM to report diagnoses is required to establish __________.
   a. medical necessity
   b. reimbursement
   c. history of the patient
   d. none of the above
10. Coding correctly helps providers avoid __________.
   a. being accused of inflating their fees
   b. being accused of fraud
   c. being sued
   d. having to send in appeals

WEB LINKS

Centers for Medicare and Medicaid Services: www.cms.gov

American Health Information Management Association: www.ahima.org

American Association of Professional Coders: www.aapc.com

Unit

8

Billing and Payment for Medical Services

The medical assistant has a great deal of responsibility to ensure that the provider is paid for the services performed on all patients within the medical office. Ultimately, all charges incurred by the patient are the responsibility of the patient. Third parties such as insurance companies, employers, government programs, and so on will play a role in the payment process; however, this never removes the patient's responsibility for services that have been received. The medical assistant is involved in virtually every aspect of collecting for the services the provider has provided the patient.

Certification Connection

	Ch. 16	Ch. 17	Ch. 18
CMA (AAMA)			
Daily reports, charge slips, receipts, ledgers, etc.	X	X	X
Coding systems		X	
Third-party billing		X	X
Billing procedures			X
Aging/collection procedures			X
RMA (AMT)			
Insurance		X	
Patient billing	X		X
Collections			X
Fundamental medical office accounting procedures	X	X	X
Financial mathematics	X		
CMAS (AMT)			
Insurance processing		X	
Insurance billing and processing		X	
Fundamental financial management	X		
Patient accounts	X		X
Medical office computer applications	X	X	X

Chapter

16 Patient Accounts

OBJECTIVES

In this chapter, you will learn the following:

KB KNOWLEDGE BASE

1. Spell and define, using the glossary at the back of the text, all the Words to Know in this chapter.
2. Explain the differences between debit and credit.
3. Describe the daysheet and the patient ledger.
4. Explain a business associate agreement.
5. List the components of an encounter form.
6. Understand the components of the pegboard method used in posting patient accounts.
7. Describe the information that should be captured on a cash control sheet.
8. Name the advantages and disadvantages of the computerized method of bookkeeping.
9. List the advantages of the double-entry system over the single-entry system of bookkeeping.
10. List some circumstances when you might need to discuss payment planning with a patient.
11. Define a professional discount.

S SKILLS

1. Record charges, credits, and adjustments in a manual system.

WORDS TO KNOW

account
accountant
accounts receivable (a/r)
adjustment
assets
bookkeeper
Business Associate Agreement (BAA)
credit
credit balance
daysheet
debit
debit balance
double-entry bookkeeping system
encounter form
journalizing
ledger
posting
single-entry bookkeeping system
trial balance

THE BOOKKEEPING PROCESS

The medical assistant's role might be that of a bookkeeper. A **bookkeeper** is one who records the financial transactions of a business, keeping a record of **accounts receivable (A/R)** and accounts payable (A/P). This differs from the role of an **accountant**, who analyzes these transactions and prepares reports that not only tell the present status of accounts receivable and payable but compare current reports with other years or periods of time. A breakdown of the most cost-efficient and least cost-efficient procedures are revealed in such a summary. In addition, the accountant might be the person designated to prepare payroll checks and pay the quarterly amounts due to government agencies for taxes withheld.

The following list provides some of the basic terminology used in recording office financial transactions:

- ***Account** or **ledger***. A record for each patient, which shows charges, payments, and balance due.
- ***Daysheet**, also called a daily journal*. All patient charges and receipts are recorded here each day. (Today, most data is entered in computerized practice management software rather than on a hardcopy sheet.)
- ***Posting***. Transfer of information from one record to another. This might be an automated process, depending on the electronic system in place.
- *Accounts receivable*. All the outstanding accounts (amounts due to the office). This type of report can be generated as needed.
- ***Debit***. A charge added to existing balance.
- ***Credit***. A payment subtracted from existing balance.
- *Balance*. Difference between debit and credit.
- ***Adjustment***. Professional courtesy discounts, write-offs, or amounts not paid by insurance. If no adjustment column is included, discounts are listed in red in the debit column.
- ***Debit balance***. Reflects that the amount paid is less than the total due.
- ***Credit balance***. Reflects that the amount paid is greater than was due, or the account is being paid in advance of service provided. Manually, a credit balance is usually written in red ink, circled, or noted in parentheses. Today, this is typically highlighted in red in the electronic format.

If it is decided that an outside company will provide your office bookkeeping needs, you should execute a signed **Business Associate Agreement (BAA)**, thereby ensuring that the company understands your expectations of what it will do with the privileged information it will have access to. The BAA also establishes guidelines regarding what will occur if an inappropriate disclosure of protected health information (PHI) occurs.

CLINICAL PEARL

When you are responsible for bookkeeping, you must be accurate in every detail. There is no almost right in bookkeeping. The work either is 100 percent correct, or it is incorrect and must be corrected. Employees have been fired from their jobs because of carelessness with figures in simple math.

POSTING PROCEDURES TO PATIENT ACCOUNTS

It is essential to post accurately the actual procedures performed on the patient on the given medical visit day so the bookkeeper can maintain close track of services rendered and payments due to the doctor or medical facility. Several methods can be used to post patient procedures to their respective patient accounts, including both manual and computerized methods. In the past, the pegboard system was exclusively to record financial transactions. Today, most offices and clinics use computerized systems to perform the bookkeeping process.

Encounter Forms

An **encounter form** lists the procedures performed in that medical office, with their respective codes (see Figure 16–1). This form is also known as a charge slip or a superbill. When the provider completes the patient's examination or treatment, the charges are entered on the encounter form, and the patient is given instructions to return it to a designated person on the way out of the office. The administrative medical assistant might be given the responsibility of preparing this form, which accompanies the patient's chart.

The encounter form has a space for the patient's name and date and can in
Larger clinics might prepa
generated encounter form
name and account number
puterized practice manage
designed to be compatible

Patient Ledger

The patient **ledger** is a re
rendered, any payments ma
ance carrier, and any adjustm
dates of these entries. In c
ment software, all charges ar
directly in the software. The
play the patient's financial s
charges, ledger notes, billin
(Figure 16–2). In the manual
are posted on a patient ledger card (Figure 16–3A-B).

PLEASE RETURN THIS FORM TO RECEPTIONIST

NAME ______________________

Receipt No: ______________________

PLACE OF SERVICE:
( ) OFFICE
( ) NEW YORK COUNTY HOSPITAL
( ) COMMUNITY GENERAL HOSPITAL
( ) RETIREMENT INN NURSING HOME
( ) ______________________

DATE OF SERVICE ______________

A. OFFICE VISITS - New Patient

	Code	History	Exam	Dec.	Time	
____	99201	Prob. Foc.	Prob. Foc.	Straight	10 min.	______
____	99202	Ex. Prob. Foc.	Ex. Prob. Foc.	Straight	20 min.	______
____	99203	Detail	Detail	Low	30 min.	______
____	99204	Comp.	Comp.	Mod.	45 min.	______
____	99205	Comp.	Comp.	High	60 min.	______

B. OFFICE VISIT - Established Patient

	Code	History	Exam	Dec.	Time	
____	99211	Minimal	Minimal	Minimal	5 min.	______
____	99212	Prob. Foc.	Prob. Foc.	Straight	10min.	______
____	99213	Ex. Prob. Foc.	Ex. Prob. Foc.	Low	15 min.	______
____	99214	Detail	Detail	Mod.	25 min.	______
____	99215	Comp.	Comp.	High	40 min.	______

C. HOSPITAL CARE

	Dx	Units	Code	
1. Initial Hospital Care (30 min)	____	____	99221	______
2. Subsequent Care	____	____	99231	______
3. Critical Care (30-74 min)	____	____	99291	______
4. each additional 30 min.	____	____	99292	______
5. Discharge Services	____	____	99238	______
6. Emergency Room	____	____	99282	______

D. NURSING HOME CARE

	Dx	Units	Code	
Initial Care - New Pt.				
1. Expanded	____	____	99322	______
2. Detailed	____	____	99323	______
Subsequent Care - Estab. Pt.				
3. Problem Focused	____	____	99307	______
4. Expanded	____	____	99308	______
5. Detailed	____	____	99309	______
6. Comprehensive	____	____	99310	______

E. PROCEDURES

		Code	
1. Arthrocentesis, Small Jt.	____	20600	______
2. Colonoscopy	____	45378	______
3. EKG w/interpretation	____	93000	______
4. X-Ray Chest, PA/LAT	____	71020	______

F. LAB

		Code	
1. Blood Sugar	____	82947	______
2. CBC w/differential	____	85031	______
3. Cholesterol	____	82465	______
4. Comprehensive Metabolic Panel	____	80053	______
5. ESR	____	85651	______
6. Hematocrit	____	85014	______
7. Mono Screen	____	86308	______
8. Pap Smear	____	88150	______
9. Potassium	____	84132	______
10. Preg. Test, Quantitative	____	84702	______
11. Routine Venipuncture	____	36415	______

F. Cont'd

	Dx	Units	
12. Strep Screen	____	87081	______
13. UA, Routine w/Micro	____	81000	______
14. UA, Routine w/o Micro	____	81002	______
15. Uric Acid	____	84550	______
16. VDRL	____	86592	______
17. Wet Prep	____	82710	______
18. ________	____		______

G. INJECTIONS

		Code	
1. Influenza Virus Vaccine	____	90658	______
2. Pneumoccocal Vaccine	____	90772	______
3. Tetanus Toxoids	____	90703	______
4. Therapeutic Subcut/IM	____	90732	______
5. Vaccine Administration	____	90471	______
6. Vaccine - each additional	____	90472	______

H. MISCELLANEOUS

1. ______________ ____ ______
2. ______________ ____ ______

AMOUNT PAID $ ______

Mark diagnosis with (1=Primary, 2=Secondary, 3=Tertiary)

DIAGNOSIS NOT LISTED BELOW ______________________

DIAGNOSIS	ICD-9-CM 1, 2, 3	
Abdominal Pain	789.0_	______
Allergic Rhinitis, Unspec.	477.9	______
Angina Pectoris, Unspec.	413.9	______
Anemia, Iron Deficiency, Unspec.	280.9	______
Anemia, NOS	285.9	______
Anemia, Pernicious	281.0	______
Asthma w/ Exacerbation	493.92	______
Asthmatic Bronchitis, Unspec.	493.90	______
Atrial Fibrillation	427.31	______
Atypical Chest Pain, Unspec.	786.59	______
Bronchiolitis, due to RSV	466.11	______
Bronchitis, Acute	466.0	______
Bronchitis, NOS	490	______
Cardiac Arrest	427.5	______
Cardiopulmonary Disease, Chronic, Unspec.	416.9	______
Cellulitis, NOS	682.9	______
Congestive Heart Failure, Unspec.	428.0	______
Contact Dermatitis NOS	692.9	______
COPD NOS	496	______
CVA, Acute, NOS	434.91	______
CVA, Old or Healed	438.9	______
Degenerative Arthritis (Specify Site) ______	715.9	______

DIAGNOSIS	ICD-9-CM 1, 2, 3	
Dehydration	276.51	______
Depression, NOS	311	______
Diabetes Mellitus, Type II Controlled	250.00	______
Diabetes Mellitus, Type II Controlled	250.02	______
Drug Reaction, NOS	995.29	______
Dysuria	788.1	______
Eczema, NOS	692.2	______
Edema	782.3	______
Fever, Unknown Origin	780.6	______
Gastritis, Acute w/o Hemorrhage	535.00	______
Gastroenteritis, NOS	558.9	______
Gastroesophageal Reflux	530.81	______
Hepatitis A, Infectious	070.1	______
Hypercholesterolemia, Pure	272.0	______
Hypertension, Unspec.	401.9	______
Hypoglycemia NOS	251.2	______
Hypokalemia	276.8	______
Impetigo	684	______
Lymphadenitis, Unspec.	289.3	______
Mononucleosis	075	______
Myocardial Infarction, Acute, NOS	410.9	______
Organic Brain Syndrome	310.9	______
Otitis Externa, Acute NOS	380.10	______

DIAGNOSIS	ICD-9-CM 1, 2, 3	
Otitis Media, Acute NOS	382.9	______
Peptic Ulcer Disease	536.9	______
Peripheral Vascular Disease NOS	443.9	______
Pharyngitis, Acute	462	______
Pneumonia, Organism Unspec.	486	______
Prostatitis, NOS	601.9	______
PVC	427.69	______
Rash, Non Specific	782.1	______
Seizure Disorder NOS	780.39	______
Serous Otitis Media, Chronic, Unspec.	381.10	______
Sinusitis, Acute NOS	461.9	______
Tonsillitis, Acute	463.	______
Upper Respiratory Infection, Acute NOS	465.9	______
Urinary Tract Infection, Unspec.	599.0	______
Urticaria, Unspec.	708.9	______
Vertigo, NOS	780.4	______
Viral Infection NOS	079.99	______
Weakness, Generalized	780.79	______
Weight Loss, Abnormal	783.21	______

ABN: I UNDERSTAND THAT MEDICARE PROBABLY WILL NOT COVER THE SERVICES LISTED BELOW

A. ______________ B. ______________ C. ______________

Date ______________ Patient Signature ______________________

Doctor's Signature ______________________

RETURN: ________ Days ________ Weeks ________ Months

DOUGLASVILLE MEDICINE ASSOCIATES
5076 BRAND BLVD., SUITE 401
DOUGLASVILLE, NY 01234
PHONE No. (123) 456-7890
EIN# 00-1234560

❑ L.D. HEATH, M.D. NPI# 9995010111
❑ D.J. SCHWARTZ, M.D. NPI# 9995020212
❑ SARAH O. MENDENHALL, M.D. NPI #9995030313

Figure 16–1: Example of an encounter form, or charge slip. *Delmar/Cengage Learning.*

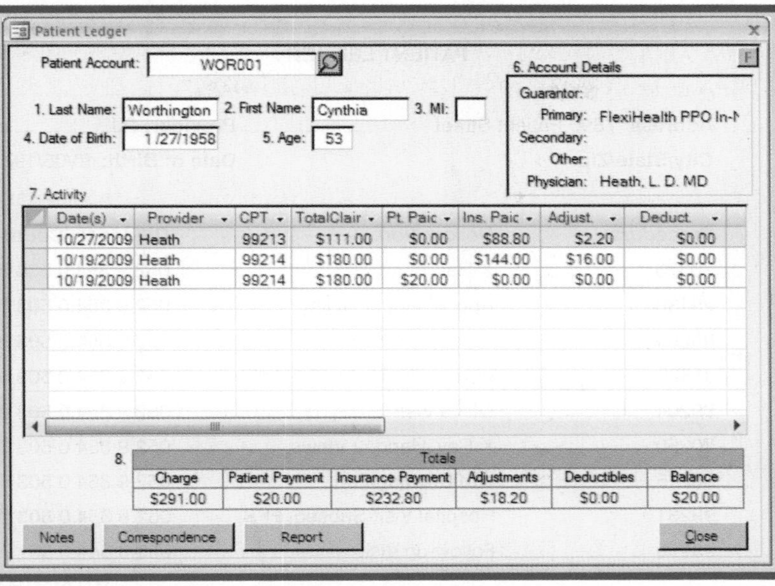
Patient Ledger

Patient Account: WOR001

1. Last Name: Worthington 2. First Name: Cynthia 3. MI:
4. Date of Birth: 1/27/1958 5. Age: 53

6. Account Details
Guarantor:
Primary: FlexiHealth PPO In-N
Secondary:
Other:
Physician: Heath, L. D. MD

7. Activity

Date(s)	Provider	CPT	TotalClair	Pt. Paic	Ins. Paic	Adjust.	Deduct.
10/27/2009	Heath	99213	$111.00	$0.00	$88.80	$2.20	$0.00
10/19/2009	Heath	99214	$180.00	$0.00	$144.00	$16.00	$0.00
10/19/2009	Heath	99214	$180.00	$20.00	$0.00	$0.00	$0.00

8. Totals

Charge	Patient Payment	Insurance Payment	Adjustments	Deductibles	Balance
$291.00	$20.00	$232.80	$18.20	$0.00	$20.00

Notes | Correspondence | Report | Close

Figure 16–2: Example of a computerized patient ledger. *Delmar/Cengage Learning.*

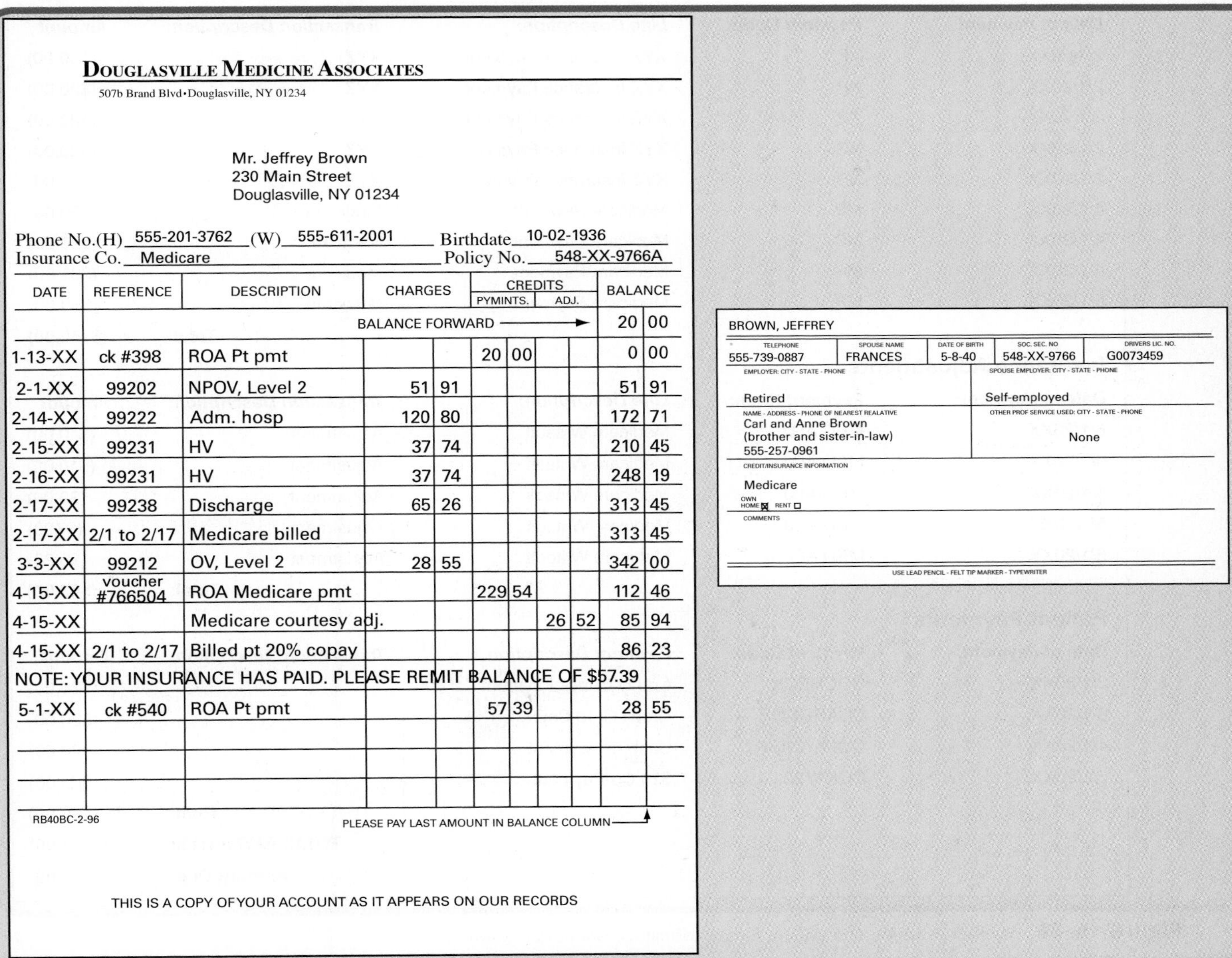
Douglasville Medicine Associates
507b Brand Blvd•Douglasville, NY 01234

Mr. Jeffrey Brown
230 Main Street
Douglasville, NY 01234

Phone No.(H) 555-201-3762 (W) 555-611-2001 Birthdate 10-02-1936
Insurance Co. Medicare Policy No. 548-XX-9766A

DATE	REFERENCE	DESCRIPTION	CHARGES	CREDITS PYMNTS.	CREDITS ADJ.	BALANCE
		BALANCE FORWARD →				20 00
1-13-XX	ck #398	ROA Pt pmt		20 00		0 00
2-1-XX	99202	NPOV, Level 2	51 91			51 91
2-14-XX	99222	Adm. hosp	120 80			172 71
2-15-XX	99231	HV	37 74			210 45
2-16-XX	99231	HV	37 74			248 19
2-17-XX	99238	Discharge	65 26			313 45
2-17-XX	2/1 to 2/17	Medicare billed				313 45
3-3-XX	99212	OV, Level 2	28 55			342 00
4-15-XX	voucher #766504	ROA Medicare pmt		229 54		112 46
4-15-XX		Medicare courtesy adj.			26 52	85 94
4-15-XX	2/1 to 2/17	Billed pt 20% copay				86 23
NOTE: YOUR INSURANCE HAS PAID. PLEASE REMIT BALANCE OF $57.39						
5-1-XX	ck #540	ROA Pt pmt		57 39		28 55

RB40BC-2-96 PLEASE PAY LAST AMOUNT IN BALANCE COLUMN

THIS IS A COPY OF YOUR ACCOUNT AS IT APPEARS ON OUR RECORDS

BROWN, JEFFREY

TELEPHONE	SPOUSE NAME	DATE OF BIRTH	SOC. SEC. NO	DRIVERS LIC. NO.
555-739-0887	FRANCES	5-8-40	548-XX-9766	G0073459

EMPLOYER: CITY - STATE - PHONE: Retired
SPOUSE EMPLOYER: CITY - STATE - PHONE: Self-employed
NAME - ADDRESS - PHONE OF NEAREST REALATIVE: Carl and Anne Brown (brother and sister-in-law) 555-257-0961
OTHER PROF SERVICE USED: CITY - STATE - PHONE: None
CREDIT/INSURANCE INFORMATION: Medicare
OWN HOME ☒ RENT ☐
COMMENTS

USE LEAD PENCIL - FELT TIP MARKER - TYPEWRITER

Figure 16–3A: An example of a patient ledger card, front and back. *Delmar/Cengage Learning.*

PATIENT LEDGER

Date: 05/31/XX

MR#: 123456	**Address:** 7890 Patient Street	**Provider:** RJ	
Name: Doe, John	**City/State/Zip:**	**Date of Birth:** 10/05/19XX	**Sex:** Male

Charges

Date of Service:	*Procedure:*	*Description:*	*Diagnosis Codes*	*Amount*
2/1/20XX	70373	X-Ray	052.9 354.0 503 847.2	$75.00
2/1/20XX	29130	App. of Finger Splint	052.9 354.0 503 847.2	$30.00
2/1/20XX	99204	Office Visit New	052.9 354.0 503 847.2	$75.00
3/1/20XX	J1820	Inj, Insulin, Up to 100 Units	052.9 354.0 503 847.2	$20.00
3/1/20XX	99204	Office Visit	052.9 354.0 503 847.2	$65.00
4/1/20XX	70250	X-Ray, Hand, 2 Views	052.9 354.0 503 847.2	$55.00
4/1/20XX	36215	Lab Drawing Fee	052.9 354.0 503 847.2	$10.00
4/1/20XX	99231	Hospital Visit-Subseq. FFS	052.9 354.0 503 847.2	$80.00
5/1/20XX	99999	Follow-up Visit	052.0 344.0 501 847.2	$65.00
			TOTAL CHARGES:	**$470.00**

Insurance Payments

Date of Payment:	*Payment Code:*	*Line Description:*	*Transaction Description:*	*Amount*
2/1/20XX	XP	XYZ Insurance Payment	XYZ	($40.00)
2/1/20XX	XP	XYZ Insurance Payment	XYZ	($20.00)
2/1/20XX	XP	XYZ Insurance Payment	XYZ	($20.00)
2/1/20XX	XP	XYZ Insurance Payment	XYZ	($20.00)
2/1/20XX	XP	XYZ Insurance Payment	XYZ	($5.00)
4/1/20XX	MP	Medicare Payment	Medicare	$0.00
4/1/20XX	MP	Medicare Payment	Medicare	($20.00)
4/1/20XX	MP	Medicare Payment	Medicare	($35.00)
5/1/20XX	MP	Medicare Payment	Medicare	$0.00
			Total:	**($160.00)**

Insurance Adjustments

Date of Payment:	*Payment Code:*	*Line Description:*	*Transaction Description:*	*Amount*
5/1/20XX	MED ADJ	Medicare Writeoff	Adjustment	($10.00)
5/1/20XX	MED ADJ	Medicare Writeoff	Adjustment	($10.00)
5/1/20XX	MED ADJ	Medicare Writeoff	Adjustment	($8.00)
5/1/20XX	MED ADJ	Medicare Writeoff	Adjustment	($7.00)
5/1/20XX	MED ADJ	Medicare Writeoff	Adjustment	($8.00)
			Total:	**($43.00)**

Patient Payments

Date of Payment:	*Payment Code:*	*Payment Description:*	*Transaction Description:*	*Amount*
2/1/20XX	COCHECK	Copay Check Payment		($20.00)
3/1/20XX	CCARDCOP	Credit Card Copay		($20.00)
4/1/20XX	COPAYCASH	Cash Copayment		($20.00)
5/1/20XX	COPAY20	$20 Co-Payment		($20.00)
			Total:	**($80.00)**
			TOTAL PAYMENTS:	**($283.00)**
			Amount Due:	**$187.00**

Figure 16–3B: Another example of a patient ledger format. *Delmar/Cengage Learning.*

PRACTICE MANAGEMENT SOFTWARE SYSTEMS

Computerized practice management software (PMS) systems are most commonly used today in clinics and medical offices to record financial transactions. This software decreases errors and increases efficiency and speedy posting of procedures to patient accounts. It also enables minute-to-minute and up-to-date financial information related to patient accounts and procedures rendered.

Electronic health records software programs are available that link directly to the financial records of the practice management software. This software allows providers to enter precoded encounter data directly in the practice management software while working in the patient's electronic medical record in the exam room, by a simple point and click on each procedure and diagnosis.

In offices with practice management systems without added electronic health records software, encounter forms are still used. The checked-off procedures on the form are entered in the practice management software, which is built to perform all necessary calculations. Note that the coding of these procedures can occur at this time or at a later date; however, the sooner the coding, the quicker the turn-around time for billing and payment to the provider or medical facility. Overall, there are far fewer steps, calculations, and paperwork involved in using computerized methods when compared to the pegboard system.

PEGBOARD SYSTEM

The pegboard system uses an actual board as a base with pegs that attach the daysheet, the ledger, and the encounter form (Figure 16–4A–B). The daysheet holds all the daily entries, listing patients seen as well as a complete financial record of charges made and payments received. All amounts are calculated at the end of the day by adding each column and posting totals in the spaces provided.

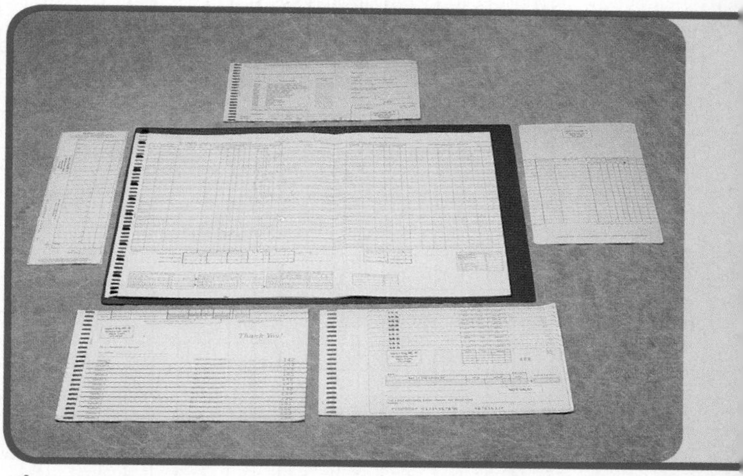

Figure 16–4A: The pegboard system. *Delmar/Cengage Learning.*

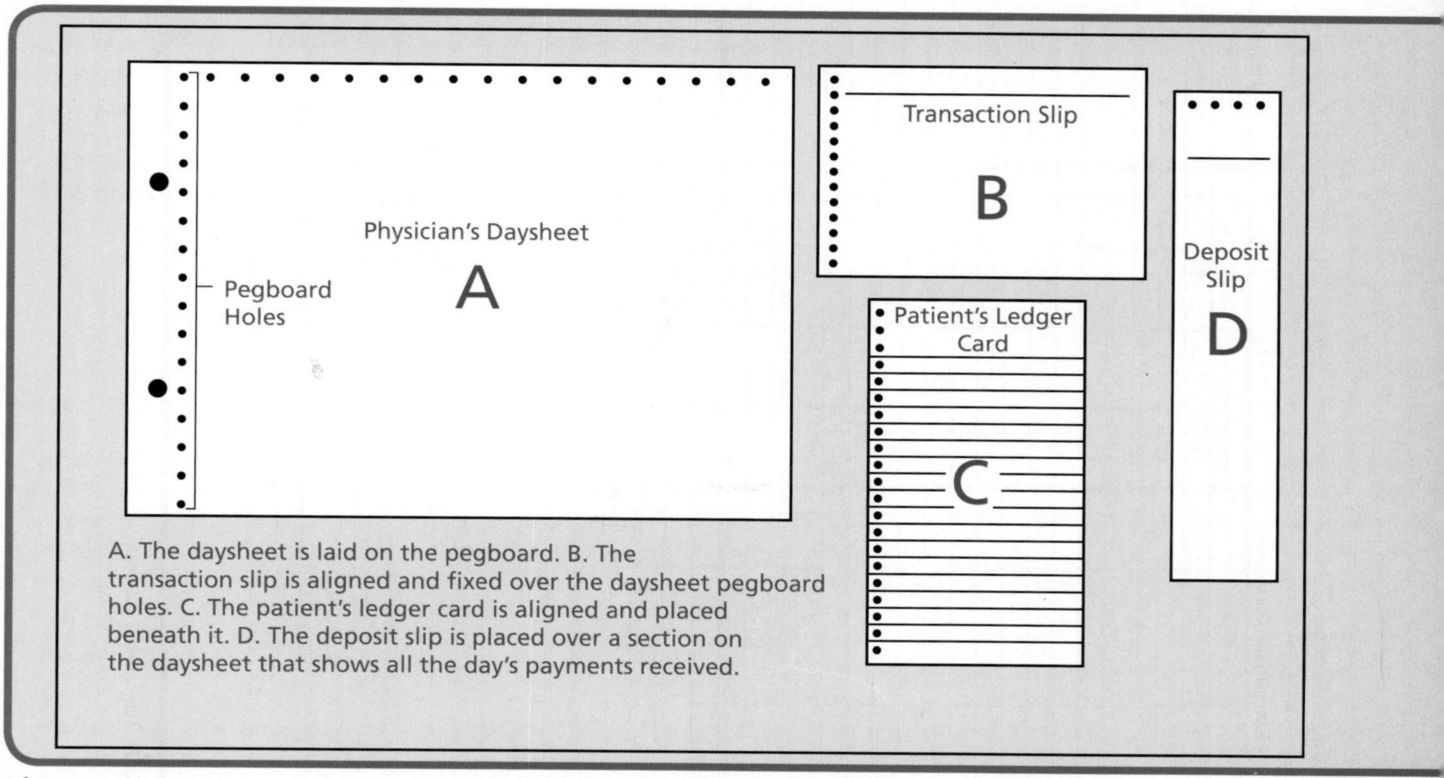
Physician's Daysheet
A
Pegboard Holes
Transaction Slip
B
Patient's Ledger Card
C
Deposit Slip
D
A. The daysheet is laid on the pegboard. B. The transaction slip is aligned and fixed over the daysheet pegboard holes. C. The patient's ledger card is aligned and placed beneath it. D. The deposit slip is placed over a section on the daysheet that shows all the day's payments received.

Figure 16–4B: Components of the pegboard system, illustrated. *Delmar/Cengage Learning.*

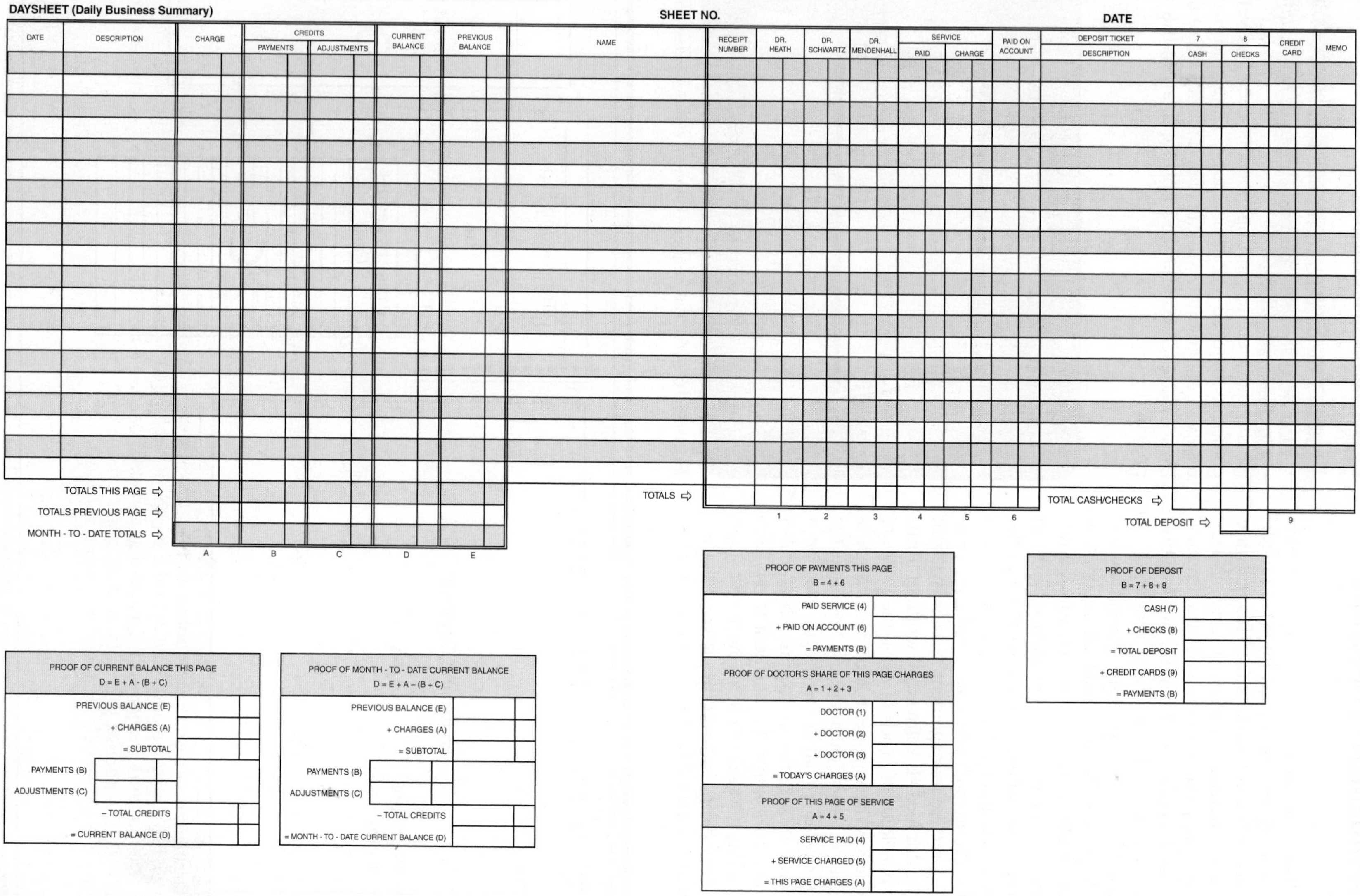

Figure 16–5: Example of a daysheet. *Delmar/Cengage Learning.*

When using the pegboard system, you must make clear, legible figures using a fine-point, black ink pen. Care must be taken to record figures in correct columns as debit or credit and always in straight columns. The decimal point must also be placed carefully and correctly; always double-check figures on a calculator or adding machine. An adding machine tape is helpful for double-checking figures easily.

This process was considered a simple way to have an up-to-date account of accounts receivable at all times. The total owed to the provider by all patients is increased by the day's charges and reduced by the day's receipts. The total of the receipts should be the amount of the bank deposit each day. This system, although felt to be very efficient, was also very time consuming and required several steps. Currently, many user-friendly and affordable software packages are available to replace the pegboard system.

Daysheet / Daily Journal / Daily log

If using a manual method, the charges or no-charge visits for each patient are recorded on the daysheet (Figure 16–5). If using the pegboard system, the patient ledger card is layered over the daysheet, and the entry is recorded on both the ledger card and the daysheet. Charges should be itemized, and a total should be put in the charge column. Payments should be placed in the credit (paid) column. Payment types should be noted in the paid column for ease of balancing the daysheet. Note the check or money order number, type of credit card used, or whether cash was paid. When a patient pays in any form, a receipt should be given so the patient has a record of the payment.

> **CLINICAL PEARL**
>
> A receipt must be given to the patient after a cash payment especially, and patients should be informed that it is not safe to pay accounts by mailing cash payments.

The daysheet will reflect the names of all patients treated in the office each day as well as record any payments received in the mail or from patients who come to the office just to pay the bill. Unassigned columns on the daysheet may be used to distribute charges or receipts among providers or to distribute charges by departments (such as laboratory, X-ray, or physical therapy) or by medication type (in cases such as chemotherapy).

When an entry is made on the daysheet, it is called **journalizing**. The entries should be kept in chronologic order. The total amount of cash and checks, including credit and debit card payments, should be recorded on a cash control sheet. This can be a daily record sheet or a monthly record showing an entire month with a line for each day to show income in cash and checks, any deposits made, and any amounts not deposited and therefore carried over to the next day.

When the balance is carried forward, it is important to record it under "previous balance" for the next day, where it will be added to the total received to calculate total on hand. This kind of record is also helpful in double-checking your bank deposit slips. The cash and checks should equal the amount shown on the cash control sheet (Figure 16–6). This amount should also equal the amount of the bank deposit for the day.

> **CLINICAL PEARL**
>
> Make sure you double-check your entries by proofreading for errors. Note that it is easy to transpose numbers as well as letters.

BOOKKEEPING AND ACCOUNTING SYSTEMS

An accounts receivable record should be kept daily. This record represents the total amount owed to the provider for services rendered. The total should be the same as the total of balances on all the active patient ledger records. The process of running such a total is called a **trial balance**. The accounts receivable balance is carried forward from month to month and added to the daily charges. The payments made by patients and any adjustments are subtracted to determine the true account receivable each day.

Cash Control Sheet

Day	Total Rec'd	Total Cash	Total Charges	Total Checks	Previous Balance	Total Available	Deposit	Balance Carried Forward
2	$2820.00	260.00	2820.00	2560.00	–0–	2820.00	2820.00	–0–
3	$ 600.00	–0–	600.00	600.00	–0–	600.00	–0–	500.00
4	$4750.00	650.00	4750.00	4100.00	500.00	6000.00	6000.00	–0–

Figure 16–6: Example of a cash control sheet. *Delmar/Cengage Learning.*

PROCEDURE 16–1 Record Charges and Credits

PURPOSE: Accurately record charges, payments, and adjustments on a patient ledger or computer accounting program

EQUIPMENT: Computerized system or pegboard system with ledger cards, daysheet, and black and red ink pens

S SKILL: Record charges, credits, and adjustments in a manual system.

Procedure Steps	Detailed Instructions and/or *Rationales*
1. Pull patient ledger card or pull up patient account on the computerized program.	
2. Post charges with descriptions. Add charges for a new total.	Charges are posted in the debit column. If a balance is shown on the patient ledger, add the new debit to get a new balance. *A computerized system will automatically calculate the totals.*
3. Post insurance payments with descriptions. Add payments for a new total.	If the credit is greater than the balance due, the difference is a credit balance and is shown in red.
4. Post insurance adjustments with descriptions. Add adjustments for a new total.	
5. Post patient payments with descriptions. Add payments for a new total.	
6. Post and calculate total charges.	
7. Post and calculate total payments.	
8. Post and calculate amount due.	The balance column should always reflect the current status of the account.
9. Check off each posted item on the encounter form.	

The single-entry method of bookkeeping records all increases and decreases in the **assets** of the practice. Assets are anything that holds value that is owned by a business. Examples of assets are accounts receivable, equipment, the building itself, and the land on which the building stands. In addition, accounts receivable and bank accounts are considered assets to a practice. The **single-entry bookkeeping system** in its most basic form is similar to a checkbook register. The journal for each transaction is recorded in one column, or on a single line, to account for either a positive or negative amount to demonstrate the receipt or disbursement of cash (Figure 16–7).

With the simple single-entry method, only the revenues and expenses are totaled, not individual values of each one. Knowing the individual amounts of revenues and expenses is important to a business. In this single-entry system example, the medical assistant can determine the revenue and expenses only by sorting each line

Date	Description	Amount
July 1	**Beginning Balance**	2,000.00
July 5	Purchased office supplies	(125.00)
July 15	Paid office rent	(1,000.00)
July 20	Patient payment (Harriet Ford – Account #56789)	100.00
July 31	**Ending Balance**	975.00

Figure 16–7: Single-entry bookkeeping system. *Delmar/Cengage Learning.*

Date	Description	Revenues	Expenses
July 5	Purchased office supplies		125.00
July 15	Paid office rent		1,000.00
July 20	Patient payment (Harriet Ford – Account #56789)	100.00	
July Totals		100.00	1,250.00

Figure 16–8: Separating revenues and expenses in the single-entry bookkeeping system. *Delmar/Cengage Learning.*

item and then calculating each total to get an ending balance. This process can be demonstrated more specifically still by using a single-entry system and including a separate column for revenues and expenses (Figure 16–8). Although this design involves more than one column or line, it is still considered a single-entry system because only one line records the cash amount transaction.

Even with columns that easily identify the revenues and expenses, single-entry bookkeeping has disadvantages:

- Asset and liability accounts (inventory, accounts receivable or accounts payable) are not tracked. These must be tracked separately in another system.
- There is no direct linkage between income and the balance sheet.
- Undetected errors can occur and might be discovered only through bank statement reconciliation.

These disadvantages make it impractical for many businesses, including medical offices. A more sophisticated method is the **double-entry bookkeeping system**. This system has two notable characteristics:

- Each transaction is recorded in two accounts.
- Each account has two columns.

In this system, two entries are made for each transaction; one entry as a debit in an account and one entry as a credit in another account. In a double-entry system, the transaction would be recorded as in Figure 16–9.

For each debit, there is an equal and opposite credit, and the total of all debits must equal the total of all credits. This method is useful in identifying errors in the process of recording transactions. Double-entry bookkeeping holds the following advantages over single-entry bookkeeping:

- Accurate calculation of profit and loss in complex businesses
- Inclusion of assets and liabilities in bookkeeping accounts
- Ability to prepare financial statements directly from the accounts
- Detection of errors and fraud are more visible

The double-entry method of bookkeeping is what most financial accounting is based upon and is the bookkeep-

Date	Description	Accounts	Debit	Credit
July 20	Patient payment (Harriet Ford – Account #3456789)	Cash	100.00	
		Revenue	100.00	
July 29	Patient Physical Exam, with no payment made, due in 30 days (Morgan, Olivia – Account #1121314)	Receivable	200.00	
		Revenue		200.00
July Totals			300.00	300.00

Figure 16–9: Double-entry bookkeeping system. *Delmar/Cengage Learning.*

ing system most often used in the large and busy medical setting. This system allows the office bookkeeper a better understanding of the medical facility's financial status.

CLINICAL PEARL

In the double entry bookkeeping system, the two entries allow for balance in the accounting equation:

Assets = Liabilities + Owner's Equity

This equation is introduced here but will be discussed in detail in Unit 9.

COMPUTERIZED ACCOUNTING SYSTEMS

Throughout this chapter, much mention has been made of the many available computerized accounting programs versus manual accounting systems. It is important to note that the concepts of bookkeeping are still used within a computerized system.

Advantages of Computerized Systems

- *Speed:* Formatted screens and built-in databases of patient accounts and vendors allow actions to be performed faster.
- *Efficiency:* Better use is made of resources and time; cash flow should improve through better debt collection and inventory control.
- *Automation:* Fast and accurate generation of accounting documents such as invoices, credit notes, statements of accounts, purchase orders, and even payroll documents can all be done automatically.

- *Calculations:* Account calculations are performed automatically for greater accuracy.
- *Accuracy:* Less room for errors exists because only one accounting entry is needed for each transaction rather than two or three with a manual system.
- *System integration:* Programs come with a computerized ledger system, which is fully integrated, so when a business transaction is entered, it is recorded or linked to a number of accounting records at the same time.
- *Concurrent information:* As information is entered in the system, the accounting records are automatically updated; therefore, account balances of patient or vendor accounts remain up-to-date.
- *Availability of information:* Information may be accessed almost instantly and made available to different users in different locations at the same time.
- *Management information:* Many types of useful reports can be produced, which helps management monitor and control the business by making wise decisions based on financial gains and losses. For example, the aging accounts will show which customer accounts are overdue.
- *Legibility:* The data input on a screen displays legible printed data and prevents errors that might be caused by poorly written numbers and documentation.
- *Staff motivation:* These systems require staff to be trained to use new skills, which can make them feel more motivated with their office abilities.
- *Reduction of frustration:* Management and providers can be on top of their accounts and thereby reducing stress levels associated with the financial unknowns.
- *Cost savings:* These programs reduce staff time in preparing accounts and audit expenses because records are neat, accurate, and up-to-date. Also, because there are so many programs to choose from, the cost to purchase a system has decreased over the years and has become more affordable for medical facilities, both large and small.

Disadvantages of Computerized Systems

- *Computer system problems:* Power failure, computer viruses, and hackers are possible problems when using computerized systems.
- *Garbage in, garbage out:* After data has been entered in the system, the output is automatically obtained; hence, the data being entered must be validated for accuracy and completeness.
- *Proper accounting system:* The accounting program must be properly set up to meet the requirements of the business; poorly programmed or inappropriate software or hardware or personnel problems can cause more problems.
- *Computer fraud:* Proper levels of control and security, both internal and external, must be instituted to prevent dangerous instances of Health Insurance Portability and Accountability Act (HIPAA) violations.

COMMUNICATING FEES TO PATIENTS

It is fairly common for the medical assistant to be the office member who answers the questions on patient accounts. If it appears that the patient will need to pay a substantial sum out of pocket, the medical assistant should discuss with the patient the manner in which payments will be made, prior to patient care. Even if patients have medical insurance, there could be a substantial amount their particular insurance company does not pay, or the co-pay is a sizable amount. Often, the costs accumulate over a long period of time, as with physical therapy, and the amount the patient owes can be quite significant.

When the patient knows in advance that there will be costly medical expenses, such as elective surgery, pregnancy, or extensive therapy, the medical assistant will be expected to review the patient's health insurance coverage. Some providers use a cost estimate sheet to give the patient an idea of the cost for surgery or long-term treatment (Figure 16–10). The estimate can include the approximate cost of the anesthesiology, any consultants, and hospital charges.

CLINICAL PEARL

It is important for the patient to understand that the anticipated costs provided on the estimate are just that—an *estimate*. In the event of unforeseen complications or additional problems, expenses are likely to be higher than the estimate. Covering this topic thoroughly prior to the care being provided allows the patient to understand financial responsibility and aids the medical assistant in future collection efforts. (Patient Collections is covered in Chapter 18.)

Assisting the patient in planning a reasonable payment schedule for these expenses helps the patient be more at ease and worry less about financial matters. The patient can concentrate on getting well. If the patient does not have current resources to pay the full amount in one payment, the medical assistant might offer the option of a fixed sum as a down payment and regular payments of a fixed amount on specified dates. *Remember, this all depends on office policy.*

If a patient is unhappy about medical costs, it is important to listen and try to explain why the charges are as stated. The provider should be told when a patient is unhappy with the cost of treatment because it might be necessary for the provider to talk with the patient about the concern regarding cost of care. However, in most instances, the provider will refer the patient to the medical assistant or the respective billing manager regarding cost and itemized billing.

SURGERY COST ESTIMATE

Catherine R. Lang
123-789-0123

Patient ______________________________ Date __________

Scheduled surgery time: ___________

At ______________________________ Hospital/Medical Center

On the day of your scheduled surgery you should arrive at _____ AM/PM and go to the _____ floor.

Check with your insurance company for the cost that you are expected to pay (your co-pay) unless your insurance covers the total cost. Plan for budgeting payments or coinsurance for this service.

For your information, in addition to the hospital costs for your surgery without complications, you will be charged for the following:

- Operating Surgeon _______________ $______ to $______
- Assisting Surgeon _______________ $______ to $______
- Anesthetist _______________ $______ to $______

The total cost of the surgery and related charges are based on the length of time for the procedure. Your costs also will vary with the procedure's complexity and length of time of your hospital stay. For the surgical procedure that you are having, the average length of stay in the hospital is ____ days. The hospital room charges depend on your preference of a semi-private or private room. Be sure to bring your insurance information with you the day of your surgery. You will be telephoned ahead of time by a hospital admissions clerk to discuss specific information and to give you a confirmed time for your surgery. This person may also ask you to come to the hospital a few days or a week before your surgery to do a series of blood tests and a preadmission exam.

If you have any questions or concerns, please call us at 999-123-4567

Figure 16–10: Example of a surgery cost estimate and information sheet. *Delmar/Cengage Learning.*

Discounts

Discounts are not as prevalent as in the past; however, they still do exist primarily for professional and significant financial hardship reasons. In all instances, the provider will notify you about these discounts for a particular patient. A professional discount is one that is authorized by the provider to discount fees to another medical professional, such as a nurse, medical assistant, another provider, or other healthcare providers. Also, when patients might have significant financial hardships, the provider can consider a discount. These discounts will vary in amounts, depending on the provider's decision. Do not take it into your own hands to provide discounts to a patient without the authorization of the provider or authorized financial management personnel.

CHAPTER SUMMARY

- Debit is a charge added to existing balance, whereas credit is a payment subtracted from existing balance.
- A daily journal or daysheet includes recordings of all patient charges and receipts.
- The daily log sheet reflects the names of all patients treated in the office each day and any payments received from them.
- The encounter form, also known as a charge slip, lists the procedures, with the respective codes, that are performed in a medical office on a given patient.
- The patient ledger is a record of all charges or services rendered, any payments made by the patient or the insurance carrier, and any adjustments, included with the specific dates of these entries.
- The pegboard system uses an actual board as a base with the use of pegs that attach the ledger, the daysheet, and the encounter form. A computerized system involves far fewer steps, calculations, and paperwork when compared to the pegboard system.
- The single-entry bookkeeping system in its most basic form is similar to a checkbook register, recorded in one column, or a single line, demonstrating the receipt or disbursement of cash.
- The double-entry bookkeeping system has two notable characteristics: Each transaction is recorded in two accounts, and each account has two columns.
- Advantages of a computerized accounting system include speed, efficiency, automation, system

integration, concurrent data, legibility, staff motivation, fewer accounting frustrations, and cost effectiveness.

- Disadvantages of a computerized accounting system include system problems and fraud; garbage in, garbage out theory; and potential for an improper and poorly programmed system.
- A cost estimate sheet gives the patient an idea of the cost for surgery or long-term treatment.
- Discounts are not as prevalent as in the past; however, they still exist primarily for professional and significant financial hardship reasons.

STUDY TOOLS

Workbook	Activities for Chapter 16
Premium Website StudyWARE	Activities and Quizzes on the **StudyWARE™ Software** for Chapter 16
	Complete the following **Competency Challenge 2.0** activity: • Monday, 11 AM, Perform Accounts Receivable Procedures
	Audio Library of medical terms
	Online access to the **Critical Thinking Challenge 2.0**
CourseMate	Activities and Quizzes for Chapter 16
WebTutor	Activities and Quizzes for Chapter 16

CHECK YOUR KNOWLEDGE

1. A(n) _________ records the financial transitions of a business; a(n) _________ analyzes these transactions and prepares current reports and comparison reports with other periods of time.
   a. daysheet; accountant
   b. daysheet; bookkeeper
   c. accountant; bookkeeper
   d. bookkeeper; accountant
2. In which of the following bookkeeping systems are all necessary forms generated with one posting?
   a. Single-entry
   b. Double-entry
   c. Pegboard
   d. Standard
3. This is a record of all charges or services rendered, any payments made by the patient or the insurance carrier, and any adjustments; it is:
   a. a daysheet.
   b. a patient ledger.
   c. accounts receivable.
   d. a credit balance.
4. When an entry is made on the daysheet, it is called:
   a. journalizing.
   b. journaling.
   c. posting.
   d. accounting.
5. An encounter form is also known as a:
   a. cost estimate sheet.
   b. patient ledger.
   c. business associate agreement.
   d. charge slip.
6. For each debit, there is an equal and opposite credit, and the total of all debits must equal the total of all credits. This describes which bookkeeping system?
   a. Single-entry bookkeeping
   b. Double-entry bookkeeping
   c. Computerized bookkeeping
   d. Trial balance bookkeeping

WEB LINKS

American Academy of Medical Management: www.epracticemanagement.org

Bankers Training and Consulting Company: www.btcc.com

Chapter 17

Preparing Insurance Claims and Posting Insurance Payments

OBJECTIVES

In this chapter, you will learn the following:

KB KNOWLEDGE BASE

1. Spell and define, using the glossary at the back of the text, all the Words to Know in this chapter.
2. Understand the history of claim forms.
3. List five common errors made when filing claims.
4. Describe the differences between filing electronic claims and filing paper claims.
5. Explain the role of a clearinghouse.
6. Describe the differences between manual and electronic claims tracking.
7. Name four pieces of information to have before calling to follow up on a delinquent insurance claim.
8. List five pieces of information contained in an explanation of benefits form.
9. Explain the purpose of a remittance advice form.
10. Describe the process of billing a secondary insurance company.

S SKILLS

1. Accurately complete a CMS-1500 claim form.
2. Accurately apply insurance payments and adjustments to patient accounts.

WORDS TO KNOW

Administrative Simplification Compliance Act (ASCA)
carrier
Centers for Medicare and Medicaid Services (CMS)
clearinghouse
CMS-1500 form
electronic claims tracking (ECT)
electronic data interchange (EDI)
electronic media claims (EMC)
Explanation of Benefits (EOB)
national provider identifier (NPI)
reimbursement
secondary insurance
third-party reimbursement

THE HISTORY OF CLAIMS

The preparation of claims for the purpose of **reimbursement** for medical services is a fairly recent development when considering the history of health care. For centuries, providers were paid directly by patients with some form of money, bartered goods, or exchange of services. With industrialization and the advancement of medicine, medicine has evolved into a very sophisticated science.

The phrase **third-party reimbursement** was coined to indicate payment of services rendered by someone other than the patient. With this came the need for some form of paperwork as the means of reporting the health care provided to the source of payment, and the claim form was developed. Today, the most common third-party reimbursers are federal and state agencies, insurance companies, and workers' compensation (see Chapter 14).

Since 2005, providers have been urged to send claims electronically, in compliance with HIPAA, to receive their payment reimbursement. In the past, patients would give the provider forms obtained from their employer's benefits office for their insurance coverage. The patient completed his or her portion of the form and either signed or did not sign the section that authorized payment for services to be made directly to the provider. If it was not signed, the patient paid the charges, and then the insurance company sent the payment to the patient. It was customary for providers to charge a small fee to complete forms after the first one was done. Patients often had multiple coverages and could even make money with covered conditions. Medical findings, diagnoses, and treatments were described verbally in medical terminology, and fees were paid as requested if they were reasonable.

COMPLETING THE CLAIM FORM

Today, and in most instances, a **CMS-1500 form**, shown in Figure 17–1, is completed and filed by the medical office for reimbursement; see Procedure 17–1. The CMS-1500 form is the standard claim form for billing in medical offices and is accepted by the Medicare and Medicaid systems as well as by most other health insurance groups for provider reimbursement.

Computerized insurance claims can greatly improve cash flow and efficiency; a claim can be completed in a matter of seconds for every patient visit. Prior to sending any claims to a third party to acquire reimbursement, be certain that you have a copy of the patient's insurance card and have secured his or her signature on a form to permit release of information and then file the claim on the patient's behalf. This is known as *signature on file*. It is a good idea to get the patient's signature annually for filing purposes. You should retain the paperwork containing the signature in the patient's medical record.

This form also has an *assignment of benefits* clause that authorizes benefits to be paid directly to the provider. Obtaining the appropriate signatures for releasing patient information to any third-party payer should be a priority when the patient completes his or her initial new-patient information paperwork. The form should be signed and dated by the patient.

EXAMPLE

The paperwork could include a statement similar to the following:

I request payment of authorized Medicare benefits to be made on my behalf to Dr. ____________ for any service furnished to me by that provider. I authorize release of medical information about me needed to determine these benefits or benefits payable for related services.

Common Claim Errors

When claim form errors are identified by the third-party payers, the claim is then rejected with a request sent to the medical facility to resubmit with corrections. This rejection and resubmission causes delay in payment to the doctor or medical facility. In a survey of insurance companies, the following common errors were listed as causes of claim payment delays:

1. The patient's—not the policy holder's—Social Security number or identification number used as the insurance plan ID number. The claim would be rejected for lack of membership in the insurance plan.
2. The Coordination of Benefits section not completed. This would suspend the claim for additional information.
3. Use of incorrect ICD codes or ICD codes that are incongruent with the CPT codes.
4. Use of incorrect or outdated CPT codes. This could result in a decreased payment or a rejection.
5. Use of an incorrect **national provider identifier (NPI)**. This could result in misdirection of payment.

CLINICAL PEARL

NPI is the acronym for national provider identifier, a unique 10-digit number identification for covered health care providers. Covered health care providers and all health plans and health care clearinghouses must use the NPIs in the administrative and financial transactions (including the CMS-1500 form) adopted under HIPAA.

Certain type of providers will not have an NPI number. Another type of identifying number might be required. The shaded area in Box 24J of the CMS-1500 claim form is provided to report this number.

1500

HEALTH INSURANCE CLAIM FORM

APPROVED BY NATIONAL UNIFORM CLAIM COMMITTEE 08/05

PICA | PICA

CARRIER

1. MEDICARE (Medicare #) | MEDICAID (Medicaid #) | TRICARE CHAMPUS (Sponsor's SSN) | CHAMPVA (Member ID#) | GROUP HEALTH PLAN (SSN or ID) | FECA BLK LUNG (SSN) | OTHER (ID)

1a. INSURED'S I.D. NUMBER (For Program in Item 1)

2. PATIENT'S NAME (Last Name, First Name, Middle Initial)

3. PATIENT'S BIRTH DATE MM DD YY SEX M F

4. INSURED'S NAME (Last Name, First Name, Middle Initial)

5. PATIENT'S ADDRESS (No., Street)

6. PATIENT RELATIONSHIP TO INSURED Self Spouse Child Other

7. INSURED'S ADDRESS (No., Street)

CITY STATE

8. PATIENT STATUS Single Married Other

CITY STATE

ZIP CODE TELEPHONE (Include Area Code) ( )

Employed Full-Time Student Part-Time Student

ZIP CODE TELEPHONE (Include Area Code) ( )

9. OTHER INSURED'S NAME (Last Name, First Name, Middle Initial)

10. IS PATIENT'S CONDITION RELATED TO:

11. INSURED'S POLICY GROUP OR FECA NUMBER

a. OTHER INSURED'S POLICY OR GROUP NUMBER

a. EMPLOYMENT? (Current or Previous) YES NO

a. INSURED'S DATE OF BIRTH MM DD YY SEX M F

b. OTHER INSURED'S DATE OF BIRTH MM DD YY SEX M F

b. AUTO ACCIDENT? YES NO PLACE (State)

b. EMPLOYER'S NAME OR SCHOOL NAME

c. EMPLOYER'S NAME OR SCHOOL NAME

c. OTHER ACCIDENT? YES NO

c. INSURANCE PLAN NAME OR PROGRAM NAME

d. INSURANCE PLAN NAME OR PROGRAM NAME

10d. RESERVED FOR LOCAL USE

d. IS THERE ANOTHER HEALTH BENEFIT PLAN? YES NO *If yes*, return to and complete item 9 a-d.

READ BACK OF FORM BEFORE COMPLETING & SIGNING THIS FORM.

12. PATIENT'S OR AUTHORIZED PERSON'S SIGNATURE I authorize the release of any medical or other information necessary to process this claim. I also request payment of government benefits either to myself or to the party who accepts assignment below.

SIGNED ______ DATE ______

13. INSURED'S OR AUTHORIZED PERSON'S SIGNATURE I authorize payment of medical benefits to the undersigned physician or supplier for services described below.

SIGNED ______

PATIENT AND INSURED INFORMATION

14. DATE OF CURRENT: MM DD YY ◀ ILLNESS (First symptom) OR INJURY (Accident) OR PREGNANCY(LMP)

15. IF PATIENT HAS HAD SAME OR SIMILAR ILLNESS. GIVE FIRST DATE MM DD YY

16. DATES PATIENT UNABLE TO WORK IN CURRENT OCCUPATION FROM MM DD YY TO MM DD YY

17. NAME OF REFERRING PROVIDER OR OTHER SOURCE

17a.

17b. NPI

18. HOSPITALIZATION DATES RELATED TO CURRENT SERVICES FROM MM DD YY TO MM DD YY

19. RESERVED FOR LOCAL USE

20. OUTSIDE LAB? YES NO $ CHARGES

21. DIAGNOSIS OR NATURE OF ILLNESS OR INJURY (Relate Items 1, 2, 3 or 4 to Item 24E by Line)

1. ___ . ___ 3. ___ . ___

2. ___ . ___ 4. ___ . ___

22. MEDICAID RESUBMISSION CODE ORIGINAL REF. NO.

23. PRIOR AUTHORIZATION NUMBER

24. A. DATE(S) OF SERVICE From MM DD YY	To MM DD YY	B. PLACE OF SERVICE	C. EMG	D. PROCEDURES, SERVICES, OR SUPPLIES (Explain Unusual Circumstances) CPT/HCPCS	MODIFIER	E. DIAGNOSIS POINTER	F. $ CHARGES	G. DAYS OR UNITS	H. EPSDT Family Plan	I. ID. QUAL.	J. RENDERING PROVIDER ID. #
1										NPI	
2										NPI	
3										NPI	
4										NPI	
5										NPI	
6										NPI	

25. FEDERAL TAX I.D. NUMBER SSN EIN

26. PATIENT'S ACCOUNT NO.

27. ACCEPT ASSIGNMENT? (For govt. claims, see back) YES NO

28. TOTAL CHARGE $

29. AMOUNT PAID $

30. BALANCE DUE $

31. SIGNATURE OF PHYSICIAN OR SUPPLIER INCLUDING DEGREES OR CREDENTIALS (I certify that the statements on the reverse apply to this bill and are made a part thereof.)

SIGNED DATE

32. SERVICE FACILITY LOCATION INFORMATION

a. NPI b.

33. BILLING PROVIDER INFO & PH # ( )

a. NPI b.

PHYSICIAN OR SUPPLIER INFORMATION

NUCC Instruction Manual available at: www.nucc.org

APPROVED OMB-0938-0999 FORM CMS-1500 (08/05)

Figure 17-1: Health insurance claim form, CMS-1500. *Centers for Medicare and Medicaid Services.*

6. Superbills attached to a claim form sometimes illegible. This error is less common today because most claims are submitted electronically.
7. Lack of operative report if procedure is unusual or complicated or fee is unusual.
8. Incorrect spelling of patient's name.
9. Inconsistent use of patient's name; for example, the middle name is used as first name; nicknames are used instead of correct first name (i.e., Bill instead of William).
10. Incorrect patient birthdate.
11. Incorrect place of service code.

PROCEDURE 17–1 Complete a Claim Form

PURPOSE: Accurately complete a claim form for processing

EQUIPMENT: CMS-1500 form, patient record, account ledger or information, computer, and software

S SKILL: Complete an approved claim form without error.

Procedure Steps	Detailed Instructions and/or *Rationales*
1. Check for a photocopy of the patient's insurance card.	
2. Check the chart to see whether the patient signature is on file for release of information and assignment of benefits.	If one is not on file, the patient must sign the form before the claim form is completed and submitted to the third-party payer.
3. Correctly complete boxes 1 to 3. **(The remaining steps of the procedure correspond to the box numbers on the CMS-1500 form.)**	Box 1: Check the appropriate box. Box 2: Enter the patient's name, ensuring that the name used on the form is the same as that on the identification card. Box 3: Enter the date of birth, using eight digits to write the date (e.g., 08/23/1961).
4. Enter the insured's name.	
5. Enter the patient's full address and telephone number.	
6. Enter the patient's relationship to the insured.	
7. Enter the insured's full address and telephone number.	
8. Enter the patient's status.	
9. Enter the other insured's name and necessary information.	• Other insured's policy or group number • Other insured's birthdate and check box for male or female • Employer's name or school name • Insurance plan name or program name • Fill in None or N/A, for not applicable, so there is no doubt that you have observed this section.
10. Check the appropriate box regarding employment and accident.	Do not leave any of these boxes blank.
11. Enter the insured's policy number and other necessary information.	• Insured's birthdate and check box for male or female • Employer or school name • Insurance plan name or program name • Is there another health benefit plan?
12. Obtain the patient's or authorized person's signature.	

Procedure Steps	Detailed Instructions and/or *Rationales*
13. Obtain the insured's signature or stamp "signature on file" if you have the record to prove it.	
14. Record the date the current illness began.	
15. Record the date the patient was first treated for the same or similar illness.	
16. Enter the dates the patient is unable to work or leave blank.	
17. Complete with the name of the referring provider or leave blank.	17a. Enter the non-NPI number of the referring provider. 17b. Insert the NPI number of the referring provider.
18. Complete with dates of hospitalization or leave blank.	
19. Leave blank.	
20. Mark the appropriate box regarding lab services.	
21. Enter an ICD code on a separate line for each diagnosis.	
22. Complete if for Medicaid.	
23. Complete if applicable with medical authorization code.	
24. Complete A through H with appropriate CPT or HCPCS codes for services.	List each service separately, with the most important listed first. 24a. Enter the rendering provider's non-NPI (legacy) number in the shaded area. Enter the provider's NPI number in the unshaded area.
25. Add the provider's federal tax ID number: Social Security number or practice tax identification number and mark the appropriate box.	
26. Add the patient's account number if applicable.	
27. Check one box regarding assignment.	This must be marked Yes to accept assignment.
28. Enter the total charged.	
29. Enter the amount paid.	
30. Enter any balance due.	The form will be rejected if this is not completed.
31. Obtain provider's signature and date.	Medicare *will* accept a stamped signature. All carriers will accept providers' typed name and credentials as indication of their signature.
32. Enter the name and address of the facility where services were rendered if other than home or office.	32a. Enter the NPI number of the facility. 32b. Enter the non-NPI number of the facility.
33. Enter the provider's name, address, and telephone number.	Do not use punctuation in the address. If you supply a nine-digit ZIP code, it is acceptable to use a hyphen to separate the last four digits. 33a. Enter the NPI number of the provider. 33b. Enter the non-NPI number of the provider.

FILING CLAIMS

Filing Claims Electronically

Many offices electronically process claim forms to the insurance **carrier**. The turnaround time is shortened, and preparation time is reduced for the claims processor responsible for filing claims. Your system must have the software required for filing claims electronically. An **electronic data interchange (EDI)** must be in place. Use of EDI transactions allow a medical facility or a provider's office to submit transactions faster and therefore be paid for claims faster while accomplishing this at a lower cost than is generally the case for paper or manual transactions.

The **Centers for Medicare and Medicaid Services (CMS)** standard electronic data interchange (EDI) enrollment form must be completed prior to submitting **electronic media claims (EMC)** or other EDI transactions to Medicare. The agreement must be executed by each provider of health care services or supplier that intends to submit EMC or use EDI, either directly with Medicare or through a billing service or clearinghouse.

Filing Paper Claims

Although claims are most often submitted electronically, there are limited situations when paper claim forms may be submitted for payment, and there are specific reasons the provider must meet to do this and receive CMS payment. These specifications are set forth by the **Administrative Simplification Compliance Act (ASCA)**. The reasons are quite detailed and require the provider to file in writing a *waiver* proving the provider qualifies for the ASCA requirement for electronic submission of claims. When approved, the institutional provider may submit a paper claim form, the CMS-1450 form (also known as the UB-40 form). The noninstitutional provider under a waiver may use the CMS-1500 form as a paper claim form when submitting for payment to CMS.

Clearinghouses

A **clearinghouse** is a private or public company that often serves as the middleman between providers and billing groups, payers and other health care partners for the transmission and translation of electronic claims information into the specific format required by payers.

Typically, a program is run on your system to flag claims that need to be billed to the carriers. The clearinghouse provides a downloadable claim form for filing claims. The claims processor completes the entries for each claim. The claims are put into batches, and the batches are sent electronically to a clearinghouse. The clearinghouse runs a claims scrubber on all the claims to check for missing or invalid data by sorting, formatting, and translating the information into the standard format. Clean claims are forwarded to the appropriate payer for processing. Any claims that are not clean are returned through a status report. These claims must be reviewed, and any errors must be corrected to be resubmitted.

Clearinghouses generally charge the providers for their services, with fees that might include a start-up fee, a monthly flat fee, or a per-claim transaction fee based on volume. The cost of the service is considered money well spent because the claims are clean when submitted, and reimbursement is received within a few weeks' time.

CLAIMS TRACKING

A method for monitoring the status and payment of insurance claims should be established, either by a manual or an electronic system. It is easy to forget about filed claims, and soon, a huge amount of money is owed to the provider. Tracking the following is helpful in monitoring claim status.

- The date the claim is filed
- The insurance company's name
- The patient's name
- The amount of the claim
- The amount paid
- The secondary company's name
- The date filed
- The amount billed
- The amount paid
- The date the patient was billed
- The follow-up date

Electronic Claims Tracking

Today, most offices use computer software designed for monitoring insurance claims. The information can be entered electronically and brought up on the screen for review or printed out so it is possible to see the total file at once.

There are numerous **electronic claims tracking (ECT)** systems to choose from that best suit your office size and needs. The ECT system allows you to know at your fingertips the status of a claim or group of claims. These systems allow the claims processor to search any claim sent and ensure quickly that it was properly received by the insurance payer. In addition, with adoption of the Functional Acknowledgment (an ASCA standard), every EDI-capable and HIPAA-compliant provider will be informed when electronically transmitted claims are received by the payer.

Advantages of ECT features usually include the following:

- Payment is quicker, with claims usually received by a payer within 24 hours.
- Claims can be entered from anywhere with Internet access with real-time response.

- Claims can be tracked online by using quick search options to check for current status receipt and provide rejection reports.
- Reduction of lost time with 24-hour rolling claims problem alerts.
- Results can be viewed easily on a computer screen and information printed as needed.
- Follow-up time and phone calls to track unpaid claims are greatly reduced.
- Office cost is reduced by eliminating the need for stamps, forms, and excess office staff labor.

Manual Claims Tracking

Although not commonly used today, some practices use a manual insurance log (a book in which a list of insurance claims is kept). When a claim is filed, it is noted on a log. The log should have columns for recording pertinent information.

Manual claims tracking is a time-consuming process that frequently causes payment delays. With manual claims processing, payers typically do not inform providers of the status of their claims, requiring office collection staff to perform the extra task of making phone calls to key payers to determine whether claims are being processed. Seldom does an office have enough staff to phone all payers and track all claims. With this system, providers can face a lengthy collection period with considerable cash tied up in accounts receivable.

Delinquent Claims

If a claim has not been paid within the appropriate time period, and you have not received a denial, it is time to follow up.

CLINICAL PEARL

Follow up on electronically submitted claims three weeks after submission; follow up on paper claims six weeks after submission.

Most carriers provide a toll-free number on the insurance card provided to the patient. Before you make the call, be sure you have the following information available:

- Your practice's tax identification number
- The patient's name, identification number, and group name or number
- If the patient *is not* the insured, the insured's (e.g., spouse's) name

After the account is identified, the carrier will request the dates of service and the total amount submitted. The carrier will then give you the status of the claim. If it is still in process, request an anticipated date of payment. If the claim is delayed pending additional information, be sure to follow up quickly and return the material requested. If the company has no record of receiving a claim, ask whether you may submit a *copy* of the claim previously submitted and verify the mailing address. Also ask whether you could direct the claim to a specific person to accelerate the process. It is helpful to have a specific contact person in case further discussion is necessary.

If the claim is close to the filing statute date, inquire about faxing the claim. If the carrier indicates that the claim has been paid, ask when the payment was made and to whom it was sent. If it was sent to the patient, you must send the patient a statement.

INSURANCE PAYMENTS

Insurance payments involve several pieces to take into consideration by the responsible staff members. **Explanation of benefits (EOB)** and remittance advice forms are two important forms to become familiar with concerning insurance payments. In addition, posting adjustments and insurance payments are two vital actions of importance when working with patient accounts.

Explanation of Benefits Document

An explanation of benefits (EOB) form or document might be sent to the patient by his or her insurance company several months after he or she has had a health care service that was paid by the insurance company (Figure 17–2). The patient should receive an EOB if he or she has private health insurance, a health plan from his or her employer, or Medicare. These may be either mailed to the home or sent to by email. An EOB provides the patient with information about how an insurance claim from a health provider (such as a doctor or hospital) was paid on his or her behalf.

A typical EOB contains the following information:

- *Patient:* The name of the person who received the service. This can be the patient or one of his or her dependents.
- *Insured ID number:* The identification number assigned to the patient by his or her insurance company. This should match the number on the patient's insurance card.
- *Claim number:* The number that identifies or refers to the claim that either the patient or his or her health provider submitted to the insurance company. Along with the patient's insurance ID number, the patient will need this claim number if he or she has any questions about the health plan.
- *Provider:* The name of the provider who performed the services for the patient or his or her dependent. This might be the name of a doctor, a laboratory, a hospital, or other health care provider.

DATE OF FORM	DATE OF SERVICE	SOURCE OF FORM	PROVIDER OF SERVICE	SERVICE PROVIDED—CODE	CHARGE	MEDICARE APPROVED	MEDICARE PAID	SECONDARY INSURANCE PAID	PATIENT RESPONSIBILITY	COMMENTS
2005										
10/9	9/27	Medicare	Radiologist #1	Mammogram—7609L XA Both Breasts	$135.00	$65.91	-0-	-0-	$65.91	$65.91 applied to '05 deductible
11/2	10/3	Medicare	Surgeon	Office Consult—99242	$105.00	$89.56	$36.38	-0-	$53.18	$44.09 applied to '05 deductible
11/10	10/11	Medicare	Primary physician	Office Consult—99243 ECG—93000 Chest x-ray—71020-XA Blood draw—36415	$130.00 54.00 69.00 7.00 $260.00	$119.40 25.68 34.71 3.00 $182.79	$95.52 20.55 27.77 2.40 $146.24	-0- -0- -0- -0-		$36.55 to be billed to insurance
11/30	10/17	Medicare	Radiologist #2	Place needlewire—19290 X-ray needlewire placement in breast—76096-26 X-ray specimen—76098-26	$275.00 140.00 22.00 $437.00	$152.40 28.73 8.21 $189.34	$121.92 22.99 6.57 $151.48	-0- -0- -0-	$30.48 $5.74 $1.64 $37.86	
11/30	10/17	Medicare	Surgeon	Excision breast lesion—19125	$800.00	$428.42	$342.74	-0-		$85.68 to be billed to insurance
11/20	10/17	Medicare	Anesthesia #1	4.3 Anesthesia—00400 Chest skin surgery QKQS	$350.40	-0-	-0-	-0-	-0-	Requested information had not been received.
11/20	10/17	Medicare	Pathologist	1 Tissue exam—88305-26 1 Tissue exam—88307-26 1 Consult in surgery—88329	$165.00 230.00 70.00 $465.00	$41.26 86.65 49.61 $177.52	$41.26 86.65 49.61 $177.52	-0- -0- -0-	-0- -0- -0-	Lab services are paid at 100% of the Medicare allowable. Patient does not owe any copay or coinsureace on lab work.
11/20	10/17	Medicare	Anesthesia #2	4.3 Anesthesia—00400 Chest skin surgery QKQS	$111.25	-0-	-0-	-0-	$111.25	Charges denied, other insurance may pay.
11/20	10/17	Insurance	Surgeon	Procedure—excision				$68.55	$17.13	Insurance paid 80% of $68.55
12/2	10/11	Insurance	Prmy Phys	Medical x-ray, testing	$260.00			$29.24	$7.31	Insurance paid 80% of $36.55
12/14	10/3	Insurance	Surgeon	Medical	$105.00	$89.56	$36.38	$42.55	$10.63	Insurance paid 80% of $53.18
12/15	10/17	Medicare	Hospital	Laboratory Radiology Pharmacy Surgical service	$155.00 399.00 182.88 2,317.92 $3,054.80	$1,527.40	$916.44	-0-	$610.96	Deductible met.
2006 1/5	10/3 and 10/17	Statement	Surgeon	Balance after insurance payments		—	—		$24.44	Pt bal after Medicare and insur.
1/16	10/11	Statement	Prmy Phys	Balance after insurance payments					$7.31	Pt bal after Medicare and insur.
1/27	10/17	Insurance	Hospital	Surgical services	$3,054.80	$1,527.40	$916.44	$610.96	-0-	Paid in full by insurance.
1/26	10/17	Insurance	Radiologist #2	X-ray services balance after insurance payments	$437.00	$189.34	$151.48	$30.29	$7.57	
2/12	10/17	Statement	Radiologist #2	X-ray services balance after insurance payments	$437.00	$189.34	$151.48		$7.57	Remaining balance due.

Figure 17-2: Summary of insurance Explanation of Benefits (EOB) form and medical expenses received in connection with one routine breast incisional biopsy procedure.

Delmar/Cengage Learning.

- *Type of service:* A code and brief description of the health-related service the patient received from the provider.
- *Date of service:* The beginning and end dates of the health-related service the patient received from the provider. If the claim is for a doctor visit, the beginning and end dates will be the same.
- *Charge* (also known as *billed charges*): The amount the patient provider billed the patient's insurance company for the service.
- *Not covered amount:* The amount of money the patient's insurance company did not pay the provider. Next to this amount might be a code that gives the reason the doctor was not paid a certain amount. A descriptions of these codes are usually found at the bottom of the EOB, on the back of the EOB, or in a note attached to the EOB.
- *Total patient cost:* The amount of money the patient owes as his or her share of the bill. This amount depends on the health plan's out-of-pocket requirements, such as an annual deductible, copayments, and coinsurance. Also, the patient might have received a service that is not covered by his or her health plan, in which case, the patient is responsible for paying the full amount.

Additional information might include the amount of payment actually made to the patient's provider and how much of the patient's annual deductible has been met.

Remittance Advice

The Remittance Advice form, and FCC Form 159-C (Continuation Sheet), is a multipurpose form that must accompany any payment to the Federal Communications Commission. The information on this form is collected to ensure credit for full payment, to ensure that the patient receives any refunds due, to service public inquiries, and to comply with the Debt Collection Improvement Act of 1996. This form can be found online as an electronic version for downloading and use by your provider's office.

INSURANCE PAYMENTS

Posting insurance payments includes applying insurance payments as well as insurance adjustments to patient accounts. This type of posting is just as vital as posting patient payments. All information is expected to be entered accurately by the data enterer of the medical office. Correct data entry provides accurate financial records for the medical facility and maintains business viability.

Applying insurance payments and adjustments to patient accounts are most commonly done with the use of a computerized system; see Procedure 17–2. The information required to post on the patient account includes the following:

- Date of the insurance payment or adjustment
- Insurance payment or adjustment amount
- Check number of the insurance payment or adjustment
- Name of the insurance company sending the payment or adjustment

PROCEDURE 17–2 Apply Insurance Payments and Adjustments to Patient Accounts

PURPOSE: Accurately record payments and adjustments on patient ledgers (accounts) or enter this information in a computerized system

EQUIPMENT: Ledger card (account), checks received, black and red ink pens, or a computer system

S SKILL: Record payments and adjustments to patient accounts.

Procedure Steps	Detailed Instructions and/or *Rationales*
1. Pull the patient ledger or pull up the patient account from the computerized accounting program.	
2. Post the amount of the insurance payment in the credit column.	Place the payment in parentheses ( ).
3. Post the amount of the insurance adjustment in the credit column.	Place the adjustment in parentheses ( ).

(continues)

(continued)

Procedure Steps	Detailed Instructions and/or *Rationales*
4. Note on the patient ledger or within the computerized program the name of the insurance company making the payment and adjustment.	
5. Note on the patient ledger or within the computerized program the date the insurance payment and adjustment are processed.	
6. Note on the patient ledger or within the computerized program the check number of each insurance payment and adjustment processed.	
7. Check that the balance reflects the current status of the account..	
8. Check all entries for accuracy and compare the amount of the checks with the amount of the payment and adjustment indicated on the patient ledger (account) or computerized program.	
9. Make a photocopy of the checks for the accounts receivable record.	
10. Return the ledger (account) to the file or save and close the account on the computerized program.	

BILLING SECONDARY INSURANCE

Secondary insurance coverage is more common today because most households now have two income earners and, likely, insurance coverage by each of their respective employments. Billing a secondary insurance company is fairly similar to billing a primary insurance company, as discussed in the previous unit. After payment is received from the primary insurance, you must create a new bill with the secondary insurance information.

CLINICAL PEARL

The primary insurance information will be placed in block 9 of the CMS-1500 form for secondary billing.

This new claim should have a copy of the EOB from the primary carrier attached and then be sent to the patient's secondary insurance company. The EOB form explains what the primary insurance company covered and what remains for the secondary insurance company to pay for the patient. At this point, the secondary insurance carrier will review the balance unpaid by the primary group to determine what it is required to pay.

In many instances, secondary insurance will pay most, if not all, of the balance left over from the primary insurance to your provider and will leave little out-of-pocket expenses for the patient. This type of dual insurance coverage makes it financially easier for a patient to follow through with medical treatment plans, with less worry about the cost of treatment when making medical choices.

CHAPTER SUMMARY

- The preparation of claims for the purpose of receiving payment for medical services is a fairly recent development when considering the history of health care.
- The CMS-1500 form is the standard claim form for billing and accepted by the Medicare and Medicaid systems as well as by most other health insurance groups.
- Electronic claims filing involves the following:
  - Electronic data interchange (EDI) with completion of an EDI enrollment form.
  - Submission of electronic media claims (EMC).
- Paper claims filing involves the following:
  - In limited situations, paper claim forms may be submitted for payment
  - Specifications are set forth by the Administrative Simplification Compliance Act (ASCA), providing reasons a provider must meet to file paper claims.
  - A provider must file in writing a waiver proving the site qualifies for an ASCA requirement and then must obtain ASCA approval.
- A clearinghouse is a private or public company that often serves as the middleman between providers and billing groups, payers, and other health care partners for the transmission and translation of electronic claims information into the specific format required by payers.
- Electronic claims tracking is the method of choice over the manual claims tracking system because it is more efficient and less time consuming for the office claims processor.
- Delinquent claims are those claims that have been electronically submitted without payment in three weeks after submission, six weeks for a paper claim, without a received denial.
- An explanation of benefits (EOB) is a form or document that provides the patient with information about how an insurance claim from a health provider was paid on his or her behalf.
- The Remittance Advice form is a multipurpose form that must accompany any payment to the Federal Communications Commission. The information on this form is collected to ensure credit for full payment, to ensure that the patient receives any refunds due, to service public inquiries, and to comply with the Debt Collection Improvement Act of 1996.
- Applying insurance payments and adjustments to patient accounts is most commonly done with a computerized system.
- Billing a secondary insurance company is fairly similar to billing a primary insurance company. The secondary insurance will pay most, if not all, the balance left over from the primary insurance to the provider and will leave little out-of-pocket expenses for the patient.

STUDY TOOLS

Workbook	Activities for Chapter 17
Premium Website	
StudyWARE	Activities and Quizzes on the **StudyWARE™ Software** for Chapter 17
	Complete the following **Competency Challenge 2.0** activity: • Monday, 3 PM, Process Insurance Claims
	Audio Library of medical terms
	Online access to the **Critical Thinking Challenge 2.0**
CourseMate	Activities and Quizzes for Chapter 17
WebTutor	Activities and Quizzes for Chapter 17

CHECK YOUR KNOWLEDGE

1. What is the term that describes payment by someone other than the patient for services rendered?
   a. Remittance advice
   b. EOB
   c. Claims tracking
   d. Third-party reimbursement
2. The most common claim form used in the medical office is the:
   a. CMS-1450.
   b. CMS-1500.
   c. UB-04.
   d. CPT-1450.
3. Which of these claims would be considered delinquent?
   a. Electronically submitted claim after two weeks
   b. Electronically submitted claim after three weeks
   c. Paper claim after four weeks
   d. Paper claim after five weeks
4. What does the acronym NPI stand for?
   a. National provider identification
   b. National provider identifier
   c. National physician identifier
   d. National physician information
5. A company that often serves as the middleman between providers and billing groups, payers, and other health care partners for the transmission and translation of electronic claims information into the specific format required by payers is known as:
   a. a clearinghouse.
   b. electronic claims tracking.
   c. electronic data interchange.
   d. a remittance advice.

WEB LINKS

CMS Electronic Billing and EDI Transactions: www.cms.gov/ElectronicBillingEDITrans

National Uniform Claim Committee: www.nucc.org

RESOURCES

Lindh, W., Pooler, M., Tamparo, C., and Dahl, B. (2010). *Delmar's Comprehensive Medical Assisting: Administrative and Clinical Competencies* (4th ed.). Clifton Park, NY: Delmar Cengage Learning.

Chapter

18

Patient Billing, Posting Patient Payments, and Collecting Fees

OBJECTIVES

In this chapter, you will learn the following:

KB KNOWLEDGE BASE

1. Spell and define, using the glossary at the back of the text, all the Words to Know in this chapter.
2. List the items the account statement contains.
3. Name and define the two methods of billing.
4. List the types of services practice management software related to patient billing and collections can offer a medical facility.
5. Name the three required information pieces needed when posting payments on a patient account.
6. List the general steps in posting a nonsufficient funds (NSF) check.
7. Explain the aging account process.
8. Describe the collection laws discussed in this chapter.
9. Understand the process in making the collection call.
10. List the words to avoid and the words to use when preparing a collection letter.
11. Describe the role of the collection agency.
12. Name and define the three special collection circumstances that most commonly exist in the medical field.
13. Explain two common exceptions to the usual billing and collection procedures.

S SKILLS

1. Accurately post NSF checks.
2. Accurately post collection agency payments.
3. Accurately process a credit balance for refund.

WORDS TO KNOW

account history
accounts receivable (A/R)
aging of accounts
alpha search
antagonize
at the time of service (ATOS)
bankruptcy
date of service (DOS)
expended
idle
nonsufficient funds (NSF)
outsourcing
practice management software (PMS)
skip
termination
Truth in Lending Act (TILA)
third party
viability
year-to-date (YTD)

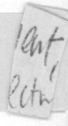

PATIENT BILLING

Patient billing requires patient account statements. These statements must be accurate in every detail, from the name of the patient to the figures for charges and payments (Figure 18–1).

The account statement contains the following patient information:

- Statement date and account number
- Name and address
- Date of services
- Description of services
- Total charges by service
- Patient payment
- Insurance payment
- Adjustments
- Deductibles
- Current balance
- Aging information
- Comment section or important notes
- Doctor's office or medical company's name and contact information

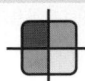

Douglasville Medicine Associates
5076 Brand Blvd., Suite 401
Douglasville, NY 01234
Ph: (123) 456-7890
Fax: (123) 456-7891
E-mail: admin@dfma.com
Web site: www.dfma.com

STATEMENT OF ACCOUNT

MANUEL RAMIREZ
1211 Gravel Way
Douglasville, NY 01234

Date: 1/3/20XX
Account No: RAM001

Date	Patient	Description of Service	Total Charges	Patient Payment	Insurance Payment	Adjust-ments	Dedu-ctible	Current Balance
18-Oct-XX	Manuel Ramirez	Established Patient - Level 3 99213	$78.00	$0.00	$47.20	$19.00	$0	$11.80
29-Oct-XX	Manuel Ramirez	Colonscopy 44389	$750.00	$0.00	$0.00	$0.00	$0	$750.00
29-Oct-XX	Manuel Ramirez	Established Patient - Level 5 99215	$176.00	$0.00	$0.00	$0.00	$0	$176.00
		Totals:	**$1004.00**	**$0.00**	**$47.20**	**$19.00**	**$0**	**$937.80**

0 to 30 Days Current	31 to 60 Days Past Due	61 to 90 Days Past Due	91+ Days Past Due
$0.00	$0.00	$937.80	$0.00

BALANCE DUE	**$937.80**

Important Note:

Figure 18–1: Computerized patient statement. *Delmar/Cengage Learning.*

These itemized statements are printed and mailed to the patients by the office or outsourced electronically to a billing service. **Outsourcing** is generally viewed as contracting out a specific business function to another company rather than having your own company manage that specific work. Outsourcing by a provider's office typically results in cost savings and higher quality because the office might not have the staff or equipment to complete the services effectively and efficiently.

The outsourced billing service will print, sort, stuff, add postage to, and mail the statements for you. Another service the outside company might offer is updated address information for your patients. This saves your practice valuable time and money by not having to deal with skip trace efforts.

If your practice processes statements in house, the office manager might inquire about purchasing, renting, or leasing envelope-stuffing machinery to complete this task. The machinery folds, stuffs, and inserts statements quickly, saving valuable time of the office staff.

METHODS OF BILLING

The two common methods of billing are monthly billing and cycle billing. Patients are more likely to pay if statements are received on a regular basis.

Monthly Billing

Monthly billing typically is more efficient in smaller medical practices. One to two days should be set aside for processing and mailing the statements. It is important for statements to be mailed in a timely manner so patients receive them by the first of each month. It is usually safe to mail five to seven business days in advance to ensure timeliness. Check with your post office on mail turn-around times.

Cycle Billing

Cycle billing is commonly used in large medical practices with a large number of statements sent out each month. With this system, accounts are divided into groups to correspond to the number of times you will be billing. The same cycle is maintained each month so that patients learn when to expect your statement. You might send A through F on the tenth of each month, G through M on the twentieth, and N through Z at the end of the month. With the statements processed on the same monthly schedule, this method allows office staff to handle the accounts in a more efficient manner and with more flexibility.

Computerized Billing

Billing is one of the most common uses for a computer in the medical office. Many computerized systems and software packages are available. Today, statements or itemized bills are most often generated through a **practice management software (PMS)** system. This category of software provides the medical office the electronic component to deal with day-to-day financial operations of a medical practice. The PMS is often connected to an electronic medical record (EMR) system. This allows information to be pulled from the EMR and populated in the financial components of the patient account of the PMS.

Practice management software offers a variety of services such as posting electronic claims and providing statistics on the number of patients seen per day (week, year), the diagnoses, and monthly and year-to-date billing information. The software should also provide Current Procedural Terminology (CPT) and International Classification of Diseases (ICD) codes for processing insurance claims efficiently. Although the system might provide CPT and ICD codes, care must be taken to ensure that the most current codes are used because these are updated annually.

If the billing system software is self-contained for the practice, patients' questions can be answered by the administrative medical assistant who handles the billing. Backing up the software on a daily basis might be necessary to keep billing records secure. Patients can have more personalized service if all transactions are done on site. If the billing is outsourced to a billing service, patients must be prepared to deal with outside billing individuals for any billing questions or problems. With planning, each method can be equally efficient.

A patient ledger within a practice management system may be called an **account history**. Generally, account histories follow the same organized plan used for ledger records of patients. The account history automatically shows the balance of the account and the number of days the account has been due. The entire account activity is available to view on the screen or to produce a printout for the patient.

You might have a choice in determining how you will find an account entered in the PMS system. The easiest and fastest method is called an **alpha search** (Figure 18–2). You type in the first few letters of the name, and the screen automatically lists all names of

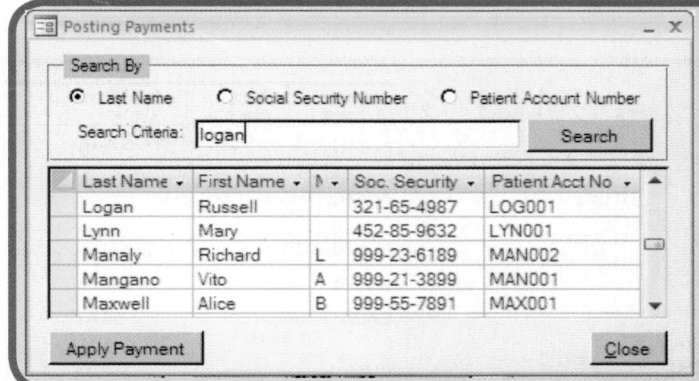

Figure 18–2: Searching for a patient account with practice management software. *Delmar/Cengage Learning.*

patients starting with those letters. You select the name attached to the correct date of birth you wish to make an entry for and type in the appropriate entry. When the system accepts a number only, you must maintain a cross-reference file of an alphabetical listing of patients along with their account numbers. The system should allow you to filter inactive accounts from the computer just as you remove inactive ledger cards.

When a provider's office uses PMS, it is important to choose the CPT codes commonly used in the practice. They are then programmed into the computer along with the descriptions of the codes and the fees to be charged for each. The ICD diagnostic codes can also be programmed into the computer for insurance claims use (Figure 18–3).

The system can be coded to indicate the source of the payment: insurance, cash, check, money order, or credit or debit cards. Adjustment codes can be used for returned checks, contractual adjustments, and any cancelled account balances.

Some PMS systems can be programmed to create encounter forms or charge slips. When the patient hands a computer-generated or handwritten encounter form (also referred to as a superbill) to the administrative medical assistant, the charge and payments can be entered in the account history. In some offices, the administrative medical assistant would check to be sure the services rendered were indicated on the charge slips and then send the slip to the business office for processing in the practice management system. All encounter forms or charge slips must be accounted for each day. The computer can create a statement or receipt to be handed to the patient before he or she leaves the office.

Some PMS systems can be programmed to lead you through the entry of every transaction by means of question or field prompts flashed on the screen or statements telling you what to do next.

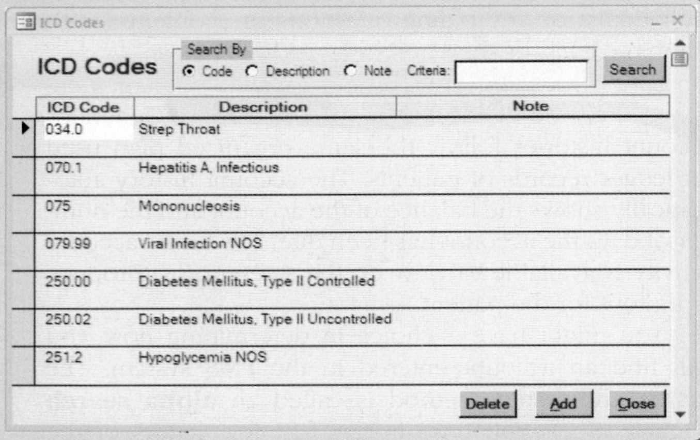

Figure 18–3: Procedure and diagnostic codes can be programmed into the practice management system for easy selection. *Delmar/Cengage Learning.*

CLINICAL PEARL

When posting charges to a patient account, take care to be accurate in entering the data the first time. However, if an error is posted on a transaction, you can reverse the transaction and start over again with a correct entry.

The computerized system can speed up monthly billing and can be programmed to withhold statements on accounts for which you do not need or wish to send statements.

EXAMPLE

Some reasons statements might be withheld include workers' compensation claims and the accounts of government-assisted patients or of families of patients who have recently passed away.

The computerized statement is considered to be an efficient collection method for the office because it not only shows an itemized account of all transactions but the age of the account. The statement should show the portion of the amount due that is current, over 30 days, over 60 days, and over 90 days. (See Figure 18–4.)

Account Number	Patient Name	0 to 30 Days Current	31 to 60 Days Past Due	61 to 90 Days Past Due	91+ Days Past Due	Total Due
ALB001	Josephine A. Albertson	($20.00)	$0.00	$0.00	$0.00	($20.00)
ALV001	Francisco B. Alvarez	$0.00	$0.00	$0.00	$475.00	$475.00
BLA002	Donald Blair	$1,832.00	$0.00	$0.00	$0.00	$1,832.00
BLA001	Francois Blanc	$60.00	$0.00	$0.00	$0.00	$60.00
CAL001	Megan E. Caldwell	$0.00	$0.00	$20.00	$0.00	$20.00
CHA001	Xao Chang	$60.00	$0.00	$0.00	$0.00	$60.00

Figure 18–4: Computerized statement showing account aging. *Delmar/Cengage Learning.*

The PMS system can also furnish you with a daily journal report. This report can be a record of cash control, also, because a listing of checks and cash can be shown separately. All computer systems should be set up to record deleted transactions as a printed safeguard against anyone tempted to steal money by entering a transaction and then deleting it.

PMS systems can print out monthly summaries of charges, payments, and accounts receivable. **Year-to-date (YTD)** reports can be produced easily. You can print out a record of all outstanding accounts with an analysis of account aging.

Some PMS systems can provide a detailed list of patients seen by each provider in a large clinic and the services rendered. It can be used to determine the number of patients seen with a specific diagnosis or for a particular procedure for research summaries.

The PMS system can also print a list of hospital and nursing-home patients to be seen. Such a list improves the accuracy in recording all out-of-office patient charges.

When you have a PMS system with many of the aforementioned printout possibilities, you will find the business management of the office much more efficient. You will also find that you can complete all these procedures in a fraction of the time required to do them by more conventional methods.

PATIENT PAYMENTS

Patient payments are vital for the financial success of a medical facility. It is important for specific payments to be requested of the patient at the time services are rendered or are accurately and appropriately billed for by the office according to the billing method the office uses. Requesting payments and posting these payments to patient accounts are essential steps in the **viability** of a medical business. Follow the credit and collection policies established by your medical facility. It is also important for the office staff to educate the patient to clearly understand the office billing and payment policies so there are no surprises when it comes to collecting payment.

Payments at the Time of Service

The patient's gratitude for the services received is highest **at the time of service (ATOS)**; that is why you should collect any amount of money that is appropriate at that time. If the patient's provider participates with the patient's insurance plan and the patient owes a co-pay at the time of service, collect only the co-pay. If the patient is uninsured (self-pay), collect the total of charges in full ATOS or follow your office policy.

CLINICAL PEARL

Remember, the best opportunity for collecting fees is when you have the patient in the office. This is true for both ATOS balances and past-due balances.

Verifying and Accepting Checks

It is usually acceptable for patients to pay by check. Details for accepting checks are covered in more depth in Chapter 19, but basic concepts are presented here. Be certain to take time to examine the check. When accepting patient checks, here are some guidelines and best practices:

- Be sure the check is valid and that no corrections have been made.
- Generally, it is not a good policy to accept checks written for more than the amount due (with the patient expecting cash back).
- Do not accept a check marked "paid in full" or "payment in full" unless it does pay the account in full, including charges incurred on the day the check is written. If a balance remains, the office would be unable to collect if the check is accepted and deposited.
- When you receive a check, stamp it with the office's deposit endorsement to protect against theft.
- Do not accept a **third-party** check (a check made out to the patient by an unknown party) unless the check is from an insurance company.
- Do not accept a postal money order with more than one endorsement. (Two is the limit honored.)

Posting Patient Payments

Posting payments to patient accounts is most commonly done with the use of a PMS system (Figure 18–5). The information required to post on the patient account includes the following:

- Date of the payment
- Payment amount
- Form of payment (cash, credit card, or check [include check number])

CLINICAL PEARL

One hundred percent accuracy is essential when entering payments in the patient's account. Remember, garbage in, garbage out. Correct data entry provides accurate financial records for the medical facility and, again, maintains business viability.

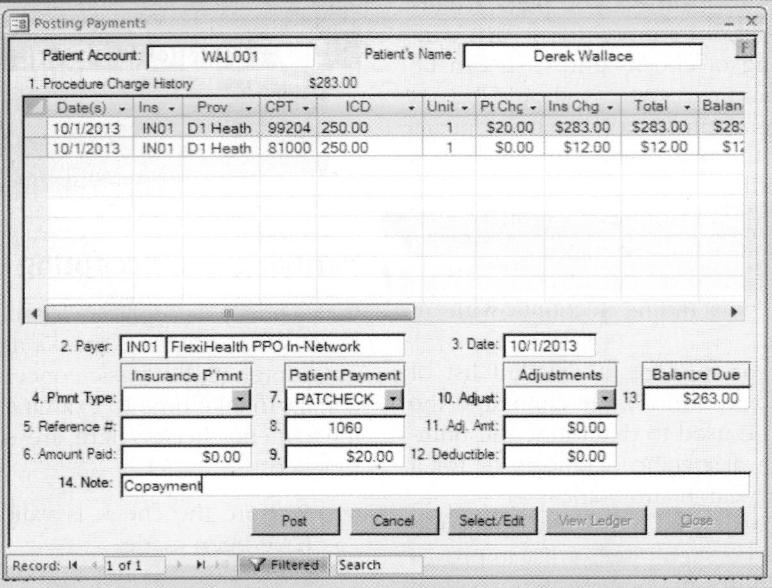

Figure 18–5: Posting a payment to a patient's account with a PMS system. *Delmar/Cengage Learning.*

Nonsufficient Funds Checks

At times, a check appropriately accepted from a patient and then deposited can be returned to the office by the bank, marked **nonsufficient funds (NSF)**, meaning the patient does not have enough money in the bank account to cover the amount of the check. It is important to notify the bank that returned the check to verify availability of funds. If the funds are available to cover the amount, immediately redeposit the check for reprocessing. Today, depending on banking processes and agreements between the bank and the medical office, the bank might reprocess the check the following day, hoping to recover the funds. If the check is returned a second time marked NSF, the administrative medical assistant dealing with this patient account would generally follow these steps:

1. Deduct the amount of the NSF check from the medical office's checking account balance.
2. In the patient's account, add the amount of the NSF check back into the account by entering the amount in parentheses in the paid column.
3. In addition, increase the patient's account balance by the same NSF amount.
4. Add a brief explanation in the description column, such as, "NSF 10/09/XX."

Be certain to follow the specific policy and procedure in the medical office in which you are employed when dealing with NSFs.

PROCEDURE 18–1 Post Nonsufficient Funds (NSF) Checks and Collection Agency Payments

PURPOSE: Post NSF checks and collection agency payments on the patient ledger or in a computerized account history

EQUIPMENT: Patient ledger (account history), returned NSF checks from the bank, checks from the collection agency, pen with black ink, calculator, or practice management software

S SKILL: Accurately post NSF checks.

S SKILL: Accurately post collection agency payments.

Procedure Steps	Detailed Instructions and/or *Rationales*
1. Pull the patient ledger or bring up the patient account history in the practice management software.	

Procedure Steps	Detailed Instructions and/or *Rationales*
2. Post the NSF check under the debit/charges column, adding back into the account the amount the check was originally issued for.	Debit the account the amount that was originally credited to the account. You originally *de*creased the account balance for the amount the check was written for. Now you want to *in*crease the account balance for this same amount because the check did not clear the bank.
3. Date the entry, noting NSF on the description portion of the patient ledger or account history.	The balance that was created by adding back in the NSF check amount must be placed with the collection agency.
4. Review the check sent from the collection agency.	
5. Post the amount of the check received in the credit column on the patient ledger or account history. Compute the new balance.	• If your practice's protocol is to adjust all balances from the accounts with a notation indicating "placed with outside collections" at the time you turn the account over to the agency, you might need to make an additional adjustment to the account. Make certain you do not reflect a credit on the account by posting the collection agency payment. • If your practice's protocol is to reflect the amount of the payment the collection agency withheld as their fee for collecting on outstanding balances, an additional adjustment might be required.

CREDIT BALANCE AND REFUNDS

A credit balance exists when an account is overpaid and a refund must be made back to the patient or to a health insurance plan by the medical facility. This situation occurs when the patient or the insurance company overpays on a patient account. It is your responsibility to identify this and issue a refund check to the patient or the insurance company. In doing so, be sure to verify the patient's or the insurance company's correct mailing address.

PROCEDURE 18–2 Process a Credit Balance and Refund

PURPOSE: Accurately process a credit balance and refund on a patient ledger or in a computerized account history

EQUIPMENT: Patient ledger (account history), company check, envelope, pen with black ink, or a computerized accounting system

S SKILL: Accurately process a credit balance for refund.

Procedure Steps	Detailed Instructions and/or *Rationales*
1. Pull the patient ledger or bring up the patient's account history in the practice management software.	Review the credit on the patient ledger (account) to determine which date of service the credit is from. Be certain the credit is from an actual overpayment, not an adjustment taken incorrectly, before refunding any money.
2. Post the amount of the overpayment in the credit column, preceded by a negative (–) sign.	*This indicates the amount that will be refunded and the amount added back into the account, bringing the balance to a zero status instead of a negative status.*

(continues)

(continued)

Procedure Steps	Detailed Instructions and/or *Rationales*
3. Indicate on the patient ledger (account history) the date the refund is being processed and to whom the refund is being issued.	• If the refund is due to the patient, verify that you have the current address before mailing a check. Sometimes, addresses are updated in the charts and not on the patient ledger (account) or computerized account. • If the refund is due to an insurance company, verify where the refund is to be mailed. Often, the claims address and refund address differ from one another.
4. Correctly complete the refund check to the patient.	• Enter the date the check is being issued in the appropriate field on the check. • Enter the name of the person or company and his or her address in the *Pay to the Order of* section of the check. • Enter dollar amount to be refunded in the appropriate field of the check (example: $32.75). • Enter the same dollar figure, spelling out the number values (example: $32.75 would be reflected as "Thirty-two and 75/100").
5. Check all entries for accuracy and compare the refund amount with the amount indicated on the patient ledger or account history.	
6. Obtain the proper signature(s) on the check.	Depending on your medical facility, checks might be signed only once a week, twice each month, daily, and so on. Keep the refund check in a safe or under lock and key until you are able to obtain the necessary signature(s).
7. Make a copy of the check for the accounts payable record.	
8. Address an envelope to the payee and mail the check.	
9. Return the patient ledger to the file or save and close the account in the PMS.	

COLLECTING FEES

To stay on top of **accounts receivable (A/R)** due from your patients, you need some type of reporting system to see who has not paid on his or her account. **Aging of accounts** is actually a way to identify accounts according to the length of time the accounts have been delinquent. It is basically a means of dividing accounts into categories according to the amount of time since the first billing date, usually breaking them down by 60, 90, and up to 120 days.

Accounts are considered current if within 30 days of the billing date. Aging dates usually appear at the top or bottom of a patient statement when mailed out to the patient as a bill. This allows the patient to understand the actual time that has passed since the services were rendered and the overdue payment time that has lapsed.

CLINICAL PEARL

PMS systems can help rapidly in analyzing accounts receivable for accounts past due. The PMS should allow you to request reports by different parameters: accounts older than 60 days without any patient payment, accounts that have not had any patient payments posted in the last 30 days, and so on.

Each practice will have its own set of guidelines for when it considers an account to be delinquent. No account should be referred to a collection agency unless the provider has given approval for this to be done or as stated in your office policy. However, federal law requires that when you have stated you will turn the account over for collection, you must follow through and do so if the bill is not paid. You cannot make **idle** threats.

COLLECTION LAWS

The Federal Trade Commission (FTC), the nation's consumer protection agency, enforces the Fair Debt Collection Practices Act (FDCPA), which prohibits debt collectors from using abusive, unfair, or deceptive practices to collect from a patient or customer. Three important instated acts are explained in this unit, which will affect the process by which you make collections.

Truth in Lending Act

The **Truth in Lending Act (TILA)**, which is enforced by the Federal Trade Commission, specifies that when there is an agreement between the provider and a patient to accept payment in more than four installments, the provider is required to provide disclosure of finance charges (Figure 18–6). The patient must sign this form in your presence, and the disclosure statement must be kept on file for two years. If the provider makes no specific arrangement for more than four payments and bills each month for the full amount, rather than installment amounts, the signed statement is not necessary.

Catherine R. Lang, MD
431 S. Water Street
Bluestone, MI 12345-6789
123-789-0123

Federal Truth in Lending Statement
For Professional Services Provided

Patient ______________________ Date __________

Address ______________________

Parent/Guardian ______________________

1. Fee for Service $________
2. Downpayment $________
3. Unpaid Balance $________
4. Amount Financed $________
5. Finance Charge $________
6. Annual Percentage Rate of Finance Charge ________
7. Total Amount of Payments (#s 4 + 5) $________
8. Deferred Payment Price (#s 1 + 5) $________

Total payment due (#7) is payable to Dr. Catherine R. Lang at the above address in monthly payments of $________, the first of which is payable on __________, 20XX. Each subsequent payment is due on the 15th of each month until paid in full.

________ ______________________

Date Signature of Patient/Parent/Guardian

Figure 18–6: An example of a federal truth in lending form.
Delmar/Cengage Learning.

Fair Debt Collection Practice Act

Under the Fair Debt Collection Practice Act (FDCPA), the patient is protected in a number of areas. The Act covers personal, family, and household debts, including money owed on a personal credit card account, an auto loan, a mortgage, and a medical bill. Under this act, every collector must send a written validation notice, explaining to the patient how much money is owed by him or her to the medical facility. This notice must be sent within five days after the patient is first contacted, must include the name of the creditor (medical facility or provider) to whom the patient owes the money, and must state how to proceed if the patient does not think he or she owes the money.

The FDCPA also outlines specific time guidelines for making collection calls. In most states, collection calls can be made between the hours of 8:00 AM and 9:00 PM. Calling for collection purposes outside of these hours can cause consequences for the medical office or collection agency. In addition, collectors may not contact patients at work if patients have indicated (either orally or in writing) that they are not allowed to get calls there. Threatening collection phone calls described as repeated calls made over and over to the patient by the medical office or a collection agency can be considered harassment. State and local governments can have additional statutes concerning the telephone and debt collection.

Statute of Limitation Laws

Each state has laws (called *statutes of limitations*) that establish the number of years during which legal collection procedures may be filed against a patient. If a patient is being treated for a chronic illness, there is no **termination** of the illness or treatment unless the patient dies or changes providers. The last date of debit or credit on the patient account card is the starting date for that particular debt.

EXAMPLE

If the statute of limitations is two years and the last date on the patient account was June 2011, it could be collected through June 2013.

In written contracts, the statute of limitations starts from the date due. Some states have a shorter time limit on the statute of limitations of single-entry (single-charge) accounts.

STRATEGIES FOR COLLECTON

A few strategies are used for collecting payment from a patient. Remember, collecting payments ATOS from a patient is the ideal time to collect money owed to the doctor or medical facility. After the patient has left the office, after insurance reimbursements have been made to the doctor, a balance usually exists as the patient's responsibility to pay. This is when mailing statements under an aging account system assists in this collection effort. There will certainly be times when the patient does not pay on time or the bill becomes delinquent, which then calls for collection strategies by the office.

Making the Collection Call

The best collection opportunity after the time of service is by telephone. The challenge with telephone collection is getting the patient to the phone with technology advances such as caller identification and call blocking,. When a person other than the patient answers the telephone and asks who is calling, the patient can refuse to take the call if he or she realizes that the medical office is making the call.

Prior to making collection calls for your practice, obtain permission to do so from your office or business manager or the provider and follow office policy. Again, check the laws in your state for appropriate calling hours. Do not call before or after stated times, or you can be liable for harassment. Calls should be made from an area of the office where neither other patients nor visitors to the office can overhear what you are saying; this is also a requirement of HIPAA.

Prior to making the collection call, review the account to verify whether any payments have been posted since the collection report was run from your practice management system. Review the notes on the account. If notes are made in more than one area of an account, review the notes in each area. Know where the patient balance is coming from—which **date of service (DOS)**.

Verify that the insurance company has been billed and has responded to any DOS in question. Have an idea of what you are going to say to the patient before placing the call. Attempt to reach the patient at the home number first. Try the cell phone and work number next (if appropriate). If the patient requests you not to call him or her at work again, you must honor the request and document this in the patient's account file. Review Table 18–1 for beginning the collection call.

Answer any questions the patient might have. If the patient indicates dissatisfaction with the results of medical care, be sure to convey this information to the provider. On occasion, patients do not pay the bill because they have questions about the service or how it was billed. After you have answered any questions, the patient might be willing to pay the bill with a credit or debit card while you are on the phone. If the patient is unable to pay the entire bill all at once, offer a payment plan that follows office policy. Ten percent of the balance on a monthly basis is usually the lowest amount a practice will agree to. After you agree on an amount, agree on a specific date each month that the patient will *mail* the payment.

EXAMPLE

If the balance is $250 and the patient agrees to pay $25 a month on the twelfth of each month, it will take 10 months to pay the bill in full. *$250 (balance of account) divided by $25 (monthly payment) = 10 months.*

Typically, payment plans are set up to have the account paid in full within 12 months, but extremely large balances from costly surgeries can take much longer than 12 months to pay. Follow office policy when setting up payment plans with patients.

Table 18–1 Steps in Beginning the Collection Call

Step	Example
1. Ask for the patient by full name when placing your call.	"May I speak with Olivia Felix, please?"
2. When you are certain you are speaking with the correct person, identify yourself and where you are calling from.	"This is Sabrina Holton calling from the office of Dr. Martin Silva."
3. Get right to the point of your call.	"I am calling today regarding your past-due balance with Dr. Silva."

At the end of the call, repeat everything the patient has agreed on during the call.

EXAMPLE

"Ms. Felix, you agree to pay $25 each month, on the twelfth of the month, for the next 10 months to pay your balance in full."

Note the account to reflect the agreement and any other pertinent information from the call. You should also note within a comment section of the patient's account about the agreed payment plan. This informs other staff members about the agreement in case the patient questions something at his or her next visit, and other medical assistants will know not to attempt to collect on the old balance when the patient is in the office.

Each month, run the report that reflects accounts with delinquent balances. You can check the report for payments that have been received on the accounts where payment plans have been established. PMS systems might offer a report specifically for accounts that have been set up on a budget payment plan and a specific field in the demographic or collection screen to note this fact.

Collection Letters

Some providers feel that collection cards or stickers are a sufficient reminder, but others prefer the use of collection letters. Consult the office procedure manual or your employer regarding preferences for follow-up on the collection of accounts. You might compose or purchase a series of standardized letter templates that you can personalize as needed (Figure 18–7A–C).

CLINICAL PEARL

When composing collection letters, avoid words that tend to **antagonize**, such as *neglected*, *ignored*, and *failure*. Words such as *missed*, *overlooked*, and *forgotten* are not quite so negative and seem more respectful.

Decide whether you are going to use a series of two or three letters. The last letter in the series usually informs the patient that you must resort to a collection agency if you do not receive payment by a *specified* date. Use your knowledge of the patient to decide which type of letter to use. You would use a stronger-sounding first letter for someone with a poor payment record. For a patient who has an excellent payment record, your first letter would be a gentle reminder.

Douglasville Medicine Associates
5076 Brand Blvd., Suite 401
Douglasville, NY 01234
Ph: (123) 456-7890
Fax: (123) 456-7891
Email: admin@dfma.com
Website: www.dfma.com

June 14, 20XX

John O'Keefe
12 Gravers Lane
Douglasville, NY 01234

Dear Mr. O'Keefe:

Your account with our office is three months past due, and you have not responded to our previous requests for payment. Please pay your balance of $852 at this time or contact us with a plan for payment.

Please call me at (123) 456-7890 if you have a question about your account or a plan for payment. Otherwise, we expect your payment immediately.

Sincerely,

Marilyn Johnson

Marilyn Johnson
Office Manager

Figure 18–7A: First collection letter. *Delmar/Cengage Learning.*

Douglasville Medicine Associates
5076 Brand Blvd., Suite 401
Douglasville, NY 01234
Ph: (123) 456-7890
Fax: (123) 456-7891
Email: admin@dfma.com
Website: www.dfma.com

July 15, 20XX

John O'Keefe
12 Gravers Lane
Douglasville, NY 01234

Dear Mr. O'Keefe:

Your son, Chris, was seriously ill in March when he was seen by Dr. Heath. Dr. Heath used her experience and education to treat Chris, believing you would pay your account within a reasonable amount of time.

Four months have passed and you still have not remitted the $852 balance on your account. We cannot continue to keep your unpaid account on our books. If you are experiencing financial difficulties, please call the office at (123) 456-7890 so we can arrange a payment schedule that is agreeable to both of us.

Sincerely,
Marilyn Johnson
Marilyn Johnson
Office Manager

Figure 18–7B: Second collection letter. *Delmar/Cengage Learning.*

Douglasville Medicine Associates
5076 Brand Blvd., Suite 401
Douglasville, NY 01234
Ph: (123) 456-7890
Fax: (123) 456-7891
Email: admin@dfma.com
Website: www.dfma.com

August 17, 20XX

CERTIFIED MAIL

John O'Keefe
12 Gravers Lane
Douglasville, NY 01234

Dear Mr. O'Keefe:

This is our final attempt to collect your account of $852, which is five months past due. You have not responded to all our previous letters, so we have no alternative but to turn over your account to a collections agency.

Your account is being assigned to Bonham Medical Collection Service, which will pursue whatever legal means is necessary to collect this debt. If you contact me at (123) 456-7890 within seven days, we can prevent the account from this assignment and resolve the balance.

Sincerely,
Marilyn Johnson
Marilyn Johnson
Office Manager

Figure 18–7C: Third collection letter. *Delmar/Cengage Learning.*

Collection Agencies

Every effort must be **expended** to collect as many accounts as possible without resorting to a collection agency, which charges a percentage of everything collected. Most offices avoid collection agencies if at all possible because they are a costly service to the provider or medical facility.

Your employer is likely to have arrangements with a reputable collection agency. Collection agencies generally come into play when a bill is delinquent for more than six months. They can charge up to 50 percent of the bill owed; however, recovery of this money owed the provider is better than receiving none at all. The provider or medical office can then write off the loss when filing for taxes.

When the decision to refer an account for collection has been made by your employer or the business or office manager, send the collection agency the full name of the patient, name of spouse or person responsible for the bill, last known address, full amount of debt, date of last entry on patient ledger or computerized account, occupation of debtor, and business address. Send no further statements, and refer any calls regarding the account to the collection agency. If you receive any information regarding the account or any payments, forward them to the collection agency.

After you have turned the account over to a collection agency, the patient's account should be identified in this way or filed separately from other accounts. Make a notation on the file that it is under a collection agency service. If the collection agency efforts or the facility attempts to collect on a highly delinquent account are unsuccessful, a lawsuit is the last resort.

SPECIAL COLLECTION CIRCUMSTANCES

Special circumstances exist for the medical assistant concerning collections. These circumstances include dealing with **skip** patients, those individuals under bankruptcy situations, and deceased patients, which might fall under estate claims. Understanding the management of these types of circumstances shows the medical assistant the most appropriate manner by which to handle these situations in the medical office.

Skips

When statements you have mailed are returned marked *moved, no forwarding address*, you have to consider the possibility that the patient is a skip (a person who has disappeared or moved to avoid payment of bills). The first step is to check your records to make sure you mailed to the correct name, address, and ZIP code. If these are all correct, place a telephone call to see whether the old phone number was transferred to a new address. You might call referring individuals to try to obtain a new address for the patient, although you must not indicate your reason for needing the new address other than that you need to verify it. You might call the patient's employer for information regarding address change, identifying yourself by name only and asking for the patient to return your call. You might find the patient simply forgot to inform the post office of an address change. You might also find that the patient has left his or her place of employment, in which case you should check with your employer about referring the account for collection. The longer you wait, the less chance you have to collect payment from the patient.

As soon as the skip is identified, the medical assistant should begin the task of locating the patient. With the Internet, it is much easier to find such a skip patient. Bear in mind, when making phone calls to locate the individual, never discuss what the call is regarding because this is a violation of HIPAA and other collection rules and privacy laws.

Bankruptcy

Bankruptcy is a petition to a court by an individual who is stating that he or she cannot pay any debt incurred. When your office receives an official notice that a patient has filed for bankruptcy, you may send no more statements and can make no attempt to collect the account. The patient who has filed a wage earner's bankruptcy will pay a fixed amount to the court to be divided among the creditors. Your office might receive only a dollar at a time. Accept this and credit the account. You will be notified of a creditors' meeting in a straight petition for bankruptcy, but it is usually best just to be sure the court has a copy of the statement and wait to see whether you will receive any money. Sometimes the patient wishes to continue seeing the provider and will make payments on the account independently on a cash basis.

Estate Claims

When it is necessary to collect a bill owed by a deceased patient, the statement is sent to the estate of the deceased in care of any known next of kin at the patient's last known address. Do not address the statement to a relative unless you have a signed agreement that that person will be responsible for the bills. You might need to contact the probate court to obtain the name of the administrator of the estate if the patient expired in a nursing home and had no known next of kin.

Exceptions to Usual Billing and Collection Procedures

There are a number of exceptions to the usual billing and collection procedures. Some providers complete physical examinations for individuals applying for insurance coverage. In this case, the bill is sent to the insurance company. Providers who specialize in sports medicine and examine athletes might be paid by the school or team referring the patient.

The provider might examine a patient in consultation in a legal claim and, in this case, the person or agency requesting the consultation is responsible for the charges. The statement is sent with the consultation report. Other examples of third-party billing are auto accidents, workers' compensation, and Medicaid.

Some offices use outside billing services to handle all aspects of their accounts receivable, insurance, and patient billing as well as collections. In this case, be sure all charges and payments are sent so that the statements will be accurate and complete. The disadvantage of this system is that you do not have records in your office of current balances for your patients. If patients ask you a question about their account, refer them to the outside billing service directly.

CHAPTER SUMMARY

- An accurate patient account statement is a required document in the patient billing process.
- Outsourcing is contracting out a specific business function to another company rather than having your own company manage that specific task. It usually results in cost savings and higher quality.
- The monthly billing cycle is typically more efficient in smaller medical practices, whereas cycle billing is commonly used in large medical practices.
- A practice management software (PMS) system is most commonly used today to deal with day-to-day financial operations of a medical practice. This computerized system might allow for information to be pulled from the electronic medical record and populated in the financial components of patient accounts for an accurate and efficient billing process.
- Posting patient payments requires the date of the payment, the payment amount, and the form of payment (cash, credit card, or check).
- A patient's check marked "NSF" returned to the office by a bank indicates insufficient funds to cover the amount of the check.
- A credit balance exists when an account is overpaid and a refund must be made back to the patient or a health insurance company by the medical facility.
- The best opportunity for collecting a patient payment is at the time of service (ATOS).
- Written communication is the least effective means of collecting patient fees, and the best collection opportunity after face-to-face contact is by telephone.
- Aging the account is a process that identifies accounts according to the length of time they have been delinquent. Accounts are usually divided by 60, 90, and up to 120 days of delinquency.
- The Federal Trade Commission (FTC) enforces the Fair Debt Collection Practices Act (FDCPA)., which protects the consumer by outlining guidelines for the debt collector to follow during the collection process.
- The Truth in Lending Act (TILA) is enforced by the FTC and specifies that when there is an agreement between the provider and a patient to accept payment in more than four installments, the provider is required to provide disclosure of finance charges.
- Statutes of limitations establish the number of years legal collection procedures may be filed against a patient.
- A collection agency is usually used for accounts delinquent more than six months. The collection agency can charge up to 50 percent of the bill for its services. After an account is turned over to the collection agency, the medical office cannot attempt to collect from the patient on that particular account. Any information regarding the account should be forwarded to the agency.
- A skip patient is one who has moved to avoid payments—skipped town. Typically, statement mailings are returned to the office marked *moved* or *no forwarding address* on these identified skip accounts.
- Bankruptcy is a petition to a court by an individual who is stating that he or she cannot pay any debt incurred, including medical bills.
- An estate claim involves sending a bill owed by a deceased patient to any known next of kin at the *patient's* last known address.

STUDY TOOLS

Workbook	Activities for Chapter 18
Premium Website	
StudyWARE	Activities and Quizzes on the **StudyWARE™ Software** for Chapter 18
	Complete the following **Competency Challenge 2.0** activity: • Monday, 1 PM, Perform Billing and Collection Procedures and Post Accounting Transactions
	Audio Library of medical terms
	Online access to the **Critical Thinking Challenge 2.0**
learninglab	Module 8: Billing and Payment for Medical Services
CourseMate	Activities and Quizzes for Chapter 18
WebTutor	Activities and Quizzes for Chapter 18

CHECK YOUR KNOWLEDGE

1. In this billing system, accounts are divided into groups to correspond to the number of times you will be billing.
   a. Computerized billing
   b. Monthly billing
   c. Cycle billing
   d. Electronic billing
2. What is PMS?
   a. Practice monitoring software
   b. Practice management software
   c. Payment management software
   d. Payment management system
3. All the following bits of information are required to post a payment to a patient account, except:
   a. date of payment.
   b. time of payment.
   c. payment amount.
   d. form of payment.
4. When is the best opportunity for collecting patient fees?
   a. When the patient is in the office
   b. Over the phone
   c. When the patient declares bankruptcy
   d. With a collection agency
5. A patient's account history is also referred to as a:
   a. monthly summary.
   b. fee statement.
   c. patient journal.
   d. patient ledger.
6. Of the following terms, which word should be avoided when composing a collection letter?
   a. Missed
   b. Neglected
   c. Overlooked
   d. Forgotten

WEB LINKS

American Academy of Medical Management: www.epracticemanagement.org

Fair Debt Collection Practices Act: www.ftc.gov/os/status/fdcpa/fdcpact.htm

REFERENCES

Lindh, W., Pooler, M., Tamparo, C., and Dahl, B. (2010). *Comprehensive Medical Assisting: Administrative and Clinical Competencies* (4th ed.). Clifton Park, NY: Delmar Cengage Learning.

Unit

9

Banking and Accounting Procedures

The medical assistant might become involved with financial transactions in the medical office, including handling cash, checks, and credit cards. This unit presents the most common banking terms and their definitions to help you understand financial transactions. The medical assistant who deals with financial situations must have a strong working knowledge of banking and basic accounting procedures. These skills are not only important in the provider's office but also in the management of your own personal finances. Knowledge of banking terms helps you communicate with the bank officials where the office has its account as well as with the accounting firm personnel who prepare the office's financial forms.

Certification Connection

	Ch. 19	Ch. 20
CMA (AAMA)		
Accounting and banking procedures	X	X
RMA (AMT)		
Banking procedures	X	
CMAS (AMT)		
Fundamental financial management	X	X
Banking	X	

Chapter

19 Banking Procedures

OBJECTIVES

In this chapter, you will learn the following:

KB KNOWLEDGE BASE

1. Spell and define, using the glossary at the back of the text, all the Words to Know in this chapter.
2. Differentiate between savings and checking accounts.
3. Explain the handling of currency in the office.
4. Differentiate among types of checks, including personal, cashiers, certified, limited, postdated, stale, traveler's, and voucher checks.
5. Identify the seven components of a check that make it negotiable.
6. List the five essential factors that must be included when writing a check.
7. Compare types of endorsements.
8. Discuss precautions to take when receiving checks from patients.
9. Identify the five most common check writing errors.
10. Describe the process of preparing a deposit slip and check register.
11. Explain the stop payment process for checks.
12. Describe the information contained on a bank statement.

S SKILLS

1. Prepare a check.
2. Prepare a deposit slip.
3. Reconcile a bank statement.

WORDS TO KNOW

agent
authorization
automated teller machine (ATM)
bank statement
currency
denomination
deposit
deposit record
deposit slip
direct deposit
endorsement
endorser
e-statement
mobile banking
negotiable
online banking
outstanding check
overdraft
payee
payer
reconciling
register
stop payment
third-party
transaction
void
withdrawal

BANKING

Banks are financial institutions in which individuals or companies may set up accounts to hold and disburse money. A **deposit** is money (cash or checks) put into an account, increasing the account balance. A **withdrawal** occurs when money is removed from the account (by check, electronic fund transfer, withdrawal slip, or passbook), thus decreasing the account balance.

Due to technology, and the Internet in particular, we no longer have to be physically present at the bank to perform banking transactions. **Online banking**, or electronic banking, is the practice of performing **transactions** by the Internet. **Mobile banking** allows account holders to perform banking transactions by a mobile device such as a smart phone or personal digital assistant (PDA). In both of these methods of banking, all information and records related to the account are tracked and can be viewed online.

An **automated teller machine (ATM)** is a banking machine operated by inserting a debit, credit, or bank card and entering a personal identification number (PIN) code. Deposits, transfers, withdrawals, and other banking functions can be performed at ATM locations.

Telephone banking allows account holders to perform banking transactions over the telephone. This method of banking offers nearly all the banking functions of an ATM, such as account balance information, lists of latest transactions, fund transfers, and electronic bill payments.

Mail banking allows account holders to deposit checks into their account by mail. This method of banking is primarily used by virtual banks (banks that do not have a physical branch location) and by account holders who live too far from a branch.

Types of Bank Accounts

The most common types of bank accounts are the checking account and the savings account. These types of accounts can be specific to the needs of an individual or a company holding the account. The medical assistant can be responsible for accurately maintaining these types of accounts for the medical office.

- *Checking account*: A bank account in which money may be deposited and checks written against. The bank issues the checks and deposit slips. A written check by the patient is a common form of payment to the provider. In addition, the medical assistant responsible for accounts payable will likely use the office checking account to make payments toward various office expenses.
- *Savings account:* A bank account from which the depositor can earn interest. The amounts deposited can be recorded in a passbook. This passbook contains a record of deposits, withdrawals, and interest earned, with the dates of all the transactions. On a monthly basis, interest earnings are credited to the account. (Many banks now also give interest on checking accounts if a minimum balance is maintained.)
- *Overdraft checking account:* A bank account that allows checks to be written for a larger amount than is currently in the account. The **overdraft** is covered by the bank in the form of a loan for which interest is charged.
- *Special checking account:* Many names and definitions apply, depending on the area of the country. It can be an account on which interest is paid if an established minimum balance is maintained in the account, an account for senior citizens for which no handling charges are incurred, or an account that charges fees for checks only. Banks are continually offering new plans to attract depositors.

CURRENCY

Currency is the name given to the cash we use in our society. It is made up of paper bills in \$1, \$2, \$5, \$10, \$20, \$50, \$100, and larger denominations issued by the Federal Reserve. Cash also comes in the form of coins in denominations of 1, 5, 10, 25, 50, and 100 cents (although 50-cent pieces are no longer made and are disappearing from circulation).

Because currency and coin are instantly expendable, care must be taken to keep it secured at all times in the medical office. All cash should be placed out of sight as soon as received, in a cash box, file drawer, or some other secure (locked) location. Usually, all daily proceeds are either locked in a safe or deposited at the close of the day.

CHECKS

A check is an order for a bank to pay money to the person or company named on the check from the account holder. Checks have a long history. The first recorded use of a check was in 1374. They were rare before 1700 but became common after World War II. The Federal Reserve reports that billions of checks are processed in the United States every year.

There are many types of checks besides a personal check, and you should be familiar with them when dealing with finances:

- *Cashier's check:* The purchaser pays the bank the full amount of the check. The bank then writes a check on its own account payable to the party specified. This type of check guarantees the recipient that the full amount of money indicated on the check will be paid on processing.

- *Certified check:* The bank stamps the customer's own check *certified* and then holds the certified amount in reserve in the customer's account until the check is cashed. This is a guaranteed check and so is always acceptable when a personal check is not.
- *Electronic check:* A check paid directly from a checking account through the Internet. The account owner establishes a list of recurring payees, their corresponding account numbers, and the electronic or actual addresses. To pay a bill, the list is called up, the payee identified, the amount of payment entered, and the payment command given. The bank electronically completes the transaction within a day or two without the need for a paper check, envelope, or stamp.
- *Limited check*: A check that will be marked void if written over a certain amount. These checks are often used for payroll or for insurance payments. A check can also list a time limit by which it must be cashed. It must be cashed within the time limit, or it is not **negotiable**.
- *Money order:* Negotiable instrument often used by individuals who do not have checking accounts or to meet the requirement for purchasing an item or service. Money orders may be purchased for a fee from banks, credit unions, post offices, and many other money order service locations.
- *Postdated check:* A check made out with a future date. You might have patients who wish to pay while they are in the office but will not have the money in their account until next payday, which is the date they will put on the check. Never deposit these checks until the date for which they are made out. The practice of writing a postdated check is illegal in some states; be sure you know the law in your state.
- *Stale check:* A check presented too long after it was written to be honored by the bank. Some checks specify that they must be cashed within 90 days and, if presented after that date, the bank will not honor payment. A period of six months is generally considered enough time for a check to be presented for payments.
- *Traveler's check:* A special check used by individuals who are traveling and do not wish to carry a large amount of cash. Personal checks are sometimes not accepted outside of the area of the bank upon which they are drawn. Therefore, in exchange for cash, banks will issue traveler's checks. These must be signed individually at the time of purchase at the bank and again when they are used for payment on goods and services. They are usually considered the same as cash, but some merchants still require some identification before they accept a traveler's check. Lost traveler's checks can usually be replaced if you can produce a list of their serial numbers. Traveler's checks are listed as checks on a deposit slip.
- *Voucher check:* A check with a detachable voucher form that shows the reason for which the check was drawn. This kind of check is often used by insurance companies. The voucher form is removed before the check is endorsed and deposited.

Check Components

Seven components, or features, must be present on a check for it to be valid (Figure 19–1):

1. *Date:* Watch for a postdate (a future date), a stale date (six months or older), or a preprinted date requirement such as *void after 60 days*. A check with these features is not valid before or after a specific period of time.
2. *Words of negotiability: Negotiable* refers to something that can be transferred or exchanged. On a check, the words "Pay to the order of" are considered to make the check negotiable. In other words, the amount written can be transferred from the account

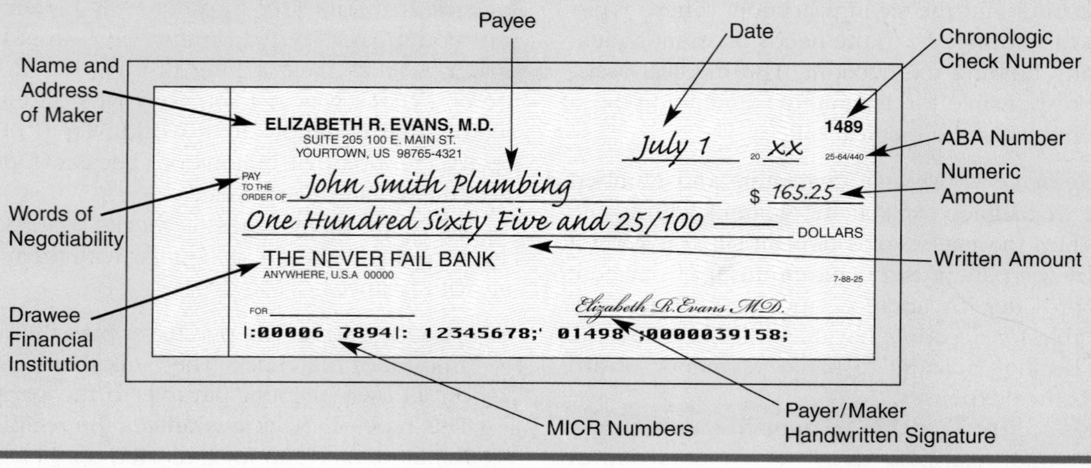

Figure 19–1: Components of a check. *Delmar/Cengage Learning.*

of the payer to the payee. A check must say, "Pay to the order of," or "Pay to the bearer," to be negotiable.

3. ***Payee:*** The check must identify to whom the check is written. In the office, this will be the provider or the medical clinic that receives checks as payment for care provided. A payee can also be a person or company that has provided services to the practice, for which a check is written out by the office.
4. *Numeric amount:* This is the amount of the check written in numbers.
5. *Written amount:* This is the amount written in words. It must agree with the numeric amount.
6. *Drawee financial institution:* This identifies where the check is payable. Checks issued by the government, traveler's checks, corporate checks, and money orders do *not* have a drawee institution printed on them because *they* are the drawee.
7. *Signature:* The signature is usually handwritten but can also be a reproduced facsimile. A reproduced type of signature is commonly seen on paychecks of large companies that employ and generate checks for a great number of employees.

Banks have instituted five other features to guard against fraud, but they are not necessary for validity. If they are missing, it is best to scrutinize the check very carefully.

1. *Name and address of the maker:* This is usually preprinted by the check printer.
2. *Chronologic check number:* This is printed at the right upper corner of the check.
3. *Check routing symbol or ABA number:* A code number found in the right upper corner of a printed check. It might be above the check number on a business check or below the check number on a personal check. It is in fractional form and identifies the institution involved in the clearing process. This number was originated by the American Bankers Association (ABA). The purpose is to have a method of identifying the area where the bank on which the check is written is located and to identify the bank within the area. It may be written as a fraction (44/119) on a business check or hyphenated (25–61) on a personal check.
4. *Magnetic ink character recognition (MICR) numbers:* These are numbers that aid in the clearing process. This technique consists of characters and numbers printed in magnetic ink at the bottom left side of checks and deposit slips. The numbers are printed with special magnetic ink and identify:
   - The Federal Reserve district and branch.
   - The drawee financial institution.
   - The maker's account number.
   - Usually the check number.

   This information is specific to each checking account and is imprinted on each check and deposit slip by the company printing the checks. The first series of numbers is the routing information that identifies the bank and area. The second series identifies the account numbers. The last series corresponds to the check number.

   When the bank processes the check, additional magnetic ink numbers are printed across the bottom identifying the amount of the check. These characters and numbers can be read by high-speed technology, which greatly enhances the bookkeeping procedures in the bank by simplifying check sorting and individual monthly statement printing.
5. *One rough or perforated edge:* This is where the check is separated from a book or sheet of checks. This will not be found on government or traveler's checks.

Check Endorsement

An **endorsement** is the payee's signature on the back of a check (Figure 19–2). It is a transfer of title on the check to the bank in exchange for the amount of money on the face of the check. The endorsement of a check transfers all rights in the check to another party. Endorsements

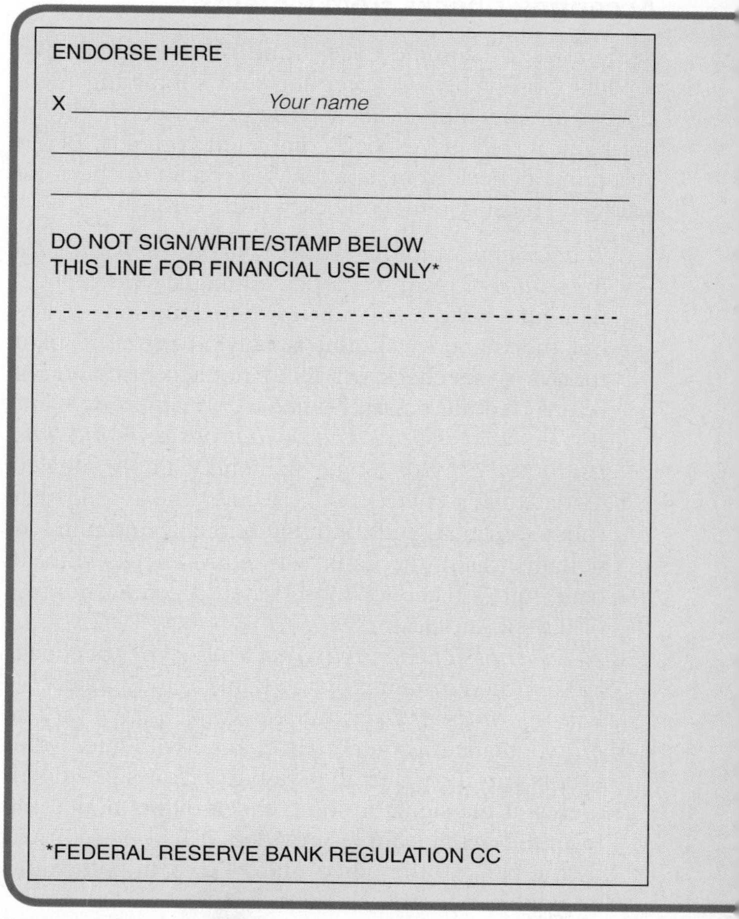
ENDORSE HERE
X Your name
DO NOT SIGN/WRITE/STAMP BELOW
THIS LINE FOR FINANCIAL USE ONLY*
*FEDERAL RESERVE BANK REGULATION CC

Figure 19–2: Proper placement of a check endorsement.
Delmar/Cengage Learning.

should always be made in ink or with a pen or rubber stamp. The end of the check to be endorsed can be identified by holding the check on the right end as you look at it, turning it over, and endorsing the opposite or left end. All checks received in the office, whether in person or through the mail, should be protected by endorsement at the time received.

The two commonly used kinds of endorsement are blank endorsement and restrictive endorsement. A *blank endorsement* is a signature only. It should not be used until the check is to be cashed because, if the check is stolen with such an endorsement, someone else could endorse the check below your name and cash the check. A *restrictive endorsement* is used to endorse checks when they are received. It is a stamp or written information that states, "PAY TO THE ORDER OF (name of bank where check is to be deposited)" followed by the name of the provider. If such a check is stolen, it could not be used in any way.

If the name of the **endorser** or payee is spelled incorrectly on the face of the check, it should be endorsed the same way, followed by the correct signature directly below.

Accepting Checks from Patients

Remember to examine checks and other banking documents closely before accepting and submitting them. Checks are much more likely to be processed quickly by the bank if they have been completed correctly. Before accepting a check from a patient, be certain to check the following most common check writing errors:

1. *The written amount does not match the numeric amount.* For example, a person might write a check with the written amount as one hundred dollars, but the numeric amount is only $10.00. The bank receiving this check will likely not accept it and will return it to the doctor's office.
2. *A check that is not dated or that has a wrong date, usually the year.* Some patients simply neglect to date their checks. Others enter the wrong date (post- or stale dated) both intentionally and unintentionally. Again, the bank will return checks with no date, future dates, or those dated a certain number of days in the past.
3. *A check not signed by the payer.* These types of checks are returned instantly by the bank to the office.
4. *The signature of the payer does not match the one on file.* Signatures generally change with age. Other events can also alter the way a person signs documents. If the signature on a check differs noticeably from the initial sample provided, it will be returned by the bank to the office. Many times, the office has no control over this situation.
5. *Modified or altered checks.* Checks that appear to have been altered with scratch-outs, write-overs, use of correction fluid, different colored inks, or multiple handwriting styles are considered altered. Even if the cause is a simple mistake, these changes look suspicious to the bank and can cause the check to be returned to the office. If a mistake absolutely must be corrected, ask the payer of the check to use *one* line to cross out the error and initial the changes. This does not guarantee that the check remains valid, but it can lower the level of suspicion.

CLINICAL PEARL

Other precautions to be observed when accepting checks include the following:

- Be sure the check has the seven components that make a check valid and that no corrections have been made.
- Do not accept a **third-party** check unless the check is from an insurance company that is authorized by your employer. A third-party check is generally one made out to the patient by someone unknown to you. Because you do not know how credit-worthy the check writer is or have any personal information about the individual, it is unwise and poor practice to accept a third-party check that another person has written.
- You might have patients who want to write a check for more than the amount due so they can have some cash in hand. This is generally not a good policy, and it would be advisable to refuse such a check. When you accept the check as payment and give out an additional amount in office cash, you risk not only the check not being honored by the bank but also that your office will lose the cash that was given to the patient.
- Do not accept a check marked "paid in full" or "payment in full" unless it does pay the account in full, including charges incurred on the day the check is written. If there is still a balance, you will be unable to collect if you accept and deposit such a check. People often write "paid in full" or "payment in full" on the memo line on the front of a check. Be sure to check this line because it is easy to overlook. When you receive a check, stamp it with the deposit endorsement (see the next section) to protect against theft.
- Do not accept a postal money order with more than one endorsement because two is the limit honored.

Preparing Checks

As the medical assistant dealing with the office finances, you might be required to write checks to pay for equipment, supplies, or wages. It is very important to perform this task with complete accuracy. The office will receive statements from utility companies, medical suppliers, periodical publishers, perhaps a rental agency or mortgage company, and various other businesses. Each statement must be checked to be certain it is for services or materials you receive. Checks may also be written for employee salaries, tax payments, provider's expenses, the office petty cash fund, and other needs. Checks can be processed traditionally, like your own personal account, or be computer generated in the office. If the latter is the case, you must learn how to use the particular software program; many programs allow you to bring up the check form on the screen and complete the entries. With software, your balance is automatically adjusted for you each time you add a deposit or write a check. Whether using either a traditional or computerized method, the same entries are required.

You must include five essential factors when writing a check:

1. *Date:* The month can be written or numerical.
2. *Payee:* The person to whom a check is written. The name of the payee is listed on the check after the words "Pay to the order of."
3. *Numeric amount:* The amount of the check in numbers. Keep the numbers close to the dollar sign so other numbers cannot be inserted to increase the amount of the check.
4. *Written amount:* The amount of the check written in terms of dollars and fractions of dollars. For example, a check for $25.89 is written, "Twenty-five and 89/100." Fill in the remainder of the space with a line to prevent insertion of words to increase the amount.
5. *Payer signature:* Signature of the person owning the account or other designated individuals. The **payer** is the person who signs the check or the corporation that pays it. The payer is also known as the maker.

Completing the Check Register

In addition to writing the check, the corresponding check stub or **register** must also be accurately completed (Figure 19–3). It is a record showing the check number, person to whom the check is paid, amount of the check, date, and balance. It is kept by the person writing the check as a record of the transaction. When using computer software, the check is recorded electronically and the register updated automatically. This supplies a record of the expenditure as well as a running balance of the account. In a traditional checkbook, it is a good practice to complete the stub or register before writing the check to avoid accidental overdraft or forgetting and then mailing the check without remembering the payee or the amount to deduct from the balance. Some traditional checkbooks have a duplicate feature that imprints a copy of each check when it is written, therefore preventing this situation.

To complete the stub or register properly:

1. Use black or blue ink.
2. Enter the check number if it is not preprinted.
3. Enter the date.
4. Identify the payee.
5. Bring forward the balance from the previous stub.
6. List any deposits.
7. Enter the amount of the check being written.
8. Enter the new balance.

When the check is finished, it is attached to the billing statement and given to the provider for signature prior to mailing.

Providers might give check-signature power to the medical assistant or office manager dealing with the finances to eliminate the need for their personal signature. A signature **authorization** card obtained from the bank must be completed to allow someone other than the recorded owner of the account to execute checks. Some offices, as a means of monitoring expenditures and preventing employee embezzlement, require two signatures on a check or have a policy requiring the individual writing the check (e.g., bookkeeper) to have another authorized person (often the office manager) sign the check. This also provides an opportunity to question expenditures and maintain a sense of cash flow. This authorized office member is considered the **agent**,

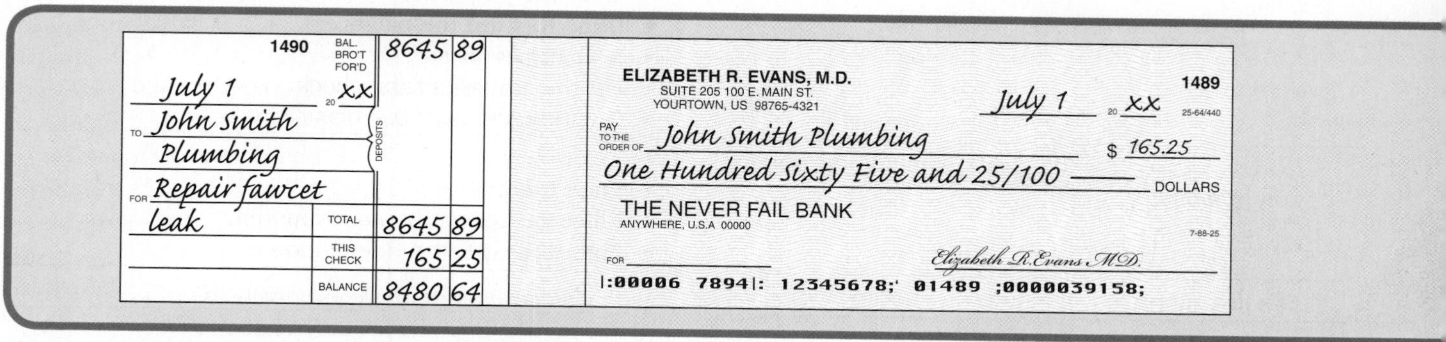

Figure 19–3: Check register and check. *Delmar/Cengage Learning.*

or the person authorized to act for another person. You are the agent for your employer, the provider, in the office. Bank officials are agents for the bank.

If a mistake is made in writing a check, it is necessary to write "**VOID**" across the check and stub and write a new one. File this voided check with your canceled checks because this check must be available for auditing purposes. Do not erase, cross out, use correction fluid, or change parts of a check because this type of check can be refused by the bank. Practice preparing checks by following Procedure 19–1 and using the workbook samples.

BANK DEPOSITS

As the medical assistant in charge of finances, you might be required to deposit cash and checks received in the office. This usually a daily task, or it can be as infrequent as once a week for a provider with a limited practice. Recall that a deposit is an amount of money (cash or checks) placed in a bank account. Deposits should be prepared in a secure place out of people's view. A **deposit slip** is an itemized list of cash and checks deposited in a checking account (Figure 19–4). It is important to keep a copy of all deposit slips to verify deposits.

Currency should be sorted as follows:

- Put all bills of the same **denomination** together.
- Face bills the same direction, portrait side up.
- Stack in order from highest to lowest denomination (for example, 50s, 20s, 10s, and 5s, with 1s at the top of the stack).

Count and enter the total amount of the bills on the currency line of the deposit slip. Next, count and enter the total amount in coin on the coin line. If there is a large amount of coin, it should be placed in wrappers. There are specific amounts to be rolled for each type of coin: $.50 for pennies, $2.00 for nickels, $5.00 for dimes, and $10.00 for quarters. Most banks also want bills in bill bands or grouped for ease of handling if in larger quantities. Assistants should check with their banks for requirements.

Ensure that all the checks have been endorsed. Arrange them facing up from the largest amount to the least. List checks by number, last name of maker, and amount on deposit slip.

A computer-generated list or an additional sheet of check listings is acceptable if a deposit slip is attached. If a money order (MO) is received, identify it as MO and the payee's name. If there are more checks than

PROCEDURE 19–1 Prepare a Check

PURPOSE: Prepare a check and stub without error

EQUIPMENT: Checkbook, pen with black or blue ink, computer, and computer checks

S SKILL: Accurately prepare a stub or register and a check.

Procedure Steps	Detailed Instructions and/or *Rationales*
1. Assemble equipment and supplies.	
2. Correctly complete the check stub with all appropriate components and then calculate the new balance.	• Enter the check number if it is not preprinted. • Enter the date. • Enter the payee name. • Bring forward the balance. • Add any deposits. • List the amount of the check. • Compute the new balance.
3. Correctly complete the check with all appropriate components.	• Enter the date. • Enter the payee. • Enter the correct numeric amount. • Enter the correct written amount.
4. Obtain authorized signature on check.	

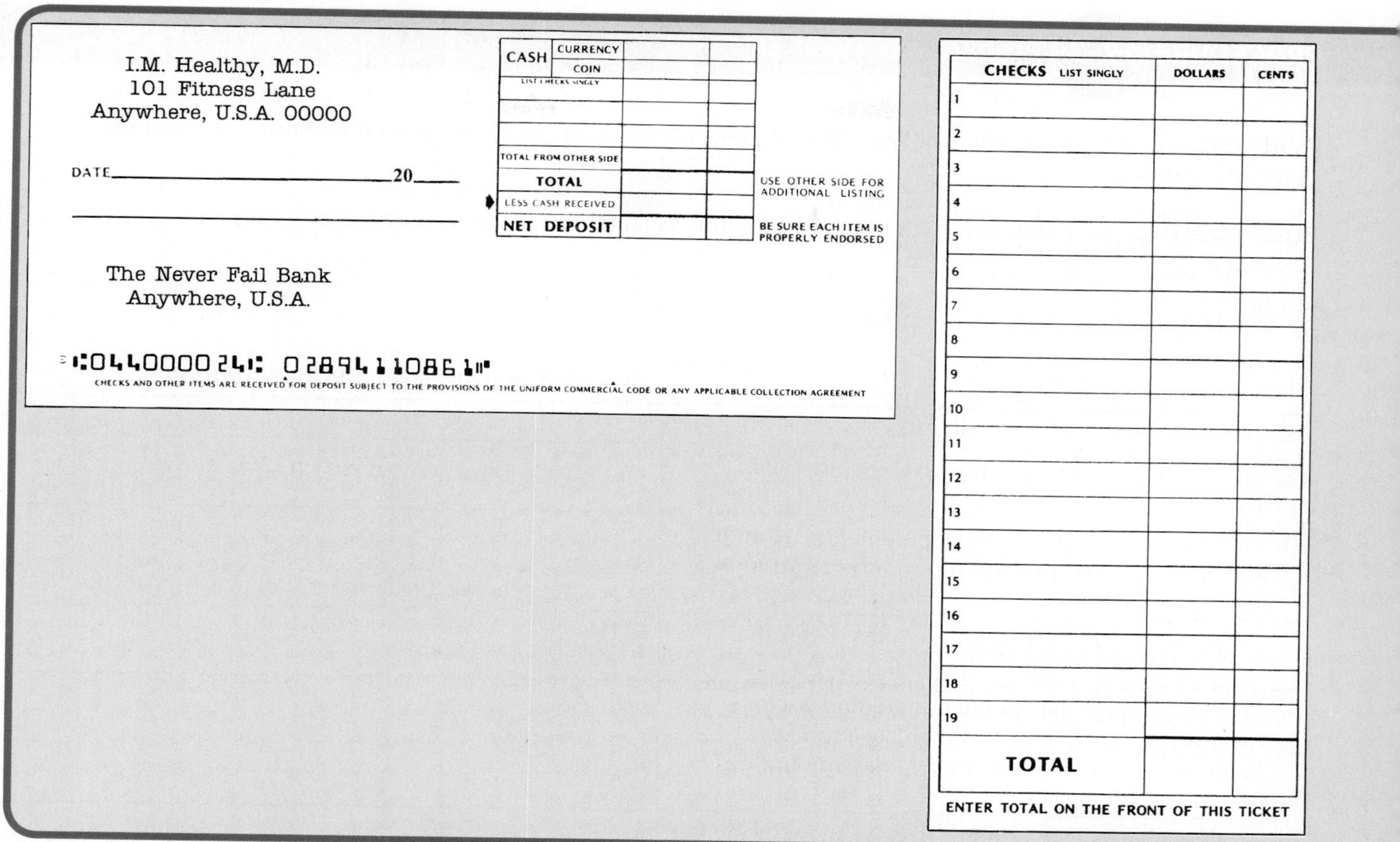

I.M. Healthy, M.D.
101 Fitness Lane
Anywhere, U.S.A. 00000

DATE ____________ 20____

CASH CURRENCY
COIN
LIST CHECKS SINGLY
TOTAL FROM OTHER SIDE
TOTAL
LESS CASH RECEIVED
NET DEPOSIT

USE OTHER SIDE FOR ADDITIONAL LISTING
BE SURE EACH ITEM IS PROPERLY ENDORSED

The Never Fail Bank
Anywhere, U.S.A.

⑆044000024⑆ 02894110861⑈

CHECKS AND OTHER ITEMS ARE RECEIVED FOR DEPOSIT SUBJECT TO THE PROVISIONS OF THE UNIFORM COMMERCIAL CODE OR ANY APPLICABLE COLLECTION AGREEMENT

CHECKS LIST SINGLY	DOLLARS	CENTS
1		
2		
3		
4		
5		
6		
7		
8		
9		
10		
11		
12		
13		
14		
15		
16		
17		
18		
19		
TOTAL		

ENTER TOTAL ON THE FRONT OF THIS TICKET

Figure 19–4: Deposit slip, front and back. *Delmar/Cengage Learning.*

can be listed on the front of the deposit slip, use the back, total the amount, and bring it forward to the correct line. Total the amount of the checks and enter it on the slip. To avoid errors, total the actual checks and compare with the total listed amount. Total the deposits and enter the amount on the deposit slip. Make a copy of both sides of a deposit slip in case any question about the deposit should arise. When the deposit slip is finished, enter the amount in the checkbook and add it to the existing balance, enter it on the daily log sheet, or post it on the appropriate computer screen.

Deposit slips are imprinted with the account number in MICR numbers that match those on the checks. These numbers make it possible for checks and deposit slips to be sorted and recorded by computer. Banks will accept a list of deposited items on something other than the bank-provided deposit slip as long as the bank deposit slip is attached.

It is important to perform a quality check by having a second reliable office staff member count the checks and cash being deposited and verified by their signature along with yours. You will need to make a copy of each deposit slip for your financial records and then match it up with the **deposit record** received by the bank. This deposit record is a record of a deposit that is given by the bank to the customer at the time of the deposit. It is important to keep the deposit record as proof of the deposit in case the bank fails to list the deposit on the monthly bank statement. Bear in mind, the deposit record from the bank should match the copied deposit slip filed behind before you left the office.

Deposits are usually placed in a zippered bank bag to be taken to the bank. They can be taken inside and given to a merchant teller (for more immediate service) or deposited in the night depository. Care should always be taken when transporting money. Be aware of your surroundings and do not put yourself in a questionable situation. If there is any chance you are being watched, do not leave your car. It probably is a good idea to vary the deposit day and time if possible so you do not become predictable.

Following the steps in Procedure 19–2, complete a deposit slip correctly. The workbook has a page of checks with stubs on which you can practice.

PROCEDURE 19–2 Prepare a Deposit Slip

PURPOSE: Prepare a bank deposit slip. All cash, checks, and coin must be entered without error and the deposit accurately totaled.

EQUIPMENT: Deposit slip, pen with black or blue ink, calculator, cash, currency, checks, and coin wraps to be deposited

S SKILL: Accurately prepare a deposit slip.

Procedure Steps	Detailed Instructions and/or *Rationales*
1. Assemble equipment and supplies.	
2. Separate money to be deposited by coin, bills, and checks.	
3. Arrange dollar currency by denomination, portrait, and direction. Total the currency and record it on the deposit slip.	
4. Count the coins; wrap large amounts. Enter the amount of coins on the deposit slip.	
5. Check to ensure that all checks are endorsed. Arrange checks face up from greatest to least. Enter checks by number, maker, and amount on the deposit slip.	
6. Total all checks listed on the back of the deposit slip and enter the total in the appropriate space on the back of the deposit slip; bring the total to the front of the deposit slip, writing in the appropriate space.	
7. Total the currency, coin, and checks and enter it on the deposit slip.	
8. Make a copy of the deposit slip for your office files.	
9. Enter the deposit total on the check stub in the checkbook.	
10. Deposit at the bank and obtain a receipt for records.	

Other Types of Deposits

A **direct deposit** is when an amount is sent electronically by the payer directly into a savings or checking account of the payee. A form of this method is known as an electronic fund transfer (EFT), which credits or debits accounts by computer without the involvement of checks or deposit slips. Direct deposit is very common in the United States. Many businesses offer their employees the option of using direct deposit to receive their paychecks. The IRS allows taxpayers to receive refunds by direct deposit.

Money can be transferred electronically by a wire transfer from the payer's account to another account overnight if the name and number of the receiving account and the name and identification number of the receiving bank are given. A fee is charged for the service, which varies by bank and location.

Checks may also be deposited by mail. Although you should avoid sending cash or currency by mail, if you must, send it by registered mail. The deposit slip and money are prepared as for any deposit. The checks should be endorsed by restrictive endorsement only. If no stamp is available, the handwritten notation, "for deposit only to the account of (name of your employer)," or "to the account number," will suffice. You should request a receipt because this record is necessary to prove that a deposit was made. It is extremely important to have an accurate record of all checks deposited with the check number, whom the check is from, and the amount of the check so that you can follow up if necessary. It is a good idea to photocopy all mailed checks. If checks become lost in the mail, it will be necessary to notify all payees to **stop payment** and issue you new checks.

Stop Payment on Checks

Stop payment is a method by which the maker of a check may stop payment. The bank charges a sizable fee for this service. Some banks will accept a stop order by phone if it is promptly followed by completion of a form, which the bank furnishes. The payer must furnish the number of the check, date issued, name of payee, amount of check, and the reason for stopping payment. The bank will then refuse to honor the check. A stop payment order is used when a check is discovered as missing or thought to be stolen or lost or if there is a disagreement regarding a product or service received. As a precautionary measure, the bank can consider placing a warning message on the account, which advises bank representatives to check signatures carefully to detect any attempt at a forged signature. Remember, when stop payment is placed on a check, the amount of the check should be added to the checking account balance.

BANK STATEMENTS

A **bank statement** is a record of an account sent to the account holder, usually on a monthly basis, showing the beginning balance, all deposits made, all checks drawn, all bank service charges and interest earned, and the closing balance. The account holder's cancelled checks are reported monthly with your bank statement and may be viewed online as a check image (a front side picture of the check). If needed, a copy of a cancelled check may be ordered from the bank.

With the increased use of online banking, **e-statements** and images of canceled checks are available online or sent by email to the account. In addition, banks offer the ability to request a bank statement through an ATM, which usually contains the last ten transactions made on an account.

Reconciling a Bank Statement

An important part of banking is the reconciliation each month of the bank statement with the office records. When a bank statement is received, you should verify that the amounts on the bank statement are consistent or compatible with the amounts contained in the office's check register. This process of confirming the amounts is referred to as **reconciling** the bank statement, bank statement reconciliation, or bank reconciliation. The statement will show all banking transactions concerning the account along with the checks the bank has received and processed. If bank statements are received in the mail as hard copies, reconciliation may be done with use of a standard form sent with the statement. If the office uses online banking, usually this electronic option offers a simple click to reconcile each check on the e-statement against checks as documented in the office check register. Most statements contain a section similar to Figure 19–5 that allows you to list outstanding checks and do other calculations to reconcile the amounts.

An **outstanding check** is one you have written that does not appear on your bank statement because the payee has not yet cashed the check. Look at the statement and put a check mark on each stub or register entry that matches a bank statement entry. A check stub or registry entry not checked indicates an outstanding check. The total of the outstanding checks is entered on the worksheet.

Items withdrawn from the account by the bank for charges, automatic payments, purchase of checks, and such that appear on the statement but are not in your checkbook must be totaled and entered on the appropriate line on the worksheet. Check the statement for deposits and compare the statement with your checkbook record. If you made a deposit since the statement was printed, it will not appear. Be certain an earlier deposit was not omitted from the statement.

Finally, the account might have earned interest that you have not recorded in the checkbook. Enter that on the form. When you have all the amounts and do the math, the corrected checkbook amount should reconcile (be consistent with) the bank statement.

With the convenience of online banking, some recurring expenses might be paid by electronic check. Unless a record is made in the traditional checkbook, there will be a difference in the balance. Be certain to check for these expenditures when you are reconciling the monthly statement. The statement will list the transaction as a bill pay and identify the payee. Other funds could be added or withdrawn by electronic transfer to and from other accounts or as automatic deposits or withdrawals.

Follow Procedure 19–3 and the workbook exercises to practice reconciling a bank statement.

RECONCILING THE BANK STATEMENT

Bank Statement Balance $ ________

(+) Plus Deposits not shown

____

____

Total ________ $ ________

(-) Less Outstanding Checks

____

____

____

____

Total ________ $ ________

CORRECTED BANK STATEMENT BALANCE	$ ________

Checkbook Balance $ ________

(-) Less Bank Charges $ ________

CORRECTED CHECKBOOK BALANCE	$ ________

Figure 19–5: Reconciliation form. *Delmar/Cengage Learning.*

PROCEDURE 19–3 Reconcile a Bank Statement

PURPOSE: Reconcile a bank statement so that the checkbook balance equals the bank statement balance

EQUIPMENT: Bank statement and canceled checks or photocopies, reconciliation worksheet, pen or pencil, and calculator or adding machine

S SKILL: Accurately reconcile a bank statement.

Procedure Steps	Detailed Instructions and/or *Rationales*
1. Assemble equipment and supplies.	
2. Compare the opening balance on the new statement with the closing balance on the previous statement. List the bank balance in the appropriate space on the reconciliation worksheet.	If the statement balances do not agree, contact the bank.
3. In the checkbook, check off all deposits credited to the account. Add to the bank statement balance any deposits not shown on the bank statement.	*Such as, amounts deposited since the statement was prepared.*
4. Put checks in numeric order and compare the check entries on the statement with the returned checks. Check off all returned checks in the checkbook. Determine whether you have any outstanding checks and, if so, list them on the reconciliation worksheet and total them.	• Mark stub or entry on register if check was returned. • List those not checked on reconciliation worksheet. • Total outstanding checks.

Procedure Steps	Detailed Instructions and/or *Rationales*
5. Subtract from your checkbook balance items such as withdrawals, automatic payments, or service charges that appear on the statement but not in the checkbook.	These items are indicated by a code such as *AP* for automatic payment or *SC* for service charge.
6. Add to your checkbook balance any interest earned as indicated on your statement.	*Some banks pay interest if a specified minimum amount is maintained in the account.*
7. Make sure the balance in your checkbook and the balance on the bank statement agree.	If they do not agree, subtract the smaller figure from the greater for a possible clue to the error and recheck all figures.

CHAPTER SUMMARY

- With the advent of electronic technology, it is no longer necessary to be physically present at a bank to perform transactions. Some common banking methods include online, mobile, ATM, telephone, and mail banking.
- Checking and savings accounts are the most common types of bank accounts.
- There are various types of checks, including personal checks, cashier's, certified, electronic, limited, postdated, stale, traveler's, voucher checks, and money orders.
- The seven components you must examine to ensure that a check is valid include the date, words of negotiability, payee, numeric amount, written amount, drawee, and signature.
- The five features banks have instituted to guard against fraud include name and address of the maker, chronologic check number, check routing symbol or ABA number, magnetic ink character recognition (MICR) numbers, and a rough or perforated edge.
- The most common check writing errors include the written and numeric amounts not matching, the check not dated, check unsigned by payer, signature of payee not matching that on file, or a modified or altered check.
- The five essential factors you must include when writing a check are the date, payee, numeric amount, written amount, and the payer signature.
- A stop payment order is used when a check is discovered to be missing or thought to be stolen or lost or if there is a disagreement regarding a product or service received.
- Currency and checks received by the medical office are totaled and entered on a deposit slip. Deposits are usually placed in a zippered bank bag to be taken to the bank. Other deposit types include direct deposit, wire transfers, and mail deposits.
- A bank statement is a summary of all financial transactions occurring over a given period of time, usually a month, for an account. They are typically mailed monthly to account holders and include service charge fees and interest earned.
- An important part of banking is the reconciliation each month of the bank statement with the office records. When a bank statement is received, you should verify that the amounts on the bank statement are consistent or compatible with the amounts in the company's cash account in its general ledger and vice versa.

STUDY TOOLS

Workbook	Activities for Chapter 19
Premium Website	
StudyWARE	Activities and Quizzes on the **StudyWARE™ Software** for Chapter 19
	Audio Library of medical terms
	Online access to the **Critical Thinking Challenge 2.0**

(continues)

CourseMate	Activities and Quizzes for Chapter 19
WebTutor	Activities and Quizzes for Chapter 19

CHECK YOUR KNOWLEDGE

1. A ___________ increases the balance of an account, whereas a __________ decreases the balance.
   a. deposit, withdrawal
   b. withdrawal, deposit
   c. transaction, withdrawal
   d. deposit, transaction
2. The person to whom the check is written is the:
   a. payer.
   b. payee.
   c. maker.
   d. third party.
3. Which person signs the front side of the check?
   a. Payer
   b. Payee
   c. Receiver
   d. Endorser
4. All the following are essential factors that must be included when writing a check, except:
   a. payee.
   b. numeric amount.
   c. written amount.
   d. endorsement.
   e. date.
5. To make sure the office and the bank agree on the amount in the account, a(n) _____ is performed.
   a. audit
   b. reconciliation
   c. trial balance
   d. accounts receivable

WEB LINKS

American Academy of Medical Management:
www.epracticemanagement.org

Bankers Training and Consulting Company:
www.btcc.com

RESOURCES

Federal Reserve Bank Services. "2007 Federal Reserve Payments Study." www.frbservices.org/communications/payment_system_research.html. (Retrieved 11/9/2010)

Brownell, M. "The Fall of the Checkbook." Mainstreet. www.mainstreet.com/article/moneyinvesting/credit/debt/fall-checkbook. (Retrieved 11/9/2010)

Krager, D., and Krager, C. (2005). *HIPAA for Medical Office Personnel*. Clifton Park, NY: Delmar, Cengage Learning.

Lindh, W., Pooler, M., Tamparo, C., and Dahl, B. (2010). *Delmar's Comprehensive Medical Assisting: Administrative and Clinical Competencies* (4th ed.). Clifton Park, NY: Delmar, Cengage Learning.

Chapter 20

Accounts Payable and Accounting Procedures

OBJECTIVES

In this chapter, you will learn the following:

KB KNOWLEDGE BASE

1. Spell and define, using the glossary at the back of the text, all the Words to Know in this chapter.
2. Identify three types of supplies or services considered accounts payable by a medical office.
3. Explain why comparing shipments to packing lists or invoices is important.
4. List and explain the required fields of a typical invoice.
5. Explain the purpose of a petty cash fund.
6. Differentiate between accounting and bookkeeping.
7. Compare operating information and managerial accounting information.
8. Identify the various accounting formulae presented in this chapter.
9. Describe the importance of calculating net worth, accounts receivable ratio, collections ratios, and cost ratio.
10. Explain and give examples of write-offs.
11. Identify the three steps of cost–benefit analysis.
12. Name and explain the two most common financial records of a medical office.

S SKILLS

1. Create and maintain a petty cash fund.

WORDS TO KNOW

accounting
accounting formula
accounts payable (A/P)
accounts receivable (A/R) ratio
assets
balance sheet
collections ratio
cost ratio
cost–benefit analysis
depleted
equity
expenditure
financial records
gross collection ratio
income statement
invoice
liabilities
managerial accounting
net collection ratio
net worth
operating information
petty cash
voucher
write-offs

ACCOUNTS PAYABLE

Accounts payable, also known as A/P or payables, refers to the total amounts owed by the practice to suppliers and other service providers for regular business operating expenses. It is the obligation or the promise that a business, in this case the medical office, owes to its creditors for buying goods or services. This includes unpaid invoices, bills, or statements for goods or services provided by outside contractors, vendors, or suppliers. In a medical office, some of these suppliers might be for medical office supplies and equipment, office rental, utilities (gas and electric, water, telephone, and Internet services), and even office staff salaries. Payments for these services are made to these suppliers by written checks so that there is a clear and concise paper trail of all money disbursed by the office. These records are likely maintained within an office financial software program.

The job of the accounts payable office personnel is a serious responsibility. Not paying bills on time and according to the specific terms and conditions can affect the office's credit ratings and ultimately business relationships. The medical assistant working in accounts payable should be highly organized and attentive to details. Good communication skills are also a plus because this individual might have to answer questions from vendors, the doctor, or coworkers in other parts of the medical facility about A/P.

PURCHASING SUPPLIES AND EQUIPMENT

Expenditure is acquired material, property, or labor in exchange for money. One area of expenditure that must be carefully monitored is payment of invoices for office equipment and supplies. When a statement is received from a supplier, it is essential to know that everything on the invoice and the amount or number of each item has in fact been received. The shipment must be compared with packing slips or invoices at the time it is received and notification of any discrepancy should be brought immediately to the attention of the supplier. Frequently, partial shipments are sent and some items are on back order. Payment of the total amount of the invoice would represent payment for goods not received, and some difficulty can also arise in trying to obtain materials not sent after you have paid in full for the shipment. The provider assumes everything was shipped as stated on the invoice because no questions were raised when the shipment was received. Be certain to maintain files to hold these invoices, usually alphabetized by the supplier's name. These records may also be scanned into a system and kept under specific vendor files within the office computerized software program.

An **invoice** is a document that includes itemization of goods and purchases or services provided together with the charges and terms of the agreement, as shown in Figure 20–1. Companies and vendors that provide services to your office email or mail invoices with the expectation of timely payment of the written charges. If you are requesting an invoice by email, it is useful to request it in PDF format so that it cannot be altered. Table 20–1 shows required fields of an invoice you should expect from a company or vendor or if producing your office's own invoice.

PETTY CASH

Medical facilities have a need for a **petty cash** fund to use when small payments are required, and it is just that—a small amount of stored cash ranging from $25 to $75. Because it is not reasonable to write checks for small office transactions, most providers have a petty cash fund. The provider determines the amount of the fund and for what it will be used. It is established by writing a check payable to Cash or Petty Cash. The check is then cashed and the money kept in a separate locked cash box. The money is often used for postage stamps, inexpensive office supplies, and small charitable donations.

A **voucher** form or expenditure list should be completed each time payment is made from this fund. When the amount in the fund is nearly **depleted**, another check is written for the difference between the established original fund amount and the remaining amount. The expense records are kept in a file to verify the use of the petty cash fund. Figure 20–2 shows a petty cash fund ledger form to monitor expenditures. Practice completing a petty cash form by referring to Procedure 20–1.

ACCOUNTING

Cr Dr adds

According to Merriam-Webster, **accounting** is "the system of recording and summarizing business and financial transactions and analyzing, verifying, and reporting the results" and provides information about the financial position of a company or organization. Accounting is different than bookkeeping, although the two are sometimes mistakenly used interchangeably. Recall that bookkeeping is the recording of financial transactions of a business, and, thus, it is only one aspect of accounting. Accounting reviews and interprets the transactions, which helps the business understand the financial impact of decisions made in the past, and provides guidance on future decisions. Accounting has a language of its own—a language that provides information about the financial position of a company or organization. In this case, the financial position of the doctor's office or medical facility is the concern. By learning this language, you can communicate and understand the financial operations of any and all types of organizations.

This section covers two integral aspects of accounting, **operating information** and **managerial accounting** information. Operating information is needed on a day-to-day basis for a company to conduct business. Employees need to get paid, patient services and fees need to be accounted for, the amounts owed to other suppliers and

ABC OFFICE SUPPLIES

INVOICE

BILL TO	My MD Office 5 Wellpoint Lane Stillwater, XY 00012	SHIP TO	My MD Office 5 Wellpoint Lane Stillwater, XY 00012

Invoice #	A65624
Invoice Date	11/16/20XX

Date Order Initiated: 11/15/20XX
Date Order Shipped: 11/16/20XX

QTY	UNITS	ITEM	DESCRIPTION	TAXABLE	UNIT PRICE	TOTAL
1		76761	Tele Message Book	Y	10.00	10.00
2	Boxes	76411	Black Pens	Y	6.00	12.00
5	Boxes	76330	Staples	Y	2.00	10.00
					Subtotal	32.00
					Tax (8.75%)	2.80
					Shipping	8.00
					BALANCE DUE	$ 42.80

PAYMENT TERMS
Payment within 30 days via check or money transfer, via online banking, only to the following account:

ABC Office Supplies, Account No: 9696

Late Fee: A late fee of 10% will be added to the next statement if not paid on the specified due date.

ABC Office Supplies
1234 Office Road
Supplier, XY 99911
Location #: 99-22

PHONE	(800) 999-9999
FAX	(866) 999-1234
E-MAIL	abcofficesupplies@internet.com
WEB SITE	http://www.abcofficesupplies.com

Figure 20–1: Sample invoice. *Delmar/Cengage Learning.*

TABLE 20–1 Information on an Invoice

Information	Description
Company details	Includes company name, company address, company telephone number, and email address.
Invoice number	Each of your invoices should have a unique invoice number. Although it is called a number, it can include letters, for example, A65624.
Dates	*Date*: The date the invoice was initiated. *Due date*: The date by which payment should be made. The due date is typically 30 days after the invoice date.
Client details	The name of the company or client contracted with the company or vendor. In this case, this would be your office name because you are the client of the company offering its services to your medical facility.
Fees	A description of the services provided and the total amount due.
Payment terms	This specifies how the company would like to receive the money from the medical office. For example: • Payment should be made within 30 days by check or money transfer, through online banking, from the date of this invoice. • Checks should be made payable to Company AAA. • Money transfers should be sent to The Vendors Bank. • Acc#012345678 (if applicable). • Reference: Use invoice number.

PETTY CASH FORM

Date	Bill/Voucher Description	Amount	Balance
10/1/20XX	Fund established		$25.00
10/5/20XX	Bill: Postage	$8.80	$16.20
10/8/20XX	Bill: Parking fee	$5.00	$11.20
10/10/20XX	Voucher: Coffee	$2.98	$8.22

Figure 20–2: Petty cash form. *Delmar/Cengage Learning.*

vendors or individuals need to be tracked, the amount of money the office has needs to be monitored, the amounts customers owe the doctor's office need to be checked, any inventory needs to be accounted for, and the list goes on. Operating information is what makes up the greatest amount of accounting information, and it provides the basis for managerial accounting.

Managerial accounting, also known as cost accounting, is the study and analysis of financial data as it applies to operational issues within a company. Good office managers should be aware of how the accounting in their medical office is being handled. Managerial accounting formulas help managers assess the financial health of different areas in their business. This information helps them make informed business decisions when it comes to salary adjustments, benefits, office purchases, and other expenses required in maintaining a well-functioning office.

Basic Accounting Formula

The basis for all financial accounting is the **accounting formula**. This basic accounting formula is:

Assets – Liabilities = Net Worth

Assets are the money and items of value in a business. In a doctor's office, this could mean patient finan-

PROCEDURE 20–1 Establish and Maintain a Petty Cash Fund

PURPOSE: Given an initial amount of cash, a petty cash form, vouchers, bills, and a pen, correctly enter the items and compute the balance accurately

EQUIPMENT: Pen with black or blue ink, calculator, vouchers, receipts, petty cash form, and computer

S SKILL: Establish and accurately maintain a petty cash fund.

Procedure Steps	Detailed Instructions and/or *Rationales*
1. Assemble equipment and supplies.	
2. Enter the opening balance on the petty cash form.	
3. Refer to a voucher and enter the description, number, and amount disbursed and compute the balance.	
4. Refer to a bill and enter the description and amount disbursed and compute the balance.	
5. Continue until all items are listed and the remaining balance is computed.	
6. Notify the provider or manager to write a new check for the difference between the balance and the established fund amount when it reaches the agreed-upon level.	

cial payments and medical equipment. **Liabilities** are debts or accounts payable (A/P) owed by the business. So, subtract liabilities from assets, and what is left is known as the **net worth** of the business. This net worth demonstrates the value of a business.

EXAMPLE

Basic Accounting Formula Using Simple Amounts

$1,500 (assets) – $500 (liabilities) = $1,000 net worth

Accounts Receivable Ratio

To begin, accounts receivable (A/R) are all the outstanding accounts, or amounts still due from the patient or customer to the doctor. The **accounts receivable ratio** or A/R ratio formula, when calculated, helps you understand how quickly outstanding accounts are paid as well as the effectiveness of the office collection process. This A/R formula is:

Current A/R Balance ÷ Average Monthly Gross Production = A/R Ratio

The current A/R balance is the total dollar amount of the outstanding payments due to the office from patients and customers. The average monthly gross production can be calculated by taking approximately six months of monthly receipts divided by the number of months—in this case, total value of receipts divided by six. So, if your receipts for six months add up to $300,000, and you divide that total amount by the number of months (6), you get $50,000 as your average monthly gross production. If you are a newly established office, you might start out with three months of data and, using the same calculation process, divide by three.

The turnaround time, or A/R ratio, has a goal of two months or less. In the following example, you see that this office has a three-month turnaround time for payment on an account, which is considered one month too long. Remember, the longer an account is past due, the less likelihood is the success of making the account collection.

EXAMPLE

Accounts Receivable Ratio (A/R Ratio) Using Simple Amounts

$150,000 (current A/R balance) ÷ $50,000 (average monthly gross production) = 3.0
This means there is a three-month turnaround time for payment on an account (A/R ratio).

Collection Ratios

Collection ratios are important for nearly every medical office or facility. Understanding both the gross and the net collection ratios remains valuable in determining how efficiently your office is collecting payments for services rendered by the providers. Today, many contracts hold doctors to maximum allowable fees, more denials, capitation rate contracts, significant overhead increases, and ongoing practice mergers. With all these factors, it is difficult for the practitioner to determine how his or her practice is doing and whether its employees are working to their fullest capacity and doing the best they can to enhance business. These types of ratios are not required to be calculated monthly but, instead, should be reviewed quarterly and annually. Now let's take a closer look at what these ratios measure.

Gross Collection Ratio

The **gross collection ratio** includes the total payments received by a practice for a specific period of time, *not* including any write-offs. The gross collection ratio can be calculated by taking the total payments for the specific period divided by the total charges, again *without* considering write-offs.

EXAMPLE

Gross Collection Ratio Using Simple Amounts

$300,000 (your total payments, A/R) ÷ $600,000 (your total charges) = 0.5
Converting this to a percentage (multiplying 0.5 by 100) = 50% gross collection ratio.

With this type of ratio, the higher the ratio the better because this shows the percentage of money-flow back into the office. In this example, this means that for every dollar charged, the practice is collecting 50 cents. Note that the ratio presented in the example box is not a good collection ratio. This might be the best a medical facility can do if the practice has a high payer mix consisting of Medicaid, Medicare, and managed care contracts, which is very common these days in most practices.

EXAMPLE

Net Collection Ratio Using Simple Amounts

$400,000 (your total payments, A/R) ÷ [$500,000 (your total charges) minus $50,000 (write-offs) = $450,000] = 0.888
Converting to a percentage (0.888 × 100) = 88.8% or 89% net collection ratio.

Net Collection Ratio

The **net collection ratio** is also known as the adjusted collection ratio. It is calculated by taking the total payments for a specific period of time divided by the total charges, *with* the write-offs deducted from the total charges.

Net collection rates should be between 90 and 100 percent *after* write-offs are taken. If net collection rates are low, a more in-depth evaluation of your business practices might be warranted.

Write-Offs

Write-offs are charges that are deemed uncollectible by any business. In the medical setting, for example, a bad debt write-off would be if a patient owes the office $200, and the patient dies unexpectedly, leaving the remaining balance of $200 uncollectible. There are various types of write-offs, and each write-off should be identified by type, such as bad debt, professional courtesy discounts, contractual discounts, and so on. Professional courtesy discounts and other discounts are credited, usually, by using special codes created by your practice. Each code is specific for each type of write-off. This enables your office to track the categories in which most of the write-offs have occurred. The providers in the practice should remain involved in monitoring the write-off activities for the group on an ongoing basis to ensure that inappropriate insurance denials are not routinely being written off in error.

Cost Ratio

The **cost ratio** formula demonstrates the cost of a specific procedure or service. This value helps identify the cost effectiveness of a service offered at the office. For instance, maintaining radiology services in a medical facility: Would it be cost-effective to continue this service in-house or to have patients go outside for radiological services? This cost ratio formula is:

Total Expenses ÷ Total Number of Procedures for One Month = Cost Ratio

EXAMPLE

Cost Ratio Using Simple Amounts

- The total radiology expenses for August were $100,000.
- The total number of procedures performed for August was 250.
- Plugging those numbers into the cost ratio formula: $100,000 (total radiology expenses for August) ÷ 250 (total number of procedures performed for August)
- $100,000 ÷ 250 = $400 (cost ratio)

The total radiology expenses can include the expenses of the radiology technologist and radiologist salaries, equipment usage, radiology products and supplies, and office space rental. Let's say each procedure is billed at $250; this would conclude that radiology services provided in this office is much too costly because it is costing the office $400 per procedure. In this case, this would be a $150 loss per procedure ($400 – $250 = $150). Bear in mind, this is for one month. A decision to maintain the services in-house should be made over a period of months to see a better picture of an actual loss or gain for the office.

A multitude of affordable software packages can calculate all these ratios at your fingertips. These figures may be converted and displayed in bar graph and chart formats for you to present to your office management team and doctors so appropriate decisions may be made for the financial benefit of the medical facility.

Cost–Benefit Analysis

Cost–benefit analysis allows for program evaluation by demonstrating whether the benefits received outweigh its costs. Considering a doctor's office, this analysis is part of good budgeting and accounting practices and enables management teams to determine the true cost of providing services. This is used because it is considered a simpler accounting cost analysis for lack of a better alternative. Although simplistic in the accounting world, there is still much involved with cost–benefit analysis and would likely be the responsibility of an accountant. Again, software packages are available for calculations of these involved methods. A basic idea of cost–benefit analysis involves three steps:

- Identify costs (one-time costs and recurring costs)
- Identify benefits (tangible benefits and intangible benefits)
- Compare costs and benefits (net present value method and payback method)

Again, pulling these values together is likely to be the accountant's responsibility to produce for the providers and office management team; however, it is your responsibility to ensure that these numbers are accurately reflected in your financial software program or in filed financial records.

FINANCIAL RECORDS

To calculate the various ratios discussed in this chapter, accurate **financial records** must be maintained by the office; these financial records reflect its financial status. The two most common financial statements are the income statement and the balance sheet. Both of these financial records are likely to be computerized with the use of a software package purchased for your medical facility.

Income Statement

An **income statement** demonstrates the profit and expenses for a given month and includes year-to-date information for a given year. Information found on this statement includes:

- Revenue (A/R for patient payments and other outside sources)
- Overhead expenses (office and medical supplies, lab fees, postage, utilities, office space rental, occupancy insurance, property taxes, janitorial services)
- Provider's compensation and benefits (payroll, bonuses, benefits, retirement plan, seminars, uniforms, professional expenses)
- Employees' compensation and benefits (payroll, bonuses, benefits, retirement plans, malpractice insurance, seminars, uniforms)
- Marketing expenses
- Outside resources (accounting, legal, consulting, retirement plan administration)
- Withholding taxes

Figure 20–3 shows a sample income statement, which is the most commonly generated year-end report.

Balance Sheet

The **balance sheet**, also known as a statement of financial position, reveals a company's assets, liabilities, and owner's **equity** (net worth). The purpose of the balance sheet is to give users an idea of the medical facility's financial position along with a picture of what the company owns and owes. These summary numbers come from information entered in a financial software system or information found on documents of financial records.

A medical office can display a balance sheet in various ways. One way is to show the assets on the left side of the balance sheet with the liabilities and equity shown on the right side of the sheet, as Figure 20–4A shows. Other balance sheets are displayed as report forms, which show assets at the top, followed by liabilities and equity at the bottom, as seen in Figure 20–4B. Balance sheets are often more detailed than the basic examples shown in these figures. Many times, balance sheets separate assets and liabilities into long-term and short-term categories.

The changes in assets and liabilities you might find on the balance sheet are also reflected in the revenues and expenses you see on the income statement, which result in the office's gains or losses. No one financial statement tells the complete story; however, examining these tools together might provide very powerful information from which your providers and management team can make decisions on financial matters.

Practice Income Statement	Month of ______, 20xx	Year-to-Date	Budget for Year	Overhead Percentages
Revenue				
A. Revenue				
Office 1	$	$	$	$
Office 2	$	$	$	$
B. Total Revenue:				
Expenses				
C. Expenses				
Non-provider (staff) salaries, gross	$	$	$	$
Staff fringes				
Payroll taxes	$	$	$	$
Employment benefits	$	$	$	$
Employment seminars	$	$	$	$
Uniforms	$	$	$	$
Retirement plans	$	$	$	$
Occupancy costs				
Rent, Office 1	$	$	$	$
Rent, Office 2	$	$	$	$
Property taxes	$	$	$	$
Insurance	$	$	$	$
Utilities	$	$	$	$
Janitor/grounds	$	$	$	$
Medical expenses				
Medications	$	$	$	$
Supplies	$	$	$	$
Lab Fees	$	$	$	$
Office expenses				
Office supplies	$	$	$	$
Postage	$	$	$	$
Telephone/Internet	$	$	$	$
Malpractice insurance	$	$	$	$
Professional expenses				
Auto expenses (provider)	$	$	$	$
Dues/subscriptions	$	$	$	$
Books and videos	$	$	$	$
Memberships	$	$	$	$
Entertainment	$	$	$	$
Professional development	$	$	$	$
Travel	$	$	$	$

Figure 20–3: Sample income statement. *Delmar/Cengage Learning.* (*continues*)

Equipment costs				
Depreciation/amoritization	$	$	$	$
Rent	$	$	$	$
Service/maintenance	$	$	$	$
Interest	$	$	$	$
Marketing expenses				
Advertising	$	$	$	$
Other fees	$	$	$	$
Professional Expenses				
Accounting	$	$	$	$
Legal	$	$	$	$
Consulting	$	$	$	$
Retirement plan admin.	$	$	$	$
D. Total Non-Provider Expenses	$	$	$	$
Operating New Income Before Providers' Costs				
E. Operating New Income Before Providers' Costs (B minus C)	$	$	$	$
Associate Providers' Costs				
F. Associate Providers' Costs				
Salaries, gross	$	$	$	$
Benefits	$	$	$	$
-	$	$	$	$
-	$	$	$	$
G. Total Non-Owner Providers' Costs	$	$	$	$
New Income Available to Owner-Providers				
H. New Income Available to Owner-Providers (E minus G)	$	$	$	$
Owner-Providers' Costs				
I. Owner-Providers' Costs				
Salaries, gross				
Dr. X	$	$	$	$
Dr. Y	$	$	$	$
Bonuses, gross				
Dr. X	$	$	$	$
Dr. Y	$	$	$	$
Retirement contributions				
Dr. X	$	$	$	$
Dr. Y	$	$	$	$
Semi-personal expenses				
Dr. X	$	$	$	$
Dr. Y	$	$	$	$
J. Total Owner-Provider Costs	$	$	$	$
Net Income				
K. Net Income (H minus J)	$	$	$	$

Figure 20–3: Sample income statement. *Delmar/Cengage Learning.*

ABC Medical Office
Balance Sheet
June 30, 20XX

Assets		**Liabilities**	
Cash	$7,000.00	Accounts Payable	$2,000.00
Inventory	500.00	**Owner's Equity**	
Land	6,500.00	John Doe, capital	12,000.00
Total Assets	**$14,000.00**	**Total liabilities and owner's equity (net worth)**	**$14,000.00**

(A)

ABC Medical Office
Balance Sheet
June 30, 20XX

Assets	
Cash	$7000.00
Inventory	500.00
Land	6,500.00
Total Assets	**$14,000.00**
Liabilities	
Accounts Payable	$2,000.00
Owner's Equity	
John Doe, capital	$12,000.00
Total liabilities and owner's equity	**$14,000.00**

(B)

Figure 20–4: Two different balance sheet formats. *Delmar/Cengage Learning.*

CHAPTER SUMMARY

- Accounts payable, also known as A/P or payables, refers to the total amounts owed by the practice to suppliers and other service providers for regular business operating expenses.
- Expenditure is acquired material, property, and labor in exchange for money.
- An invoice is a document that includes itemization of goods and purchases or services provided together with the charges and terms of the agreement.
- The following are required fields of an invoice: company details, invoice number, dates (initiation and due dates), client details, fees, and payment terms.
- Petty cash is a small amount of stored cash ranging from $25 to $75, often used for postage stamps, inexpensive office supplies, and small charitable donations.
- A voucher form or expenditure list should be completed each time payment is made from the petty cash fund.
- Two integral aspects of accounting are operating information and managerial accounting information.
- Operating information is needed on a day-to-day basis for a company to conduct business.
- Managerial accounting, also known as cost accounting, is the study and analysis of financial data as it applies to operational issues within a company.
- The basis for all financial accounting is the accounting formula. This basic accounting formula is

  Assets − Liabilities = Net Worth.
- The accounts receivable ratio or A/R ratio formula, when calculated, helps you understand how quickly outstanding accounts are paid as well as the effectiveness of the office collection process.
- The two types of collection ratios are gross collection ratio and net collection ratio.

- The cost ratio formula demonstrates the cost of a specific procedure or service.
- Cost–benefit analysis enables program evaluation by demonstrating whether the benefits received outweigh its costs.
- Write-offs are charges that are deemed uncollectible by any business.
- The two most common financial statements are the income statement and the balance sheet.

STUDY TOOLS

Workbook	Activities for Chapter 20
Premium Website	
StudyWARE	Activities and Quizzes on the **StudyWARE™ Software** for Chapter 20
	Audio Library of medical terms
	Online access to the **Critical Thinking Challenge 2.0**
learninglab	Module 9: Banking and Accounting Procedures
CourseMate	Activities and Quizzes for Chapter 20
WebTutor	Activities and Quizzes for Chapter 20

CHECK YOUR KNOWLEDGE

1. The R in A/R stands for ____________ and the "P" in A/P stands for ____________.
   a. receipts, purchases
   b. receipts, payable
   c. receivable, payable
   d. receivable, purchases
2. This type of accounting is the study and analysis of financial data as it applies to operational issues within a company.
   a. Managerial accounting
   b. Operational accounting
   c. Cost ratio accounting
   d. Expenditure accounting
3. All the following is information contained on an invoice, except:
   a. company details
   b. invoice details
   c. packing slip
   d. fees
4. Another term for net worth is:
   a. owner's equity.
   b. assets.
   c. financial position.
   d. gross collections.
5. This ratio is calculated by dividing the total payments for a specific period of time by the total charges, *with* the write-offs deducted from the total charges.
   a. Cost ratio
   b. Accounts receivable ratio
   c. Gross collection ratio
   d. Net collection ratio
6. This demonstrates the profit and expenses for a given month and includes year-to-date information for a given year.
   a. Balance sheet
   b. Income statement
   c. Cost–benefit analysis
   d. Net worth
7. These are debts or accounts payable (A/P) owed by the business.
   a. Assets
   b. Liabilities
   c. Owners equity
   d. Cost ratio

WEB LINKS

American Academy of Medical Management: www.epracticemanagement.org

Bankers Training and Consulting Company: www.btcc.com

RESOURCES

Averkamp, Harold. "*Explanations for 30 Accounting Topics*." www.AccountingCoach.com. (Retrieved 11/11/2010)

Lindh, W., Pooler, M., Tamparo, C., and Dahl, B. (2010). *Comprehensive Medical Assisting: Administrative and Clinical Competencies* (4th ed.). Clifton Park, NY: Delmar, Cengage Learning.

Unit

10

Managing the Medical Office Environment

As a medical assistant, you will be called upon in numerous capacities and assist your provider in many aspects of the medical practice. These duties include facilities management and emergency preparedness. You must take an active role in not only the day-to-day patient care activities but in planning and preparing the facility for smooth and seamless operations during normal and emergency situations. Many of the procedures you need to follow fall under regulatory compliance of a variety of agencies. You must familiarize yourself with policies, procedures, and regulations (such as for OSHA) and create, implement, and participate in employee training programs.

Many duties performed in a medical office can be categorized under the broad classification of general management duties. This unit identifies a wide range of duties to acquaint you with those behind-the-scenes activities needed to operate a successful medical practice efficiently.

A medical assistant is expected to exercise leadership, professionalism, and good judgment. It is critical to understand management duties because every medical assistant holds some type of leadership role. You could be a manager, supervisor, office coordinator, super-user, or designated to any other administrative role.

Certification Connection

	Ch. 21	Ch. 22
CMA (AAMA)		
The physical environment	X	
Maintaining liability coverage		X
Equipment and supply inventory	X	
Time management		X
RMA (AMT)		
Employee payroll		X
Financial mathematics		X
Supplies and equipment management	X	X
Office safety	X	
CMAS (AMT)		
Human resources		X
Office communication		X
Business organization management		X
Physical office plant	X	X
Risk management and quality assurance	X	X
Business organization management		X
Safety	X	
Supplies and equipment		X

Chapter 21

Facilities Management and Emergency Preparedness

OBJECTIVES

In this chapter, you will learn the following:

KB KNOWLEDGE BASE

1. Spell and define, using the glossary at the back of the text, all the Words to Know in this chapter.
2. Name things to check to ensure safety in the reception area, at the front desk, and in examination and lab rooms.
3. List tasks to perform to prepare the front desk for the day.
4. List key elements of procedures to close a medical office.
5. List and describe the governmental agencies and regulations involved in the promotion of safety and security in the health care industry as presented in this chapter.
6. Identify and comply with safety signs, symbols, and labels.
7. Describe the importance of Materials Safety Data Sheets (MSDS) in the health care setting.
8. List safety hazards of spills (dropped objects) and identify six items that are considered to be protective barriers to prevent skin and mucous membrane exposure to pathogens.
9. Discuss requirements for responding to hazardous material disposal.
10. Name three elements necessary for fire and list ways a fire might start.
11. Discuss potential roles of the medical assistant in emergency preparedness.
12. Discuss critical elements of an emergency plan for response to a natural disaster or other emergency.
13. Identify emergency preparedness plans in your community.
14. Recognize the effects of stress on all persons involved in emergency situations.
15. List evacuation procedures for emergencies.

S SKILLS

1. Maintain medical facility.
2. Evaluate the work environment to identify safe versus unsafe working conditions.
3. Perform an inventory of supplies.
4. Select appropriate barrier/personal protective equipment (PPE) for potentially infectious situations
5. Respond to and document a mock exposure event.
6. Develop a personal safety plan and an environmental safety plan.
7. Demonstrate methods of fire prevention in the health care setting.
8. Demonstrate proper use of a fire extinguisher.

B BEHAVIORS

1. Demonstrate self-awareness in responding to emergency situations.

WORDS TO KNOW

assault
atmosphere
barrier
biohazard
emergency
emergency preparedness
environment
evacuated
extinguisher
hazard
intervention
inventory
irrational
materials safety data sheet (MSDS)
prevention
reception
threshold
volatile

OPENING THE OFFICE

Staff should arrive at the office in time to make preparations for receiving patients (Figure 21–1). A well-prepared, organized, and tidy office **environment** is immediately noticed by patients, providers, and visitors. The surroundings set the tone for the office and the first impression and level of professionalism anticipated. Preparation procedures can differ according to the type of practice, number of providers, weekly schedules, and many other variables. A checklist, specific to your office, should be created and followed to ensure that you cover all daily functions of opening, operating, and closing the office. Before the first patient arrives, several things need attention. Procedure 21–1 addresses many of these tasks.

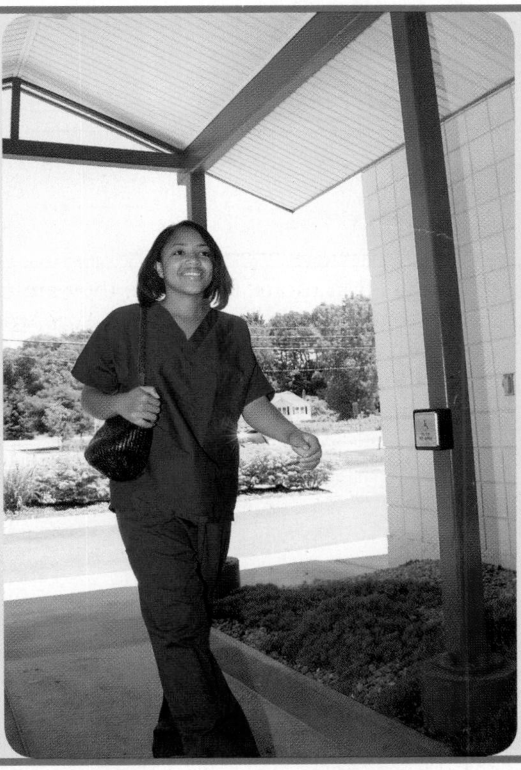

Figure 21–1: The medical assistant arrives at work. *Delmar/Cengage Learning.*

Security in the Medical Office

Safety and security is of high concern in a medical office. A criminal can target cash from daily receipts or drugs kept on site. Unfortunately, physical or sexual **assault** can also occur when the interior office is accessible from unlocked outside access or the reception area. The U.S. Department of Justice, Civil Rights Division, National Task Force on Violence Against Health Care Providers has recommended that medical facilities "install dead bolt locks on office doors leading to hallways and other public areas, consider installing a 'buzzer' entry door system (on door between waiting room or reception area and examination rooms or office areas) [and] managers should issue and control keys, conduct semi-annual inventories, and have locks changed when keys are missing." These locks provide a degree of security. Any opening between two areas, such as a window, should also be fitted with a security device to prevent unauthorized access. If there are private entry doors, be certain they are kept locked at all times. If you must enter or leave the office when dark, be especially alert. The outside area should be well lit. If building security people are available, ask for an escort.

Many offices are equipped with electronic security systems. In addition to the private records of patients, they contain many valuable items (computers and medical and office equipment), cash receipts, drugs, and medications. Systems can vary from keypad entry with alarm to a sophisticated alarm with camera system. If you are the first staff member to arrive at work, it will be necessary to enter the code before opening the door or enter the code on an internal key pad before the entrance delay period expires. Both these systems lend a feeling of safety and security, but, be aware: It takes only a few seconds for someone to grab your purse or wallet or force you to hand over office money or drugs. Never enter the office if you see evidence of forced entry or if it appears that someone might either be inside or has been inside. Leave at once and call building security or the police.

PROCEDURE 21–1 Open the Office and Evaluate for Safety

PURPOSE: Role-play the actions necessary to prepare a medical office to see patients.

EQUIPMENT: A simulated office, if available; in a classroom or lab setting, role-play, explaining the procedure

S **SKILL:** Maintain medical facility.

S **SKILL:** Evaluate the work environment to identify safe versus unsafe working conditions.

Procedure Steps	Detailed Instructions and/or *Rationales*
1. Unlock the reception room door.	
2. Evaluate and prepare the reception room for cleanliness, comfort, and safety.	• Adjust heat or air conditioning. • Check for safety hazards: Check for frayed electric wires, damaged furniture, or objects on the floor that might cause patients to fall. • Check magazines for condition and date.
3. Prepare the front desk area.	• Turn on computers, printers, and scanners. • Check the telephone answering device or call the answering service for any messages.
4. *If working in a paper-based office*: Pull the charts of patients to be seen. Check each patient's previous visit to see whether any studies were ordered and place results into chart. *If working in an EHR office*: Review the patient schedule, check for previously ordered studies, and scan to chart. (Provide original copy to provider for review and validation prior to scanning.)	Check the patient's previous visit to see whether any studies were ordered and attach to (or place into) chart. *Results must be filed in the chart before the patient is seen.*
5. If it is the policy of the office, prepare a list (or print from electronic system) of the patients to be seen and the times of their appointments and place copies in designated areas.	
6. Inspect and prepare exam and lab rooms for cleanliness and safety.	• Check examination rooms to be sure they are clean, safe, and stocked with supplies. *Check exam rooms in case the provider saw a patient after office hours.* • Fill and turn on sterilizer. • Prepare hazardous waste disposal containers.
7. List three to five safe working conditions identified: 1. ____________________ 2. ____________________ 3. ____________________ 4. ____________________ 5. ____________________	

8. List three to five unsafe working conditions identified:

1. ______________________________

2. ______________________________

3. ______________________________

4. ______________________________

5. ______________________________

Evaluating the Reception Area

A safe environment begins at the front door. The **reception** room requires a safety check every morning to ensure that it presents no hazards for patients and visitors:

- *Observe the physical environment of the reception room.* Studies have shown that the reception room **atmosphere** can be an **intervention** or a reflection of the encounter, which can affect the outcome of the office visit. Atmosphere affects how people experience their environment and can have a relationship to their response to treatment.
- *Check the temperature.* The room temperature should ensure the patients' comfort.
- *Look at the room's appearance* (Figure 21–2). The presence of large plants and attractive paintings soften the office environment. The choice of color and lighting affects behavior. Soft colors and subdued light are calming. The use of relaxing background music has become commonplace in medical and dental offices. Aquariums can provide diversion and an enjoyable bubbling sound. Try standing in the reception room and looking around. Be conscious of the sights, sounds, and even smells you perceive.
- *Observe the condition of the furniture carefully.* Pay attention to chair and table legs—they must be stable and able to support appropriate weight.
- *Perform a safety check.* Remember to make a daily visual check of electrical devices, furniture, floors, and lighting before any patients arrive. Lamps and electrical cords should be examined. Bulbs should not dim or flicker, and cords should be in good condition with no evidence of fraying. Be sure lighting is adequate. Check the floor to be certain there are no carpet wrinkles or tears or anything lying on the floor that might cause someone to fall. Do not use decorative or throw rugs.
- *Check the reading material.* Neatly arrange magazines. Clean and sanitize reading materials that are shared by patients. Make them accessible in several seating areas. Remove torn and outdated material. Many providers have a prepared brochure that describes their practice, discusses the office policies, and provides information regarding appointments, office hours, and other useful details. An assortment of informative, health-related pamphlets may also be offered in a display rack. Copies of professional medical journals or similar technical material are not appropriate for general display.
- *Check the toys and books.* If children's toys or books are provided, they require constant monitoring. All toys should be washable and of a safe design and material with no sharp edges or parts small enough for a child to swallow. The toys should be cleaned and sanitized regularly. During daily inspection, remove any broken or visibly soiled toys or books.

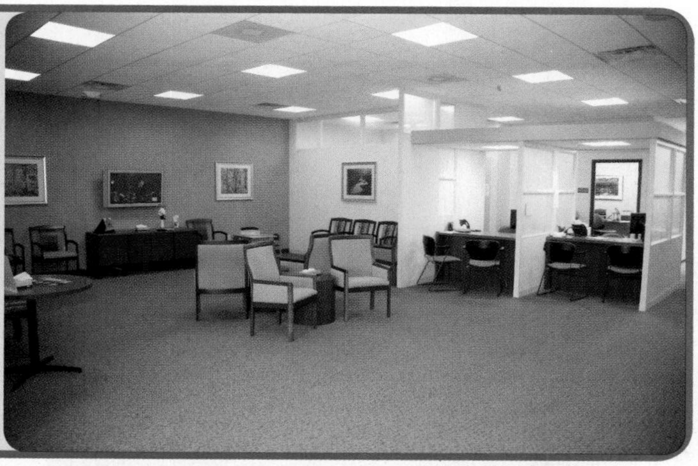

Figure 21–2: The reception area should appear pleasant, clean, and well maintained. *Delmar/Cengage Learning.*

If at all possible, the children's play area should be situated in a corner or within a half-walled space to contain things within a controlled area to reduce the possibility of adults falling over objects on the floor. In pediatricians' offices, there are usually two reception rooms, or at least a room with a separate section, each with its own play area. One is considered the well area, and the other is the "sick" area to separate children with fevers, coughs, nausea and vomiting, diarrhea, and other disease conditions from the well children.

- *Display the smoking policy.* Be certain the Smoke-Free sign is displayed and that it is enforced.

Preparing the Front Desk

When preparing the front desk at the beginning of the day:

- *Turn on computers, scanners, printers (and other electronic equipment).* Offices with electronic health records (EHR) must have all computers and tablets operational before the first patient can be checked in and encounter started.
- *Retrieve telephone messages.* Retrieve and record all messages on the answering machine. If an outside service is used, call and obtain the messages.
- *Retrieve faxes.* Sort per office protocol.
- *Retrieve printed lab and hospital reports.* Sort per office protocol.
- *Place charts for check-in.* At least one day before, you should pull charts (or review schedule if EHR) and look at the appointment book or run a hard copy from the computer of all patients who have appointments that day. You will need to attach reports of any previously ordered studies (labs, consults) to the chart. Have materials ready for initiating charts for scheduled new patients. This process should be done at least the day before to reduce morning preparation duties. Many offices like to post a copy of the day's schedule and place it on the provider's desk for his or her personal use and reference.
- *Prepare sign-in sheets, cash balance forms, and so on.* Have daily forms available along with pens and other basic equipment.

CLINICAL PEARL

When working in the receptionist or business office area during the day, pay special attention to file drawers and cupboard doors. NEVER open more than one file drawer in a vertical file at a time because the unbalanced weight could cause the cabinet to tip forward. You could sustain a back or extremity injury from the automatic reaction to catch a cabinet. Also, be careful with opened bottom drawers, which can easily be tripped over. Wall cupboards pose another safety hazard. If the door is left open, you could strike your head quite forcefully when you stand up or rise up from underneath. All electrical cords must be kept behind desks and other office furnishings so that they cannot be tripped over. All equipment should operate properly and show no evidence of electrical shorts or damage.

Inspecting Examination Rooms and Lab Areas

At the beginning of the day, visually inspect all rooms for cleanliness (Figure 21–3). Even if they were cleaned the previous day, the provider might have seen a patient after hours. Replace examining paper and be certain waste receptacles are emptied. Observe room temperature and plug in any disconnected electrical equipment. Be certain everything is in working condition. Restock

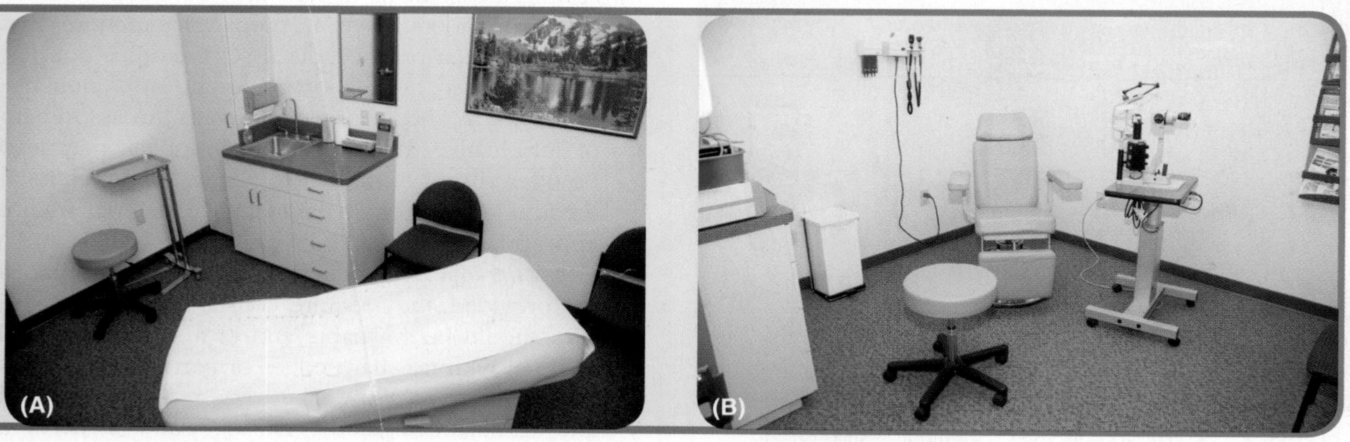

Figure 21–3: (A) Examination room. (B) Procedure room. *Delmar/Cengage Learning.*

supplies so that needed materials are available. Maintain an inventory control sheet (check list) and select a set day of the week as restocking day. Of course, you will restock as necessary on a daily basis.

Check common areas for cleanliness and be certain everything is in order. Check the water level in the autoclave and turn it on. Be sure hazardous waste disposal containers are available for use in all areas where needed.

During the course of the day, the examination table must be cleaned after each patient. The table must operate properly, and you must be thoroughly competent in its use. Assist patients as necessary to sit or lie on the table. If the use of a stool is necessary, be especially cautious to guard against the patient's stepping on the edges, which could cause it to tip. Very ill patients, elderly patients, and children should not be left alone on an examination table from which they could fall.

Children, and some adults, also have a natural curiosity about things in the examination room cabinets or on counters. Anything that might be hazardous or could become contaminated should be kept out of sight. Prescription pads should not be left lying around; they should be kept in a secure, locked area. Secure all electrical cords in the examination rooms so that they will not interfere with movement or walking in the room.

Chemicals kept in the office for laboratory work must be properly labeled and stored. Chemicals that could become **volatile** when kept beyond their expiration date must be monitored carefully. Testing patients' urine, blood, and other specimens requires special procedures. Containers for the disposal of used equipment and **biohazardous** waste must be readily accessible. A strict adherence to standard precautions is essential to the maintenance of a safe and healthy lab environment.

Supply Inventory

The office manager or, in some offices, the medical assistant is expected to maintain an **inventory** of clinical and administrative supplies. Some of your duties can include inventory and ordering of office (clerical) supplies, clinic supplies (exam room orders), and medication orders. Careful monitoring of inventory is vital. You do not want to run out of needed supplies, yet you also do not want to over-order items, especially because many can have an expiration date and are often quite costly. Good inventory control and cost comparison is essential in your position. Be sure to coordinate your activities with the provider to avoid duplication and to be aware of any updates or changes to items or medications.

A minimum amount of supplies to be maintained should be determined and will depend on the type of office practice and the number of patients seen on an average day, known as a **threshold** (sometimes referred to as par level). It would be better to err on excess than not have adequate supply. All staff should sign out for supplies and medications so an accurate inventory can be kept (Figure 21–4). Some offices perform this function electronically with the use of scanners and bar codes (Figure 21–5).

Maintain a binder with current information and create an electronic file system using spreadsheets (for example, Microsoft Excel) to track your inventory and purchases. Keep a current list of all the suppliers of goods and services compiled by category, such as administrative, laboratory, clinical, and general. By using a spreadsheet, you can sort this information and create an alphabetical list as well. Entries of vendors (businesses) should name the company, the address and phone number, and a contact person if possible. A list of what products or services they provide should be entered for each company.

Some items require special storage, such as a locked cabinet for narcotics or refrigeration for some laboratory items and medications (Figure 21–6). All items need to be inventoried or counted on a regular basis to be sure adequate supply is on hand to operate the office. If items are time sensitive (date expirations), store in order of expiration, with the first to expire in front. Discard expired items properly. If your office uses linens requiring laundering, be sure to factor in the turnaround time with getting fresh linens delivered.

ITEM	QUANTITY	REORDER POINT	LOCATION
Black felt-tip pens	6 bx. 5 4 3 2 1	2	Drawer #2
9 x 12 manila file folders (center cut)	6 bx. 5 4 3 2 1	2	Cupboard #4
Blue adhesive file folder labels	8 bx. 7 6 5 4 3 2 1	5	Cupboard #4
3" center metal fasteners	6 bx. 5 4 3 2 1	3	Drawer #3

Figure 21–4: Inventory card for office supplies. *Delmar/Cengage Learning.*

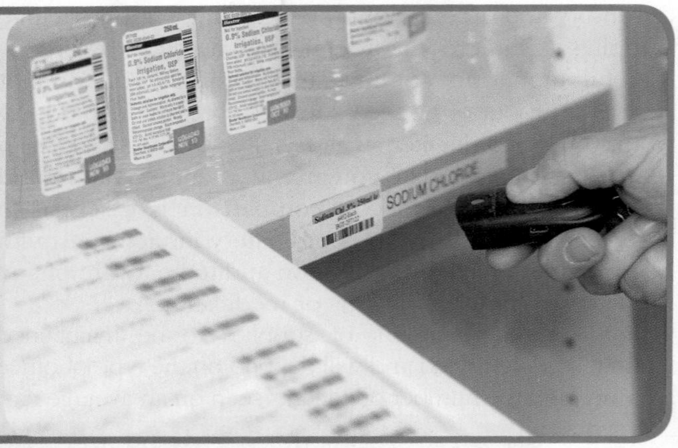

Figure 21–5: In an electronic system, the bar code is scanned when an item is removed from the storage area. *Delmar/Cengage Learning.*

An example of a small practice supply to be used to check supplies for an examination room might look something like Figure 21–7. It could include the date and initials of the person performing the inventory. By noting the items on hand, it is easy to see what needs to be ordered. After completing the form, give it to the person responsible for ordering supplies. Procedure 21–2 describes performing a basic inventory of supplies.

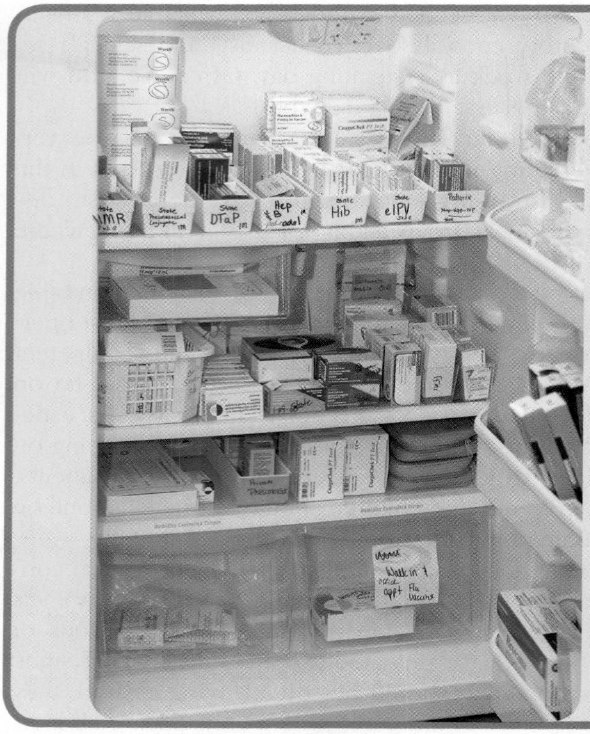

Figure 21–6: Refrigerator with medications and immunizations. *Delmar/Cengage Learning.*

Examination Room Supply Inventory

Date: 6-28-20XX Taken by: G Stone, MA

	Item	Supply minimum	Amount on hand	Place order
1.	Table paper	2 Rolls	1	✓
2.	Cover sheets	1 Box	2	
3.	Pillow covers	2 Boxes	2	
4.	Examination vests	1 Box	1 1/2	
5.	Examination gowns	1 Box	0	✓
6.	Tissues	6 Boxes	10	
7.	Examination gloves	2 Boxes	4	
8.	Alcohol wipes	2 Boxes	1	✓
9.	Otoscope covers	2 Boxes	3	

Figure 21–7: Sample supply inventory checklist. *Delmar/Cengage Learning.*

PROCEDURE 21–2 Perform an Inventory of Supplies

PURPOSE: Perform a supply inventory; arrange any items that are time sensitive in front; count the number of items in storage and accurately record on the list.

EQUIPMENT: Clipboard, supply inventory checklist, paper, and pen

S SKILL: Perform an inventory of supplies.

Procedure Steps	Detailed Instructions and/or *Rationales*
1. Enter the date on the form.	
2. Check the package dates on time-sensitive materials. Arrange the supplies with the first to expire in front.	
3. Count each category of items on the inventory list and complete the form.	• Enter the number of items left in storage in the appropriate place. • Note on the form the supplies below the minimum amount. • Sign the form.
4. Give the completed form to the appropriate person to order supplies (if you are not the designated person).	

CLOSING THE OFFICE

At the end of the day, the examination rooms should be restocked and cleaned, and discarded material should be placed for pickup. This saves time the next morning. Charts must be collected, checked for completeness, and filed in a locked cabinet. If there is not time to file, place charts in a separate area (basket, file cabinet, and so on) designated for charts to be filed and place them in the cabinet to be filed the next day. Some doctors dictate their notes, which must first be typed onto the chart before it can be filed. EHR offices will reduce (or eliminate) the use of paper charts and the file-back required.

All electrical appliances and the autoclave must be turned off, including computers. If you are using a network computer system supported by a larger health care facility or IT department, you need to know the requirements for computer shutdown at the end of the day. It is the office manager's responsibility to confirm (or develop) IT policy concerning computer usage and enforce compliance that is so critical to patient privacy and HIPAA guidelines, and it is each staff member's responsibility to follow this policy. At the very least, all providers and staff will be required to log off all applications and software programs at day's end. In some cases, the computer may be left powered on for patches and updates to be pushed through.

Receipts collected during the day can be taken to the bank for deposit or locked in the office safe. Tidy the reception area and sanitize it. (If you have a cleaning service, be sure to inspect for proper cleaning of the entire office suite and report any deficiencies.) Pull and prepare charts for the next day. Place lab, consultations, and hospital reports with the charts and then place at the front desk (reception area) for check-in.

Always take a walk through the office to complete your checklist of things to do (see Procedure 21–3). Activate your answering system, securely lock all the doors and windows, close blinds, activate the alarm system, and turn off the lights. Be aware of your surroundings as you leave the office. Try always to leave with a coworker, rather than leave alone, for safety reasons. If you must leave the office after dark or alone, ask a building attendant for assistance if available.

SAFETY IN THE MEDICAL OFFICE

The medical office, like the home, is a place that should feel safe and secure. But just like a home, it takes conscious effort to ensure that the office has a protective, healthy environment. As a medical assistant, you are a vital part of the team responsible for recognizing any safety, security, or operational **hazards**; helping eliminate them; and warning coworkers and patients of any dangers.

PROCEDURE 21–3 Close the Office

PURPOSE: Role-play the actions required to close the office.

EQUIPMENT: A simulated office if available; otherwise, role-play, explaining the procedure

S SKILL: Maintain the medical facility.

Procedure Steps	Detailed Instructions and/or *Rationales*
1. Check to see that records are collected and filed in locked cabinets.	
2. Place any money in the safe or take to the bank to be deposited.	
3. Turn off all electrical appliances and computers.	Many offices also ask you to unplug electrical appliances. *Eliminates the chance of electrical fire.* Note: Depending on your IT support center, computers might need to be left turned on but logged off so that software patches and updates can be installed.
4. Check that rooms are cleaned and supplied for the next day. Straighten reception room if time allows.	
5. *For paper offices*: Pull charts for the next day if time allows and prep with lab reports, consults, or available hospital reports. *For paperless offices (EHR)*: Review the next day's schedule for previously ordered studies. Scan to patient EHR chart; provide original to provider for review and validation prior to scanning.	
6. Activate the answering device on the phone or notify the answering service and indicate when you will be back in the office.	
7. Close and lock all access doors to office. Check that all windows are closed and locked and blinds shut. Turn off lights. Activate alarm system if available.	
8. Set the lock and close the door; check to ensure that it is locked.	

You should be able to evaluate the work environment to identify safe versus unsafe working conditions. Some examples of evaluating the work environment can include:

- Using a checklist, perform a safety inspection at your facility at intervals according to institution policy and preparing a report on the findings. Figure 21–8 shows a checklist of some of the safety considerations in a medical office.
- Verifying that needlestick prevention devices (safety needles) are used and proper disposal is performed.

Care should be taken to make the whole office accident-proof. If anyone is injured in the medical office, no matter how insignificant it might seem, you must have the individual examined by the provider. If the patient should claim he or she was not injured and refuse examination, the incident must still be care-

ITEM	YES	NO	N/A	ACTION REQUIRED
General Safety				
Are all walking surfaces clean, clear of debris, and dry?				
Are stairs, steps, and handrails in good condition?				
Are all rooms well lit?				
Is all furniture in a good state of repair?				
Exam Room Safety				
Are all surfaces clean and disinfected?				
Are all sharps containers in proper locations and not filled past the "fill line"?				
Is the eyewash station in working order?				
Is the room appropriately stocked with supplies?				
Are biohazard containers properly marked?				
Chemical Safety				
Are all hazardous chemicals are stored properly?				
Are all chemicals are properly labeled?				
Is PPE readily available and accessible for all employees?				
Evacuation Safety				
Are exits properly identified and lighted?				
Are exit paths clear, and all exit doors operable?				
Are evacuation floor plans posted?				
Fire Safety				
Are fire extinguishers available and serviced annually?				
Do smoke, heat & other detection alarm systems work?				
Are flammable items properly stored in cabinets?				
Is there any evidence of electrical wiring overheating, blown fuses, frayed cords, or worn insulation?				

Figure 21–8: Safety inspection checklist (partial). *Delmar/Cengage Learning.*

fully recorded on his or her chart and the refusal of care noted. The quality assurance (QA) (also known as risk management) department might require any type of accident to be reported on an Unusual Occurrence Report form. Some providers might require a signed release of responsibility to protect against a later claim of injury. Documenting incident reports are discussed further in Chapter 36.

The medical office environment must ensure the health and safety of the provider, staff, and all persons being treated as well as those accompanying them. This refers not only to the physical surroundings in the office but also to the general maintenance of the facility, the mechanical condition of the equipment, and the procedures used to control the presence of harmful microorganisms.

Federal and State Regulations

For the protection of employers and employees, federal and state agencies have established legislation dealing with policies, procedures, and guidelines to reduce disease transmission. A number of governmental agencies and regulations are involved in the promotion of safety and security in the health care industry, such as the Occupational Safety and Health Administration (OSHA), the Centers for Disease Control and Prevention (CDC), the Americans with Disabilities Act (ADA), the Clinical Laboratory Improvement Amendments (CLIA), and fire regulations.

OSHA

The United States Department of Labor established regulations through OSHA that require employers to provide employees with safe working conditions to protect them from harmful exposure and substances. An example of this regulation is the provision of protective gloves to safeguard employees during patient contact. There are mandatory reporting requirements and compliance provisions. More information can be found in Chapter 36 and online at OSHA's website, www.osha.gov.

CDC

The United States Public Health Department operates the CDC in Atlanta, Georgia. It is the CDC's responsibility to collect data on pathogens and diseases and establish guidelines to prevent their spread. The CDC has developed a system of classifications or categories of infectious diseases related to their method of spread. It was this agency that established guidelines concerning contact with blood and body fluids, referred to as universal precautions. These guidelines were developed to control the spread of hepatitis and AIDS. Universal precautions have since been incorporated into guidelines called standard precautions. These expanded precautions are set infection control guidelines to be used by all health care professionals when caring for patients. Standard precautions are discussed in more depth in Chapter 36. Additional information can be found on the CDC's Website, www.cdc.gov.

ADA

The American with Disabilities Act (ADA) is enforced by the United States Department of Justice. Regulations affecting medical offices can be found on its Website, www.ada.gov. You should include ADA on your list of safety and planning resources. It offers a guide to disability rights laws, ADA question and answers, medications, guide for small businesses, and regulations.

An example of an ADA requirement is to protect its citizenry from harm, including helping people prepare for and respond to emergencies. Making local government emergency preparedness and response programs accessible to people with disabilities is a critical part of this responsibility. Another requirement is to identify accessible modes of transportation that might be available to help evacuate people with disabilities during an emergency. For instance, during floods, some communities have used lift-equipped school or transit buses to evacuate people who use wheelchairs.

CLIA

The Clinical Laboratory Improvement Amendments (CLIA) of 1988 established federal regulatory standards regulating all laboratory testing (except research) performed on humans in the United States. This governmental agency also establishes regulations for the safety of patients and health care workers. It is their responsibility to ensure that the public is safeguarded by regulating all testing of specimens coming from the human body. All clinical laboratories must adhere to the strict regulations set forth by the legislation. CLIA is discussed in more depth in Chapter 44. Additional information about CLIA can be found on the CMS's Website, www.cms.gov/clia.

Fire Regulations

The local fire department will conduct routine walk-throughs of the facility to verify compliance with fire codes. This should be done when first moving into an office, prior to seeing patients. In addition, you should receive an annual inspection. A courtesy inspection is often available by contacting your local fire department. At all times, fire extinguishers should be inspected and labeled, smoke alarms should work properly, and any other safety hazards addressed. Be sure to evaluate the fire extinguisher(s) rating in your office and be able to operate it according to the manufacturer's instructions.

TABLE 21–1 Common Safety Signs

	Biohazard		Poison
	Flammable		Radiation hazard
	No smoking	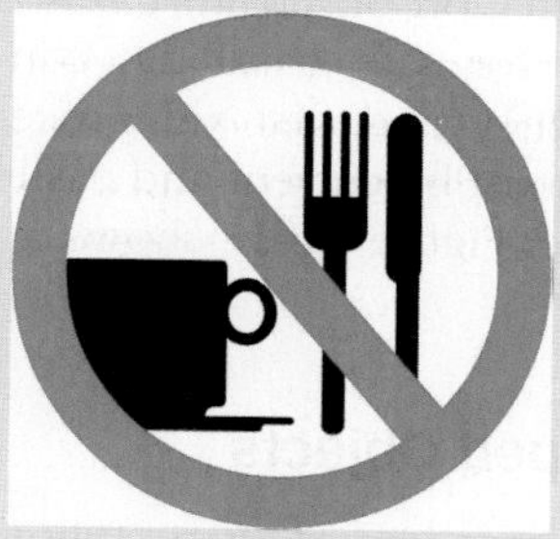	No eating or drinking

Source: Delmar/Cengage Learning.

Safety Signs, Symbols, and Labels

It is important to monitor the compliance of proper storage and disposal of supplies and specimens according to standard precautions and OSHA guidelines. It is important to be able to recognize and comply with posted signs, symbols, and labels. Table 21–1 reviews some common signs and their meanings.

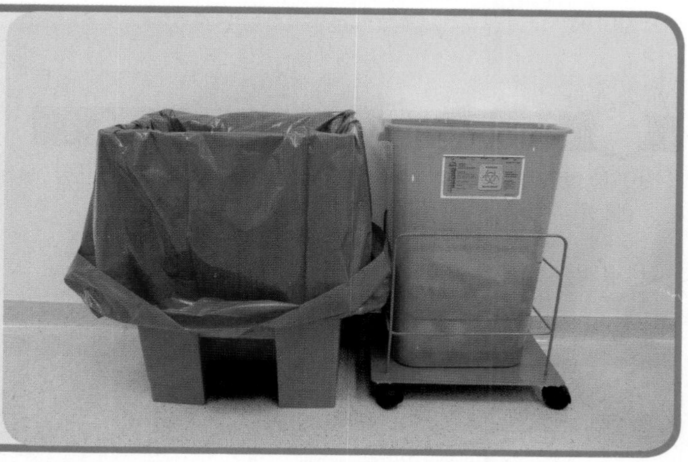

Figure 21–9: Biohazard waste receptacles.
Delmar/Cengage Learning.

Perform a review of the facility to ensure the following:

- Refrigerators used to store reagents, test kits, or biological specimens are labeled with a biohazard symbol and bear the legend, "Not for Storage of Food or Medications."
- Biohazard waste receptacles bear the biohazard symbol and are lined with red plastic bags (Figure 21–9). Biohazard waste should be disposed of in an appropriate receptacle only.
- Chemicals and reagents are evaluated for hazard category classification and labeled with the National Fire Protection Association's color and number coding (Figure 21–10).

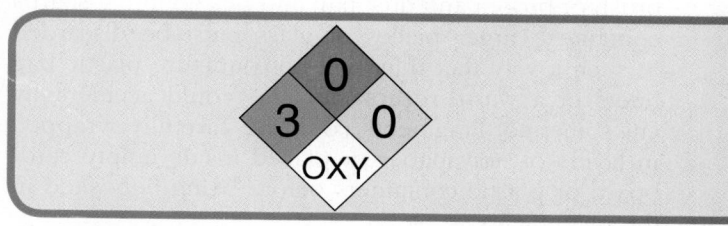

Figure 21–10: NFPA's color and number coding.
Delmar/Cengage Learning.

- Signs are clearly posted in appropriate places for prohibiting smoking, eating, drinking, or application of cosmetics or contact lenses in the facility.

Material Safety Data Sheets

Material safety data sheets (MSDSs) provide information about working with or handling a particular chemical substance. The United States Department of Labor, through OSHA, created MSDSs "to ensure that the hazards of all chemicals produced or imported are evaluated, and that information concerning their hazards is transmitted to employers and employees. This transmittal of information is to be accomplished by means of comprehensive hazard communication programs, which are to include container labeling and other forms of warning, material safety data sheets and employee training" (USDOL/OSHA).

These forms provide information on health hazards of the substance, precautions for safe handling, control measures to take, emergency and first aid procedures, and more. MSDS forms must be current and easily accessible in the medical office. Figure 21–11 shows an example of an MSDS.

Cleaning Spills and Dropped Objects

In the event of a spill, it is very important to follow proper procedure and see that spilled liquids are cleaned up immediately (Figure 21–12). When the spill involves bodily fluids such as blood or urine, universal precautions must be observed by using gloves and eye protection and placing materials in a biohazard waste bag. Your office should have a standard spill kit on hand. Properly bag contaminated clothing and materials in a leak-proof, labeled biohazard bag. Place a second bag around the first and dispose of it in the proper method (licensed waste disposal service). After the spill is cleaned, the area must be thoroughly cleaned with an effective disinfectant or a 10 percent solution of household bleach. The soiled paper towels or cloths should also be discarded in the hazardous waste container. See Procedure 21–4 for the steps to take when cleaning a spill.

Be aware of any objects dropped on the floor and be sure they are picked up immediately to prevent falls. Glass fragments are best picked up using a brush or broom and dust pan and placed into a sharps container. Larger pieces of glass must be discarded in such a way that they will not puncture plastic bag liners of a waste receptacle—this could accidentally cut someone. Fragments could be carefully wrapped in layers of newspaper or placed inside empty cardboard or plastic containers before being deposited in the receptacles.

Personal Safety

In addition to safety precautions taken in the workplace, it is a good idea to develop a personal safety plan, both as an employee in a medical office as well as in your personal life. Safety precautions should be regularly practiced so you will be equipped to respond to an actual emergency.

As an employee, develop a safety checklist that includes:

- Always using appropriate personal protective equipment (PPE). The type of PPE will vary according to the procedure performed, and you will need to be able to select the correct types of PPE for the procedure.
- Knowing where MSDS sheets are and how to read them.
- Knowing where fire extinguishers and eyewash stations are located and how to use them. Fire extinguishers should be present, easily accessible, in good working order, and labeled with inspection date. Operate a fire extinguisher by using the PASS acronym (discussed later in this chapter). Eyewash stations should be present and have documentation of performance of routine maintenance/inspection (Figure 21–13).
- Always disposing of sharps in puncture-proof, labeled sharps containers. Do not overfill sharps containers.
- Knowing the proper protocols for use of biohazard and standard waste receptacles.
- Being aware of your physical surroundings at all times for general safety. Ensure that electrical cords are not frayed; floors have no rolled edges, cracks, or damage; and electrical outlets are not present near water and have ground fault interrupter (GFI) rating.

It is also helpful to research methods and tools to prepare for safety in your personal life. For example:

- Develop a plan for your family in case of an environmental emergency such as tornado or flood.
- Develop an evacuation plan for your family in case of fire.

CLINICAL PEARL

There are many resources on the web to help you develop safety plans for your home and personal life. Some Websites include:

Business & Legal Reports: http://safety.blr.com

Home Safety Council: www.homesafetycouncil.org (click the link for Personalized Checklist)

National Resource Center for Health and Safety in Child Care and Early Education: www.healthykids.us/checklists/checklist_main.htm

MATERIAL SAFETY DATA SHEET

I – PRODUCT IDENTIFICATION

COMPANY NAME: We Wash Inc.

ADDRESS: 5035 Manchester Avenue
Freedom, Texas 79430

Tel No: (314) 621-1818
Nights: (314) 621-1399
CHEMTREC: (800) 424-9343

PRODUCT NAME: Spotfree

Product No.: 2190

Synonyms: Warewashing Detergent

II – HAZARDOUS INGREDIENTS OF MIXTURES

MATERIAL:	(CAS#)	% By Wt.	TLV	PEL
According to the OSHA Hazard Communication Standard, 29CFR 1910.1200, this product contains no hazardous ingredients.		N/A	N/A	N/A

III – PHYSICAL DATA

Vapor Pressure, mm Hg: N/A
Evaporation Rate (ether=1): N/A
Solubility in H_2O: Complete
Freezing Point F: N/A
Boiling Point F: N/A
Specific Gravity H_2O=1 @25C: N/A

Vapor Density (Air=1) 60–90F: N/A
% Volatile by wt N/A
pH @ 1% Solution 9.3–9.8
pH as Distributed: N/A
Appearance: Off-White granular powder
Odor: Mild Chemical Odor

IV – FIRE AND EXPLOSION

Flash Point F: N/AV

Flammable Limits: N/A

Extinguishing Media: The product is not flammable or combustible. Use media appropriate for the primary source of fire.

Special Fire Fighting Procedures: Use caution when fighting any fire involving chemicals. A self-contained breathing apparatus is essential.

Unusual Fire and Explosion Hazards: None Known

V – REACTIVITY DATA

Stability—Conditions to Avoid: None Known

Incompatibility: Contact of carbonates or bicarbonates with acids can release large quantities of carbon dioxide and heat.

Hazardous Decomposition Products: In fire situations heat decomposition may result in the release of sulfur oxides.

Conditions Contributing to Hazardous Polymerization: N/A

Figure 21–11: A material safety data sheet. *Delmar/Cengage Learning.*

(*continues*)

Spotfree

VI – HEALTH HAZARD DATA

EFFECTS OF OVEREXPOSURE (Medical Conditions Aggravated/Target Organ Effects)

A. ACUTE (Primary Route of Exposure) EYES: Product granules may cause mechanical irritation to eyes.
SKIN (Primary Route of Exposure): Prolonged repeated contact with skin may result in drying of skin.
INGESTION: Not expected to be toxic if swallowed, however, gastrointestinal discomfort may occur.

B. SUBCHRONIC, CHRONIC, OTHER: None known.

VII – EMERGENCY AND FIRST AID PROCEDURES

EYES: In case of contact, flush thoroughly with water for 15 minutes. Get medical attention if irritation persists.
SKIN: Flush any dry Spotfree from skin with flowing water. Always wash hands after use.
INGESTION: If swallowed, drink large quantities of water and call a physician.

VIII – SPILL OR LEAK PROCEDURES

Spill Management: Sweep up material and repackage if possible.
Spill residue may be flushed to the sewer with water.

Waste Disposal Methods: Dispose of in accordance with federal, state and local regulations.

IX – PROTECTION INFORMATION/CONTROL MEASURES

Respiratory: None needed — Eye: Safety glasses — Glove: Not required

Other Clothing and Equipment: None required

Ventilation: Normal

X – SPECIAL PRECAUTIONS

Precautions to be taken in Handling and Storing: Avoid contact with eyes. Avoid prolonged or repeated contact with skin. Wash thoroughly after handling. Keep container closed when not in use.
Additional Information: Store away from acids.

Prepared by: D. Martinez — Revision Date: 04/11/XX

Seller makes no warranty, expressed or implied, concerning the use of this product other than indicated on the label. Buyer assumes all risk of use and/or handling of this material when such use and/or handling is contrary to label instructions.

While Seller believes that the information contained herein is accurate, such information is offered solely for its customers' consideration and verification under their specific use conditions. This information is not to be deemed a warranty or representation of any kind for which Seller assumes legal responsibility.

Figure 21–11: *(continued).*

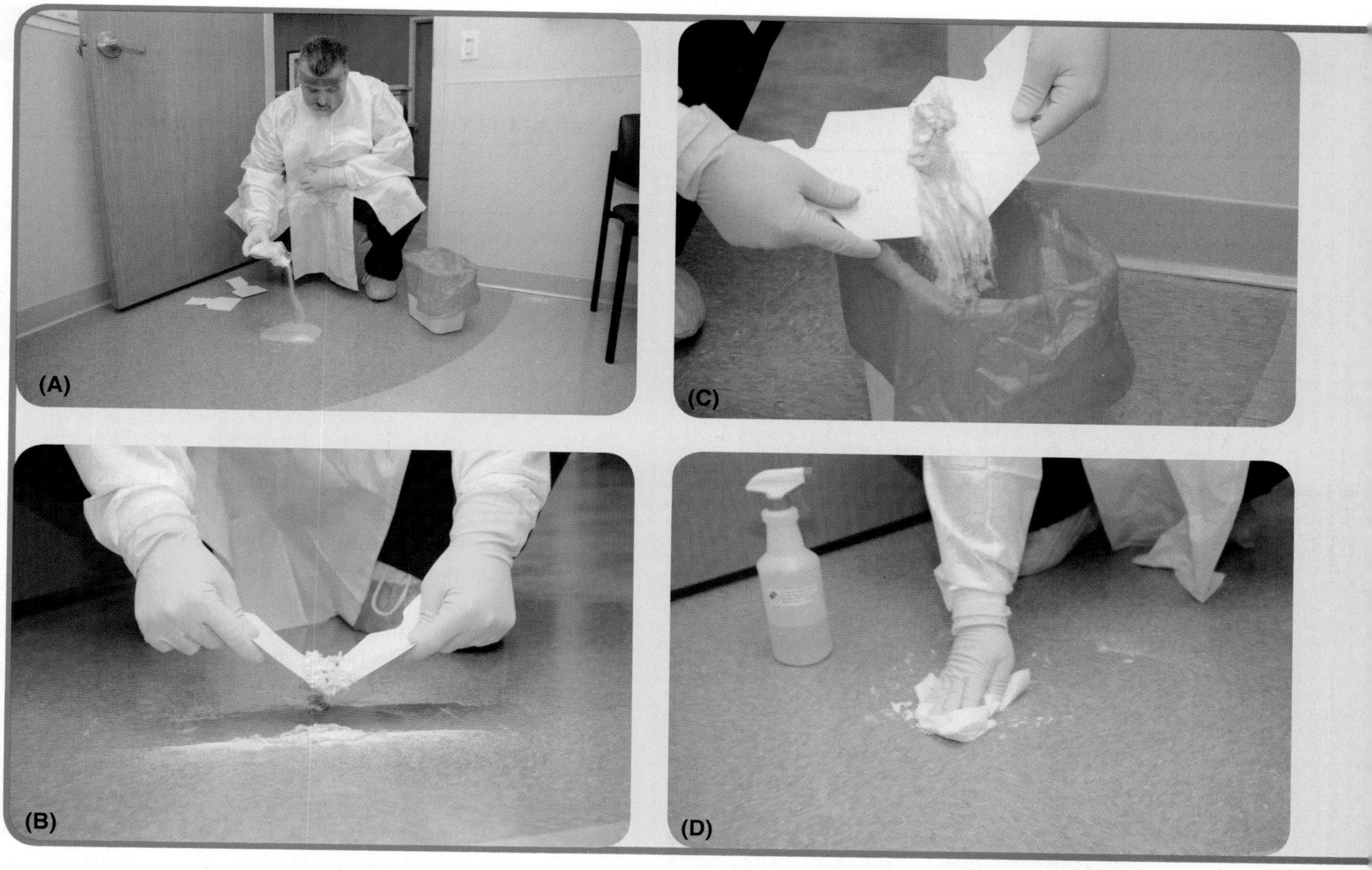

Figure 21–12: Cleaning a spill. (A) Open spill kit and pour coagulating powder on spill. (B) When spilled materials have been absorbed, use scoop to remove. (C) Place in an appropriate biohazard container. (D) Clean the area with a 10% bleach solution. *Delmar/Cengage Learning.*

PROCEDURE 21–4 Clean a Spill

PURPOSE: Clean a spill (when blood or other body fluids are involved), observing universal precautions

EQUIPMENT: Gloves, eye protection, plastic apron with sleeves, hair and shoe covers, biohazard bags, disinfectant, and paper or cloth towels

S **SKILL:** Select appropriate barrier or personal protective equipment (PPE) for potentially infectious situations.

S **SKILL:** Respond to and document a mock exposure event.

Procedure Steps	Detailed Instructions and/or *Rationales*
1. Select appropriate barrier or personal protective equipment.	• Wear eye protection (mask and face shield). • Wear protective plastic apron with sleeves. • Wear protective hair and shoe covers. • Wear gloves.
2. Locate the office spill kit and follow office protocol for cleaning spills. Follow instructions on the spill kit appropriate to the hazard.	Be sure to leave cleaning fluids on the affected area for the appropriate amount of time.

(continues)

(continued)

Procedure Steps	Detailed Instructions and/or *Rationales*
3. Thoroughly clean area with an effective disinfectant or a 10 percent solution of household bleach.	
4. Dispose of materials in biohazard waste container.	Place any paper or cloth towels in the biohazard container for disposal.
5. Document the incident, findings, and actions taken and then date and sign.	

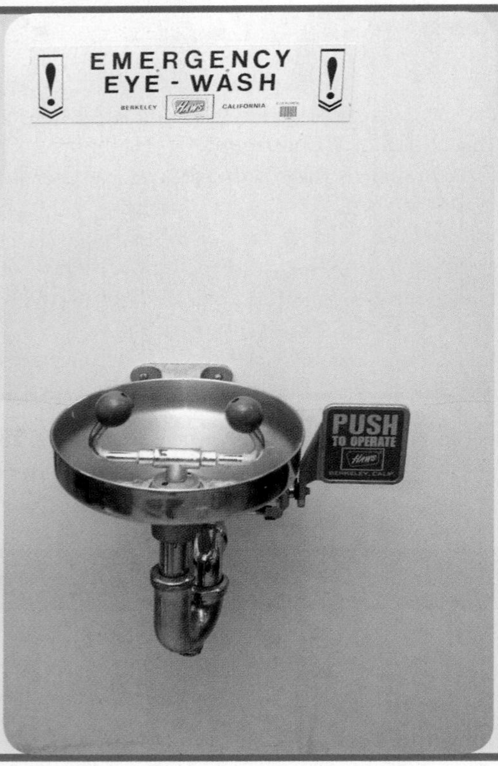

Figure 21–13: Eyewash station. *Delmar/Cengage Learning.*

Infection Control and Personal Safety

The effort to reduce or eliminate exposure to harmful organisms is known as *infection control*. All types of health care settings and personnel must maintain procedures to control the transmission of organisms. By the very nature of the services provided, health care workers are constantly coming into contact with patients who are ill or who might have contagious diseases. The patients in this setting are also exposed to organisms from other patients. It is extremely important for the health and safety of all concerned to prevent the spread of these organisms. All health care workers must practice standard precautions to protect themselves against acquiring HIV, hepatitis B, or other infectious diseases. This means the appropriate use of gloves, face shields, masks, protective eyewear, aprons, and gowns as needed. Persons likely to be in an emergency situation also need to use mouthpieces, ventilation bags, and other ventilating devices to avoid direct contact with saliva or possible blood due to an injury. Standard precautions are discussed in depth in Chapter 36.

FIRE PREVENTION

Fire prevention is very important to everyone's safety. Only three elements need to be present for a fire to start: heat, fuel, and oxygen (Figure 21–14). Fires can be started in many ways. A few examples include:

- A defective outlet or frayed wires on any electrical appliance or office equipment.
- Coffee pots and water sterilizers that boil dry and cause a fire. It is a good policy to unplug all electrical appliances whenever the office is closed.

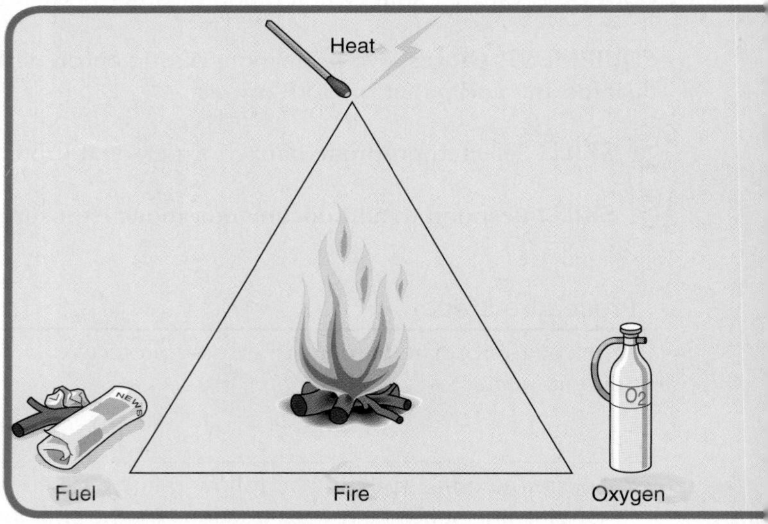

Figure 21–14: The fire triangle. *Delmar/Cengage Learning.*

- A carelessly discarded match or cigarette ash dropping onto furniture or being discarded in a trash container.

The office should have an established policy regarding the procedure to follow in case of fire. All patients and office staff must be **evacuated** from the building, and the fire department must be notified. Exit signs should be clearly posted. All stairways and hallways should be free from clutter to allow quick, safe passage.

You must know the location and proper use of the fire **extinguishers** to aid in preventing a fire from spreading (Figure 21–15). Remember the acronym PASS when operating a fire extinguisher:

- **P**ull the pin at the top of the extinguisher.
- **A**im at the base of the fire.
- **S**queeze the handle slowly, to release the extinguishing agent in the fire extinguisher.
- **S**weep from side to side until the fire is completely out.

Procedure 21–5 discusses fire safety and operating a fire extinguisher.

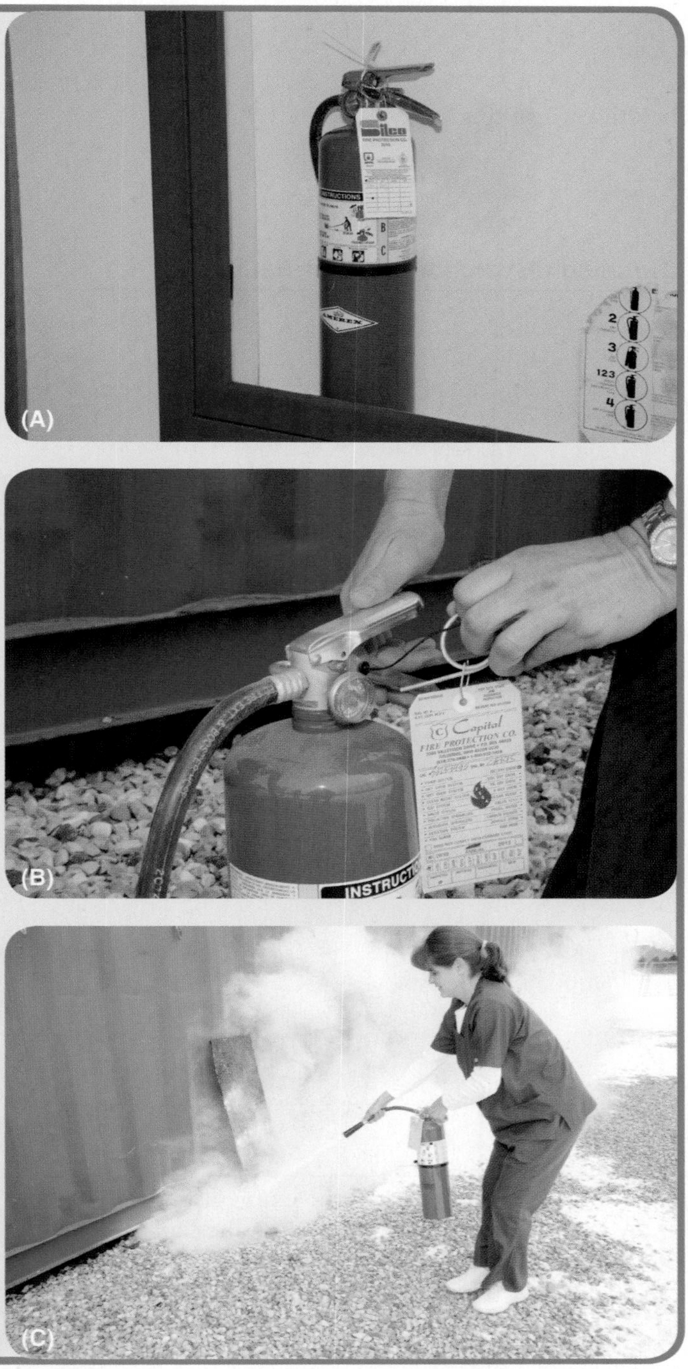

Figure 21–15: Operating a fire extinguisher. (A) Know the location of the fire extinguisher. (B) Pull the pin. (C) Point the hose at the base of the fire, squeeze the handle, and sweep from side to side. *Delmar/Cengage Learning.*

EMERGENCY PREPAREDNESS AND EVACUATION

Every business, including the medical office, should have plans for **emergency preparedness**. Use the available United States Department of Homeland Security resources to create office preparedness and emergency plans (www.ready.gov). On this Website, you will find the brochure and templates for a business emergency plan, computer inventory, insurance coverage, and emergency supplies. Refer to the "Web Links" section at the end of the chapter to find these resources.

Development of emergency plans, assignment of duties, and practice drills are usually the responsibility of the office manager, but everyone is responsible for becoming familiar with and executing the plan if an emergency situation occurs.

Emergency evacuations can be required for any number of situations. A planned route of escape should be prominently posted (Figure 21–16). Follow all emergency preparedness policies and procedures. Table 21–2 presents considerations when developing an example emergency evacuation plan. Part of the emergency evacuation plan should address how to assist patients with special needs in various situations, such as:

- Hearing-impaired patients in the waiting room.
- Sight-impaired patient with an escort in an exam room.
- Personnel working in the laboratory.
- Wheelchair-bound patient in an exam room.

CLINICAL PEARL

The CDC's Emergency Preparedness and Response site (http://emergency.cdc.gov) is another excellent resource. It provides resources for specific hazards, such as natural disasters, health outbreaks, bioterrorism, chemical emergencies, and more. There are also tools for training, education, and coping with these disasters.

PROCEDURE 21–5 Fire Preparedness

MEDIA LINK: View the "Fire Safety" video for this chapter on the Premium Website.

PURPOSE: Identify and respond to fire hazards; describe and demonstrate how to operate a fire extinguisher correctly, using the PASS acronym

EQUIPMENT: Fire extinguisher

S SKILL: Demonstrate methods of fire prevention in the health care setting.

S SKILL: Demonstrate proper use of a fire extinguisher.

Procedure Steps	Detailed Instructions and/or *Rationales*
1. Read the following scenarios and identify the fire hazards presented. Then describe how to respond to (correct) each hazard. A. Multiple pieces of equipment are plugged into extension cords (copy machine, fax machine, computer station with printer, coffee pot). ____________________________ ____________________________ ____________________________ B. Keyboard cleaning fluid and spray is located next to the outlet strip on the counter. ____________________________ ____________________________ ____________________________ C. During the course of the day, Sally Medstudent spilled a cup of coffee on the keyboard. ____________________________ ____________________________ ____________________________	
2. Describe how to operate a fire extinguisher, explaining what the PASS acronym means.	
3. Correctly operate the fire extinguisher, using the PASS method.	• **P**ull the pin at the top of the extinguisher. • **A**im at the base of the fire (not at the flames). • **S**queeze the handle slowly. • **S**weep from side to side until the fire is completely out.

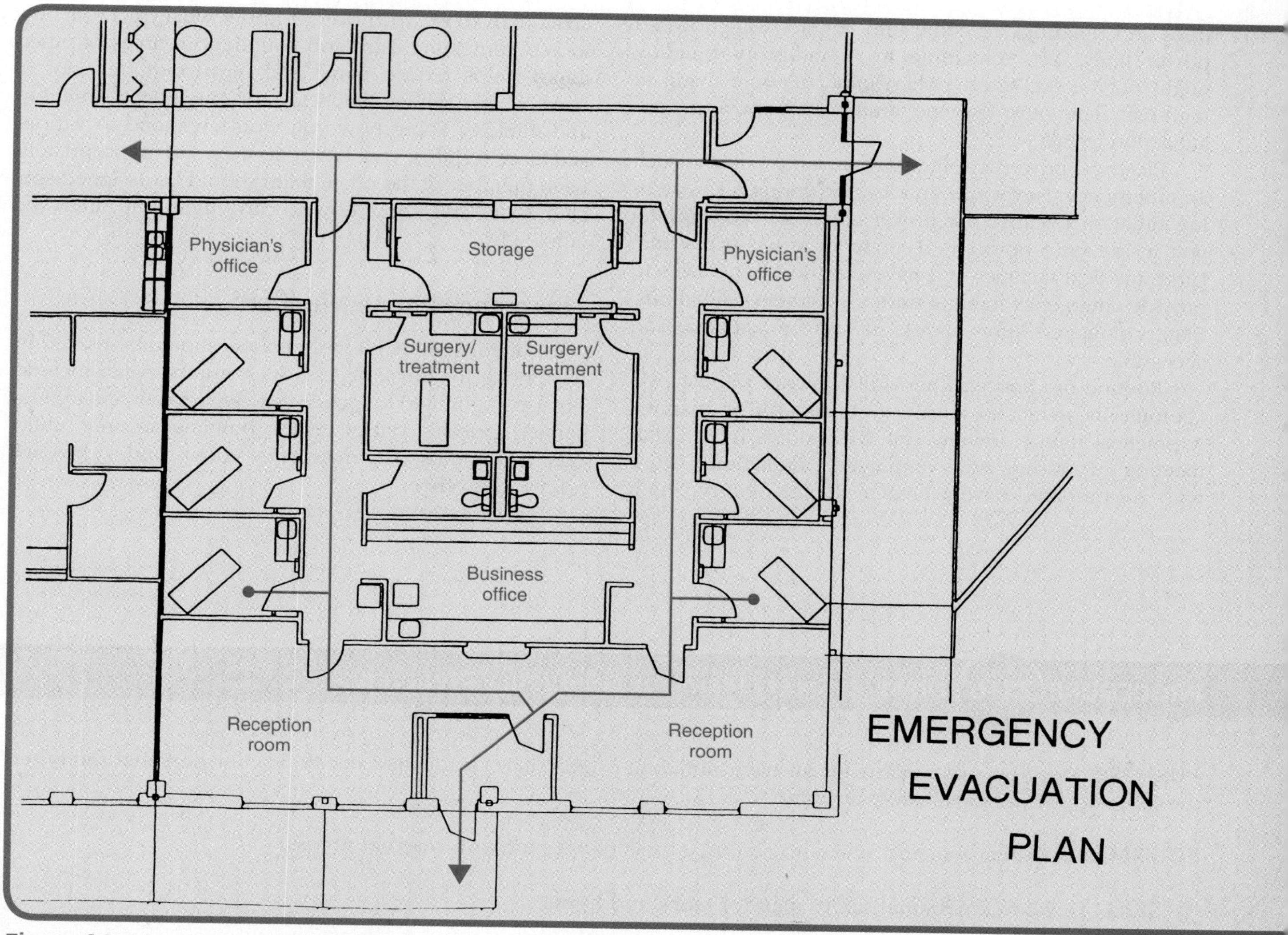

Figure 21–16: Emergency evacuation plan. *Delmar/Cengage Learning.*

TABLE 21–2 Emergency Evacuation Planning

1. Inspect facility for all possible evacuation routes.
2. Create or copy a floor plan of the office with evacuation routes and assembly area clearly marked.
3. Determine who is responsible for informing emergency response services and other building occupants if necessary.
4. For each area of the office, assign a staff member to be responsible for ensuring evacuation of patients, personnel, and visitors.
5. After reaching the assembly point, verify that all patients, visitors, and staff are present.
6. Instruct all parties to remain in place until authorities have cleared the building for re-entrance.

In addition to fire, a severe weather warning is another event that requires an established policy for what to do in case it occurs. Natural disasters such as strong electrical storms and tornados are unpredictable and can claim lives if necessary steps are not taken. In these instances, people must remain inside and take shelter in the predetermined safest area. In areas where there is danger from earthquakes, it is wise to stand in doorframes or beneath a sturdy structure. It may be dangerous to go outside where you could be struck by falling trees and buildings or come into contact with downed power lines. Yet, remaining in a multistory building might not be the safest policy, either. People living in high-risk areas must become familiar with the appropriate action to take.

Electrical power is sometimes disrupted during such an emergency. Never use an elevator during a threatening situation because the power could go off, trapping you inside until power is restored or you are rescued. Large medical facilities can have electrical generators to provide emergency lighting during emergency situations. Battery-powered lights should always be available and accessible.

Routine fire and weather drills prepare people psychologically to act in a safe and responsible manner. A practical time to review drill procedures is at a staff meeting or during new employee orientation. Those who are prepared have a greater chance of surviving a crisis than those who do not know what to do or how to act. Remaining calm and confident in times of emergency helps reduce panic and **irrational** behavior in yourself and others. Practicing for emergency situations and thinking about how you would respond to various situations equips you better to respond appropriately. Each member of the office team should be assigned specific duties and know how to carry them out safely and efficiently.

Emergency Phone Numbers

A list of emergency phone numbers should be posted by the phone for quick access. Such numbers can include, but are not limited to, police, fire department, emergency service, poison control center, building security, utility companies, hospital emergency room, and a hospital admissions office.

PROCEDURE 21–6 Develop Safety Plans for Emergency Preparedness

PURPOSE: Develop safety plans for an environmental event (such as a tornado or flood), for personal safety on the job, and for personal safety at home

EQUIPMENT: Paper, pen, and access to resource tools (computer with Internet access)

S SKILL: Develop a personal safety plan for work and home.

Procedure Steps	Detailed Instructions and/or *Rationales*
1. Develop a personal plan for yourself and your family in case of environmental emergency, such as tornado or flood.	Include evacuation routes, emergency meet-up locations, items to bring, and so on.
2. Find local telephone numbers of organizations and include these in your personal plan.	Include numbers for the fire department, police, poison control center, provider, hospital, and so on.
3. Verbalize (explain) an evacuation plan out of your home in case of fire.	Include evacuation routes, emergency meet-up locations, items to bring, and so on.
4. Develop a typed safety plan in the case of a chemical spill in the office.	Discuss appropriate PPE, actions to take, and how to document.
5. Verbalize (explain) an evacuation plan for a medical office in the event of an emergency.	

CHAPTER SUMMARY

- Opening the office requires attention to detail and being well prepared, organized, and tidy. The surroundings set the tone and first impression for the office and the level of professionalism anticipated. Safety and security must be evaluated each and every day, including a walk-through evaluation of the reception area, exam rooms, and lab.
- The front desk is the point of first impression. Make sure all computers and office equipment are turned on and operational prior to receiving patients. Retrieve telephone messages, faxes, and lab and hospital reports. Sort and file appropriately. Place charts in a designated area for check-in and prepare sign-in sheets, cash balance forms, and so on.
- Key elements of closing the medical office include cleaning and restocking exam rooms, filing charts, preparing charts for the next business day, and turning off electrical appliances as appropriate. Receipts collected during the day should be reconciled, prepared for bank deposit, and locked in a secure safe if not banking until the following day. Perform a final walk-through, checking for answering service activation; security of all doors and windows; blinds closure; and alarm activation.
- Numerous governmental agencies and regulations are involved in the promotion of safety and security in the health care industry. Be familiar with the agencies and regulations such as those from OSHA, CLIA, DEA, CDC, and ADA and how they are applied and enforced by your office.
- In the medical office are many safety signs, symbols, and labels. Learn to identify the safety signs and how they apply to your office in creating a safe, hazard-free environment.
- Materials safety data sheets (MSDSs) provide information about working with or handling a particular chemical substance. These sheets are to be maintained in a visible location for easy reference and provide information about health hazards of the substances, precautions for safe handling, control measures, and emergency and first aid procedures.
- In the event of a hazardous spill, you must follow universal precautions to protect yourself and others and see that spills are cleaned up immediately. Follow office procedures, wear personal protective equipment (PPE), and use the office spill kit.
- The requirement for responding to hazardous material disposal is that all universal (standard) precautions are followed and contaminated materials are properly disposed of. This means you must wear gloves, face shield, protective eyewear, aprons, gowns, and hair and shoe coverings.
- Three elements necessary for fire: heat, fuel, and oxygen. Ways a fire might start include smoking, a defective outlet, and frayed wires on an electrical appliance or office equipment. Coffee pots and water sterilizers can also boil dry and cause a fire.
- The medical assistant is often the first responder in an emergency or disaster. Preparation for such emergencies is known as emergency preparedness. You must be aware of emergency plans and participate in preparation, assignment, drills, and evacuations. There are a number of resources for creating and preparing plans such as those found at www.ready.gov.
- Critical elements of an emergency plan for response to a natural disaster or other emergency include inspection of the facility for all possible evacuation routes; creating or copying a floor plan with evacuation routes clearly marked; determining who is responsible for informing emergency response services; taking role and assignment to ensure evacuation of patients, personnel, and visitors; confirming that everyone is accounted for after an evacuation; and instructing all parties to remain in place until authorities have cleared the building for entrance.
- In addition to the policies and procedures of your office, learn to identify emergency preparedness plans in your community, including personal safety plans and using resources such as www.ready.gov, sponsored by the U.S. Department of Homeland Security.

STUDY TOOLS

Workbook	Activities for Chapter 21
Premium Website	
MEDIA LINK	View these **Media Links** for Chapter 21: • Fire Safety
StudyWARE	Activities and Quizzes on the **StudyWARE™ Software** for Chapter 21

	Complete the following **Competency Challenge 2.0** activity: • Thursday, 10 AM: Complete Inventory and Maintenance • Thursday, 11 AM: Prepare for Emergencies
	Audio Library of medical terms
	Online access to the **Critical Thinking Challenge 2.0**
CourseMate	Activities and Quizzes for Chapter 21
WebTutor	Activities and Quizzes for Chapter 21

CHECK YOUR KNOWLEDGE

1. Preparing to open the office involves creating a checklist and performing which of the following functions?
   a. Checking the waiting room temperature
   b. Performing a visual check of electrical devices, furniture, floors, and lighting
   c. Locking the outside access doors
   d. All of the above
   e. a and b only
2. To prepare the front desk for opening the office, which of the following is NOT a function?
   a. Retrieving faxes
   b. Retrieving messages
   c. Retrieving superbills
   d. Turning on computers and office equipment
3. Inspection of the examination rooms entails which of the following responsibilities?
   a. Replacing examining paper
   b. Plugging in electrical equipment
   c. Restocking supplies
   d. All of the above
   e. a and b only
4. Which of the following is NOT part of the inventory supply duties?
   a. Printed schedule of patient appointments
   b. Medication
   c. Office (clerical) supplies
   d. Laboratory
   e. Checklist of exam room supplies
5. Safety in the medical office is regulated and promoted by which of the following agencies?
   a. Occupational Health and Safety Administration (OSHA)
   b. Drug Enforcement Agency (DEA)
   c. American with Disabilities Act (ADA)
   d. Center for Medicare and Medicaid Services (CMS)
   e. All of the above
   f. a, b, and c
6. Which agency created the guidelines called universal precautions?
   a. Centers for Disease Control and Prevention (CDC)
   b. Occupational Health and Safety Administration (OSHA)
   c. Drug Enforcement Agency (DEA)
   d. Center for Medicare and Medicaid Services (CMS)
7. The objective of the Clinical Laboratory Improvement Amendments (CLIA) is?
   a. To receive Medicare payments
   b. To ensure quality laboratory testing
   c. To promote universal precautions
   d. To comply with OSHA regulations
8. Proper use of safety signs, symbols, and labels would be used in which of the following?
   a. A refrigerator used to store reagents, test kits, or biological specimens is labeled with a biohazard symbol and bear the legend "Not for Storage of Food or Medications."
   b. Biohazard waste receptacles bear the biohazard symbol and are lined with red plastic bags. Biohazard waste is not disposed of in inappropriate receptacles.
   c. Chemicals and reagents are evaluated for hazard category classification and labeled with the National Fire Association's color and number coding.
   d. Signs are clearly posted in appropriate places for where smoking is allowed and where to eat or drink.
   e. All of the above
   f. a, b, and c
9. In response to a fire, your first responsibility is to:
   a. Wedge open doors.
   b. Warn others in a frantic tone.
   c. Evacuate patients and staff by using the closest elevator.
   d. Sound the alarm.
   e. All of the above

10. When closing the office, it is your responsibility to:
    a. Cancel appointments.
    b. Turn off fax machine.
    c. Deposit receipts (cash) to bank or in safe.
    d. Collect charts for review the following day.
    e. Both c and d.

WEB LINKS

Americans with Disabilities Act: www.ada.gov

Clinical Laboratory Improvement Amendments: www.cms.hhs.gov/clia/

American Academy of Medical Management: www.epracticemanagement.org

Occupational Safety and Health Administration: www.osha.gov

CDC's Emergency Preparedness and Response: emergency.cdc.gov

Ready.gov: www.ready.gov

Informational Downloads from Ready.gov: www.ready.gov/business/publications/index.html

Chapter 22

Managing the Office

OBJECTIVES

In this chapter, you will learn the following:

KB KNOWLEDGE BASE

1. Spell and define, using the glossary at the back of the text, all the Words to Know in this chapter.
2. Describe at least six responsibilities the office manager has to employees.
3. Describe how HIPAA has affected office policy.
4. Identify components of an office policy manual and office procedure manual.
5. Explain the purpose of W-4, W-2, and I-9 forms.
6. Differentiate between gross and net salary.
7. Describe six examples of benefits that may be offered to employees.
8. Discuss the importance of liability insurance for the office as well as for the medical assistant.
9. Describe the office manager's role in staff meetings, employee evaluation and review, and terminating employment.
10. Describe the office manager's responsibility to providers.
11. List general facility responsibilities of managers.
12. Identify components of a practice information brochure.
13. List organizations that might perform site visits at a medical office.

S SKILLS

1. Prepare employee payroll.
2. Manage a provider's professional schedule and travel.

WORDS TO KNOW

accountant
benefits
bereavement time
complimentary
deductions
disability
evaluations
exemption
expenditure
fiscal
fringe benefits
gross
hourly wage
Internal Revenue Service (IRS)
longevity
net
productivity
profit sharing
reimbursement
salary
vested

MANAGEMENT ROLES AND RESPONSIBILITIES

Medical assistants often advance into administrative roles in the medical office, so it is good practice to understand the management role and responsibilities to employees, providers, and the facility. You will find that understanding, creating, and relying on practice policies and procedures assist in management of the practice.

Managers can provide research and insight and make inquires to present to the providers. When managers have been promoted from medical assistant, administrative, or clinical positions, they have a valuable understanding of the patient care requirements.

In large practices, clinics, and corporations, decision-making responsibilities can be divided among the providers according to their area of interest or expertise or to a designated managing provider. When decisions need to be made, the manager has to confer with only that provider or two instead of the total partnership. An example of division of responsibility is:

- Employment and personnel concerns.
- Purchasing and office facility concerns.
- Lab and radiology issues.
- Fees, investments, and other financial matters.
- Productivity trends.

Decisions made by designated providers are then usually discussed at a general providers' meeting. The manager can also be involved in the review and negotiations involved in the practice management.

RESPONSIBILITIES TO EMPLOYEES

The manager in large practices often has the following responsibilities related to the support staff employees:

- Interview, hire, discipline, and terminate employees in coordination with providers.
- Supervise or personally train employees. This applies to new personnel as well as to updating current staff.
- Conduct staff meetings to inform, discuss, and exchange information.
- Create, implement, and enforce work schedules.
- Arrange vacation schedules and coverage.
- Conduct performance evaluations, establishing probationary periods as deemed necessary.
- Consult providers concerning performance evaluations, salary increases, and benefits. (In a larger group practice or association with a health care facility, an HR department might set the policy for salary increase, probationary periods, and benefits.)

Office Policy Manual

The office manager is responsible for developing and maintaining the policy manuals for the office. Office policy manuals include the following characteristics:

1. Manuals define roles and responsibilities, including instructions (instructional material).
2. Manuals provide standard operating procedures, so disputes can be avoided and proactively addressed through the implementations of standard practice and procedures.
3. Productivity can be enhanced when the processes are clearly identified and laid out in a manner that makes them second nature.

Table 22–1 shows a partial list of topics that can be included in the office policy manual, and Figure 22–1 is an example of a time record policy.

HIPAA and Office Policy

When the HIPAA rulings began in 1996, policy manuals required updating to include the new directives for protecting patient information and providing security measures and specific instruction for electronically transmitting patient data. Dealing with patient information to families, other health care entities, insurance companies, and business associate contacts requires following strict guidelines.

The legislation also created three roles to be established. A HIPAA compliance officer must be designated to coordinate and oversee compliance with the rules. A security officer must also be designated and is responsible for the security of the patients' records. A third position is for a privacy officer, who is to keep track of who has access to the protected information. The three positions can be filled by as few as two people, with a third as backup, or several people can be designated in large practices. The office manager most often fills the role of at least one of these positions.

The manager has the responsibility to ensure compliance in all HIPAA-related areas. One method is to conduct audits and present an analysis of protected health information (PHI) security. In addition to the audit, the manager must review policy and procedure, update if necessary, and develop training materials and implement training and education for employees as needed. HIPAA

TABLE 22–1 Office Policy Manual Topics

Shredding policy	Disease management
Prescription refill	Nondiscrimination/harassment
Information technology	Facsimile (fax)
Artificial nails	Infection control
Human resources	Visitors in the workplace
Absenteeism	Paid time off (PTO)
Confidentiality	Continuing education
Chain of command	Expected performance
Employee evaluation	Employee termination

Time Record Policies and Procedures

It is a requirement that all staff adhere to scheduled work times. Utilize time management and prioritize your work. **REMEMBER:** You are **only** to clock in when you are ready to **begin work, *not just when you are arriving at the office.***

Time and staffing issues have been addressed at multiple staff meetings, individual summaries, and counsel. This memo will serve as a formal/final notice for compliance.

1. Arrive ready to work at your scheduled time.
2. Lunches are one hour.
3. Clock out at your scheduled time, not to exceed 8 hours.
4. No overtime is authorized.
5. Do not clock in earlier than your time scheduled. Schedules are made to accommodate providers and office hours/coverage.
6. If you are found to be over your assigned hours, you will be scheduled off enough time to balance your clock-out time (including extending your lunch hour).
7. You will not be authorized overtime to complete your assignments. Buddy coverage is available as assigned. Use time management and prioritize your workflow.
8. Avoid disruption of staff working during lunch hour/break times, respecting their work time.
9. Avoid activities and personal calls not related to your specific job duties. This should be done on your break/lunch time.
10. Keep your activities and tone of voice professional at all times, avoiding HIPAA violations and personal chatter, unbecoming to the office.

If the provider you are assigned to is off, be prepared for:

1. Assignment to complete immediate/urgent tasks at hand.
2. Being scheduled to cover other providers, assignments, duties; performing/completing all duties for that position (including buddy coverage).
3. Being scheduled to Float Pool.

Other requirements:

1. All paid time off (PTO) requests must be submitted at least two (2) weeks in advance and will not be approved if you do not have PTO available in your "bank."
2. Do not exceed six (6) unscheduled absences in a 12-month (rolling) period.
3. It is your responsibility to notify manager in advance of any schedule changes.

Your time card is a legal record of your hours worked and is the basis for completing your paycheck. All employees are required on a daily basis to keep an accurate record of all time word, as well as PTO and excused absences, and to sign in and out for all meal periods. Falsification of time cards can be grounds for termination.

Under no circumstances should an employee request or allow anyone else to sign in or out on the time card for him/her. Altering, falsifying, tampering with time records, or recording time on another employee's time record will subject both parties to immediate disciplinary action, up to and including termination. Any changes to the time card must be authorized by your supervisor's initials or signature. Correction fluid may not be used on time cards under any circumstances. All corrections should be made by crossing out the incorrect information and substituting the correct information. Time cards must bear the employee's signature.

Failure to adhere to these work practices will result in disciplinary action.

I acknowledge receipt of this memo:

______________________________ ______________________

Employee signature Date

Figure 22–1: Example of a time record policy. *Delmar/Cengage Learning.*

discussions should be included at every staff meeting to heighten awareness. Enforcement of policies, including disciplinary action for HIPAA violations, is another responsibility of the practice manager.

HIPAA has transformed how the medical office handles PHI. The HIPAA security officer is responsible for overseeing development and enforcements of all policies and procedures necessary to protect the confidentiality, integrity, and availability of the practice information system and data. Areas affected are:

- Check-in process
- Medical charts (cover patient information)
- Secured fax machine (document confidentiality)
- Confidential phone lines
- Covering medical information in unsecured areas (e.g., the hallway)
- Computer screen
- Disposal of documents containing PHI
- Reporting a security incident
- Password unique

Risk Adjustment Factor—Medical Problem List Workflow

1. The medical records clerk prepares the charts for the next day's visits and attaches the overlay to the chart with a RAF diagnosis list if the patient is 65 years of age or older (65+) and highlights the patient's age on the overlay.
2. If a RAF Medical Problem List for patient has been provided, the medical records clerk will insert in chart.
3. Physician examines the patients and sees the code sheet on the outside of the chart, and the Medical Problem List insert in chart, which is a flag to discuss the noted medical problem and document the date of visit and code on the overlay, and in chart notes.
4. A laminated RAF code sheet list will be kept in the exam rooms for the MD/NP's for quick reference as well.
5. Office staff (medical assistant and/or receptionist) will attach the RAF Medical Problem list in the chart per provider preference.
6. Overlays get turned into the batchers, with RAF diagnosis noted on overlay by provider. RAF diagnosis list that was attached to the chart will be returned to the batcher with overlay, unmarked, for recycling to medical records for placement onto all 65+ patient charts with overlays.
7. Batcher works the overlays for the day and if there is one marked/tagged 65+, the batcher will verify the diagnoses selected are coded to the highest 4th or 5th digit specificity. If codes are not listed on overlay by provider, the batcher will retrieve chart and review against the codes listed on the Medical Problem List and confirm with provider.

Figure 22–2: Example of a Risk Adjust Factor (RAF) Workflow procedure. *Delmar/Cengage Learning.*

The amount of PHI used or disclosed should be the minimal necessary to do the job.

Office Procedure Manual

An office procedure manual identifies the common procedures performed in the office and includes directions for performing them (Figure 22–2). The manual can include such procedures as:

- Opening and closing the office.
- Laboratory tests.
- Documentation requirements.
- OSHA and CLIA requirements.
- Basic clinical procedures.
- Basic administrative procedures.
- Emergency procedures.
- Risk adjust factor (RAF) as related to insurance billing and reimbursement rates.

The office manager should address these manuals during the employee's orientation. Employees should always sign a statement that they have read and fully understand the information included in the manuals.

The office manager is usually responsible for maintaining and updating the policy manual annually. When a new operational policy is adopted, it must be put into writing and added to the manual. As new procedures become necessary, the manager should also develop the written procedure guidelines and add them to the procedure manual.

Employee Records

federal govt

All employees in a provider's office must have a Social Security number, the nine-digit number obtained from the Social Security Administration. Each employee must also complete an Employee's Withholding Allowance Certificate (W-4 form) indicating the number of **exemptions** claimed (Figure 22–3). Any employee who fails to complete a W-4 form will have withholding figured on the basis of being single with no exemptions. A new W-4 form must be completed if there is a change in marital status or the number of exemptions.

Federal legislation requires employees to complete an Employment Eligibility Verification, Form I-9 (Figure 22–4). The form is issued by the Department of Justice, Immigration, and Naturalization Service. Its purpose is to ensure that all persons employed are United States citizens, lawfully admitted aliens, or aliens authorized to work in the United States. By law, this form must be completed before an individual can be officially hired. Payroll will not be issued to individuals who do not have an I-9 form on file.

In addition to these federal requirements, forms must also be processed for state and local tax records. Local government tax is paid to the city and state (if applicable) where employment occurs regardless of where the employee lives.

All employees should have the following documents or information available when filling out initial payroll forms:

- Driver's license or other state picture identification
- Social Security card and a copy of Social Security numbers of all dependents
- If not a United States citizen, a green card or equivalent

Other documentation needed for each employee's personnel file includes:

- Immunization records.
- Copies of any professional license, registration, or certification.
- Evidence of pertinent diplomas, degrees, or certificates.
- Evidence of professional liability insurance (if applicable).
- Verification of Occupational Safety and Health Administration and Clinical Laboratory Improvement Amendments (OSHA and CLIA) training.
- Exposure classification record.

The very nature of work in a medical office brings staff into contact with pathogens. Because of the chance of

Form W-4 (2011)

Purpose. Complete Form W-4 so that your employer can withhold the correct federal income tax from your pay. Consider completing a new Form W-4 each year and when your personal or financial situation changes.

Exemption from withholding. If you are exempt, complete **only** lines 1, 2, 3, 4, and 7 and sign the form to validate it. Your exemption for 2011 expires February 16, 2012. See Pub. 505, Tax Withholding and Estimated Tax.

Note. If another person can claim you as a dependent on his or her tax return, you cannot claim exemption from withholding if your income exceeds $950 and includes more than $300 of unearned income (for example, interest and dividends).

Basic instructions. If you are not exempt, complete the **Personal Allowances Worksheet** below. The worksheets on page 2 further adjust your withholding allowances based on itemized deductions, certain credits, adjustments to income, or two-earners/multiple jobs situations.

Complete all worksheets that apply. However, you may claim fewer (or zero) allowances. For regular wages, withholding must be based on allowances you claimed and may not be a flat amount or percentage of wages.

Head of household. Generally, you may claim head of household filing status on your tax return only if you are unmarried and pay more than 50% of the costs of keeping up a home for yourself and your dependent(s) or other qualifying individuals. See Pub. 501, Exemptions, Standard Deduction, and Filing Information, for information.

Tax credits. You can take projected tax credits into account in figuring your allowable number of withholding allowances. Credits for child or dependent care expenses and the child tax credit may be claimed using the **Personal Allowances Worksheet** below. See Pub. 919, How Do I Adjust My Tax Withholding, for information on converting your other credits into withholding allowances.

Nonwage income. If you have a large amount of nonwage income, such as interest or dividends, consider making estimated tax payments using Form 1040-ES, Estimated Tax for Individuals. Otherwise, you may owe additional tax. If you have pension or annuity income, see Pub. 919 to find out if you should adjust your withholding on Form W-4 or W-4P.

Two earners or multiple jobs. If you have a working spouse or more than one job, figure the total number of allowances you are entitled to claim on all jobs using worksheets from only one Form W-4. Your withholding usually will be most accurate when all allowances are claimed on the Form W-4 for the highest paying job and zero allowances are claimed on the others. See Pub. 919 for details.

Nonresident alien. If you are a nonresident alien, see Notice 1392, Supplemental Form W-4 Instructions for Nonresident Aliens, before completing this form.

Check your withholding. After your Form W-4 takes effect, use Pub. 919 to see how the amount you are having withheld compares to your projected total tax for 2011. See Pub. 919, especially if your earnings exceed $130,000 (Single) or $180,000 (Married).

Personal Allowances Worksheet (Keep for your records.)

A Enter "1" for **yourself** if no one else can claim you as a dependent . . . . **A** ______

B Enter "1" if:
- You are single and have only one job; or
- You are married, have only one job, and your spouse does not work; or
- Your wages from a second job or your spouse's wages (or the total of both) are $1,500 or less.

. . . **B** ______

C Enter "1" for your **spouse.** But, you may choose to enter "-0-" if you are married and have either a working spouse or more than one job. (Entering "-0-" may help you avoid having too little tax withheld.) . . . . **C** ______

D Enter number of **dependents** (other than your spouse or yourself) you will claim on your tax return . . . . **D** ______

E Enter "1" if you will file as **head of household** on your tax return (see conditions under **Head of household** above) . . **E** ______

F Enter "1" if you have at least $1,900 of **child or dependent care expenses** for which you plan to claim a credit . . . **F** ______
(**Note.** Do **not** include child support payments. See Pub. 503, Child and Dependent Care Expenses, for details.)

G **Child Tax Credit** (including additional child tax credit). See Pub. 972, Child Tax Credit, for more information.
- If your total income will be less than $61,000 ($90,000 if married), enter "2" for each eligible child; then **less** "1" if you have three or more eligible children.
- If your total income will be between $61,000 and $84,000 ($90,000 and $119,000 if married), enter "1" for each eligible child plus "1" **additional** if you have six or more eligible children . . . . **G** ______

H Add lines A through G and enter total here. (**Note.** This may be different from the number of exemptions you claim on your tax return.) ► **H** ______

For accuracy, **complete all worksheets that apply.**
- If you plan to **itemize** or **claim adjustments to income** and want to reduce your withholding, see the **Deductions and Adjustments Worksheet** on page 2.
- If you have **more than one job** or are **married and you and your spouse both work** and the combined earnings from all jobs exceed $40,000 ($10,000 if married), see the **Two-Earners/Multiple Jobs Worksheet** on page 2 to avoid having too little tax withheld.
- If **neither** of the above situations applies, **stop here** and enter the number from line H on line 5 of Form W-4 below.

Cut here and give Form W-4 to your employer. Keep the top part for your records.

Form **W-4** Department of the Treasury Internal Revenue Service

Employee's Withholding Allowance Certificate

► **Whether you are entitled to claim a certain number of allowances or exemption from withholding is subject to review by the IRS. Your employer may be required to send a copy of this form to the IRS.**

OMB No. 1545-0074 **2011**

1 Type or print your first name and middle initial.	Last name	**2** Your social security number
Home address (number and street or rural route)	**3** ☐ Single ☐ Married ☐ Married, but withhold at higher Single rate. **Note.** If married, but legally separated, or spouse is a nonresident alien, check the "Single" box.	
City or town, state, and ZIP code	**4** If your last name differs from that shown on your social security card, check here. You must call 1-800-772-1213 for a replacement card. ► ☐	

5 Total number of allowances you are claiming (from line **H** above **or** from the applicable worksheet on page 2) **5** ______

6 Additional amount, if any, you want withheld from each paycheck . . . . **6** $ ______

7 I claim exemption from withholding for 2011, and I certify that I meet **both** of the following conditions for exemption.
- Last year I had a right to a refund of **all** federal income tax withheld because I had **no** tax liability **and**
- This year I expect a refund of **all** federal income tax withheld because I expect to have **no** tax liability.

If you meet both conditions, write "Exempt" here . . . . ► **7** ______

Under penalties of perjury, I declare that I have examined this certificate and to the best of my knowledge and belief, it is true, correct, and complete.

Employee's signature
(This form is not valid unless you sign it.) ► **Date ►**

8 Employer's name and address (Employer: Complete lines 8 and 10 only if sending to the IRS.)	**9** Office code (optional)	**10** Employer identification number (EIN)

For Privacy Act and Paperwork Reduction Act Notice, see page 2. Cat. No. 10220Q Form **W-4** (2011)

Figure 22–3: Form W-4, Employee's Withholding Allowance Certificate. *U.S. Internal Revenue Service.*

Form W-4 (2011) Page **2**

Deductions and Adjustments Worksheet

Note. Use this worksheet *only* if you plan to itemize deductions or claim certain credits or adjustments to income.

1 Enter an estimate of your 2011 itemized deductions. These include qualifying home mortgage interest, charitable contributions, state and local taxes, medical expenses in excess of 7.5% of your income, and miscellaneous deductions . . . . **1** $______

2 Enter: { $11,600 if married filing jointly or qualifying widow(er) / $8,500 if head of household / $5,800 if single or married filing separately } . . . . . **2** $______

3 **Subtract** line 2 from line 1. If zero or less, enter "-0-" . . . . . **3** $______

4 Enter an estimate of your 2011 adjustments to income and any additional standard deduction (see Pub. 919) **4** $______

5 **Add** lines 3 and 4 and enter the total. (Include any amount for credits from the *Converting Credits to Withholding Allowances for 2011 Form W-4 Worksheet* in Pub. 919.) . . . . . **5** $______

6 Enter an estimate of your 2011 nonwage income (such as dividends or interest) . . . **6** $______

7 **Subtract** line 6 from line 5. If zero or less, enter "-0-" . . . . . **7** $______

8 **Divide** the amount on line 7 by $3,700 and enter the result here. Drop any fraction . . . **8** ______

9 Enter the number from the **Personal Allowances Worksheet,** line H, page 1 . . . **9** ______

10 **Add** lines 8 and 9 and enter the total here. If you plan to use the **Two-Earners/Multiple Jobs Worksheet,** also enter this total on line 1 below. Otherwise, **stop here** and enter this total on Form W-4, line 5, page 1 **10** ______

Two-Earners/Multiple Jobs Worksheet (See *Two earners or multiple jobs* on page 1.)

Note. Use this worksheet *only* if the instructions under line H on page 1 direct you here.

1 Enter the number from line H, page 1 (or from line 10 above if you used the **Deductions and Adjustments Worksheet**) **1** ______

2 Find the number in **Table 1** below that applies to the **LOWEST** paying job and enter it here. **However,** if you are married filing jointly and wages from the highest paying job are $65,000 or less, do not enter more than "3" . . . . . **2** ______

3 If line 1 is **more than or equal to** line 2, subtract line 2 from line 1. Enter the result here (if zero, enter "-0-") and on Form W-4, line 5, page 1. **Do not** use the rest of this worksheet . . . . **3** ______

Note. If line 1 is **less than** line 2, enter "-0-" on Form W-4, line 5, page 1. Complete lines 4 through 9 below to figure the additional withholding amount necessary to avoid a year-end tax bill.

4 Enter the number from line 2 of this worksheet . . . . . **4** ______

5 Enter the number from line 1 of this worksheet . . . . . **5** ______

6 **Subtract** line 5 from line 4 . . . . . **6** ______

7 Find the amount in **Table 2** below that applies to the **HIGHEST** paying job and enter it here . . . . **7** $______

8 **Multiply** line 7 by line 6 and enter the result here. This is the additional annual withholding needed . . **8** $______

9 Divide line 8 by the number of pay periods remaining in 2011. For example, divide by 26 if you are paid every two weeks and you complete this form in December 2010. Enter the result here and on Form W-4, line 6, page 1. This is the additional amount to be withheld from each paycheck . . . . . **9** $______

Table 1

Married Filing Jointly		**All Others**	
If wages from **LOWEST** paying job are—	Enter on line 2 above	If wages from **LOWEST** paying job are—	Enter on line 2 above
$0 - $5,000 -	0	$0 - $8,000 -	0
5,001 - 12,000 -	1	8,001 - 15,000 -	1
12,001 - 22,000 -	2	15,001 - 25,000 -	2
22,001 - 25,000 -	3	25,001 - 30,000 -	3
25,001 - 30,000 -	4	30,001 - 40,000 -	4
30,001 - 40,000 -	5	40,001 - 50,000 -	5
40,001 - 48,000 -	6	50,001 - 65,000 -	6
48,001 - 55,000 -	7	65,001 - 80,000 -	7
55,001 - 65,000 -	8	80,001 - 95,000 -	8
65,001 - 72,000 -	9	95,001 -120,000 -	9
72,001 - 85,000 -	10	120,001 and over	10
85,001 - 97,000 -	11		
97,001 -110,000 -	12		
110,001 -120,000 -	13		
120,001 -135,000 -	14		
135,001 and over	15		

Table 2

Married Filing Jointly		**All Others**	
If wages from **HIGHEST** paying job are—	Enter on line 7 above	If wages from **HIGHEST** paying job are—	Enter on line 7 above
$0 - $65,000	$560	$0 - $35,000	$560
65,001 - 125,000	930	35,001 - 90,000	930
125,001 - 185,000	1,040	90,001 - 165,000	1,040
185,001 - 335,000	1,220	165,001 - 370,000	1,220
335,001 and over	1,300	370,001 and over	1,300

Privacy Act and Paperwork Reduction Act Notice. We ask for the information on this form to carry out the Internal Revenue laws of the United States. Internal Revenue Code sections 3402(f)(2) and 6109 and their regulations require you to provide this information; your employer uses it to determine your federal income tax withholding. Failure to provide a properly completed form will result in your being treated as a single person who claims no withholding allowances; providing fraudulent information may subject you to penalties. Routine uses of this information include giving it to the Department of Justice for civil and criminal litigation, to cities, states, the District of Columbia, and U.S. commonwealths and possessions for use in administering their tax laws; and to the Department of Health and Human Services for use in the National Directory of New Hires. We may also disclose this information to other countries under a tax treaty, to federal and state agencies to enforce federal nontax criminal laws, or to federal law enforcement and intelligence agencies to combat terrorism.

You are not required to provide the information requested on a form that is subject to the Paperwork Reduction Act unless the form displays a valid OMB control number. Books or records relating to a form or its instructions must be retained as long as their contents may become material in the administration of any Internal Revenue law. Generally, tax returns and return information are confidential, as required by Code section 6103.

The average time and expenses required to complete and file this form will vary depending on individual circumstances. For estimated averages, see the instructions for your income tax return.

If you have suggestions for making this form simpler, we would be happy to hear from you. See the instructions for your income tax return.

Figure 22–3: Form W-4, Employee's Withholding Allowance Certificate. *U.S. Internal Revenue Service.*

OMB No. 1615-0047; Expires 08/31/12

Department of Homeland Security
U.S. Citizenship and Immigration Services

Form I-9, Employment Eligibility Verification

Read instructions carefully before completing this form. The instructions must be available during completion of this form.

ANTI-DISCRIMINATION NOTICE: It is illegal to discriminate against work-authorized individuals. Employers CANNOT specify which document(s) they will accept from an employee. The refusal to hire an individual because the documents have a future expiration date may also constitute illegal discrimination.

Section 1. Employee Information and Verification *(To be completed and signed by employee at the time employment begins.)*

Print Name: Last | First | Middle Initial | Maiden Name

Address *(Street Name and Number)* | Apt. # | Date of Birth *(month/day/year)*

City | State | Zip Code | Social Security #

I am aware that federal law provides for imprisonment and/or fines for false statements or use of false documents in connection with the completion of this form.

I attest, under penalty of perjury, that I am (check one of the following):

- ☐ A citizen of the United States
- ☐ A noncitizen national of the United States (see instructions)
- ☐ A lawful permanent resident (Alien #) ____________
- ☐ An alien authorized to work (Alien # or Admission #) ____________
  until (expiration date, if applicable - *month/day/year*) ____________

Employee's Signature | Date *(month/day/year)*

Preparer and/or Translator Certification *(To be completed and signed if Section 1 is prepared by a person other than the employee.) I attest, under penalty of perjury, that I have assisted in the completion of this form and that to the best of my knowledge the information is true and correct.*

Preparer's/Translator's Signature | Print Name

Address *(Street Name and Number, City, State, Zip Code)* | Date *(month/day/year)*

Section 2. Employer Review and Verification *(To be completed and signed by employer. Examine one document from List A OR examine one document from List B and one from List C, as listed on the reverse of this form, and record the title, number, and expiration date, if any, of the document(s).)*

	List A	OR	List B	AND	List C
Document title:					
Issuing authority:					
Document #:					
Expiration Date *(if any)*:					
Document #:					
Expiration Date *(if any)*:					

CERTIFICATION: I attest, under penalty of perjury, that I have examined the document(s) presented by the above-named employee, that the above-listed document(s) appear to be genuine and to relate to the employee named, that the employee began employment on *(month/day/year)* ________ **and that to the best of my knowledge the employee is authorized to work in the United States. (State employment agencies may omit the date the employee began employment.)**

Signature of Employer or Authorized Representative | Print Name | Title

Business or Organization Name and Address *(Street Name and Number, City, State, Zip Code)* | Date *(month/day/year)*

Section 3. Updating and Reverification *(To be completed and signed by employer.)*

A. New Name *(if applicable)* | B. Date of Rehire *(month/day/year) (if applicable)*

C. If employee's previous grant of work authorization has expired, provide the information below for the document that establishes current employment authorization.

Document Title: ____________ Document #: ____________ Expiration Date *(if any)*: ____________

I attest, under penalty of perjury, that to the best of my knowledge, this employee is authorized to work in the United States, and if the employee presented document(s), the document(s) I have examined appear to be genuine and to relate to the individual.

Signature of Employer or Authorized Representative | Date *(month/day/year)*

Form I-9 (Rev. 08/07/09) Y Page 4

Figure 22–4: Form 1-9, Employment Eligibility Verification. *U.S. Department of Homeland Security, U.S. Citizenship and Immigration Services.*

exposure to hepatitis B in blood and other body fluids, OSHA regulations require employees to have a series of vaccinations, provided by your employer, for your protection. If the employee's particular office responsibilities make it unlikely to come in contact with the virus, the employee might be permitted to decline the vaccine. In that case, the employee would need to sign a form stating that the vaccine was declined and that if the employee comes upon a spill of blood or body fluids, he or she will avoid contact and notify a properly trained person to handle the material. If the job responsibilities change at any time, the vaccine might have to be administered.

Employee Payroll

The medical office must have a federal tax reporting number (called the Employer Identification Number or EIN), which is obtained from the **Internal Revenue Service (IRS)**. In states that require employer reports, a state employer number must also be obtained.

When payroll checks are prepared, a record must be kept showing Social Security, federal taxes, any state and city taxes, and insurance amounts deducted from earnings. Employees may be paid an **hourly wage** or a **salary** (a fixed amount paid on a regular basis for a prescribed period of time). The Federal Fair Labor Standards Act regulates the minimum wage and requires overtime to be paid to hourly wage earners at a minimum rate of one and one-half times the regular rate for hours above 40 hours per week. It is necessary to keep records of hours worked, total pay, and all **deductions** withheld for all employees. A number of electronic time card systems, in addition to a time clock (punch type) and custom time record, are available (refer to Figure 22–5).

All employees are expected to work the assigned number of hours per day, week, and month. Any time off must be reconciled on the payroll records and the wages adjusted according to office policy.

Forms are available from office supply businesses (and often online) for payroll recordkeeping. Office management may be used for recording payroll data. There should be a page for each employee's payroll record. The heading should give the following:

- Name
- Address
- Social Security number (or employee ID number)
- Date of employment

WEEKLY TIME SHEET

Employee:

Manager:

Week Ending:

Day		Regular Hours	Overtime	Sick	Vacation	Total
Monday						
Tuesday						
Wednesday						
Thursday						
Friday						
Saturday						
Sunday						
	Total Hours					
	Rate per Hour					
	Total Pay					

Employee Signature: **Date:**

Manager Signature: **Date:**

Figure 22–5: Sample weekly time card. *Delmar/Cengage Learning.*

Medical Office One
1234 Main Street
Anytown, US 12345-6789

3/23/2010

Pay to: SALLIE MED STUDENT $781.91
****************Seven hundred eighty one & 91/100*****************

Sally Med Student
1234 Healthcare Lane
Anytown, US 12345-6789

Medical Office One 1234 Main Street Anytown, US 12345-6789	Sally Med Student 1234 Healthcare Lane Anytown, US 12345-6789
CHECK DATE: 03/23/2010 PERIOD START: 03/14/2010 PERIOD END: 03/20/2010 EMPLOYEE ID: ***-**-6789	NET PAY: $781.91

EARNINGS:				TAXES:		DEDUCTIONS:		YEAR TO DATE	
Type	Hours	Rate	Amount	Type	Amount	Type	Amount	Type	Amount
Wage	40	$25.00	$1000.00	FED WTH	$111.59			Wages	$5,000.00
				FICA	$62.00			Fed Wth	$557.95
				MED FICA	$14.50			FICA	$310.00
				ST WTH	$30.00			Med Fica	$72.50
								St Wth	$150.00

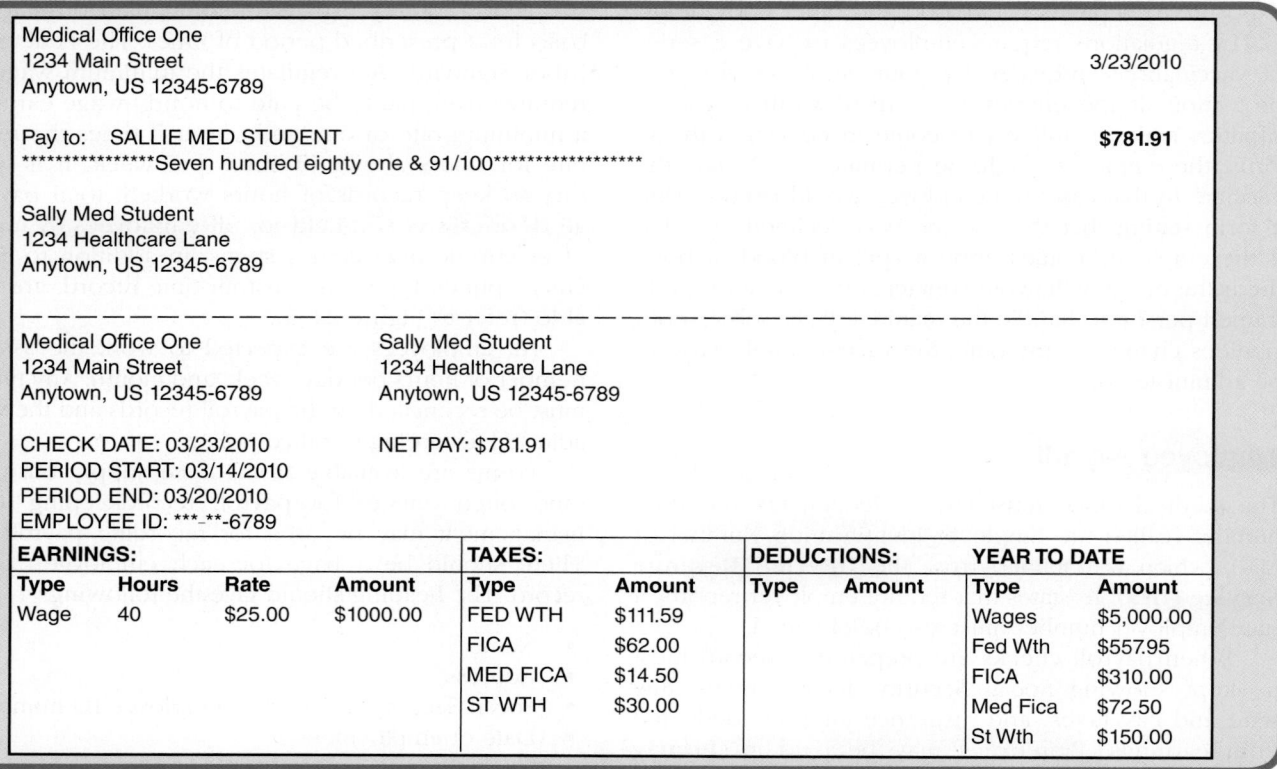

Figure 22–6: Sample payroll check. *Delmar/Cengage Learning.*

There are columns in which the following information can be recorded:

- Date of check
- Hours worked (regular and overtime)
- **Gross** salary
- Individual deductions: federal income tax, Social Security tax, state tax, local tax, insurance, and other deductions (perhaps uniforms)
- **Net** pay (the actual amount of the paycheck after deductions).

Refer to Figure 22–6 for an example of a payroll check.

When an **accountant**, management firm, payroll (or HR) department is employed to prepare payroll, office records must be given to them by a designated date each pay period (weekly, bi-weekly, or monthly) so that payroll can be prepared on time and records maintained on file.

The amount of federal tax withheld is based on the amount earned, marital status, number of exemptions claimed, and length of the pay period. The IRS provides the charts used to figure deductions for federal income tax and Social Security tax. State and local taxes are usually a percentage of gross earnings. Payroll software programs automatically calculate deductions and are updated with new tax tables each calendar year or if tax rates change.

The net pay (pay actually given to the employee) is the gross earnings minus taxes and other deductions. The provider or employer must provide the employee with a statement of gross pay and deductions along with the check each pay period. The tax deductions withheld must be deposited within the specified time frame by IRS regulation. If the tax deposit or report is late, substantial penalties are assessed. Be sure to check with your accountant or access the IRS Website for the most current information (www.irs.gov). You must also comply with reporting requirements (often quarterly and annually) to the federal, state, and local governments.

A W-2 form (Figure 22–7), which is a summary of all earnings for the year and all deductions withheld for federal, state, and local taxes, must be provided to each employee by January 31st of each year. The Social Security Administration must also receive a report of W-2 forms each year. If you collect state or local taxes, you must also provide a copy of the W-2 to these entities as well. Other reporting taxes and reporting requirements include the state and federal government for unemployment taxes and state disability. Procedure 22–1 lists the steps to take when preparing employee payroll.

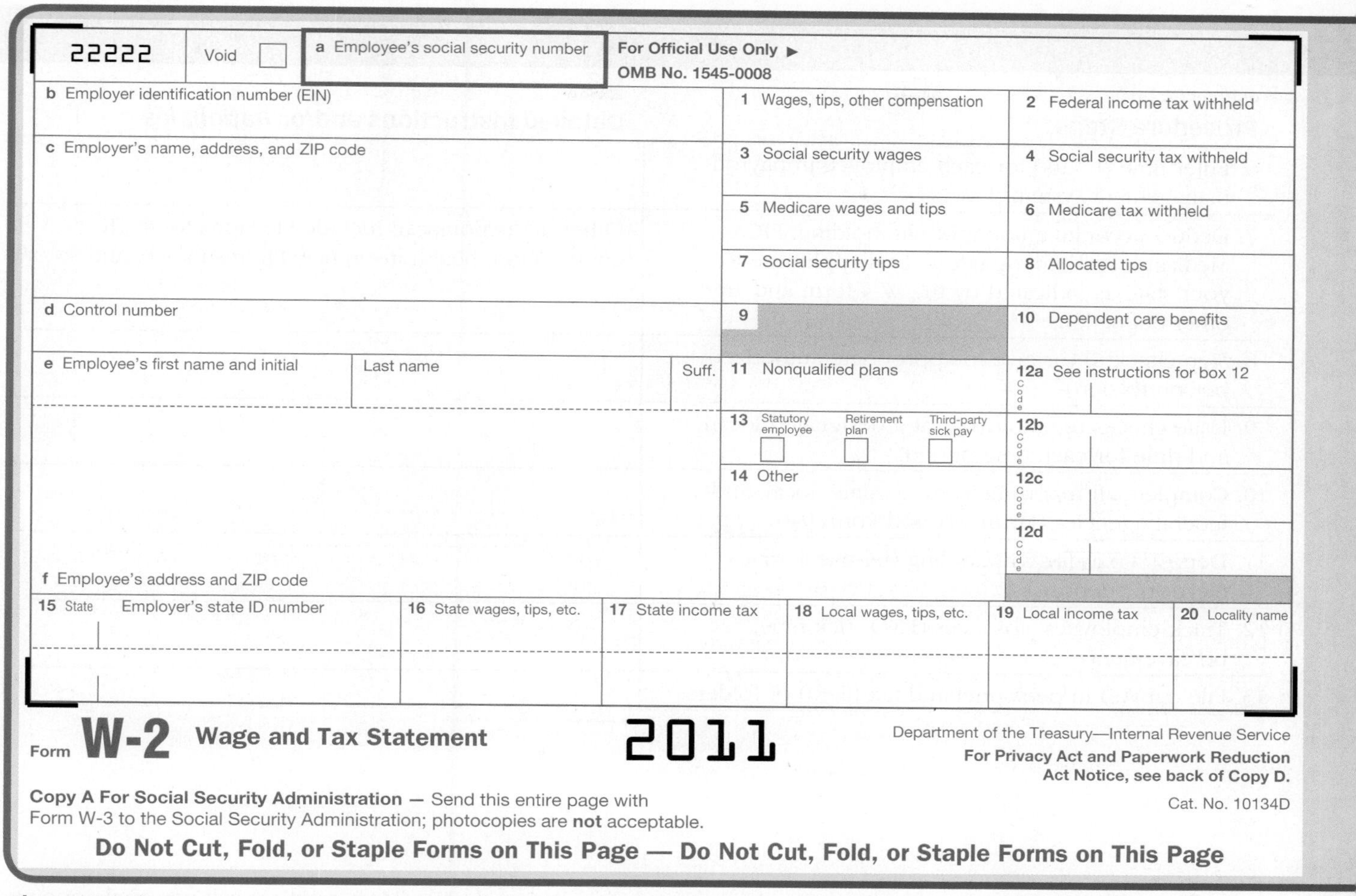

22222 | Void ☐ | a Employee's social security number | For Official Use Only ▶ OMB No. 1545-0008

b Employer identification number (EIN)

c Employer's name, address, and ZIP code

d Control number

e Employee's first name and initial | Last name | Suff.

f Employee's address and ZIP code

1 Wages, tips, other compensation
2 Federal income tax withheld
3 Social security wages
4 Social security tax withheld
5 Medicare wages and tips
6 Medicare tax withheld
7 Social security tips
8 Allocated tips
9
10 Dependent care benefits
11 Nonqualified plans
12a See instructions for box 12 — Code
13 Statutory employee ☐ Retirement plan ☐ Third-party sick pay ☐
12b Code
14 Other
12c Code
12d Code

15 State	Employer's state ID number	16 State wages, tips, etc.	17 State income tax	18 Local wages, tips, etc.	19 Local income tax	20 Locality name

Form **W-2** **Wage and Tax Statement** **2011**

Department of the Treasury—Internal Revenue Service
For Privacy Act and Paperwork Reduction Act Notice, see back of Copy D.
Cat. No. 10134D

Copy A For Social Security Administration — Send this entire page with Form W-3 to the Social Security Administration; photocopies are **not** acceptable.

Do Not Cut, Fold, or Staple Forms on This Page — Do Not Cut, Fold, or Staple Forms on This Page

Figure 22–7: Form W-2 summarizes all earnings and deductions for the year and must be prepared for each employee by January 31. *U.S. Internal Revenue Service.*

PROCEDURE 22–1 Prepare Employee Payroll

PURPOSE: Given a list of employees, time cards, and personnel files with withholding information, prepare payroll and associated tax reports.

EQUIPMENT: Pen, time cards, time clock, calculator, computer, printer, paper, checks (unless outsourced).

S SKILL: Prepare employee payroll.

Procedure Steps	Detailed Instructions and/or *Rationales*
1. Assemble supplies and equipment.	Assemble time cards, employee personnel file(s), calculator, pen, paper, checks, forms, computer, and printer.
2. Review all personnel files and collect copies of employee W-4 and I-9 forms.	
3. Issue time cards (or badges), depending on time and attendance system selected.	
4. Collect time cards (sheets) at end of pay period.	
5. Verify hours and employee signature.	

(continues)

(continued)

Procedure Steps	Detailed Instructions and/or *Rationales*
6. Enter time (hours) for each employee in payroll management system.	
7. Deduct accurate amount of withholding, FICA, Medicare, and other payroll taxes applicable to your state as indicated by the W-4 form and any other deductions.	Other deductions can include elections for 401K contribution, health insurance, life insurance, and so on.
8. Sign check(s) (or give to appropriate authorized person to sign).	
9. Issue checks to employees at a designated location and time for each time period.	
10. Complete all reporting forms to state, local, and federal agencies (Form 941 and Form 940).	
11. Deposit taxes for withholding (by check or electronic deposit).	
12. Track employees' absences (PTO, sick time, bereavement)	
13. File copy(s) in personnel and tax file(s) or folders.	

Benefits

Full-time medical office employees can expect **benefits** in addition to their wages. These are sometimes known as **fringe benefits**. Benefits vary according to the size of the practice. The following are examples of benefits that might be offered.

- *Paid time off (PTO):* Some practices group holidays, personal days, sick, and vacation time into one category called PTO benefits. Using a mathematical equation based upon the employee's date of hire, a percentage of PTO is accrued each pay period.

If your practice does not use PTO, you can expect:

- *Vacation:* Often an average of two weeks with pay after completing a year of full-time employment; increases with **longevity**.
- *Holidays:* Usually six paid holidays per year—New Year's, Memorial Day, Fourth of July, Labor Day, Thanksgiving, and Christmas.
- *Sick time (if not included as part of your PTO or vacation):* Some practices will pay employees when they need to be out of the office because of illness for a limited number of days (three to five sick days per year).
- *Personal time:* (Most practices ask personal appointments to be made during lunch or after hours or when your provider is not seeing patients.) If not included in a PTO package, this time is for an employee to take off for medical or dental appointments and other personal matters without having to use vacation or sick time. There is a limit on personal time (usually not more than three days per year), and it can also be used for family care matters.
- **Bereavement time**: This is time an employee can take off when a family member dies. The amount of time is usually based on the relationship of the employee with the deceased.
- *Jury duty:* Some practices will pay employees when they are summoned to appear in court. The amount of time granted is based on the court order. It is possible to be excused from duty if your position is considered critical to your employer.
- *Health insurance:* Options are usually available (but might require some copayment). If the employee is covered by insurance through the spouse's employment, he or she might not be covered, or larger organizations might offer a cafeteria option by which he or she can choose benefit coverage with a set amount of money for the package.

- **Disability** insurance: This benefit covers a percentage of the salary if the employee is unable to work because of a disabling condition.
- *Life insurance:* Usually for a set amount such as equal to a year's salary.
- **Profit sharing** (retirement): A form of pension plan to employees who meet certain requirements such as being at least 21 years old, working a minimum of 1,000 hours in a year, and remaining employed for at least a year to establish eligibility. Each plan has its own requirements. For example, an amount equal to a certain percentage of the employee's salary is deposited annually into the plan by the employer. This amount accumulates interest and grows tax free until it is withdrawn. The employee is normally responsible for the taxes due. There is usually a period of time, five years for example, before an employee becomes **vested** in the plan. This means the person must be employed at least five years before being eligible to receive the money in the account if employment is terminated.

Sometimes medical care is offered to employees (referred to as **complimentary** health care); however, some practices prohibit employee–provider PCP relations due to potential conflicts of interest. It can be a benefit to be a practice's employee when a referral to another provider or medical specialist is needed. This is something the manager should discuss with providers and set an office policy about.

Medical practices that offer a good benefit package and competitive salary usually have less turnover in staff, resulting in more reliable long-term relationships. This results in reduced expense of training new employees and maintains of a high level of **productivity** for the office and practice.

Office Liability Insurance

Risk management is a fundamental piece of the medical practice. The individual provider or the providers within a group practice purchase insurance to protect their personal and professional assets in case they are found liable for some action or lack of action (commonly referred to as malpractice insurance). Cost of such coverage varies greatly in relation to the type of practice. Other types of insurance need to be in place, such as general liability coverage, workers' compensation insurance, structure coverage (from loss due to theft, fire, other damage), and so on. If you as manager are responsible for acquiring necessary insurance coverage, it is imperative to find a reputable insurance broker experienced in medical practices. If your practice is part of a medical group, the risk management or quality assurance department most likely handles all insurance and claims on behalf of the practice.

Many providers are likely to provide coverage for their employees, who can also be named in a lawsuit. The names of the covered persons are identified within the policy, and the manager might be required to maintain an up-to-date list of employees to ensure that everyone is covered. Depending on the wording of the policy, it might state that all persons receiving wages from the practice are covered, and the listing of individuals would therefore not be necessary. All employees should be informed of their exposure to suit when they are hired. This includes managers and the risk of being named in a harassment or hostile work environment complaint.

It is also important to see that premiums are paid when due to keep the policy in effect. If liability is not offered by the practice, medical assistants should purchase their own policy to protect their personal assets.

Staff Meetings

Figure 22–8 shows the health care team gathered to discuss important in-house matters, decisions regarding patient care, in-service scheduling, and other topics at a staff meeting. The purpose of staff meetings was addressed in Chapter 7. Issues critical to successful staff meetings and the efficient flow and operation of a medical office require further elaboration.

The office manager is responsible for setting staff meeting schedules, the agenda, and conducting the meetings but often delegates and rotates this responsibility with office staff, which promotes shared responsibility and teamwork. Staff meetings should last from 30 minutes to one hour and be held at least once a month. Often, they are associated with lunch or a continental breakfast to use time more effectively. Employees should receive pay for staff meeting time.

To have a successful meeting, create the agenda to organize the topics to be covered and distribute it to

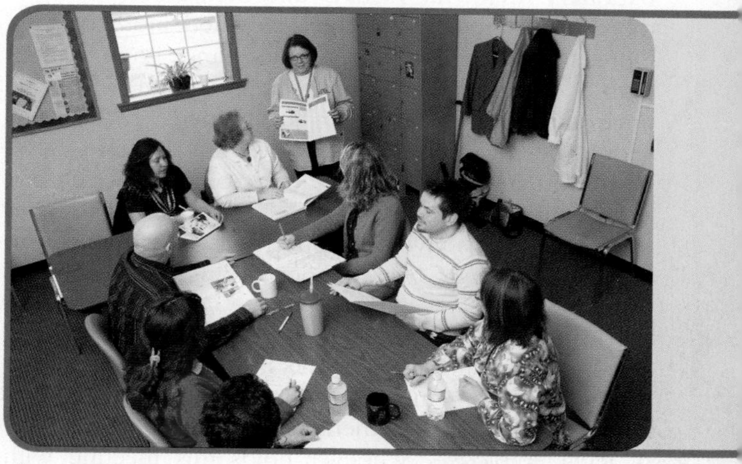

Figure 22–8: Staff meeting. *Delmar/Cengage Learning.*

staff in advance. If decisions are made that will affect office operation, be sure a written record in the form of minutes is kept so there is a reference for any necessary changes in the policy and procedure manual. The meetings should be informative and beneficial and should concern the operation of the office. The meeting should never be allowed to turn into a gripe session. Discussing personal issues associated with individual employees should be avoided when the total staff is present. If an employee wants to discuss an issue that might be considered controversial, the manager should schedule a private meeting to determine the appropriateness of how the issue might affect the practice.

Although one or more of your office providers often attend the staff meetings, in large practices with several providers, physician assistants, and nurse practitioners, separate providers' meetings are held monthly as well. This is in addition to the support staff meetings yet also require an agenda, scheduled times, and distribution in advance to providers.

It is important for all employees to attend staff meetings to learn about any new procedures, policies, or decisions that will affect them. A memo requiring sign-off by each person validates notification. Noting attendance at meetings confirms that each staff member received the information and identifies anyone who did not. Use a sign-in sheet at each staff meeting with the date and employee name or title and attach the agenda.

Employee Evaluation and Review

It is vital to have private meetings between manager and employees to discuss personal goals, performance, expectations, wage adjustments, and educational pursuits. Most employers require employees to have regular, routine, or periodic reviews or **evaluations** regarding their work performance. The time schedule can vary from place to place, but usually there is a probationary review at 90 days and then annual reviews thereafter. A review can be scheduled more often if there is a problem. (Often, a performance improvement plan is developed and implemented with a specific time frame for progress to be attained.) Evaluations should be regarded as an opportunity to share views on performance and expectations. Some employers ask each employee to submit a self-evaluation and peer evaluations. This gives an opportunity to provide input and perception of performance during the evaluation process.

Evaluations are generally conducted by the supervisor, the office manager of the facility, and sometimes by the physician-employer. When complete, the evaluation becomes a permanent part of the personnel file of each employee. Whoever holds this meeting with the employee offers insightful observations about the person. This is done to point out positive performance and areas that might need improvement. A form similar to the one shown in Figure 22–9 (or a much more detailed evaluation) can be used. Upon completion, the evaluation is made available to the employee in a private meeting with the presenter (usually manager or provider on occasion). The employee will be asked to sign it at the bottom, indicating it has been read, discussed, and understood. A copy is given to the employee and the original filed with all the other employee personnel documents.

The performance review presents a good time and opportunity to highlight achievements, outline necessary improvements, and create performance goals (Figure 22–10). For the employee, performance goals mean finding a way to contribute and feel comfortable. For the manager, if expectations of the employees are clear, they can work without constant supervision and in line with the priorities of the practice.

If a special review or performance improvement plan is indicated, the expression "constructive criticism" usually elicits a note of negativity that, even though spoken with good intentions, immediately shuts down the communication process. Although the manager must clearly indicate the deficiency in performance, be sure to keep discussions on a professional level. Give the employee ample, uninterrupted time to tell his or her side of the

Employee's name Job title/position Date hired

Supervisor Title Date of evaluation

Scheduled evaluation/review: ___Initial ___3 month ___6 month ___annual ___*other

*Explain ___

Previous review date ___ Rating ___

Comments ___

Total days/times: absent___ Tardy___ Left early___

Rate the following areas of the employee appropriately using the scale from 1 to 10:
1 2 3 4 5 6 7 8 9 10

Job knowledge: very little / limited / adequate / average / good / superior / outstanding ___

Quality of work: very poor / fair / good / acceptable / excellent / superior / outstanding ___

Quantity of work: inferior/ inadequate/ does just enough/ average/superior/outstanding ___

Speed: very slow / below average / average / above average / outstanding ___

Initiative: lacking / needs pushing / adequate / good / excellent / outstanding ___

Judgment: poor / unreliable / limited / reliable / superior / outstanding ___

Cooperation: very uncooperative / difficult / cooperative / excellent / outstanding ___

Adaptability: poor / slow / satisfactory / good / excellent / superior / outstanding ___

Appearance: poor/unprofessional/avg/reluctantly complies with dress code/outstanding___

Attendance: poor / average / good / excellent / superior / outstanding ___

Total ___

Since last evaluation the employee has:
___improved ___made no noticeable change ___regressed

Recommendation for pay raise: ___Yes ___No

Overall impression:
___unsatisfactory ___fair ___satisfactory ___excellent ___outstanding

Comments about employee's strengths and weaknesses:___

Supervisor's signature___

Employee's signature___

Figure 22–9: An example of an employee evaluation form, which employers may use in documenting employment progress. *Delmar/Cengage Learning.*

Performance Goals

CATEGORY 1: *INNOVATIVE*

- What are you going to do that has never been done in this organization before?
- What new technique, product, tool, service, formula, or any other resource will you create and develop?

CATEGORY 2: *PROBLEM SOLVING*

- What crises do we need to prevent from recurring?
- What problems periodically occur, causing everyone to stop pro-acting and react by putting out these fires?

CATEGORY 3: *OPERATIONAL*

- What needs to be done to keep the operation going?
- What operations, administrative, or ongoing results need doing again this year?
- What are the *key* ongoing results that need to be addressed to keep the operations going?

CATEGORY 4: *PERSONAL AND PROFESSIONAL GROWTH*

- What are you going to do to keep growing so as to prevent yourself from becoming obsolete?
- How are you increasing your human asset value to yourself, your organizational unit, and to the organization?
- What new knowledge, skill, or behavior will you acquire in the upcoming rating/evaluation period?

Figure 22–10: Sample performance goals by category. *Delmar/Cengage Learning.*

story and be an active listener during the meeting. Carefully document the incident and spend time to work on solutions such as asking how could that situation have been handled differently. By using questions, it gives an opportunity for the employee to problem-solve the issue along with assistance of the manager.

Even employees who have excellent work performance can be surprised or even insulted that a supervisor would bring up a trivial weakness (food or drink at the work station). Supervisors who see potential in others are obligated to encourage professional performance, teamwork, growth, and development. This type of meeting can be very difficult for both the manager and employee, so remain open-minded and calm and discuss the problem. Chances are it can be a misunderstanding that can be talked out easily. End the meeting on a positive note of accomplishments and goals. Open dialogue and clear communication works wonders and leads to a better working relationship between managers and employees (Figure 22–11). Many positive results are achieved from reviews of both employee and employer.

Terminating Employment

An employee might leave his or her job for any number of reasons—relocation, advancement to a more responsible position, a higher-paying job, illness, educational pursuits, pregnancy, or a change in lifestyle. The employee, however, has a major responsibility: to give as much advance notice as possible but no fewer than two weeks (Figure 22–12). The manager and employer expect this of all employees to allow the practice to continue running smoothly during the transition of personnel. Receiving notice allows time for the employer to fill the position that is being vacated. However, it often takes much longer than two weeks to advertise, interview, and train a replacement. The employee should direct the notice, a letter of resignation, to the immediate supervisor, the provider-employer, or HR department, if appropriate for the organization, and it should include the date of his or her last working day. This presents a good opportunity to review and update the job description for each employee's position, providing enough detail to help a new employee perform the job with a minimum amount of difficulties.

Employment can also be terminated by the employer. It is often the responsibility of the manager to terminate support staff after discussion and coordination with the provider(s) and HR department. The usual cause for termination initiated by the employer is failure of an employee to perform his or her job responsibilities satisfactorily. Deficiencies can include tardiness, high absenteeism, failure to get along with coworkers and patients, poor work habits, undependability, dishonesty, poor attitude, and uncooperativeness. The manager must synchronize the termination with the payroll department to comply with Department of Labor regulations for providing final payroll within the specified period of time. Consult your local labor department for up-to-date regulations.

In some situations, through employer–employee negotiation, it is possible to change the situation from a termination to accepting a letter of resignation. Depending on the circumstances, it is usually much

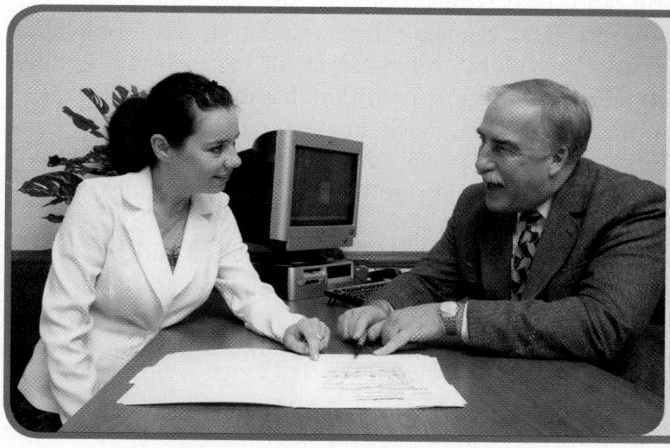

Figure 22–11: Employer discussing evaluation in an open communication manner. *Delmar/Cengage Learning.*

Date

Marlene Blackstone, CMA
Office Manager
Sports Medicine Center
7386 Canyon Road
Anywhere, U.S.A. 10000

Dear Ms. Blackstone:

It is with much regret that I submit this letter as my notice of resignation. My employment over the past five years in sports medicine has been an interesting experience for me. I have learned much in working with such a fine group of professionals. I am grateful for having had this opportunity.

My husband has taken a new position with his company; we are being transferred out of state. I will miss working with everyone at the center. I am giving my two week notice from the date of this letter. My last day will be (insert date).

My thanks to all of you for making my years of employment at the center something that I can look back on with fond memories.

Sincerely,

Patsy J. Keene, RMA

Date

Maxwell S. Mitchell, M.D.
472 Circle Drive
Anywhere, U.S.A. 10000

Dear Dr. Mitchell:

Please accept this as my letter of resignation. During my employment in your practice I have learned a great deal, and I have greatly enjoyed working for you. However, (at this point the writer may choose to add a sentence or two elaborating on the specific reason for leaving).

My X years of employment with you have been a valuable experience for me; thank you for the opportunity to work and learn.

In accordance with your personnel regulations, this letter is my two week notice; my last day in the office will be (at least two weeks hence).

Sincerely,

Your name and title or position with your signature

Figure 22–12: Sample letters of resignation. *Delmar/Cengage Learning.*

better for an employee to resign from a position than to be terminated. As manager, you must check with the employer to see whether a resignation will be accepted.

RESPONSIBILITIES TO PROVIDERS

Providers need to be kept informed and aware of conditions affecting the practice, including financial, staffing, and legal issues; budgets; security; and technology support. The manager has a great deal of obligation to the providers and must at all times listen to their concerns. With most providers having such busy schedules, it is best to check in personally on a daily basis to see whether special issues need attention (such as a change in schedule due to a hospital meeting). Advise the provider if any staff changes, site visits, or IT interruptions are scheduled. Routine items (budget, facility maintenance, and so on) can wait until monthly provider meetings. Communication is essential, as is taking the appropriate action to address and follow up on their concerns.

Some areas the manager must address are:

- Assisting in creating or updating business policies to increase efficiency.
- Attending meetings pertaining to office management such as those sponsored by the medical association and other professional organizations.
- Updating providers on Medicare, health plans, and insurance company policy changes, fee schedules, and reimbursement rates (for example, changes in Current Procedural Terminology [CPT] and International Classification of Diseases [ICD] codes or descriptors or reduction in Medicare coverage affecting reimbursement when accepting assignment). It is critical for providers to learn how coding their services can affect their practice and revenue reimbursement.
- Ordering CPT and ICD books annually and reviewing for deleted or added numbers.
- Holding provider meetings to discuss practice concerns.
- Managing staff in the most efficient and effective manner for provider productivity.
- Maintaining safety and security of patients, office, and staff.
- Ensuring legal compliance (OSHA, QA, HIPAA, ADA, DEA, and so on).
- Selecting, training, and implementing software programs and updates; maintaining hardware and security (the information technology component of a medical practice).

- Creating budgets, FTE usage, revenue grids, and billing and coding analysis (financial status of the practice).

Provider's Professional Meetings

The provider might ask the manager for assistance with all office scheduling, including travel arrangements to attend or make presentations at professional meetings. The schedule can be marked (blocked) so that no patients are booked if it is known far enough in advance. If patients have already been scheduled, they will have to be contacted and offered alternative times. Providers might also want another provider to be contacted to cover during his or her absence. When providers practice within a group, it is usually possible to schedule patients with another group member.

If arranging travel, ask the provider for personal preference. Sponsors of a medical meeting such as the American Medical Association (AMA) will send a conference information flyer that identifies the hotel or hotels in which rooms have been blocked for the attendees. Conference headquarters and meeting rooms can be held in one of the hotels or at a nearby convention center. It is usually convenient to be as close to the meetings as possible. Other activities are sometimes arranged for family members to enjoy during the meetings. Registration for the conference consists of completing the form, selecting a lodging preference, indicating any additional activities, and submitting the registration fee.

There are many things to be considered before you make travel plans:

- Dates
- Will the provider combine the conference with personal time off before or after the meetings?
- Will the provider attend all or part of the conference?
- Is the provider attending alone or with family?
- Hotel and room style preference; compare prices among identified hotels.
- Airline reservations: Is the provider a frequent flyer member with one or more airlines?
- Air transportation to the conference is often contracted at a special rate with one or two airlines and is available by using a special code identifier when booking.
- Compare flight times and prices.
- Will you use a travel agent instead of the association's arrangements? Note that it is not always possible to get room reservations if associations have all the rooms blocked.
- Will you make your own arrangements online?

After you have all the details, you can proceed with making arrangements. Have the practice credit card available on which to charge the reservation and tickets. Many variables are possible when making travel plans. Follow the steps in Procedure 22–2 as one way to manage a provider's professional schedule and travel.

PROCEDURE 22–2 Manage a Provider's Professional Schedule and Travel

PURPOSE: Given all necessary equipment and information, arrange the office schedule, complete and send an event registration, make a lodging reservation, and schedule travel to meet a provider's specifications

EQUIPMENT: Computer, practice credit card, event information, and provider's preferences

S SKILL: Manage a provider's professional schedule and travel.

Procedure Steps	Detailed Instructions and/or *Rationale*
1. Obtain all event, lodging, and travel details from the provider (including provider's preferences).	
2. Arrange the office schedule for the absence: a. Block appointment matrix. b. Arrange coverage as needed.	
3. Complete the event registration information, including extra events and activities.	• Make a lodging selection on the registration form (or select from provider's preferences). • Total the registration and extra event charges. • Copy the registration form.

(continues)

(continued)

Procedure Steps	Detailed Instructions and/or *Rationale*
4. Prepare a check for the amount or charge on the office credit card.	
5. Book the flight, using the practice credit card; print out the e-ticket.	• Go online to contact the preferred conference airline. • Select the most convenient flight schedule. • Process a ticket request, using the identifying code and credit card payment.
6. Record the itinerary specifics for quick reference and make a copy.	
7. Give the provider the itinerary, a copy of the registration, and e-tickets; ensure that the arrangements meet the provider's needs.	

After arrangements have been completed, prepare an itinerary sheet that lists dates, airline, flight numbers and times, hotel name, phone numbers, and any other pertinent information for the provider's quick reference. Tickets obtained online list all the flight numbers, departure times, connecting flights, arrival times, and meal information and can be printed out. This becomes an e-ticket, and no paper tickets will be mailed or need to be picked up. Give the itinerary, reservation information, and e-tickets to the provider. Maintain a copy for office reference.

RESPONSIBILITIES FOR THE FACILITY

The manager has many responsibilities related to the facility, including maintaining the physical structure as well as maintaining the organization's well-being as a whole, as outlined in the following paragraphs.

Regarding the physical structure of the office, the manager assumes responsibility for:

- Maintenance of office services such as cleaning and laundry.
- Subscribing to magazines and health-related literature.
- Monitoring and paying utilities.
- Suggesting improvements: repairs, decorating, and organization of rooms.
- Security (locks, alarm, and so on), privacy, HIPAA-compliant staff, and vendors.
- Information technology support: hardware and software (security and operability)
- Grounds and parking maintenance (unless included in building lease; if so, responsibility can include lease negotiations of the facility).
- OSHA and other regulatory compliance of the facility.
- Proper licensing and insurance of the facility.

A manager who has served successfully in the position can also be given the responsibility to handle renewals of business and professional insurance policies. This could also involve researching different providers and making comparisons of coverage and benefits to obtain the most coverage for the amount spent. Another area that is often the responsibility of the manager is the negotiation of leases and prices for equipment and supply contracts. Careful comparisons of equipment features, supply packaging amounts, and price determine the best purchase option.

Practice Information Brochure

The office manager might be asked to compose an information brochure (also known as a patient information booklet). This brochure can be created using word processing, graphic design, or publishing software. It should be printed on good-quality paper and, if the practice has a logo, this can be placed on the cover of the brochure. The brochure can be as simple as a single sheet neatly folded or as complex as a booklet. An added touch would be a picture of the provider(s) and a map showing the office location. A brochure can be sent to a new patient as confirmation of an appointment or given to the patient at the initial appointment. The brochure must be updated as providers or services are added or deleted from the practice.

The brochure can also contain the following information:

- Brief overview of the practice (name, address, phone/fax numbers)
- Brief description of provider's education and practice interests
- Hospital affiliation
- Practice information and policies
- Office hours
- After-hours policy (nonemergency care)
- Appointment policy (missed and cancellation)
- Financial and payment policies
- Referrals

Daily and Monthly Account Records

As discussed in Unit 9, medical offices use a variety of bookkeeping and accounting systems to maintain a sense of **fiscal** status. An essential component is to identify expenditures and income totals to ensure that the practice is earning sufficient income to meet office expenses, employee salaries, taxes, insurance premiums, and benefits payments in addition to providing an income for the provider. Proper recordkeeping and revenue is necessary to build assets for equipment purchases, investments, and perhaps the hiring of additional employees when needed.

Close monitoring of fiscal matters and active collection of fees and services are vital to the financial health of the practice. With most of the income being billed to third-party payers, it is necessary to keep a record of accounts receivable. You can do this with a record page that begins the month with the amount carried over from the preceding month or with an accounting and bookkeeping software program. Each day, you list charges and receipts and increase or decrease your total accounts receivable balance, depending on whether your receipts or charges were greater. A trial balance, or total of all outstanding accounts, should be calculated each month. The total should agree with the accounts receivable balance.

The accounts payable records include all invoices for purchases, the checks (banking), and the disbursement record. All **expenditures** must be carefully entered. Office expenses must be separated from the provider's personal expenses. Office expenses are tax deductible, but not all personal expenses are.

Practice management software should allow calculations of daily, weekly, and year-to-date figures to provide reports for analyzing the complicated nature of income sources (co-pays, HMO capitation, PPO third-party payments, Medicare, Medicaid, all at contracted rates usually much lower than billed service rates). The accounting software should also provide lists of outstanding receivables and generate a list of delinquent accounts.

Many offices send their billing and invoices to an accounting service through a telephone-linked terminal. Still other offices prepare all accounting records in a batch and take them to an accounting service computer center to be processed. When a personal accountant is employed, the records are maintained and a report provided to the medical practice each month that indicates the expenditures, balances, and accounts receivable. In addition to those already mentioned, the 1099 payment reporting forms issued by third-party payers, which indicate the total amount paid directly to the provider during the year, must be saved and given to the accountant for inclusion with the tax forms.

Once again, software programs offer the most efficient methods for accounting. Consultation with the IT department (or an expert in medical software) for programs that offer the most functionality and interoperability or ones that actually interface with your scheduling and EHR applications should be considered. Managers must spend time with the providers, IT department, and field analysts to determine the most appropriate program(s) for the office.

Fee Schedules

The office manager may be asked to research and contribute to the determination of fee schedules for patient care. The manager will have a continuing awareness of the costs involved for the provider to perform certain diagnostic studies or the cost of disposable products and supplies involved in certain procedures. As costs of products and supplies increase, the fees may have to be adjusted to accommodate the increased expense. The manager will need to refer to the Centers for Medicare and Medicaid Services (CMS) Website for updated (annually) information regarding approved procedures and approved reimbursement rates for reference and guidance.

Patient Accounts

Many medical offices have outside billing services to handle patient accounts. If this is the case, it is still the responsibility of the provider and office staff to ensure accurate ICD and CPT coding. In addition, the office (provider, manager, and staff) is still responsible for recoding rejected claims. The practice is required to collect current insurance and demographic information from patients and update on a regular basis. If your office bills directly, then as manager, you must follow billing guidelines as discussed in Unit 8.

Patient Refunds

Managers usually assume the responsibility of verifying overpayment to a patient's account before approving **reimbursement**. This situation occurs when both the patient and the insurance company pay the provider or an error in the amount due is made and a refund is due the patient (see Chapter 18).

Missed or Late Cancelled Appointments

A related area that a manager might need to address is missed or late cancelled appointments. A missed appointment policy should be distributed in new-patient packets either prior to or during the first office visit. If a patient does not show or late cancels, the provider or practice receives no payment for that scheduled time of the day. In addition, another patient who needed to see the provider was either scheduled at another time or referred out if necessary. As an example, say there is one no-show for an average charge of $50. If this occurs three days in a week for 48 weeks during a year, $7,200 of income is lost. A policy of calling to remind patients of upcoming appointments can be established to reduce the incidence of missed or late cancelled appointments, in addition to a fee assessed.

Any time a patient calls to cancel an appointment, it is critical to record it in the patient's chart or entered in the computer system, documenting the reason for the cancellation. This demonstrates that the patient failed to keep an appointment and generates a no-show or late cancel charge. A courtesy letter can be sent reminding patients of the policy and charge (Figure 22–13). This creates a record of warning if the patient habitually misses or late cancels appointments, and the provider determines to dismiss the patient from the practice.

Dear [Patient Name]:

This letter is to inform you that you missed your last appointment scheduled for [DATE] and did not cancel without giving at least an eight–business hour notice. Please understand that our goal is to provide all our patients with quality medical care. Please call the office in advance if you have to cancel your appointment. It is the policy to charge for no-show appointments without proper notice. Thank you in advance for your cooperation.

Sincerely,

Figure 22–13: Sample letter to patient about a missed appointment. *Delmar/Cengage Learning.*

Preparing for Site Reviews

It is the responsibility of the manager to prepare the office for site reviews, which might need to be delegated to the office staff. Many insurance companies announce their visits in advance. Inspections for compliance with regulations such as Clinical Laboratory Improvement Amendments (CLIA), Occupational Safety and Health Administration (OSHA), and boards of health do not always give advance notification. It is imperative for office managers to familiarize themselves with the latest guidelines regarding these regulations. Keep current handbooks, licenses, policies, and procedure manuals up to date and readily accessible. Good teamwork is essential when preparing for site visits.

Many organizations inspect providers' offices from time to time, including:

- Insurance companies.
- Commission on Office Laboratory Accreditation (COLA).
- OSHA.
- Local or state board of health.
- Drug Enforcement Administration (DEA).
- Fire department.

Many areas are examined during site reviews. They can be divided into categories such as:

- Site guidelines.
- Building and facility.
- Service accessibility.
- Pharmaceuticals.
- Laboratory.
- Equipment.
- Medical records, general.
- Medical records, content, and structure.
- Staffing issues.
- Radiology.
- Patients' rights.
- Medical records, preventive medicine items.

Moving the Office

Medical offices change locations for many reasons. Some offices outgrow their space. Others find a facility that is more economical or in a better and more convenient location. The office manager is usually the one who coordinates the move. Prior to the change, communication with the practice owner is essential. Goals need to be clearly defined. When the date of the move is known, patient schedules should be adjusted to allow for any last-minute changes. It is also recommended for schedules to be reduced to 50 percent for the first day at the new office because, often, there

TABLE 22–2 Responsibilities at Existing Facility

• Purging medical records	• Preparing current medical records (charts) for move
• Purging X-rays	• Arranging for storage of purged records (approved HIPAA storage facility)
• Discarding or cleaning and storing items that are no longer relevant	• Obtaining a minimum of three written estimates from moving companies (must be HIPAA compliant and approved vendors)
• Reviewing lease and complying with any terms stated upon vacating premises	• Notifying vendors and utility companies
• Performing IT assessment, arranging for coordinated time to power off, move, and reinstall at new location	

are technical issues with equipment, computers, EHR programs, software, hardware, and so on. Table 22–2 represents many of the responsibilities that arise as a result of an office move.

You must notify many businesses of your move. This is a good time to evaluate carefully which businesses you wish to continue to work with and which you want to replace. The following is a partial list of businesses you must notify several weeks prior to your move:

- Gas company
- Electric company
- Telephone company
- Waste management
- Vending machine company
- Security company
- Grounds maintenance (landscaping and snow removal services)
- Background music provider
- Equipment leasing companies
- Post office
- Directory assistance
- White business and yellow pages
- Biohazardous waste removal
- Medical bureau
- Cleaning company
- Periodicals companies
- Lab
- Pharmacy(ies)
- Support service group (e.g., IT support services)

If there is more than one provider in the practice, each one must be listed with the post office, phone company, medical bureau, and so forth. If the practice has a name, information for that too must be changed. All companies that provide services must be notified and work together to make certain that the office has uninterrupted service throughout the entire move.

Other businesses that need to be notified of your move include the hospitals and insurance companies with which the practice has current contracts, state medical boards, laboratories, CLIA, COLA, X-ray board, and all providers who send referrals or to whom the practice sends referrals.

The patients are the most important group to be notified of an office relocation. This is most effectively done by sending a form letter (or email notice for offices with a patient email database) to each one. The database in the computer should be able to produce names and addresses to merge into form letter text to make it seem more personal. Names and addresses can be printed directly on the envelope or onto mailing labels, which can be affixed to the envelope. The move should be announced to patients coming to the office as soon as it is known because of the need to make follow-up appointments. The move also can become part of the office's recorded phone message. An announcement in the local newspaper would also be beneficial.

Preparing the New Facility

Many things must be taken care of at the new facility prior to the move. If the facility is new or requires some remodeling, it can be necessary to work with construction contractors. During the construction phase, it will be important to involve the IT department to install necessary wiring for computers, telephones, and wireless systems (in addition to security systems). The manager is responsible for verifying the contractor who is building the site to meet OSHA, CLIA, fire, and other regulatory compliance. A building inspection is normally required prior to occupancy. Confirm this with the contractor and local building department. Interior designers can take care of the decorating. Furniture, window coverings, and other items for the new facility must be ordered. Equipment and supplies must be stocked, utilities turned on, and the phone system installed to operate properly. Moving an office is a very involved task that must be organized and coordinated to the very last minute to be as efficient and smooth as possible. There are often delays in construction, supplies, and equipment, so careful planning with enough allotted time is essential when planning a move. Moving also requires things to be up and running the same day, which is why a reduced schedule is often recommended.

The Day of the Move

There are times the staff should be divided on the day of the move; part of the staff will remain at the old location, and part will go to the new location. If professional movers have coordinated the move and all equipment is installed, office is functional, and patients have been notified, then everyone could be assigned to the new facility. Assign each staff member specific responsibilities. After everything has been moved from the old facility, make a thorough inspection of the old office, arrange for the cleaning, and join the other staff members at the new facility.

CHAPTER SUMMARY

Medical assistants often advance into administrative roles in the medical office. Some of the managerial responsibilities will include:

- Responsibilities to employees of the interview, hire, supervision, training, work and vacation schedules, performance evaluations, discipline and termination.
- Preparing and maintaining up-to-date policy and procedure manuals. Examples include the understanding of HIPAA and office policy, employee records, employee payroll, staff meetings, and employee evaluation and review.
- The administrative medical assistant also has responsibilities to the providers. You must understand and prepare a provider's processional schedule, meetings, and travel arrangements as necessary.
- You will also be responsible for the facility, including duties to create and update practice information brochures; establish, update, and enforce patient accounts policies (missed appointments, daily and monthly account records, patient refunds); maintain office liability insurance; and prepare for site reviews (site visits and insurance site review).
- The responsibility for decision making will fall to the administrative medical assistant. Your role is to work in collaboration with the practice management team and providers for decision making in the medical office.
- Moving and relocating a medical office are large tasks assigned to the office manager. Medical offices relocate for many reasons: They outgrow existing space, or a new facility is more economical or in a better or more convenient location. These responsibilities are paramount to the success of the move: IT assessment of current and new facility; review of lease; record purging; vendor contact; and patient notification, all of which must provide a smooth and seamless transition.

STUDY TOOLS

Workbook	Activities for Chapter 22
Premium Website StudyWARE	Activities and Quizzes on the **StudyWARE™ Software** for Chapter 22
	Audio Library of medical terms
	Online access to the **Critical Thinking Challenge 2.0**
learninglab	Module: Managing the Medical Office Environment
CourseMate	Activities and Quizzes for Chapter 22
WebTutor	Activities and Quizzes for Chapter 22

CHECK YOUR KNOWLEDGE

1. The manager has which of the following responsibilities?
   a. Conduct staff meetings to inform, discuss, and exchange information
   b. Create, implement, and enforce work schedules
   c. Arrange vacation schedules and coverage
   d. Conduct performance evaluations, establishing probationary periods as deemed necessary
   e. a, b, and d
   f. All of the above
2. Ensuring compliance with HIPAA regulations is the manager's responsibility by:
   a. discussing HIPAA at providers' meetings.
   b. discussing HIPAA at staff meetings.
   c. conducting an audit of PHI.
   d. updating computer passwords.
   e. b, c, and d.
   f. b and c.
3. The office policy manual does NOT include policies regarding:
   a. paid time off (PTO).
   b. harassment.
   c. information technology.
   d. opening and closing the office.
4. The office procedure manual includes procedures regarding:
   a. confidentiality.
   b. continuing education.
   c. employment evaluation.
   d. emergency procedures.
5. All employees should have the following documents or information available when filling out initial payroll forms.
   a. Driver's license or other state picture identification
   b. Major credit card
   c. Social Security card and a copy of Social Security numbers of all dependents
   d. All of the above
   e. a and c
6. Documentation needed for personnel files includes:
   a. immunization record.
   b. copies of any professional license, registration, degree, diplomas, or certification.
   c. verification of Occupational Safety and Health Administration and Clinical Laboratory Improvement Amendments (OSHA and CLIA) training.
   d. all of the above.
7. When preparing a payroll check, which of the following should NOT be included?
   a. Date of check
   b. Employee telephone number
   c. Gross salary
   d. Individual deductions: federal income tax, Social Security tax, state tax, local tax, insurance, and other deductions
   e. Net pay (the actual amount of the paycheck after deductions)
8. In addition to wages, employees can often expect to receive which of the following benefits?
   a. Paid time off (PTO)
   b. Health insurance
   c. Auto insurance
   d. All of the above
   e. a and b
9. Staff meetings are a method to accomplish what?
   a. Personality conflict resolution
   b. Employee evaluations
   c. Policy implementation
   d. Employee salaries
10. Employee evaluations achieve which of the following?
    a. Two-week termination notice
    b. Performance goals
    c. Achievement recognition
    d. Necessary improvements
    e. All of the above
    f. b, c, and d
11. Responsibilities to the providers do NOT include:
    a. grounds maintenance.
    b. financial and budgeting issues.
    c. staffing.
    d. security.
    e. technology support.
12. Responsibilities to the facility include which of the following?
    a. Monitoring and paying (approving) bills
    b. Staff meetings
    c. OSHA and other regulatory compliance
    d. a and c

WEB LINKS

American Academy of Medical Management: www.epracticemanagement.org

Americans with Disabilities Act: www.ada.gov

Clinical Laboratory Improvement Acts: www.cms.hhs.gov/clia/

Internal Revenue Service: www.irs.gov

Occupational Safety and Health Administration: www.osha.gov

RESOURCES

Krager, D., and Krager, C. (2005). *HIPAA for Medical Office Personnel*. Clifton Park, NY: Delmar Cengage Learning.

Lindh, W., Pooler, M., Tamparo, C., and Dahl, B. (2010). *Comprehensive Medical Assisting: Administrative and Clinical Competencies* (4th ed.). Clifton Park, NY: Delmar Cengage Learning.

Simmers, L. (2001). *Diversified Health Occupations* (5th ed.). Clifton Park, NY: Delmar Cengage Learning.

United States Department of Homeland Security, United States Department of Justice, Civil Rights Division, National Task Force on Violence against Health Care Providers, *Security Tips*. Retrieved 4/7/01. *www.justice.gov/crt/about/crm/faceweb.php*

Section

3

Structure and Function of the Body

Unit

11

Anatomy and Physiology of the Human Body

The human body is a fantastic combination of parts that function in an organized manner, far more efficiently and effectively than any machine ever developed. This unit begins with the body's fundamental structure and function. It continues with the organization of the body into its systems of function that work together to provide a state of homeostasis (or normal state). This means that all the complicated parts are working together appropriately.

The diseases and disorders affecting the human body are a result of impairment, deterioration, or malfunction of one or more of its component parts. These chapters present the anatomy of each body system and how that system physiologically functions within itself and with the other body systems. Following the presentation of each system will be a discussion of characteristic pathophysiologic conditions and disorders, many of which result from the body's inability to adapt or defend itself.

A basic discussion of the critical role of the immune system in maintaining a healthy state will help you to correlate your knowledge of the body's complex interrelationships. With this understanding, you will be able to see how the patient's concerns and complaints, the physician's examination, and the clinical findings fit together to indicate the diagnosis and the plan of treatment the physician prescribes.

In addition, there is content regarding the characteristics of the body's structure and function as it relates to an individual's age, as well as a look at the interaction of the systems that are involved in a disease condition.

Material relating to the structure and function of the human body is exciting yet at times quite technical. The inclusion of diagnostic examinations, diseases and disorders, and usual methods of treatment further complicates the content. In order to obtain the most recent information available, the National Institutes of Health, medical newsletters and health-related association publications have been utilized. Professional colleagues reviewed the content and provided information. Almost daily, the print and electronic media releases information on new research findings and results of studies that are rapidly changing the manner in which health care is provided. All these data are beyond the capability of any one individual to fully acquire or use. The speed at which scientific discovery occurs can be explosive once a specific "piece of the puzzle" is found. Before this material is published, another discovery may cause the information to be inaccurate or obsolete. You must be alert to information about new findings. Evaluate it carefully. Look for *fact,* not "seems-to-be" results. Observe the persons studied in any research to see if it makes a reported finding seem valid for the total population. It is hardly significant when the findings are shown to be in a small group of people who are living in the same area or are all about the same age and gender. You live in a time when scientific capability is raising many ethical, moral, and legal questions. The possibility of altering our very cellular structure is at hand. Be inquisitive, be excited, be informed, and you will be knowledgeable.

Certification Connection

	Ch. 23–35
CMA (AAMA)	
Body as a whole, including multiple systems	X
Systems, including structure, function, related conditions and diseases, and their interrelationships	X
RMA (AMT)	
Body systems	X
Disorders and diseases	X
CMAS (AMT)	
Basic structures and functions of body systems	X
Various disorders of the body (diseases, conditions, syndromes)	X

Chapter

23 Anatomic Descriptors and Fundamental Body Structure

OBJECTIVES

In this chapter, you will learn the following:

KB LEARNING OBJECTIVES

1. Spell and define, using the glossary at the back of the text, all the Words to Know in this chapter.
2. Describe the anatomical position.
3. Apply the appropriate terminology to anatomical directional references on the human body.
4. Locate the eight body cavities on an illustration.
5. Name the major organ(s) located within each body cavity.
6. Identify the regions of the abdomen.
7. Describe the basic characteristics of the cell.
8. Explain the condition of hemostasis and what happens when it is not maintained.
9. Explain what happens when a mutation occurs.
10. Name the patterns of inheritance and explain how they affect a trait.
11. Describe the six ways molecules pass through cell membranes.
12. Describe the identifying characteristics of the following genetic conditions: cleft lip, cleft palate, Down syndrome, spina bifida, Klinefelter's syndrome, talipes, and Turner's syndrome.
13. Explain why age-related characteristics usually do not occur with congenital and genetic disorders.
14. Identify the three systems that interact in cystic fibrosis.
15. Explain DNA "fingerprinting."
16. Describe the four main types of body tissues.
17. Name the 10 systems of the body.

WORDS TO KNOW

abdominal
abdominopelvic
anatomic
anatomy
anterior
biochemistry
buccal
cardiac
carriers
caudal
cavities
cell membrane
centrioles
chromosomes
congenital
connective
coronal
cranial
cytology
cytoplasm
cytotechnologist
dehydration
diaphragm
diffusion
distal
DNA
dominant gene
dorsal
edema
elements
endocytosis
endoplasmic reticulum
epigastric
epithelial
etiology
exocytosis
extremities
filtration
frontal
gene
Golgi apparatus
gross anatomy
histology
histotechnologist
homeostasis
horizontal
hypertonic
hypochondriac
hypogastric
hypotonic
iliac
inferior
inguinal
involuntary
isotonic
keloid
lateral
lumbar
lysosomes
medial
membrane
microscopic anatomy
midline
midsagittal
mitochondria
mitosis
muscle
mutation

myelin
nasal
nerve
neurilemma
neuron
normal saline
nucleolus
nucleus
orbital
organ
organelles
osmosis
osseous
pathophysiology
pelvic
peritoneum
phagocytosis
physiology
pinocytosis
posterior
proximal
pubic
quadrant
recessive gene
retroperitoneal
ribosome
skeletal
smooth
spinal
stem cells
striated
superior
syndrome
system
thoracic
tissue
trait
transverse
umbilical
ventral
voluntary
X-linked

ANATOMY AND PHYSIOLOGY DEFINED

Two terms are used in discussing the study of the human body: **anatomy**, which is the study of the physical structure of the body and its organs, and **physiology**, which is the science of the function of cells, tissues, and organs of the body. In other words, anatomy describes the framework and physical characteristics, whereas physiology explains how everything works together to support life.

Anatomy can be subdivided into various areas of study. For instance, the term **gross anatomy** refers to the study of those features that can be observed with the naked eye by inspection and dissection. As an example, the pathologist, when examining a tissue specimen, will describe its gross **anatomic** surface appearance and then proceed with the dissection and its description.

An area of study known as **microscopic anatomy** deals with features that can be observed only with the use of a microscope. Referring again to the pathologist, a fragment of a specimen can be properly prepared on a slide and observed with a microscope to complete the description of the specimen's characteristics and formulate an opinion as to its identity or state of condition.

There are two related areas of microscopic anatomy, **cytology**, the study of cell life and formation, and **histology**, the study of the microscopic structure of tissue. **Cytotechnologists** and **histotechnologists** are laboratory specialists who precisely prepare cells and tissue for microscopic examination and diagnosis by the pathologists.

Physiology is the study of the interrelationships of all the functioning structures of the body. When everything is in harmony and all biological indicators are within acceptable limits, the individual is referred to as being in a "steady state" or "normal." This state is also known as **homeostasis**. When the normal physiology is disrupted to the point of instability and begins to deteriorate, pathophysiologic mechanisms are likely to occur and may result in the development of a disease condition. **Pathophysiology** is the study of mechanisms by which disease occurs, the responses of the body to the disease process, and the effects of both on normal function.

Pathophysiology attempts to bring together the clinical signs and symptoms present with the knowledge of the effects of the disease processes on the body, from the cellular level to the total human being. Often close observation of the clinical signs of a disease state has led to the discovery of physiologic functions previously unknown. This is currently apparent in the great effort to understand the immune system to find a way to effectively control and eventually eliminate acquired immunodeficiency syndrome (AIDS) and cancer.

Fortunately, the healthy body has an enormous capacity to protect itself by compensating, defending, and adapting to the pathophysiologic effects of disease. However, when this fails, appropriate medical intervention can often correct or at least control the disease process.

LANGUAGE OF MEDICINE

The members of the health care team must be able to accurately communicate information, findings, and instructions among themselves. Much of the language of medicine is precise and is specific to the field of health care. For instance, it is necessary to not only know about the human body but also to be able to physically and verbally locate body structures and be able to describe the site of a patient's complaint or injury. The following fundamental descriptive terminology will be essential to the understanding of body references.

ANATOMIC DIRECTIONAL TERMS

Certain directional terms are universally used in describing anatomic structures. A body is said to be in the anatomic position when standing erect, with arms down at the sides, and the palms of the hands facing forward (Figure 23–1). This means that when the person is facing you, his or her right side is on your left, as if you were looking in a mirror. When reference is made to a body structure or a specific area, it is in relationship to this anatomical position. The same is true when you are studying illustrations in this textbook or labeling a drawing in the workbook.

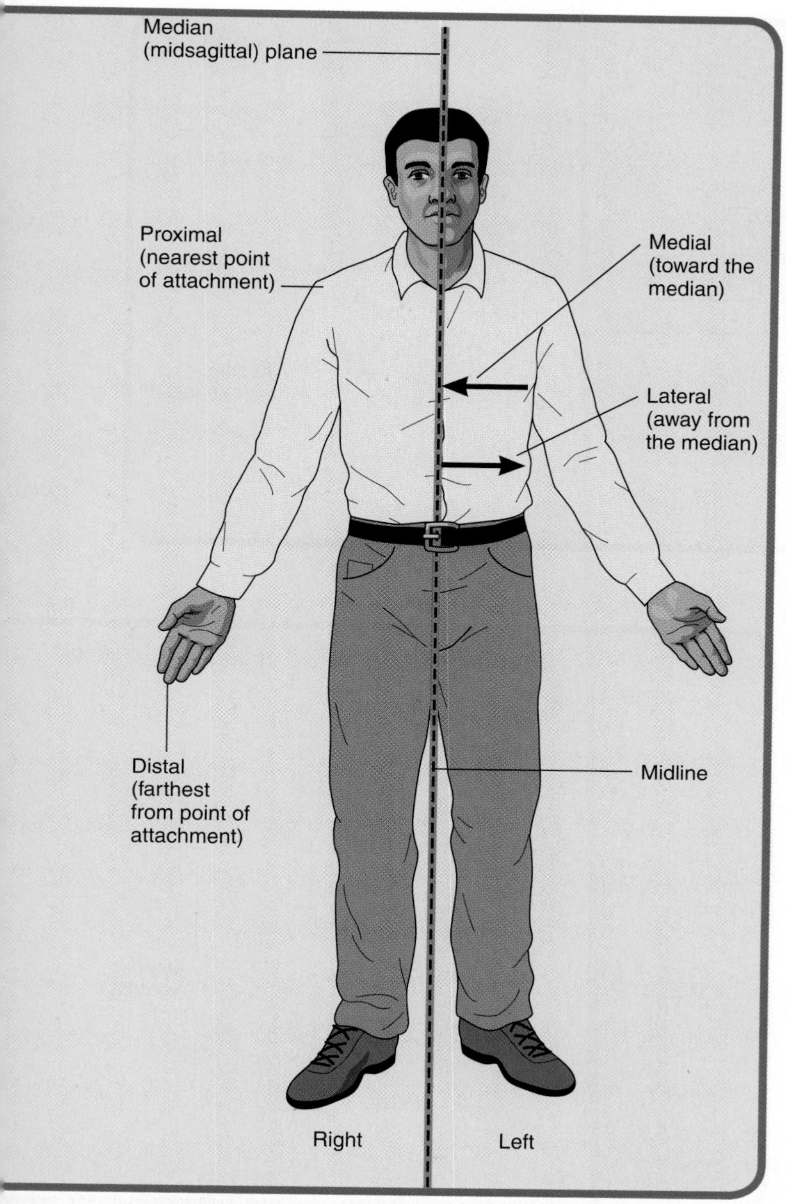

Figure 23–1: Anatomic position with directional references. *Delmar/Cengage Learning.*

Dividing the body vertically down the front will result in a right and left half. This imaginary line is known as the median or **midsagittal** plane. The right and left designations always refer to right and left in anatomic position. Anything located toward the **midline** is said to be **medial**, whereas anything away from the midline is said to be **lateral**.

Two other terms are used to describe the relationship of the **extremities** or ends of the body, such as the arms and legs, to the trunk of the body. **Proximal** indicates nearness to the point of attachment, whereas **distal** indicates distance away from the point of attachment. These terms are also applicable when describing parts of the arms, legs, fingers, or toes. For example, the thumb and great toe have proximal and distal sections, whereas the other fingers and toes have proximal, middle, and distal sections (Figure 23–2).

If you draw a line vertically through the side of the body from the top of the head to the feet, you will make a front and back section (Figure 23–3). This line is known as the **frontal** or **coronal** plane. The front is known as the **anterior** or **ventral** section; the back is called the **posterior** or **dorsal** section.

Finally, drawing an imaginary line **horizontally** (across) the body creates a **transverse** plane. The portion of the body above the line is known as **superior** or **cranial**. The portion below the line is called **inferior** or **caudal**. It is not necessary that the body be divided into equal parts. The terms superior and inferior refer to any relationship of structures above or below a "line" and depend on where it is drawn. For example, with a transverse line at the waist, the chest is superior to the abdomen, but if at the neck, the chest is inferior to the head. All anatomic directional terms are appropriate only when describing the relationship of one structure to another.

These planes or sections can be applied to internal structures and to the body as a whole. *Incisions* (cuts) made on the body surface or into organs are often made along a plane. The surgeon's description of the operation will identify the location of the incisions made using referencing planes. A tissue specimen cut along the transverse plane is known as a *cross section.*

BODY CAVITIES AND ORGANS

The body is divided into two main **cavities**, an anterior or ventral cavity and a posterior or dorsal cavity (Figure 23–4). A dome-shaped **muscle** known as the **diaphragm** divides the anterior cavity into an upper **thoracic** cavity and a lower **abdominopelvic** cavity. The thoracic cavity (chest) has a wall of ribs that protects its vital organs—the heart, lungs, and the great blood vessels (Figure 23–5).

The diaphragm alternately contracts and relaxes to move the lungs, causing breathing to occur.

The abdominopelvic cavity has two parts, an upper **abdominal** portion and a lower **pelvic** portion. The abdominal portion extends from the diaphragm to the top edge of the pelvic girdle (bones). The organs found in the abdomen are the stomach, small intestines, most of the large intestine, the liver, spleen, pancreas, and gallbladder. The kidneys are located in the dorsal abdominal area but are behind the peritoneal **membrane** that lines the cavity and thus are technically outside the abdominal cavity. This space is referred to as **retroperitoneal**, behind the **peritoneum**. The pelvic cavity is surrounded by the pelvic girdle, which provides

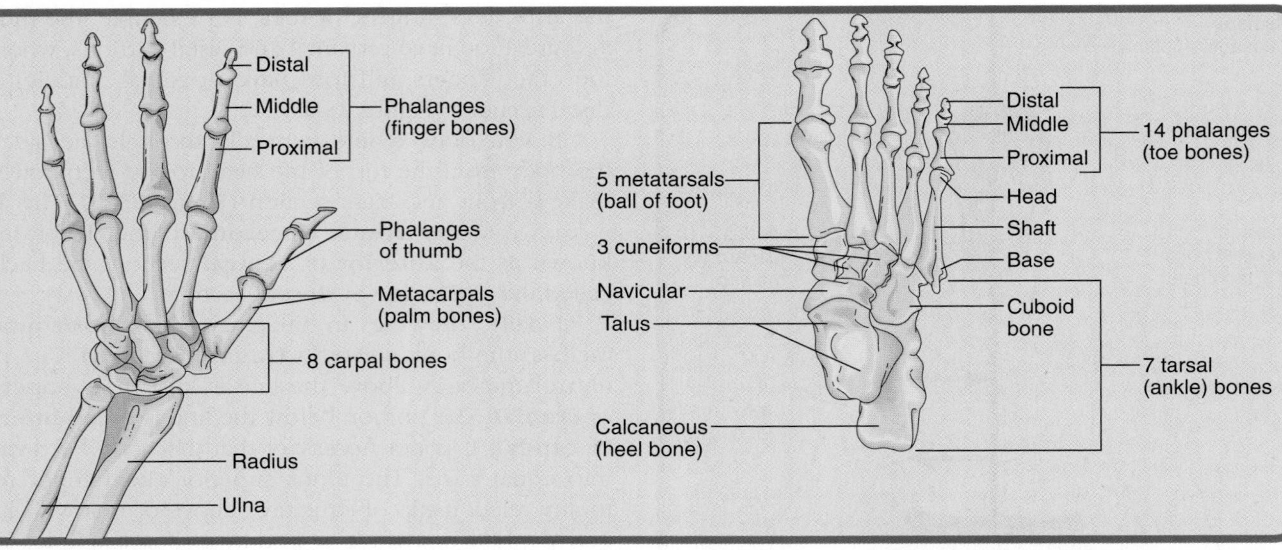

Figure 23–2: Phalanges of the hand and foot. *Delmar/Cengage Learning.*

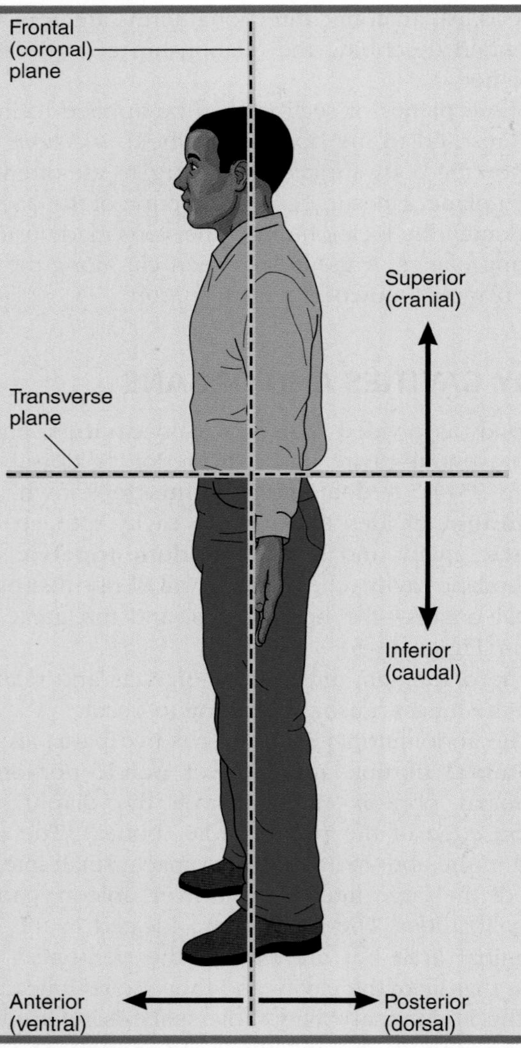

Figure 23–3: Anatomic directional references. *Delmar/Cengage Learning.*

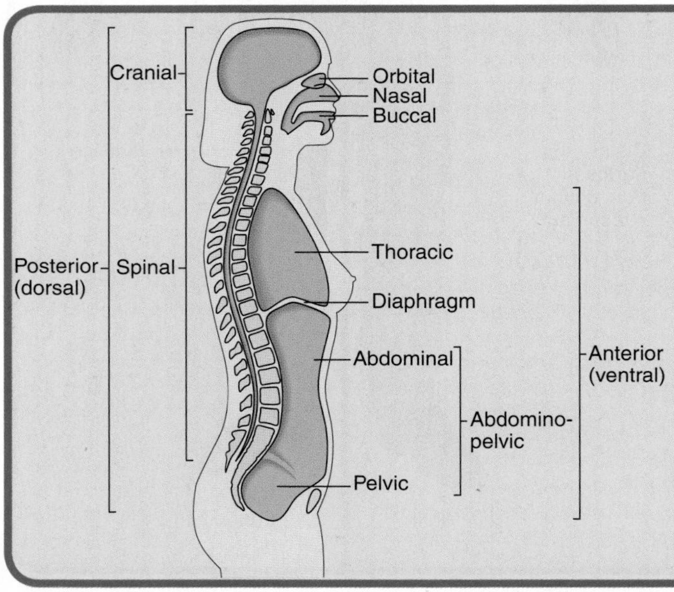

Figure 23–4: Body cavities. *Delmar/Cengage Learning.*

protection for the urinary bladder, the last portion of the large intestine, and the internal reproductive organs. Since organs of the digestive system are found in both cavities, frequently the term abdominopelvic is used to describe this area.

The posterior dorsal body cavity includes a cranial and a spinal section. The cranial cavity is totally encased by the bones of the skull, which provides protection for the brain. The cranial cavity is joined at its base by the **spinal** cavity, which extends through the center of the column of vertebrae (bones). This bony structure contains the spinal cord and protects it from injury.

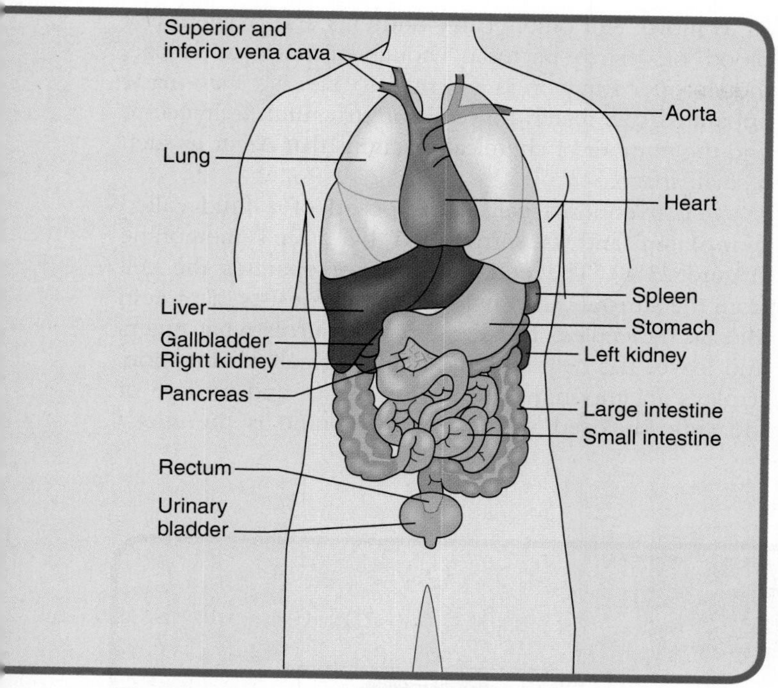

Figure 23–5: Thoracic and abdominal organs. *Delmar/Cengage Learning.*

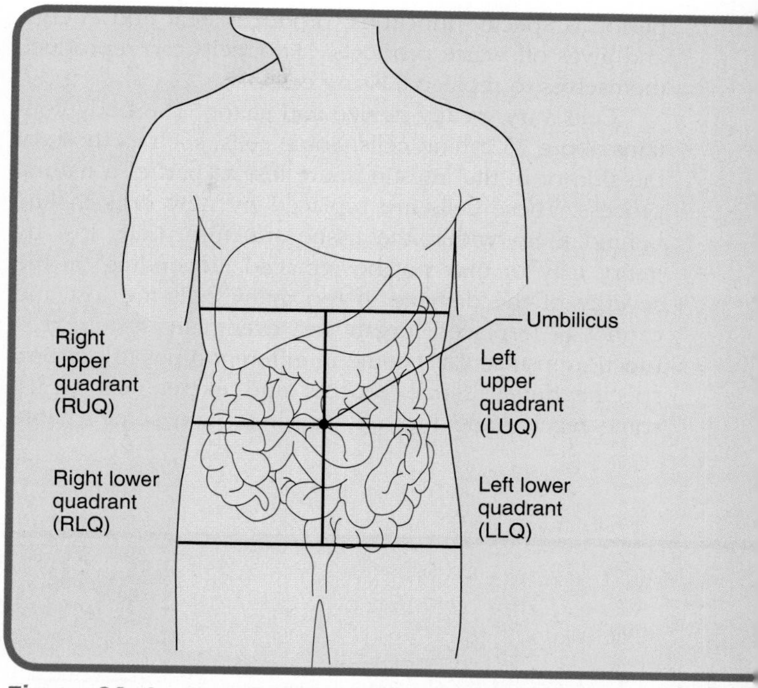

Figure 23–6: The four abdominal quadrants. *Delmar/Cengage Learning.*

There are three other small cavities, the **orbital** for the eyes, the **nasal** for the structures of the nose, and the **buccal** or mouth.

Abdominal Regions

The abdomen is such a large area of the body that it is necessary to divide it into quadrants or regions for purposes of identification or reference. There are two recognized methods. One creates **quadrants** known as the right and left upper quadrants (RUQ and LUQ) and the right and left lower quadrants (RLQ and LLQ) (Figure 23–6).

A more exacting division results in nine regions identifiable by location and an anatomical reference point. The divisions create three central areas:

- **Epigastric** (over the stomach)
- **Umbilical** (around the umbilicus)
- **Hypogastric** (below the stomach; also known as **pubic**)

These are surrounded by six side areas:

- Right and left **hypochondriac** (below the cartilage, referring to the ribs)
- Right and left **lumbar** (loin or side region; also called lateral)
- Right and left **iliac** (referring to the ileum portion of the pelvic bone; also known as the **inguinal**, meaning groin, region)

Figure 23–7 shows these nine regions of the abdomen.

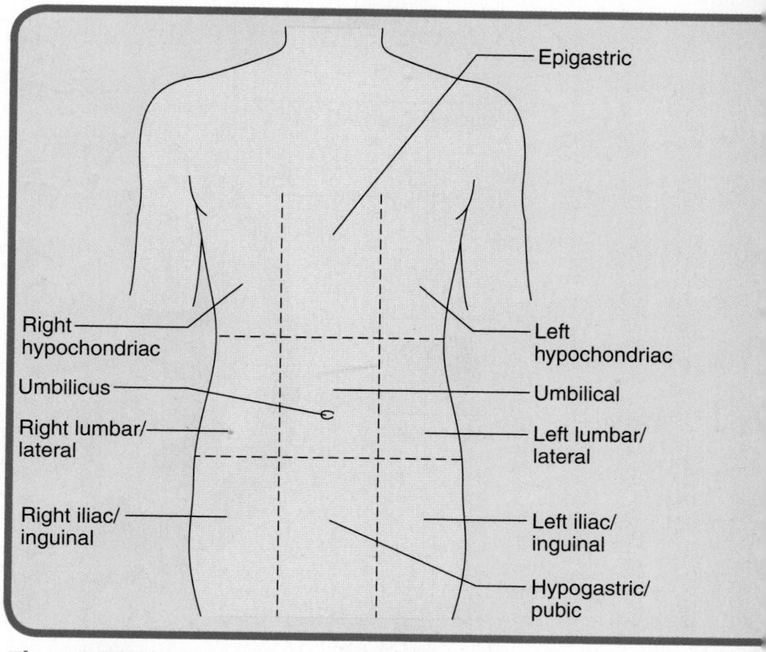

Figure 23–7: Nine regions of the abdomen. *Delmar/Cengage Learning.*

THE CELL

To understand the structure of the body, you must first learn about its basic building block, the cell. This fascinating wonder is a living, working, microscopic image of the body. It requires nutrients and oxygen to survive, performs specific functions, produces heat and energy, and gives off waste products. Many cells can reproduce themselves to replace missing cells.

Cells vary greatly in size and shape. The body contains about 75 trillion cells. Some cells, such as those of the skin or in the intestines, are lost as part of a natural process. These cells are replaced by new cells in line behind them within the tissue structure. Cells lost by injury may or may not be replaced, depending on the severity of the damage. If too many cells are lost and cannot be replaced, organ and eventually system dysfunction results. Cells come in different types to perform specific duties. Some process and excrete chemicals, some receive and transmit impulses, and some enable us to move. Still others carry nutrients and oxygen, clot blood, or destroy bacteria. Though microscopic in size, their proper function is essential to life. No man-made apparatus can match the cell for structural architecture and the number of chemical reactions that occur in such a small space.

A conventional cell is composed of a fluid called **cytoplasm** and is surrounded by a cell membrane (Figure 23–8). The **cell membrane** separates the cell from the surrounding environment. It consists of protein and fat molecules. The membrane controls what enters and leaves the cell, thereby regulating cellular function. It plays an important role in the health and welfare of the cell. Enclosed within the membrane is the sticky

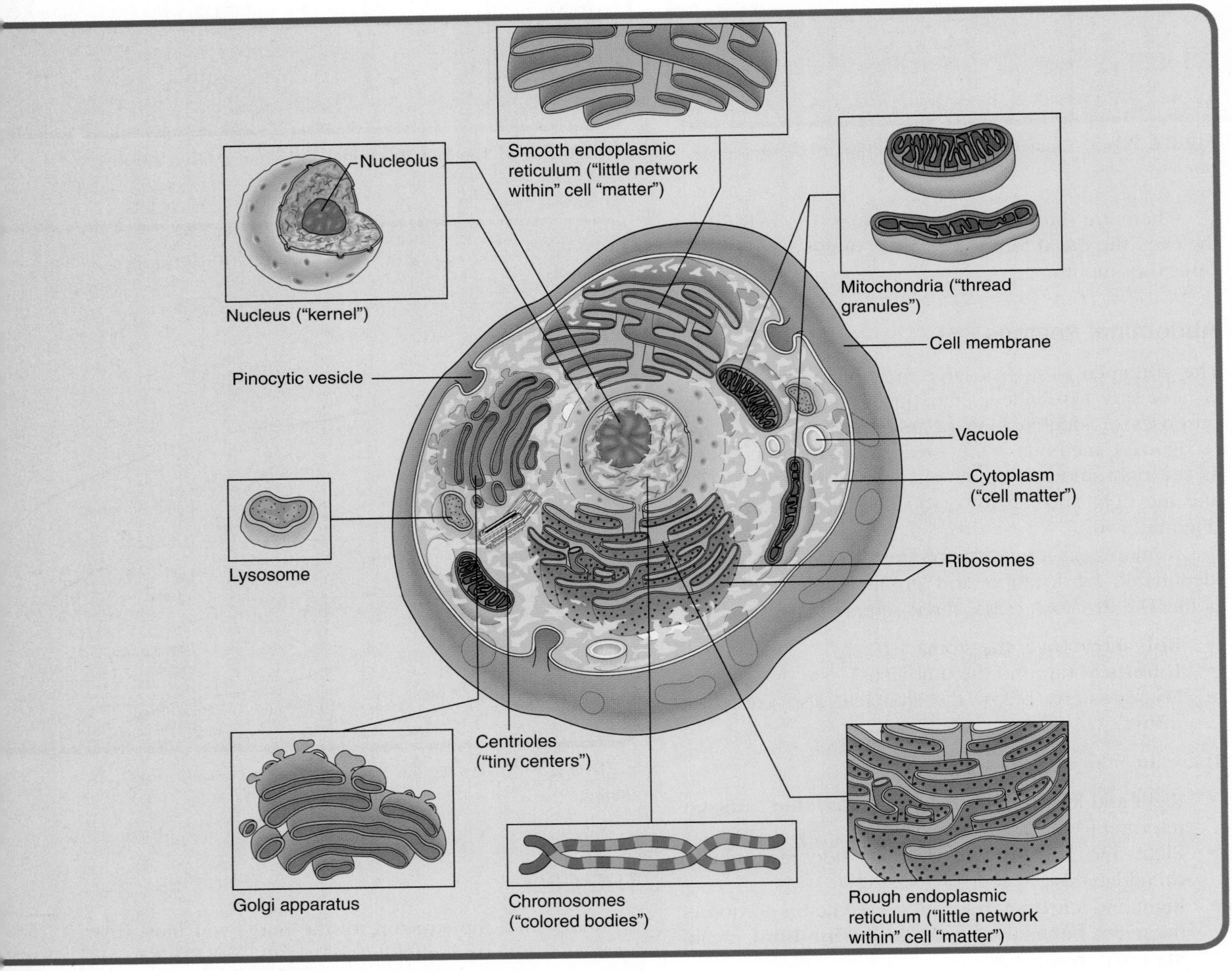

Figure 23–8: Structure of a basic cell. *Delmar/Cengage Learning.*

semifluid material known as cytoplasm. It is a combination of protein, lipids (fat), carbohydrates, minerals, salts, and water (over 70%). Chemical reactions such as cellular respiration and protein synthesis occur in the cytoplasm.

MEDIA LINK

Go to the Premium Website and watch the animation, "Anatomy of a Typical Cell," for this chapter.

The Organelles

Within the cytoplasm of the cell are many minute bodies called **organelles** that perform amazing tasks. The organelles are the **nucleus**, **mitochondria**, **ribosomes**, **centriole**, **endoplasmic reticulum**, **Golgi apparatus**, and **lysosomes**. Refer to Table 23–1 for a summary of the organelles' functions. Scientists still do not understand how some functions are carried out, but they do know some organelles physically separate the chemical reactions occurring in the cytoplasm because many reactions are not compatible. Organelles also control the time when reactions take place, such as producing or processing a molecule in one organelle and then later using the molecule in another reaction.

Organelle Structure and Function

The *nucleus* is a dense mass within the cytoplasm and is the control center of the cell. It is surrounded by its own nuclear membrane. Materials pass in and out of the nucleus from the cytoplasm through pores in the membrane. The membrane is continuous with the endoplasmic reticulum, which often has ribosomes attached. It regulates the chemical reactions and controls the process of mitosis (cell division) for reproduction.

Within the nucleus are the structures called **chromosomes**. Each member of a species has a specific number of chromosomes. Human beings have 46 individual or 23 pairs of chromosomes that store the hereditary material passed on from one generation to the next. Twenty-two pairs of chromosomes are autosome (same in number and kind), and one pair are sex chromosomes, either both X if female or an X and a Y if male. One chromosome from each of the 23 pairs is contributed by the mother and one by the father. When the egg and sperm unite at fertilization, their chromosomes are united so that the new cell, a zygote, will also contain 23 pairs. The sex of the child is determined by whether it is combined with a father's cell carrying an X or a Y chromosome.

Chromosomes are rod-shaped structures composed of long strands of molecules known as deoxyribonucleic acid (**DNA**). DNA is the material within the chromosome that encodes the **genes** that are located at specific sites on the chromosome. The DNA carries all of the genetic information necessary for cellular functions. DNA is composed of sugar, phosphate, and four bases: adenine, cytosine, guanine, and thymine. These bases join together as pairs to form the double helix structure of the

TABLE 23–1 Cell Organelles

Organelle	Function
Cell membrane	Regulates transport of substances into and out of the cell.
Cytoplasm	Provides an organized watery environment in which life functions take place by the activities of the organelles contained in the cytoplasm.
Nucleus	Serves as the "brain" for the control of the cell's metabolic activities and cell division; has DNA and genes.
Nuclear membrane	Regulates transport of substances into and out of the nucleus.
Nucleoplasm	A clear, semifluid medium that fills the spaces around the chromatin and the nucleoli.
Nucleolus	Functions as a site for RNA synthesis.
Ribosomes	Serve as sites for protein synthesis.
Endoplasmic reticulum	Provides passages through which transport of substances occurs in cytoplasm.
Mitochondria	Serve as sites of cellular respiration and energy production; the "powerhouse" of the cell.
Golgi apparatus	Manufactures carbohydrates and packages secretions for discharge from the cell.
Lysosomes	Serve as centers of cellular digestion.
Pinocytic vesicles	Transport large particles into a cell.
Centrosome	Contains two centrioles that are functional during animal cell division.
Centrioles	Provide spindle fibers for attaching chromosomes during cellular division.

DNA. It is estimated the human genome has 3 billion of these base pairs. The genetic coding makes it possible for the exact duplication of the cell.

Genes

Every individual has a different DNA code, but the code in all cells of the same individual are identical. It is the arrangement of the base pairs of the DNA code that makes for the differences. The genes are the units of instruction that produce or influence particular characteristics or traits and the capabilities of an organism. Genes are specific segments of DNA molecules that are located on the chromosomes in the cell nucleus. They act in pairs to dictate traits from eye color to the chemical reactions that determine not only cell structure but also function and, therefore, heredity. A gene consists of sequences of thousands of DNA base pairs. Originally, scientists estimated there were over 100,000 pairs or more of genes, but while the exact number of genes encoded by the genome is still unknown, 2004 findings by the International Human Genome Sequencing Consortium reduce the number of human protein-coding genes from 35,000 to only 20,000–25,000 genes that compose the DNA of a cell. Genes coding for proteins make up about 2% of the human genome. The remaining 98% are in non-coding regions thought to be involved in chromosomal structure and regulating gene activity. This great number of genes helps explain why there is so much variety in the human race, and yet each individual's structure is uniquely and identifiably their own. Consider that during meiosis, each parent's chromosomes are halved, "shuffled," and then combined at fertilization. The father and mother each contribute half of the child's total number of genes to their offspring. The new being now has a unique combination of genes and, consequently, traits.

The nucleus itself will have at least one **nucleolus**. In a nucleolus, portions of ribonucleic acid (RNA) are assembled with proteins to make subunits of the ribosomes, which then pass through the nuclear pores of the nuclear membrane into the cytoplasm, to become a complete two-part ribosome to synthesize protein. Ribosomes are found circulating in the cytoplasm or attached to the endoplasmic reticulum.

Centrioles are the two cylinder-shaped organelles near the nucleus. During mitosis, the centrioles separate and form spindle fibers that attach to the chromosomes to ensure their equal distribution to the two new daughter cells.

Endoplasmic reticulum crisscrosses the cytoplasm in a network fashion. When attached to the nuclear membrane, it serves as a passageway for the transportation of materials in and out of the nucleus. If grouped together, they can store large amounts of protein. The difference between rough and smooth endoplasmic reticulum is the presence of *ribosomes* on the membrane. Ribosome sites of protein synthesis give the membrane a rough appearance.

Mitochondria are round or rod-shaped organelles that supply the cell's energy. There may be one to over a thousand in each cell depending on how much energy that type of cell requires. Mitochondria have a double-membraned structure with the inner membrane folding into ridges. The cell is capable of cellular respiration because the enzymes located in the ridges break down nutrient molecules and oxygen to provide carbon dioxide, ATP (adenosine triphosphate; energy for the cell), and water.

The *Golgi apparatus* is a stack of membrane layers that synthesize carbohydrates and combine them with molecules of proteins. The organelle appears to store and prepare secretions to excrete from the cell. Therefore, the cells of the gastric, salivary, and pancreatic glands have large numbers of Golgi apparatus.

Lysosomes are round or oval structures. They have a strong digestive enzyme that consumes protein molecules such as those found in old worn cells, bacteria, or foreign matter. This is a very important function of the body's natural immune system.

Pinocytic vesicles are pocket-like formations in the cell's membrane. These structures permit large molecules like protein and fat, which cannot pass through the pores of the cell membrane, to enter with the extracellular fluid into the vesicle. Then the "pocket" closes, forming a vacuole (bubble) in the cytoplasm. This process is called **endocytosis**. When liquid droplets, instead of protein or fat molecules, are enclosed, the process is known as **pinocytosis**, which means "cell drinking." A related term, **exocytosis**, refers to a similar process whereby substances are moved from the cell to the outside. On entering the cytoplasm, most vesicles fuse with lysosomes, and their contents are digested. Special white blood cells known as phagocytes rely on endocytosis to destroy harmful bacteria in the body. As you learn more about your body, you will begin to appreciate what a magnificent piece of "equipment" it is and how important it is that you care for it properly. You have the physical and mental power to have a great impact on your health and your life.

PASSING MOLECULES THROUGH CELL MEMBRANES

As stated before, the cell membrane controls materials entering and leaving the cell. This is necessary for the cell to acquire substances from its environment to be processed for its use, for secretion, and for excretion of waste materials. There are six processes by which materials pass through a cell membrane: **diffusion**, **osmosis**, **filtration**, active transport, **phagocytosis**, and pinocytosis.

Diffusion is a process whereby gas, liquid, or solid molecules distribute themselves evenly through a medium. When the medium is a fluid and the molecules are solid, they are called solutes (Figure 23–9). When solutes and water pass across a membrane to distribute themselves, they will move from an area of higher concentration to an area of lesser concentration. Diffusion plays a vital role in the body. For example, higher concentrations of oxygen in the alveolus (air sac) of the lung cross the membrane into the lesser concentrated area of the red blood cell in the capillary (see Figure 23–9). The blood cell, now with a high concentration of oxygen, circulates in the blood to a body cell with lower oxygen concentration and exchanges its oxygen for the cell's higher concentration of waste products. Hence, the body's cells "breathe" in a process called *internal respiration*.

Osmosis is a process of diffusion of water or another solvent through a selective permeable membrane, one through which some solutes can pass but others cannot (Figure 23–10). In the illustration, the membrane will only allow the salt and water to pass through; therefore, the salt leaves the greater concentrated area within the membrane to go to the lesser concentrated water. At the same time, the water leaves its higher concentrated area to enter the lesser concentrated area within the membrane. When the water molecules are equal on both sides, the diffusion will stop. The pressure of the water molecules inside the membrane is then said to be at *equilibrium,* a state known as the *osmotic pressure*.

The osmotic characteristics of solutions are classified by their effect on red blood cells (Figure 23–11). If the solution is of the same osmotic pressure as blood serum, it is known as an **isotonic** solution. A 0.9% salt (NaCl) solution has the same salt concentration as that of the red blood cell and is called **normal saline**. If the osmolality is lower, the solution is **hypotonic**, and the blood cell will swell with water and burst. In a **hypertonic** solution, the cell will release its water and shrink.

Filtration is the movement of solutes and water across a semipermeable membrane as a result of a

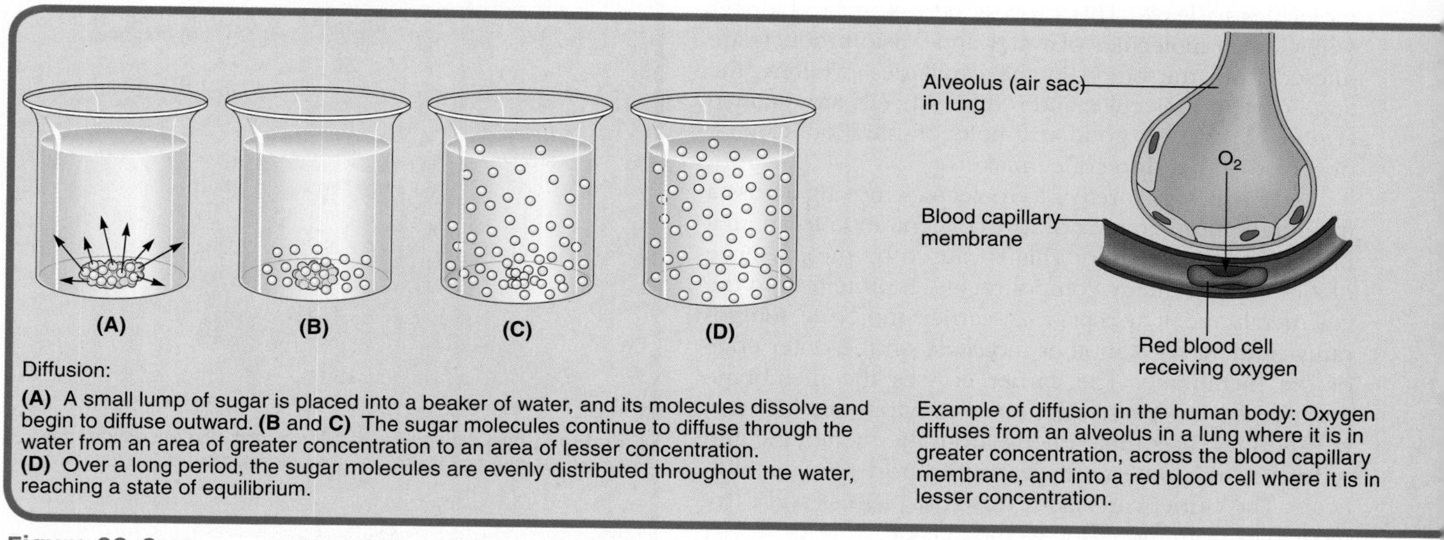

Alveolus (air sac) in lung
O_2
Blood capillary membrane
(A)
(B)
(C)
(D)
Red blood cell receiving oxygen
Diffusion:
(A) A small lump of sugar is placed into a beaker of water, and its molecules dissolve and begin to diffuse outward. **(B** and **C)** The sugar molecules continue to diffuse through the water from an area of greater concentration to an area of lesser concentration.
(D) Over a long period, the sugar molecules are evenly distributed throughout the water, reaching a state of equilibrium.
Example of diffusion in the human body: Oxygen diffuses from an alveolus in a lung where it is in greater concentration, across the blood capillary membrane, and into a red blood cell where it is in lesser concentration.

Figure 23–9: The process of diffusion. *Delmar/Cengage Learning.*

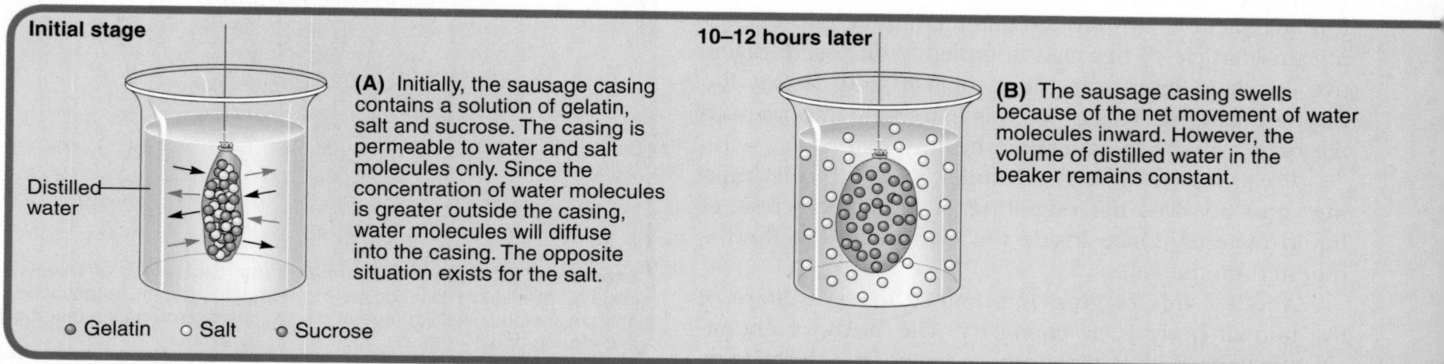

Initial stage
Distilled water
(A) Initially, the sausage casing contains a solution of gelatin, salt and sucrose. The casing is permeable to water and salt molecules only. Since the concentration of water molecules is greater outside the casing, water molecules will diffuse into the casing. The opposite situation exists for the salt.
10–12 hours later
(B) The sausage casing swells because of the net movement of water molecules inward. However, the volume of distilled water in the beaker remains constant.
Gelatin
Salt
Sucrose

Figure 23–10: Osmosis is the diffusion of water through a selective permeable membrane. A sausage casing is an example of a selective permeable membrane. *Delmar/Cengage Learning.*

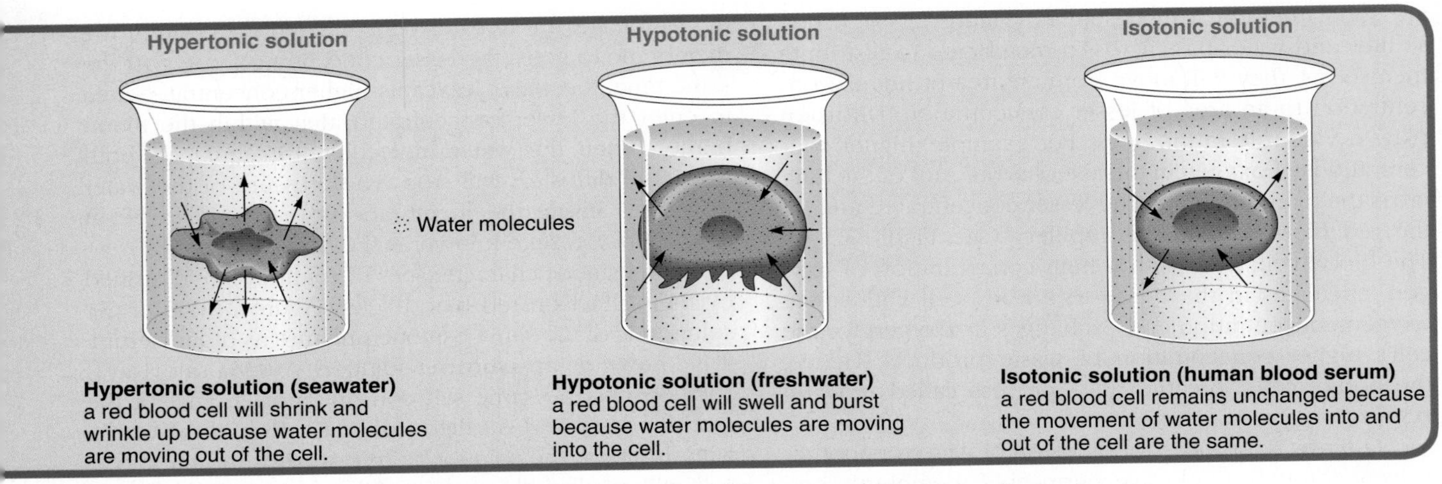

Hypertonic solution
Hypotonic solution
Isotonic solution
Water molecules
Hypertonic solution (seawater) a red blood cell will shrink and wrinkle up because water molecules are moving out of the cell.
Hypotonic solution (freshwater) a red blood cell will swell and burst because water molecules are moving into the cell.
Isotonic solution (human blood serum) a red blood cell remains unchanged because the movement of water molecules into and out of the cell are the same.

Figure 23–11: Movement of water molecules in solutions of different osmolalities. *Delmar/Cengage Learning.*

force such as gravity or blood pressure. The particles move from a higher to a lower area of pressure. The size of the pores of some membranes allow only small molecules to leave. This process occurs in the kidneys where small molecules of water and waste products are filtered from the blood in the capillaries, whereas the large protein molecules and red blood cells are retained (Figure 23–12). A good example of filtration can be observed with a drip coffee maker.

Active transport refers to molecules moving across a membrane from an area of low concentration to an area of higher concentration. This is caused by the presence of ATP, a high-energy compound and a protein from the cell membrane. It appears as a "carrier" molecule, temporarily binding with another molecule on the outer edge of the membrane. The carrier crosses the membrane and releases its "passenger" into the cytoplasm. The carrier then receives more energy from the membrane and returns to the outer surface to transport another molecule. The carrier can also reverse the process and carry molecules from the inside to the outside.

Phagocytosis is known as "cell eating." White blood cells become phagocytes and engulf bacteria, cell fragments, or damaged cells (Figure 23–13). The white cell forms a vacuole by enfolding its membrane and enclosing the particle. When it is completely enclosed, digestive enzymes enter from the cytoplasm and destroy the trapped material. This process is extremely important to the body's ability to maintain a healthy state.

Pinocytosis, as discussed earlier, is called "cell drinking" and involves the engulfing of large molecules of liquid material. Once inside the cytoplasm, the fluid is digested by the cell.

Another area of great importance to the welfare of the human body is its chemistry. The study of chemical reactions within the body is called **biochemistry**. The basic building blocks of all matter are the **elements**, substances in their simplest form. There are 92 natural

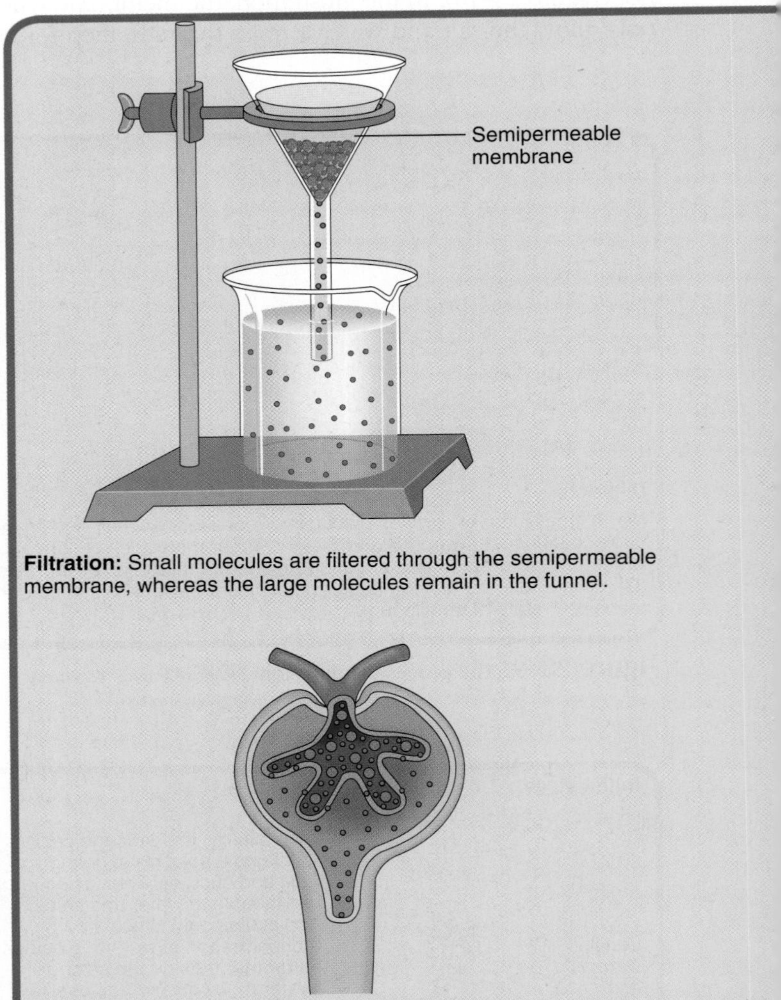

Semipermeable membrane
Filtration: Small molecules are filtered through the semipermeable membrane, whereas the large molecules remain in the funnel.
Example of filtration in the human body: Glomerulus of kidney; large particles like red blood cells and proteins remain in the blood, and small molecules like urea and water are excreted as a metabolic excretory product—urine.

Figure 23–12: Filtration is a passive transport process. *Delmar/Cengage Learning.*

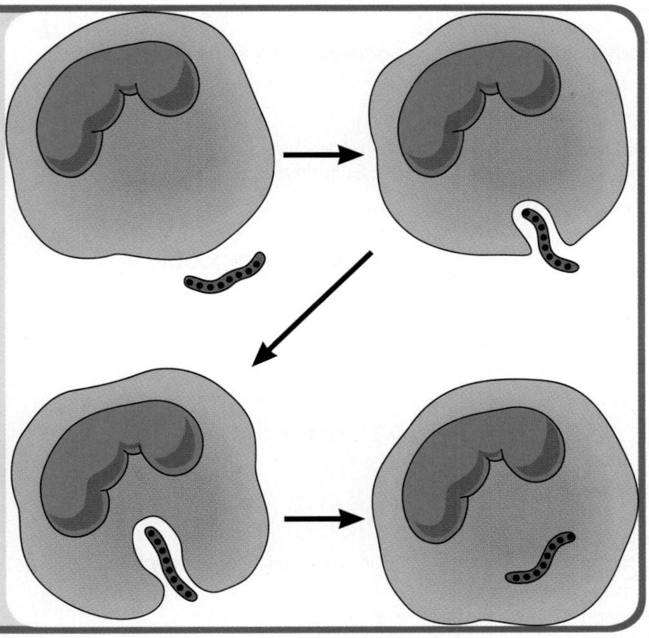

Figure 23–13: Phagocytosis of bacteria by a white blood cell. Phagocytosis can occur in the bloodstream, or white cells may squeeze through capillary walls and destroy bacteria in the tissues. *Delmar/Cengage Learning.*

and at least 13 man-made elements. Of these, about 20 are in all living things. Four of these 20 elements make up 97% of all living matter. They are carbon, oxygen, hydrogen, and nitrogen. The remaining 16 elements are sodium, chlorine, magnesium, phosphorus, sulfur, calcium, potassium, iron, copper, manganese, zinc, boron, tin, vanadium, cobalt, and molybdenum. Because the last four elements occur in the body in such minute amounts, they are known as *trace elements.*

Many elements combine together in specific amounts to form new substances known as *compounds.* Some common compounds are water (hydrogen and oxygen), carbon dioxide (carbon and oxygen), salt (sodium and chloride), hydrochloric acid (hydrogen and chlorine), and sodium bicarbonate (sodium, hydrogen, carbon, and oxygen). Compounds can be classified in one of three groups: acids, bases, or salts. An acid compound will have positively charged ions of hydrogen and negatively charged ions of some other element. They have a sour taste such as is found in some citrus fruits (limes and lemons). However, an unknown substance should not be tasted to determine its acidity; it should be tested by the special dyes contained in litmus paper. If acid is present, blue litmus paper will turn red.

A base compound is also called an alkali. A base substance will have negatively charged hydroxide ions and positively charged ions of a metal. Bases have a bitter taste and will turn red litmus paper blue. Table 23–2 lists some common acids and bases and identifies where they are found.

When an acid and a base are combined, they form a salt and water. A common example is sodium chloride (table salt), which is the result of combining hydrochloric acid with sodium hydroxide. When the water evaporates, the salt remains.

Frequently, the determination of acidity or alkalinity of a body fluid or solution is desired. This measurement is referred to as the pH. A pH value of 7.0 on the pH scale indicates the solution has the same amount of hydrogen ions as hydroxide ions and therefore is neutral. An example of a neutral solution is water. A pH value between 0 and 6.9 indicates an acidic solution. The lower the number, the stronger the acid or hydrogen ion concentration. A pH value of 7.1 to 14.0 indicates the solution is basic or alkaline. The higher the number is above 7.0, the stronger the base or hydroxide ion concentration. The pH inside most cells is maintained between 7.2 and 7.4. The pH values of some common acids, bases, and human body fluids and their effect on a pH testing strip are shown in Figure 23–14.

CELLULAR DIVISION

The division of cells is known as mitosis and is controlled by the nucleus of the cell (Figure 23–15). When a cell is preparing to divide, the two pairs of centrioles, just outside the nucleus, move to opposite sides of the cell (A). Spindle fibers form and attach to the chromosomes, which

TABLE 23–2 Names, Location, or Use of Some Common Acids and Bases

Name of Acid	Where Found or Used	Name of Base	Where Found or Used
Acetic acid	Vinegar	Ammonium hydroxide	Household liquid cleaners
Boric acid	Weak eyewash	Magnesium hydroxide	Milk of Magnesia
Carbonic acid	Carbonated beverages	Potassium hydroxide	Caustic potash
Hydrochloric acid	Stomach	Sodium hydroxide	Lye
Nitric acid	Industrial oxidizing acid		
Sulfuric acid	Batteries and industrial mineral acid		

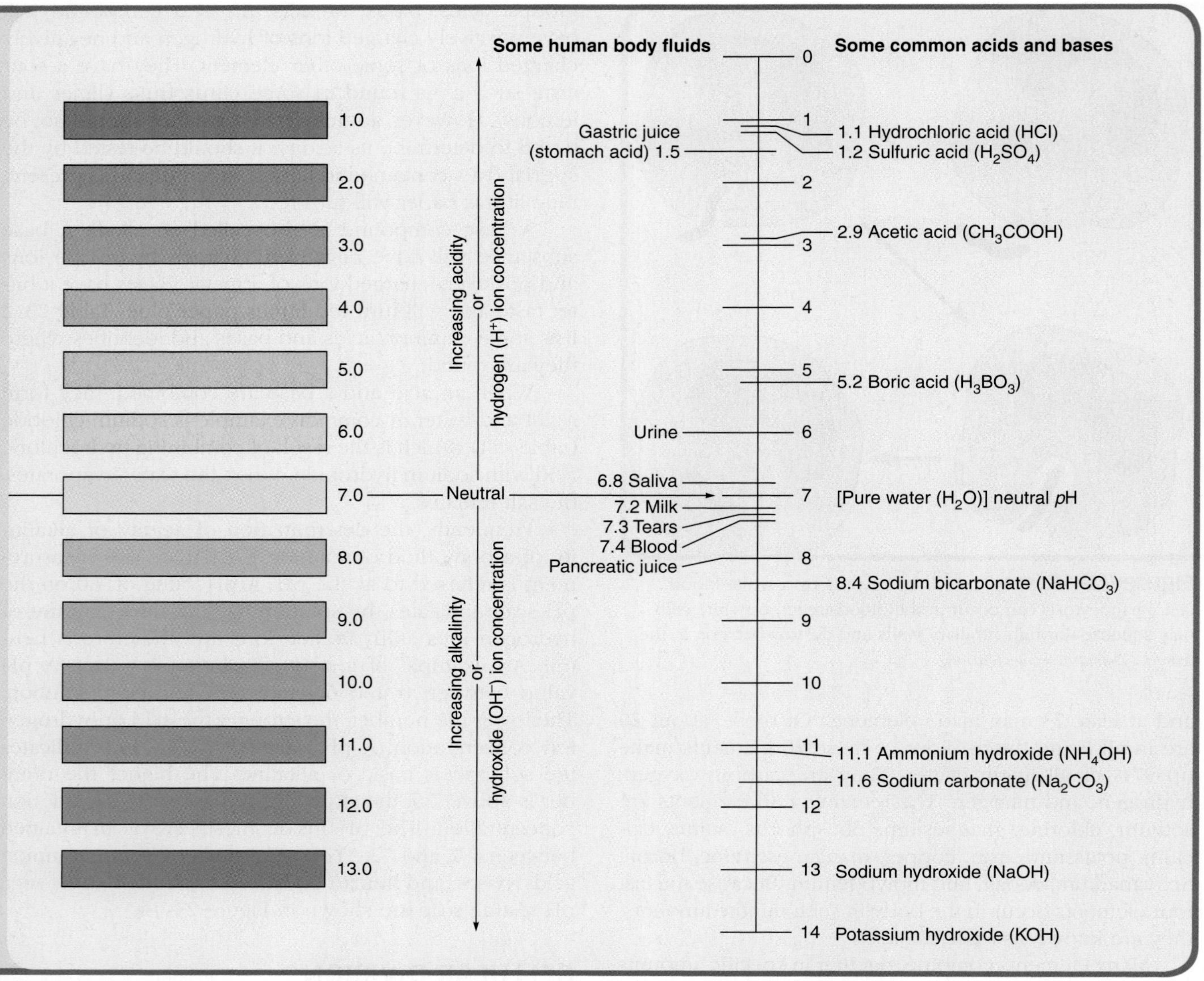

Figure 23–14: pH values of some common acids, bases, and human body fluids and the collar changes that can occur to a pH strip when tested. *Delmar/Cengage Learning.*

"line up" in the center (B). The chromosomes divide and move toward the centrioles at different ends of the cell (C). The spindles then dissolve, and a nuclear membrane develops around each new set of chromosomes (D). For unknown reasons, the cell then pinches itself in two, thereby making two new cells (E) called daughter cells. Mitosis results in the formation of two daughter nuclei with the exact same genes as the mother cell nucleus. The purpose of cell division is to provide exact duplication of cells for growth and repair of the body. In the unit on immunity, you will discover what happens when an antigen (foreign matter) interferes with this copying process.

All cells do not reproduce at the same rate. The bloodforming cells of the bone marrow, the cells of the skin, and the cells of the intestinal lining reproduce continuously. Muscle cells only reproduce every few years; however, muscle tissue formed of voluntary muscle cells may be hypertrophied (enlarged) with exercise. This is apparent from the great increase in muscle size produced by body builders who use weights and repetitions of routines to achieve muscle definition and enlargement. Cells of the **nerve** tissue, or **neurons**, do not increase in number after birth, and some cannot be regenerated if damaged or destroyed.

There are many kinds of cells with different shapes and sizes. The characteristics shown previously in Figure 23–8 are common to most cells. However, cells like those in the blood (red, white, and platelets) and the nerve cells are very different and perform specialized functions. With this specialization, some of the other cell functions may be lost, such as the ability of some

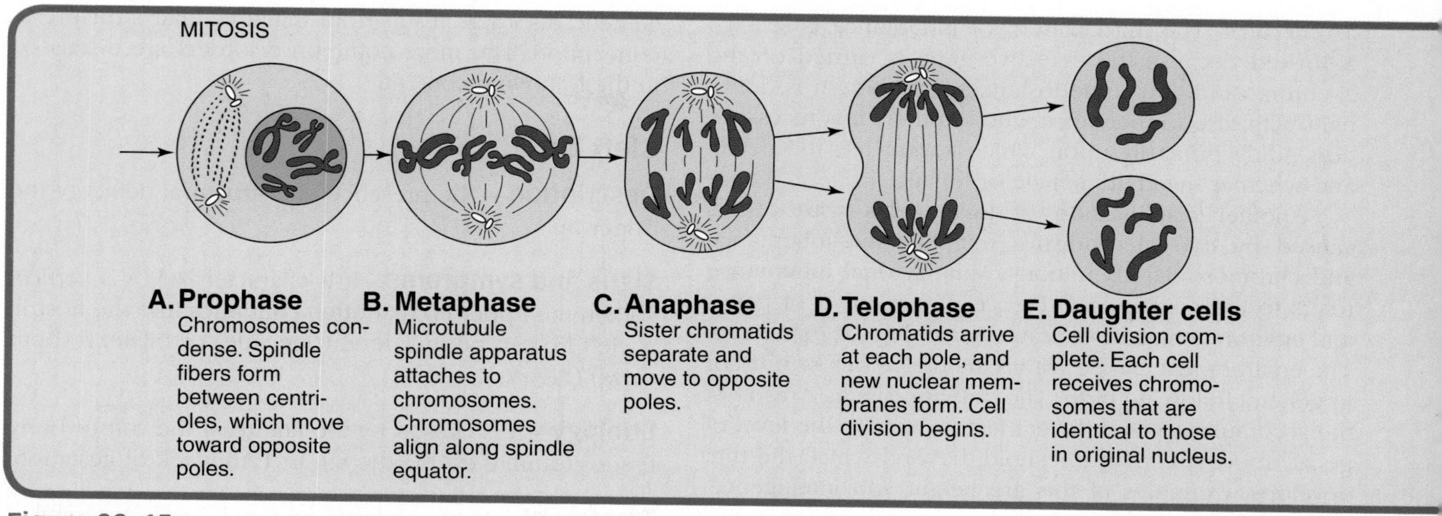

MITOSIS
A. Prophase
Chromosomes condense. Spindle fibers form between centrioles, which move toward opposite poles.
B. Metaphase
Microtubule spindle apparatus attaches to chromosomes. Chromosomes align along spindle equator.
C. Anaphase
Sister chromatids separate and move to opposite poles.
D. Telophase
Chromatids arrive at each pole, and new nuclear membranes form. Cell division begins.
E. Daughter cells
Cell division complete. Each cell receives chromosomes that are identical to those in original nucleus.

Figure 23–15: Stages of mitosis in cells. *Delmar/Cengage Learning.*

nerve cells to reproduce. Specialization also results in an interdependence among cells to enable them to carry out their activities. One type of cell that is very different is the sex cell (gamete), which is responsible for reproduction. During a process known as meiosis, the ovum from the female and the spermatozoon from the male each reduce their respective 46 chromosomes to 23, one half the normal amount. When fertilization occurs, the two cells combine to form a single cell called a zygote, which will then have the full set of 46 chromosomes, 23 from each parent. The zygote will subsequently, by mitosis, divide again and again until the new being is fully developed. This cellular activity will be more fully discussed in the unit on the reproductive system.

HOMEOSTASIS

The body has many control systems, some of which operate within the cell. It is important that the fluid within the cell (*intracellular fluid*) maintains the proper chemical and pH balance for the cell to maintain life. The fluid surrounding the cells (*extracellular fluid*) mixes with the fluid of the blood to supply the cell with food and other substances. When the internal environment is functioning properly and all the organs and tissues of the body are performing their appropriate tasks, a condition of *homeostasis* exists. This is a stable condition of the internal environment. This condition continues until one or more of the control systems loses the ability to maintain it. When this occurs, all cells of the body suffer. A moderate dysfunction causes illness; a severe dysfunction leads to death.

MUTATIONS AND TRAITS

Remember that the DNA is a code that provides information to the cell. It has been compared with the dots and dashes of the Morse code or the "0s" and "1s" of the computer binary code. When these symbols are arranged in different sequences, they form different words. The same is true of DNA. When DNA is being replicated, if some is lost, rearranged, or paired in error, the resulting change in instruction of the genetic code could lead to an improperly functioning or missing protein when the DNA's code is translated. This is known as **mutation**. Genetic mutations can be caused by internal or external factors. Internal factors are those that occur during replication and abnormal metabolism. The amount of background or natural mutations occurring at birth is estimated to be around 3%. External causes include chemicals, X-rays, sunlight, and other radiations. A mutation is a change in a cell resulting from a chemical and/or viral change in the structure of the gene. It is first reflected in the RNA copy, then in the enzyme or protein, and finally in the appearance of new **trait**. A trait is the recognizable result of the effect of a gene or group of genes. Mutations may be either dominant or recessive. They may result in no change or can produce minimal or drastic alterations. They can be beneficial or cause diseases and loss of critical cell function. Mutations provide an essential key for part of evolutionary change, even among humans.

Single genes may be involved in one of three patterns of inheritance as they produce recognizable traits. These are known as dominant, recessive, and X-linked. A **dominant gene** can produce a trait without regard to the nature of its pair member. (Remember: There are two genes, one each from the mother and father.) Dominant disorders are usually milder and result in structural defects rather than abnormalities in function. A **recessive gene** is one whose presence within the pair does not result in a recognizable trait *unless* both members of the gene pair are of a similar mutation; in this case, a recessive disorder would occur. People who have one dominant and one recessive gene are known as **carriers**. The third pattern of inheritance is sex- or **X-linked** because the defective gene is carried on the X chromosome. In some instances, the pattern is dominant with direct inheritance, and in others it is recessive, depending primarily upon which parent has the defect and whether the child is male or female.

Another classification of traits deals with results caused by two mechanisms: multifactorial inheritance and chromosomal aberrations. Multifactorial inheritance refers to the combined influence of a number of genes and environmental factors causing a trait to be expressed. The environment can be within the uterus before birth or in general following birth. The trait appears as a result of the accumulation of sufficient factors to raise the level of genes above a certain threshold, beyond which the trait develops. Examples of this are height and intelligence. Both are influenced prenatally by parental influence and postnatally by environment. Another example is pyloric stenosis, a narrowing of the opening from the stomach into the small intestines that interferes with the passage of food. It is linked to the possibility of a viral infection during pregnancy, and it is known that the child's sex is a factor. Development of the disorder is *influenced* by the fact that the threshold of the factor is lower in the male than in the female. Examples of environmental exposures that are classified as toxins include the use of alcohol (which results in small birth weights), liver dysfunction, and the condition known as fetal alcohol syndrome. Another toxin is the drug diethylstilbesterol (DES), which can adversely affect sex organ development.

Chromosomal abnormalities are the result of either a group of genes occurring in excess or as a deficit of genetic materials. There is a difference in the general effects depending on whether the abnormality affects pairs numbered 1-22, called autosomes, or the X and Y chromosomes of the 23rd pair. Autosome genetic imbalance is invariably associated with mental retardation and exerts influence on the development of the physical structure of the early embryo and fetus. Incorrect numbers of X and Y chromosomes are among the most common chromosomal abnormalities. Chromosomal abnormality can occur as the result of abnormal cell division and from exposure to toxins.

GENETIC AND CONGENITAL DISORDERS

As we have learned, genetic and **congenital** disorders can result from improper sex cell division at the time of fertilization, from the inheritance of an altered gene or genes, from environmental factors, or from toxins. They cause structural defects, retardation, and physiologic disorders. These are collectively called genetic or congenital disorders.

There is a difference between the two. The word congenital is defined as "occurring during fetal life; not hereditary." In other words, it is a "born with" condition. Genetic disorders result from initial cellular structure at conception. The more common disorders are discussed in the following content.

Cleft Lip

Description—The presence of a structural defect of the upper lip.

Signs and symptoms—It is characterized by a vertical split in the upper lip that often continues into the nostril. A cleft lip can be unilateral (one side) or bilateral (both sides) (Figure 23–16A).

Etiology—It is caused by the failure of the soft or bony tissues to unite during the 8th to 12th week of gestation.

Treatment—Modern plastic surgery is very successful at closing the clefts and normalizing the infant's appearance.

Cleft Palate

Description—The presence of a structural defect in the roof of the mouth.

Signs and symptoms—It is characterized by an opening or hole to a total split of the palate. It is often associated with a cleft lip (Figure 23–16B).

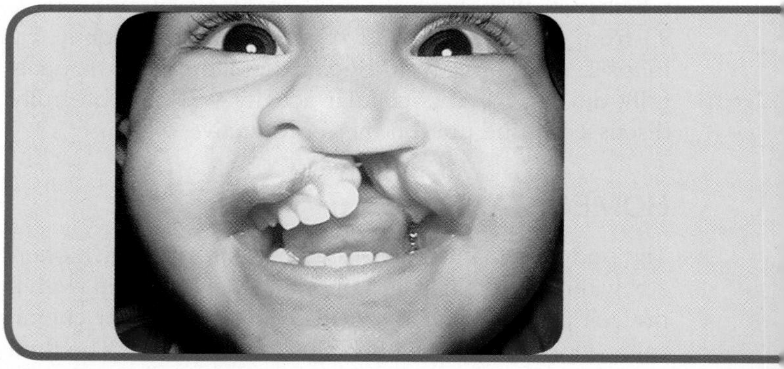

Figure 23–16A: Cleft lip. *Courtesy of Dr. Joseph Konzeiman, School of Dentistry, Medical College of Georgia.*

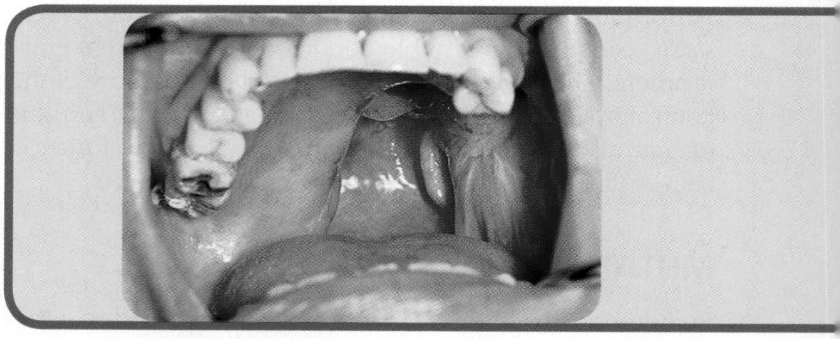

Figure 23–16B: Cleft palate. *Courtesy of Dr. Joseph Konzelman, School of Dentistry, Medical College of Georgia.*

Etiology—It is caused by the failure of the soft and bony tissues to unite during the 8th to 12th week of gestation.

Treatment—Surgical intervention is necessary. The cleft can cause feeding problems for an infant because liquid is able to get into the nose and breathing passages. A temporary solution to the problem involves the use of various types of nipples or an inverted "spoon-like" feeder with a nursing nipple, which provides an artificial roof in the mouth. This allows the infant to suck milk until surgical repair can be done.

Color Vision Deficiency

Description—An inherited trait that makes perception of colors inaccurate. It is erroneously called "color blindness" because most people see some color; rarely do people see only black, white, and gray (monochromatism).

Signs and symptoms—Most affected people see colors and do not realize they have a deficiency until they have a color vision test. The most common problem is distinguishing reds and greens, which can be a problem when driving an automobile. (See Ishihara color vision acuity color plates, Chapter 40.)

Etiology—The deficiency is caused by a defective gene carried on the X chromosome and occurs most frequently among men. Because men have only one X chromosome, it is more likely to be expressed. Women have two X chromosomes and are likely to have a normal gene that will dominate the defective one. Rarely the condition is caused by a severe lack of vitamin A or by retinal disease or cataracts.

Treatment—There is no treatment to correct the problem. Individuals with the deficiency must learn to compensate. It is estimated that seven million drivers in North America have the condition. The difficulty in recognizing traffic light colors and red taillights on cars accounts for some accidents. Studies have shown color defective drivers take much longer to respond to color signals. Traffic lights have been redesigned so red is at the top, amber in the middle, and green at the bottom. Experts suggest that adding a distinctive shape for each color would also be beneficial. White borders have been added to red stop signs to make them more visible. It has also been suggested that taillights be changed to green because it is the least sensitive color. Drivers must learn to compensate for their deficiency by allowing more distance from the car ahead and approaching intersections with extra caution.

Cystic Fibrosis (Sis′-tic Fi-bro′-sis)

Description—A generalized dysfunction of the exocrine glands, affecting multiple organ systems. It is the most common fatal genetic disease of Caucasian children. It is an inherited chronic disease that affects the lungs and digestive system. It affects about 30,000 children and adults in the United States. In the 1950s, few children lived to attend school. Today the predicted median age of survival is more than 37 years due to advances in medical treatments.

Signs and symptoms—These include sweat gland dysfunction resulting in salty-tasting skin; wheezing; dry, nonproductive cough; dyspnea; clubbed fingers; bulky, foul-smelling stools; and excessive appetite but poor weight gain.

Etiology—It is caused by an autosomal recessive trait that probably causes an alteration in a protein or an enzyme.

Treatment—All states require infant screening before leaving the hospital in order to identify cystic fibrosis. Treatment is aimed at helping the child lead as normal a life as possible. Salt is prescribed generously, and pancreatic enzymes and vitamins A, D, E, and K are added to food. Breathing exercises, aerosol therapy, postural drainage, and oxygen assist with breathing. Antibiotics are used aggressively when episodes of acute pulmonary infection occur. There is no cure, but research by Dr. Jeffrey Bartlett at Children's Hospital in Columbus, Ohio, may lead to a strategy to permit delivery of a normal copy of a gene to replace a defective one. He has been able to modify a nonpathogenic virus so that it will carry a "treated" gene to the epithelium of the airway cells. Patients with cystic fibrosis have defective fibrocystic genes that result in the development of the disease. This discovery will not only benefit these patients but will affect many other gene therapy processes.

Down Syndrome (Sin′-drom)

Description—A well-known genetic **syndrome** (group of features) caused by improper cell division. Incidence in North America is about 1 in every 1,000 live births, depending on the mother's age.

Signs and symptoms—It is characterized by slanting eyes, a fold at the inner eye, a large tongue, pug nose, and microcephaly (small head). Other distinguishing features are a simian crease (a single transverse palmer crease), slow dental development, small external ears, and a short neck. Most people with Down syndrome have IQs that fall in the mild to moderate range of intellectual disability (formerly known as retardation) (Figure 23–17).

Etiology—Improper cell division results in the number 21 chromosome occurring in triplicate rather than as a pair, so the individual has 47 instead of 46 chromosomes

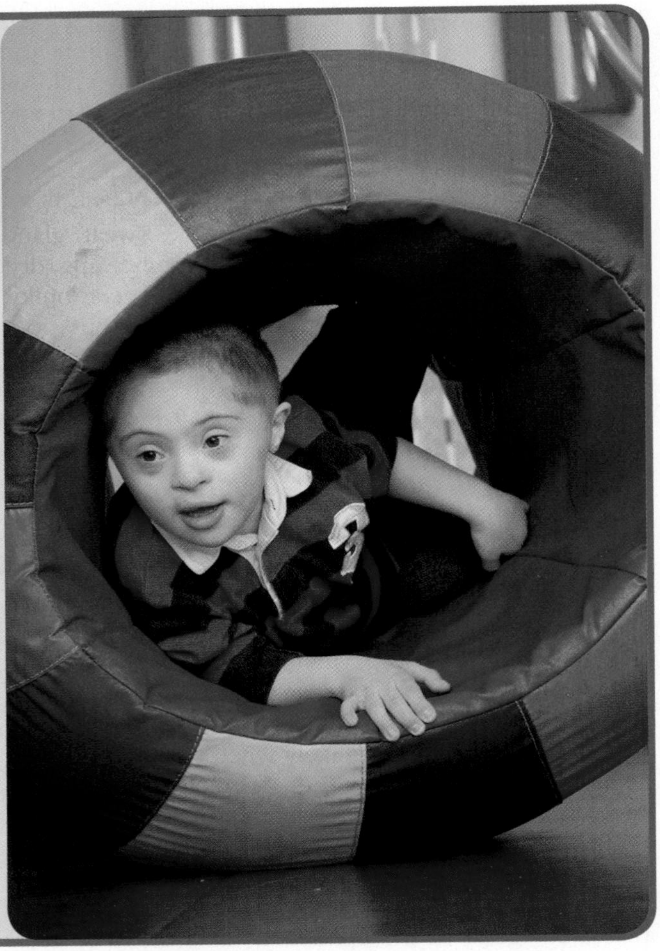

Figure 23–17: Child with Down syndrome features. *Delmar/Cengage Learning.*

per cell. Another form occurs when the long arm of chromosome number 21 breaks and attaches to another chromosome.

Treatment—There is no treatment to correct the disorder. Amniocentesis, a diagnostic test, is recommended when prenatal interviews indicate the possibility of a genetic problem (see Chapter 35). It is also indicated in pregnancies of women older than age of 35. At 20 years of age, a woman has about 1 chance in 2,500 of having a child with Down syndrome, but by age 45, the risk rises to 1 in 40. Amniocentesis requires a small amount of amniotic fluid, which surrounds the fetus, to be withdrawn from the pregnant uterus. Skin cells from the fetus can be found floating in the amniotic fluid and can be grown in a culture for examination. The test can either relieve parental anxiety or can allow them time to prepare for managing a Down syndrome child. Early pregnancy termination can be achieved if findings are a cause of great concern for the parents.

Within a few years another option may be open to parents. In May 2000, one of the scientific groups of the consortium working to decode the human genome completed the DNA sequence of the 21st chromosome. They learned it has only 225 genes and approximately 33,827,477 decodable units of DNA. When scientists can identify the location and function of each gene on the chromosome, perhaps gene therapy could be devised to correct the abnormality. (See Discoveries in Human Genetics and New Genetic Techniques in this unit.) Other medical conditions have also been traced to this chromosome, such as acute myeloid leukemia, Alzheimer's disease, epilepsy, Lou Gehrig's disease, and schizophrenia. This widely diverse group of seemingly unrelated diseases demonstrates the complexity of the human body.

Dwarfism

Description—Dwarfism is a condition that causes an abnormally short or undersized person. There are about 200 conditions that result in dwarfism, most of which are genetic in origin. Dwarfism can also result from an endocrine dysfunction (lack of growth hormone), a deficiency disease, or from renal insufficiency. Achondroplastic dwarfism accounts for about 70% of all cases of short stature. This genetic type results from an autosomal dominant gene. It affects 1 in every 26,000 to 40,000 births.

Signs and symptoms—Achondroplastic dwarfism is characterized by a normal-sized trunk but shortened extremities, particularly shortened upper arms and thighs; an enlarged head; bowed legs; shortened hands and fingers; and prominent buttocks. The average height for adult males is 52 inches (4 feet, 4 inches) and adult females is 49 inches (4 feet, 1 inch).

Etiology—Achondroplastic dwarfism results from a newly mutated *FGFR3* gene. It is random and unpreventable. In fact, 85% of children with the condition are born to parents of average size. One copy of the altered gene in each cell is sufficient to cause the disorder. Other cases are the result of an inherited *FGFR3* gene from a parent with the condition. No environmental or other factors have been identified. Depending on the cause of short stature, little people can have average-sized children.

Treatment—Supplemental growth hormone and other treatments that are indicated with some forms of dwarfism are not effective with achondroplastic dwarfism. Because the etiology is genetic, no form of drug therapy would be beneficial. A degree of additional height can be achieved through a surgical procedure known as limb-lengthening, which is usually performed on the lower extremities. Upper arm lengthening can also be performed in situations in which shortness causes difficulty with performing personal care or if desired for a more balanced appearance.

Figure 23–18 shows extremely rare 13-year-old identical twin achondroplastic dwarfs with a 13-year-old average-size friend. The twins were born to average-size parents and have two older average-size siblings. Neither parent could identify any family history of either dwarfism or the occurrence of twins. At age 9 the boys decided they wanted leg-lengthening surgery after seeing a program on television. At this time they were only 38 inches tall. They were experiencing difficulty in managing routine things at school such as climbing stairs and using the drinking fountains and bathroom facilities. Boarding the school bus presented an additional challenge.

Limb lengthening involves cutting the femur, tibia, and fibula of both legs. The bones are held in line with an external fixator (a scaffold-like frame) with metal pins or wires into the bone (Figure 23–19). The frame allows for tension and "distraction" by slowly turning attached mechanisms a few times each day to pull apart the cut bone. The tension on the bone stimulates it to grow gradually, filling in the gap as it is widened. The surrounding muscles, nerves, skin, and blood vessels also grow. Periodic X-rays measure the degree of growth of new bone and determines the rate at which lengthening can be achieved. The maximum rate for children is 1 mm per day, or an inch per month. After the bone is lengthened, it must heal completely in the lengthened position before the frame can be removed. The process usually takes between 2 1/2 to 3 months per inch depending upon age, general health, and rehabilitation success. A cast may be applied after the frame is removed to give temporary support if necessary. An additional lengthening procedure can be performed after several years if desired.

The procedure is not without discomfort and is prone to infection at the pin sites. The twins' mother turned 8 fasteners 1/4 turn, three times per day per child for 2 months to separate the bones. They achieved a 2-inch lengthening at the femur and another 2 inches at the tibia and fibula for a total of 4 inches in leg length. After the maximum length was achieved, it took 2 months for their bones to harden and another 2 months in rehabilitation to regain leg strength and

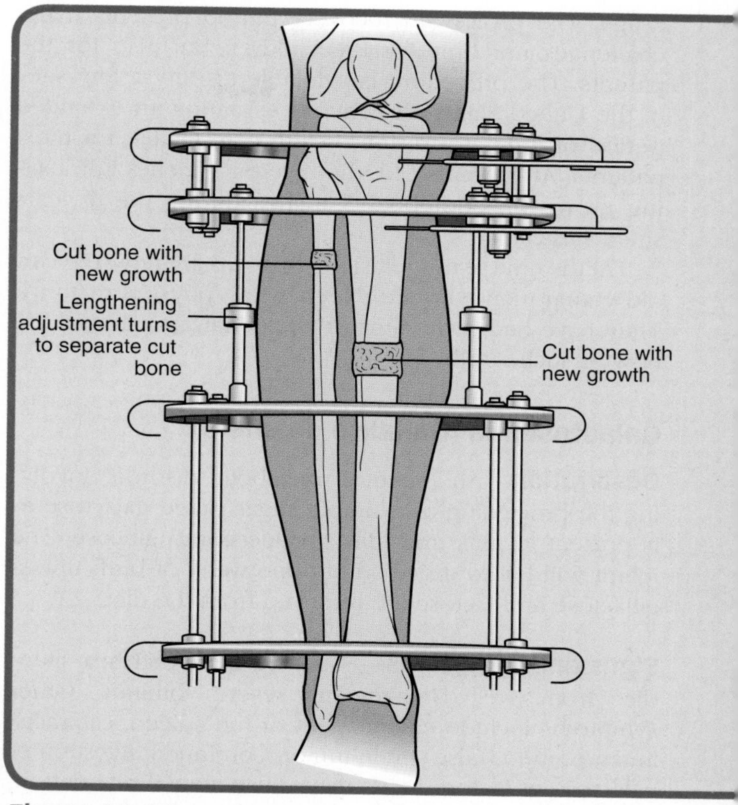

Figure 23–19: External fixator attached to tibia and fibula after limb-lengthening surgery. *Delmar/Cengage Learning.*

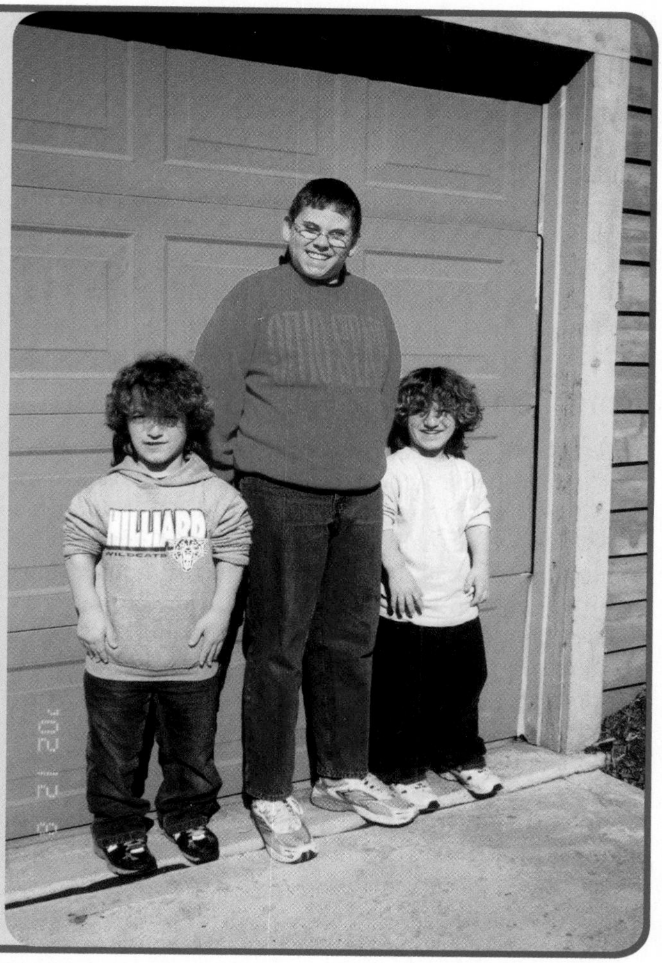

Figure 23–18: 13-year-old identical twin males with achondroplastic dwartfism next to an average-size 13-year-old male. *Courtesy of Barbara A. Wise.*

usage. The prolonged recovery period presents many challenges not only for the children but also for the parents. The procedure is available at only a few sites in the United States, thereby necessitating an extended period of time at a distant health care facility for most patients. At 13 years old, they were 47 inches tall, having grown an additional 5 inches during the 4 years since surgery.

At the time of this revision, the twins are now 17-year-old young men who are experiencing physical maturity. They have had some limited additional growth and are now 52 inches tall.

Galactosemia (Ga-lakto-se′-me-a)

Description—An inherited metabolic disorder involving the processing of a simple sugar called galactose as is present in milk and milk products, into glucose. The infant will fail to thrive within one week of birth unless galactose and lactose are removed from the diet.

Signs and symptoms—Usual signs are diarrhea, jaundice from liver damage, and severe vomiting. Other symptoms include enlargement of the spleen, cataracts, and a pseudo (false) brain tumor. Continued ingestion of galactose or lactose foods may cause mental retardation, progressive liver damage, and death.

Etiology—A recessive gene causes an inability to normally metabolize the sugar galactose, which is formed by the digestion of lactose in milk.

Treatment—Elimination of galactose and lactose from the diet will cause the side effects to subside. Infants must have breast or cow's milk replaced with a soybean-based formula. A galactose-free diet must be maintained throughout life. Screening of newborns is required in every state in the United States. Standard blood tests on newborns include testing for galactosemia to provide for early identification to prevent the unnecessary consequences of the disease.

Hemochromatosis (He-mo-kro-ma-to′-sis)

Description—A genetic condition of iron overload in the body. It is a common genetic disorder, affecting approximately 5 out of every 1,000 people. It is most prevalent in Caucasians of northern European descent. It has been overlooked in the past by physicians, but now more attention is being paid to its presence. Screening for the disorder is being recommended for all family members of diagnosed persons, but a team researching the disorder believes all young adult Caucasians should be screened at least once before age 40. The screening involves an inexpensive, simple blood test that detects the presence of a marker for iron status. Researchers found 70% to 80% of first-degree relatives (siblings, children, and parents) of diagnosed individuals were affected. Complications of cirrhosis of the liver, arthritis, diabetes, and congestive heart failure can be avoided by early intervention.

Signs and symptoms—Unfortunately, early signs are not observable. When complications arise, the signs and symptoms of those disorders are recognizable. Other signs may include increased skin pigmentation, usually bronze from increased melanin accumulation, but a metallic gray may also be visible from iron deposits in the skin. Other common abnormalities include depressed secretions from the pituitary gland, calcium deposits in cartilage, and iron deposits in the synovial fluid of the joints. Males may also have testicular atrophy and loss of libido.

Etiology—Complications arise because the body absorbs too much iron from foods as a result of a faulty metabolism. The absorbed iron is deposited in the tissues of the body. The slow accumulation of iron deposits in the cells causes tissue damage and the typical clinical features.

Treatment—The primary treatment is the removal of excess iron by withdrawing blood frequently until serum iron levels drop within normal range. It may take up to 3 years to obtain acceptable results. A drug, deferoxamine, mobilizes iron stores and promotes their excretion, but it is only about half as effective as blood withdrawal. Other systemic diseases that have developed must also be treated.

Hemophilia (He-mo-fil′e-a)

Description—A sex-linked inherited pattern caused by a defect in the gene located on the X chromosome that is involved in the production of blood clotting factor VIII or IX. A male with the abnormal gene on his X-chromosome will have hemophilia. A female must have the gene on both her X chromosomes to have the disease. The female is a carrier of hemophilia if she has the gene on one of her X chromosomes. Even though she does not have the disease, she can pass it on to her male children. Incidence is approximately 5 in every 40,000 live births.

Signs and symptoms—It is characterized by abnormal bleeding, which may be mild to severe, depending upon the degree of clotting deficiency. Typically there is easy bruising, hematomas, a tendency for nosebleeds, bleeding gums, and prolonged bleeding after injury or dental or surgical procedures. In severe cases, internal bleeding into joints, organs, and from major blood vessels is a cause for great concern. It is very dangerous when bleeding occurs within the brain, throat, or heart; this can lead to shock and death.

Etiology—An inherited X-linked recessive trait with known transferral percentages. Female carriers have a 50% chance of transmitting the gene to each daughter, who then becomes a carrier, and a 50% chance of transmitting the gene to each son, who would develop hemophilia. The trait causes abnormal bleeding through the absence or deficiency of a clotting factor. A diagnosis is made following evidence from a clotting factor profile and a positive family history.

Treatment—The disorder is not curable but can be controlled to prevent anemia and severe deformities. Bleeding must be quickly stopped by administering the deficient clotting factors to raise the plasma levels so that the individual can form clots. Fresh, frozen plasma may be used if factors are not immediately available.

Klinefelter's Syndrome (Kline′-fel-ters)

Description—A sex-linked disorder caused by chromosome abnormality affecting, in varying degrees, approximately 1 in every 600 males.

Signs and symptoms—Mild cases probably go undetected. It usually becomes apparent at puberty when the penis and testicles fail to mature fully, often leading to sterility. Other symptoms are breast enlargement, mental retardation, sparse body hair, abnormal body build (long legs with a short, obese trunk), a tendency toward alcoholism, and often personality disorders.

Etiology—This is caused by one or more extra X chromosomes resulting from abnormal meiosis. The severity depends on the number of extra X chromosomes—the more extra chromosomes, the more severe the disorder.

Treatment—If begun early, treatment with testosterone (the male hormone) may help reverse the feminine characteristics but will not reverse the sterility or mental retardation. Psychotherapy is indicated when sexual dysfunction causes emotional maladjustment.

Phenylketonuria (Fenil-keto-nure-a) (PKU)

Description—A devastating, genetic metabolic disease, requiring early intervention to prevent its development and progress. It is characterized by the presence of phenylpyruvic acid in the urine due to the failure of the body to oxidize the amino acid phenylalanine.

Signs and symptoms—The warning symptoms are not readily observable, so early detection and prevention are necessary. PKU disorders can be diagnosed from blood and urine tests. All states require PKU testing after birth.

Etiology—The inability of the newborn's body to act upon an amino acid called phenylalanine. The newborn lacks the necessary liver enzyme, so the amino acid builds up in the blood and tissues, causing brain damage, which results in profound retardation, seizures, and stunted growth.

Treatment—A restrictive diet is indicated to keep levels of phenylalanine low. This requires elimination of natural proteins from the diet and a milk substitute that has a normal amount of other amino acids, carbohydrates, and fat until at least age 5 or 6. The child must avoid breads, cheese, eggs, meat, poultry, fish, nuts, flour, and legumes. This must be carefully monitored to avoid brain damage.

Spina Bifida (Spi′-na Bi′-fid-a)

Description—A structural malformation of the spine in which the posterior portion of the spinal tissues fails to close during the first three months of pregnancy. These malformations occur in three forms: spinal bifida occulta, meningocele, and myelomeningocele. (See Spinal Cord Defects, Chapter 24, for more information. See also Figure 24–17.)

Talipes (Tal′i-pez)

Description—A structural malformation of the feet, commonly called clubfoot (Figure 23–20).

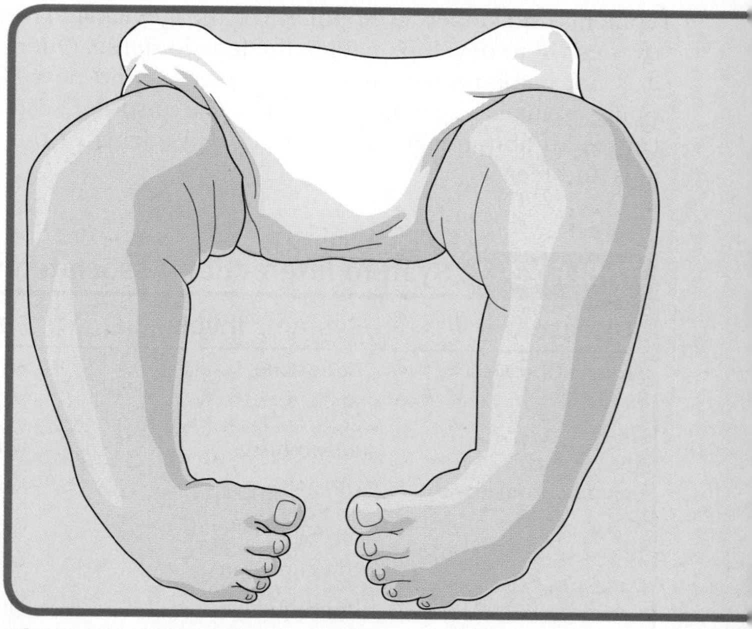

Figure 23–20: Talipes. *Delmar/Cengage Learning.*

Signs and symptoms—It is characterized by varying degrees of inward, outward, downward, or upward turning of one or both feet.

Etiology—The result of a deformed talus (foot bone) and a shortened Achilles tendon, apparently caused by a combination of genetic and in utero environmental factors. There is a strong heredity factor in some instances and an apparent arresting of development during the 9th and 10th weeks of life when the feet are formed.

Treatment—A distinction needs to be made between true and apparent clubfoot. X-ray reveals whether the talus and calcaneus bones of the foot are superimposed. Correction involves three stages: correcting the deformity, maintaining the correction, and long-term observation. Surgical correction is done shortly after birth. Repositioning is maintained by a cast. After correction, proper alignment must be maintained through exercise, night splints, and special shoes. A deformity that resists manual correction or a neglected clubfoot will require surgical adjustment of the bone and tendons.

Turner's Syndrome (Turn-ers Sin′-drom)

Description—A sex-linked disorder with a group of structural defects that affects about 1 in 10,000 newborn females.

Signs and symptoms—It is characterized by short stature, webbing of the neck, a low hairline, a wide chest with broadly spaced nipples, poor breast development, and underdevelopment of the genitalia. The ovaries fail to develop, making the female sterile. Often it is not recognizable until lack of menses and developing genitalia become apparent. The disorder also causes an abnormality of the aorta and edema of the legs and feet.

Etiology—The affected individual has only 45 chromosomes because the sex cells fail to divide correctly in meiosis, causing only one sex chromosome to be present in the cells.

Treatment—The use of estrogen (female hormone) after age 13, to prevent growth from stopping, will induce sexual maturation but doesn't reverse the sterility. Psychotherapy may be indicated to deal with the emotional adjustment required to deal with the disorder.

System Interaction Associated with Disease Conditions

Because the body is so dependant upon all its separate "parts" to function together, when disorders or diseases develop, there is usually interaction of more than one body system. Table 23–3 summaries the systems involved and the pathology that is present in two examples of genetic disease or disorder. It is possible to see that the pathology present relates to the symptoms the patient exhibits with the condition.

AGE-RELATED BODY CHARACTERISTICS

Persons with genetic or congenital disorders may have age-related characteristics associated with their disorder; however, often their life expectancy is shortened so aging is not a significant factor. Early diagnosis and intervention prevents the development of many of the devastating effects of the disorders; however, the long term effects of Down syndrome, for example, may become apparent. As these individuals age, they tend to become overweight and experience difficulty with balance and posture due to the lack of muscle tone in their limbs. Because they are prone to have congenital heart disease, leukemia, and other chronic infections, these may also cause changes in their bodies.

TABLE 23–3 System Interaction Associated with Disease Conditions

Disease	Systems Involved	Pathology Present
Cystic fibrosis	Endocrine	Sweat gland dysfunction
	Digestive	Excessive appetite but poor weight gain, foul-smelling stools
	Respiratory	Difficulty breathing, wheezing, acute pulmonary infections
Hemochromatosis	Circulatory	Excess iron in the blood, congestive heart failure
	Musculoskeletal	Calcium deposits in cartilage and iron deposits in synovial fluid
	Integumentary	Skin pigmentation, iron deposits
	Reproductive	Male testicular atrophy

DISCOVERIES IN HUMAN GENETICS

In 2003, a 13-year federally funded study called "The Human Genome Project" was completed, which analyzed human genetics at the molecular level. The project was launched because it seemed to promise the best hope for ultimately defeating not only diseases long known to be inherited but also those with more subtle links, like cancer. The planners estimated it would take several tens of thousands of technician years to find the sequence of all the DNA bases and the human genes and 390,000 pages to list them. The sequencing, it was believed, would reveal the possible functions and location of the then human genes. But first it was then necessary to devise "a genetic map," or diagram, that describes how thousands of known marker sequences in the chromosomes separate and recombine. They also needed physical maps to show the order along a chromosome of recognizable sequence sites. Using the maps, a researcher could compare a given condition's pattern of inheritance with that of the marker sequences. This makes it possible to determine where a gene that causes the condition might be located. Computers can then "match" the reams of data coming from sequencing machines onto the sites on a physical map. By comparing the two maps, it is possible to quickly find genes associated with an illness.

Completing the gene sequencing has revolutionized the understanding and treatment of disease. The genome is the approximate 3 billion letter code of the human DNA that is the chemical sequence containing the basic information for building and running a human body. This chemical sequence determines every characteristic in the human body, from eye color to vulnerability to disease. (For the current status, go to http://genomics.energy.gov/.)

The sequencing of the human genome was completed earlier than expected because of the significant development of new technologies. These same technologies are now being used to help diagnose human diseases, design custom treatments, and even identify criminals.

It is predicted that science will be able to zero in on the genetic factors involved in diabetes, heart disease, and other common disorders within the next few years. Cancer drugs are already being targeted at the molecular level of the disease. Companies have been formed that are taking blood samples from volunteers with known diseases to compare the codes and to identify the responsible genes.

In the course of the genome project, other genetic technologies like gene therapy and gene transplantation have been developed that will hopefully permit treatment of faulty genes in the future. Although science is much closer to understanding defects in genes and the diseases that result, cures based upon changes in the genetic code may lead to new drugs and ways to deliver corrected genes into defective cells are developed.

The exciting new technology is not without its critics. There is a potential problem with protecting against the misuse of individual genetic information. Discrimination in employment and life and health insurance has already surfaced. People with a genetic condition, or who are at risk for one, are often turned down for employment or insurance, and some have lost their current jobs and coverage. There is concern that insurers might even classify the mutations as a pre-existing condition and refuse to cover any treatments related to that condition. Several states have enacted laws to limit descrimination based on genetic data. Congress is working on federal legislation to discourage or prevent insurance discrimination nationally.

On the positive side, mutated genes have now been identified for some diseases such as cystic fibrosis, polycystic kidney disease, some forms of Alzheimer's and cardiovascular diseases, and hereditary forms of breast, ovarian, and colon cancers. Tests are becoming more commonplace. If someone is identified as having the mutated gene, the known percentages for its disease probability can be provided. An example using this technology is BRAC analysis for breast and ovarian cancer. Blood cells are tested to determine if a woman has a certain type of mutation in the BRAC gene. This information can help determine the woman's risk for cancer. With the near certainty for contracting specific inherited malignancies, some people have gone so far as to elect surgical removal of both breasts and entire colons in order to save their lives. This new information can be used to personalize health care to prevent the onset of a disease. Understanding defects in a person's genes will be important in the emerging field of personalized medicine.

Some researchers worry about uncontrolled testing and the interpretation of results. Many physicians are not well enough informed to be giving genetic advice. The psychologic harm from DNA testing is also receiving growing attention. Governments around the world are working on legislation to protect individual rights and confidentiality.

In the United States, the Presidential Commission for the Study of Bioethical Issues studies the ethical, legal, and social questions surrounding these issues. For instance: Just how far should scientific technology go to alter the human? Where does relieving human suffering end and manipulation for personal desire begin? This area of science will be a topic for discussion for years to come. Read more about current studies and research at www.bioethics.gov. Former presidential commission documents are available at www.bioethics.gov/cms/former-commissions.

NEW GENETIC TECHNIQUES

Polymerase Chain Reaction

Polymerase chain reaction is a technique being used in molecular biology to allow scientists to isolate, characterize, and produce large quantities of specific pieces of DNA from very small amounts of starting material that would otherwise be undetectable. Practical applications are applied to prenatal and postnatal diagnosis of genetic diseases, infectious disease (such as AIDS), and cancer. It assists in the matching of transplant recipients with donors, in the study of human genetic history and evolution, and in DNA fingerprinting by forensic scientists.

DNA Fingerprinting

DNA fingerprinting is a detection and identification method that was first announced by a British geneticist in 1985. Except for identical twins, the DNA code for each individual is unique. Examination of blood, semen, and other body fluids at a crime scene can render positive identification when compared with the DNA molecules of the suspect. The evidence of a DNA match, in view of the great variance among the population, is considered to be a positive identification.

Genetic Counseling

Genetic counseling provides information to a couple regarding their risks of having a child with a genetic disorder. Even "normal" couples face some risk with any pregnancy. About 3% of all live-born infants have a significant birth defect. Counseling is available to those couples who perceive their risk to be greater than the population in general. Information provided should include known risk statistics and offer available alternatives such as amniocentesis, pregnancy termination, adoption, artificial insemination (if the male has the risk factor), or information to permit understanding and acceptance of a pregnancy situation for which the parents agree no termination action will be taken.

Gene Therapy

Gene therapy is a technique for correcting defective genes responsible for disease development. In most gene therapy studies, a perfect gene is inserted into the genome to replace the disease-causing gene. Current gene therapy is experimental and the Food and Drug Administration (FDA) has not approved any gene therapy product for sale. The first clinical trial for gene therapy began in 1990 when genetically engineered cells were infused into a 4-year-old girl with a life-threatening immune deficiency. The infused cells were from her own blood into which researchers had inserted copies of a missing gene that produces the missing immune product.

Genetic Engineering

Genetic engineering is being used in the prenatal diagnosis of inherited diseases. The DNA pattern of cells from the parents, who may carry a gene for a congenital disorder, and the pattern of the fetus are compared. The disease status of the fetus can currently be determined in the following instances: thalassemia, Huntington's disease, cystic fibrosis, and Duchennes' muscular dystrophy.

Genetic engineering has allowed discoveries that could not otherwise have been made. An example is the discovery of oncogenes and tumor suppressor genes that play a role in causing some cancers. Scientists were able to cut the cancer-causing DNA into segments and identify the specific segments that were responsible for transforming normal cells into cancer cells. Much research remains to be done to achieve the promise of gene therapy and genetic engineering, but its value could be enormous.

There is always controversy when new techniques are introduced, but manipulating human cellular structure appears to have many ethical and moral issues to be resolved. On one hand is the opportunity to eliminate the devastating physical and mental conditions resulting from defective genes, and few people would deny the social and economic advantages of this capability. On the other hand, there are those who say man is playing "God," and that is not right. There is also the criticism that if you have enough money, you could "buy" perfect children of the sex, color, intelligence, and projected size you desired. When technology is known, regardless of ethical controls (which have yet to be developed), someone will always be operating outside the accepted practice for a price.

The reality of genetic identification discrimination hangs in the balance. Only the future will determine that outcome. As the director of the National Center for Human Genome Research said in *Scientific American,* "as the number of genetic tests grow, we are going to see it [genetic identification discrimination] happen on a larger scale, since we're all at risk for something."

Stem Cell Research

A stem cell possesses the ability to develop into many different types of cells and possesses two properties: the ability to self-renew (through cell division), as well as the ability to specialize into tissue- or organ-specific cells with special functions. Scientists believe that offered the possibility of stem cell research, they could regenerate any tissue in the human body and therefore cure many medical conditions such as Parkinson's disease, diabetes, paralysis, and heart failure.

Stem cells can be embryonic or adult. The embryonic cells are obtained from the inner cell mass of a week-old embryo. Usually, these are excess cells created during infertility treatment in standard in vitro fertilization practices. The participants donate the excess cells for research purposes rather than have them destroyed. Embryonic stem cells have the potential to develop into all or nearly all of the tissues of the body. The cells are cultured and can grow and divide indefinitely. The cells develop into a stem cell line, descended from the original. Batches of cells are then separated and distributed to researchers in the United States, Australia, India, Israel, and Sweden. Private research has developed more than 60 genetically diverse stem cell lines.

Adult stem cells are unspecialized, can renew themselves, and become specialized to yield cells from the tissue from which they originated. However, adult stem cells are thought to be limited to differentiating into different cell types based on where they are harvested from.

In 2006, researchers were able to identify some specialized adult cells which could be "reprogrammed" to function similar to embryonic stem cells. These cells are called induced pluripotent stem cells, meaning they have the potential to develop into all or nearly all of the tissues of the body.

The use of federal money to fund embryonic stem cell research has become a topic of debate. While some wanted unlimited support to find cures for many diseases, others condemned the research because it involves prohibiting the development of the embryo, thereby violating the sanctity of human life. In August 2001, the Bush Administration announced that federal funds could be used only on the *existing* embryonic stem cell lines. Other decisions were made regarding the research criteria, the denying of funds for additional cells, embryos, or cloning. On March 9, 2009, President Obama repealed a ban on federal funding enacted under President Bush, thus allowing federal funds to be applied beyond what was previously authorized. Congress then passed the Omnibus Appropriations Act of 2009, which still contained the longstanding provision that bans federal funding of "research in which a human embryo or embryos are destroyed, discarded, or knowingly subjected to risk of injury or death." This effectively prevents federal funding being used to create new embryonic stem cell lines by many of the known methods. Presidents Obama's policy allows the potential of applying for funding for research involving the hundreds of existing stem cell lines as well as any further line created using private funds or state level funding.

TISSUES

As you are already aware, not all cells are alike. They may be transparent, as in the eye, or transmit electrical impulses or nutrients. Some have long, thin fibers, and others produce secretions. When cells of the same type group together for a common purpose, they form a **tissue**. Tissues are composed of 60% to 99% water. The essential substances needed by the body are either dissolved or suspended in the tissue fluids. Therefore, water is indispensable to cell life, and lack of it causes death more rapidly than lack of any other substance, except oxygen.

Two common medical terms describe the opposites of tissue fluid balance. When there is too little fluid, the condition is known as **dehydration**. An abnormal accumulation of excess fluid, causing puffiness of the affected tissues, is known as **edema**.

Tissue Classifications

Tissues can be classified into four main types: **epithelial**, **connective**, nerve, and muscle.

Epithelial

Epithelial tissues form the body's glands, cover the surface of the body, and line the cavities. Epithelium is the main tissue of the skin, which serves as a protective covering for the body. Epithelium also covers all the organs and lines the intestinal, respiratory, and urinary tract and uterus. Some epithelial tissues secrete fluids, such as mucus and digestive juices. Others selectively absorb nutrients, chemical elements, and water. The epithelium of the urinary bladder is uniquely arranged in folds to allow for expansion as the bladder fills.

Epithelial tissues in glands specialize to provide specific secretions for the body. Glands that secrete directly into the blood in the capillaries are known as *endocrine* or ductless glands.

Glands that produce secretions through ducts within the body are classified as *exocrine* (Figure 23–21). Two glands, the liver and pancreas, produce both endocrine and exocrine secretions.

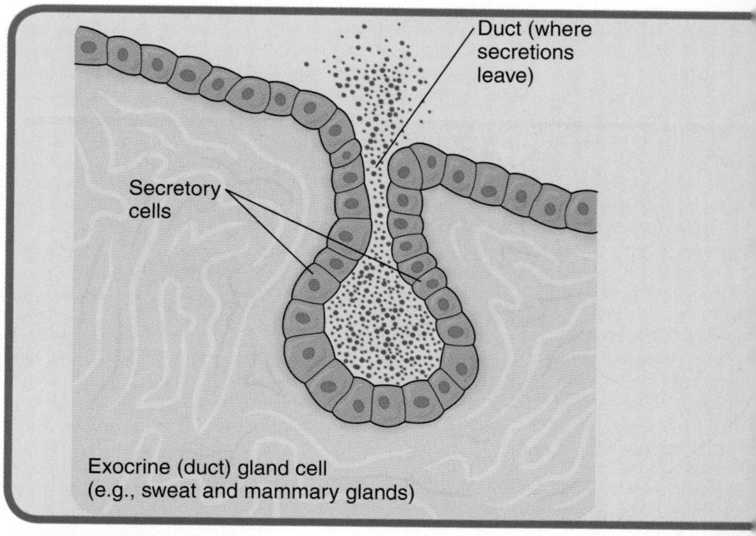

Figure 23–21: Epithelial cell tissue of an exocrine gland. *Delmar/Cengage Learning.*

Connective

Connective tissue forms the supporting structure of the body, connecting other tissues together to form the organs and body parts. There are three categories of connective tissue: (1) connective tissue proper, (2) supportive connective, and (3) fluid connective tissue. Connective tissue in the form of adipose or fat tissue, stores the body's reserve of food, fills the area between tissue fibers, insulates against heat and cold, and pads the body structures (Figure 23–22). Supportive connective tissue is stretchable and forms the subcutaneous layer of the skin. A dense supportive connective tissue in the form of tendons, ligaments, and organ capsules serves to support and protect organs and lend elasticity to the walls of arteries (Figure 23–23).

Blood and lymphatic vessels, lymph, the blood, and blood cells are forms of fluid connective tissue. Cells in the blood carry nutrients and oxygen to the cells and pick up metabolic wastes for elimination. Lymph fluid consists of water, glucose, fats, and salt and is present in the spaces between the cells of the tissues and within the lymph vessels. Connective tissue plays a major role in the repair of damaged body tissue. The repair process involves new blood vessel formation and the growth of new connective tissue known as scar tissue. Excessive blood vessel development in the early stages may result in a condition called "proud flesh." In instances of surgery or suturing (sewing) of a clean wound, the need for tissue regrowth and therefore the resulting scar are reduced because the cut edges are brought together closely by the surgical process. An excessive growth of scar tissue is called a **keloid**.

Supportive connective tissue can be found in the cartilage and bones of the body. Cartilage is located between the bones of the spine (where it acts as a shock absorber and allows for flexibility) and in the ear, nose, and voice box (to provide shaping). Bone tissue is actually cartilage with the addition of calcium salts. This addition takes place gradually from birth until the tissue becomes hardened (Figure 23–24).

Bone is a form of supportive connective tissue that is also called skeletal or **osseous** tissue. It is not a lifeless material. Within most bone is a medullary cavity filled with yellow marrow, which is composed of fat, connective tissue, and blood vessels. Some long bones contain cavities filled with red marrow, which manufactures red blood cells. Because bone is a living tissue with a blood supply and nerves, it can easily repair itself when it is damaged.

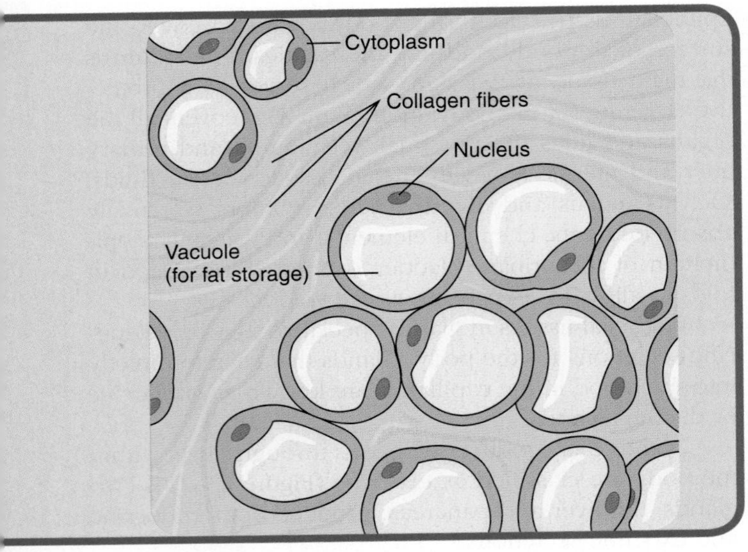

Figure 23–22: Connective (adipose) tissue throughout the body. *Delmar/Cengage Learning.*

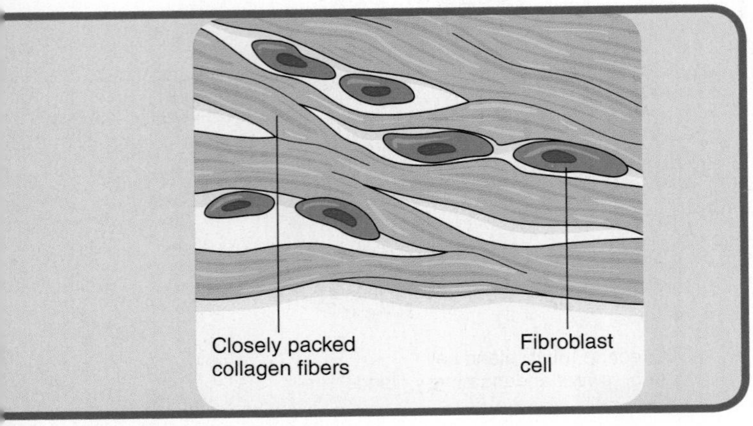

Figure 23–23: Dense supportive connective tissue in ligaments and tendons. *Delmar/Cengage Learning.*

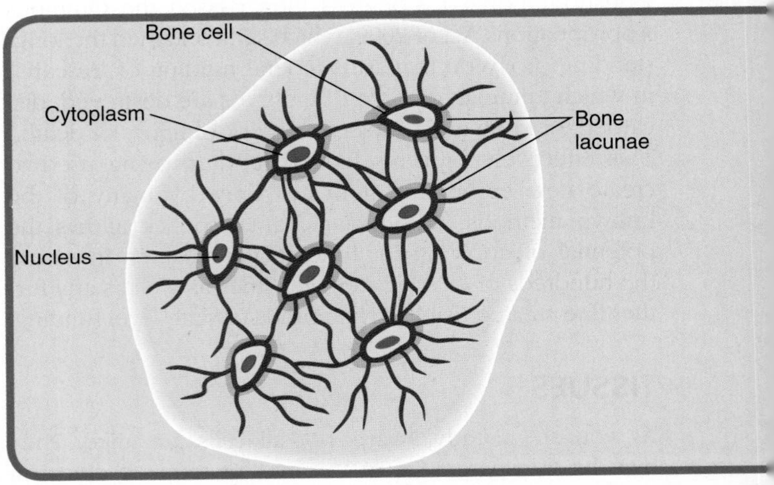

Figure 23–24: Supportive connective tissue found in bone. *Delmar/Cengage Learning.*

Nerve

Nerve tissue is found throughout the body. It serves as the body's communication network. The basic structural unit of the tissue is the neuron, which consists of a nerve cell body and fibers that resemble tree branches (Figure 23–25). The dendrites bring impulses to the cell body; the axon conducts impulses away. Neurons range from a fraction of an inch up to 3 feet in length.

There are three types of nerve cells or neurons. A *sensory neuron* in the skin or sense organs picks up a stimulus and sends it toward the spinal cord and brain. An *interneuron,* or *connecting neuron,* carries the impulse to another neuron. A *motor neuron* receives an impulse and sends a message, which causes a reaction.

Clusters of neurons form the nerve tissue. Nerves throughout the body join together to form the spinal cord, which in turn transmits electrical impulses to and from the brain. Nerves outside the brain and spinal cord are called *peripheral nerves*. Most of the fibers of these nerves are covered with a fatty insulating material called a **myelin** sheath, which is then covered with a thin membrane called **neurilemma**. If a sheathed nerve fiber is damaged or cut, it can be surgically repaired, and a new fiber may form within the sheath, but nerve tissue recovers very slowly. Unfortunately, fibers of the brain and spinal cord lack sheaths and cannot be restored by surgery when damaged or cut.

Muscle

Muscle tissue is designed to contract on stimulation. Tissue that can be controlled at will with impulses from the brain is called **voluntary** muscle tissue. This type is found connected to the bones of the body and is called **skeletal** or **striated** muscle (Figure 23–26A). It gives us the ability to move our bodies.

Involuntary muscle action occurs without control or conscious awareness. There are two types of involuntary muscle tissue. One type, called **smooth** muscle tissue, is found within the walls of all the organs of the body except the heart. This type of tissue moves food and waste material through the digestive tract and changes the size of the iris of the eye and the diameter of arteries (Figure 23–26B). The other type of involuntary muscle tissue, called **cardiac** muscle tissue, is found only in the heart. Cardiac muscle fibers are joined in a continuous network and must contract together in a forceful, rhythmic action to pump blood throughout the body (Figure 23–26C).

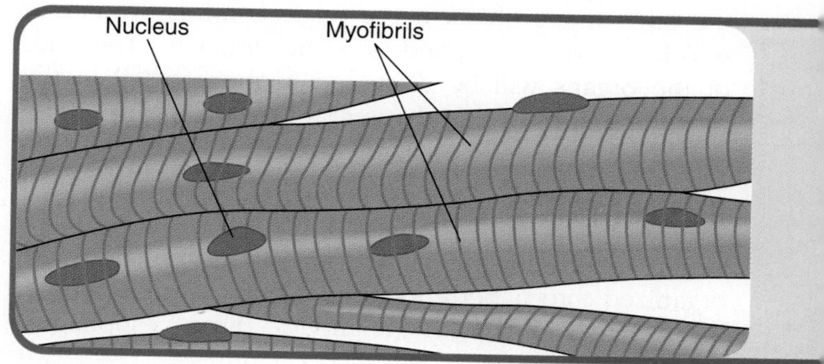

Figure 23–26A: Skeletal muscle tissue (striated voluntary) attached to bone. *Delmar/Cengage Learning.*

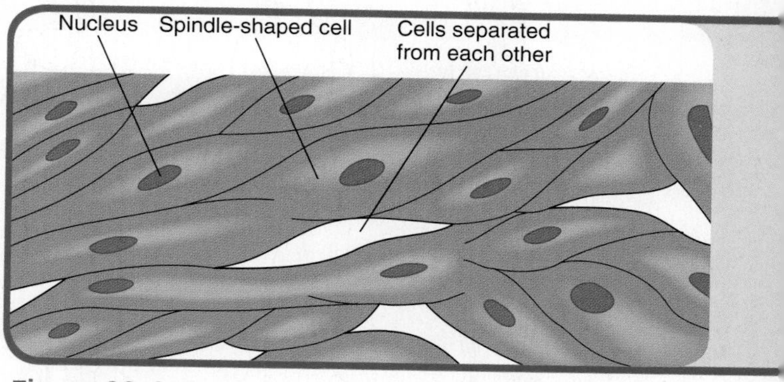

Figure 23–26B: Smooth muscle tissue in the walls of organs and blood vessels. *Delmar/Cengage Learning.*

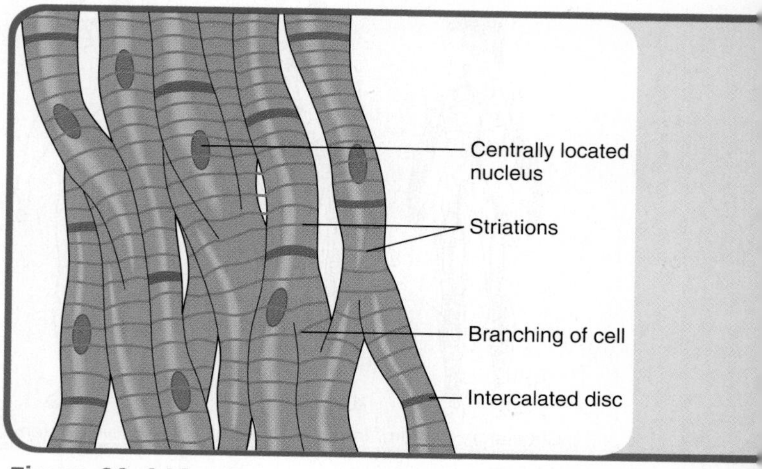

Figure 23–26C: Cardiac muscle tissue of the heart. *Delmar/Cengage Learning.*

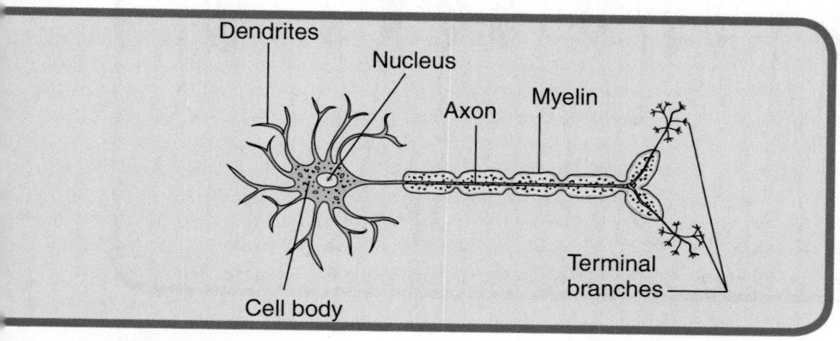

Figure 23–25: A motor neuron. *Delmar/Cengage Learning.*

ORGANS

The **organs** of the body are made of two or more types of tissue that work together to perform a specific body function. For example, the stomach is constructed with walls of smooth muscle tissue to "churn" the food; it is lined with one type of epithelial tissue, which secretes gastric juices, and covered with another type, which protects the organ; connective tissue fills the spaces between the other tissue fibers; nerve tissue controls the rate at which material is emptied from the stomach. (The roles of the organs will be discussed in more detail in the remaining units of this chapter.)

SYSTEMS

Organs of the body that perform similar functions are organized into a body **system**. Again, as an example, the stomach joins with the mouth, throat, esophagus, and small and large intestines to make up the alimentary tract of the digestive system. The alimentary tract combines with the teeth, tongue, salivary glands, liver, pancreas, and gallbladder to form the total digestive system. The other systems of the body, which will be discussed individually, are the integumentary, skeletal, muscular, respiratory, circulatory, urinary, nervous, endocrine, and reproductive systems.

One additional "system" will also be discussed later in this chapter. The immune system is not considered to be a system. However, because the body's health and well-being directly depend on an intact and effective immune response, you should have a basic knowledge of its role in disease response. As scientists begin to better understand how it functions and what can be done to correct its malfunction, perhaps we can solve the mysteries of cancer, AIDS, and many other immunologically based disorders. The basics of the complex subject of immunology are discussed in Chapter 31.

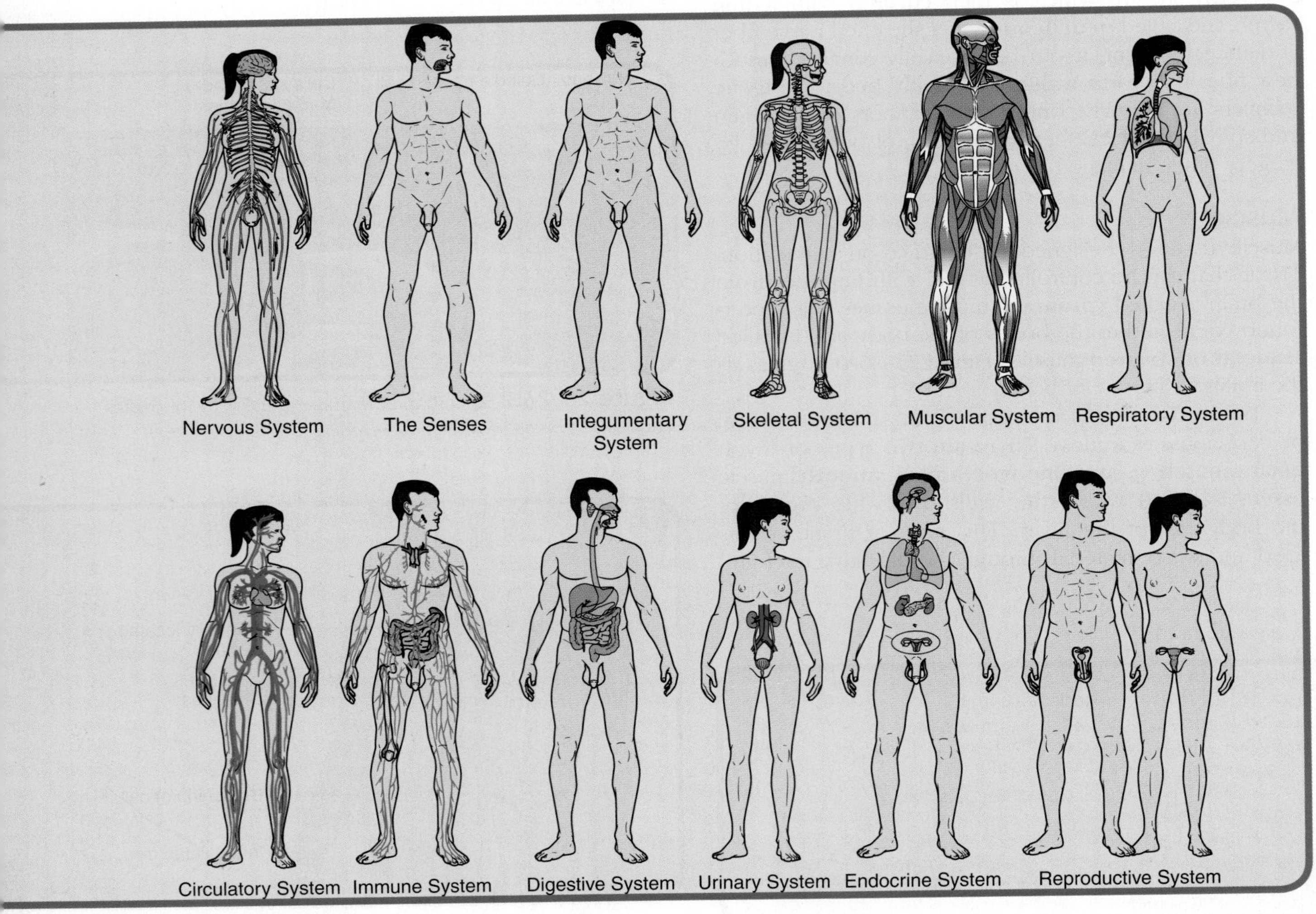

Figure 23–27: The body systems. *Delmar/Cengage Learning.*

Even a body system cannot function alone. All systems must combine their individual contributions for the health and well-being of the total human body. Figure 23–27 illustrates the systems of the body.

The following is a summary of the fundamental structure of the human body: it is composed of billions of cells, which are grouped together to form tissues that bind together to form organs to perform the functions of a system that cooperates with other systems to become the human body (Figure 23–28).

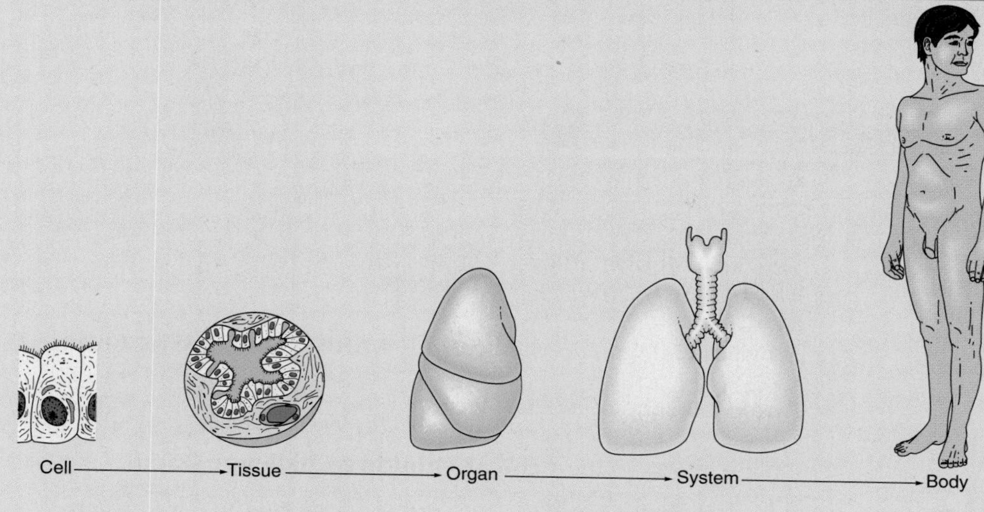

Figure 23–28: Fundamental cell to human body structures sequence. *Delmar/Cengage Learning.*

CHAPTER SUMMARY

- Anatomy is the study of the physical structure of the human body. Physiology is the science of the function of cells, tissues, and organs of the body.
- Anatomical directions terms are used universally to describe anatomic structures.
- The body is divided into two main cavities, the anterior and the posterior. These are further divided into the upper thoracic cavity and the lower abdominopelvic cavities.
- The abdomen can be referred to as having either four or nine regions.
- The cell is the basic building block of the body. Cells come in different types to perform specific duties. Cells have a membrane and are filled with cytoplasm. There are seven organelles within the cell.
- Genes are specific segments of DNA molecules located on the chromosomes in the cell nucleus.
- Molecules pass through cell membranes by six processes: diffusion, osmosis, filtration, active transport, phagocytosis, and pinocytosis.
- Biochemistry is the study of chemical reactions within the body. This involves the 92 natural and 13 man-made elements. The main natural elements are carbon, oxygen, nitrogen, and hydrogen. Some elements combine into compounds that are classified as an acid, base, or a salt.
- Cells divide by a process known as mitosis, which results in two new daughter cells. Cells from different types of tissue reproduce at different rates.
- When all tissues and organs of the body are performing their appropriate tasks and the internal environment is functioning properly, the body is said to be in a condition of homeostasis.

- Cellular mutation occurs when DNA is lost, rearranged, or paired incorrectly during replication. A trait is the recognizable result of a gene or group of genes and can be dominant, recessive, and x-linked.
- Congenital and genetic disorders result from improper cell division, inheritance of altered gene or genes, environmental factors and toxins.
- The Human Genome Project analyzed the human genetic structure to determine the location of genes causing disease. Other genetic technologies such as DNA fingerprinting, gene therapy, and genetic engineering have developed.
- Stem cell research has great potential as well as great controversy. The government is trying to establish medical, legal, ethical, and moral guidelines.
- Cells combine to form tissues, which join together to become organs that function together as systems to form the human body.

STUDY TOOLS

Workbook	Activities for Chapter 23
Premium Website	
MEDIA LINK	View this **Media Link** for Chapter 23: • Anatomy of a typical cell
StudyWARE	Activities and Quizzes on the **StudyWARE™ Software** for Chapter 23
	Audio Library of medical terms
	Online access to the **Critical Thinking Challenge 2.0**
learninglab	Module 11: Fundamental Body Structures
CourseMate	Activities and Quizzes for Chapter 23
WebTutor	Activities and Quizzes for Chapter 23

CHECK YOUR KNOWLEDGE

1. The science of the function of cells, tissues, and organs of the body is called:
   a. anatomy.
   b. physiology.
   c. pathophysiology.
   d. homeostasis.
2. An individual is standing erect, with arms down to the sides and the palms of the hands facing forward. What is this position?
   a. Midsagittal
   b. Frontal
   c. Anatomic
   d. Anterior
3. What are the names of the two main cavities of the body?
   a. Abdominal and pelvic
   b. Abdominal and ventral
   c. Anterior and ventral
   d. Anterior and posterior
4. RUQ, RLQ, LUQ, and LLQ refer to what?
   a. The abdominal quadrants
   b. The regions of the abdomen
   c. The thoracic cavity
   d. The abdomenopelvic cavity

5. Diffusion is:
   a. the movement of water or a solvent through a selected permeable membrane.
   b. the movement of solutes and liquid molecules evenly within a medium.
   c. the engulfing of bacteria or damaged cells.
   d. the movement of water across a membrane as a result of gravity or pressure.
6. When the internal environment is functioning properly and all the organs and tissues of the body are performing their appropriate tasks, this is known as:
   a. mutation.
   b. osmosis.
   c. hemostasis.
   d. equilibrium.
7. What are the four main types of tissues?
   a. Epithelial, connective, nerve, and muscular
   b. Endocrine, exocrine, muscular, and nerve
   c. Muscular, bone, nerve, skin
   d. Connective, osseous, nerve, muscular

WEB LINKS

Centers for Disease Control and Prevention: www.cdc.gov

Human Genome Project Information: www.ornl.gov/sci/techresources/Human_Genome/home.shtml

Information about Achrondroplastic Dwarfism: www.nlm.nih.gov/medlineplus/dwarfism.html

Chapter

24 The Nervous System

OBJECTIVES

In this chapter, you will learn the following:

KB LEARNING OBJECTIVES

1. Spell and define, using the glossary at the back of the text, all the Words to Know in this chapter.
2. Name the two main divisions of the nervous system.
3. Identify the two types of peripheral nerves and explain the function of the spinal nerves.
4. Describe simple and complex reflex actions.
5. Describe a synapse and the effects of various substances on its action.
6. Describe the purpose of the automatic nervous system, and explain the action of its two divisions.
7. Identify the main parts of the brain and their functions.
8. Name the coverings of the brain and spinal cord and describe their purpose.
9. Describe the function of cerebrospinal fluid.
10. Name common diagnostic tests used to identify neurologic disorders and possible reasons for their use.
11. List the functions of the hypothalamus.
12. Describe 25 diseases or disorders of the nervous system.
13. Identify three body systems that interact in cerebral palsy.

WORDS TO KNOW

action potential
angiography
arachnoid
arteriography
auditory
autonomic
axon
central
cerebellum
cerebrospinal fluid
cerebrum
coma scale
computerized axial tomography (CAT or CT scan)
cranium
dendrite
dura mater
electroencephalography (EEG)
electromyography
frontal
ganglion
hypothalamus
interneurons
longitudinal fissure
lumbar puncture
magnetic resonance imaging (MRI)
medulla oblongata
meninges
midbrain
migraine
motor
myelography
occipital
olfactory
optic
parasympathetic
parietal
peripheral
pia mater
plexuses
pons
positron emission tomography (PET scan)
sciatica
sensory
skull x-ray
spina bifida occulta
subarachnoid
subdural
sympathetic
synapse
syndrome
temporal
thalamus
thorax
ventricle

THE NERVOUS SYSTEM

The nervous system is the communication network that organizes and coordinates all the body's functions. It is a complex and somewhat difficult system to understand, and in most texts, it is not usually discussed early in the study of the body systems. However, in this text, it is being presented first. Hopefully, this will help you to better understand the involvement of the nervous system's regulatory action in the functioning of the other body systems as they are discussed.

You might think of the system as being something like your telephone system. You can make local, in-state, national, and international calls. You can easily call next door, but the further away you wish to call, the more number messages and the more "routing" of signals you need to complete your call. The phone picks up your voice (stimulus), converts it to impulses, and sends it along a charged line to a bundle of lines and on to phone company switching equipment. Every so often, the impulse is "boosted" to maintain your "voice." It may even be given special treatment and sent through space and bounced off a satellite, but the message is forwarded to its destination. Your nervous system operates in a similar but much more complicated manner. The system has two main divisions: the **central** nervous system (CNS), which consists of the brain and the spinal cord, and the **peripheral** nervous system, which includes all the nerves that connect the CNS to every organ and area of the body. The **autonomic** nervous system is a specialized part of the peripheral system and controls internal organs and other self-regulating body functions.

Like in all systems, the basic functioning unit is the cell; in this system the unit is a nerve cell or neuron. As described in Chapter 23, there are three types of neurons in nerve tissue: **sensory**, connecting, and **motor**. They receive stimuli or impulses, transmit impulses to other neurons, and deliver response actions to the muscles and glands. Connecting neurons are also called *associative* or *internuncial neurons*. Figure 24–1 illustrates the three types of neurons.

All nerve cells have a nucleus, cytoplasm, and a cell membrane. Scattered throughout the cytoplasm are little microscopic granular "dots" called Nissl bodies. They are involved in protein synthesis and metabolism. The cell body has processes that are extensions of cytoplasm called **dendrites** and **axons**. A neuron may have many dendrites but only one axon. These extensions are also called *fibers*. Around the long, thin axons of peripheral nerves are the Schwann cells. They form a tight protective covering called the myelin sheath and also play a part in the transmission of messages. The myelin is then surrounded by the neurilemma, an elastic sheath covering.

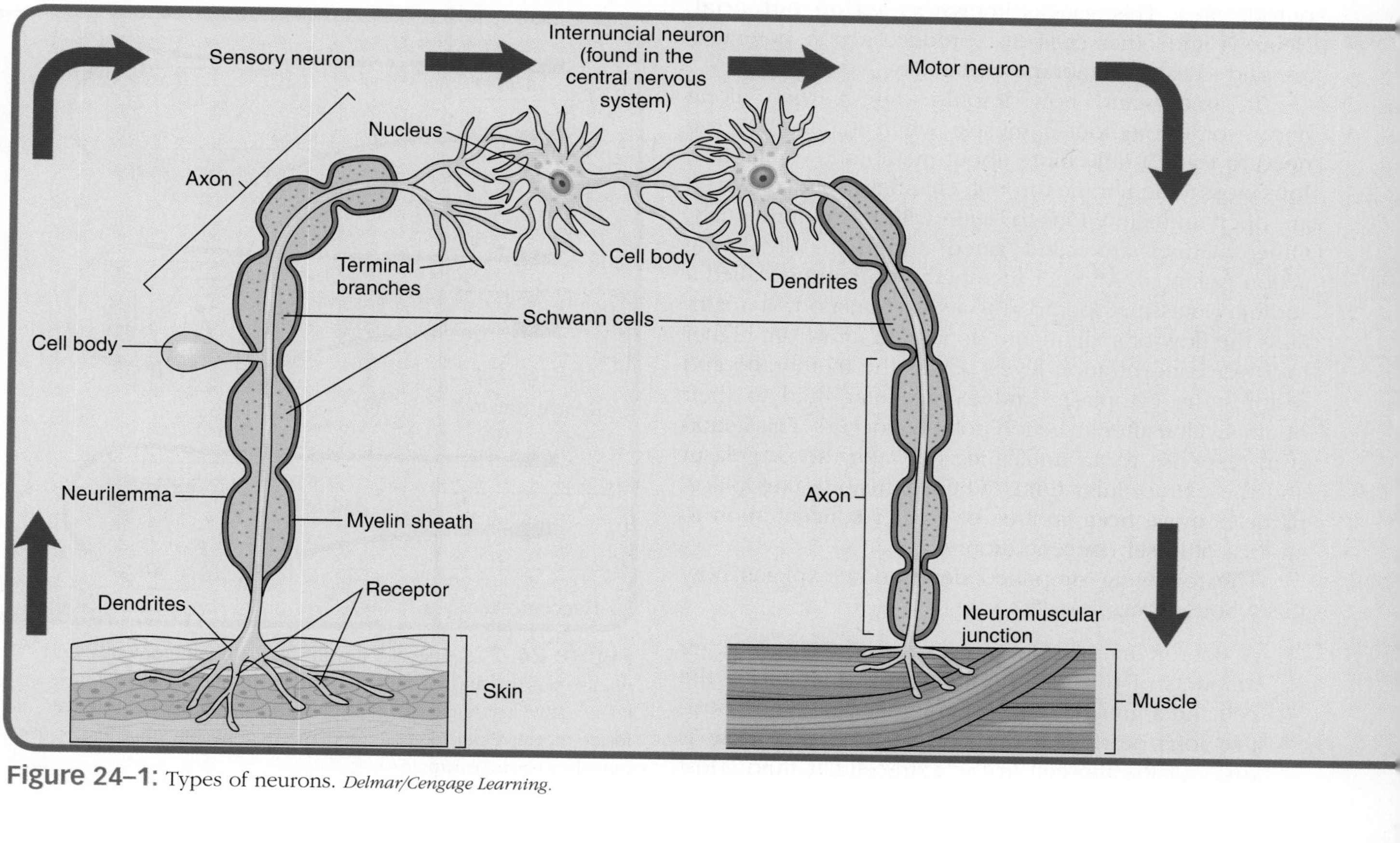

Figure 24–1: Types of neurons. *Delmar/Cengage Learning.*

A nerve is composed of bundles of nerve fibers bound together by connective tissue. If a nerve is composed of fibers going from the sense organs to the spinal cord or brain, it is a *sensory* or *afferent nerve*. If it is carrying impulses from the brain or spinal cord to a muscle, organ, or gland, it is known as a *motor* or *efferent nerve*. Some nerves have both kinds of fibers and are known as *mixed nerves*.

MEDIA LINK

Go to the Premium Website and watch the animation, "Firing of a Neuron," for this chapter.

MEMBRANE EXCITABILITY

Nerves carry impulses by creating electric charges in a process known as membrane excitability. Neurons have a membrane that separates the cytoplasm inside from the extracellular fluids outside the cell, thereby creating two chemically different areas. Each area has differing amounts of potassium and sodium ions and negative charged ions (anions) and positive charged ions (cations), with the inside being the more negatively charged. When a neuron is stimulated, ions move across the membrane, creating a current that, if large enough, will briefly change the area inside of the neuron to be more positive than the outside area. This state is known as **action potential**. Neurons and other cells that produce action potentials are said to have membrane excitability.

To understand how impulses are carried along nerves or throughout a muscle when it contracts, we need to learn a little more about membrane excitability. Ions cross a membrane through channels, some of which are open and allow ions to "leak" (diffuse) continuously. Other channels are called "gated" and open only during action potential. Another membrane opening is called a sodium-potassium pump. By active transport, it maintains the flow of sodium and potassium ions from higher to lower concentration levels across the membrane and restores the cytoplasm and extracellular fluid to their original value after an action potential occurs. This action is in response to an imbalance between the cytoplasm and the extracellular fluid. When diffusion takes place, particles move from an area of greater concentration to an area of lesser concentration.

The following simplified description explains how this whole process works.

1. A neuron membrane is "at rest." There are larger amounts of potassium and negative ions inside the cell and a greater concentration of sodium and positive ions outside in the cytoplasm. The reverse is true outside the cell in the extracellular fluid. Most of the open channels are for potassium (K+) to pass through, so it leaks out of the cell.
2. As the K+ ions leave, the inside becomes relatively more negative until some K+ ions are attracted back in, the electrical force balances the diffusion force, and movement stops. The inside is still more negative, and the amount of energy between the two differently charged areas is ready to work (carry an impulse). This state is called *resting membrane potential* (Figure 24–2A). The membrane is now polarized. The sodium ions (NA+) are not able to move in because their channels are closed during the resting state; however, if a few leak in, the membrane pump sends an equal number out.
3. Now suppose a sensory neuron receptor is stimulated by something, such as a sound. This will cause a change in the membrane potential. The stimulus energy is converted to an electrical signal, and, if it is strong enough, it will depolarize a portion of the membrane and allow the gated sodium ion channels to open (Figure 24–2B).
4. The sodium and positive ions move through the gated channels into the cytoplasm, and the inside becomes more positive until the membrane potential is reversed and the gates close to sodium ions.
5. Next, the potassium gates open, and large amounts of potassium and negative ions reenter the cell, resulting in the repolarization of the membrane (Figure 24–2C). After repolarization, the

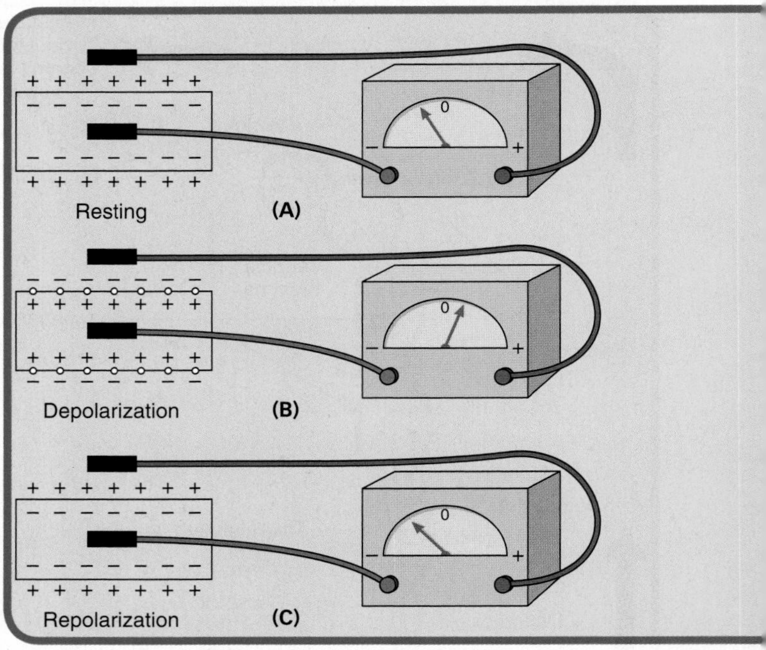

Figure 24–2: Sequence of events in membrane potential and relative positive and negative states: (A) Normal resting potenital–negative inside, positive outside. (B) Depolarization–positive inside, negative outside. (C) Repolarization–negative inside, positive outside. *Delmar/Cengage Learning.*

sodium-potassium pump restores the initial concentrations of sodium and potassium ions inside and outside the neuron.

This whole process occurs in a few milliseconds. When this action occurs in one part of the cell membrane, it spreads to adjacent membrane regions, continuing away from the original site of stimulation, sending "messages" over the nerve. This cycle is completed millions of times a minute throughout the body, day after day, year after year.

But what happens when the impulse reaches the end of the neuron? You will recall that impulses travel across a neuron from the dendrites to the cell body and then to the axon. Here there is a minute space between the dendrites of the next neuron called a **synapse**, which the impulse must "jump" chemically. This space is technically called a *synaptic cleft*. Impulses from the sending cell release chemical messengers called neurotransmitters into the cleft. These substances are signaling molecules that can cause a rapid change in the membrane potential of the receiving cell. These chemicals can either speed up or slow down the transmission. Normally nerve impulses travel about 200 miles per hour. The intake of alcohol, for instance, seems to aid the chemical that causes impulses to be blocked, and our reactions are therefore slowed down. Other chemicals, such as stimulant drugs and wartime nerve gases, cause the release of a chemical that allows the transmission of impulses to speed up, even to the point of causing a flood of impulses to the brain resulting in the possible breakdown of the body's ability to function.

Scientists have discovered that a number of mental disorders are the result of imbalances in brain chemistry. This has resulted in the design of new medications for treating specific mental disorders and behavior problems. The best known of the drugs is probably fluoxetine (Prozac). It inhibits the sending cell from reabsorbing the chemical serotonin. Research has indicated that depressed people have less serotonin than people who are not depressed, so by blocking its reuptake, the effect of a small amount of serotonin on the receiving cell is boosted (Figure 24–3).

There are now new classes of drugs that affect the neurotransmission of both serotonin and norepinephrine. These include venlafaxine (Effexor) and duloxetine (Cymbalta). These same chemicals (serotonin and norepinephrine) have been found to play a critical part in the transmission of pain so that the same drugs used to treat depression may be used to modify pain. These two families of drugs are called SSRIs (selective serotonin reuptake inhibitors) or SSNRIs (selective serotonin norepinephrine reuptake inhibitors).

A disease condition called tetanus results from the effects of the bacterium *Clostridium tetani* on the nervous and muscular systems. Bacteria invade the body through a puncture wound from a contaminated object or an animal bite. The tissues deep in the puncture do not receive oxygen, so they die off and the bacteria multiply. A substance is released by the bacteria that is toxic to the motor neurons that innervate the muscles. A neuron normally stimulates muscle tissue through *balanced chemical messages,* which alternately contract and relax the muscle tissue. This balance is essential to our ability to maintain erect stature and movement. However, with the release of the neurotoxin from the bacteria, excitation is unbalanced, and the inhibitory synapses of the motor neurons of the brain and spinal cord are affected, thereby allowing excessive contraction of the muscles.

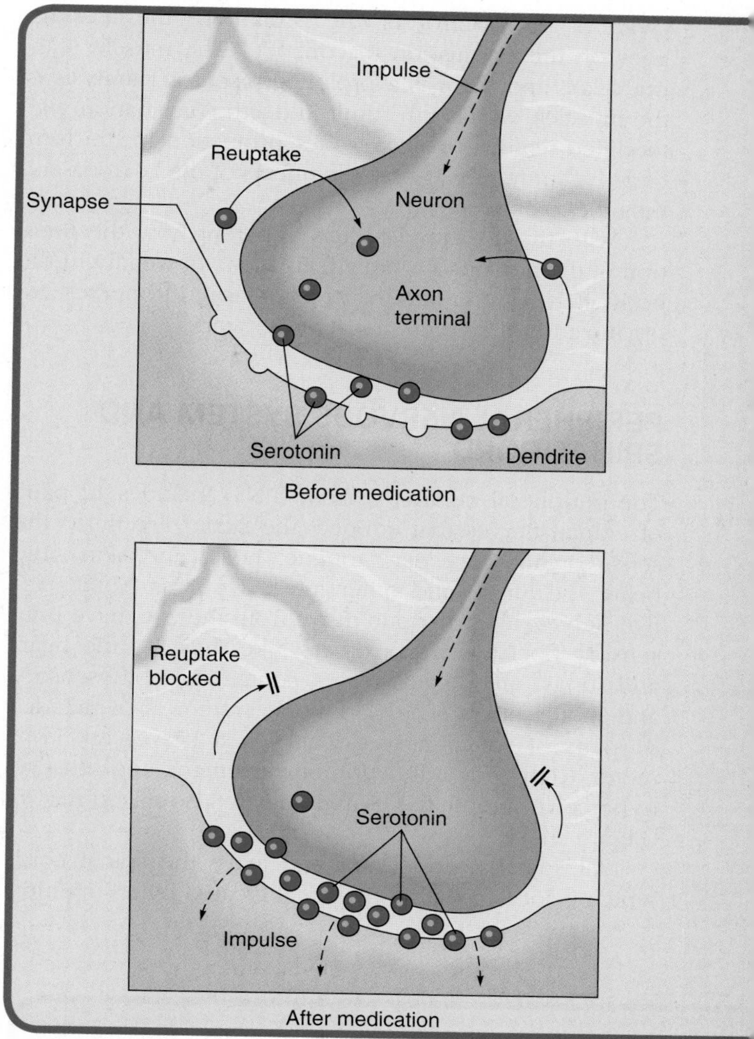

Figure 24–3: Transmission of a nerve impulse across a synapse is chemical. People who are depressed have less of the neurotransmitter serotonin and/or norepinephrine. *Note*: The serotonin is released from the axon before the medication is reabsorbed by the sending cell. With the presence of a serotonin uptake inhibitor, such as fluoxetine (Prozac), the reabsorption is blocked or slowed to increase the effect of serotonin of the receiving call. *Delmar/Cengage Learning.*

(Without the control of the "inhibitor," the message goes on full permission to contract.) The muscles cannot relax, and there is a prolonged, spastic paralysis of the muscles, which can result in death. Vaccination with modified tetanus toxin provides protection in the form of active immunity against the effects of the bacteria and thus the toxins.

With these examples, it is apparent how the function of the nervous system affects the total welfare of the body. It is now important to learn how the nerves are organized in the communication network.

PERIPHERAL NERVOUS SYSTEM AND SPINAL CORD

The peripheral nervous system (PNS) includes 12 pairs of cranial nerves that connect the brain directly to the sense organs (eye, ear, tongue, nose, and skin), the heart, the lungs, and other internal organs. Some cranial nerves, like the optic nerve from the eye, have only sensory fibers, whereas others, like those to the heart and lungs, are mixed nerves containing both sensory and motor fibers. The peripheral system also includes 31 pairs of spinal nerves. The spinal nerves are both motor, to provide a function or movement, and sensory, to perceive stimuli; therefore, they are also mixed nerves (Figure 24–4).

All spinal nerves enter and leave the spinal cord, which is located within the canal created by an opening in each of the bones (vertebrae) of the spinal column. A cross section of the cord would reveal a rounded white mass of myelinated nerve fibers with a notched area on the anterior surface (Figure 24–5). The white matter is mainly comprised of axons of **interneurons**. Some axons are grouped together into major sensory nerves going to a specific section of the brain. Others are grouped into major motor nerves going to their muscle or organ destination. Still others connect with each other up, down, and within the gray matter to provide control over activities that occur within the cord itself. In the center of the white area is a gray area in the shape of an H, which includes the nerve cell bodies and their fibers without the myelin covering. The gray matter is involved mainly with reflex connections in the spinal cord that deal with the reflexes involved in such things as walking or blinking.

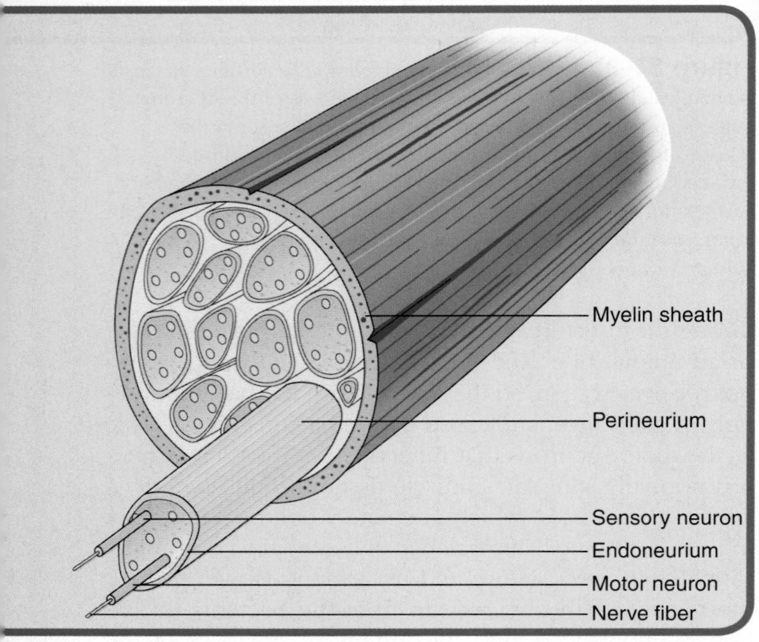

Figure 24–4: Cross section of a spinal nerve showing both sensory and motor nerves (greatly enlarged). *Delmar/Cengage Learning.*

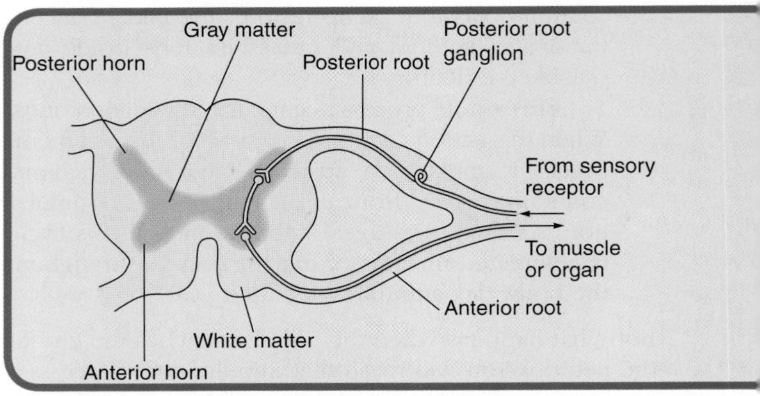

Figure 24–5: Cross section of the spinal cord. *Delmar/Cengage Learning.*

A spinal nerve splits into two roots as it enters the cord. The posterior root carrying sensory fibers to the cord enters at the posterior horn of the H. The bulge on the posterior root contains the sensory nerve cell bodies and is called a **ganglion**. The anterior root of the nerve leaves at the anterior horn of the H, carrying motor nerve fibers that have their cell bodies inside the gray matter of the cord. Neurons within the cord connect sensory to motor nerves.

Sensory neurons transmit messages from millions of special receptor cells to the spinal cord and on to the brain for interpretation and decisions. If a reaction is needed, impulses from the central nervous system (CNS) are transmitted to the appropriate muscle or organ over the motor neurons. Connecting interneurons route impulses throughout the body, permitting any nerve to communicate with any other nerve.

In very simple reflex actions in which no interpretation or decision is required, the nerve impulse travels only to the spinal cord and back. The knee jerk test often used by physicians illustrates such a simple reflex and provides an evaluation of the nervous system. When the knee is hanging completely relaxed, the leg should kick up sharply when the tendon below the kneecap is lightly tapped (Figure 24–6). If there is no response, a nervous system disease or disorder can be suspected.

In more complicated reflex actions, such as the body coming into contact with something harmful, the sensory impulse is relayed through nerve cells to the spinal cord and up to the brain (Figure 24–7). There the impulse is interpreted, and the motor neurons carry the message back down the spinal cord and out the appropriate motor nerves to the muscles and the legs move the body away.

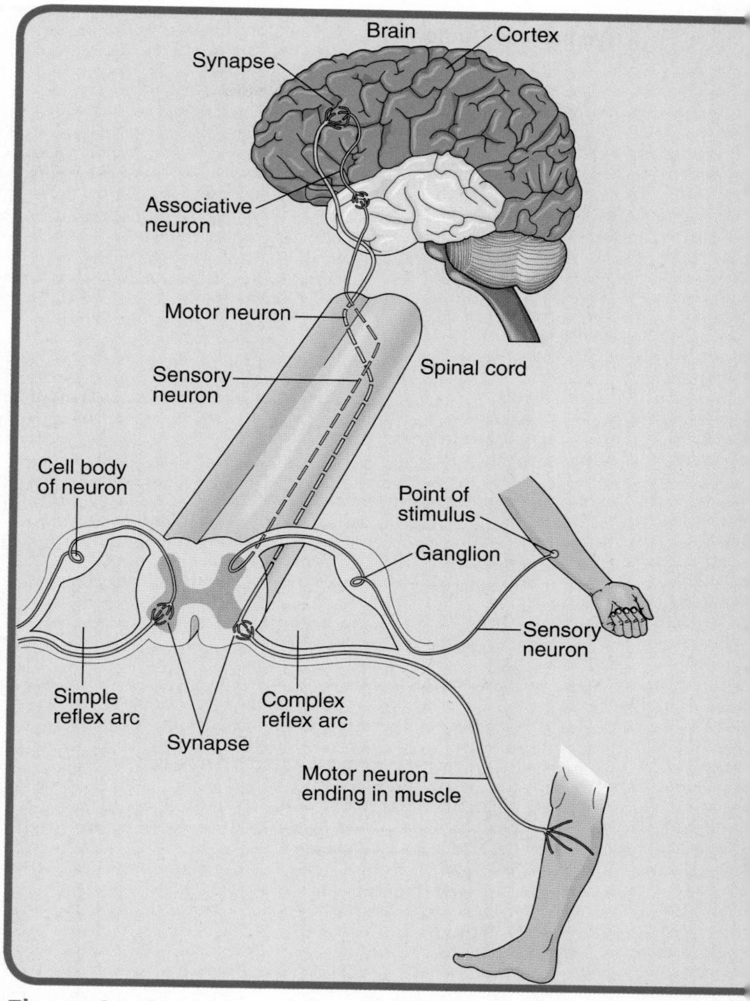

Figure 24–7: Complex reflex action. *Delmar/Cengage Learning.*

Autonomic Nervous System

The autonomic nervous system (ANS) is part of the peripheral nervous system. These nerves are involuntary and regulate functions such as breathing, heartbeat, and digestion. The system consists of nerves, ganglia, and **plexuses** (networks of nerves). There are two divisions of the autonomic system. The **sympathetic** division accelerates activity in the smooth, involuntary muscles of the body's organs, and the **parasympathetic** division reverses the action and slows down activity. For example, the sympathetic nerves constrict blood vessels and speed up the heartbeat; the parasympathetic nerves dilate the blood vessels and slow down the heartbeat. These activities continuously balance each other to maintain homeostasis in the body. However, this on and off mechanism does not apply to all organs, because some do not have a dual nerve supply. Also, nerves in both divisions can have excitatory or inhibitory effects. At any given time, the actual effect depends on the net outcome of the two opposing signals.

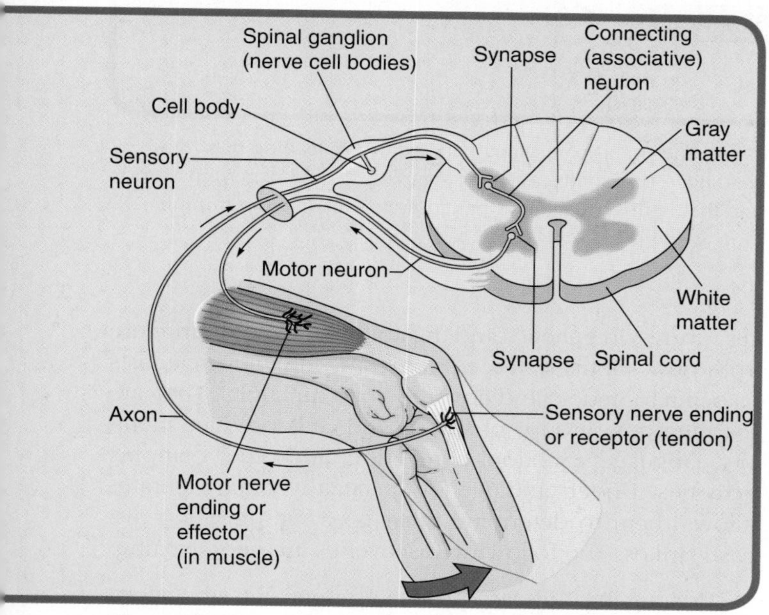

Figure 24–6: Reflex action. In this example, tapping the patellar tendon of the knee results in extension of the leg, producing the knee jerk reflex. *Delmar/Cengage Learning.*

The *sympathetic nervous system* begins at the base of the brain and runs down both sides of the spinal column in two tracts. These tracts consist of nerve fibers and ganglia. The sympathetic nerves extend to all the vital internal organs, the blood vessels, the iris of the eye, and even to the sweat glands (Figure 24–8).

The *parasympathetic system* has two important nerves, the vagus and the pelvic nerve. The vagus extends from the medulla oblongata of the brain and branches to the neck, chest, and upper abdominal organs. The pelvic nerve exits the spinal cord around the hip area and branches into the lower abdominal and pelvic organs. Both systems are strongly affected by emotions such as fear, anger, and stress.

The action of the autonomic system is extremely important to our ability to react in an emergency. It is frequently called our "flight-fright mechanism" because

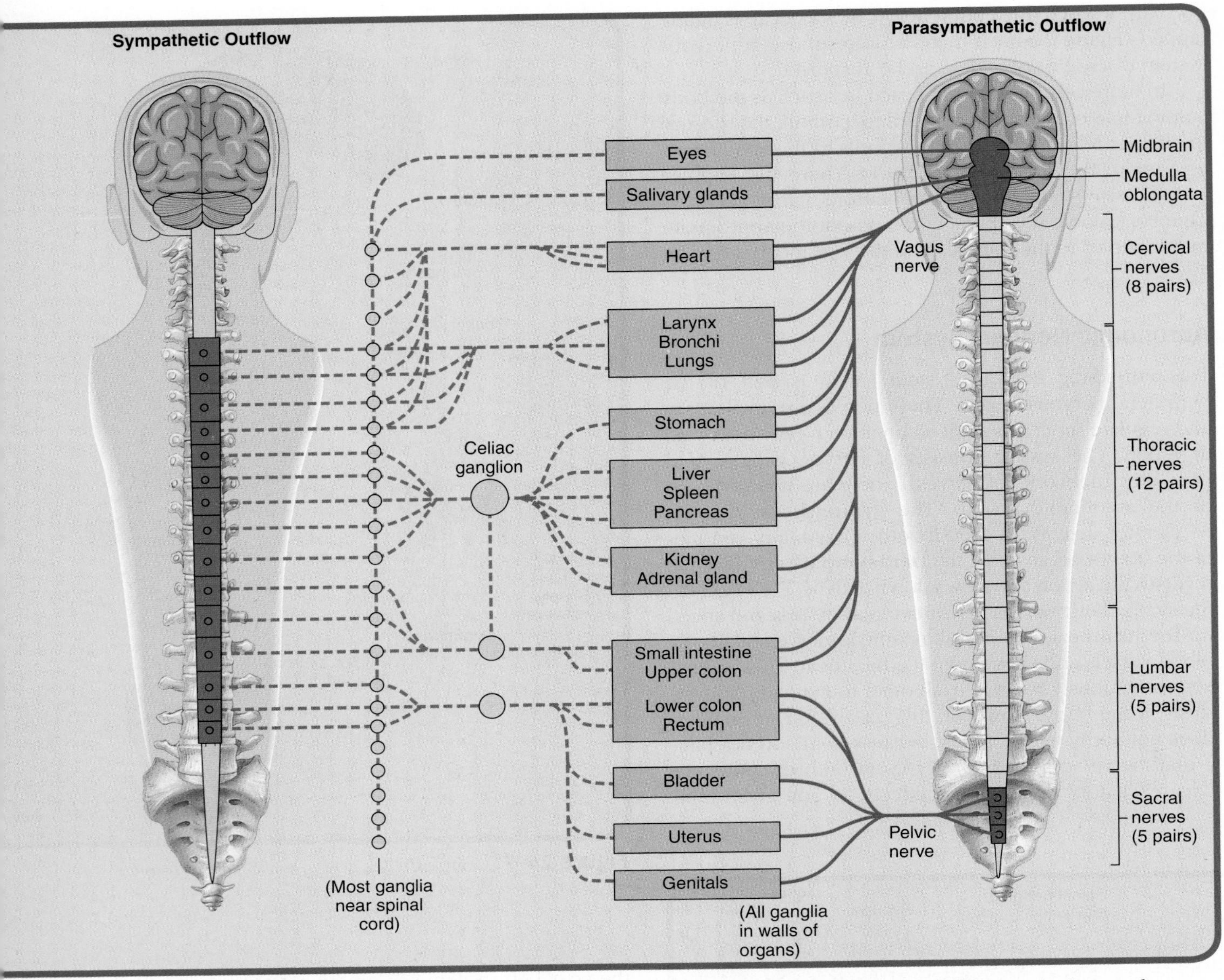

Figure 24–8: Autonomic nervous system. Shown here are the main sympathetic and parasympathetic pathways leading out from the central nervous system to some major organs. As the lists of examples suggest, in some cases, the sympathetic and parasympathetic nerves operate antagonistically in their efforts on the organ. Keep in mind that both systems have paired nerves leading out from the brain and spinal cord. *Delmar/Cengage Learning.*

it accelerates our body functions to permit escaping or otherwise dealing with danger.

CENTRAL NERVOUS SYSTEM

The Brain

The brain is a large mass of nerve tissue with about 100 billion neurons. Scientists call it the most complex and challenging structure ever studied. This small organ, weighing only about 3 pounds, is a mass of interconnecting nerve cells that "talk" to each other continuously in both chemical and electrical language. The new discoveries in genetics and the ability to view its structure with new sophisticated equipment is allowing scientists to begin to understand how the brain functions. They are learning how groups of specialized cells produce memory, language, emotion, perception, and other complex activities. Understanding how a healthy brain operates allows them to determine what goes wrong when disease strikes. The following discoveries are very exciting:

- Identifying disease-producing genetic mutations allows diagnosis of some inherited disorders and the ability to predict who will develop them. This knowledge will permit new therapies to alter the genes.

- Beginning to understand the programmed death of nerve cells that leads to degenerative diseases or expands the damage after a stroke may lead to new drugs to interfere with the destructive process.
- Using the naturally occurring chemicals that protect nerve cells from environmental destruction may prevent disease or reverse nerve injury.
- Understanding how brain chemistry affects mood and mental health is helping not only the patient with depression but hopefully others as well.

Scientists have found abnormal genes associated with Huntington's disease, Alzheimer's disease, amyotrophic lateral sclerosis, epilepsy, and muscular dystrophy.

The Structure and Function of the Brain

The brain is protected and supported by surrounding membranes known as **meninges** (Figure 24–9). It is further protected by the **cranium** (skull). The brain surface has extensive deep furrows and folds and is divided into two hemispheres by a **longitudinal fissure**. The hemispheres are connected internally with nerve fibers and share information. The cerebral surface is covered with ridges and furrows known as *fissures* if they are deep or *sulci* if they are shallow. The elevated ridges between the sulci are called *convolutions*.

The brain is divided into five parts. The largest is the **cerebrum**, which controls sensory and motor activities. The cerebrum is further divided into lobes (Figure 24–10 A and B). The **frontal** lobe behind the forehead seems to be related to emotions, personality, moral traits, and intellectual functions. The frontal lobe is also the motor area for active voluntary muscle movements and two areas that control speech. The **occipital** lobe is the far back portion of the cerebrum. This area is associated with vision. The impulses of color and light received by the eyes are transmitted by the **optic** nerve fibers to the occipital lobe for interpretation. Between the frontal and occipital lobes is the **parietal** lobe; the motor area governing speech lies at its junction with the frontal lobe. It is the parietal lobe that receives impulses from receptors in the hands, feet, and tongue, among others, and sends impulses that cause movement in all these parts in response. This area also receives nerve impulses from sensory receptors for pain, touch, heat, and cold. A small **temporal** lobe lies on the side of the cerebrum. The **auditory** nerve association area is here, which provides us with the sense of hearing. The **olfactory** area, which provides our sense of smell, is within a small projection under the temporal lobe. It is connected by nerve fibers to receptors in the nasal cavity.

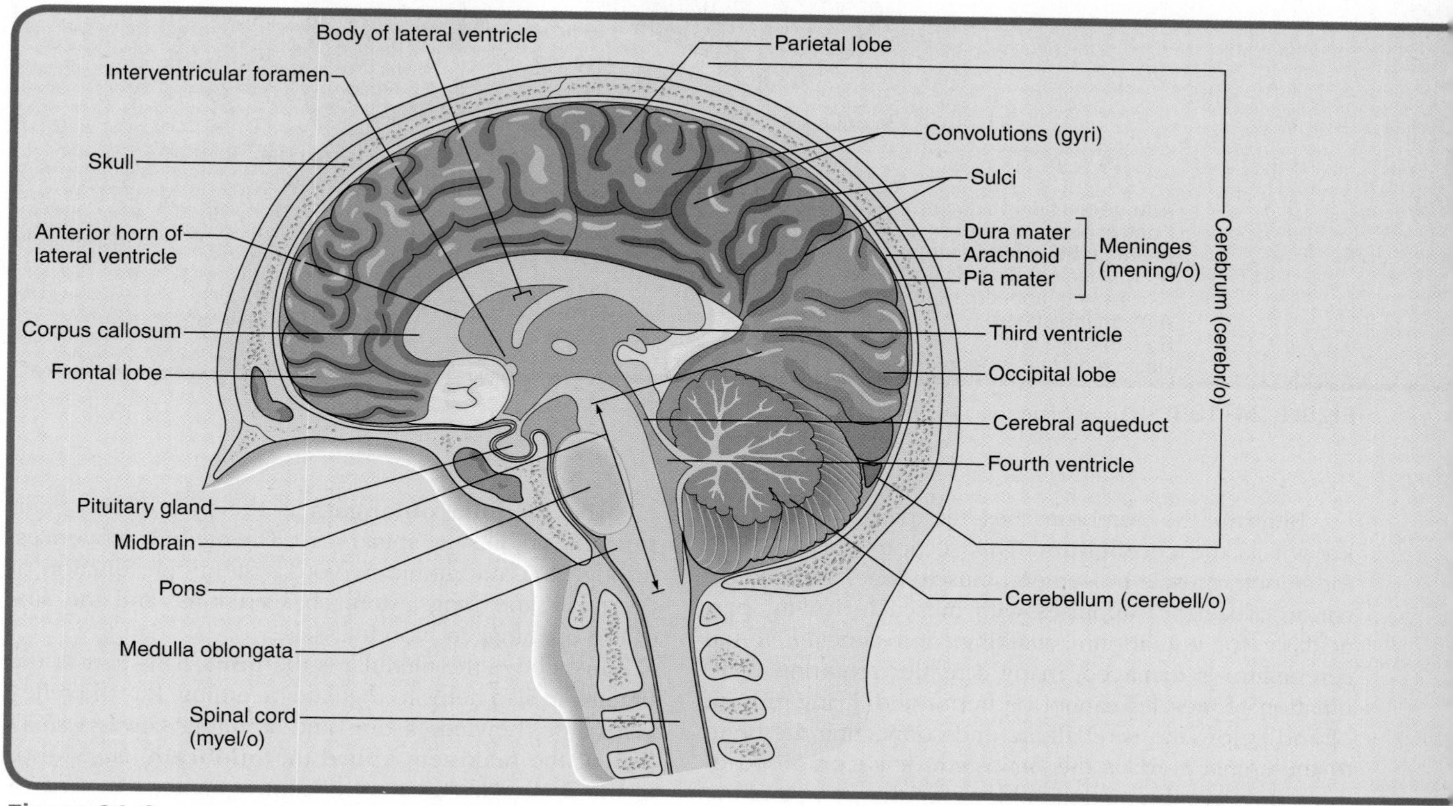

Figure 24–9: Cross section of the brain. *Delmar/Cengage Learning.*

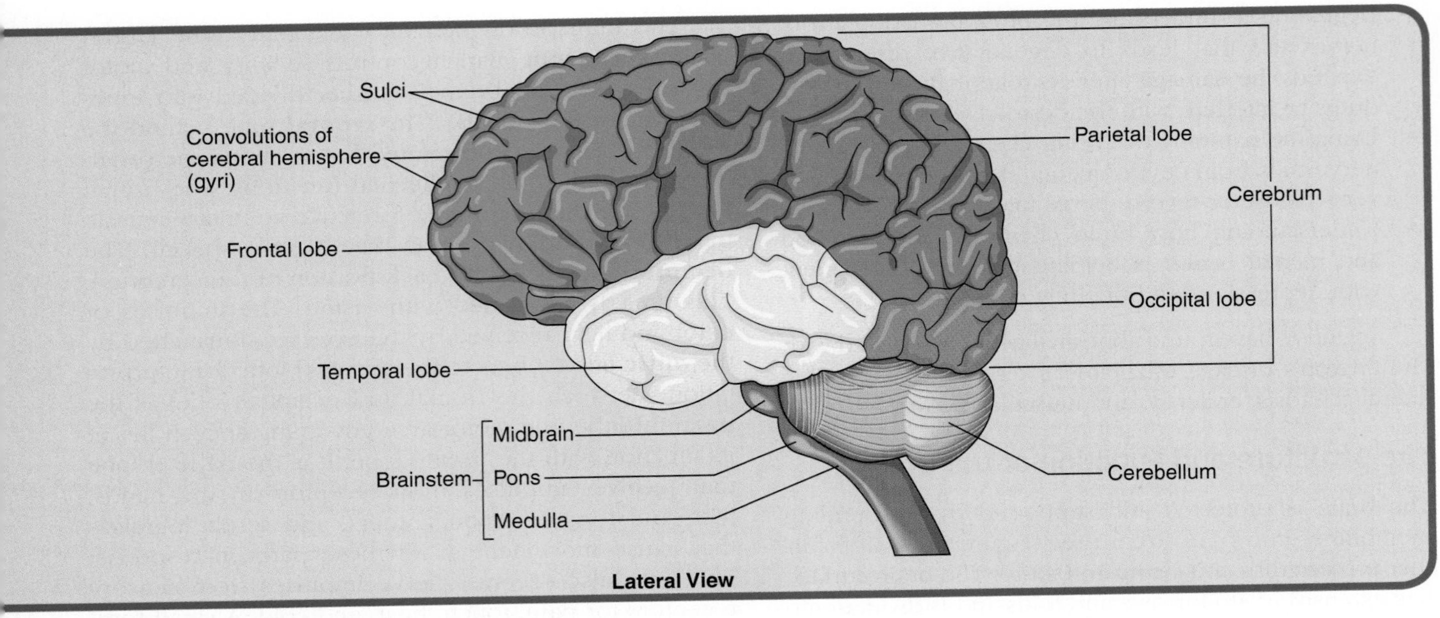

Figure 24–10A: The parts of the brain. *Delmar/Cengage Learning.*

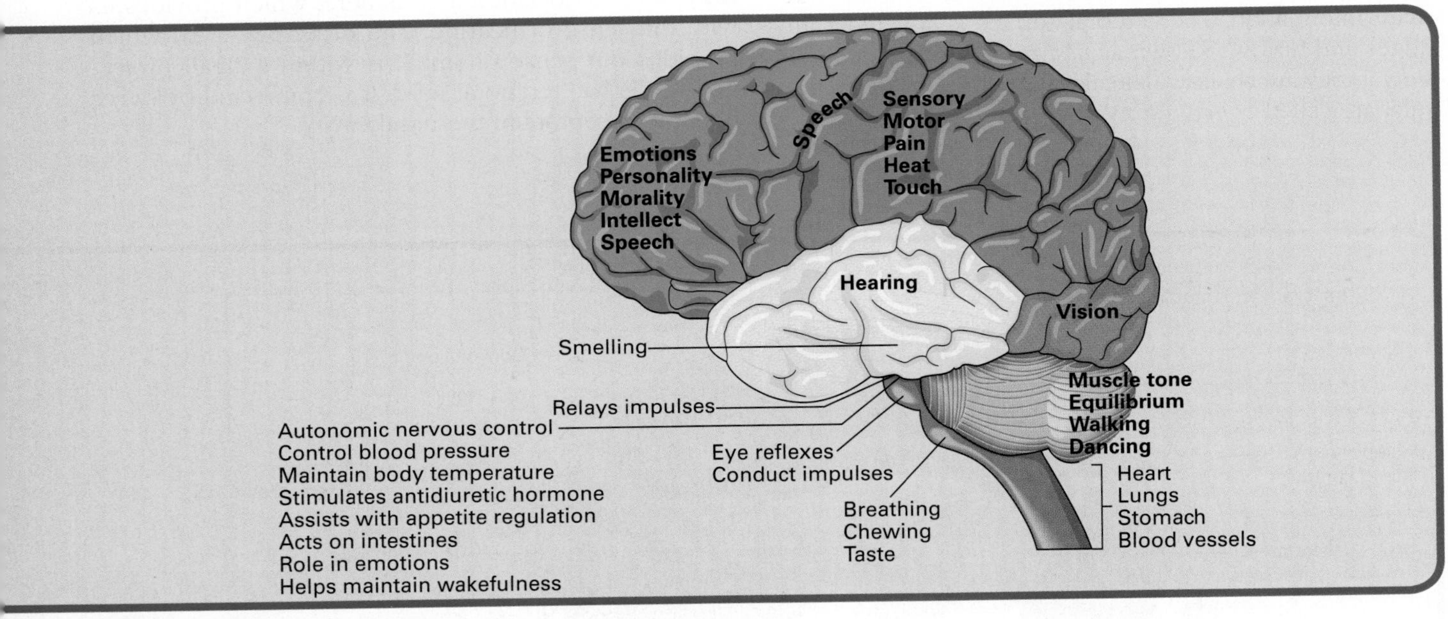

Figure 24–10B: Areas of brain function. *Delmar/Cengage Learning.*

Beneath the cerebrum lies the part of the brain known as the **cerebellum**. This section is responsible for smooth muscle movement, muscle tone, and coordination of sensory impulses with muscular activity, particularly for equilibrium, walking, and dancing. If the cerebellum is damaged, many activities requiring coordination of muscles cannot be performed. Lying in front of and below the cerebellum, and connecting the brain to the spinal cord, is the brainstem. It is composed of three sections: the medulla oblongata, the pons, and the midbrain.

The **medulla oblongata** is the part of the brain stem that adjoins the spinal cord. The medulla influences, through the autonomic nervous system, the function of the heart and lungs, stomach secretions, and the size of the openings in blood vessels.

Just above the medulla is the **pons**. This part of the brainstem also helps to regulate breathing. It is the reflex center for chewing, tasting, and secreting saliva. A small part of the brainstem, called the **midbrain**, is superior to the pons. This area is the control center for some of the reflex movements of the eyes, such as blinking and changing the size of the pupil. It also conducts impulses between the brain parts above and below it.

Doctors learned long ago that nerve fibers from the right side of the body cross over in the brainstem to the left side of the brain. The body's left side is likewise controlled by the right side of the brain. Therefore, when a person is paralyzed on the right side, there may be damage to the left side of the brain.

In an area between the cerebrum and the midbrain are two major structures, the **thalamus** and the **hypothalamus**. The thalamus acts as a relay station for impulses going to and from the brain and those impulses from the cerebellum and other parts of the brain. The hypothalamus lies below the thalamus and is connected to the pituitary gland, midbrain, and thalamus by a bundle of nerve fibers. The hypothalamus performs many vital functions:

1. Controlling the autonomic nervous system.
2. Controlling blood pressure by regulating the heartbeat and blood vessel constriction and dilation.
3. Maintaining body temperature.
4. Stimulating the production of an antidiuretic hormone to conserve water in the body and to cause thirst to maintain normal water balance.
5. Assisting in the regulation of appetite.
6. Increasing secretions and motility in the intestinal tract.
7. Playing a role in emotions such as fear and pleasure.
8. Helping maintain wakefulness when it is necessary.

Meninges

Because of their common origin, the brain and the spinal cord are covered with the same membranes, the meninges (Figure 24–11). Three membrane layers make up the meninges. The innermost layer is called the **pia mater**, a delicate, tight-fitting covering containing blood vessels to nourish the nerve tissue. The middle layer, the **arachnoid**, is a delicate, lacelike membrane. The outer layer, called **dura mater**, is a tough, fibrous tissue that protects the CNS from being damaged from contact with the bony surfaces of the skull and spine. The space between the dura mater and the arachnoid is called the **subdural** space. The **subarachnoid** space is between the arachnoid and the pia mater.

Cavities of the Brain and Spinal Cord

Within the brain are several spaces or cavities called **ventricles**. They extend into the lobes of the cerebrum and into contact with the other sections of the brain by

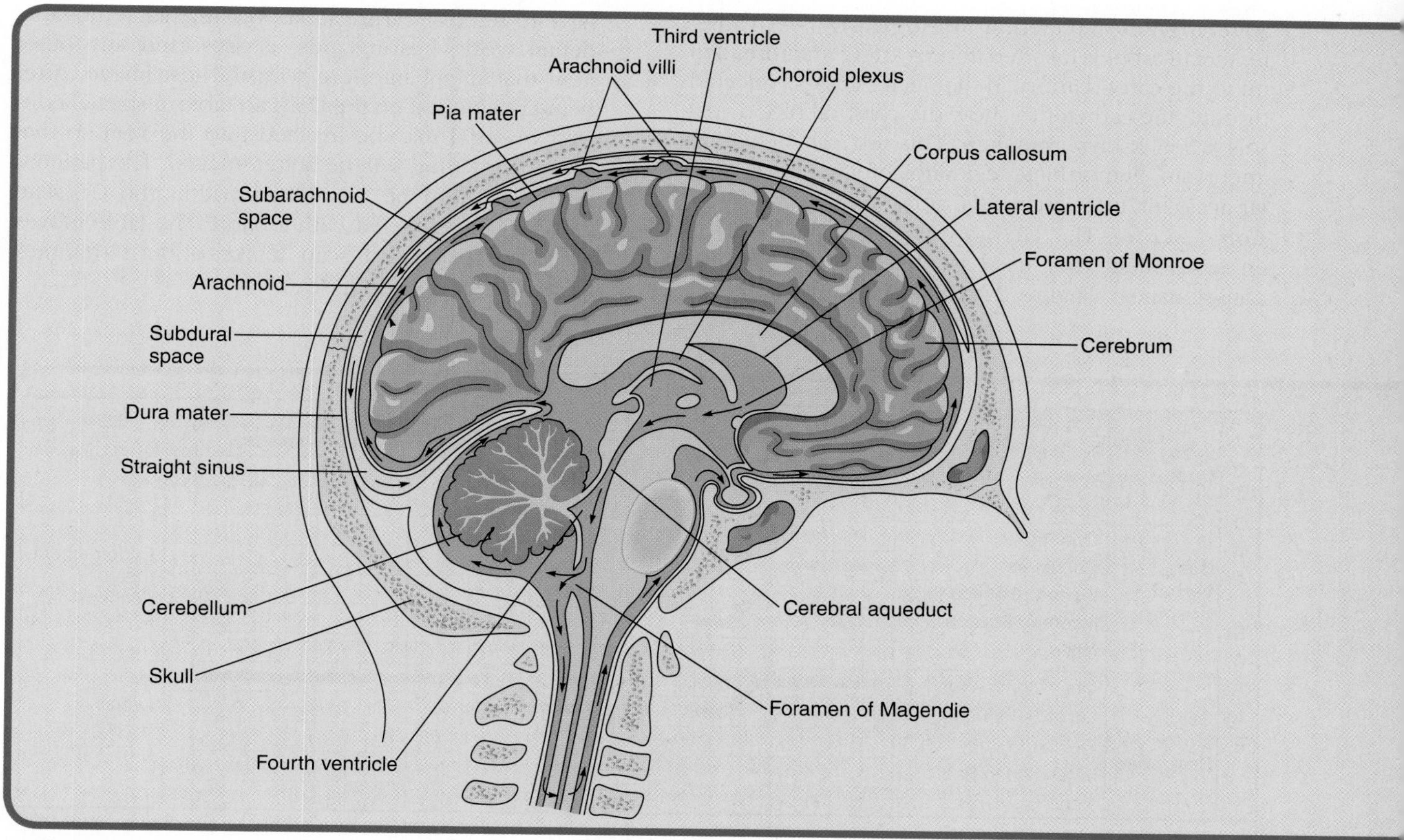

Figure 24–11: A diagrammatic representation of the meninges and the circulation of the cerebral spinal fluid from its formation in the choroid plexus until its return to the blood in the cranial sinus. *Delmar/Cengage Learning.*

means of small passageways. The central canal of the spinal cord is directly connected to the most inferior ventricle. There are also connections from the ventricles into the subarachnoid space of the meninges.

Cerebrospinal Fluid

The cavities within the brain and spinal cord are filled with a liquid called **cerebrospinal fluid** (CSF). This fluid acts as a watery cushion or shock absorber to provide additional protection for the delicate tissues of the CNS. The fluid transports nutrients, primarily proteins and carbohydrates, to the brain and spinal cord. CSF is formed continuously within the ventricles of the brain at the rate of 450 mL (15 oz) per day. Only 150 mL are present at any one time in a normal adult. The fluid circulates within the cavities of the brain and spinal cord and the subarachnoid space, being reabsorbed into the blood vessels in special structures called *arachnoidal villi*.

DIAGNOSTIC TESTS

Diagnosis of neurologic disorders and diseases may require the use of specific tests. Some of the more common tests and a few possible findings are as follows:

- ***Arteriography*** (cerebral **angiography**)—A catheter (small tube) is inserted into an artery and threaded up to the carotid artery in the neck. A dye is injected through the catheter to show the cerebral blood vessels when X-rays are taken. This test can detect an aneurysm, hemorrhage, evidence of a cerebrovascular accident, arteriosclerosis, and a tumor.
- ***Coma scale***—The Glasgow Coma Scale (GCS) is an assessment tool used to describe the level of consciousness (Figure 24–12). Terms often used to indicate this state are semicomatose, stupor, lethargic, comatose, vegetative, and others. The tool was developed in 1974 at the University of Glasgow to standardize what observers were reporting as evidence of the state of "coma" with head injury patients. The method is now acceptable in both European and American neurologic centers as a quick, accurate, and simple tool for evaluating neurologic status. The scale assesses three things: eye movement, verbal response, and motor response. The scale is based upon the need for more stimulation to induce a response in the patient. Paramedics may be trained to perform the grading at the accident scene or en route to alert the emergency room staff to the severity of the injury of the incoming patient. (This probably would not be encountered in the physician's office, but knowledge of the scale will be helpful in personal understanding and patient teaching.)
- ***Computerized axial tomography (CAT or CT scan)***—A series of X-rays of layers of the brain to construct a three-dimensional picture. It is useful for identifying tumors, bleeding, blood clots, decrease in brain size, and brain edema. The machine is doughnut-shaped and was developed in the early 1970s. Today, CT scans can be equipped with spiral imaging to make images in seconds. The patient will have to remove earrings, hair ornaments, removable dental work, hearing aids, glasses, and any other item that might interfere with the test image. After being positioned on the CT scan table, a special contrast material may be injected into the vein so that certain structures will be better imaged. The patient's head will then be positioned within the CT scan ring and immobilized with a band. The table moves slightly between each scan. It takes about 15 minutes to complete a head CT scan.

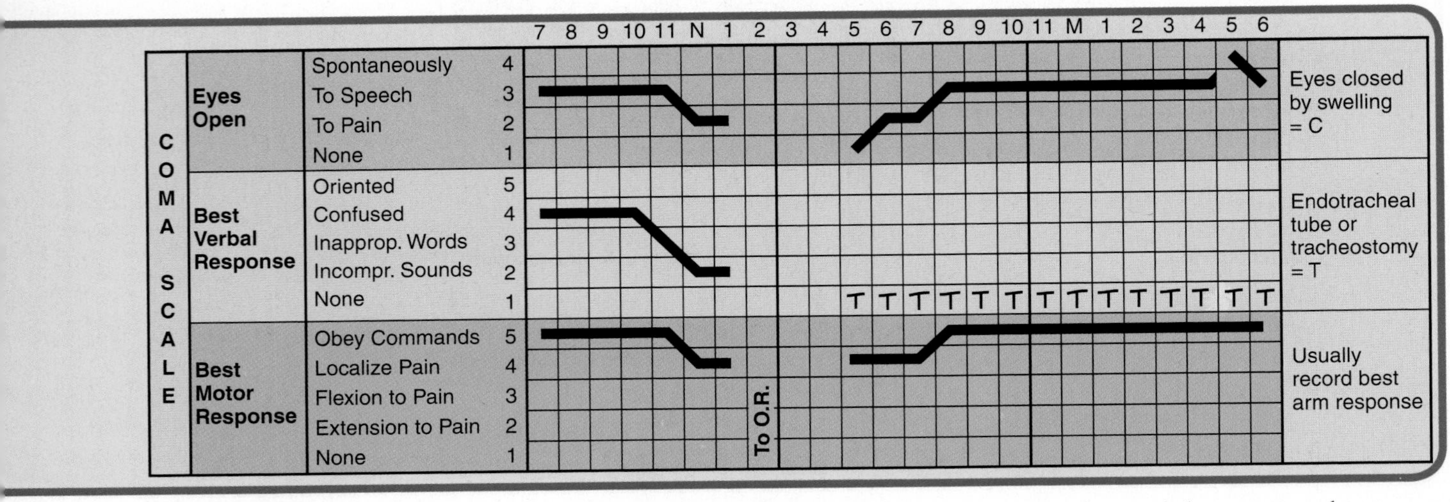

Figure 24–12: The Glasgow Coma Scale (GCS) includes three parts: assessment of eye opening, verbal response, and motor response. Each can be assessed hourly, given a numerical value, and plotted graphically. *Delmar/Cengage Learning.*

- ***Electroencephalography (EEG)***—A brain wave test that measures the brain's electrical signals, both normal and abnormal. It can pick up abnormalities caused by epilepsy, a tumor, a stroke, a head injury, or infection. It can also document sleep disorders. It cannot detect mental retardation unless it is associated with seizures or brain atrophy. An EEG in retardation as well as in psychologic disorders is normal unless they are caused by a disease such as lupus. New technology has developed an ambulatory EEG monitor that helps diagnose neurological conditions, including fainting "spells" and seizures, by permitting continuous monitoring.
- ***Electromyography (EMG)*** and nerve conduction studies (NCSs)—Electromyography (EMG) demonstrates the electrical activity of the peripheral muscles at rest and when activated. A small needle is inserted into the muscle. NCSs are done in conjunction with an EMG to measure the speed of nerve conduction. EMGs/NCSs can help diagnose disorders like radiculopathy (pinched nerve), ALS (amyotrophic lateral sclerosis), peripheral neuropathy (including diabetic neuropathy) and carpal tunnel syndrome.
- ***Lumbar puncture***—A spinal needle is inserted into the subarachnoid space between the vertebrae of the lower back, and CSF is removed for examination (Figure 24–13A and B). The procedure is indicated when infection is suspected (e.g., meningitis), when there is hemorrhage from injury, or when the fluid pressure must be measured. When measurement is desired, a calibrated glass tube is attached to the needle, and the level of the fluid is observed and recorded.

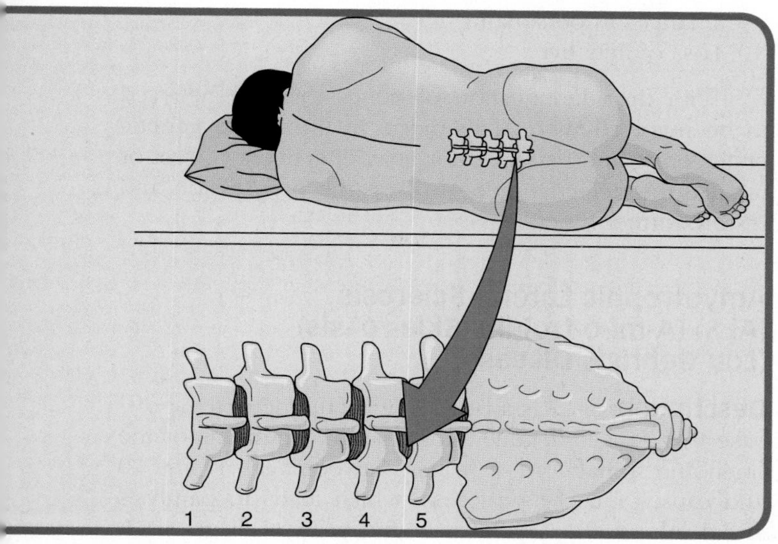

Figure 24–13: (A) Positioning of patient for limbar puncture; (B) site of lumbar puncture. *Delmar/Cengage Learning.*

- ***Magnetic resonance imaging (MRI)***—MRI was pioneered in 1977. The machine resembles a large white tube and uses powerful magnets to generate pictures. When images of the brain and spine are needed, MRI is the method of choice as long as the patient has no ferrous (iron) metal implants or pacemakers. Its advantages are that it can image from numerous angles, and it imparts no radiation. MRI can be combined now with MRA (magnetic resonance angiogragraphy) where dye is used, to help diagnose cerebral aneurysms, bleeds, or tumors.
- ***Myelography***—A lumbar puncture is performed to remove CSF and instill a dye to outline the spinal structures on X-ray. This will show irregularities or compression of the spinal cord. It is less frequently used since the advent of MRI. It is used most often in postoperative spinal evaluations where metal implants may impair magnetic MRI signals.
- ***Positron emission tomography (PET scan)***—A newer form of imaging that allows visualizing the physiologic performance of the body. An "agent" is labeled or "mixed with" a radioactive substance. Agents can be many things, such as glucose or any number of hormones. After the material is injected into the blood, images are recorded to measure where the material ends up in the body. The images are further enhanced by the use of color, which can be selected by the operator. The brighter the shade of the color, the greater the amount of uptake. The PET scan has been most useful with evaluating and staging malignancies.
- ***Skull X-ray***—To identify fractures and abnormal bone structures that may indicate a tumor or increased pressure within the skull.

DISEASES AND DISORDERS

Alzheimer's Disease (Alts′-hi-merz)

Description—This is a progressive, degenerative disease that attacks the brain and results in impaired memory, thinking, and behavior. It affects an estimated 4 million American adults. It is the most common form of dementia (loss of mental function). Alzheimer's is the 6th leading cause of death in United States, with 74,632 deaths recorded in 2007 by the Centers for Disease Control and Prevention.

Signs and symptoms—Evidence of the disease includes a gradual memory loss, a decline in ability to perform routine tasks, impairment of judgment, disorientation, personality change, difficulty in learning, and loss of language skills. The individuals eventually become totally incapable of caring for themselves. Unfortunately, these are the same symptoms of other neurologic disorders.

Etiology—The exact cause is unknown. Suspected causes include a genetic predisposition, a slow virus or other infectious agent, environmental toxins, and immunologic changes. The underlying cause of Alzheimer's disease is the gradual extinction of certain brain cells. Brains from people who have died from Alzheimer's have been studied and show abnormalities called amyloid plaques and neurofibrillary tangles. About 20% of all cases are inherited, and these people tend to develop symptoms earlier in life than others. Scientists have also recently discovered several mutated genes that can cause the inherited form.

Treatment—There is no cure for Alzheimer's disease. Scientists are working on preventing the death of nerve cells. Unlike other types of cells, nerve cells cannot reproduce themselves—they were meant to last a lifetime. It is normal for some brain cells to be gradually lost, but when a large population of a certain type die over time, it causes problems. Researchers are looking at neuroprotectors to keep cells alive even when there is a stroke or spinal cord injury. Cells manufacture several neuroprotectors on their own. It is their hope to develop neuroprotective drugs that could guard brain cells against damage and death or perhaps even help them regenerate. In the meantime, appropriate medication continues to be used to lessen agitation, anxiety, and unpredictable behavior; improve sleeping; and treat depression. Physical exercise, social activity, good nutrition, and health maintenance are important. A calm and well-structured environment may help maintain the patient's sense of well-being. It is especially important to support and assist the family in dealing with this devastating disease. The course usually runs from 2 to 10 years, but it can take as long as 20 years. The role of the caretakers is difficult and exhausting.

Currently, positive diagnosis of Alzheimer's is not possible until after death, when the brain can be examined for the telltale signs of amyloid plaque; therefore, there is no way to rule out other degenerative diseases. Recently, a cell abnormality in Alzheimer's patients has been found and may lead to early diagnosis and treatment. The cells were grown and tested in the laboratory and showed collapsed potassium channels in their membranes, a finding that occurred only in the Alzheimer's patients. Preliminary results are fairly reliable, and if after extensive clinical tests it appears to be diagnostic, it could save millions of dollars annually in diagnostic evaluations. Within the next 20 years, as the population ages, the incidence of the disease is expected to rise from the current level of about 4 million to approximately 12 million.

There is as yet no proven way to reverse or stop the disease. Current research on Alzheimer's suggests three "keys to cognitive vitality": (1) build reserve brain capacity, (2) acquire more knowledge, and (3) protect your brain from various forms of damage. It is possible to reduce the risk of Alzheimer's by following the eight steps to keep the brain function sharp:

1. Establish a brain reserve; think of it as a brain bank.
2. Exercise the body; it improves blood supply to the brain.
3. Eat well; it will protect against four potential causes: inflammation, oxidative stress, elevated homocysteine levels, and small strokes.
4. Consider a daily aspirin; some studies have identified it as a link to reduced risk.
5. Get enough folic acid through fortified foods or supplements because it keeps down serum levels of homocysteine. Alzheimer's patients have a higher than normal level.
6. Maintain a positive attitude, because it may help hold off cognitive decline.
7. Avoid tobacco and excess alcohol. Smokers are more than twice as likely to develop Alzheimer's. Alcohol appears to be protective if only consuming one to two drinks per day.
8. Treat chronic conditions that can affect cognitive function such as hypertension, heart disease, high cholesterol, diabetes, or depression.

The Alzheimer's Association publishes a list of 10 warning signs of the disease of which you should be aware. They are as follows:

1. Recent memory loss that affects job skills
2. Difficulty performing familiar tasks
3. Problems with language
4. Disorientation of time and place
5. Poor or decreased judgement
6. Problems with abstract thinking
7. Misplacing things (putting things in an inappropriate place, such as an iron in the refrigerator)
8. Changes in mood or behavior
9. Changes in personality
10. Loss of initiative

With the identification of genes that are believed to be involved with Alzheimer's, in the future genetic engineering and manipulation may effectively correct or replace the defective gene to stop the progression and restore former function.

Amyotrophic Lateral Sclerosis (ALS) (A-mi-o-trof'ik) (Skle-ro'-sis) (Lou Gehrig's Disease)

Description—ALS is a progressive, fatal neurologic disease that causes degeneration of motor neurons of the brain and spinal cord. It strikes between ages 40 and 70 and causes muscle weakness, which leads to paralysis and death usually within two to five years of diagnosis. It affects 5,600 new people each year, with approximately 25,000 Americans having the disease at any given time.

ALS is 20% more common in men than women, but with increasing age, it is more equally represented. About 10% of ALS cases are familial and can be passed on to children. The remaining 90% are known as sporadic ALS.

Signs and symptoms—The onset is insidious (slow and unnoticed) with muscle weakness or stiffness as the early symptoms. As the weakness progresses, leg and arm paralysis begins and muscle atrophy can occur. Problems may include difficulties with speech, chewing, and swallowing and if the brain stem is involved, breathing difficulty. Occasional choking and excessive drooling will result. Bowel and bladder function is not affected and mental deterioration does not usually occur; therefore, the patient is acutely aware of the progressive physical deterioration, so depression caused by the consequences of the disease may develop.

Etiology—The cause of sporadic ALS is unknown. There is much speculation about a combination of genetic and environmental factors that perhaps cause a mutation that leads to the disease. On the other hand, some cases of familial ALS (FALS) have been shown to be linked to a defective gene on chromosome 21 that produces excessive copper-containing enzymes that appear to lead to the death of nerve cells in the brain and spinal cord. Studies have indicated that over 60 mutations can interfere with the enzyme's ability to protect against free radical damage. FALS seems to run in families and can be passed on to children; however, there is no definite hereditary pattern. Scientists hope to soon identify what causes the mutant proteins to produce chemicals (oxidants) that interfere with the cell's ability to protect itself.

Treatment—There is no cure for ALS, only methods to control symptoms and provide emotional and physical support. Rehabilitation techniques, assistive devices, and respiratory support can enhance the quality of life. The FDA approved the drug riluzole (Rilutek); it has been shown to prolong the life of persons with ALS by at least a few months. The drug, the first to alter the course of the disease, slows the progress of ALS, allowing the patient more time in the higher functioning state of the disease.

Bell's Palsy (Pawl′-ze)

Description—This disease affects the seventh cranial nerve of the face. It occurs suddenly and will usually spontaneously subside within one to nine weeks.

Signs and symptoms—The affected nerve causes weakness or paralysis on one side of the face, which causes the mouth to droop on the affected side, resulting in the drooling of saliva. There is a distorted sense of taste and an inability to close the affected eye. Occasionally, pain in the area of the jaw's angle may be present.

Etiology—The cause is unknown, but many scientists believe it results from a viral infection that inflames the facial nerve.

Treatment—Early treatment with steroids and an antiviral medication, such as valacyclovir (Valtrex), may shorten the course. Prednisone is usually prescribed in a high dose and then quickly reduced over seven to 10 days. Moist heat applied to the face and jaw helps relieve pain, but care must be taken to avoid burning the skin. It may be advisable to protect the eye with an eye patch while outdoors, or if exposed to dust or pollutants, and while sleeping.

Cerebral Palsy (Se-re′-bral)

Description—This disorder is a nonprogressive brain injury that occurs during fetal development, perinatally, or in early infancy. Its incidence is 2.5 per 1,000 live births, or about 8,000 per year. There are four forms of the disorder: spastic (50% to 75% of the cases), athetoid (15% to 20%), atonic (10%), and mixed.

Signs and symptoms—Characteristics of the spastic form are hyperactive tendon reflexes, rapid alteration between muscular contraction and relaxation, contracture tendency (permanent muscle shortening), and underdevelopment of the affected extremities. Approximately 40% of the children affected are also intellectually impaired, 25% have seizures, and 80% have speech impairment.

Etiology—Cerebral palsy is probably caused by conditions that resulted in a lack of oxygen to the brain, hemorrhage, infection, or trauma. Prenatal conditions that may be associated with cerebral palsy include rubella (German measles), toxemia, maternal diabetes, and malnutrition. There is a higher incidence in low birth weight and premature infants. Maternal smoking and alcohol are risk factors.

Treatment—There is no cure for cerebral palsy, only supportive treatment including physical, occupational, and speech therapy; psychologic assistance; braces or splints; perhaps orthopedic surgery for severe contractures; muscle relaxers; and, when indicated, barbiturates and anticonvulsants to control seizures.

Encephalitis (En-sef-a-li′tis)

Description—This is a severe brain inflammation that causes edema and nerve cell destruction. The onset is sudden and acute.

Signs and symptoms—Symptoms include fever, headache, and vomiting with progression to stiff neck and back, drowsiness, and eventually restlessness, convulsions, and coma.

Etiology—It is usually caused by a virus-bearing mosquito or tick. It can also be contracted from viruses that cause chickenpox, herpes, or mumps or following measles, rubella, or mononucleosis.

Treatment—The disease is treatable with supportive drug therapy to control restlessness and convulsions, reduce edema, and relieve headache. Antiviral agents are ineffective except against herpes virus encephalitis.

Epilepsy (Ep′-i-lep-se)

Description—This seizure disorder affects 1% to 2% of the population. It is associated with abnormal electrical impulses from the neurons of the brain.

Signs and symptoms—The disorder is characterized by either petit or grand mal seizures. Petit mal seizures are of short duration and mild. Grand mal seizures may last up to 5 minutes with convulsions, loss of control of bodily functions, and unconsciousness.

Diagnosis is made based on evidence of seizure characteristics, a positive EEG, and various X-ray procedures.

Etiology—It may be caused by either abnormal brain chemistry or several other possibilities, including prematurity, anoxia (lack of oxygen), meningitis, encephalitis, ingestion of toxins (mercury, lead, carbon monoxide), certain medications, brain tumor, PKU, head injury, or stroke.

Treatment—Treatment consists of drug therapy to control the seizures and psychological support.

Essential Tremor

Description—This is the most common movement disorder: an involuntary shaking of the hands and head, which is made worse by action or movement. It affects between 3 and 4 million people in the United States, usually beginning in the 30s or 40s with mild symptoms that may become troublesome by the 50s. This common and benign condition is often confused with Parkinson's disease even though symptoms differ.

Signs and symptoms—Initially, mild shaking is noticed when trying to hold silverware to eat, thread a needle, drink from a glass, or perform writing tasks. The hands shake when trying to make movements, and the head may move in a yes-yes or no-no motion. The voice may also become shaky. Symptoms may worsen, but can be partially controlled with medication. With Parkinson's disease, the hands shake at rest, and head motions are very infrequent. Also, writing with essential tremor results in large and scrawled letters, whereas Parkinson's causes progressively smaller and shakier handwriting within a piece of correspondence.

Etiology—The cause is unknown, but it is generally accepted to be a disorder of the nervous system. It is usually inherited, and each child of a person with essential tremor has a 50% chance of developing the disorder.

Treatment—The disorder can be treated with the beta-blocker propranolol (Inderal) or an antiseizure medication such as primidone (Mysoline). These can be taken daily or may be used only on occasions such as dining out. The severity of tremors is reduced about 60% by the drugs. Other antiseizure drugs and tranquilizers can also be tried. If the tremors become severe, a device can be implanted in the brain that delivers a mild electrical stimulation to block the signals causing the tremor. An unusual treatment may be the therapeutic use of alcoholic beverages. Essential tremor is usually relieved by alcohol and in fact alcohol can be used as a low-tech way to rule out other causes of tremor. Some doctors hesitate to recommend alcohol as a treatment because of the potential for abuse, but with no history of alcoholism, liver, or kidney disease, one to two drinks a day can relieve the tremor.

Headache

Headaches are commonly classified as vascular, muscle contraction (tension), or traction-inflammatory. Both muscle contraction and traction-inflammatory types cause dull, persistent aching and a feeling of a tight band around the head, with tender spots on the head or neck. Most chronic headaches result from tension that may be caused by emotional stress, fatigue, or environmental conditions. Other causes include inflammation of the sinuses, diseased teeth, and muscle spasms of the neck and shoulder.

Vasodilators, such as nitrates, alcohol, and histamine, expand arteries, causing pressure against the brain's nerve endings, and may be causative factors of headaches. Some people are sensitive to anything aged or fermented, such as cured or processed meats and wine, especially red wine. Other foods or additives cause headaches by the vasoconstricting action of amines in such things as MSG, chocolate, and aspartame. A condition known as hypoglycemia (low blood sugar) can result in vasodilation and headaches but can be avoided by eating more frequent, smaller meals a day.

Headache—Migraine (Mi′-grayn)

Description—This is a severe throbbing vascular headache that occurs frequently within families. About 16 to 18 million Americans suffer from **migraines**; approximately 75% are women. Although less common, children as young as two years old can have migraines.

Signs and symptoms—Migraines are frequently characterized by prodromal (beginning) symptoms, which may include fatigue, visual disturbances (such as zigzag lines and bright lights), sensory symptoms (such as tingling of the face and lips), and sometimes motor symptoms like staggering. This is referred to as an aura. Usually the extreme pain is accompanied by sensitivity to light, nausea, and vomiting. Symtoms are usually on one side of the head, can occur suddenly, and will last from a few hours to a few days.

Etiology—The headache is caused by the initial constriction and then dilation of the blood vessels in the brain. There are "triggers" that seem to initiate migraines that must be avoided if possible. They include chocolate, red wine, bright light, and sleeping late.

Treatment—Migraine incidence and severity can be decreased by diet and exercise. Medication can also reduce frequency and intensity. Some medications are preventive, some abortive, and some "rescue." Preventive medications are taken daily and may include beta blockers such as propranolol (Inderal) or timolol (Blocadren) or neuronal stabilizing agents such as divalproex (Depakote) or topiramate (Topamax). Many other categories of medications may help various migraine sufferers including tricyclic antidepressants, antihypertensives, antihistamines, muscle relaxants, and even Botox injections. There are additional herbals and minerals such as Coenzyme Q, B2, and magnesium.

Abortive migraine medications attempt to limit the severity and duration of an attack and may include the triptans (Imitrex, Maxalt, Zomig, or Relpax), ergotamines (nasal spray or injection), or other compounds like Midrin.

Rescue medications are for when the abortives fail. They include pain medications, anti-nauseants, and muscle relaxants.

When an attack occurs, some people benefit from lying quietly in a darkened room with an ice bag to the head and a wet cloth over the eyes and forehead. Usually, it is just a matter of waiting out the episode.

When headaches are frequent, unusual (such as causing awakening in the middle of the night), persistent, or become increasingly more intense, medical attention should be sought. It is important to rule out the presence of pathology such as an aneurysm, abscess, intercranial bleeding, or tumor.

Herpes Zoster (Her′-pez Zos′-ter) (Shingles)

Description—This is an acute usually unilateral inflammation of the dorsal root ganglion (see Chapter 26).

Signs and symptoms—It is characterized by fluid-filled vesicle lesions on the skin and severe pain from the affected nerve. The onset is characterized by fever and discomfort followed by severe deep pain, itching, and abnormal skin sensations. The vesicles erupt in about two weeks, spreading around the **thorax** or vertically on the extremities or even involving the cranial nerves. The episode may last from 1 to 4 weeks.

Etiology—Shingles is caused by the same herpes virus that causes chickenpox. The virus has reactivated after lying dormant in the ganglion since a previous episode of chickenpox. Why this occurs is not clear; however, it may follow trauma, malignancy, and local radiation and is common in individuals with diabetes. Occasionally, there is no known factor.

Treatment—Treatment consists of medication, sometimes even narcotics, to relieve the pain and itching, plus an antiviral to reduce the length of viral shedding and steroids to minimize post-herpetic neuralgia.

There is a vaccine for herpes zoster, Zostavax. It is recommended for individuals over age 60 or those who may be immunologically compromised, e.g., chemotherapy patients.

Hydrocephalus (Hi-dro-sef′-a-lus)

Description—This excessive accumulation of CSF within the ventricles of the brain occurs most frequently in newborns. The increased fluid compresses the brain tissue against the skull, which can result in brain damage unless treated soon after birth.

Signs and symptoms—Hydrocephalus is characterized by an abnormally enlarged head; distended scalp veins; fragile, shiny scalp skin; a high-pitched, shrill cry; irritability; and vomiting.

Etiology—Hydrocephalus results from either the overproduction of CSF or the lack of its absorption. Either results in excessive fluid and the enlargement of the brain. Because the newborn skull is not completely hardened, it expands to accommodate the extra fluid, resulting in the characteristic appearance.

Treatment—Surgery is the only treatment for hydrocephalus. A shunt (passageway) is inserted into a ventricle in the brain to drain off excess fluid into either the peritoneal cavity of the abdomen or the atrium (upper chamber) of the heart for absorption by the body (Figure 24–14A). The ventriculoperitoneal (VP) shunt is the most common (Figure 24–14B).

Meningitis (Men-in-ji′-tis)

Description—This is an inflammation of the meninges of the brain and spinal cord. It may be viral or bacterial. Mortality is 70% to 100% if bacterial meningitis is left untreated. Viral meningitis is a much more benign disease.

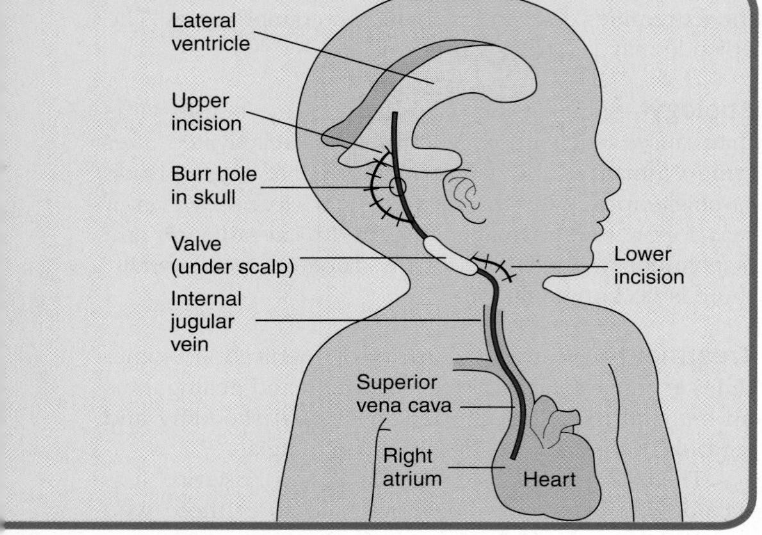

Figure 24–14A: The ventriculoatrial shunt drains spinal fluid into the circulation in the heart. *Delmar/Cengage Learning.*

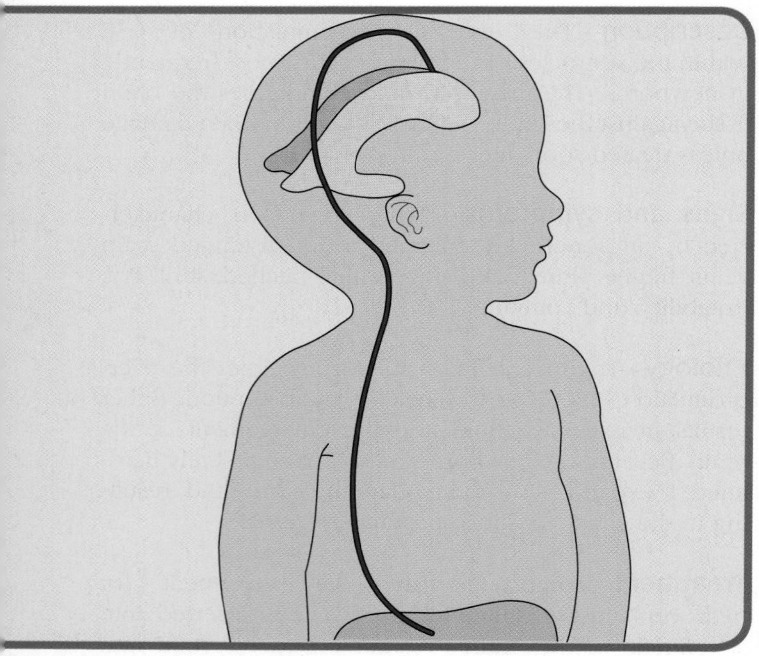

Figure 24–14B: The ventriculoperitoneal (VP) shunt drains spinal fluid into the peritoneum. *Delmar/Cengage Learning.*

Signs and symptoms—Meningitis is characterized by a high fever, chills, headache, vomiting, and specifically by positive Brudzinski's and Kernig's signs (Figure 24–15) in adults. Brudzinski's sign is demonstrated by the flexing of the hips and knees when the head and neck of a dorsal recumbent person are raised and pulled forward. Kernig's sign is demonstrated by pain and resistance when the knee is straightened after flexing at the thigh and knee.

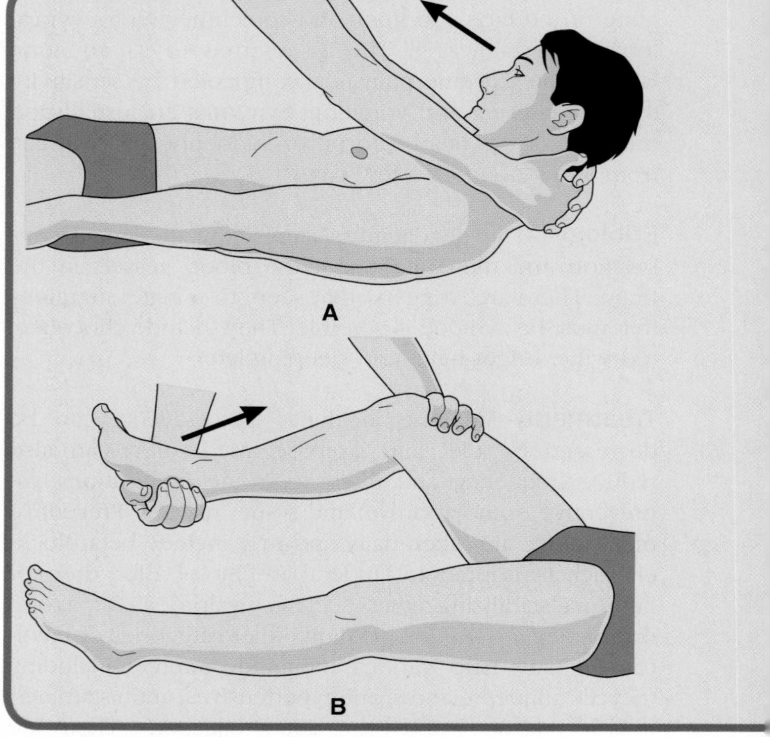

Figure 24–15: Two telltale signs of meningitis in adults: (A) Brudzinski's sign; (B) Kernig's sign. *Delmar/Cengage Learning.*

Diagnosis of meningitis is confirmed by a lumbar puncture that shows elevated pressure, cloudiness from the excess white cells, and identification of the causative organism after culturing.

Etiology—Meningitis is usually caused by a bacterial infection from the ears, sinuses, or lungs (pneumonia) or an abscess of the brain. Aseptic meningitis may result from a virus or other microorganism. At times, the cause is unknown.

Treatment—Treatment consists of antibiotics if bacterial, medication to reduce cerebral edema, pain relievers for headache, and an anticonvulsant. Isolation may be indicated in certain instances of bacterial meningitis.

AGE-RELATED BODY CHARACTERISTICS

Infants less than 12 months of age who develop *bacterial* meningitis have typical signs and symptoms of fever, irritability, change in feeding patterns, lethargy, vomiting, high pitched cry, seizures, and purpura (a purple rash). An older child may exhibit severe headache, stiff neck, and photophobia (light sensitivity).

Young children with *viral* meningitis may have similar symptoms but it is rare to see purpura. Accurate diagnosis requires a lumbar puncture to determine the type.

Young adults are at increased risk of meningitis from age 13 to age 25. There is a vaccine available to prevent one type of bacterial meningitis.

Multiple Sclerosis (MS) (Skle-ro′sis)

Description—This is a demyelinating disease of the nervous system that attacks young men and women in the prime of life. It affects the central nervous system and is usually first diagnosed between the ages of 20 and 40. It is estimated that 500,000 Americans have MS or a related disorder. It causes a heavy economic burden on affected families because a great many people with MS are unable to work.

Signs and symptoms—The symptoms depend upon the site of nerve damage but may include paralysis, numbness, double vision, foot dragging, loss of balance, extreme weakness, hand tremors, speech and hearing difficulties, bladder and bowel problems, and "pins and needles" sensations. Multiple sclerosis patients may go into remission after just one episode, but most patients have a history of remissions and exacerbations with eventual progressive worsening.

Etiology—The disease attacks the myelin sheaths of the nerves, destroying patches that are replaced by scar tissue that distorts or interrupts the passage of nerve impulses. Much of the current research is based upon the idea that the disease is probably the result of a reactivated, dormant, slow-acting virus; an autoimmune response; or both. There is evidence that environmental factors play a role, but genetic factors may also determine a predisposition to MS.

Treatment—Treatment for an acute exacerbation (increase in severity) may include IV ACTH (adrenocorticotropic hormone), however, many new medications have entered the market to decrease the frequency of exacerbations and relapses. The new drugs include interferons, e.g., Avonex, Biogen, and Betaseron, and anti-cancer chemotherapy drugs such as azathioprine and Cytoxan. Drugs to help with emotional swings and muscular spasticity are used as required. Prevention of fatigue is important during acute phases.

The use of physical and occupational therapy is helpful. They optimize strength, help relieve some of the stiffness in the muscles, enhance balance and endurance, and help with functional adaptation in the home and workplace.

Neuralgia (Nu-ral′-je-ah)

Description—This is a term used to describe general nerve pain. It is further classified in relation to the area of the body that is affected.

Signs and symptoms—Neuralgia causes severe pain along the course of the involved nerve or nerves.

Etiology—This results from pressure on nerve trunks, faulty nerve nutrition, toxins, inflammation of the nerve, or changes in the root ganglia.

Treatment—Medications, the use of heat, physical therapy, rest, or stretching, depending upon the nerve involved, help relieve the pain.

Paralysis

Paralysis is a term used to describe the temporary or permanent loss of voluntary function in a portion of the body. Any voluntary movement depends on the integrity of the motor neurons—the upper motor neurons in the brain, the lower motor neurons in the spinal cord, and those axons passing to the muscle. Paralyses are divided into two general groups: spastic, if caused by upper motor neurons, and flaccid, if caused by lower motor neurons. There are many forms of paralysis, but for the purpose of this unit, the term is being used to identify the condition following an injury or destruction of nerve tissue in the brain or spinal cord. Three general classifications will be discussed: hemiplegia, paraplegia, and quadriplegia. *Caution:* It is extremely important to prevent damage to the brain and spinal cord. The possibility of a stroke, which damages the brain, can be reduced with proper exercise, healthy blood pressure and cholesterol, refraining from smoking, and the reduction in stress. Injury can be prevented with proper instruction, applying safety principles, the use of protective gear, not driving after drinking, and using seat belts. Unfortunately, once damage has occurred, it is usually irreversible. Spinal cord damage and head injuries are devastating and change one's life *forever.*

Hemiplegia (Hem-e-ple′je-ah)

Description—Hemiplegia is unilateral (one-sided) paralysis that follows damage to the brain. Because nerves cross in the brainstem, damage to the right side of the brain causes left-sided paralysis, whereas damage to the left side causes right-sided paralysis.

Signs and symptoms—Hemiplegia may involve weakness or paralysis of the arm, leg, face, and tongue. It may be sudden, if caused by a stroke or injury, or gradual, if caused by a tumor or disease. The paralysis begins as flaccid but often progresses to spastic. Hemiplegics often have difficulty understanding oral or written language, may develop muscle shortening and foot drop, have a decreased level of consciousness, and may experience problems eating.

Etiology—Hemiplegia is caused by any injury to the brain or one side of the spinal cord, such as cerebrovascular accident (CVA or stroke), a tumor, CNS infection, a degenerative disease, or trauma (see CVA, Unit 8). If the damage is less severe, weakness instead of paralysis may result.

Treatment—Early treatment involves preventing further involvement and lessening the effects of the damage, which varies with the cause. Later treatment focuses on prevention of complications such as muscle contractions, foot drop, and spastic muscular movements. The use of physical, occupational, and speech therapy; orthopedic devices; and modifications in the surroundings are important to rehabilitation and promoting independence (Figure 24–16). At age 44, the man in Figure 24–16 suffered a near-fatal rupture of a cerebral aneurysm, which severely damaged the left side of his brain. Initially he was not expected to survive, but with time he regained some physical functions. He was unable to stand. With therapy he managed to go from a wheelchair to a walker and then to a cane. Now six years later, he can walk alone and wears only a small brace on his right ankle. He has lost most of the use of his right hand.

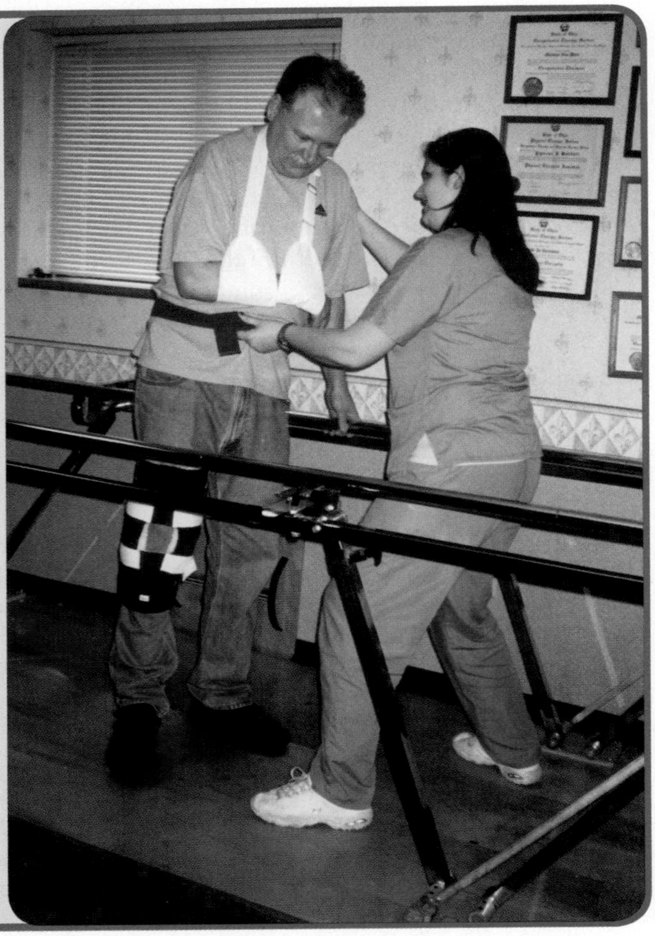

Figure 24–16: Physical therapy can be helpful for the hemiplegic patient following a stroke on the left side of his brain that affected the right side of the body. *Courtesy of Barbara A. Wise.*

Paraplegia (Par-a-ple′-je-ah)

Description—This is the loss of motor or sensory function in the lower extremities, usually from trauma, with or without involvement of the abdominal and back muscles. The paralysis may be permanent or temporary, spastic or flaccid. Almost half of the 10,000 to 12,000 spinal cord injuries each year result in paraplegia. It occurs twice as often in males as in females, with the highest incidence between the ages of 16 and 35.

Signs and symptoms—The onset of total or partial paralysis is immediate in most patients, with the loss of motion, sensation, and reflexes below the level of damage. With complete spinal cord injury, there is lack of sensation or voluntary muscle control that persists for 24 hours; any return of functional muscle activity below the injury is unlikely. There is usually loss of bladder, bowel, and sexual function. With incomplete damage, the patient can still sense the perianal area, flex the toes, and control the bladder and bowels.

Etiology—Paraplegia usually results from trauma that occurs with automobile, motorcycle, and sporting accidents; gunshot wounds; and falls. Conditions such as spina bifida and cerebral palsy may also cause paralysis.

Treatment—It is important that treatment starts at the time of the accident. The patient must be strapped on a board before any movement occurs to prevent additional spinal cord injury. The spine must be realigned and any fractures reduced. Compression of the cord and nerves must be relieved. Surgery may be required to repair fracture dislocations and remove bone fragments. A urinary catheter is installed to drain urine. Extensive care to maintain the skin, monitor fluids, and promote good nutrition and medications to prevent infection and control muscle spasms are required. Rehabilitation to promote as much activity as is possible begins early. Psychological support is very important. The final extent of paralysis cannot be accurately evaluated until at least two years following the injury.

Quadriplegia (Quah-drih-plee′-je-ah)

Description—The devastating permanent paralysis affecting all body systems, the arms, the legs, and all of the body below the level of the injury to the spinal cord. The injury is usually the result of a trauma. It affects about 150,000 Americans, most being men between the ages of 20 and 40.

Signs and symptoms—Quadriplegia is evidenced by the flaccid or spastic appearance of the arms and legs and the loss of sensation and movement below the level of the injury. If the cord is damaged above the fifth cervical vertebrae of the neck, body systems also will be dramatically affected. This type of injury would produce symptoms such as:

- Low blood pressure from the blocking of the sympathetic nervous system
- Low body temperature caused by dilated surface blood vessels, which allows heat to escape
- Slow heart rate caused by absence of sympathetic system inhibiting action
- Respiratory system involvement, which may require mechanical support

Etiology—Paralysis results from spinal cord injury in the cervical vertebrae. It is usually the result of automobile, motorcycle, or sporting activities accidents; gunshot wounds; or falls. Diving and gymnastics are common causes. The dangers of horseback riding became apparent in 1995 with the extensive injury to the late actor Christopher Reeve, which in a few seconds changed his life forever.

Treatment—Again, treatment begins at the scene of the accident with immobilization of the neck and spine. Following hospitalization, tongs or a halo traction are attached to the skull to pull the neck into alignment and stabilize the spine. Treatment is aimed at reducing the edema (swelling) of the spinal cord, thereby relieving pressure on the spinal nerves. An artificial airway will be required if injury is above the 5th vertebra, and ventilation assistance will be necessary. After about 10 days, surgery is done to fuse vertebrae and remove any fragments. Unfortunately, many functional problems will occur. Some of the more common are:

- Maintaining open airway and adequate respiration
- Providing adequate fluids and nutrition
- Excessively slow heart rate and resulting low blood pressure
- Low body temperature, perhaps to less than 90°F, which will require warming with blankets
- Extremely high blood pressure, which may lead to heart failure and intracranial bleeding when injury is above the 4th vertebra

The greatest challenge comes from the enormous change in the individual's life. If there is an artificial airway, the patient may not be able to even speak. Paralysis requires extensive emotional, physical, and social support, not only for the affected individual but also for the entire family and circle of friends.

Extensive research continues to find ways of restoring function to damaged nerves. A great deal of discussion regarding the possibilities of stem cell applications is giving these individuals some glimmer of hope.

Parkinson's Disease

Description—This is a common progressive, sometimes crippling disease affecting about one in every 100 people over age 50, which translates to about 60,000 new cases annually in the United States. It affects men more often than women. It may progress for about 10 years until pneumonia or another infection results in death.

Signs and symptoms—The main symptoms are muscle rigidity and tremor of the hand, described as "pill-rolling." The disease produces a high-pitched, monotone voice and a masklike expression. As it progresses, the condition is characterized by severe muscle rigidity, a peculiar gait, drooling, and a progressive tremor. The body becomes bent forward, with head bowed. The steps become faster and faster with increasing forward body inclination, which often results in falling.

Etiology—The cause of Parkinson's disease is unknown; however, it has been established that a deficiency in dopamine prevents affected brain cells from functioning properly. Some researchers have noted some forms may be caused by a viral infection experienced many years earlier.

Treatment—There is no known cure for the disease, although a drug called levodopa relieves most of the symptoms until the necessarily increased dosage begins to cause serious side effects. In selected patients, surgical procedures can either freeze, electrically coagulate, or radioactively destroy a small area of the brain to prevent the involuntary motions.

Surgical options are appropriate only for those in good health, who are relatively young (under age 70), no longer able to tolerate medication, and have specific symptoms. A thalamotomy, which destroys a specific group of cells in the thalamus, is appropriate for 5% to 10% of patients with severe tremor of the hand and arm. It results in immediate improvement in 80% to 90% of the patients. A pallidotomy destroys a specific group of cells within the globus pallidus (movement center of the brain). It is used for patients with slow movement, tremor, imbalance, and drug side effects. The results are about the same as with thalamotomy. *Note:* The surgery will not cure the disease; it only relieves the symptoms and decreases need for medication. The disease will progress.

Again, a well-known person is giving urgency to research into treatment and a cure for this debilitating disease. Popular actor Michael J. Fox was diagnosed with Parkinson's disease in 1991, many years before he reached the "average age" of incidence. The involvement of well-known people like the late Christopher Reeve and Michael J. Fox in forming foundations for research and education into these tragic conditions is having a very positive impact on the urgency for answers and treatments.

Reye's Syndrome

Description—This acute childhood illness is characterized by fatty infiltration of the liver and increased intracranial pressure (ICP). Further damage from fat infiltration occurs in the kidneys and possibly the muscle of the heart. The **syndrome** (group of symptoms) affects children from infancy to adolescence, occurring equally in males and females, but affects whites more than blacks. It is rare, affecting about one in a million.

The syndrome prognosis depends on the degree of CNS depression from ICP. At one time, mortality was 90%; now with early treatment and ICP monitoring, the rate has been reduced to 20%. Death usually results from cerebral swelling, respiratory arrest, or coma.

Signs and symptoms—The symptoms occur in stages of severity, beginning with vomiting, lethargy, and liver dysfunction and then progressing to hyperventilation, delirium, hyperactive reflexes, and coma. The condition worsens as symptoms of rigidity; deepening coma; large, fixed pupils; seizures; and eventual respiratory arrest occur.

Etiology—Reye's syndrome almost always follows within one to three days of an acute viral infection, such as upper respiratory infection, type B influenza, or chickenpox. A correlation was found between the use of aspirin in children and the development of Reyes. Since aspirin is now contraindicated in the treatment of children with infections, the incidence of Reye's has nearly disappeared.

Treatment—Proper treatment is essential. With increased ICP, the prime concern is to reduce the pressure and brain edema to prevent damage. Aggressive action involves medications to reduce body fluid, prevent seizures, and maintain appropriate levels of vitamin K and glucose. If the condition worsens, the ICP is monitored, and mechanical ventilation may be necessary. As a final effort, coma may be induced with barbiturates, dialysis may be used to extract fluids and built-up elements, and a section of skull may be removed to relieve brain compression.

Sciatica (Si-at′-i-ka)

Description—**Sciatica** is a generic term for neuritic leg pain along the sciatic nerve. It is usually unilateral and is more common in males and in middle age.

Signs and symptoms—A sharp, shooting pain that may begin gradually or abruptly and runs down the back of the thigh and into the lower leg. It may seem to originate deep within the buttocks. It is often intensified with movement. The pain may become worse at night or when the atmosphere changes with the approach of a storm. It may be difficult to achieve comfort while sitting or standing.

Etiology—The nerve roots that comprise the sciatic nerve may have been injured or irritated by impingement by spinal arthritis or a herniated disk. The nerve may become damaged by accidental stretching during strenuous activities or pelvic tumors or scarring.

Treatment—Activities causing discomfort will need to be curtailed temporarily. Treatment consists of trying to maintain activities as tolerated, heat or cold applications, medication for pain and/or inflammations; and sometimes the use of traction. Often, the use of specific stretching exercises, begun gently, will gradually solve the problem. The discomfort may persist for an extended period of time. Most cases improve with time and conservative care. Some cases may become chronic and cause atrophy (wasting away) of the affected muscles, although that is unusual. Surgery may be indicated in severe cases that do not respond to conservative measures.

Spinal Cord Defects

Description—Spinal cord defects result from failure of tissues to properly close during the first three months of pregnancy. They occur most frequently in the lumbosacral area.

The incidence is approximately 5% of live births or about 100,000 infants per year.

Signs and symptoms—**Spina bifida occulta** (spi′-na bif′-i-da oc-cult′-ah) is the most common type of the defects. It is characterized by the incomplete closure of one or more vertebra but without protrusion of the spinal cord or meninges (Figure 24–17A). It is usually asymptomatic and is an incidental finding on an X-ray. There may be a depression, a tuft of hair, a port wine nevus, or a combination of these signs over the lower back. In spina bifida with meningocele (men-in′-go-sel), (Figure 24–17B) a protruding sac contains meninges and CFS. With myelomeningocele (mie-lo-men-in′-go-sel), the meninges, CFS, and a portion of the spinal cord or distal nerve roots are within the sac (Figure 24–17C). The defects usually occur in the lumbosacral area but are occasionally found in the thoracic and cervical areas. Neurologic symptoms of myelomeningocele range from minimal weakness of the feet and some bladder and bowel problems to permanent neurologic dysfunction, such as paralysis, inability to control the bladder and bowels, hydrocephalus, clubfoot, and sometimes mental retardation.

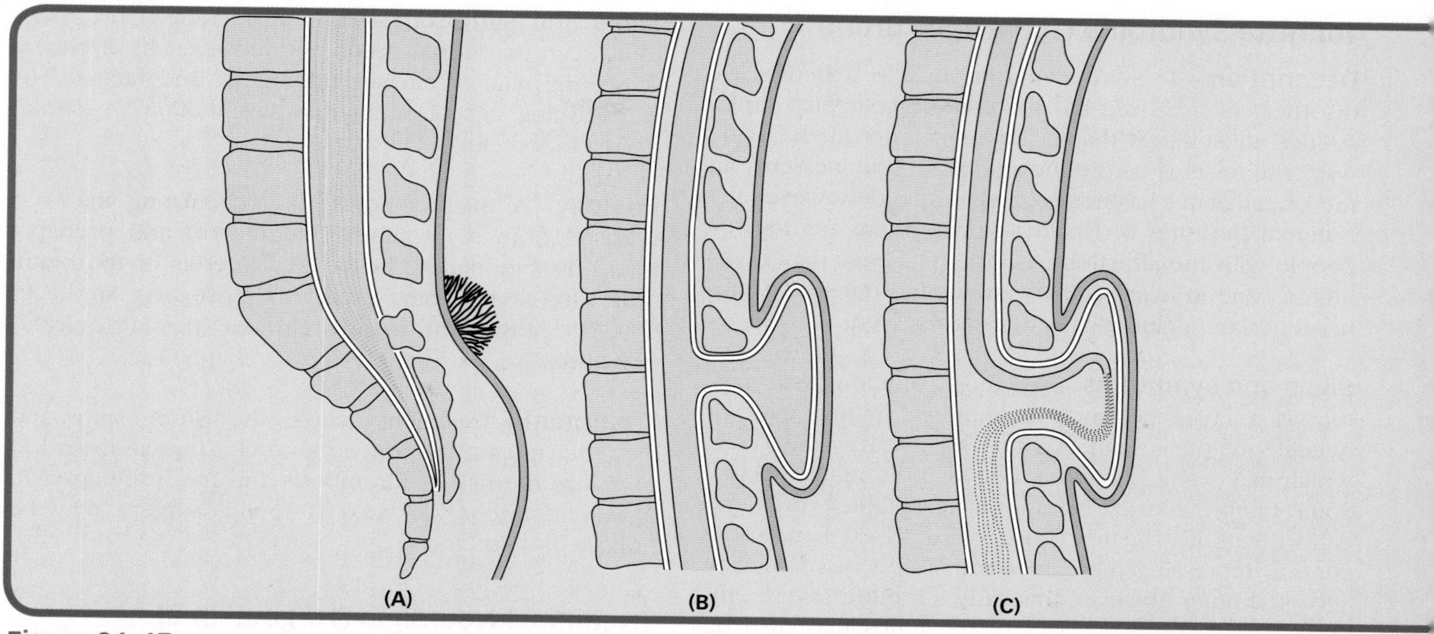

Figure 24–17: Spinal cord defects: (A) spina bifida occulta, (B) meningocele, (C) myelomeningocele. *Delmar/Cengage Learning.*

Etiology—A congenital defect caused by the failure of the neural tube of the embryo, which becomes the brain and spinal cord, to close properly. The neural tube usually closes by the 23rd day of gestation. Research found that folic acid deficiency was a major factor in neural tube defects. All prenatal vitamins now include large amounts of folic acid, and all pregnant women should be encouraged to take adequate folate as early in pregnancy as possible. Viruses, radiation, the environment, and genetic factors may also be responsible for neural tube defects.

Treatment—Treatment and prognosis depend on the extent of the defect. Spina bifida occulta usually requires no treatment. If CSF and meninges are involved, surgical closure is required to prevent further injury. Unfortunately, the neurologic conditions with myelomeningocele cannot be reversed. If hydrocephalus is also present, a shunt will be implanted to relieve the fluid pressure. Supportive measures to promote independence may involve leg braces, crutches, walkers, and wheelchairs. *Note:* With paralysis and spinal cord defects, there are bladder and bowel concerns.

Subarachnoid Hemorrhage (Sub-a-rak′-noyd)

Description—This is a collection of blood in the subarachnoid space, usually caused by the spontaneous rupture of a weakened blood vessel.

Signs and symptoms—The patient may complain of a sudden, severe headache and experience nausea and projectile vomiting. This may be accompanied by motor disturbances, seizures, and deviations in sensory perception, particularly in vision.

Etiology—Precipitating factors include hypertension, oral contraceptives, malformations of cranial blood vessels, trauma, and family history.

Treatment—Treatment varies with the causative factor. With hypertension, efforts would be made to lower the blood pressure. If contraceptives are suspected, they would be discontinued.

Subdural Hematoma (Sub-dur′-al He-ma-to′-ma)

Description—This is a collection of blood within the subdural space. It is usually a slow process in which the gradually accumulating blood causes progressive symptoms.

Signs and symptoms—There are disturbances in motor activities and a progressive facial weakness on the side opposite the hematoma. With progression, there may be seizures and a decreased level of consciousness. Because the blood accumulates slowly, symptoms may not occur until days after the injury.

Etiology—Hematoma results from blood leaking into the subdural space as the consequence of a head injury.

Treatment—Surgical intervention is indicated to remove the pressure on the brain tissues caused by the hematoma when symptoms and intracranial pressure reach a significant level.

Tourette Syndrome (Tur′-et)(Sin′drom)

Description—Tourette syndrome (TS) is a neurologic disorder characterized by "tics"—the involuntary, rapid, sudden movements that occur repeatedly in the same way. The onset is before the age of 21. The incidence in the United States has not been determined; however, the National Institutes of Health estimate there are 100,000 people with the affliction, and the incidence may be as high as one in every 200 if chronic and transient childhood tics are included. Most tics are benign.

Signs and symptoms—The most common first symptom is a facial tic, such as rapidly blinking eyes or twitches of the mouth. Another tic involves the voice, which may result in barking noises and tongue clicking. Some people vocalize socially unacceptable words and echo things just heard. People with TS do have some control, repressing the symptoms until a more socially accepted time; however, this causes a more severe outburst when expressed. Tics of the limbs may also be an initial sign. Motor tics may cause jumping, touching other people or things, twirling about, and self-injurious actions such as hitting or biting oneself. There is no diagnostic test to confirm TS; only history and observation can be used to diagnose.

Etiology—The cause of TS has not been definitely identified. There is evidence that it is caused by the abnormal metabolism of at least one brain chemical called dopamine. Others are suspected. Genetic studies show that TS is from an inherited dominant gene that can produce different symptoms in different family members.

Treatment—Most persons are not sufficiently affected to require treatment. There are medications to control the outbursts when necessary. The dosage must be determined individually. Psychotherapy can assist persons and their family to cope with the strange condition. Relaxation techniques and biofeedback help reduce stress that causes tics to increase. Affected people may be ridiculed and rejected. Children can be excluded from school activities and experience difficulty in interpersonal relationships.

Transient Ischemic Attack (Trans′-e-ent Is-ke-mick)

Description—A transient ischemic attack (TIA) is a recurring strokelike event that lasts from a few seconds to hours, then disappears after 12 to 24 hours. It is considered to be a warning sign of impending stroke. The age of onset varies but rises dramatically after age 50. It is highest among blacks and men. TIAs have occurred in 50% to 80% of patients who experience a stroke from a blood vessel blockage.

Signs and symptoms—It is characterized by symptoms such as double vision, slurred speech, dizziness, staggering gait, weakness, numbness, and falling. TIA is a warning sign of impending thrombotic CVA (stroke from a blood clot).

Etiology—A microembolus (tiny circulating mass) is released from a thrombus (blood clot) and probably interrupts blood flow in the tiny arteries of the brain. This causes symptoms similar to those of a stroke to develop; however, they are transient (passing quickly) in nature.

Treatment—Treatment includes the use of aspirin and an anticoagulant to reduce blood clot formation and to minimize the risk of thrombosis and the resulting CVA. If carotid artery blockage is found, surgery may be indicated.

Trigeminal Neuralgia (Tri-gem′-in-al Nu-ral′-je-ah) (Tic Douloureux) (tick dol-o-roo′)

Description—This is a disorder of the 5th cranial nerve, usually on one side of the face.

Signs and symptoms—It produces episodes of excruciating facial pain. It frequently follows exposure to heat or cold, a draft from air, smiling, or drinking hot or cold liquids. The episodes may last from 1 to 15 minutes, recurring from several times daily to a few times a year. Persons with the disorder live in fear of the next attack. It occurs mostly in people over the age of 40, in women more than men, and more frequently on the right side of the face.

Etiology—The exact cause is still under investigation. However, such things as compression on nerves by tumors, an aneurysm, and an afferent reflex condition can cause it. Occasionally, it is associated with multiple sclerosis or herpes zoster. The pain is probably the result of an interaction or short-circuiting of touch and pain fibers.

Treatment—Treatment consists of oral medication or the injection of alcohol or phenol into the nerve branch. With frequent, severe attacks, a surgical procedure is indicated that severs the nerve, thereby relieving the pain but also resulting in loss of sensation to the innervated area. Care must be taken afterward to protect the affected eye, avoid burns from hot food, guard against dental decay, and avoid biting the inner cheek and lip.

Tumor

Description—Tumors can occur anywhere in the body. However, those in the brain that are malignant are especially difficult to treat. There are several types with differing age and sex preferences, but almost all limit life from six months to six years following diagnosis. They are slightly more common in men than women, with an incidence of 4.5 per 100,000 people. They are most prevalent between the ages of 40 and 60 in adults and between 2 and 12 in children. They are one of the most common causes of death from cancer in children.

Signs and symptoms—Tumors cause changes in the CNS because of the destruction of tissue; the compression of the brain, cranial nerves, and blood vessels; cerebral swelling; and increased intracranial pressure. Specific symptoms vary with the type of tumor, its location, and the extent of involvement. Common symptoms are nausea, vomiting, headache, seizures, facial nerve palsies, dizziness, visual and hearing changes, weakness, and many others. The symptoms are usually insidious (slow) and often misdiagnosed.

Etiology—The cause of brain tumors is unknown.

Treatment—A resectable tumor is removed; a nonresectable tumor is debulked if possible. The type of therapy depends upon the cellular structure, its sensitivity to radiation, and its location. Surgery, radiation, chemotherapy, and relief of increased intracranial pressure (ICP) by diuretics or shunting are the usual treatments.

System Interaction Associated with Disease Conditions

The nervous system interacts with all other systems to control the body's functions. Table 24–1 summarizes some of the interaction present in two examples of neurological disorders.

TABLE 24–1 System Interaction Associated with Disease Conditions

Disease	System Involved	Pathology Present
Cerebral Palsy	Sketetal	Body degeneration, loss of bone density due to lack of weight bearing
	Muscular	Muscle wasting from sedentary lifestyle, contractures
	Digestive	Difficulty eating, swallowing
	Integumentary	Pressure ulcers from body weight
Spina Bifida	Skeletal	Loss of bone density
	Muscular	Muscle wasting if paralysis
	Integumentary	Pressure ulcers, skin breakdown if loss of bladder and bowel control

Note: Teenagers may have significant psychosocial difficulties and problems with adjustment due to poor self image with physical disabilities.

CHAPTER SUMMARY

- The nervous system is a communication network. It has two main divisions, the central nervous system (CNS), consisting of the brain and spinal cord, and the peripheral nervous system (PNS), consisting of all the nerves that connect the CNS to every organ and area of the body.
- There are three types of neurons: motor, sensory, and associative or internuncial neurons.
- Action potential refers to the brief electrical change inside the neuron and is known as membrane excitability.
- A synapse is the minute space between the axon of one neuron and the dendrites of the next neuron across which an impulse must travel. The space is technically the synaptic cleft.
- Various drugs affect the speed of impulse travel and help with treatment of mental, emotional and pain management.
- The peripheral nervous system (PNS) includes 12 pairs of cranial nerves that connect the brain to the sense organs, the heart, the lungs and other internal organs. The PNS also has 31 pairs of spinal nerves which have both sensory and motor as well as mixed nerves.
- A ganglion is the cell body of a sensory spinal nerve.
- The autonomic nervous system (ANS) is part of the peripheral nervous system and is involuntary. The system controls functions such as breathing, heartbeat and digestion.
- The ANS has a sympathetic and a parasympathetic division.
- The brain consists of 100 billion neurons that control the body. It is protected by membranes called meninges. The brain is divided into five parts: the cerebrum, which is made up of the frontal, the occipital, the parietal, temporal lobes; the cerebellum; the brainstem, which consists of the medulla

oblongata; the pons and the midbrain; the thalamus and the hypothalamus.

- The meninges cover both the brain and spinal cord. The meninges consists of the pia mater, the arachnoid, and the dura mater. The spaces between the membrane layers are called the subdural and subarachnoid spaces.
- The brain has connecting cavities known as ventricles. The spinal cord also has a central cavity and connects to the brain. Cerebral spinal fluid circulates within these cavities.
- Diagnostic tests include, arteriograph, CAT or CT scan, EEG, EMG, and MRI.
- The Glasgow Coma Scale is an assessment tool to evaluate neurological status.
- The diseases discussed in the chapter are Alzheimer's, amyotrophic lateral sclerosis, Bell's palsy, cerebral palsy, encephalitis, epilepsy, essential tremor, headache, migraine, herpes zoster, hydrocephalus, meningitis, multiple sclerosis, neuralgia, paralysis, Parkinson's, Reye's syndrome, sciatica, spinal cord defects, subarachnoid hemorrhage, subdural hematoma, Tourette syndrome, transient ischemic attack, trigeminal neuralgia, and tumor.

STUDY TOOLS

Workbook	Activities for Chapter 24
Premium Website	
MEDIA LINK	View this **Media Link** for Chapter 24: • Firing of a Neuron
StudyWARE	Activities and Quizzes on the **StudyWARE™ Software** for Chapter 24
	Audio Library of medical terms
	Online access to the **Critical Thinking Challenge 2.0**
CourseMate	Activities and Quizzes for Chapter 24
WebTutor	Activities and Quizzes for Chapter 24

CHECK YOUR KNOWLEDGE

Select the most appropriate answers to the following multiple choice questions:

1. The space between a neuron dendrite and the next neuron axon is called:
   a. membrane potential.
   b. synapse.
   c. axon terminal.
   d. neurotransmitter.
2. A ganglion is:
   a. a collection of nerve endings.
   b. a type of nerve cell.
   c. part of the gray matter of the spine.
   d. the sensory nerve cell bodies in the posterior root.
3. The autonomic nervous system include all but:
   a. the sympathetic division.
   b. the parasympathetic division.
   c. nerves, ganglia, and plexuses.
   d. motor and sensory nerves.
4. The largest part of the brain is:
   a. the cerebellum.
   b. the cerebrum.
   c. the frontal lobe.
   d. the parietal lobe.
5. The outermost meninges is:
   a. the arachnoid.
   b. the pia mater.
   c. the duramoid.
   d. the dura mater.
6. The cavities and hollow spaces within the brain are called the:
   a. ventricles.
   b. subarachnoid space.
   c. subdural space.
   d. hypothalamus.
7. The electroencephalography:
   a. measures peripheral muscle activity.
   b. shows irregularities of the spinal cord.

c. measures the level of spinal fluid.
d. measures the brain's electrical signals.

8. Alzheimer's disease is characterized by:
   a. gradual memory loss, personality change, inability to care for self.
   b. wasting away of the muscles.
   c. a sudden onset with weakness or paralysis.
   d. involuntary shaking of the hands and head.
9. Multiple sclerosis is the result of:
   a. abnormal brain chemistry, premature birth or brain injury.
   b. acute inflammation of the dorsal root ganglion.
   c. destruction of the myelin sheath of the nerves.
   d. excessive accumulation of cerebral spinal fluid.
10. Parkinson's disease causes:
   a. severe headache, sensitivity to light, and nausea.
   b. permanent muscle contracture and underdevelopment.
   c. muscle rigidity, drooling, and hand tremors.
   d. weakness and paralysis on one side of the face.

WEB LINKS

Disease Conditions in A-Z Topic List: www.emedicinehealth.com

Chapter

25 The Senses

OBJECTIVES

In this chapter, you will learn the following:

KB LEARNING OBJECTIVES

1. Spell and define, using the glossary at the back of the text, all the Words to Know in this chapter.
2. Name the senses of the human body, identifying the corresponding organ(s) responsible for perception.
3. Identify on an anatomical illustration the structures of the eye, ear, nose, tongue, and skin.
4. Trace the path of a visual image from the cornea to the visual center of the brain.
5. Explain the effects of the lens and cornea upon the focusing of images.
6. Trace the path of sound from the entrance of the ear to the auditory center of the brain.
7. Explain the balance function of the inner ear.
8. Describe the anatomy of the olfactory organ, and explain how an odor is perceived.
9. Name the types of contact receptors found in the skin.
10. Describe 17 diseases or disorders of the eye, eight of the ear, three of the nose, and three of the mouth and tongue.
11. Discuss the age-related changes that occur with the senses.
12. Identify the body systems involved in diabetic retinopathy and, Ménière's disease.

WORDS TO KNOW

accommodation
amblyopia
aqueous humor
astigmatism
auditory
cataract
cerumen
choroid
cochlea
conjunctiva
cornea
enucleation
epistaxis
eustachian tube
fovea centralis
glaucoma
hyperopia
incus
insidious
iris
lacrimal
lens
malleus
Ménière's disease
myopia
optic disc
organ of Corti
otitis
otosclerosis
polyps
presbycusis
presbyopia
pupil
receptor
retina
retinopathy
sclera
semicircular canals
sensorineural
stapes
strabismus
tinnitus
tympanic membrane
vitreous humor

THE FIVE SPECIAL SENSES

The human being is able to communicate with the surrounding environment because of a miraculous network of nerves coordinated with the organs of the five special senses, which allow us to see, hear, taste, smell, and touch. Knowledge of the environment requires the cooperation of three factors: the sense organs to perceive, intact cranial nerves to transmit, and a functioning area of the brain to interpret the received stimuli.

A stimulus is anything the body is able to detect by means of its **receptors**. Receptors are the peripheral nerve endings of sensory nerves that respond to stimuli. They are not all alike and do not respond to the same kinds of stimuli. Some respond to environmental chemical energy from ions or molecules that are dissolved in body fluids. These are chemoreceptors and are associated with the sense of taste and smell. Changes in position or pressure or the effects of acceleration create mechanical energy, which is detected by mechanoreceptors. These are associated with touch, hearing, and equilibrium. The detection of energy from light is possible as a result of the photoreceptors in the eyes. Thermoreceptors detect radiant energy from heat and are in the skin or connective tissue.

The stimulus, regardless of its form, is converted into energy. If the stimulus is sufficient enough to cause an action potential in the neuron, the message will travel along the sensory nerve to the brain. The reason messages are interpreted differently (such as being hot, a color, or an odor) is that certain nerves always end up in the same specific part of the brain. In other words, the sensation of heat or pain and the "seeing" of a color actually occurs in the brain, not at the point of stimulus. The ability to distinguish between hot, cold, red, or blue, for example, is the outcome of messages being received in an appropriate section of the brain, undergoing routing, being compared with stored past experiences, and producing the interpretation of the stimulus.

The primary organs of the senses are familiar: the eye and the sense of sight; the ear and the sense of hearing; the tongue and the sense of taste; the nose and the sense of smell; and the skin and the sense of touch. However, these organs cannot perform their functions without the cooperation of the corresponding nerves and the section of the brain.

THE EYE AND THE SENSE OF SIGHT

The structure of the eyeball is frequently compared with that of a camera. The outside of the camera is made of a strong plastic or metal to protect its interior structures. Well-protected, the eye is located within the bony orbital cavity of the skull. For additional protection, the outside of the eye is covered with tough, white fibrous tissue called the **sclera** (Figure 25–1). The sclera helps maintain the shape of the eyeball. Six extraocular or extrinsic (outside) muscles are attached to the sclera and are anchored in the walls of the orbital cavity; these contract or relax as pairs to move the eyeball within its cavity. This permits the eyes to roll up and down, in and out, and in combinations of these directions, thereby permitting a large field of vision without moving the head (Figure 25–2). A seventh muscle, the superior levator palpebrae, does not move the eyeball but is attached to and moves the eyelid. Under the sclera is another covering called the **choroid**. The choroid consists of a collection of blood vessels that form the blood supply to the outer portions of the retina. The retinal vessels supply the inner portion of the retinal tissue.

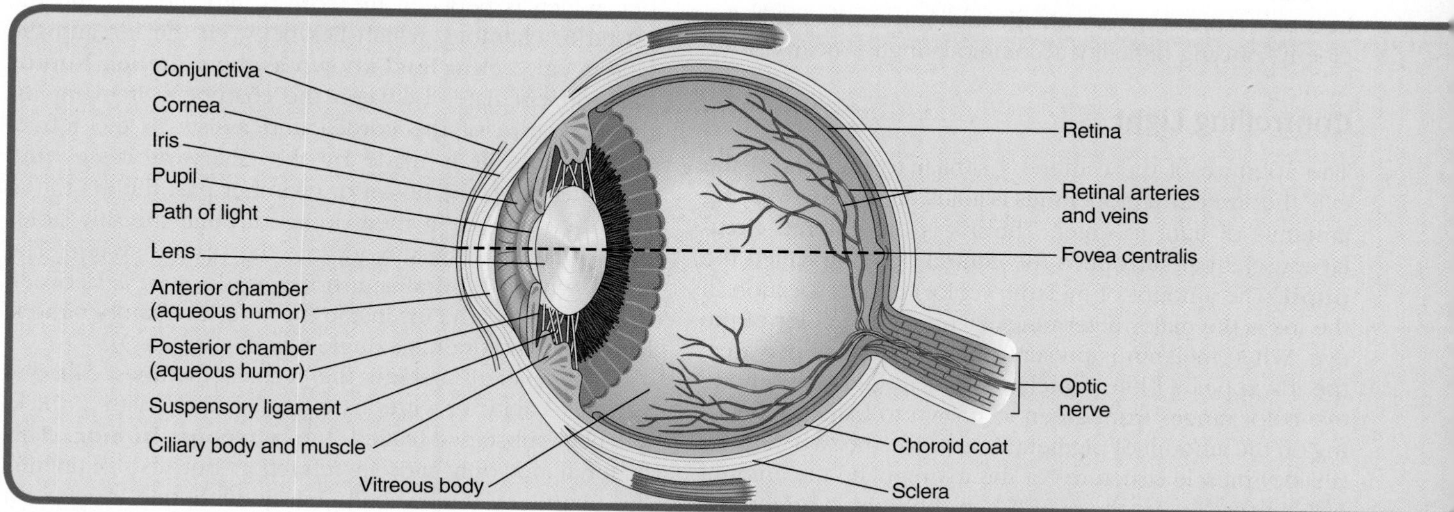

Figure 25–1: Cross-section of the eye. *Delmar/Cengage Learning.*

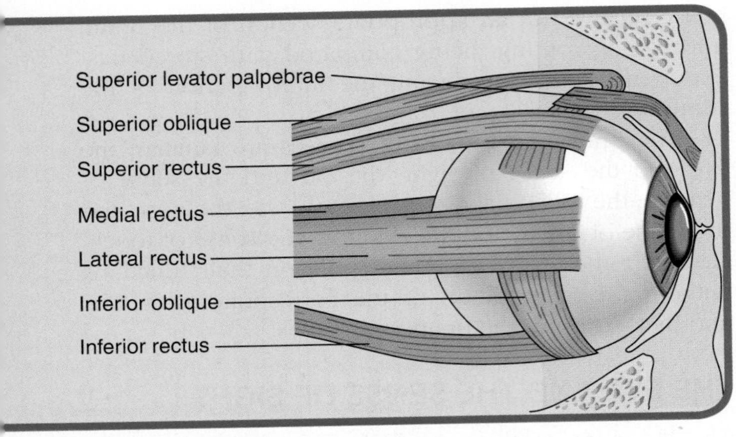

Figure 25–2: Extraocular (extrinsic) muscles of the eye. *Delmar/Cengage Learning.*

MEDIA LINK

Go to the Premium Website and watch the animation, "Vision," for this chapter.

Focusing the Image

Both the eye and the camera have a lens to focus an image onto a surface for "recording." In the camera this surface is the film or the sensors in a digital camera. In the eye it is the **retina**. In the camera, the distance between the film and the camera lens is adjusted to bring the picture into focus before it is recorded on the film. In the eye, the shape of the crystalline **lens** is automatically altered by the actions of the ciliary muscles of the ciliary body to focus objects onto the retina. When the ciliary body contracts, the lens becomes rounder in a process known as **accommodation** to permit near vision. With relaxation, the lens thins out to allow focusing on distant objects. The shape of the lens is convex on both the anterior and posterior surfaces. The shape is quite rounded in childhood but becomes more convex with age until it is nearly flat in the elderly, causing difficulty accommodating for near vision.

Controlling Light

The aperture of the camera is similar to the **iris** of the eye; the size of their openings is adjusted to allow varying amounts of light to enter. The iris is the colored circular muscle that surrounds the central opening called the **pupil**. The amount of melanin (color) and its location in the iris is the major determines factor for the color of the eye. When melanin is present only in the posterior area, the iris appears blue; if melanin is scattered throughout, eye color ranges from green to brown to black, depending on the amount of pigment. In the eye, the two intrinsic (inside) muscle structures of the iris regulate the amount of light that enters the eye. When the light is bright, the circular muscle fibers of the iris contract, reducing the size of the pupil, thereby permitting less light to enter. If it is dark or dimly lit, the pupil will dilate (enlarge) as the radial muscle fibers of the iris contract to pull it outward, permitting more light to enter.

The Cornea

The **cornea** is a transparent extension of the sclera that lies in front of the pupil. This covering has no blood vessels to interfere with vision, so the tissue is nourished by lymph fluid circulating through the cellular spaces. It has both pain and touch receptors, which cause it to be extremely sensitive to any foreign body that touches its surface. If an injury to the cornea results in scarring, vision will be impaired.

The curvature of the cornea "corrects" some of the unclear image that the edge of the lens projects. If the cornea develops an abnormal shape, vision becomes blurred, and the result may be a disorder known as **astigmatism**.

Surface Membranes

A mucous membrane called the **conjunctiva** lines the inner surfaces of the eyelids and covers the anterior sclera surface of the eye. At the margin of the cornea, the conjunctiva merges with the transparent epithelium covering that protects the cornea. The conjunctiva and cornea are lubricated by tiny glands that secrete an oily substance. Further protection for the eye is provided by **lacrimal** glands, which secrete tears to moisten and cleanse the surface of the membrane.

Cavities and Humors

The eyeball is divided into two main areas separated by the lens and its supporting ciliary body structures. The more anterior area is subdivided into the anterior chamber, which is between the cornea and the iris, and the posterior chamber, which lies between the iris and the lens. A salty, clear fluid known as the **aqueous humor** fills and circulates between the chambers. It maintains the curvature of the cornea and assists in the refraction process. It is made by the ciliary processes and circulates from the posterior chamber past the iris to the anterior chamber. It then drains through the tiny holes of the trabecular meshwork into the venous system. The space where the drainage holes are located is between the cornea and the iris inside the anterior chamber and is known as the drainage angle (see Figure 25–9).

The eyeball behind the lens, sometimes called a vitreous cavity or vitreous body, is filled with a thick, jellylike substance called the **vitreous humor**. This material not only aids in refraction but also maintains the shape of the eyeball. Injury with the loss of an appreciable amount of the vitreous may cause damage to the eyeball, which could necessitate surgical removal of the eye by a procedure called **enucleation**.

The Retina

The inside layer of the eyeball is the retina, a multilayered nervous tissue. Specialized nerve cells called rods and cones transmit the stimuli focused on the retinal surface through the optic nerve to the visual center in the brain where the image is "seen." The cones, about 7 million in number, are sensitive to colors and function only in well-lighted environments. Most of them are located in a depression on the posterior surface of the retina called the **fovea centralis**, the area of sharpest vision. There are about 100 million rods in the more peripheral areas of the retina. The rods are very sensitive to light and permit us to see, without color, in dimly lit or nearly dark surroundings.

Optic Disc

Two other types of nerve cells in the retina relay impulses from the rods and cones. The axons of one type form the fibers of the optic nerve. Where the optic nerves exit the retina, there are neither rods nor cones, so this area is referred to as the **optic disc** or blind spot.

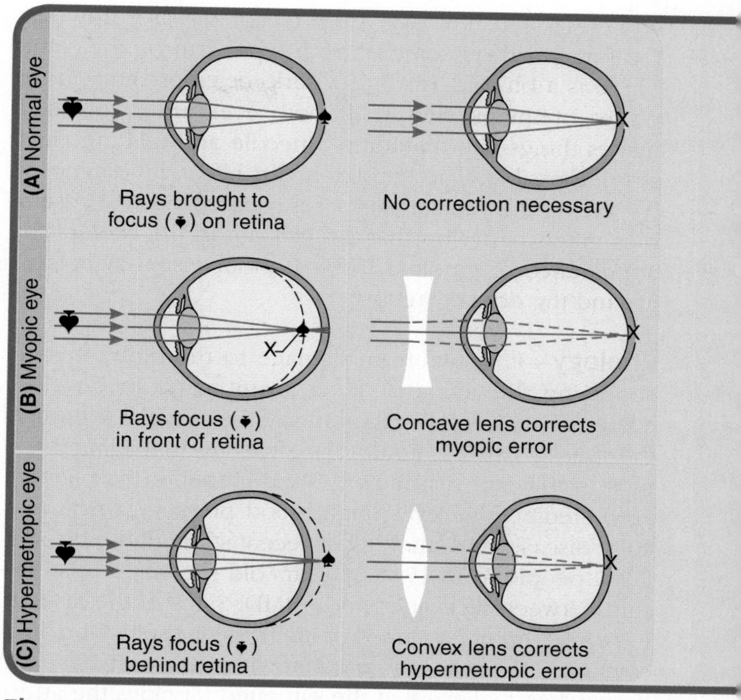

Figure 25–3: The refraction of an image in (A) normal vision, (B) nearsightedness, (C) farsightedness and the type of lens required to correct the vision. *Delmar/Cengage Learning.*

The Path of Light

The process of sight begins with the passage of light rays through the cornea; on through the aqueous humor, the pupil, and the lens into the vitreous humor; and finally focusing at the back of the eyeball on the retina. Here the image is picked up by the rods and cones, transformed into nerve impulses, and transmitted over the optic nerve to the thalamus. Here some of the fibers cross over to the nerve tract of the other eye. From the thalamus, other neurons relay the impulses to the visual center in the occipital lobe of the cerebrum, where the impulses are "developed" into pictures and "seen."

Refraction Error

Each part of the eyeball refracts (deflects) the light to cause the image to focus on the retina (Figure 25–3A). However, this does not always occur correctly. When the image is improperly refracted and focuses in front of the retina (B), the person is said to be nearsighted, or to have **myopia**. When the image focuses behind the retina (C), the person is said to be farsighted, or to have **hyperopia**. These conditions may result from abnormal curvature of the lens or cornea or from an abnormally shaped eyeball. Note that images are inverted when they pass through the lens because of the curvature deflecting the image. Eyeglasses provide a means of refracting light to correct abnormal deflection of the image. They perform artificially what the eyes' structures fail to do.

DIAGNOSTIC TESTS

All vision acuity tests are included in Chapter 40 with the physical examination discussion. They include the Snellen, Jaeger, Ishihara, and Pelli-Robson. The major instruments used to assess the condition of the eye, the ophthalmoscope, tonometer, and slit lamp microscope are mentioned but the tonometer and microscope are used primarily in an ophthalmology practice.

DISEASES AND DISORDERS OF THE EYE

Age-Related Macular Degeneration (ARMD) (Mak′-u-lar De-jen-er-a′-shun)

Description—A disease that affects the macula, the small central point of light-sensing retina in the back of the eye. It causes loss of central vision. Two types of ARMD exist: dry ARMD and wet ARMD. Ten million Americans have some loss of vision from age-related macular degeneration (ARMD). It causes 90% of new legal blindness in the United States.

Signs and symptoms—ARMD is painless. Central vision is lost; however, side or peripheral vision is often maintained. Vision loss can be rapid with the "wet" form and slow with the "dry" form of the disease; however, the functional outcome of both types can be the same. There is a blurred, distorted, dark, or empty area in the center of things viewed. If both eyes are involved, it makes things like threading a needle and reading virtually impossible. The condition can be easily diagnosed by having the patient look at a square grid that resembles graph paper but has a small dot in the center. The appearance of crooked lines or other visual symptoms around the dot is diagnostic.

Etiology—It results from damage to the blood vessels supplying the retina. It takes many years to develop, eventually causing the thinning of the macula. Although the specific cause is not known, it seems that aging is the most significant risk factor. Other identified risk factors are heredity, blue eyes, high blood pressure, cardiovascular disease, and smoking. A recent study of the diets of 2,000 people from 45 to 84 years old showed a relationship between dietary fat and ARMD. Signs of the disease were 80% more common with those people who had consumed the most saturated fat within the past 10 years. Researchers believe that the saturated fat clogs the arteries and reduces the amount of blood that reaches the retina. This form of degeneration is also known as "dry," or "atropic," macular degeneration and represents about 90% of the macular-related disease.

Another form known as "wet" macular degeneration accounts for the remaining 10% of cases. Although wet ARMD is less common, it is more serious. Abnormal blood vessels grow in a layer beneath the retina. They leak blood and fluid, creating distorted vision or a large blind spot of scar tissue in the center of the visual field.

Treatment—There is no cure for ARMD. The basis for treatment is modification of risk factors and interventional measures. Recent studies have shown that using antioxidant dietary supplements such as vitamin C, E, beta-carotene and zinc can lower the risk of disease progression. Smoking cessation, hypertension control, and adoption of a "heart-healthy" diet are encouraged for good cardiovascular and ocular health. Sunglasses that block exposure to ultraviolet light from the sun are advised to decrease potential damage to the macula.

Nonsurgical intervention is mainly optical. There are various optical devices including magnifying lenses and telescopes, closed circuit TV, large-print reading materials, and special lighting sources to assist with vision.

Surgical intervention is available for wet ARMD where subretinal blood vessels are leaking. Imaging techniques such as fluorescein angiography and ocular coherence tomography are used to search for treatable forms of ARMD. The aim of treatment is to halt the progression of the leaky blood vessels.

In the past, lasers have been applied directly to the retina to destroy the abnormal vessels. This leaves a blind spot at the site of the laser treatment. Photodynamic therapy was used next because it caused less retinal damage. In this technique, a chemical dye is injected in the arm and it collects in the abnormal vessels of the retina. A special laser is then used to activate the chemical in the abnormal vessels, and they are destroyed. The most recent injection technique consists of injecting chemicals directly into the vitreous cavity. These chemicals inhibit vascular endothelial growth factors and can therefore produce regression of abnormal new growth of blood vessels.

Scientists are perfecting an artificial retina that will permit limited vision of light and large objects. The technology involves the use of a bionic silicon chip and is being used in patients with retinitis pigmentosa, a genetically induced form of blindness. It is anticipated that it may also be applicable to macular degeneration.

Amblyopia (Am-ble-o′-pe-a) (Lazy Eye)

Description—**Amblyopia** is a condition known as lazy eye. It can occur when the eyes aren't aligned properly (misaligned). The "lazy" eye does not develop normal 20/20 vision acuity. Amblyopia occurs in children while the visual system is still developing and persists into adulthood if not treated.

Signs and symptoms—Ocular misalignment can manifest as an eye that turns in toward the nose, outward toward the ear, or it can be in straight and proper alignment. Blurred vision results, regardless of which alignment is present, and the brain suppresses the visual impulses from the affected eye.

Etiology—Amblyopia is caused by any condition that affects normal use of the eyes and their development. The three major causes are strabismus because of misaligned eyes, unequal focus caused by refractive errors, and cloudiness in the normally clear eye tissues. Strabismus is the most common cause because the crossed eye "turns off" to avoid double vision and becomes amblyopic. (See Strabismus on page 487 in this unit.)

Treatment—Treatment of amblyopia depends upon the cause. Misaligned eyes must be aligned either with surgery or eyeglasses or a combination of both. Unequal focus is corrected with eyeglasses. Cloudiness to the parts of the eye involved in the path of light, such as a cataract, must be corrected surgically. Occlusion therapy is used in conjunction with the above treatments. The "good eye" is covered with a patch, thereby stimulating the development of the "lazy eye." For a good prognosis, therapy should begin before the age of 8; otherwise, eventual blindness of the affected eye may result. Sometimes surgery is required to correct the eye.

Arcus Senilis (Are′-cuss Se-nill′-us)

Description—The condition accompanies normal aging and is included in this discussion because it is so prevalent. It results in a thin grayish-white arc or circle not quite at the edge of the cornea. If it is present in young people, it may suggest hypercholesterolemia (high level of cholesterol in the blood).

Blepharitis (Blef-ar-i′-tis) (Lid Margin Disease)

Description—This is a persistent inflammation of the edges of the eyelids involving the hair follicles and glands. The condition is usually associated with seborrhea of the scalp (dandruff), oily skin, or dry eyes.

Signs and symptoms—The person experiences itching and burning sensations, which causes continuous blinking and rubbing of the eyes, resulting in red-rimmed eyelid margins. The person develops greasy scales and sticky, crusted eyelids. Ulcerated lid margins, loss of lashes, and the presence of nits (eggs of lice) with pediculosis are possible.

Etiology—There are bacteria and excess secretions from the hair follicles of the eyelids. It may also develop from pediculosis of the brows and lashes.

Treatment—Treatment depends on the cause. It consists of frequent shampoos of the hair and daily cleansing of the eyelids with a mild baby shampoo to remove the scales. Placing warm wet washcloths over closed eyelids at least twice daily helps soften scales and other debris. It also helps liquefy the oily secretions so a chalazion, a painful, inflamed lump in an oil gland, can be prevented. Also gently scrubbing at the base of the eyelashes for about 15 seconds with a cotton swab or washcloth helps remove scales.

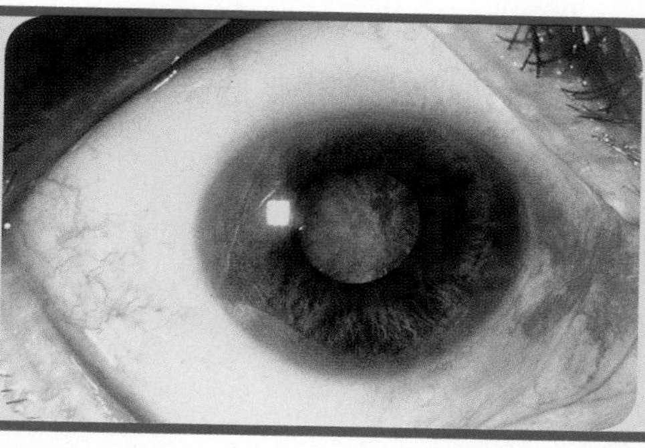

Figure 25–4: Cataract. *Courtesy of National Eye Institute, NIH.*

If necessary, artificial tears will relieve dry eye symptoms. Antibiotic medication or topical ointment will decrease the bacteria. Occasionally, short-term use of a steroid is necessary to reduce the inflammation. If pediculosis is present, the parasite must be removed.

Cataract (Kat′a-rakt)

Description—This gradually developing opacity (cloudiness) of the lens occurs most frequently in persons over 70 years of age as part of the aging process.

Signs and symptoms—The condition causes a painless, gradual blurring and loss of visual acuity. The pupil turns from black to a milky white as the lens becomes cloudy (Figure 25–4). People with cataracts frequently complain of seeing halos around lights or being blinded at night by oncoming automobile headlights. This is because as the lens becomes cloudy, it no longer sharply focuses light on the retina (Figure 25–5A), but instead the cataract either blocks or scatters the light coming into the eye around the retina (Figure 25–5B), causing blurring of the vision.

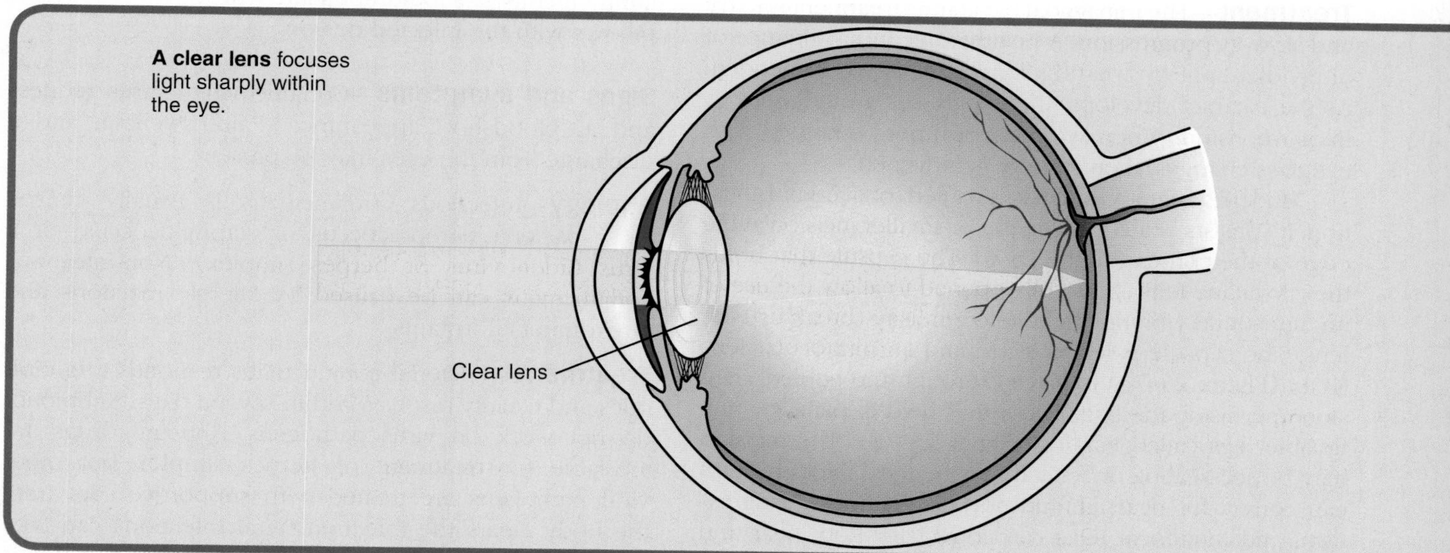
A clear lens focuses light sharply within the eye.
Clear lens

Figure 25–5A: Light through clear lens focuses on retina. *Delmar/Cengage Learning.*

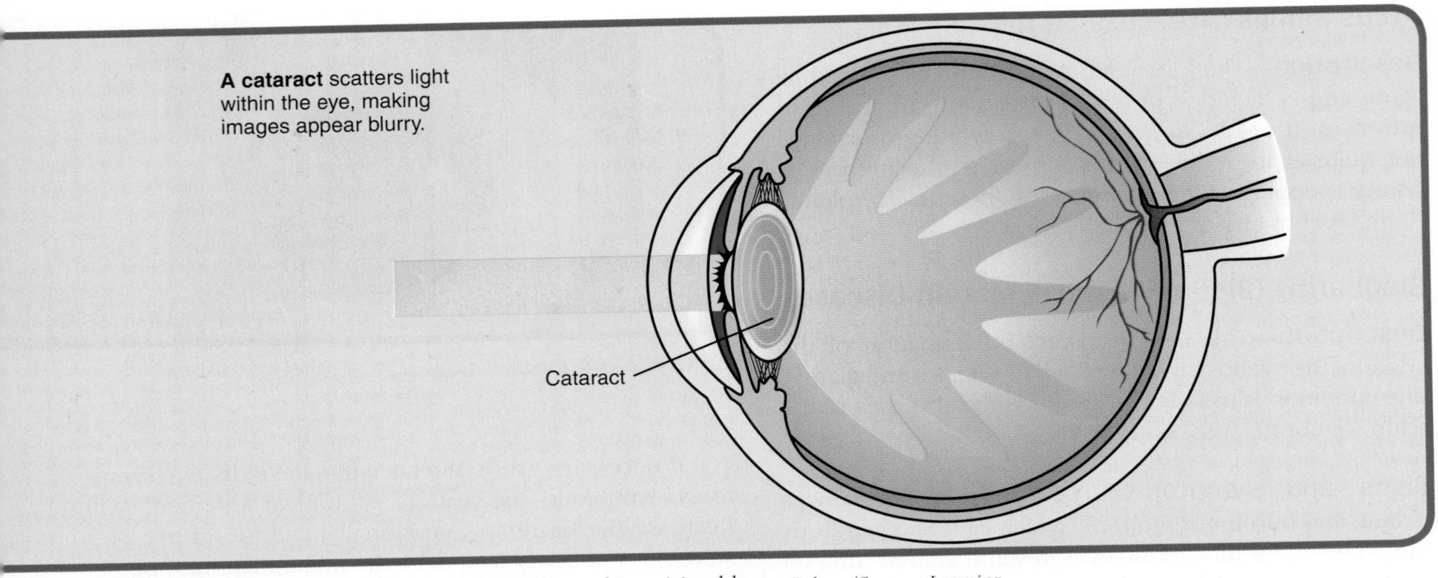
A cataract scatters light within the eye, making images appear blurry.
Cataract

Figure 25–5B: Light through cataract scatters, making vision blurry. *Delmar/Cengage Learning.*

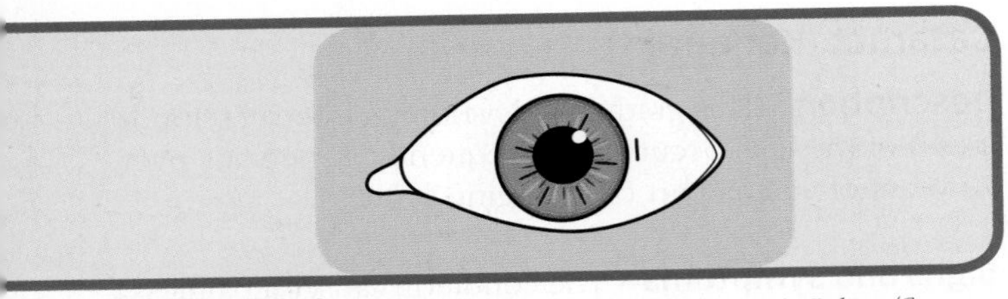

Figure 25–6: Incision size to remove a cataract. *Delmar/Cengage Learning.*

Etiology—The probable cause of **cataracts** is a change in the composition of the proteins of the lens. Aging is the underlying cause. Other things such as trauma, medications such as steroids, systemic diseases such as diabetes, and prolonged exposure to ultraviolet light can cause cataracts. Babies are occasionally born with a cataract.

Treatment—The initial goal of cataract treatment is to try and slow its progression. A healthy diet and avoidance of ultraviolet light by wearing sunglasses is recommended. As the cataract develops, the eyeglasses are adjusted to improve vision. When symptoms cannot be helped with eyeglass changes, then surgery is indicated.

Modern cataract surgery is called phacoemulsification. It consists of a 2.4 millimeter or smaller incision at the edge of the cornea (Figure 25–6). The capsule that holds the crystalline lens is carefully opened to allow the use of an ultrasound vibrating needle to emulsify (break up) the lens. The capsule is left in place and an intraocular lens (IOL) (Figure 25–7A) is placed through the corneal incision and inside the bag. The IOL is held in place by tiny flexible legs called haptics (Figure 25–7B). The incision may be self-sealing or a stitch may be used. Modern IOLs can correct for nearsightedness, farsightedness, astigmatism, and multifocal IOLs can correct for both near and far vision. Visual recovery after modern cataract surgery is very quick with most patients seeing well the following day. Cataract surgery is now done on an outpatient basis, with the patient detained only an hour or two.

Sometimes after surgery, the posterior capsule, which is now supporting the IOL, may become clouded, once again obstructing the path of light into the eye. This problem can be easily solved without invasive surgery, using a laser beam to make a tiny opening in the capsule, which lets in light and restores vision.

Conjunctivitis (Kon-junk-ti-vi′tis) (Pinkeye)

Description—This condition is caused by inflammation of the conjunctiva. It usually begins in one eye, spreading rapidly to the other from contamination by a washcloth or by the hands. Because it is highly contagious, other family members should not share towels, washcloths, or pillows with the infected person.

Signs and symptoms—Conjunctivitis causes redness and a "bloodshot" appearance. Pain, swelling, and a discharge from the eyes may be present.

Etiology—Infectious conjunctivitis is usually caused by a bacteria (streptococcus or staphylococcus) or a virus (adenovirus or herpes simplex). Non-infectious conjunctivitis can be caused by allergic reactions and environmental irritants.

Treatment—Bacterial conjunctivitis responds to antibiotics and usually resolves within several days. Antibiotics do not work on virus pathogens. Antiviral drugs are available for treatment of herpes simplex but other viral pathogens are treated with supportive care until the body clears the infection. Viral infections can take weeks to resolve in some cases. Allergic conjunctivitis

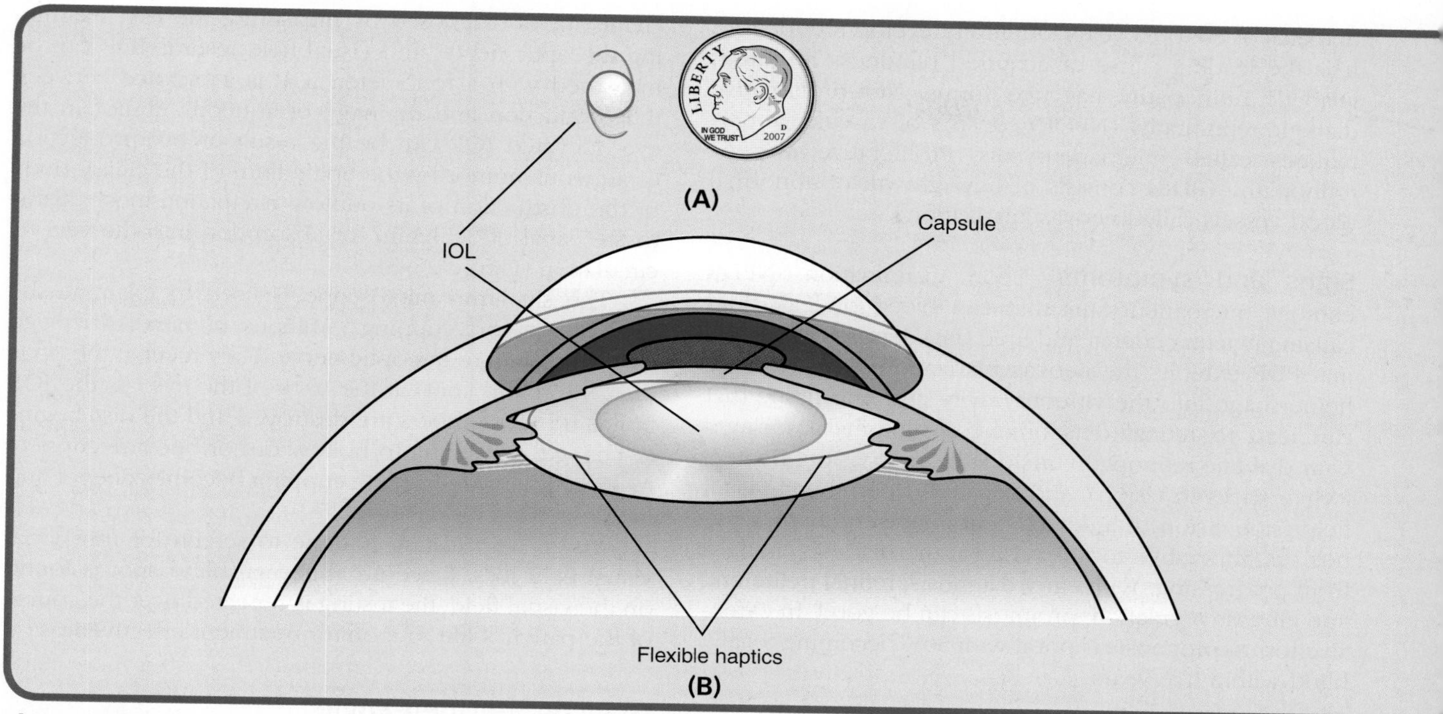

Figure 25–7: The intraocular lens (IOL) size (A) and location (B). *Delmar/Cengage Learning.*

is treated with anti-allergy eye drops and avoidance of the environmental irritants, if possible. Oral allergy medications rarely help with eye conditions.

Corneal Abrasion (Kor′ne-al A-bra′-zhun)

Description—A scratch or trauma to the cornea, usually from a foreign body in the eye. Even if the eye waters profusely to cleanse the surface, the scratch (abrasion) remains. Vision may be affected if the location and extent of injury are significant.

Signs and symptoms—The presence of redness, tearing, and irritation that causes excessive blinking.

Etiology—It is most often caused by dirt or small pieces of wood, metal, or paper that become embedded under the eyelid or an injury from a fingernail. Abrasions may also occur from falling asleep while wearing contact lenses.

Treatment—Foreign bodies embedded in the cornea require removal following application of a topical anesthetic. Treatment consists of antibiotic eyedrops or ointment. Corneal epithelium heals rapidly within 24 to 48 hours.

Corneal Ulcers (Kor′ne-al Ul′-ser)

Description—An acute disease caused by an infectious infiltration into the cornea of the eye.

Signs and symptoms—The signs are a painful red eye, excessive tearing, sensitivity to light, and blurred vision. The diagnosis is made using a slit lamp microscope, which shows the presence of various sizes of white corneal infiltrates. The corneal surface can appear irregular or smooth with an intact surface depending on the severity of the infection.

Etiology—Corneal ulcers result from bacterial, viral, or fungal infections. They are commonly associated with contact lens wear.

Treatment—A culture of the drainage to determine the causative organism will indicate appropriate medication. Broad-spectrum antibiotics are used initially to prevent corneal scarring and the resulting impairment of vision. Certain bacterial ulcers progress so rapidly that, without proper treatment, the cornea will perforate (develop a hole), and vision in the eye will be lost unless the perforation is sealed or an corneal transplant is performed.

Diabetic Retinopathy (Di-a-bet′ik Retin-op′a-the)

Description—This form of vascular **retinopathy** results from juvenile or adult diabetes. Approximately 75% of patients with juvenile diabetes develop diabetic retinopathy within 20 years after the onset of diabetes. Incidence in adults with diabetes increases with the length of time a person is diabetic. About 80% of patients with diabetes of 20 to 30 years' duration develop retinopathy. It is the leading cause of acquired blindness in adults. Diabetic retinopathy has two forms. Non-proliferative diabetic retinopathy (NPDR) consists of vascular abnormalities called microaneurysms. Proliferative diabetic retinopathy (PDR) consists of new growth of abnormal blood vessels called neovascularization.

Signs and symptoms—Upon examination, NPDR exhibits microaneurysms that can bleed or leak fluid causing macular edema and lipid (fat) deposits in the retina. PDR exhibits the neovascularization, which causes hemorrhage into the vitreous cavity and scar tissue that can lead to retinal detachment. Symptoms associated with diabetic retinopathy include blurred vision, floaters (white specs in vision), and decreased peripheral visual field (side vision) if a detachment is present. Early diagnosis is imperative to help control the diabetic changes from progressing. With early diagnosis, retinal treatment, and glucose regulation, prognosis can be good. In extensive forms, prognosis is poor, with 50% becoming legally blind within five years.

Etiology—Excess glucose in the blood is processed through an alternate glucose metabolism pathway called the sorbitol pathway. Sorbitol gets deposited in the walls of the retinal blood vessels and prevents diffusion of oxygen to the retina. The retinal vessels become leaky and develop dilations, microaneurysms, and make new blood vessels (neovascularization) in an attempt to get adequate oxygen to the retina.

Treatment—The most important form of initial treatment is to obtain strict blood glucose and blood pressure control. NPDR is treated by frequent ophthalmic examinations until the presence of vision-threatening vascular changes or edema appear. Laser treatments and intraocular injections of drugs into the vitreous cavity are used to treat leaky microaneurysms and macular edema. PDR is treated with large amounts of laser therapy to the retina. If vitreoretinal scarring is severe, then vitrectomy (removal of the vitreous cavity contents) surgery is performed.

Glaucoma (Glaw-ko′-ma)

Glaucoma is a disease associated with intraocular eye pressure (IOP) and atrophy of the optic nerve. Glaucoma causes severe visual impairment and eventually complete blindness if uncontrolled. It is believed that damage to the optic nerve in glaucoma is a result of a combination of the force from compression by elevated IOP and poor blood flow. It occurs in 2% of adults over age 40 and accounts for 15% of all blindness in the United States.

There are two types of glaucoma—open-angle (most common) and closed-angle—both have elevated IOP. Glaucoma is diagnosed by measuring the IOP, examining the optic nerve, and visual field testing. IOP can be measured with a tonometer. IOP is a balance between the production and drainage of aqueous humor in the eye. Elevated IOP can be the result of overproduction of aqueous humor by the epithelium of the ciliary body or the obstruction of its outflow circulating mechanisms to the canal of Schlemm for absorption into the venous circulation (Figure 25–8).

The slit lamp microscope is used to examine the optic nerve for "cupping." Millions of nerve fibers go from the retina to the optic nerve. They meet at the optic disc, the "blind spot" at the back of the eye. As the IOP builds up, nerve fibers are destroyed and the disc begins to change, appearing to hollow out or become cupped. As more fibers are lost, the cupping becomes deeper and more vision is lost (Figure 25–9).

Visual field testing is done to screen for functional visual field loss. Once an abnormal blind spot is found on the visual field, the testing is repeated over the course of the patient's life to monitor treatment effectiveness.

Glaucoma—Open-angle

Signs and symptoms—The symptoms are **insidious** (gradual), bilateral, and often not recognized until late in the disease. They include painless loss of peripheral (side) vision, seeing halos around lights, and difficulty seeing at night or in darkened places.

Etiology—In open-angle glaucoma, the drainage angle is open. With high IOP, the production of aqueous fluid is either too high or the outflow is obstructed in the trabecular meshwork, the canal of Schlemm, or the aqueous veins. It is thought to be more of a blood flow issue.

Treatment—Treatment is aimed at lowering the IOP to prevent further optic nerve damage. Medical therapy consists of eye drops and oral medication that decrease aqueous humor production or increase the outflow by way of an accessory pathway. Laser to the trabecular meshwork can be used to lower IOP. By applying the laser directly to the meshwork, flow can be increased by either creating new drainage holes in the meshwork or by stimulating macrophages to "clean out" the existing meshwork. If laser is insufficient, then a surgical procedure is performed to create a shunt (passageway) from inside the eye to the subconjuntival space. This procedure is called a trabeculectomy.

Glaucoma—Closed-angle

Signs and symptoms—There is pain and redness of the affected eye with a feeling of pressure. The pain can be so intense that a patient has nausea and vomiting. The pupil is moderately dilated and nonreactive to

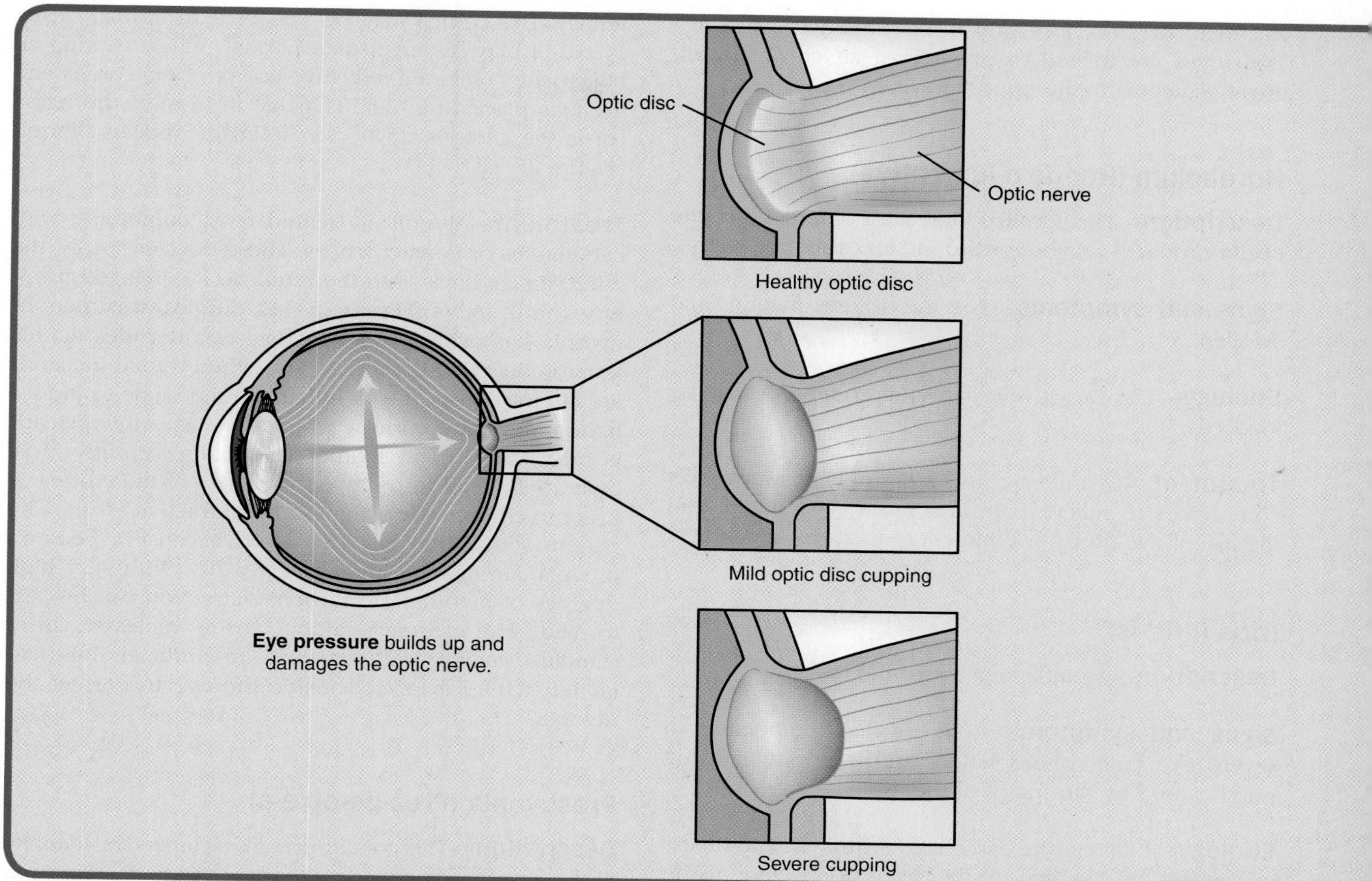

Figure 25–8: How glaucoma affects the optic disc. *Delmar/Cengage Learning.*

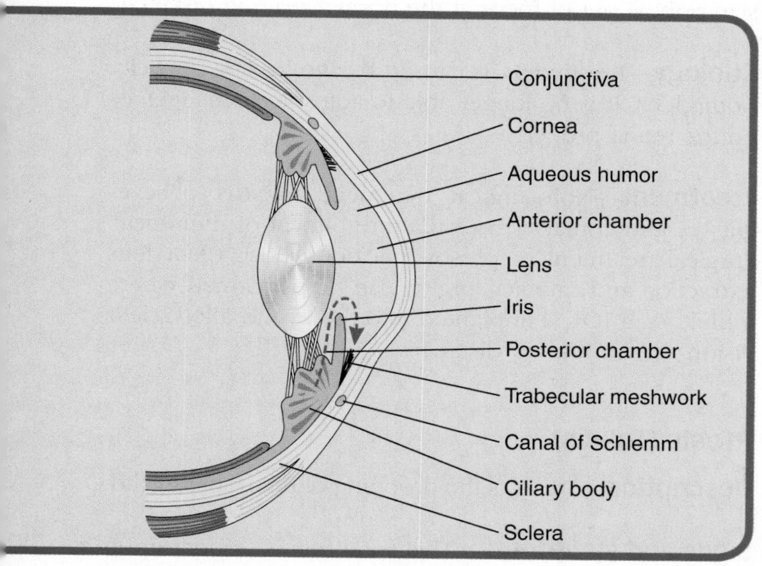

Figure 25–9: Normal flow of aqueous humor. *Delmar/Cengage Learning.*

light. There is blurred and decreased visual acuity and sensitivity to light. Unless the pressure is relieved quickly, blindness may occur within 24 hours.

Etiology—This type of glaucoma results from physical obstruction of the trabecular meshwork openings by the iris. An anatomically shallow or narrow angle becomes "closed" when the iris physically blocks the drainage holes. This commonly happens when the pressure behind the iris is greater than in the front. The pressure causes the iris to bow forward closing off the already narrow angle, thus covering up the meshwork. There is a rapid onset of symptoms, and this is considered an ocular emergency.

Treatment—Usual treatment consists of aggressive drug therapy and a peripheral iridotomy. The laser is applied to the peripheral iris to make a small hole to allow the pressure in the anterior chamber (in front of the iris) to equalize with the posterior chamber (behind the iris) (see Figure 25–8). This allows the iris to flatten out and thus uncover the trabecular meshwork. A second treatment may be necessary in closed-angle glaucoma. Both eyes are treated to prevent an attack of closed-angle glaucoma in the opposite eye.

Hordeolum (Hor-de′o-lum) (Stye)

Description—This localized infection of a gland of the eyelid produces an abscess around an eyelash.

Signs and symptoms—The eye is red, painful, and swollen.

Etiology—The causative organism is commonly staphylococcus.

Treatment—Treatment consists of applying warm, wet compresses to relieve pain and promote drainage and the use of eye drops or ointment to treat the infection.

Iritis (I-rit′-is)

Description—An inflammation of the iris.

Signs and symptoms—Iritis produces moderate to severe eye pain, photophobia, and a poorly reacting pupil caused by the spasm of the iris.

Etiology—Iritis can be associated with systemic illness or caused by trauma to the eye. Connective tissue diseases such as rheumatoid arthritis, lupus, and other autoimmune diseases are commonly associated with iritis. Traumatic iritis can occur after minor blunt trauma to the eye or with other corneal problems including abrasion or infectious ulcer.

Treatment—Prompt treatment is required to prevent complications. The pupil is dilated with mydriatics to allow the eye to rest to prevent the formation of posterior synechiae (adhesions of the iris to the lens). Corticosteroid drops are used to reduce the inflammation.

Myopia (Miop′-e-a)

Description—This condition is a defect in vision that is also known as nearsightedness. Objects can be seen distinctly only when close to the eyes. The rate of incidence is believed to be around 11 million Americans.

Signs and symptoms—There is a blurring of vision when looking at objects beyond immediate surroundings.

Etiology—The primary cause of myopia can be found in the shape of the eye. In myopia, the eye is larger or longer than normal in its axial length (front of cornea to retina). The cornea may be steeper than normal or the eye itself may be larger than normal. When viewing an object, the combined refractive power of the cornea and the lens places the "20/20" image in from of the retina (or in the vitreous cavity) so the image appears blurred (Figure 25–3B).

Treatment—Myopia is treated most commonly with eye glasses or contact lenses. These devices "push" the 20/20 image back onto the retina so it is imaged properly and in focus (Figure 25–3A). Surgical treatment of myopia has evolved over the last two decades. Radial keratotomy (RK) is a procedure where radial incisions are cut into the cornea with a diamond blade to induce flattening of the cornea, which decreases myopia. RK is rarely used now. Eximer lasers are currently most commonly used to remove thin layers of the cornea in order to correct myopia and other refractive errors. The patient should be past childhood because a person's myopia can change into the early 20s. With very high degrees of myopia, a clear lens extraction can be performed. The clear crystalline lens is removed, as in standard cataract surgery, and an artificial intraocular lens (IOL) is placed inside the eye to correct the myopia.

Presbyopia (Prez-be-op′e-a)

Description—This condition is characterized by inability of the lens to accommodate for near vision. **Presbyopia** occurs as part of the normal aging process.

Signs and symptoms—The first symptom is usually the inability to read smaller print without straining and the use of a bright light. With advancement, all normal size print is out of focus at the normal reading distance.

Etiology—Presbyopia is caused by the loss of elasticity of the lens. It is no longer able to adjust to focus images on the retina properly.

Treatment—Non-surgical treatment consists of eyeglasses and contact lenses that are bifocal or multifocal. Surgical treatment of presbyopia does exist. Clear lens extraction and cataract surgery can be performed where a multifocal IOL is implanted into the eye to allow clear vision at near and far distances.

Ptosis (To′-sis)

Description—Ptosis is the drooping of the upper eyelid.

Signs and symptoms—This condition is evident upon observation. Eyes appear to be only partially open. The individual has a "sleepy" appearance.

Etiology—Ptosis may be a congenital condition or the result of aging, the presence of an excess fatty fold, or a neurologic factor.

Treatment—Treatment may be required if vision is restricted or the appearance is cosmetically undesirable. A surgical procedure on the eyelid muscles is the most common treatment to correct ptosis. If surgery is not desired, a device can be attached to the eyeglasses to help elevate the lid.

Retinal Detachment (Ret′-i-nal)

Description—This disorder is characterized by the separation of the retina from its underlying support layers. There are three main types of retinal detachment (RD): rhegmatogenous, exudative, and traction.

Signs and symptoms—Diagnosis can be made from the patient's complaints of seeing floating spots, flashes of light, and a gradual vision loss. Confirmation is possible after pupil dilation and ophthalmoscopy reveal a gray and opaque retina with indefinite margins in the affected areas. Folds, tears, and a ballooning inward of the retina may be seen.

Etiology—Rhegmatogenous RD can happen due to normal aging. As the eye naturally ages, the vitreous humor shrinks—it pulls away from its attachments to the retina and can cause a tear or hole that allows fluid to seep underneath the layers of the retina. Trauma is another source of tears. Exudative RDs can occur due to build up of fluids underneath the retina. This can be associated with diseases such as hypertension and inflammatory conditions. Traction RDs are caused by the traction of "pulling" on the retina by scar tissue. The most common cause is severe diabetic retinopathy.

Treatment—Treatment of RDs depends on the cause. If a hole or tear is found when the detachment is very small, then a coagulation laser beam can be used to seal or "spot weld" the retina to prevent progression of the detachment. If significant detachment is already present, then surgical therapy is necessary to reattach the retina. A combination of heat, cold, and gas can be used to assist the surgical correction. Laser (heat) and cryotherapy (cold) are used to create a sterile inflammatory response that scars the retinal tissues back together. A scleral buckle is a silicone band that is sewn around the outside of the eyeball in order to push the retina against the tear. A combination of the therapies can be used to seal the break.

Virectomy is a procedure used to remove the vitreous humor from the inside of the eye, thus allowing gas to be placed in the vitreous cavity to compress the retinal layers together from the inside of the eye. Vitrectomy is required for repair of traction RDs so the scar tissue causing the traction can be removed.

Treatment—Treatment consists of limiting eye movements with a patch, bed rest, sedation, and appropriate positioning of the head. Spontaneous reattachment is rare. A coagulation laser beam can repair simple tears in the retina by "spot welding" the area with several rows of "welds," but once separation has occurred, other treatment will be necessary. Both heat and cold therapies are used to create a sterile inflammatory reaction that causes the retina to readhere. A tight band is placed around the eyeball, inside the sclera layer, which makes the choroid "indent" against the retina to maintain its closeness. Various surgical procedures to reattach the retina to the choroid can be performed.

Strabismus (Stra-biz′-mus)

Description—This is a condition in which one eye deviates with the gaze being abnormally inward or outward, higher or lower than the other eye (Figure 25–10). An abnormally inward gaze (convergent or "crosseye") is also called esotropia, and an abnormally outward gaze (divergent or "walleye") is also known as exotropia.

Signs and symptoms—This condition is obvious upon examination. The deviation and absence of coordinated eye movement cause complaints of double vision and the inability to see objects clearly. **Strabismus** is frequently associated with Down syndrome, cerebral palsy, and mental retardation.

Etiology—The disorder results from eye muscle imbalance or attempts to compensate for extreme farsightedness.

Treatment—Conservative initial treatment consists of a patch on the normal eye, corrective glasses, and specific eye exercises. Surgery to adjust the muscles that control eye placement and movement may be indicated. If strabismus is not corrected prior to the age of 12 to 13, the deviated eye may be suppressed, resulting in ambylopia, which could cause permanent loss of vision.

Eye Protection

The Prevent Blindness America Association promotes many programs stressing the importance of protecting eyes from injury. Many occupations require the use of goggles or safety glasses. The association recommends the

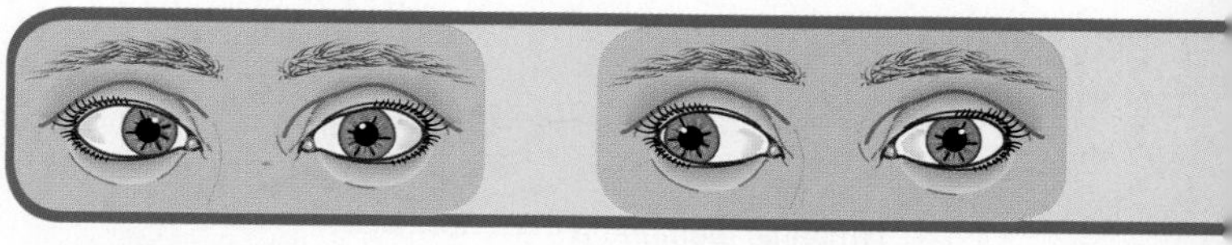

Figure 25–10: Strabismus: (left) convergent or esotropia; (right) divergent or exotropia. *Delmar/Cengage Learning.*

use of impact-resistant glass or plastic in all eyeglasses and sunglasses. A 1972 federal ruling requires that the lens be able to withstand the impact from a 5/8-inch-diameter steel ball dropped from a height of 50 inches. Individuals with sight in only one eye should use industrial-quality safety lenses and frames. When engaging in do-it-yourself work, sports, or hobbies that involve visual hazards, protective eye wear should be worn. It should be noted that contact lenses do not provide protection for the eyes, and the use of protective eye wear is necessary.

If injury should occur, initial treatment is important in order to prevent further damage. If something is splashed or blown into the eye, it should be rinsed thoroughly, with the eye held open. If caustic, rinse for several minutes. A physician should examine the eye as soon as possible. Foreign bodies that are not embedded may be removed with a fold of a wet tissue or a moistened cotton swab. Objects that are embedded into the surface require medical attention. See Foreign Bodies, Chapter 55.

THE EAR AND THE SENSE OF HEARING

The ear is capable of receiving vibrations in the air and translating them into the sounds we recognize: the more vibrations per second, the higher the frequency, or pitch, of the sound; the stronger the vibration, the louder the sound.

The Outer Ear

Vibrations are picked up by the pinna (auricle) of the outer ear and directed down the external **auditory** canal to the **tympanic membrane** (eardrum) (Figure 25–11).

The Middle Ear

The sound waves vibrate the membrane and the **malleus** (hammer) attached to its inner surface. The malleus in turn "strikes" the **incus** (anvil), which moves the **stapes** (stirrup). These three small bones and the space around them are called the middle ear. The middle ear communicates the vibrations to the inner ear by the stapes pushing against the fluid in the vestibule of the inner ear through the oval window.

The middle ear is connected by means of the **eustachian tube** to the throat. The eustachian tube is responsible for equalizing air pressure in the middle ear with the outside atmospheric pressure. Unfortunately, infections from the throat often pass through the tube into the middle ear. Rapid changes in altitude, harsh blowing of the nose, or a forceful sneeze may cause temporary air pressure imbalances resulting in pain, effusions, and hearing loss.

The Inner Ear

The vibrations from the middle ear continue through the coiled **cochlea**, which contains the **organ of Corti**, a collection of specialized nerve cells (Figure 25–12). These cells transmit the impulses to the auditory nerve, which passes them on to the auditory center of the temporal lobe of the cerebrum for interpretation.

The inner ear also contains three **semicircular canals**. These structures are responsible for maintaining equilibrium (balance). Inside the canals, hairlike nerve cell receptors are embedded in a gelatin-like material.

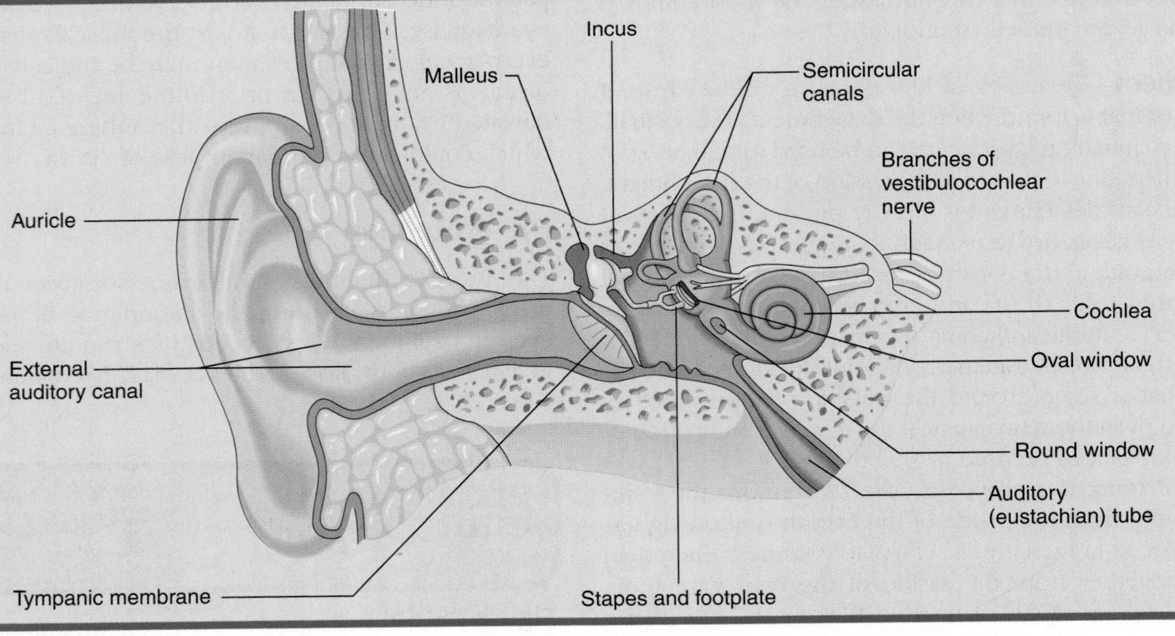

Figure 25–11: The ear. *Delmar/Cengage Learning.*

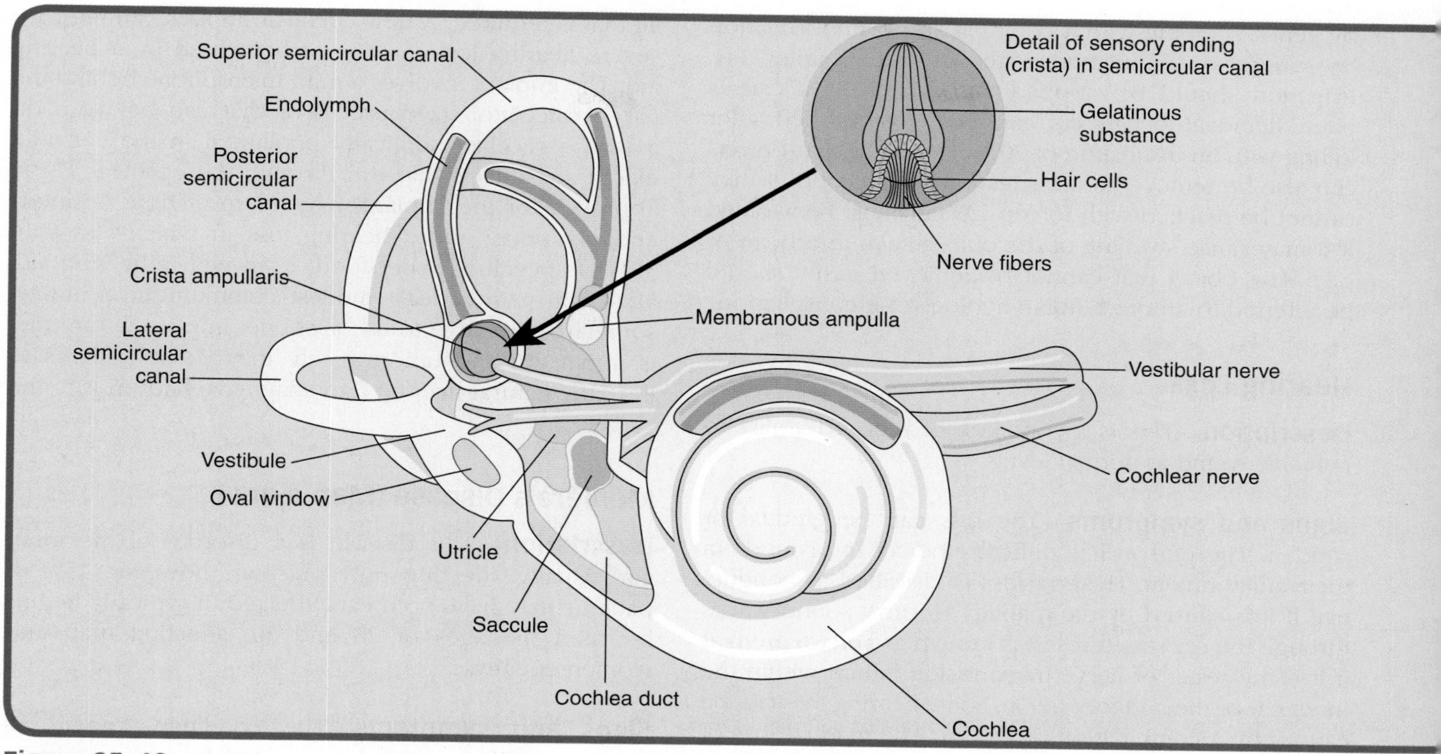

Figure 25–12: The inner ear. *Delmar/Cengage Learning.*

When the head moves, the material pushes against the receptors, which transmit to the brain the change in position.

Another nerve receptor network in the semicircular canals is similarly constructed inside two small sacs. The gelatin surface here is covered with a layer of tiny limestone grains. When the head moves, the grains shift, causing the hair cells to send out impulses.

The inner ear, therefore, carries out two important functions for the body: It transmits vibrations to the auditory nerve so that we can hear, and its semicircular canals allow us to maintain our balance.

DIAGNOSTIC TESTS

Routine diagnostic examinations for the ear, such as audiometry, Weber, and Rinne, are discussed in Chapter 40.

Videonystagmograph

The videonystagmograph (VNG) is a special examination that evaluates balance function. Because eyes and ears work together through the nervous system, measurement of eye movements are used to evaluate the balance system. The test is performed with the patient wearing special goggles that record eye movement. Cables from the goggles attach to a recording machine. Warm and cool water or air are gently introduced into each ear canal. Patients are asked to identify locations of visible objects when shown. Coordination is evidence of balance function and will be affected by the involved ear.

MRI

MRI of the brain with special emphasis on the inner ear can be used to identify pathology.

DISEASES AND DISORDERS OF THE EAR

Auditory Canal Obstruction

Description—This refers to anything in the ear canal that in some manner occludes the opening.

Signs and symptoms—Symptoms vary with the obstruction. Insects may produce sounds or movement, or objects can cause discomfort, a degree of hearing loss, or annoyance.

Etiology—The auditory canal can be obstructed by impacted **cerumen** (ear wax) or a foreign body such as a bean, pea, pebble, bead, or insect. Children often put objects into their ears.

Treatment—Treatment consists of a removal technique appropriate to the obstruction. Cerumen can be removed by gentle scraping with a cerumen spoon and irrigation by syringe or an aerated water jet (see Chapter 14). Irrigation should be stopped immediately if it causes pain. Removal of insects can be accomplished after killing with an instillation of 70% alcohol. Similar objects can also be removed after irrigation with alcohol if they cannot be reached with forceps. Water must be avoided if it may cause swelling of the object, such as a bean or pea. Any object that cannot be removed easily should be referred to an otorhinolaryngologist for consultation.

Hearing Loss

Description—This is a condition of reduced ability to perceive sound at normal levels.

Signs and symptoms—The loss can be gradual or sudden. The person has difficulty perceiving sounds in their environment. Hearing loss is classified as conductive if it is caused by the inability to carry sound waves through the ear structures. It is known as **sensorineural** if it is the result of nerve transmission failure within the inner ear or the auditory nerve. Some hearing loss can be caused by a combination of factors. The gradual loss of hearing that occurs normally as part of the aging process is known as **presbycusis**.

Etiology—Conductive loss may be caused by an obstruction from a buildup of cerumen (wax), a foreign body, swelling within the auditory canal, middle ear infection, or otosclerosis.

Sudden loss of hearing without prior impairment is considered a medical emergency, because prompt treatment may restore hearing. Common causes are acute infection, head trauma, brain tumor, toxic drugs, or metabolic and vascular disorders.

Hearing loss can also be noise-induced and can be temporary or, over time, permanent. It follows prolonged exposure to noise in excess of 85 to 90 db (see Chapter 40). It is common among people who work in constant industrial noise, military personnel, and rock musicians. This loss is preventable with the enforcement of the use of protective devices, such as ear plugs, as mandated by law in occupational exposure.

Bone and air conduction hearing loss is assessed by the Rinne and Weber tests. An audiometer can be used to give a pure tone audiometry examination to measure the threshold and degree of loudness at which sound can be perceived (see Chapter 40).

Treatment—The form of treatment depends upon the causative factor. Removal of obstructions will correct the related conductive loss. With sudden loss, treatment may involve medication, surgery, or antidotes to toxins. Loss caused by aging can usually be improved with the use of modern hearing aids; providing sound amplification is all that is required. A new cochlear implant can improve severe hearing loss that is not benefitted by a hearing aid. The implant involves a mini-microphone behind the ear, a calculator-sized processor that can be worn on a belt, a receiver surgically implanted in the ear, and electrical contacts that run through the cochlea. To be approved for the implant, patients must have an intact auditory nerve and a hearing loss in which less than 30% of speech is understood, even with a hearing aid. Most will gain at least modest communication ability; some are even able to use a phone. Implant failure rate is about 2% and unfortunately may cause patients to lose any natural hearing they may have had prior to the surgery.

Ménière's Disease (Man-e-arz′)

Description—This disease is a disorder of the inner ear, usually affecting only one ear; however, 15% of patients may have both ears affected. It typically begins between the ages of 20 and 50, affecting men and women equally.

Signs and symptoms—The condition known as **Ménière's disease** is characterized by severe vertigo (dizziness) and **tinnitus** (ringing in the ears). Violent attacks may last from 10 minutes to hours and cause severe nausea, vomiting, and perspiration. Occasionally, the vertigo causes loss of balance and results in the person falling. There is intermittent hearing loss early in the disease, but over time a fixed loss may develop, probably as a result of the degeneration of hair cells in the cochlea.

Etiology—The cause is unknown, but it probably results from an abnormality in the fluids of the inner ear.

Treatment—Treatment consists of drugs to reduce fluid, antihistamines, and mild sedation. Anti-vertigo and anti-nausea medications may be used. Patients are advised to avoid caffeine, salts, smoking, and alcohol. Excessive fatigue and stress may aggravate the disease. Patients who experience vertigo without warning are advised not to drive or engage in any type of potentially hazardous activity because of the possibility of an accident. If attacks are not controlled conservatively and become disabling, a surgical procedure may be indicated. Options range from a shunt to remove excess fluid to the cutting of the balance nerve (which will usually control the vertigo while still maintaining hearing) to a labyrinthectomy (which destroys both the balance mechanism and hearing on the affected side, but will control the attacks). Medical labyrinthectomy with vestibule-toxic drugs is appropriate in some cases. There is only a cure for vertigo, not for Ménière's disease.

Motion Sickness

Description—A condition that occurs when engaging in activities involving movement, such as riding in automobiles, boats, planes, or amusement rides.

Signs and symptoms—This is characterized by loss of equilibrium, perspiration, headache, nausea, and vomiting brought on by irregular motion.

Etiology—The disorder probably results from excessive stimulation of the inner ear receptors or confusion in the brain between the visual stimulus and movement perception.

Treatment—Treatment consists of avoiding the causative motions, lying down, and closing the eyes. When avoidance is not possible, the head should be kept still and vision focused on distant and stationary objects. Medications to prevent nausea and vomiting, such as valium, scopolamine, and antihistamines, are usually beneficial if taken prior to the trip. Symptoms can also be controlled by applying medication (scopolamine) in a patch form to the skin behind the ear.

Otitis Externa (O-ti′-tis)

Description—An infection of the external auditory canal.

Signs and symptoms—**Otitis** causes pain and hearing loss.

Etiology—Otitis externa can result from contaminated swimming water (swimmer's ears); cleaning the canal with bobby pins or introducing an organism on a cotton swab; regular use of earphones or plugs, which can trap moisture, creating optimal growing conditions; and scratching the ear canal with a fingernail.

Treatment—It is best treated with pain medication and antibiotic ear drops, following thorough cleaning. Fungal otitis acterna may also occur. It will require debridement and antifungal ear drops.

Otitis Media

Description—An infection of the middle ear often associated with respiratory infections.

Signs and symptoms—Otitis media is characterized by a severe, deep, and throbbing pain; fever; and hearing loss. The tympanic membrane may be reddened and bulge into the external canal. Excessive pressure may cause it to rupture, resulting in drainage into the canal. Recurring episodes may scar and thicken the membrane, causing a conductive hearing loss. Holes and tears from a rupture will also cause a loss of hearing.

Etiology—Otitis media usually occurs from an organism that has caused a sore throat or cold. However, it can also be caused by obstruction of the eustachian tube that results in a negative pressure within the ear that "pulls" serous fluid from the blood vessels into the middle ear.

Treatment may require antibiotics, such as amoxicillin or erythromycin (with a sulfa drug if allergic to penicillin), in addition to pain medication. A myringotomy (incision of the tympanic membrane) may be indicated if bulging and severe pain are present.

Note: Young children and infants are prone to ear infections. Anatomically, their eustachian tubes lie horizontally, which makes it more difficult for them to open and ventilate the middle ear. Infants who are allowed to take a bottle while lying down may get fluid and bacteria into their eustachian tubes from reflux or from obstruction, causing negative pressure to extract fluid. Children will have ear pain, fever, and be irritable.

Treatment—With chronic fluid collection caused by obstruction, it may be necessary to insert a tiny polyethylene tube through the tympanic membrane to temporarily equalize the pressure. This procedure is known as a tympanostomy. Tubes usually fall out after about 6 to 12 months. *Caution:* Untreated middle ear infection can lead to severe complications, such as mastoiditis, brain abscesses, or meningitis. With today's antibiotics, these complications are rare. Sudden hearing loss, headache, dizziness, chills, and fever are possible warning signs.

Otosclerosis (O-to-skle-ro′sis)

Description—The most common cause of conductive deafness is **otosclerosis**. It is characterized by the formation of spongy bone that immobilizes the stapes in the oval window of the vestibule, disrupting the conduction of vibrations from the tympanic membrane to the cochlea.

Signs and symptoms—Otosclerosis is a condition characterized by the slow and progressive loss of hearing and may be accompanied by tinnitus.

Etiology—It appears to result from a genetic factor and often occurs among family members. Incidence in Caucasians is at least 10%, affecting twice as many females as males, usually between 15 and 30 years of age.

Treatment—Treatment for otosclerosis consists of surgically removing the stapes (stapedectomy) and inserting an artificial substitute, which results in partial to complete return of hearing. An appropriate hearing aid is helpful if a stapedectomy is not possible.

Presbycusis (Prez-bi-ku′-sis) (Senile Deafness)

Description—This hearing loss is an effect of aging. It is sensorineural in nature.

Signs and symptoms—The deafness normally manifests itself through the loss of high-frequency sounds. It is usually accompanied by an annoying tinnitus. The patient has difficulty understanding the spoken word and may become depressed because of inability to communicate.

Etiology—The loss is caused by the deterioration of the auditory system and a loss of the hair cells in the organ of Corti.

Treatment—Presbycusis is irreversible but can be helped with an effective and properly fitting hearing aid.

THE NOSE AND THE SENSE OF SMELL

The sense of smell is due to the olfactory organ in the top of the nasal cavity (Figure 25–13). The nerve fibers in the organ are chemoreceptors that respond to stimuli from ions or molecules dissolved in the moisture from the mucous membranes. The organ is connected by nerve fibers, which run through tiny holes in the skull bone above the nasal cavity, to the olfactory center in the brain. The nerve fibers connect with receptor cells in the mucous membrane of the nose. These odor detectors can "smell" something only after it is dissolved in the mucus secretions.

DISEASES AND DISORDERS OF THE NOSE

Epistaxis (Epi-stak′-sis) (Nosebleed)

Description—Bleeding from the nose.

Signs and symptoms—The presence of blood coming from the nose is evidence of epistaxis. However, blood originating from the nose may be expectorated from the mouth or swallowed into the throat. Symptoms other than visible blood may be lightheadedness, a drop in blood pressure, rapid pulse, dyspnea, pallor, and other indications of shock.

Etiology—This usually occurs after injury, either external or internal, such as a blow to the nose, nosepicking, or foreign body insertion. Less frequent causes of **epistaxis** are chronic conditions, such as nasal or sinus infection that results in capillary congestion and bleeding, or the inhalation of irritating substances. Predisposing systemic factors include high blood pressure; anticoagulation drugs; chronic aspirin use; and blood diseases, such as anemia, hemophilia, and leukemia.

Treatment—Treatment varies depending on the cause, location, and severity. Even moderate bleeding is considered serious if it persists longer than 10 minutes after pressure is applied. Initial first aid treatment may consist of elevating the head, compression of nostrils against the septum continuously for 5 to 10 minutes, application of ice or cold compresses to nose, preventing the swallowing of blood (to determine the amount lost), avoiding talking or blowing the nose, and observing for amount of blood loss and signs of shock.

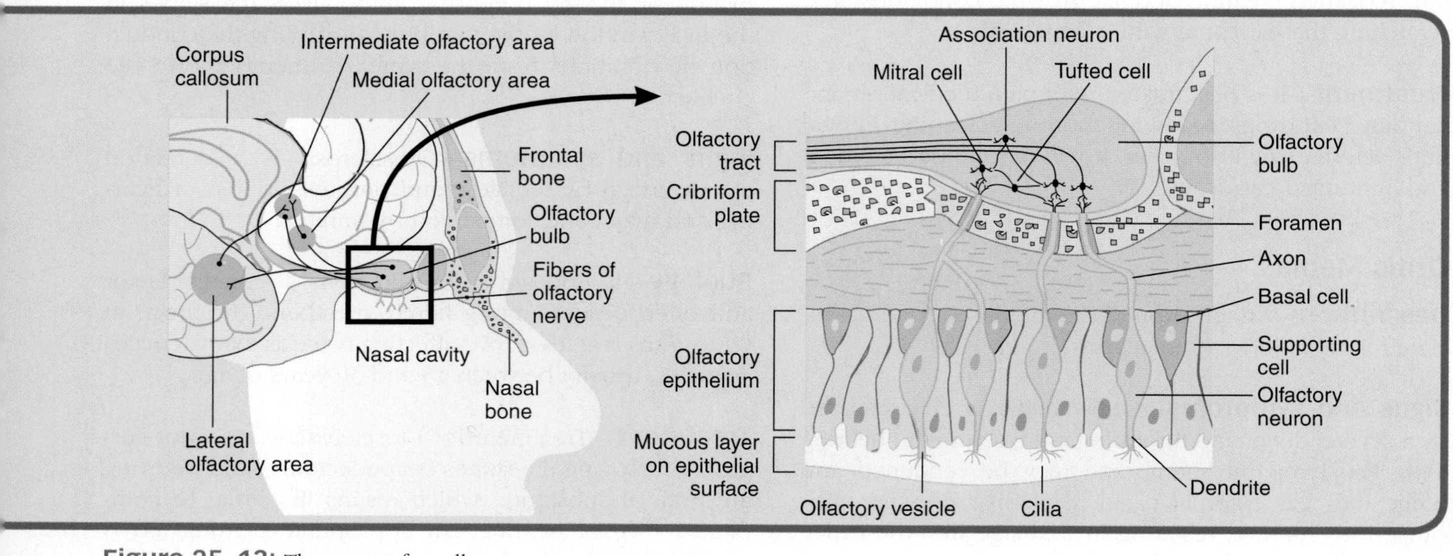

Figure 25–13: The sense of smell. *Delmar/Cengage Learning.*

Advanced treatment depends on location. For anterior bleeding, apply an epinephrine-saturated cotton ball or gauze to the bleeding site and use external pressure. For chronic anterior, bleeding cauterization by electric cautery or silver nitrate may be indicated. For posterior bleeding, the insertion of a nasal balloon for 48 to 72 hours may be required. Small catheters with balloons are passed through the bleeding side of the nose into the nasopharynx. The ballons are inflated, creating pressure against the leaking blood vessels. If necessary, anterior bleeding can be treated by packing for 24 to 48 hours. Other treatment may include supplemental vitamin K, blood transfusions, and surgical ligation (tying) of the bleeding artery. Embolization of blood vessels (clotting) by X-ray guided catheters is also effective.

Nasal Polyps (Pol′ips)

Description—These usually benign growths most often multiple, and in both sides of the nose, may occur in large enough numbers and size to obstruct the airway.

Signs and symptoms—Patients usually complain of obstruction and "something" in the nose. They experience difficulty breathing and loss of smell. Diagnosis is made by visual observation through a nasal speculum or by X-rays of the nasal passages and the sinuses.

Etiology—They are thought to be related to prolonged mucous membrane edema associated with allergies, chronic sinusitis, rhinitis, and recurrent nasal infections.

Treatment—If infected, treatment with steroids and antibiotics will temporarily reduce the size of the **polyps**. However, surgical removal is the treatment of choice and is usually necessary.

Rhinitis (Allergic) (Ri-ni′-tis)

Description—Allergic rhinitis is a reaction to airborne allergens.

Signs and symptoms—It causes sneezing, profuse watery discharge, itching of the eyes and nose, conjunctivitis, and tearing. Many symptoms are the result of the body's attempt to dilute or remove irritants coming into contact with its mucous membranes.

Etiology—Any antigen occurring in the environment can be an irritant and cause allergic rhinitis. Some of the most common are dust, ragweed, pollens, and cat and dog dander.

Treatment—Treatment consists of eliminating environmental antigens when possible and the use of antihistamines and topical corticosteroids. Long-term management includes injections of the offending allergens to cause desensitization, the use of air conditioning, and, if severe and persistent, relocation to a safe environment.

THE TONGUE AND THE SENSE OF TASTE

The ability to taste flavors is located in the receptors of the taste buds on the tongue. They are located at the tip, sides, and back. Like the sense of smell, taste is possible because of the chemoreceptors that receive stimuli from ions or molecules and initiate the impulses. As with smell, taste is not possible unless the substance is moistened. This moisture is supplied by the salivary glands in sufficient quantities to affect taste.

DISEASES AND DISORDERS OF THE MOUTH AND TONGUE

Candidiasis (Kan-di-dia′-sis) (Thrush)

Description—This disease is a fungal infection of the mucous membranes of the mouth and throat. The organism can cause infection in other locations, such as nails, skin (diaper rash), vagina, and the gastrointestinal tract.

Signs and symptoms—Evidence of the disease is cream-colored or white patches of exudate on the tongue, mouth, or throat that cannot be scraped off. The infected areas may swell, causing respiratory distress in infants. Occasionally, they are painful, but they usually cause a burning sensation in the throat and mouth of adults.

Etiology—It is usually caused by a fungal organism of the *Candida* species. These organisms are normally present in the body but cause infection when their sudden growth is permitted by some change, such as an illness, a suppressed immune system, drug abuse, or from the use of broad-spectrum antibiotics that alters the body's normal flora, which permits candida to increase. Infants may acquire thrush during birth.

Treatment—Initial treatment is aimed at improving the underlying cause, then swabbing the mouth with an oral nystatin suspension or oral antifungal medication.

Note: If the mother is breast-feeding, she must also treat her nipples with an antifungal medication.

Glossitis (Gloss-i′-tis)

Description—Inflammation of the tongue.

Signs and symptoms—The condition results in a red, swollen tongue, pain on chewing, difficult speech, and occasionally an obstructed airway.

Etiology—It is caused by an organism, irritation, injury, or nutritional deficiencies. Agents such as tobacco, alcohol, spicy foods, and jagged teeth may cause glossitis.

Treatment—Treatment includes topical anesthetic mouthwash, systemic pain medication, good oral hygiene, and the avoidance of alcohol and hot, cold, or spicy foods.

Oral Cancer

Description—In recent years, a significant increase in the incidence of oral cancer has been noted. There seems to be evidence that some people have switched from cigarettes to smokeless forms of tobacco in an effort to avoid the development of lung cancer. Oral cancer is linked to alcohol and tobacco ingestion.

Signs and symptoms—Any lesion or growth within the mouth is not normal and should be examined by a physician or dentist. They can be of varying shapes and types and may present no evidence of pain or discomfort.

Etiology—No one knows for certain the exact cause for cancer, but there are strong correlations between substances and the development of malignant lesions. Normal cells are affected by something in their environment that causes their normal growth-limiting control to fail and excessive cell production to begin. The use of products such as chewing tobacco and snuff causes extensive disease of the gums, tongue, and other oral structures and often results in the development of cancer within the oral cavity.

Treatment—The use of surgical excision as a treatment depends upon the form of cancer developed. Quite disfiguring results arise from removal of part of the mouth, and often speech is affected when the tongue is involved. Chemotherapy and radiation are appropriate in selective cases.

THE SKIN AND THE SENSE OF TOUCH

The sense of touch requires direct contact with the body through contact receptors (Figure 25–14). The sense of touch involves mechanical energy, such as pressure or traction, which activates mechanoreceptors. Radiant energy, such as heat or cold, activates thermoreceptors. The design of the receptor varies with its location on the body. Touch receptors are most concentrated in the fingertips. Pain receptors are simply bare nerve endings in the skin and other organs. Separate skin receptors perceive heat and cold. Each of the contact receptors in the skin has its own perceptive function, enabling us to feel the many different sensations of pain, touch, pressure, heat, cold, traction, and tickle. This sense aids us in protecting ourselves, identifying injury, feeling pleasure, and maintaining contact with our environment. The skin is the subject of the next chapter.

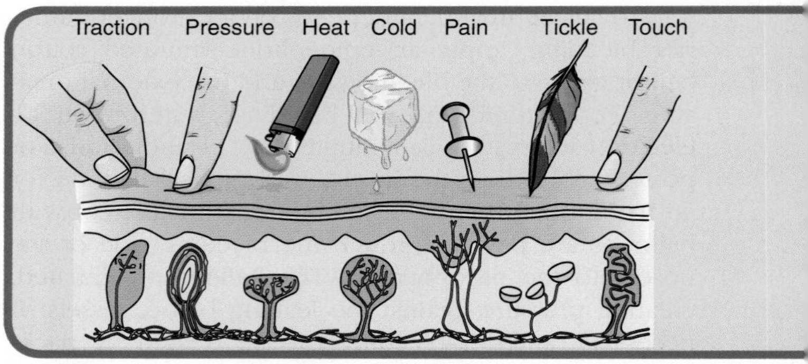

Figure 25–14: The sense of touch. *Delmar/Cengage Learning.*

AGE-RELATED BODY CHARACTERISTICS

There are many age-related conditions of the senses. Children tend to have myopia and have difficulty seeing clearly at a distance, but it may change by adulthood. Older people will develop presbyopia and cannot clearly see smaller print up close. Vision is also affected in older adults by atheriosclerosis and athrosclerosis due to the change in blood vessels. Cataracts and glaucoma are primarily diseases that develop with aging.

The sense of hearing also changes with age. Children normally have an acute hearing ability while the older adult may experience a gradual loss, perhaps to a point of needing a hearing aid in order to communicate. Young children commonly are affected by otitis media, especially infants, due to the anatomical structure of their Eustachian tubes.

Even the sense of touch and taste tends to be less acute in older persons. Many relate that things do not have as much taste as they formerly did. Because of the reduction in the sense of touch, older persons must be careful with handling hot items to prevent burns. Often numbness and tingling of the fingers make it difficult for the elderly to pick up small items and do some tasks. Injuries can occur without awareness until the evidence is seen.

System Interaction Associated with Disease Conditions

The senses are actually a part of the nervous system and allow the person to perceive and respond to his or her environment. As with all systems, the senses interact by way of the nerves with the muscles, blood vessels, digestive, respiratory and other systems. Table 25–1 summarizes the systems involved and the pathology present in an example of a disease of the senses.

TABLE 25–1 System Interaction Associated with Disease Conditions

Disease	System Involved	Pathology Present
Diabetic retinopathy	Nervous/senses	Blurred vision, floaters, decreased peripheral vision, neuropathy
	Circulatory	Retinal blood vessel changes, edema
	Endocrine	Hyperglycemia

CHAPTER SUMMARY

- Receptors enable the body to perceive its environment.
- Primary organs of the senses are the eyes, ears, nose, tongue, and the skin.
- The eyeball compares to a camera.
- The structure of the eye includes the sclera, six extraocular muscles, the choroid, retina, crystalline lens, ciliary body, the iris, pupil, cornea, conjunctiva, lacrimal glands, aqueous and vitreous humor.
- The retina is a multilayered nervous tissue with nerve cells called rods and cones.
- The path of light travels from the cornea through the aqueous humor, the pupil, the crystalline lens, the vitreous humor on to the retina.
- The eye refracts light onto the retina. If the retina is too short, it is myopia; if too long, it is hyperopia.
- The diseases of the eye are age-related macular degeneration, amblyopia, arcus senilis, blepharitis, cataract, conjunctivitis, corneal abrasion, corneal ulcer, diabetic retinopathy, glaucoma (open and closed angle), hordeolum, iritis, mopia, presbyopia, ptosis, retinal detachment, and strabismus.
- The outer ear consists of the auricle, auditory canal, and tympanic membrane.
- The middle ear carries sound waves to the malleus, incus, and stapes.
- The Eustachian tube connects the middle ear to the throat.
- The inner ear continues the vibrations through the cochlea and the organ of corti, to the temporal lobe of the cerebrum.
- Semicurcular canals maintain equilibrium.
- The videonystagmograph evaluates balance.
- Auditory canal can be obstructed causing a degree of hearing loss.
- Hearing loss can be sensorineural or presbycusis.
- Diseases and disorders of the ear include Ménière's disease, motion sickness, otitis externa and media, otosclerosis, and presbycusis.
- The nose has the olefactory organ, which is the sense of smell.
- Nasal diseases are epistaxis, polyps, and rhinitis.
- The tongue has taste buds that permit the sense of taste.
- Diseases of the mouth are candidiasis, glossitis, and oral cancer.
- The skin has seven different receptors to perceive the environment.

STUDY TOOLS

Workbook	Activities for Chapter 25
Premium Website	
MEDIA LINK	View this **Media Link** for Chapter 25: • Vision
StudyWARE	Activities and Quizzes on the **StudyWARE™ Software** for Chapter 25
	Audio Library of medical terms
	Online access to the **Critical Thinking Challenge 2.0**
CourseMate	Activities and Quizzes for Chapter 25
WebTutor	Activities and Quizzes for Chapter 25

CHECK YOUR KNOWLEDGE

1. The outside of the eye is covered with a tough membrane called the:
   a. retina.
   b. sclera.
   c. choroid.
   d. cornea.
2. When the ciliary body focuses the lens for near or far vision, it is known as:
   a. refraction.
   b. astigmatism.
   c. ciliary contraction.
   d. accommodation.
3. The amount of light entering the eye is controlled by the muscles of the:
   a. iris.
   b. cornea.
   c. lens.
   d. pupil.
4. The area of the retina where vision is sharpest is called the:
   a. optic disc.
   b. fovea centralis.
   c. vision receptor.
   d. myopia.
5. When a cataract develops,
   a. a grayish-white circle appears around the cornea.
   b. the lens becomes cloudy.
   c. the macula has thinned.
   d. the pupil dilates.
6. Glaucoma is the result of:
   a. improper drainage of the vitreous humor.
   b. increased pressure against the sclera.
   c. increased interocular pressure.
   d. excessive of blood supply to the eye.
7. The middle ear contains the:
   a. tympanic membrane, malleus, and stapes.
   b. cochlea, malleus, and incur.
   c. malleus, stapes, and semicircular canals.
   d. malleus, incus, and stapes.

8 Ménière's disease is characterized by:
   a. ringing in the ears and vertigo.
   b. pain and redness of the tympanic membrane.
   c. loss of hearing.
   d. motion sickness.

9. The most common cause of conductive deafness is:
   a. presbycusis.
   b. otitis media.
   c. tinnitus.
   d. otosclerosis.
10. Nasal polyps are:
   a. developed from infected hair follicles.
   b. benign growths in the nose.
   c. malignant growths in the nose.
   d. the main cause of nosebleeds.
11. Candidiasis:
   a. can lead to oral cancer.
   b. causes a red, swollen, and painful tongue.
   c. interferes with the sense of taste.
   d. causes cream-colored patches of exudate on the tongue.
12. Oral cancer may be caused by:
   a. use of alcohol and cigarettes.
   b. use of chewing tobacco and snuff and alcohol.
   c. eating spicy foods.
   d. the lack of vitamins C and E.
13. A trabeculoplasty:
   a. instills a tiny tube through the tympanic membrane.
   b. reshapes the trabecula of the eye.
   c. removes the lens of the eye.
   d. makes an opening to drain aqueous tumor.
14. The videonystagmograph diagnostic test:
   a. evaluates balance.
   b. determines the need for a hearing aid.
   c. measures the intraocular pressure.
   d. determines the strength of the impulse in the auditory nerve.
15. Diabetic retinopathy involves the:
   a. sense of vision and muscular system.
   b. sense of vision and urinary system.
   c. sense of vision and endocrine system.
   d. sense of vision and respiratory system.

WEB LINKS

The American Cancer Society, information about cancer of the organs of the senses: www.cancer.org

National Library of Medicine, discussion of aging changes in the senses: www.nlm.nih.gov/medlineplus/ency/article/004013.htm

Chapter

26 The Integumentary System

OBJECTIVES

In this chapter, you will learn the following:

KB LEARNING OBJECTIVES

1. Spell and define, using the glossary at the back of the text, all the Words to Know in this chapter.
2. List the five functions of the skin.
3. Explain how the skin regulates body temperature.
4. Describe how the body cools its surface.
5. Name the three layers of skin tissue and the characteristic structures of each layer.
6. Describe the process that causes wrinkles.
7. Explain what causes a suntan to develop.
8. Describe the distinguishing features of basal cell and squamous cell carcinoma lesions.
9. Identify the ABCDE rules and other warning signs of melanoma and the factors that contribute to its development.
10. Explain what causes blushing, birthmarks, moles, and albinism.
11. Identify 20 diseases or disorders of the skin.
12. Discuss how the skin changes with age.
13. Identify the body systems that interact with Lyme disease.

WORDS TO KNOW

acne
albino
alopecia
carbuncle
constrict
dermatitis
dermis
dilate
eczema
epidermis
erythema
follicle
folliculitis
furuncle
herpes simplex
herpes zoster
integumentary
keloid
lesion
Lyme disease
macule
melanin
melanocytes
papule
pediculosis
perception
pigment
psoriasis
pustule
receptors
sebaceous
sebum
slough
subcutaneous
transdermal
urticaria
verrucae
vesicle
viral shedding
wheals
whorl

THE INTEGUMENTARY SYSTEM

The word **integumentary** refers to an external covering or skin. You may never have thought of the skin as a "body system," but according to the definition of a system in Chapter 23, the skin with all its structures qualifies: it is many tissues (nerve, connective, muscle, epithelial), forming organs (sweat and oil glands), to perform a function. The skin is not usually listed as one of the body's systems, however. Most anatomists classify the skin as an organ. When listed in this category, it becomes the largest organ of the body. An average adult has about 3,000 square inches of skin surface. The skin makes up about 15% of the total body weight, which would be approximately 20 pounds of a 145-pound person. The skin varies in thickness from very thin on the eyelids to quite thick on the soles of the feet.

The skin is so important to survival that the loss of even a small percentage of its vital function is a cause for concern. If about one third of the skin of a healthy young adult is lost, death may result. Skin covers all the body's surface, preventing the tissue fluids from escaping and foreign materials in the environment from entering. At the openings to the body, such as the nose, mouth, or anus, it joins with the mucous membranes that line the openings into the respiratory and digestive systems to make a continuous internal and external covering.

FUNCTIONS

The skin performs five important functions for the body: protection, perception, temperature control, absorption, and excretion. The skin protects against the invasion of bacteria by serving as a barrier. It is effective, however, only as long as it remains intact. A cut or scrape of the surface allows bacteria to enter. It also protects the delicate underlying tissues from injury by the damaging rays of the sun. Equally important, it protects the body's tissues from loss of fluid. This is of great concern when large areas of skin are lost as a result of burns, for example, which allows fluids to escape and bacteria to enter.

The skin serves as an organ of **perception** in cooperation with the nervous system and the sense of touch. A square inch of skin contains about 72 feet of nerves and hundreds of **receptors** registering pain, heat, cold, and pressure.

In that same square inch are about 15 feet of blood vessels, which provide nutrients and oxygen and also regulate the body's temperature. This function is of such importance to the body that the skin receives approximately one third of the blood circulating throughout the body. When the body's temperature control center in the brain senses the body is becoming too warm, the nervous system sends messages to the surface vessels to **dilate**, which allows heat from the blood to escape through the skin's surface and therefore cool the body. If heat must be retained, the vessels are ordered to **constrict** to reduce the loss of heat so that body temperature can be maintained at an adequate level. This important function is discussed in greater detail in Chapter 38.

The skin also contains sweat glands, which are likewise controlled by the heat regulator in the brain. When the air temperature rises, the body produces sweat, which evaporates from its surface to provide a cooling effect and thereby reduce the amount of heat within the underlying blood vessels.

The skin is capable of absorbing some materials from its surface through the hair **follicles** and the glands. This function can be of use to the physician in treating certain conditions. Perhaps the two most common applications are anti-motion sickness medication in a patch form, which is placed on the skin's surface behind the ear, and in a medicated paste form, which is placed on the chest to treat certain heart conditions. A trend seems to be developing toward a greater amount of medications being administered through the skin. Primarily the advantages are "timed release," which spreads medication evenly over a long period, thereby eliminating repeated dosage and the digestive system side effects from certain oral drugs. This form of drug administration is called **transdermal**.

Several substances known as lipid-soluble (e.g., vitamins A, D, E, and K and the sex hormones) and almost all gases (e.g., oxygen, hydrogen, and nitrogen) can pass through the skin. It is interesting to note that carbon monoxide cannot pass.

The skin's function of excretion consists primarily of eliminating water and salt plus a minute amount of other waste products. Excessive fluid loss as a result of strenuous activity or a highly elevated temperature can be a matter of concern. Fluid must be replaced to maintain a proper fluid balance. The skin also combines the ultraviolet rays from sunlight with compounds normally present in the skin to produce vitamin D.

A great number of microscopic skin structures are located within an area of only 1 square centimeter. This is illustrated in Figure 26–1 as a small circle on the back of the hand. It seems inconceivable that this large group of anatomical structures could be located in such a small area. These microscopic wonders perform an invaluable service for the body.

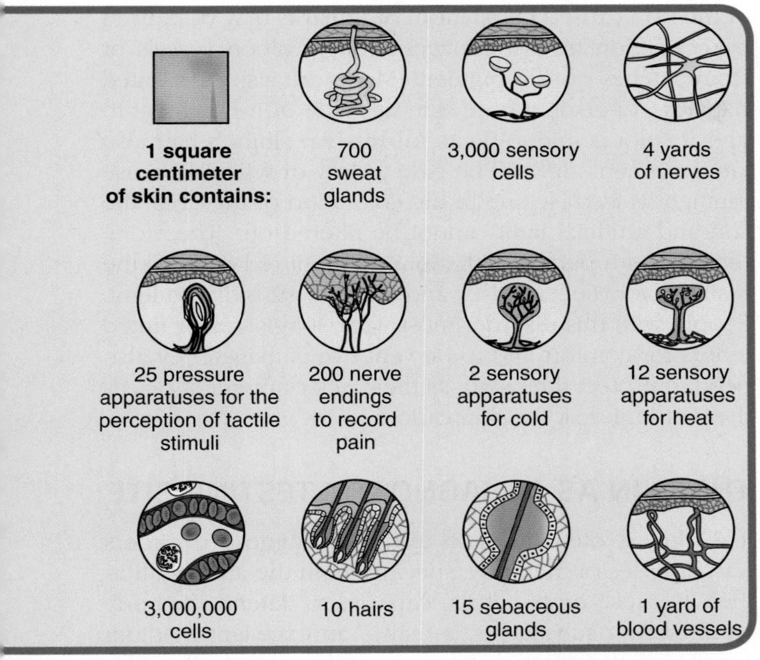

Figure 26–1: Structures of the skin. *Delmar/Cengage Learning.*

STRUCTURE OF THE SKIN

The skin is composed of three layers: the **epidermis** on the top, the **dermis** in the middle, and the **subcutaneous** layer on the bottom (Figure 26–2). The subcutaneous layer is filled with fat globules, blood vessels, and nerves. The dermis contains blood vessels, nerves, hair follicles, and sweat and oil glands. This layer is usually referred to as the "true skin." The top of the dermis is covered with cone-shaped papillae, which create an uneven surface. The epidermis is full of ridges that fit snugly over the papillae on top of the dermis. These ridges form the **whorls** and patterns on the fingertips that we call fingerprints. Because no two people have exactly the same pattern of ridges, they will not have the same fingerprints, making this characteristic a suitable means of identification. Similar patterns of ridges appear on the soles of the feet and are used for identification of newborns. New cells are formed deep in the epidermis. Here rapid cell division pushes cells toward the surface of the skin to replace those that wear away, die, and flake off. The process from division to flaking off takes about 28 to 60 days. Because of the skin's ability to reproduce cells rapidly, it can repair itself quickly following cuts and abrasions.

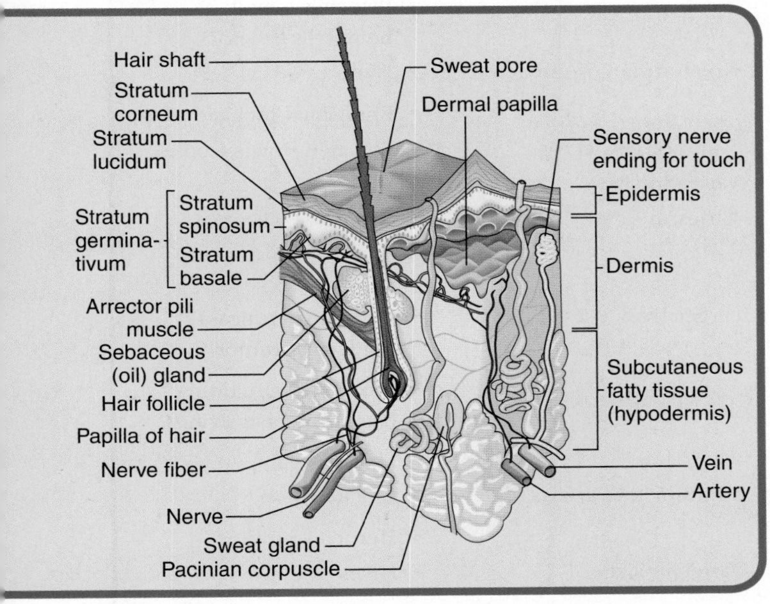

Figure 26–2: Cross-section of skin. *Delmar/Cengage Learning.*

The skin is strong, soft, flexible, and elastic in young people because of the presence of keratin in the epidermis and collagen fibers in the dermis. With age, elastic fibers in the dermis increase in size, and collagen in the dermis degenerates. The support for the epidermis is decreased, and as a result, wrinkles occur. This is especially noticeable in areas where there is more facial movement, such as around the eyes and mouth.

The skin has four appendages. These are the sweat glands, oil glands, hair, and nails. The dermis contains the sweat and **sebaceous** (oil) glands. Sweat glands are tiny coiled tubes deep in the dermis and corkscrew tubules leading to the surface. Oil glands are located in or near hair follicles over the entire skin surface, except for the palms of the hands and the soles of the feet.

A sebaceous gland produces an oily substance that helps prevent the hair and skin from becoming dry and brittle. Unfortunately, oil glands often become plugged by cell overgrowth. The gland continues to produce oil, which fills the duct and results in development of a blackhead or pimple. This results in a condition known as **acne**.

Every hair has a root, which is inside a follicle (shaft) that extends deep into the dermal layer. With long hair, the root extends into the subcutaneous layer. Attached to each follicle is a small involuntary muscle. With certain emotions or sensations of coldness, the muscle contracts, causing the hair to stand erect and producing what we call "goose flesh." An inner layer of cells in the shaft of hair contains a **pigment** that gives the hair its color. Hair that is white has cells that contain little pigment.

The hair and nails are composed of hard keratin (soft keratin is found in the epidermis). The keratins are similar, but the hard keratin is more permanent and does not **slough** (drop) off, which means they must be cut occasionally.

MEDIA LINK

Go to the Premium Website and watch the animation, "The Skin," for this chapter.

Skin Color

A brown-black pigment called **melanin** is produced by cells called *melanocytes,* which are present in the epidermis. They protect the underlying tissues from damage by the sun. The amount of melanin affects the color of the skin, as does another pigment, carotene, which is yellow. In light-skinned people, melanin is found at the bottom of the epidermis. In people with darker skin, it is found throughout the epidermis. The presence of blood vessels in the dermis also contributes to the coloration of the skin. When the skin is exposed to the sun, it may become reddened because of dilation of the superficial blood vessels. The condition is known medically as **erythema**, but it is commonly known as sunburn. If it is not severe, the skin will acquire a brown coloration or suntan, which is produced by the melanin pigment increasing and moving to the surface to protect the underlying tissues. New melanin will replace the old in the lower cell layer. Freckles are actually small areas of melanin pigment.

Skin coloration is affected by many factors. When we blush, the rich supply of blood vessels causes reddening of the skin caused by dilation. Birthmarks may be caused by coloration from a concentration of blood vessels or from patches of skin pigment. Moles are also pigmented patches. A person whose skin has little or no pigment to give it color is said to be an **albino**. An albino's hair also lacks pigment and will be pale yellow or white. Because pigment is also lacking in the coloration of the eyes, the sun and artificial light cannot be filtered out. Therefore, the eyes of a person with albinism are a red color as the result of translucent irises and are very sensitive to light. People with this disorder must wear sunglasses or tinted lenses for comfort and to prevent eye damage.They also need to protect their skin, as their lack of pigment places them at high risk for skin cancer.

THE SKIN AS A DIAGNOSTIC TESTING SITE

The skin is often used to test and diagnose disorders and diseases of the body, specifically in the area of allergies. Because of its natural capacity to defend the body from foreign substances, it makes an excellent medium for testing the reaction to minute amounts of allergens.

TABLE 26–1 Types of Skin Lesions, Their Characteristics, Size, and Examples

Type of Skin Lesion	Characteristics	Size	Example
Bulla (blister)	Fluid-filled area	Greater than 5 mm across	• A large blister
Crust	A collection of dried serum and debris	Varies in size	• Impetigo or eczema
Excoriation	Area missing the epidermal layer	Varies in size	• Scrape or burn
Fissure	Linear crack from epidermis to dermis	Varies in size	• Athlete's feet, hand dermatitis
Macule	A round, flat area usually distinguished from its surrounding skin by its change in color	Smaller than 1 cm	• Freckle • Petechia (small hemorrhage spot)
Nodule	Elevated solid area, deeper and firmer than a papule	Greater than 5 mm across	• Wart • Epidermal inclusion cyst
Papule	Elevated solid area	5 mm or less across	• Elevated nevus (mole)
Pustule	Discrete, pus-filled raised area	Varies in size	• Acne
Ulcer	A deep loss of skin surface that may extend into the dermis that can bleed periodically and scar	Varies in size	• Venous stasis ulcer
Tumor	Solid mass of cells that may extend deep through cutaneous tissue	Larger than 1–2 cm	• Benign (harmless) epidermal tumor • Basal cell carcinoma (rarely metastasizing) • Lipoma
Vesicle	Fluid-filled raised area	5 mm or less across	• Chickenpox • Herpes simplex
Wheal	Itchy, temporarily elevated area with an irregular shape formed as a result of localized skin edema	Varies in size	• Hives • Insect bites

Following injection of common substances, usually on the patient's back or the inner surface of the forearm, the skin will form various-sized areas around the injection sites, reacting to those materials that initiate an allergic response. Besides injecting allergens, the skin can also be used for patch tests. Tiny amounts of allergens are placed on stainless steel discs and applied to the back. Forty-eight hours later the skin under the discs is assessed for reaction. Based upon these findings, physicians can then identify causative substances and recommend measures to reduce the problems associated with the allergic disorder. (See Chapter 45).

Skin Appearance

Conditions of the skin cause changes in its appearance. These changes are known as **lesions** and manifest themselves as specific eruptions. Table 26–1 identifies the most common types of lesions.

DISEASES AND DISORDERS

Acne Vulgaris (Ak′ne Vul-gar′is)

Description—This inflammatory disease of the follicles of the sebaceous glands mainly affects adolescents.

Signs and symptoms—The acne may appear as a closed comedo or whitehead if it does not protrude from the follicle and is covered by the epidermis. If it protrudes and has black coloration caused by the melanin or pigment from the follicle, it is known as a blackhead or open comedo. Eventually, the enlarged plug leaks or ruptures, spreading into the dermis and resulting in inflammation and the development of pustules and **papules**.

Etiology—The cause is multifactorial (many factors). Research has determined that dietary habits appear to be less of a factor than originally thought. Present findings seem to suggest that hormonal dysfunction and an oversupply of **sebum**, oil from the sebaceous glands, are the probable underlying causes. It collects at the openings to the glands, hardens, and closes off the natural flow of oily secretion, causing blackheads or cysts to develop. Sometimes the area will become filled with leukocytes that cause pus to accumulate and pimples develop. Trapped bacteria within the follicle are also a contributing factor.

Treatment—Usual treatment for severe acne includes a topical antibacterial product either alone or in combination with a topical retinoid product. Antibiotics applied to the skin are helpful. Systemic antibiotics decrease bacterial growth within follicles. Isotretinoin (Accutane) is reserved for use in those patients with severe scarring acne. Oral contraceptives are used in women.

Alopecia (Al-o-pe′she-a)

Description—This is loss of hair, usually occurring on the scalp. There are two types of **alopecia**: a scarring type, which causes irreversible hair loss, and a nonscarring type, which usually is reversible.

Scarring Alopecia

Signs and symptoms—The main symptom is the continous loss of hair, resulting in gradual thinning and the eventual absence of hair.

Etiology—This is usually an irreversible loss of hair resulting from the destruction of the hair follicles. It is caused by chronic inflammation or chemical trauma or the chronic tension on the hair shaft from braiding or tight rolling of the hair. Certain diseases like lupus erythematosus, bacterial or viral infections, and skin tumors may also cause this type.

Treatment—This depends upon the cause. A change in the way the hair is cared for and the control of infection could prevent further loss but may not restore lost follicles.

Nonscarring Alopecia (Several Forms)

Male-pattern baldness

Signs and symptoms—The most common form of nonscarring alopecia is the evidence of hair loss with male-pattern baldness. It often begins around age 30 with a receding front hairline and loss of hair on the top and back. In some men, the areas eventually meet, leaving hair only on the sides (Figures 26–3).

Etiology—It seems to be primarily caused by aging and the level of androgen (male hormone). There is a tendency for genetic influence, and it will often be displayed among male family members. Women may also exhibit the male pattern but at a lesser degree.

Treatment—There is no known "cure"; however, the use of minoxidil (Rogaine) and finasteride (Propecia)

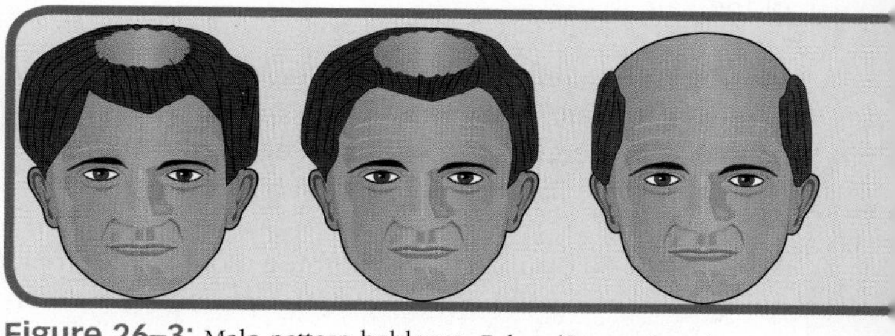

Figure 26–3: Male-pattern baldness. *Delmar/Cengage Learning.*

seems to prevent further loss and encourage regrowth in some men. Surgical grafting of hair follicles from other parts of the scalp have proved successful.

Physiologic

Signs and symptoms—A normal temporary hair loss that may occur immediately following or up to four months after giving birth.

Etiology—Prolongation of the growing phase.

Treatment—None required.

Areata (idiopathic)

Signs and symptoms—This type is mostly self-limiting and reversible, occurring among both sexes from young to middle-age adults. It usually causes small patches but can involve the entire scalp and body.

Etiology—Unknown, but some feel it may be linked to stress and changes in the immune system.

Treatment—None. Regrowth is normally spontaneous. Solutions and local injections of triamcinolone (Kenalog) as well as topical steroid creams may also be used.

Trichotillomania

Signs and symptoms—This hair loss is characterized by patchy, incomplete areas of hair loss with many broken hairs, primarily on the scalp, but can also involve other areas, such as the eyebrows. It is more common in children.

Etiology—This loss is the result of it being pulled out or twisted because of compulsive behavior.

Treatment—Some form of psychotherapy may be necessary. Dressings over the areas aid in behavior change to encourage normal growth.

Chemotherapy related

Signs and symptoms—There is a sudden loss of most of the hair.

Etiology—Certain chemical agents destroy the cells of the hair, which result in the massive loss of hair over a two- or three-day period soon after the initiation of the drug. Normally, some fine hair will remain but is very sparse.

Treatment—Fortunately, about three months after treatments end, hair will begin regrowth, sometimes a different color or texture.

Cancer

Description—The skin may be the site of different forms of cancerous lesions, such as basal cell carcinomas, squamous cell carcinomas, and malignant melanomas. Nevi (moles) are considered to be potentially malignant and require careful observation.

Signs and symptoms—Bleeding; itching; or a change in color, size, shape, or texture of a mole suggests a possible conversion to a malignant state. A new, nonhealing lesion that bleeds easily should also raise suspicion.

Basal Cell Carcinoma

This is a slow-growing, locally destructive skin tumor. They occur where there are abundant sebaceous follicles, especially on the face. It is more prevalent in persons over the age of 40, especially those who are blond, blue-eyed, and fair skinned. It is the most common malignant tumor affecting Caucasians. There are basically three types of basal cell carcinoma lesions, each with its own distinctive characteristics and usual location. They are diagnosed by appearance and surgical biopsy.

1. *Nodulo-ulcerative* lesions occur most often on the face and are small, smooth, pinkish, and translucent papules. As they enlarge, the centers become depressed and the borders elevated and firm.
2. *Superficial* basal cell carcinomas are often multiple and commonly occur on the chest and back. They are oval or irregularly shaped with sharply defined, threadlike borders that are slightly elevated.
3. *Sclerosing* basal cell lesions occur on the head and neck. They appear yellow to white, are waxy, and do not have distinct borders.

Etiology—Basal cell carcinoma is caused primarily by prolonged exposure to the sun.

Treatment—Treatment depends upon the extent of the lesion. It can include surgical excision, irradiation, chemosurgery, or curretage and electrodesiccation.

Squamous Cell Carcinoma (Skwa′-mus)

Description—This is an invasive tumor with metastatic potential. Its incidence is highest in fair-skinned Caucasian males over the age of 60. Living in sunny climates, working in outdoor employment, and smoking greatly increase the risk of development.

Signs and symptoms—This form of carcinoma is commonly found on the face, the ears, the back of the hands, and other sun-damaged areas. The lesions rarely metastasize, with those located on unexposed skin having the greater incidence. Lesions of the lower lip and ears are more likely to metastasize (Figure 26–4).

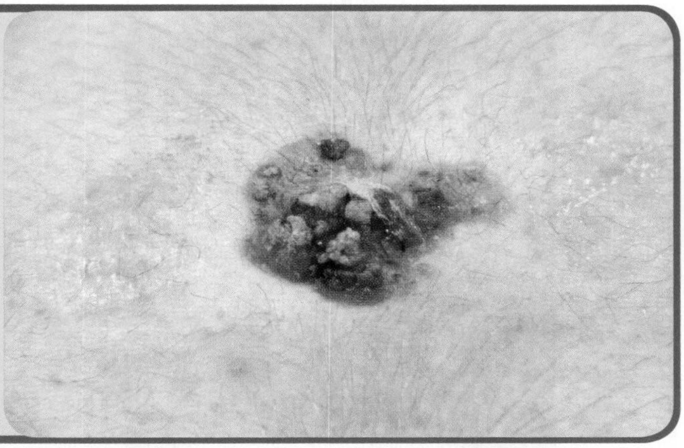

Figure 26–4: Squamous cell carcinoma. *CDC/Bob Craig.*

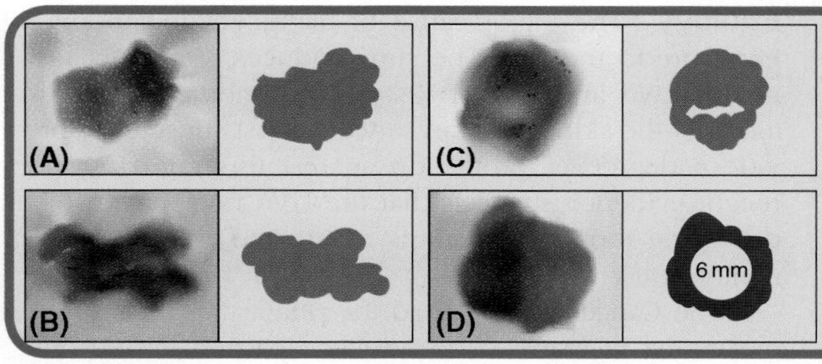

Figure 26–5: The signs of melanoma: (A) asymmetry; (B) border irregularity; (C) color; (D) diameter. See Table 26-2. *Delmar/Cengage Learning.*

Etiology—This type is predisposed by sunlight, the presence of premalignant lesions, X-ray therapy, environmental carcinogens, and chronic skin irritation.

Treatment—The treatment varies with the size, location, and invasiveness of the lesion. Options include wide surgical excision, scraping and electrodesiccation, radiation, and chemosurgery.

Malignant Melanoma (Ma-lig′-nant Mela-no′ma)

Description—A neoplasm that develops from the pigment-producing **melanocytes**. The peak of incidence occurs between 50 and 70 years of age. The incidence is more common in women. There are four clinical types: superficial spreading melanoma, nodular melanoma, lentigo maligna melanoma, and acral lentiginous melanoma. Superficial lesions may be curable with wide local excision. Deeper lesions may metastasize through the lymphatic and circulatory systems. Prognosis depends on the depth of the lesion, as measured in millimeters by the pathologist.

The American Cancer Society releases facts about the incidence of malignant melanoma. In 1993, 32,000 people were diagnosed; about 6,500 died. This translated into a lifetime risk of 1 in every 105 United States residents (compared with only 1 in every 1,500 in 1935). The lifetime risk of developing melanoma is now about 1 in every 50 people for white people, 1 in 1000 for African Americans, and 1 in 200 for Hispanics. The rate has gone down since 1990 for people younger than 50; however, it has remained stable or increased for those over 50. The American Academy of Dermatology views this prevalence as an undeclared epidemic. The American Cancer Society, in its most recent release, estimated that there would be 68,720 new cases and 8,650 deaths in 2009.

Signs and symptoms—The information and photos in Figure 26–5 and Table 26–2 shows the appearance signs of melanoma.

TABLE 26-2 Ordinary Moles versus Melanoma

	Ordinary Mole	Melanoma
Shape	Symmetrical, round, or oval	**Asymmetrical**—one side does not match the other (Figure 26–5A)
Border	Sharply defined **borders**	Edges are irregular ragged, notched, or blurred (Figure 26–5B)
Color	Evenly **colored** brown, tan, or black	Varies from one area to another; shades of brown, tan, and black. May also have shades of red, white, or blue (Figure 26–5C)
Diameter	Generally less than 6 mm in diameter	Usually greater than 6 mm in **diameter** (Figure 26–5D)
Development	Once developed, remains the same size, shape, and color. Moles may fade with age.	**Evolving.** The surface of a mole may change to be scaly, oozing, or bleeding. A bump may appear. Pigmentation may spread past the mole border into the surrounding skin, and redness or swelling may occur. The mole may itch, swell, and feel tender. The person may even experience pain.

Adapted from The American Academy of Dermatology.

Etiology—The major cause of malignant melanoma is exposure to the sun. The sun produces ultraviolet rays, mainly UVA and UVB. UVBs cause sunburn, premature aging of the skin, and skin cancers. Most sunscreens provide a degree of protection against this ray. However, recent evidence suggests that the UVA rays may also be damaging the skin, perhaps aiding the cancer-forming ability of UVB.

The Cancer Society cited the primary reasons for the melanoma increase to be weekend-packed leisure time, which results in intense bursts of exposure to UVB; the loss of the ozone layer protection; UVA rays not being blocked by sunscreens; and the tendency of people to purposely lie flat in the sun for hours at a time, which allows deeper penetration of the rays. People most at risk are those who have had severe blistering sunburns prior to age 20.

Other contributing factors are blond or red hair, fair skin, blue eyes, and a tendency to sunburn. Persons who work or spend many hours outdoors or who live in places with intense year-round sunshine are also at risk. Arizona has the highest incidence reported in the United States.

Treatment—Surgical resection is always required with a melanoma. If it is deep, the resection is at least 1 cm beyond the primary lesion's borders and into the deep tissues. Closure often requires a skin graft. Large lesions may also require chemotherapy. If there is metastasis, radiation may be used to relieve pain, but it will not prolong survival.

The best treatment for melanoma is prevention. Skin cancer is preventable. Sun avoidance is the best defense.

Dermatologists recommend avoiding sun altogether from 10:00 AM to 3:00 PM (perhaps from 8:00 AM to 6:00 PM if the ozone condition worsens), and using a sunscreen of at least 30 SPF that will block both UVA and UVB during exposure. Sunlamps, tanning pills, and tanning salons should be avoided.

The practice of monthly self-examination should be established to observe for any developing lesion so that it can be caught in the early stages. While standing in a brightly lit room in front of a full-length mirror and using a hand mirror, completely examine the body. Check under arms, on backs of legs, on feet, and between toes. Examine the back of the neck, and part the hair to check the scalp. If any growth, mole, sore, or discoloration appears suddenly or begins to change, it needs to be seen by a physician.

Cellulitis (Sel-u-li′-tis)

Description—The acute diffuse or spreading inflammation of the skin and subcutaneous tissue.

Signs and symptoms—It is characterized by localized swelling, pain, heat, and redness (Figure 26–6).

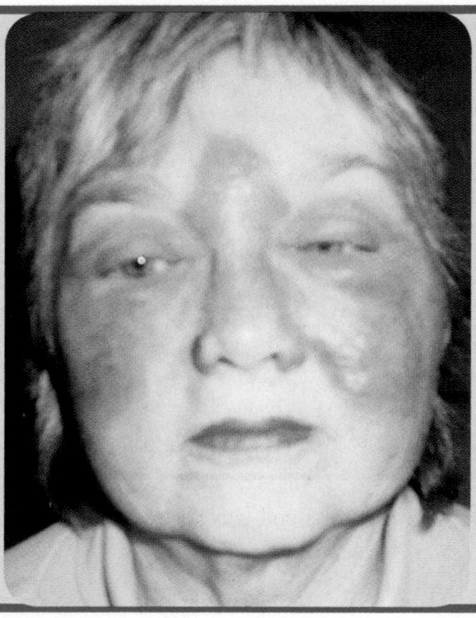

Figure 26–6: Cellulitis. *Delmar/Cengage Learning.*

Etiology—The cause of cellulitis is usually the *Streptococcus* or *Staphylococcus aureus* bacteria. It is potentially dangerous and may be deadly. There are antibiotic-resistant strains that require prompt treatment. Methicillin-resistant *Staphlococus aureus* (MRSA) is one of these antibiotic-resistant strains that produce serious wounds and ulcers and poses the risk of sepsis.

Treatment—It is usually treated successfully with oral antibiotics if diagnosed early. Severe cases require hospitalization and IV antibiotics.

Dermatitis (Der-ma-ti′-tis)

Description—The term means inflammation of the skin and can refer to any form of skin condition such as seborrhea, eczema, contact **dermatitis** (from irritants), allergic contact dermatitis (from allergens), exfoliative dermatitis (large pieces of peeling skin), or stasis (from lack of blood supply).

Signs and symptoms—Common symptoms are dry skin, redness, itching, edema, formation of lesions, and scaling.

Etiology—Dermatitis is often caused by allergens, such as wool; detergent; cosmetics; pollen; or foods, such as eggs, milk, seafood, or wheat products. Irritants to the skin; lack of moisture in the environment; harsh soaps; and long, hot showers also contribute to dermatitis and inherited skin conditions like eczema.

Treatment—It is treated by avoiding known allergens and irritants; using emollients, hydrocortisone creams and ointments, systemic steroids, and antihistamines; and taking other dermatitis-specific measures.

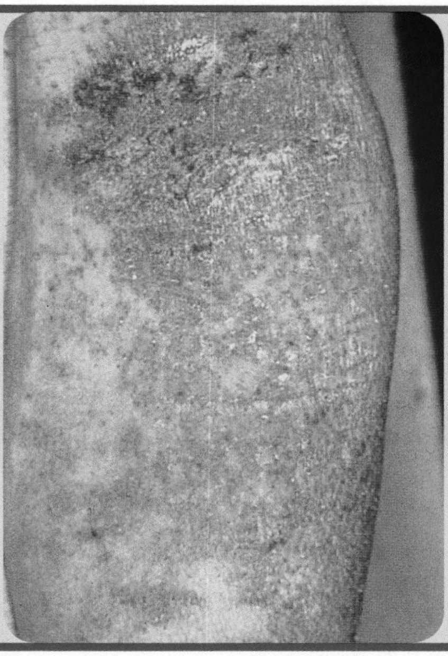

Figure 26–7: Eczema. *Courtesy of the Centers for Disease Control and Prevention, Atlanta, GA.*

Eczema (Ek′-ze-ma)

Description—This noncontagious dermatitis that can be acute or chronic. Some forms of eczema are inherited. It can also be associated with environmental allergies or asthma.

Signs and symptoms—This condition is characterized by dry, red, itchy, and scaly skin. There may be the presence of a watery discharge if it becomes chronic (Figure 26–7).

Etiology—Several things may initiate **eczema**, such as diet, cosmetics, clothing, medications, soaps, occupational or environmental substances, and emotional stress.

Treatment—Treatment consists primarily of removal of the causative agent where possible and the local application of ointments to alleviate the symptoms. Topical steroids are indicated to reduce inflammation, and antibiotics are used if secondary infection is present. The noncortisone cream tacrolimus (Protopic) and pimecrolimus (Elidel) are effective remedies considered relatively safe to use long term. This and other eczema medications are available by prescription only.

Folliculitis (Fo-lik-u-li′tis)

Description—**Folliculitis** is an infection of the hair follicle with the formation of a pustule. It can be of a superficial form, involving only the surface area around a single follicle, or deep, involving the total hair follicle.

Signs and symptoms—The presence of redness and pustules around a single follicle on the scalp, arms, and legs, and on the face of bearded men.

Etiology—The most common cause is *Staphylococcus aureus.*

Treatment—Treatment consists of thorough cleansing of the area, the application of moist heat to promote drainage from the lesion, and the use of topical antibiotics. Systemic antibiotics are usually indicated in severe cases.

Furuncles (Fu′rung-kls)

Description—Folliculitis may lead to the development of **furuncles** (boils).

Signs and symptoms—They are hard, painful nodules that enlarge over several days' time until they rupture, releasing pus and dead cells through one draining point. The area remains red and swollen for a short time, but the pain lessens.

Etiology—Furuncles may be caused by irritation, pressure, friction, or infection with *Staphylococcus aureus.*

Treatment—Treatment consists of the measures used for folliculitis with moist heat to relieve pain and encourage "ripening" of the lesion. Often, incision and drainage are required to allow complete expulsion of the purulent material. Patients must be cautioned not to squeeze a boil because it may rupture into the surrounding tissues. Systemic antibiotics are necessary if there is surrounding erythema or a fever. A patient with recurring furuncles should see a physician to rule out any underlying cause, such as diabetes.

Carbuncles (Kar′-bung-kls)

Description—A **carbuncle** begins as a nodule, then enlarges to involve several adjacent hair follicles.

Signs and symptoms—It is characterized by deep follicular abscesses of several follicles with multiple draining points. It is extremely painful and usually associated with fever and general malaise.

Etiology—Usually caused by a persistent staphylococcal infection and often follows a furuncle.

Treatment—Carbuncles require treatment with systemic antibiotics in addition to the localized heat applications and drainage. Washcloths, towels, bed sheets, and clothing used by the infected person must not be shared with other family members to prevent spreading the bacteria.

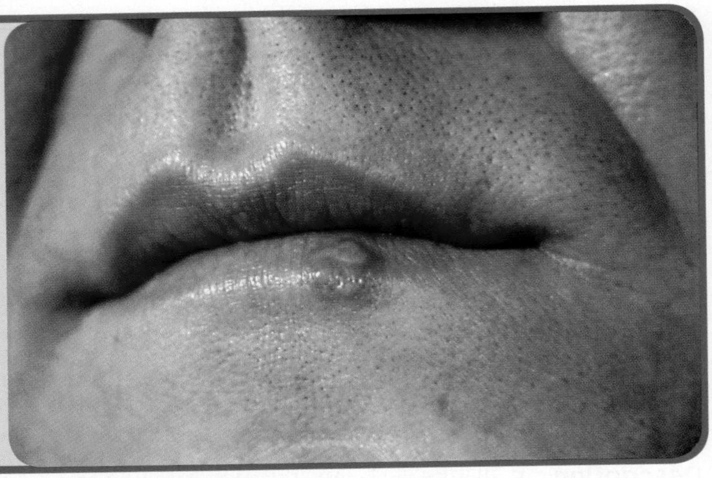

Figure 26–8: Herpes simplex of the lower lip. *CDC/Dr. K.L. Hermann.*

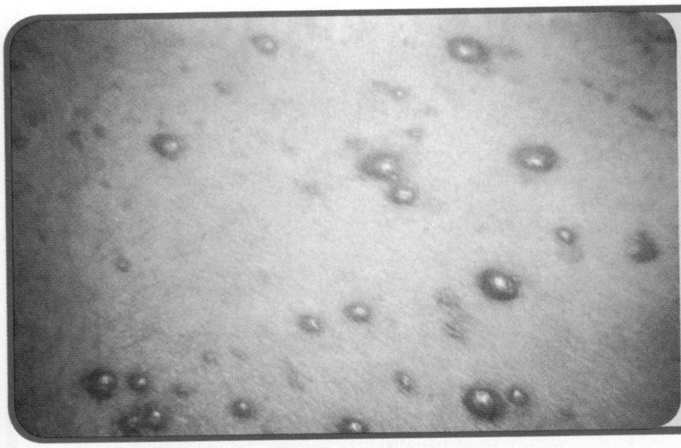

Figure 26–9: Herpes Zoster (shingles). *CDC/Dr. K.L. Hermann.*

Herpes Simplex (Her′-pez)

Description—This viral infection is equally prevalent among males and females and occurs throughout the world. **Herpes simplex** I is most often associated with lesions in the oral and nasal area. Herpes simplex II is associated with genital lesions. The incubation period following exposure is from four to 10 days. A prodrome (symptom of approaching disease) of pain, tingling, and itching signals the oncoming **vesicle**.

Signs and symptoms—The presence of small, grouped, painful, clear vesicles on an erythematous base (Figure 26–8).

Etiology—It is caused by the herpes virus.

Treatment—The most effective treatment is an oral antiviral medication. It has shown some decrease in pain and new lesion formation and a shortened period of viral shedding and healing time. Some relief from minor outbreaks may occur with the application of various over-the-counter topical preparations.

(*Note:* The term **viral shedding** refers to that period of time when a virus is the most active and most contagious.)

Herpes Zoster (Her′-pez Zos′-ter)

Description—**Herpes zoster** is an acute infectious process also known as shingles (Figure 26–9).

Signs and symptoms—It causes severe neuralgic pain along the area of the involved nerves. It is characterized by fever, malaise, and the eruption of vesicles in the painful area, which spread unilaterally around the back, chest, or back of neck or vertically on the extremities. (See Chapter 24.)

Etiology—It is caused by the varicella zoster virus, which also causes chickenpox.

Treatment—Usually the patient requires an analgesic and antipyretic to reduce fever and relieve pain. Antiviral drugs decrease acute pain, new lesion formation, viral shedding, healing time, and rates of dissemination (spreading), and incidence of post-herpetic pain.

Hirsutism (Hur′-sut-izm)

Description—This disorder usually appears in women and children. Excessive body hair develops in an adult male pattern of growth.

Signs and symptoms—The most common symptom is growth of facial hair, but other masculinization signs, such as deepening voice, increased muscle mass, menstrual irregularity, and breast size reduction, may be exhibited.

Etiology—There may be a family history of the disorder, or it could be related to an endocrine problem resulting from either pituitary dysfunction, ovarian lesions, or adrenal gland enlargement.

Treatment—Treatment consists of hair removal by shaving, depilatory creams, or waxing as well as bleaching to minimize the appearance of hair. Electrolysis will permanently destroy the hair follicles but is slow and expensive. Laser hair removal may be effective. A new topical cream is available to treat increased hair growth on the face. If hormonal causes are evident, treatment may involve counteracting or controlling endocrine secretions in specific situations.

Referral of female children to an endocrinologist is necessary to reduce or prevent masculinization and encourage appropriate sexual development.

Impetigo (Im-pe-ti′go)

Description—This is a contagious, superficial skin infection that is usually seen in young children.

Signs and symptoms—If the cause is streptococcal, the small red **macule** (flat area with definite edges) turns into a vesicle (raised lesion containing serous fluid) and then to a **pustule** (lesion with purulent material) within a relatively short time. (The terms macule, vesicle, and pustule refer to any skin lesion that demonstrates these descriptive characteristics, not just impetigo alone.) When the lesions break, a characteristic yellow crust develops from the exudate (drainage). Other sites develop from contact with the lesions or the drainage. The staph lesion is characterized by a thin-walled vesicle that forms a thin, clear crust from the exudate. Both forms characteristically have a clear central area and definite outer rims. The lesions appear primarily on the face, neck, and other exposed areas of the body. Contamination of others is prevented by avoiding contact through washcloths, towels, and bed linens. Scratching of the lesions must be prohibited.

Etiology—It is caused by *Streptococcus* or *Staphylococcus aureus* bacteria.

Treatment—Good hygiene is essential. The exudate can be removed by washing with soap and water two to three times a day. An oral systemic plus a topical antibiotic is indicated.

Keloid

A scar that developed excess dense tissue as it progressed through the healing process is known as a **keloid**. Excessive keloiding may require surgical revision by a plastie surgeon.

Lyme Disease (Lime)

Description—A tick-borne disease named after Old Lyme, Connecticut, where it was first reported in 1975. It has since been reported in 45 states, but over 90% of the cases occur within distinct areas: the East Coast from Massachusetts to Maryland, the upper midwest, the South and Southeast, and northern California and Oregon. Incidence is increasing dramatically. In 1986, only 700 cases were reported. In 1988, there were 5,000 reported. In 1994, New York alone reported 3,098 new cases. The most recent incidence reports issued for 2008 showed 28,921 confirmed and 6,277 probable cases. This was a 5% increase over the number of cases reported in 2007. The disease is spreading primarily because people are moving into suburban and rural areas, and the explosive deer population is moving into habitated areas. Both humans and pets can become infected. *Note:* If you live or work in one of the high-incidence areas, find out more about Lyme disease.

Signs and symptoms—The early stage of **Lyme disease** is usually marked by flu-like symptoms: fatigue, chills, fever, headache, muscle and joint pain, and swollen lymph nodes. In 60% of the cases, there is a characteristic circular, red skin lesion caused by the spirochete (corkscrew-shaped bacterium) migrating through the skin in all directions. This can appear from three days to one month after a bite. It enlarges to as much as several inches across and develops a clear center, giving it the appearance of a bull's eye; hence the name, "bull's eye rash" (Figure 26–10). Diagnosis is difficult in the remaining 40% who do not develop the rash and therefore may not get diagnosed and treated early. Their first symptoms are usually arthritis, fatigue, and memory loss. Later, nervous system symptoms develop. These may include numbness and pain, Bell's palsy, poor motor coordination, insomnia, irritability, heart arrythmia, headaches, and depression.

Etiology—Lyme disease is caused primarily by the bite of a spirochete-infested deer tick. It is an unusual three-host tick with a two-year life cycle. It begins when adult

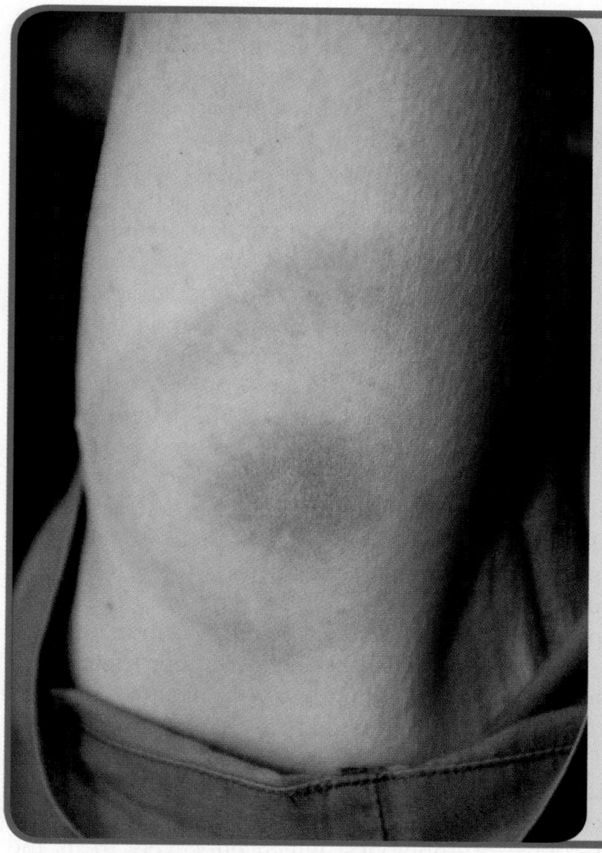

Figure 26–10: A rash in the pattern of a "bull's eye" is a sign of Lyme disease. *CDC/James Gathany.*

ticks feed and mate on deer and then drop off to lay eggs. The eggs hatch and the young ticks, called nymphs, attach and feed on small rodents that carry the spirochete and infect the tick. The mice carry the nymphs through the woods and fields and into human habitats: the grass, shrubs, wood piles, garages, and homes. From contact they attach and feed on dogs, squirrels, and humans. Bites seem to occur most often between May and September. The tick, in its unfed state, is about the size of a pinhead. It looks like a pear-shaped crab and has eight legs. Ticks insert their barbed mouth parts into the skin, deposit spirochetes, suck blood until satisfied (usually two to four days), and then drop off. The longer a tick feeds, the larger it becomes and the greater the chance for infection. If the tick is removed before the first 24 hours, infection is unlikely. (Not all ticks carry the spirochete; approximately 30% to 60% of northeastern ticks test positive.)

Treatment—The best treatment is prevention. Avoid tick-infected areas especially from May through September. Dress in light-colored clothing to make ticks more visible—they are not easily seen. Long sleeves and long pants tucked into light-colored socks or boots are highly recommended. Spray clothing with a tick repellent, and allow to dry before wearing. Applying a repellent containing up to 30% DEET directly to the skin (according to directions) is advisable for adults but unsafe for children because of its chemical composition. Check your entire body at the end of the day, paying particular attention to ankles, knees (especially backs), groin, armpits, under breasts, scalp, ears, and the back. Check all pets *before* bringing them into the house. *Do not* let pets sleep in or on the bed. Before washing, put outdoor clothing in the clothes dryer on the highest temperature for 30 minutes to kill hiding ticks. They can survive laundering.

If a deer tick is found, remove it and show it to a doctor, or send it to health authorities for positive identification. (See "How to Remove a Tick.") Its size is important because it is evidence of the length of time attached. Ticks that are to be tested should be put in a clean glass container and placed in the refrigerator until they are sent to health authorities. Results take about two weeks. Ticks, dead or alive, can be tested using a polymerase chain reaction test that detects the DNA of the spirochete, which will identify the type of tick, confirm the spirochete's presence, and therefore determine treatment. If identification can be made without testing, dispose of the tick by dropping it in 70% alcohol or diluted bleach. Do not "treat" ticks that are going to be tested.

If symptoms or a positive test result indicate Lyme disease, a course of antibiotics are prescribed for three weeks, with one week off, and then another three-week course of antibiotics, which effectively treats the infection. If diagnosis is not made until later-stage disease, then other systemic conditions require treatment in addition to antibiotics. Recent discovery of a specific antibody in patients with the disease may lead to immediate diagnosis and earlier treatment. Current blood tests are not conclusive. Dogs, cats, cattle, and horses can also become infected and treated with antibiotics if detected early. Prevention in dogs is possible with a good tick collar and a vaccine. Two human vaccines have been tested that may provide protection for uninfected people when available.

PATIENT EDUCATION

HOW TO REMOVE A TICK

Removal is done with forceps or tweezers at the mouth parts. Pull gently until it releases its hold. The entire head should be removed. If tweezers are not available, cover with a tissue. Never use bare fingers. A ruptured tick can release infectious material onto a cut in the skin and transfer its disease. If a part remains, see a physician immediately. After removal, wash the area and your hands thoroughly and treat the area with 70% alcohol. Monitor the site for signs and symptoms; if any develop, see a physician immediately.

Pediculosis (Pe-dik-u-lo′-sis)

Description—There are three types of **pediculosis** resulting from three varieties of parasitic lice: capitis from head lice, corporis from body lice, and pubis from pubic lice. The lice feed on human blood and lay eggs known as nits on body hairs or fibers of clothing. The nits hatch and will die in 24 hours unless they feed on a host. Nits mature in two to three weeks.

Pediculosis Capitis

Description—It is the most common form and is found primarily among children, especially girls. It spreads through shared combs, brushes, clothing, and hats.

Signs and symptoms—It is identifiable as an oval, grayish, dandruff-like fleck that cannot be shaken off. Its symptoms are itching and scalp abrasions, with matted, foul-smelling hair in severe cases.

Etiology—Pediculosis is caused by parasitic forms of lice that are found in overcrowded conditions and with poor personal hygiene.

Treatment—Treatment consists of gamma benzene hexachloride (GBH) cream rubbed into the scalp at night, then rinsed out with GBH shampoo the next morning. Treatment is repeated the second night. A fine-toothed comb dipped in vinegar helps remove nits from the hair.

Parents have the option of purchasing over-the-counter medication if they choose; it is similar to prescription medication and provides effective treatment.

Pediculosis Corporis

Description—Pediculosis corporis lives in clothing seams, except when feeding on the host.

Signs and symptoms—Initially, small red papules appear, which itch. The resulting scratching causes rashes and wheals to develop.

Etiology—Prolonged wearing of the same clothes, overcrowding, and poor hygiene. It is spread through shared clothing and linens.

Treatment—Pediculosis corporis can be removed by bathing unless infestation is severe. Clothing and bed sheets must be washed, ironed, or dry cleaned. A prescription medication may be ordered if necessary.

Pediculosis Pubis

Description—Pediculosis pubis, commonly called crabs, is found attached primarily to pubic hair.

Signs and symptoms—The lice cause itching, which results in skin irritation from scratching.

Etiology—It is transmitted through sexual intercourse or contact with infected clothes, bedding, or towels.

Treatment—Pediculosis pubis is treated with a prescription medication and left on for 24 hours or with shampooing the affected area. Treatment must be repeated in one week. The sexual partner must also be treated or reinfestation will occur. This type of infestation is also treated with a prescription drug.

Poison Ivy

Description—This is the most common allergic contact dermatitis and is caused by the poison ivy plant.

Signs and symptoms—Initially, poison ivy causes moderate itching and burning that is soon followed by small blisters. As blisters increase, some break and skin is covered with a coating of serum. Marked discomfort and intense itching may be present (Figure 26–11).

Etiology—It is caused by the sap of the three-leafed poison ivy plant, fresh or dry.

Treatment—The best treatment is prevention. Learn to recognize and avoid contact with the plant. Especially susceptible people can be given injections to prevent its development. Different preparations are available to control the itching and to dry up the lesions. Treatment depends upon the extent of involvement. Oral steroids or topical steroid cream is usually sufficient.

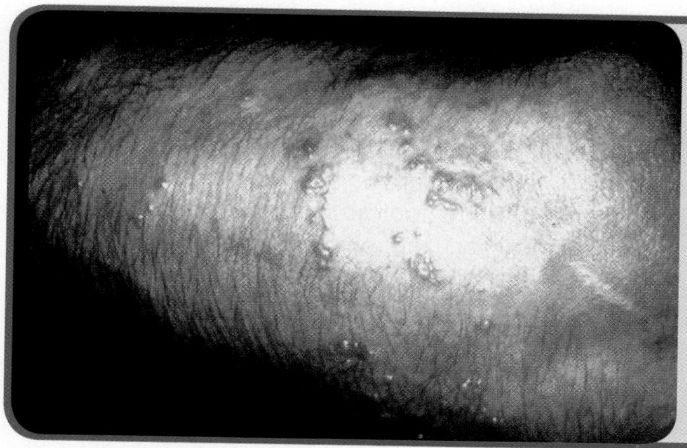

Figure 26–11: The fluid-filled vesicles of poison ivy. *Courtesy of the Centers for Disease Control and Prevention, Atlanta, GA.*

Psoriasis (So-ri′-a-sis)

Description—This is a chronic inflammatory condition that is recurrent, with alternating periods of remission or increased severity. The episodes are affected by the environment (cold weather causes flare-ups), endocrine changes, pregnancy, and emotional stress.

Signs and symptoms—**Psoriasis** is a chronic disease characterized by red papules that are covered with silvery scales (Figure 26–12). The lesions are dry, cracked, and encrusted, sometimes covering large areas of the body. The scales either flake off or build up, covering the lesion.

Etiology—The appearance is caused by the overgrowth of skin cells. Normally, a cell takes 14 days to move from the basal layer to the surface, where after another 14 days of wear it is sloughed off. The life cycle of

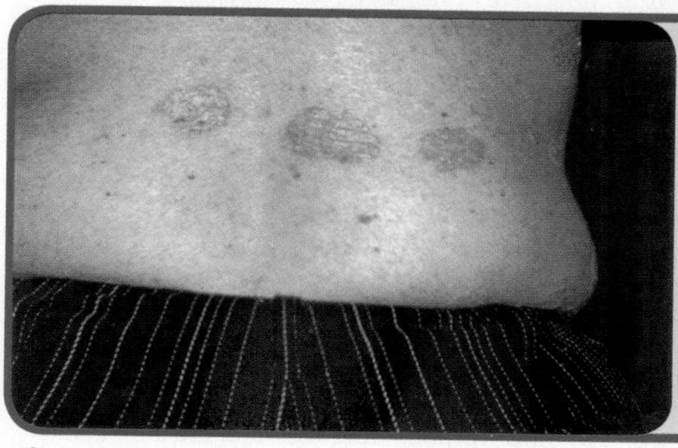

Figure 26–12: Psoriasis. *Delmar/Cengage Learning.*

a psoriatic skin cell is only four days, during which it produces a surface of immature cells causing a thick and flaky appearance.

Treatment—Psoriasis cannot be cured, but it may be controlled. Initial therapy is with topical hydrocortisone preparations. Then, topical retinoids, vitamin A or D creams, topical tar, and salicylic acid preparations are also used. Ultraviolet light in a controlled, prescribed setting slows the cell turnover. Oral medications in the form of antimetabolites, retinoids, and immunosuppressives are used in extensive severe cases. The new eximer laser is effective in treating localized psoriasis.

The most effective medications are called biologicals, which are systemic drugs capable of slowing down specific immunologic factors that cause psoriasis. These drugs include Enbrel, Remicade, Stelara, and Humira.

Ringworm

Description—This fungus may affect the scalp (tinea capitis), the body (tinea corporis), or other areas, such as the groin, beard, or feet (tinea pedia, or athlete's foot).

Signs and symptoms—On the body, it is characterized by flat lesions, which are dry and scaly or moist and crusty. When they enlarge, clear central areas develop, leaving an outer ring from which it gets its name (Figure 26–13). On the scalp, small papules occur causing scaly patches of baldness.

Etiology—Fungi dermatophytes.

Treatment—Treatment consists of systemic medication or the topical applications of antifungals. Because the disease is contagious, care must be taken to prevent its spread by refraining from sharing bed linens, combs, and towels.

Rosacea (Ro-za′-se-a)

Description—It is a chronic skin eruption that makes the face, especially the nose and cheeks, look flushed. It occurs most often in Caucasian women between 30 and 50 years old. It also occurs in men but is usually more severe and associated with rhinophyma (dilated follicles with an enlarged red nose).

Signs and symptoms—There is the characteristic coloration of the face that may also exhibit papules and pustules like acne but without the comedones.

Etiology—The condition results from the dilation of small blood vessels that causes the flushed, red appearance. The exact cause is unknown. Stress, infection, vitamin deficiency, and endocrine problems do aggravate the condition. Certain foods, such as spicy things and hot beverages, also cause problems. It is also affected by alcohol, physical activity, sunlight, and extreme temperatures.

Treatment—Topical use of metronidazole gel ointment to reduce erythema may be helpful. Oral doses of tetracycline given in decreasing amounts as symptoms subside and electrolysis may destroy the large or dilated blood vessels.

Figure 26–14 shows a female who has had rosacea for 20 years. Her skin will react to temperature changes and becomes flushed with drinking hot liquids or alcohol. She also tends to develop pustules, and her skin becomes very sensitive. She uses metronidazole gel (MetroGel) to alleviate her symptoms.

Scabies (Ska′-bez)

Description—This skin infestation is caused by the itch mite.

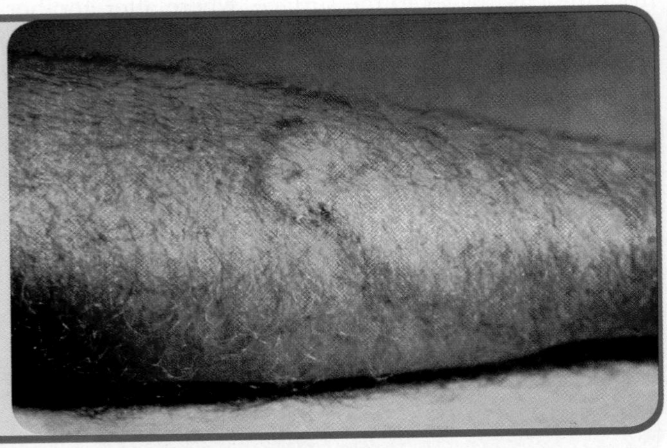

Figure 26–13: Tinea corporis (ringworm) on the arm. *CDC.*

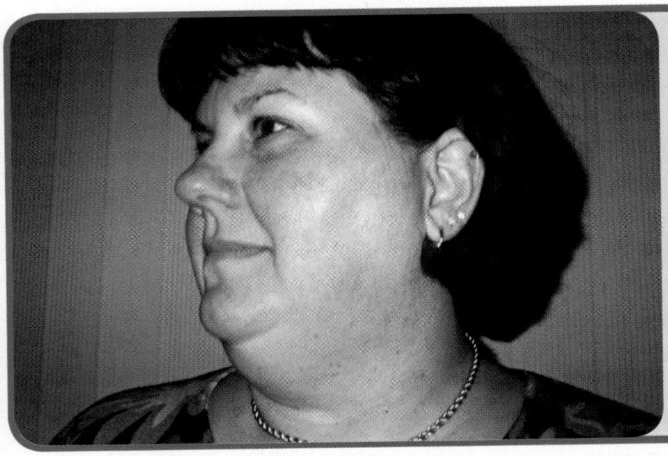

Figure 26–14: Female with rosacea. *Courtesy of Barbara A. Wise.*

Signs and symptoms—The condition causes an itching that becomes intense at night. The lesions are characteristically threadlike red nodules, approximately 3/8-inch long. They occur between fingers, at the inner wrist area, on the elbows, in axillary folds (armpit), around the waist, on genitalia (external sex organs) of males, and on the nipples of females. The infestation is spread by skin contact or sexual activity.

Etiology—It is caused by the itch mite, which burrows into the skin to lay eggs. The larvae emerge to mate and then reburrow under the skin. It can be associated with overcrowding and poor personal hygiene.

Treatment—Treatment consists of an application of pediculicide such as the prescription drug Elimite, which must remain on the skin from six to eight hours or overnight. The treatment is then followed with a bath. An antipruritic (against itching) or steroid may be applied topically to help reduce the itching.

Urticaria (Ur-ti-ka′re-a) (Hives)

Description—This is a self-limiting reaction to allergens. **Urticaria** often occurs during especially stressful or emotional times or during a viral infection.

Signs and symptoms—The reaction produces distinct, raised **wheals** surrounded by a reddened area. They may be few in number or cover the entire body. They may or may not cause itching, burning, and tingling.

Etiology—Urticaria are caused by allergy to drugs, food, insect stings, and occasionally inhaled allergens from animal hair, cosmetics, and flour. Nonallergic urticaria can be caused by the body's release of histamine for unknown reasons.

Treatment—Urticaria is treated by eliminating or limiting the causative allergen or, when that is not possible, by gradual desensitization through interdermal injection of the allergen. An antihistamine is used to reduce itching and swelling. A tranquilizer may be required when the causative factor is emotional stress.

Verrucae (Ver-roo-ka) (Warts)

Description—This is a benign (noncancerous) viral infection of the skin.

Signs and symptoms—Common **verrucae** are characterized by a rough, elevated, rounded surface, usually on the extremities, especially the hands and fingers. They can also occur on the elbows, knees, and face and scalp.

Etiology—Warts are caused by a family of viruses known as human papillomavirus, which is spread by direct contact. It invades skin cells where the surface is broken and "encourages" the creation of more infected cells. In most cases, the body's immune system eventually eliminates the wart. It is estimated that a wart will die off within about five years. Plantar warts occur primarily at pressure points on the soles of the feet. Condyloma accuminatum (venereal warts) are moist, soft, pink-to-red warts occurring singly or most often in large clusters on the penis, vulva, or anus. They grow rapidly in groups, often accumulating into large clusters. Genital warts spread by sexual contact and are highly contagious. They are associated with an increased risk of cervical cancer in women.

Treatment—Treatment of warts varies with the type, size, and location. Common types often disappear spontaneously. When removal is necessary, they can be destroyed by methods using electricity, acid, liquid nitrogen, or solid carbon dioxide. Genital warts must be treated promptly. Partners must also be evaluated by a physician for evidence of the virus and treated if present or the infection will be reacquired upon renewed contact.

Wrinkles

As people age, the skin begins to develop wrinkles, particularly on the face and back of the hands. This is primarily caused by years of exposure to the sun and the diminishing layer of collagen beneath the skin. Many forms of treatment can be performed to remove or reduce their presence and at least temporarily improve the patient's appearance. Because there is such an interest in the procedures, a brief discussion of the most common forms of correction follows.

Dermabrasion

This is the controlled scraping of the top layers of the skin to remove scars from acne or accidents and to smooth out fine facial wrinkles, such as those around the mouth. It involves the use of a high-speed, hand-held rotary instrument with a rough wire brush or diamond impregnated burr. It is rarely performed since newer techniques using users and chemical peels have been developed.

Microdermabrasion This is a noninvasive, nonsurgical procedure. A controlled spray of fine aluminum oxide crystals is applied to remove the outer layer of the skin. It may improve the appearance of fine wrinkles, superficial age spots, and sun-damaged skin.

Chemical Peel

This is known as chemosurgery and can be done at three levels: light, medium, and deep. They involve the application of varying concentrations of an acid that strips away old, damaged skin cells, causing the body to replace them with healthy new ones.

Light peel This type affects only the top layer and may make the skin appear softer, reduce the size of pores, produce a more even coloring, and may reduce some fine lines.

Medium peel This type affects surface and some underlying cells. It also stimulates collagen and elastin. This results in much smoother skin and the reduction of wrinkles. Some precancerous lesions may be removed.

Deep peel This type requires a strong acid and destroys all the top layers of skin and sometimes a part of the dermal layer. This results in removing all the signs of skin aging except deep forehead furrows and the nose-to-mouth grooves from sagging. It can also result in the loss of pigment, which causes a waxy, lighter face that may not match the body; scar formation is a serious complication and risk.

Laser Resurfacing

This is the newest form of repair and involves the use of a controlled, pulsed laser beam to vaporize the skin's surface. Surface blemishes, sun-damaged skin, and the wrinkled surface are removed. It also stimulates the development of new cells and collagen for new, smoother, younger-looking skin and produces a tightening effect on the skin. The results are usually considered well worth the discomfort and temporary inconvenience.

Plastic Surgery

This term is derived from a Greek word meaning to mold or give form. Plastic surgery is also known as cosmetic surgery and involves the reshaping of the facial features to improve appearance. The procedure demands a skillful surgeon to achieve the desired results. The procedures can remove "bags" under the eyes, lift drooping upper lids, and tighten up skin around the eyes. The repair of both upper and lower lids is known as quadrilateral blepharoplasty. The procedures to raise sagging jaws and forehead and pull back the sides of the face is commonly referred to as a "face lift." These procedures can be performed under general or local anesthesia in connection with sedation. Pain, marked swelling, and bruising will require medication for a few days. The recovery time varies, but most swelling and significant bruising are sufficiently gone after two to three weeks to allow the patient to go out in public.

A face lift technique known as "thread lift" is being marketed as less invasive and less expensive. It involves using a special suture with "barbs" to stitch through subcutaneous tissue and make loops at various points to pull surface tissue upward toward the temple. The recovery time may be less, but it means the skin tissue must "reposition" itself after being "gathered up," which may ultimately take longer than the traditional face lift. Again, nothing is lifted beneath the surface, so results and length of effect are anticipated to be about five years. This technique may allow other surgeons and dermatologists to enter the field of plastic surgery without the extensive surgical training and experience.

AGE-RELATED BODY CHARACTERISTICS

The skin changes as the body ages. Infants and small children have soft, supple, beautiful skin. The teenager will probably experience a period of acne and an increase in the secretion from oil glands. As individuals age, the skin structure becomes less elastic and there is a loss of collagen, resulting in the development of wrinkles. The skin of the elderly is quite fragile and thin with an increase in pigmentation. The skin of the aged is easily damaged and will bruise and bleed from minor injury.

System Interaction Associated with Disease Conditions

The skin is composed of many kinds of tissues from nerves, blood vessels, and glands to muscles and hair, so the interaction of body systems occurs continuously even when no disease condition exists. Table 26–3 summarizes the systems involved and the pathology present in two examples of disease conditions.

Table 26–3 System Interaction Associated with Disease Conditions

DISEASE	SYSTEMS INVOLVED	PATHOLOGY PRESENT
Lyme Disease	Integumentary	Red skin lesion, bull's eye rash
	Circulatory	Swollen lymph glands, arrhythmia
	Skeletal/muscular	Muscle and joint pain, arthritis
	Nervous	Numbness, pain, Bell's palsy
Hirsutism	Integumentary	Excessive growth of body hair
	Muscular	Increase muscle mass
	Reproductive	Menstrual irregularity, reduced breast size

CHAPTER SUMMARY

- Integumentary system refers to the skin and all its structures.
- The skin serves as an organ of perception through pain, heat, cold, and pressure receptors.
- The skin regulates body temperature by constricting or dilating blood vessels and evaporating sweat.
- The skin has three layers: the epidermis, the dermis, and the subcutaneous.
- Skin color is determined by a pigment called melanin and blood vessels.
- The skin can be used as a diagnostic site.
- The diseases and disorders discussed in the chapter are acne vulgaris, alopecia, skin cancer, cellulitis, dermatitis, eczema, folliculitits, furuncles, carbuncles, herpes, pediculosis, poison ivy, psoriasis, ringworm, rosacea, scabies, urticaria, and verrucae.
- Wrinkles can be treated by dermabrasion, chemical peel, and laser resurfacing.
- Plastic surgery involves reshaping of features.

STUDY TOOLS

Workbook	Activities for Chapter 26
Premium Website	
MEDIA LINK	View this **Media Link** for Chapter 26: • The skin
StudyWARE	Activities and Quizzes on the **StudyWARE™ Software** for Chapter 26
	Audio Library of medical terms
	Online access to the **Critical Thinking Challenge 2.0**
learninglab	Module 12: Nervous, Sensory, and Integumentary Systems
CourseMate	Activities and Quizzes for Chapter 26
WebTutor	Activities and Quizzes for Chapter 26

CHECK YOUR KNOWLEDGE

1. Giving medication by applying it to the skin is called:
   a. intramuscular.
   b. subcutaneous.
   c. intradermal.
   d. transdermal.
2. Which of the following cannot pass through the skin?
   a. Oxygen
   b. Carbon monoxide
   c. Vitamins
   d. Sex hormones
3. Which layer of skin contains blood vessels, nerves, hair follicles, sweat, and oil glands?
   a. Subcutaneous
   b. Epidermis
   c. Hypodermia
   d. Dermis
4. Patchy hair loss due to the pulling out of hair from a compulsive behavior is:
   a. alopecia.
   b. areata.
   c. physiologic loss.
   d. trichotillomania.
5. Which description does not reflect melanoma?
   a. Asymmetry
   b. Defined border
   c. Irregular pigmentation
   d. A diameter larger than 6 mm
6. Herpes simplex refers to lesions that:
   a. spread around one side of the body.
   b. are located in the genital area.
   c. are located on mucous membranes.
   d. are located around the nose and mouth.

7. A disease caused by a tick is:
   a. pediculosis.
   b. scabies.
   c. Lyme disease.
   d. ringworm.
8. Verrucae is the medical term for:
   a. ringworm.
   b. hives.
   c. shingles.
   d. warts.
9. Skin wrinkles are not the result of which of the following?
   a. Loss of collagen
   b. Increased size of elastic fibers
   c. Environmental exposure
   d. Excessive rubbing of the skin
10. A temporary red, itchy spot caused by an allergic reaction or an insect bite is called a:
    a. wheal.
    b. whorl.
    c. bulla.
    d. vesicle.
11. Elderly persons have skin that is:
    a. full of collagen.
    b. supple.
    c. excessively oily.
    d. easily damaged.
12. Hirsutism involves the:
    a. urinary, muscular, and reproductive systems.
    b. integumentary, muscular, and reproductive systems.
    c. muscular, nervous, and integumentary systems.
    d. skeletal, reproductive, and integumentary.

WEB LINKS

American Cancer Society, Cancer facts and figures: www.cancer.org

WebMD Genital Herpes Health Center: www.webmd.com/genital-herpes/default.htm

Chapter

27 The Skeletal System

OBJECTIVES

In this chapter, you will learn the following:

KB LEARNING OBJECTIVES

1. Spell and define, using the glossary at the back of the text, all the Words to Know in this chapter.
2. Name the two divisions of the skeletal system and the bone groups in each division.
3. Describe the structure of the long bones.
4. Explain how long bones grow.
5. Identify the elements that make up bone tissue.
6. Identify the major bones of the body.
7. List the six functions of the skeletal system.
8. Name the divisions of the spinal column and the number of vertebrae in each division.
9. Describe fontanels and explain why they are essential.
10. Describe the structure of the rib cage and its primary function.
11. Identify three kinds of synovial joints and give examples of each.
12. List the parts of a synovial joint and identify the purpose of each part.
13. Name the seven types of fractures and the characteristics of each.
14. Outline the treatment of a fracture.
15. Describe the healing process of a fracture.
16. Define the term fatty embolus, explaining its origin and what might occur.
17. List situations predisposing to amputation.
18. Define the phantom limb sensation.
19. Describe four diagnostic examinations.
20. Explain why the symptoms of carpal tunnel syndrome occur.
21. Name the three types of spinal curvatures, describing their physical characteristics.
22. Identify 20 diseases and disorders of the skeletal system.
23. Explain the correlation between age and fractures.
24. Identify the body systems involved with rheumatoid arthritis.

WORDS TO KNOW

alignment
amputate
appendicular
arthritis
articulation
axial
bunion
bursa
callus
cancellous
carpal
cartilage
cervical
clavicle
coccyx
comminuted
compound
cranium
depressed
diarthrosis
dislocation
embolus
epiphysis
femur
fibula
fracture
greenstick
humerus
ilium
impacted
intervertebral
ischium
kyphosis
laminectomy
ligament
lordosis
marrow
metacarpal
metatarsal
osteoporosis
patella
periosteum
phalanges
phalanx
phantom limb
prosthesis
radius
reduce

sacrum
scapula
scoliosis
simple
skeletal
spinal fusion
spiral
sprain
sternum
symphysis pubis
synovial
tarsal
tibia
traction
ulna
vertebrae
xiphoid

THE SKELETAL SYSTEM

The **skeletal** system consists of organs called bones. It may be difficult to think of bones as living, functioning organs that use food and oxygen and perform functions just as other organs do.

The skeleton is divided into two sections. The spinal column, skull, and rib cage make up the **axial** skeleton. The bones of the arms, hands, legs, feet, shoulders, and pelvis make up the **appendicular** skeleton (Figure 27–1).

The primary purpose of the skeletal system is to support the body. This support must be strong yet not heavy. Bone is said to be as strong as cast iron, yet it is much lighter and more flexible. The skeleton must be flexible enough to endure pressure, stress, and shock without shattering.

BONE STRUCTURE

Over 20% of the weight of bone is water. Two thirds of the remainder are minerals and one third, organic matter. The main minerals are calcium, phosphorus,

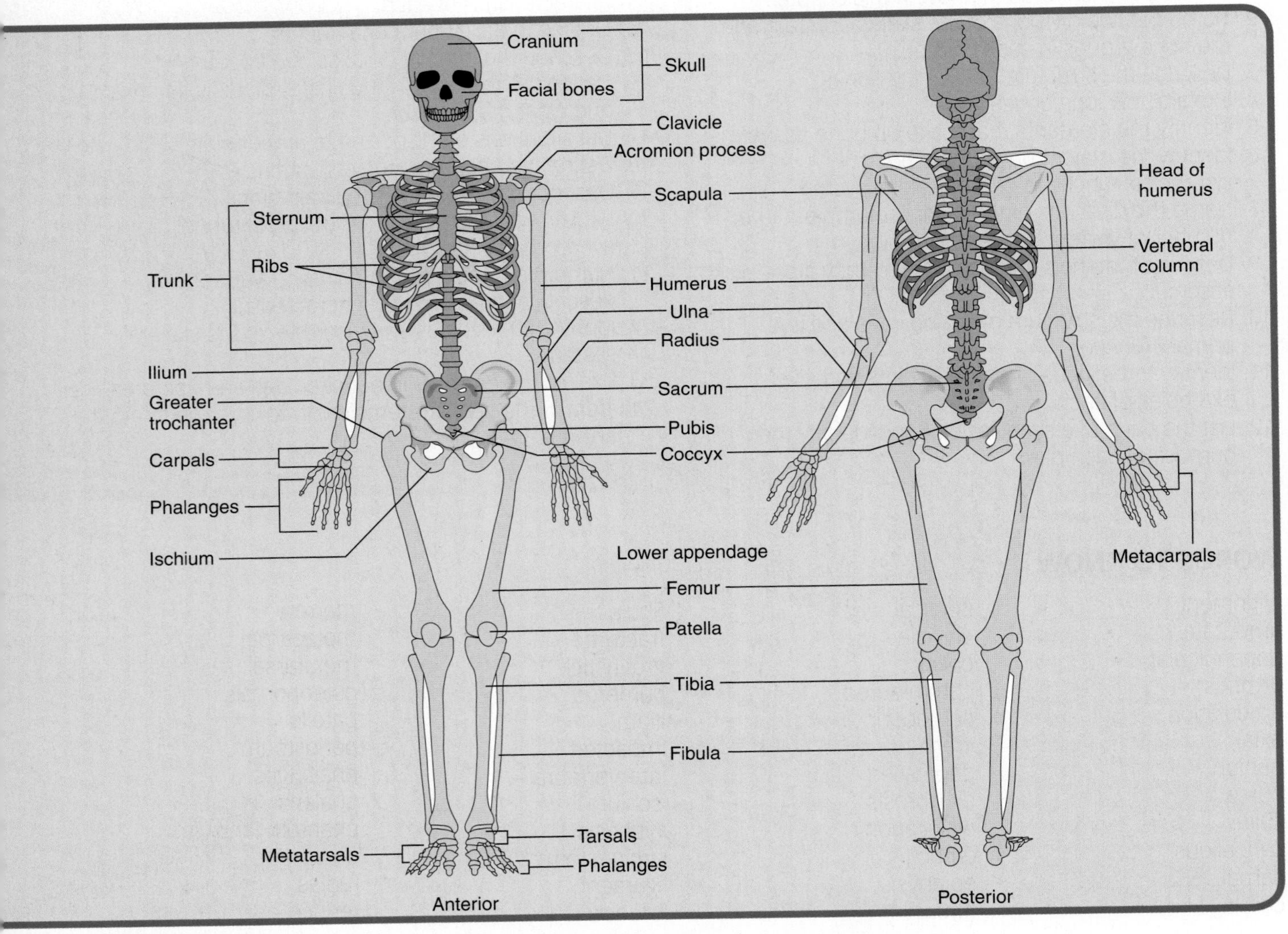

Figure 27–1: Bones of the skeleton (axial in blue, appendicular in gray). *Delmar/Cengage Learning.*

and magnesium. The organic matter is primarily collagen, a type of protein fiber that forms the matrix (intercellular substance) of the bone.

The ends of long bones have articulating (connecting) surfaces that fit together with other bones to form joints (Figure 27–2). These ends are separated by cartilage to facilitate movement. The ends and parts of the shaft are filled with a meshlike network of spongy **cancellous** bone. The openings in the spongy bone are filled with red **marrow**. The inside of the shaft of the bone is filled with a fat or yellow marrow. Dense bone called cortical bone makes up the outside of long bones.

A tough membrane called **periosteum** covers the surface of the bone. Blood vessels and nerves pass through the periosteum and into the bone through a network of openings called Haversian canals. Some larger vessels pass directly into both the yellow and red marrow.

NUMBER OF BONES

At birth, a baby has 270 bones. As the child grows, some of the bones fuse together so that in adulthood there are only 206. For example, at the lower end of the spinal column, five **vertebrae** have fused to form the **sacrum**, whereas the last four have fused into the **coccyx** (tailbone) (Figure 27–3). The smallest bones in the body are the malleus, incus, and stapes of the middle ear.

FUNCTIONS OF THE SKELETON

The skeleton serves at least six functions for the body. One, as previously indicated, is to support the body. The bones provide a framework for the distribution of the body's fat, muscles, and skin.

Two, the bones also serve to protect the body's vital organs. The brain and spinal cord are both located within bony cavities. The cranium also provides protection for

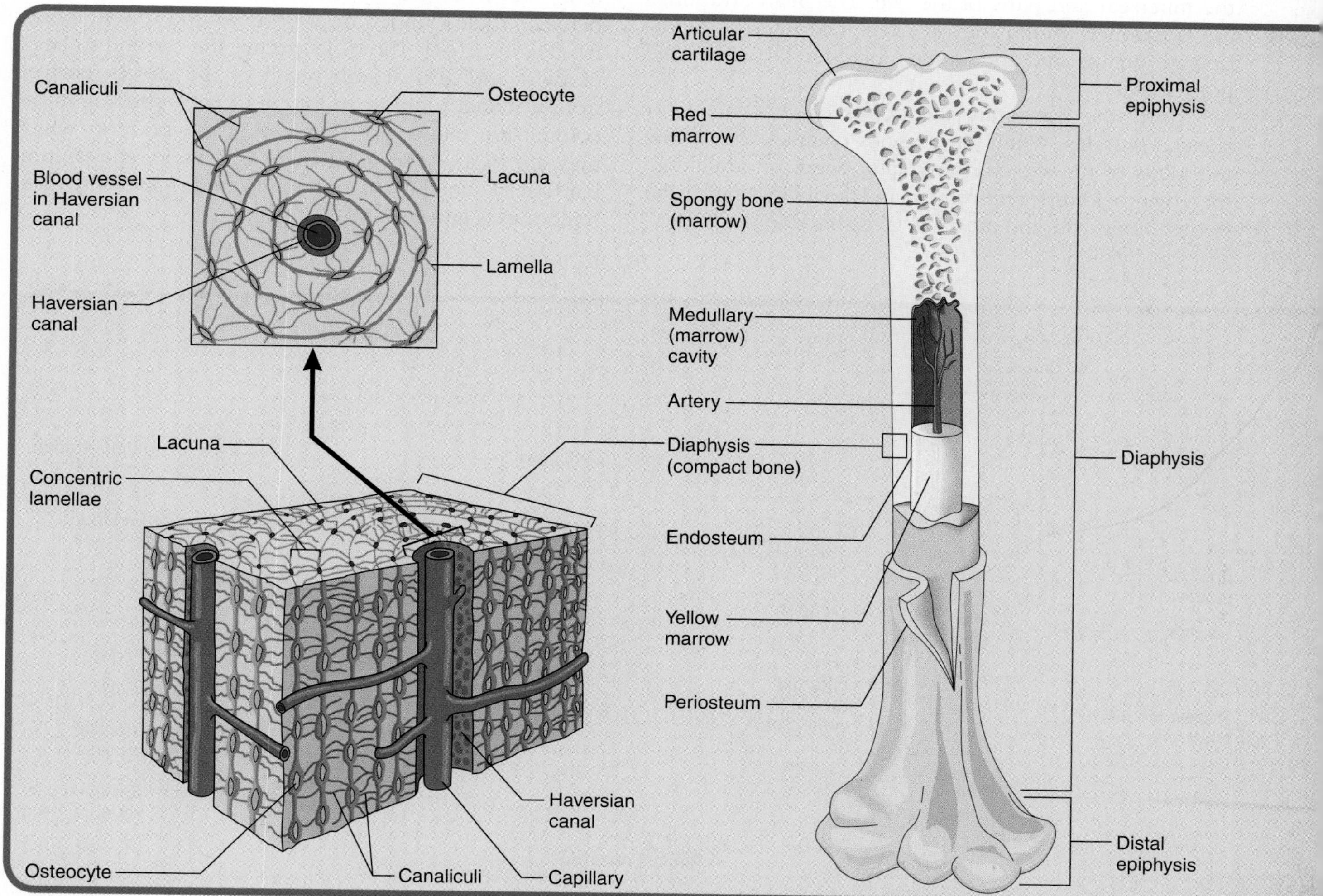

Figure 27–2: Structure of a long bone. *Delmar/Cengage Learning.*

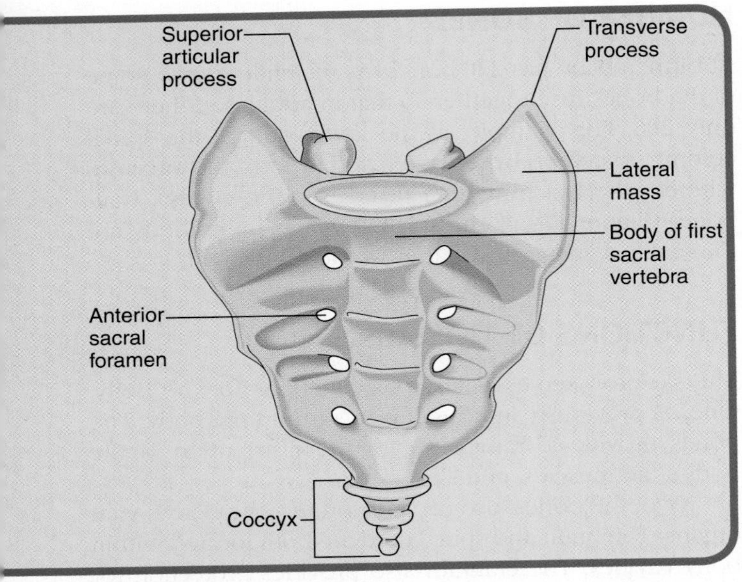

Figure 27–3: The sacrum and coccyx. *Delmar/Cengage Learning.*

the inner ear and parts of the eye. The heart and lungs are positioned within the rib cage. The internal reproductive organs and the urinary bladder lie within the bony pelvis.

Third, the bones are the points of attachment for skeletal muscles. When the muscles contract, they allow the joints of the skeleton to rotate, bend, or straighten, thereby providing for movement and flexibility. Fourth, the bones, along with the muscles, give shape to the body.

A fifth and vital function of bone is the formation of the red and white blood cells and the platelets. The red marrow in the spongy areas of the long bones, the ribs, and the vertebrae produces millions of red blood cells a minute. This rate is necessary to replace the cells, which live only a few weeks. When the body needs more red cells than the red marrow can produce, some of the yellow marrow is converted to red.

Finally, bones store most of the body's supply of calcium. Calcium is needed by the heart to beat, by the muscles to contract, and by the blood to clot. When the calcium in the body is inadequate for all its needs, the blood takes calcium from its storage in the bone. The bone minerals are constantly being borrowed and replaced through the blood flow within the body.

SPINAL COLUMN

The spinal column is a stack of vertebrae that supports the head and keeps the trunk erect. As noted earlier, it provides protection for the spinal cord, which descends from the brain through its canal. The bones of the column are separated by **intervertebral** cartilage disks between their rounded front portions, the vertebral bodies (Figure 27–4). The disks permit the column to bend or twist and also absorb much of the shock received from walking, running, or jumping. The vertebrae in the column are named for the area of the body in which they are located: **cervical** (neck), thoracic (chest), lumbar (back), sacral (posterior pelvic girdle), and coccygeal (tailbone) (Figure 27–5).

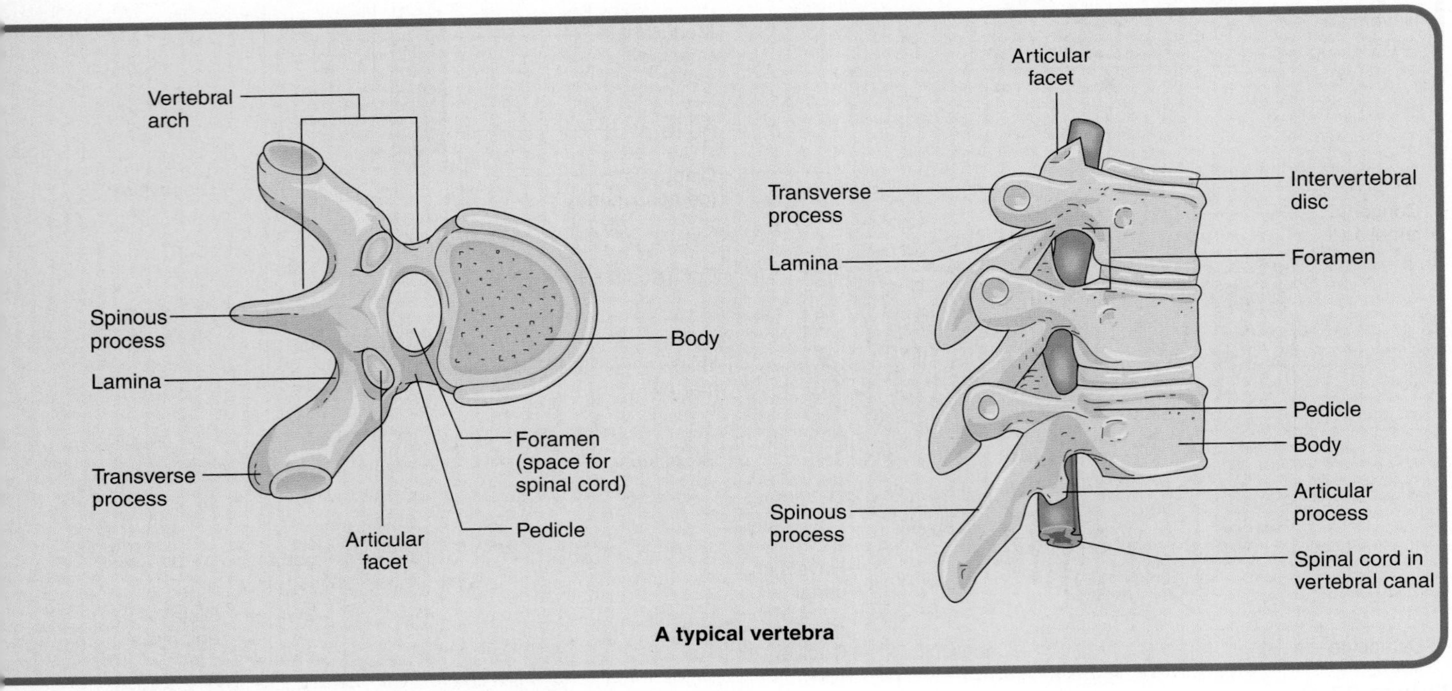

Figure 27–4: Vertebrae structure. *Delmar/Cengage Learning.*

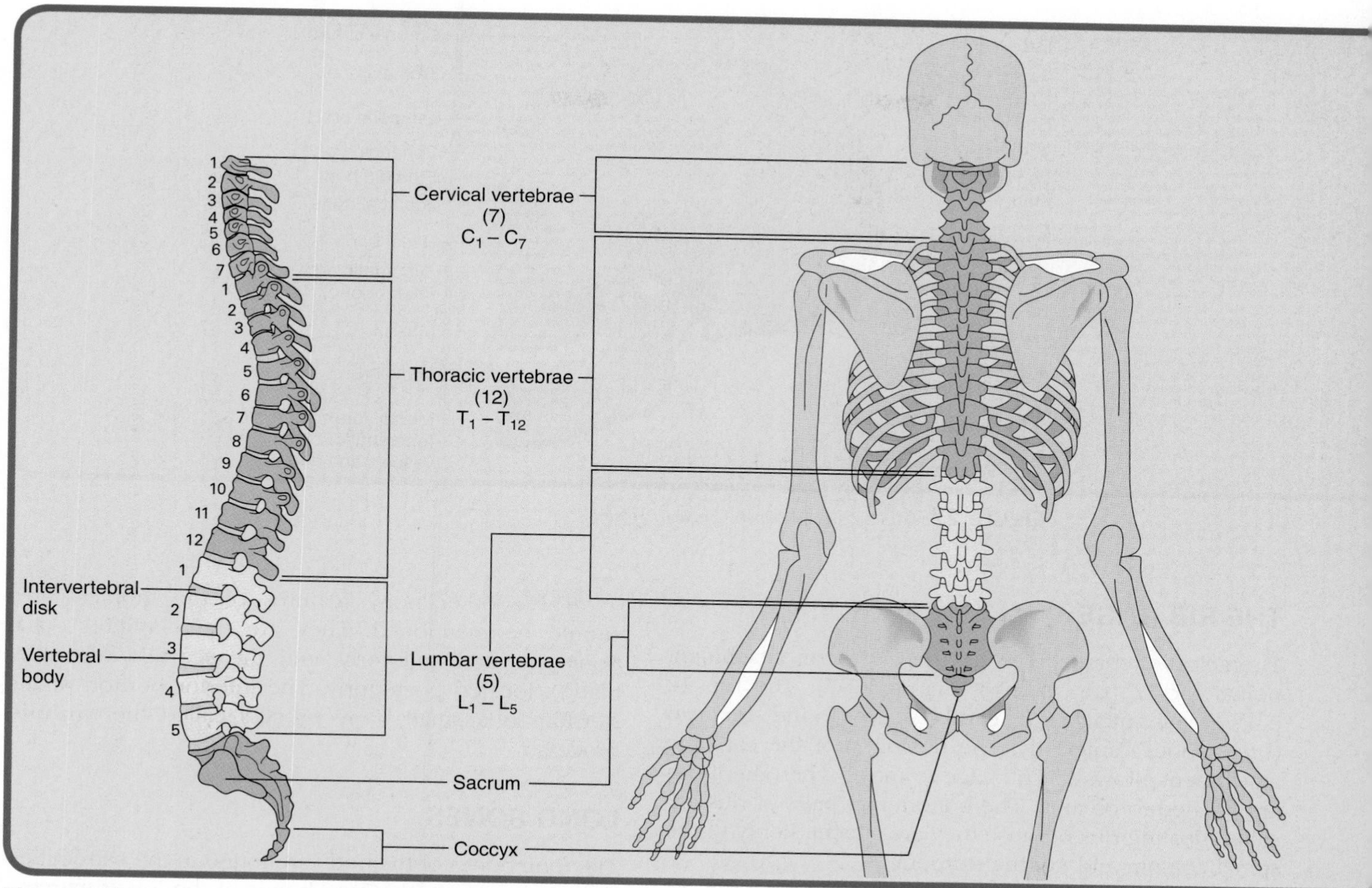

Figure 27–5: The spinal column. *Delmar/Cengage Learning.*

The spinal nerves enter and leave the spinal cord through foraminae (openings) between the vertebrae. The disks maintain adequate spacing between vertebrae to prevent damage to the spinal nerves from bone-to-bone contact.

Typical vertebrae, as shown in Figure 27–4, have descriptive parts, mainly the large solid part called the *body,* the winglike side projections called the *transverse processes,* a posterior projection called a *spinous process* (the part you can feel if you arch your back), and the *foramen* through which the spinal cord passes. Other processes called *articular* facets are where parts of two vertebrae touch.

THE SKULL

The skull is the bony structure of the head. It consists of a cranial and a facial portion. The **cranium** is actually a fusion of eight cranial bones, with the vital function of protecting the brain from injury (Figure 27–6). The main bones of the cranium are the frontal (the forehead and upper eye sockets), two parietal, two temporal, and the occipital (back of the skull). The facial bones are the mandible (lower jaw), the maxillae (upper jaw), the zygomatic (cheek bones), and the several small bones around the eyes, nose, and palate.

The cranium is not solid bone at birth. Spaces between the bones are soft, incomplete bone to allow for the molding of the skull during the birth process and for enlargement of the skull as growth occurs. A large, diamond-shaped anterior area where the frontal and parietal bones meet and a triangular space posteriorly where the occipital bone meets the parietals are known as *fontanels,* or "soft spots," and can easily be felt. Other smaller fontanels are located along the sides of the skull. Without these areas for growth, the brain could not increase in size during late pregnancy and early infancy. The fontanels gradually close, turning the membrane and cartilage into solid bone after about two years. The irregular lines marking the former growth areas are called *sutures.*

The skull does not grow remarkably when compared with the rest of the body. It makes up about one fourth of the total length of the infant's body but only one eighth of the adult's total length.

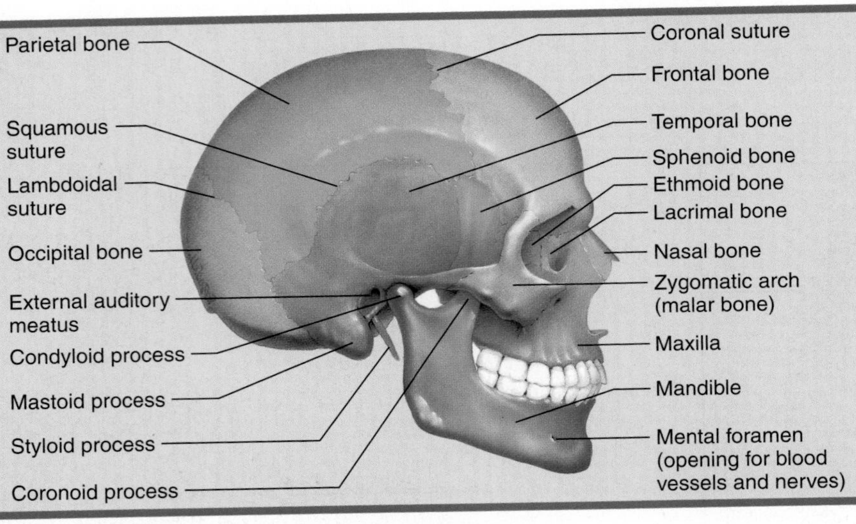

Figure 27–6: The skull. *Delmar/Cengage Learning.*

THE RIB CAGE

Thoracic vertebrae serve as the posterior attachment points for 12 pairs of ribs (Figure 27–7). The top 10 pairs are also attached by cartilage strips to the **sternum** (breast bone) anteriorly. The flexibility of the cartilage attachment allows the rib cage to move when the lungs are inflated to breathe. The bottom two pairs of ribs are called floating ribs because they are attached only to the spinal column and not the sternum.

The rib cage is sometimes described in terms of true and false ribs. When this division is made, the first seven pairs of ribs are considered "true" ribs because of their posterior and direct anterior attachment. The last five pairs are "false" ribs because they attach anteriorly to the cartilage of the rib above or have no anterior attachment.

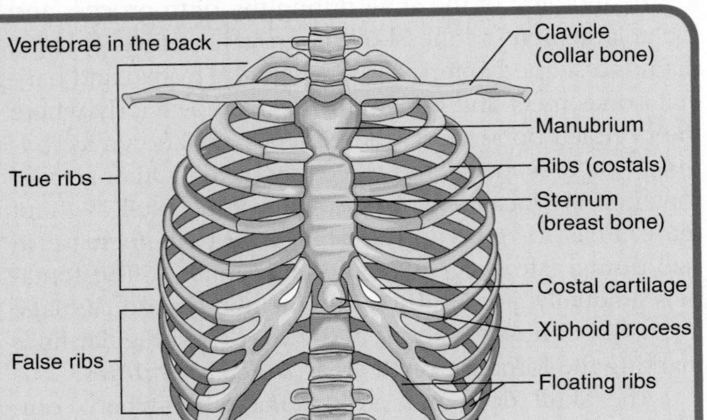

Figure 27–7: The rib cage. *Delmar/Cengage Learning.*

Three other bony features of the thoracic area should be mentioned. They are the **clavicle** (collar bone), located anteriorly, and the **scapula** (shoulder blade), located posteriorly. The inferior portion of the sternum is a small bony process called the **xiphoid** process.

LONG BONES

The long bones of the body are found in the extremities. To a great extent, the long bones of the lower extremities determine height. Long bones are generally shaped like hollow cylinders to be strong with the least amount of weight. A typical long bone has three distinct regions: diaphysis, epiphysis, and metaphysis. The middle shaft (diaphysis) is connected to the ends (**epiphysis**) by a transitional segment (metaphysis). Early in life the epiphysis is mainly **cartilage**. Later the cartilage becomes a strip or "growth plate" that permits new tissue growth and bone length. At maturity, growth stops and the cartilage is replaced by bone.

The **femur** (thigh bone) is the longest bone in any species, extending from the hip joint to the knee. (Refer to Figure 27–1.) The thickness of the femur wall depends on the size and needs of the species. For example, large animals, such as the bear, have a thick, heavy femur to support their weight and accommodate slow movements, whereas the deer has a very thin and light femur to permit speed. The **tibia** (shin bone) and **fibula** complete the long bones of the leg. The small bone at the knee is known as the **patella**.

The long bones of the upper extremities are the **humerus** of the arm and the **radius** and **ulna** of the forearm. The radius extends from the thumb side of the wrist to the elbow, whereas the ulna extends from the little finger side to the elbow joint.

BONES OF THE HANDS AND FEET

The bones of the hands and feet are similar in structure (Figure 27–8). The wrist has eight bones, known as **carpals**, whereas the ankle has seven, called **tarsals**. In the palm area of the hand, there are five **metacarpals** that correspond to the five **metatarsals** of the instep of the foot. The **phalanges** (fingers and toes) are further subdivided into individual sections called a **phalanx**. There are three phalanx sections in each finger and toe, except in the thumb and great toe, which have only two. The section of a phalanx is identified as distal, middle, or proximal by its relationship to the metacarpals or metatarsals.

THE PELVIC GIRDLE

The pelvic girdle provides the structure for the hip area. Two large bones called *os coxae* (hip bones) are joined posteriorly with the sacrum. The top blade-shaped portion is called the **ilium** (Figure 27–9). The anterior lower portion is called the pubis, and the point of attachment (right and left pubis) is called the **symphysis pubis**. The posterior lower portion of the bone is called the **ischium**. The hip bone provides the recessed area where the head of the femur fits. The anatomical name for the socket is *acetabulum*.

JOINTS

The place where two or more bony parts join together is known as an **articulation** or joint. Strong, flexible bands of connective tissue called **ligaments** hold long bones together at joints. Ligaments can stretch and often become torn as a result of injury.

There are three main types of joints, classified primarily by their degree of movement. A movable joint, such as the knee or elbow, is called a **diarthrosis** or **synovial** joint. A partially movable joint, like where the ribs attach to the spine or between the vertebrae, is known as *amphiarthrosis* or *cartilaginous*. An immovable joint, such as a cranial suture, is called *synarthrosis* or *fibrous*.

Most of the body's joints are diarthrotic. They may have three distinct parts: articular cartilage, a **bursa** (saclike capsule), and a synovial cavity. The articulating joint surfaces of bones are covered with the articular cartilage, which provides a slippery, smooth surface and enables the joint to absorb shock. An articular capsule of tough, fibrous tissue encloses the articulating surfaces and is lined with a synovial membrane, which secretes synovial fluid into the cavity, lubricating the joint and reducing friction.

The joint is surrounded by ligaments, tendons, and muscles that hold the joint together but still allow for movement. Some synovial joints have cushionlike sacs called bursa, which form from the synovial membrane and are filled with synovial fluid. These are generally located between tendons and bones. In addition, synovial membranes may also form sheaths that wrap around the tendons. Bursae and tendon sheaths cushion and lubricate tendons and help reduce friction between the tendons and the bone.

The synovial joints of the body have been copied by man to develop many useful devices (Figure 27–10). The ball and socket joint found in the hip or shoulder can be seen in the movement of a desk pen set. The action of the fingers, knees, and elbows is like that of a hinge. An unusual pivot joint appears at the wrists and elbows. When the palm of the hand is up, the radius and ulna are side by side. As the palm is turned down, the radius crosses

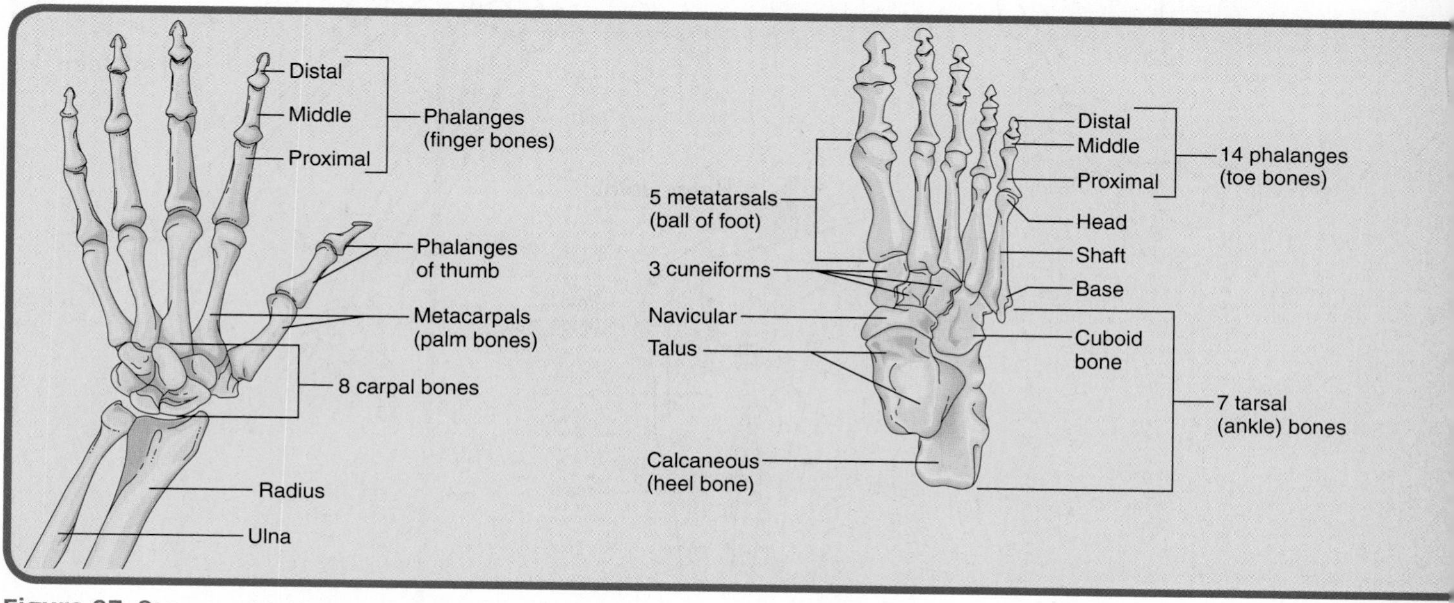

Figure 27–8: Bones of the hand and foot. *Delmar/Cengage Learning.*

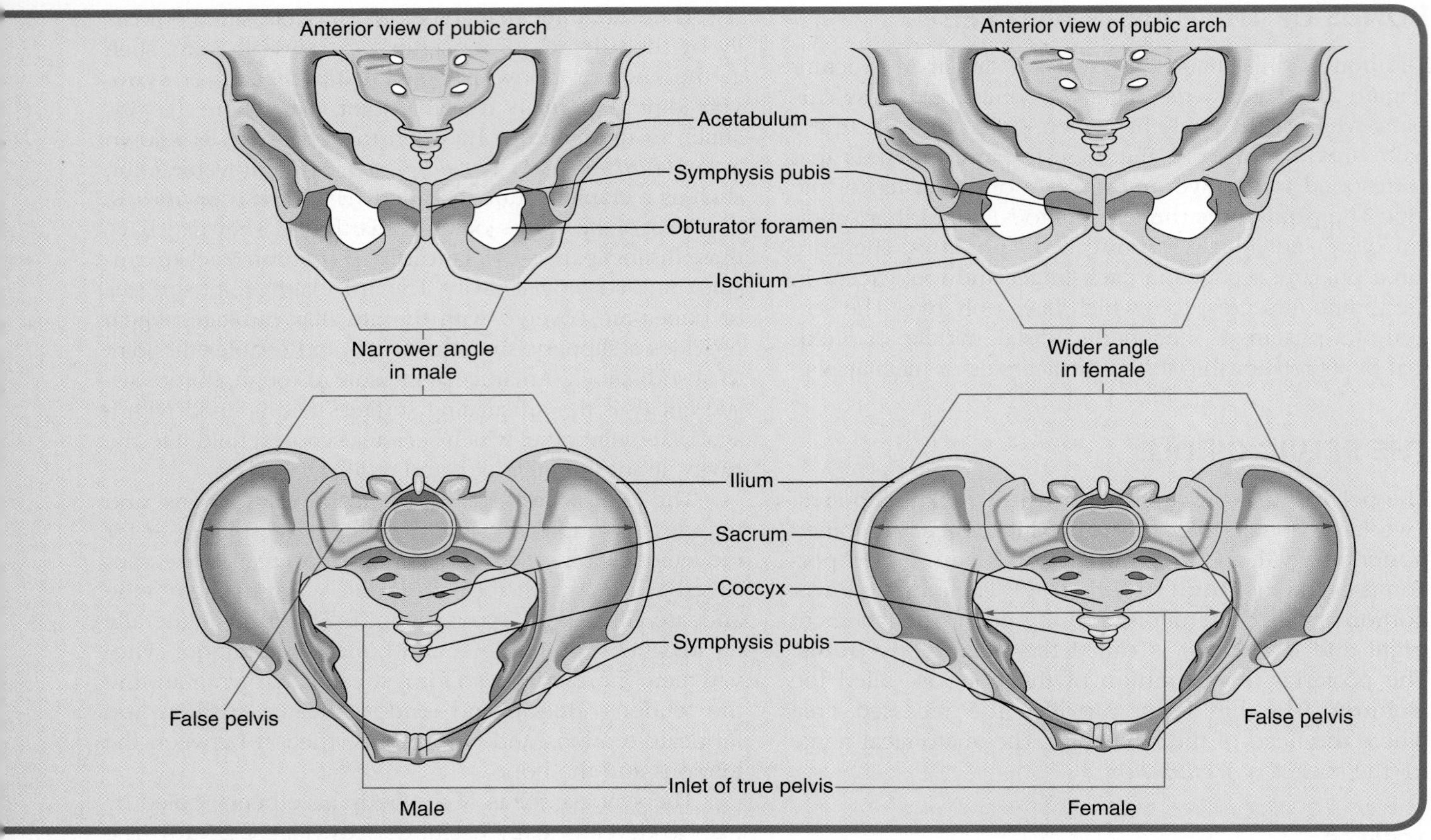

Figure 27–9: The pelvic girdle. *Delmar/Cengage Learning.*

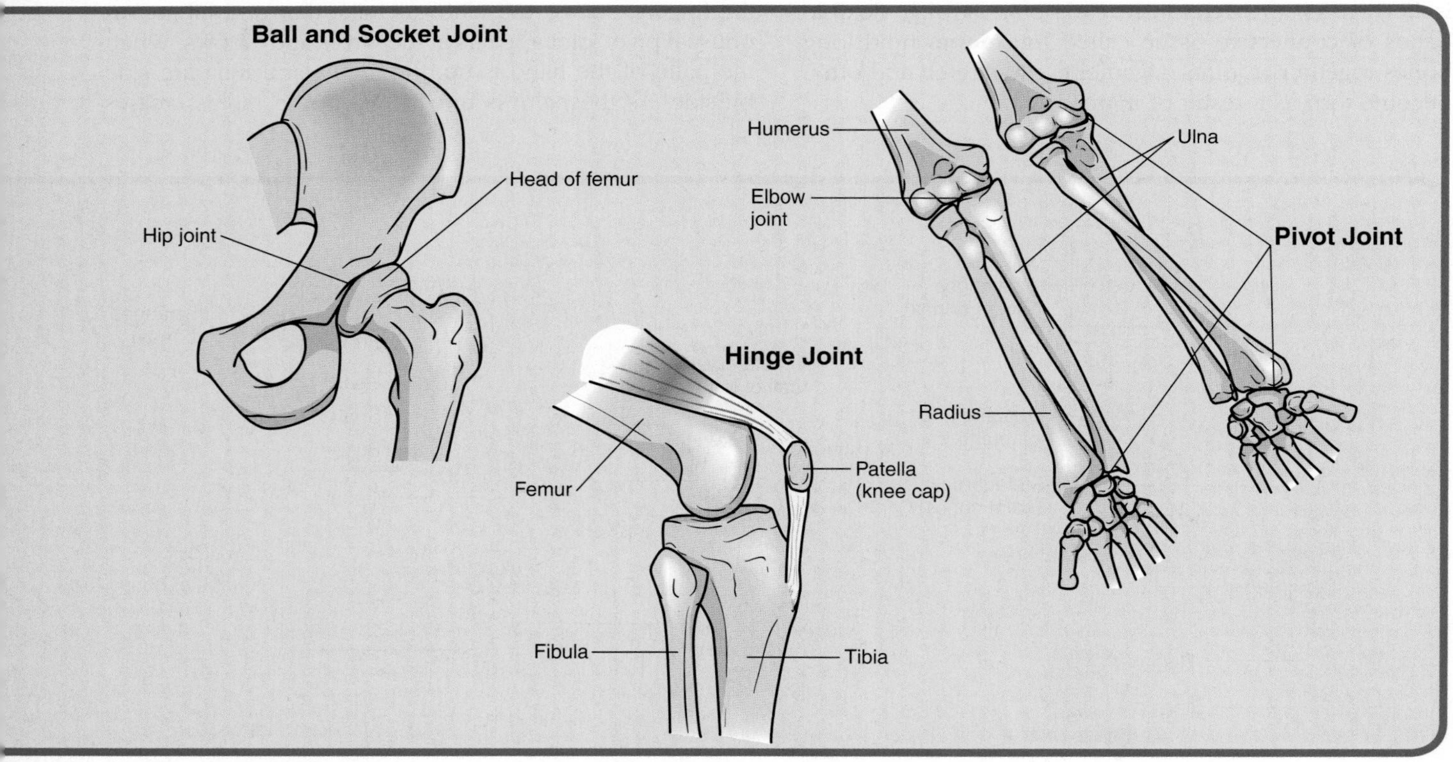

Figure 27–10: Types of joints. *Delmar/Cengage Learning.*

over the ulna in a pivoting action. This type of motion is independent of the elbow's hinge action. Joints found in the wrists and ankle are formed by bones with curved surfaces, which allow for various angular movements.

FRACTURES

The bones of children contain a high percentage of cartilage and are much more flexible than those of an adult. Frequently, the bone will crack under pressure but will not break all the way through. This type of break is known as a **greenstick fracture**.

A complete bone break in which there is no involvement with the skin surface is known as a **simple** or "closed" fracture (Figure 27–11). When broken bone protrudes through the skin's surface, it is known as an open fracture, formerly called a **compound** fracture. This causes additional concerns because of the possibility of infection to the area. A more involved type of fracture is called **impacted**, which indicates that the broken ends are jammed into each other. A **comminuted** fracture is one with more than one fracture line and several bone fragments. A **depressed** fracture may occur with severe head injuries in which a broken piece of skull is driven inward. A **spiral** fracture may occur with a severe twisting action, such as in a skiing accident, causing the break to wind around the bone.

MEDIA LINK

Go to the Premium Website and watch the animation, "Head Injuries," for this chapter.

A common injury among children is the Colles' fracture. This involves the breaking of the distal end of

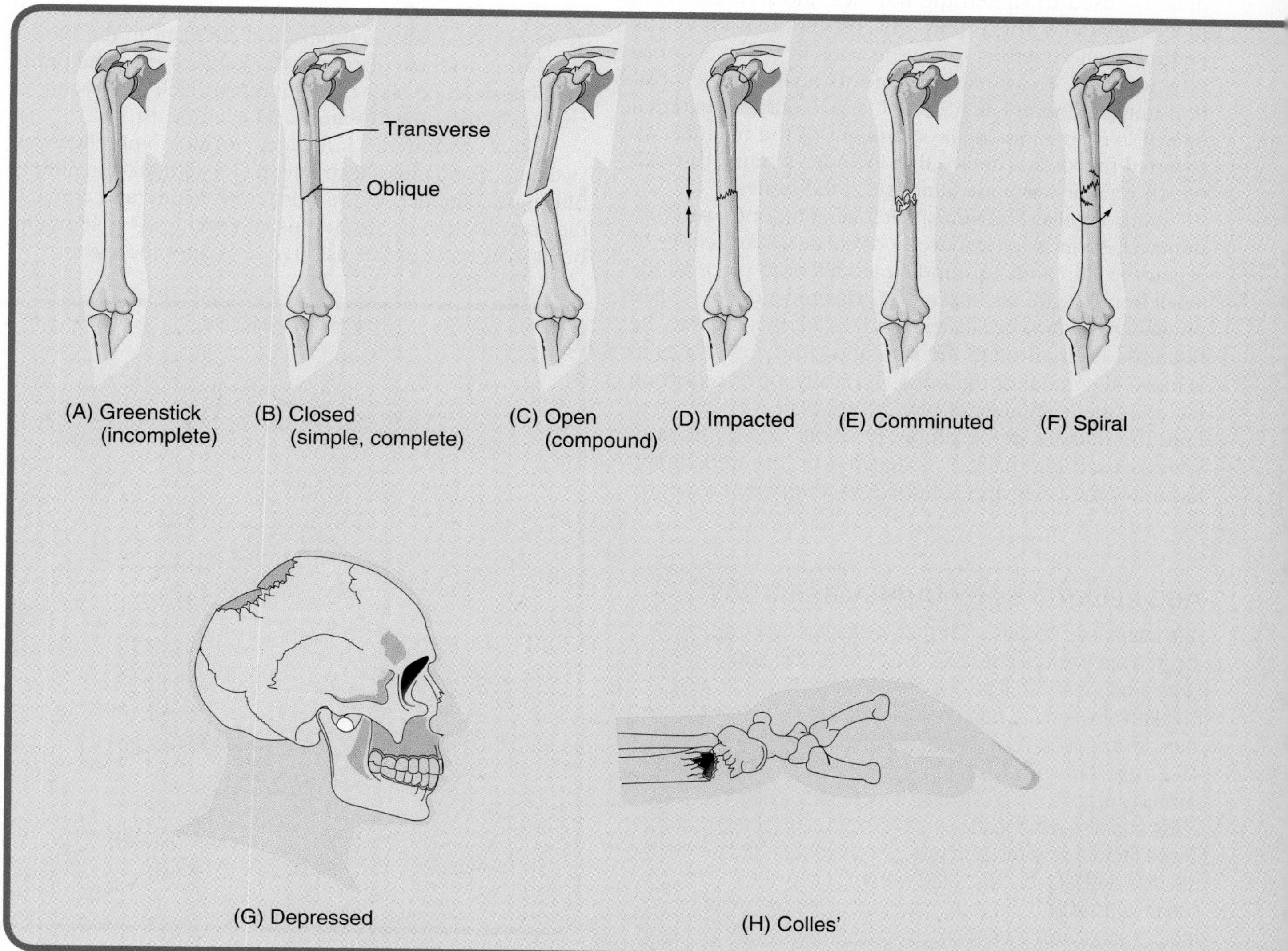

Figure 27–11: Types of fractures. *Delmar/Cengage Learning.*

the radius, causing a characteristic bulge at the wrist. Often, the ulna is also fractured, resulting in a greater wrist deformity and a limply hanging hand. It is a common fracture of children from injuries while skating, riding bikes, and climbing. It is generally the result of falling on an outstretched hand.

In treating fractures, immobilization of the affected part and prevention of shock are the main concerns. The extremity is splinted, extending above and below the area of fracture. Elevation of the part and application of a cold pack or ice help prevent swelling. When there is also extensive damage to the surrounding tissues, especially to the exterior, control of bleeding may be indicated. This may require direct pressure over the wound.

When long bones are broken, they are usually pulled by the muscles attached to their surfaces into abnormal positions, often causing overlapping of their broken parts. Before the bone can be set, **traction** (pulling)—either manually or by a system of ropes and pulleys—must be used to stretch the muscles and pull the bone pieces back into **alignment**. This procedure is known as **reducing** the fracture. Once the ends fit together properly, a splint or cast can be used to maintain the position until the bone has healed. Occasionally, an external fixator is used to maintain alignment of the fracture. An external fixator is a device that includes a frame through which pins or wires are attached to the bones.

With involved fractures, such as compound or comminuted, surgical procedure is often necessary either to repair the skin and surrounding tissues or to place all the small bone fragments in position. This procedure is called an *open reduction* because it involves an opening into the fractured bone through the skin and overlying tissues to achieve alignment of the bone. Typically, open reduction includes the placement of pins, wires, plates, or screws to hold the fracture in the proper position. When the hardware is used internally, it is covered by the normal soft tissues of the body and is known as an internal fixation.

AGE-RELATED BODY CHARACTERISTICS

Age influences fractures. Children have greenstick or incomplete fractures because their bones still have a large amount of cartilage and are therefore rather flexible. Children also tend to fracture their arms more than the lower extremities. The Colles', fracture is a good example. As we age, our cartilage is replaced with bone and the flexibility is gone. As adults age, they tend to lose muscle mass and also experience some loss of vision and balance. These factors may result in falls, which fracture primarily the hips and long bones of the extremities. These fractures can be closed or open with many variations and often require surgical intervention.

Bone Healing Process

When a fracture occurs, a collection of blood (hematoma) forms around the fracture site. The hematoma begins an inflammatory reaction that initiates the healing process. A fibrous bridge is formed between the fracture fragments. Some of the cells in this fibrous mesh differentiate into cartilage cells and begin to accumulate calcium, forming a **callus** (Figure 27–12). As time passes, the callus turns first to cartilage and then to bone. Certain bone cells build the new bone tissue, whereas others remove the cartilage and then slowly smooth the repaired section back to its approximate original size.

A complication that may occur after the fracture of a long bone is a fat **embolus**. An embolus is a mass of foreign material circulating within the blood vessels. This potentially fatal complication may follow the release of fat droplets from the marrow of the long bones. The trauma of the event can also cause the body to release catecholamines (organic compounds and hormones), which in turn activate fatty acids. The fatty acids can develop into a fatty embolus and circulate in the blood, interfering with circulation in the lungs or even the brain. This interference may cause hypoxia (lack of oxygen), a change in the mental status, and even death.

Usual symptoms and signs include apprehension, sweating, fever, rapid heart rate, pallor, difficulty breathing, bluish discoloration of the skin, convulsions, and coma. If the complication occurs, it is usually within 24 to 48 hours, but it may occur as late as three days after the fracture.

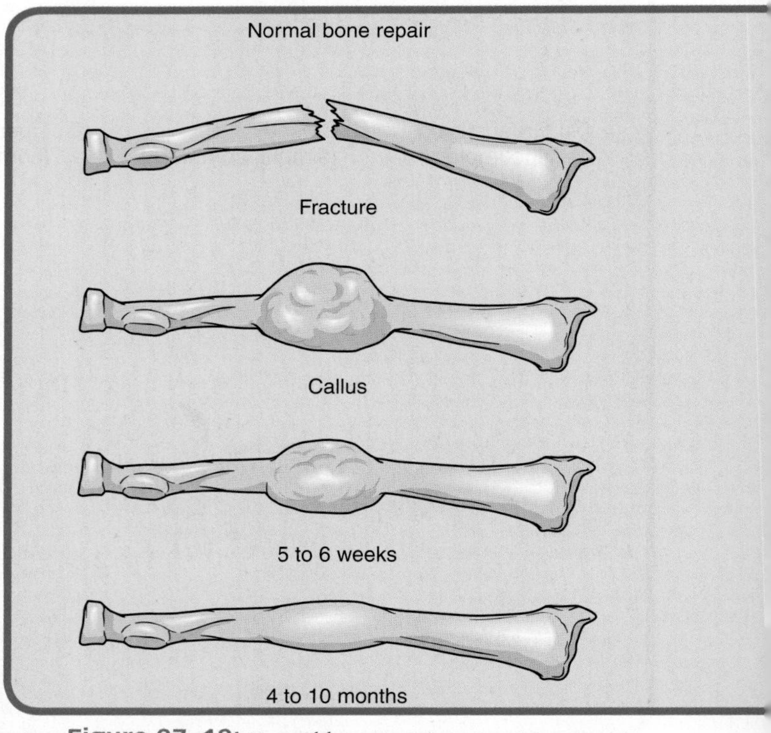

Figure 27–12: Normal bone repair. *Delmar/Cengage Learning.*

AMPUTATION

Severe trauma, a malignant tumor, lack of circulation, or complications of other conditions, such as diabetes, may result in the need to **amputate** an extremity. The change in the patient's body image and function causes emotional and physical difficulties in coping with daily activities. Following amputation, a condition often occurs known as **phantom limb**, the sensation that the missing extremity is still present. It is often described as an itching or tingling sensation. This may last for quite some time but will usually subside eventually. It is considered normal to experience the sensation.

When the amputated stump has healed sufficiently, a **prosthesis** (artificial part) may be fitted. Lower limbs are either attached directly to the remaining extremity, fastened by means of straps or belt to the waist, or hung from the shoulder. The method depends to a great extent on the amount of the remaining extremity. Upper limbs may be replaced by a "hook" device that can be opened and closed to grasp objects. A prosthesis that closely resembles a real arm and hand cosmetically is often desired, even though it lacks the flexibility of the "hook."

DIAGNOSTIC EXAMINATIONS

- *Arthroscopy*—This endoscopic procedure permits direct visual inspection of a joint, most often the knee (Figure 27–13). In an arthroscopic examination, a surgeon makes a small incision in the patient's skin and then inserts pencil-sized instruments that contain small lenses and lighting systems to magnify and illuminate the structures inside the joint. Light is transmitted through fiber optics to the end of the arthroscope that is inserted into the joint. By attaching the arthroscope to a miniature television camera, the surgeon is able to see the inside of the joint through this very small incision. It is frequently used to evaluate injuries suffered by athletes. Arthroscopy is useful in detecting **arthritis**, torn meniscus, cysts, or loose pieces of tissue. The display of the image on the television screen allows the surgeon to look throughout the knee to determine the amount or type of injury. Many surgical procedures can be performed through the scope, thereby eliminating open surgery.
- *Bone scan*—This is a precise nuclear medicine procedure using small amounts of a radioactive substance that are injected into a vein to help diagnose the presence of disease based on structural appearance. A scintillation or gamma camera positioned over the area obtains images by detecting the substance in the bones and recording it on a computer or film. Usually, the procedures is done in two parts. The injection is given first, and the medium is carried in the blood to the skeleton and distributed throughout the bones. After the injection, the patient may leave the area for about two hours while the bones thoroughly absorb the medium. After the time has passed, the patient returns and is placed on the imaging table, and the camera is positioned over the patient. It slowly moves up or down a framework over the body, taking the images for at least

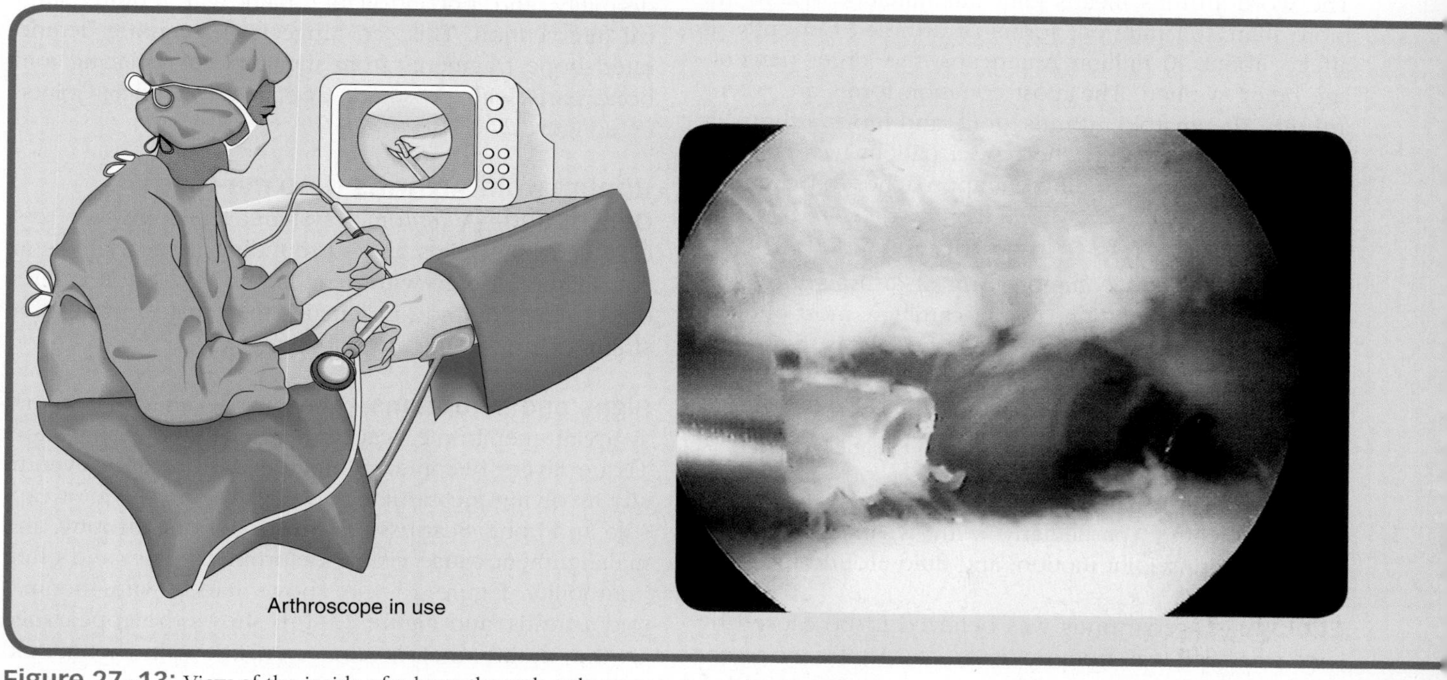

Figure 27–13: View of the inside of a knee through arthroscope. *Delmar/Cengage Learning.*

30 minutes. It is important that the patient remains still throughout the scanning process.

- *Computed tomography (CT) scan*—This is a special X-ray in that the X-ray tube moves around the patient. A computer takes the information and reconstructs a cross-sectional (axial) "slice" of the patient. Multiple slices are taken that allow the physician to determine the anatomy in three dimensions.
- *Magnetic resonance imaging (MRI)*—This process uses strong magnets that cause all of the protons in the field to "line up." Radio waves are then passed through the patient, causing the protons to resonate. A computer takes this information and constructs images in any plane. This technology has three advantages over CT scans: (1) There is no ionizing radiation (X-ray) used, (2) soft tissues are seen in more detail, and (3) images can be constructed in any plane (not just axial). The major disadvantage is that the technique is expensive. There are also some factors that prevent many patients from being candidates for the procedure, such as obesity or claustrophobia.
- *X-ray*—This is a frequently used test that evaluates the condition of bones in cases such as dislocations, sprains, and fractures. X-ray can also be used to determine bone structure changes like those occurring in some metabolic conditions such as acromegaly (gigantism) and **osteoporosis** or with Paget's disease.

DISEASES AND DISORDERS

Arthritis (Ar-thri′-tis)

The word arthritis means joint inflammation. There are more than 100 different forms of arthritis. Currently, it affects about 40 million Americans, the larger percentage being women. The most common forms are osteoarthritis, rheumatoid arthritis, gout, and lupus arthritis. It is important to identify the type a patient has, because different types require different approaches to treatment.

Osteoarthritis (Os-te-o-ar-thri′tis)

Description—This common form of arthritis results in progressive deterioration of joint cartilage, most often at the hips and knees. It affects many people as they grow older. Symptoms result from the breakdown of cartilage between bones and of the bones themselves. It is also known as degenerative joint disease. There is no cure.

Signs and symptoms—It is accompanied by joint pain, stiffness, aching (particularly with weather changes), "grating" during joint motion, and fluid around the joint.

Etiology—Osteoarthritis was believed to be caused by joint wear-and-tear from years of use. However, recent research suggests that a mild, slow-moving inflammation or a metabolic disorder is the root of the problem. There is a familial component to osteoarthritis.

Treatment—Osteoarthritis is best treated with aspirin and other nonsteroidal anti-inflammatory drugs (NSAIDs), intraarticular joint injections of steroids, and reducing pressure on joints through weight loss and the use of a cane, crutches, or a cervical collar. One popular drug used to treat arthritis is Celebrex. It is from a class of drugs called COX-2 inhibitors, which means they block an enzyme that causes inflammation but not the enzyme that controls production of a prostaglandin that protects the lining of the stomach. They are effective in relieving discomfort without the significant risks of the gastric side effects of NSAIDs (e.g., ibuprofen, naproxen, and Feldene).

If the COX-2 drugs and intraarticular steroid injections do not work, new injectable drugs containing hyaluronic acid can be used. The acid is a gooey fluid found in joint cavities that normally lubricates and absorbs shock. A series of several injections may be necessary and can provide relief for months. Initially, the injections were approved for the knee joint only. Other promising therapies involve transplanting cartilage cells harvested from the patient's own healthy knee cartilage. They are grown in a culture and then injected into the injured area to make new tissue. A third therapy uses stem cells harvested from the patient and grown and implanted in defects where cartilage is worn. A fourth removes a cylindrical plug of cartilage and bone from a healthy area within the knee and fits it into a drilled hole in the damaged cartilage. All these rely on the body's ability to repair itself if given the necessary materials. Occasionally, disability and uncontrollable pain will require surgical intervention. This can range from scraping deteriorated bone fragments from the joint to replacing joint bone parts with prosthetic appliances (artificial joints). (See Figure 27–17B.)

Rheumatoid Arthritis (Roo′ma-toyd)

Description—A chronic systemic inflammatory disease attacking joints and surrounding tissues, this is an intermittent disease with periods of remission. It is three times more common in females than males, most often striking between the ages of 35 and 45.

Signs and symptoms—The disease attacks the joint synovial membrane, causing edema and congestion. Tissue layers become granulated and thicken, eventually involving the cartilage and destroying the joint capsule and bone. Scar tissue formation, bone atrophy, and malalignment cause visible deformities, pain, and often immobility. Figure 27–14A shows hands with rheumatoid arthritis, and Figure 27–14B shows the appearance of the thumb that is characteristic with rheumatoid arthritis.

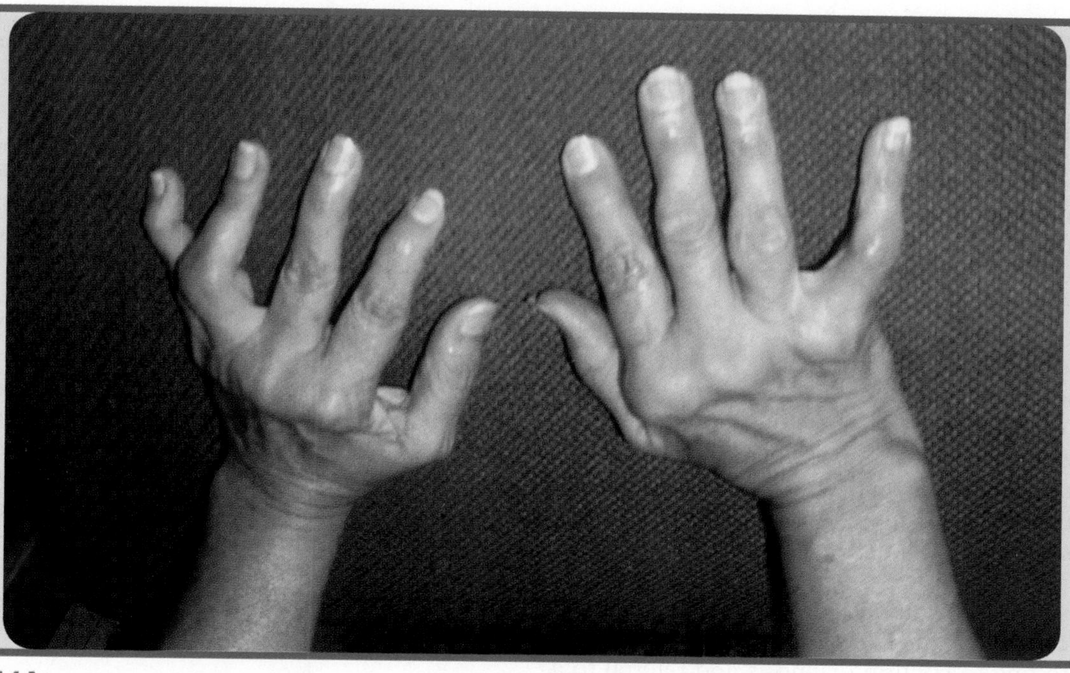

Figure 27–14A: Rheumatoid arthritis of the hands. *Courtesy of Barbara A. Wise.*

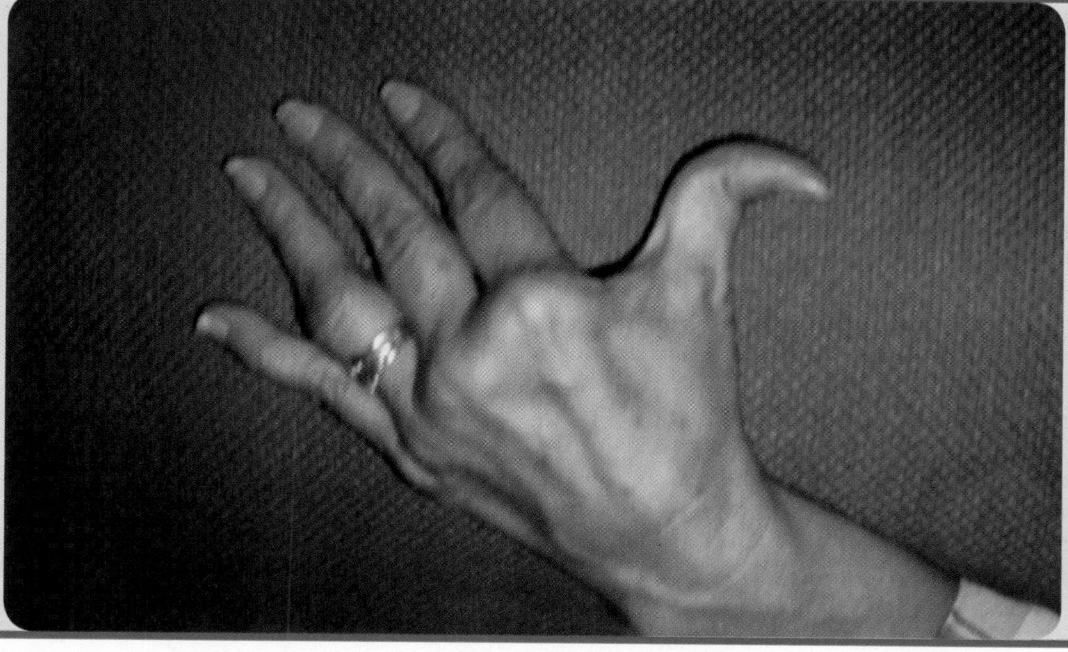

Figure 27–14B: Characteristic thumb position of rheumatoid arthritis. *Courtesy of Barbara A. Wise.*

Etiology—Rheumatoid arthritis is caused by a fault in the immune system that causes it to attack the joint membranes. The attack not only triggers inflammation but also stimulates the abnormal growth of cartilage and bone. It can affect persons of all ages.

Treatment—Treatments include anti-inflammatory and disease-modifying drugs, exercise, heat or cold, saving energy, joint protection, and sometimes surgery. Injections of cortisone directly into the joint may help to relieve pain and swelling; however, repeated frequent injections into the same joint can produce undesirable side effects. Researchers using genetic engineering techniques developed a drug called cA2 that blocks the immune system action. Maintaining a normal weight lessens stress on joints. Range of motion and low-impact aerobic exercise is beneficial and helps maintains flexibility. Warm water exercise is especially easy on joints. The woman whose hands are pictured in Figure 27–14A and B was diagnosed with rheumatoid arthritis 16 years ago at 34 years of age. She initially experienced debilitating pain with marked swelling and heat in her joints and considerable deformity. Current treatments have greatly improved her condition. One day a week she takes six tablets of methotrexate, and she also gets injections of Enbrel twice a week, plus daily prednisone. These medications require frequent lab work due to the possibility of liver damage. Her treatments cost her approximately $14,000 a year.

Children can also be affected with this disease. Juvenile rheumatoid arthritis (JRA) is characterized by fevers, joint pain, and redness over the joint areas. Laboratory testing to confirm diagnosis and referral to a specialist provides the best outcomes for the child with rheumatoid arthritis.

Gout (Gouty Arthritis)

Description—This metabolic disease results in severe joint pain, especially at night. It most often affects the great toe but can involve other joints. The pain results from deposits of urates (uric acid salts), which are overproduced or retained by the body. Often gout is associated with another disease, such as leukemia or because of cell destruction by chemotherapy. Gout may also follow drug therapy that interferes with urate excretion.

Signs and symptoms—Gout can be a progressive disease, initially causing severe pain and a hot, tender, inflamed joint. This attack will be followed by a symptom-free period of approximately six months to two years, when a second episode will occur. Additional attacks usually involve other joints of the feet and legs. Eventually, the condition becomes chronic (ongoing), involving many joints that are persistently painful and become degenerated, deformed, and disabling.

Etiology—The exact cause of gout is unknown, but it seems linked to a genetic defect in purine metabolism that causes overproduction of uric acid, retention of uric acid, or both. This interferes with urate excretion, leading to urate deposits that cause local tissue destruction.

Treatment—Gout is best treated with medication to suppress uric acid formation and promote excretion of the urates. Dietary restrictions such as avoiding alcohol, primarily beer and wine, and purine-rich foods, such as liver, sardines, kidneys, and lentils, can lessen symptoms.

Bursitis (Bur-si′tis)

Description—This is a painful inflammation of the bursa. A bursa is a sac located around a joint containing lubricating fluids that allow muscles and tendons to move freely over bony surfaces. Bursitis occurs most frequently at the hip, shoulder, or knee.

Signs and symptoms—The most common sign is pain upon movement and limited motion of the affected joint. The pain can be gradual or sudden. Symptoms vary according to the joint involved.

Etiology—It usually occurs in middle age and is the result of recurring trauma that stresses or pressures a joint. It can also be the result of an inflammatory joint disease. A chronic form develops from repeated attacks of acute bursitis or repeated trauma and infection.

Treatment—Treatment consists of joint rest, often immobilization, a pain medication, and bursal injection with a steroid combined with an anesthetic. It may be necessary to remove bursal fluid by aspiration (withdrawal through a needle) and the institution of a program of physical therapy to preserve joint motion.

Carpal Tunnel Syndrome

Description—This condition results from the compression of the median nerve at the wrist. The carpal tunnel is a passageway for nerves, blood vessels, and flexor tendons to the fingers and thumb. The carpal canal is formed by the carpal bones and the transverse ligament. The tendon sheaths become inflamed, causing swelling, which presses the median nerve against the transverse ligament.

Signs and symptoms—There is pain, tingling, numbness, and weakness of the hand. It usually involves only the thumb and index and middle finger. The patient will be unable to make a fist.

Etiology—People who develop the syndrome come from a variety of industries and job types, but is especially common in those performing assembly-line work, such as manufacturing, sewing, cleaning, and meat packing. Systemic conditions that cause the carpal tunnel to swell are diabetes mellitus, pregnancy, menopause, hypothyroidism, and benign tumors.

Diagnosis can be made based on an examination that reveals decreased sensitivity of the first two fingers and the thumb on pricking with a pin and an electromyogram showing delayed motor nerve conduction. Patients may also have *atrophy* (shrinking) of the muscle on the palm side of the thumb because of decreased innervation.

Treatment—If the syndrome is of short duration, treatment will consist of immobilizing the hand and forearm in a splint, local injections of corticosteroids, and systemic anti-inflammatory medication. It may be necessary to seek new employment if a work-related connection is determined. If conservative treatment does not correct the problem, a surgical procedure may be indicated to section the transverse ligament and "free-up" the nerve.

Congenital Hip Dysplasia (Kon-jen′-i-tal Dis-pla′-je-a)

Description—This abnormality of the hip joint is present at birth. It is the most common hip disorder of children, affecting one or both joints. It is present in three forms: unstable, with the hip in place but easily dislocated by manipulation; incomplete dislocation, with the head of the femur on the edge of the acetabulum; and complete dislocation, with the head totally outside the hip socket.

Signs and symptoms—Signs of hip dysplasia include the appearance of one leg being shorter than the other or one hip being more prominent. The child has a characteristic "duck waddle" if both hips are involved, or, if one hip only, a limp.

Etiology—The exact cause of dysplasia has not been proven. It is believed that hormones that relax maternal ligaments at the time of labor may also cause the infant ligaments to relax around the hip joint capsule. There is also an association of dislocation and a breech delivery.

Treatment—Early treatment is essential to normal development. In infants, a splint device is used for three to four months to maintain proper positioning. Older babies may be placed in traction, or the hips may be reduced and a cast applied for a period of four to six months.

Dislocation

Description—Displacement of bones at a joint so that the regularly articulating surfaces are no longer in contact is a **dislocation**. This occurs most frequently at joints of the finger, shoulder, knee, and hip.

Signs and symptoms—It is extremely painful and is often accompanied with joint surface fractures. Dislocation produces deformity around the joint, changes the length of the involved extremity, interferes with motion, and causes joint tenderness.

Etiology—Dislocation can be congenital, or it may follow trauma or disease of the surrounding joint.

Treatment—Prompt reduction (relocation) is essential to limit damage to surrounding tissues. Following reduction, a splint, cast, or traction (depending on the joint involved) to immobilize the area is indicated. Two to eight weeks will be needed to allow surrounding ligaments to heal completely.

Epicondylitis (Ep-i-kon-dil-i′-tis) (Tennis Elbow)

Description—This is an inflammation of the forearm extensor tendon at its attachment to the humerus or, less commonly, the flexor tendon at its attachment to the humerus.

Signs and symptoms—Pain occurs at the elbow and becomes intense. There is tenderness over the area where the radius articulates with the humerus.

Etiology—The condition probably begins as a tear and is common among people who grasp things forcefully or twist the forearm. Untreated epicondylitis can become disabling.

Treatment—The condition is best treated with an injection of a steroid and a local anesthetic, aspirin, an immobilizing splint, heat, or cold and physical therapy. Epicondylitis usually resolves with or without treatment.

Hallux Valgus (Hal′-uks Val′-gus)

Description—Common in women, this is a lateral deviation of the great toe with enlargement of the first metatarsal head and a **bunion** formation. A bunion may be associated with a painful bursa.

Signs and symptoms—The bursa becomes inflamed, filled with fluid, and tender. The overlying skin is red.

Etiology—It may be congenital but is usually acquired from degenerative arthritis or the prolonged pressure on the foot from narrow, high-heeled shoes. Hallux valgus will cause bone deformity, and the change will alter the person's weight-bearing pattern.

Treatment—Early treatment with proper shoes, the use of padding and straightening devices, and exercises may correct the situation. A severe deformity and disabling pain will require surgical removal of the bunion.

Herniated Disk (Her-ne-a′-ted) (Ruptured Disk)

Description—In this situation, the soft gel-like material within an intervertebral disk has been forced through the disc's outer surface. The extruded material may cause pressure on a spinal nerve exiting the spinal cord or may impinge on the spinal cord itself.

Signs and symptoms—The classic symptom is severe lower back pain, frequently radiating deep into the buttocks and down the back of the leg. It is usually unilateral (one sided). Sensory loss results from nerve compression, and the patient experiences numbness, muscle spasm, motor difficulty, and eventually weakness and atrophy of the leg muscles.

Etiology—A herniated disk may result from severe trauma or strain, but it is frequently related to degeneration of the intervertebral joints. It occurs most often in the lumbar or lumbosacral regions. Herniated disk usually occurs in adults, mainly men, under age 45. In elderly people with disk degeneration, herniation can occur from a minor trauma.

Treatment—Conservative treatment consists of avoidance of painful activities, light exercises, frequent resting, analgesics as appropriate for pain, and anti-inflammatory medications, both steroidal and nonsteroidal. A **laminectomy** is indicated if there is neurologic involvement that does not improve with conservative therapy. This procedure involves removing a portion of the lamina (flattened portion of the vertebral arch) to remove the protruding disk material.

If symptoms persist, a surgical procedure, **spinal fusion**, is performed to stabilize the adjoining vertebrae. A spinal fusion is typically accomplished by placing a screw and rod assembly into the spine to achieve a stable internal fixation. A piece of bone for a graft can be harvested from the pelvis or obtained from the bone bank. It is placed within a prepared space in the vertebra in conjunction with the hardware to achieve a solid fusion. When the bone heals, the joined vertebrae can no longer move independently to impinge on the nerve or spinal cord.

Kyphosis (Ki-fo′-sis) (Roundback, Humpback)

Description—This is a bowing of the back, usually at the thoracic level, resulting from improper vertebral alignment (Figure 27–15A). There are two types of **kyphosis**: adolescent and adult.

Signs and symptoms—With adolescent kyphosis, the condition is essentially without symptoms except for the visible curving of the back. Some adolescents may have mild pain, fatigue, localized tenderness, stiffness in the involved area, and tightening of the hamstring muscles of the posterior thighs because of compensating posture. In adult kyphosis, there is the characteristic

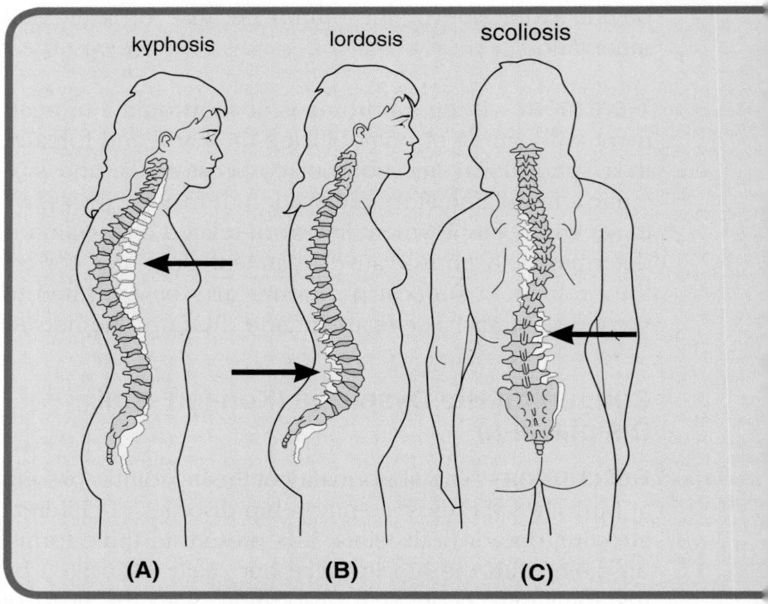

Figure 27–15: Abnormal curvatures of the spine: (A) kyphosis, (B) lordosis, (C) scoliosis. *Delmar/Cengage Learning.*

rounded back, possible pain, weakness of the back, and fatigue.

Etiology—In children and adolescents, kyphosis may be caused by growth retardation or the result of rapid growth periods with improper epiphysis development. Poor posture and excessive sports activity can also result in curvature. In the adult form, it is caused by aging and the degeneration of intervertebral disks or the actual collapse of vertebrae resulting from osteoporosis.

Treatment—Kyphosis as a result of poor posture during childhood can be treated by therapeutic exercise, a firm mattress, and a Milwaukee brace to straighten the spine until spinal growth is complete. If neurologic damage or disabling pain occurs in adolescents and adults (which happens rarely), a surgical procedure may be indicated, which involves posterior spinal fusion, bone grafting, and casting to straighten the severe curvature. With full skeletal maturity and debilitating curvature, a posterior spinal fusion can be accomplished with the use of a stainless steel Harrington rod mechanism to align the vertebrae.

Lordosis (Lor-do′-sis)

Description—This abnormal anterior convex curvature of the lumbar spine is commonly referred to as swayback (see Figure 27–15B). The body's spine normally curves in at this point; however, if it is exaggerated, it is considered to be **lordosis**.

Signs and symptoms—The obvious visual symptom is the excessive inward curvature of the lumbar portion of the back.

Etiology—It is usually caused by poor posture. The wearing of high heels causes the inward positioning of the lower back to counteract the position of the feet to maintain balance.

Treatment—This condition can be improved, or at least prevented from progressing, by appropriate exercises, improving posture, and wearing proper footwear.

Lumbar Myositis (Lum-bar Mi-o-si′tis)

Description—An inflammation of the lumbar region muscles of the back.

Signs and symptoms—Low back pain.

Etiology—It is common and is primarily caused by a straining of the back muscles.

Treatment—The condition is best treated with rest, mild analgesics, and muscle relaxers. When improved, a program of stretching exercises is prescribed to condition and strengthen the muscles.

Osteoporosis (Os-te-o-por-o′-sis)

Description—A metabolic bone disorder, characterized by acceleration of the rate of bone resorption while the rate of bone formation slows down, which results in a loss of bone mass. The loss of calcium and phosphate from the bone allows it to become porous, brittle, and prone to fracture. There are two forms of osteoporsis: primary and secondary. Primary is also known as senile or postmenopausal osteoporosis because it affects primarily elderly, postmenopausal women. Of the 25 million older Americans with osteoporosis, only 5 million are men. Secondary osteoporosis can occur following prolonged steroid therapy, bone immobilization or lack of use (with paralysis), malnutrition, excessive alcohol intake, scurvy, and hyperthyroidism. It is usually discovered following injury from bending to lift something.

Signs and symptoms—The individual feels instant pain in the mid thoracic to lumber spine. The pain is from the collapse of a vertebra. Other common signs of osteoporosis are slowly developing kyphosis with loss of height, fractures of the forearm or hip from minor falls, and additional spontaneous vertebral fractures. Figure 27–16 illustrates the progression of spinal curvature caused by osteoporosis and the resulting loss of height. (Note height measurements.)

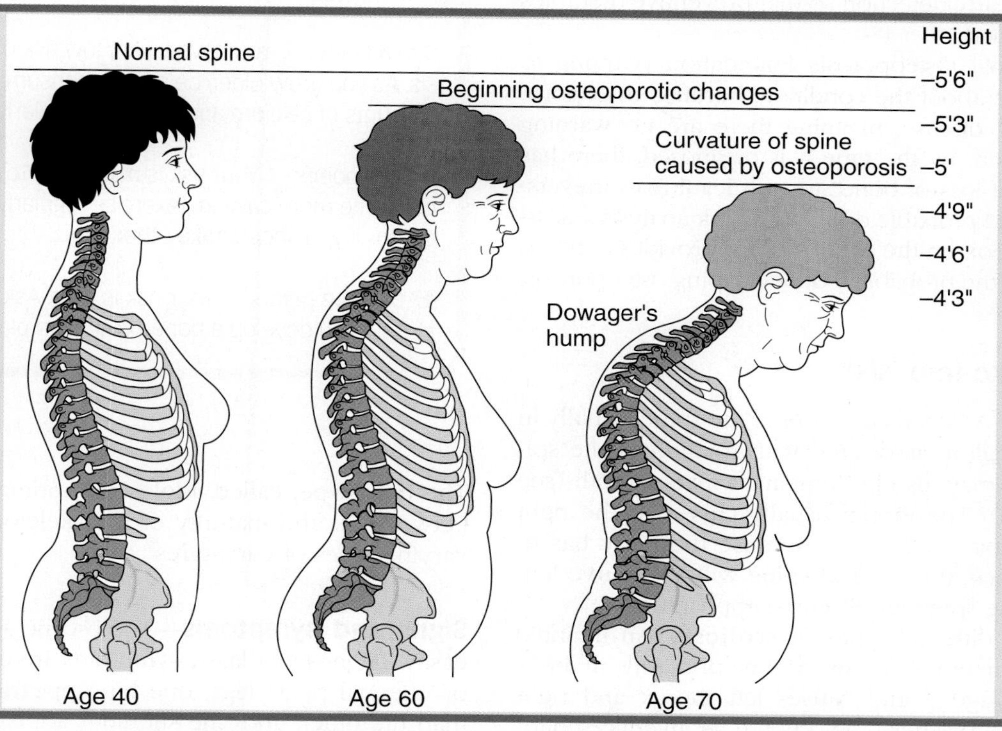

Figure 27–16: Osteoporosis: loss in height and the Dowager's hump. *Delmar/Cengage Learning.*

Etiology—The cause of primary osteoporosis may be the combination of aging, prolonged inadequate dietary intake of calcium, faulty metabolism because of estrogen deficiency, or a sedentary lifestyle. Females with small, thin frames are more likely to develop it. Males with low levels of testosterone are also more prone. The use of tobacco and a family history of osteoporosis also increases the risk.

Treatment—The condition is treatable to prevent additional fracturing by increasing exercise, giving an estrogen supplement, and taking calcium and vitamin D to support normal bone metabolism.

Today there are several approved treatments, including bisphosphonates (some examples are Fosamax, Boniva, and Reclast); estrogen therapy; estrogen agonists/antagonists (also called selective estrogen receptor modulators or SERMS); parathyroid hormone; hormone therapy; and RANK ligand (RANKL) inhibitor.

The most significant development is the ability to determine the disease before fractures occur. There are seven different techniques for measuring bone density in various body locations. The most used form of densitometry is called dual energy X-ray absorptiometry (DEXA). It can measure bone density and also estimate fracture risk. The procedure is relatively fast, uses a low level of radiation, and is fairly inexpensive. Another even simpler method screens for the rate of bone loss with a urine test called Osteomark, or the NTX test. The purpose of all procedures is early detection so that preventive therapies can be prescribed.

The National Osteoporosis Foundation is trying to educate people about the condition, because osteoporosis is a "silent" disease, meaning there are no warning symptoms. Often, by the time it is diagnosed, there has been significant loss of bone strength leading to irreversible damage and probable disability. A risk analysis assessment (see the box on the next column) provides a means of determining the probability of developing osteoporosis.

PATIENT EDUCATION

RISK ANALYSIS FOR OSTEOPOROSIS

Yes (4)_____	No (0)	I smoke cigarettes.
Yes (4)_____	No (0)	I drink alcoholic beverages [3 oz. or more a day].
Yes (2)_____	No (0)	I drink alcoholic beverages [1 to 2 oz. a day].
Yes (0)_____	No (3)	I often drink/eat dairy foods.
Yes (0)_____	No (3)	I exercise regularly.
Yes (4)_____	No (0)	I have an eating disorder.
Yes (2)_____	No (0)	My diet is high in red meat.
Yes (2)_____	No (0)	I often drink three or more cups of coffee or two or more cola beverages a day.
Yes (4)_____	No (0)	There's a history of osteoporosis in my family.
Yes (4)_____	No (0)	I have a small-boned frame.
Yes (2)_____	No (0)	I am older than 40.
Yes (4)_____	No (0)	I am older than 70.
Yes (3)_____	No (0)	I am a post-menopausal woman who began menopause before age 45.
Yes (4)_____	No (0)	I have taken steroid (cortisone) medications.
Yes (4)_____	No (0)	I have had or have an overactive thyroid gland.
Yes (3)_____	No (0)	I have chronic kidney disease.
_____	Total Risk Points	

0 to 8 points You have a very low risk of osteoporosis. As you grow older, be sure to consume adequate amounts of calcium and exercise regularly.

9 to 16 points Your risk is moderate. To reduce it, consume more calcium, exercise regularly, and ask your doctor if you should take other steps.

17 or more points Your risk is high. Ask your doctor to help you develop a bone-protection plan.

Scoliosis (Sko-le-o′-sis)

Description—A lateral curvature of the spine, usually in the thoracic region, associated with rotation of the spinal column. It may also be lumbar or involve both (see Figure 27–15C). The thorax usually curves to the right while the lumbar curves left. Because the body has to maintain balance, the cervical spine will also curve left, which gives the spine an "S" curve appearance.

There are different types of **scoliosis**. An infantile type of transmitted scoliosis occurs primarily in boys from birth to age 3 and causes left thorax and right lumbar curves. Another type, known as juvenile scoliosis, affects both sexes between the ages of 4 and 10. The third type, called adolescent, primarily affects girls between 10 and maturity of the skeleton and results in varying types of curvatures.

Signs and symptoms—Adolescent scoliosis can be easily diagnosed. Classic symptoms are uneven hemlines or unequal pants legs, one hip appearing to be higher than the other, and one shoulder appearing higher and perhaps the scapula more pronounced.

Etiology—Different types have different causes. Some are from congenital defects of the vertebra, muscular dystrophy, paralysis, or a transmitted trait that develops during the growth process. Others are the result of poor posture or uneven leg lengths. Most scoliosis is of idiopathic (without apparent cause) origin.

Treatment—Treatment includes observation, exercises, and a brace. With curvature beyond 60 degrees, an immobilizing cast or preoperative traction system is followed by surgical correction using posterior spinal fusion and insertion of a Harrington rod for stabilization.

PATIENT EDUCATION

HOW TO DETECT SCOLIOSIS

Parents:
To check your child for scoliosis (abnormal curvature of the spine) perform this simple test. First, have your child remove his or her shirt and stand up straight. As you look at the child's back, answer these questions:

- Is one shoulder higher than the other, or is one shoulder blade more prominent?
- When the child's arms hang loosely at his or her sides, does one arm swing away from the body more than the other?
- Is one hip higher or more prominent than the other?
- Does the child seem to tilt to one side?

Ask your child to bend forward, with arms hanging down and palms together at knee level. Can you see a hump on the back at the ribs or near the waist?

If your answer to any of these questions is yes, your child needs careful evaluation for scoliosis. Notify your doctor.

Sprain

Description—The complete or incomplete tear in the supporting ligaments of a joint.

Signs and symptoms—**Sprains** are characterized by pain, swelling, and a black-and-blue discoloration. The ankle is the most common site.

Etiology—Sprains follow a severe twisting action of a joint.

Treatment—Care of sprains should follow the easy to remember R.I.C.E. method—Rest, Ice, Compression, and Elevation. Treatment consists of (1) controlling pain and swelling by elevating the joint and applying ice intermittently for the first 12 to 24 hours, (2) immobilization using an elastic wrap or, if very severe, a soft cast, and (3) the use of crutches to eliminate stress on the joint. If healing does not occur normally in three to four weeks, the torn ligaments may require surgical repair, especially if sprains recur.

Subluxation (Sub-luks-a′-shun)

Description—The partial or incomplete dislocation of the articulating surfaces at the joints.

Signs and symptoms—There is joint deformity, impaired motion, pain, and change in length if an extremity is involved. Common sites are shoulders, elbows, wrists, knees, fingers and toes, hips, and ankles. Diagnostic X-ray is usually indicated to rule out or confirm accompanying joint fracture.

Etiology—Subluxation is caused by an injury or a disease process of a joint. Often with an injury there is also involvement of the surrounding nerves, blood vessels, ligaments, and soft tissues that results in pain, swelling, and joint deformity.

Treatment—Treatment consists of reduction as soon as possible to minimize swelling and muscle spasms, which make reduction difficult. The use of medication to control muscle spasm and pain and possibly a splint or cast to provide joint immobilization and support while ligaments heal depend on the joint involved.

Temporomandibular Disorders (TMD) (Tem-po-ro-man-dib′-u-lar)

Description—This is a condition of the jaw that is described as a feeling that the jaw has come unhinged. For unknown reasons, 90% of sufferers are women.

Signs and symptoms—The symptoms include a grinding or clicking sound and pain and discomfort when opening the mouth. Jaw muscles become sore, chewing is difficult, and pain spreads to the facial and neck muscles. Symptoms persist continuously. Headaches, toothaches, and earaches may also be part of the disorder.

Etiology—The cause is not certain. Some feel it is emotional stress; others feel that the joint is very complicated and TMD is a matter is a of many factors adversely affecting the joint. Teeth grinding and clenching cause muscle spasm and can be caused by it. A malocclusion of the teeth can throw the jaw out of line. Bad posture that thrusts the chin forward can strain the neck and jaw muscles. Certain orthopedic problems, such as arthritis and bone degeneration, can contribute. Other causes may be excessive chewing of gum or chewy foods or a blow to the jaw. A common cause is prolonged gripping of a phone between the shoulder and cheek or carrying a heavy shoulder bag that strains neck and shoulder muscles.

Treatment—First is self-treatment, such as a soft diet and an analgesic for the pain, and eliminating activities known as causes. Hot or cold compresses, gentle exercises, controlling yawns (with the hands), and resting of the jaw may help. If malocclusion is present, a simple grinding of teeth surfaces by a dentist may correct the problem. Bite splints or plates fitted over the teeth can also stabilize the bite and eliminate night grinding. Taking muscle relaxers and eliminating the source of stress may be necessary.

REPLACING BONE AND JOINTS

When bone is destroyed by injury, cancer, or an infectious process, doctors may use bone taken from other places in the body. However, there is a limit to the amount that can be "borrowed." When desperate, bone can be salvaged from cadavers, but the problems of inflammation and infection are a concern. Surgeons have discovered that coral from the ocean is uniquely compatible with bone and makes an excellent framework upon which bone cells can construct new bone. Certain species of coral have an almost identical physical makeup as bone. It unites, almost without seams, with the human skeleton. In addition, it does not activate the body's inflammation or immune responses. Once the surgery has healed, the strength of the resulting bone composite is excellent. The coral is available in blocks of different sizes, which doctors carve into the shapes they need for surgery.

Replacing worn or damaged joints is a commonly performed procedure. The knees and hips are the joints most often affected by the wear and tear of movement and supporting the body. Articulating surfaces at joints normally have protective coverings of cartilage that allow the surfaces to move against each other easily. When this cartilage wears thin, is damaged, or breaks up, it causes pain within the joint from the fragments and the bones rubbing together. Figure 27–17A shows a knee with the loss of cartilage from rheumatoid arthritis. Note the bones at the joint have no space between them and are therefore painful upon movement. In Figure 27–17B, the damaged knee is replaced with an artificial joint. The ends of the natural bone are modified to attach and insert the new metal surfaces.

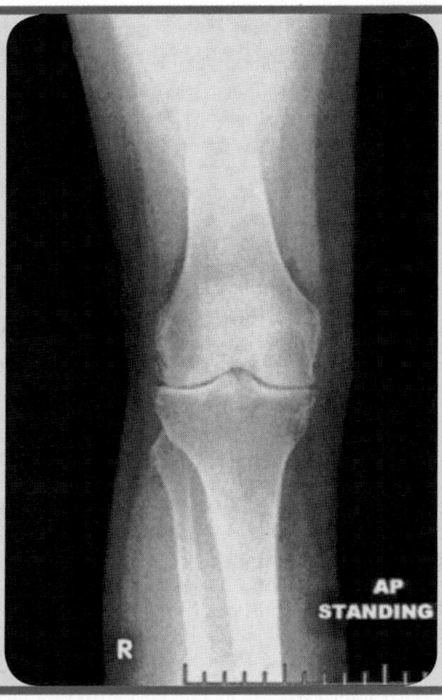

Figure 27–17A: Preoperative knee with cartilage destroyed by rheumatoid arthritis. *Delmar/Cengage Learning.*

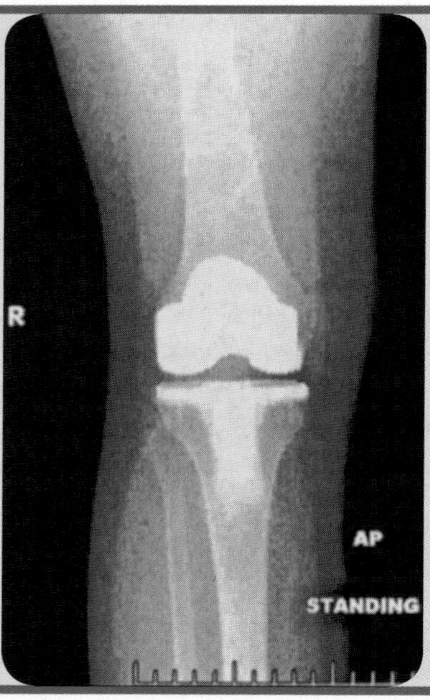

Figure 27–17B: Postoperative knee with replacement artificial joint. *Delmar/Cengage Learning.*

In Figure 27–17C, the head of the femur is damaged. Usually, the head will not stay within the socket of the pelvis due to years of movement and the weakening of the supporting joint structures. In Figure 27–17D, the head of the femur has been removed and a metal shaft inserted into the femur. The corresponding socket has

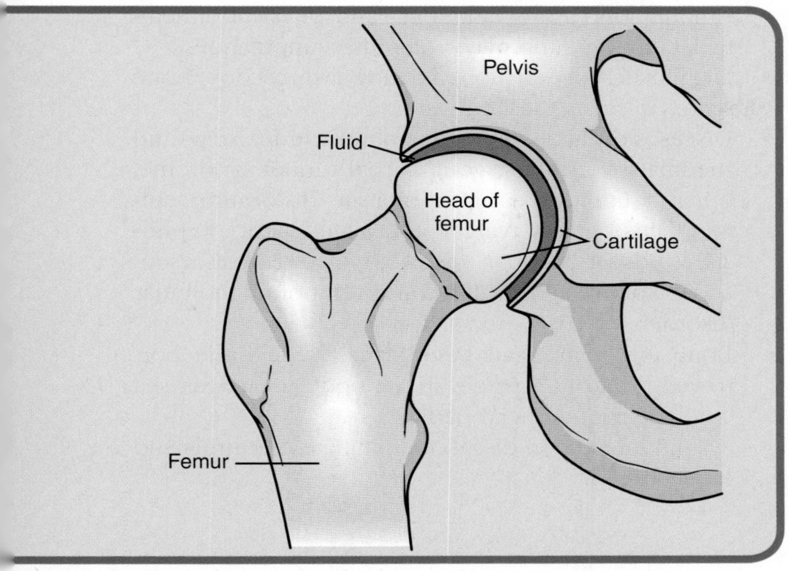

Figure 27–17C: Preoperative hip joint. *Delmar/Cengage Learning.*

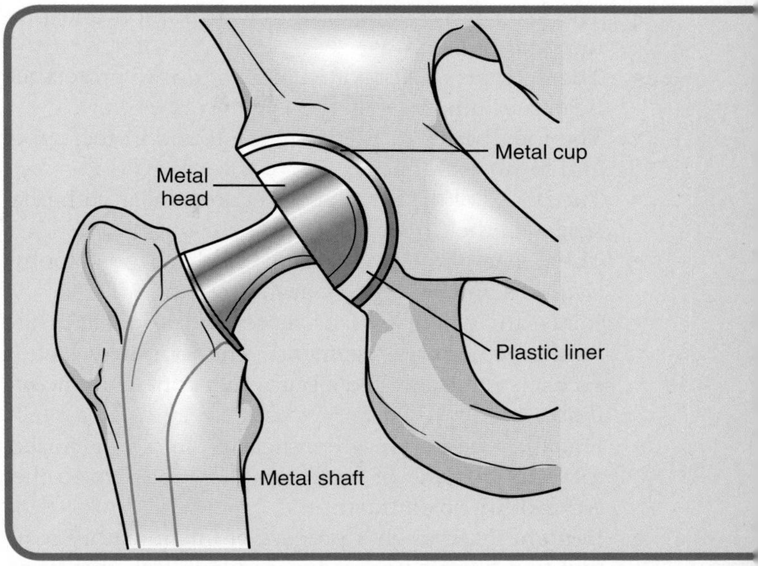

Figure 27–17D: Postoperative artificial hip joint. *Delmar/Cengage Learning.*

TABLE 27–1 System Interaction Associated with Disease Conditions

Disease	System Involved	Pathology Present
Rheumatoid arthritis	Skeletal	Swelling and deformity of joints
	Immune system	Destruction of joint membranes
	Circulatory system	Inflammation
Osteoporosis	Skeletal	Porous bone structure, fracture prone
		Kyphosis, loss of height
	Digestive	Inadequate calcium intake
	Reproductive	Inadequate estrogen

been implanted into the pelvic bone. This new joint will last for 10 to 15 years but will eventually wear or loosen and require replacement.

Research continues to identify new materials and techniques to prolong the life of artificial joints. Replacement is usually delayed as long as possible, particularly in younger people. Joints can be redone, but the risk of complications increases with repeat operations.

System Interaction Associated with Disease Conditions

The skeletal system provides the framework upon which the body structure is supported. However, as we know, bones are alive and functioning as is true with other systems, they do not function alone in either a healthy or diseased condition. Table 27–1 summarizes two skeletal disease interactions.

CHAPTER SUMMARY

- The skeletal system has two sections, the axial and the appendicular skeleton.
- Bone structure is 20% water with the remainder being minerals and organic matter.
- The body contains 270 bones at birth that reduce through fusion to 206 by adulthood.
- The skeleton has six functions: support, protection, attachment for muscles, providing shape for the body, formation of blood cells, and storing calcium.
- The spinal column has 24 cervical, thoracic, and lumbar vertebrae plus the sacrum and coccyx.

- The skull has a cranial and facial portion and protects the brain.
- The rib cage consists of 12 pairs of ribs to protect the heart and lungs.
- The long bones of the body are found in the upper and lower extremities.
- The bones of the hand and feet are similar with phalanges in the fingers and toes.
- The pelvic girdle is joined anteriorly at the symphysis pubis and posteriorly at the sacrum.
- Joints are where two or more bones join and are held together with ligaments. The joint may have a saclike structure called a bursa that contains synovial fluid.
- Fractures vary from greenstick to simple or closed, to various forms of compound or open and other types of involved fractures.
- Bone heals through a process of inflammatory reaction to a fibrous bridge and cartilage cells that accumulates calcium to form a callus.
- Amputation causes emotional and physical difficulties. Phantom limb may occur after amputation.
- Diagnostic examinations include arthroscopy, bone scan, CT scan, MRI, and X-ray.
- Diseases discussed in the chapter include osteo- and rheumatoid arthritis, gout, carpal tunnel syndrome, bursitis, congenital hip dysplasia, dislocation epicondylitis, hallux valgus, herniated disk, kyphosis, lordosis, lumbar myositis, osteoporosis, scoliosis, sprain, subluxation, and temporomandibular disorder.
- Bone and joints can be replaced with bone borrowed from other places in the body, a cadaver, sea coral, or with artificial parts.
- System interaction diseases: rheumatoid arthritis and osteoporosis.

STUDY TOOLS

Workbook	Activities for Chapter 27
Premium Website	
MEDIA LINK	View this **Media Link** for Chapter 27: • Head injuries
StudyWARE	Activities and Quizzes on the **StudyWARE™ Software** for Chapter 27
	Audio Library of medical terms
	Online access to the **Critical Thinking Challenge 2.0**
CourseMate	Activities and Quizzes for Chapter 27
WebTutor	Activities and Quizzes for Chapter 27

CHECK YOUR KNOWLEDGE

1. An adult has how many bones?
   a. 207
   b. 270
   c. 206
   d. 260
2. The bone covering is called:
   a. marrow.
   b. cancellous.
   c. cortical.
   d. periosteum.
3. Sacral vertebrae are located in the:
   a. neck.
   b. chest.
   c. back.
   d. posterior pelvic girdle.
4. The place where two or more bony parts join together is called a(n):
   a. diarthrosis.
   b. bursa.
   c. amphiarthrosis.
   d. articulation.
5. Arthroscopy is:
   a. a surgical procedure to view inside a joint.
   b. the injection of radioactive substance into a vein.
   c. a special X-ray of a joint.
   d. an imaging test using radio waves.

6. Rheumatoid arthritis is caused by:
   a. a fault in the immune system.
   b. a virus.
   c. an injury to the joint.
   d. wear and tear on the joint.
7. Carpal tunnel syndrome:
   a. develops after acute bursitis.
   b. causes symptoms in the thumb and first two fingers.
   c. causes deformities of the joint.
   d. is an inflammation of the forearm extensor tendon.
8. Lordosis refers to:
   a. the bowing of the back at the thoracic level.
   b. a lateral curvature of the spine.
   c. a backward curvature of the cervical area.
   d. the abnormal anterior convex curvature of the lumbar spine.
9. Subluxation is:
   a. a feeling the jaw is unhinged.
   b. the incomplete dislocation of a joint.
   c. the incomplete tear in the supporting ligaments of a joint.
   d. the deposit of urates at a joint.
10. Bones of the spinal column are separated by:
    a. marrow.
    b. ligaments.
    c. synovial fluid.
    d. cartilage disks.
11. Osteoporosis involves:
    a. skeletal, circulatory, and immune systems.
    b. skeletal, digestive, and reproductive.
    c. immune, digestive, and skeletal.
    d. digestive, circulatory, and skeletal.

WEB LINKS

Arthritis Foundation; provides information on all forms of arthritis: arthritis.org

National Osteoporosis Foundation; provides information on osteoporosis: www.nof.org

Centers for Disease Control and Prevention: www.cdc.gov

Chapter

28 The Muscular System

OBJECTIVES

In this chapter, you will learn the following:

KB LEARNING OBJECTIVES

1. Spell and define, using the glossary at the back of the text, all the Words to Know in this chapter.
2. Explain how muscular activity increases body heat.
3. List six functions of skeletal muscles.
4. Name and describe the three types of muscular tissue and the purpose of each.
5. Describe the purpose of a muscle team and give an example.
6. Explain what muscle tone means.
7. Describe the structure and function of a tendon and identify the body's strongest tendon.
8. Explain the terms *origin* and *insertion*.
9. Describe a muscle sheath and a bursa and the purpose of each.
10. Identify the muscles of respiration and describe how their function results in breathing.
11. Name the major skeletal muscles of the body.
12. Describe the smooth muscle action of peristalsis.
13. Explain the structure and function of a sphincter.
14. Describe four disorders or diseases of the muscular system.
15. Discuss how muscle changes with age.
16. Identify the body systems involved with fibromyalgia.

WORDS TO KNOW

abduction
Achilles' tendon
adduction
anchor
aponeurosis
atrophy
biceps
contracture
cramp
deltoid
dystrophy
extensor
fascia
flexor
gastrocnemius
gluteus maximus
hamstring
hiccough
insertion
intercostal
latissimus dorsi
muscle team
muscle tone
musculoskeletal
origin
pectoralis major
peristalsis
quadriceps femoris
sartorius
sheath
spasm
sphincter
sternocleidomastoid
strain
tendon
tendonitis
tibialis anterior
torticollis
trapezius
triceps

MUSCLES

There are approximately 600 muscles in the human body. Muscles are composed of muscular tissue, which is constructed of bundles of muscle fibers about the size of a human hair. The larger the muscle, the greater the number of fibers. Muscles perform their duties by alternately contracting and relaxing. All muscle activity is influenced by the nervous system. Motor neuron axons innervate several muscle cells within a muscle. Signals from the brain go through the axons and cause all the cells under their control to contract at the same time. That group of cells and its motor neuron are called a *motor unit*. When only one stimulus acts on the unit, causing a contraction, it is called a *twitch*. This quick, simple contraction naturally occurs occasionally as a spontaneous event in a muscle. Scientists can study these units by using an electrical stimulus, which will also activate the motor unit. A muscle contraction is a quick progression of events following a stimulus—a very brief interval before the contraction begins, then it intensifies to a peak, and decreases to relaxation. If a second stimulus is received before the first is completed, the contraction will strengthen. When repeated stimulation occurs without a relaxation time, the muscle is maintained in a state of contraction called *tetanus* (not to be confused with the disease of the same name). This occurs when we experience muscle **cramps** and **spasms**.

At all times, motor units are alternately either contracted or relaxed; there is no other state in which they exist. The units that make up the muscles are contracted in sufficient number to meet whatever need is necessary. During sleep, for instance, only a few would be contracted at a given time, yet during strenuous activity, a great number would be called on to contract, a process known as *muscle recruitment*.

Some muscles work in partnership with the bones and can be controlled voluntarily by the motor nerves of the peripheral nervous system to achieve movement. Other muscles function continuously without the slightest conscious concern. The autonomic nervous system directs their activities to provide the body with essential services. It is the action of these muscles that causes us to breathe and our blood to circulate.

MUSCLE FUEL

All body tissues must have food and oxygen to survive. The muscles receive an ample supply of both because of their importance to the body's safety and well-being. The body stores carbohydrates in its muscles in the form of a starch called *glycogen*. When muscles function, they use the stored glycogen, changing it to glucose, as their source of energy. Heat is released as this fuel is used, thereby warming the body. Strenuous exercise burns a great deal of stored glycogen and therefore often results in overheating the body.

FUNCTIONS OF MUSCLE

In addition to providing heat and the ability to move, muscles support the structures of the body and hold the body upright. The muscles along the back, shoulders, and neck hold the trunk and head erect while permitting great flexibility in movement.

The structure of the skeletal muscles protects the blood vessels and nerves that lie throughout the body. The contraction of lower leg muscles aids in the return flow of blood to the heart by squeezing the veins of the legs. Muscles also provide protective padding to shield delicate internal organs and structures from injury.

Visually, the muscles add greatly to our appearance by giving shape to the body. Body-building enthusiasts spend years developing the degree of muscle enlargement and definition they feel is desirable. Muscle fiber, and therefore the muscle, hypertrophies (grows larger) with exercise; the number of fibers does not increase, however.

AGE-RELATED BODY CHARACTERISTICS

Muscle tissue changes slightly with age. During infancy, muscles have little connective tissue, often being attached to the bone directly. With maturity, the connective tissue increases, as do the elastic fibers. Muscles grow in relation to the structures to which they are attached. Muscles of the eye, for example, grow very little, whereas the large muscles of the lower extremities grow considerably.

TYPES OF MUSCLE TISSUE

There are three types of muscle tissue (Figures 28–1A-C). First, there is the *skeletal* type. Skeletal muscles are attached to bones and therefore permit movement. Because we have some control over movements, this type of muscle tissue is also called voluntary. Skeletal muscle cells are long and strong, some reaching lengths up to 12 inches. These cells are held together by connective tissue to form a muscle bundle. The bundles in turn are enclosed in a tougher connective tissue **sheath** to form the muscle organs such as the **biceps** of the arm. The larger the muscle organ, the greater the number of fibers.

The second type of muscle tissue is *smooth*. Smooth muscle tissue is made of small, delicate muscle cells and is found throughout the internal organs of the body, except for the heart. Smooth muscle activity occurs continuously in such actions as breathing, moving food through the intestinal tract, changing the size of the pupil of the eye, and dilating or constricting blood vessels. These muscles function without conscious direct control, so they are also called involuntary.

The third type is *cardiac* muscle tissue. As the name implies, this type is found in the heart. These cells are joined in a continuous network without sheath

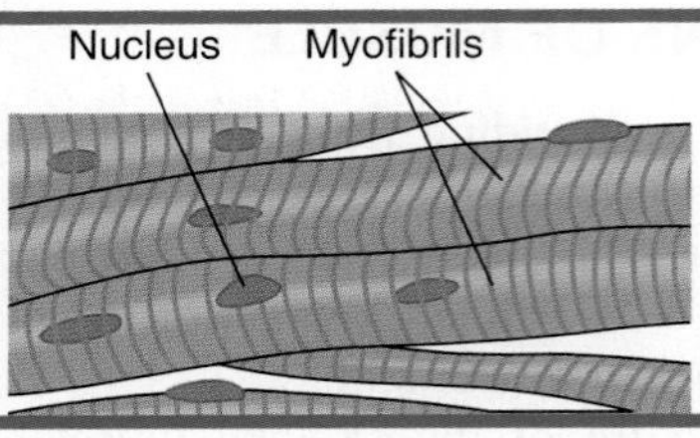

Figure 28–1A: Skeletal muscles are attached to the skeleton (bones, tendons, and other muscles). *Delmar/Cengage Learning.*

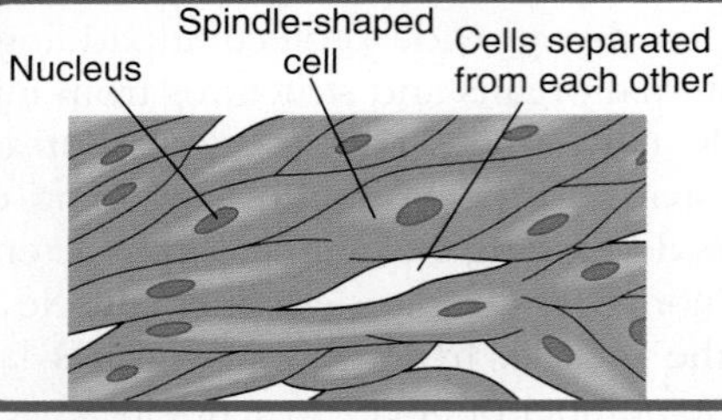

Figure 28–1B: Smooth muscles make up the walls of the digestive, genitourinary, and respiratory tracts; blood vessels; and lymphatic vessels. *Delmar/Cengage Learning.*

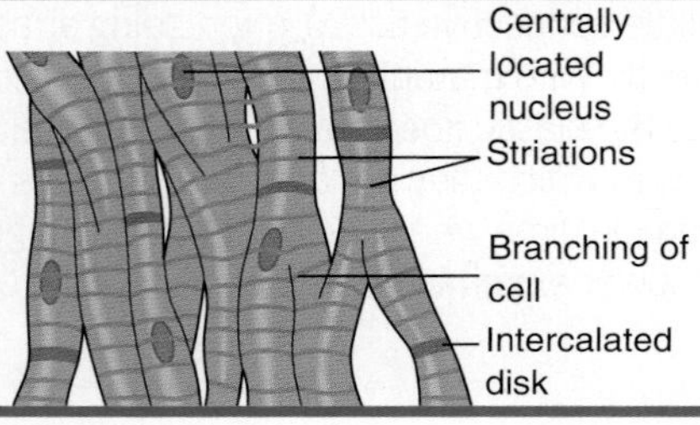

Figure 28–1C: Cardiac muscles make up the walls of the heart. *Delmar/Cengage Learning.*

separation. The membranes of adjacent cells are fused at places called *intercalated disks.* A communication system at the fused areas will not permit independent cell contraction. When one cell receives a signal to contract, all neighboring cells are stimulated and they contract together to produce the action of a heartbeat. This type of muscle tissue is also involuntary, which is fortunate. It would be a full-time job to consciously contract the heart muscle 70 times a minute, 100,800 times a day.

MEDIA LINK

Go to the Premium Website and watch the animation, "Types of Muscles," for this chapter.

SKELETAL MUSCLE ACTION

When muscles contract, they become shorter and thicker. A good example is the skeletal muscle of the upper arm, the biceps. When the biceps contracts to bend the elbow, the shorter and thicker muscle causes a bulge in the upper arm (Figure 28–2).

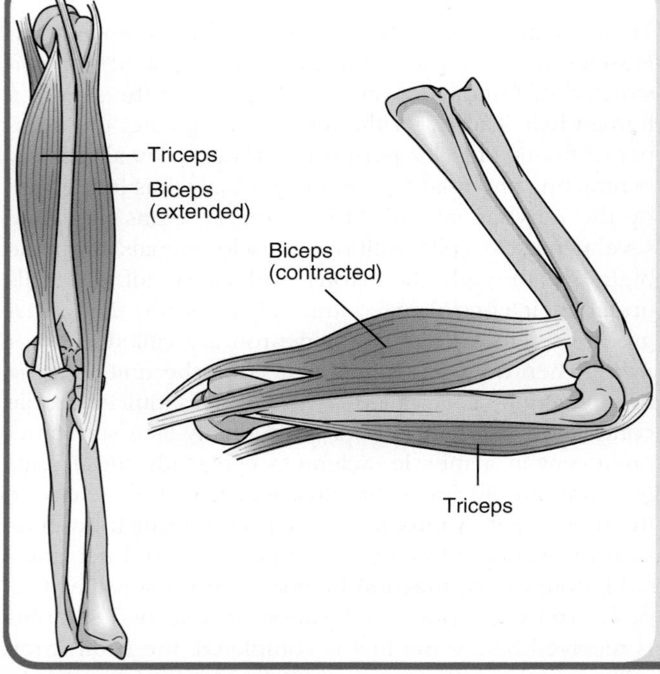

Figure 28–2: Action of the biceps/triceps muscle team. *Delmar/Cengage Learning.*

The skeletal muscle that bends a joint is called a **flexor**, whereas the action of straightening the joint is done by the **extensor** muscle. The extensor muscle that straightens the elbow is the **triceps**. The flexor and its partner, the extensor muscle, form what is known as a **muscle team** to bend and straighten joints (Figure 28–3). Muscles also contract to move extremities away from the body's center line, (**abduction**), or toward the center line (**adduction**) (Figure 28–4).

MUSCLE TONE

Most skeletal muscles are partially contracted at all times to maintain the body's erect position. It is believed that some fibers contract while others rest and that they then exchange roles. This constant state of contraction is known as **muscle tone**. Physicians frequently refer to muscle tone when examining patients. Evaluation of muscle tone aids in determining the status of the CNS and the motor function of the peripheral nerves.

Loss of muscle tone can occur when muscles are not used, as with severe illness, elderly people, paralysis, or temporarily when an extremity has been immobilized in a cast. With prolonged lack of use, muscles will **atrophy**, which is a progressive wasting away of the muscle tissue. Another muscular condition that develops from lack of use is called **contracture**. Here flexor muscles become shorter and permanently bend the joints. This is a common condition with paralyzed or unconscious patients. The most common sites are the fingers, elbows, knees, and hip joints.

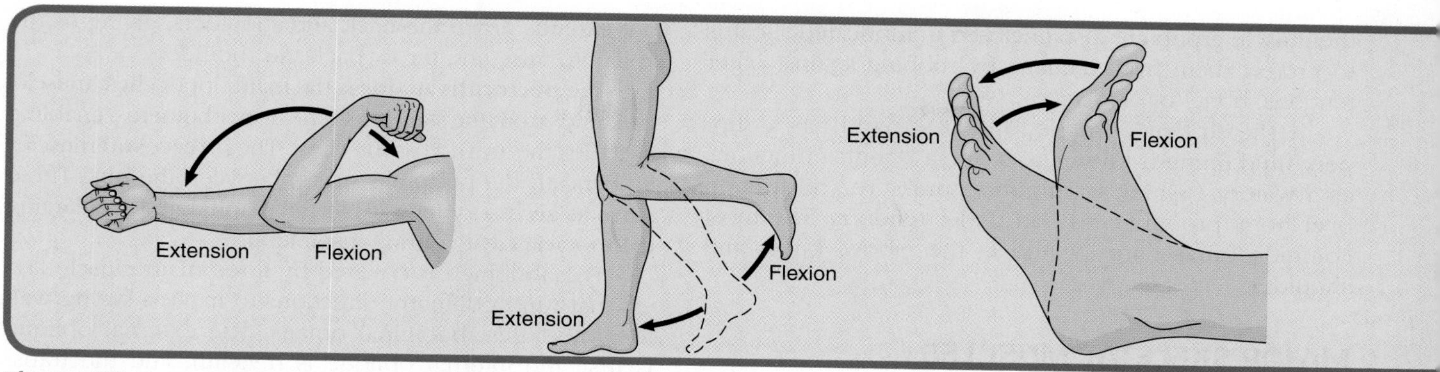

Figure 28–3: Flexor/extensor muscle team action. *Delmar/Cengage Learning.*

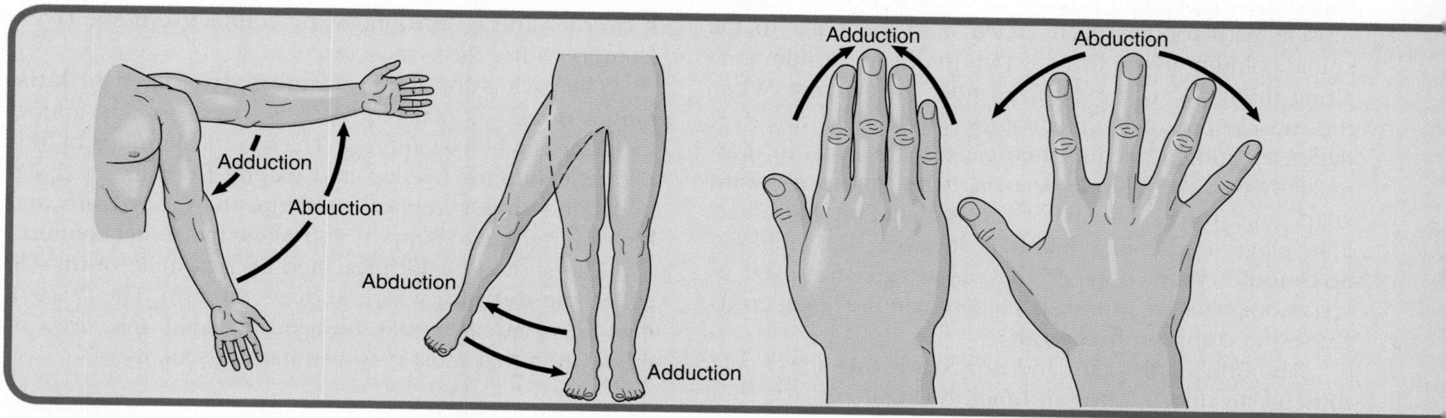

Figure 28–4: Abduction/adduction muscle team action. *Delmar/Cengage Learning.*

MUSCLE ATTACHMENT

Skeletal muscles are attached to bone in various ways. In some instances the connective tissue within the muscle is attached directly to the bone periosteum. Some muscular connective tissue sheaths extend to form a strong fibrous structure known as a **tendon**, which is attached to rough surfaces on a bone. Tendons are extremely strong and do not stretch. A 1-inch thick tendon reportedly will support 9 tons of weight. Because of this characteristic, a bone will sometimes fracture before the tendon attached to it will separate. The thickest and strongest tendon in the human body is the **Achilles tendon**, which attaches the **gastrocnemius** muscle in the calf of the leg to the heel bone.

A similar type of connective tissue is called a ligament, but it does not perform the same function. A ligament is a flexible, fibrous tissue that supports organs and connects bone to bone at joints. Ligaments, unlike tendons, do stretch.

Another form of muscular attachment is by **fascia**, a sheetlike, tough membrane that forms sheaths to cover and protect the muscle tissue. The term **aponeurosis** designates either a fascia or a flat tendon type of muscle attachment.

Origin or Insertion

When skeletal muscles join bones that meet at joints, one of the bones becomes the **anchor** on which the muscle has its **origin**. The bone to be moved becomes the **insertion** end for the muscle. For example, the biceps has its origin at the shoulder and its insertion on the radius. When the biceps contracts, being firmly anchored at the shoulder, it pulls upon the insertion location on the forearm, and the arm flexes (bends).

The terms origin and insertion can also apply to muscle attachments other than at joints. Essentially, the end nearest the center of the body is described as the origin, whereas the distal end is referred to as the insertion. Usually, the origin is relatively immobile, whereas the insertion is into a movable structure.

SHEATHS AND BURSAE

To protect the moving parts of the muscles, muscle groups are separated from each other by membranes called *sheaths* to reduce the friction from movement. Within muscle groups, individual muscles are also separated by membranes. The tendons that extend from the muscle group are also enclosed in lubricated sheaths to protect them from damage by rubbing against other tendons, bone, or cartilage.

A sheath that is shaped like a sac and has a slippery fluid lining is known as a bursa. A bursa functions as a watery cushion to minimize pressure and friction over bony prominences and under tendons. The most common bursae are located at the elbow, knee, and shoulder.

MAJOR SKELETAL MUSCLES

The muscle most important in breathing divides the chest cavity from the abdominal cavity. This muscle is called the *diaphragm* (Figure 28–5). It is a dome-shaped muscle with tendons that attach it in the back to the spinal column, in the front to the tip of the sternum, and along the sides to the cartilage edge of the ribs. When the muscle contracts, it becomes shorter and therefore flatter, creating a vacuum that causes the lungs to draw in air. When the muscle relaxes, it returns to its dome shape and forces air out of the lungs. The diaphragm also plays a role in coughing, sneezing, or laughing. Spasmodic contractions of the diaphragm, followed by spasmodic closure of the space between the vocal cords, cause the common **hiccough**.

The orbicularis oculi and orbicularis oris are circular muscles around the eye and mouth (Figure 28–6). Their contraction enables us to squint or wink and to whistle or pucker the mouth. The **sternocleidomastoid** and the **trapezius** are the major muscles of the neck and upper back that hold the head erect and assist with its movement (Figure 28–7). The trapezius not only supports the head but extends down the back and shoulders, giving us the ability to raise and throw back the shoulders.

The **pectoralis major** is the main upper chest muscle. It extends from the sternum to the upper humerus, enabling us to flex the arm across the chest. The **intercostal** muscles lie beneath the pectoralis major, between the ribs. These serve as accessory muscles to the diaphragm by enlarging the thoracic cavity during inspiration.

The abdomen is covered by three main muscle layers that run in different directions to make a strong wall to protect the abdominal organs. The external oblique is first, the internal oblique is beneath, and the transversus abdominis is the innermost layer. A long, narrow muscle, the rectus abdominis, extends from the pubis to the bottom of the rib cage in the center of the abdomen. It overlies and is surrounded by connective tissue layers from the other three muscles.

The back is covered by a large muscle called the **latissimus dorsi**. Its main function is to extend and adduct the arm, as when swimming. Thick vertical groups of four different muscles overlap and extend from the occipital bone and upper cervical vertebrae to the sacrum and lower vertebrae to support and move the spinal column.

The shoulders are protected by a triangle of muscle called the **deltoid**, which abducts the arm. The deltoid, if of adequate size, may be used for small injections of medication that must be given intramuscularly.

Lower Extremity Muscles

The muscles of the lower extremities involve about half of the body's total muscle mass. The buttocks are formed by the large **gluteus maximus** muscles, which support

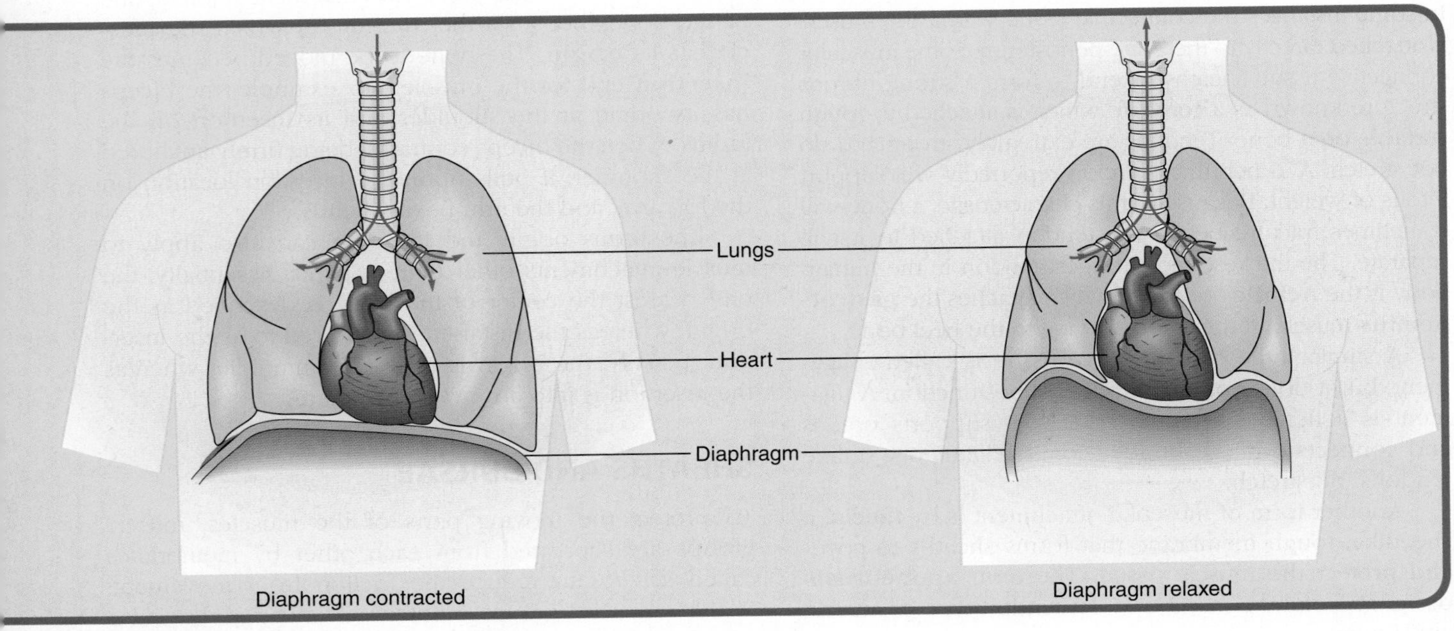

Figure 28–5: The action of the diaphragm muscle. *Delmar/Cengage Learning.*

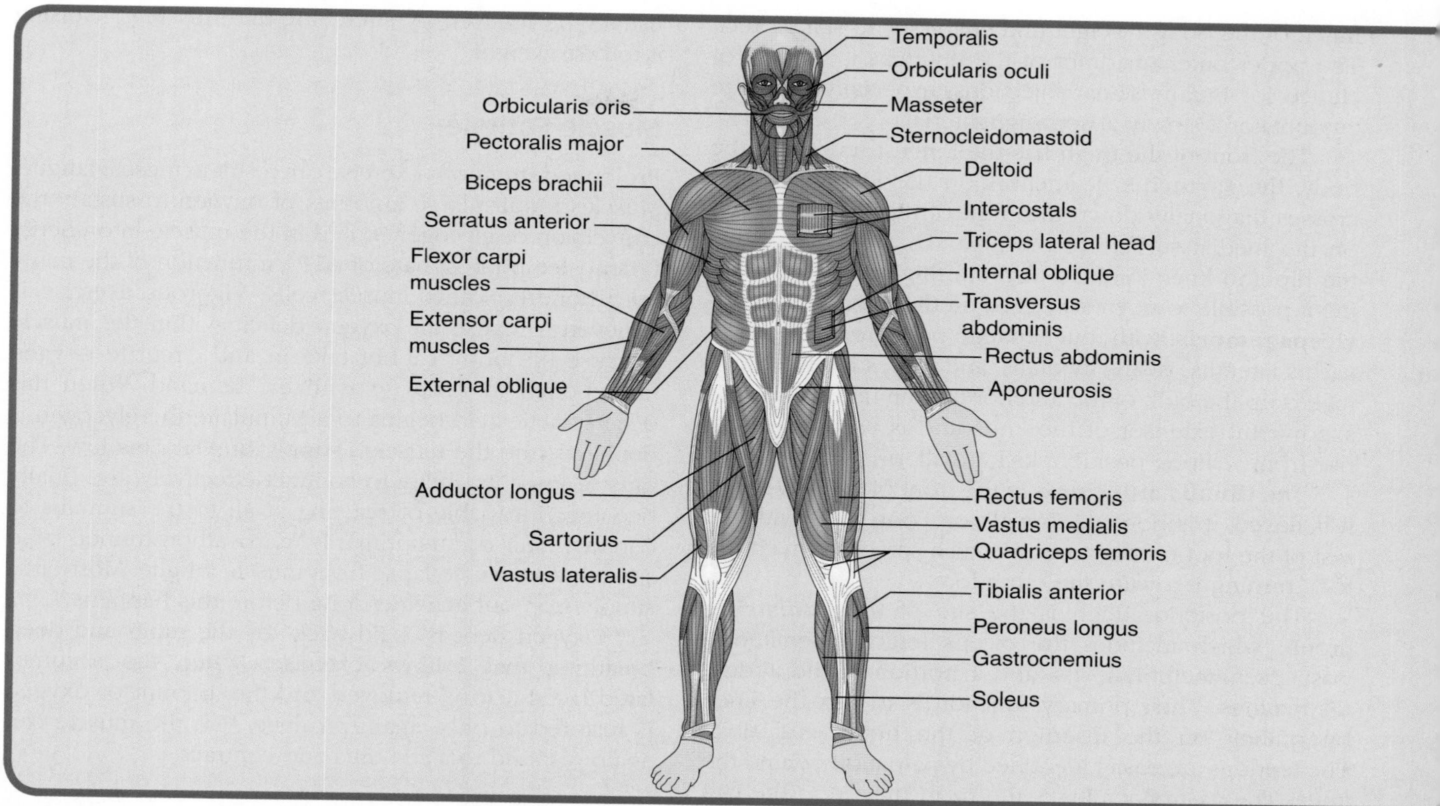

Figure 28–6: Principal muscles (anterior view). *Delmar/Cengage Learning.*

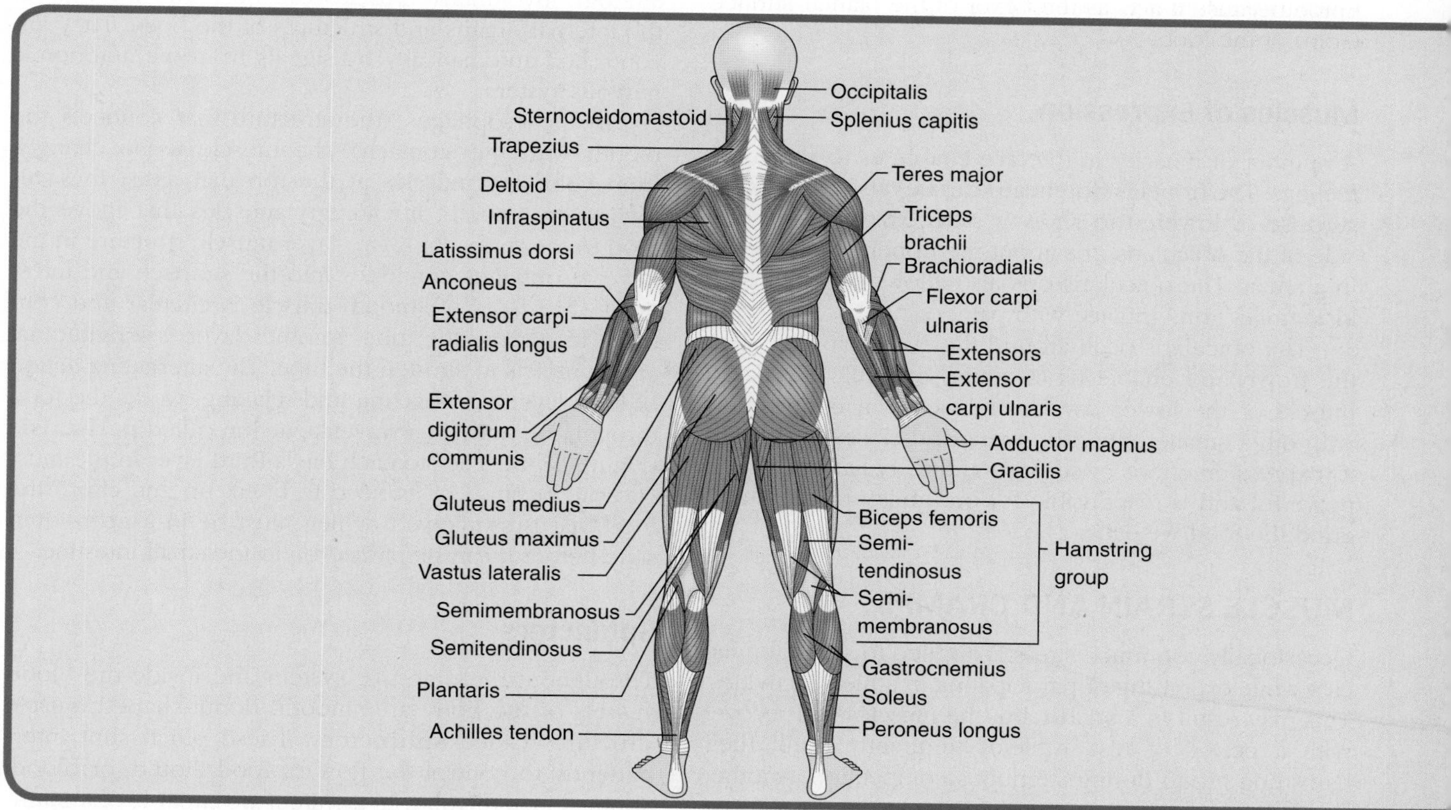

Figure 28–7: Principal muscles (posterior view). *Delmar/Cengage Learning.*

much of the body's weight and enable us to stand erect. The upper outer quadrant of the buttocks is the site of choice for intramuscular injections, especially for large amounts of a slowly absorbing material.

The front of the thigh has the longest muscle of the body, the **sartorius**. It anchors on the iliac spine and crosses diagonally down the front of the thigh to insert on the medial surface of the tibia. The sartorius flexes the hip and knee joints to turn the thigh outward, making it possible to sit cross-legged on the floor. The **quadriceps femoris**, with four separate parts (rectus femoris, vastus lateralis, vastus medialis, and vastus intermedius), makes up the bulk of the anterior thigh musculature. It is a powerful extensor of the knee and is used when we rise from a sitting position, kick a ball, or swim.

The **tibialis anterior** is in the front of the leg. When it is flexed, it is possible to walk on your heels with the rest of the foot off the ground. It also serves to invert the foot, turning it toward the other foot.

The posterior thigh is the site of the **hamstring** group, which includes the biceps femoris, semitendinosus, semimembranosus, and a portion of the adductor magnus. Their primary function is to flex the knee by pulling on the insertion at the fibula and tibia. The tendons are easily identified by palpation behind the knee. The gastrocnemius is the main muscle in the calf of the leg. Its tendon, the Achilles, has been mentioned. Contraction of the gastrocnemius permits you to stand to tiptoe because it acts as the flexor of the plantar surface (sole) of the foot.

Muscles of Expression

A number of muscles in the face enable us to show our feelings. The frontalis (forehead) can be raised to express surprise or lowered to show a stern gaze. Raising one side of the obicularis oris about the upper lip will result in a sneer. The obicularis oris also allows us to whistle, kiss, smile, grin, grimace with pain, or pout.

The obicularis oculi around the eyes help complete the frown and enable us to squint or wink. The large muscle of the lower jaw, the masseter, in cooperation with other smaller muscles, opens and closes the mouth to express emotions of surprise and disbelief but also is powerful and is responsible for our ability to chew and grind the food we eat.

MUSCLE STRAIN AND CRAMPS

Occasionally, too much stress is applied to skeletal muscles while exercising or participating in athletic activities. This may result in a **strain**, but the muscles will recover with a period of rest. Athletes frequently "pull" their hamstring group during strenuous competition. Another frequent occurrence is a muscle cramp or spasm, caused by a muscle that has contracted but cannot relax. It can usually be relieved by stretching the muscle or causing it to bear weight.

Muscle Fatigue

Prolonged strenuous exercise can result in muscle fatigue. Muscles require large amounts of oxygen to sustain the conversion of glycogen stored in the muscle into energy (adenosine triphosphate or ATP), a function of the many mitochondria within muscle cells. Vigorous exercise is believed to cause an oxygen deficit within the muscle because the body cannot take in and circulate oxygen fast enough to keep up with the demand. When this occurs, lactic acid begins to accumulate, the glycogen is depleted, and the muscle's supply of ATP runs low. The muscle loses its ability to contract effectively and finally becomes incapable of reacting at all to the stimulus to contract. This occurs primarily in marathon runners who sometimes even collapse from muscle fatigue. Most of us simply stop our activities long before this happens.

Oxygen debt is "paid back" by the rapid and deep breathing that follows exercise. When the accumulated lactic acid is removed and the amount of oxygen is restored to once again produce ATP, the muscle can again respond to a stimulus and contract.

SMOOTH MUSCLE ACTION

Smooth, involuntary muscles can be found throughout the internal organs and structures of the body. They are controlled automatically by signals from the autonomic nervous system.

In the esophagus (the structure that connects the mouth with the stomach), the muscle tissue changes from voluntary muscles at the top that assist in swallowing, to smooth, involuntary muscles that move the food to the stomach. A two-layer muscle structure in the lower esophagus continues into the stomach and intestines. One layer of smooth muscle is circular and contracts to narrow the tube. Another layer is longitudinal and contracts to shorten the tube. The alternating action of both layers, contracting and relaxing, works the food through the body in a wavelike action called **peristalsis** (Figure 28–8). The stomach has a third layer in the muscle wall because of its need to break up and churn the food that is swallowed, which must be in a near-liquid state before it can be passed on to the small intestine.

Sphincters

Throughout the digestive system and inside the blood vessels of the body are smooth, donut-shaped muscle structures called **sphincters**. These pinch shut intermittently to control the flow of food, liquid, or blood. Sphincters in the digestive system are capable of remaining contracted for hours if necessary. Both ends of the

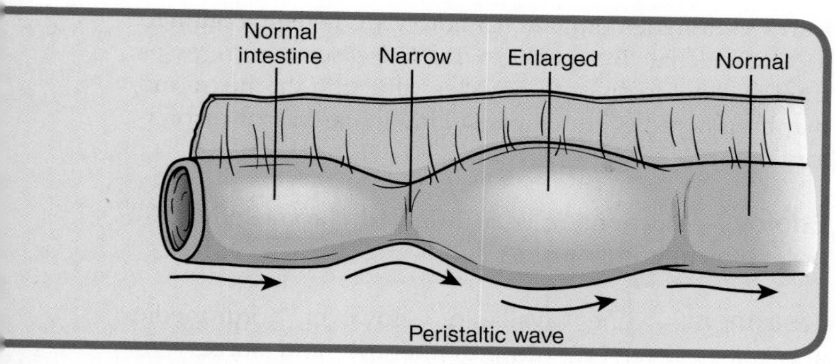

Figure 28–8: Peristaltic action. *Delmar/Cengage Learning.*

stomach have sphincter muscles to hold the contents securely inside while muscular action and chemical processes digest food. When the food is in the proper state, the lower sphincter opens slightly to allow small amounts of the liquid to escape into the small intestine.

An example of smooth muscle sphincter action that can be easily observed is the pupil of the eye. When available light is decreased, the radial muscles of the iris contract to enlarge the pupil, permitting more light to enter, thereby increasing the ability to see. When light is focused on the eye, the circular sphincter muscles of the iris that surround the pupil contract, making the pupil smaller, thereby limiting the amount of light striking the retina. The physician will usually check light reflex action of the eyes in assessing the condition of the brain and autonomic nervous system.

DISEASES AND DISORDERS

Bursitis/Tendonitis (Bur-si′-tis/Ten-dun-i′-tis)

Description—**Tendonitis** is a painful inflammation of the tendon and tendon-muscle attachments to bone, usually at the shoulder, hip, heel, or hamstrings. Bursitis is an inflammation of the bursa that covers and lubricates the muscles and tendons and occurs most often at the shoulder, elbow, or knee.

Signs and symptoms—Pain at joints or at the muscle attachment that results in limited motion.

Etiology—Tendonitis normally follows a sports-related activity that damages the muscle-tendon structure. It can also result from misaligned posture and other **musculoskeletal** disorders.

Treatment—With injury, apply ice initially for the first 12 to 24 hours. Later, applications of heat will usually aid in relief of the joint pain. If calcium deposits have formed within the tendon, it becomes weak, and the condition will be aggravated by heat. The calcium deposits are visible on X-ray to confirm the diagnosis. Application of ice packs will help relieve discomfort from calcified tendonitis.

Both conditions may be treated by resting the joint, oral doses of pain medication, and injections of a mixture of corticosteroid and a local anesthetic. If fluid has accumulated within the area, it may require aspiration prior to the injection treatment. When pain has subsided, a physical therapy regimen may be indicated to maintain joint function and prevent muscular atrophy.

Epicondylitis (Epi-kondi-li′tis) (Tennis Elbow)

Description—This is inflammation of a forearm tendon at the attachment on the humerus at the elbow.

Signs and symptoms—The initial elbow pain gradually worsens and often involves the forearm and the back of the hand when an object is grasped or the elbow is twisted. There is tenderness over the head of the radius and the projection of the humerus at the elbow joint.

Etiology—Epicondylitis probably begins as a partial tear of the tendon from its attachment.

Treatment—Injection of the area, as with tendonitis, is effective. Immobilization, heat therapy, and manipulation of the tendon attachment are used before resorting to surgical excision of the tendon for recurring and continual inflammation.

Fibromyalgia Syndrome (Fibro-mi-al′-ja)

Description—Fibromyalgia is a chronic musculoskeletal condition characterized by widespread pain. It was once called fibrositis. It affects people of all ages. It is estimated that at least 3.7 million people have the syndrome. Fibromyalgia occurs frequently in people with autoimmune and arthritis disorders.

Signs and symptoms—The prime symptom is widespread pain and the presence of tender points or trigger points at specific sites on the body (Figure 28–9). Diagnosis is considered positive when 11 of the 18 points are painful. Besides pain and muscle stiffness, patients may experience fatigue, an inability to concentrate, sleep disturbances, dry eyes and mouth, frequent urination, irritable bowel syndrome, headaches, numbness or tingling in the arms or legs, bursitis, tendonitis, and depression. All are symptoms of an alteration in the body's sympathetic nervous system.

Etiology—The cause is unknown. There seems to be some familial tendency, but a genetic connection has not been proven. It appears to be affected by many things, such as the weather, stress, and a poor state of physical fitness. Symptoms come and go, but the syndrome persists.

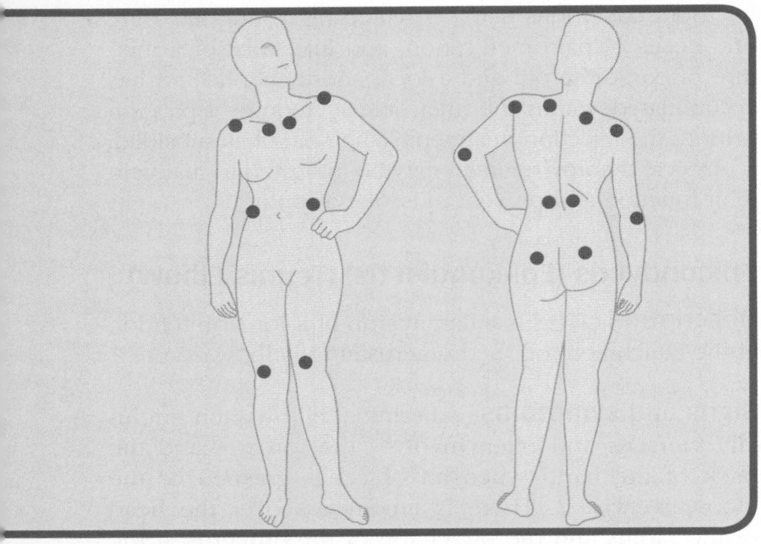

Figure 28–9: The tender point sites of fibromyalgia. *Delmar/ Cengage Learning.*

Treatment—There is no cure, only methods to make it possible to cope with the symptoms. The use of biofeedback, massage, warm showers or baths, gentle aerobic exercise, and adjustments to reduce stress are helpful. Other treatments include injection of the tender points, spraying the skin with ethyl chloride and then stretching the muscles, physical therapy, ultrasound, heat and cold applications, a jacuzzi, and medication to relax muscles and relieve pain. Currently used drugs include low doses of tricyclic medications, such as Elavil and Flexeril. Other similar drugs are used that increase the level of serotonin, a neurotransmitter. Newer approved medications for fibromyalgia pain include Cymbalta, Neurontin, and Lyrica. When the serotonin level is low, there is an increase in depression, sensitivity to pain, and difficulty with sleeping. The best course of treatment is becoming physically fit, achieving a good body weight, and acquiring restful sleep.

Muscular Dystrophy

Description—This group of congenital disorders results in progressive wasting away of skeletal muscles. There are several types of muscular **dystrophy**.

Duchenne's Dystrophy

This disorder represents about 50% of all the cases. In this genetic disease, the gene is carried by the female but affects only males; it can affect multiple members of the family. The onset is in early childhood, with death occurring after 10 to 15 years. It is usually first recognized when the child is about 1 year of age.

Signs and symptoms—Initially, the leg and pelvic muscles are affected, making all activities involving the lower extremities difficult. Children are usually confined to a wheelchair by ages 9 to 12. The disease progresses from skeletal to smooth muscles, affecting the heart and diaphragm and eventually resulting in cardiac or respiratory failure.

Etiology—Duchenne's is an X-linked chromosome disorder affecting only males.

Treatment—None available. However, orthopedic appliances, exercise, physical therapy, and surgery to correct muscle contractures can help preserve mobility.

Erb's or Juvenile Muscular Dystrophy

This type progresses slowly and occurs later in childhood or adolescence. It affects both sexes. It does not reduce life expectancy.

Signs and symptoms—Erb's main symptoms are weakness of the upper arm and pelvic muscles. Other symptoms include winging of the scapulae, lordosis with protruding abdomen, waddling gait, poor balance, and the inability to raise the arms.

Etiology and treatment—Same as Duchenne's.

Torticollis (Torti-kol'is) (Wryneck)

Description—This neck deformity bends the head to the affected side and rotates the chin toward the opposite side. It can be congenital or acquired.

Signs and symptoms—The obvious positioning of the head.

Etiology—Torticollis is caused by shortening or spasm of the sternocleidomastoid neck muscle. The congenital form usually follows a difficult (breech) birth and occurs mostly in firstborn females. It is thought to develop from malposition before birth, prenatal injury, or the rupture of muscle fibers with resulting scar tissue development. Acquired **torticollis** results from muscle damage by disease, a cervical spine injury, or muscle spasms. Torticollis has increased in infants since they are now placed on their backs to prevent SIDS. The sternocleidomastoid muscle shortens due to the position. Physical therapy is used to treat the deformity.

Infants younger than 6 months of age with poor neck control can rupture the sternocleidomastoid muscle. The muscle heals over time. Pain relievers, such as Tylenol, can be used.

Treatment—Treatment of the congenital type consists of stretching the shortened muscle through passive exercises and positional arrangement of the head

TABLE 28–1 System Interaction Associated with Disease Conditions

Disease	System Involved	Pathology Present
Fibromyalgia syndrome	Muscular	Muscle stiffness
	Nervous	Pain, numbness, tingling, trigger points, headache
	Digestive	Irritable bowel syndrome
	Urinary	Urinary frequency

during sleeping. Surgical correction of the muscle can be accomplished if conservative methods are not effective. Acquired torticollis is treated by correcting the underlying cause whenever possible. Application of heat, cervical traction, a neck brace, exercise, psychotherapy, and massage are indicated.

System Interaction Associated with Disease Conditions

There are few diseases that involve only the muscles of the body, with the exception of muscular dystrophy. Fibromyalgia, however, affects others systems and produces symptoms listed in Table 28–1.

CHAPTER SUMMARY

- The body has 600 muscles. Muscle activity is produced by motor neurons that innervate the muscle cells.
- Muscles need food and oxygen to contract. They receive an ample supply because of the responsibility of muscles to keep the body safe.
- Muscles provide heat, the ability to move, support the body's structures, store glycogen, protect the blood vessels and nerves, aid in the return of blood to the heart, add to our appearance, and provide protective padding of vital organs.
- Muscles change slightly with age, beginning with little connective tissue and developing elastic fibers. Muscles grow in relation to their attached structures.
- There are three types of muscle tissue: skeletal, smooth, and cardiac.
- Muscles are attached to bones to provide movement. Flexing a muscle bends a joint while the extensor muscle straightens the joint.
- Muscle tone refers to the state of contraction.
- Skeletal muscles are attached to bone by connective tissue and tendons that can stretch. Ligaments connect bone to bone at joints and do not stretch.
- The origin of the muscle is the anchor while the insertion is the where it attaches to the bone to be moved.
- Muscle groups are separated by membranes called sheaths.
- The major skeletal muscles are identified on Figures 28–6 and 28–7.
- Muscles of expression enable us to show feelings.
- Muscle strain results when too much stress is applied. Muscle fatigue happens following prolonged strenuous exercise.
- Smooth muscle action is involuntary and can be found throughout the organs and structures of the body.
- A sphincter is a donut-shaped muscle that opens and closes to control the flow of blood, liquids or food.
- The diseases discussed are bursitis/tendonitis, epicondylitis, fibromyalgia, muscular dystrophy, and torticollis.
- Fibromyalgia involves four body systems: muscular, nervous, digestive and urinary.

STUDY TOOLS

Workbook	Activities for Chapter 28
Premium Website	
MEDIA LINK	View this **Media Link** for Chapter 28: • Types of muscles
StudyWARE	Activities and Quizzes on the **StudyWARE™ Software** for Chapter 28
	Audio Library of medical terms
	Online access to the **Critical Thinking Challenge 2.0**

learninglab	Module 13: The Skeletal and Muscular Systems
CourseMate	Activities and Quizzes for Chapter 28
WebTutor	Activities and Quizzes for Chapter 28

CHECK YOUR KNOWLEDGE

1. Tendonitis is:
   a. an inflammation of the coverings of the muscles and tendons at a joint.
   b. a tear in the tendon attachment.
   c. a chronic condition of the joint structures.
   d. an inflammation of the tendon–muscle attachment.
2. Bursitis is:
   a. an inflammation of the tendon–muscle attachment.
   b. an inflammation of the coverings of the muscles and tendons at a joint.
   c. an inflammation of the smooth muscle.
   d. the result of misaligned posture.
3. Epicondylitis is:
   a. inflammation of the condyles at the knee.
   b. widespread pain in muscles.
   c. inflammation of the forearm tendon at the elbow.
   d. a congenital muscle disease.
4. Muscular dystrophy is:
   a. a temporary muscle disorder.
   b. a group of muscles that are inflamed.
   c. a muscle-wasting disorder.
   d. characterized by trigger points.
5. The Achilles tendon:
   a. attaches the quadriceps femoris to the knee.
   b. permits a person to sit cross-legged.
   c. permits flexion of the biceps.
   d. attaches the gastrocnemius to the heel.
6. A sphincter is:
   a. the permanent flexor muscle shortening.
   b. a painful muscle contracture.
   c. a smooth muscle found in the opening of the heart.
   d. a circular-shaped muscle.
7. Food is moved throughout the body by:
   a. contracture.
   b. peristalsis.
   c. the conversion of glycogen to ATP.
   d. intercostal muscle contractions.
8. The term *flexor* refers to:
   a. straightening a joint.
   b. bringing the legs together.
   c. raising the arm at the side of the body.
   d. bending the joint.
9. Abduction means to:
   a. move an extremity away from the body's center.
   b. move an extremity toward the body's center.
   c. flex the muscle to bend a joint.
   d. flex muscles to straighten a joint.
10. Hiccoughs are caused by:
    a. a lack of oxygen.
    b. the contraction of the intercostal muscles.
    c. spasmotic contractions of the diaphragm and vocal cord space.
    d. the rhythmic contraction of the muscles of the throat.
11. Fibromyalgia syndrome involves:
    a. nervous, respiratory, and urinary systems.
    b. reproductive, nervous, and muscular systems.
    c. digestive, circulatory, and muscular systems.
    d. muscular, urinary, and digestive systems.

WEB LINKS

NINDS Muscular Dystrophy Page: www.ninds.nih.gov/disorders/md/md.htm

WebMD, Understanding Muscular Dystrophy Basics: www.webmd.com/parenting/understanding-muscular-dystrophy-basics

Chapter

29 The Respiratory System

OBJECTIVES

In this chapter, you will learn the following:

KB KNOWLEDGE BASE

1. Spell and define, using the glossary at the back of the text, all the Words to Know in this chapter.
2. Describe the source and importance of oxygen.
3. Trace the path of oxygen to an internal cell.
4. Describe the structure and function of the nose, pharynx, epiglottis, larynx, trachea, bronchus, bronchiole, and alveolus.
5. Explain how voice sounds are produced.
6. Differentiate between external and internal respiration.
7. Describe the structure and function of the pleural coverings of the lungs and chest cavity.
8. Describe the relationship of the diaphragm and brain to breathing.
9. Describe five normal occurrences that alter breathing patterns and explain why they occur.
10. Identify diagnostic examinations for respiratory assessment.
11. Explain the role of surfactant in the lungs.
12. Differentiate between perfusion and ventilation scans.
13. Describe the diseases or disorders of the respiratory tract.
14. Describe the age-related changes occurring with asthma.
15. Identify the body systems involved with COPD.

WORDS TO KNOW

allergic rhinitis
alveoli
angiography
apnea
arteriography
asthma
atelectasis
bleb
bronchi
bronchiole
bronchitis
carbon dioxide
chronic obstructive pulmonary disease (COPD)
cilia
cyanosis
diaphoresis
dyspnea
emphysema
empyema
epiglottis
epistaxis
expectorated
expiration
fibrosis
hemothorax
hiccoughs
hiccup
histoplasmosis
hypoxia
influenza
inspiration
intubation
laryngectomy
laryngitis
larynx
legionnaires' disease
liter
lung
orthopnea
oxygen
perfusion
pharynx
pleura
pleurisy
pneumonia
pneumonoconiosis
pneumothorax
pulmonary
pulmonary edema
pulmonary emboli
respiratory
rhinitis
septum
sinusitis
spirometer
spontaneous
sputum
sudden infant death syndrome (SIDS)
surfactant
trachea
tracheotomy
tuberculosis
upper respiratory infection
ventilation
vital capacity

In the environment, **oxygen** (O_2) is provided continuously by plants on land and in the sea. Plants use sun, water, and **carbon dioxide** (CO_2) to make oxygen, which they release into the air. Humans breathe O_2 and exhale CO_2 and water. This cycle provides the means for supporting life.

Oxygen in the air is essential to the survival of living cells. An adult human being carries 2 quarts of O_2 in the blood, lungs, and tissues. This supply is adequate to sustain life for about 4 minutes. The respiratory system is responsible for taking in air, removing the oxygen, and sending it through the blood to the cells of the body. The oxygen concentration of inhaled air is about 21%.

The respiratory system must also take from the blood the waste product CO_2 and exhaust it from the lungs. Exhaled air still contains about 16% oxygen. When the level of CO_2 in the blood rises to a certain point, the respiratory center in the brain is triggered and a breath is taken. This function is so vital to life that its interruption for just a few minutes will result in death.

THE PATHWAY OF OXYGEN

The Nose

Air enters the body through the nose (Figure 29–1). Here the air is filtered, warmed, and moistened by the structures within the nasal cavity. The nose is divided by a wall of cartilage called the **septum**. Near the middle of the nasal cavity, on each side, are a series of three scroll-like bones called conchae or turbinates. The conchae are covered with mucus-producing epithelium, which adds moisture to the air, and are supplied with abundant blood vessels, which warm the air. Just inside the nostrils are hairs called **cilia**, which trap particles in the air so that they do not enter the lungs.

The mucus from the lining also helps trap dust and bacteria. When irritating substances come in contact with the lining, extra mucus is produced to dilute the irritant. This is why sneezing occurs and the nose "runs." Both actions are methods of removing irritants.

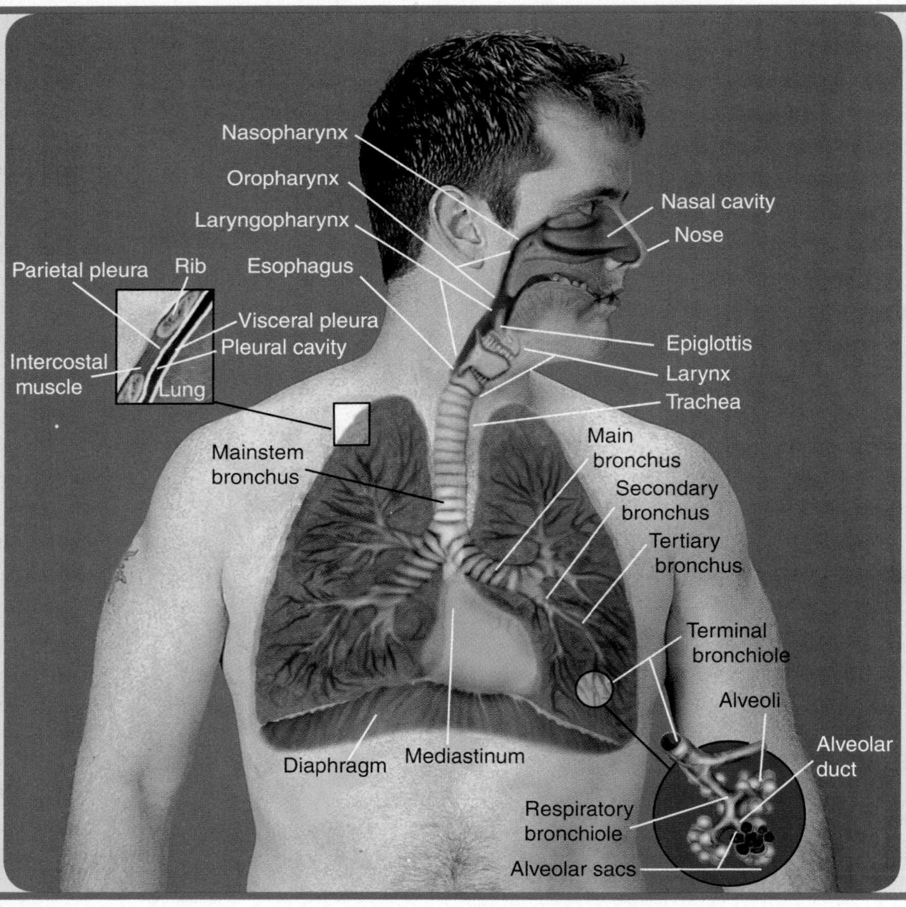

Figure 29–1: The respiratory system. *Delmar/Cengage Learning.*

Ciliated mucosa in the posterior portion of the nose and in the pharynx (throat) help propel inhaled particles into the back of the pharynx to be swallowed. Particles inhaled into the trachea and bronchi must first be propelled upward past the epiglottis, in an action called *mucus streaming*. The particles can then be directed toward the esophagus and swallowed. The constant beating action of the cilia and the flow of the mucus secretions cleanse the air passages. This beneficial function is temporarily halted by the effect of smoking, which paralyzes the cilia and mucus streaming action, thereby allowing foreign particles to enter the lungs. The paralysis lasts for several minutes.

The sinuses of the head are lined with the continuation of the nasal membranes (Figure 29–2). This explains why **sinusitis** occurs frequently with nasal infections.

The Pharynx, Larynx, and Epiglottis

After the air is filtered, warmed, and moistened in the nose, it enters the **pharynx**. The pharynx serves as a passageway for both air and food. Except for an occasional mistake, it is not possible to swallow food and breathe at the same time. When this does occur, the result is choking, which can be very serious.

Normally, when food is swallowed, a cartilage "lid" called the **epiglottis** is pushed by the base of the tongue to cover the opening into the **larynx**. At the same time, the larynx moves up to help close the opening. With the opening to the larynx covered by the epiglottis, food is directed down the esophagus into the stomach.

When air passes under the open epiglottis, it enters the larynx, commonly called the voice box. The larynx is a tube with a series of nine separate cartilages to maintain its opening (Figure 29–3A). The thyroid cartilage is the largest and is located anteriorly. Its prominent projection is known as the Adam's apple, and its action can be observed when a person swallows. The larynx is lined with mucous membrane, which also forms two folds called the vocal cords. The cords are attached to the front of the larynx wall by cartilage. Muscles attach to the cartilage, and when they contract or relax, the vocal cords move either toward or away from the center of the larynx (Figure 29–3B).

During breathing, the vocal cords are near to the wall of the larynx so that air can pass freely in and out. During speaking, the vocal cords move across the larynx and are held tense by the contracting muscles. The degree of tension and the length of the cords determine the pitch of the voice. The tighter and longer the cords the

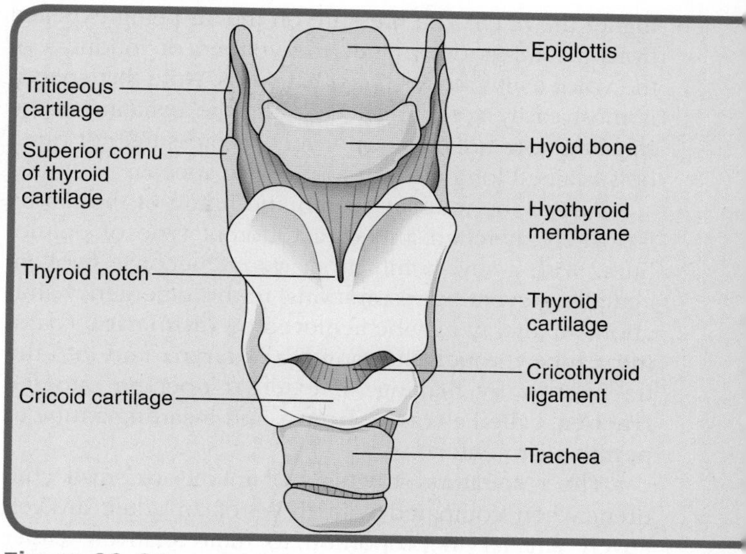

Figure 29–3A: Larynx (anterior view). *Delmar/Cengage Learning.*

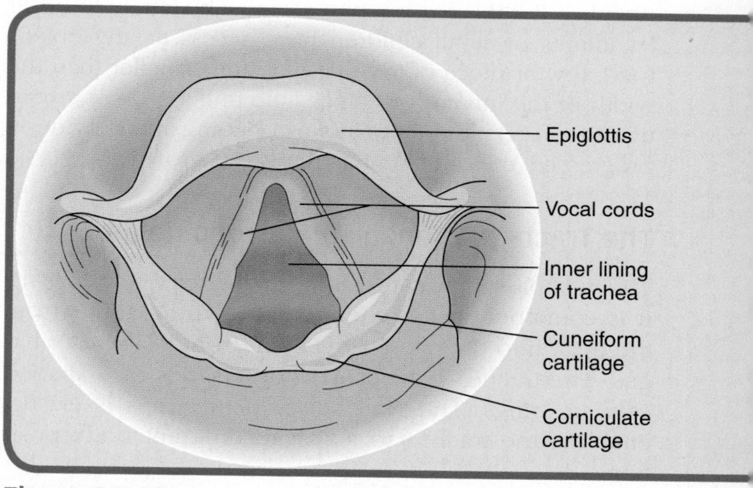

Figure 29–3B: The vocal cords in the larynx. *Delmar/Cengage Learning.*

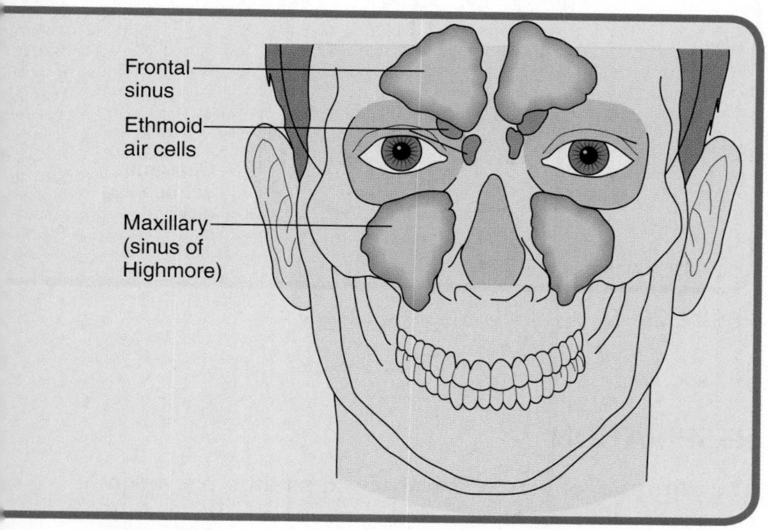

Figure 29–2: Paranasal sinuses (frontal view). *Delmar/Cengage Learning.*

higher the pitch. The pressure on the air being expelled from the lungs determines the volume or loudness of the voice as it vibrates the vocal cords. Note that speech is most easily accomplished during the exhaling of air. Inhaling does not create sufficient air pressure, nor can it be sustained long enough to produce speech.

Part of the mucous membrane lining of the larynx is loosely attached and of a different type of epithelium. With a severe infection, it may become swollen, actually preventing respirations. In this emergency situation, an airway may be achieved by **intubation** (passing a tube through the mouth and larynx and into the trachae) or by making an external opening into the **trachea**, called a **tracheotomy**, and inserting a tube to permit air to enter.

The respiratory structures of infants or small children, when compared with those of an adult, are relatively smaller in proportion to their relatively larger tongue and epiglottis. This difference results in a much easier obstruction of their airway. It takes a much smaller object or amount of material to completely occlude the opening. For this reason, parents must be taught to never let infants or small children have access to any object, food, toy, or piece of toy that measures smaller than the width of the infant's or child's little finger. This is a relative size in relation to the airway opening and provides a progressive measurement as the infant grows.

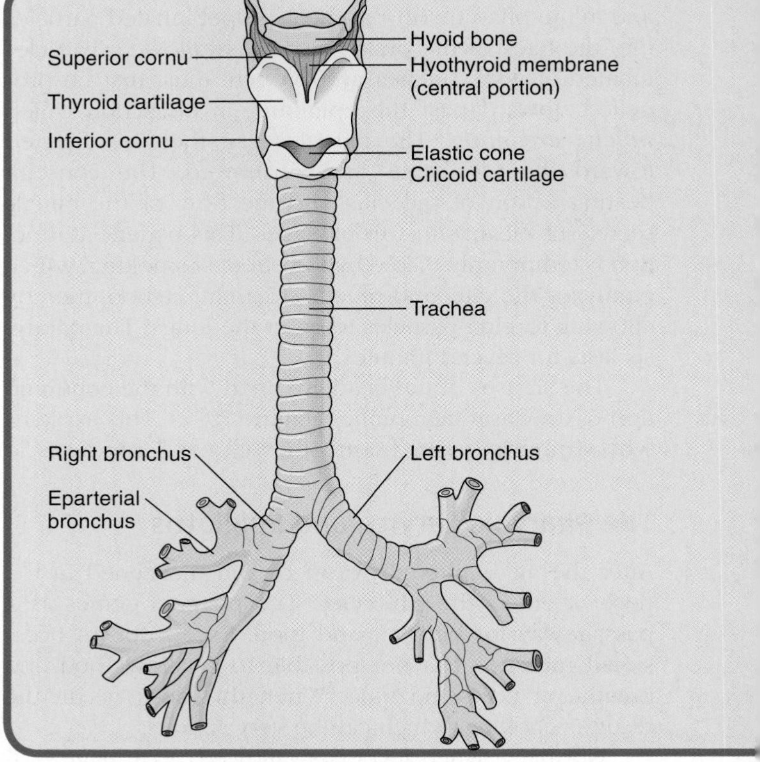

Figure 29–4: The larynx, trachea, and bronchi. *Delmar/Cengage Learning.*

The Trachea, Bronchi, and Bronchioles

The next passageway for air is the trachea (Figure 29–4). It is commonly called the windpipe and extends from the neck into the chest, directly in front of the esophagus. The trachea is held open by a series of C-shaped cartilage rings. The wall between the rings is elastic, enabling the trachea to adjust to different body positions.

About the middle of the sternum, the trachea divides into two sections called the right and left **bronchi**. The structure of the two main bronchi is similar to that of the trachea, with incomplete cartilage rings to maintain the air passageway. Each bronchus divides and subdivides into many increasingly smaller bronchi, each with the cartilage-ringed structure, until they are barely visible without a microscope. These tiny air passageways have walls of muscle cells and are called **bronchioles**.

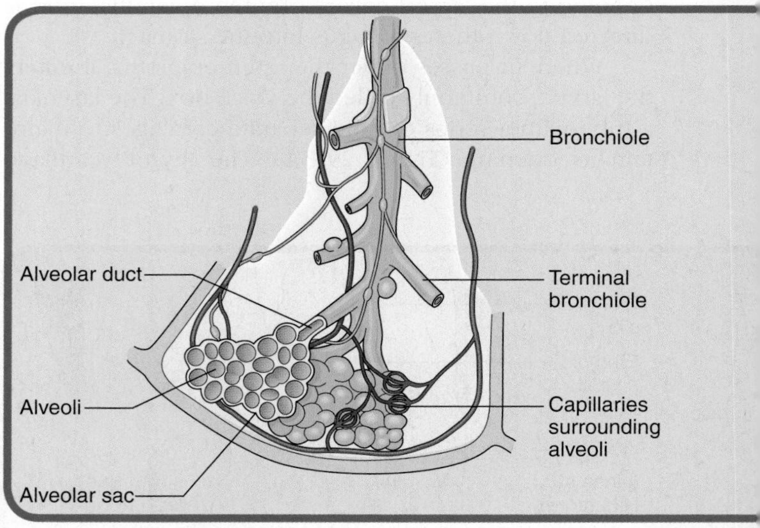

Figure 29–5: Alveoli. *Delmar/Cengage Learning.*

The Alveoli

Each bronchiole ends in a grapelike cluster of microscopic air sacs called **alveoli**. It is estimated that the body contains about 500 million alveoli, approximately three times the amount necessary to sustain life. The membrane walls of the alveoli are only one cell thick and are surrounded by a network of microscopic blood vessels called capillaries (Figure 29–5).

RESPIRATION

The structure of the **respiratory** apparatus has been compared with an upside-down tree, with the trunk, branches, twigs, and leaves corresponding to the trachea, bronchi, bronchioles, and alveoli.

On **inspiration**, air enters the body, eventually arriving in an alveolus. Here O_2 passes through the wall of the alveolus into the surrounding capillary as CO_2 leaves the capillary and enters the alveolus. When **expiration** occurs, CO_2 exits from the bronchial tree and is exhaled from the body. The process of getting O_2 from the nose to the alveolus and into the capillary and the return of CO_2 to the nose is known as *external respiration* (Figure 29–6A).

At the same time, oxygen from the alveolus is circulating through the body to every cell. First, the oxygen enters the capillary surrounding the alveolus, then it circulates through a venule, a vein, back to the heart, out an artery, to an arteriole, and into a capillary next to a tissue cell. Here the O_2 in the blood is given to the cell while CO_2 from the cell is picked up by the capillary. The exchange of O_2 and CO_2 at the cell is known as *internal respiration* (Figure 29–6B).

Oxygen and carbon dioxide in the alveolus and the cell exchange by the process of *diffusion*. Remember that materials move across a membrane from an area of higher concentration to an area of lower concentration. In the alveoli of the lung, O_2 concentration is greater than in the surrounding capillary, so it diffuses into the blood. At the same time, CO_2 is in higher concentration in the blood than in the alveolus, so it leaves the blood, enters the alveolus, and is exhaled during the next respiration. At the tissue cell, the O_2 content in the capillary is greater than that within the cell, so the O_2 leaves the blood and enters the cell. On the other hand, the CO_2 level within the cell is greater than in the capillary, so CO_2 diffuses out of the cell into the blood. This process of external and internal respiration is continuous throughout the life span of a person.

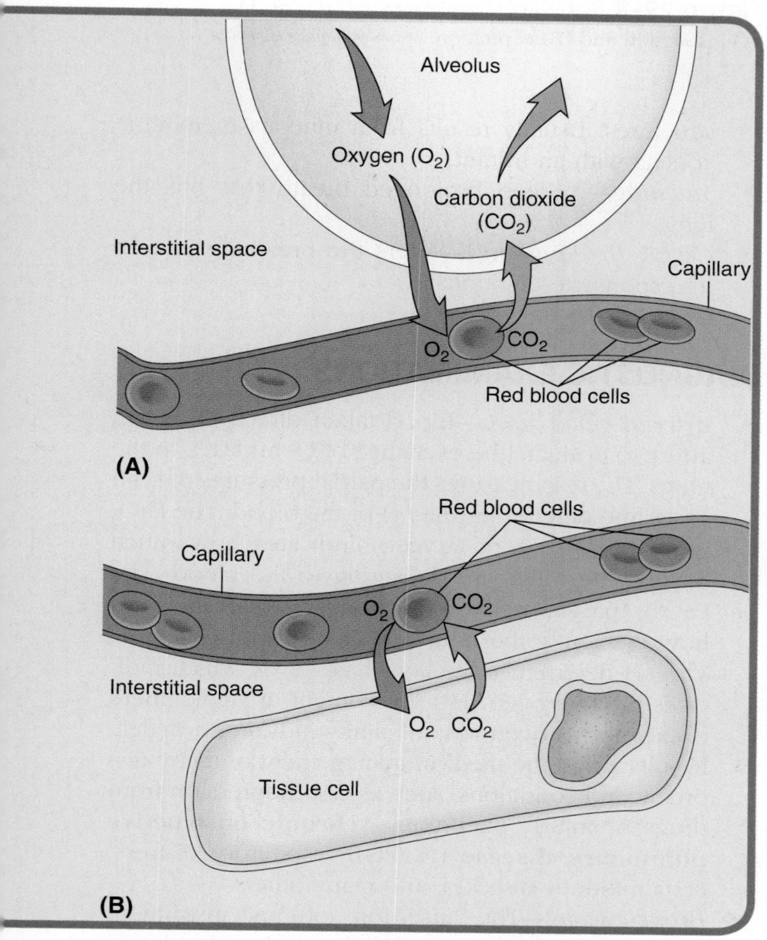

Figure 29–6: Simplified external and internal respiration: (A) external respiration in the lungs and (B) internal respiration at the cell. *Delmar/Cengage Learning.*

MEDIA LINK

Go to the Premium Website and watch the animation, "Respiration," for this chapter.

THE LUNG AND THE PLEURA

The structures of the bronchial tree are contained in an organ known as the **lung**. The tissue of the lung is so filled with the alveoli that it is spongy and extremely light. It will float if placed in water. Prior to birth and breathing, the lung is solid and will sink in water. At birth, the lungs begin to fill with air, inflating the alveoli. The degree of inflation depends on the presence of **surfactant**, a fatty molecule on the respiratory membrane. The surfactant maintains the inflated alveolus so that it does not collapse between breaths. Surfactant is not present in sufficient amounts to cause adequate inflation in premature infants and sometimes also in those born with other conditions. This results in *respiratory distress syndrome* (RDS) or hyaline membrane disease (described in detail later). The lungs continue to mature throughout childhood, with additional alveolar formation. Smoking at an early age retards the maturing of the lungs, and the additional alveoli are never developed.

The lung is divided into a right and left lung (Figure 29–7). The right lung has three lobes: upper, middle, and lower. The left lung has two: upper and lower. The heart lies on the medial surface of the left lung in a space called the *cardiac notch*. Each lung with its blood vessels and nerves is enclosed in a membrane called the visceral **pleura**. A membrane also lines the thoracic cavity and is called the parietal pleura. The airtight space between the pleural membranes is known as the pleural space or cavity. It contains a lubricating fluid to prevent friction as the membranes rub together during respiration. The space is virtually nonexistent in healthy lungs because the lungs fill the thoracic cavity within the rib cage, pressing the visceral against the parietal pleura. However, as will be discussed later, certain conditions and diseases cause an abnormal presence of fluid or air within the pleural space.

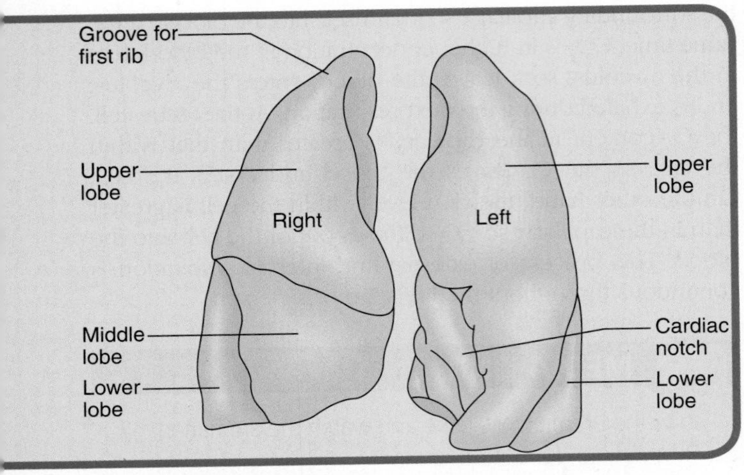

Figure 29–7: Anterior lung surface. *Delmar/Cengage Learning.*

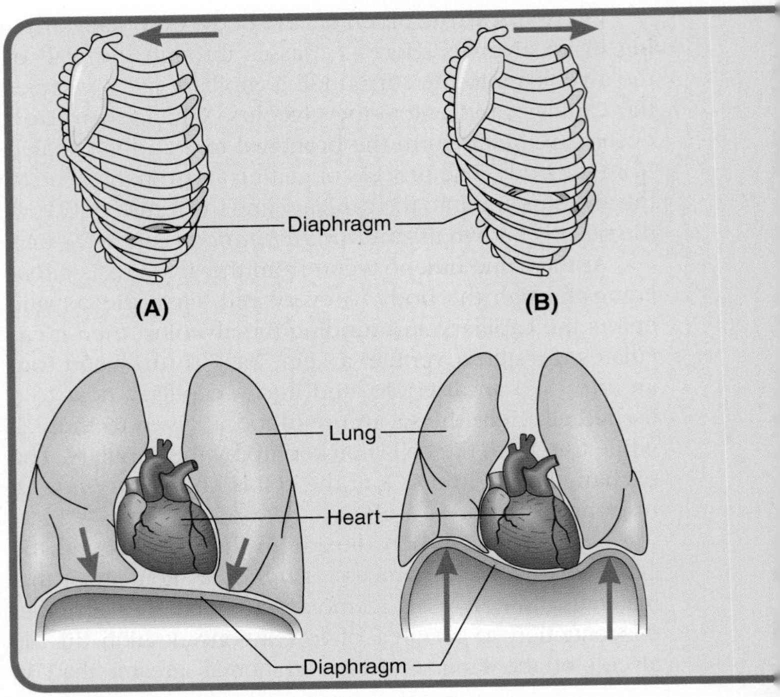

Figure 29–8: Position of diaphragm and ribs during (A) inspiration and (B) expiration. *Delmar/Cengage Learning.*

THE MUSCLES OF BREATHING

The action of the diaphragm and the muscles of the rib cage were discussed in Chapter 28. The diaphragm is the principal breathing muscle, and when it contracts, it produces a vacuum within the thoracic cavity, causing air to be drawn in. When this begins, there is a negative pressure within the lungs; the pressure inside is less than the atmospheric pressure outside. When the inside pressure exceeds outside atmospheric pressure, it becomes positive and causes expiration to again equalize inside and outside pressure. When the diaphragm returns to its relaxed state, air is forced out of the lungs (Figure 29–8).

Breathing action is controlled by the respiratory center in the brain. An increase of CO_2 or a lack of O_2 in the blood will trigger the center. Because we can somewhat voluntarily control breathing, it is possible to force rapid respirations, temporarily interrupting breathing and possibly losing consciousness. Children will occasionally hold their breath to frighten their parents and receive concessions. Usually, there is no need to be overly concerned, because sooner or later a breath has to be taken. If consciousness is lost, the automatic system resumes control, and breathing returns to normal.

Other situations can alter a breathing pattern for perfectly normal reasons, such as:

- *Coughing*—When a deep breath is taken followed by a forceful exhalation from the mouth to clear something from the lower respiratory structures.
- ***Hiccoughs*** (also spelled **hiccups**)—Caused by a spasm of the diaphragm and a spasmodic closure of the glottis (space between the vocal cords). It is believed to be the result of an irritation to the diaphragm or the phrenic nerve, which innervates the diaphragm.
- *Sneezing*—Occurs like a cough except air is forced through the nose to clear the upper respiratory structures. Usually results from mucous membrane contact with an irritant.
- *Yawning*—A deep prolonged breath that fills the lungs.
- *Crying (or laughing)*—Alters the breathing pattern in response to emotions.

DIAGNOSTIC EXAMINATIONS

- *Arterial blood gases*—Blood taken directly from an artery to evaluate the exchange of O_2 and CO_2 in the lungs. The test measures the partial pressures of both gases and determines the *p*H of the blood. The PaO_2 (partial pressure of oxygen) indicates how much oxygen the lungs are delivering to the blood. The $PaCO_2$ (partial pressure of carbon dioxide) indicates how efficiently the lungs eliminate carbon dioxide. The *p*H determines the acid–base level, which indicates the hydrogen (H^+) ion content. If acidic, there is excess hydrogen ion; alkalinity indicates a deficit. Results aid in the medical management of many disorders and conditions, such as CNS depression from drugs or injury, pneumonia, **chronic obstructive pulmonary disease** (COPD), respiratory distress, certain kidney diseases, and many others.
- *Bronchoscopy*—The insertion of an instrument called the bronchoscope into the trachea and bronchial tree to view the airways, obtain a secretion or tissue sample, or remove a foreign body.

- *Chest CT scan*—A very sensitive computer-generated image that gives much more detail of the lungs and other structures in the chest than a chest X-ray. The scan is done with an electron beam tomography scanner (Figure 29–9A). The examination is four times more sensitive in detecting lung cancer than conventional X-rays. It can be used as a screening examination to identify disease long before symptoms occur. Unfortunately, about 85% of lung cancer is discovered after it has begun to spread. The high-speed scan takes only a few seconds and does not require removal of clothing. Figure 29–9B is a photo of a lung scan showing a nodule in the left upper lobe.
- *CT scan of pulmonary arteries*—Also known as a CT angiogram of the chest. This is a scan accompanied by injection of an IV contrast media. It is typically used to evaluate for pulmonary embolus. High-resolution CT scan (HRCT) is used to evaluate lung tissue in greater detail than a standard CT scan. This is useful in evaluating pulmonary fibrosis.
- *CT-guided needle biopsy*—Done by a trained radiologist. Using the CT scan as a guide, the radiologist inserts a needle into the chest cavity to biopsy a lung mass.
- *Chest X-ray*—A radiologic examination to determine the general health of lung and surrounding tissues or to identify a disease process, such as pneumonia.
- *Lung* ***perfusion*** *scan*—An examination of the lung following intravenous (IV) injection of a radioactive contrast medium to provide a visual image of pulmonary blood flow. It is useful in diagnosing blood vessel obstruction, such as **pulmonary emboli** (blood clot in an artery), but not as sensitive as a CT scan of the pulmonary arteries.
- *Lung* ***ventilation*** *scan*—An examination following the inhalation of a mixture of air and radioactive gas from a mask and bag. The test indicates the areas of the lung that are ventilated during respiration. It is used in conjunction with a lung perfusion scan to evaluate for a possible pulmonary embolus. This can also be used to determine the amount each lobe of the lung is perfusing, for example, before performing a lobectomy.
- *PET (positron emission tomography) scan*—A nuclear medicine examination to determine cellular uptake in parts of the body. It is often fused with a CT scan of the chest. From a pulmonary perspective, PET scans are used for:
  1. Determination of lung cancer metastasis, such as bone, mediastinal lymph nodes, and abdominal organs
  2. Evaluation of a solitary pulmonary nodule that is greater than 1 cm in patients that are a high risk for biopsy
  3. Early detection of recurrent cancer. Areas of the body that are positive for uptake of the injected material are consistent with a potential malignancy and warrant further evaluation.

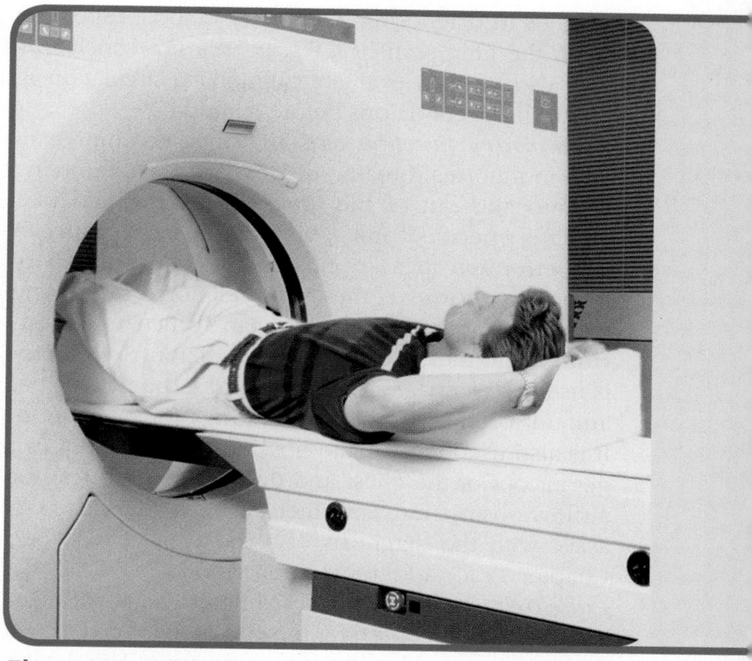

Figure 29–9A: High-speed CT scanner. *Courtesy of CAT SCAN 2000.*

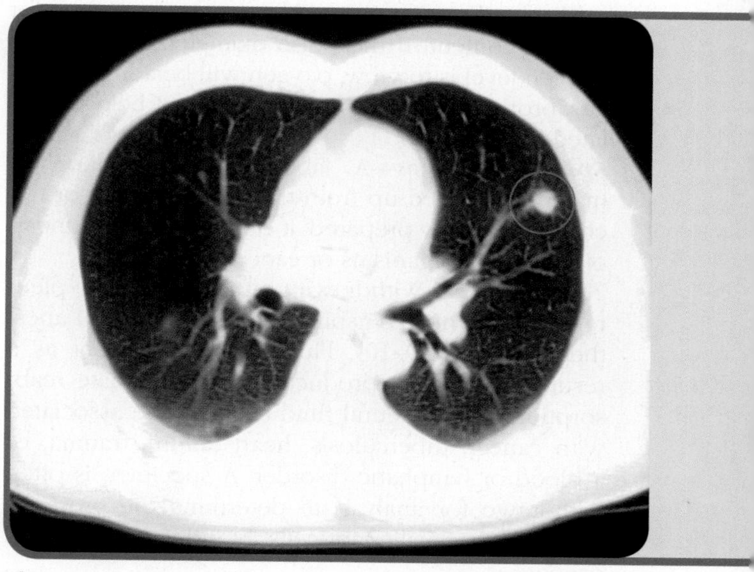

Figure 29–9B: Lung scan showing a nodule in the left upper lobe. *Courtesy of CAT SCAN 2000.*

- *Pulmonary* ***angiography/arteriography***—A radiologic examination of the pulmonary circulation following the injection of a radiopaque iodine material through a catheter that is placed in the pulmonary artery or one of its branches. The catheter is inserted into a vein at the inner surface of the elbow or in the groin and passed through the veins and through the first half of the heart into the pulmonary artery. The test aids in diagnosing pulmonary emboli, especially when the lung scan or CT scan was not conclusive. It is also used to evaluate pulmonary circulation in certain heart conditions before surgery.

- ***Pulmonary** function tests*—To measure lung volume in a normal breath, lung capacity when forcing air into and out of the lungs, and other variables within a specified time. Many noninvasive tests can be performed in a specialized hospital pulmonary laboratory; however, the most common test and one that is appropriate to the physician's office uses a **spirometer** to measure ventilation function. Spirometry is used to evaluate a patient's **vital capacity**, or the amount of air available in the lungs for respiration. It is also used to evaluate how quickly a patient can get air out of the chest and thus is useful to test for airflow obstruction. Spirometry is most often used to assist with the diagnosis of asthma or COPD. (See Chapter 14 for additional information.)
- *Pulse oximeter*—The pulse oximeter is a small electronic device that fits over the end of the index finger and is connected by a wire to a machine. The device determines the amount of oxygen in the blood and displays it digitally in the window of the machine. Frequently, postoperative patients and patients with cardiac and respiratory conditions are monitored for oxygen content. If the pulse oximeter indicates the oxygen level is too low, oxygen will be administered at a proper amount to supplement that being circulated by the body.
- ***Sputum** analysis*—A laboratory examination of material coughed up from the bronchial tree or trachea. If properly prepared, it can aid in the diagnosis of infectious organisms or cancer cells.
- *Thoracentesis*—Withdrawing of fluid from the pleural space by needle aspiration following local anesthetic (Figure 29–10). Fluid may be present as a result of excessive production or inadequate reabsorption of the pleural fluid that may be associated with cancer, tuberculosis, heart failure, trauma, or a blood or lymphatic disorder. A specimen is often withdrawn for analysis to determine the presence of organisms, malignant cells, blood, or lymph fluid properties.

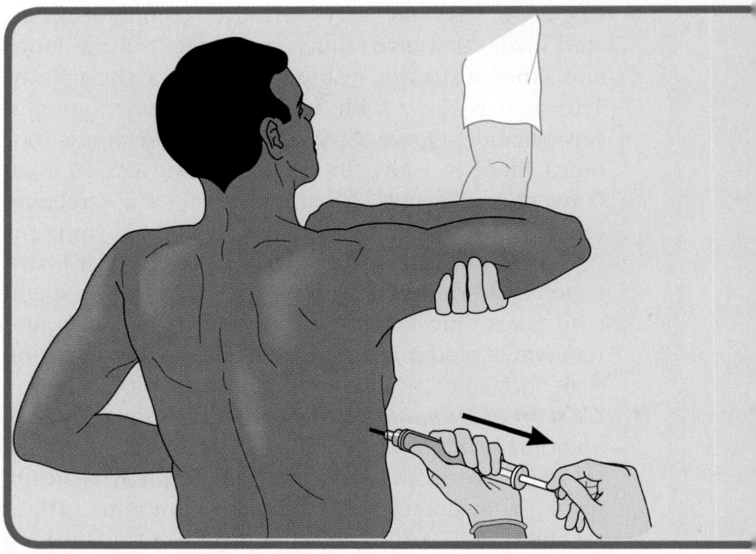

Figure 29–10: Thoracentesis. Fluid is being removed from the pleural cavity. *Delmar/Cengage Learning.*

DISEASES AND DISORDERS

Allergic Rhinitis (Ri-ni′-tis)

Description—A reaction of the eyes, nose, and sinuses to airborne allergens.

Signs and symptoms—Sneezing, profuse watery nasal discharge, itching of the eyes and nose, red and swollen eyelids, and nasal congestion.

Etiology—**Allergic rhinitis** may be seasonal, as with hay fever, or perennial, caused by dust, mold, cigarette smoke, and animal mites.

Treatment—Treatment consists primarily of administering antihistamines, topical nasal steroids, and decongestants and avoiding the allergens. The use of air conditioning filters allergens, keeps down dust, and removes excess moisture from the air. The use of steroid nasal sprays to reduce inflammation may also be helpful. Desensitizing injections of the allergens before or during the season may be indicated for long-term management. In severe or persistent cases, it may be necessary to relocate to a relatively pollen-free environment.

Asthma (Az′-ma)

Description—**Asthma** is a chronic disorder characterized by swelling, inflammation, and constriction of the bronchi and bronchioles.

Signs and symptoms—Wheezing, coughing, and shortness of breath are the most common symptoms. With a severe attack, there can be significant bronchospasm (narrowing of the bronchioles) and mucous production, markedly limiting airflow. This can result in respiratory distress, causing anxiety and a feeling of suffocation. Following an acute episode, accumulated mucus is coughed up and **expectorated**.

Etiology—Asthma is commonly caused by an allergic reaction to allergens, such as pollen, dust, animal hair, certain foods, and a number of other substances.

However, it can also result from nonspecific irritants to the airway, such as cigarette smoke and other unknown causes. It can develop at any age.

Treatment—Determination of the offending allergens can sometimes be accomplished with a series of skin tests. Minute amounts of the most common causative agents are introduced just below the skin by a needle prick or applied as patches to the skin surface. The presence of a reddened area around a site after a specified time is evidence of sensitivity. (See Chapter 45.)

The treatment of choice for allergic asthma is prevention by eliminating allergens. Drugs to prevent or control attacks, such as inhaled steroids, long-acting bronchiodilators, and leuketriene modifiers block asthma response to allergen and exercise triggers. Other drugs are used to provide quick relief of an episode. The bronchodilating drugs albuterol and ipratropium open airways almost instantly and are considered rescue medications. The goals of asthma treatment are to prevent or reduce symptoms, maintain normal activity levels, and prevent flare-ups of asthma. During severe attacks, O_2 may be administered at approximately 2 **liters** per minute to ease breathing and increase O_2 within the arteries. In addition, an albuterol nebulizer treatment and an oral, IM, or IV steroid burst may be required.

Atelectasis (Ate-lek′-ta-sis)

Description—This is the lack of air in the lungs caused by the collapse of the microscopic structures of the lung; **atelectasis** may occur following abdominal or thoracic surgery or with pressure from pleural effusion (fluid, air, pus, blood, or lymph) in the pleural cavity.

Signs and symptoms—Symptoms vary with the cause of collapse and the degree of hypoxia. There is generally some **dyspnea**. With extensive collapse there is severe dyspnea, anxiety, **cyanosis, diaphoresis** (profuse perspiration), tachycardia (rapid pulse), and retraction of intercostal muscles.

Etiology—It can be chronic, caused by mucous plugs in the bronchial tree in patients with cystic **fibrosis** and in heavy smokers with obstructive pulmonary disease. Bronchial occlusion can also result from cancer or inflamed tissues. Acute (sudden) atelectasis may occur with any condition that causes pain on deep breathing, such as rib fractures, traumatic injury, surgical procedures, or pleurisy.

Treatment—Treatment includes chest percussion, postural drainage, frequent coughing, and deep breathing exercises or intermittent positive pressure breathing (IPPB).

Bronchitis (Brong-ki′-tis)

Description—**Bronchitis** can be an acute or chronic disease with inflammation of the bronchial walls with distortion and narrowing of the airways. Chronic bronchitis is a condition in which excessive mucus is secreted in the bronchi during several months a year for several years in a row. The typical patient is middle-aged or older, often with a long history of cigarette smoking. Acute bronchitis is associated with an infection. It occurs abruptly and lasts several days or weeks.

Signs and symptoms—The presence of a cough that produces yellowish-gray or green mucus is one of the main symptoms of acute bronchitis. Other symptoms may include those common with upper respiratory disease such as sore throat, slight fever, soreness or feeling of constriction in the chest, and general malaise. Chronic bronchitis sufferers also produce thick mucus with a constant "smoker's cough," have recurring respiratory infections, and may have weakness and weight loss. Wheezing and prolonged expiration time may be observed.

Etiology—Acute bronchitis is caused by a viral or bacterial respiratory infection. You can also develop bronchitis from exposure to your own or someone else's cigarette smoke and even pollutants such as household cleaners and smog. Bronchitis can also occur when acids from the stomach consistently back up into the esophagus, a condition known as gastroesophageal reflux disease (GERD, see Chapter 32), which causes a reflex mechanism. Chronic bronchitis is caused by damaged cilia, enlarged mucous glands, and chronic inflammation. The severity of chronic bronchitis is related to the amount and duration of smoking.

Treatment—Acute bronchitis is managed with expectorants to help remove excessive mucus and by avoiding smoking. Antibiotics such as azithromycin are sometimes needed if bacterial infection is suspected. Chronic bronchitis requires bronchodilators, such as ADVAIR, respiratory therapy to loosen mucous secretions, smoking cessation, and corticosteroids in some cases. Adequate fluid intake is important.

Chronic Obstructive Pulmonary Disease (COPD)

Description—This is a condition characterized by chronic obstruction of the airways. COPD is an umbrella term that includes conditions such as emphysema, chronic bronchitis, and asthma. It is a progressive disease. Symptoms occur gradually and become worse with age. COPD is the most common chronic lung disease, affecting an estimated 17 million Americans. It affects males more often than females, probably because until recently men were more likely to smoke heavily. COPD is a leading cause of death in both men and women; however, there has been a significant increase recently in the number of women with the disease.

Signs and symptoms—The first signs are a decline in the ability to exercise or do strenuous work. A productive cough will begin to develop. These symptoms worsen with time, and eventually the patient develops dyspnea on minimal exertion and has frequent respiratory infections, wheezing, hypoxemia (lack of oxygen in the blood), and grossly abnormal pulmonary function studies. Difficulty with breathing makes eating difficult, so weight loss and lack of appetite is common. With advanced disease, the patient must work so hard to breathe that he or she may consume up to 20% of their resting energy. Thoracic deformities develop (usually a barrel chest from muscular changes caused by struggling to breathe). Eventually, there is overwhelming disability, severe respiratory failure, and death.

Etiology—The primary cause of COPD (80% to 90%) is long-term cigarette smoking, which impairs the ciliary action, causes inflammation in airways, destroys alveolar walls, and results in the formation of scar tissue around the bronchioles. COPD is the result of emphysema, chronic bronchitis, asthma, or any combination of these disorders. It can also develop from chronic respiratory infections and allergies.

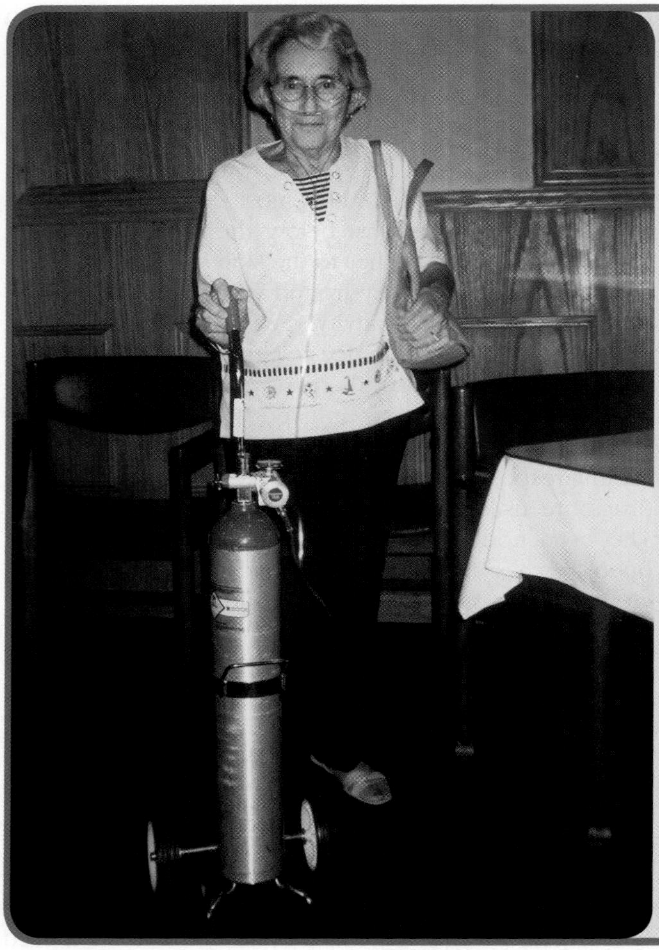

Figure 29–11A: Individuals with COPD often need a portable oxygen tank to assist with breathing, allowing them to leave home. *Courtesy of Barbara A. Wise.*

Treatment—Treatment consists of methods to halt the progression of the disease and control symptoms. Prime emphasis is placed on stopping smoking and avoiding other respiratory irritants. The main focus of treatment involves the use of bronchodilators, like ADVAIR, prompt treatment of respiratory infections, effective breathing and coughing instructions, proper diet, the use of O_2 as indicated, and exercise rehabilitation programs. Lung volume reduction surgery and lung transplant are options for a select group of patients. The woman in Figure 29–11A began having significant respiratory problems about 10 years ago, experiencing severe acute episodes of asthma. Her condition became chronic and is now considered COPD. She requires the use of oxygen continuously. While at home, she uses a machine called an oxygenator, which concentrates oxygen from the room, but when she leaves, she must use a portable tank to provide her with supplemental oxygen.

Another option for portable oxygen is shown in Figure 29–11B. This woman has had diabetes since childhood and now has multiple problems including severe leg ulcers, inadequate oxygen intake, a history of heart attacks, and multiple mild strokes. She needs a small amount of supplemental oxygen and therefore her smaller oxygen supply is adequate and will last for about two hours. It can be carried easily in the case on her right arm or strapped across the handles of her wheelchair. She also uses an oxygenator at home and must carry additional small tanks whenever she leaves.

Emphysema (Em-fi-se′-ma)

Description—This is the irreversible enlargement of the air spaces in the lungs caused by the destruction of the alveolar walls. **Emphysema** results in the inability to exchange O_2 and CO_2 in the affected areas and to exhale stale air from the lungs. The lungs may actually be enlarged, but at the same time they are not efficient because of the decreased surface area for exchanging oxygen and carbon dioxide. Figure 29–12 is a photo of a CT scan showing the **blebs** (bubbles) of destroyed alveoli around the outer lung areas of a patient with emphysema. These are visible as large white-edged black areas.

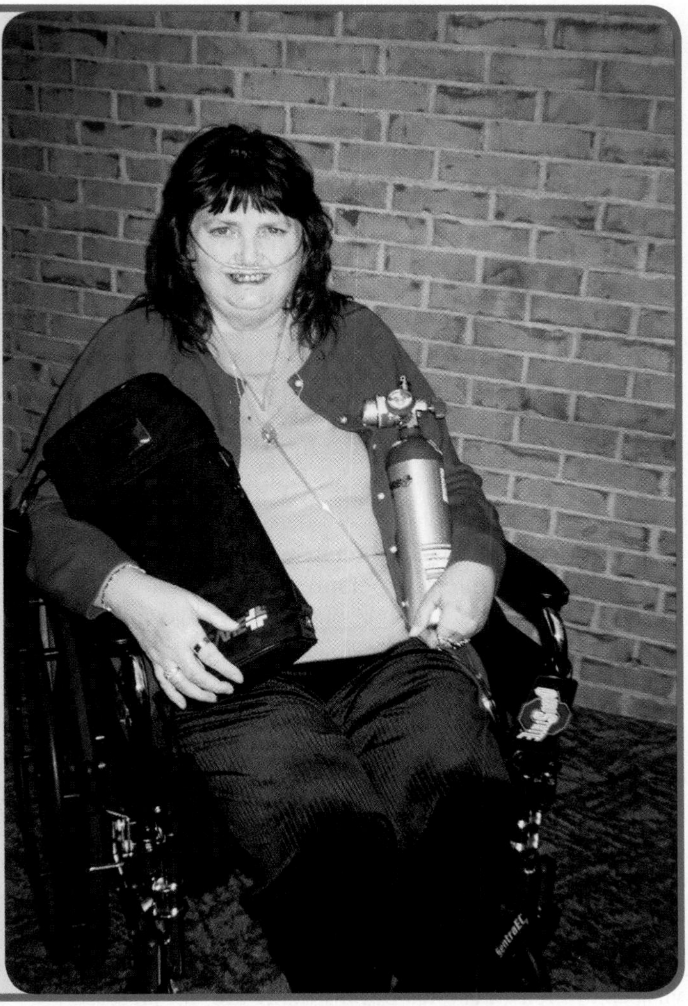

Figure 29–11B: Woman with small portable oxygen tank. *Courtesy Barbara A. Wise.*

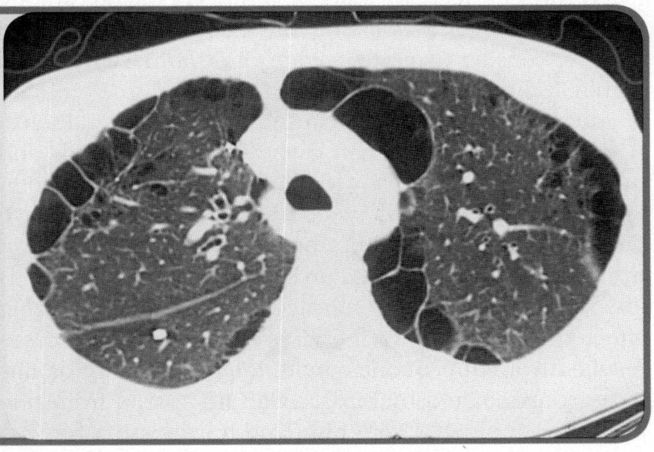

Figure 29–12: CT scan showing the large blebs (bubbles) of emphysema. They are identifiable as the large dark areas with white borders on the outer edges of the lungs. *Courtesy of Philip T. Diaz, MD, pulmonologist.*

Signs and symptoms—Emphysema is characterized by a chronic cough, weight loss, fatigue, barrel chest, the use of accessory muscles to breathe, pursed lips, cyanosis, and eventually respiratory failure, heart enlargement and failure, and death.

Etiology—The prime cause is cigarette smoking. Emphysema can also develop from chronic infection or irritation from environmental factors.

Treatment—The treatment is the same as for COPD: smoking cessation, the use of bronchodilators, prompt treatment of respiratory infections, effective breathing and coughing instructions, proper diet, and the use of O_2 as indicated.

Epistaxis (Epi-stak′-sis) (Nosebleed)

Description—Epistaxis is the loss of blood through the nose. (See Chapter 25.)

Signs and symptoms—The visible presence of blood coming from the nose or the patient experiencing bleeding posteriorly into the throat.

Etiology—Nosebleeds usually follow injury, either external or internal, such as a blow to the nose, nosepicking, or foreign body insertion. Less frequent causes of **epistaxis** are chronic conditions, such as nasal or sinus infection that results in capillary congestion and bleeding, or the inhalation of irritating substances. Predisposing systemic factors include high blood pressure; anticoagulation drugs; chronic aspirin use; and blood diseases, such as anemia, hemophilia, and leukemia.

Treatment—Treatment varies depending on the cause, location, and severity. Even moderate bleeding is of concern if it persists longer than 20 minutes after pressure is applied. Symptoms of severe blood loss may include lightheadedness, a drop in blood pressure, rapid pulse, dyspnea, pallor, and other indications of shock. Initial first aid treatment may consist of elevating the head, compressing the nostrils against the septum continuously for 5 to 10 minutes, applying ice or cold compresses to the nose, preventing the swallowing of blood (to determine the amount lost), avoiding talking or blowing the nose, and observing for the amount of blood loss and signs of shock.

Advanced treatment for anterior bleeding includes applying an epinephrine-saturated cotton ball or gauze to the bleeding site and the use of external pressure, followed by cauterization by electric cautery or silver nitrate. For posterior bleeding, the insertion of a nasal balloon for 48 to 72 hours may be required. If necessary, anterior bleeding can be treated by packing for 24 to 48 hours. Other treatment may include supplemental vitamin K to aid in blood clotting, blood transfusions, and surgical ligation (tying) of the bleeding artery.

Histoplasmosis (His-to-plaz-mo′-sis)

Description—This is a fungal infection that occurs worldwide. In the United States, histoplasmosis occurs in three forms: primary acute, progressive disseminated, and chronic pulmonary.

Signs and symptoms—Symptoms vary with the form contracted. The primary acute form resembles a severe cold. The progressive form involves the liver, spleen, and lymph glands, and it may cause inflammation of the heart muscle, the pericardium (covering membrane), and the meninges of the brain and spinal cord. The chronic form resembles tuberculosis, causing a productive cough, dyspnea, weakness, hemoptysis (spitting up blood), fever, and cyanosis.

Etiology—**Histoplasmosis** is caused by an organism found in droppings from birds or bats, or in soil near their roosts, as in barns, caves, chicken coops, around buildings, and under bridges. It may also come from cat feces because of ingested birds.

Treatment—The acute form generally does not require treatment. With the progressive disseminated or chronic pulmonary forms, a high dose or long-term treatment with an antifungal such as amphotericin B or itraconazole is indicated. Surgery to remove pulmonary nodules and a shunt to relieve intracranial pressure may be necessary. Oxygen can be given to reduce respiratory distress. Additional treatments are indicated if other severe conditions develop.

Hyaline Membrane Disease (HMD) (Hi′-a-lin)

(See Respiratory Distress Syndrome.)

Influenza (In-flu-en′-za) (Flu)

Description—This acute, highly contagious respiratory infection usually occurs in colder months and in infrequent epidemics (widespread incidence, not of local origin). It is more prevalent in school children aged 6 to 14 and adults over age 40. **Influenza** can be fatal to the elderly or people with chronic heart, lung, or kidney disease. Influenza viruses have the ability to alter their influence on the population. As people develop immunity to a virus after coming into contact with it, the virus alters its composition and a new strain results to which people have little or no resistance. Hence an epidemic or pandemic (present in many areas of the world at the same time) can develop.

Influenza viruses are classified into three types:

- *Type A*—The most lethal, occurring every two to three years, with a major new strain developing every 10 to 15 years
- *Type B*—Occurring every four to six years, resulting in epidemics (types A and B combined are responsible for 50% of viral pneumonia cases.)
- *Type C*—Endemic (of local origin) and causing infrequent cases

Signs and symptoms—Symptoms of flu are the sudden onset of chills and a fever of 101° to 104°F (38° to 40°C), headaches, muscle aches, a nonproductive cough, and **rhinitis**. Pneumonia is the most common complication, developing three to five days after infection begins.

Etiology—The disease is directly transmitted by droplets inhaled from an infected person's sneezing or coughing or by indirect contact with contaminated objects, such as a drinking glass.

Treatment—Treatment consists of bed rest, adequate fluid intake, and aspirin or similar medication to relieve the pain and fever. Antibiotics have no effect on the virus and should not be used unless there is secondary bacterial infection. Flu immunizations, which provide protection for three to six months, are recommended for the high-risk population. However, the vaccine is only 75% effective. Avian influenza is an infection caused by a flu virus that occurs naturally in birds. Wild birds carry the viruses in their intestines but normally are not affected by it. Infected birds shed the viruses in feces, nasal drainage, and saliva. Other birds become infected by coming into contact with the secretions; infected fowl; or contaminated surfaces, feed, or water. It is very contagious among birds and can infect *domestic* birds, chickens, ducks, and turkeys, causing a mortality rate of 90% to 100%, often within 48 hours.

One type of bird flu is caused by the avian influenza A (H5N1) virus, which can cause infection in birds and humans. There are many different subtypes of type A viruses; to date 16 HA types and 9 NA subtypes have been identified, and all can be found in birds. Infection from these viruses can occur in humans, but the risk is low. There have been confirmed cases of humans being affected by subtypes of the virus since 1997. Most cases resulted from direct contact with infected poultry or surfaces contaminated by birds. Avian flu spread from one person to another is very rare, and transmission has not occurred beyond one person.

To date all cases have occurred in Asia, Africa, the Pacific, Europe, and the near East. Since first reported in 2003, there have been 228 confirmed cases with 130 deaths. The World Health Organization has responded immediately to any new case, and the spread has been contained. There is a ban on all poultry and eggs from any country having any disease. Symptoms of avian flu in humans are like typical human flu: fever, cough, sore throat, and muscle aches. In addition, eye infections, pneumonia, severe respiratory diseases, and other life-threatening complications may occur depending upon which virus causes the infection. Because these viruses are not common among humans, there has been no buildup of immunity in the population.

Viruses are capable of change and may mutate, possibly causing infection and spreading among humans. When this happens, a pandemic may occur. (Pandemic means that the infection is epidemic in different parts of the world at the same time.) The 2009 H1N1 influenza virus (swine flu) produced such a pandemic. According to the Centers for Disease Control and Prevention (CDC), from 43 to 89 million cases of 2009 H1N1 infection occurred between April 2009 and April 2010. The CDC estimated that between 195,000 to 403,000 H1N1 cases required hospitalization and between 8,870 to 18,300 H1N1-related deaths occurred in the United States during the same one-year period.

An H1N1 vaccine became available during the pandemic, initially in a limited supply, and was reserved to vaccinate high-risk groups who were at risk to develop severe complication from the H1N1 infection. These groups included children younger than 2 years old, adults 65 years of age or older, pregnant women, and persons with chronic medical conditions such as asthma, COPD, neurological disorders and developmental delays, and kidney, liver and metabolic disorders. Health care providers were also considered to be in a high at-risk group because of their contact with infected people.

Currently, it is recommended that all persons receive a seasonal flu vaccine, which as of this writing, contains a vaccine for three viruses that are most likely to cause the seasonal flu, including the H1N1 infection. In patients that do develop the flu, antiviral medications such as oseltamivir (Tamiflu) and zanamivir (Relenza) may make symptoms milder and shorten the length of illness. Antivirals may also diminish the risk of developing serious complications.

Laryngectomy (Larin-jek′to-me)

This is not a disease or disorder but a surgical solution to a life-threatening situation. It is the surgical removal of the larynx and is usually performed to treat throat cancer caused by smoking. The earliest symptom of internal disease of the larynx is persistent hoarseness. With involvement externally, it is a lump in the throat or pain, or burning when drinking hot liquids or citrus juices.

Diagnosis can often be made by viewing the larynx with a laryngoscope. This examination is often followed with radiological studies to confirm the diagnosis. With positive diagnosis, the larynx may be partially or totally removed. With total removal, a permanent opening called a stoma is made in the neck through which air can be taken in and exhaled (Figure 29–13). Coughing results in material being expelled through the stoma.

A great deal of patient support is necessary to assist in developing alternative methods of communication prior to surgery. The patient may need psychiatric assistance to cope with the loss of speech, sense of smell, ability to blow the nose, and related problems. Much support can be obtained from organizations established to aid in rehabilitation of **laryngectomy** patients. Local chapters of the "Lost Chord Club," made up of persons who have lost their larynx, volunteer their services to speak with new patients and help them learn techniques of producing speech. The American Cancer Society and the International Association of Laryngectomies also provide assistance with speech methods that use esophageal air that is swallowed and released slowly, the artificial larynx, and other mechanical devices.

The individual in Figure 29–13A has a Blum finger voice prosthesis inserted into the stoma (Figure 29–13B shows an inserter). By placing his finger over the opening in the prosthesis, he is able to produce a good quality of speech. A "patch" of thin foam is worn over the opening to prevent inhaling foreign materials. The foam is porous and permits easy exchange of air.

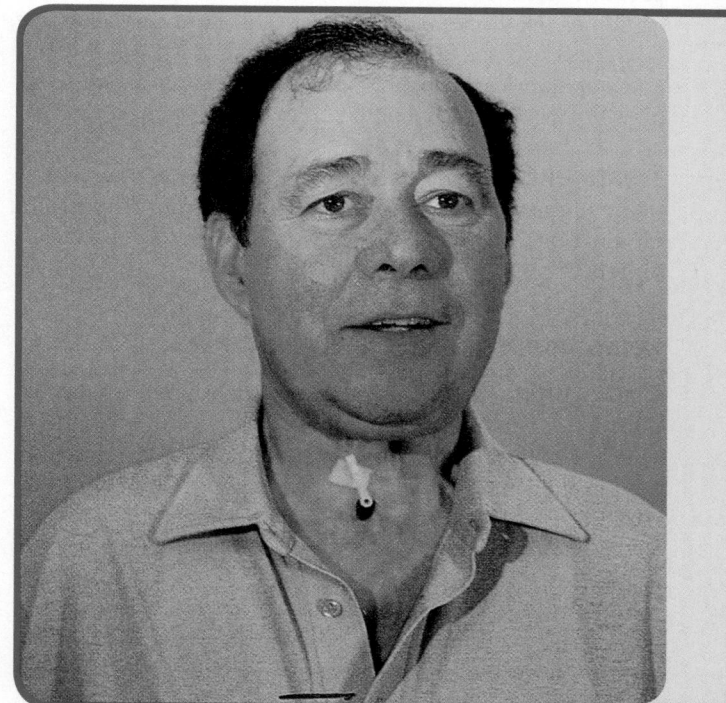

Figure 29–13A: Laryngeal stoma following laryngectomy with an inserted Blum finger prosthesis. *Delmar/Cengage Learning.*

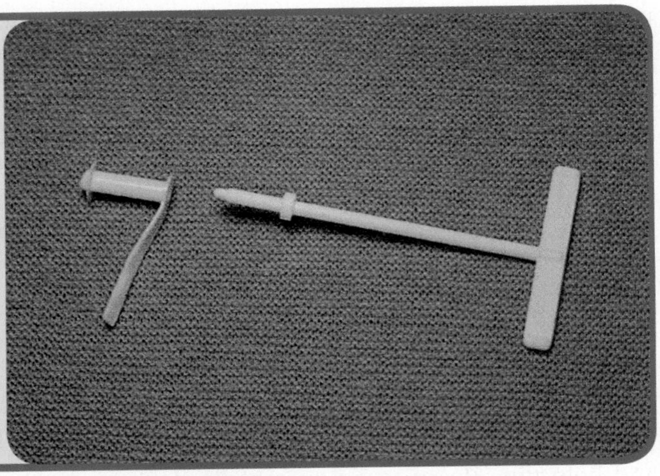

Figure 29–13B: An inserter. *Delmar/Cengage Learning.*

Laryngitis (Lar-in-ji′-tis)

Description—This inflammation of the vocal cords occurs in both acute and chronic forms.

Signs and symptoms—Acute **laryngitis** usually begins as hoarseness, with either minimal or complete loss of voice. There may be some pain when talking or swallowing, a dry cough, fever, and malaise. With chronic laryngitis, the only symptom is persistent hoarseness.

Etiology—Acute laryngitis usually results from an infectious process, excessive use of the voice, inhalation of smoke or fumes, or accidental aspiration of chemicals. Chronic laryngitis develops from other preexistent chronic conditions (such as sinusitis, bronchitis, and allergies) or from smoking, abuse of alcohol, or continual exposure to irritants.

Treatment—Laryngitis is treated by resting the voice, using medication for underlying infection, if present, and eliminating coexistent causes (in the case of chronic laryngitis).

Legionnaires' Disease (Le′-jun-airs)

Description—This is an acute bronchopneumonia that derived its name from a highly publicized incident in which 182 people developed the disease at an American Legion Convention in Philadelphia in 1976. **Legionnaires' disease** usually occurs in late summer or early fall.

Signs and symptoms—Symptoms are nonspecific and include diarrhea, lack of appetite, headache, chills, weakness, and an unremitting fever that develops within 12 to 48 hours. Temperature may reach 105°F (40.5°C). A cough then develops, which becomes productive, with grayish sputum. Other symptoms are nausea, vomiting, confusion, dyspnea, and chest pain. Severe symptoms are evidence of complications and include low blood pressure, irregular heartbeat, respiratory failure, kidney failure, and shock (which is usually fatal). Smokers are three to four times more likely to develop legionnaires' disease than nonsmokers.

Etiology—It is caused by the bacteria *Legionella pneumophilia* and is transmitted through water that is contaminated with the bacteria. In past epidemics, it was spread through air-conditioning systems and cooling towers. It does not spread person to person.

Treatment—Treatment consists of antibiotics, medication to reduce the fever, maintaining fluid balance, and measures to support adequate respiration, such as oxygen and mechanical ventilation.

Lung Cancer

Description—This is the leading cause of cancer deaths among men and women, despite the fact that it is largely preventable. It is the progressive cellular degeneration of lung tissue. It usually develops within the wall or lining of the bronchial tree. There are different types of lung cancer: squamous cell, small-cell, adenocarcinoma, and large-cell. Approximately 222,000 new cases of lung cancer were estimated in 2010. This represents 14.5% of all cancer diagnoses. Lung cancer is still the leading cause of cancer-related deaths, with an estimated 157,300 deaths, or 20% of all cancer deaths, in 2010.

Signs and symptoms—There are often minimal symptoms that are usually not associated with cancer, such as cough, fatigue, and shortness of breath. This frequently results in diagnosis at the late stages when the disease is far advanced, offering little hope for survival. The symptoms of squamous and small-cell carcinomas are smoker's cough, sneezing, dyspnea, hemoptysis, and chest pain. Symptoms of adenocarcinoma and large-cell types include fever, weakness, weight loss, and anorexia. Unfortunately, there is no proven screening test for lung cancer.

Etiology—It is attributed to inhalation of carcinogens in tobacco and the environment. The inhalation of carcinogens causes damage to the cells of the lungs, which then causes uncontrolled abnormal growth when these cells become cancerous. There is a correlation between the risk of cancer and the number of cigarettes smoked daily, the depth of inhalation, the age at which smoking began, and the nicotine content of the tobacco. An individual over 40 who began smoking as a teenager and has averaged a pack a day for at least 20 years is most susceptible. Lung cancer can take 20 to 30 years to develop. Less than 10% of lung cancers occur among nonsmokers.

Other inhalants that increase *susceptibility* to cancer are industrial air pollutants, such as asbestos, arsenic, iron oxides, chromium, radioactive dust, vinyl chloride, and coal dust. There also is an indication that there is a familial tendency link to lung cancer. The combination of industrial pollutants and cigarettes is very risky. For example, asbestos workers who also smoke increase their risk of developing lung cancer by 60 times.

Involuntary smoking, which the nonsmoker receives "second hand" from a spouse or others, is less concentrated but still contains the same harmful substances. For example, wives exposed to husbands who smoke 20 or more cigarettes a day at home have double the risk of lung cancer when compared with wives of nonsmokers. Cancer caused by second-hand smoke kills 3,400 nonsmokers per year. Children of smoking parents are also affected. They are more prone to respiratory and middle ear infections, asthma, and sudden infant death syndrome (SIDS).

The prognosis for lung cancer patients is very poor because by the time a diagnosis is made, two thirds of the patients have passed the stage where it might be curable. Only 13% of all lung cancer patients (all races and all stages) live five or more years after diagnosis. This is primarily the result of delayed diagnosis because of lack of symptoms. The disease metastasizes to many other sites within the thoracic cavity and throughout the entire body.

Treatment—Treatment consists primarily of surgical excision when appropriate, radiation, and chemotherapy. Often the disease is advanced before treatment begins, and little more than alleviation of symptoms is possible. The best treatment is obviously prevention. Quitting smoking or never starting is the best defense against lung cancer.

Pleurisy (Ploo′ris-e)

Description—This is an inflammation of the visceral and parietal pleura in the thoracic cavity. **Pleurisy** develops as a complication of viral infections, pneumonia, tuberculosis, chest injury, and other factors.

Signs and symptoms—Sharp, stabbing pain is experienced on respiration because of irritation of the pleural nerve endings as the lungs move, rubbing against the inner chest wall. As a result, lung movement on the affected side may be limited, and dyspnea occurs.

Etiology—Pleurisy pain is caused by the inflammation or irritation of sensory nerve endings in the parietal pleura. It begins suddenly as a complication of pneumonia, a viral infection, or other causes.

Treatment—In the case of a viral infection, treatment is generally symptomatic, with bed rest and medications to reduce the inflammation and relieve the pain. If fluid collects within the pleural space (see Pleural Effusion), a thoracentesis is indicated to prohibit lung compression by the fluid or to determine, by laboratory examination, a causative agent (see Figure 29–10).

Paroxysmal Nocturnal Dyspnea (PND) (Parok-sizmal Nok-turn-al)

Description—This is a symptom associated with chronic lung disease or left ventricular failure (heart disease).

Signs and symptoms—It occurs at night. Individuals awaken from sleep with a feeling of suffocation. They often run to open a window and gasp for air. Just sitting upright will help some people because of the effect of gravity on fluid in the lungs.

Etiology—This is associated with chronic lung disease and left ventricular heart failure probably caused by the accumulation of fluid in the lungs.

Treatment—The episode will often resolve within a few minutes; however, the symptom of PND indicates a serious underlying condition that requires treatment.

Pleural Effusion (Plooral E-fu′-zhun)

Description—This is the presence of excess fluid in the pleural space (Figure 29–14).

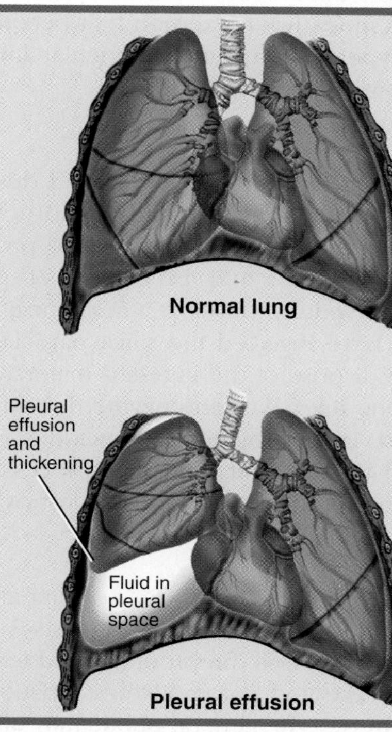

Figure 29–14: Comparison of a normal lung with pleural effusion. *Delmar/Cengage Learning.*

Signs and symptoms—When the effusion becomes symptomatic, it compresses lung tissue and reduces the lungs' ability to exchange O_2 for CO_2, and **hypoxia** (lack of O_2) results. If the fluid is a result of an infectious process, exudate (pus) and dead tissue may be present, and the effusion is known as **empyema**.

Etiology—Pleural effusion results from the overproduction or the inadequate reabsorption of the pleural fluid. Some effusions result from chronic diseases, such as congestive heart failure, liver disease, tuberculosis, malignancy, lupus, and rheumatoid arthritis.

Treatment—Oxygen is administered to increase concentration to the remainder of the lung. Drainage of the material by thoracentesis and insertion of chest tubes may be necessary. Antibiotics may be required if the effusion is infectious in origin. Effusion that contains blood is called a **hemothorax** and will require drainage to prevent fibrothorax (scar tissue) formation.

Pneumonoconiosis (Nu-mo-kone-o′sis)

Description—These are lung diseases developed after years of contact with environmental or occupational causative agents. Basically, there are three types of **pneumonoconiosis**: silicosis, asbestosis, and black lung disease.

Signs and symptoms—Some symptoms, common to all forms of pneumonoconioses, are rapid respirations, dry cough, dyspnea upon exertion that becomes worse, pulmonary hypertension, right ventricular involvement, and recurrent respiratory infections.

Silicosis

This occurs from exposure to silica sand dust in occupations such as sand blaster and foundry worker; in manufacturing of ceramic and sandstone products and construction materials; and in mining of gold, lead, zinc, and iron. Nodules develop where specific disease-fighting cells have ingested the silica particles but then are unable to dispose of the ingested material. The cells die, causing the release of an enzyme that attracts more cells to assist in destroying the invading material. A fibrous (scar) tissue results, and the process continues until large areas of the lung tissue are destroyed.

Asbestosis

This condition can develop 15 to 20 years after regular exposure to asbestos has ended. Asbestosis is most prevalent in the construction, fireproofing, and textile industries and in brake and automotive occupations dealing with clutch linings. The general public may also develop the condition from exposure to fibrous dust or the waste piles of asbestos factories. Asbestosis is the result of inhaling minute asbestos fibers, which enter the bronchioles and penetrate the alveolar walls. The fibers become encased, and fibrosis of the lung tissue develops, obliterating the air passages. Fibers also cause fibrotic changes in the parietal pleura.

Coal Worker's or Black Lung Disease

This is a progressive nodular type found in two forms: simple, which produces small lung lesions, or complicated, which produces masses of fibrous tissue. The development usually occurs after 15 years or more of exposure and depends to some extent on the amount of dust, the type of coal mined, the silica content, and the location of the mine.

Initially, the body's fighting cells ingest the dust and become filled, forming macules in the terminal bronchioles, which are surrounded by dilated alveoli. The supporting tissue atrophies (wastes away), resulting in permanent dilation of the small airways. When the disease changes from a simple to a complicated form, one or both lungs can become involved. The fibrous tissue masses enlarge, causing destruction of the alveoli and airways.

Treatment—Treatment of all types is essentially the same: avoid respiratory infections, use bronchodilators to aid in respiration, supplement oxygen when indicated, and other use respiratory therapy to improve removal of bronchial secretions.

Pneumonia (Nu-mo′-ne-a)

Description—This is an acute infection of the principal tissues of the lungs, which may impair the exchange of O_2 and CO_2. Chances for recovery from **pneumonia** are good for persons with normal lungs, but pneumonia is a very common cause of death in debilitated (weakened) patients.

Pneumonia is classified in several ways: by microbiological origin (bacterial, viral, or fungal), by location (bronchial or lobar), or by type (primary or secondary).

Signs and symptoms—Symptoms include coughing, sputum production, pleural chest pain, chills, and fever.

Etiology—Pneumonia can be caused by inhaled pathogens, an inhaled chemical, or an infection spread from another area of the body. It often occurs with a chronic weakening illness (such as cancer or AIDS) or following surgery. It is also associated with malnutrition, smoking, COPD, advanced age, and with a decreased level of consciousness.

Treatment—Treatment consists of bed rest, antibiotics for bacterial pneumonia, adequate fluid intake, respiratory support measures (such as oxygen or mechanical breathing therapy), and medication for pain.

Pneumothorax (Nu-mo-tho′-raks)

Description—In this condition, air or gas has accumulated between the parietal and visceral pleurae, causing some degree of collapse of the lung tissue. Figure 29–15A shows an accumulation of air at the mid portion of the left chest, which has collapsed a portion of the upper lobe. This space is identifiable by the darkened area on the film. You will also notice the ECG leads placed on the chest wall. Another interesting feature of the film is the sternal wires along the right sternal edge. This woman has had open heart surgery and the sternal wires were used to reattach the ribs to the sternum. In Figure 29–15B, you can see the outline of the inserted chest tube around the eighth rib on the left side. With the tube connected to a suction device, the air has been mostly removed and the lung structure is again visible.

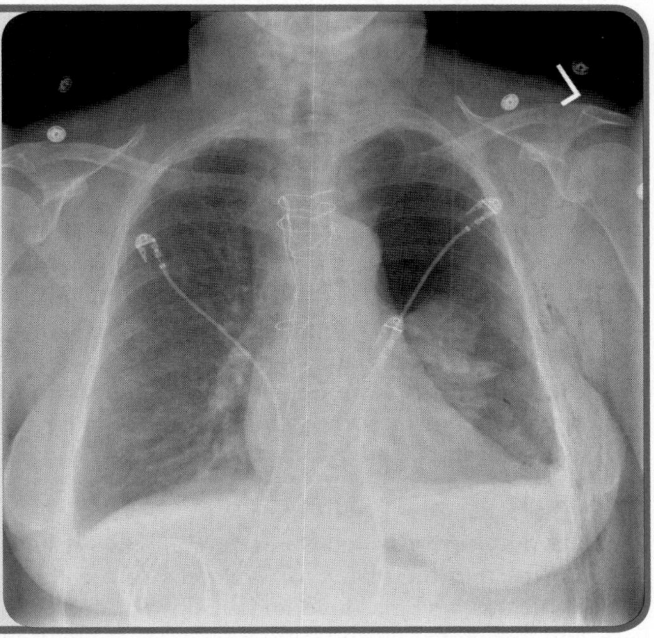

Figure 29–15A: An example of pneumothorax. Pneumothorax of the left lung. *Courtesy of Paul R. Beery II, MD, MS, FACS, trauma surgeon.*

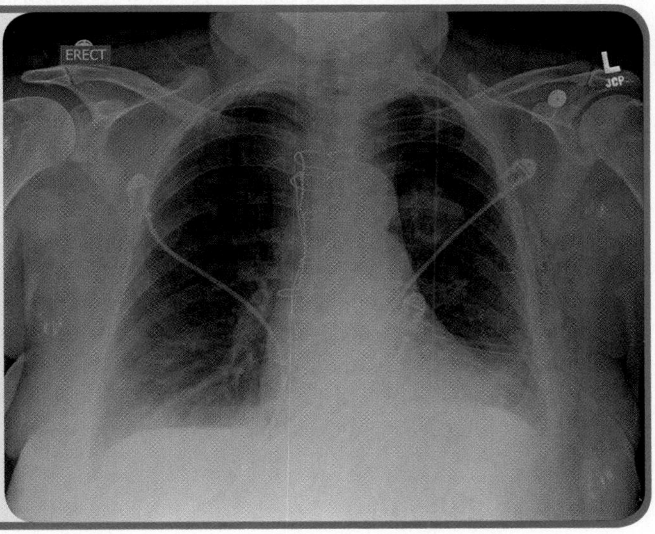

Figure 29–15B: Post pneumothorax *Courtesy of Paul R. Beery II, MD, MS, FACS, trauma surgeon.*

Signs and symptoms—The primary symptoms of pneumothorax are sudden, sharp pain made worse by breathing or coughing and shortness of breath. As the degree of collapse increases, respirations become more stressful, the pulse becomes rapid and weak, and the patient becomes pale or cyanotic. Death may result without prompt treatment.

Etiology—If it is **spontaneous**, air has leaked from the lung tissue as the result of a disease process or a ruptured blisterlike lesion. A traumatic **pneumothorax** results from a penetrating chest wound (as by a knife or gunshot), from thoracic surgery, or as a complication from the insertion of tubing into the blood vessels of the chest. Fractured ribs can penetrate the thorax, causing collapse of the lung. Because the atmospheric pressure outside is greater than that within the pleural cavity, the air compresses the lung tissue as it enters. Frequently, blood is also present with an injury, and if it is located between the pleura, it is referred to as a hemothorax.

In tension pneumothorax, air enters the pleural space but is unable to leave by the same route. Each inspiration results in additional trapped air being sucked in. Eventually, pressure is exerted against the large chest veins, interfering with blood flow returning to the heart. If severe, the great vessels of the chest and the heart may be pushed toward the uninjured side of the chest. This is a medical emergency.

Treatment—Treatment varies with the degree of collapse. If the pneumothorax is spontaneous, small in size, and not associated with dyspnea, or if there are apparent signs of increasing difficulty, it may be treated with bed rest and careful monitoring of vital signs. With greater than 30% collapse, the lung is reexpanded by low suction through a tube inserted into the chest. In some cases of recurrent pneumothorax or inadequate re-expansion with chest tube placement, surgery may be required.

Pulmonary Fibrosis (Pul′mo-ne-re Fi-bro′-sis)

Description—Scarring of the lung tissue, making the lungs stiff and small. This condition is often progressive and usually fatal. If scaring is advanced, oxygen cannot enter the alveoli, resulting in hypoxia.

Signs and symptoms—The most common symptom is shortness of breath on exertion. As the disease progresses, even minimal exertion such as talking causes dyspnea. A dry cough is also common. Signs include tachypnea, cyanosis, and a crackling sound when auscultating the lungs, like velcro being pulled apart.

Etiology—Chronic exposure to dust (see pneumoconiosis); inhalation of certain allergens; and connective tissue diseases such as rheumatoid arthritis, scleroderma, and lupus can cause fibrosis. It also results from some medications, especially chemotherapeutic agents and radiation therapy to treat cancer in the chest. Often no cause can be found, and the etiology is called "idiopathic."

Treatment—Steroids and immunosuppressive agents are used to slow the progression. Oxygen is often needed. Lung transplant offers hope for a cure, but the condition is often fatal.

Pulmonary Edema (E-de′ma)

Description—This is the accumulation, within the tissues of the lungs, of fluid that has escaped from the blood vessels caused by increased pressure in these vessels. **Pulmonary edema** is common in these vessels, with heart disorders causing left ventricular failure.

Signs and symptoms—Symptoms include dyspnea on exertion, coughing, **orthopnea** (ability to breathe only in an upright position), and rapid pulse and respiration. With progression, respirations become more labored, noisy, and rapid. A cough that produces frothy, bloody sputum may develop. As the condition worsens, the patient becomes cold, clammy, and cyanotic. Confusion and a depressed level of consciousness occur in cases of severe heart failure.

Etiology—Pulmonary edema usually results from left ventricular heart failure resulting from arteriosclerosis, hypertension, or a faulty valve that causes increased pressure within the left atrium and blood vessels of the lungs. The pressure causes fluid to "squeeze" out of the blood and into the lung tissue.

Treatment—Treatment consists of procedures to decrease the accumulated fluids and improve the exchange of O_2 and CO_2. Diuretics (water pills), nitroglycerin, and high concentrations of oxygen may be indicated.

Pulmonary Embolism (Em′bo-lizm)

Description—Obstruction of a pulmonary artery or arteriole by a circulating thrombus (blood clot) is called a pulmonary embolism.

Signs and symptoms—The obstruction causes dyspnea, chest pain, rapid heart rate, a cough, and a low-grade fever. The symptoms vary with the extent of obstruction. In massive embolism, with over 50% obstruction of arterial circulation, death can occur rapidly.

Etiology—Predisposing factors include long-term immobility, which permits slow-moving blood to clot within the vessels; varicose veins; surgery; pregnancy; vascular injury; obesity; fractures; cancer; clotting disorders; and many chronic pulmonary and circulatory diseases.

Treatment—Treatment consists of measures to maintain adequate heart and lung function while the obstruction is being resolved, usually within 10 to 14 days. Medication is given to inhibit the blood from forming additional clots and to break up the present occlusion. Supportive oxygen therapy is used as needed. If the embolus is caused by purulent material from an infectious process, aggressive antibiotic therapy is indicated. Filters are sometimes placed in the vena cava to prevent clots from entering the heart and lungs.

Respiratory Distress Syndrome (RDS)

Description—Formerly known as hyaline membrane disease, this is a mysterious condition that kills apparently healthy infants. Those between birth and 8 months of age are at highest risk. The death is unexplainable even after autopsy. RDS attributes to approximately 40,000 newborn deaths annually in the United States. The condition occurs more frequently in infants born to smoking or diabetic mothers. Other maternal conditions, such as hemorrhage and infection, may also precipitate RDS.

Signs and symptoms—RDS most commonly presents symptoms within the first 3 to 5 minutes of breathing. Normal breaths become rapid and shallow. The nostrils flare, and the intercostal and substernal muscles are used to help with respirations, as evidenced by the retraction of the sternum. A "grunting" type of noise generated by the infant's attempt to breathe signals respiratory failure.

Etiology—RDS is caused by the lack of a lipoprotein called surfactant in the lungs. This substance maintains the openness of the alveoli at the end of expiration. Without adequate surfactant, many of the alveoli collapse, resulting in poor oxygenation of the infant.

Treatment—Urgent aggressive treatment is needed, preferably in a large hospital's neonatal intensive care unit to improve the outcome. Oxygen therapy, insertion of an endotracheal (breathing) tube, a ventilator, and the use of artificial surfactant are treatment priorities. Infants who have had RDS are more likely to have an increased incidence of respiratory infections after discharge from the hospital.

Sinusitis (Si-nus-i′tis)

Description—Sinusitis is the inflammation of the paranasal sinus cavities.

Signs and symptoms—Symptoms include nasal congestion, low-grade fever, headache, pain over cheeks and upper teeth, pain over eyes or eyebrows, and a nonproductive cough.

Etiology—It usually results from the common cold organism or chronically from persistent bacterial infection.

Treatment—Treatment consists of analgesics for pain, medication to decrease secretions, steam inhalations to encourage drainage, and application of heat to relieve pain and congestion. Antibiotics are sometimes required in severe or chronic cases. Surgical drainage of the affected sinus cavity may be necessary in persistent, severe conditions.

Snoring

Description—The presence of noisy breathing while asleep. About 45% of normal adults snore at least occasionally, and 25% are habitual snorers. It is more prevalent among males and people who are overweight. It tends to grow worse with age.

Signs and symptoms—The snorer breathes loudly during sleep, particularly when lying on the back. It not only disturbs the sleep of the snorer but also disturbs other family members. An exaggerated form is known as obstructive sleep apnea, when loud snoring is interrupted by frequent episodes of totally obstructed breathing. If this lasts over 10 seconds and occurs more than seven times an hour, it is considered a serious problem. Some patients have 30 to 300 obstructed events a night, resulting in a low blood oxygen level that causes more forceful heartbeats to "catch up" circulation. This can lead to irregular heart rhythm, elevated blood pressure, and heart enlargement.

Etiology—The noisy sounds of snoring occur when there is an obstruction to the flow of air through the back of the mouth and nose. This is the collapsible portion of the airway where the tongue and upper throat meet the uvula and soft palate. These structures strike against each other and vibrate during breathing. People who snore have at least one of the following:

- Poor muscle tone in the tongue and throat muscles, which allows the tongue to fall backward into the airway. Often this occurs after the use of alcohol or sleep medication.
- Excessive bulkiness of throat tissues, such as tonsils and adenoids. Rarely, cysts or tumors can be the cause. Overweight persons also have bulky neck tissues.
- Excessive length of the soft palate and uvula may narrow the opening into the throat. A long uvula makes matters worse.
- Obstructed nasal airways, as when the nose is stuffy or blocked, cause the person to pull in air harder, creating an exaggerated throat vacuum that pulls the floppy throat tissues together and makes noise. Allergy season causes many to snore because of blocked nasal passages. The deformity of a deviated septum may also be the contributing factor.

Treatment—The majority of snorers can be helped by trying the following:

1. Lose weight and exercise daily to develop good muscle tone.
2. Avoid tranquilizers, sleeping pills, and antihistamines before bedtime.
3. Avoid alcohol within four hours of retiring.
4. Avoid heavy meals within three hours of retiring.
5. Avoid getting overtired.
6. Establish regular sleeping patterns.
7. Tilt the entire head of the bed up 4 inches on blocks.
8. Allow the nonsnorer to get to sleep first.

The very heavy snorer who interrupts family life needs a thorough physical examination. Sleep lab studies help determine how serious the snoring is and how much the person's health is being affected. Treatment may be only the management of an allergy or infection. Corrective surgery can alter contributing nasal and throat structures. Using a nasal mask overnight to deliver air pressure into the throat is helpful if other measures are not possible.

Sudden Infant Death Syndrome (SIDS)

Description—This is a mysterious condition that kills apparently healthy infants. It is unexplainable even after autopsy. **Sudden infant death syndrome** kills about 8,000 infants annually in the United States. It occurs more frequently in winter, in poorer families, to mothers under 20, and among underweight babies. There is a slight increased risk to twins or triplets, those who received no prenatal care, and with mothers who smoked or took drugs during pregnancy. Death occurs rapidly, silently, and unexpectedly, usually during sleep.

Etiology—Study of the syndrome suggests that the infant may have had undetected respiratory dysfunctions that caused prolonged periods of **apnea** (absence of breathing), resulting in extreme hypoxemia (lack of oxygen in the blood) and serious irregular heartbeat. Although the true cause is unknown, there is an increased risk of SIDS occurring with infants who sleep on their stomachs. In 1992, the American Academy of Pediatrics advocated a program called "Back to Sleep" that simply referred to placing babies on their backs to sleep. Since the acceptance of the sleeping position, the incidence of SIDS has declined by almost 50%. Several characteristics of the syndrome are diagnostic of SIDS, but an autopsy must be performed to rule out other causes of death. Child abuse must always be ruled out.

Treatment—The use of the proper sleep positioning and ongoing research to find other causes is the only thing that will save lives. Parents need a great deal of support to deal with the death because they often feel they were somehow to blame. There is a National Sudden Infant Death Foundation with local chapters of parents whose babies have died of the syndrome. Many local health organizations provide counseling and information services. These resources can be of great assistance.

Tuberculosis (Tu-ber-ku-lo′-sis) (TB)

Description—An acute or chronic, highly contagious infection causing nodular lesions and patchy infiltration of the lung tissue is known as **tuberculosis** (TB). The body reacts to the invading causative organism by converting the destroyed tissue into a cheese-like material. This material may localize and become fibrotic, or it may develop into cavities within the lung tissue. The cavities are filled with the multiplying bacilli, and the infected debris spreads throughout the tracheobronchial tree.

On initial contact with the tubercular bacillus, most people's immune defense system kills the organism or walls it off in a nodule. These dormant organisms may become active later, causing an acute phase.

Signs and symptoms—Symptoms of primary infection include fatigue, weakness, lack of appetite, weight loss, night sweats, and low-grade fever. On reactivation, symptoms may also include a productive cough characterized by purulent mucus, which is occasionally mixed with blood, and chest pains.

Etiology—Tuberculosis is caused by the bacillus organism *Mycobacterium tuberculosis.* Currently, there is an increase in incidence of TB primarily because of the relationship of AIDS, the use of drugs, and the influx of third world immigrants. Certain conditions tend to increase the incidence of TB, such as low income, homelessness, alcoholism, being a prisoner, being HIV positive, and being a resident in a long-term care facility.

Treatment—Treatment consists of isolation until the contagious phase has passed. Care must be taken in handling the nasal and expectorated discharges. Bed rest and an adequate diet are very important. Medication specifically for TB, such as rifampin (Rifadin), must often be continued for 6 to 12 months or more to effect a cure. After two to four weeks, the disease is no longer infectious, and the person can resume a normal lifestyle.

Upper Respiratory Infection (URI)

Description—This term is used to refer to symptoms associated with the common cold.

Signs and symptoms—The disease is usually self-limiting after a one- to four-day incubation period. It is characterized by sore throat, nasal congestion, headache, burning and watery eyes, fever, and general lethargy. A cough may be present, which is nonproductive and hacking, often at night. Symptoms usually persist for a week before subsiding. Secondary bacterial infections affecting the lower respiratory tract are uncommon.

Etiology—An **upper respiratory infection** (URI) may be caused by several different viruses and be transmitted by respiratory droplets, contaminated objects, or hands. Children are the main transmitters of the organism.

Treatment—There is no cure for the common cold. Symptomatic treatment includes aspirin, fluids, and rest. Decongestants can relieve congestion, and throat lozenges can relieve soreness. Antibiotics are not indicated unless there is a chronic illness or complications.

Is It a Cold, Allergy, or the Flu?

It is sometimes difficult yet always important to determine whether symptoms suggest a common cold, an allergy, or the flu, because treatment and the course of the disease vary according to the diagnosis. Review Table 29–1. It summarizes the differences between a common cold, the flu, and an allergy. The main symptoms to compare are fever, cough, muscle aches, nasal discharge, and fatigue.

AGE-RELATED BODY CHARACTERISTICS

An example of the long-term effects of a disease upon the body is evident with asthma. Childhood asthma can be mild to rather severe, but it is often outgrown or greatly improved as children grow older. However, if not, repeated inflammation and bronchial constriction contribute to the alveoli progressively losing function. Bronchitis and pneumonia become more frequent. Without adequate treatment and due to the effects of adult lifestyles with exposure to tobacco, environmental pollutants, and irritants, the alveoli remodel similar to the changes seen with COPD.

System Interaction Associated with Disease Conditions

As with other body systems, diseases of the respiratory system also effect many parts of the body. Table 29–2 summarizes the system interaction occurring with COPD.

TABLE 29–1 How to Tell a Cold from the Flu or an Allergy

Symptoms	Common Cold	Influenza (Flu)	Allergy
Fever	Uncommon; slight	Prominent; high (typically 102°–104°F); sudden onset; lasts 3–4 days	None
Headache	Rare	Prominent	Common
Muscle aches	Slight	Prominent, often severe	None
Fatigue, weakness	Mild	Extreme; sudden onset; may last several weeks	None
Runny, stuffy nose	Common	Occasional	Common
Sneezing	Common	Occasional	Common
Sore throat	Common	Occasional	Occasional
Cough	Sometimes; mild to moderate	Common; often severe	Occasional
Red, itchy eyes	Rare	Uncommon	Common
Itchy nose	No	No	Common
Nasal discharge	Thick and clear to yellowish green	Uncommon	Watery and clear
Response to antihistamines	Poor	Poor	Good to excellent

TABLE 29–2 System Interaction Associated with Disease Conditions

Disease	Systems Involved	Pathology Present
Chronic Obstructive	Respiratory	Productive cough, dyspnea, frequent infection, wheezing
Pulmonary Disease (COPD)	Circulatory	Hypoxia
	Digestive	Poor appetite, weight loss
	Muscular	Difficulty eating
		Barrel chest

CHAPTER SUMMARY

- Oxygen and carbon dioxide provide the means for supporting life.
- Oxygen enters the body through the nose. The septum, conchae, and epithelium add moisture and warm the air. Cilia trap particles.
- Mucus streaming cleanses the bronchi and trachea.
- The pharynx serves as a passageway for both air and food.
- The epiglottis covers the opening of the larynx.
- The larynx contains the vocal cords that affect speech.
- The trachea extends from the throat to the bronchi. It is held open with cartilage rings.
- The right and left bronchi further divide into bronchioles carrying oxygen into the lungs.
- The alveoli are microscopic clusters of air sacs where oxygen and carbon dioxide are exchanged.
- Respiration is the combination of inspiration and expiration. There is both external and internal respiration.
- The lungs are spongy tissue and contain the structures of the bronchial tree. They are divided into

three lobes on the right side and two lobes on the left.

- Surfactant maintains the inflated alveolus at birth.
- Pleura membranes cover the lungs and line the thoracic cavity.
- The action of the diaphragm and intercostal muscles cause breathing to occur. It is controlled by the respiratory center in the brain.
- Breathing is altered by coughing, hiccoughs, sneezing, yawning, and crying.
- Diagnostic examinations include, arterial blood gases, bronchoscopy, chest CT scan, CT scan of the pulmonary arteries, CT-guided needle biopsy, chest X-ray, lung perfusion scan, lung ventilation scan, PET scan, pulmonary angiography, pulmonary function tests, pulse oximeter, sputum analysis, and thoracentesis.
- Diseases and disorders discussed include allergic rhinitis, asthma, atelectasis, bronchitis, COPD, emphysema, epistaxis, histoplasmosis, influenza, laryngectomy, laryngitis, legionnaires disease, lung cancer, pleurisy, paroxysmal nocturnal dyspnea, pleural effusion, pneumonoconiosis, pneumonia, pneumothorax, pulmonary fibrosis, pulmonary edema, pulmonary embolism, respiratory distress syndrome, sinusitis, snoring, sudden infant death syndrome (SIDS), tuberculosis, and upper respiratory infection.
- Age-related body characteristics associated with asthma include more frequent bronchitis and pneumonia. If treatment is inadequate, the alveoli will remodel similar to the changes seen with COPD.
- COPD involves the respiratory, circulatory, digestive, and muscular systems.

STUDY TOOLS

Workbook	Activities for Chapter 29
Premium Website	
MEDIA LINK	View this **Media Link** for Chapter 29: • Respiration
StudyWARE	Activities and Quizzes on the **StudyWARE™ Software** for Chapter 29
	Audio Library of medical terms
	Online access to the **Critical Thinking Challenge 2.0**
CourseMate	Activities and Quizzes for Chapter 29
WebTutor	Activities and Quizzes for Chapter 29

CHECK YOUR KNOWLEDGE

1. Mucus streaming is:
   a. what makes your nose run.
   b. the cause of post-nasal drip.
   c. watery discharge after breathing in an allergen.
   d. propelling particles upward past the epiglottis.
2. The epiglottis:
   a. vibrates to make speech.
   b. is attached to the upper pharynx.
   c. covers the opening to the larynx when swallowing.
   d. is above the tongue.
3. The bronchoscope can be used for all the following except:
   a. removing a foreign body.
   b. delivering oxygen into the lungs.
   c. obtaining a sample tissue of secretion.
   d. viewing the airways.
4. The pulse oximeter:
   a. measures the amount of oxygen in the blood.
   b. measures pulse.
   c. determines the rhythm of the pulse.
   d. can detect pulse irregularities.
5. Emphysema causes:
   a. enlarged alveolar spaces in the lungs.
   b. large amounts of mucus.
   c. slower respirations due to enlarged alveoli.
   d. more efficient exchanges of oxygen and carbon dioxide.

6. Which of the following is not a symptom of influenza?
   a. Vomiting and diarrhea
   b. Chills and fever
   c. Coughing
   d. Fever
7. A pneumothorax is:
   a. the collection of air in the lungs.
   b. air in the thorax.
   c. air in the pleural space.
   d. air between the lung and the diaphragm.
8. Pulmonary edema occurs when:
   a. fluid accumulates within the tissues of the lung.
   b. the pulmonary artery becomes enlarged.
   c. blood pressure decreases within the blood vessels.
   d. tissue fluids leak out of the alveoli.
9. A pulmonary embolus is:
   a. a mysterious condition that kills healthy infants.
   b. a blood clot obstructing an arteriole in the lungs.
   c. the result of years of smoking.
   d. something that can occur after an extended period of running.
10. The incidence of tuberculosis is increasing because of all of the following except:
    a. its relationship with AIDS.
    b. an influx of immigrants.
    c. the organism mutating to a stronger strain.
    d. the use of drugs.
11. Asthma:
    a. primarily affects adults.
    b. can progress to a condition similar to COPD.
    c. is not affected by environmental conditions.
    d. is not associated with the incidence of bronchitis and pneumonia.
12. COPD involves:
    a. respiratory, skeletal, and immune systems.
    b. muscular, circulatory, and urinary systems.
    c. respiratory, digestive, and circulatory systems.
    d. circulatory, muscular, and endocrine systems.

WEB LINKS

Centers for Disease Control and Prevention, COPD: www.cdc.gov/copd

Cleveland Clinic Center for Continuing Education, Pulmonary Diseases: clevelandclinicmeded.com/medicalpubs/diseasemanagement/pulmonary

Chapter 30

The Circulatory System

OBJECTIVES

In this chapter, you will learn the following:

KB KNOWLEDGE BASE

1. Spell and define, using the glossary at the back of the text, all the Words to Know in this chapter.
2. Name the four main parts of the circulatory system.
3. Describe the anatomy of the heart, identifying the internal and external structures.
4. Differentiate between pulmonary, systemic, and portal circulation.
5. Describe the heart sounds, including the actions producing the sounds and where they can be auscultated.
6. Locate the pacemaker, explain its action, and tell how the heart rate is influenced by the body.
7. Explain how the cardiac conditions of heart block and fibrillation relate to the pacemaker.
8. Explain the purpose of an artificial pacemaker and how it functions.
9. Name the five types of blood vessels and their purpose and structure.
10. Describe the function of a capillary bed.
11. Trace the pathway of blood through the pulmonary and systemic circulation.
12. Explain the function and structure of the lymphatic system.
13. Name the components of whole blood and the role of each.
14. Describe the clotting process.
15. Name the blood types and explain their importance to recipients of transfusions.
16. Explain the importance of the Rh factor in pregnancy and transfusions.
17. Identify nine cardiovascular tests and the reasons for giving them.
18. Describe 26 diseases or disorders of the circulatory system.
19. Explain the purpose of collateral circulation.
20. Identify the system relationships with congestive heart failure.

WORDS TO KNOW

accelerator
acute phase
adenitis
ambulatory
anemia
aneurysm
angina
angioplasty
anticoagulant
aorta
arrhythmias
arterioles
arteriosclerosis
artery
atherosclerosis
atrium
AV node
bicuspid
bradycardia
capillary
cardiac
cardiovascular
cerebrovascular accident
cholesterol
chronic leukemia
compatible
congestive heart failure
coronary
cross-match
diastole
electrocardiograph (ECG)
embolism
endocardium
erythrocyte
exudate
fibrillation
heart block
hemoglobin
hemorrhage
Holter monitor
hypertension
hypotension
infarction
ischemia
leukemia
leukocyte
lubb dupp
lymph

lymphatic system
lymphocyte
metastasize
mitral
MUGA scan
murmur
myocardial infarction (MI)
myocardium
nodes
pacemaker
papillary muscles
pericardium
phlebitis
plasma
platelet
portal
Rh factor
SA node
semilunar
septum
sickle cell anemia
spleen
stasis ulcer
systole
tachycardia
thrombophlebitis
thrombosis
transfusion
transient ischemic attack
tricuspid
triglycerides
vagus
valve
varicose
vein
vena cava
ventricle
venule

The circulatory system transports oxygen and nutrients to the body's cells, and it transports carbon dioxide and other waste products from the cells to be eliminated from the body. The blood, which flows through a closed circuit of vessels, is the transportation vehicle. A very efficient muscle, the heart, is the force behind the system. A few minutes' interruption of the circulatory system can result in death.

The circulatory system is composed of four main parts: (1) a pump, the heart; (2) the plumbing, the blood vessels; (3) the circulating fluid, the blood; and (4) an auxiliary fluid system, the **lymphatic system**. Each day the heart pumps the equivalent of 4,000 gallons of blood, at 40 miles per hour, through an estimated 70,000 miles of blood vessels. To achieve this, the heart must forcefully contract, squeezing out blood, at an average rate of 72 times per minute or about 100,000 times each day. In a year's time, the heart will contract 40 million times, resting only a fraction of a second between beats. To appreciate this phenomenal organ, alternately open and close your fist a little more often than once a second for just 1 minute by the clock. You will notice that not only your hand but also your forearm muscles begin to tire. Scientists have estimated that the work of the heart is about equal to the energy needed to lift a 10-pound weight 3 feet off the floor twice a minute for a lifetime. The condition of the blood vessels and the composition of the blood are major factors in the amount of force the heart must exert to circulate the blood.

THE HEART

The heart is about the size of a clenched fist and is located behind the sternum, between the lungs, with two thirds of it on the left side of the chest. It is constructed of several layers of muscles arranged in both circular and spiral fashion. When the muscles contract, blood is squeezed out of the heart chambers. During the relaxation phase, the heart fills with blood entering from the great **veins**. There is a considerable difference in the size of the heart during the phases, as shown in Figure 30–1.

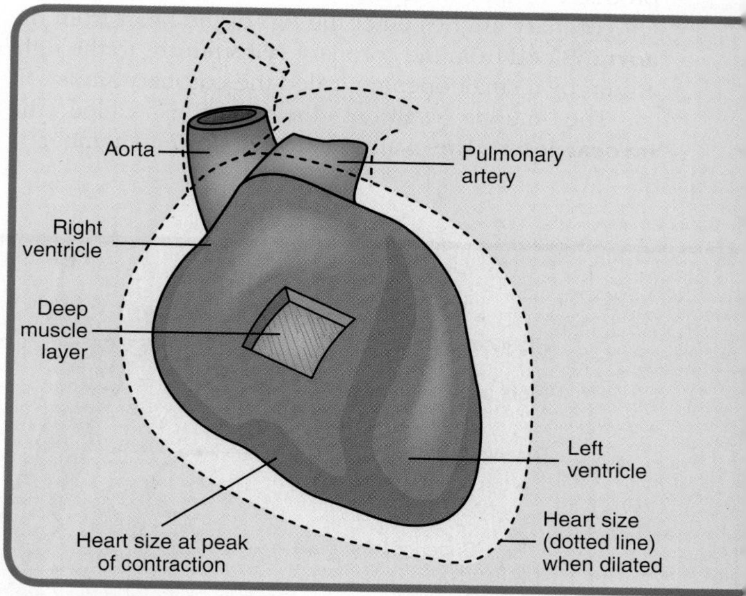

Figure 30–1: Heart size during contraction and filling actions. *Delmar/Cengage Learning.*

The contraction phase is known as **systole**, and the relaxation phase is called **diastole**. Systole is the period when the heart exerts the greatest pressure on the blood. This corresponds to the beat phase of the heart and can be heard over the heart with a stethoscope or felt as the pulse in an **artery**. The systolic pressure can be determined by measurement with blood pressure equipment and is represented by the larger or top number of the blood pressure reading. Diastole is the period of least pressure and is the time when the heart rests. This phase cannot be felt as a beat, but the diastolic pressure can be heard and determined by measurement. It is represented by the smaller or bottom number of the blood pressure reading.

MEDIA LINK

Go to the Premium Website and watch the animation, "The Heart," for this chapter.

External Heart Structures

The outer wall of the heart is surrounded by a sac called the **pericardium**. Like the pleura of the lungs, the pericardium has one layer called the parietal, which lines the sac, and another layer called the visceral, which covers the heart itself. The pericardial fluid between the layers prevents friction when the heart beats. The heart structure does not receive its blood supply from the blood pumped through its interior but from a number of small blood vessels that cover the surface of the heart (Figure 30–2). These blood vessels, called the **coronary** arteries and veins, carry oxygen, nutrients, and waste products to and from the heart muscle. The right and left coronary arteries enter the top of the heart from the **aorta**. Blood from the coronary veins returns to the right atrium by a small opening called the coronary sinus.

The muscle wall of the heart is called the **myocardium**. The wall of the left lower chamber is thicker because it must pump blood through the entire general or systemic circulation, as discussed later.

Internal Heart Structures

A tissue known as **endocardium** lines the interior surface of the heart (Figure 30–3). The lining also covers the heart valves and the interior surface of the blood vessels to allow for the smooth flow of blood. Internally, the heart is a double pump, divided into a right and left side by a muscular wall called a **septum**. The septum prevents the blood on the right side from mixing with that on the left. The sides are further divided into upper and lower chambers. The right upper chamber is called the right **atrium**, and the lower is the right **ventricle**. The left side is similarly divided into a left atrium and left ventricle.

The chambers are separated by one-way **valves** that keep the blood flowing in the right direction. The **tricuspid** valve is between the right atrium and ventricle,

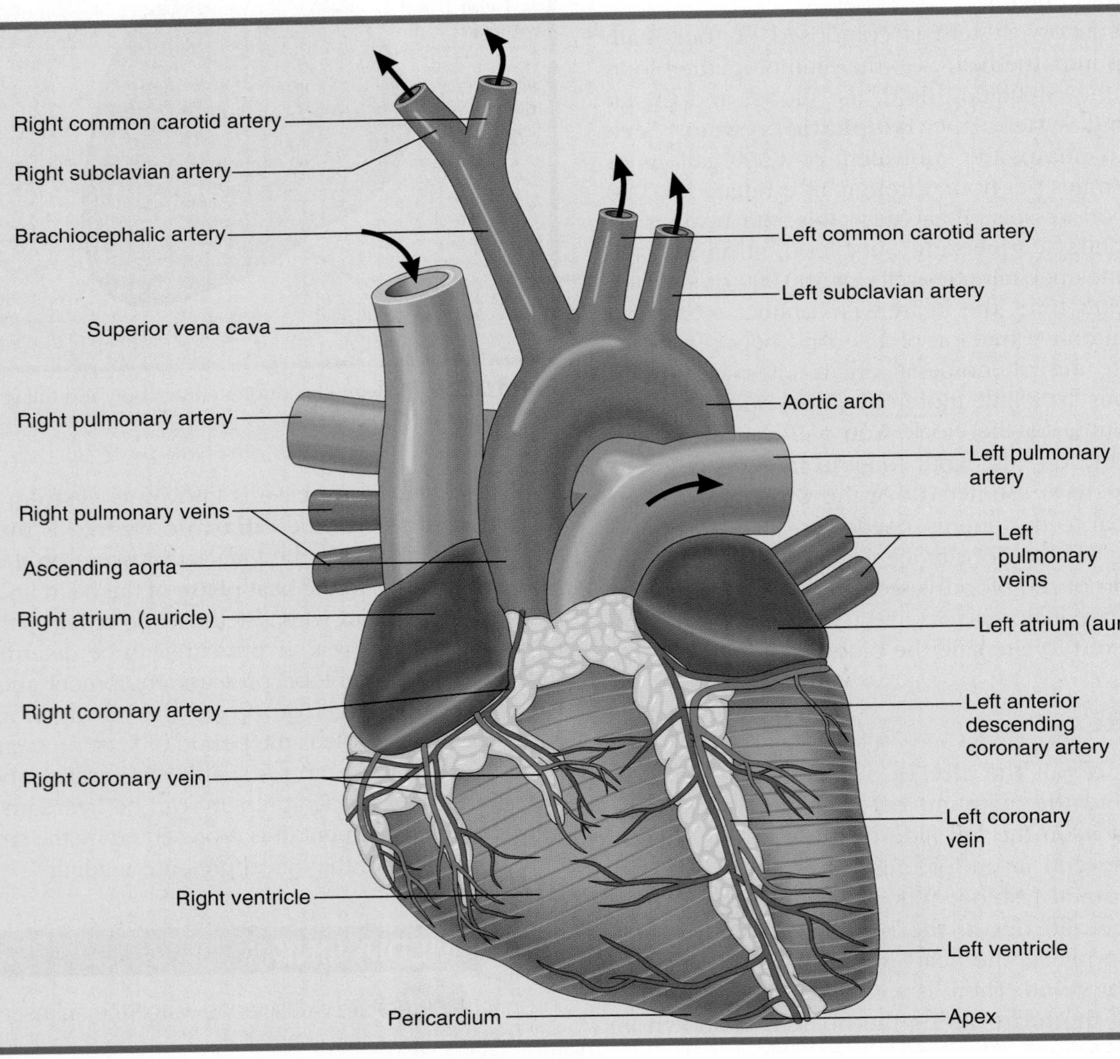

Figure 30–2: External heart structures. *Delmar/Cengage Learning.*

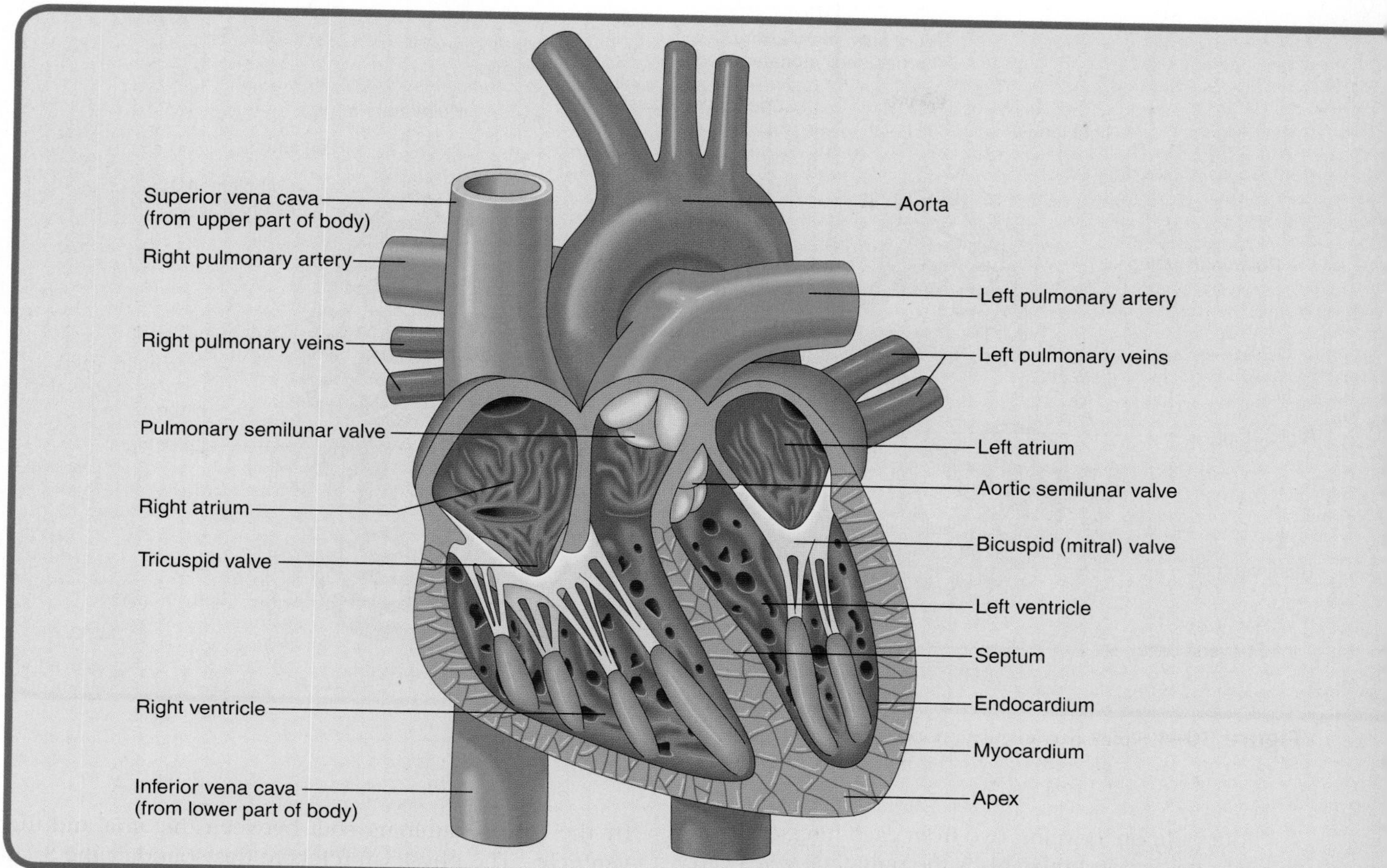

Figure 30–3: Internal heart structures. *Delmar/Cengage Learning.*

and the **bicuspid** or **mitral** valve is between the left atrium and ventricle. **Papillary muscles** are attached by cords to the undersurfaces of the valve cusps or leaflets. When the atria contract, the papillary muscles also contract to pull open the valves, allowing the blood from the atria to enter the empty ventricles. Then the muscles relax, which allows the valves to close as the atria refill. The closed valves prevent the blood from reentering the atria when the ventricles contract.

When the ventricles contract, blood is forced out to the great arteries of the body. The right ventricle sends the blood through a **semilunar** (pulmonic valve) valve into the pulmonary artery on its way through the pulmonary circulation in the lungs for a supply of oxygen. The left ventricle forces the blood past a semilunar valve (aortic valve) into the aorta to be distributed throughout the general or systemic circulation of the body.

A specific sequence of events occurs within the body as the blood is circulated. Blood flow occurs in two distinct patterns: *pulmonary circulation* between the heart and the lungs and *systemic circulation* between the heart and the rest of the body. Figure 30–4 and the following material describe the flow of blood through the pulmonary system.

Pulmonary Circulation

1. Deoxygenated (without oxygen) blood is brought to the superior vena cava from veins of a person's arms, head and neck. The inferior vena cava receives blood from the lower extremities and internal organs. Both the superior and inferior vena cava empty into the right atrium.
2. The right atrium contracts, squeezing blood through the tricuspid valve, which is opened by the papillary muscles, into the right ventricle. Then the valve closes.
3. The right ventricle contracts, sending blood out through the pulmonic semilunar valve into the pulmonary artery. (Remember, this artery carries deoxygenated blood but is still an artery because it is leaving the heart.)
4. The pulmonary artery divides into a right and left branch, one going to each lung. The division continues into smaller arteries, arterioles, and then to the capillaries in the alveolar sacs. Here the deoxygenated blood gives up its CO_2 and picks up O_2.
5. With a fresh supply of O_2, the capillaries join the venules, then become veins and reenter the heart as

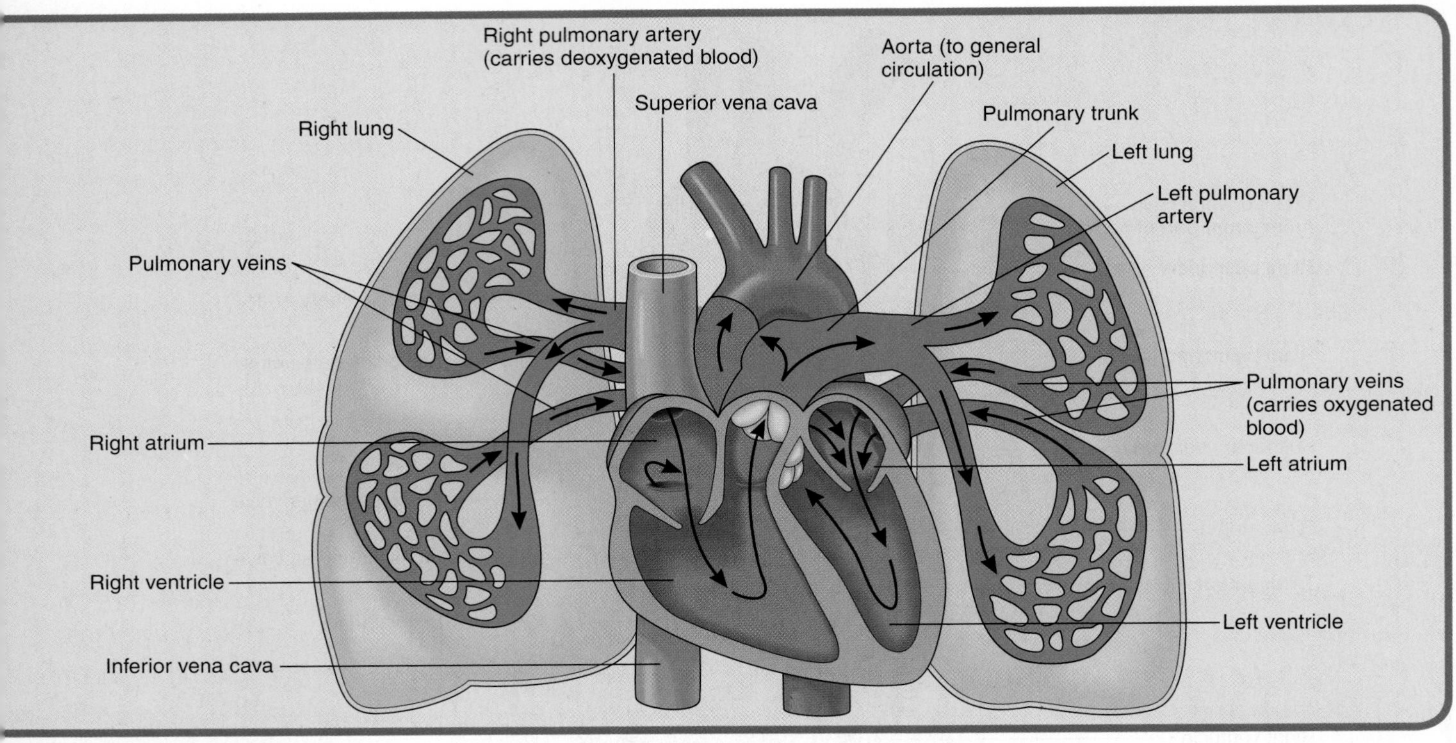

Figure 30–4: Pulmonary circulation. *Delmar/Cengage Learning.*

four pulmonary veins, two from each lung, emptying into the left atrium. (This is the only time veins carry oxygenated blood, but they are still veins because they are returning to the heart.)

6. The left atrium contracts, forcing blood through the mitral or bicuspid valve into the left ventricle, and the valve immediately closes.
7. The left ventricle contracts forcefully, sending blood racing out of the heart past the aortic semilunar valve into the aorta.

The action of the chambers of the heart just described occurs simultaneously in both sides of the heart. In other words, both atria contract at the same time, as do the ventricles. The chambers must work in unison, or blood being pushed forward would have no place to go (this situation does occur in certain cardiovascular disorders and will be discussed later). The total action just described occurs each time the heart beats.

Heart Sounds

The physician listens at specific locations on the chest wall to hear specific functions of the heart. Figure 30–5 illustrates the anatomical location of the valves and the corresponding auscultatory areas. When a stethoscope is used to listen to the heartbeat, two distinct sounds can be heard. They are referred to as the **lubb dupp** sounds. The lubb sound, which is heard first, is caused by the valves slamming shut between the atria and the ventricles. The physician refers to this sound as the S_1. It is heard loudest at the apex of the heart.

The dupp, heard second, is shorter and higher pitched. It is caused by the semilunar valves closing in the aorta and the pulmonary arteries. This sound is

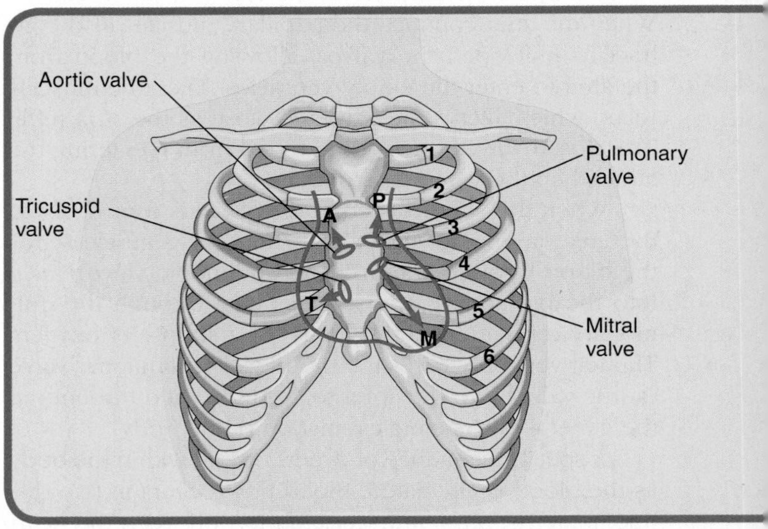

Figure 30–5: Anatomical location of the heart valves and the corresponding auscultatory location. Valves are shown as oval structures and the auscultatory locations by the letters A, T, M, and P. The rib levels are numbered. *Delmar/Cengage Learning.*

known as the S_2. It is loudest at the second intercostal space on each side of the sternum. With a little practice, the valves' condition and level of function can be evaluated from their sounds.

Certain conditions cause changes in the action of the heart valves. Normally, the right heart valves close a fraction of a second after the left. When the ventricles are distended, an audible vibration may occur, which is referred to as an S_3 or a ventricular gallop. Occasionally, just before S_1 at the end of diastole, the atria may contract, forcing blood into an already filled ventricle. This causes a rise in the ventricular pressure and vibrations known as atrial gallop or S_4.

The Pacemaker

The normal heart beats rhythmically as long as the cells receive the correct balance of sodium, calcium, and potassium and an adequate supply of oxygen and nutrients. Another essential element is the "spark" from the group of nerve cells in the right atrium called the sinoatrial or **SA node**, also called the **pacemaker** (Figure 30–6). The node generates the electrical impulse that starts each wave of muscle contraction in the heart. The impulse in the right atrium spreads over the muscles of both atria, causing them to contract simultaneously, sending blood into the ventricles. The impulse apparently triggers the atrioventricular or **AV node**, located between the atria and the ventricles, even though there is no direct connection between the nodes. The AV node has nerve fibers that extend through the septum and are called the *bundle of His*. The bundle divides into a right and left branch, infiltrating the muscles of each ventricle with a system of Purkinje fibers, which cause contraction of the ventricles.

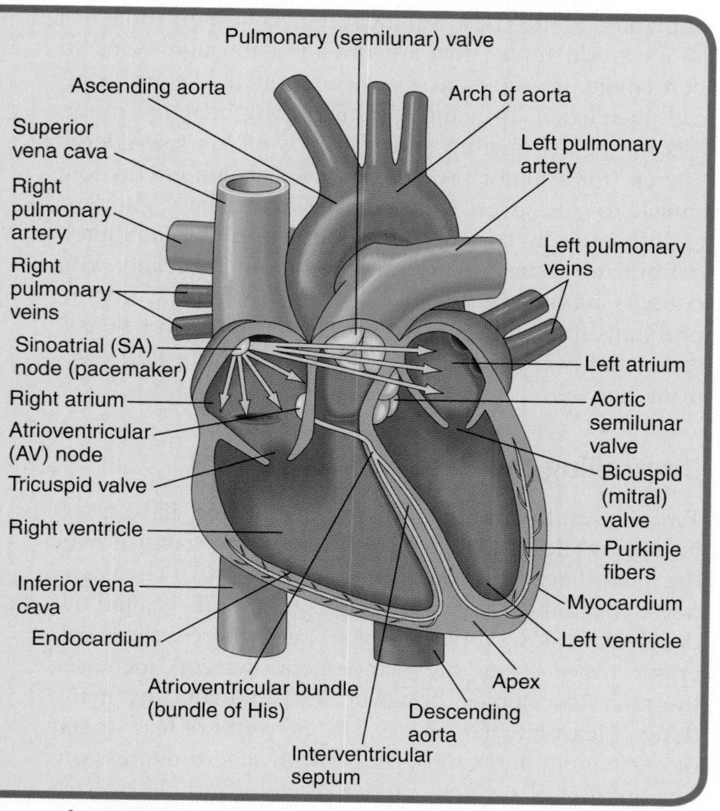

Figure 30–6: SA and AV nodes and the conduction pathway of the heart's electrical impulse. *Delmar/Cengage Learning.*

Rhythm Disorders

The self-generating impulse of the heart is one of the body's miracles. Even if the heart were removed from the body, it would continue to beat as long as it was supplied with the necessary nutrients. In a **cardiac** condition known as **heart block**, there is an interruption in the message from the SA node to the AV node. The interruption can occur in varying degrees. The abnormal rhythm patterns can be viewed on an **electrocardiograph** (**ECG**, heart action recording). *First degree block* is characterized by a momentary delay at the AV node before the impulse is transmitted to the ventricles. *Second degree block* can be of two forms. One occurs in cycles of delayed impulses until the SA node fails to conduct to the AV node, then returns to near normal. A second form is characterized by a pattern of only every second, third, or fourth impulse being conducted to the ventricles. This causes a marked decrease in heart output and usually progresses to the third degree. *Third degree heart block* is known as "complete heart block." There is no impulse carried over from the pacemaker. Because the heart is essential to life, there is a built-in safety factor. The atria continue to beat at 72 times per minute while the ventricles contract independently at about half the atrial rate; this is adequate to sustain life but results in a severe decrease in cardiac output.

Other rhythm disorders are known as **arrhythmias** (any deviation from the normal electrical rhythm of the heart). Premature contractions cause arrhythmia and occur when an area of the heart (not the SA node) "sparks" and stimulates a contraction of the rest of the myocardium. This area is known as an ectopic (abnormal place) pacemaker. There are three types of premature contractions, each identified by the area of its location: atrial, ventricular, or AV junctional.

Atrial contractions are known as *premature atrial contractions* (PACs) and cause the atria to contract ahead of the anticipated time. *Premature junctional contractions* (PJCs) have the ectopic pacemaker focused at the junction of the AV node and the bundle of His. Usually, PACs and PJCs are of no clinical significance and are caused by nicotine, caffeine, fatigue, or tension.

Premature ventricular contractions (PVCs) are a different matter. They originate in the ventricle and cause contraction ahead of the next anticipated beat. They can be benign or deadly. If frequent (five to six per minute) or in pairs, they may require immediate intervention to decrease the irritability of the cardiac muscle to maintain cardiac output. If the PVCs occur every other beat, it is a *bigeminal rhythm;* if they occur every third beat, it is a *trigeminal rhythm*. PVCs can be caused by electrolyte and acid-base imbalance, drug therapy, myocardial infarction (see diseases), or oxygen deficit.

Artificial Pacemaker

When the natural pacemaker of the heart fails to maintain a normal heart rate and cardiac drug therapy designed to cause effective, regular beats fails to correct the situation, an artificial pacemaker may be indicated. The device consists of a small battery-powered pulse generator with electrode catheters (Figure 30–7). The electrodes are inserted into a vein and threaded through the vena cava, one to the right atrium, the other into the right ventricle at the apex. The procedure is accomplished while observing the path of the electrodes by fluoroscopy. The action of the heart throughout the procedure, and for at least the first 24 hours following, is monitored carefully by frequent ECG tracings. The stimulation threshold of the pacemaker to maintain myocardial contractions is determined by noting the number of milliamperes (MA) that produce the desired QRS complex (ECG tracing of contraction). This MA and the desired rate can be set in the pacemaker with a hand-held radio transmitter.

It should be noted that when the heart is totally dependent on artificial pacing, the heart rate may always be that which is artificially set. Newer artificial pacemakers can increase the rate to meet the needs of increased activity by sensing body motion.

A pacemaker is permanently inserted surgically into a muscular pocket on the chest wall. Permanent units are self-contained and will operate for about 3 to 12 years. Pacemakers can also be of either the fixed or the demand type. Fixed units fire continuously at a predetermined rate. Demand types sense the person's own rate and fire only when required. An external unit can be programmed to change the mode of firing of some implanted types. Battery failure requires replacement of the entire generating unit.

Pacemakers are of benefit to patients with a slow, irregular heart rhythm, complete heart block, or a slow ventricular rate resulting from congenital or disease conditions.

In another malfunction of the impulse mechanism known as ventricular **fibrillation**, the rhythm breaks down and the muscle fibers contract at random without coordination. This results in very ineffective heart action and is a life-threatening condition. An electrical device called a *defibrillator* is used to discharge a strong electrical current into the patient's heart through electrode paddles held against the bare chest wall. The shock should interfere with the uncoordinated action and allow the SA node to resume its control.

A type of artificial pacemaker, known as an implantable cardioverter defibrillator, can also affect the rhythm of the heart. The defibrillator is used to re-establish effective heart action with patients who have episodes of potentially fatal ventricular fibrillation. This device consists of a small power pack about the size of a pager. It is implanted in the chest wall near the clavicle and attaches to electrode tubes that are threaded through veins to permanent positions in the heart, much like an artificial pacemaker. It includes a microcomputer that monitors the heart's rhythm and responds with a low-energy "shock" for a minor problem or gives a high energy jolt, similar to one given with external defibrillator paddles, to automatically correct fibrillation. Use of the implanted defibrillator is becoming more common, especially with patients who have an increased risk of heart rhythm problems following a heart attack. In 2001, over 60,000 Americans were implanted with the sophisticated electronic device.

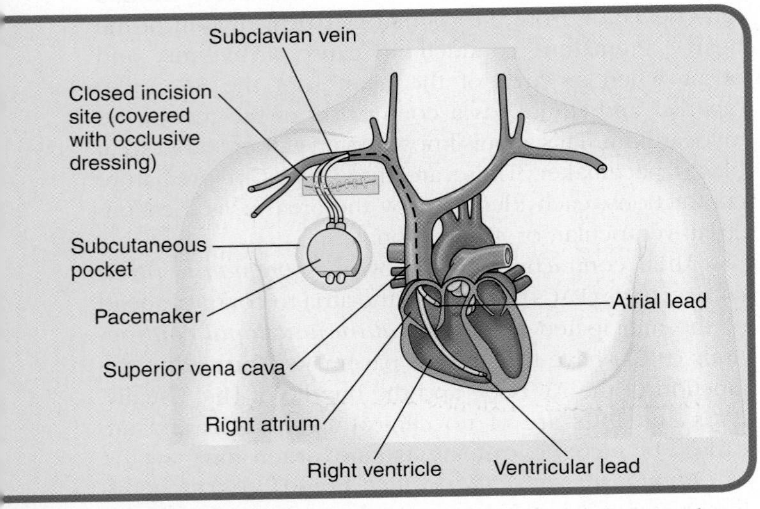

Figure 30–7: Artificial pacemaker with atrial and ventricular leads. *Delmar/Cengage Learning.*

Controlling the Rate

Two nerves, the **vagus** and the **accelerator**, have fibers in the muscle of the heart and have some control over the natural rate of the heartbeat (Figure 30–8). The vagus nerve (from the parasympathetic system), also called the decelerator, slows down the heart rate, whereas the accelerator nerve (from the sympathetic system) increases the rate. The nerves, however, are stimulated by many things. Heart rate can increase as the result of fear, anger, or excitement and can decrease with severe depression. The amount of oxygen, carbon dioxide, and electrolytes (sodium, potassium, magnesium, phosphates, and chlorides) present in the blood affect the rate of the heart.

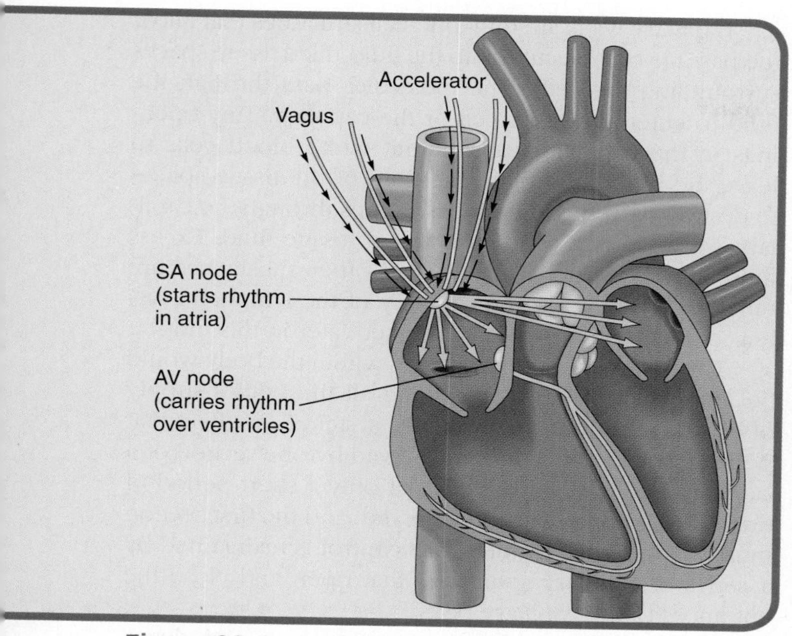

Figure 30–8: Nerves influencing the heart rate. *Delmar/Cengage Learning.*

A heart rate that is consistently rapid (over 100 beats per minute) is known as **tachycardia**. When the rate is consistently slow (less than 60 beats per minute), it is referred to as **bradycardia**.

THE BLOOD VESSELS

Blood vessels are divided into three main types: arteries, veins, and **capillaries** (Figure 30–9).

Arteries

An artery always carries blood *away* from the heart and usually carries fresh, oxygenated blood. The one exception is the pulmonary artery, which leaves the right ventricle of the heart on its way *to* the lungs to pick up oxygen. Arteries are constructed with layers of elastic fibers that allow the walls to expand and recoil in response to the enjection of blood when the ventricles contract. In the systemic circulation, this action causes a wavelike effect within the arteries, which can be felt as the pulse at the pulse points of the body. Figure 30–10 shows the main arteries of the human body. In areas where arteries lie over firm or bony structure, such as at the wrist, the side of the neck, or the inner elbow surface, the pulse can be felt if the artery is pressed against the underlying structure.

The major arteries of the body are:

- *Aorta*—The large artery exiting the left ventricle of the heart and extending down the center of the body. All other arteries branch off the aorta. The abdominal aorta branches off to the hepatic, splenic, gastric, and renal arteries.

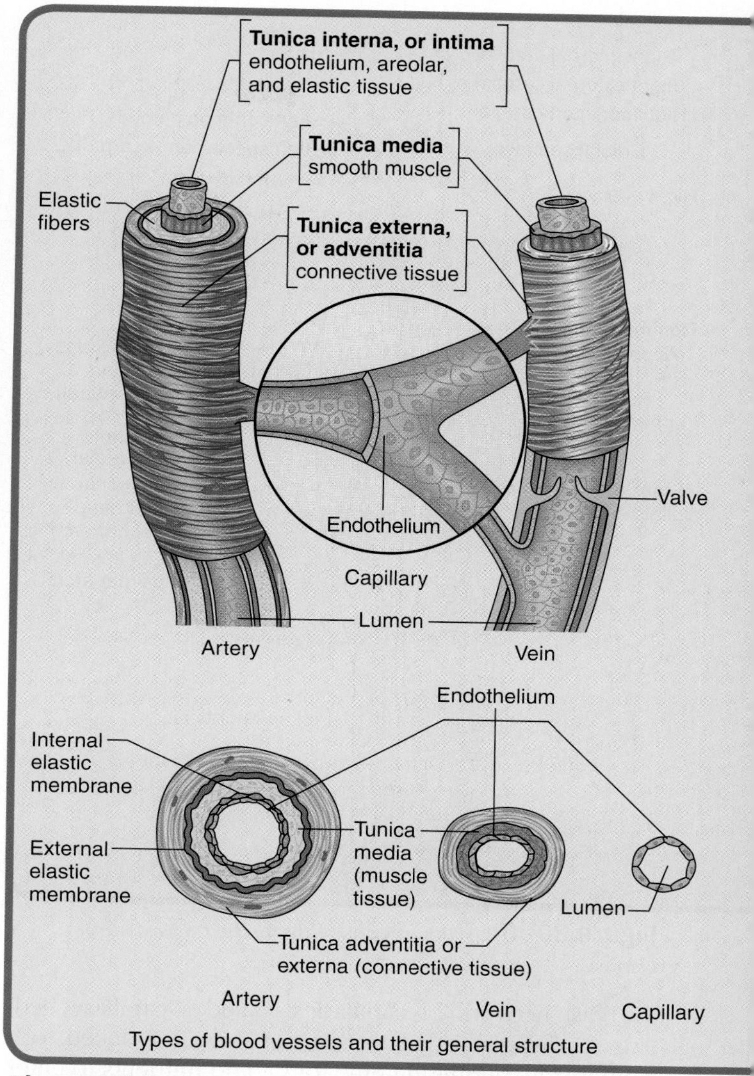

Figure 30–9: Comparative structure of blood vessels. *Delmar/Cengage Learning.*

- *Carotid*—Extends up the side of the neck into the head
- *Pulmonary*—Extends from the right ventricle to the lungs
- *Brachial*—Extends down the arm
- *Radial*—Extends on the thumb side of the forearm
- *Ulnar*—Extends on the little finger side of the forearm
- *Common iliac*—Branches off the abdominal aorta and extends down through the pelvis
- *Femoral*—Extends to the thigh
- *Tibial*—Extends from the femoral through the lower leg
- *Dorsalis pedis*—Extends along the top of the foot

As the arteries divide and branch off into smaller and smaller vessels, they become known as **arterioles**. Eventually, the arterioles join the microscopic blood vessels known as capillaries. When the blood enters

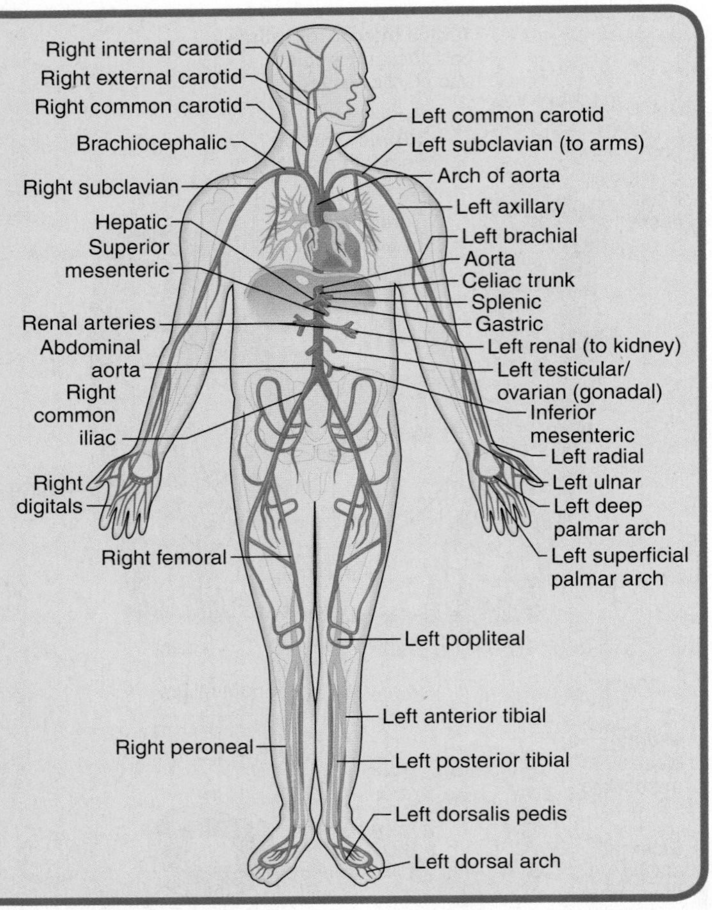

Figure 30–10: Major arteries of the body. *Delmar/Cengage Learning.*

the vast network of capillaries, called a capillary bed, it is so dispersed that the rate of flow is reduced to a slow trickle, permitting time for O_2 and nutrients to enter the tissue cells in exchange for CO_2 and waste products (Figure 30–11).

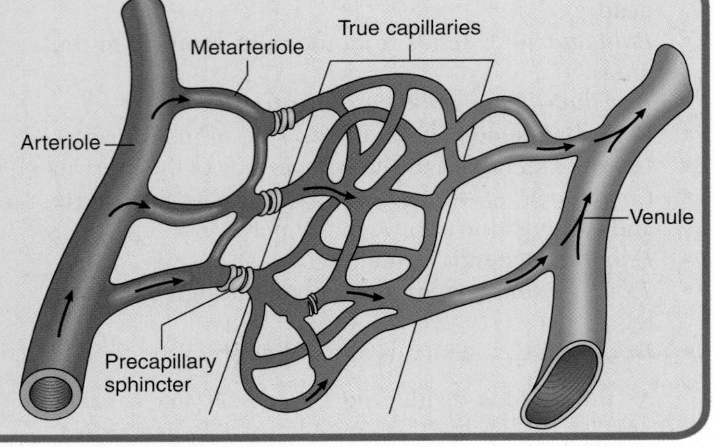

Figure 30–11: Capillary bed connecting an arteriole with a venule. *Delmar/Cengage Learning.*

Capillary walls are thin, one-cell structures that allow the passage of molecules into the fluid-filled tissue spaces surrounding the cells. The molecules pass through the fluid to enter either the cell or the capillary. Tiny openings in the capillary walls permit white blood cells to leave the blood and enter the fluid of the tissue spaces to destroy bacteria. **Plasma** also seeps through the capillary walls, adding to the amount of tissue fluid. Excess fluid, certain waste products, and other substances are removed by an adjoining capillary of the lymphatic system, an action that will be discussed later in this unit.

The vast number of capillaries within the body would be more than capable of holding all the body's supply of blood. Therefore, an automatic system is in effect that permits a group of cells being served by one section of a capillary bed to receive blood for only a short period of time. Then another section is served, and the first section must wait for another turn. This control is maintained by a series of capillary sphincters that open and close the entrances to the capillary beds.

Body cells, in order of importance, have a predetermined priority for receiving the available blood supply. At any given time, only two of the three major body functions can be served. The brain and other central nervous system structures always have first priority. Next come the skeletal muscles that enable us to move and therefore provide a degree of protection to the body with the flight/fight options. Last is the supply to the internal organs of the digestive system. This means that if you have eaten recently and you decide to run, swim, or exercise strenuously, your stomach may complain with cramps because the muscles are not getting enough blood supply to digest its contents.

When the blood leaves the capillary bed, it carries CO_2 and waste products from the cells to be circulated to the proper organ for disposal. Capillaries join with **venules**, which are tiny branches of the veins. As they return blood toward the heart, venules join together, forming veins that eventually enter the heart from the lower body by the inferior **vena cava** and from the upper body by the superior vena cava.

Veins

Veins are similar to arteries in construction, except the walls are thinner and they lack the elastic fiber lining that lets arteries alter the size of their openings. The pressure that is present in arteries is absent in veins, and therefore they can collapse when they are not filled. The major veins of the body are shown in Figure 30–12.

The major veins of the body are:

- *Tibial*—From the feet to the thigh
- *Saphenous*—In the thigh from the knee into the pelvis
- *Femoral*—In the thigh from the knee into the pelvis

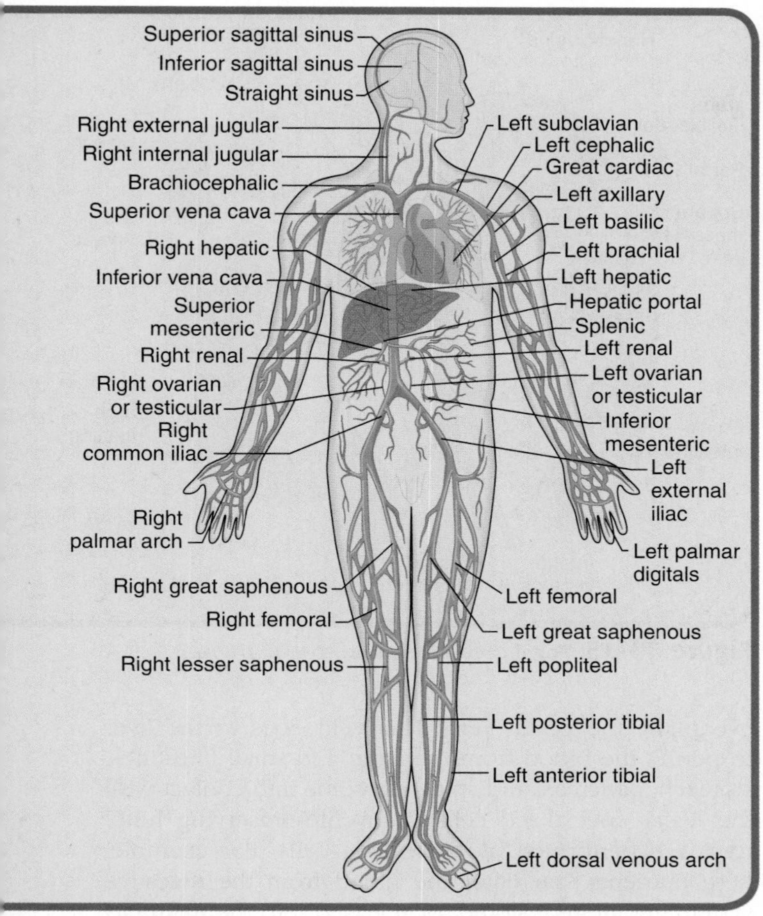

Figure 30–12: Major veins of the body. *Delmar/Cengage Learning.*

- *Common iliac*—From the saphenous and femoral to the inferior vena cava
- *Inferior vena cava*—All lower body veins to the right atrium of the heart
- *Jugular*—From the head and neck
- *Brachial*—From the arm to the brachiocephalic
- *Cephalic*—From the arm to the brachiocephalic
- *Superior vena cava*—All upper body veins to the right atrium of the heart
- *Pulmonary veins*—From the lungs to the left atrium

Veins carry deoxygenated blood back to the heart to be sent to the lungs for exhaling of CO_2 and to pick up a new supply of O_2. Every time the heart beats, blood is forced through the arteries and arterioles to the capillaries, where the pressure from the heart is dissipated in the vast capillary network. With each successive beat, additional blood is forced through the capillaries into the venules and veins, which move it back toward the heart. Special valve structures are located throughout the veins to maintain the flow of blood in the proper direction (Figure 30–13). Veins in the lower extremities especially contain many valves because they are returning blood "uphill" so to speak. During the relaxation phase of the heartbeat, the venous blood could flow back toward the capillaries, but the valves close as relaxation begins, and the blood is trapped in the veins until the following beat forces it to move forward.

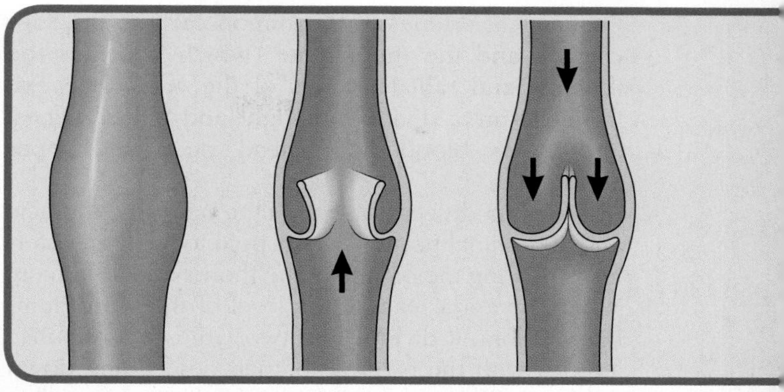

Figure 30–13: Vein valves: (left) external view showing dilation at site of valve, (middle) veins opened and valves opened, and (right) valves closed to prevent backflow of blood. *Delmar/Cengage Learning.*

Another factor helps move blood in veins back to the heart. The veins of the extremities are located in and around the large skeletal muscles. When the muscles contract, they squeeze the veins, thereby aiding in the movement of the blood (Figure 30–14).

Blood flows to every cell in the body through the systemic circulation. Refer to Figures 30–10 and 30–12 as you read the following description of the flow through the major arteries and veins.

Systemic Circulation

1. As the blood leaves the left ventricle, it enters the huge aorta. Immediately, the right and left coronary arteries to the heart exit from the aorta at its arch.

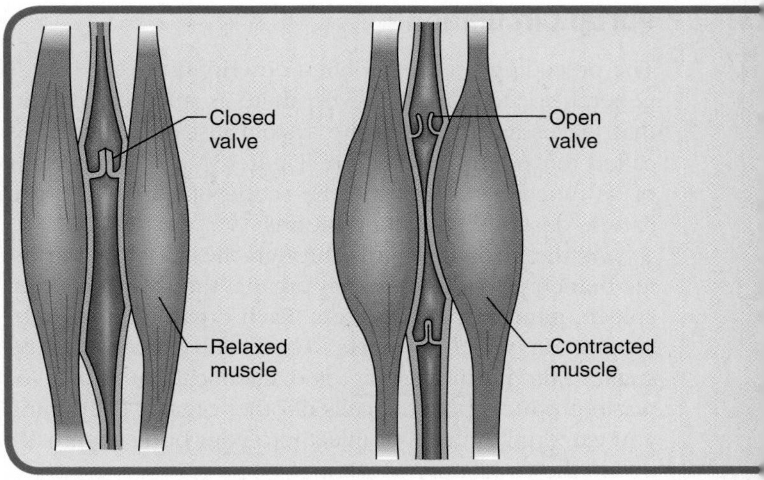

Figure 30–14: How muscles help move blood through internal veins. *Delmar/Cengage Learning.*

Other great arteries, the common carotid, the subclavian, and the innominate (which becomes the brachial and radial arteries of the arm), also exit from the arch, divide into right and left branches, and supply blood to the head, neck, and upper extremities.

2. As the aorta descends through the body, the thoracic and abdominal portions give origin to the large arteries supplying the organs of the thorax and abdomen.
3. When the aorta reaches the level of the fourth lumbar vertebra, it divides into two large common iliac arteries with the external branch descending down the legs and the internal branch leading to the pelvic organs and genitalia (external sex organs).
4. The external branch of the iliac artery becomes the femoral artery in the thigh and continues down the leg as the tibial branch.
5. Eventually, all systemic arteries throughout the body subdivide until they become arterioles and then join the capillaries. In this circuit, the capillaries deliver the O_2, water, and nutrients to the body's cells and pick up the cells' CO_2 and wastes.
6. Upon leaving the capillaries, the blood is considered deoxygenated. The capillaries join venules, which eventually become veins.
7. The major lower extremity veins are the anterior and posterior tibial, the lesser and great saphenous, the popliteal, and the femoral. These join with pelvic veins and enter the inferior vena cava.
8. The major veins of the upper extremities are the basilic, median, and cephalic. These join with the subclavian, internal and external jugular, the innominate, and the sinuses from the head to enter the superior vena cava.
9. The superior vena cava and inferior vena cava empty into the right atrium of the heart, and systemic circulation is completed.

Portal Circulation

The preceding was a simplified description of the body's general circulation. However, there is another "circuit" that leaves and reenters the system just described. It is called the **portal** circulation (Figure 30–15). The details of its function are beyond the scope of this text, but it can be described in general terms.

As the aorta descends through the abdomen, arteries branch off to the internal organs: the stomach, liver, spleen, pancreas, kidneys, etc. Each organ receives substances on which it reacts. These substances may be sugar, salt, hormones, a toxic chemical, nutrients, or waste products from the cells of other organs. Everything you eat, drink, inhale, or inject into your body eventually enters the circulatory system.

The blood leaving certain organs (ones without a pair) empties into the special portal circulation and

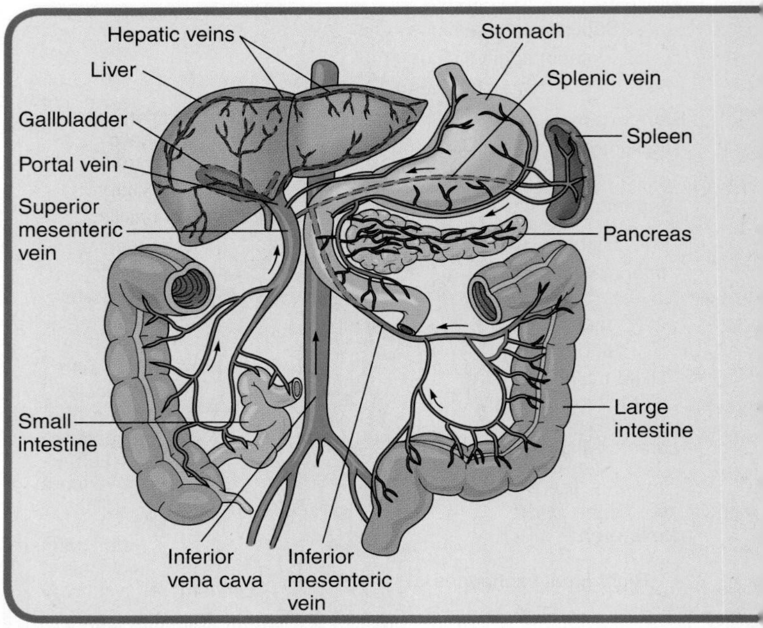

Figure 30–15: Portal circulation. *Delmar/Cengage Learning.*

eventually the portal vein. This vein goes to the liver to permit the blood from the large and small intestines, stomach, pancreas, and spleen to come into contact with the liver's specialized cells. Many life-preserving functions are performed by these liver cells. For example, here nutrients that enter the blood from the digestive system are altered, stored, or released into the main circulatory system as needed. After passing through the liver, the blood is carried by the venous system to the inferior vena cava and is recirculated.

THE LYMPHATIC SYSTEM

The lymphatic system consists of **lymph** (a straw-colored fluid similar to blood plasma), lymph **nodes**, lymph vessels, and the **spleen**. In addition, the lymphatic tissue, which produces **lymphocytes** (a type of blood cell), is often considered to be part of the system. This includes the tonsils, the thymus gland, and the intestinal lymphoid tissue.

Lymph

Lymph is composed of blood plasma that filters out of the capillaries, lymphocytes, hormones, and many other substances that are the products of cellular activity, such as water, digested nutrients, salts, oxygen, carbon dioxide, and urea (Figure 30–16). It is a continuous-forming process. Lymph fills the spaces between the cells and is also referred to as intercellular or *interstitial fluid*. Lymph acts as the "bridge" between cells and capillaries. Lymph is moved through the lymph vessels primarily by contraction of the skeletal muscles. There is no pump

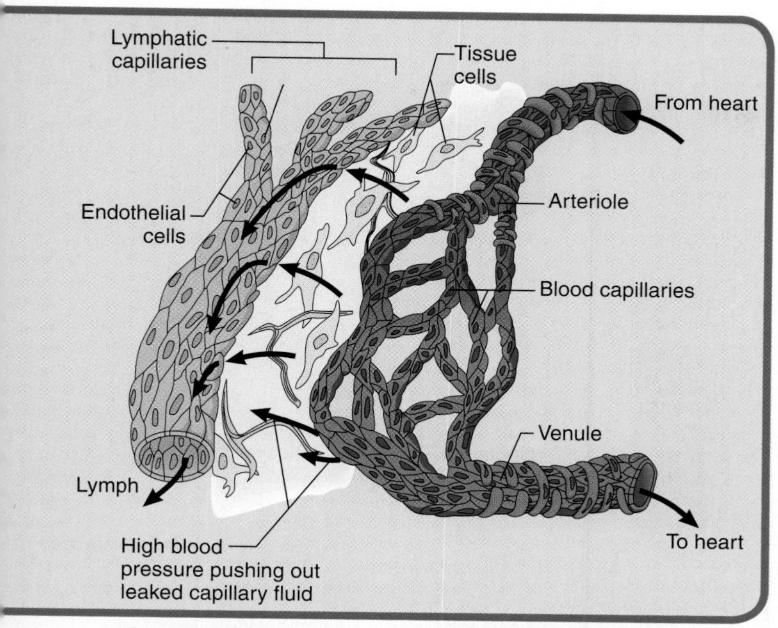

Figure 30–16: Leaked blood capillary fluid enters the lymphatic capillaries and becomes lymph. *Delmar/Cengage Learning.*

like the heart to move lymph. Lymph vessels are constructed like veins, however, with valves to prevent the backflow of fluid.

Lymph Vessels

Vessels carrying lymph are located throughout the body, somewhat like veins. Lymphatic capillaries absorb fluid and other substances from the tissues and return them to the circulatory system (Figure 30–17). However, it is a one-way system only, from the cells toward the heart. There are no separate vessels bringing lymph to the cells.

The vast network of lymph capillaries joins to form small lymph vessels that in turn form larger vessels called *lymphatics*. Lymphatics eventually form two main ducts. The right lymphatic duct receives lymph from the right side of the head, the right arm, and the upper right trunk. The thoracic duct receives lymph from the rest of the body (Figure 30–18).

The thoracic and right lymphatic duct empty into the large veins near the heart and become part of the body's circulating blood. It is gradually filtered back out of the capillaries as interstitial fluid and begins its journey back to the lymphatic vessels and ducts.

Lymph Nodes

Lymph nodes are small, round or oval structures located usually in clusters along the lymph vessels at various places in the body. Lymph enters the nodes from four afferent lymph vessels, filters through a mesh of sinuses, and leaves by way of a single efferent vessel. Lymphocytes, a type of white blood cell, are derived from stem cells in the bone marrow. They enter the bloodstream and go to the lymph tissue to "live." Their action is essential to the immune system of the body. When needed, they divide by mitosis, greatly increasing in number. The structure of the nodes and the cell's function purify the lymph by removing harmful substances, such as bacteria or malignant cells. The nodes increase and decrease in size in relation to the amount of material being filtered. In acute infections, they become swollen

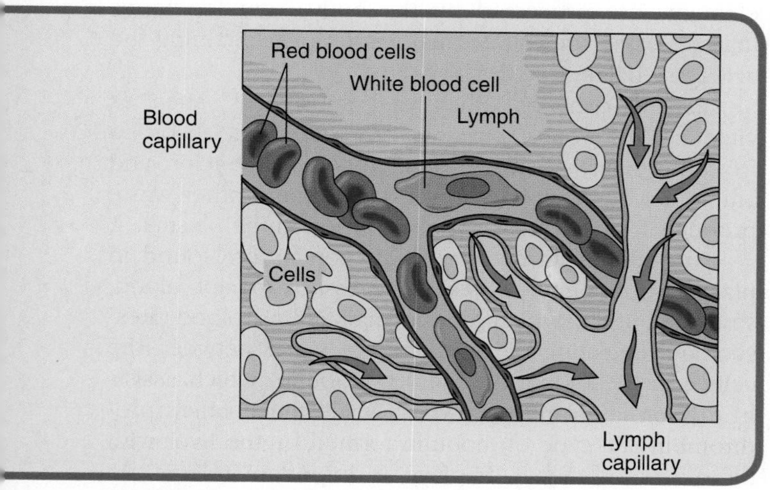

Figure 30–17: Lymph capillary. *Delmar/Cengage Learning.*

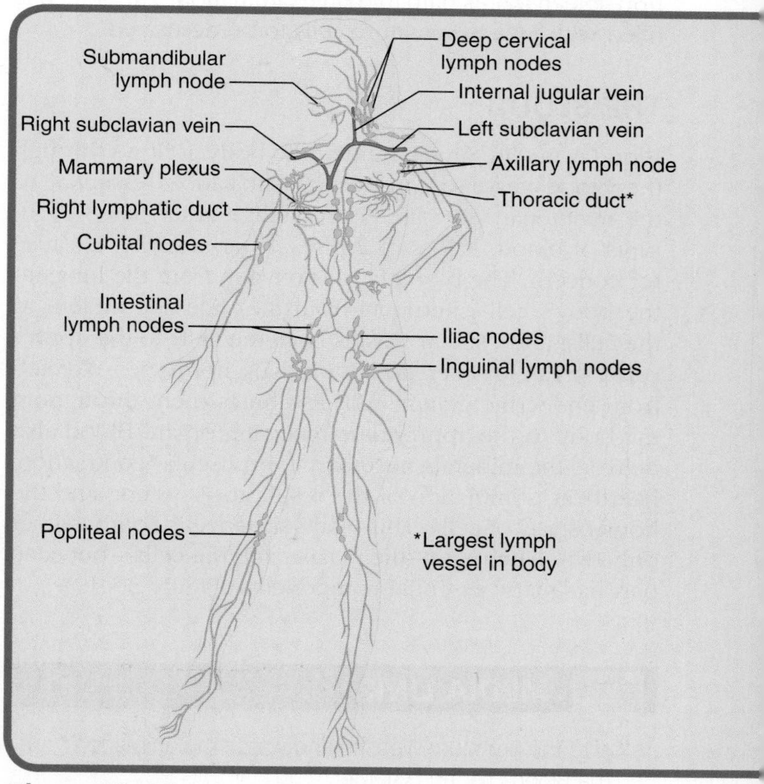

Figure 30–18: The lymphatic system. *Delmar/Cengage Learning.*

and tender because of the collection of cells gathered to destroy the invading substances. This condition is known as **adenitis**. With extensive involvement, the node may break down, and an abscess will form.

Physicians palpate for nodes when patients have infectious conditions or when a malignancy is known or suspected. With malignancy, the cancer cells are abnormal and so are identified by the cells in the lymph node to be removed from the circulating fluid. As more cells accumulate, the node becomes enlarged and is therefore palpable. Early detection of lymph node involvement is critical to the prognosis of patients with cancer, for it is through the lymphatic system that a malignancy often **metastasizes** (spreads) to other sites. The extent of lymph node involvement is an important indicator of the ultimate prognosis of the patient.

The Spleen

The spleen is an organ composed of lymphatic tissue that lies just beneath the left side of the diaphragm, in back of the upper portion of the stomach. The spleen produces lymphocytes, stores red blood cells, keeps the appropriate balance between cells and plasma in the blood, and removes and destroys worn-out red cells. The organ functions like a large lymph node. It is soft and elastic and varies in size according to the flow of blood through the organ. During an acute infection, it will become enlarged and tender. Patients with leukemia may have an enlarged, firm spleen that is palpable on examination. The spleen is filled with excess immature cells to be destroyed.

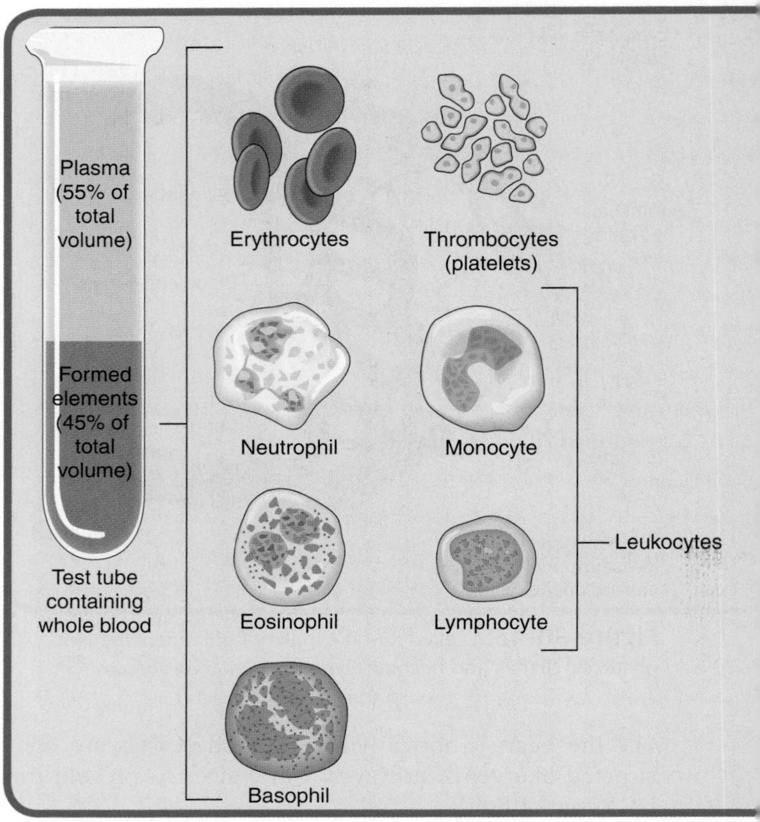

Figure 30–19: Major components of the blood. *Delmar/Cengage Learning.*

THE BLOOD

Blood is the life-giving fluid of the body. It flows through the blood vessels, transporting substances essential to the maintenance of life. The average adult has 8 to 10 pints of blood. A loss of 2 pints, or about 20%, is cause for concern. The blood carries oxygen from the lungs to the body's cells, nutrients from the digestive system to the cells, and cellular wastes from the cells to the appropriate organ for excretion. It picks up hormones excreted from endocrine glands and distributes them throughout the body to the appropriate receiving organ. Blood also delivers the minerals necessary for muscular contraction, heartbeat, stimulation of the respiratory system, and the homeostasis of cells. This vital substance is composed of only two main parts—the plasma and the cells—but each part has many essential components (Figure 30–19).

MEDIA LINK

Go to the Premium Website and watch the animation, "The Blood," for this chapter.

Plasma

Plasma is a straw-colored liquid that makes up a little over half the volume of blood. It is about 90% water, the remainder consisting of minerals, such as calcium, sodium, potassium, phosphorus, and bicarbonates. The minerals are commonly referred to as *electrolytes*. These elements are processed by the body from the foods that are eaten and play a major role in maintaining the acid-base balance of the blood.

Plasma contains other vital substances, such as vitamins, hormones, enzymes, and nutrients absorbed from the digestive system (i.e., glucose, fatty acids, and amino acids). Oxygen, carbon dioxide, and other waste products from the cells are also carried in the plasma.

In addition, three important proteins are found in plasma: fibrinogen, which is necessary to clot blood; serum albumin, which aids in maintaining blood pressure by regulating the exchange of water between the cells and the blood; and serum globulin, which assists in the formation of antibodies. A substance called prothrombin is a type of globulin formed by the liver with the aid of vitamin K. It plays an important role in the clotting of the blood.

Cells

The cellular portion of the blood can be divided into three types of cells: red, white, and platelets.

Red Blood Cells

Erythrocytes (red blood cells) are biconcave disks with very thin centers to enable them to fold over if necessary to pass through a narrow opening. Red cells number about 25 trillion in the body or about 5 million to a cubic millimeter of blood. It is the red cells that give blood its color. A red blood cell lives about four months. They are produced in the bone marrow at a rate of about 1 million a second, the same rate at which they wear out.

Erythrocytes obtain their color from **hemoglobin**, which is a combination of a protein and an iron pigment. It is hemoglobin that attracts and carries the oxygen and carbon dioxide in the blood. When hemoglobin is carrying a lot of oxygen, it is bright red in color. As the oxygen is given up to the cells and exchanged for carbon dioxide, the color changes to the dark reddish blue that is visible in surface veins.

White Blood Cells

White blood cells are called **leukocytes**. Leukocytes are present in the blood at approximately 5,000 to 9,000 per cubic millimeter, or about one white cell for every 600 to 700 red blood cells. White cells are about twice the size of red blood cells. Leukocytes play a vital role in defending the body against invasion, moving through capillary walls into the tissue fluid to chase down bacteria.

Leukocytes are divided into two major groups, granulocytes and agranulocytes, depending upon the presence of granules and certain staining characteristics.

Granulocytes are produced in red bone marrow and live for only a few days. There are three types. *Neutrophils* phagocytize (destroy) bacteria by surrounding, swallowing, and digesting them. *Eosinophils* are thought to consume the toxic substances in tissues because they are found in increasing numbers when the body has had a foreign protein injected, has an allergic reaction, or has been infected by a parasite. The third type, the *basophils,* are also thought to participate in phagocytosis because their numbers increase with chronic inflammation or during healing from an infection.

Agranulocytes are of two types: *lymphocytes,* which are produced by bone marrow and lymphoid tissues (such as the nodes and spleen), and *monocytes,* which are formed in the bone marrow. Lymphocytes primarily specialize in providing immunity for the body by attaching themselves to foreign bodies and destroying them and by developing antibodies. The monocyte assists with phagocytosis. Some enlarge greatly when they enter tissue and become fixed.

When an inflammation occurs, white cells can divide and proliferate into capsule-like structures around foreign objects that cannot be digested, such as silica dust and carbon particles, or causative organisms of infections, such as tuberculosis. This action effectively walls off involved tissue in an attempt to contain the foreign material or prevent the spread of disease. The evidence of a phagocytic reaction to invading bacteria or a foreign object is the presence of **exudate** (pus). Exudate is composed of lymph, bacteria, and dead white blood cells.

Platelets

The third kind of cell is the **platelet**. These cells are the smallest of the three and are present in the blood at a rate of 200,000 to 400,000 per cubic millimeter. They are also formed in the bone marrow from cell fragments.

Platelets function in the life-saving process of clotting blood. When a blood vessel is cut or damaged, it is believed that the rough surface may catch or attract platelets to the area. This reaction occurs only when there is an incidence of bleeding; otherwise, the clotting process would stop circulation within the blood vessels. When there is a cut, platelets pile up at the site to form a small mass. Once attached firmly to the damaged area, they release the chemical serotonin, which causes the blood vessel to spasm, resulting in a narrowing of the vessel and a decrease in blood loss until the clot can be formed (Figure 30–20). At the same time, platelets and injured tissues release thromboplastin, which triggers the clotting process to begin. The thromboplastin cooperates with calcium ions and other blood clotting factors in the blood to convert prothrombin (present in plasma) into thrombin. The thrombin acts on another protein in the plasma called fibrinogen. This reaction results in the formation of fibrin, tiny threads that form a network of fine mesh fibers over the cut. This net begins to catch the red blood cells, other platelets, and plasma, forming the clot. It should be remembered that unless the cut blood vessel is small, a clot may not be able to form. The force of the flow of blood will wash away the body's efforts to form fibrin nets and therefore will be unable to collect the ingredients of the clot. Clotting can be assisted by applying pressure over the area to stop the blood flow until a clot can form. When major vessels are cut, it may be necessary to surgically close the opening with sutures to control the bleeding. Fortunately, internal bleeding vessels can also undergo the clotting process. Complications can occur from the clotted mass, especially if the clot or its fragments break loose and enter the circulation before the body's natural "housekeeping" function can gradually remove it from the blood vessel.

Bleeding Time

The length of time required for blood to clot from an induced puncture wound is useful information when preparing a patient for a surgical procedure or evaluating

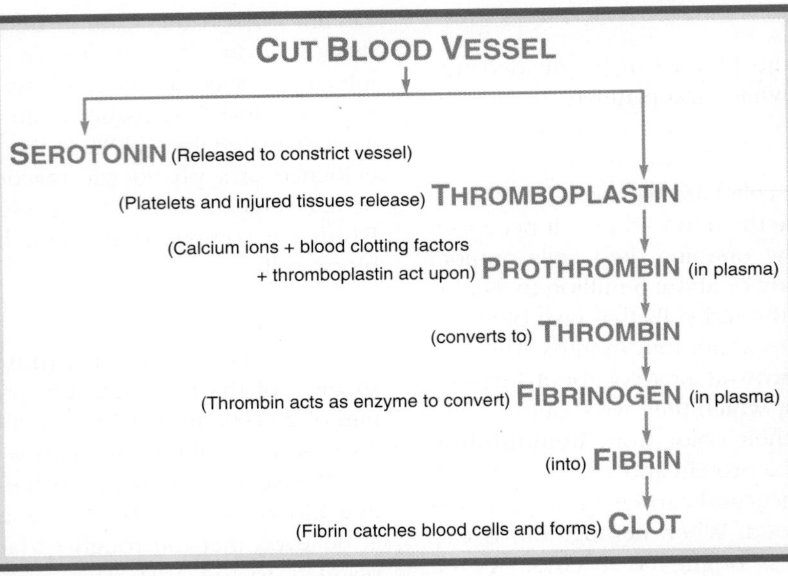

Figure 30–20: Process of blood clot formation. *Delmar/Cengage Learning.*

the effects of certain disorders or medications. The normal range of bleeding time for the template puncture method is from 2 to 8 minutes. The length of time varies with the method used.

Blood Types

There are four types of blood: A, B, AB, and O. The type of blood a person has depends on the presence of a protein factor called agglutinogen or antigen on the surface of the red blood cell. Type A blood has an A agglutinogen, type B has a B agglutinogen, type AB has both agglutinogens, and type O has neither (Figure 30–21).

Similarly, a protein known as agglutinin or antibody is present in blood plasma. Type A blood has a *b* agglutinin, type B blood has an *a* agglutinin, type AB has no agglutinins, and type O has both *a* and *b*.

The term *agglutinate* refers to the process of clumping or sticking together. Blood clumps and forms clots in the blood vessels if agglutinins and agglutinogens of the same type are mixed together. This reaction can be fatal. Therefore, it is extremely important to determine the blood types of both the recipient and the donor when blood **transfusions** are required. A laboratory test known as type and **cross-match** is necessary to make this determination prior to the administration of either whole blood or packed cell transfusions. Not only is the blood typed, but it is also mixed and observed to ensure that agglutination does not occur. Cross-matching will also detect the presence of subtypes and an agglutinogen known as H.

Figure 30–22 shows how the different types of blood would be distributed through 100 people as identified by the American Red Cross. The need for blood from donors is a constant concern for patients and their physicians. Information from the central area of a midwestern state indicates that 550 donors are needed each day. That translates to 16,775 per month or over 200,000 a year. A recent survey showed that 33% of Americans feel there is a great risk of getting AIDS or hepatitis from a

Blood Type	Percent of Population	Antigen/Agglutinogen on Red Blood Cells	Antibody/Agglutinin in Plasma	Can Receive	Can Donate To
A	41%	A	Anti-B	A or O only	A or AB only
B	12%	B	Anti-A	B or O only	B or AB only
AB	3%	A and B	None	A, B, AB, O Universal recipient	AB only
O	44%	None	Anti-A and B	O only	A, B, AB, O Universal donor

Figure 30–21: Blood types. *Delmar/Cengage Learning.*

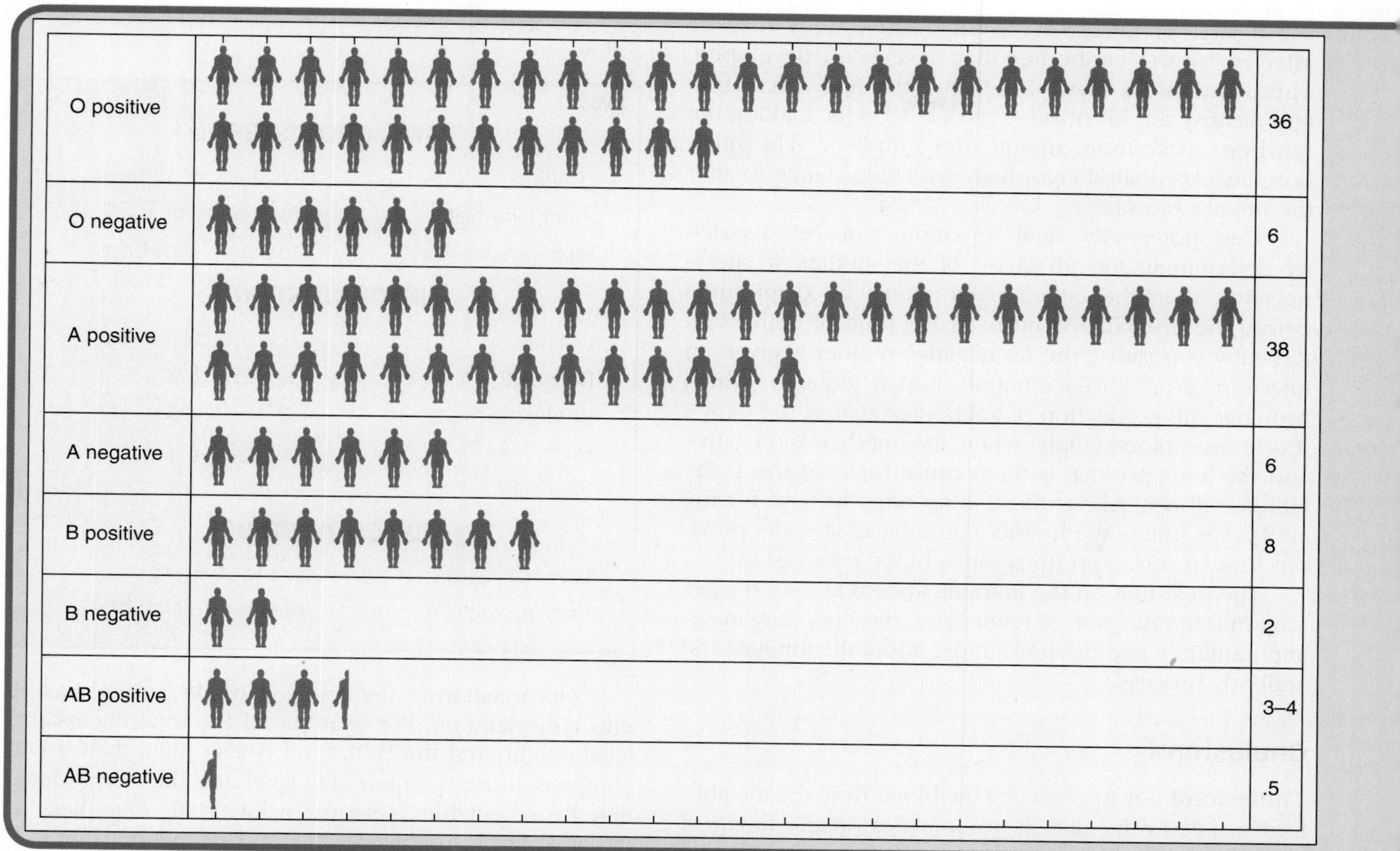

Figure 30–22: The occurrence of blood types within 100 people as identified by the American Red Cross. *Delmar/Cengage Learning.*

transfusion. Currently, with the methods used to screen donors and the tests performed on the blood, it is highly unlikely. The risk of blood-borne AIDS is now only one in 420,000 units of blood; hepatitis is far smaller. A new form of hepatitis called hepatitis "G" has now been identified, so testing for it will be developed. To this point, six types have been found, and more are suspected. Scientists have been trying to develop an artificial blood as a substitute. One firm is now ready to test its product. Another research project has led to the creation of three pigs that carry genes that produce human hemoglobin that can be extracted, chemically modified, and then pasteurized for human use. It has a longer storage life, does not require refrigeration, avoids the risks of human viral diseases, and works in all blood types. At this point, it is in the testing stage.

Rh Factor

Red blood cells may have another factor known as the **Rh factor**. It is an antigen that was first detected in the blood of a Rhesus monkey (thus the name Rh). If the red blood cell has the factor, it is said to be Rh positive, or Rh+. If the factor is absent, then the blood is said to be Rh negative, or Rh–. Blood must also be checked for the presence of this antigen when a transfusion is to be given. If an Rh– negative person receives Rh-positive blood, the antigen is "foreign" to the recipient's bloodstream. Within two weeks, the individual will produce antibodies in response to this invasion of a foreign substance. Usually, no problems occur unless at a later date the person receives another Rh-positive transfusion. This time the developed antibodies will react to the antigen being received and may cause serious complications.

It should be noted that persons who are Rh positive can receive either Rh-positive or Rh-negative blood, provided it is properly typed and cross-matched, because they already have the factor, and the Rh-negative blood is without the antigen. When the two blood samples can mix without evidence of any clumping and the Rh factor is appropriate, the blood is said to be **compatible**.

The Rh factor is also of concern with pregnancy. If a female who is Rh negative becomes pregnant with an Rh-positive baby, a few positive cells may enter the mother's blood at delivery and cause the production of antibodies. The firstborn will not be affected, but if later pregnancies are Rh positive, they may be affected by the antibodies that have been developed. These antibodies slowly filter into the fetal circulation and destroy the Rh-positive red blood cells, making the newborn profoundly anemic and jaundiced. The situation must be treated vigorously with steps taken to alter the infant's blood.

This potentially fatal situation can be avoided by determining the Rh factor of the mother. If she is negative, then the father's factor must be determined before the first child is born. At the time of delivery, if the baby is positive, the Rh-negative mother is given an injection of an Rh(D) immune human globulin, which prohibits the production of antibodies against the baby's Rh-positive blood. Only when the mother is negative and the fetus positive is there cause for concern. If the father is also negative, there is no need to treat for the antibodies unless the mother could have, at some previous time, received an Rh-positive blood transfusion.

The next unit on the immune system takes a deeper look into the function of leukocytes and how they maintain immunity and discusses more about the antigen and antibody process.

Cholesterol

Cholesterol is a substance in the blood from the metabolism of fats in the diet. It accumulates on the lining of blood vessels in the form of plaque. This narrowing of the opening results in decreased blood flow to the tissues and an increase in blood pressure to pump blood through the restricted arteries. It is important to monitor the level of cholesterol present in the blood in order to reduce the development of coronary heart disease. High levels of cholesterol promote heart attacks, strokes, and death. Cholesterol can often be controlled with a combination of healthy eating, exercise, weight control, limiting alcohol intake, and refraining from smoking. When lifestyle changes alone are not sufficiently effective, cholesterol-lowering drugs may be required.

Cholesterol evaluation is divided into three classifications: total cholesterol; low-density lipoprotein (LDL), the "bad" form; and high-density lipoprotein (HDL), the "good" form. Total cholesterol levels matter less than the HDL and LDL levels. In the 2006 guidelines issued by the American Heart Association, the acceptable levels were changed because of continued high incidence of heart disease. A new emphasis was placed on the protective factor of high levels of HDL. There is also a lowering of acceptable levels of LDL in certain circumstances, such as having a previous heart attack; being a diabetic; and being at risk for a vascular event because of age, smoking, high cholesterol, hypertension, family history, and obesity. Diabetes is now considered such a potent risk factor that it automatically places an individual in the high-risk category.

The general guidelines for cholesterol levels are as follows:

TOTAL CHOLESTEROL	
Desirable	Less than 200 mg/dL
Borderline-high	200–239 mg/dL
High	240 mg/dL and above
LDL CHOLESTEROL	
Optimal	Less than 100 mg/dL
Desirable	100–129 mg/dL
Borderline-high	130–159 mg/dL
High	160–184 mg/dL
Very high	190 mg/dL and above
HDL CHOLESTEROL	
Low (risk factor)	Less than 40 mg/dL
High (protective)	More than 60 mg/dL

Interpretation of the results can take several factors into consideration. For example, if the total cholesterol level is high and the HDL level is also high, then it will compensate for a higher LDL level and the overall level may be acceptable. However, a low HDL, regardless of the other levels, is considered a major concern. High LDL cholesterol levels respond well to a group of drugs called statins. The most common are Lipitor, Zocor, Mevacor, Pravachol, Crestor, and Lescol. They have proven to reduce the risk of coronary artery disease. Many people take drugs as a preventive measure when family history of heart disease is present.

Drug therapy may be considered at certain levels of cholesterol, for example:

- People without coronary heart disease but with two risks factors or less and an LDL level of 190 or higher
- People without coronary heart disease and two or more risk factors with a level of 160 mg/dL or higher
- People with heart disease may begin with a level of 130 mg/dL

Triglycerides

Triglycerides are common types of fats that are good for you in normal amounts. They are present in food and are also manufactured by the body. Abnormally high levels are associated with some common diseases and disorders such as diabetes cirrhosis of the liver, underactive thyroid, and inflammation of the pancreas. High levels are also known to be associated with high LDL cholesterol, low HDL cholesterol, and obesity, risk factors for heart disease. It is believed triglycerides contribute to the thickening of arterial walls, which is a predictor of atherosclerosis.

High triglyceride levels are a warning sign of heart disease risk. It is important to lose weight, exercise, stop smoking, limit alcohol intake, control diabetes, and follow a diet low in saturated fat and with a limited intake of carbohydrates. The U.S. National Heart, Lung, and Blood Institute guidelines for triglyceride levels are as follows:

TRIGLYCERIDE LEVEL	CLASSIFICATION
Less than 150 mg/dL	Desirable
150–199 mg/dL	Borderline high
200–499 mg/dL	High
500 mg/dL and higher	Very high

CARDIOVASCULAR TESTS

Many sophisticated tests can be performed on the circulatory system, but most of them are best studied at a more advanced level. A few of the more frequently encountered **cardiovascular** diagnostic procedures will be discussed briefly here. Common studies done on blood are discussed in Chapter 15.

- *Arteriography (angiography)*—A radiologic examination of an artery or arteries after the injection of a contrast medium. The test is used to indicate the status of blood flow, collateral circulation, malformed vessels, an aneurysm, or the presence of **hemorrhage**. Figure 30–23 is an example of an artery following injection. A heart catheterization is very helpful in diagnosis of coronary artery disease. It can reveal faulty motion of the heart wall, leakage of blood back through diseased valves, or a hole between the right and left sides. In the coronary arteries, angiography can help locate blockages, which can then be treated with an angioplasty procedure or identified for bypass surgery. About 1 million angioplasties are performed in the United States each year.
- *Cardiac catherization*—A catheter to the right side of the heart is inserted into a vein at the antecubital space of the right or left arm. A catheter to the left side of the heart is inserted into the brachial artery at the left or right antecubital space. The femoral artery or vein can also be used. The catheter is passed through the blood vessels until it reaches the heart. When it is determined by fluoroscopy that the catheter is properly positioned, a contrast medium is injected to permit visualization. The heart's chambers and valves and the coronary arteries or the pulmonary artery may be viewed, depending on the site being catheterized. The procedure can also be used to measure blood pressure within the pulmonary artery and some portions of the heart. It is used in connection with coronary angiography. Figure 30–24 illustrates the usual points of insertion of the cardiac catheter. Notice the different shapes of the catheter tips that help to guide the catheter into the desired position.
- *Dobutamine stress test*—This is a variation of the cardiac stress test that also combines the information from an echocardiogram. A resting state echocardiogram is performed first to evaluate the myocardium, the valves, the blood flow, and the action of the heart. Then, dobutamine is given intravenously in ever-increasing amounts to "stress" the heart chemically without the need for exercise. During the test, additional echocardiogram findings are

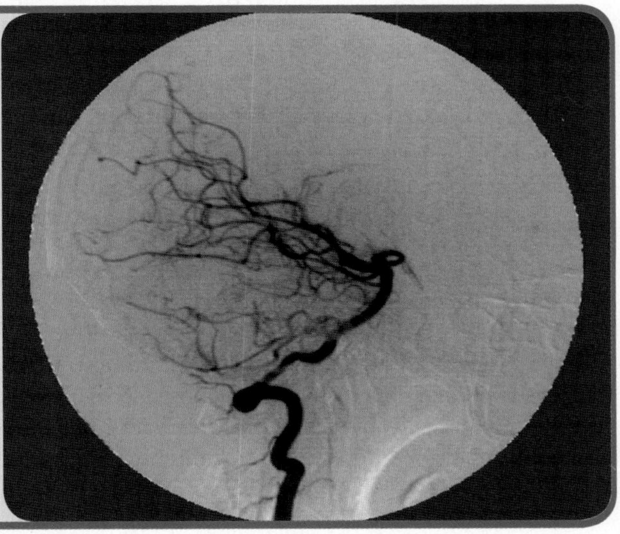

Figure 30–23: Example of an angiogram (angiograph) of the brain. *Delmar/Cengage Learning.*

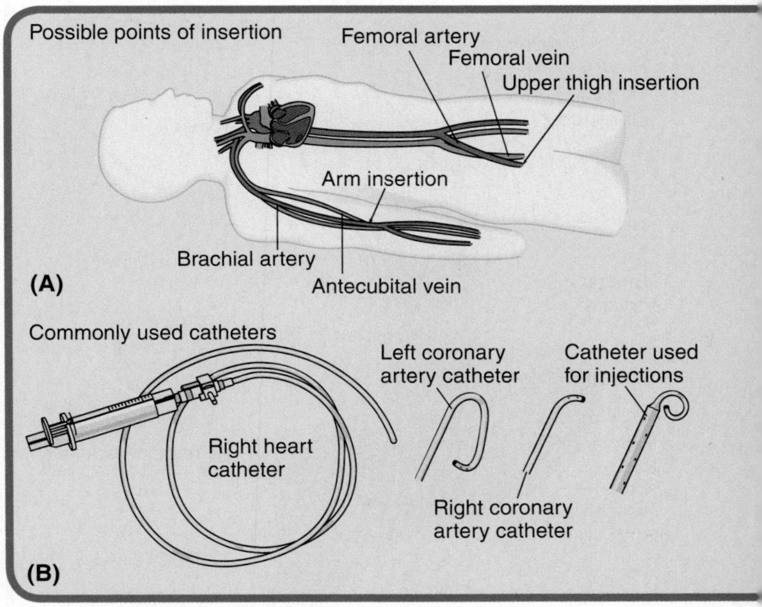

Figure 30–24: (A) Points of insertion for a cardiac catheter, (B) commonly used catheters. *Delmar/Cengage Learning.*

taken and the blood pressure is monitored. At peak stress, additional echocardiogram pictures are taken. A continuous ECG records the activity of the heart throughout the examination. Upon completion, the effects of dobutamine gradually subside, and the patient's heart rate returns to normal. This combination of diagnostic tools gives the cardiologist a fairly complete picture of structural and functional aspects of the heart. Other drugs, such as Persantine or Adenostine, are used with a radioactive tracer (such as Cardiolite) and a special camera to produce similar studies of the heart.

- *Doppler ultrasonography*—Sound waves are transmitted through the skin and are reflected by the cells in the blood moving through the blood vessels (Figure 30–25). This diagnostic tool can evaluate the major blood vessels of the body to determine deep vein **thrombosis** (DVT), peripheral arterial **aneurysms**, and occluded carotid arteries.
- *Echocardiogram*—This is a noninvasive test that uses ultrasound (high-frequency sound waves) to make images of the internal structures of the heart. A special gel is applied to the chest wall, and a hand-held device called a transducer is maneuvered over the heart area. Sounds waves are transmitted through the skin and strike the structures of the heart, sending echoes back to the transducer. The machine converts the information into images that are displayed on the screen and produce an image or picture of the structures of the heart and its chambers. The test evaluates cardiac function and structure and can reveal valve irregularities, abnormalities of the heart muscle, and the presence of fluid between the layers of the pericardium.

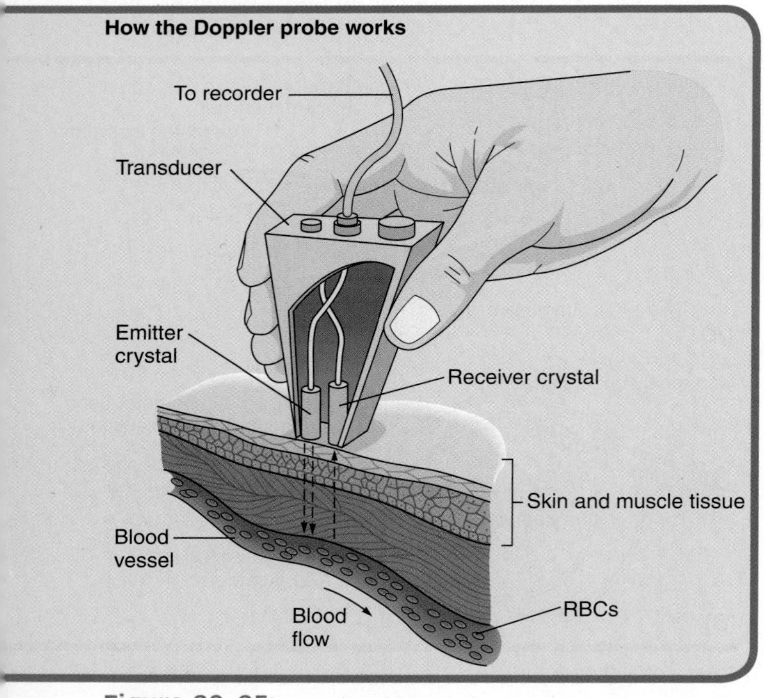

Figure 30–25: Doppler ultrasound. *Delmar/Cengage Learning.*

- ***Electrocardiograph (ECG)***—This test is also called EKG. It is perhaps the most common tool used to evaluate heart performance. The ECG is a graphic recording of the electrical activity of the heart. It identifies rhythm, abnormalities in conduction, and electrolyte imbalance. The graph is useful in documenting diagnosis and provides a method of measuring progression of cardiac disease conditions. The ECG also helps evaluate the effectiveness of an artificial pacemaker and cardiac medications.

The test may be taken while the patient is lying in a comfortable position or in an exercise mode, such as bicycling or walking a treadmill. The exercise mode measures the effects of controlled physical stress and is referred to as a *stress ECG.* Frequently, abnormalities of cardiac action are more evident upon exertion.

Another type of ECG is called the **Holter monitor** or **ambulatory** (walking) ECG. The ECG electrodes are attached to the patient's chest wall and a portable cassette recorder (monitor) is placed in a belt about the waist. For a 24-hour period, the patient's heart action is recorded, and a diary is kept of daily activities and any associated symptoms. At the end of the test, the recording is analyzed by computer, and a report is printed. This type of test is most beneficial for symptoms that occur irregularly or to evaluate the status of recovering cardiac patients. Another version permits the patient to activate the recording device only when experiencing symptoms. This patient-activated monitor can be worn for several days. (See Chapter 47.)

- *Heart scan*—This noninvasive test using a high-speed scanner takes accurate pictures of the heart in less than a second. The technology is known as ultra-fast CT scan and is done by an electron beam tomography scanner. (This same technology can also scan the chest, abdomen, and pelvis.) The scanner sweeps electron beams across the patient so quickly that it actually freezes the beating motion of the heart. The scan is helpful in screening for calcified plaque in coronary arteries. The amount of calcification is measured and given a score that is an indicator of the degree of coronary artery occlusion. The scan is a screening tool and provides a baseline assessment of coronary artery condition. It can identify coronary disease before symptoms of artery blockage occur, thereby permitting lifestyle changes and treatment to prevent a heart attack. Typically, blockage must be about 50% or more before it can be detected by a stress test.
- ***MUGA scan***—MUGA is an acronym for MUltiple Gated Acquisition; it is a test to evaluate the condition of the myocardium of the heart. The test can be done in a resting or exercise mode. Isotopes are injected

intravenously and the scintillation camera records the motion of the heart. The test permits measurement of ventricular contractions to evaluate the strength of the heart muscle. Patients who receive a chemotherapeutic drug that has cardiac toxicity side effects are monitored periodically by MUGA scans because of the drug's tendency to damage the myocardium.

- *Myocardial perfusion imaging*—This is a test to measure the passage of blood through the coronary arteries to the myocardium. The first part of the test involves "stressing" the heart by dilating the arteries with a special IV medication. This is done over a six-minute period. (Normal arteries will dilate more than partially or completely blocked arteries.) The heart is monitored during the test by ECG. After dilation, a radioactive imaging material is injected into the IV. The material concentrates in those parts of the myocardium that have the best blood flow. For about 45 minutes, the camera records images that identify any part of the heart that is not getting enough blood. Later, after the dilating drug has worn off, a series of images will be taken to show perfusion of the heart "at rest." The two series are compared to identify the differences in blood flow. A healthy heart will show little difference.
- *Stress cardiolyte ECG*—This test evaluates myocardial blood flow and the condition of the heart muscle. The ECG electrodes are attached to the patient before performing the stress test on either a treadmill or a bicycle. The blood pressure and pulse rate are carefully monitored. When the patient reaches peak stress, the tracer material is injected intravenously into the antecubital vein and the exercise continued for an additional minute to ensure circulation of the isotope to the heart. The ECG electrodes are removed, and within three to five minutes the patient is positioned under the scintillation camera. The scanner records the amount of cardiolyte uptake by the heart over the next several minutes. Areas of the heart with normal blood supply and healthy cells rapidly take up the isotope. Areas of poor blood flow or damaged cells do not take up the material and appear as dark spots on the scan; these are known as cold spots.

  The test is indicated for assessing myocardial condition, demonstrating the location and extent of a **myocardial infarction (MI)**, diagnosing coronary artery disease, and determining the effectiveness of artery grafts and angioplasty procedures. Persantine cardiolyte is also a type of stress test. It is used for patients with arthritis or any other condition that prevents a patient from exercising. It determines the presence of coronary artery disease.
- *Transesophogeal echocardiography (TEE)*—In this procedure a transducer device is inserted into the esophagus behind the heart to more thoroughly view portions of the heart. In about 10% of patients, external echocardiography cannot provide a clear enough picture. Chest deformities, chronic lung disease, and obesity are the main reasons for poor-quality imaging. TEE is particularly helpful when valve abnormalities, blood clots, tumors, growths, and aortic dissection (tears in the artery) are suspected. It may also be beneficial in detecting valve hardening, stenosis, and fungus or bacterial infections.
- *Venogram*—This radiographic examination uses a contrast medium to determine the condition of the deep veins of the legs. It is especially useful in determining the presence of deep vein thrombosis (DVT), which may occlude the vein systems and lead to pulmonary embolism, a potentially lethal situation. DVT may result from vein injury, prolonged bed rest, surgery, childbirth, irregularity in th... on process, or the use of oral cor...
- *Ultrasound, cardiac*—(See Ech...
- *Ultrasound, carotid artery*—T... t measures the thickness of the ... neck using sound waves to cr... discovered that the risk of hea... increased in direct proportion to... artery walls. The thicker the wa... buildup of atherosclerotic plaqu... the thickest walls had more than... stroke and heart attack as those w...

DISEASES AND DISORDERS

Anemia (A-ne′me-a)

Description—This term indicates that ce... lacking in the blood. There are various ty...

Iron Deficiency Anemia

This is the most common form of anemia.

Description—This form is characterized by an inadequate supply of iron to form normal red blood cells. When the body's supply of iron decreases, so does the number of red blood cells and, as a result, the hemoglobin. This reduces the body's ability to carry oxygen to the cells.

Signs and symptoms—Symptoms include fatigue, listlessness, pallor, inability to concentrate, and difficulty in breathing on exertion.

Etiology—Iron deficiency anemia develops from an inadequate dietary intake of iron or inability of the body to absorb iron as the result of diarrhea, partial or total removal of the stomach, or certain diseases. It can also be caused by intestinal bleeding, heavy menstruation, colon cancer, or bleeding ulcers. It is most common among premature infants, children, adolescents (especially girls), and women before menopause.

Treatment—Iron deficiency is treated by first identifying the underlying cause. Once determined, iron replacement can begin. Oral preparations of iron sulfate or iron combined with ascorbic acid are given. Intramuscular injections are possible but not desirable because of the discomfort produced. Intravenous infusion is relatively painless and requires fewer injections.

Aplastic Anemia

Description and causes—Aplastic anemia results from injury or destruction of the blood cell formation by the bone marrow.

Signs and symptoms—This disease generally produces symptoms of weakness and fatigue.

Treatment—Treatment for aplastic anemia must first rule out any identifiable cause and follow with transfusions of blood products. Recovery may take months. Bone marrow transplant is the treatment of choice in severe aplastic anemia and with those needing constant RBC transfusions. The use of corticosteroids and bone marrow stimulants is appropriate in some cases. Patients with aplastic anemia should be referred to a hematologist for treatment.

Blood Loss Anemia

Description and causes—This term describes conditions of low red blood cell count occurring over extended periods of time. However, low red blood cell count can also occur following an acute blood loss and is referred to by some as acute blood loss anemia.

Signs and symptoms—In this instance, there is a sudden loss of red blood cells and therefore hemoglobin and iron. The rapid loss of blood volume can be fatal.

Etiology—Acute blood loss can result from severe trauma, the inability to coagulate the blood, ruptured gastric or intestinal ulcers, postoperative bleeding, postpartum (after birth) hemorrhage, or a ruptured aneurysm. A loss of 20% to 30% of blood volume causes circulatory insufficiency with symptoms of shock, restlessness, low blood pressure, rapid pulse, perspiration, and cool, clammy skin. With a loss greater than 30%, the circulatory system may fail and be followed by shock and then coma. Blood loss beyond 40% is life threatening, and the patient will die unless blood volume is immediately replaced.

Treatment—The treatment goal in acute blood loss anemia is to control the hemorrhage and restore blood volume. Prevention of shock is very important. Immediate infusion of IV fluids, electrolyte solutions, and plasma can increase the circulating volume while packed cells or whole blood are being typed and cross-matched for infusion.

Aneurysm (An′u-rism)

Description—This is the ballooning out of the wall of an artery. Often an aneurysm is associated with **atherosclerosis** or **arteriosclerosis** and hypertension.

Etiology—A slight break or weakness in the muscular layer of an artery allows the pressure of the blood to push the walls of the blood vessel out (Figure 30–26). The larger the bulge, the thinner the arterial wall becomes. Eventually, the wall gives way and a hemorrhage occurs. The extent of the bleeding and its effects on the body depend to a great extent on the location of the aneurysm and the size of the involved blood vessel.

Aneurysms are found primarily in cerebral arteries, the thoracic or abdominal section of the aorta, and the femoral and popliteal arteries of the leg. Some aneurysms are without symptoms and are discovered by accident or an X-ray.

Cerebral Aneurysm

This type occurs within the brain.

Description—Depending on its location, it may rupture and cause bleeding within the subarachnoid space, or an artery within the brain tissue itself may rupture. If the hemorrhage is not too massive, the blood clots. Later, the body will slowly reabsorb the blood clots, and function will return. Hemorrhage may be fatal, however, because of increased intracranial pressure from the blood, which compresses and damages brain tissue. Remember, the skull does not stretch; therefore, when bleeding occurs, the delicate tissues of the brain are displaced and damaged. Cerebral aneurysms are graded from I to V depending on the amount of bleeding. Rebleeding after seven to 10 days is not uncommon. When the initial blood has clotted, the body resumes its normal function of removing clotted material, which may lead to a renewed and often fatal recurrence.

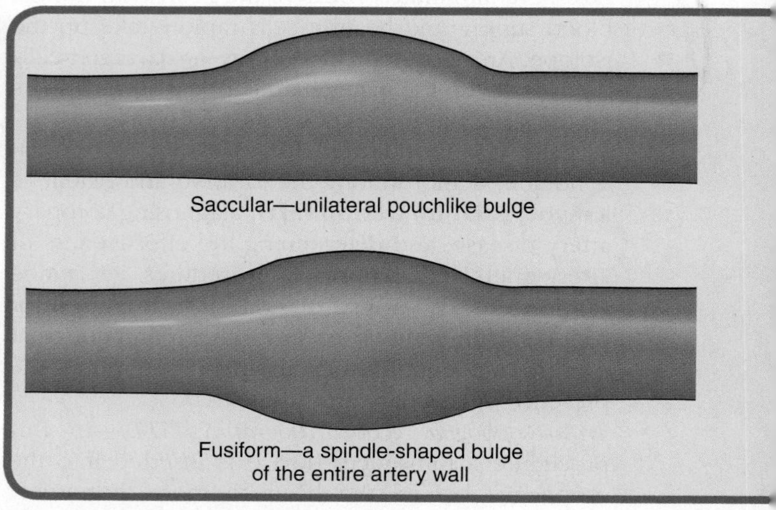

Figure 30–26: Types of aneurysms. *Delmar/Cengage Learning.*

Signs and symptoms—Usually the onset is without warning, but headache, nuchal (back of neck) rigidity, stiffness in the back and legs, and intermittent nausea may be present for several days preceding the rupture. Upon rupture, there is a sudden severe headache, nausea, vomiting, and maybe some altered level of consciousness, including coma. Following bleeding, there may be back and leg pain, restlessness, fever, irritability, and occasionally seizures and blurred vision. If there is bleeding into the tissues, there may be paralysis, sensory deficits, difficulty speaking, and visual defects.

Treatment—Treatment is directed toward reducing the risk of rebleeding by repairing the aneurysm surgically. When the patient's condition will not withstand the surgery, a conservative treatment is indicated. This involves bed rest for four to six weeks; avoidance of coffee, other stimulants, and aspirin; analgesics as needed; a hypotensive drug if there is hypertension; corticosteroids to reduce edema; a drug to delay blood clot destruction; and sedatives to reduce stress.

Thoracic Aortic Aneurysms

Description—These occur as a result of great pressure in the artery. Rupture of the aorta is usually fatal. If the thoracic aneurysm begins by "splitting" of the wall, the person may experience a tearing or ripping sensation accompanied by chest pain, pallor, rapid pulse, shortness of breath, loss of pulses below the neck, and other symptoms.

Treatment—Surgery can remove the damaged segment of the aorta and replace it with a Dacron or Teflon graft.

Abdominal Aortic Aneurysms

Description—Usually without symptoms, this type is detectable on palpation as a pulsating mass in an area around the umbilicus (navel). If it ruptures, the patient may experience pain similar to that of kidney stones. About 20% of such patients die immediately; however, if the bleeding is in the retroperitoneal space (behind the peritoneal lining of the abdomen), the limited space puts pressure on the tear as it fills with blood, closing off the opening.

Treatment—An abdominal aneurysm is repaired like an aneurysm of the thoracic aorta. In addition, an external Dacron prosthesis (artificial part) may be applied around the aneurysm and sutured into place to support the weakened wall. A new procedure to repair abdominal aortic aneurysms involves placement of a stent graft in suitable individuals. This is a much lower-risk procedure.

Aneurysms in the lower extremities may interfere with circulation and result in severe **ischemia** (lack of blood) and gangrene (tissue death), which may require amputation of the extremity. This can also be treated with stent grafts with improved outcomes.

Angina (An′ji-na)

Description—This heart condition causes severe chest pain that radiates down the inner surface of the left arm, usually associated with emotional stress or physical exertion. The episode may last from a few seconds to several minutes.

Signs and symptoms—Symptoms, in addition to the pain, include irregular heart rate, lowered blood pressure, anxiety, and perspiration.

Etiology—The pain is believed to be caused by a spasm or blockage of one or more coronary arteries, which results in ischemia to a portion of the heart muscle.

Treatment—The treatment consists of nitroglycerin, in a tablet form, placed under the tongue. The nitroglycerin dilates the constricted artery or arteries to permit the flow of blood to the heart tissue. When **angina** pain persists after 10 minutes and the use of three sublingual tablets, the patient should go directly to the nearest hospital emergency room.

The patient must be instructed to have nitroglycerin available at all times. Tablets must be kept in a dark, tightly closed bottle, without cotton, and be protected from heat and sunlight. Tablets over six months old should be discarded. Nitroglycerin is also available as an oral spray or in the form of a paste that is applied to the skin to permit prolonged release of the drug in measurable doses. Other medications, such as calcium channel blockers and beta blockers, are also used to prevent angina.

A new little-known procedure is being used in specific centers in the United States. It is thought useful in about 5% to 15% of angina sufferers who are *not* candidates for established alternatives. It is called Enhanced External Counterpulsation. It involves the use of "cuffs" positioned around the legs, thighs, and hips. The apparatus is operated by a computer that synchronizes pulsations to the heartbeat and a compressor that inflates the cuffs, forcing blood to the arteries when the heart muscle is relaxed. This increases blood flow to the heart and decreases the workload. It requires daily one-hour treatments for 35 days. At present, the treatment is limited to patients with stable angina who are not candidates for other treatments. The patients treated have shown a decrease in the frequency and intensity of pain and an increase in exercise tolerance. Some have been able to resume work and even exercise. The treatment is noninvasive but does require a considerable investment in time. At present, insurance will not cover the costs because it is considered experimental.

Arrest (Cardiac)

Description—This is complete, sudden cessation of heart action. The condition is rapidly fatal, producing irreversible brain damage after five minutes.

Signs and symptoms—The major symptom is the sudden ending of heart function, hence the absence of heartbeat and pulse.

Etiology—It is believed to result from a failure in the body's ability to transport calcium, which interferes with its electrical and mechanical functions. It is associated with a severe lack of blood to the myocardium. Cardiac arrest can also be caused by heart failure, electrical shock, fibrillation, drowning, anesthetics, respiratory failure, and severe electrolyte imbalances.

Treatment—Arrest is treated initially by external cardiac massage (cardiopulmonary resuscitation [CPR] technique), then supplemented by defibrillation, IV drug therapy, and ventilation procedures. Death is certain if function cannot be restored quickly.

Arrhythmia (A-rith-me-a)

Description—This term is used to identify any abnormal changes in the heart rhythm. Arrhythmias vary in severity from mild to life threatening, as with fibrillation. They are classified according to the origin of the irregularity (e.g., PVC or atrial flutter). The more the heart action is affected, the greater the consequences on the cardiac output and the blood pressure, which in turn determines the clinical significance.

Signs and symptoms—The presence of an irregular heart rate and palpitations.

Etiology—Arrhythmias may be congenital or may result from myocardial ischemia, infarction, hypertrophy of muscle fiber from hypertension, or degeneration of conductive tissue required to maintain normal rhythm.

Treatment—Treatment varies in relation to the cause and severity of the irregularity from no treatment to medication, eliminating known causes, CPR, the insertion of a pacemaker, and a defibrilator.

Arrhythmia that produces extra beats, delayed beats, or missed beats often results from caffeine, amphetamine, or a medication reaction and can usually be treated by removing the causative factor.

The choice of treatment depends upon the type of arrhythmia and whether there is underlying structural heart disease. Amiodarone can treat atrial or ventricular arrhythmias as can a beta blocker.

Arteriosclerosis (Ar-te-re-o-skle-ro′-sis)

Description—In this "hardening" of the arteries and arterioles, the muscular and elastic tissue is gradually replaced by fibrous tissue and calcification. Because the vessels are no longer capable of expanding and recoiling with each heartbeat, the heart must exert more pressure on the blood to pump it through the more rigid vessels. Arteriosclerosis results in high blood pressure and may lead to an aneurysm and cerebral hemorrhage.

Signs and symptoms—The major sign is hypertension.

Etiology—The artery and arteriole walls become fibrous and contain calcium deposits.

Treatment—The prime focus of treatment is aimed at preventing the rupture of an aneurysm or a CVA (stroke) by reducing blood pressure.

Atherosclerosis (Ath-er-o-skle-ro′-sis)

Description—This condition is characterized by the deposit of fatty material along the linings of the arteries (Figure 30–27). As the material builds up, the opening of the artery may become partially or totally closed, thereby reducing or eliminating the flow of blood to the area. Atherosclerosis can also result in elevated blood pressure, but the greatest danger is a blocked coronary artery and heart attack. There is also danger from the

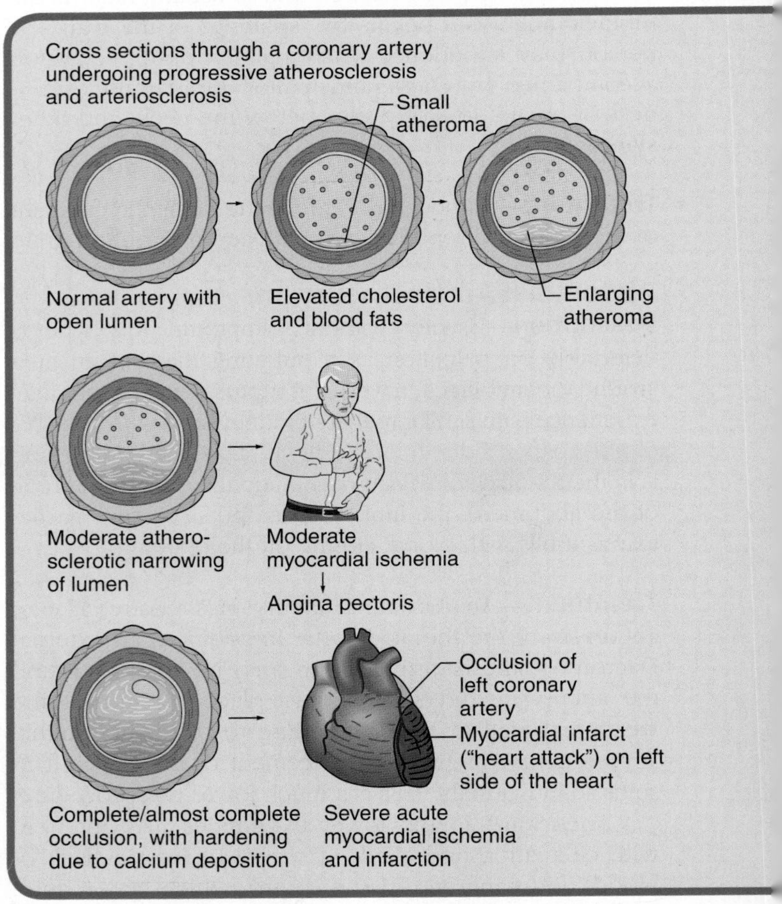

Figure 30–27: The natural history of coronary heart disease. *Delmar/Cengage Learning.*

atherosclerotic plaque deposits that can break loose and circulate through the bloodstream as emboli.

Signs and symptoms—The major symptom is determined by the territory affected by the blocked blood vessel. Examination of the interior of arteries would show plaque of lipids and fat deposits. Decreased circulation symptoms are particularly observable in the carotid, coronary, and lower extremity arteries.

Etiology—Atherosclerosis is linked to many risk factors: family history, hypertension, obesity, smoking, diabetes, stress, sedentary lifestyle, and high serum cholesterol and triglyceride levels.

Treatment—If there is coronary involvement, the goal of treatment is to prevent occlusion of the arteries and prevent myocardial infarction. Dietary restrictions to reduce intake of salt, fats, and cholesterol; abstaining from smoking; and reducing stress are indicated. Angioplasty is used to open the blocked arterial segment. With complete obstruction, bypass surgery may be indicated.

Athletic Heart Syndrome

Description—This is a series of cardiac changes resulting from strenuous exercise. Primarily, the heart enlarges (cardiomegaly), particularly the ventricles, because of its adaptive ability to meet the body's need for increased output. Because the heart is a muscle, it reacts just as the biceps do to physical endurance training. This syndrome is increasing because of the emphasis on physical fitness.

Signs and symptoms—The athletic heart usually produces no symptoms except perhaps pounding or irregularity after strenuous activity. Bradycardia of 40 beats per minute is common and may be considered "normal" because of the heart's increased efficiency upon contraction.

Etiology—The syndrome is probably a physiologic response to maintaining optimal cardiac performance during physical endurance training. The stress placed on the heart causes the left ventricle to enlarge and thicken in order to meet the demand for more oxygen and hence more blood flow.

Treatment—Nothing is required unless there is underlying cardiac disease, which will necessitate discontinuing training.

Carditis (Kar-di′tis)

Description—Literally, it is inflammation of the heart. The term is usually used with one of three prefixes that define the portion of the heart that is involved. The inflammation results from an infectious process caused by a viral, fungal, or bacterial invasion. Other causes vary with the form of inflammation, as follows.

Pericarditis (Per-i-kar-di′tis)

Description—An inflammation of the pericardium, the fibroserous tissue sac that covers the heart.

Signs and symptoms—It may result in a purulent or bloody exudate forming within the sac, or the tissue may become thickened and fibrous, constricting the filling action of the heart. Pericarditis can follow injury to the heart, an infarction, or cardiac surgery.

Acute pericarditis typically causes sharp, sudden pain that begins at the sternum and radiates across the back to the shoulders and arms. It is similar to pleurisy, becoming more intense on inspiration but decreasing when sitting upright and leaning forward. A very serious condition known as tamponade will occur if the collection of fluid within the pericardium is rapid. Pressure within the sac prevents ventricular filling during diastole, thereby severely decreasing cardiac output and resulting in pallor, hypotension, and eventually cardiovascular collapse and death.

Etiology—Acute pericarditis is caused by bacterial, fungal, or viral infections. It can be caused by noninfectious etiologies as well.

Treatment—With tamponade, emergency treatment to remove the fluid by needle aspiration or surgical incision will result in a dramatic improvement.

Pericarditis that causes a gradual fluid accumulation allows time for the pericardium to stretch, often to hold 1 to 2 liters of fluid. Chronic pericarditis that results in constriction or recurrent collection of fluid may necessitate partial removal of the pericardium to allow escape of the fluid or, if constriction, a total pericardectomy (removal of the pericardium). Anti-inflammatory agents, nonsteroidal medications, colthicine and steroids, may be used.

Myocarditis (Mio-kar-di′tis)

Description—An inflammation of the myocardium (heart muscle). It can occur in both acute and chronic forms.

Signs and symptoms—Symptoms produced are generally nonspecific, such as fatigue, palpitations, fever, and dyspnea. It is usually an uncomplicated disease and is self-limiting in nature. Normally, it is associated with a recent upper respiratory infection (URI) and fever.

Myocarditis may produce mild chest soreness and a feeling of pressure, but not the anginal type of pain. Occasionally, myocarditis may initiate a degenerative process of the tiny fibrils (small fibers) in the muscular tissue. This may result in heart failure, enlargement, and arrhythmia.

Etiology—Myocarditis is caused by a viral or bacterial infection, an immune reaction (rheumatic fever), radiation therapy to the chest, and effects of chemicals, such as in chronic alcoholism.

Treatment—Myocarditis is treated with bed rest and appropriate measures for complications that may develop.

Endocarditis (En-do-kar-di′tis)

Description—This is infection of the endocardial lining, heart valves, tissue adjoining artificial valves, or the blood vessel linings. In the infectious process, fibrin and platelets collect where the invading circulating organisms have produced wartlike vegetations on the valves and often the surrounding structures. The vegetative growths may cause serious complications if they embolize to the spleen, kidneys, lungs, or brain.

Etiology—The infecting organism in acute endocarditis is usually a streptococcus, staphylococcus, or pneumococcus. The gonococcus is also capable of causing endocarditis. Intravenous drug abuse may lead to infections from staph or fungi normally present on the skin surface. A subacute form may affect persons with valve or other cardiac lesions that may be acquired or congenital.

Treatment—If endocarditis is left untreated, it usually results in death. Recovery is improved to 70% with proper treatment. The choice of drug therapy depends upon the organism causing the infection. When severe valve damage occurs, resulting complications may include insufficient cardiac action and congestive failure caused by improper valve function. Damaged valves can be surgically removed with open heart surgery and replaced with artificial valves. If the infection involves an artificial valve, surgery to replace the prosthesis will be required. Often valves from pigs or cows are used to replace damaged human heart valves and function very effectively.

Cerebrovascular Accident (CVA) (Se-re-bro-vas′-ku-lar)

Description—A condition commonly known as a stroke, CVA is the sudden impairment of the flow of blood to the brain, thereby diminishing or interrupting the supply of oxygen and causing serious damage or destruction of brain tissue. Because of the urgency for intervention and treatment, strokes are now being referred to as "brain attacks." The phrase "time is brain" also emphasizes the importance of immediate treatment. Strokes are the third leading cause of death and the leading cause of serious long-term disability in the United States. The risk of stroke doubles each succeeding decade of life, beginning at age 55. More men than women have strokes, but women are more likely to die. African Americans and Hispanics have a higher rate than whites. Strokes are often referred to as the silent killer because usually no symptoms are noticed in advance.

CVAs are classified according to their cause and effect. **Transient ischemic attacks** (TIAs) are small, temporary interruptions of blood flow. These are referred to as "warning strokes" because they may happen before a major stroke. The symptoms usually last only a few minutes. The most common major stroke is an ischemic stroke, meaning a blood vessel is blocked by a clot and stops all flow of blood to a portion of the brain. A rarer but more dangerous type of stroke is called hemorrhagic, meaning a blood vessel has ruptured, and the escaping blood is damaging brain tissue either by pressure against it or from lack of circulation through the tissue.

Signs and symptoms—Symptoms vary with the area of the brain that is involved. CVAs involving posterior cerebral arteries affect the vision and often result in coma. Anterior artery involvement results in confusion, weakness, loss of coordination, personality changes, and numbness, especially in the legs. If the CVA occurs in the right hemisphere of the brain, symptoms are produced on the left side of the body, and if in the left hemisphere, on the right side. A CVA may leave the patient with many varied symptoms that may include slurred speech, amnesia, dizziness, paralysis (one extremity, one side, or total), inability to speak, coma, double vision, incontinence (inability to control bladder and bowels), and rigidity. In addition, hemorrhagic stroke usually causes severe headache, difficulty breathing, nausea, and vomiting.

Etiology—A **cerebrovascular accident** is the result of high blood pressure, which ruptures an artery; atherosclerosis, which occludes an artery; or thrombosis (a blood clot), which interrupts the flow of blood. When a large enough area is involved, death may result.

All medical personnel should be familiar with the warning signs of stroke as listed in Table 30–1.

Table 30–1 The Warning Signs of Stroke

The development of difficulty in speaking or in understanding simple statements.
Sudden blurred or decreased vision.
Loss of balance or coordination when combined with another warning sign.
Numbness, weakness, or paralysis of face, arm, or leg—especially on one side of the body.
Loss of consciousness or severe drowsiness.
A sudden, severe headache.

These signs could represent a stroke; call 911 or other emergency assistance immediately.

Treatment—Remember, with stroke every minute counts. Patients should go to the emergency room immediately either by EMS services, or, if it is quicker, by private car. The patient must NOT drive him- or herself. Upon arrival, a CT scan or MRI will be ordered to identify the type of stroke, the location, and the extent of the damage. With ischemic stroke, a clot buster called tissue plasminogen activator (tPA) is administered intravenously (IV) or directly into the brain by catheter for about one hour. It can dissolve about 60% to 80% of the clots and effectively prevent brain damage but ONLY if given within three hours of the onset of symptoms. A clot-busting chemical called prourokinase is being tested and has shown to minimize brain damage up to six hours after a stroke. Also, a nontoxic form of snake venom was accidentally discovered that is being investigated in clinical trials as stroke treatment. There is always danger from any clot-buster because the blood rushes back in after the blockage is cleared, and the weakened arteries can result in life-threatening bleeding in about 6.5% of patients. An experimental device is being researched as an alternative treatment. It is a tiny pump called an AngioJet that vacuums up a clot almost instantly and without chemicals. It is hoped this proves to be a safer, more effective treatment.

A hemorrhagic stroke is treated differently. Administering tPA could cause life-threatening brain hemorrhage. These patients are treated with methods to control heart rhythm, stabilize blood pressure, and monitor brain function. Unfortunately, little can be done to quickly solve the effects of the hemorrhage.

Research has found that administering neuroprotective materials within 24 hours helps protect the damaged cells. Enzyme-blocking chemicals may be effective for more than a week to prevent damaged cells from dying. After approximately one year, little additional progress toward recovery is anticipated.

Scientists have developed many exciting devices to help maximize the patient's ability to function. A "Handmaster" uses voice activation to duplicate brain impulses to move extremities. A minute computer chip has been implanted in the brain to allow brain signals to form a readout on a computer screen so that a person who is paralyzed and mute can communicate. Also, encouraging results are being achieved from infusion of millions of fresh lab-grown neurons into the damaged brain. It was discovered that when cancerous cells in a lab were treated with retinoic acid, they transformed into healthy neurons. Initially, lab rats were induced to have strokes, and following neuron injection, they regained function. A few humans have received these neuron transplants and are showing improvements for the first time since their devastating strokes.

Perhaps the best treatment is prevention. The strongest predictors of stroke are hypertension, irregular heartbeat, diabetes, a sedentary lifestyle, and use of tobacco. Some protective measures may be beneficial. The use of vitamins B_6 and B_{12} and folic acid seems to help because they lower homocysteine levels. It appears that drinking up to two alcoholic drinks per day offers protection against ischemic stroke by increasing HDL cholesterol and tPA levels to keep clots from forming. Higher intake increases risk for hemorrhagic stroke.

Congestive Heart Failure (CHF)

Description—This group of cardiac dysfunctions results in poor performance of the heart with related congestion of the circulatory system. Usually the myocardium of the left ventricle is affected, often as a result of prolonged high blood pressure. **Congestive heart failure** can also be a complication of coronary artery disease or a result of a mechanical disorder involving the heart's valvular functions. It may also be caused by myocarditis and left ventricular dysfunction.

Left-Sided Heart Failure

Description—Cardiac output is decreased; however, the left atrium continues to force blood into the ventricle, resulting in increased pressure and volume within the ventricle. As this backup continues, the left atrium becomes congested, backing up blood into the pulmonary veins and then the pulmonary capillary beds. The fluid in the capillaries fills the alveolar spaces, resulting in pulmonary edema. There is a lack of oxygen exchange and a decrease in the emptying capability of the right ventricle.

Signs and symptoms—Symptoms of left-sided failure are shortness of breath, inability to breathe while lying down, periods of gasping for air, weak and rapid pulse, cool and clammy skin, and an ashen gray or cyanotic skin coloring. Often a cough produces pink, frothy sputum.

Etiology—Congestive heart failure is caused by the increased pressure of blood within the heart, primarily from the poor emptying of the ventricles, which causes fluid from the blood to collect in the tissues. With left-sided heart failure, blood backs up into the lungs, releasing fluid into the alveoli.

Right-Sided Heart Failure

Description—Returning blood flow becomes congested in the systemic circulation, eventually causing fluid to enter the interstitial spaces.

Signs and symptoms—Initially, the fluid can be viewed as edema in the lower extremities, but as the failure continues, edema is present in the upper extremities and in various organs throughout the system. Right-sided failure symptoms include swelling of the extremities, enlarged liver and spleen, and ascites (fluid in the abdominal cavity) caused by filtration from portal circulation venous pressure.

Etiology—When the right ventricle fails to move blood forward into the lungs, the blood backs up into the atrium, which therefore cannot accept incoming blood, so congestion occurs in the lower extremities and abdomen.

Treatment—Heart failure is extremely serious. Treatment involves the use of drugs to quickly increase cardiac output and remove congested fluids. Arterial vasodilators increase the efficiency of heart action. Bed rest is enforced and antiembolism stockings are used to prevent thromboembolism resulting from venous stasis. Continued treatment involves the use of cardiac drugs, frequent periods of rest, the use of elastic support stockings, skin care of the lower extremities, and dietary adjustments to reduce sodium intake and ensure proper nutrition.

Treating the underlying cause of congestive heart failure is the best first step. This may involve diseased heart valves, blocked coronary arteries, or toxins that directly damage heart muscle. Often there is no way to correct the cause, so doctors use an angiotensin-converting enzyme inhibitor (ACE inhibitor), such as Prinivil, Vasotec, or Zestril, to take some workload off the heart. These vasodialators work to relax stiffened blood vessels to make it easier for the weakened heart to push blood through the circulatory system. Diuretics or thiazide diuretics, such as Hydrodiuril, work to decrease edema in the lungs and legs. A weak diuretic, spironolactone, is given to some CHF patients because it helps the body hold on to potassium, whereas Lasix (a powerful diuretic) makes the patient lose potassium, which then causes other problems. Doctors are now using beta blockers, such as Coreg and Toprol-XL, that significantly reduce the risk of hospitalization and death in patients with mild to severe heart failure. This type of medication is the standard of care for most patients with heart failure, as well as the ACE inhibitors and angiotensin receptor blocking agents. In some patients, digitalis is used, which helps improve the contractibility of the heart muscle.

Coronary Artery Disease

Description—This is a disease of the arteries that surround the heart, carrying oxygen and nutrients to the myocardium.

Signs and symptoms—The lack of oxygen causes the typical symptoms of angina: tightness of the chest and crushing substernal chest pains radiating to the left arm, neck, and shoulder blades. Other symptoms may be nausea, vomiting, fainting, and perspiring. When angina pain persists, it suggests an infarction.

Coronary artery disease may be diagnosed by the ECG during an attack or during a treadmill or exercise bicycle test. A heart catheterization, also called a coronary angiogram, allows visualization by X-ray examination of the coronary arteries following injection of a contrast medium into the blood vessels.

Etiology—Characteristically it is caused by atherosclerosis that narrows the blood vessel opening, thereby reducing the volume of blood flow to that portion of the heart muscle served by the arterial branch and resulting in angina symptoms.

Treatment—Narrowed, clogged arteries can be treated by three methods. First is the use of nitrates to dilate the vessel. Nitroglycerin in tablet form is placed under the tongue, can be applied in a paste form to the skin surface, or is given in oral form. Beta blockers and calcium blockers can also be used. When medication does not relieve symptoms and arterial openings are considerably narrowed, other treatments are required. Second, an **angioplasty** can be performed during catheterization of the heart. A balloonlike device is inflated to compress the fatty deposits against the arterial walls, thereby opening the constricted vessel. This is called a balloon angioplasty (Figure 30–28A). About 54% of the vessels clog again within three years and require a second angioplasty or bypass surgery. Another similar procedure is known as directional coronary atherectomy. It is performed like the conventional balloon procedure except that one side of the tip has a metal cylinder with a cutting blade that is attached to an external motor that rotates the cutter, grinding up the deposits and sucking them out of the catheter (Figure 30–28B). This method is believed to better control the reformation of deposits. A third type of artery procedure is called a coronary stent (Figure 30–28C). A balloon catheter with a stent (stainless steel mesh tube) is inserted into the artery. The balloon is inflated, compressing the deposits toward the sides of the artery and opening up the stent, which expands and stretches the arterial wall. The balloon is deflated and the catheter removed, leaving the stent to keep the vessel open. So far it has produced the best results.

In total, about 700,000 angioplasties are performed each year, often on two or three vessels at a time. Stents are used the majority of the time. Research has shown that six months after an angioplasty with a stent in place is performed, patients suffered less pain and less clogging and were less likely to need bypass surgery or additional angioplasty. However, there are some other results. The stent does not seem to decrease the risk of subsequent heart attacks or stroke, primarily because the stents

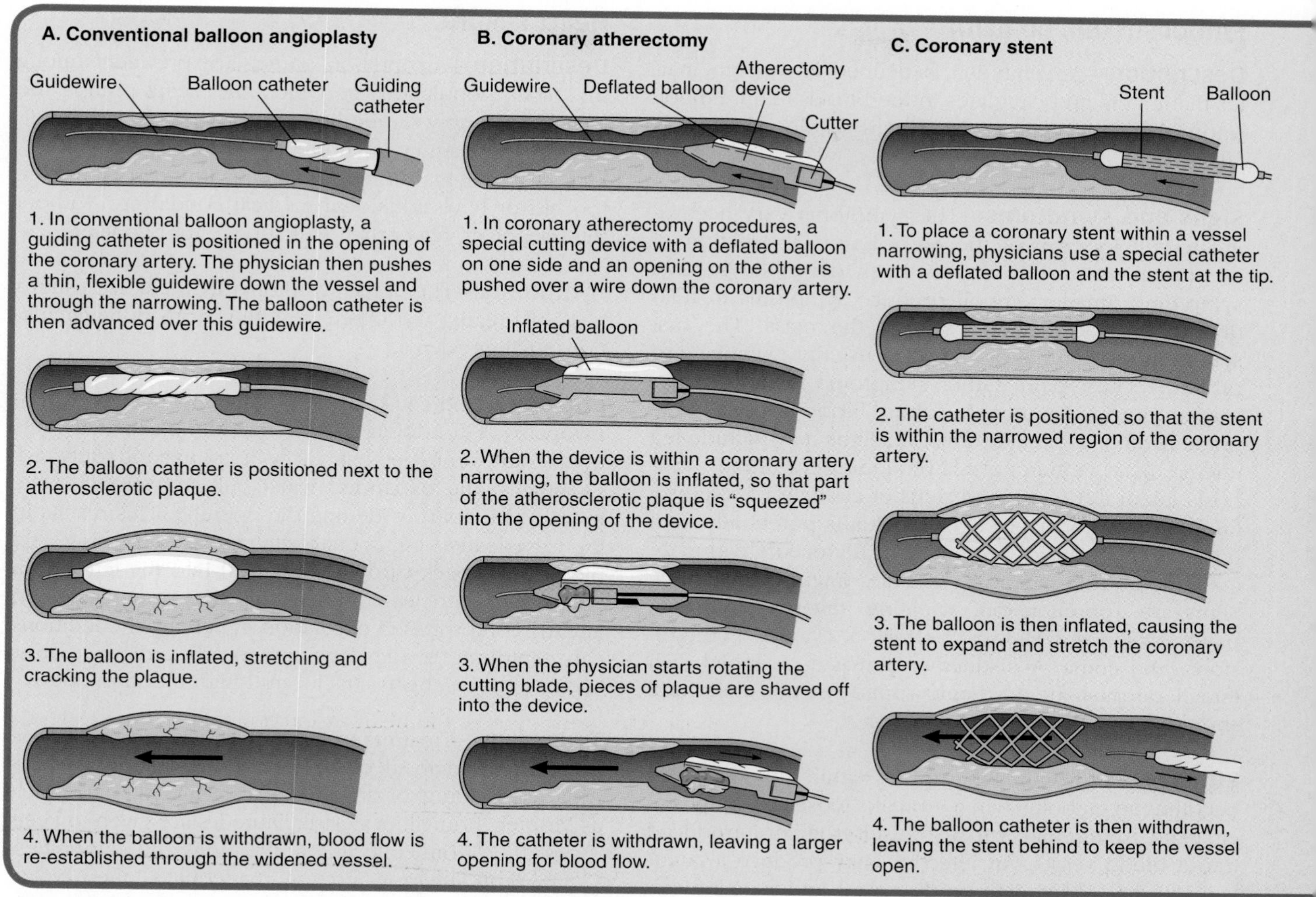
A. Conventional balloon angioplasty
Guidewire
Balloon catheter
Guiding catheter
1. In conventional balloon angioplasty, a guiding catheter is positioned in the opening of the coronary artery. The physician then pushes a thin, flexible guidewire down the vessel and through the narrowing. The balloon catheter is then advanced over this guidewire.
2. The balloon catheter is positioned next to the atherosclerotic plaque.
3. The balloon is inflated, stretching and cracking the plaque.
4. When the balloon is withdrawn, blood flow is re-established through the widened vessel.
B. Coronary atherectomy
Guidewire
Deflated balloon
Atherectomy device
Cutter
1. In coronary atherectomy procedures, a special cutting device with a deflated balloon on one side and an opening on the other is pushed over a wire down the coronary artery.
Inflated balloon
2. When the device is within a coronary artery narrowing, the balloon is inflated, so that part of the atherosclerotic plaque is "squeezed" into the opening of the device.
3. When the physician starts rotating the cutting blade, pieces of plaque are shaved off into the device.
4. The catheter is withdrawn, leaving a larger opening for blood flow.
C. Coronary stent
Stent
Balloon
1. To place a coronary stent within a vessel narrowing, physicians use a special catheter with a deflated balloon and the stent at the tip.
2. The catheter is positioned so that the stent is within the narrowed region of the coronary artery.
3. The balloon is then inflated, causing the stent to expand and stretch the coronary artery.
4. The balloon catheter is then withdrawn, leaving the stent behind to keep the vessel open.

Figure 30–28: Opening clogged arteries: (A) balloon angioplasty, (B) coronary atherectomy, and (C) coronary stent. *Delmar/Cengage Learning.*

can become blocked with clots, scar tissue, or new fatty deposits. Stents have been shown to decrease anginal symptoms. In an effort to improve the results with stents, intracoronary radiation has been used when patients have developed restenosis. The radiation technique called brachytherapy reduces the risk of new obstructions. Some researchers feel that perhaps radiation alone might be the most effective because blood clots do not seem to appear later. Stents are also being coated to improve their effectiveness. Heparin (an anticlotting agent) and paclitaxel (drug-eliciting stents) have been used. The drug-elicting stents have remained open for eight months in all 30 patients studied, and none have had an additional heart attack, needed a repeat procedure, or died.

Another way to correct clogged arteries is coronary bypass surgery. This entails bypassing clogged arteries by redirecting blood through vein grafts surgically transplanted from the legs to the heart's surface. The replacement vessels, however, are subject to the same disease as the original vessels. Currently, 10% to 15% of bypass surgeries are repeat procedures. A new procedure uses the internal thoracic artery for the graft because it tends to remain free of atherosclerosis longer. Heart surgeons can now operate without opening the chest cavity. The method is called the daVinci Computer-Enhanced Surgical System. Basically, the surgeon sits at a computer keyboard with a monitor and joystick. The doctor controls robotic arms holding specially designed surgical instruments and tiny cameras. The robot performs the surgery through tiny incisions in the chest. The bypass graft is taken from the inside wall of the chest, thereby eliminating harvesting it from the leg. This new minimally invasive procedure greatly reduces pain, postoperative scarring, and recovery time, which can be significant with the open-chest method.

Coronary artery disease is best treated by prevention. That includes weight control; a diet low in salt, fats, and cholesterol; regular active exercise; reduction of stress; and refraining from smoking.

Embolism (Em′bo-lizm)

Description—An embolus is defined as foreign matter that enters and circulates in the bloodstream. Emboli (more than one) can be composed of blood, exudate, fat, or air.

Signs and symptoms—The symptoms vary according to the location of the **embolism**. Obstruction of a cerebral artery has already been described in CVA symptoms. Smaller emboli produce symptoms in relation to the location and size of the mass. The first symptom of pulmonary emboli is usually dyspnea and probably chest pain. Other symptoms include tachycardia, productive cough (often blood-tinged), low-grade fever, and pleural effusion. Signs may include leg edema; massive hemoptysis (coughing up blood); cyanosis; pleural friction; and signs of circulatory collapse, fainting, and coma. A fatty embolus is potentially fatal if it is in the brain or lung. It typically occurs within 24 to 72 hours following an extremity fracture or trauma. Signs are apprehension, sweating, fever, tachycardia, pallor, dyspnea, pulmonary effusion, cyanosis, convulsions, and coma. A distinctive sign is a petechial rash (small purplish hemorrhagic spots) on the chest and shoulders.

Etiology—A thrombus that forms within a blood vessel becomes an embolus when it breaks loose and begins to circulate. An embolus can also result from air introduced into a blood vessel. An infection may produce a circulating clump of exudate, as discussed under endocarditis. Skeletal fractures cause the formation of fat emboli. One theory holds that minute fat globules from the bone marrow enter the damaged blood vessels at the fracture site. The greatest danger of fat emboli is that they may circulate to the capillary beds in the lungs and block the alveolar exchange, resulting in an insufficient supply of oxygen.

An embolus of any type is potentially lethal if the circulating mass is of adequate size to obstruct the blood supply to a significant portion of an organ. The resulting **infarction** (interference with circulation) is especially rapid when it occurs within a major pulmonary artery or in one of the coronary arteries, and it can be fatal. Infarction of a kidney, the spleen, or the brain will produce symptoms related to the degree of tissue damage. If a nonvital organ is extensively destroyed, surgical removal may be indicated.

Treatment—Depending upon the location of the embolus, treatment can include administering oxygen, use of heparin, reduction of pulmonary edema, intubation to restore and support breathing, medications to cause the mass to disintegrate, antibiotic with an exudate, and other supportive measures.

Heart Failure

Description—A condition, particularly prevalent among the older population, in which the heart pumps too weakly to supply the body with blood. With severe failure, life expectancy is shortened. A transplant will correct the problem, but most patients with heart failure are too old or have additional medical conditions. Without the transplant, fewer than half survive for two years.

Symptoms—The prime symptoms are weakness, shortness of breath, and others resulting from poor circulation, such as edema.

Etiology—One cause of heart failure is dilated cardiomyopathy, a condition characterized by weakened walls of the left ventricle that allow it to expand outward. Eventually, the expanded walls pull the edges of the mitral valve apart, widening the opening. This results in the valve leaflets being unable to cover the opening, and blood flows backward (regurgitates) into the left atrium when the ventricles contract. This only complicates an already compromised circulation. A variety of conditions can contribute to the development of cardiomyopathy, such as viruses, heart attacks, and high blood pressure.

Treatment—Treatment of regurgitation and the loss of pumping strength involves specific medication, such as Aldactone, Coreg, or digoxin, and an ACE inhibitor, such as Vasotec, Prinivil, or Zestril. Diuretics are given to keep excess fluid from collecting in the lungs and extremities.

If drug therapy proves inadequate, then valve replacement or repair may be indicated. Artificial or animal heart valve replacements have been used for quite some time. Replacement procedures involve a temporary but substantial loss of pumping function because left ventricular tissue around the valve is lost when the valve is removed. This procedure is considered too risky for people with severe failure because their function is already critical. A new procedure called annuloplasty repairs the leaky valve by narrowing the expanded valve opening, which greatly reduces or eliminates regurgitation. The surgeon simply sews a plastic ring around the edge of the mitral valve opening, "cinching" it tighter so that the leaflets overlap. In one study of the procedure, only one patient out of 91 died as a result of the surgery. After one year, 80% were still alive, and 70% survived two years. Additional study is continuing, and the results are encouraging.

Heart Replacement

Perhaps the ultimate treatment for severe heart problems is heart transplant. This procedure involves an enormous amount of physical, financial, legal, emotional, and ethical preparation. Usually, the patient is not a good operative risk because of the extent of disease. There is always an emotional rollercoaster of events while waiting to obtain a donor heart match. Many patients do not survive the wait. Even with the best odds possible, transplantation is not always successful. Some patients have transplant rejections and have been fortunate enough to receive and survive a second successfully. The ability to mentally and emotionally accept the placement of another person's heart into your body can be very difficult. The realization that someone had to die for you to get a chance to survive can be a life-changing experience. Fortunately, trained professionals provide support and counseling to assist in this procedure.

In spite of all the odds, the American Heart Association has reported rather impressive results from heart transplants. There were 2,210 transplants reported in the United States in 2007 and 2,163 reported in 2008. Data from June of 2009 showed a one-year survival rate of 88% for males and 77.2% for females. Rates for five years were equally impressive with 73% for males and 67.4% for females.

There have been attempts made to manufacture an artificial heart to provide a solution to serious heart failure. In the mid-1980s, Robert Jarvik developed the Jarvik 7 heart that kept a man alive for more than 600 days. However, this was a large external device to which the patient was attached, so it was not very practical.

In July 2001, a totally implanted mechanical heart was developed and tested in five patients, all of who were extremely ill, not eligible for transplants and very poor operative risks. All were expected to die of their disease within 30 days. The anticipated survival with the artificial heart was only 60 days. The first patient survived for five months. A total of 14 people were eventually permitted to participate in the trials. One patient was able to return home and live a somewhat normal life, surviving for 17 months. The trials were suspended by the FDA in June 2005 because it was thought the device was not ready for additional use. All the patients had suffered in their final days and eventually died. The participants had all volunteered for the trials, even knowing the eventual outcome, just for the chance to be with their families for a little while longer.

Hypertension (Hiper-ten′-shun)

Description—In this condition, blood pressure is consistently elevated above 140/90. In the diabetic population, blood pressure greater than 130/85 is considered hypertensive. These both represent systolic and diastolic hypertension and both need treatment.

Signs and symptoms—The presence of elevated blood pressure readings is the only observable sign of hypertension. Some people may sense that their blood pressure is high and experience headache or "feel" pressure.

Etiology—*Hypertension* may be classified as *essential* (unknown cause) or *secondary* (resulting from another disease or disorder). Essential hypertension is correlated with family history, race, obesity, stress, a diet high in saturated fats and salt, oral contraceptives, and aging.

Secondary hypertension may be the result of kidney disease; thyroid, pituitary, or parathyroid dysfunction; or neurologic disorders that interfere with blood pressure regulation. Treatment of the primary cause will reduce the blood pressure.

Hypertension may also be classified as *benign* or *malignant*. In the benign form, the pressure rises moderately over a fairly long period. Malignant hypertension is characterized by an accelerated, rapid, and severe increase, which may not respond to treatment.

Hypertension is the foremost contributing factor to CVAs, kidney damage, and various cardiac conditions.

Treatment—Treatment of hypertension is directed at reducing the elevated pressure and maintaining an acceptable level of blood pressure. It is of great importance to prevent complications of the disease. Treatment focuses around diet, the control of sodium (currently being questioned), the use of diuretics to encourage elimination of retained body fluids, and antihypertensive drugs from diuretics to renin antagonists and angiotensive-converting enzyme inhibitors to reduce vasoconstriction or increase kidney filtration. It is of the utmost importance that the patient maintain the treatment regimen because hypertension is not curable, only treatable. Patients must be encouraged to continue with their medication even if they have no symptoms of hypertension. Compliance with dietary and drug therapy is the only means of preventing life-threatening complications.

Hypertrophic Cardiomyopathy (Hi-per-tro′-fik Kar-de-o-mi-op′-a-the)

Description—This is a disease in which the walls of the ventricles of the heart are markedly thickened, sometimes to three times their normal width. The "muscle-bound" heart is stiff and cannot fill with blood and pump efficiently. It affects an estimated one in every 2,000 people in the United States. It is recognized as an important cause of heart failure and sudden death. Some prominent victims have been young athletes who collapse and die during sports events. The enlargement is for no apparent reason and is not caused by increased workload as with hypertension or aortic narrowing. (Those problems result in left ventricular hypertrophy.) This disease is not to be confused with athletic heart syndrome.

Signs and symptoms—Some signs include lightheadedness, fainting, shortness of breath, heart palpitations, and occasionally chest discomfort like angina. Many patients have a heart murmur. There may also be arrhythmia of the atria and sometimes of the ventricles as well. Rapid ventricular arrhythmia or fibrillation causes fainting and sudden death in about 2% of patients annually.

Etiology—In some cases the disease is caused by a defective gene located on the 14th chromosome. This form results in a 50% chance their children may develop the condition. Other causes are unknown. Diagnosis is confirmed by echocardiogram.

Treatment—Most patients are placed on medication to slow the heart to encourage a relaxation phase using beta and calcium channel blockers. Some patients also require medication to control arrhythmia. Defibrillation treatment may be indicated. Often, strenuous activity is to be avoided. A new therapy involves the use of a permanent pacemaker and defibrilator to change the heart contraction to prevent sudden death.

A surgical procedure, which has shown improvement of symptoms, is also used in specialized centers to remove a portion of the ventricular septum.

Hypotension (Hi-po-ten′-shun)

Description—Defined as blood pressure below the normal range, **hypotension** may become life-threatening when the circulation of blood becomes impaired and the exchange of gases is inadequate.

Etiology—Hypotension can result from an acute blood loss, heart failure, shock, kidney failure, thyroid disease, and other infectious conditions.

Treatment—The treatment of hypotension is determined by the underlying cause. Options include transfusion and intravenous fluid replacement, cardiac stimulants, thyroid medication, and other appropriate drugs.

Leukemia (Loo-ke′-me-a)

Description—This is a malignant disease of the bone marrow (myelogenous) or lymphatic tissue (lymphocytic). **Leukemia** can be present in either an acute or chronic form. Leukemia will strike 94,200 Americans this year and will cause the death of 51,650.

Signs and symptoms—In the **acute phase**, a great number of immature white blood cells are produced in the bone marrow or lymph tissue. The excessive amount of white blood cells causes pressure and discomfort within the bones, swelling and pain in the lymph nodes, and greatly elevated white blood cell count in the blood. The earliest symptoms of the disease are fever, pallor, fatigue, swelling of lymphoid tissue (spleen, liver), and a tendency toward large bruises.

Even in the presence of great numbers of leukocytes and lymphocytes, the body has little defense against infection because of the immaturity of the cells. The major complication of leukemia is infection. The disease process may progress to produce bleeding within the brain and other vital organs. In acute leukemia, the onset is rapid, and death occurs within a few months unless treated aggressively with chemotherapy. Acute lymphocytic leukemia is the form common in children. Typically, it is approximately 30% into its course before it is diagnosed. Acute myelogenous leukemia is more common in adults. Both acute forms are ultimately fatal, but long-term remissions in the childhood form and approximately 70% cures are now being reported.

Chronic leukemia differs from acute only in that its onset is more insidious (slow), and its course is more prolonged. The median survival rate is three to four years.

Signs and symptoms—Often the first symptoms are a general malaise (vague discomfort, feeling "bad") and weight loss. Anemia, fatigue, and greatly enlarged spleen and lymph nodes are typical symptoms. Chronic myelogenous leukemia is almost always associated with a chromosome irregularity known as the Philadelphia chromosome. Chronic myelogenous leukemia is characterized by two distinct phases: the chronic phase, which is insidious, lasting an average of three to four years, and the eventual acute phase, an immature cell crisis, lasting only a few weeks or months before death occurs.

Diagnosis can be confirmed initially by blood studies in addition to typical clinical findings. Differentiation of type and positive identification of acute or chronic forms is possible through cellular and chromosomal analysis of bone marrow aspirates. The bone marrow sample can be withdrawn through a large-gauge needle introduced into the sternum or preferably the posterior superior iliac spine.

Treatment—Treatment varies with the type and form of leukemia. Systemic chemotherapy is used to destroy abnormal white blood cells and induce a remission so that more normal function of the bone marrow will occur. The side effects of the drugs are loss of hair, nausea, vomiting, gouty arthritis, and a number of other complications. Some success has been achieved with bone marrow transplants among siblings, particularly twins. This procedure is especially indicated in treatment of children and younger adults. Before the marrow is given, the patient is medicated with large doses of drugs to completely suppress the body's ability to react to foreign material. Total bone radiation treatments are used to induce marrow aplasia (lack of function) and aid in lowering the body's resistance to the transplant. Approximately 1 liter (1,000 mL) of bone marrow is removed from the pelvic bones of the donor. The marrow is processed and then given to the recipient intravenously. To prevent contact with any microorganisms, the patient is placed in a reverse isolation unit. The patient is in an extremely vulnerable state, and a prolonged hospital stay is inevitable. Barring complications, which are numerous, chances for recovery are good.

Murmur

Description—The abnormal sound of blood flowing through a heart valve can be heard with a stethoscope and is known as a **murmur**. The murmur is named for the valve which is "leaking" or stenotic.

Signs and symptoms—The mitral valve is the one most frequently affected, and the gurgling or swishing sound is called a mitral murmur. Murmurs are further identified as systolic or diastolic. This classification specifies whether the sound is heard during the contraction or relaxation phase of the heartbeat.

Etiology—Valve damage that results in murmurs can be caused by rheumatic fever, an inflammatory disease that follows a streptococcal infection. The valves may become inflamed and in time thicken and develop scar tissue. Hence, the valves lose their flexibility and no longer close completely.

Endocarditis is another condition that may lead to valve damage. As previously discussed, bacteria circulating through the heart collect on the valvular surfaces, causing the growth of vegetation and resulting in ulceration and death of some tissue. In its damaged state, the valve is no longer capable of normal function. Preexisting valve damage from rheumatic fever, especially of the mitral valve, is quite common in endocarditis. Another etiology of heart murmurs is the thickening of the aortic valve which can occur secondary to a congenital abnormality of the bicuspid valve. This can also occur secondary to rheumatic heart disease or just aging of the patient and can lead to aortic stenosis.

Treatment—Artificial or pig valve replacement may be indicated to alleviate the problem if severe enough to interfere with circulation.

Myocardial Infarction (MI) (Mi-o-kar′-de-al In-fark′-shun)

Description—MI is a complication of coronary artery disease that results from occlusion (partial or complete) of the artery, causing myocardial tissue destruction. MIs are one of the leading causes of death in the United States. Mortality is high when treatment is delayed; approximately 50% of patients will die within an hour after symptoms develop.

Signs and symptoms—It is characterized by severe, crushing pain, which radiates through the chest to the neck and jaw and down the left arm. It is not relieved by rest, as with angina, and is accompanied by nausea, perspiration, a change in blood pressure, hypotension or hypertension, and dyspnea.

Etiology—Predisposing factors include sedentary lifestyle, stressful occupation, obesity, cigarette smoking, hypertension, aging, positive family history, and elevated levels of cholesterol and triglycerides in the blood. An attack can often be precipitated by a heavy meal, physical exertion, or exposure to cold weather.

Treatment—Treatment of MI is directed at relieving the pain with strong analgesic drugs, such as demerol or morphine, and administering extra oxygen to maintain an adequate supply to the tissues. It is important to prevent complications. Heart rhythm must be stabilized to prevent arrhythmia, which can lead to congestive heart failure. Complete bed rest must be enforced to decrease cardiac workload and a possible additional infarction. **Anticoagulant** drugs, such as heparin, are given to reduce the tendency to develop thromboembolism. One treatment includes the immediate use of a clot-busting drug such as tPA or Retavase to open the narrowed or blocked coronary artery in order to restore circulation to the myocardium. In about 20% of cases this fails to work, and if there are associated bleeding ulcers or a stroke, it is prohibited. An angioplasty is now being performed on these selective patients and with other MI patients. Immediate accessibility to qualified surgeons and angioplasty within one hour is a problem in many areas. In contrast, clot-busting drugs can be administered immediately almost anywhere, possibly even by specially trained emergency vehicle personnel in the future.

Severe complications may occur in the damaged ventricular area in addition to the systemic threat of embolism and heart failure. Unusual and potentially lethal conditions may develop. The ventricular septum may rupture, causing a circulatory defect in which blood flows between the ventricles. The ventricular wall may weaken because of necrosis following infarction. The wall may develop an aneurysm, leading to a ventricular rupture.

The patient who survives an MI will be faced with a lengthy recovery period. Lifestyles may need to be altered and dietary and smoking habits changed. An exercise rehabilitation program should be initiated and adhered to for optimum recovery and maintenance of a healthy state.

PATIENT EDUCATION

HOW TO RECOGNIZE A HEART ATTACK

Any of the following symptoms lasting more than 2 minutes may signal the start of a heart attack.

- A sensation of uncomfortable pressure, fullness, squeezing, aching, or pain, usually located in the center of the chest.
- Pain, aching, or heaviness in the shoulders, neck, jaw, arms, or upper back or spreading to those areas from the chest.
- Pain accompanied by lightheadedness, fainting, sweating, nausea, vomiting, or shortness of breath.

Taking a 325-mg aspirin tablet while waiting for help will help prevent clots from getting any larger.

Clot-dissolving drugs, given intravenously within an hour of the first signs of a heart attack, could prevent about 90% of deaths. Unfortunately, half of all people wait more than two hours before getting to a hospital, often because they do not realize they are having a heart attack.

Phlebitis (Fle-bi′-tis)

Description—This localized inflammation of a vein causes an alteration in the epithelial lining, which predisposes to the formation of a thrombus. **Phlebitis** can occur in deep or superficial veins (see Thrombophlebitis for more information).

Sickle Cell Anemia

Description—Sickle cell anemia is an inherited condition due to an autosomal recessive trait. It is a condition in which there aren't enough healthy red blood cells to carry adequate oxygen throughout the body. It is most common in people of African descent. When two people who are carriers of the trait have children, there is a 25% chance that each child will have the disease. When two persons with **sickle cell anemia** have children, all children will have the disease. If only one has the disease and the other is normal, all children will be carriers of the trait.

Signs and symptoms—Sickle cell disease is detected at birth by newborn universal screening. Sickle cell trait is also detected by the screening. Sickle cell anemia is characterized by red blood cells with a hemoglobin defect in their molecular structure that causes the cells to become sickle-shaped. Cells of this shape cannot pass easily through blood vessels and they tend to interfere with circulation.

Symptoms may include tachycardia, cardiomegaly, cardiac murmurs, chronic fatigue, unexplained dyspnea, chest pain, enlarged liver, jaundice, pallor, swollen joints, aching bones, and leg ulcers.

The most common feature of the disease is a painful crisis, which usually appears first at about age 5. Sickled red blood cells become tangled, causing blood vessel obstruction and a lack of oxygen to the tissues, with possible destruction of the involved area. This tissue infarction causes severe pain to the affected area. Usual sites are the lungs, liver, bones, and spleen. The spleen, particularly, is affected so frequently that the resulting damage and scarring cause it to shrink and become useless. A crisis usually lasts from four days to several weeks and recurs cyclically.

Diagnosis can be made from a positive family history and the typical clinical features. It is confirmed by a blood smear that shows the sickled cell structure. At present, research has failed to discover a means to prevent the sickling alteration.

The disease produces long-term complications, such as delayed puberty and a tendency toward delayed growth.

Etiology—It is an inherited condition due to an autosomal recessive trait.

Treatment—Treatment focuses on alleviating the symptoms of the disease and on transfusions with packed red blood cells when an aplastic crisis occurs (depression of the bone marrow activity and destruction of RBCs). The most successful treatment may be prevention through genetic counseling of persons known to be carriers. Information is provided to allow individuals to arrive at informed decisions regarding the conception and birth of children.

There is no known cure for sickle cell anemia. However, recently, a cancer drug has been shown to help prevent the attacks. Hydroxyurea (Hydrea) can cut the rate of painful episodes and complication in half, but the drug poses risks, so only adults with the most severe form are advised to take it. The average life expectancy is now in the mid-40s age range.

Stasis Ulcer (Sta′-sis Ul′-ser)

Description—This is a secondary condition resulting from chronic venous insufficiency. The most common site of **stasis ulcers** is the ankle at the internal malleous area.

Signs and symptoms—Varicosities and edema are common. Early signs are dusky red deposits in the skin with itching and dimpling of the tissue. Later, there is redness and scaling of large areas of the legs. Then, cracks develop with crusts and ulcers. Figure 30–29A shows edema of the lower legs, ankles, and feet as a result of inadequate *return* of blood by the veins, causing fluid to

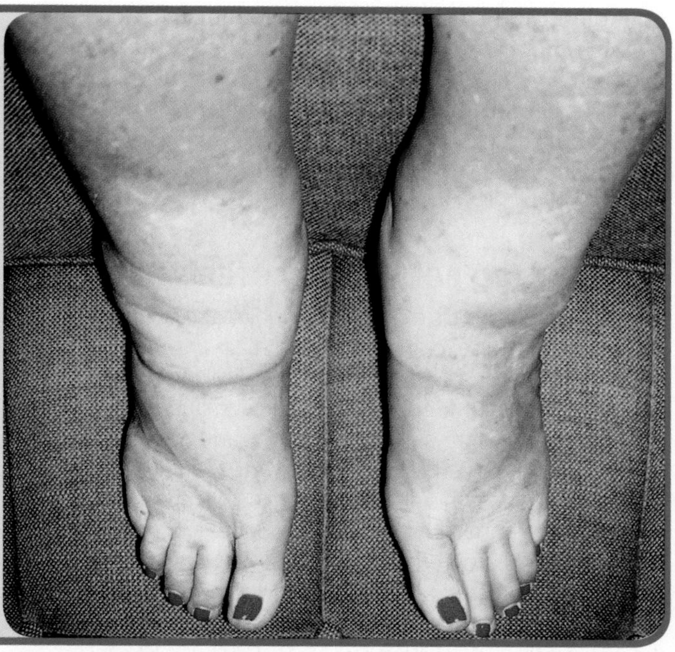

Figure 30–29A: Marked edema of the lower legs, ankles, and part of the feet due to venous insufficiency. Also note skin coloration. *Delmar/Cengage Learning.*

escape into the tissues. There are also red spots developing on the skin. This woman has venous insufficiency, which may lead to a stasis ulcer if not treated. Currently, she wears 40-mm compression hose to the knees, which assist the veins to return fluids and control most of the edema. By contrast, in Figure 30–29B, the dark skin is caused by inadequate blood supply *to* the legs due to

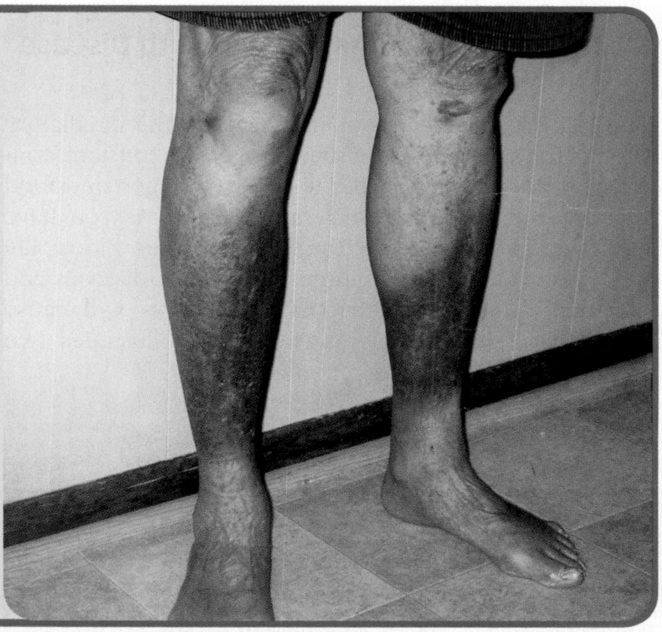

Figure 30–29B: Marked discoloration of lower legs from chronic arterial insufficiency. *Delmar/Cengage Learning.*

chronic arterial insufficiency. This man injured his legs, causing an interruption of the flow of blood. His skin is even hard to the touch.

Etiology—Stasis ulcers develop following deep vein thrombophlebitis that destroys the valve structures. Communicating veins in the affected area fail to compensate for the damaged vein. The venous pressure increases, causing fluid to enter the interstitial tissues and produce edema. The tissue swelling leads to fibrosis and skin discoloration from blood entering the subcutaneous tissues. The poor condition of the skin and the inadequate circulation from the area lead to a breakdown of the surrounding tissues. They can also be caused by lower extremity trauma or a skin irritation.

Treatment—Treatment of small ulcers involves elevation of the affected extremity, warm soaks, bed rest, and the use of drugs to counteract infection. When the swelling subsides, pressure is applied by a sponge rubber dressing or an Unna's boot (zinc gelatin boot). Large stasis ulcers not responding to treatment may require removal of the ulcer site followed by a skin graft.

Thrombophlebitis (Throm-bo-fle-bi′-tis)

Description—This is an acute condition in which the lining of the vein wall becomes inflamed and a thrombus forms. **Thrombophlebitis** can develop within small superficial veins and is usually self-limiting. Deep vein thrombosis (DVT) can affect small or large veins. When there is an alteration of the vein lining, platelets begin to collect at the area. The platelet fibrin catches red blood cells, white blood cells, and additional platelets, forming a blood clot. The thrombus enlarges rapidly, particularly if the blood flow is slow, causing an inflammation that becomes fibrotic. The enlarging clot may completely fill the vein opening, occluding the vessel, or it may break loose, becoming an embolus.

Signs and symptoms—Symptoms of deep thrombophlebitis include severe pain, fever, chills, and possibly edema, with discoloration of the affected extremity. When superficial veins are involved, visible and palpable signs may include heat, swelling, tenderness, redness and discoloration, and induration (hardening) along the affected portion of the vein.

Etiology—DVT usually results from lining damage, but it can also follow accelerated blood clotting and a slow, reduced flow of blood. Conditions that precipitate thrombophlebitis are prolonged bed rest, trauma, childbirth, surgery, and the use of oral contraceptives.

Treatment—Treatment is directed toward preventing complications, controlling the development of thrombi, and relieving the discomfort. The patient is maintained on bed rest, with the affected extremity elevated to aid circulation. Warm, moist soaks are applied to the affected area. Medication is given to relieve pain, and anticoagulants are frequently used to reduce the blood's clotting ability. Antiembolism stockings (tight-fitting, elastic, knee- or thigh-length hose) are indicated to assist the return of blood from the legs to the heart. Individuals who are prone to develop thrombophlebitis should avoid prolonged periods of sitting or standing, especially with little movement, to help eliminate pooling of blood in the lower extremities. When sitting, the legs should be resting on a support that does not cause pressure to interfere with return circulation.

Varicosities (Va-ri-kos′-i-tes)

Description—Veins that become dilated, twisted, and inefficient are known as **varicose** veins. The condition usually results from weakness of the valves in the saphenous vein and its branches, which permits blood to leak backward as a result of incomplete closure. As the blood accumulates, the veins become dilated, the valve is no longer capable of reaching across the opening of the vein, and the situation becomes worse.

Signs and symptoms—Symptoms include a feeling of heaviness, night leg cramps, aching, and a feeling of fatigue. With deep vein involvement, edema may accumulate in the feet and ankles, often associated with the discoloration that precedes stasis ulcers. Superficial varicosed veins can often be seen or palpated behind the knees or on the medial surface of the calf. Varicosed veins are not to be confused with the tiny purplish red surface veins seen on the skin of most adults. These are commonly referred to as spider veins and are evidence of increased venous pressure. They are often associated with varicosities.

Etiology—This stasis (stagnation) of blood is often the result of occupations requiring long periods of standing or of other factors interfering with circulation, such as pressure against the veins during pregnancy.

Treatment—Treatment for mild to moderate varicosities includes an exercise program to improve circulation; use of antiembolism stockings; attention to sitting position; and the elimination of tight-fitting or constricting clothing, such as girdles, garters, elastic bands of clothing, and knee-high or thigh-high hose. More severe varicosities may require injection of a sclerosing agent into small venous areas to scar and harden the vein. Larger involvement will necessitate surgical ligation (tying off) of the involved vein from its branches and stripping the vein from the leg.

AGE-RELATED BODY CHARACTERISTICS

Collateral circulation is a process by which the body can establish circulation to an area after a main artery is obstructed by using small connecting vessels to distribute blood. Development of collateral circulation appears to be the result of pressure building in a major artery that leads to dilation of the side branches of the artery and the connecting capillaries. This ability changes as we age.

Infants are born with a limited amount of collateral circulation. This is demonstrated by the fact that if a foot or hand is compressed for even a short period of time, the part will become pale, cool, and somewhat cyanotic until the compression is relieved.

As a person ages, the increase in the collateral circulation network allows for improved circulation and function of the major organs. Aerobic exercise is thought to improve the collateral circulation network.

In the elderly, however, collateral circulation does not seem to be as much of a benefit as it is with young or middle-aged persons. This may be due to the development of arteriosclerosis, which decreases the elasticity of the vessels.

System Interaction Associated with Disease Conditions

The body is especially dependent upon the circulatory system for survival. All tissue must be in constant contact with the blood in order to receive oxygen and food and give off carbon dioxide and wastes. As you have read, without the force of the heart to pump blood, life will cease within a few minutes. Therefore, diseases and disorders affecting the circulatory process will cause symptoms in other systems. Table 30-2 illustrates two examples of system interaction.

Table 30–2 System Interaction Associated with Disease Conditions

Disease	Systems Involved	Pathology Present
Congestive heart failure	Circulatory	Decreased cardiac output, rapid pulse, cyanosis, circulatory congestion, enlarged spleen, ascites
	Respiratory	Pulmonary edema, cough, shortness of breath, can't breathe lying down, pink frothy sputum

Disease	Systems Involved	Pathology Present
	Integumentary	Cool, clammy skin, dependent edema, stasis ulcers
	Digestive	Enlarged liver
Leukemia	Circulatory	Abnormal WBC, enlarged spleen and liver, bruising, swollen lymph glands, anemia
	Integumentary	Huge areas of bruising, palor
	Immune	Infections
	Skeletal	Pain due to swelling within from excess WBCs

CHAPTER SUMMARY

- The circulatory system transports oxygen and nutrients to the body's cells and carbon dioxide and waste products from the cells.
- The system has four main parts: the heart, the blood vessels, the blood, and the lymphatic system.
- The heart has a contraction or systole phase and a relaxation or diastole phase.
- The heart is surrounded by the pericardium. Surface vessels on the heart are called coronary arteries and veins.
- Internally the heart has four chambers: the right and left atriums, and the right and left ventricles. The biscuspid and tricuspid valves are between the atria and ventricles. The semilunar pulmonic and semilunar aortic valves are between the heart ventricles and the pulmonary vein and aorta.
- Pulmonary circulation sends blood from the right atrium through the tricuspid valve into the right ventricle. It then goes through the pulmonic semilunar valve into the pulmonary artery and to the lungs to pick up oxygen and give up carbon dioxide.
- From the lungs it is carried by the pulmonary vein into the left atrium, through the mitral or biscuspid valve into the left ventricle.
- Blood leaves through the aortic semilunar valve into the aorta to the body.
- Heart sounds known as lubb dupp are caused by the closing of the heart valves.
- The pacemaker is the SA node in the right atrium. This electrical impulse carries over to the AV node causing the ventricles to contract.
- Rhythm disorders may involve interruption in the electrical impulse or a deviation in the regularity.
- Artificial pacemakers can cause the heart to contract effectively when drugs therapy is ineffective.
- The vagus and accelerator nerves control the rate of the heart.
- Blood vessels consist of three types: arteries, veins, and capillaries.
- The main arteries of the body carry oxygenated blood to the body's cells. They are the aorta, gastric, splenic, renal, carotid, pulmonary, brachial, radial ulnar, femoral, tibial, and dorsalis pedis.
- Arteries become arterioles, which connect to capillaries and then join venules to begin returning blood to the heart.
- The main veins of the body carry deoxygenated blood from the cells. They are the tibial, saphenous, femoral, common iliac, inferior and superior vena cava, jugulár, brachial, cephalic, and pulmonary.
- Systemic circulation begins with the aorta leaving the heart, one branch goes to the coronary arteries, one to the head, and another to the upper extremities. Blood descends through the abdominal aorta, common iliac, femoral, and tibial branches to arterioles and the capillaries.
- When blood leaves the capillaries of the lower extremities, it enters venules that join the tibial, saphaneous, popliteal, and femoral veins, eventually emptying into the inferior vena cava returning to the heart.
- Blood leaving the head and upper extremities enters the basilica, median, cephalic, subclavian, internal and external jugular, and the innominate to enter the superior vena cava returning to the heart.
- Portal circulation serves only the internal organs. It carries substances upon which the organ react.
- The lymphatic system consists of lymph nodes, lymph (fluid), lymph vessels, and the spleen. Lymphatic tissue in the tonsils, thymus, and intestines is also a part of the system.
- Lymph is a fluid that fills spaces between cells and transports the products of cellular activity. The fluid circulates through vessels similar to veins in a one-way system to the larger vessels called lymphatics

eventually forming two main ducts that join the veins near the heart.

- Lymph nodes are structures that filter harmful substances and malignant cells from the lymph. They become swollen and tender with infections.
- The spleen produces lymphocytes, stores red blood cells, destroys old red cells, and maintains the cellular-plasma balance on the blood.
- Blood consists of plasma, red, white, and platelet cells. There are four types: A, B, AB, and O. An average adult has between 8 to 10 pints of blood.
- Blood given by transfusion must be typed and cross-matched to the recipient to assure compatibility.
- The Rh factor is an antigen. If a person has the antigen, he or she is Rh+; if not, he or she is Rh–.
- Cholesterol is a product of metabolism of fats. Total, low-, and high-density lipoprotein levels are evaluated in relation to the probability of or a vascular event.
- Trigylcerides are fats normally present in the body. High levels are associated with heart disease and atherosclerosis.
- Cardiovascular tests discussed are arteriography, cardiac catheterization, stress testing, Doppler ultrasound, echocardiogram, ECG, heart scan, MUGA scan, stress cardiolyte, transesophogeal echocardiography, venogram, and cardiac and carotid artery ultrasound.
- Diseases covered are anemia (iron deficiency and aplastic), aneurysm (thoracic and abdominal), angina, arrest, arrhythmia, arteriosclerosis, atheriosclerosis, atheletic heart syndrome, carditis (pericarditis, myocarditis, endocarditis), cerebral vascular accident, congestive heart failure (left and right sided), coronary artery disease, embolism, heart failure, heart replacement, hypertension, hypertrophic cardiomyopathy, hypotension, leukemia, murmur, myocardial infarction, phlebitis, sickle cell anemia, stasis ulcer, thrombophlebitis, and varicosities.
- CHF involves the circulatory, respiratory, integumentary, and digestive systems; leukemia involves the circulatory, integumentary, immune, and skeletal systems.

STUDY TOOLS

Workbook	Activities for Chapter 30
Premium Website MEDIA LINK	View these **Media Links** for Chapter 30: • The heart • The blood
StudyWARE	Activities and Quizzes on the **StudyWARE™ Software** for Chapter 30
	Audio Library of medical terms
	Online access to the **Critical Thinking Challenge 2.0**
learninglab	Module 14: The Respiratory and Circulatory Systems
CourseMate	Activities and Quizzes for Chapter 30
WebTutor	Activities and Quizzes for Chapter 30

CHECK YOUR KNOWLEDGE

1. Cholesterol is:
   a. a by-product of fat metabolism in the blood.
   b. caused by being overweight.
   c. developed from a lack of exercise.
   d. due to decreased blood flow in the arteries.
2. Triglycerides:
   a. are common with diabetes.
   b. are believed to contribute to the thickening of arterial walls.
   c. are beneficial in high levels.
   d. are a combination of three fats high levels.
3. A heart catheterization can:
   a. permit visualization of the coronary arteries.
   b. measure the amount of oxygen in the heart.
   c. remove blood for analysis.
   d. accurately measure electrical activity of the heart.

4. The Dobutamine stress test:
   a. is done on a treadmill.
   b. uses a drug to stress the heart.
   c. allows visualization of the coronary arteries.
   d. requires instillation of a radioactive material and a special camera.
5. The Doppler ultrasound:
   a. can diagnose coronary artery disease.
   b. determines leaking heart valves.
   c. measures cardiac output.
   d. evaluates disease in major blood vessels.
6. Arrhythmia is a term that can mean any of the following except:
   a. absence of heartbeat.
   b. a rhythm with extra beats.
   c. a rhythm with missed beats.
   d. the presence of delayed beats.
7. Atherosclerosis is the:
   a. replacement of muscular artery tissue by fibrous tissue and calcification.
   b. presence of fatty deposits on the artery lining.
   c. scarring of the arterial lining.
   d. thickening of the lining of the arterial wall.
8. A cerebrovascular accident is not caused by:
   a. high blood pressure rupturing an artery.
   b. athersclerosis occluding an artery.
   c. a thrombus that clogs an artery.
   d. an accidental injury to the cerebral artery.
9. A heart murmur is:
   a. an additional flutter of the heart valves.
   b. a soft, barely audible extra heartbeat.
   c. a sound caused by inadequate blood flow.
   d. an abnormal sound of blood flowing through a closed valve.
10. What will most likely contribute to death when an MI occurs?
    a. Taking an aspirin tablet
    b. Waiting to see if the symptoms improve
    c. Taking a dose of nitroglycerin
    d. Taking a strong pain medication
11. Collateral circulation:
    a. is absent at birth.
    b. increases more rapidly in the aged.
    c. is between arteries and veins.
    d. is best in young and middle aged.
12. Leukemia affects:
    a. circulatory, integumentary, and immune systems.
    b. circulatory, digestive, and respiratory systems.
    c. digestive, respiratory, and urinary systems.
    d. respiratory, urinary, and circulatory systems.

WEB LINKS

The following four sites have articles pertaining to the discovery and existence of collateral circulation:

www.ncbi.nlm.nih.gov/pmc/articles/PMC1648418/

content.onlinejacc.org/cgi/content/full/44/1/28

American Heart Association, provides information on heart diseases, blood pressure, cholesterol and vascular diseases: www.heart.org

National Heart, Lung and Blood Institute: www.nhlbi.nih.gov

Chapter 31

The Immune System

OBJECTIVES

In this chapter, you will learn the following:

KB KNOWLEDGE BASE

1. Spell and define, using the glossary at the back of the text, all the Words to Know in this chapter.
2. List the body's three main lines of defense against antigens.
3. Define the function of the immune system.
4. Identify the three basic services of the immune system.
5. Describe the origin of blood cells.
6. List the organs of the immune system, and identify their locations.
7. Describe the purpose of MHC.
8. Explain the role of the B cell.
9. Identify the four types of T cells.
10. Tell how NK cell action differs from phagocytic action.
11. Explain what causes an inflammatory response.
12. Tell how immunizations and vaccines work.
13. Explain how the acquired immunodeficiency syndrome (AIDS) virus destroys the immune system.
14. Identify five ways to acquire the AIDS virus.
15. List four high-risk behaviors to avoid.
16. Name the three most common opportunistic diseases.
17. Define cancer.
18. Name the classifications of cancer.
19. Identify six characteristics of a cancerous cell.
20. Identify the basic cause of cancer.
21. Describe grading and staging of cancer.
22. List four types or categories of carcinogens.
23. Identify the three categories of diagnostic testing.
24. List the four major cancer treatment methods.
25. List five symptoms of chronic fatigue syndrome.
26. Explain how lupus affects the immune system and the major body organs it may affect.
27. Identify the symptoms of rheumatoid arthritis.
28. Tell how immunity changes through the years.
29. Identify the body systems affected by AIDS.

WORDS TO KNOW

abstinence
acquired immunodeficiency syndrome (AIDS)
allergens
allergies
anaphylaxis
antibody
antibody-mediated
antigen
autoimmune
basophils
benign
biopsy
brachytherapy
cancerous
carcinoembryonic antigen (CEA)
carcinogens
carcinoma
cell-mediated
chemotherapy
clonal
complement
corticosteroids
cytokine
cytotoxic
debilitating
desensitization
discoid
eosinophils
extracellular
histamine
humoral
immune
immunoglobulin
immunosuppressed
interferon
interleukin
intracellular
leukemia
lupus erythematosus
lymphedema
lymphocyte
lymphokine
lymphoma
macrophage
malignant
metastasis
monoclonal
monocyte
monogamous

monokine
mutation
neoplasm
neutrophils
oncogenes
opportunistic
permeable
phagocyte
prostaglandin
psychoneuroimmunology
radiation
Raynaud's phenomenon
remission
retrovirus
sarcoma
staging
suppressor
surveillance
thymus
transmission
vaccine
virus

The **immune** system is not usually given the distinction of being identified as a body system. The function of immunity is primarily provided by specific cells and organs of the circulatory system, so it is usually included in that system's discussion. The role of immunity is essential to the health and well-being of humans. When the system misfires or is crippled, a whole host of diseases can develop, such as AIDS, allergy, arthritis, and cancer. Because its function is of such importance, it is being given significance equal to a body system in this text.

We live in an environment full of **antigens**, things that the immune system recognizes as nonself and responds to by destroying or rendering them ineffective. All antigens carry markers that identify them as foreign to the immune system. Foreign materials, bacteria, **viruses**, fungi, and parasites are antigens. Foreign material can be a cell, tissue, a protein, the food we eat, and even particles in the air. Blood from a transfusion or cells and tissue from a transplant are prime examples of foreign material. In abnormal situations, the immune system can mistake self for nonself and attack. This results in the development of an **autoimmune** disease, such as rheumatoid arthritis, diabetes, and lupus. Sometimes, the system responds inappropriately to harmless substances, such as ragweed pollen or cat hair. This kind of antigen is called an **allergen**, and the result is known as an allergy. When one's own cells become **malignant**, their structure changes, making them "different," and a response occurs. Many antigens can cause serious reactions, infections, diseases, and even death.

The body has three main lines of defense against antigens: barriers, the inflammation process, and **antibodies**. The first line of defense are the three types of barriers that prevent entry of antigens. (1) Anatomic barriers are the skin, which covers the body, and the mucous membranes, which line the respiratory, gastrointestinal, and genitourinary tracts. (2) Biochemical barriers are located within the anatomic barriers. Sebaceous glands in the skin secrete antibacterial and antifungal fatty acids and lactic acid. Tears, perspiration, and saliva contain enzymes that attack the cellular walls of gram-positive bacteria. Secretions from certain glands make the skin acidic, which is hostile to bacteria. (3) Mechanical barriers work to eliminate substances. Skin sloughs off, and irritated membranes cause coughing. The acts of urinating and vomiting expel materials.

The second and third lines of defense involve cooperation of various components of the immune response that require additional specific explanation before the defense can be understood. For now, inflammation, the second line, occurs when the barriers have been penetrated. This response begins within seconds of an injury or invasion and results in the familiar warm, red, and swollen area that we recognize as an infection. The third line, antibody defense, is a dual-response system involving the actions of specific cells and other immune system components to attack the antigen. This is our immunity and is our last line of defense.

The function of the immune system is to create effective immune responses to continually defend the body against antigens. To do this, the immune system must be able to provide three basic services: (1) identify self and destroy nonself substances, (2) maintain homeostasis, and (3) conduct continual **surveillance**. To understand how these services work, it is necessary to learn about the way each part of the system contributes to the services. The system includes a variety of cells, the organs, the **complement** system, antibodies, cytokines, and the process of surveillance.

ORIGIN OF CELLS

In the last unit, it was stated that cells within the blood are of three types—red, white, and platelets. The leukocytes (white blood cells) were identified as playing a vital role in defending the body. It is these cells in cooperation with protein molecules that are responsible for immunity.

All blood cells originate in the bone marrow and initially develop from stem cells. They progress through different stages of maturation and differentiation until they become mature, functioning cells. Refer to Figure 31–1 as the origin and maturity of cells is explained. Erythrocytes (RBCs) develop from erythroid stem cells and mature in the bone marrow. White blood cells (WBCs), which become the granulated **eosinophils**, **neutrophils**, and

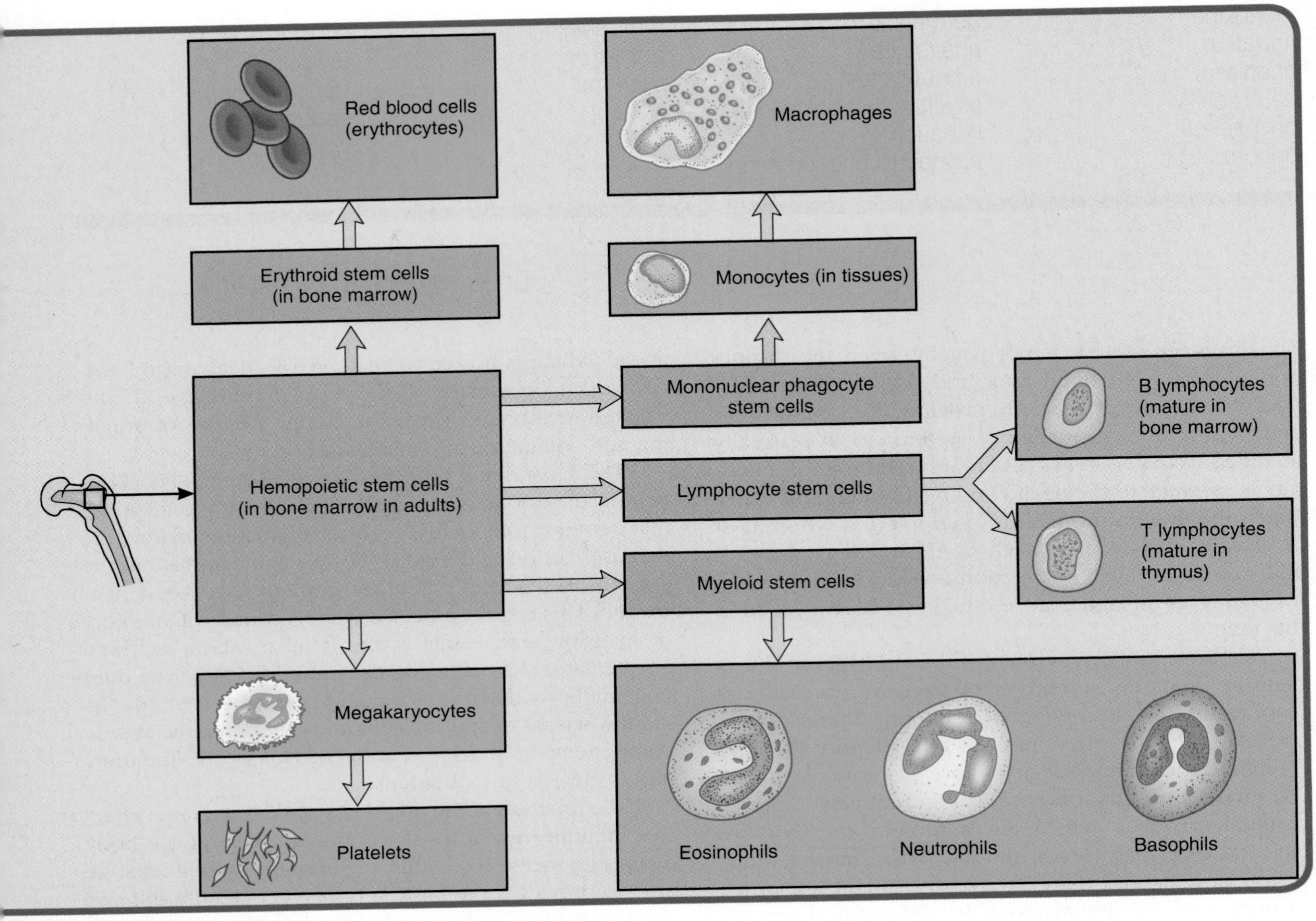

Figure 31–1: Origin of cells. *Delmar/Cengage Learning.*

basophils, develop from myeloid stem cells. One type of agranulocyte, the **lymphocyte**, develops from a lymphocyte stem cell into two major classes: B cells that mature in the bone marrow and T cells that mature in the **thymus**. A granulated cell means that it has granules within its cytoplasm. If no granules are present, the cell is agranulated. Mononuclear phagocyte stem cells become the **monocytes**.

Monocytes are immature cells that have little ability to fight infection. However, once they enter the tissue, they sometimes swell to as large as 80 micrometers, large enough to be seen by the naked eye. At this stage, they are called **macrophages** and are very effective at fighting infection. The most important function of macrophages is phagocytosis, the ability to engulf and destroy antigens. They can phagocytize as many as 100 bacteria and large organisms or cells, such as whole red blood cells and some parasites. Neutrophils are also phagocytic, but in addition, they carry granules of potent chemicals to destroy microorganisms. They can only engulf small particles, such as bacteria.

Neutrophils make up about 40% to 60% of all white blood cells. They are also known as segmentals (segs) and polymorphonuclear neutrophils (PMNs). They attack and destroy invading bacteria, viruses, and other antigens. Eosinophils make up about 2% to 3% of white blood cells. They are weak **phagocytes** when fighting common infections but are produced in large amounts in response to certain parasitic infections. A high number of eosinophils will be found when there is inflammation or an allergic reaction. Basophils release heparin and histamine, which are essential components of the inflammatory process. Eosinophils and basophils are also granulated cells. They release their chemicals onto harmful cells or microbes in their environment.

ORGANS OF THE IMMUNE SYSTEM

The organs of the immune system are located throughout the body and are generally known as lymphoidal organs because they are where lymphocytes develop, grow, and perform their functions. These organs include the bone marrow, the thymus, lymph nodes, spleen, tonsils, adenoids, appendix, and clumps of lymphoid tissue in the small intestine called Peyer's patches (Figure 31–2). The lymph tissue organs house large numbers of lymphocytes and are located strategically throughout the body. The lymph tissue in the Peyer's patches is exposed to antigens invading the intestinal tract. The lymph tissue of the tonsils and adenoids intercept antigens invading the upper respiratory tract. The tissues in the spleen and bone marrow are involved in fighting antigens that reach the blood vessels. When the B and T lymphocytes leave the bone marrow and the thymus, they travel throughout the body in the blood. They exit the capillaries and enter the **extracellular** fluid surrounding the cells to patrol the environment. As the lymph flows around the cells and through the body, it carries the lymphocytes, macrophages, and the antigens into the lymph capillaries and vessels. All along the lymphatic vessels are clusters of lymph nodes. A node functions somewhat like a filter. Immune cells and antigens enter the nodes through incoming afferent lymph vessels. Each node contains specialized compartments that store large numbers of B and T cells and others. The antigens are trapped and presented to the T cells for destruction (Figure 31–3). After the response is completed, the lymphocytes leave the lymph nodes in the outgoing efferent lymph vessels that eventually return them to the blood, where they begin the patrolling cycle once again.

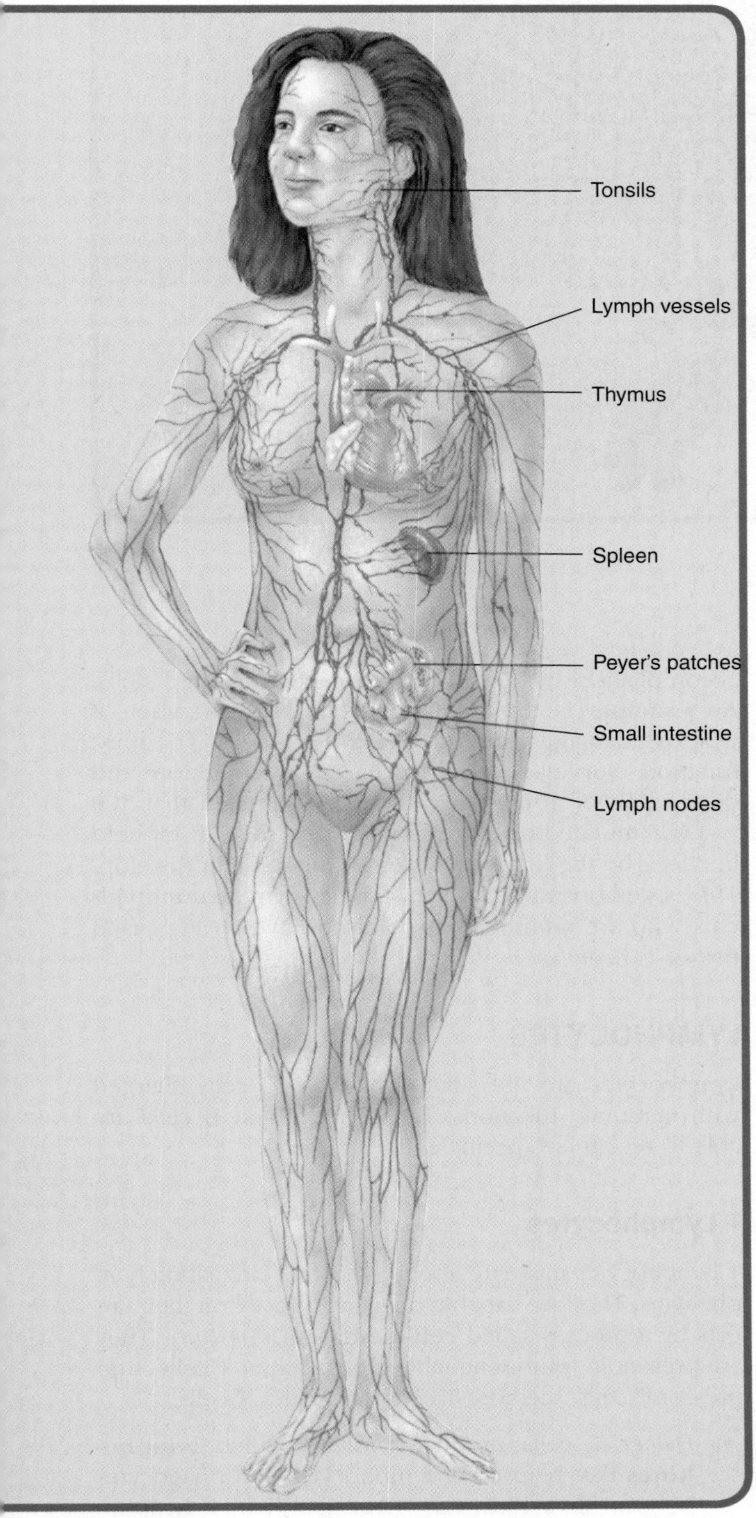

Figure 31–2: Organs of the immune system. *Delmar/Cengage Learning.*

Now that you know how lymph nodes function, it is easy to understand why they become swollen and tender during periods of infection. It is because of the increased amount of cellular activity within the nodes. In the same manner, when malignant cells break away from the primary tumor and begin to circulate in the lymph fluid, they become trapped in the nearest nodes. When the nodes cannot contain all the malignant cells, the cells are able to circulate to another body site and begin to produce another area of malignancy. This is known as metastasis. The amount of lymph node involvement is one of the criteria for determining the extent of the cancer. This assessment is called **staging** and is determined by the size of the tumor, the number of involved lymph nodes, and the metastatic progress. As an example, when a mastectomy is performed for breast cancer, the surgeon also removes the lymph nodes that drain from that area of the breast. The nodes are tested for cancer cells, and the results become one factor in determining the staging of the cancer and the plan of treatment.

MEDIA LINK

Go to the Premium Website and watch the animation, "The Immune System," for this chapter.

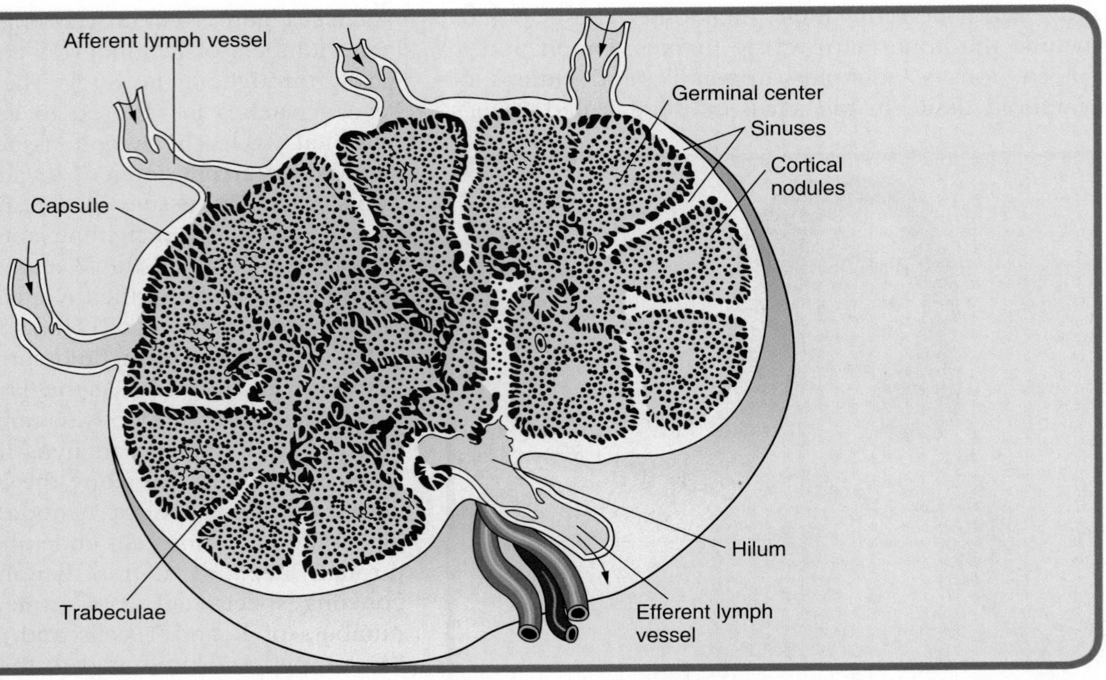

Figure 31–3: Lymph node. *Delmar/Cengage Learning.*

CELL MARKERS

Basic to the immune system is the ability of immune cells to determine initially the self or nonself status of encountered cells and molecules. All body cells carry molecules that are encoded by a group of genes known as the *major histocompatibility complex* (MHC). This is like a biochemical "fingerprint" that serves as the "ID" for cells so that they are marked as "self." This allows immune cells to recognize and communicate with each other. The body's immune defenses do not normally attack cells carrying this "self" marker. In addition, the millions of lymphocytes have approximately 100 million different surface receptor molecules that can "read" the surface patterns of virtually all nonself molecules that might invade the body. When they meet molecules carrying foreign markers, they move quickly to destroy them. Any nonself substance capable of triggering an immune response is considered to be an antigen. An antigen announces its foreignness by carrying different kinds of characteristic shapes called *epitopes,* which stick out from its surface. The immune system is capable of recognizing millions of these nonself molecules, or it can produce matching molecules that can counteract and destroy the antigen.

The MHC markers enable the immune system to achieve its function of recognizing self from nonself. The second function, homeostasis, involves the maintenance of the steady state of the system. This is accomplished by destroying damaged or dead cells. An example is the function of the spleen when it destroys damaged and dead red blood cells. The third function, surveillance, involves the recognition and destruction of abnormal cells. It is estimated that 100 to 1,000 mutated cells are formed every day. If not held in check by the immune system, cancer might develop. This is demonstrated by statistics showing that individuals who are immunocompromised have an increased risk of cancer.

LYMPHOCYTES

Lymphocytes are the small white blood cells charged with immunity functions. Both T cells and B cells are able to recognize specific antigen targets.

T Lymphocytes

T lymphocytes make up about 80% of all circulating lymphocytes. They are capable of acting directly on their targets by a process called **cell-mediated** *immunity*. They are present in four identifiable types: helper T cells, suppressor T cells, memory T cells, and killer T cells.

- *Helper* T cells produce proteins called **lymphokines** that help other lymphocytes and phagocytes perform their functions. They also help B lymphocytes make antibodies. Helper T cells are identifiable by the CD4+ cell marker. The HIV virus affects the function of the helper T cells, and the severity of the disease is measured by the CD4+ blood counts.

- *Suppressor T* cells stop or turn off the actions of the T cells when the "battle" is under control.
- *Killer T* cells can directly kill infected or malignant cells and those cells carrying a target antigen. They are also known as **cytotoxic** T cells and carry the CD8+ cell marker. One type of killer T cell can attach tightly to its target and secrete perforin and other chemicals, which make holes in the target cell's membrane, destroying it before it can reproduce. Unfortunately, killer T cells will also attack the nonself marker cells of transplant tissues and organs, causing rejection.
- *Memory T* cells have a memory from a previous experience with specific antigens and so are prepared to act immediately upon recontact.

B Lymphocytes

B lymphocytes represent about 20% of the total lymphocytes. They act upon their targets by producing antibodies in a process called humoral immunity. When B cells are maturing, they go through two stages of development. The first begins with the cell inserting numerous molecules of one specific kind of antibody into its cytoplasmic membrane. Each type of B lymphocyte is capable of making only one type of antibody, and only one specific antigen can activate it. There are about 100,000 antibodies on the cell membranes of B lymphocytes. These each have a "combining site" with specific characteristics that will match the same characteristic site on the surface of a specific antigen.

When B cells with their antibody molecules come into contact with antigens, they undergo a second change. When the combining site of a B cell's surface "fits" one of the variety of antigen's surface shapes, they join and are changed into an antigen-antibody complex, and the antibody begins to perform its duties. It causes the antigen to stick to other antigens, forming clumps so the large macrophages can destroy large numbers of them at one time.

It also causes the B cell to begin to divide, rapidly producing many clone cells with the same antibody. Later the cells divide into memory or plasma cells (Figure 31–4). The memory cells go to the lymph nodes to stand by for the next same-antigen invasion while the plasma cells continue to secrete millions of identical antibody molecules.

The immune system stockpiles a huge arsenal of cells, some for general defense, others for specific invaders. To be able to match millions of antigens, the system stores a few of each kind but can produce millions of the type to match the antigen within a very short period.

Antibodies

The antibodies from the B cells are protein substances belonging to a family of large molecules known as **immunoglobulins**. Five classes of human immunoglobulins have been identified and are classified by "Ig" for immunoglobin and a capital letter. The classes are: IgA, IgD, IgE, IgG, and IgM. Their presence in the body can be measured by a blood test called *serum protein electropheresis*. The role of antibodies is summarized in Table 31–1, which lists the antibody classes and key points of their function.

COMPLEMENT SYSTEM

Antibodies may change their shape slightly when they bind with antigens. This change will expose two regions called complement-binding sites. Complement is a group of about 20 *inactive* enzyme proteins normally present in the blood and involved in humoral immunity. When one complement protein meets an antibody-antigen complex, it will *activate* and begin a chain reaction of attracting the others to "complement" the activity of the antibodies in destroying bacteria. Complement proteins circulate in the blood in

TABLE 31–1 Antibody Class and Function

Class	Function
IgA	Concentrated in body fluids, such as tears, saliva, and respiratory and gastrointestinal secretions, to guard the entrances of the body
IgD	Located on B cell membranes. Believed to regulate B cell activity
IgE	Very effective against parasites but also involved in allergic responses, such as hayfever, asthma, and urticaria
IgG	The most plentiful antibody. It coats microorganisms in the tissues to speed up the uptake by other immune system cells. It carries out both antibacterial and antiviral activity. It can cross the placenta barrier.
IgM	Found in the bloodstream and very effective in killing bacteria. It is responsible for initial formation of antibodies once exposed to an antigen.

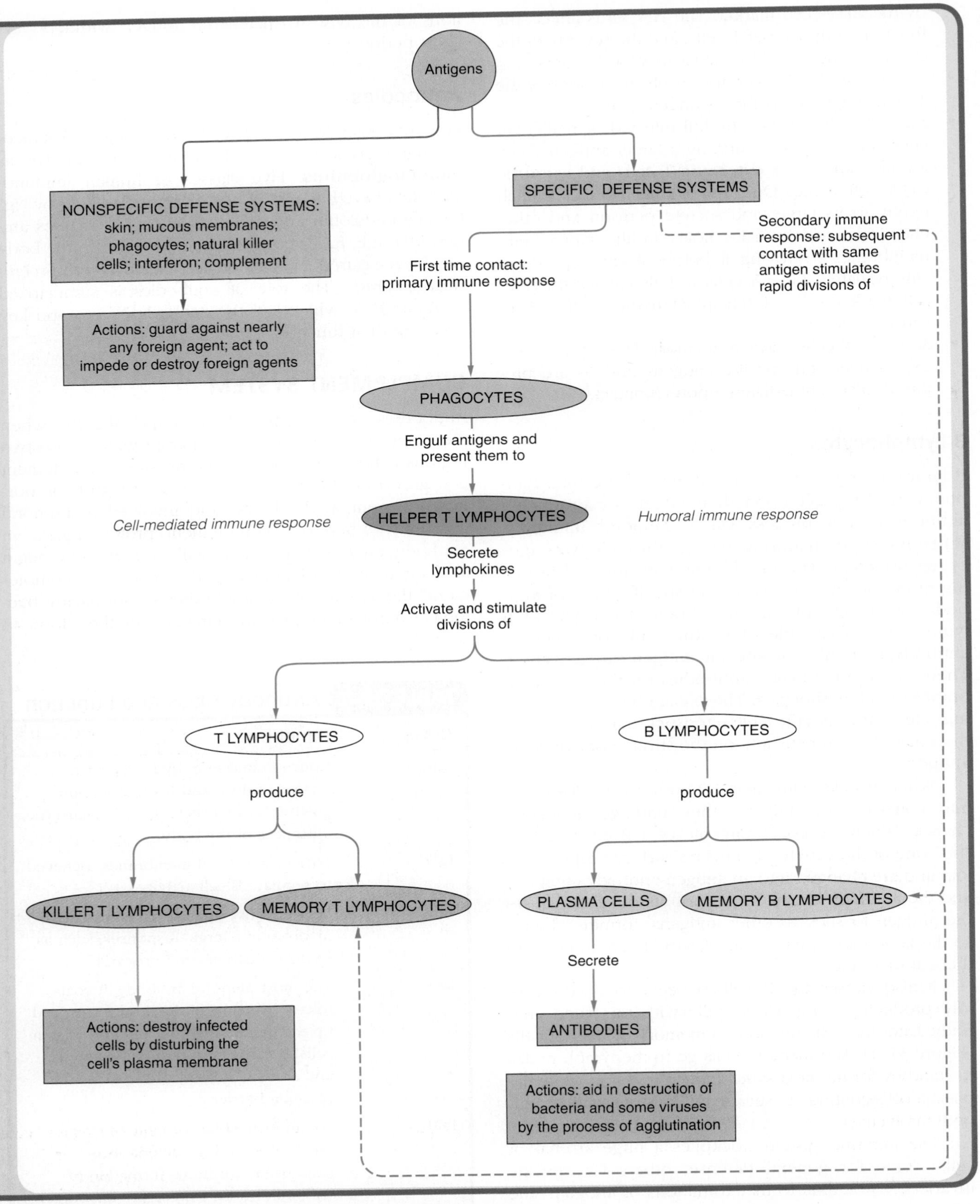

Figure 31–4: The body's defense mechanisms. *Delmar/Cengage Learning.*

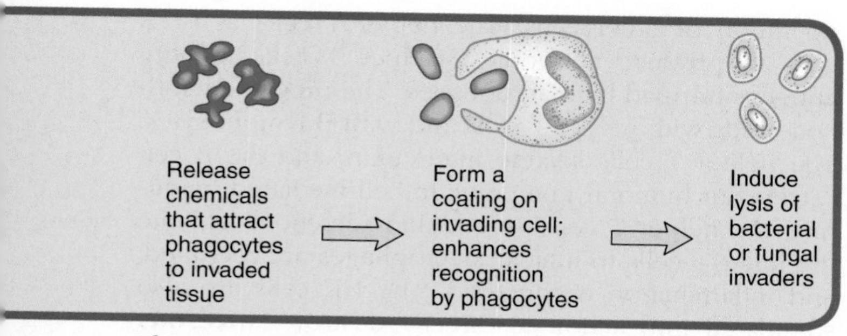

Figure 31–5: Function of proteins in the complement system. *Delmar/Cengage Learning.*

an inactive form. When the first of the complement substances is triggered—usually by an antibody interlocked with an antigen—it sets in motion a ripple effect. As each component is activated in turn, it acts upon the next in a precise sequence of carefully regulated steps known as the "complement cascade." This results in the creation of lethal chemicals to attract the phagocytes to the scene, coat the target cell to make it more recognizable, or destroy the antigen by puncturing its membrane. In this way, antibodies and the complement system work together to destroy antigens by the **antibody-mediated** response also known as **humoral** immunity (Figure 31–5).

Inflammation

The events set off by antibody-mediated response and the other chemicals help to develop an inflammatory response. When complement proteins begin to act, basophils and mast cells are also activated. Both cells release the substance called **histamine**, which dilates blood vessels, slowing down the rate of flow. The vessel walls become more **permeable,** which allows fluid to seep into the surrounding tissues. The result is localized warmth, redness, and swelling. The complement proteins and other factors in the fluid can easily leave the blood vessels and attract the phagocytes in the tissues to fight the intruders.

CYTOKINES

Cytokines are nonantibody proteins that regulate the immune response. These substances are diverse and potent chemical messengers. Cytokines produced by T cells are called *lymphokines*. Those produced by macrophages/monocytes are called **monokines**. Another group of cytokines are produced by both lymphocytes and macrophages/monocytes. Lymphokines bind to specific receptors on target cells and set off other actions, such as getting other cells and substances involved, encouraging cell growth, and stimulating macrophages. Two other cytokines are lymphotoxin from lymphocytes and tumor necrosis factor from macrophages. Both of these cytokines kill tumor cells. Many cytokines have been renamed as **interleukins** (IL), which means "messengers between leukocytes." IL-1 from macrophages helps to activate B and T cells. IL-2 is produced by antigen-activated T cells and promotes rapid growth of mature B and T cells and the development of different types of T cells. There are six types of interleukins identified at present.

Some of the first cytokines discovered were **interferons**. They are produced by T cells, macrophages, and some cells outside the immune system. Interferons are a family of proteins that can fight viruses. Interferon from immune cells activates macrophages. The cytokine called tumor necrosis factor, which also comes from macrophages, kills tumor cells and inhibits parasites and viruses. Scientists have genetically engineered genes with cytokines to attack cancer cells. The tumor necrosis factor is measured to determine the effects of chemotherapy on certain cancers.

A summary of the 14 groups of cytokines is included in the Components of the Immune System, a color-treated section of the text following the discussion on immune response.

Natural Killer (NK) Cells

Natural killer (NK) cells are non-T and non-B lymphocytes. NK cells are numerous in the bloodstream and the reticuloendothelial system. (The tissue macrophages and phagocytes in the blood and lymph.) NK cells kill cancer cells and cells infected with viruses without using antibodies or having prior exposure to the antigen. Like the killer T cell, they contain granules filled with potent chemicals. They bind to their targets and deliver a lethal burst of their chemicals to produce holes in the target cell's membrane, leading to its destruction. NK cells get the name "natural" because they do not need to recognize a specific antigen like other T cells in order to kill the invading antigen. The killing function of NK cells can be boosted by the administration of alpha interferon (a cytokine, nonantibody protein that is produced by T cells). Treatment with alpha interferon is used for many types of cancer, including chronic myelogenous leukemia and renal cell cancer, to increase the ability of NK cells to kill the cancer cells.

IMMUNE RESPONSES

The organs of the immune system, immune cells, cell markers, complement system, and related activities have been discussed. It is time to put it all together in an immune response as it would occur in the body.

The immune response system has two branches, one resulting from B cell activity, the humoral or antibody-mediated immune response, and one resulting from T cell activity, the cell-mediated immune response (review Figure 31-4). The response can also be primary when it is the first encounter with the antigen or a secondary response with subsequent encounters.

Primary Humoral (Antibody-Mediated) Response

In primary humoral response, an antigen enters the body and goes undetected past "virgin" desensitized B cells until it meets one with matching antibody sites. The B cell connects (becomes sensitized) and processes the antigen to attract helper T cells. When the sensitized B cell and the helper T combine, interleukins are released, which cause the cell to begin mitosis. At the same time, other similar antigens have been engulfed by the macrophages. Helper T cells bind with the macrophages, and interleukins are secreted. The secretion of interleukin stimulates the helper T cells to mature and secrete lymphokines to cause a rapid growth and division of the B cells. Some of the differentiated B cells become plasma cells and release identical antibodies in order to bind with more antigens for recognition and destruction. Some B cells convert to memory B cells. They do not produce antibodies at the time of the initial exposure, but they "remember" the encounter until the next exposure to the same antigen.

The immunoglobulins get other cells and substances involved. IgM and IgG activate macrophages and the complement system. IgE stimulates mast cells to release histamine. IgA causes secretions in the first line of defense in the saliva, tears, lungs, and intestines to protect the body's entrances. IgD works in the cell's membranes to regulate activity. A full primary immune response requires five to six days to develop.

Humoral antibody-mediated responses act against bacteria and extracellular viruses, fungi, and parasites. They *cannot* react to an invader already within a cell's cytoplasm, only those in circulation or attached to a cell's surface.

Secondary Response

In a secondary response, the reaction is much faster, taking only two to three days. This is possible because left-over **clonal** lymphocytes with memory are able to attack the antigen. Once one of the cells meets the same antigen, mitosis is immediate, and large numbers of appropriately matched cells and antibodies are produced to destroy the antigen.

Primary Cell-Mediated Response

Primary response of T cells in cell-mediated response is both quick and direct. Some T cells are vital to the operation of other cells. The helper T cells assist B cells to produce antibodies. Helper T cells identify antigens trapped by macrophages. The processed antigen binds with helper T cells and with B lymphocytes. The helper T cells secrete interleukin, and the B cell carries out humoral immunity. In cell-mediated immunity, the helper T cells' interleukin secretions activate the killer T cells to attack. Macrophages are recruited, and inflammation is triggered. The NK cells are also stimulated into action to directly destroy **cancerous** and virus-infected cells before they can divide and begin growing.

Some T cells will also develop memory and are held in reserve for subsequent invasions. Cell-mediated immune responses attack **intracellular** viruses, fungi and protozoans, cancer cells, and transplant tissue cells.

Killer cells that cause rejection of organ transplants do so because the MHC markers of the donor cells are not identical self-markers unless they are from an identical twin. Individuals who are to receive organs are given drugs to destroy the killer T cells to prevent rejection; however, that leaves the recipient without the ability to have a full immune response to other invaders and can lead to death from infections such as pneumonia.

Both antibody-mediated and cell-mediated immune responses are controlled reactions. When the "battle" is won, the binding sites are saturated with antibodies, and the **suppressor** T cells stop the attack. Without this feedback, immune reactions would go out of control.

The complexity of the immune system makes it very difficult to understand. The two features on the following pages provide summaries, one of the components and another of the surveillance process, to make the immune system a little clearer. This material is taken from a presentation by Elaine Glass, RN, MS, OCN; Clinical Nurse Specialist in Medical Oncology and Hematology. She explains the functions of the components of the immune system and relates them to the familiar roles of a police and military force (shown in italics). The cell-mediated responses are the duties of the police, whereas the antibody response is the job of the army. There is even one firefighter who is involved. Note that there are also statements in italics and parentheses concerning emotions, exercise, and personal interactions and their effect upon the immune system. This connection is now being recognized as important and as evidence of the impact of diet. Because these effects are often based on multiple and difficult to measure factors and usually cover long periods, studies require long-term commitments from participants and extended time to identify and validate apparent cause and effect relationships in the development of disease.

COMPONENTS OF THE IMMUNE SYSTEM

AGRANULOCYTES

A. Macrophages/Monocytes

The cop on the beat

Monocytes circulate in the blood; macrophages infiltrate the tissues. They engulf antigens and summon other cells to analyze them.

(Stress causes release of cortisol that renders the macrophage unresponsive.

Exercise increases endorphins [natural brain analgesic], which may increase macrophage activity.)

B. Lymphocytes

A collective label for T and B immune cells

1. T CELLS
   Involved in the cellular immune system response. Mature in the thymus gland.
   a. Helper T cell
      The detective
      Identifies the antigens trapped by macrophages or monocytes and stimulates other cells to destroy them. Does not attack or destroy by itself.
   b. Activated helper T cell
      Helps destroy identified antigens by producing interleukin-2, which stimulates other helper and killer T cells to multiply.
   c. Killer T cell
      SWAT team member
      Destroys cells that have been invaded by antigens. They can trigger a process that punctures a cell membrane and destroys it before the invading virus inside has a chance to grow.
   d. Natural killer T cell
      Rambo or a vigilante
      Attacks cancerous or virus-infected cells without previous exposure to the antigen. NKs are stimulated by interferon. They can recognize artificial antigens created in a lab to which humans have never come into contact.
      (In one study, patients with a lot of support from their "significant others" and doctors had higher levels of NK cells.)
   e. Suppressor T cell
      The police chief
      Slows down or stops other immune cell activity after antigens are destroyed.
2. B CELLS
   Produces antibodies against antigens; involved in the humoral immune response.
   a. Plasma cell
      The army sergeant
      Descends from B cells to produce antibodies. They make thousands of antibodies per second.
   b. Antibodies
      The foot soldiers
      Proteins that neutralize antigens and destroy other cells where the antigen has invaded.
      1) IgG
         The most common protein antibody in the blood and tissue spaces, where it coats antigens, speeding their uptake by other immune cells.
      2) IgM
         A protein antibody that circulates in the bloodstream in star-shaped clusters; very effective in killing bacteria.
      3) IgA
         A protein antibody in body fluids (tears, saliva, respiratory and digestive tracts) to guard body entrances.
         (College students who watched a video of Mother Teresa had higher levels of IgG and IgA than students who watched a video that did not stimulate positive emotions.)
      4) IgE
         A protein antibody that attaches itself to mast cells and basophils. When it encounters its matching antigen, it stimulates the cell to pour out its contents. It provides protection by coating bacteria and viruses.
      5) IgD
         A protein antibody that inserts itself into the membrane of the B cell to regulate the activation of the cell.
   c. Complement
      Flying Aces
      A series of 20 proteins that circulate in the blood in an inactive state until they are triggered by contact with antigen-antibody complexes or by contact with the cell membrane of an invading organism.

T cells = Police chief with a history on the force
B cells = Army sergeant with a history in the service

T and B cells that have been activated by an antigen and continue to circulate within the body, ready to attack an antigen if it reinvades. (These cells are the basis of how vaccines work.)

GRANULOCYTES

A group of immune cells filled with granules of toxic chemicals that enable them to digest microorganisms.

A. Neutrophil

Like cop on beat but more heavily armed

A circulating WBC that destroys foreign matter and cell debris by phagocytosis, by digesting cellular membranes, and by releasing chemotactants and pyrogenic substances that cause a fever.

B. Basophil

A firefighter

A circulating WBC that is responsible for allergy symptoms by releasing heparin, histamine, bradykinin, and serotonin from its granules, to cause vasodilation and permeability.

C. Eosinophil

A circulating WBC that can digest microorganisms, especially parasites, and assists in allergic reactions by detoxifying some of the inflammation-inducing substances to prevent the spread of the local inflammatory process.

D. Mast cells

Special member of police force that is armed with chemicals.

Special cells found in tissues that contain granules of chemicals that produce redness, warmth, and swelling (allergy symptoms).

CYTOKINES

All nonantibody proteins that regulate the immune response. Cytokines produced by T cells are called *lymphokines*. Cytokines produced by macrophages/monocytes are called *monokines*.

A. Lymphokines

A number of proteins produced by T cells

1. Granulocyte-macrophage colony-stimulating factor (GM-CSF)

   GM-CSF stimulates the growth of neutrophils, eosinophils, and macrophages. It increases the ingestion of bacteria and the killing of tumors coated with antibody. It activates mature granulocytes and macrophages.

2. Interferons

   A class of lymphokines with important immunoregulatory functions, especially improving the activities of macrophages and NK cells. *Exercise may increase the production of interferon.*

   a. Alpha (IFN-α)

      Is produced by leukocytes in response to viral infections. It also increases NK activity and the numbers of cytotoxic T cells and starts the tumoricidal activity of macrophages.

   b. Beta (IFN-β)

      Its activity is similar to IFN-α.

   c. Gamma (IFN-γ)

      Is produced by T and NK cells. It (1) activates killer T cells; (2) increases the ability of B cells to produce antibodies; (3) keeps macrophages at the site; and (4) assists them in digesting bacteria and cancerous cells they engulf. IFN-γ also regulates other lymphokines, increases NK activity, and starts the production of T cell suppressor factor.

3. IL-2 (Interleukin-2)

   Is produced by helper T cells and NK cells, which stimulates other helper, killer, and suppressor T cells to multiply. It starts cytokine production by T cells and monocytes. It improves NK cell activity.

4. IL-3

   Is produced by activated T cells. It is a growth factor for mast cells and most bone marrow progenitor (after stem) cells.

5. IL-4

   Is called B cell growth factor and causes B cells, mast cells, and resting T cells to multiply. It increases toxicity of killer T cells and macrophages. It is produced by helper T cells.

6. IL-5

   Is produced by activated T cells. It is an important factor in the final differentiation of eosinophils and activated B cells. It increases IgA, IgM, and IgE development and secretion. It begins the appearance of IL-2 receptors on B cells.

7. Soluble immune response suppressor (SIRS)

   SIRS is released by suppressor T cells and may slow down immune cell activity.

B. Monokines

Proteins produced primarily by monocytes

1. Granulocyte colony-stimulating factor (G-CSF)

   G-CSF stimulates the growth and activity of neutrophils. It is produced by monocytes and some other nonblood cells.

2. Macrophage colony-stimulating factor (M-CSF)

   M-CSF stimulates the growth and activity of macrophages. It is also produced by monocytes and other nonblood cells.

   (GM-CSF, G-CSF, IL2, and interferon are now produced synthetically and are being used as anticancer drugs. They have shown promise in the treatment of some types of malignancies.)

C. Other cytokines

(Produced by both lymphocytes and macrophages/monocytes)

1. IL-1

   Is produced by macrophages, T cells, granulocytes, and NK cells. It activates helper T cells and raises the body's temperature. (Fever increases immune cell activity). It stimulates the production of lymphokines and activates macrophages to immobilize cancer cells. It starts the differentiation of stem cells and activated B cells and increases the number of activated B cells. Exercise may increase IL-1 production.

2. IL-6 (B cell differentiation factor)

   Is called BCDF and causes some B cells to stop dividing and to start making immunoglobin and antibodies. Improves the differentiation of killer T cells. Is produced by helper T cells, monocytes, and fibroblasts. It also stimulates the production of platelets.

3. Tumor growth factor-beta (TGF-β)

   TGF-β is produced by T cells, macrophages, and tumor cells. It suppresses T and B cell growth and differentiation and antibody secretion.

4. Tumor necrosis factor-B (TNF-B)

   TNF-B, also known as lymphotoxin, is produced by B cells, T cells, mast cells, and macrophages. It makes some cells more vulnerable to lysis by NK cells.

5. Tumor necrosis factor (TNF)

   TNF is produced by monocytes, activated macrophages, NK cells, and mast cells. It can kill tumors or retard their growth. It causes some tumors to bleed and die. It stimulates the production of lymphokines and activates macrophages.

By now, you must be amazed at the complexity and function of the immune system. The previous outline of the duties of its components causes one to wonder how all that coordinated effort ever gets accomplished. And yet, so much more is not understood.

To give a brief overall picture of what happens when an immune system cell comes into contact with an antigen, consider the box to the right and on the next page. In italics within parentheses are descriptions of the cartoon slides Glass uses to summarize her discussion of the surveillance process of the immune system. She again uses the police and military roles in the scenarios. If you can visualize the scene, it may help you to get an understanding of the immune process.

IMMUNE SYSTEM SURVEILLANCE PROCESS

1. A macrophage (or complement protein, NK cell, or memory cell) recognizes an antigen (alien).
   (A cop begins to struggle with an alien.)
2. Helper T cells bind to the macrophage and become activated by the cytokine, IL-1, which also causes a fever.
   (The detective sees the cop and alien struggling and calls for help.)
3. Activated helper T cells produce a lymphokine, IL-2, which stimulates other helper and killer T cells to multiply.
   (Help arrives as detectives, SWAT team, and a few army sergeants.)
4. Helper T cells also secrete a lymphokine, IL-4, which causes B cells to multiply.
   (The detective decides more army personnel are needed and calls in the troops. The army comes marching in.)
5. Helper T cells also secrete a lymphokine, IL-6, which causes some B cells to stop dividing and start making antibodies.
   (The sergeant calls the foot soldiers into duty.)
6. Helper T cells also produce the lymphokine interferon, which activates killer T cells, increases the ability of B cells to produce antibodies, and keeps macrophages at the site and assists them in digesting the cells they engulf.
   (The detective calls out words of encouragement to the SWAT team, the sergeants, and the street cops.)
7. Killer T cells destroy the cells where antigens have invaded.
   (The SWAT team member nails an alien inside a phone booth.)
8. Antibodies neutralize the antigen and destroy other cells that have also been infected.
   (A foot soldier punches out an alien.)
9. Complement proteins, triggered by antigen-antibody complexes, or the cell membranes of some invading microorganisms:
   (The flying aces come into the action.)
   - Cause movement of macrophages and neutrophils to the area. *(An ace calls in the street cop.)*
   - Increase phagocytosis by macrophages and neutrophils. *(The street cops look mean and ugly.)*
   - Activate basophils and mast cells to release immobilizing chemicals and other products that increase inflammation. *(The firefighters and cops with chemicals soak the aliens.)*

- Change the invader's cell surface, causing them to stick together. *(The aliens get stuck.)*
- Attack the invader's structure and make it inactive. *(The aces crop-dust the aliens.)*
- Rupture the invader's cell membrane. *(The ace's gunner blows a hole through the alien.)*

10. Suppressor T cells halt the immune response after the antigen is destroyed. *(The police chief enters the scene and halts the action once the aliens are destroyed.)*
11. Memory T and B cells are left in the blood and lymph system to defend against another attack. *(The detectives and the army sergeants have the alien's ID in case future attacks occur.)*

Note: Scientists have made great progress in understanding the functions of the many components of the immune system, but a great deal still remains a mystery. It is an unbelievably complicated interaction of cells, antibodies, and proteins against antigens and allergens. Recently, it has been recognized that the brain, nervous system, and hormones also have a relationship with the immune response. A new science called **psychoneuroimmunology** involves researching the connection between the brain, behavior, and immunity. Scientists have discovered that the brain produces over 50 neuropeptides that have receptors on WBCs and can affect the cell's activity. For example, people who feel hopeless have sluggish macrophages. Laughter increases NK activity, lymphocyte proliferation, migration of monocytes, and the production of IL-2 and IgA. It would seem we may have the power to influence our own immune system if we can learn how.

IMMUNIZATION

With the knowledge of immune reactions, it is easy to understand how immunizations (shots) and vaccinations provide protection against antigens. The smallpox **vaccine**, for instance, was the deliberate introduction of the smallpox antigen into the body in a state that caused only minor reaction but was sufficient for the body to produce an antigen-antibody complex and eventually memory cells against the disease. Other examples of purposeful antigen introduction are measles, mumps, diphtheria, poliovirus, varicella, hepatitis A and B, pneumonia, pertussis, and tetanus toxoid (given routinely to infants and children).

Vaccines are given in initial and in "booster" doses to provide memory cells and antibodies for longer periods. These methods provide active immunity because the recipients make their own immunity. Another form is known as passive immunity and is given to people already exposed to a disease, such as tetanus. Antibodies from another source are injected into the person to provide a temporary immunity to counter the immediate attack of pathogens. This immunity is short lived. The tetanus antitoxin given after certain injuries or animal bites is an example of this type of vaccine.

DISEASES AND DISORDERS

Acquired Immunodeficiency Syndrome (AIDS) (I-mu-no-de-fish′-en-se)

Description—**Acquired immunodeficiency syndrome (AIDS)** is a worldwide epidemic caused by the human immunodeficiency virus (HIV). The term AIDS refers to the most advanced stages of HIV infection. It is estimated that there are 60 million people in the world living with HIV infection. The AIDS epidemic is greatest in sub-Saharan Africa. In Zimbabwe the prevalence is estimated at 20% of the population. The impact is great on the work force and families, especially the large number of orphans. In South Africa in 2004, over one in five teachers between 25 and 34 years of age were HIV positive. The epidemic has slowed somewhat from 1.5 million new HIV infections per year in the 1990s to 1.1 million for the next three years.

Globally, HIV prevalence is still increasing over time as the epidemic spreads to different countries. Data are very difficult to obtain in developing countries due to lack of contact with the medical community and ineffective means of collection. Also, intense and even life-threatening stigma and discrimination in some cultures leads to denial and underreporting.

The Joint United Nations Program on HIV/AIDS maintains data on global infection. In 2008, it was estimated that since first diagnosed, 60 million people have acquired HIV with 25 million having died. For 2008 alone, estimates are 33.4 million people living with HIV, with 2.7 million new cases and 2.0 million deaths due to AIDS. There were 430,000 children born with AIDS in 2008. It is easy to see why AIDS is considered an epidemic.

The beginning of AIDS in the United States is well documented. Between October 1980 and May 1981, five young, previously healthy homosexual men were treated for a pneumonia caused by *Pneumocystis carinii*. They were treated at three different hospitals in Los Angeles. Doctors and health care professionals were curious because usually *P. carinii* pneumonia occurred only in immunosuppressed patients, especially those receiving cancer therapy. At the same time, a rare and unusual blood vessel malignancy called Kaposi's sarcoma was being diagnosed with increasing frequency in young homosexuals in California and New York (Figure 31–6). By July 1981, 26 cases of Kaposi's sarcoma had been diagnosed. Seven of these men also had serious infections; four had *P. carinii* pneumonia. These cases were an early indication of an epidemic of a previously unknown disease. Later it was called the acquired immunodeficiency syndrome, or AIDS.

In 2008, a total of 1,073,128 cases were reported with 851,974 being male and 211,804 female, with 9349 cases being children younger 13 years of age. The number of adult deaths during this time was 571,453 or about 67% of those infected. Deaths among children were 4931 or about 53%.

The data in Tables 31–2, 31–3 and 31–4 are adapted from CDC HIV/AIDS Surveillance Report: HIV Infection and AIDS in the United States, 2008.

The incidence of AIDS varies considerably by race and ethnicity. The CDC tracks information on seven groups of people. Table 31–2 list the estimated cases of AIDS in the United States for 2008 and the cumulative numbers through 2008.

Table 31–3 lists the estimated cumulative AIDS cases by age. Observe that a very large number of patients, 809,830 (approximately 75%), are younger than 45 years old. This translates into a lifelong battle against the disease for a lot of people. It also translates into billions of dollars needed for their care.

The Centers for Disease Control and Prevention estimated at the end of 2006 that 1,106,400 persons in the United States were living with HIV/AIDS, and another 21% were undiagnosed and unaware of their HIV infection.

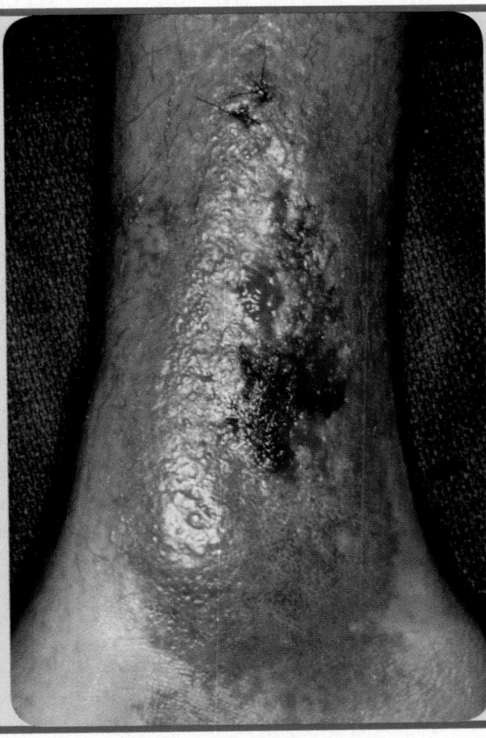

Figure 31–6: Typical skin lesions of Kaposi's sarcoma.
CDC/Dr. Steve Kraus.

Table 31–2 Estimated Number of AIDS Cases in 2008 by Race or Ethnicity

Race or Ethnicity	Estimated # of AIDS Diagnoses 2008	Cumulative Estimate # AIDS Diagnoses Through 2008
American Indian/Alaska Native	199	3,741
Asian	525	8,253
Black/African American	18,328	452,916
Hispanic/Latino	7,043	180,061
Native Hawaiian/Other Pacific Islanders	51	830
White	10,570	419,905
Multiple Races	435	7,054

Table 31–3 Estimated Number of AIDS Cases by Age in 2008

Age	New AIDS Cases in 2008	Number of AIDS Cases, through 2008 (Estimated)
<13	41	9349
13–14	48	1,220
15–19	497	6,685
20–24	1,976	40,735
25–29	3,616	125,755
30–34	4,461	209,554
35–39	5,719	229,111
40–44	6,683	187,421
45–49	5,920	121,111
50–54	3,946	68,560
55–59	2,242	36,987
60–64	1,140	19,669
65	862	16,972

Etiology—AIDS is an infectious disease caused by the human immunodeficiency virus (HIV), which renders the body's immune system ineffective. The virus has been found in many body fluids but survives well only in those with numerous WBCs, such as in blood, semen, and vaginal secretions. The virus invades the helper

T cells and macrophages, hiding within their membranes. Because both stimulate one another at different times in the immune response, when the helper Ts are "disabled," they do not cause the macrophages to act, which results in the diversion of B cell antibody production and the absence of NK cell formation. HIV is a **retrovirus**: its genetic material is RNA instead of DNA. It wraps itself in components from the host helper T cell membrane. Once inside the host, an enzyme uses the viral RNA as a "pattern" for making DNA and inserts these new instructions into the host's chromosome.

The virus hides in the cells for months or even years. It is difficult to determine its average or maximum incubation period. The onset of AIDS following infection with the HIV virus has been observed from as little as six months to as many as 10 years or more. The average onset of symptoms of AIDS appears to be 10 years. At some time, the body makes a secondary response, and the infected cells are activated. They copy their new DNA with the viral RNA, and new virus particles are assembled. They form "buds" on the helper T cell membrane and separate. This process continues until the helper T cells are depleted and the immune system is destroyed, leaving the person vulnerable to opportunistic infections that may eventually cause death.

The HIV virus requires certain conditions to be able to transfer to a new host. Avoiding these situations will decrease the risk of becoming infected. The virus can be transmitted by the following methods:

- Unprotected sex with an infected partner. **Transmission** can occur through the vagina, vulva, rectum, penis, and mouth during sex.
- Sharing drug needles or syringes with a person infected with HIV.
- Women with HIV can transmit the virus to their babies during pregnancy, birth, and breastfeeding. Twenty-five to thirty-three percent of infected mothers will transmit the infection to their babies. (The medication AZT [zidovudine] and delivery by cesarean section can significantly reduce the transmission rate.)
- The risk of getting HIV from blood transfusions is extremely low. All blood in the United States is screened for HIV.
- The risk to health care professionals of obtaining HIV from accidental needle sticks and contact with blood and body fluids are eliminated by following protective standard precautions when providing care.

Table 31–4 identifies the method of contact for the estimated number of cases of AIDS in 2008. At best these are estimates, because there is a considerable lapse of time between exposure and development of AIDS.

Table 31–4 Estimated Number of AIDS Cases by Exposure Category in 2008

Exposure Category	Male	Female	Total
Male-to-male sexual contact	17,758	—	17,758
Injection drug use	3,555	2,256	5,811
Male-to-male sexual contact and injection drug use	1,704	—	1,704
Heterosexual contact	4,301	7,112	11,413
Other (includes hemophilia, blood transfusion, perinatal, and risk not reported)	225	199	424

There are some people who fear that HIV can be transmitted in other ways, but it has not been proven by research. The most common misconceptions are:

- Casual contact with an infected person through sharing food utensils, towels, toilet, telephones, bedding, or swimming pools.
- Closed-mouth kissing. The CDC does recommend eliminating open-mouth kissing, although the risk is very low.
- Mosquitoes, bedbugs, or other biting insects.
- Tattooing and body piercing could theoretically transmit the virus if the open skin area comes into contact with the organism or if contaminated instruments are used. There have been no instances of HIV transmission in the United States from either activity.

Early signs and symptoms—Many people who are infected with the virus do not have any symptoms when first infected. Within a month or two after exposure, however, they may have a flulike illness that includes headache, fever, fatigue, and enlarged lymph nodes. The symptoms usually subside within a week. During this flulike period, the HIV virus is present in high concentrations in genital fluids, and infected persons are highly contagious.

Later signs and symptoms—Severe symptoms of HIV infection may not appear for 10 or more years in adults and two or more years in children. However, during this asymptomatic period, the infected person is still capable of passing on the virus, and the T helper cells are being systematically destroyed. The numbers decline (as measured by the CD4 [T4] counts) and infections and other symptoms begin to occur, such as:

- Enlarged lymph nodes
- Fatigue
- Pelvic inflammatory disease
- Fever, sweats
- Weight loss
- Yeast infections
- Rashes, dry skin
- Short-term memory loss

Late signs and symptoms of AIDS—The signs and symptoms of AIDS are related to the effects of infections and cancer.

The presence of the opportunistic infections, such as *Pneumocystis carinii pneumonia,* are indicated by a fever, cough, and difficulty breathing; by *Kaposi's sarcoma,* a form of cancer appearing as purplish blotches on the skin (see Figure 31–6); by *candidiasis,* a yeast infection that is sometimes present in the mouth, esophagus, and vagina; and by the usual infections. There are over 20 opportunistic infections that people with AIDS may experience, such as other forms of pneumonia, meningitis, encephalitis, esophagitis, persistent diarrhea, and skin inflammation. These are often resistant to treatment. About 60% of AIDS patients have neurologic symptoms, including motor problems, inability to concentrate, memory loss, and progressive mental deterioration. They are believed to be caused by brain infection or cancer.

Diagnosis of HIV Infections

Early HIV infection usually has no signs or symptoms; therefore, it can only be detected by a blood test or by testing saliva. Blood tests detect antigens found on the virus or detect antibodies made against HIV. The antibodies may not be detectable for one to four months after infection, and it may be as long as six months before enough antibodies are present in the blood to test positive.

There are two different tests for HIV antibodies, the *ELISA* (enzyme-linked immunosorbent assay) and the *Western blot.* A general guideline used is if the ELISA test is reactive, it is repeated two more times. If it is positive three times, a Western blot test is performed. The Western blot is used to confirm the diagnosis because a small number of ELISA tests may show a false positive. Another test called the Coulter HIV-p24 Antigen Assay can detect the presence of HIV antigens. In the clinical setting, it is used when patients are highly suspected to be positive but show negative tests on both the ELISA and Western blot tests.

Home testing for HIV is available and is increasing the process of testing, primarily because it protects the patient's identity. Some tests use a blood sample, whereas another, called the Orasure, uses a treated cotton pad to collect an oral sample between the gum and cheek.

Physicians can now predict the risk of HIV progressing to AIDS by monitoring the HIV virus levels in the blood. The test is based on studies that have shown that higher levels of the virus in the blood correlate with an increased risk of the disease progressing to AIDS and AIDS-related infection or death.

Diagnosis of AIDS

The CDC diagnosis for AIDS requires a positive confirmed test for HIV and at least one of the following:

- CD4 count less than 200 per cubic millimeter of blood or a CD4 count of less than 14% of the total number of lymphocytes. The CD4 count measures the number of helper T lymphocytes.
- The presence of an **opportunistic** infection, such as pneumocystis pneumonia.
- An AIDS-related cancer, a severe wasting, or dementia.

Table 31–5 lists the clinical conditions in patients that indicate AIDS.

AIDS Prevention

AIDS can be prevented by practicing personal measures to protect oneself. The disease is contracted primarily through contact with an infected person's blood, semen, or vaginal secretions. The virus enters through the vagina, penis, rectum, or mouth (in oral sex). The safest lifestyle is sexual **abstinence** or a faithful **monogamous** relationship. If these conditions are not absolutely certain, then precautions must be taken.

1. Avoid high-risk sexual activities. Behaviors that may cause you to acquire the virus are very clear:
   - Having unprotected sex, homosexual or heterosexual, with an HIV-infected person (oral, vaginal, or anal).
   - Using IV drugs and sharing needles.
   - Having many sexual partners; risk increases with number of partners.
   - Having other sexually transmitted diseases, such as gonorrhea, syphilis, or genital herpes.
2. Use a latex condom *properly* to maintain a barrier to the transmission of the virus. It must stay intact and be in place from the beginning to the end of vaginal, anal, or oral sex. The use of a spermicide provides additional protection. The condom must be carefully removed and disposed of properly. Condoms must never be reused.

Treatment—Unfortunately, no vaccine, antitoxin, or drug "cures" AIDS. In 1981, when AIDS was first diagnosed in the United States, there were no effective

Table 31–5 Clinical Conditions in Patients with AIDS

AIDS Indicator Diseases
Opportunistic Infections
Candidiasis: bronchi, esophageal, trachea, lungs
Coccidiomycosis
Cryptococcosis, extrapulmonary
Cryptosporidiosis, chronic intestinal greater than one month in duration
Cytomegalovirus, other than liver, spleen, or nodes
Cytomegalovirus retinitis with loss of vision
Disseminated histoplasmosis
Herpes simplex: chronic ulcers more than one month in duration or bronchitis, pneumonitis, or esophagitis
HIV encephalopathy
Isosporiasis, chronic
Mycobacterium avium complex or *M. kansasii*, disseminated or extrapulmonary
Mycobacterium of other species
Pneumocystis carinii pneumonia
Pneumonia, recurrent in 12-month period
Progressive multifocal leukoencephalopathy
Salmonella septicemia
Toxoplasmosis of the brain
Tuberculosis, extrapulmonary
Tuberculosis, pulmonary
AIDS-Related Cancers
Burkitt's lymphoma
Immunoblastic lymphoma
Lymphoma, primary brain
Invasive cervical cancer
Kaposi's sarcoma
Other
HIV wasting syndrome

medications to treat the disease. A number of medications to treat HIV infection have been approved by the Food and Drug Administration (FDA). The virus can become resistant to any of these drugs; therefore, combinations of medications are used. All medications and combinations used to treat HIV have numerous side effects, including bone marrow suppression, nausea, and nerve damage. The side effects decrease the individual's compliance to taking the medications.

Medications to Treat HIV and AIDS

The following medications are used to treat HIV and AIDS.

- *Nucleoside reverse transcriptase (RT) inhibitors*—These drugs were the first to be approved to treat HIV infection. They are incorporated into the DNA of HIV and stop the building process. They can slow the spread of HIV and delay the onset of opportunistic infections. Examples are AZT (zidovudine or ZDV), ddl (didanosine), and d4T (stavudine).
- *Non-nucleoside reverse transcription inhibitors (NNRTIs)*—These drugs prevent HIV replication by inhibiting a viral protein. Examples include efavirenz (Sustiva), nevirapine (Viramune), and delavirdine (Rescriptor).
- *Protease inhibitors*—The inhibitors interrupt virus replication at a later stage in the life cycle. Examples include ritonavir (Norvir), saquinavir (Invirase), and indinavir (Crixivan).
- *Entry inhibitors*—These newer drugs prevent HIV from entering healthy T cells. The first drug approved in this class is enfuvirtide (Fuzeon).
- *Highly active antiretroviral therapy (HAART)*—HAART is a treatment regimen that combines reverse transcriptase inhibitors and protease inhibitors. It is considered highly effective and is believed to be responsible for reducing the number of deaths from AIDS by almost half in the United States. Patients who are newly infected with HIV and those with AIDS can take HAART. It has been found to decrease the amount of circulating virus to almost undetectable levels. However, it still cannot eliminate HIV from the body.

Treatment of Opportunistic Infections and Cancer

A variety of at least 22 FDA-approved medications are available to prevent and treat the many opportunistic infections and cancers experienced by patients with AIDS. Table 31–6 lists some of the most common.

HIV Vaccines

Research is being conducted in the United States and throughout the world to develop a safe and effective vaccination against HIV infection. The vaccines are designed to induce the development of antibodies to different strains of HIV.

Needless to say, AIDS must be prevented. To obtain a free brochure, materials, and confidential AIDS counseling, call the toll-free National AIDS Hotline (800–342–AIDS). Information is also abundant on the Internet. Search under various sites, such as CDC, AOL Health, and AIDS organizations.

Table 31–6 Management of Opportunistic Infections in AIDS

Acyclovir	Herpes infection
Amphotericin B	Candida and aspergillus fungal infections
Fluconazole	Candida infections
Foscarnet	Cytomegalovirus infections of the eye
Gancyclovir	Cytomegalovirus infections of the eye
Interferon alfa-2a	Kaposi's sarcoma
Interferon alfa-2b	Kaposi's sarcoma
Pentamidine	*Pneumocystis carinii* pneumonia
Trimethoprim/ sulfamethoxazole	*Pneumocystis carinii* pneumonia

Allergies (Al′er-jees)

Description—Sometimes the immune system can damage instead of protect the body. A secondary response to a normally harmless substance is seen in **allergies** and may actually damage tissues. About 15% of humans are predisposed to become sensitive. Allergies may affect different areas of the body.

In the nose—as hay fever or allergic rhinitis
In the lungs—as asthma
In the eyes—as conjunctivitis
On the skin—as eczema, contact dermatitis, or hives
In the digestive tract—as cramps, vomiting, and diarrhea

When exposed to the sensitive allergens, the antibody IgE is produced, resulting in allergic symptoms. With each additional exposure to the allergen, IgE antibody is produced and becomes attached to the mast cells or basophils, which in turn release histamine and **prostaglandins** (Figure 31–7).

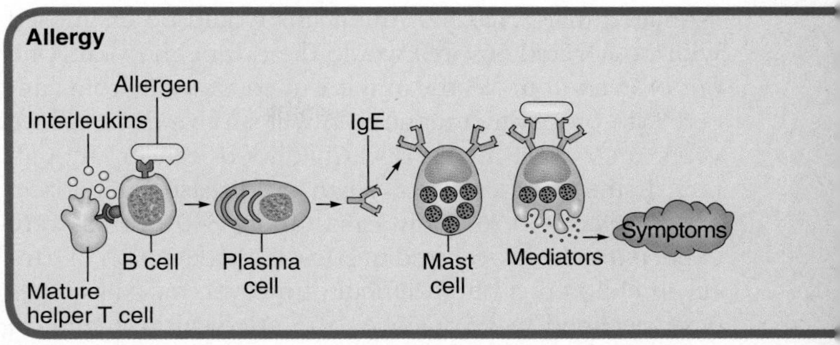

Figure 31–7: Response to allergens. *Adapted from the United States Department of Health and Human Services.*

Signs and symptoms—The histamine causes the mucous membranes to secrete and capillaries to become more permeable. Prostaglandins constrict smooth muscle in some organs, such as the bronchioles of the lungs. The two initiate a local inflammatory response. With hay fever or asthma, for example, there is sneezing, runny nose, congestion, and difficult breathing.

Exaggerated reactions to allergens can be life-threatening. For instance, some people are very sensitive to bee stings and certain drugs. The histamine and prostaglandins cause extensive bronchial constriction, mucus production, and excessive capillary permeability. Breathing is difficult, and extensive loss of blood plasma drastically lowers the blood pressure, leading to circulatory collapse and death. This reaction is known as **anaphylaxis**, and the situation is called *anaphylactic shock*.

Etiology—The most common causative substances are dust, animal hair, certain foods, pollen, insect stings, and drugs. Other factors, such as emotional state, air pressure or temperature change, and infections, can either trigger or complicate allergic reactions.

Diagnostic procedures—To confirm allergies consist of blood counts to determine eosinophil numbers (an increase denotes allergy), chest X-ray to determine congestion and perhaps focal atelectasis (mucous plugs with asthma), and pulmonary function test to evaluate lung condition. Often there is a family history of sensitivity. A series of skin tests can identify allergic substances (see Chapter 45).

Treatment—Treatment consists of eliminating contact with allergens and other causative factors as much as possible. **Desensitization** to specific allergens may be helpful. By injecting minute amounts of the allergen intradermally and gradually increasing the amount, the body can be caused to produce IgG antibodies that circulate and bind with the allergen, prohibiting its interaction with IgE. In addition, antihistamines, bronchodilators, antibiotics for secondary infection, and sometimes corticosteroids are helpful.

Cancer

Description—Cancer is a group of diseases characterized by uncontrolled growth of abnormal cells. These cells accumulate and form tumors that may compress, invade, or destroy normal tissue. Cells have the potential to break away from a tumor and travel to other areas of the body. The spread of a tumor to a new site is called **metastasis.** Cancer is the second leading cause of death in adults and children ages 1 through 14 in the United States. The American Cancer Society statistics for 2010 estimated that 1,529,560 Americans would be diagnosed with cancer and 569,490 would die during the year. One out of every four deaths in the United States is from cancer. With proper treatment, 63% will survive five or more years after their diagnosis. Childhood cancer, though rare, is the chief cause of death by disease in children. An estimated 10,700 new cases and 1,340 deaths were expected to have occurred in 2010. Early detection of cancer in children is often difficult; however, mortality rates have declined by 55% since 1975. Medical and surgical oncologists, physicians with specialized education in the management and treatment of cancer, are best suited to deal with this complicated disease. Figures 31–8A and B illustrate the leading sites of new cancer and deaths estimated for the year 2010 by the American Cancer Society.

Characteristics of Cancer Cells

The word **neoplasm** is defined as new growth and can refer to both **benign** and malignant tumors. Both types of tumors contain growing tumor cells, connective tissue, and blood vessels. Benign tumors are usually slow growing, do not invade other tissues, and do not spread

Men	
1. Prostate	217,730
2. Lung and bronchus	116,750
3. Colon and rectum	72,090
4. Urinary bladder	52,760
5. Melanoma of the skin	38,870
6. Non-Hodgkin's lymphoma	35,380
7. Kidney and renal pelvis	35,370
8. Oral cavity and pharynx	25,420
9. Leukemia	24,690
10. Pancreas	21,370

Women	
1. Breast	207,090
2. Lung and bronchus	105,770
3. Colon and rectum	70,480
4. Uterine corpus	43,470
5. Thyroid	33,390
6. Non-Hodgkin's lymphoma	30,160
7. Melanoma of the skin	29,260
8. Ovary	21,880
9. Pancreas	21,770
10. Urinary bladder	17,770

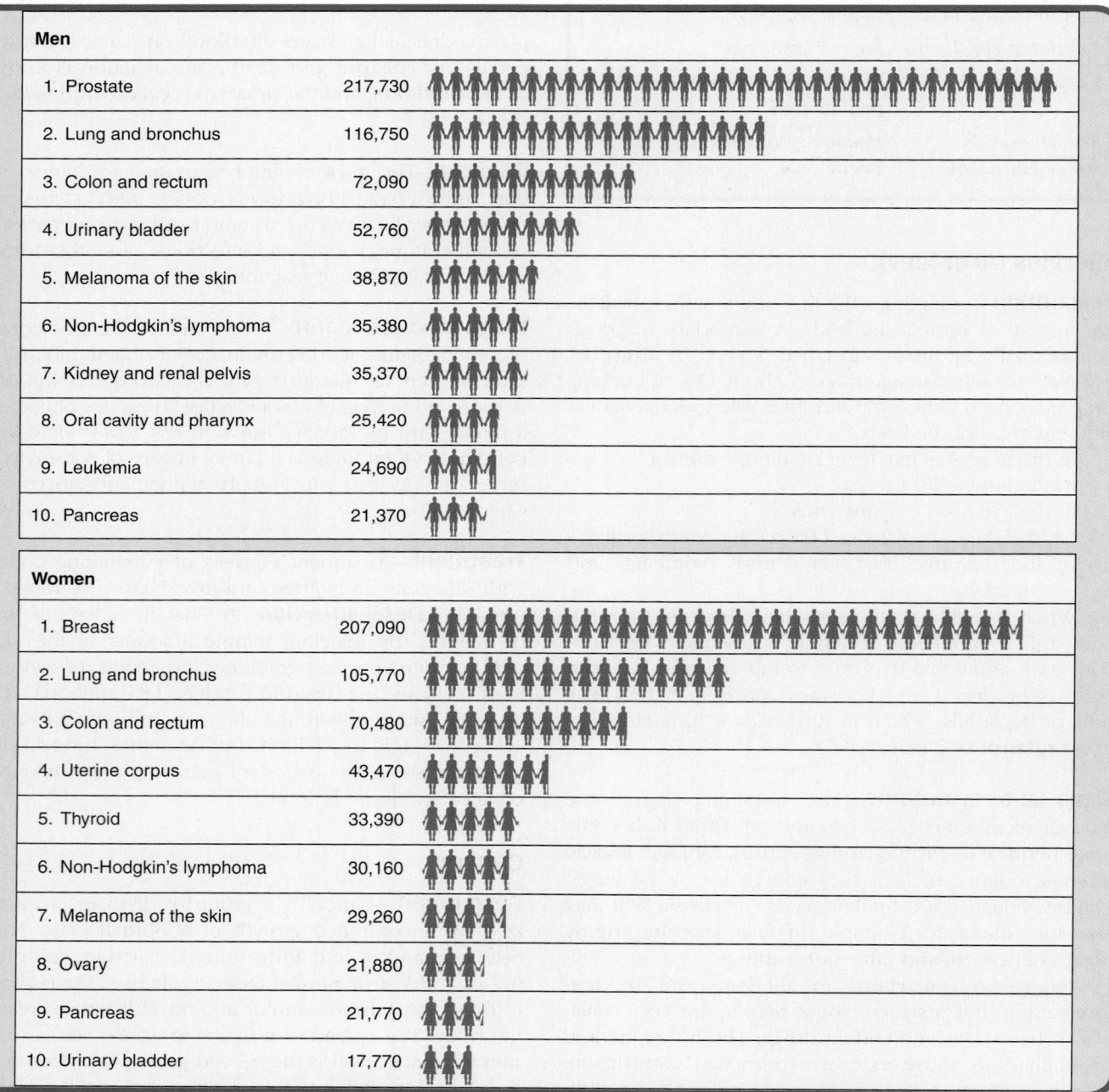

Figure 31–8A: Leading sites of new cancer cases and deaths–2010 estimates. *Adapted from the American Cancer Society, Inc.*

Men	
1. Lung and bronchus	86,220
2. Colon and rectum	26,580
3. Prostate	32,050
4. Pancreas	18,770
5. Leukemia	12,660
6. Liver and intrahepatic bile duct	12,720
7. Esophagus	11,650
8. Non-Hodgkin's lymphoma	10,710
9. Urinary bladder	10,410
10. Kidney and renal pelvis	8,210

Women	
1. Lung and bronchus	71,080
2. Breast	39,840
3. Colon and rectum	24,790
4. Pancreas	18,030
5. Ovary	13,850
6. Leukemia	9,180
7. Non-Hodgkin's lymphoma	9,500
8. Uterine corpus	7,950
9. Brain and other nervous system	5,720
10. Multiple myeloma	4,890

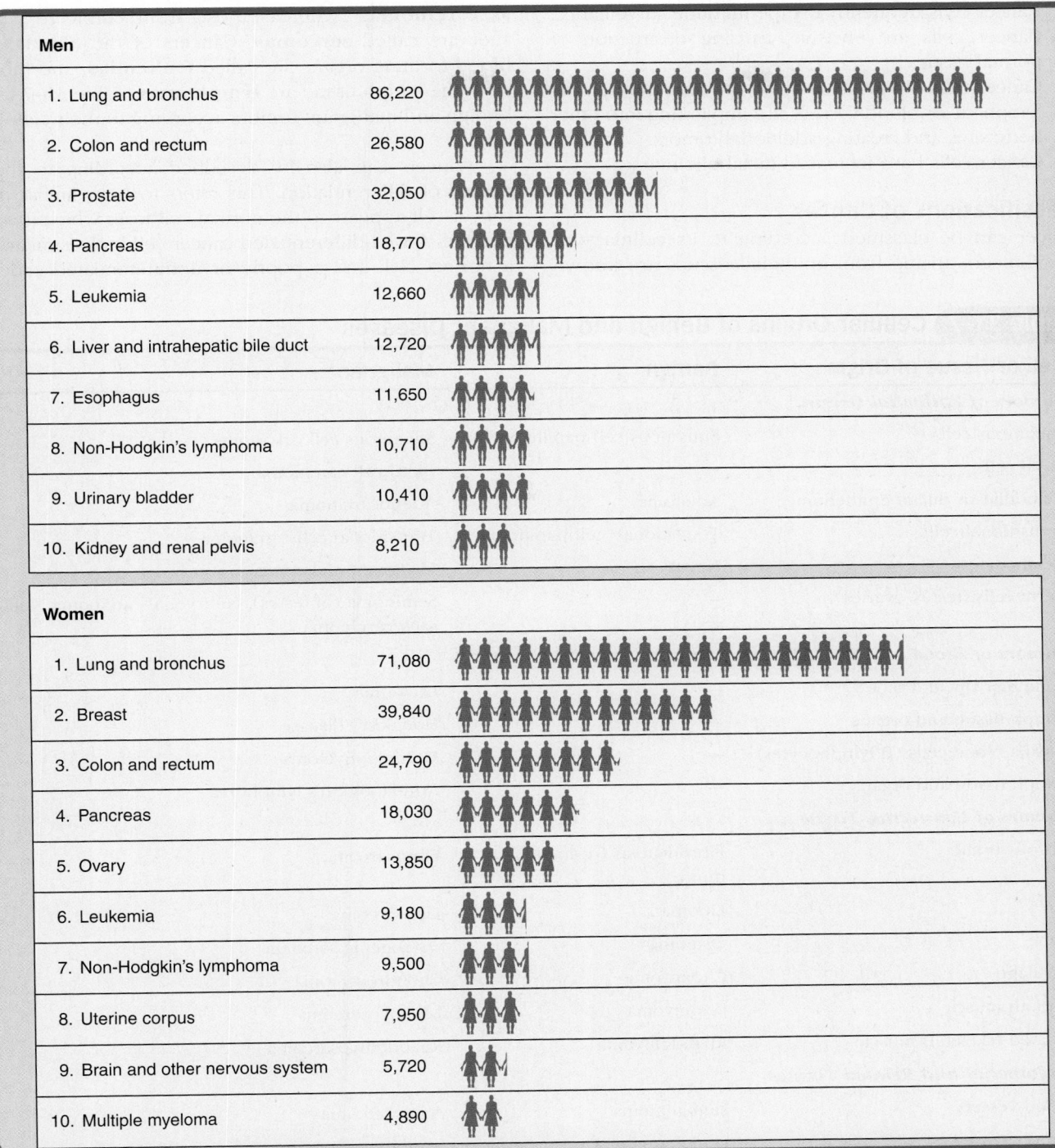

Figure 31–8B: Ten leading sites of cancer deaths–2010 estimates. *Adapted from the American Cancer Society, Inc.*

to other parts of the body. Usually they do not cause any problems unless they are growing in a confined space, such as in the brain. Malignant tumors are cancerous and differ from benign in several ways:

- Cancer cells have an altered cell structure that includes an increased nuclear size, irregular chromatin distribution, and prominent nucleoli.
- Cancer cells lack normal growth controlling mechanisms; growth is unorganized and disorderly.
- Cancer cells lack contact inhibition (normal cell growth stops when other cells are contacted). They continue to grow and invade into other tissue.
- Cancer cells do not respond to growth factors that stimulate or inhibit growth of normal cells. They can grow rapidly with reduced growth factors.

- Cancer cells frequently escape immune surveillance.
- Cancer cells are invasive, causing destruction of normal tissue.
- Cancer cells can metastasize by traveling through the lymphatic or blood vessels and implanting into other body sites and creating additional tumors.
- Cancer cells have increased metabolic rate.

Classifications of Cancer

Cancer can be classified according to its cellular origin. Cancers arising from epithelial tissues are known as **carcinomas**, whereas those from connective tissues are called **sarcomas**. Cancers of the blood and blood-forming organs are called **leukemias**, and those from the lymph tissue are **lymphomas**. Table 31–7 lists benign and malignant tumors according to their cellular origins.

Cancers can also be described according to their degree of differentiation. This refers to how similar the cancer cell appears to the normal cell from which it was derived. A well-differentiated cancer cell looks similar to a normal cell, and a poorly or undifferentiated cancer

Table 31–7 Cellular Origins of Benign and Malignant Diseases

Cell or Tissue of Origin	Benign	Malignant
Tumors of Epithelial Origin		
Squamous cells	Squamous cell papilloma	Squamous cell carcinoma
Basal cells	—	Basal cell carcinoma
Glandular or ductal epithelium	Adenoma	Adenocarcinoma
Transitional cells	Transitional cell papilloma	Transitional cell carcinoma
Melanocytes	Nevus	Malignant melanoma
Germ cells (testes/ovaries)	—	Seminoma (of testes), embryonal carcinoma, yolk sack carcinoma
Tumors of Blood and Blood-Forming Organs/Lymphoid Tissue		
Bone marrow and blood	—	Leukemia
Lymph tissue and organs	—	Hodgkin's disease
Plasma blood cells (B lymphocytes)	—	Multiple myeloma
Lymph tissue and organs	—	Non-Hodgkin's lymphoma
Tumors of Connective Tissue		
Fibrous tissue	Fibromatosis (desmoid tumor)	Fibrosarcoma
Fat	Lipoma	Liposarcoma
Bone	Osteoma	Osteogenic sarcoma
Cartilage	Chondroma	Chondrosarcoma
Smooth muscle	Leiomyoma	Leiomyosarcoma
Striated (skeletal) muscle	Rhabdomyoma	Rhabdomyosarcoma
Endothelial and Related Tissues		
Blood vessels	Hemangioma	Angiosarcoma
Lymph vessels	Lymphangioma	Lymphangiosarcoma
Synovium	—	Synovial sarcoma
Mesothelium	Meningioma	Malignant mesothelioma
Meninges	Meningioma	Malignant meningioma
Neural and Retinal Tissue		
Nerve sheath	Neurilemoma neurofibroma	Malignant peripheral sheath tumor
Nerve cells	Gangioneuroma	Neuroblastoma
Retinal cells (cones)	—	Retinoblastoma

cell appears very abnormal. Sometimes it is so poorly differentiated that it is difficult to tell from what type of cell it originated, these cancers are termed "carcinomas of unknown primary." Grading refers to the degree of differentiation of the cancer cell. The grading system goes from Grade 1, which is a well-differentiated cell, to Grade III or IV, which is undifferentiated. The grading and staging findings predict prognosis.

Cancer Staging

Staging is a term used to identify the extent of spread. It is a system that is accepted worldwide for primary site evaluation. It provides a standardized description for planning treatments, evaluating outcomes, and estimating prognosis. It is also a criterion for patient eligibility for individual clinical trials. The method is known as the TNM system and uses standardized measurement criteria:

(T)—the size or extent of local spread of the primary tumor
(N)—the presence or absence and extent of regional lymph node metastasis
(M)—the presence or absence of distant metastasis

Numbers are added to the three components to indicate the clinical extent of the disease to show an increase in tumor size, local involvement, regional lymph node spread, or distant metastasis:

Tumor size	T0	T1	T2	T3	T4
Nodal involvement	N0	N1	N2	N3	
Metastasis	M0	M1			

In addition to the letters and numbers, four staging classifications are also used:

c—Clinical based on acquired evidence from exams and studies
p—Pathologic based on information after a surgical procedure
r—Retreatment based on disease-free interval with planned new treatment
a—Autopsy based on pathology after death

In the future, multiple biologic factors, such as hormone receptors, genetic markers, cellular proliferation, and metastasis potential, will probably be used to further classify cancer.

Signs and symptoms—The signs and symptoms vary according to the type of cancer, its location, and the individual affected. The American Cancer Society has developed the warning signals for cancer in adults and children (Tables 31–8 and 31–9). Unfortunately, these are often signs of fairly advanced disease. Many individuals have no symptoms; however, cancer can sometimes be detected through routine cancer screening tests. (Chapters 40 and 41, discuss recommended screening tests.)

Table 31–8 The Seven Warning Signals of Cancer

- Change in bowel and bladder habits
- A sore that does not heal
- Unusual bleeding or discharge
- Thickening or lump in a breast or elsewhere
- Indigestion or difficulty swallowing
- Obvious change in a wart or mole
- Nagging cough or hoarseness

Table 31–9 Warning Signals of Childhood Cancer

- Unusual mass or swelling
- Unexplained paleness and loss of energy
- Sudden tendency to bruise
- Persistent, localized pain or limping
- Prolonged, unexplained fever or illness
- Frequent headaches, often with vomiting
- Sudden eye or vision changes
- Excessive, rapid weight loss

Etiology—Cancer is believed to be caused by cellular **mutations** or abnormal activation of cellular genes that control cell growth and division. Cancer occurs from the abnormal growth of a single mutated cell. These abnormal genes are called **oncogenes**. In cells, proto-oncogenes and tumor suppresser genes are normal genes that regulate the growth and repair of cells. If a proto-oncogene is mutated, it may be left permanently in the "on position," causing continuous cell growth. If the tumor suppresser gene is mutated, it may be left permanently in the "off" position, also allowing continued cell growth.

One of the most common known mutated genes in human cancers is the *p53* tumor suppresser gene. This gene normally stops cell proliferation and promotes DNA repair of damaged cells. Some clinical trials using gene therapy are looking at ways to interact with the *p53* tumor suppresser gene. There is evidence that some tumor suppressor gene defects are inherited. Patients with inherited retinoblastoma, a rare pediatric tumor of the eye, are known to have a defective tumor suppressor gene.

Only a small fraction of cells that mutate ever lead to cancer (remember it is estimated that 100 to 1,000 mutated cells are formed every day). Many of the mutated cells cannot survive because they are so defective. Others are destroyed by the immune system, particularly the NK cells. The probability of mutations is increased when a person is exposed to certain chemical, physical, or biologic factors called **carcinogens**. Carcinogens are usually categorized under chemical, viral, physical, and familial headings. Table 31–10 lists the types of known carcinogens and the resulting cancers.

Some other reasons for failure of the immune system to destroy mutated cells have been suggested:

- A decrease in antibodies and lymphocytes caused by cytotoxic drugs or steroids
- Stress, which stimulates production of *cortisol,* a lymphocyte destroyer
- Severe infection, which depresses the immune system
- Cancer itself causes suppression of the immune system and predisposes to other cancers
- Increased infection caused by radiation, toxic drug therapy, and bone marrow depression, which interferes with leukocyte production

Table 31–10 Types of Known Carcinogens and the Resulting Cancers

Carcinogen	Type of Cancer
Chemical Carcinogens	
Alkylating chemotherapy agents (e.g., nitrogen mustard, cyclophosphamide)	• Leukemia
Arsenic	• Liver • Lung • Skin
Benzene	• Leukemia
Chewing tobacco	• Oral cancer
Cigarette smoking	• Oral cancer • Head and neck cancer • Lung cancer • Bladder cancer • Cervical cancer
Vinyl chloride	• Liver cancer
Viral Carcinogens	
Epstein–Barr virus	• Burkitt's lymphoma in Africa • Nasopharyngeal cancer
Hepatitis B virus	• Hepatocellular liver cancer
Human T cell leukemia/ lymphoma virus (HTLV-1)	• T cell leukemias and lymphomas
Human papilloma virus (HPV-16 or HPV-18)	• Found in at least 70% of cases of cervical cancer
Physical Carcinogens	
Asbestos	• Bronchogenic lung cancer • Mesothelioma
Ionizing radiation	• Leukemia • Lymphoma • Potentially all solid tumors
Ultraviolet radiation	• Melanoma • Skin cancers
Familial Carcinogenesis	
Dysplastic nevus syndrome	• Melanoma
Fanconi's anemia	• Leukemia
Familial polyposis	• Colorectal cancer
Gardner's syndrome	• Colorectal cancer
Neurofibromatosis	• Brain tumors • Endocrine cancers
Xeroderma pigmentosum	• Melanoma • Skin cancer

Diagnostic Tests

Additional tests are indicated when a patient has a positive screening test or has symptoms of cancer. The diagnosis of cancer can only be considered 100% accurate if a sample of cells are removed and examined microscopically. The major goals of the diagnostic evaluation are to determine:

- The primary site (e.g., breast)
- The tissue type of the cancer (e.g., carcinoma, sarcoma)
- The grade of the cancer (the degree of differentiation)
- The extent of the disease in the body (stage)

Diagnostic tests for cancer can be categorized into biopsies, laboratory tests, and tumor imaging.

Biopsies. A **biopsy** is the removal of a sample of tissue from the body for microscopic examination to determine a diagnosis. Treatment decisions for cancers arising from the same organ differ based upon the type of cell involved. For example, adenocarcinoma of the lung is treated very differently than a sarcoma of the lung. Common techniques for biopsies are needle, incisional, excisional, and bone marrow aspiration. During a needle biopsy, a needle is inserted into the tumor and cells are withdrawn. Incisional biopsy involves removing a portion of the tumor for testing. The entire tumor is removed during an excisional biopsy. A bone marrow aspiration is used to test for leukemia and cancers that involve the bone marrow. A local anesthetic is injected over the iliac crest, and a long needle is inserted through the bone and into the marrow where blood cells are made.

Sentinel lymph node biopsy is a technique used to remove and sample lymph nodes that may be cancerous. It is most commonly used for breast cancer and melanoma. The sentinel lymph node (SLN) is the first lymph node that drains the area of the cancerous tumor. The patient is injected with a radioactive material. SNLs will have a higher uptake of the material than other lymph nodes, identifying them for removal. A blue dye is also simultaneously injected for visual correlation at the time of surgery. The advantage of SLN biopsy is that fewer nodes are removed, resulting in fewer complications.

Stereotactic breast biopsy is used for breast tumors that are difficult to locate. The biopsy is done while the patient is having a mammogram or ultrasound, allowing the surgeon to see the location of the tumor in order to obtain the biopsy.

Laboratory Tests. Different laboratory tests of the blood, serum, urine, and other body fluids help establish the diagnosis of cancer. In addition to standard tests, tumor markers and genetic testing can be done for different types of cancer.

Tumor markers are proteins, antigens, genes, hormones, or enzymes produced by the tumor and released into the blood. Tumor markers can help establish the diagnosis of cancer but primary indication is measuring response to treatment. For example, if a patient has an elevated tumor marker, then the number should decrease with cancer treatment. Tumor markers, however, are not always specific for cancer and can be affected by other factors. **Carcinoembryonic antigen (CEA)** is a tumor marker often elevated in patients with colon cancer; however, it can also be elevated in smokers.

Genetic Testing. Conducting genetic testing is appropriate for some types of cancer and for individuals at high risk for developing inherited cancers. The ethical, social, and legal issues need to be considered. Most genetic tests are performed by drawing blood samples. For example, Breast Cancer (BRCA) genes 1 and 2 are abnormal in just fewer than 5% of all breast cancers. Defects in these genes are believed to be responsible for up to 80% of *inherited* breast cancers. *BRCA1* and 2 are present in everyone; however, when the genes mutate, the risk for breast and ovarian cancer increases. *BRCA1* and *BRCA2* mutations have also been linked to prostate cancer and possibly to colon cancer. Both men and women can inherit and pass on the genes. Women who inherit the *BRCA1* and *BRCA2* mutated gene have a 50% to 80% chance of developing breast cancer.

Tumor Imaging. A variety of different radiology and imaging tests are used to aid in the diagnosis and staging of cancer, including X-rays, CT scans, MRIs, endoscopy, ultrasound, and nuclear medicine. X-rays include mammography used to screen for breast cancer. CT scans are commonly used to aid in the diagnosis of lung, liver, and head and neck cancers. MRIs are used to diagnose and stage cancers such as brain and musculoskeletal cancers (e.g., sarcomas).

Endoscopy is used to visualize the interior of hollow organs. After a hollow tube is inserted into the organ, images may be taken, and tissue samples can be obtained through the scope. Bronchoscopy is used for diagnosis of lung cancers. Sigmoidoscopy and colonoscopy are used for the screening and diagnosis of colorectal cancer. Ultrasound is used to distinguish between a fluid-filled cyst and a solid tumor.

Nuclear medicine imaging involves the injection or ingestion of radioactive substances, followed by imaging of the organ or organs that concentrate the radioactive material. Common nuclear medicine scans include bone, liver, spleen, brain, thyroid, and kidney.

Positron emission tomography (PET) scan is a type of nuclear medicine test that has only recently been used to detect cancer. PET scans are computerized images of the metabolic activity of the body tissues by measuring glucose uptake and can suggest the presence of cancer.

Radiolabeled **monoclonal** *antibodies* include Prosta-Scint scans used for the early detection of prostate cancer. With this technology, antibodies are made for specific tumor types and labeled with a radioactive substance. The radioactive antibody searches for the specific tumor antigen and is detectable by the scan. *Radiolabeled peptides* are most commonly used to detect neuroendocrine tumors.

Treatment—The treatment of cancer is primarily based upon the type, grade, and stage of the cancer. In addition, treatment considerations include the risk or probability that the cancer will metastasize or recur after treatment. The treatment after surgical removal of the cancer to reduce the recurrence rate is termed "adjunct therapy." The planning sequence for treatment is as follows:

The patient presents with a symptom or has a positive screening test
↓
History, physical examinations, laboratory work
↓
Biopsy
↓
Biopsy positive for cancer
↓
The cancer is classified according to cell type and is graded according to the degree of differentiation
↓
The extent of the disease is determined (staging)
↓
Cancer treatment
↓
Cancer re-evaluated
↓
Need for additional therapy evaluated

Goals of Cancer Therapy

The goals of therapy—cure, control, or palliation—are based on the patient's type and stage of cancer. Cure means that there will be no evidence of disease for a specified time. Control indicates that the disease cannot be cured but can be controlled for a period using the identified therapy. Palliation means that the disease cannot be cured or controlled, and palliative treatments will be used to control symptoms only.

Local Versus Systemic Treatment

The major treatment methods for cancer are surgery, **radiation**, **chemotherapy**, and biologic response modifiers. Treatments can have local or systemic effects. A local treatment effects only the area of the therapy and any side effects that occur within that area. An example of local therapy is surgery. Systemic therapy travels throughout the body to treat cancer cells in different locations. Side effects will be systemic as well. An example of systemic therapy is chemotherapy. Most patients receive a combination of local and systemic therapies, especially if they already have or are at increased risk for metastasis. Table 31–11 lists the types of treatment and their key points.

- *Surgery* is the oldest form of treatment for cancer. About 60% of all patients with cancer will have some type of surgery. It can be used for the purpose of diagnosis, treatment, or palliation of symptoms.
- *Radiation therapy* is the use of high-energy particles or waves, such as X-ray or gamma rays, to destroy or damage the DNA or RNA of cancer cells. It is most effective on dividing cells. Radiation therapy can be delivered by external beam or brachytherapy. External beam therapy is delivered externally through the skin to the area. **Brachytherapy** uses radioactive isotopes that are placed directly on or very near the tumor. Brachytherapy can be delivered interstitially, using seeds "planted" into the tissues, or intracavitary, using a tube or catheter that is later removed, to instill the material. This is commonly used for prostate and

Table 31–11 Types Of Cancer Treatment

Type	Key Points
Surgery	• Most common treatment • Local treatment • Diagnosis and staging • Treatment • Palliation of symptoms
Chemotherapy	• Most routes: systemic treatment • Affects cell division in cancer and normal cells • Most effects, seen in rapidly dividing normal and cancer cells • Side effects: nausea, vomiting, bone marrow depression, hair loss, stomatitis (mouth sores)
Radiation: external beam therapy	• Local treatment • Affects cell division of cancer and normal cells • Side effects: fatigue, skin reactions, other side effects dependent upon site treated
Radiation: brachytherapy	• Local treatment • Radioactive isotope placed near site of cancer • Most common uses: cervical cancer, lung cancer, prostate cancer
Radiation: radiosurgery	• Radiation used to directly target a small area • Most common uses: brain tumors
Biologic response modifiers	• Also called immunotherapy • Examples: alpha interferon, interleukins, monoclonal antibodies, tumor necrosis factor, colony-stimulating factors • Side effects: fatigue, fever, chills, muscle and joint aches, anaphylaxis
Gene therapy	• Investigational • Affects growth-controlling factors of tumors
Complementary therapy	• Complements standard therapies • Examples: massage therapy, biofeedback, music therapy, art therapy
Alternative therapy	• Not approved by the Food and Drug Administration • Examples: shark cartilage, laetrile, megadoses of vitamins, herbs

breast cancer. General side effects of radiation therapy include fatigue and weakness.

- *Chemotherapy* involves the use medications to treat cancer cells by altering cell growth and division; therefore, it effects both rapidly dividing cancer cells and normal tissues. It can be administered orally, intravenously, subcutaneously, intramuscularly, intra-arterially, topically, intraperitoneally, and into the central nervous system.

  The route is dependent upon the type of chemotherapy and the type of cancer. Patients can receive one type of chemotherapy or combinations of chemotherapy. The patient in Figure 31–9 is receiving one of a combination of chemotherapeutic agents.

  Although drug specific, common side effects of chemotherapy include hair loss, skin changes, mouth sores, and bone marrow depression. Bone marrow depression can lead to anemia and increased risk of infection due to low white blood cell counts and increased risk for bleeding if platelets are low.
- *Biologic response modifiers* (BRM) are defined as any substance that is capable of altering the immune system by either stimulating or suppressing its action. BRMs are also referred to as immunotherapy or biotherapy. The action of BRMs can be divided into three categories:

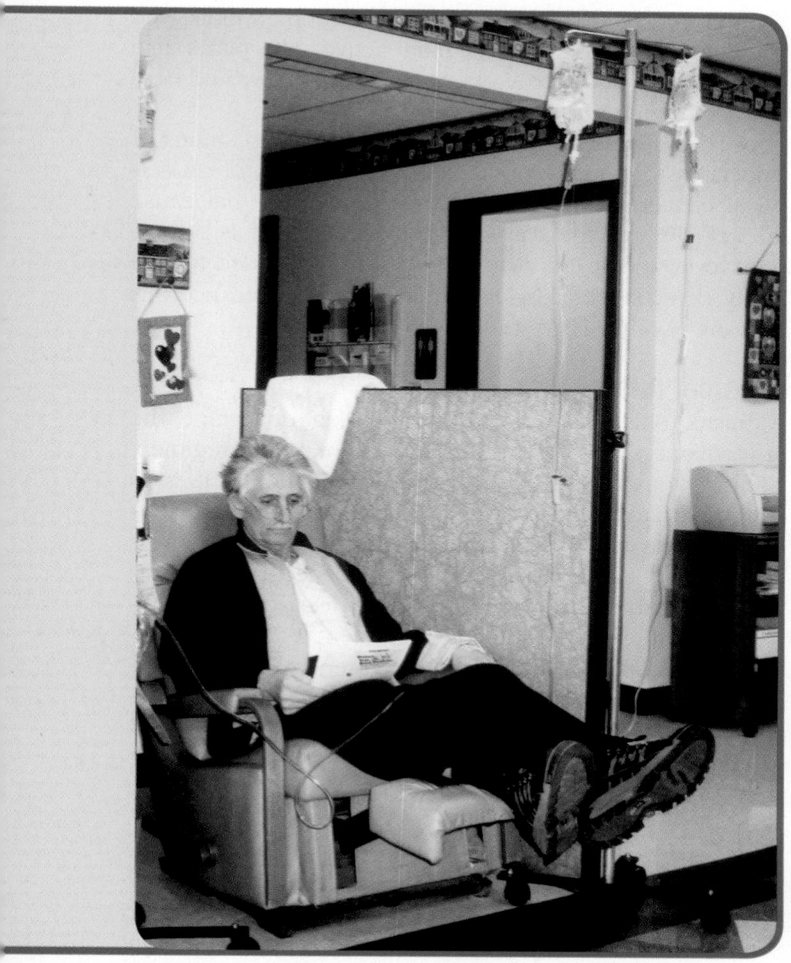

Figure 31–9: Patient receiving intravenous chemotherapy.
Courtesy of Carol A. Martin.

1. Agents that restore, augment, or modulate the host's immune response
2. Agents that have direct antitumor activity
3. Agents that have other biologic effects, such as affecting tumor growth, differentiation, or the ability of the tumor to metastasize

There are numerous BRMs. Examples include colony-stimulating factors, interferons, interleukins, monoclonal antibodies, and tumor necrosis factor.

Colony-stimulating factors (CSFs) are cytokines that regulate hematopoiesis, the growth and maturation of blood cells. The CSFs work on different blood cell lines. For example, granulocyte colony-stimulating factor (GLSF) works to promote the maturation of granulocytes, important white blood cells for fighting infection. Erythropoetin targets only red blood cell maturation. Other CSFs regulate stem cell growth and platelet growth. GLSF is used to treat granulocytopenia (lack of granulocytes) and allow increased doses of chemotherapy to be given without the risk of long-term low white blood cell counts. GLSF is administered subcutaneously.

Interferons are naturally occurring cytokines that have antiviral, immunomodulatory, and antiproliferative effects. Interferon interacts with T cells to increase the activity of NK cells to have direct cytoxic affects on cancer cells. Alfa interferon is used to treat a variety of cancers, including renal cell cancer, hairy cell leukemia, melanoma, lymphomas, and Kaposi's sarcoma. It is administered intravenously or subcutaneously. Side effects include flulike symptoms, such as fever, chills, fatigue, rigors, and headache.

Interleukins are important regulatory proteins produced naturally by lymphocytes and monocytes. The most commonly prescribed interleukin is interleukin-2 (IL-2). It is produced by helper T cells. An important function of IL-2 is to stimulate and activate NK cells, which have a cytotoxic affect on cancer cells. IL-2 has been used to treat renal carcinoma, melanoma, and lymphoma. It is administered intravenously or subcutaneously. IL-2 has numerous side effects, including severe flulike symptoms and a change of fluids, which can lead to hypotension, ascites (fluid in the abdomen), and pleural effusion.

Monoclonal antibodies are antibodies directed at specific tumor antigens. They can be used alone to directly activate the host's immune system or can be attached to a chemotherapeutic agent for direct delivery to the cancer cell. Monoclonal antibodies are currently being used to treat a variety of cancers, including breast, B cell lymphoma, and melanomas.

Alternative Therapies

Alternative therapies are promoted as cancer cures; however, they have not been proven because they have not been scientifically tested or were tested and found to be statistically ineffective. Alternative therapies have not been approved by the Food and Drug Administration as treatments for cancer. Some examples include:

- Shark cartilage
- Laetrile
- Immunoaugmentive therapy
- Megadoses of vitamins
- Herbal supplements

Complementary Therapies

Complementary therapies refer to supportive methods that are used to complement or add to recognized treatments, such as chemotherapy, radiation, and surgery. They are not given to cure cancer but to help control symptoms and improve well-being. Examples of complementary therapies are:

- Art therapy
- Biofeedback
- Imagery
- Massage
- Meditation
- Music therapy
- Pet therapy
- Relaxation
- Yoga

Cancer Vaccine

Researchers have worked diligently for the past four and a half decades trying to develop a vaccine for cancer. They were hampered by the lack of knowledge about the immune system. With the mapping of the genes, much has been learned about cellular structure and function. We now know the body's natural defense from the immune system fails to work because cancer cells are mutated from normal cells and the immune system does not recognize them as "foreign."

Researchers have been able to develop vaccines to make cancer cells visible. White blood cells are withdrawn from the patient's blood through a collection process known as leukapheresis. The cells are exposed to a cancer protein then infused back into the same patient. The fused cells trigger an immune reaction, and cells are carried back to the lymph nodes. Here, the antigen-specific B and T cells are activated and increase in number. T cells go out to travel the body, identifying and destroying the tumor cells. B cells are activated to make antibodies to attack the antigens.

The first FDA-approved cancer vaccine occurred in 2010 with sipuleucel-T (Provenge) for prostate cancer. It is indicated for patients with prostate cancer that has metastasized to the bone. sipuleucel-T has been shown to improve life expectancy in patients with metastatic prostate cancer. The future of vaccines is considered to be another form of cancer treatment to supplement chemotherapy, radiation, and surgery, but with less-invasive procedures and fewer side effects.

Vaccine therapy is promising. At present, efforts are primarily aimed at preventing recurrence. However, efforts are also being made to develop a vaccine to boost the immune system to keep some cancers from forming in the first place. The thought is to have many extra immune cells to fight off the virus cells, already present in most people's bodies, which trigger tumor cell development. Scientists believe we may always have cancer, but the goal is to make it a chronic disease instead.

Infection with the human papillomavirus (HPV), a sexually transmitted disease, has been shown to be responsible for most cervical cancers. A newly approved vaccine targets HPV and will cause a dramatic reduction in the current 4,200 estimated 2010 deaths from cervical cancer. As of June 2006, a federal advisory panel recommended that all girls be routinely given the vaccine at 11 or 12 years of age. Three injections are given over a six-month period and are most effective when administered before the girls become sexually active. The panel also believes girls and women between 13 and 26 would benefit from immunization.

The vaccine appears effective against two strains of the virus that are responsible for about 70% of all cervical cancers and against two others strains that cause almost 90% of the cases of genital warts. It is important to note that PAP tests are still recommended for the early detection of cervical cancer and the precancerous lesions of other HPV strains.

Clinical Research Trials

Clinical trials are research studies that determine the effectiveness and safety of a cancer treatment regimen. Before a treatment can be used for patients, it goes through many years of investigation—first through laboratory trials and then in animal trials. If the treatment is found effective and safe, it is then tested on humans. Patients with specific criteria in their disease are permitted to participate in the trial treatment. After the studies are completed and there is evidence that the new therapy is more effective and safe, it is evaluated by the Food and Drug Administration to be used as standard therapy.

Chronic Fatigue Syndrome (CFS)

Description—This **debilitating** disorder was officially recognized and reported in 1984 by two doctors near Lake Tahoe, Nevada. It was officially declared a disease in 1988. The CDC started a surveillance program costing $1.5 million to track the frequency and impact of the disorder.

Signs and symptoms—The following guidelines have been established to help physicians diagnose the condition.

- Persistent overwhelming fatigue that lasts for at least six months and does not go away with rest
- Low-grade fever
- Sore throat or swollen lymph nodes
- Headaches
- Lingering fatigue after levels of exercise that would normally be easily tolerated
- Unexplainable muscle weakness or pain
- Pain in joints without swelling
- Forgetfulness, irritability, confusion, inability to concentrate, depression, sensitivity to light, and impaired vision
- Sleep disturbances

Patients experience varying levels of ability to perform activity, from profound fatigue to being completely bedridden. CFS affects twice as many women as men, particularly between 25 and 45 years old. However, children and senior citizens have also been diagnosed.

The disorder begins suddenly like the common flu, but the CFS symptoms last for three or four years. Only about 15% to 20% seem to recover fully; 5% are homebound or bedridden.

Etiology—The cause of the disorder is unknown. Current theories suggest that a virus, bacteria, allergen, or environment chemical enters the body but does not set off the normal immune response to fight the invasion. Instead, the system continues to make symptom-producing chemicals. A second theory suggests that some unidentified organism weakens the immune system, allowing normally dormant viruses to become activated. Recently, DNA from a virus (xenotropic murine leukemia virus-related virus – XMRV), was detected more commonly in patient's with CFS but its relation to CFS is still unknown.

Physicians still do not know much about the disorder; some deny its existence because it cannot be detected by a blood test. Diagnosis requires a thorough physical examination and laboratory tests to rule out other conditions with similar symptoms.

Treatment—Many treatments have been tried, but only cognitive behavioral therapy and graded exercise have proved effective. Cognitive behavioral therapy involves a series of one-hour sessions designed to alter beliefs and behaviors that might delay recovery. Treatment for insomnia, pain, and symptoms of depression is also important.

Lupus Erythematosus (Lu′-pus Eri-the-ma-to′-sis)

Description—**Lupus erythematosus** is a chronic disease of unknown cause in which striking changes occur in the immune system. It causes inflammation of various parts of the body. It can involve only a few body organs or cause serious life-threatening problems. Lupus can affect the skin, joints, kidneys, lungs, heart, nervous system, and other body organs and systems.

In lupus, the usually protective antibodies are produced in large quantities but react against the person's own normal tissue; therefore, it is called an autoimmune disease. There are three main types of lupus:

- Discoid lupus erythematosus (DLE)—Cutaneous or **discoid** lupus is confined to the skin and causes a persistent flush of the cheeks or discoid lesions on the face, neck, scalp, and other areas exposed to ultraviolet light. The lesions of the face are referred to as a butterfly rash. The rash is usually scaly and red but not itchy. If not treated, scarring may result, and if on the scalp, bald spots.
- Systemic lupus erythematosus (SLE) inflames the organs of the body. Some persons also have skin and joint involvement; in others, skin, lungs, kidneys, or blood may be affected. The disease is characterized by periods of **remission**, when few if any symptoms are evident, and other periods of active disease and symptoms.
- Drug-induced lupus can be caused by certain medications and is similar to SLE. The most common offenders are hydralazine for hypertension and procainamide for cardiac arrhythmia. The symptoms fade when the drugs are stopped.

The Lupus Foundation of America believes that total prevalence may be as many as 1,500,000 people in the United States. SLE affects women 10–15 times more often than men, most frequently during the childbearing years. Lupus is more common in African, Asian, and Native Americans. About 16,000 new cases are diagnosed each year.

Signs and symptoms—Symptoms of lupus are:

- fever
- weight loss
- headache
- fatigue
- swollen glands
- depression
- loss of appetite
- nausea and vomiting
- easy bruising
- hair loss
- edema

Suggestive signs of lupus include:

a rash over cheeks and bridge of nose	discoid lupus lesions ulcers inside mouth
rashes developing after being in the sun	pleurisy
	anemia
arthritis in two or more joints	**Raynaud's phenomenon** (fingers turn white or blue in the cold)
seizures	
bald spots	

Diagnosis is made from symptoms and blood tests for evidence of autoantibodies. Urine is checked for protein, RBCs, and WBCs. A specific antibody test called ANA (antinuclear antibody) looks for antibodies to the nuclei of cells. Over 99% of people with lupus will have a positive test; however, only 33% of people with a positive ANA have SLE.

Etiology—Unknown immune system change.

Treatment—Treatment of SLE consists of assuring patients they can live near-normal lives. Limits on activities are dictated by the disease. Patients are encouraged to rest when needed, but otherwise engage in normal employment and exercise. Sun exposure should be avoided at peak hours (10:00 AM to 2:00 PM), otherwise, as tolerated. Sunscreens of at least SPF 15 are advisable. No medication has been developed to cure lupus. Joint and muscle pain is controlled with anti-inflammatory and analgesic drugs, such as aspirin, ibuprofen, and naproxen. During flareups or if major organs are involved, steroids, such as prednisone, are often used to suppress inflammation. The steroid also interferes with the proliferation and interaction of the cells in the immune system and causes T cells to gather in the lymph nodes, which removes them from concentrating at the inflammation sites. The drugs chloroquine and Plaquenil (antimalarials) are valuable in managing the skin lesions and also help control arthritis symptoms.

Many new treatments are being tested, several dealing with self-antigens, immunoreplacement therapy, and even plasmapheresis (the removal of blood plasma, and hence antibodies). It is believed with further understanding of the immune system, an effective treatment of lupus will be discovered.

Lymphedema (Limf-e-de′-ma)

Description—**Lymphedema** is swelling in the tissues of the body caused by an accumulation of lymphatic fluid. Approximately 20% of women who have had breast cancer surgery develop the condition. It may begin as soon as a few months or as late as several years after surgery.

Signs and symptoms—A swelling within the fatty tissue just under the skin of the arm and hand. When it first begins, the arm may seem normal in the morning, but the hand or arm will swell during the day. If it occurs following overuse of the arm in the first year or year and one-half after surgery, it can often be reversed with aggressive treatment. If it occurs two or more years after surgery, complete reversal is unlikely, but the condition can be controlled. With chronic marked swelling in the arm, serious complications can arise, such as infection, loss of function, and skin breakdown.

Etiology—Normally, lymph fluid circulates easily through the vessels and is filtered in the nodes. However, when the system is altered or damaged, it cannot handle the amount of fluid. This is especially true when lymph nodes in the axilla are removed during surgery for breast cancer. Damage can also result from radiation therapy. The more extensive the damage, the greater the risk of developing lymphedema.

One way to reduce the risk from surgery is to perform the sentinel node biopsy procedure. A dye material is injected at the site of the tumor to identify the first node along the lymph vessel that drains the area. This node is biopsied to determine if cancer cells are present. If cancer is not found, then no other lymph nodes are removed.

Treatment—The most comprehensive treatment for lymphedema is complete or complex decongestive physiotherapy (CDP). This involves massage, exercise, hygiene training, and compression bandages or clothing. A trained therapist is required to provide manual lymph drainage. This requires daily massage over a one- to four-week period. The massage removes excess fluid by stimulating the lymph vessels to dilate to drain fluid and to open new passageways. After each massage, the affected limb is wound in compression bandages to prevent the build-up of fluid.

Exercise and skin care techniques are also used during the maintenance phase of CDP. Compression bandages may be required for 24 hours a day at the beginning, but once edema has decreased, a compression sleeve that is worn during periods of activity may be adequate. The sleeve is also necessary when exercising or traveling in a plane. CDP may not be appropriate for people under treatment for congestive heart disease. Diuretics are contraindicated because they contribute to protein build-up and may further affect the tissues.

Precautions—Physicians advise patients to take precautions to reduce the risk of lymphedema by observing the following advice:

- Avoid any injury to the arm or puncture to the skin.
- Avoid infection from cuts, burns, or insect bites by applying or taking antibiotics.
- Protect the affected arm by avoiding injections, blood withdrawal, intravenous procedures, and blood pressure readings if the other arm can be used.
- Avoid constricting clothing or jewelry.
- Avoid an activity that might cause heat in the arm or chest, such as tanning, saunas, hot tubs or baths, and vigorous exercise.
- Wear compression bandages or garments when exercising or flying.
- The woman in Figure 31–10A has lymphedema of her left arm, primarily in the forearm, following a mastectomy with lymph node removal. She stated at times it is much worse, becoming larger, warm, and sometimes developing skin lesions. The compression sleeve and glove (Figure 31–10B) helps to return lymph fluid and reduce swelling.

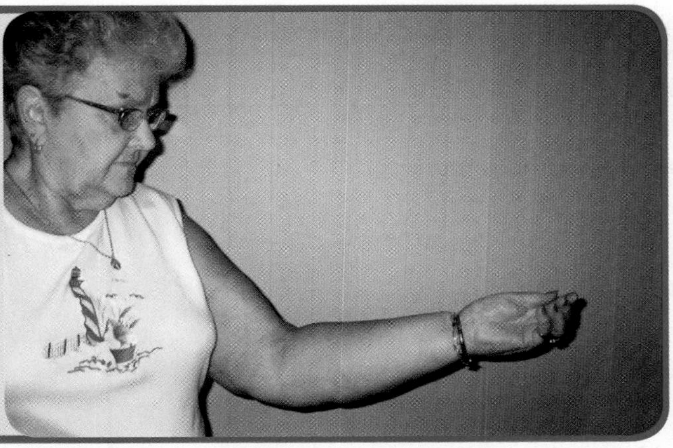

Figure 31–10A: Woman with lymphedema of the left arm following mastectomy and removal of lymph nodes.
Courtesy of Barbara A. Wise.

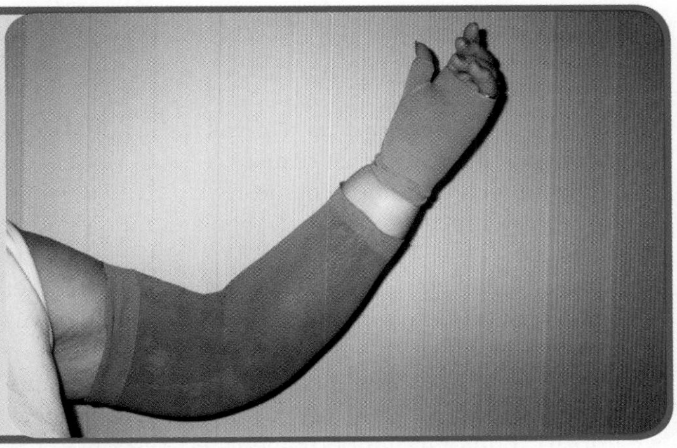

Figure 31–10B: Compression sleeve and glove.
Courtesy of Barbara A. Wise.

Rheumatoid Arthritis (Room′-a-toyd Ar-thri′-tis)

Description—This chronic systemic inflammatory autoimmune disease affects the joints and surrounding muscles, tendons, ligaments, and blood vessels. It affects women three times more often than men. It occurs primarily between the ages of 20 and 60, with a peak onset period between 35 to 45.

Signs and symptoms—The symptoms develop insidiously, then become localized in joints, usually bilaterally. Following inactivity, the affected joints stiffen, swell, and may show beginning signs of deformity. They eventually become tender, painful, hot, and enlarged and have marked deformities and decreased function.

This disease was discussed in the unit on the skeletal system; however, it is believed there is a connection to the immune system. Recent findings suggest a link to genetic defects, which cause the cells to display a specific cell marker. Patients may also have an autoantibody known as *rheumatoid factor,* which locks onto the body's own IgG molecule as if it were an antigen. These antigen-antibody complexes seem to be deposited on the synovial membranes of the joints and are the targets of the inflammatory response.

Etiology—The etiology of rheumatoid arthritis in unknown, but it results in an inflammatory response by the immune system. When the complement system is activated, the macrophages gather at the joint. The inflammatory response dilates the blood vessels, and fluid accumulates in the joint cavity. The cells of the membrane proliferate in response, thickening the joint membrane and causing more swelling. These events continue in cycles and result in the destruction of the joint.

Treatment—Treatment is varied depending on the severity of symptoms. Initially, therapy includes salicylates, **corticosteroids** (prednisone), nonsteroidal anti-inflammatory agents (ibuprofen), gold salts, and antimalarial drugs (chloroquine) and chemotherapy (methotrexate). Patients need periods of rest during the day and 8 to 10 hours of sleep every night. Activities that may be helpful are range of motion exercises, application of heat during chronic episodes, and ice packs with acute phases. Newer therapies include monoclonal antibodies such as etanercept (Enbrel), infliximab (Remicade), and adalimumab (Humira), which are anticytokine therapies that either enhance or inhibit the immune response of the disease.

AGE-RELATED BODY CHARACTERISTICS

The immune system decreases in effectiveness as we age. When born, passive immunity is transmitted from the mother to the infant. This is increased even more by the passing antibodies through breast milk. By 18 months this immunity has waned. Routine immunizations given to infants and children provide immunity to the usual childhood diseases as well as previous life threatening diseases. People with compromised immune systems, chronic diseases, or certain risk factors, as well as the aged, are routinely given a flu vaccine as a means of providing a short term resistance to influenza. The elderly and other people with chronic conditions are given a pneumonia vaccine to provide resistance to that disease. As we have just read, some new vaccines may influence the immune system to prevent us from initially developing certain cancers or many prohibit recurrence.

System Interaction Associated with Disease Conditions

The immune system is actually a function of both the circulatory and the skeletal systems. Since its function involves the lymph nodes and vessels, white blood cells, some of which come from bone marrow, it is an interactive system so any disease will at least affect both. Table 31–12 summarizes two disease conditions involving the immune system.

Table 31–12 System Interaction Associated with Disease Conditions

Disease	Systems Involved	Pathology Present
Lupus	Skeletal	Arthritis in joints
	Circulatory	Swollen lymph glands, bruises, anemia
	Integumentary	Butterfly rash, baldness
	Digestive	Nausea, vomiting, loss of appetite
AIDS	Circulatory	Lymph node enlargement
	Integumentary	Rashes, dry skin, herpes simplex
	Respiratory	Cough, breathing difficulty Pneumonia
	Nervous	Mobility problems, memory loss
	Digestive	Persistent diarrhea, yeast infection in mouth and esophagus

CHAPTER SUMMARY

- A strong immine system is necessary for well-being.
- We live in an environment of antigens: foreign materials, bacteria, viruses, fungi, and parasites.
- Immune system can self attack causing rheumatoid arthritis, diabetes, and lupus.
- The body has three main lines of defense: the skin and mucus membranes; biochemical barriers, and mechanical barriers.
- Blood cells originate in bone marrow and mature in various places.
- The lymphoidal organs of the immune system are bone marrow, the thymus, lymph nodes, spleen tonsils, adenoids appendix and Peyer's patches.
- All body cells carry molecules encoded by genes known as the major histocompatibility complex that identify themselves.
- T lymphocytes are present in four types: helper T cells, suppressor T cells, memory T cells, and killer T cells.
- B lymphocytes produce antibodies that can be activated by only one antigen.
- Antibodies are protein substances from the family of immunoglobulins. There are five types: IgA, IgD, IgE, IgG, and IgM.
- Complement is a group of about 20 inactive enzymes proteins involved in humoral immunity.
- Inflammation develops as a result of an antibody-mediated response that causes blood vessels to dilate and leak fluid into tissues.
- Cytokines are proteins that regulate the immune response.
- Natural killer cells can kill cancer cells and other cells infected with viruses without having previous exposure to them.
- Immune responses are either B cell, the humoral or antibody response, or T-cell, the cell-mediated response.
- Primary humoral, antibody-mediated response acts against bacteria and extracellular viruses, fungi, and parasites.
- Primary cell-mediated response activates the killer T cells to attack and the macrophages to assist in directly destroying the antigen.
- Review the outline explaining the Components of the Immune System.
- Review the explanation of the characters in the Immune System Surveillance Process.
- Immunizations are materials injected to activate immunity or restore its effect.
- Diseases covered in this chapter are: Acquired immunodeficiency syndrome (AIDS), allergies, cancer, chronic fatigue syndrome, lupus erythematosus, lymphedema, and rheumatoid arthritis.

STUDY TOOLS

Workbook	Activities for Chapter 31
Premium Website MEDIA LINK	View this **Media Link** for Chapter 31: • The Immune System

StudyWARE	Activities and Quizzes on the **StudyWARE™ Software** for Chapter 31
	Audio Library of medical terms
	Online access to the **Critical Thinking Challenge 2.0**
CourseMate	Activities and Quizzes for Chapter 31
WebTutor	Activities and Quizzes for Chapter 31

CHECK YOUR KNOWLEDGE

1. Persons diagnosed with cancer are best treated by a(n):
   a. personal family practice physician.
   b. internist.
   c. cytologist.
   d. oncologist.
2. A clinical trial is:
   a. a test performed in a physician's office.
   b. the discussion of a treatment by a group of attorneys.
   c. the testing of a new product to be used in a clinic.
   d. a research study to determine the effectiveness and safety of a treatment.
3. Tumor markers can:
   a. help locate sentinel lymph node.
   b. help diagnose a tumor and its response to treatment.
   c. mark the best location for focusing radiation.
   d. assist the surgeon to locate the tumor for removal during surgery.
4. A biopsy can be any of the following except:
   a. withdrawing a tissue sample through a needle.
   b. excising the whole tumor.
   c. removing a piece of the tumor by incision.
   d. focusing a laser beam on the tumor to destroy a small part at a time.
5. Genetic testing is appropriate when:
   a. a person is at high risk for developing inherited cancers.
   b. a patient wants to see if he has cancer.
   c. you want to determine if all the cancer has been removed.
   d. you need to see if a treatment has been effective.
6. Brachytherapy refers to:
   a. treatment that places radioactive material at the tumor.
   b. a treatment used only with patients who have the BRCA genes.
   c. an intravenous therapy given through the brachial artery.
   d. the administration of the drug Brachysone DX.
7. Which of the following statements does not refer to lupus?
   a. It cannot be detected by a blood test.
   b. It is an autoimmune disease.
   c. It causes changes in the immune system.
   d. It affects women more than men.
8. Lymphedema:
   a. results from the weakening of the immune system.
   b. is swelling of the tissues by accumulated lymph fluid.
   c. can be confirmed by a blood test.
   d. requires the removal of lymph nodes to stop the symptoms.
9. Rheumatoid arthritis:
   a. occurs primarily after age 65.
   b. is the wearing of cartilage at the joints.
   c. is treated with braces and splints to prevent joint movement.
   d. is an insidious chronic autoimmune disease.
10. Cancer vaccine:
    a. can make cells visible to the immune system.
    b. will eliminate all cancer cells in the body.
    c. can be developed quickly.
    d. is primarily directed toward people with BRCA1 gene mutation.
11. Immunity is strongest:
    a. in the aged.
    b. after recovering from the illness.
    c. during infancy.
    d. at 18 months of age.
12. Lupus:
    a. is a contagious disease.
    b. is limited to females only.
    c. occurs primarily after age 50.
    d. is an autoimmune disease.

WEB LINKS

NPIN HIV/AIDS Information: www.cdcnpin.org

American Cancer Society, cancer facts and figures: www.cancer.org/Research/CancerFactsFigures/index

Office of Minority Health & Health Disparities: www.cdc.gov/omhd

Chapter

32 The Digestive System

OBJECTIVES

In this chapter, you will learn the following:

KB KNOWLEDGE BASE

1. Spell and define, using the glossary at the back of the text, all the Words to Know in this chapter.
2. Name the four phases of the digestive process.
3. Define digestion.
4. Name the raw materials required for a healthy body.
5. Trace the pathway of food through the alimentary tract.
6. Describe the structures of the mouth and the digestive processes that occur there.
7. Explain the process of swallowing.
8. Describe how the esophagus propels food toward the stomach.
9. Describe the structure and function of the stomach.
10. Describe the structure and function of the small intestine.
11. Tell why the duodenum is a vital link in the digestive system.
12. List the functions of the liver, including the portal circulation connection.
13. Describe the role of the gallbladder and its association with the liver.
14. Describe the location and function of the pancreas.
15. Explain how and where nutrients are absorbed.
16. Name the sections of the colon and describe its function.
17. Describe the function of the rectum.
18. Describe the structure and function of the anal canal.
19. Describe the diagnostic examinations of the digestive tract.
20. Describe the disorders and diseases of the digestive system.
21. Discuss the presence of GERD in infants and adults.
22. Identify the body systems involved with GERD and hepatitis.

WORDS TO KNOW

alimentary canal
anal
anus
appendectomy
appendicitis
ascending
bile
bolus
bowel
cardiac sphincter
cecum
cholecystectomy
cholelithiasis
chyme
cirrhosis
colitis
colon
colostomy
common bile duct
constipation
Crohn's disease
cystic
defecate
descending
diarrhea
digestion
digestive
diverticulitis
duodenum
emesis
enzyme
esophagus
fecal
fissure
fistula
flatus
gallbladder
gastric
gastrointestinal (GI)
gastroscopy
hemorrhoidectomy
hemorrhoids
hepatic
hepatitis
hernia
herniorrhaphy
hiatus
hydrochloric acid
ileocecal
ileostomy
ileum
impaction
incontinent
insulin
intestine
jaundice
jejunum
liver
mesentery
mouth

nausea
pancreas
pancreatitis
paralytic ileus
peptic
peristalsis
polyp
proctoscope
pruritus ani
pyloric
rectum
reflux
saliva
salivary glands
sigmoid
sigmoidoscopy
stenosis
stomach
stool
tongue
transverse
ulcer
varices
vermiform appendix
villi
villous adenoma
vomit

THE DIGESTIVE SYSTEM

The **digestive** system is the group of organs that changes food that has been eaten into a form that can be used by the body's cells. The system is also known as the **gastrointestinal (GI)** tract or system, and the connecting chain of organs is sometimes referred to as the **alimentary canal**. The digestive process can be divided into four phases: *ingestion, digestion, absorption,* and *elimination*. Food that is consumed is acted on by various mechanical and chemical means as it progresses through the body. Each organ, whether main or accessory, plays an important role in physically or chemically altering the composition of the food, selectively absorbing the elements, or eliminating the remains.

The main organs of the system are those through which the food passes. These organs form a continuous tube from the entrance to the exit of the body. They are the mouth, pharynx, esophagus, stomach, small intestine, and large intestine. As important as these organs are, it is the accessory organs that play a major role in the digestive process. In the mouth, there are the teeth, salivary glands, and tongue. The liver, gallbladder, and pancreas have access to the small intestine (Figure 32–1).

Digestion is the activity performed by the organs of the digestive system, and it is defined as the process by

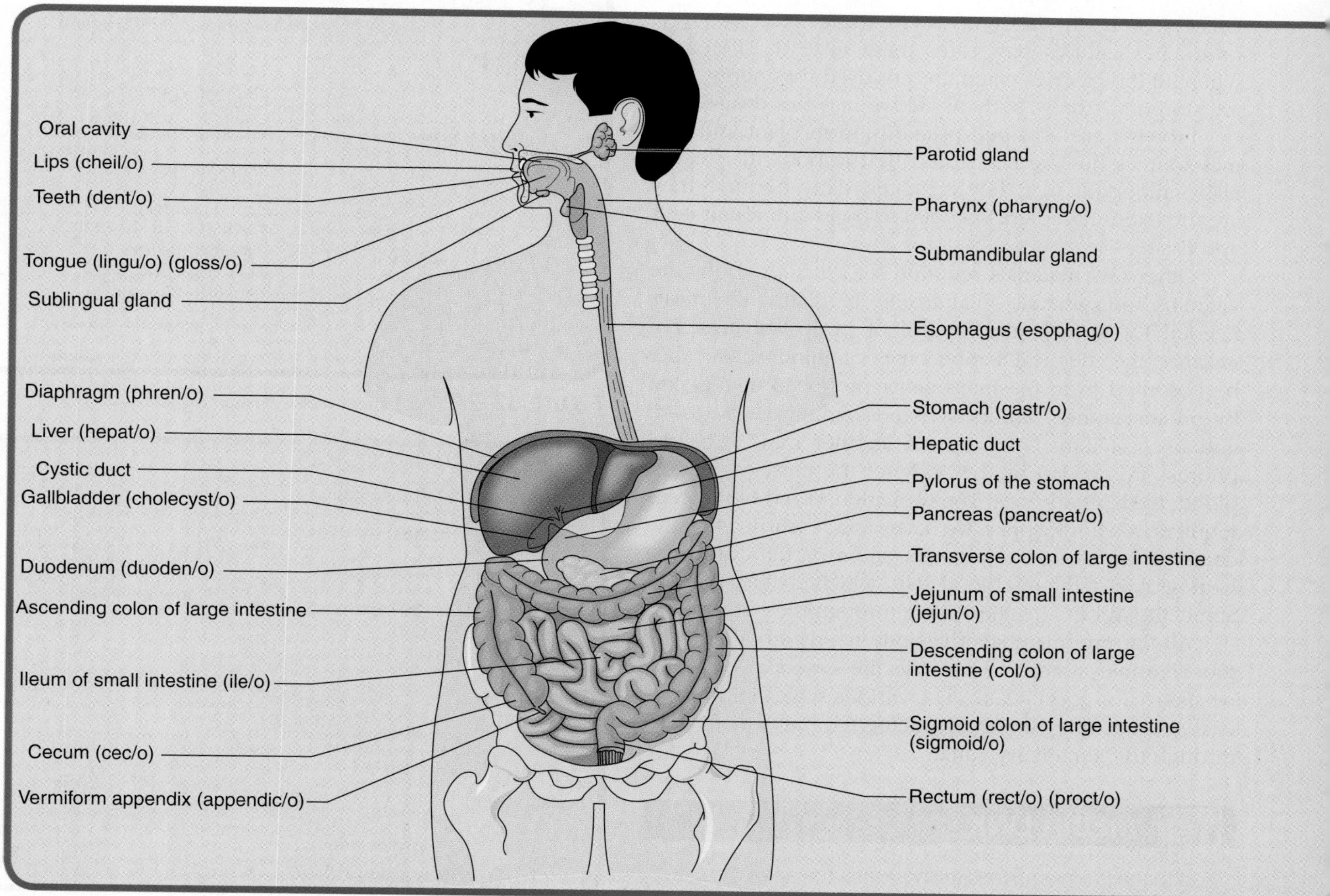

Figure 32–1: The digestive system. *Delmar/Cengage Learning.*

which food is broken down, mechanically and chemically, in the GI tract and converted into an absorbable form that can be used by the cells of the body. This process cannot occur within the digestive system alone. As with all body functions, an interrelationship of systems is required to achieve the desired results. Digestion requires cooperation from the nervous system, the muscular system, the circulatory system, and the endocrine system.

The human body can be compared with an engine that needs appropriate fuel to operate. The energy we need to function must come from the foods we eat. The right fuel will not only supply the body with energy, but also provide the materials necessary to build and repair the body so that it can operate efficiently. If the wrong fuel is used too often, the machine will eventually break down.

The human body can manufacture the appropriate fuel if it receives an adequate supply of the right raw materials, mainly carbohydrates, proteins, fats, minerals, vitamins, water, and roughage. All these raw materials are available from the basic food groups and should be eaten daily.

Carbohydrates supply about two thirds of the energy calories needed each day. Fats are also an excellent source of energy; in fact, an ounce of fat yields about three times the calories of an ounce of carbohydrate. Unfortunately, the body does not waste excess energy-producing calories but stores them instead. Therefore, when all the calories eaten are not used for energy, they are stored as excess body tissue we may not desire.

Proteins are obtained primarily from plant and animal sources but are not stored by the body. It is especially important that they be eaten daily because they are the main ingredients needed to build and repair cells and tissue.

Other raw materials required for a healthy body are vitamins and minerals. Vitamins are regulating chemicals needed for growth and control of body activities. For instance, the chemical that becomes vitamin D must either be absorbed from the intestine or produced in the skin by photosynethsis. The body needs vitamin D to absorb and use calcium. Calcium and another mineral, phosphorus, are needed by the body for the muscles, nerves, blood, teeth, and bones. The formation of red blood cells requires iron and copper. We have already learned that the combination of an iron pigment and a protein forms the hemoglobin of the red blood cells, which enables them to attract O_2 and CO_2 as they move through the body.

All the raw materials the body needs are altered by the digestive system to provide the essential elements necessary for good health. The various stages in this process will become clearer by tracing the pathway of food through the alimentary canal.

MEDIA LINK

Go to the Premium Website and watch the animation, "Digestion," for this chapter.

THE MOUTH

Food enters the body through the **mouth**. It is held in the oral cavity while the initial digestive process is begun. Teeth break up food into small pieces to make it easier to swallow and also to prepare it for more effective action by digestive enzymes. "Baby" teeth are called *deciduous* and begin to appear at about 6 months. They are gradually exchanged for permanent teeth beginning at about 6 years. Different teeth have specific duties to perform. The incisors bite food with their sharp edges. The canines or cuspids are pointed to puncture and tear. The premolars or bicuspids and the molars are for grinding and crushing (Figure 32–2A and B). The **tongue** aids in the process by moving the food around within

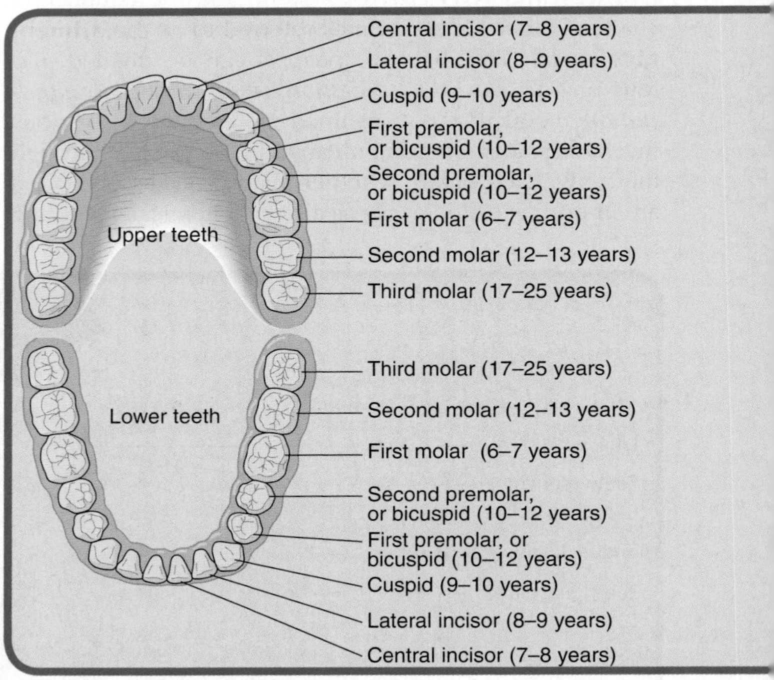

Figure 32–2A: Permanent teeth. *Delmar/Cengage Learning.*

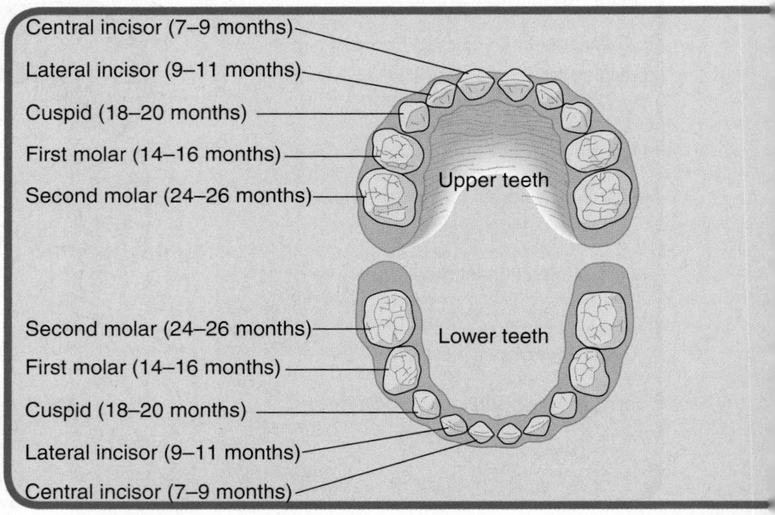

Figure 32–2B: Deciduous teeth. *Delmar/Cengage Learning.*

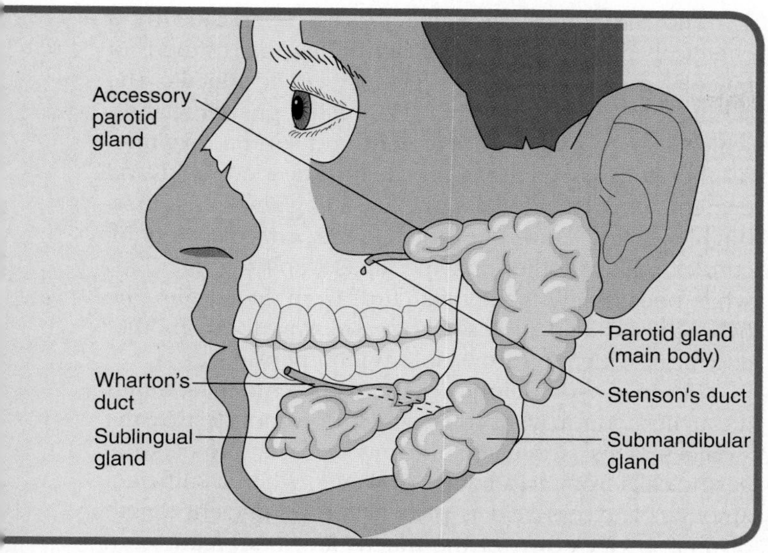

Figure 32–3: Salivary glands. *Delmar/Cengage Learning.*

the mouth, bringing it into contact with the teeth. The tongue is a muscle and can alter its shape to reach all areas of the mouth. The surface of the tongue contains the taste buds, located within the papillae projections.

The **salivary glands** excrete the fluid known as **saliva**. It is released from three pairs of glands: the parotid, the submandibular, and the sublingual (Figure 32–3). Certain foods cause the glands to excrete profusely, often producing some discomfort, as when eating something sour. The disease called mumps is the inflammation of the parotid glands. A virus causes the glands to enlarge and become painful. With mumps, mastication (chewing) causes great discomfort because the muscle action squeezes the swollen glands.

Saliva contains an **enzyme** called ptyalin. This chemical begins the break down of carbohydrates into sugar. Saliva also provides moisture that enables the taste buds to perceive the sensations of sweet, sour, bitter, and salty. In addition, saliva aids in cleansing the teeth by washing away food particles that might allow bacteria to grow. The presence of saliva in the oral cavity keeps the surfaces moist and flexible, which aids in the production of speech.

The combination of mashed food substances and saliva is called a **bolus**. When it has been mixed well and contains sufficient moisture, it can be easily swallowed. For this to occur, several muscles must work together. The tongue presses upward and backward against the palate (roof of the mouth), while the muscles in the cheeks help in the formation of a chute to direct the bolus toward the back of the mouth and into the pharynx (Figure 32–4). At this point, the bolus could go in three different directions: into the nasal cavity, down and forward into the trachea, or down into the **esophagus**.

The directing of the bolus is accomplished by a complex combination of "lids" and muscles, which operate automatically. As the bolus is swallowed, it raises the soft palate, closing off the nasal cavity. At the same time, the epiglottis, a cartilage lid attached at the top of the larynx, moves across the opening into the larynx when the tongue pushes the bolus against the palate. At the moment of swallowing, the larynx moves upward against the epiglottis to close the opening. Usually, this reflex action works perfectly, but when the timing is slightly off, food may enter the larynx, triggering the cough reflex (to remove the material). We say, "It went down the wrong pipe."

THE ESOPHAGUS

Once food is swallowed, its movement through the body is maintained by the smooth, involuntary muscle action called **peristalsis**. The esophagus has two layers of involuntary muscles. The inner layer forms circles around the esophagus, whereas the outer layer runs

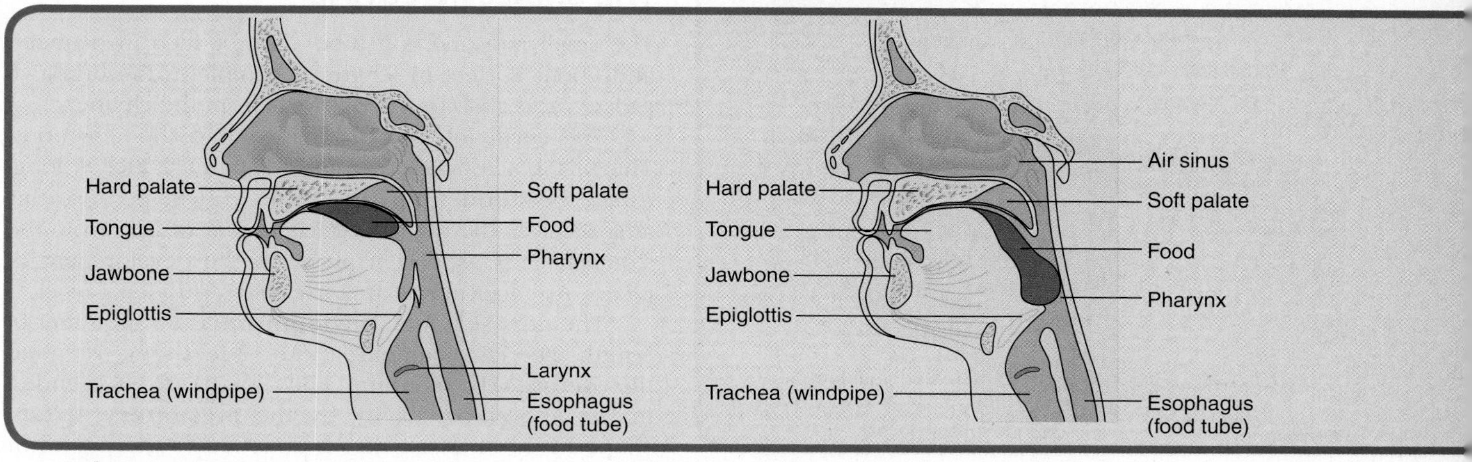

Figure 32–4: The process of swallowing. *Delmar/Cengage Learning.*

longitudinally along its approximately 10-inch length. When food enters the esophagus, the muscles alternately contract and relax, squeezing the bolus. Together they create the peristaltic "milking action," which moves the bolus to the **stomach**. The whole process only requires about 5 seconds. Because peristaltic action moves material in one direction only and this process does not depend on gravity, it is possible to drink a glass of water while standing on your head.

THE STOMACH

The upper opening to the stomach is controlled by a circular muscle called the **cardiac sphincter**. As the peristaltic wave approaches, the sphincter dilates, allowing the food to enter. Once the food is inside, this one-way "gate" closes to prevent its escape.

The stomach is a 10-inch-long, J-shaped organ constructed of three layers of strong muscle tissue (Figure 32–5). It lies just beneath the diaphragm. The inner lining of the stomach is thick and full of folds called *rugae*. Because muscle tissue is elastic and the folds in the lining can straighten out, the stomach is capable of expanding. It can hold about half a gallon of food and liquid.

Once the material has entered the stomach, the muscular layers begin to contract. A circular layer, a longitudinal layer, and an oblique layer work together in a strong rhythmic motion to break up the food into tiny particles. The stomach continues the digestive process that began in the mouth. The churning action is prolonged and made more difficult by poorly chewed food.

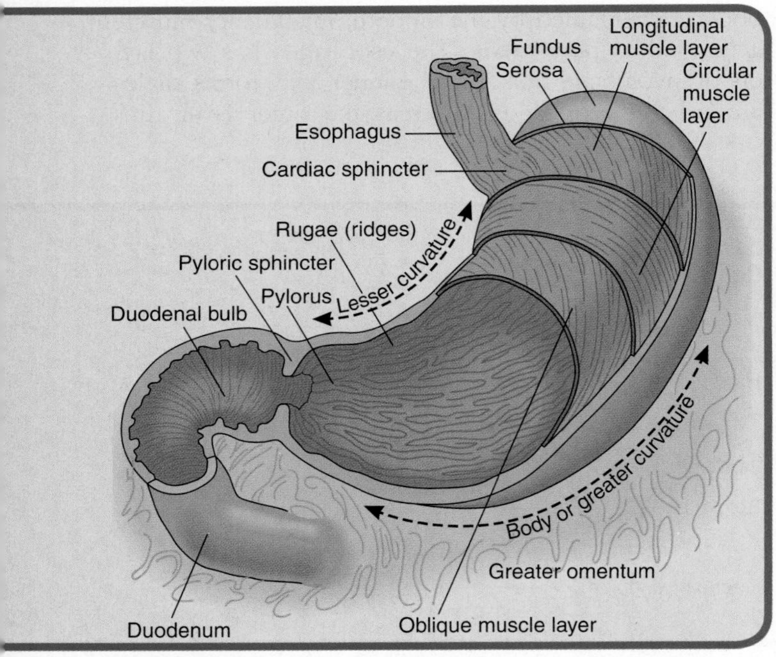

Figure 32–5: The stomach. *Delmar/Cengage Learning.*

The mechanical digestive process is assisted by a chemical process. The stomach lining is formed of mucous membrane, whose glands secrete mucus. The stomach lining also has about 35 million **gastric** glands, which secrete **hydrochloric acid** and several enzymes. As the stomach contents are being kneaded, acid and enzymes are excreted by the gastric glands and thoroughly mixed into the bolus. One enzyme, rennin, curdles milk. Another enzyme, lipase, splits certain fats, while pepsin digests the milk curds from the rennin. The hydrochloric acid unites with protein to form another chemical, which in turn is split by the pepsin.

Because hydrochloric acid burns holes in most things it touches, you may wonder why it does not destroy the stomach. This is because the mucus layer protects the gastric cells from acid injury. However, when a sufficient amount of excess acid is present for a sufficient length of time, break down of the mucus layer can lead to an **ulcer** (open sore), usually along the posterior wall near the pylorus. An ulcer in the stomach that is caused by acid is known as a gastric (stomach) or **peptic** ulcer.

The partially digested food in the stomach is changed into a semiliquid state called **chyme** in three to five hours. Liquids, on the other hand, pass through the stomach in a matter of minutes. Of the solid foods, carbohydrates are digested first, proteins second, and fats last. When the consistency of the chyme is right, the **pyloric** sphincter, at the end of the stomach, allows the chyme to spurt through the sphincter into the small **intestine**.

Because of the two sphincters, food is held in the stomach until it is properly prepared to leave. But occasionally, when you suffer from **nausea** and **vomit**, it is obvious the material did not go in the right direction. This action is accomplished by the contraction of the abdominal muscles, forcefully squeezing the stomach as it is pushed downward by the diaphragm. With this pressure and reverse peristaltic waves, the contents of the stomach are forced out and **emesis** (vomiting) occurs.

THE SMALL INTESTINE

The small intestine is a tube about 1 inch in diameter and about 20 feet in length. It completes the digestive process and absorbs the nutrients from the chyme.

The small intestine is divided into three sections. The first is a C-shaped segment, about 9 inches long, called the **duodenum** (see Figure 32–6). Because this area receives the highest concentration of acid from the stomach, it is especially prone to the development of ulcers. An ulcer in this area is called a duodenal ulcer.

The next segment, the **jejunum**, is about 8 feet in length. The last segment, about 12 feet long, is called the **ileum**. The jejunum and ileum are suspended in the abdominal cavity by the **mesentery**, a fan-shaped fold of tissue that is attached to the posterior abdominal wall.

The ileum is reduced to about half an inch in diameter by the time it joins the large intestine in the right lower quadrant of the abdomen. The junction is marked by a sphincter called the **ileocecal** valve, which allows the chyme to enter the **cecum** (first segment of the large intestine) but prohibits anything from returning to the ileum.

ACCESSORY ORGANS AND THE ABSORPTION PROCESS

The small intestine completes the digestive process with the aid of accessory organs and intestinal juice secreted by the glands of the small intestine.

The Liver and Gallbladder

The **liver** is the largest gland in the body. It lies below the diaphragm in the upper right quadrant of the abdomen, extending into the upper left quadrant (Figure 32–6). The liver is a vital organ that performs several functions for the body. It secretes **bile** at a rate of over a pint a day, and the bile is continuously excreted through bile passages to the bile duct. Unconcentrated liver bile is a bitter, yellow-orange liquid that is required to digest fats. Bile is composed primarily of water and contains pigment from red blood cells that have been destroyed (carried to the liver from the spleen in the portal vein). The pigment is changed in the intestines and excreted in **fecal** material, giving it its yellow-brown color. The iron from the destroyed cells is reabsorbed into the body.

The liver also stores glycogen, a form of glucose (carbohydrate). When the body needs additional blood sugar, it changes the glycogen back to glucose and releases it. In addition, the liver processes proteins from amino acids and either burns fats as fuel or stores them. The liver performs the life-essential service of manufacturing fibrinogen, prothrombin, and other substances required for the process of clotting blood. Antibodies to counteract certain disease organisms are produced in the liver. Also, toxins (poisons) that have been absorbed from the intestine, inhaled, injected, or otherwise taken into the body are circulated in the blood to the liver, where for the most part they are rendered harmless. The liver is also an important storage area for blood and body fluid because of its large size.

The liver receives blood from two separate systems. It receives arterial blood for its own support and preservation from the hepatic artery. It also receives blood from the portal vein that conveys absorbed nutrients and other substances from all the abdominal organs for processing.

The **gallbladder** is a small sac attached to the underside of the liver (Figure 32–7). Its sole purpose is the concentration and storage of bile. When the body needs bile to digest food, the gallbladder releases the concentrated bile to supplement that being currently produced by the liver. Concentrated bile is very bitter and is green-yellow in color. The gallbladder empties its contents via the **cystic** duct. The cystic duct from the gallbladder and the **hepatic** duct from the liver combine to form the **common bile duct**. This common duct empties the bile directly into the duodenum to be added to the chyme

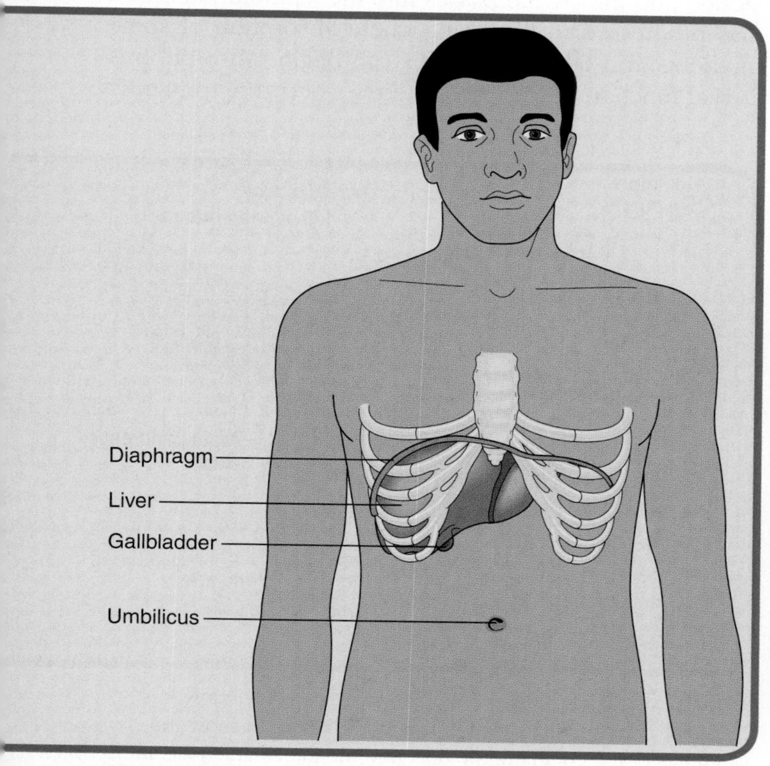

Figure 32–6: The liver and gallbladder. *Delmar/Cengage Learning.*

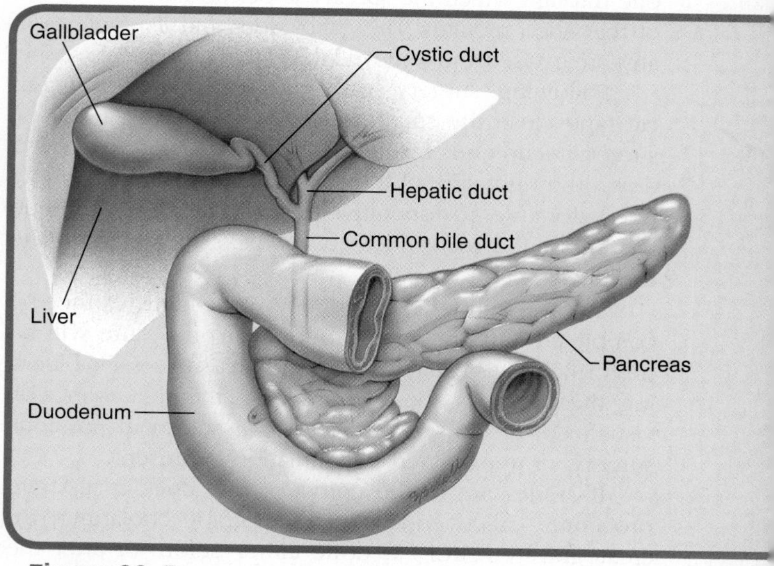

Figure 32–7: The gallbladder and cystic, hepatic, and common bile ducts on the underside of the liver. *Delmar/Cengage Learning.*

during the digestive process. The duodenum is a very vital segment of the digestive system. Not only does it receive chyme from the stomach and bile from the liver and gallbladder, but as we will soon see, it also receives pancreatic juices from the pancreas.

Obstruction of the bile ducts by **cholelithiasis** (gallstones) from the gallbladder is not uncommon. Bile contains certain mineral salts that can become crystallized into "stones" in the gallbladder, perhaps from poor drainage or extended storage. Frequently, the stones will be expelled into the cystic duct where they become lodged, causing pain and an inadequate supply of bile and frequently requiring surgical removal. If the stone reaches the common bile duct before becoming lodged, a much more serious situation results. Stones in the common bile duct are called choledocholithiasis. Now neither the gallbladder nor the liver can empty its bile. The liver maintains its production, but now the bile is absorbed into the bloodstream, producing the yellow discoloration of the sclera, mucosa, and skin known as **jaundice**. The gallbladder itself may become infected or filled with stones and nonfunctional. Periodic "gallbladder attacks" will usually prompt a **cholecystectomy** (surgical removal). The hepatic duct and the common bile duct must remain for the liver to function, however.

A newer surgical procedure to remove the gallbladder and cholelithiasis is called laparoscopic cholecystectomy. It has revolutionized the way gallbladder surgery is performed. The procedure is accomplished with the use of three or more laparoscopes (tiny telescope instruments) inserted into the abdomen. One is placed in the right upper quadrant, one near the umbilicus, and one in the mid-upper abdomen. One scope serves as the source of light and has a camera attachment and a video monitor. Another is an air supply to manipulate tissues, and the third is the one through which the surgery is performed with the aid of the video monitor. The gallbladder and its contents, if any, are excised and removed through the operative scope.

Following surgery, only a few sutures or surgical tape close the small abdominal openings. Previous surgery techniques resulted in a long incision extending down the right side of the abdomen and a considerably uncomfortable postoperative period. The new technique has shortened recovery to two weeks or less from the former six weeks period.

Occasionally, the endoscopic procedure cannot be completed and an "open" abdominal procedure will be performed. This usually occurs if there is excessive bleeding, the patient is obese or pregnant, the area cannot be visualized, there is excessive scar tissue from previous surgery, or unexpected inflammation is present.

If stones are in the common bile duct, a separate procedure called endoscopic retrograde cholangiopancreatography (ERCP) is done either before or after the laparoscopic cholescystectomy in order to remove them, or an open procedure is substituted.

The Pancreas

The **pancreas** lies behind the stomach, with its head in the curve of the duodenum (Figure 32–8). The pancreas, like the liver, is a gland, but it secretes substances in two different ways. Functioning as an *exocrine gland* (secreting through ducts), the pancreas secretes pancreatic juice via the pancreatic duct directly into the duodenum. The three powerful enzymes in pancreatic juice react chemically on all three types of nutrients to break them down for absorption into the bloodstream. Most of the chemical changes that occur in the intestinal tract are caused by pancreatic juices, which are probably sufficient to digest all foods by themselves. If pancreatic juice is absent, serious digestive problems occur.

Functioning as an *endocrine* (ductless) *gland,* the pancreas also secretes directly into the bloodstream a substance called **insulin**. This function will be covered in Chapter 34, The Endocrine System.

It should be clear now why the duodenum is such a critical segment of the digestive tract. Because it receives products from four organs—stomach, liver, gallbladder, and pancreas—it is a vital connective link. When ulceration occurs or a tumor develops in this area, it may interfere drastically with the digestive process. Involvement of the duodenum is a cause for concern.

The Absorption Function

When all the digestive juices and enzymes have been added and the chyme passes into the jejunum, digestion has progressed to the point where absorption of some nutrients and other substances can begin. Absorption is a vital function of the small intestine, occurring primarily

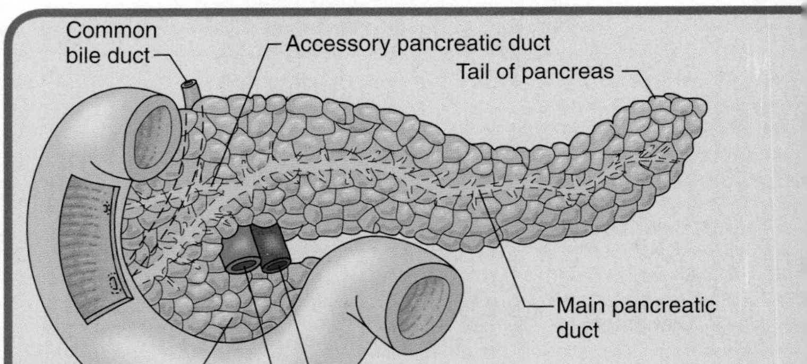

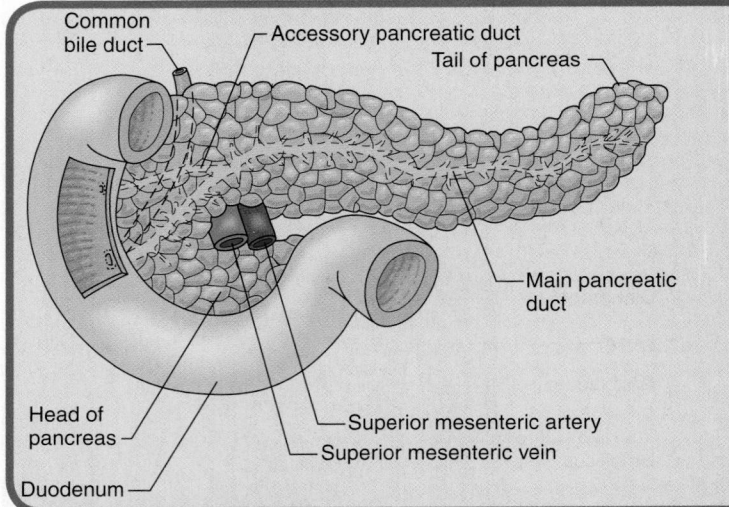

Figure 32–8: The duodenum and pancreas. A window has been cut into the anterior wall of the duodenum to show the openings of the common bile duct and the pancreatic ducts into the lumen of the duodenum. *Delmar/Cengage Learning.*

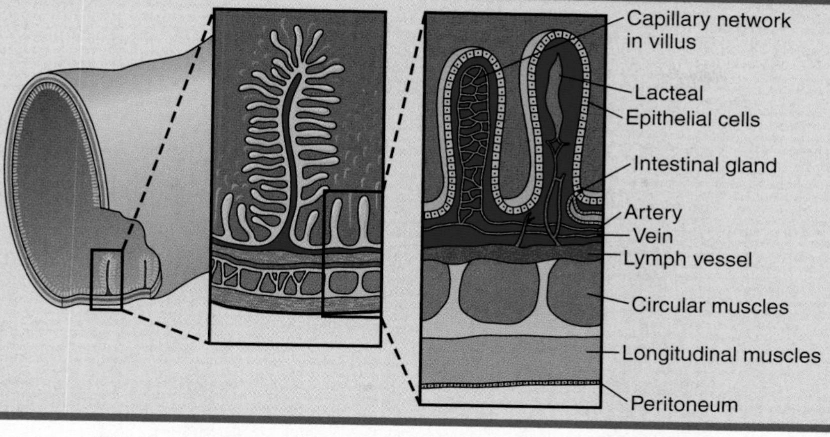

Figure 32–9: A magnified view of the inner lining of the small intestine showing the villa with blood and lymphatic capillaries for the absorption of the products of digestion. *Delmar/Cengage Learning.*

in the jejunum and gradually decreasing toward the end of the ileum.

Absorption is accomplished through millions of microscopic structures known as **villi** (Figure 32–9). The villi project from the lining of the major part of the small intestine. These fingerlike structures serve a dual purpose. First, they move continuously, swinging back and forth to keep the chyme thoroughly mixed with the digestive juices. Second, each projection is equipped with blood capillaries and a lacteal (intestinal lymphatic capillary) from the lymphatic system. The external cells of the villi absorb the nutrients, minerals, and water from the chyme. Some fats and all carbohydrates and proteins, in the form of sugar and amino acids, are absorbed into the capillaries of the villi, to be sent by way of the portal vein to the liver. Here, the products are processed and released into the body or stored in reserve. Many fats are absorbed into the lacteals of the lymphatic system to be processed through the lymph nodes and eventually returned to the circulatory system for distribution.

THE LARGE INTESTINE

With digestion completed and the useful nutrients and other substances absorbed from the chyme, the waste products, any undigestible material, and the excess water are sent on to the large intestine through the ileocecal valve. The large intestine is only about 5 feet long, but it is approximately 2 inches in diameter. The **colon**, as it is also called, frames the abdomen (Figure 32–10).

The large intestine absorbs the excess liquid from the chyme through capillaries in the lining. There are no villi in the large intestine. The absorbed water, plus some salts and proteins, are later filtered out of the blood by the kidneys to be eliminated in the urine. The remaining fibrous waste materials are formed into semisolid feces to be eliminated through the **rectum**.

The Cecum and Appendix

When material leaves the ileum, it enters a small, pouch-like segment of the colon called the cecum. A small projection, the **vermiform appendix**, extends from the cecum. The appendix is a worm-shaped structure about the size of the little finger. It tends to become filled easily but drains rather slowly. Occasionally, a substance causes irritation to the lining, resulting in a painful, inflammatory process known as **appendicitis**. If it persists or progresses, a surgical procedure called an **appendectomy** is indicated.

The Ascending, Transverse, and Descending Colon

The large intestine is divided into **ascending**, **transverse**, and **descending** sections as a means of identification. The ascending section joins the cecum at the level of the ileocecal valve and continues upward along the right side of the abdomen to the hepatic flexure (bend at the liver). It is generally a little larger in diameter than the descending section. The upper right corner, the hepatic flexure, lies in front of the right kidney and behind the right lobe of the liver. The transverse section begins at the hepatic flexure and extends in a loop across the abdominal cavity to a point below the spleen, the splenic flexure (bend at the spleen). The center section is attached to the mesentery but can move freely. Both the hepatic and splenic flexures are firmly attached to the rear of the abdominal wall, with the splenic attachment being slightly higher.

The descending section begins at the splenic flexure and extends downward along the left side of the abdomen until it reaches the edge of the pelvic cavity. This section is somewhat smaller in diameter. It is firmly anchored to the abdominal posterior wall to maintain its position.

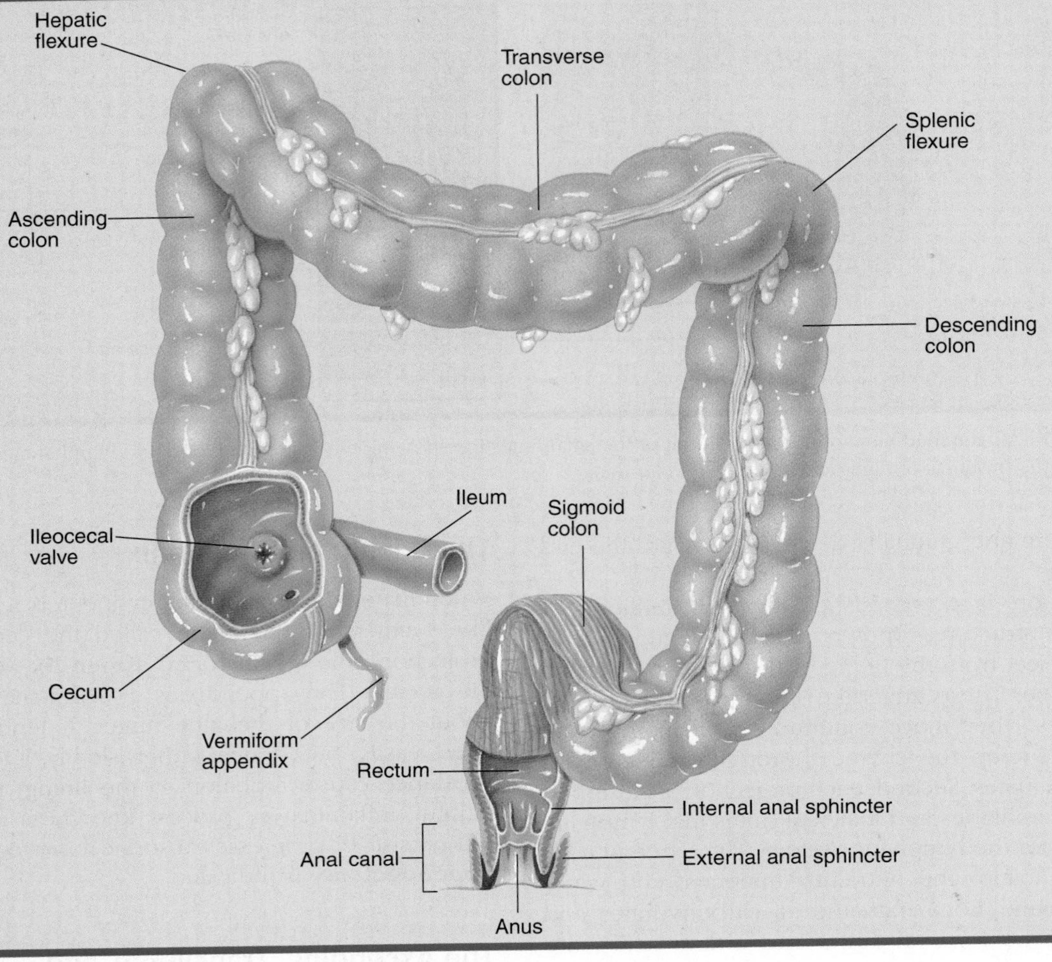

Figure 32–10: The large intestine. *Delmar/Cengage Learning.*

The Sigmoid, Rectum, and Anal Canal

After the large intestine enters the pelvic cavity, it makes two bends suggestive of an S and is therefore labeled the **sigmoid** section of the colon. The sigmoid section extends from the left iliac crest over and back to join the rectum. The rectum is 6 to 8 inches long. It serves as a collecting area for the remains of digestion. When enough material is accumulated, sensors are activated, and the urge to **defecate** is felt.

The **anal** canal is a narrow passageway about an inch long, extending from the rectum to the **anus** (opening from the body). Both ends of the anal canal are controlled by sphincter muscles. The internal anal sphincter is an involuntary muscle. When defecation occurs, the nerve endings in the rectum are stimulated to contract, and the internal sphincter is relaxed, allowing the fecal material to enter the anal canal. The external anal sphincter is a voluntary muscle and can be consciously controlled to prevent the rectum from emptying when it is inappropriate. It is unwise to make a habit of delaying defecation unnecessarily, however, as this tends to lessen the urge, which can result in **constipation**.

When a patient's condition interferes with the ability to control the anus, as in a stroke with paralysis, and the rectum empties whenever the nerve impulse is triggered, the patient is said to be **incontinent** of feces. This situation can be extremely embarrassing to a patient who is still capable of being aware of this occurrence. The opposite problem is often the result of prolonged or serious illness causing a loss of muscle tone so that the patient is too weak to expel the contents of the rectum. This results in material becoming more and more solid as fluid content is lost and the mass becoming of such size that it cannot be expelled. This condition is known as a fecal **impaction**. The best solution is manual breakup of the mass followed by an enema to irrigate the rectum and remove the material. A patient may attempt to remove the impaction by taking a laxative. Laxatives work either by increasing the rate of passage through the tract, therefore reducing the water absorption time, or by stimulating the secretion of fluid into the tract. Regardless, the results will not help an impaction but only cause an uncontrollable flow of liquid **stool** around the mass.

The proper function of the digestive system is essential to health. If raw materials cannot be digested and absorbed, the patient will starve. If waste products are not adequately removed, toxins may accumulate and cause illness and even death. This vital function requires a total of about 36 hours from the mouth to the anus. Of course, this time period is influenced by the type of foods eaten and the rate of the peristaltic action.

DIAGNOSTIC EXAMINATIONS

A great many studies can be done on blood to determine the function of the digestive organs. Also, chemical analysis can be performed on secretions withdrawn by catheter from the stomach or small intestine. However, six other types of examinations will be discussed here because they are so frequently used in diagnosis.

- *Colonoscopy*—An examination to view the entire large intestine using a flexible fiberoptic scope. It is indicated in patients with complaints of diarrhea, constipation, bleeding, or lower abdominal pain. It is especially indicated following negative or inconclusive results from barium enema studies or sigmoidoscopy examination. The American Cancer Society recommends a colonoscopy every 10 years, beginning at age 50, as a screening test for colon cancer. Persons with personal or family history of polyps or other colon diseases should follow a more frequent screening. Preparation for the examination is quite involved. Starting 24 hours prior to the examination, the patient is allowed only clear liquids or things that become liquid when eaten, such as gelatin. If bleeding is suspected, then no liquids that contain red food coloring may be consumed. In addition to the diet, the patient is instructed to take a strong dose of laxative and repeat a liquid laxative until the stool becomes nothing but liquid. Twelve hours before the procedure, nothing can be taken by mouth.

  When the procedure is performed, the patient is sedated and positioned on the left side, and the scope is guided and advanced through the large intestine. The physician may insert air to distend the walls of the intestine to facilitate passage. Manipulation of the abdomen also assists with insertion, and the repositioning of the patient facilitates passage through the splenic and hepatic flexures. It is possible to obtain tissue samples and secretions through the scope to provide cytology studies. Polyps can also be snared, and electrocautery can be performed through the instrument.
- *Gastrointestinal series* (X-rays)—Radiologic studies of the GI tract are indicated for a wide variety of reasons and concentrated on various portions of the system.

  Barium swallow—If the condition or function of the esophagus is in question, the patient may be asked to drink a radiopaque liquid called barium while the action of the esophagus is observed by fluoroscope. This test is known as a barium swallow. It aids in diagnosing conditions such as dysphagia, hiatus hernia, diverticulosis, and varices. It also detects strictures, tumors, ulcers, and functional disorders. The barium swallow is usually included as part of the more complete GI series.

  Upper GI series—A barium swallow is performed initially to evaluate the esophagus. Sixteen to twenty ounces of additional barium are drunk as the progress of the medium is observed by fluoroscope. X-ray films are taken at specific periods to permit further evaluation. The stomach is compressed to ensure that the barium coats the entire lining. As the barium enters the small intestine, the radiologist manipulates the abdomen to obtain distribution of the barium throughout the bowel loops. The patient is rotated to several positions to record pertinent areas. Spot films may be taken at 30- to 60-minute intervals until peristalsis carries the barium to the ileocecal valve.

  An upper GI series is not painful, but the chalky taste and consistency of barium are unpleasant. Preparation for the test may require a two to three day diet of low-residue foods before the examination. All oral intake must stop at least eight hours before it is scheduled. The patient must also refrain from smoking. Both a laxative and a cleansing enema may be ordered the evening before the procedure to be certain the tract is empty.

  An upper GI series aids in the diagnosis of gastric ulcers, tumors, strictures of the sphincters, inflammation of the lining, motility irregularities, duodenal ulcers, tumors, filling defects, and the like. Following the exam, another laxative may be ordered to aid in removal of the barium from the intestines. Retained barium may cause constipation, obstruction, or fecal impaction.

  Lower GI series—To permit viewing of the entire large intestine, the barium mixture is administered as an enema. The medium outlines the interior wall of the colon for detection of mucosal changes, tumors, **polyps**, ulcerated sites, **diverticulitis**, and structural irregularities. The patient must be carefully prepared with a restrictive, low-residue diet for about two days, followed by a diet of liquids only the day before examination. A cathartic (strong laxative) is ordered the afternoon preceding the test, and the colon is thoroughly emptied with tap water enemas until no more fecal material is expelled.

  A barium enema of 1000 to 1500 mL is administered through a tube inserted into the rectum. This tube is often capable of being inflated with a balloonlike section to aid in retention of the medium until the examination is completed. As the medium is instilled, the filling is observed by fluoroscope. The patient is rotated on the X-ray table to assist the flow of the barium. The patient is placed on the left side to fill the descending, on the back to fill the transverse, and on the right side to fill the ascending colon. Periodic X-ray films are taken.

When the procedure is completed, the balloon is deflated and the tube is removed. The patient is instructed to expel as much barium as possible. An additional X-ray may be taken to record the ability of the colon to empty.

- ***Gastroscopy**/esophagogastroduodenoscopy (EGD)*—Viewing of the esophagus, stomach, and upper duodenum through a flexible scope that is lighted by fiberoptics. This permits observation of the inside of the organs without an exploratory operation. If an unusual area or growth is seen, a biopsy (small piece) can be removed through the scope. The procedure is also used to remove small foreign objects, to obtain cells from the lining, and, with the attachment of a camera, to photograph suspicious areas for later study.

  The patient is prepared by spraying the back of the throat with local anesthetic to block the gag reflex and is given a sedative to produce drowsiness. The patient must be awake to swallow the scope. As it is passed into the patient, air is instilled to expand the pathway or flatten out folds. Water may also be instilled to wash off the lens and is removed, along with the air and any other secretions, by suction.

  The examination is especially helpful in diagnosing tumors, ulcers, structural abnormalities, damage from ingested chemicals, and esophageal varices. Figure 32–11 shows a fairly large tumor attached to the wall of the stomach. It is clearly visible through the scope and easily accessible for biopsy.
- *Nuclear medicine study*—Scanning of structures, such as the liver or spleen, is made possible by radioactive materials. A special camera or scanning device may be used to screen the liver for disease processes, infarcts, cysts, tumors, and organ size. The patient is given an intravenous injection of a radioactive material that the body will absorb in the cells of the liver. The scanner is positioned above the patient and passes slowly back and forth in a descending pattern over the area being examined. The resulting pictures outline the organ and indicate irregularities in its composition. A gamma camera is capable of producing images instantly without the scanning procedure.

  Similar studies are accomplished with different types of equipment. Computerized axial tomography studies (CT scans) are multiple X-ray beams passed into tissue to be interpreted and reconstructed by a computer into a three-dimensional picture on a screen. This type of study can be done on the liver, the ducts, and the pancreas.
- *Occult blood test*—When bleeding from the intestinal tract is not visible because of the small quantity, it can be detected through analysis of the feces. Occult blood studies are frequently used to identify bleeding associated with colorectal malignancy.

  Visible blood in the stool has a characteristic coloration that suggests the approximate location of the bleeding. Basically, the nearer the rectum, the brighter red the blood. Dark maroon stool is an indication of bleeding in the ileum or jejunum. Bleeding from the stomach or esophagus will be acted on by gastric juices, which cause it to turn black, resulting in a tarry-looking stool. A simple test involves the use of a occult blood slide upon which a thin smear of stool is placed. Developer is applied to the smear, and results are read within a minute. A trace or change of color to blue is positive for occult blood.
- *Proctoscopy*—An examination of the lower rectum and anal canal through a 3-inch-long **proctoscope**. It is preceded by a digital examination to determine anal sphincter condition. The proctoscope permits detection of hemorrhoids, polyps, fissures, fistulas, and abscesses. The patient may need an enema if fecal material is obstructing the view.
- ***Sigmoidoscopy***—An examination to view the lower portion of the sigmoid and rectum through a 10- to 12-inch sigmoidoscope. A longer flexible fiber optic scope is capable of manipulation into the descending colon. A digital examination to determine anal sphincter condition precedes insertion of the scope. The patient is examined, preferably on a special jackknife table, or otherwise in the less comfortable knee-chest position. Sigmoidoscopy aids in the diagnosis of inflammation, infection, or ulcerative conditions. It also permits viewing of tumors, polyps, and other disease processes. Biopsy through the scope permits confirmation of a diagnosis without surgery. The patient must be prepared for the examination

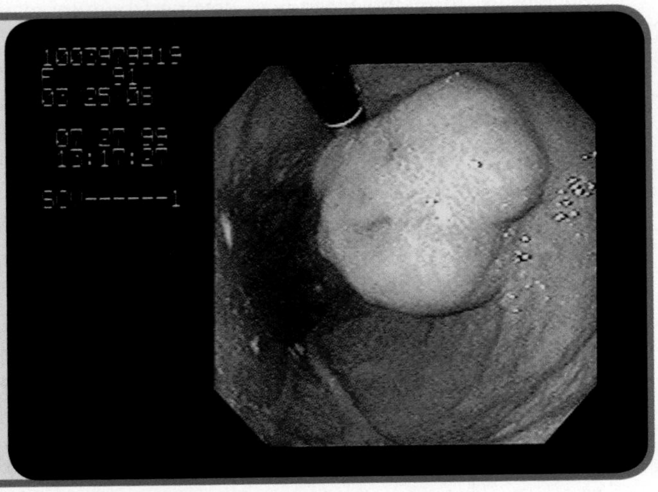

Figure 32–11: Tumor in stomach as seen during an esophagogastroadenoscopy examination. *Courtesy of Thomas C. Ransbottom, MD, Gastroenterologist.*

with an enema administered a short time before. Soap or other irritants must not be added to the water because they may affect the appearance of the lining.

- *Ultrasound*—Ultrasonography uses high-frequency sound waves directed toward the liver, gallbladder, or pancreas. The waves create echos of varying degrees, which are changed into patterns of dots on a screen. The patterns reveal the size, shape, and position of the organ being studied. Ultrasonography is especially useful when liver and gallbladder functions are impaired and the use of contrast media is ineffective.

DISEASES AND DISORDERS

Anorectal Abscess and Fistula (A-no-rek′tal Ab′-ses Fis′-tu-la)

Definition—This localized infection is a collection of exudate in the soft tissue adjacent to the anus or rectum.

Signs and symptoms—It is characterized by a throbbing, painful lump, which makes sitting and coughing very uncomfortable.

Etiology—The abscess may be initiated from within the rectum because of a sharp object in the feces, such as a piece of seashell or bone, penetrating the surrounding tissue. Because the feces contain bacteria, an infection develops and an abscess results. The exudate may develop an escape route into the rectum, anal canal, or skin surface, which will periodically relieve the pain and excess pressure. Such a tract is known as a **fistula**.

Treatment—Surgical intervention is indicated to correct the condition by incision and drainage of both the abscess and the tract (Figure 32–12).

Occasionally, an abscess occurs without a fistula. It may appear on the surface of the perineum as a large, firm, red mass, with or without a yellow center. This abscess requires incision to promote drainage and eventual expression of the solid core of material. The application of heat by sitting in a tub of warm water aids in the drainage process and relieves discomfort.

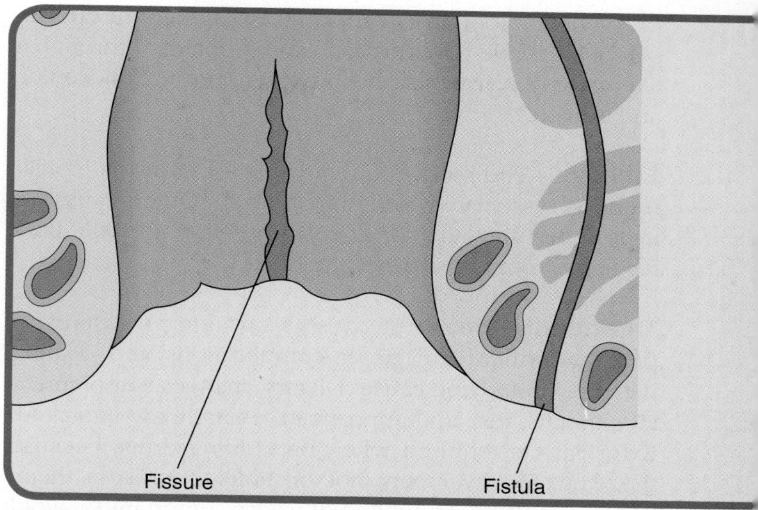

Figure 32–12: Anal fissure and fistula. *Delmar/Cengage Learning.*

Appendicitis (A-pen-di-si′-tis)

Description—An acute inflammation of the appendix probably is caused by an obstruction of the intestinal lumen.

Signs and symptoms—Symptoms of appendicitis begin with generalized abdominal pain that later localizes in the lower right abdomen at a site known as McBurney's point. Increased tenderness, anorexia, nausea, vomiting, and rebound tenderness (produced by slowly compressing the abdomen over the site, then suddenly releasing the pressure) occur. A slight fever may be present. A moderately elevated white blood cell count (12,000 to 15,000) in addition to the physical findings supports the diagnosis. The sudden cessation of symptoms is an indication of infarction or rupture.

Etiology—When obstruction occurs, an inflammatory process begins and leads to infection, thrombosis, destruction of tissue, and eventually perforation of the appendix. On rupture, the infectious material spills into the abdominal cavity and initiates peritonitis, a serious complication. If left untreated, it is fatal.

Treatment—The only effective treatment for appendicitis is surgical removal, an appendectomy. When appendicitis is suspected, abdominal heat, enemas, or laxatives must never be administered because of the risk of causing perforation. Usually pain medication is avoided to prevent masking of the symptoms. Positioning patients on their right side with the knees flexed will usually help to reduce the discomfort.

Cirrhosis (Si-ro′-sis)

Description—This chronic disease of the liver causes destruction of the liver cells. The destruction leads to impaired blood and lymph circulation and interferes with the life-preserving functions of the liver.

Signs and symptoms—Early symptoms include a variety of GI tract signs, such as lack of appetite, indigestion, nausea, vomiting, constipation, and **diarrhea**. Later, nosebleeds, bleeding gums, and anemia may develop. The liver becomes enlarged, jaundice is present, and ascites (collection of fluid) occurs within the abdomen. Because the disease interferes with portal circulation, hypertension occurs in the portal system, causing esophageal varices that eventually rupture and bleed.

Various blood tests support the diagnosis of **cirrhosis**, but positive confirmation can be obtained through a liver biopsy. A liver scan will detect abnormal thickening and a mass.

Etiology—The most frequent cause of cirrhosis is malnutrition associated with alcoholism. Other causative factors are hepatitis or the suppression of bile flow resulting from a disease of the ducts.

Treatment—Treatment consists of taking measures to prevent further damage or complications and dealing with the underlying cause. Dietary changes, supplemental vitamins, rest, and appropriate exercise are indicated. Extra care is required when prescribing drugs because the damaged liver may not be able to process them. Alcohol must be prohibited. It is also important to avoid contact with infections. Mortality is high, with many patients dying within five years of diagnosis.

Colitis (Ko-li′-tis)

Description—This inflammation of the colon causes tenderness and discomfort. It may be acute, occurring as the result of a bacterial invasion, or chronic, associated with allergy, emotional stress, or other diseases. (See ulcerative **colitis**.)

Colorectal Cancer (Kolo-rek′-tal)

Description—This is a malignancy of the colon or rectum. The American Cancer Society estimated 142,570 new cases of colorectal cancer in 2010. It is the third most common cancer in men and women. Incidence rates did decline 1% from 2006 to 2010, possibly because of increased screening and polyp removal. (Some polyps tend to become malignant over time.) The Society also estimated 51,370 deaths in 2010, which represented about 10% of all cancer deaths. The one-year survival rate is 82%, whereas the 5-year rate is 61%. When detected early at the localized stage, the five-year survival rate increases to 90%; however, only 37% are detected this early. When there is distant metastases, the survival rate drops to only 8%. Figure 32–13A illustrates the percentage of incidence in the common sites and shows that 75% are within viewing distance of the flexible sigmoidoscope. This illustration emphasizes the importance of sigmoidoscopy screening on a regularly scheduled basis as a way of identifying a large percentage of colorectal cancer in its early stage when intervention is most effective.

Signs and symptoms—Symptoms can vary in relation to the area involved. With right-side colon involvement, there may be black tarry stools, anemia, abdominal aching, pressure, and dull cramps in the beginning. As the disease progresses, weakness, fatigue, dyspnea, vertigo, and eventually diarrhea, anorexia, weight loss, vomiting, and other signs of intestinal obstruction will occur. (Because the wastes are liquid in this section, obstruction is delayed.) With left-side involvement, obstruction signs occur earlier because of the formed consistency of the fecal material. There is rectal bleeding, abdominal fullness, cramping, and rectal pressure. Later, there are diarrhea and "ribbon" or pencil-shaped stools. Bright red blood and mucus is in or on the stools. With rectal cancer, the first symptom is a change in bowel habits—often "morning diarrhea" may alternate with obstipation (constipation caused by obstruction). This will be followed by a feeling of incomplete evacuation and later pain and a feeling of rectal fullness.

Etiology—Basically the cause is unknown. However, certain risk factors have been identified.

- A personal or family history of colorectal cancer or polyps
- Inflammatory bowel disease
- Possible relationship to smoking, physical inactivity, high-fat or low-fiber diet, alcohol consumption, and low intake of fruits and vegetables

Recent studies seem to suggest that estrogen replacement therapy and the use of NSAIDs, such as aspirin, may reduce the risk.

Treatment—The most effective treatment is surgery to remove the tumor, adjacent tissues, and any lymph nodes that may be involved. The type of tumor and extent of involvement determine the surgical procedure. It may involve only the removal of a section of the colon and its supporting structures, to total resectioning of the rectum and the construction of a permanent colostomy. Chemotherapy is indicated with metastasis, residual disease, or a recurring inoperable tumor. Radiation and chemotherapy may be used before surgery to reduce the tumor size and activity and also are given following surgery to treat any missed cells.

Figure 32–13B shows a gastostomy tube inserted into a patient's abdomen and connected to a suction machine. This patient is at home after having surgery for cancer (note dressing), but extensive metastasis and lymph node involvement is suspected of causing intestinal obstruction. The tubing can be clamped to allow the patient to take oral medication and eat or drink fluids. After a period of time, the clamp is opened to remove the remaining fluid.

Colostomy (Ko-los′to-me)

Description—This is an artificial opening of the colon, allowing fecal material to be excreted from the body through the abdominal wall. **Colostomies** are classified according to the portion of the colon involved

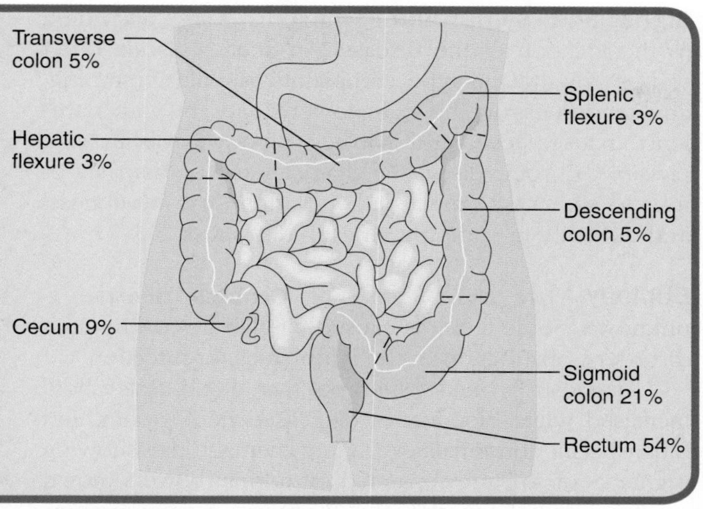

Figure 32–13A: Incidence of colorectal cancer by sites. *Delmar/Cengage Learning.*

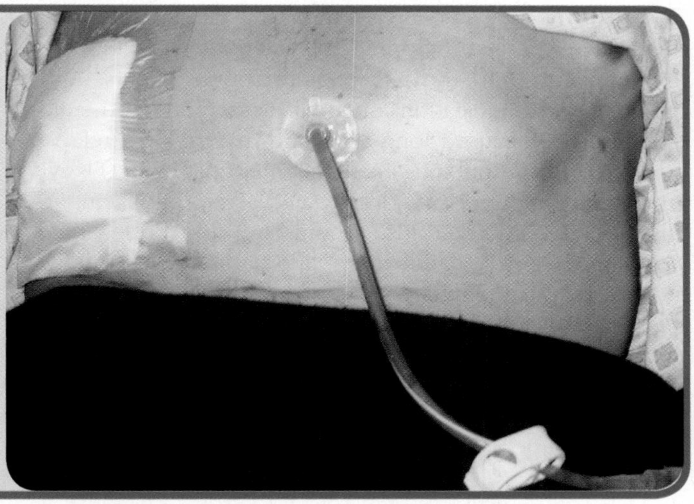

Figure 32–13B: Gastrostomy tube to remove stomach contents. *Courtesy of Barbara A. Wise.*

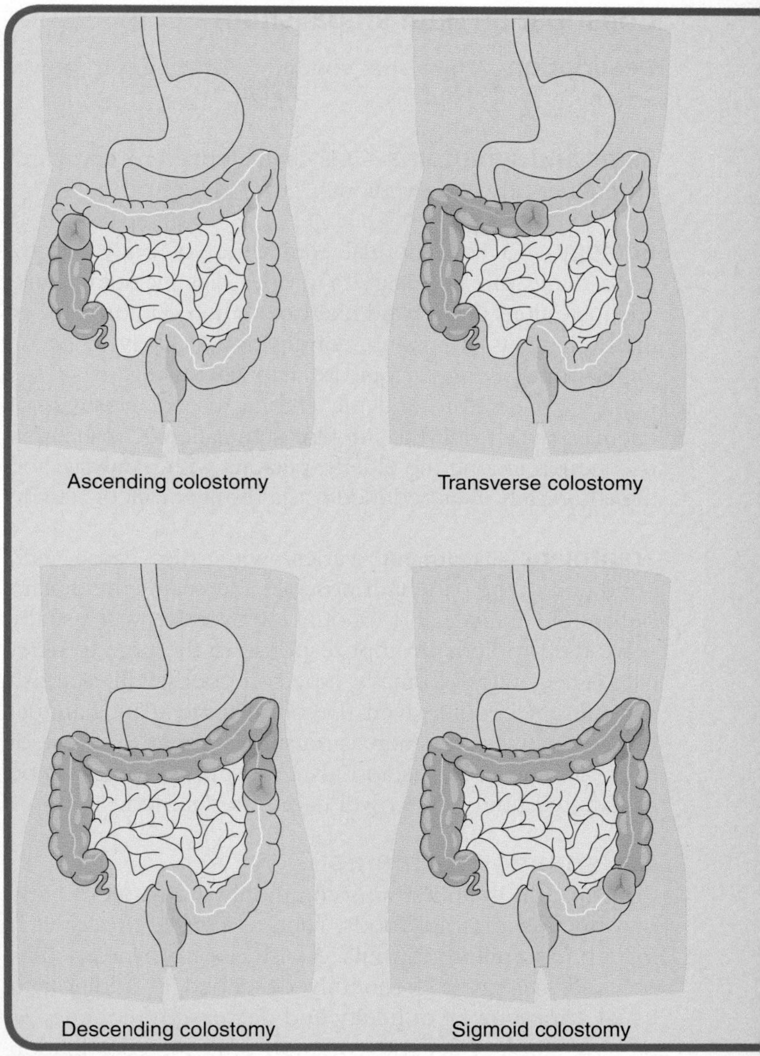

Figure 32–14: Colostomy sites. *Delmar/Cengage Learning.*

(for example, transverse colostomy, Figure 32–14). The terms *single* and *double barrel* tell whether only the proximal loop is involved or both the proximal and distal loop. A colostomy can also be temporary or permanent. If a disease process could improve if the colon were not constantly irritated by passing feces, then a temporary colostomy is indicated. By surgically providing for the fecal material to empty through an opening in the colon before reaching the affected area, the area is allowed to rest and heal. After an adequate period, surgery is performed to reattach the ends of the colon.

A colostomy is also indicated when an obstructive growth process, such as a tumor, prohibits the passage of feces. When the growth is close to the end of the rectum, there may not be enough healthy tissue remaining to which a segment of the colon can be attached. There may also be evidence that removal of the affected area, even if possible, would present no advantage. In these cases, a colostomy will be performed for elimination to occur until the disease process results in death.

The colostomy patient has a major emotional adjustment in addition to the physical adjustment to make. The alteration in body image may be difficult to accept. The thought of fecal material being expelled into a pouch attached to the abdomen may be very unappealing. Consider also that there is no control over the expulsion of **flatus** (gas) or stool, and it is easy to understand the new patient's rejection. However, with time, diet control, and the use of irrigation, a colostomy can be regulated so that its emptying is at the patient's convenience. Support groups of colostomy patients provide emotional and physical assistance to help new colostomy patients adjust to their changed lifestyle.

Constipation (Kon-sti-pa′-shun)

Description—This is a condition of sluggish bowel action.

Signs and symptoms—It is characterized by dry, hard, infrequent bowel movements.

Etiology—To have normal elimination of body wastes, three things are necessary: a proper diet including bulk, adequate fluid intake, and exercise. When one or more of these elements is missing, constipation is likely to occur. Other contributing factors are habitual disregard of the impulse to defecate and the chronic use of laxatives or enemas, which dull the impulse stimulation. Constipation is common among the elderly, persons with paralysis, and the chronically ill or bedridden, as a result of lack of activity.

Treatment—Treatment varies with the cause and condition of the patient. If possible, increasing the dietary bulk, fluid intake, and amount of exercise will usually solve the problem. Prompt response to the urge to defecate is necessary. Normally, a person's body will establish a routine schedule given the opportunity. The habitual use of laxatives and enemas must be stopped. The use of bulk-forming products and glycerin suppositories can be substituted until new bowel habits are learned.

Constipation in infants

Constipation in an infant is commonly the result of early introduction of solid foods, such as cereal, or a switch from breast milk to formula. A history of fussiness, colic, or excessive gas is frequently described in addition to usual symptoms of difficulty and decreased frequency in passing stool. A second common time for constipation to occur is with toilet training because of the pressure the parent or caregiver places on the child to defecate or urinate in the toilet.

Treatment—For infants (less than 1 year of age), adding a fruit juice, such as pear or apple, may resolve the constipation. A glycerin suppository may be needed to soften the stool to reduce the discomfort with defecation. Constipation in infants that does not respond to juice or glycerin suppository needs to be thoroughly evaluated by a physician or gastrointestinal specialist. The parents of a child who is in the process of toilet training should be advised to stop the training until the child is interested in using the toilet or potty chair.

Crohn's Disease (Kronz′)

Description—This is an inflammation of any portion of the GI tract, most common in the terminal ileum. The inflammation involves all layers of the intestinal wall leading to edema, ulceration, narrowing, and the formation of abscesses and fistulas.

Signs and symptoms—Symptoms vary according to the location of the disease. An acute episode often causes appendicitis-type complaints of pain, cramping, and tenderness in the right lower quadrant with flatulence, nausea, fever, and diarrhea. Bloody stools are also possible. Chronic disease is characterized by diarrhea of four to six stools daily, marked weight loss, weakness, and difficulty in coping with everyday stress.

Etiology—The exact cause of **Crohn's disease** is unknown. Some feel it is caused by allergies or immune disorders, obstruction of the lymphatics, or infection.

Diagnosis is made after positive blood tests show increased white blood cells, decreased hemoglobin, and other specific abnormalities. Barium enema studies showing segments of stricture separated by normal bowel, known as *string signs,* supports the diagnosis. Sigmoidoscopy, which reveals patchy areas of inflammation, helps to differentiate Crohn's disease from ulcerative colitis.

Treatment—Treatment is mainly symptomatic and may include dietary supplements, steroids to reduce the inflammation, and the use of antibacterial agents. Anti-inflammatory medications such as mesalamine and sulfasulazine can be used long term and may delay a relapse of the disease. Antibiotics, such as metronidazole (Flagyl) and immunosuppressive drugs, such as ciprofloxacin, are also used. Corticosteroids, prednisone, and budesonide, have both anti-inflammatory and immunosuppressive action, but can only be given for a short time due to potential severe side effects. Most important are changes in lifestyle to obtain more rest and dietary adjustments to eliminate contributing agents. The ingestion of fruits and vegetables must be restricted with intestinal stenosis (narrowing). Surgery may be necessary if certain conditions develop, such as a fistula, bowel perforation, hemorrhage, or obstruction. With extensive disease of the colon, a colectomy with **ileostomy** may be required (see Ileostomy).

Diarrhea (Di-a-re′-a)

Description—This is a condition of repeated passage of unformed wastes.

Signs and symptoms—It is characterized by frequent, liquid stools, which can be very serious in infants and small children because of the excessive loss of body fluid.

Etiology—Diarrhea can be caused by a bacterial, viral, or amebic organism. It can also result from a poor diet, toxic substances, foods such as prunes that stimulate peristalsis, or an irritated colon. Basically, diarrhea occurs because the chyme is moved too rapidly through the colon without sufficient time for the water to be absorbed. When the lining is inflamed, as with colitis, rapid peristalsis occurs as soon as material reaches the affected area. In addition, the lining secretes excess mucus to counteract the irritating material. This response results in a liquid stool with shreds of mucus. Diarrhea can also result from nervousness or anxiety. Again, the peristaltic action is stimulated and the waves move rapidly.

Treatment—Diarrhea is best treated by providing an adequate intake of liquids and taking care of the underlying cause. Medication to slow down peristalsis is helpful, but it will not treat the underlying cause.

Diverticulosis (Diver-tik-u-lo′-sis)

Description—This is the presence of bulging pouches in the wall of the GI tract where the lining has pushed into the surrounding muscle. The sigmoid colon is the most common site, but diverticuli can occur anywhere from the esophagus to the anus.

Signs and symptoms—Symptoms of diverticulitis (an infected diverticula) include irregular bowel movements, lower left abdominal pain, nausea, flatus, low-grade fever, and an increase in WBCs. Chronic diverticulitis may result in fibrosis and adhesions (tissues growing together) that severely limit or obstruct the lumen. Symptoms progress from constipation to ribbon-like stools, diarrhea, distention (swelling up) of the abdomen, nausea, vomiting, pain, and abdominal rigidity.

Etiology—They are believed to be caused by a high degree of internal pressure and an area of weakness in the intestinal wall. There is a theory that lack of roughage in the diet permits the bowel lumen (opening) to narrow, resulting in higher pressure developing during defecation. The disease is much less common in nations where more natural food and fiber are eaten.

Diverticulitis develops when undigested food mixes with the bacteria normal to the tract and collects in a diverticular sac, forming a hard mass. The mass shuts off the blood supply to the thin-walled sac, followed by inflammation, infection, possibly perforation (a hole), abscess, or hemorrhage.

Treatment—Treatment initially consists of preventing constipation and combating infection. A liquid diet, antibiotics, one medication to soften the stool, and another medication to relieve pain and relax muscle spasms are called for. When conservative measures fail, the affected colon section may need to be removed.

Esophageal Varices (E-sof-a-je′-al Var′-i-sez)

Description—Dilated, tortuous veins in the lower section of the esophagus are called esophageal **varices**.

Signs and symptoms—This results in fluid entering the abdominal cavity, causing ascites. With the veins dilated and therefore thinner and the number of platelets reduced, hemorrhage occurs readily and is often the first sign of the condition. Often, massive hemorrhage occurs, producing bloody emesis and stools.

Etiology—They are the result of hypertension within the portal vein. The blood flowing through the portal system in the liver meets with resistance because of cirrhosis, a tumor, thrombosis, or occlusion of the veins. As a result, blood backs up to the spleen, causing it to enlarge, and the blood flows through other veins. The number of platelets decreases, and the other veins dilate.

Treatment—Treatment is limited. To control bleeding, a tube may be inserted into the esophagus to put pressure against the bleeding site. In addition, iced salt water may be instilled into the tube. A drug may be given to control bleeding temporarily. Surgical bypass procedures to correct venous flow may cause from 25% to 50% mortality, and the patient may still die eventually from liver complications instead of hemorrhage. Blood transfusions are also temporary measures. At best, the patient can be kept comfortable until the inevitable massive hemorrhage or coma from liver damage occurs.

Fissure of the Anus (Fish′-ur)

Description—An anal **fissure** is a crack or tear in the lining of the anus (see Figure 32–12).

Signs and symptoms—Symptoms of acute fissure are a burning pain and a few drops of blood on the toilet tissue or underwear. The fissure may develop a swelling at the lower end known as a *sentinel pile.* This protrusion may ulcerate, resulting in painful anal sphincter spasms.

A fissure may heal completely or become chronic as a result of partial healing and retearing. Later, scar tissue develops in the area, narrowing the passageway. Because the anus must stretch each time stool is passed, healing is difficult.

Etiology—It is usually the result of passing large, hard stools that stretch the lining beyond its capacity.

Treatment—Treatment consists of digital dilation to prevent stricture, a low-residue diet, stool softeners, adequate liquid intake, hot sitz baths, and a local medication for pain. A chronic condition will require surgical excision of the scar tissue, providing two fresh surfaces that can heal by a gradual regrowth of tissue. Fissures can be prevented by drinking plenty of fluids (eight glasses of water a day), eating a proper diet, and passing stool promptly when indicated.

Gastroenteritis (Gas-tro-en-ter-i′-tis)

Description—This is an inflammation of the stomach and intestines. The term may be applied to such conditions as intestinal flu, traveler's diarrhea, and food poisoning. The inflammation usually subsides within several days and poses no threat to persons in good general health. However, people who are very young, elderly, and generally debilitated are at risk because of the loss of intracellular fluid.

Signs and symptoms—Gastroenteritis is characterized by fever, nausea, abdominal cramping, diarrhea, and vomiting. Other possible symptoms include fever; malaise; and a gurgling, splashing sound over the intestines.

Etiology—There are many possible causes, such as bacteria (associated with food poisoning), amoebas and parasites, viruses (usually with traveler's diarrhea), ingestion of toxic plants, drug reactions (perhaps to antibiotics), and food allergies.

Treatment—It is treated with bed rest, increased fluid intake, and diet. Antibiotics and intravenous fluids to combat dehydration may be indicated for the person at risk. Medication may be needed to control vomiting and diarrhea.

Gastroesophageal Reflux Disease (GERD) (Gas-tro-e-sof-a-je′-al Re′-fluks)

Description—This is a backflow of gastric and sometimes duodenal contents into the esophagus through the sphincter just above the stomach.

Signs and symptoms—The most common feature is heartburn, which becomes more severe with vigorous exercise, bending, or lying down. There may be esophageal spasms that mimic angina pain, radiating to the neck and arms. **Reflux** may be associated with hiatal hernia. If there is regurgitation of fluids, there may be pulmonary symptoms of aspiration, including nocturnal wheezing, bronchitis, asthma, morning hoarseness, and coughing.

Etiology—It is caused by a faulty lower esophageal sphincter (LES) that is supposed to prevent the backup of gastric contents by creating pressure, which closes the lower end of the esophagus. Normally, the sphincter relaxes after each swallow to allow food into the stomach. Reflux occurs when the pressure is insufficient or the pressure within the stomach exceeds that of the sphincter. Certain other factors may contribute to the condition, such as hiatal hernia, a position that increases intra-abdominal pressure, and any agent that lowers the LES pressure (such as food, alcohol, cigarettes, and certain drugs).

Treatment—Common treatment includes the use of common antacids, such as Alka-Seltzer, Maalox, Mylanta, Rolaids, Tums, and others. These work almost immediately after taken to suppress the symptoms and continue for about three to four hours. Another group of drugs, such as Pepcid AC, are called H_2-blockers. They suppress the secretion in the first place to prevent the heartburn. Their effects begin after about an hour but last for several. Perhaps the best treatment is prevention:

- Avoid or cut back on foods that trigger heartburn (alcohol, chocolate, fat, peppermint, and spearmint); these tend to relax the sphincter.
- Avoid caffeine; it stimulates gastric acid (caffeine is found in coffee; strong tea; soda pop; and medications, such as Anacin, Excedrin, and No Doz).
- Avoid carbonated drinks; which distend the stomach and increase the pressure.
- Lose weight if overweight.
- If a smoker, quit.
- Use gravity (don't lie down after eating, and raise the head of the bed on 4- to 6-inch blocks at night).

Hemorrhoids (Hem′-o-royds)

Description—The anal canal and the lower portion of the rectum contain vertical folds of mucous membrane called anal and rectal columns. The veins in the mucosa of the folds frequently become dilated, resulting in internal or external **hemorrhoids**.

Signs and symptoms—Hemorrhoids may be asymptomatic but characteristically cause painless, intermittent bleeding, which occurs with the passing of stool. There may also be some itching. As they worsen and prolapse, they are still painless as long as they return to the anal canal. With continued progression, constant discomfort may result because of prolapse, which must be corrected by manual reduction. If blood becomes trapped in prolapsed hemorrhoids, it causes thrombosis, which results in sudden rectal pain and a large firm lump that can be felt.

Etiology—Hemorrhoids can result from long periods of sitting or standing, diarrhea, constipation, vomiting, coughing, hepatitis, alcoholism, loss of muscle tone, pregnancy, or anorectal infections. Any condition that increases portal pressure, such as pregnancy or hepatitis, or that leads to a trapping of blood in the veins, as when stool is being expelled, interferes with the return flow of blood. As more blood enters the veins, it causes dilation, and the veins bulge into the anal canal or protrude to the outside, resulting in hemorrhoids. With protrusion comes the possibility of developing a thrombosis. The blood may become trapped externally, forming a painful, hard lump. Once this occurs, it will probably need to be incised to remove the clotted blood.

Treatment—Treatment of mild to moderate hemorrhoids involves regulating bowel habits; limiting sitting time on the toilet; increasing intake of water, raw vegetables, fruits, and fiber; and applying local heat. When swelling and discomfort persist with pain and bleeding on defecation, additional treatment is indicated. A sclerosis agent can be injected into internal hemorrhoids, which causes scar tissue to develop, thus reducing the dilation. More severe involvement requires surgical removal of the dilated vein and the surrounding stretched mucosa in a procedure called a **hemorrhoidectomy**.

Hepatitis (He-pa-ti′-tis)

Description—**Hepatitis** is an inflammation and infection of the liver that can result in cell destruction and death. It is caused by a virus that has been identified in several different forms. Hepatitis B, serum hepatitis, was the first to be identified over 20 years ago. It is very contagious with a relatively high mortality rate. A vaccine was developed to control its spread. Next, hepatitis A, infectious hepatitis, was identified. Type A is also highly contagious but seems to be self-limiting and rather benign. A vaccine also exists for type A hepatitis. After 15 years, a type C (HCV) was identified. It is the most worrisome form. It usually has a silent beginning but develops into a chronic form that causes the liver to scar.

Recently, other strains have been identified. Because they do not meet the criteria for A, B, or C, they have been called D and E. D is like A but not highly prevalent in this country. E is like B. The latest strain, G, appears to be related to C and has been recently added to the family of viruses. There is no F; however, scientists do not believe this is the end of their discoveries.

Etiology—Type A is usually transmitted by the fecal-oral route, meaning organisms from sewage, human, or animal wastes get into the food chain. It is usually transmitted through ingestion of food, water, or milk that has been contaminated, and from seafood taken from contaminated water. Type B is usually transmitted parenterally (other than by mouth). Health care workers are especially prone to it because of contact with human secretions and feces. Universal precautions are indicated when caring for all patients to prevent acquiring or spreading the disease. Like AIDS, hepatitis B can also be acquired through sexual intercourse and contaminated needles, including ear piercing and tattooing. It can be passed from mother to newborn during delivery. But it can be spread by more casual contact through cuts in the skin and in saliva.

In most patients, involved cells will repair themselves, leaving little damage, and in the case of type A hepatitis only, conferring a lifelong immunity. When other disorders are present, such as congestive heart failure, diabetes, severe anemia, cancer, and advanced age, complications are more likely and the prognosis is poor.

Type C hepatitis is acquired through blood and body fluids. It seldom causes illness when contracted, but about 75% of those afflicted develop a chronic form that goes undetected for years. Carriers never lose the virus or the ability to transmit it to others. No vaccine has been developed.

Signs and symptoms—Hepatitis produces a variety of symptoms, which appear suddenly with type A; type B symptoms are insidious. Clinical features of stage one include fatigue, malaise, headache, anorexia (lack of appetite), sensitivity to light, sore throat, cough, nausea, vomiting, frequently a fever of 100° to 101°F (37° to 38°C), and possibly liver and lymph node enlargement. These symptoms occur during the preicteric (before jaundice) stage and disappear when jaundice begins. About 6% to 10% of adults and 25% to 50% of children become chronic carriers. These individuals are infectious and can develop potentially fatal complications because of liver degeneration and cancer.

The second, icteric, stage has begun once the urine becomes dark, the stool is clay-colored, the sclera and skin is yellow, and a mild weight loss has occurred. The liver remains enlarged and tender, and the spleen and cervical nodes swell. The jaundice may continue for one to two weeks. Then, liver enlargement subsides, but the fatigue, flatulence (intestinal gas), abdominal tenderness, and indigestion continue. The third stage, posticteric, usually lasts for two to six weeks. Full recovery requires six months.

Complications may develop, leading to a chronic hepatitis, which occurs in benign or active forms. The active form, known as chronic aggressive hepatitis, has about a 25% fatality rate because of liver failure from cell destruction.

Hepatitis C may be acquired completely without symptoms. Some people, however, do experience nausea, vomiting, fever, and jaundice for a few days, but all symptoms disappear after several days of bed rest. These people are fortunate, because early diagnosis may be made. Diagnosis is made based on history that reveals recent exposure to drugs, chemicals, a jaundiced person, or a blood transfusion and the presence of typical symptoms. Blood tests revealing hepatitis B antigens and the presence of B antibodies confirm type B hepatitis. Antigens are present only in the early phase of the disease, so a false negative result may occur if the blood is drawn too late.

Presence of the antibody (anti-HAV) indicates type A hepatitis. If these antigens and antibodies are absent but the patient still exhibits appropriate symptoms, then type C hepatitis is expected. There is a test to identify antibodies for HCV (type C). People testing positive should be treated before the disease progresses.

HCV can lay dormant for decades before symptoms appear. By then it may have destroyed the liver. It is a silent, deadly virus that infects an estimated four million Americans with up to 155,000 new cases diagnosed each year. Annually about 10,000–20,000 people die. One third of all liver transplants in the United States in 1994 were done because of this virus. The new organ will become infected but will not necessarily be seriously damaged. There is no vaccine, and only 10% to 25% become inactive with medical therapy. The carriers never lose the virus or the ability to transmit it to others. Most people discover they are infected when they undergo routine lab tests or when they donate blood. Fortunately, HCV is not highly infectious. Infection is possible from shared manicure tools, toothbrushes, and razors—things that can hold blood. The largest infected group is IV drug users. Sexual activity does not seem to be a very efficient means of transmission, although it increases with the number of partners. Hepatitis G is transmitted through blood but is very rare at this time. Currently, little is known about the strain.

Prevention—Vaccines have been developed to prevent hepatitis A and B and are recommended for the following groups of people:

- IV drug users
- Health workers
- Individuals living with an infected person
- Sexually active homosexuals
- Heterosexuals with multiple partners
- Recipients of certain blood products
- Children born to immigrants from regions where hepatitis B is common, such as Southeast Asia
- Infants born to infected women (Up to 90% of children born to infected mothers become infected and suffer a high death rate.)
- Travelers spending more than six months in an area with high incidence

The main problem with the vaccine is it requires three shots over a six-month period and is relatively expensive in the United States. Many of the targeted groups of people, except for health care workers and infected mothers, are difficult to reach. It is interesting to note several developing countries are immunizing newborns and others at a cost of about $1.

Treatment—There is no cure for hepatitis B; however, there are now many drug treatments such as interferon, lamivudine, and adefovir. Patients are expected to rest and eat small meals with high calorie and protein content. Medication to help relieve nausea and vomiting may be necessary. An effort is made to determine the source of infection or contagion. Hepatitis is one of several contagious diseases that are to be reported to the local public health department.

Health care workers should protect themselves from suspected or confirmed disease by wearing gloves to handle body secretions or draw blood. Hospitalized patients are isolated, with strict techniques used to prevent the spread of the disease.

Treatment of patients with HCV who develop progressive liver scarring usually require powerful drug treatments. Two antiviral agents are the only approved drug therapies of the disease. These are interferon alpha-2b and an antiviral, ribavirin. Interferon is one of the body's lymphokines. It helps boost the immune system and attack viruses. Ribavirin works by blocking the virus's ability to multiply. When they are used together, the drugs can destroy the virus to undetectable levels in about 40% of patients. However, severe side effects of nausea, fatigue, seizures, and even heart or kidney failure make this option suitable only as a life-saving measure. The virus often comes back after treatment is discontinued. A vaccine is in the process of being developed but is not yet available.

Hernia, Hiatus (Her′-ne-a, Hi-a′-tus)

Description—The protrusion of an internal organ through a natural opening in the body wall is known as a hernia or rupture. One form of hernia involves a defect in the diaphragm that allows a portion of the stomach to move up into the chest cavity through the opening for the esophagus. It is called a **hiatus** or hiatal **hernia**. There are three types of hiatal hernias: sliding, which is most common; rolling or paraesophageal (alongside the esophagus); and mixed, which is a combination of both. This condition is found in up to 50% of the population over 50 years old. If no symptoms occur, no treatment is required.

In all forms of hiatal hernia, some portion of the stomach, the end of the esophagus, or both slip(s) through the diaphragmatic opening (Figure 32–15).

Signs and symptoms—In the paraesophageal form, a portion of the stomach "rolls" through the opening into the chest but causes few symptoms except a feeling of fullness in the chest and angina-like pain. This type of

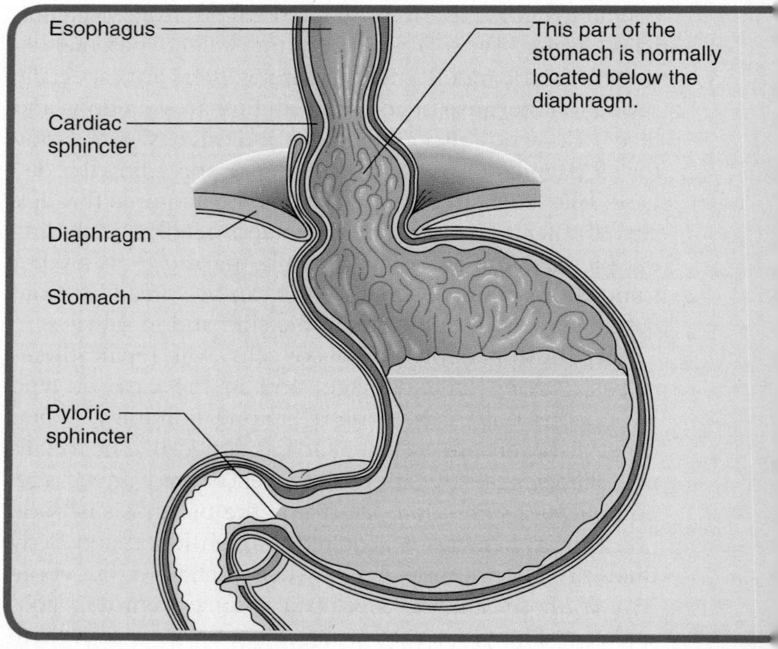

Figure 32–15: Hiatal hernia. *Delmar/Cengage Learning.*

hernia needs surgical repair. A sliding hernia may cause symptoms, such as heartburn from one to four hours after eating (which is often aggravated by reclining and occasionally results in regurgitation or vomiting), chest pain (caused by the reflux [return] of gastric juices), distention and spasms of the stomach, difficulty swallowing (caused by inflammation of the esophagus), or an ulcer. The most serious symptoms are severe pain and shock, which result from incarceration when a large portion of the stomach is trapped above the diaphragm, cutting off circulation to that part of the organ. Because strangulation leads to tissue death, immediate surgery is indicated.

Etiology—It is caused by a portion of the stomach protruding up through the diaphragm.

Treatment—Conservative treatment for uncomplicated hiatal hernia involves medication to strengthen the esophageal sphincter muscle; using gravity to decrease the reflux of gastric juices; and a diet of small, frequent, bland meals. Other helpful measures include waiting at least two hours after eating to lie down; eating slowly; and avoiding spicy foods, fruit juices, alcohol, and coffee. Smoking is discouraged because it stimulates the production of gastric acid.

Hernia, Inguinal (Her′-ne-a, In′-gwi-nal)

Description—The wall of the abdominal cavity has normal openings through which blood vessels or other body structures pass. For example, the male's spermatic cords pass through the inguinal rings of the lower abdominal wall to reach the testes, which are external to the body. When a portion of an organ protrudes through an opening, it is known as a hernia.

Signs and symptoms—Diagnosis of a smaller hernia can be made on manual examination of the inguinal ring while the patient is asked to cough. If the examiner feels something touch the examining finger, the patient has a hernia.

Etiology—When the surrounding structure of fibrous tissue, the fascia, becomes weak, it allows a loop of small intestine to protrude through the ring, following the path of the spermatic cord. This type of hernia is called an inguinal hernia, and it often extends into the scrotum when the patient stands.

Treatment—A protruding hernia is visible and can usually be reduced or pushed back into place. Some patients may wear a device called a truss, which exerts pressure directly over the herniated opening, to hold the protruding mass inside the cavity. Occasionally, the mass cannot be reduced and will remain in the hernial sac. It is then possible for additional intestine to enter the sac or the contents to become twisted or trapped, interfering with the circulation of blood to the intestine. This condition is referred to as a *strangulated hernia* and requires a surgical procedure known as **herniorrhaphy** as quickly as possible. The procedure replaces the contents of the sac within the abdominal cavity and closes the opening.

Hernias can be the result of weak abdominal muscles caused by a congenital condition or the natural process of aging. Hernias can also develop from increased abdominal pressure caused by heavy lifting, pregnancy, obesity, or straining.

Other types of hernias are femoral, which occurs where the femoral artery exits the abdomen to the legs; umbilical, involving the structure around the umbilicus; and incisional, in an area of previous surgery (Figure 32–16).

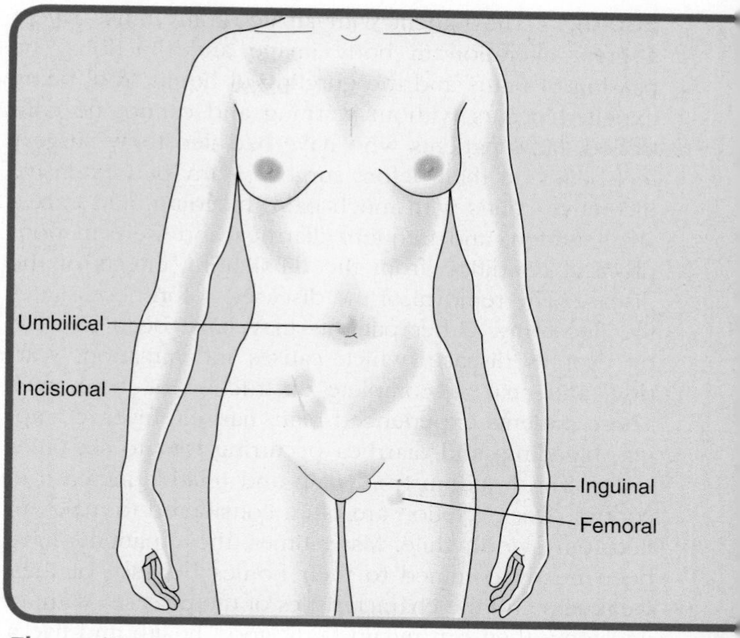

Figure 32–16: Common sites of hernias. *Delmar/Cengage Learning.*

Ileostomy (Il′e-os′-to-me)

Description—This surgical opening of the ileum allows the chyme of the small intestine to empty through the abdominal wall. This is not a disease but rather a solution to a disease process. An ileostomy is similar to a colostomy except that the chyme is liquid and highly caustic to the skin because of the digestive juices. The patient with an ileostomy has no control over its function and must wear an ostomy appliance (collection bag) attached to a donut-like disk that perfectly surrounds the stoma (mouth or opening). A protective adhesive creates a watertight seal. A belt attached to the disk supports the device. A permanent type of bag may be attached, which must be emptied and cleaned periodically. Disposable plastic bags can also be used. Some disposable types incorporate a deodorizing material; the permanent type requires instillation of a deodorizer.

Etiology—The patient with an ileostomy must accept a great alteration in body image and function. The passing of flatus and the gurgling of liquid stool being expelled occurs without warning and cannot be controlled. Most patients who have had ileostomy surgery feel better off than before surgery. Many had extensive ulcerative colitis with much pain; bleeding; and excessive, sudden, and frequent diarrhea and were in poor physical condition from the debilitating effects of the disease. The removal of the diseased colon necessitates the ileostomy. Other patients may have been affected by Crohn's disease, which causes inflammation, scarring, and near or complete obstruction of the bowel. These patients experienced pain, nausea, fever, cramping, bleeding, and diarrhea occurring four to six times a day. The freedom from pain and relative increase in control over excretion are often considered to make an ileostomy worthwhile. Many times, these patients have been nearly confined to their homes because of their weakness and the characteristics of the disease. With an ileostomy they can regain fairly good health and live a nearly normal life.

Irritable Bowel Syndrome

Description—This is a common condition marked by chronic or periodic diarrhea and alternating constipation. Irritable **bowel** syndrome is also called spastic colon.

Signs and symptoms—The syndrome is characterized by lower abdominal pain that is relieved by passing flatus or defecation and diarrhea during the day. Stools are often small and contain mucus. There may be abdominal distention and digestion difficulties.

Etiology—It is generally associated with psychologic stress, but it may result from physical factors, such as ingestion of irritants (coffee, raw fruits and vegetables), an abuse of laxatives, food poisoning, a lactose intolerance, diverticular disease, or colon cancer.

Treatment—Treatment is aimed at relieving symptoms and teaching the patient to deal with stress. Elimination of known food irritants, rest, and heat to the abdomen are helpful. The use of sedatives and antispasmodics are recommended for a limited time.

Oral Cancer

Description—The mouth should be examined for oral cancer every time a visit is made to a dentist for routine cleaning and examination. It should also be inspected by the physician as part of a physical examination. People who do not visit a dentist or physician frequently should observe their own mouths for oral cancer.

Signs and symptoms

- Swelling, lump, or growth anywhere in or around the mouth
- White scaly patches inside the mouth
- Any size sore that does not heal
- Numbness or pain anywhere in the mouth area
- Repeated bleeding in the mouth without cause

Any of these signals should be examined by a physician or dentist.

Etiology—Oral cancer strikes about 36,540 per year, with about 7,800 dying. About 90% of the cancers are squamous cell that develop in the tissue lining or covering of the mouth, lip, tongue, and throat. The single greatest risk factor is the use of tobacco, in the form of cigarettes, cigars, pipe, or chewing tobacco. The use of snuff is clearly linked with cancer of the cheek, tongue, and mouth structures. Abuse of alcohol is also a risk factor. Heavy drinkers who also smoke a pack of cigarettes per day have 24 times the amount of oral cancer risk. Overexposure to the sun is a factor in lip cancer.

Treatment—Oral cancer is usually treated with surgery or radiation or both. With advanced disease, chemotherapy in combination with surgery or radiation is being used. The choice of treatment depends upon the tumor size and location and the patient's willingness to undergo the side effects. Expected survival of five years is only 51%.

Oral cancer can result in a disabling and disfiguring condition when areas are excised. If the tongue is involved, speech and the process of eating become difficult.

Pancreatitis (Pan-kre-a-ti′-tis)

Description—This is inflammation of the pancreas, which occurs in both acute and chronic forms. **Pancreatitis** progresses in an unusual manner. The enzymes normally produced and excreted into the pancreatic duct remain and digest the pancreatic tissue. If the cells that produce insulin are destroyed, the condition will be complicated by diabetes.

Signs and symptoms—Mild pancreatitis is characterized by epigastric pain not relieved by vomiting. A severe attack causes extreme pain, persistent vomiting, a rigid abdomen, and rales (noisy, auscultated breath sounds) at the lung bases with pleural fluid on the left side. Tachycardia may occur, as may a fever of from 100° to 102°F (38° to 39°C) with cold, perspiring extremities. Rapidly progressing pancreatitis can cause massive hemorrhage, which results in shock and coma. Mortality is as high as 60% when there is tissue destruction and hemorrhage.

Etiology—The most frequent predisposing factors are alcoholism, trauma to the pancreas, reaction to certain medications, and pancreatic carcinoma. It may also develop as the result of a duodenal ulcer.

Treatment—The complicated treatment consists of methods to decrease pancreatic secretions and relieve pain while maintaining adequate fluids. Shock is treated vigorously by replacing electrolytes and proteins intravenously (IV) to prevent death. After the emergency passes, IVs containing electrolytes and proteins that do not stimulate the pancreas are continued for five to seven days. This may be followed by tubal feeding if the patient is unable to take enough nutrients by mouth. In extreme cases, a pancreatectomy, the removal of the pancreas, may be indicated.

Paralytic Ileus (Para-li′-tik Il′-e-us)

Description—A physiologic intestinal obstruction, a **paralytic ileus** usually occurs in the small intestine. Peristalsis is either drastically reduced or totally absent.

Signs and symptoms—The condition causes severe abdominal distention and distress, frequently accompanied by vomiting.

Etiology—It is often precipitated by manipulation of the bowel during abdominal surgery or the paralyzing effects of the anesthesia. The ileus usually disappears after two to three days.

Treatment—If it continues for more than 48 hours, it may be necessary to insert a weighted tube into the small intestine to remove the accumulated fluids and gas. Medication to stimulate colon action may be given.

Peptic Ulcer (Pep′-tik Ul′-ser)

Description—This is an encircled lesion in the mucous membrane lining of the stomach, lower esophagus, duodenum, or jejunum.

Signs and symptoms—*Duodenal* peptic ulcers cause heartburn, epigastric pain that is relieved by food, a weight gain (caused by extra eating), and a strange feeling of bubbling hot water in the back of the pharynx. Attacks occur whenever the stomach is empty or after drinking alcohol, juice, or coffee. *Gastric* ulcers usually cause heartburn and indigestion, pain in the left epigastrium, and a feeling of fullness. There may be weight loss and repeated episodes of serious GI bleeding. Gastric ulcers tend to cause discomfort after eating because the stomach lining is "stretched," causing pain from the lesion in the membrane lining. Either type of ulcer may develop complications, such as perforation, hemorrhage, and pyloric obstruction.

Etiology—For years, physicians thought ulcers were caused by the overproduction of gastric juices from emotional stimulation. In 1982, an Australian physician drank a concoction with millions of bacteria to prove his theory that ulcers were caused by an organism. A few days later he developed an inflamed stomach lining—the beginnings of an ulcer—and proved that even though the stomach is full of acid, the *Helicobacter pylori* (*H. pylori*) bacteria could survive. The organism itself does not cause the ulcer, but the burrowing of the corkscrew bacteria into the membranes weakens the linings, allowing the stomach acid and the digestive enzymes to create an ulcer. Not everyone who has the organism develops an ulcer, and not every ulcer is the result of the bacteria. However, at least 80% of gastric and 95% of duodenal ulcers are associated with the bacteria, and the remainder are often caused by nonsteroidal anti-inflammatory drugs. Other contributing factors are smoking, drinking alcohol, aspirin taken over long periods, and a hereditary tendency.

Treatment—With the new discovery came a new treatment. If there is bacteria and the existence of an ulcer is confirmed with endoscopy, the infection can be permanently cured with drug therapy involving two antibiotics and a bismuth preparation, such as Pepto-Bismol. Most physicians also add H_2 blocker such as Pepsid AC to relieve symptoms and hasten the healing. A new blood test for *H. pylori* antibodies is probably adequate for people with confirmed ulcer history. Newly diagnosed patients with mild to moderate symptoms may be placed on several months of treatment with newer acid-suppressing drugs and blockers. They will usually heal, and one in three sufferers will not have a recurrence. If the ulcer returns, they are then treated with the antibiotic therapy.

Polyp (Pol′-ip)

Description—This is a mass of tissue that results from an overgrowth of upper epithelial cells of the mucosal membrane of the GI tract. There are five varieties, some hereditary, others of common adenoma structure. Most are benign, but **villous adenoma** and hereditary polyps show a tendency to become malignant. Most types develop in adults over 45 years old. Predisposing factors are age, heredity, diet, and infection.

Signs and symptoms—Polyps are difficult to diagnose because they are almost always asymptomatic. They are usually discovered accidentally during a rectosigmoidoscopy or lower GI series X-ray. The most common symptom is rectal bleeding. The structure of the polyps varies from small lesions covering the surface of the rectum or sigmoid to large lesions attached by long, thin stalks. The type of polyp determines its physical characteristics.

Etiology—Overgrowth of epithelial cells. It takes about 10–15 years for abnormal cells to grow into polys that are malignant.

Treatment—Treatment consists of surgical removal often by electrocautery, especially if benign and pedunculated (on a stalk). If they are villous adenomas, which are invasive and therefore malignant, treatment usually involves abdominoperineal resection (removal of the colon and rectum, including the area around the anus), with a resulting permanent ileostomy. Each type of polyp is dealt with in relation to its current state or its tendency to become malignant.

Pruritus Ani (Proo-ri′-tis A′-ni)

Description—This is itching of the area surrounding the anus, often associated with irritation and burning.

Signs and symptoms—Classic symptoms are itching after a bowel movement or at night. Scratching can cause reddened, weeping skin, or thickened, leathery, darker tissue.

Etiology—The main contributing factors for **pruritus ani** are harsh, vigorous rubbing with soap and a washcloth; poor hygiene; spicy foods; anal skin tags (small pieces of suspended extra skin); excessive perspiration; a systemic disease, such as diabetes; the use of perfumed or colored toilet paper; coffee, alcohol, or food preservatives; a fungus or parasitic infection; an anorectal disease, such as fissure, fistula, or hemorrhoids; and certain skin cancers.

Treatment—Treatment consists of removing the underlying cause, such as a rectal tag, and eliminating irritants to the skin, such as soaps, powders, and colored tissue. The area should be kept clean and dry. Witch hazel applied on wiping pads or cotton balls is soothing. Steroid creams aid in reducing inflammation and controlling itching.

Pyloric Stenosis (Pi-lor′-ik Ste-no′-sis)

Description—This is a narrowing of the pyloric sphincter, which interferes with the emptying of the stomach. The sphincter is enlarged and often cartilagenous, causing a narrowing of the opening, which results in the dilation of the stomach.

Signs and symptoms—Adults will experience symptoms when there is a delayed action of the stomach to empty its contents, which causes distention. Because of the thickening of the pylorus and the backup of contents, the most common symptom is projectile or forceful vomiting.

Etiology—**Stenosis** can be caused by scar tissue developed during healing of a gastric ulcer.

Treatment—In adult stenosis, the patient may be able to alter the diet and use medication for some time; however, surgical correction will probably be required eventually.

Stenosis in infants

Symptoms of pyloric stenosis usually begin before 4 weeks of age and are considered to be congenital. There is forceful vomiting that may lead to serious dehydration. This condition occurs almost exclusively in infant boys. If vomiting is not too intense, the condition will be observed and may self-correct in time. Otherwise, surgical intervention to open the pyloric sphincter muscle is performed to correct the problem.

Ulcerative Colitis (Ul-ser-a-tiv Ko-li′-tis)

Description—An inflammatory disease, often chronic, that affects the mucosa of the colon. It usually begins in the sigmoid and rectum, extending upward to involve the whole colon. The small intestine is not involved. The disease produces congestion followed by edema, which makes the mucosa fragile. As the lining breaks down, ulcers are formed, which eventually develop into abscesses. The disease can be confined to one area and be known as segmented colitis, or it can spread throughout the colon. Severe colitis may cause a perforation of the colon, which can result in a life-threatening infection called peritonitis and in toxemia (blood poisoning).

Ulcerative colitis primarily affects young adults, mostly female.

Signs and symptoms—The prime symptom of ulcerative colitis is recurrent bloody diarrhea, often containing exudate and mucus. The frequency and intensity will vary with the extent of the disease. Other symptoms include weight loss, weakness, anorexia, nausea, vomiting, irritability, and abdominal pain. The disease leads to other complicating conditions, such as anemia; coagulation defects; liver damage; arthritis; loss of muscle mass; hemorrhoids from frequent stools; and stricture resulting from no solid stool, perforated colon, and toxemia.

Etiology—Predisposing factors are a family history of colitis, a bacterial infection, overproduction of enzymes that damage the mucous membrane, emotional stress, an autoimmune reaction, and allergic reactions to some foods.

Treatment—Treatment consists of controlling inflammation, maintaining nutrition and blood volume, and preventing complications. Patients are usually placed on bed rest, IV fluid replacement, and a clear liquid diet. Drug therapy is used to control the inflammatory process and combat infection. Anti-inflammatory agents, such as topical 5-ASA compound (sulfasalazine

AGE-RELATED BODY CHARACTERISTICS

Gastroesophageal reflux disease (GERD) can affect people throughout life. Infants can have GERD at an early age. The onset of symptoms such as arching of the back, crying during feeding, vomiting, and increased irritability can occur as early as 2 weeks of age. Infants are treated with H_2 blockers in a liquid form. It is also beneficial to have the parents keep the infant upright at about 30 degrees for at least 30 minutes after a feeding.

Adults, of course, can also have GERD. Oftentimes, with aging, the lower esophageal sphincter of the esophagus fails to work properly or a hiatal hernia has developed. Adults can lessen their symptoms with attention to diet, eliminating smoking, losing weight, and maintaining an upright position for 3–4 hours after eating. Adults typically demonstrate respiratory symptoms of wheezing, bronchitis, and coughing due to the irritation of the digestive acids upon the esophagus.

and mesalamine) and systemic anti-inflammatory corticosteroids and immunomodulators, such as methotrexate, cyclosporine, and azathioprine, provide some relief. Severe involvement may necessitate antispasmotics and pain medication to relieve the cramping and discomfort. If the patient fails to respond to medical treatment and the symptoms become intolerable, surgical resection (removal) of the colon is indicated, with a colostomy or ileostomy as previously described. Patients who develop colitis before age 15 and in whom the condition persists for at least 10 years are especially prone to colorectal cancer.

System Interaction Associated with Disease Conditions

Diseases of the gastrointestinal system can also cause effect with other systems and the function of the body. In Table 32–1, the pathologies present in the systems involved with GERD and hepatitis listed as examples.

TABLE 32–1 System Interaction Associated with Disease Conditions

Disease	Systems Involved	Pathology Present
GERD	Digestive	Heartburn, esophageal spasms, fluid regurgitation
	Respiratory	Coughing, wheezing, bronchitis, asthma
Hepatitis	Digestive	Anorexia, nausea, vomiting, liver enlargement and tenderness
	Circulatory	Lymph node enlargement, cellar damage, presence of antigens or antibodies in the blood
	Integumentary	Jaundice of skin
	Senses	Jaundice of eyes, sensitivity to light

CHAPTER SUMMARY

- Digestive system also known as the gastrointestinal tract, chain of organs called alimentary canal.
- Digestion is the activity by which food is broken down and converted into an absorbable form.
- Energy manufactured from carbohydrates, proteins, fats, minerals, water, and vitamins.
- The mouth begins digestion with accessory organs of teeth, tongue, salivary glands, and saliva.
- Ptyalin begins the chemical breakdown along with moisture to turn mashed food into a bolus.
- The epiglottis closes as swallowing moves the bolus to the esophagus by means of peristalsis into the stomach.
- The stomach has a cardiac sphincter at the esophageal end and a pyloric sphincter at the duodenal end.
- Mucus, hydrochloric acid, and several enzymes change the bolus into chyme.
- Contents of the stomach empty into the small intestine, which consists of the duodenum, jejunum, and the ileum.
- The liver and gallbladder contribute to digestion by adding bile to the chyme.
- The gallbladder concentrates and stores bile, which is emptied into the duodenum during digestion by way of the cystic duct.
- The cystic duct and the hepatic duct from the liver form the common bile duct.
- Gallstones are called cholelithiasis and may cause jaundice if they block the cystic or common bile duct.

- The gallbladder and gallstones can be removed by a surgical procedure called laproscopic cholecystectomy.
- The pancreas is both exocrine and endocrine in function. It produces pancreatic enzymes and digestive juices and secretes insulin.
- Nutrients are absorbed from digestive material by intestinal villi in the small intestine.
- The large intestine eliminates waste products and undigestible material. It absorbs water, salts, and protein from the chime.
- The appendix is attached to the cecum section of the large intestine.
- The large intestine is composed of the ascending, transverse, and descending sections.
- The sigmoid, rectum, and anal canal make up the last section of the colon.
- Diagnostic examinations include colonoscopy, barium swallow, upper and lower GI series, gastroscopy, nuclear medicine studies, occult blood test, proctoscopy, and sigmoidoscopy.
- Diseases and disorders discussed are anorectal abscess and fistula, appendicitis, cirrhosis, colorectal cancer, colostomy, constipation, Crohn's disease, diarrhea, diverticulosis, esophageal varices, fissure of the anus, gastroenteritis, GERD, hemorrhoids, hepatitis, hiatal hernia, inguinal hernia, ileostomy, irritable bowel syndrome, oral cancer, pancreatitis, paralytic ileus, peptic ulcer, polyps, pyloric stenosis, and ulcerative colitis.

STUDY TOOLS

Workbook	Activities for Chapter 32
Premium Website	
MEDIA LINK	View this **Media Link** for Chapter 32: • Digestion
StudyWARE	Activities and Quizzes on the **StudyWARE™ Software** for Chapter 32
	Audio Library of medical terms
	Online access to the **Critical Thinking Challenge 2.0**
learninglab	Module 15: The Immune and Digestive Systems
CourseMate	Activities and Quizzes for Chapter 32
WebTutor	Activities and Quizzes for Chapter 32

CHECK YOUR KNOWLEDGE

1. Cholecystography can detect:
   a. a properly functioning gallbladder.
   b. a non-functioning gallbladder.
   c. cholelithiasis.
   d. bile duct operation.
   e. all of these answers.
2. Barium swallow can detect all of the following except:
   a. condition and function of esophagus.
   b. esophageal varices.
   c. hiatal hernia.
   d. esophegeal stricture.
   e. cholelithiasis.
3. Upper GI series can detect a:
   a. gastric ulcer.
   b. tumor of the stomach.
   c. polyp of the colon.
   d. both a and b.
   e. both b and c.
4. Lower GI series can detect all of the following except:
   a. a duodenal ulcer.
   b. tumors of the colon.
   c. polyps.
   d. ulcerative areas.
   e. diverticula.
5. Gastroscopy makes it possible to:
   a. view growth for biopsy.
   b. remove foreign objects.
   c. obtain cells for study.
   d. both a and c.
   e. all of the above.
6. Nuclear and ultrasonography studies can:
   a. screen for disease processes.
   b. obtain cells for study.
   c. locate cysts and tumors.
   d. both a and b.
   e. both a and c.

7. Occult blood test will:
   a. detect mucus in feces.
   b. detect blood in feces.
   c. determine location of bleeding.
   d. determine enzymes in stool.
   e. all of the above.
8. Proctoscopy will permit viewing of:
   a. hemorrhoids.
   b. colitis.
   c. polyps of the sigmoid.
   d. gastric ulcers.
   e. diverticula.
9. Sigmoidoscopy will permit viewing of:
   a. duodenal ulcers.
   b. condition of ileocecal valve.
   d. gastric ulcers.
   c. tumor of the lower colon.
   e. both a and b.
10. Cirrhosis is a disease of the:
   a. stomach.
   b. pancreas.
   c. liver.
   d. gallbladder.
11. Crohn' disease affects primarily the:
   a. appendix.
   b. stomach.
   c. liver.
   d. ileum.
12. The prime symptom of ulcerative colitis is:
   a. jaundice.
   b. bloody diarrhea.
   c. constipation.
   d. hunger.

WEB LINKS

MedicineNet.com, information about ulcerative colitis: www.medicinenet.com/ulcerative_colitis/article.htm

eMedicineHealth.com, information about Crohn's disease: www.emedicinehealth.com/crohn_disease/article_em.htm

CDC, information about hepatitis C: www.cdc.gov/hepatitis

Chapter

33 The Urinary System

OBJECTIVES

In this chapter, you will learn the following:

KB KNOWLEDGE BASE

1. Spell and define, using the glossary at the back of the text, all the Words to Know in this chapter.
2. Explain the three main functions of the urinary system.
3. Identify the organs of the urinary system, and describe their physical characteristics.
4. Explain how the urinary system functions with other systems.
5. Describe the interior structure of the kidney.
6. Name the parts of a nephron and explain how each part functions.
7. Describe the process of dialysis and name two types.
8. Explain the likelihood of success with a kidney transplant.
9. List the two main categories of diagnostic examination and give examples, explaining briefly how each test is performed and for what purpose.
10. Describe 10 diseases or disorders of the urinary system.
11. Discuss the age-related characteristics of incontinence.
12. Identify the body systems that interact with chronic glomerular nephritis and renal failure.

WORDS TO KNOW

acute glomerulonephritis (AGN)
acute renal failure
anuria
bladder
Bowman's capsule
calculi
calyces
calyx
catheterization
chronic glomerulonephritis
chronic renal failure
cortex
cystitis
dialysis
dribbling
dysuria
elimination
excretion
fistula
frequency
glomerulus
graft
hematuria
hemodialysis
hesitancy
hilum
intravenous pyelography (IVP)
invasive procedure
kidney
lithotripsy
medulla
nephron
nephrotic syndrome
nocturia
noninvasive procedure
oliguria
peritoneal
polycystic kidney disease
polyuria
ptosis
pyelonephritis
renal
residual
retention
secretion
stricture
uremia
ureter
urethra
urgency
urinary
urinary meatus
urine
void

The **urinary** system removes nitrogenous waste products, certain salts, and excess water from the blood and eliminates them from the body. At the same time, it evaluates the body's acid-base balance and selectively reabsorbs the elements needed to maintain the proper ratio.

The urinary system performs three main functions. The first is **excretion**, the process of removing waste products and other elements from the blood. The second is **secretion**, by which **urine** is produced. The third is **elimination**, the emptying of the urine from its bladder storage.

The major work of the system is performed by two organs called the **kidneys** (Figure 33–1). The well-being of the human body depends heavily on the function of the kidneys. When waste products are not removed from the blood, they build up, producing potentially fatal toxicity. After the kidneys have performed their functions, the waste material, urine, is carried through the **ureters**, one for each kidney, to temporary storage in the **bladder**. When an adequate amount has been accumulated, the bladder expels the urine through the **urethra**, eliminating it from the body.

As previously stated, no system can function by itself. The urinary system is no exception. Waste products and other substances that are filtered out of the blood must first have been ingested, digested, and absorbed by the digestive system into the circulatory system, to be delivered in the blood to the kidneys. The peristalsis of the muscular system moves the urine through the ureters. The nervous system, in cooperation with a muscular sphincter, controls elimination. The respiratory system and the urinary system cooperate to control the body's acid-base balance and the amount of fluid retained. Pulmonary action influences the amount of O_2-CO_2 exchange and the amount of fluid loss through respiration. Hormones from the endocrine system also influence the amount of urine excreted. The integumentary system works in close relationship to the urinary system to remove or retain body fluid as required. Once again, it is apparent that the body is a complex, interdependent organism.

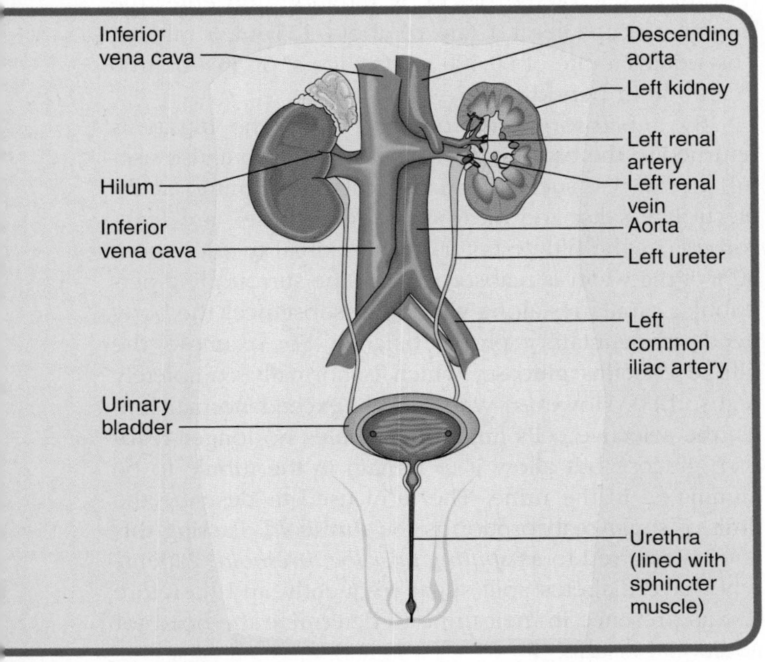

Figure 33–1: The urinary system *Delmar/Cengage Learning.*

THE KIDNEYS

The kidneys are shaped like lima or kidney beans. Each kidney is about 4½ inches long, from 2 to 3 inches wide, and about an inch thick, and it weighs about ¼ pound. The kidneys are located on each side of the vertebral column, high up on the posterior wall of the abdominal cavity, between the muscles of the back and the parietal peritoneum that covers the abdominal organs. Because they are not within the area occupied by the digestive system organs, the kidneys are said to be retroperitoneal (behind the peritoneum). The left kidney is slightly higher than the right, which is displaced by the liver. Normally, a heavy cushion of fat helps keep the kidneys in their proper position. A condition known as **ptosis** (dropping) occurs in very thin persons as a result of an inadequate fatty cushion.

Externally, the kidney is covered with a tough, fibrous capsule. The concave border has a notch called the **hilum** through which the **renal** (kidney) artery enters and the renal vein and renal pelvis of the ureter exits. Internally, the kidney is divided into two sections: an outer layer, the **cortex**, and an inner layer, the **medulla** (Figure 33–2). The medulla is divided into triangular-shaped wedges called renal pyramids with bases toward the cortex and "tops," or renal papillae, emptying into cavities called **calyces** (singular: **calyx**). The pyramids have a striated (striped) appearance; the cortex appears smooth. The cortex extends inward between the pyramids in sections called renal columns.

The Nephrons

The life-preserving service of the kidney is performed by microscopic units called **nephrons**. Each kidney has over 1 million of these units, which altogether contain roughly 140 miles of filters and tubes. Each minute, the kidneys filter over 1,000 mL of blood, producing about 60 mL of urine per hour. In an average day, a person takes in 2,500 mL of fluid (2½ quarts) and generates another 300 mL (10 ounces) of water, which is formed by the cells in the process of combining oxygen and other materials. About 1,500 mL (1½ quarts) is eliminated as urine each day. Additional fluid is lost through feces and respiration. Some moisture is also lost through the skin, especially when perspiring. Despite the amount of liquid consumed, the kidneys maintain a constant amount of fluid in the body's tissues, excreting the excess as urine. The concentration of the urine is in direct relationship to the amount of liquid consumed.

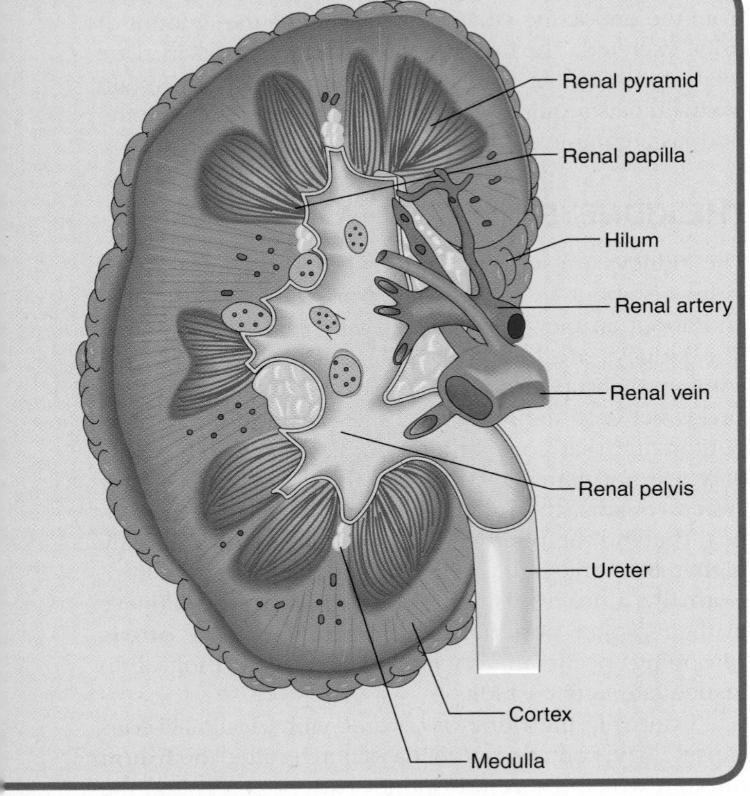

Figure 33–2: Internal structure of the kidney *Delmar/Cengage Learning*.

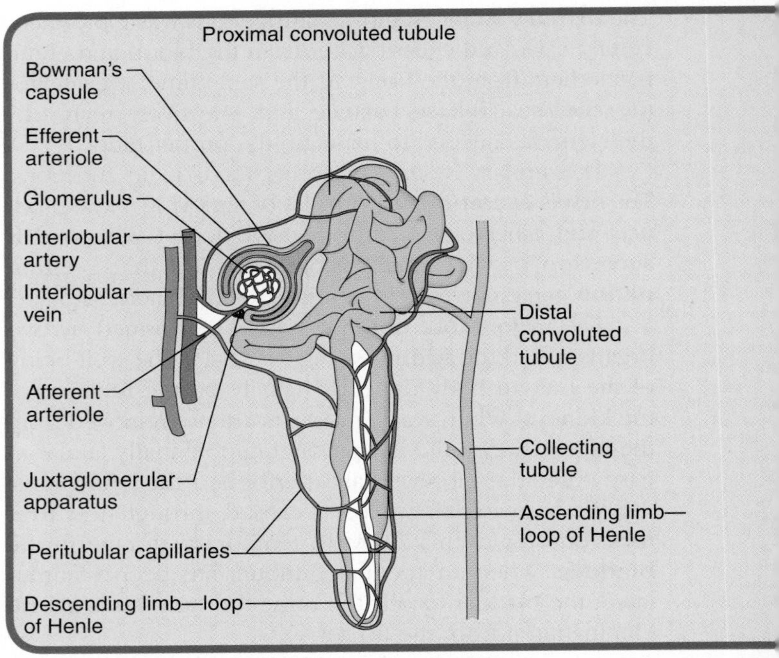

Figure 33–3: A nephron unit and related structures. The collecting tubules, which are not microscopic, give the pyramids of the medullary portion of the kidney a striated appearance. As shown, there are some collecting tubules in the cortical portion of the kidney as well *Delmar/Cengage Learning*.

The process by which the nephrons produce urine is complex. The nephron is a peculiarly shaped structure, resembling a funnel with a long, twisted tail (Figure 33–3). The top of the funnel is a double-walled hollow capsule called the **Bowman's capsule**. Each capsule contains a cluster of about 50 capillaries called the **glomerulus**. The Bowman's capsule and the glomerulus together are known as the renal corpuscle.

Blood enters the glomerulus by way of an afferent arteriole, flows through the glomerular capillaries, and leaves through the efferent arteriole. The efferent arteriole branches into capillaries that surround the renal tubule. The capillaries come back together in tiny veins, which join a branch of the renal vein.

Beyond the Bowman's capsule is a twisted section of tubule called the *proximal convoluted tubule*. The capsule and this section of tubule descend into the medulla and are called the *loop of Henle*. This loop has a straight descending and ascending limb, but when it returns to the cortex, it changes into another twisted section called the *distal convoluted tubule*. Several distal tubules join into a straight collecting tubule, which empties into the calyx.

Filtration and Reabsorption

Filtration is the first process in the formation of urine. Blood enters the capsule by way of the afferent arteriole, carrying waste products, water, salt, urea, and glucose. The afferent arteriole divides, forming approximately 50 glomerular capillaries. Because so many capillaries are then emptied by a single efferent arteriole, blood pressure increases significantly. This higher pressure forces the fluid to leave the blood by filtration and enter the Bowman's capsule at a rate of about 125 mL a minute. This equals a rate of 60,000 mL (60 liters, or 56.8 quarts) in an 8-hour period.

By a reabsorption process, 99% of the filtrate is returned to the bloodstream. Not only fluid but also useful substances, such as glucose, vitamins, amino acids, electrolyte salts, and bicarbonate ions (base), are reabsorbed. As the filtrate enters the proximal tubule, about 80% of the water is reabsorbed into the surrounding peritubular capillaries along with other substances the body needs to maintain a proper balance. For example, the filtrate contains glucose, which is normally completely reabsorbed. However, when levels exceed normal limits, the selective cells lining the tubules no longer reabsorb glucose but allow it to remain in the tubule to be eliminated in the urine. The term used to describe the limit of sugar reabsorption is the *threshold*. Passing this level is referred to as *spilling over the threshold*. Patients who have diabetes spill sugar frequently and therefore test its presence in their urine to determine the need for additional insulin.

A final reabsorption takes place in the distal tubule. The remaining 10% to 15% of water may be reabsorbed, depending on the body's need. The process is controlled by a hormone that acts upon the nephron.

Secretion

The secretion function of the nephron moves substances directly from the blood in the peritubular capillaries into the urine in the distal and collecting tubules. The substances secreted directly are ammonia, hydrogen ions, potassium ions, and drugs. The elements are selectively secreted to maintain the body's acid-base balance.

Urinary Output

Anything that increases the volume of blood in the capillaries increases the output of urine; conversely, the urine output decreases with a lessening of blood volume. For example, a large fluid intake increases the volume of blood and the output of urine. Hemorrhage or dehydration decreases blood volume and urine output.

Another factor regulating secretion is the amount of solutes in the filtrate. Again considering the diabetic, when there is an increase in the amount of glucose, it spills over into the urine, increasing the urine volume eliminated that day because more liquid is allowed to pass through to dilute the glucose content.

The functional capacity of the healthy kidney is so great that removal of one kidney poses no problem to the body in removing liquid wastes.

MEDIA LINK

Go to the Premium Website and watch the animation, "Urine Formation," for this chapter.

THE URETERS

The urine secreted by the nephrons drops out of the collecting tubules into the calyces, then enters the renal pelvis and continues down the ureters into the urinary bladder (Figure 33–4). The ureters begin with a widened upper portion, continuing as a long, slender, muscular tube approximately 10 to 12 inches in length. Peristaltic waves, at a rate of one to five a minute, move the urine down the ureter to enter the lower posterior wall of the bladder. Because of the solutes in urine, some persons tend to form renal **calculi** (stones). As the calculi form in the renal pelvis, they are washed into the ureter by the urine. When a stone is large enough to become lodged in the ureter, severe pain results. Frequently, removal of the stone may be required if it cannot be passed into the bladder. (See Renal Calculi in Diseases and Disorders.)

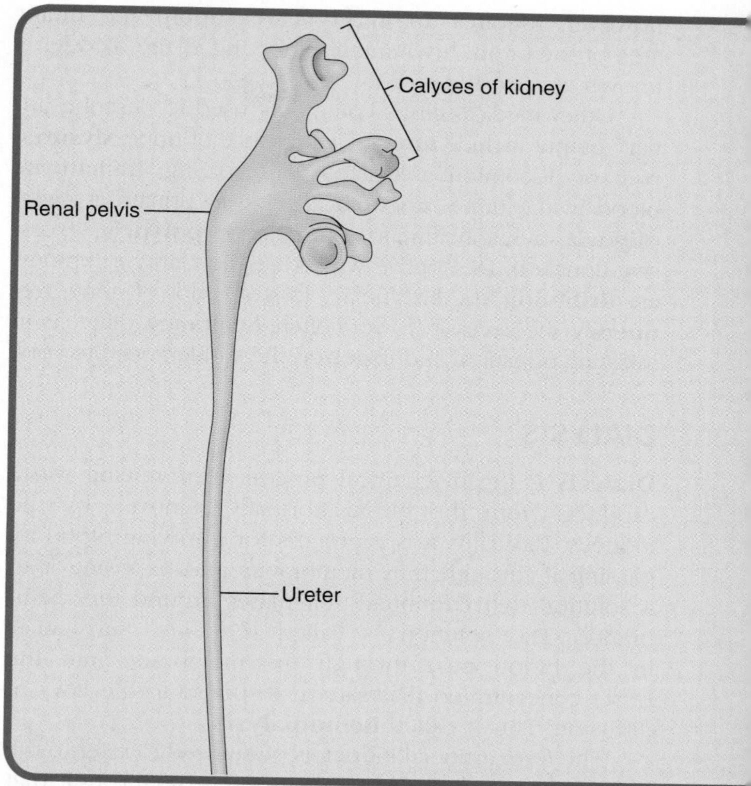

Figure 33–4: The ureter, renal pelvis, and calyces *Delmar/Cengage Learning.*

THE URINARY BLADDER

The bladder is a collapsible bag of muscular tissue lying behind the symphysis pubis. The lining has many folds, giving it the ability to expand. The bladder serves as a reservoir for urine, collecting approximately 250 mL before the urge to **void** (urinate) is felt. The capacity of the bladder is two to three times this amount, and in instances of **retention** (inability to empty bladder) may be in excess of 1,000 mL. In such instances, urine must be removed by inserting a catheter (a tube) through the urethra into the bladder to relieve the distention and discomfort. This procedure is known as **catheterization**.

THE URETHRA

The urethra is a tube leading from the bladder to an exit from the body. In the female, it is a straight tube about 1½ inches in length. It opens externally between the clitoris and the vagina within the folds of the labia minora. The opening is called the **urinary meatus**. Only urine passes through the female urethra. In the male, the urethra is about 8 inches long, extending internally from the bladder down through the prostate gland and out through the penis to the meatus. The male urethra also serves as a passageway for semen.

A circular muscle sphincter within the urethra permits voluntary control of bladder function. This control, however, requires an intact nerve supply and motor area of the brain. Involuntary emptying of the bladder is known as *incontinence*.

Other medical terms commonly used to describe urinary output include **anuria**, an absence of urine; **dysuria**, pain or discomfort associated with voiding; **hematuria**, blood in the urine; **nocturia**, having to urinate at night; **oliguria**, a scanty urinary output; and **polyuria**, excessive urination. Descriptive words used to clarify symptoms are **dribbling**, the involuntary loss of drops of urine; **frequency**, the necessity to void often; **hesitancy**, difficulty in initiating urination; and **urgency**, the sudden need to void.

DIALYSIS

Dialysis is the mechanical process of removing waste products from the blood normally removed by the kidneys. Basically, it is a process for purifying blood by passing it through thin membranes and exposing it to a solution that continually circulates around the membranes. The solution is called *dialysate*. Substances in the blood pass through the membrane into the lesser-concentrated dialysate in response to the laws of diffusion. This is called **hemodialysis**.

The term artificial kidney is often used to refer to the kidney dialysis unit. However, the part of the unit that actually substitutes for the kidney is a glass tube approximately 8 inches long and about 1½ inches in diameter. The tube, called the dialyzer, is filled with thousands of minute hollow fibers attached firmly at both ends (Figure 33–5). Blood from the patient flows through the fibers, which are surrounded by circulating dialysate. The dialysate can be individualized for each patient to provide the appropriate levels of sodium, bicarbonate, and other substances. These cross the membrane and enter the blood. At the same time, extra water and waste products leave the blood to enter the dialysate.

The patient is connected to the dialysis unit by means of needles and tubing that take blood from the patient, circulate it through the machine, and return it to the patient. New programmable dialysis management systems, as seen in Figure 33–6A, can monitor blood pressure; allow variable control of solution substances; adjust temperature, flow, and filtration rate of the blood; preset the length of treatment time; and perform other functions, all automatically. (On the system pictured in Figure 33–6A, the dialyzer is located just left of center; it has black ends with tubing attached to both ends.)

The hemodialysis unit in Figure 33–6B is a pediatric unit that is currently out of use and therefore has the "Bleach" label placed across the machine. This indicates the machine has been cleaned and contains bleach that must be removed before it is used.

Connecting the patient to the dialysis unit requires the preparation of an access to the bloodstream. There are four methods; an (1) intravenous catheter, (2) an

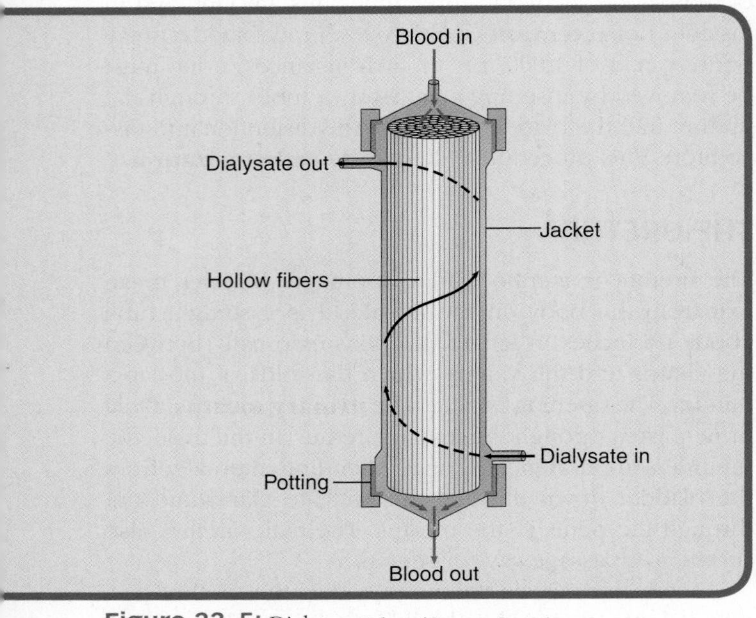

Figure 33–5: Dialyzer *Delmar/Cengage Learning.*

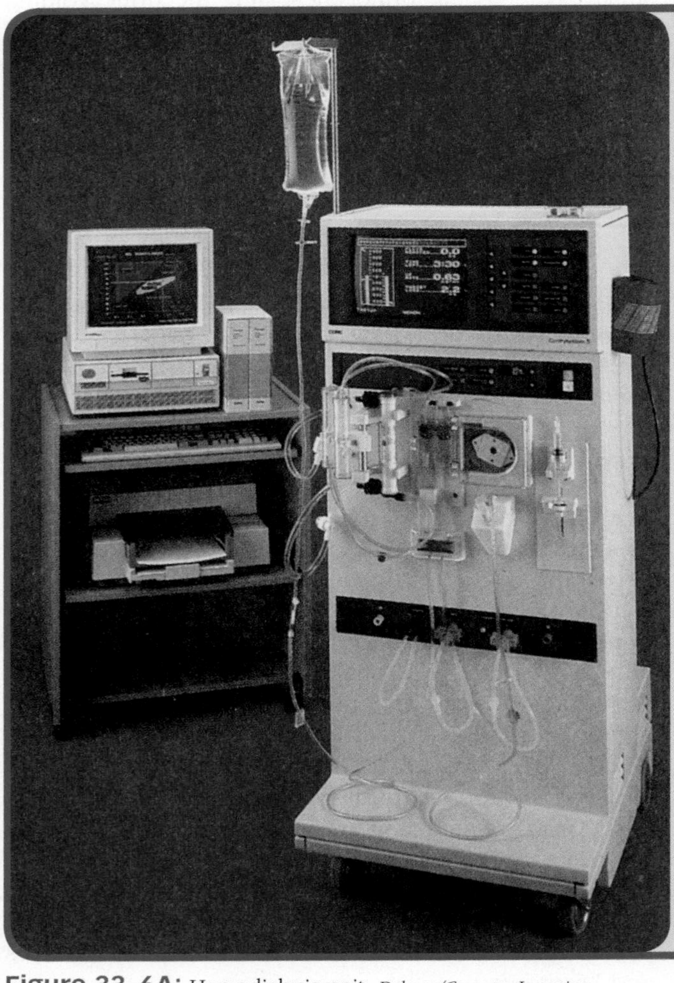

Figure 33–6A: Hemodialysis unit. *Delmar/Cengage Learning.*

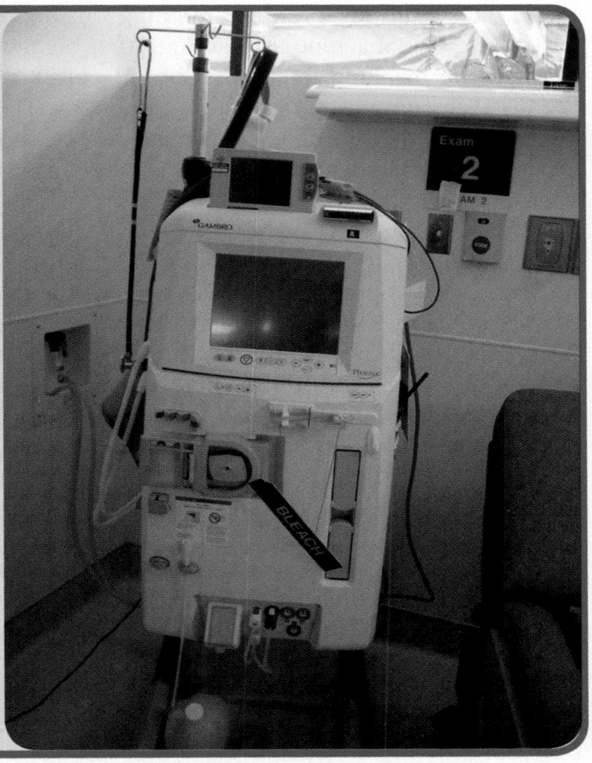

Figure 33–6B: Pediatric hemodialysis unit. *Courtesy of Barbara A. Wise.*

arteriovenous (AV) fistula, (3) a synthetic graft, and (4) a Permacath.

The catheter has two openings and is inserted into a large vein. One opening allows blood flow to be withdrawn and sent to the dialysis unit for cleansing and then returned through the other opening to the patient. Catheters are usually used for short-term dialysis because infection is a problem and venous stenosis (narrowing) occurs due to the catheter's being a foreign body, causing an inflammatory reaction in the vein.

An arteriovenous (AV) fistula, Figure 33–7A is created by a vascular surgeon who joins an artery and a vein together and makes an opening between the two so that blood flows directly from artery to vein, bypassing the capillaries. This rapid flow of blood can be felt over the fistula and is described as a "buzzing" feeling. Listening with a stethoscope at the fistula, you can hear the blood flow sound, which is called a bruit. A fistula requires about four to six weeks to mature before it can be used. Repeated needle insertions require rotation of sites, but eventually the fistula will fail and another will need to be made.

The synthetic graft, Figure 33–7B, is similar to a fistula except it is made with either a synthetic material or a treated, sterilized animal vein. The graft is inserted when the patient's blood vessels do not permit a fistula. It joins the artery and the vein, Figure 33–7B, and matures for use a little quicker than a fistula. Grafts are at risk for narrowing in the vein near where it is sewn, which causes clotting. Since they are a foreign material, infection becomes a risk.

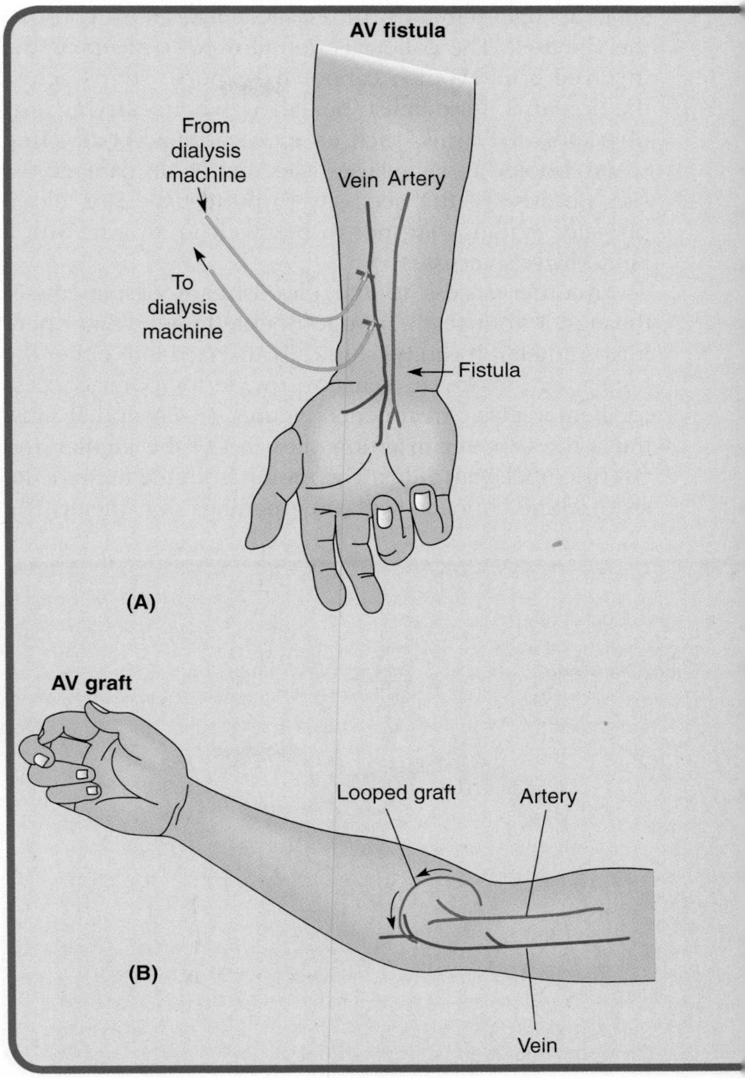

Figure 33–7: Hemodialysis sites: (A) arteriovenous fistula and (B) arteriovenous vein graft. *Delmar/Cengage Learning.*

The initial access site is the nondominant forearm, usually at the radial artery. When this begins to fail, sites are constructed at the brachial artery, then in the dominant arm, and finally grafts at the femoral artery in the groin area. Artificial veins last from three to five years. Some patients who have had a graft constructed from one of their own veins have had unusually successful sites for as long as 10 years, but this is not the norm. Because dialysis occurs so frequently, the multiple needle insertions not only affect the grafts or fistulas but the overlying skin as well. When too much damage has occurred, the site is no longer usable. The patient must learn to care for the site and protect it from damage. This is truly the lifeline for the patient with renal failure. Nothing, such as tight clothing or elastic cuffs, must constrict the site area. The patient is not allowed to sleep on the involved arm. Women cannot have purse straps across the forearm. Care must be taken when carrying any objects in the arms, such as grocery bags, boxes, firewood, books, and similar articles that could damage the site. Because of the necessity to protect the site, blood pressure readings are not to be taken in an arm with a hemodialysis access.

Another access to the bloodstream of patients is through a Permacath, a large double-lumen (two openings) catheter. It can be surgically inserted into either the jugular or subclavian vein to provide temporary access for hemodialysis treatments. Figures 33–8A and B illustrates the catheter insertion sites in (A) the jugular and (B) the subclavian veins. The tubing from the hemodialysis machine connects with the openings of catheter. The blood exits from the proximal opening on the catheter and goes to the machine for filtering. After being treated through the machine filters, the blood returns through the distal opening of the catheter to the body. The catheter is inserted to provide immediate use of a dialysis access to permit hemodialysis. It is often used while waiting for a fistula or a graft to mature.

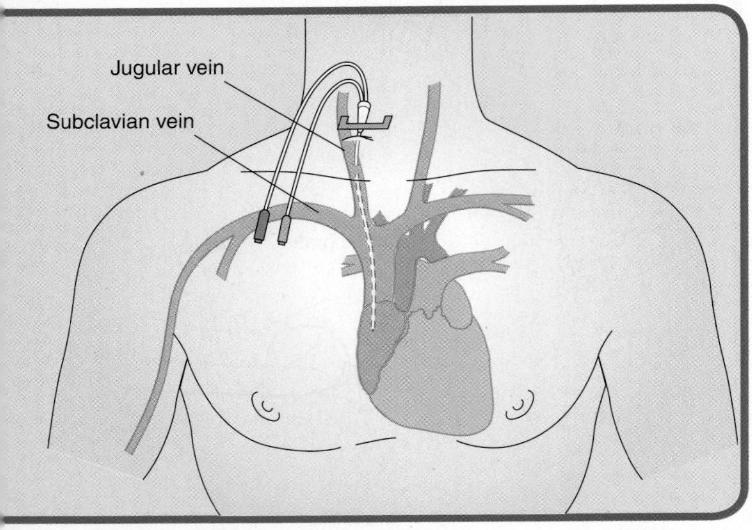

Figure 33–8A: Catheter insertion sites in the jugular vein. *Delmar/Cengage Learning.*

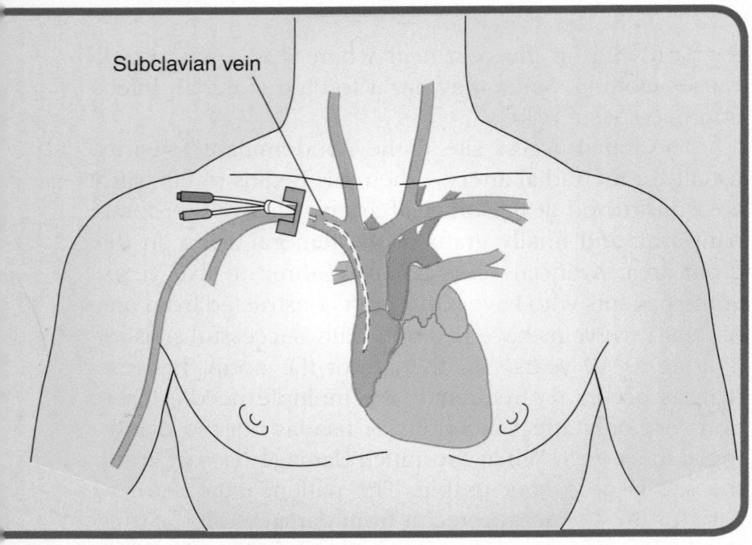

Figure 33–8B: Catheter insertion sites in the subclavian vein. *Delmar/Cengage Learning.*

Because the rest of the patient's life depends on dialysis, access to a machine becomes critical. Most patients are assigned to dialysis centers for periodic treatment. However, equipment can be obtained for home dialysis if the patient and the family are willing to assume the responsibility. The equipment is similar to that in the centers. The training may take from several weeks to a few months. There are three types of home hemodialysis processes. The conventional process is done three times a week for at least three to four hours each time. A short daily home hemodialysis can be done five to seven times a week with a new type of machine that only needs to operate about two hours because the procedure is performed nearly daily. A third process is called nocturnal home hemodialysis. This process is a long, slow treatment during the night while the patient sleeps. This type is usually done nightly or at least every other night. Usually, the patient can choose and maybe mix the treatment options, depending upon the machine used and the amount of dialysis needed.

An alternative to hemodialysis is **peritoneal** dialysis. Instead of an artificial dialyzer to cleanse the blood, the patient's own peritoneal membrane is used (the peritoneum covers the abdominal organs and lines the abdominal cavity).

There are different types of peritoneal dialysis. The most common form is continuous ambulatory peritoneal dialysis (CAPD) (Figure 33–9A and B). This type does not require a machine, and the patient is free to walk around while the solution is within the abdominal cavity. The dialyzing solution is introduced into the peritoneal cavity, where it comes into contact with blood vessels. The solution enters through a catheter permanently implanted into the abdomen. The solution tubing is aseptically attached, and approximately 2 liters of dialyzing solution are infused by the process of gravity by suspending the bag at shoulder level. Then the empty bag is rolled up and placed around the waist under the clothing. The solution attracts the waste products and water from the blood, and they are suspended in the solution. After approximately four to six hours, the bag is unrolled and placed lower than the abdomen, and the waste-bearing dialyzing solution is drained out. Another fresh bag is infused, and the dialysis continues. The exchange process of draining the solution and infusing fresh solution requires from 30 to 45 minutes. This is repeated about every four to six hours during the day and for an eight-hour period at night.

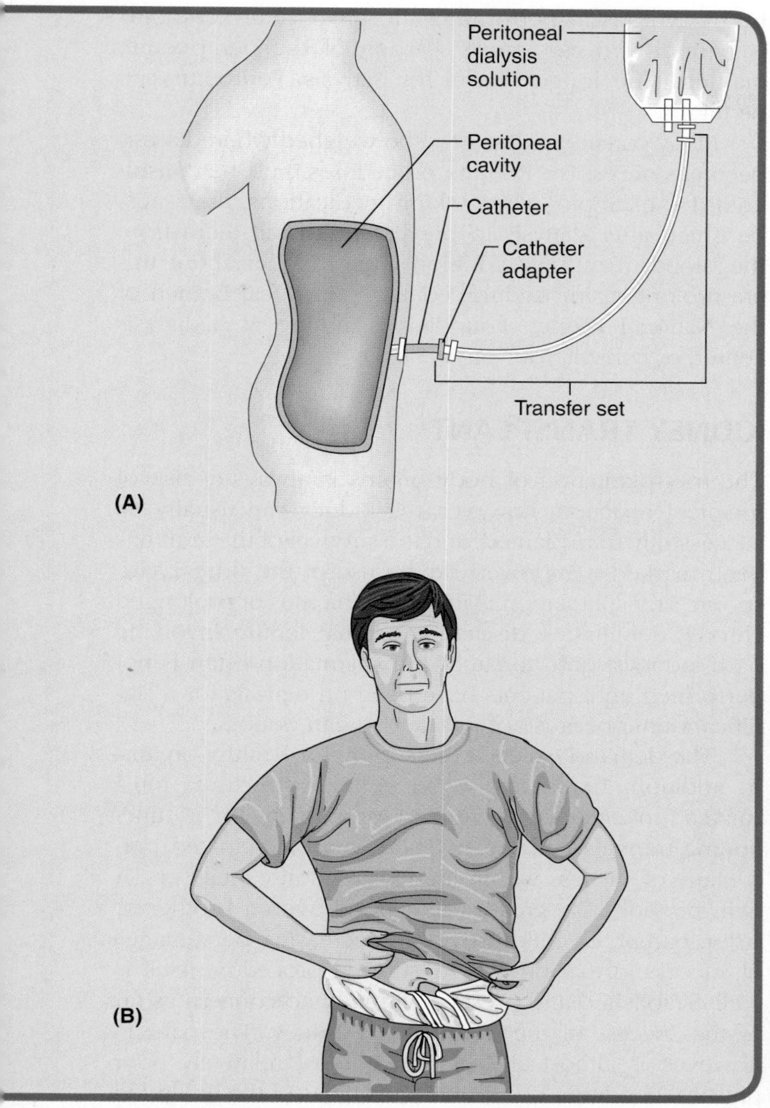

Figure 33–9: Peritoneal dialysis: (A) infusion of the solution; (B) rolled empty solution container hidden under clothing. *Delmar/Cengage Learning.*

Another form of peritoneal dialysis is called *continuous cycler-assisted peritoneal dialysis* (CCPD). This is more acceptable to some individuals because the dialysis is accomplished during 6 to 8 hours every night while they sleep. This is especially well suited for children. The patient can completely control peritoneal dialysis, permitting greater freedom of activity.

The CCPD uses an automated cycler, to perform three to five exchanges during the night. In the morning, one exchange is instilled, which stays in the abdomen all day.

Figure 33–10A shows the cycler, which automatically fills and drains the abdomen while the person sleeps. It is programmed to deliver a specific amount of dialysis solution into the abdomen where it will remain for what is called a "dwell time." At the end of the time, the fluid is drained from the abdomen into a container to be discarded in the morning. The cycler then refills the abdomen for another fluid exchange. Note the bag on top of the machine. The dialysis solution in the bag is warmed by the heating area on top of the cycler before it enters the body. In Figure 33–10B, the woman's abdomen shows where the catheter enters her body. This catheter has been surgically implanted to permit the peritoneal dialysis procedure.

This woman was initially diagnosed with kidney failure at 38 years old. Her first symptom was hypertension. She eventually underwent dialysis for three to four months and received her first kidney transplant from a sister when she was 40. After six years, blood work indicated the kidney was being slowly rejected. She had to return to dialysis, three times a week for the next eight months. She then received a second transplant from her brother and was placed on anti-rejection drugs. After five years, this transplant also began failing, so she was back on dialysis. She had a catheter placed in her carotid artery while a shunt was healing in her arm. After more catheters and four shunts failed, she decided to try ambulatory peritoneal

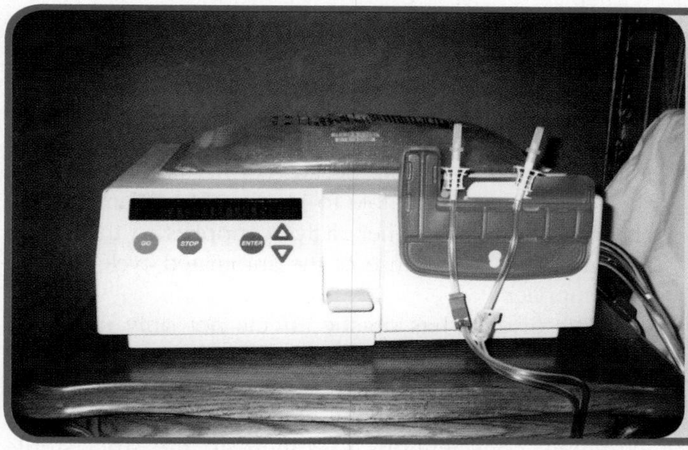

Figure 33–10A: Peritoneal dialysis automated cycler. *Courtesy of Barbara A. Wise.*

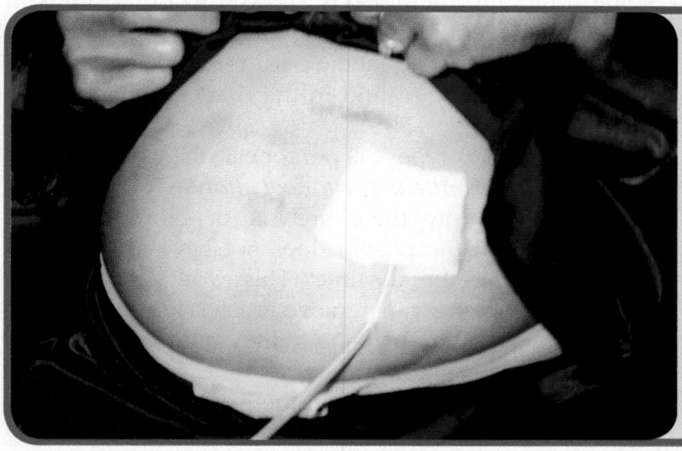

Figure 33–10B: Abdomen showing catheter insertion. *Courtesy of Barbara A. Wise.*

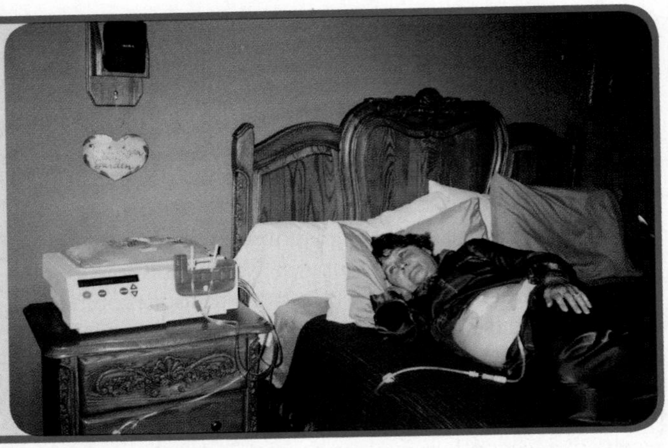

Figure 33–10C: Woman pepared for overnight CCPD.
Courtesy of Barbara A. Wise.

dialysis. After six to eight weeks, she was evaluated for the automated cycler and began, along with family members, two weeks of intensive training to perform the necessary precise sterile procedures. In Figure 33–10C, she is connected to the machine in preparation for the overnight dialysis. She will have three cycles of 1500 ml of fluid instilled and withdrawn while she sleeps. She has been doing CCPD for the past 10 months and has seen great improvement in her physical condition. Because of her family's support, she recently was even able to join her family on a trip to Hawaii by forwarding her dialysis supplies to their hotel and arranging for the use of the automated cycler from a local supplier.

This disease has drastic affects not only upon the person, but also upon the family. Like all peritoneal dialysis patients, she worries about the possibility of developing peritonitis, but her husband or sister are extremely conscientious to adhere to the strict sterile procedures when attaching the dialysis solution and tubing for the dialysis. She feels very fortunate because she still has enough kidney function that she passes some urine and therefore is allowed to drink fluids in moderation. People with little or no kidney function have very limited fluid intake because it cannot be eliminated and builds up fluid in the tissues until the next dialysis.

Yet another type of peritoneal dialysis is called *nocturnal intermittent peritoneal dialysis* (NIPD). This is like CCPD only there are six or more overnight exchanges, and the patient does not have any solution instilled during the daytime. This works for patients whose peritoneum can remove wastes rapidly or who still have adequate remaining kidney function.

The main complication of peritoneal dialysis is peritonitis, an inflammation of the peritonium from accidental contamination of the tubing when connecting and disconnecting solutions. Users of the method must be meticulous in performing the procedure. Peritonitis is painful and can cause scarring of the peritoneum, making it no longer useful for dialysis. Peritonitis can be fatal.

Many considerations must be weighed when dialysis becomes necessary. Routine procedures must be considered: for example, when taking medications, they must be timed after dialysis to prevent removing them from the bloodstream. For additional information about this life-prolonging procedure, contact your local branch of the National Kidney Foundation, inquire at a dialysis center, or consult your physician.

KIDNEY TRANSPLANT

The transplantation of body organs is always at risk of recipient rejection; however, the kidney can usually be successfully transplanted, and the survival of the graft has been markedly improved by the use of the drug cyclosporin. Transplantation is indicated in cases of prolonged chronic debilitating disease and renal failure involving both kidneys; unfortunately, transplantation often is not performed until patients have been on dialysis for a significant time because of a lack of organ donors.

The demand exceeds the supply for healthy organs. In addition, blood and other cellular structures must "match" to ensure the greatest probability for a functioning transplanted organ. There is an anticipated percentage of success within immediate family members. A twin provides the greatest likelihood, with a brother or sister, parent, or child providing decreasing percentages of success in that order. The surgical procedure itself is well established and presents virtually no concern as far as the success of the transplanted kidney. The patient, however, is almost always in a state of relatively poor physical condition because of the effects of the extended illness. This status and the tendency of the body to reject a "substance" that is foreign and not of the same cellular structure sometimes result in the organ not surviving in its new host. The use of drugs to control the body's natural defensive mechanism of rejection increases the rate of success.

Transplant patients need to take medication every day to protect their new kidney. Most patients require three drugs. The primary one will probably be cyclosporine, tacrolimus, or sirolimus. In addition, some form of steroid and either mycophenolate mofetil, azathioprine, or rapamycin will be taken. These patients require frequent medical examination at the transplant location to ensure the health of the new organ.

You might find it interesting to learn that a transplanted kidney may not physically replace the patient's own kidney. The woman in Figure 33–10B still has her own poorly functioning kidneys and both transplants are surgically attached to arteries and veins within her abdomen.

DIAGNOSTIC EXAMINATIONS

Several procedures and tests are used to determine the physical characteristics of the urinary system and assess its function. Analysis of the blood can determine levels of uric acid and the amount of urea nitrogen present. Urinalysis (analysis of the urine) can determine the presence of blood cells and bacteria; acidity level; specific gravity (weight); and physical characteristics, such as color, clarity, and odor.

- **Noninvasive procedures**—Procedures that attempt to evaluate function deal with urinary output. An *intake-output measurement* involves keeping a record of all fluid, or food that melts to liquid, that is consumed, along with all urine or other fluid loss, be it measured or estimated. For example, emesis would be measured; perspiration estimated as slight, moderate, or profuse; diarrhea indicated as to frequency; and any other loss (such as bleeding, drainage through a stoma, or excessive respiratory activity) evaluated. Hence, intake is compared with output to determine fluid balance within the body.

  A *routine specimen,* preferably the first of the morning, is simply voided into a clean container. A *clean catch specimen,* usually for culture purpose, pregnancy determination, or microscopic examination, involves specific cleaning of the meatal area and catching the specimen midstream in a sterile container. A *24-hour urine test* collects all urinary output, from a specified hour one day until the same time the next day, in a special container under specific conditions (see Chapter 46). Urine can be collected by various methods, depending to some degree on the purpose for collection. Urine analysis, which can be collected by a clean catch voided specimen or urethral catheterization, is an easy routine evaluation of the urine. It provides information about protein, glucose, signs of infection, blood, and cells which may be found in the urine.

  An *X-ray* or *plain film* of the abdomen may be taken to determine size, shape, and position of the urinary organs. It may also indicate the presence of calculi. This is usually referred to as a KUB (kidneys, ureter, and bladder) series.

  The kidney may also be examined by *ultrasound* to detect abnormalities or to clarify findings from other tests. It is a safe, painless procedure that can be used especially in cases in which sensitivity to the radiological opaque materials prohibits other tests. Examinations for kidney function that use a contrast medium are of little value when there is renal failure. Ultrasound, however, can be used to at least view the structure of the kidney in these instances.
- **Invasive procedures**—Another means of collecting a urine specimen is to withdraw it directly from the bladder through a catheter into a sterile container by strict aseptic (sterile) technique. This procedure, called catheterization, is discussed in Chapter 46 with collection of body fluid specimens. Catheterization can also be performed to determine the amount of **residual** urine left in the bladder after a patient has voided.

  One of the most common diagnostic procedures is an X-ray series called **intravenous pyelography (IVP)**. The patient is required to fast (no food or water) for approximately 10 hours beforehand. A laxative or cleansing enema removes from the colon any fecal material that might obscure the urinary organs. A contrast medium is injected into a vein, usually at the antecubital space of the arm. After a time, a film is taken to demonstrate the function, location, and position of the kidneys, as determined by the presence of the dye. Subsequent films outline the ureters and bladder as the dye is processed by the system. The film is taken at specific intervals to assess the efficiency of the kidney function. Because the contrast medium is iodine based, it is extremely important to determine if the patient has an allergic response to iodine or seafood before the injection.

  Cystourethroscopy is an examination using a lighted instrument inserted into the urethra and bladder to view the interior surface (Figure 33–11). A local anesthetic (sometimes a general) is given. The scope is lubricated, and as it is inserted, the interior of the urethra is observed. The scope is then advanced into the bladder. A solution is instilled to distend the bladder for observation and to make the ureteral openings visible. At this point, based on findings, other procedures can be performed, such as *catheterization of the kidney(s)* by inserting a catheter up through the ureter(s), *biopsy of a tumor,* or *removal of calculi* in the bladder. It may

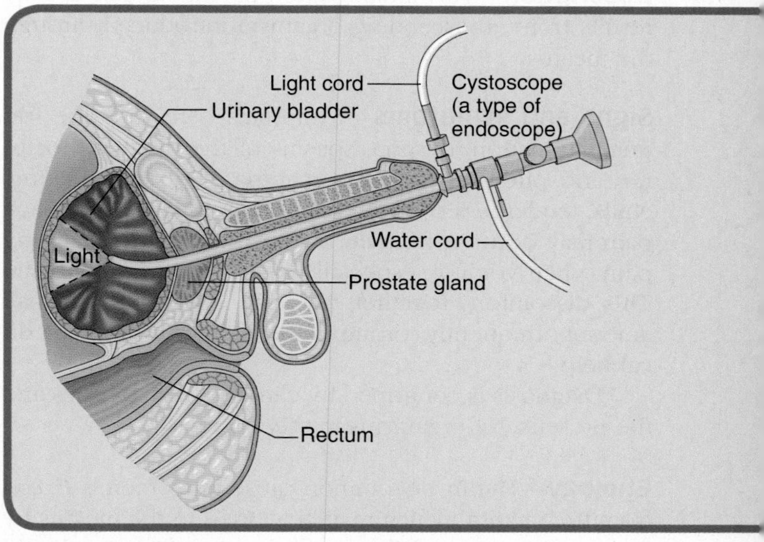

Figure 33–11: A cystoscopic examination of the male bladder *Delmar/Cengage Learning..*

be possible to crush larger calculi with an instrument and irrigate the pieces out through the scope. When examination of the bladder is completed, the scope is slowly withdrawn as the neck of the bladder and the interior of the urethra are examined.

Other standard procedures performed initially during cystourethroscopy are obtaining a sterile specimen for culture, cytology (for cancer cells), and sensitivity testing.

Other X-ray examinations can be performed in connection with endoscopic examinations. When a catheter is inserted into one of the ureters and passed into the pelvis of the kidney, a radiopaque medium can be instilled. This procedure, known as *retrograde ureteropyelography,* is especially useful for viewing the inside of the kidney when poor kidney function prohibits an IVP procedure. The structure of the ureters can be seen by an additional dye injection as the catheter is withdrawn.

Fluoroscopy and X-ray films aid in determining abnormalities. A delayed film, 15 to 20 minutes following instillation of the dye, can be taken to check for retention indicative of urinary stasis (stagnation). If an obstruction of the kidney is observed, it can be located by the film to be corrected. When an obstruction prohibits urine drainage, the catheter may be left in position temporarily to ensure adequate drainage. A kidney can be severely, if not permanently, damaged in a relatively short period if pressure from urine builds up because of the inability to drain.

DISEASES AND DISORDERS

Cystitis (Sis-ti′-tis)

Description—This inflammation of the bladder usually results from an ascending organism introduced through the meatus.

Signs and symptoms—Symptoms of cystitis are frequent urination, dysuria, spasms of the bladder, nocturia, and often fever and hematuria. Nausea, vomiting, chills, tenderness over the bladder area, and lower-back pain may occur. A frequent complaint is sharp, stabbing pain when voiding, especially at the end of the stream. This discomfort, together with the urge to void small amounts frequently, prompts the patient to seek medical help.

Diagnosis is confirmed by clinical characteristics and the presence of organisms in the urine.

Etiology—The most common cause in women is *E. coli* from the rectum, which may be carried to the meatus by improper cleansing following defecation. Women should be instructed to always cleanse from front to back when washing, wiping, or drying the perineal area. **Cystitis** can also be caused by organisms from the vagina. Women are far more prone to infection than men, presumably because the urethra is so short. Also, in men, the prostatic fluid acts as an antibacterial shield, thereby providing protection.

Treatment—Cystitis is treated with antibiotics sufficient to sterilize the urine. Usually, medication is given for approximately three days. A culture of the urine after the three days should show no organisms. If bacterial resistance to a certain medication has developed, the drug of choice will need to be changed. The sensitivity studies performed on the urine culture will identify appropriate alterations.

Women who have had cystitis a few times can identify the characteristic symptoms as soon as they begin and start to drink cranberry juice and water.

Urinary tract infections (UTI) are particularly common in patients with neurogenic bladders. The problem stems from the loss of innervation to the bladder, which can cause incontinence, urinary retention, spasticity, or flaccidness. Bedfast patients or those confined to wheelchairs are especially susceptible. The use of indwelling catheters to deal with incontinence or the inability to void frequently results in UTI as a result of the direct entrance route for bacteria into the bladder.

Prevention—Women may be able to avoid cystitis by following some simple measures:

- Drink enough water to keep urine a light straw color; this washes out bacteria.
- Drinking 4 ounces of cranberry juice daily may also decrease bacteria.
- Don't use a diaphragm for birth control if you have recurrent UTIs; it boosts the risk for repeat infections.
- Urinate immediately after sex. Often, bacteria in the vagina may be introduced into the bladder, and urination expels the bacteria and decreases the likelihood of infection.

Glomerulonephritis (Glo-mer-u-lo-ne-fri′-tis)

This inflammation of the glomerulus of the nephron occurs in both acute and chronic forms.

Acute Glomerulonephritis (AGN)

Description—**Acute glomerulonephritis (AGN)** can occur following bacterial infections of the respiratory tract, the urinary tract, or the bloodstream. It affects boys ages 3 to 7 most frequently but can strike either sex at any age. Up to 95% of children and 70% of adults recover fully, with the remainder developing chronic renal failure.

Signs and symptoms—AGN usually begins one to three weeks after an untreated throat infection. Symptoms include moderate edema, protein in the urine, hematuria, oliguria, and fatigue. Hypertension may develop because of retention of sodium or water from the decreased glomerular filtration rate. Diagnosis is made following a detailed history and clinical assessment. Laboratory findings confirm elevated electrolytes, BUN (blood urea nitrogen), creatinine in the blood, red and white blood cells, and protein in the urine. A throat culture may show a streptococcal organism.

Etiology—AGN results from a collection of antigen-antibodies from streptococcal infections that become entrapped in the glomeruli membranes. The entrapment causes interference in the glomerular function, damaging the membrane and resulting in the loss of its ability to selectively filter solutes. Red blood cells and protein molecules are allowed to filter out, and the filtration rate drops. Uremic poisoning may result. (See Uremia.)

Treatment—Treatment consists of bed rest, fluid and salt restriction, and correction of the electrolyte imbalance. Diuretics (water pills) may be used to reduce the accumulation of cellular fluid. At this time, the use of antibiotics is controversial. The course of AGN usually resolves in about two weeks.

Chronic Glomerulonephritis

Description—This is a slow, progressive disease. It causes scarring and sclerosing of the inflamed glomeruli, gradually leading to renal failure. Unfortunately, sufficient symptoms are not produced to cause early clinical investigation.

Signs and symptoms—The first symptoms are proteinuria (protein in the urine), hematuria, and a specific form of a urine cast. By the time it is diagnosed, **chronic glomerulonephritis** is usually irreversible.

The chronic stage can be asymptomatic for many years, suddenly becoming progressive and producing hypertension, proteinuria, and hematuria. In the later stages, uremic symptoms occur, such as nausea, vomiting, pruritus, dyspnea, fatigue, mild to severe edema, and anemia. Severe hypertension may cause enlargement of the heart, congestive heart failure (CHF), and eventually renal failure.

Etiology—Occasionally, the chronic form follows AGN, but most frequently it is an insidious disease precipitated by other primary renal disorders or systemic syndromes.

Treatment—Treatment consists of measures to treat the symptoms only, such as a diet to restrict sodium, antihypertensive drugs, correction of the electrolyte imbalance, reduction of edema, and prevention of cardiac failure.

Incontinence (In-con′-tin-ence)

Description—This is the uncontrollable loss of urine. It is estimated that at least 20 million people in the United States suffer from incontinence; 85% are women. It interferes with sleep, physical and sexual activity, travel, and daily activities. Many women avoid social activities and are home-bound because of the fear of an accident. Twenty-five percent of women ages 15 to 64 have incontinence. This increases to over 40% for those older than 60. It occurs basically in three forms: stress, overflow, and urge. *Stress incontinence,* the most common, occurs when a person coughs, sneezes, or laughs. Urine may also leak from the stress on muscles when exercising or rising from bed or a chair. *Overflow incontinence* occurs because the bladder never empties completely and its fullness causes leakage. *Urge incontinence* occurs unexpectedly. There is a strong, uncontrollable urge to void, requiring immediate emptying of the bladder to prevent wetting.

Males may also be affected by incontinence, but not as frequently as women. The rate among men is 1.5% to 5% but also increases with age. (It may be higher because so many prefer to be silent.) Nearly all older men have "dribbling" of urine when the prostate becomes enlarged and displaces the bladder. (The prostate, shaped somewhat like a donut, lies directly beneath the bladder, with the urethra running through its center.) If the prostate is removed, the prostatic portion of the urethra is involved, and control of urine is affected.

Signs and symptoms—The primary symptom is the involuntary loss of urine.

Etiology—Age is not a cause. There are a number of reasons for incontinence; some are specific to one of the forms previously discussed. All involve the physical structure and function of the bladder and urethra. In the female, the bladder lies beneath and is somewhat supported by the uterus and its ligaments (Figure 33–12A). As the bladder fills, a message to void goes to the brain, but if it is not convenient, the external sphincter is contracted and the bladder neck stays closed. This signals the bladder to relax (Figure 33–12B). When it is time to void, the message goes to the external sphincter to relax and it opens; this signals the bladder neck to open and the bladder to contract (Figure 33–12C). With stress incontinence, coughing, sneezing, or laughing increases pressure on the bladder, thereby increasing pressure on the bladder neck, which is not able to stay closed. The external sphincter cannot control urine alone, so it spurts out. With overflow incontinence, the bladder does not empty completely for various reasons, including prolapse of a pelvic organ or failure of the bladder muscle. The pressure builds up and overpowers the sphincter, causing leakage. In women, the displacement of the bladder during pregnancy and the pressure during the process

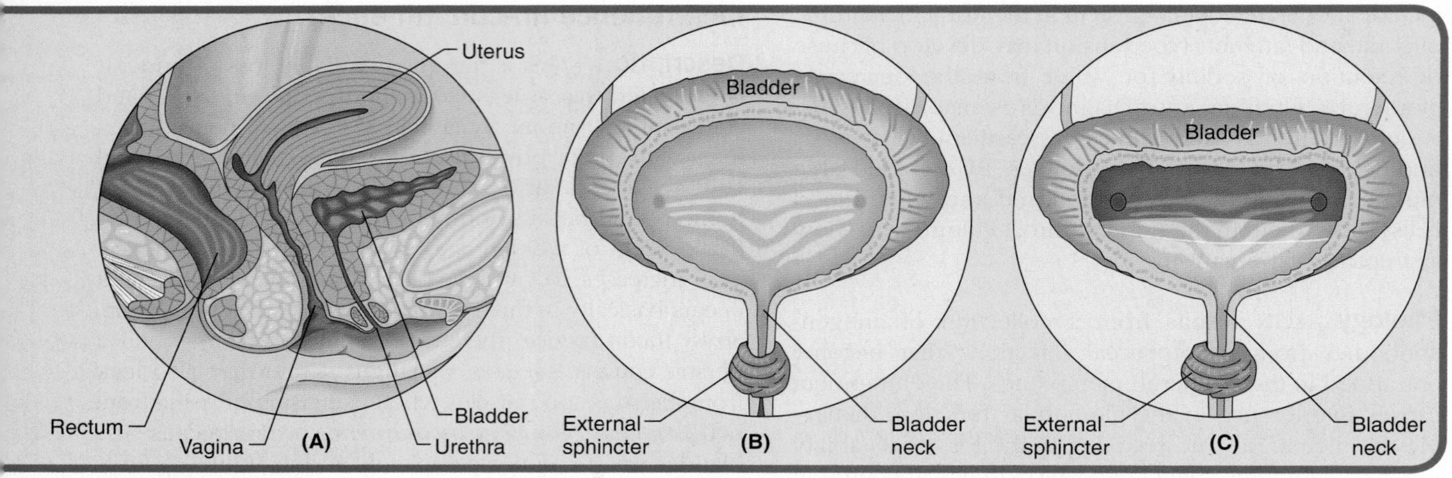

Figure 33–12: (A) Structure and function of the urinary bladder. The bladder is located beneath the uterus and in front of the vagina in a female. (B) The sphincter contracts to close the urethra and sends a message to the bladder to relax and the bladder neck to stay closed. (C) To void, the sphincter relaxes and a message goes to the bladder to contract and the bladder neck to open. *Delmar/Cengage Learning.*

of childbirth are definite factors in the development of incontinence. Often, following hysterectomy (removal of the uterus), the bladder will "drop" and protrude into the vagina, causing a cystocele and resulting in improper positioning and the inability to empty completely. With urge incontinence, the urge to urinate is received even though there is little urine, the bladder continues to contract longer than the sphincter can prevent leakage, and urine is leaked. Menopause is often responsible because the drop in estrogen weakens the urethral sphincter, causing an inability to keep it tightly closed, so a woman feels the urge to void small amounts several times an hour.

Treatment—A variety of things can be done. Many people find it necessary to wear sanitary napkins or specially designed incontinence pads in order to conceal their leakage. Others wear adult-style diapers or waterproof briefs. Some, especially men, wear an external appliance to catch the urine. For stress-related incontinence, exercises of the pelvic floor muscles may be helpful. These muscles act as a sling to keep the bladder and the bladder neck lifted and to control the external sphincter. These exercises are known as "Kegels." They involve contracting and briefly holding the muscles several times a day, which over time can tighten and strengthen the pelvic floor (Figures 33–13A and B). The recommended "workout" is 25 to 40 repetitions of 5 to 10 seconds duration. For females, topical estrogen (female hormone) therapy is also helpful. The injection of collagen into the tissue surrounding the sphincter can be very effective in narrowing the urethra. Figure 33–14 illustrates the injection into the tissue from a needle within the cystoscope. This procedure may take several injections, which often cost up to $5,000 each. It has a 69% cure rate.

Overflow incontinence can be improved with self-catheterization to remove the urine. Surgery may be indicated if there is vaginal prolapse or if the bladder has partially descended through the muscles of the pelvic floor. Urge incontinence is best treated with drugs to relax the bladder contractions and estrogen to improve the sphincter tone. The Kegel exercises are also helpful. Drug therapy costs about $40 to $50 per month and must continue throughout life.

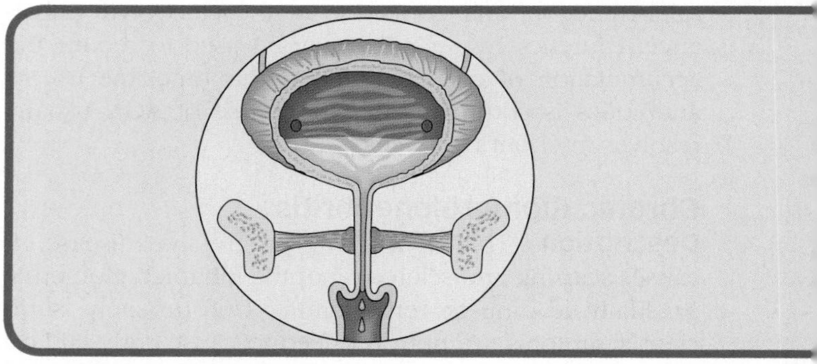

Figure 33–13A: Kegel exercises. Before pelvic muscles are thin and the sphincter is weak, so the urethra cannot close. *Delmar/Cengage Learning.*

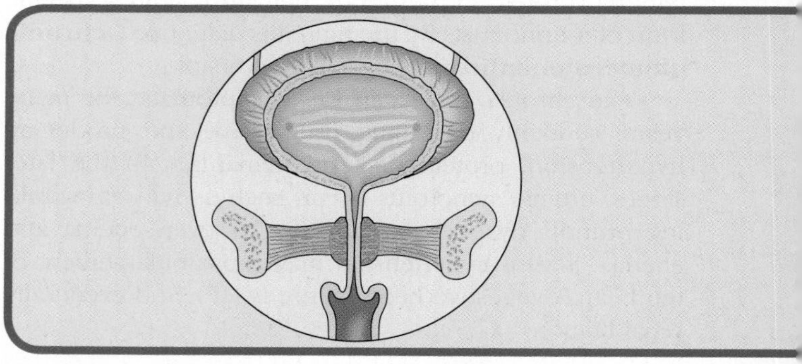

Figure 33–13B: After three months of exercises, the muscles are thicker and stronger, closing the sphincter. *Delmar/Cengage Learning.*

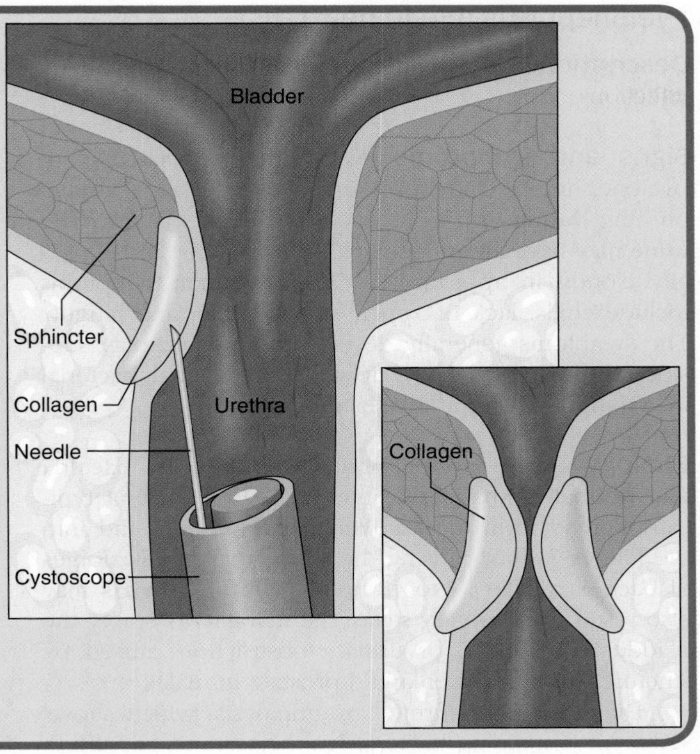

Figure 33–14: Injecting collagen near the sphincter narrows the urethra to control leakage. *Delmar/Cengage Learning.*

A change in behavior may be sufficient to control incontinence. With stress incontinence, a bathroom trip should be made every three hours. Urge incontinence requires bladder training by beginning bathroom trips every hour the first week, then every hour and a half, and eventually every three hours. Kegels are used to control the urge. The process is slow and not too successful, helping 54% to 75% but only curing 12% to 16%. Bladder surgery may achieve up to 85% success, but it often lasts only a few years and requires an extended period of time for recovery. The repaired supporting muscles tend to separate again, allowing the bladder to fall out of position.

A surgical procedure for stress incontinence known as transobturator tape (TOT) uses a piece of fabric, in a slinglike fashion, to support the bladder and urethra in their proper position. The tape is inserted through the anterior vaginal wall, then two small incisions are made through the lower groin area of the abdomen. The fabric is attached with enough tension to properly support the bladder and urethra. This repair has about a 90% rate of success to correct stress incontinence. The recovery period is from three to six weeks and has restrictions of lifting no more than five pounds and no driving, stairs, or bending over for the first three weeks.

In males, exercises following prostate surgery are very important to regain urinary control. The surgical procedure weakens the related muscles and may injure the urethral sphincter. Occasionally, incontinence persists either because of increased bladder pressure or a sphincter problem, or both. If it persists, periurethral collagen injections can be effective. A surgical procedure involving the insertion of an artificial sphincter can also be performed. This device has a valve mechanism that the person can activate to control and expel urine. A newer procedure involves placing a sling in the perineum to provide additional support to the urethra.

There are other health problems that cause incontinence for both sexes. The effects of a stroke and Parkinson's disease, for instance, can damage the nerves, making control impossible. If leakage begins suddenly, it may signify a bladder infection or a medication side effect. High blood pressure drugs called alpha blockers weaken the sphincter. Antihistamines and sleeping pills may also cause problems. Smoking can exacerbate stress incontinence and obesity is an additional risk factor for stress incontinence in females.

Nephrotic Syndrome (Ne-frot′-ik) (Nephrosis)

Description—This noninflammatory disease involving the glomerular membrane allows a large number of protein molecules to leave the blood and enter the urine. As a result, large amounts of water accumulate in the body, causing generalized dependent edema. This often leads to pleural effusion, swollen external sex organs, and ascites (fluid within the abdomen). **Nephrotic syndrome** occurs most often in children, but adults can contract the disease also.

Signs and symptoms—Symptoms range from the dominant clinical feature of edema to hypotension (especially on standing), lethargy, fatigue, lack of appetite, pallor, and depression.

Diagnosis can be confirmed from consistently elevated proteinuria over a 24-hour period, the presence of characteristic fatty casts and oval fat bodies in the urine, and increased serum cholesterol levels with decreased albumin levels.

Etiology—The underlying cause of the disease is usually glomerulonephritis (75% of the cases). The remaining 25% are associated with diabetes; circulatory diseases, such as sickle cell anemia, CHF, and renal vein thrombosis; toxins that affect the nephrons, such as mercury, bismuth, or gold; allergic reactions; and systemic infections, such as tuberculosis.

Treatment—Treatment consists of correcting the underlying cause whenever possible. Supportive treatment involves a high-protein diet, restrictive sodium intake, diuretics for edema, and antibiotics to combat infection. Some favorable results have occurred with the use of corticosteroids, but they are limited to specific uses.

Polycystic Kidney Disease (Pole-sis′-tik)

Description—An inherited disorder, **polycystic kidney disease** is characterized by bilateral, grapelike clusters of fluid-filled cysts that replace normal renal tissue (Figure 33–15). The presence of the cysts greatly enlarges the size of the kidney externally and also compresses the nephrons inside, eventually replacing the functioning renal tissue. One form of the disease appears in infants, called autosomal recessive ("infantile") polycystic kidney disease and results in stillbirth or early newborn death. Occasionally, an infant will survive for about two years before developing renal failure. The adult form has an insidious onset, usually apparent between ages 30 to 50. The deterioration of the kidney is slower but is nevertheless fatal unless treated by dialysis or transplantation.

Signs and symptoms—Symptoms of the infantile form include a pointed nose, small chin, floppy low-set ears, and folds in the inner eyelids. The kidneys become huge bilateral masses between the bottom of the ribs and the top of the ileum and are symmetrical, firm, and dense. Usually, there is evidence of CHF and respiratory distress. Adult polycystic disease initially presents nonspecific symptoms, such as hypertension, polyuria, and UTI. Eventually, additional symptoms appear relating to enlarged kidney masses, such as lumbar pain; widened body; and a swollen, tender abdomen. As the disease advances, the patient develops recurrent hematuria, life-threatening bleeding from cyst rupture, proteinuria, and pain caused by ureteral spasm from the passing of clots or calculi. Ultimately, the insufficiency of the kidney results in failure and uremia.

Etiology—This disease is an inherited disorder.

Treatment—Polycystic disease is not curable, but it can be managed, to a certain degree, by controlling hypertension and urinary infections. Treatment is like that for any chronic, destructive kidney disease.

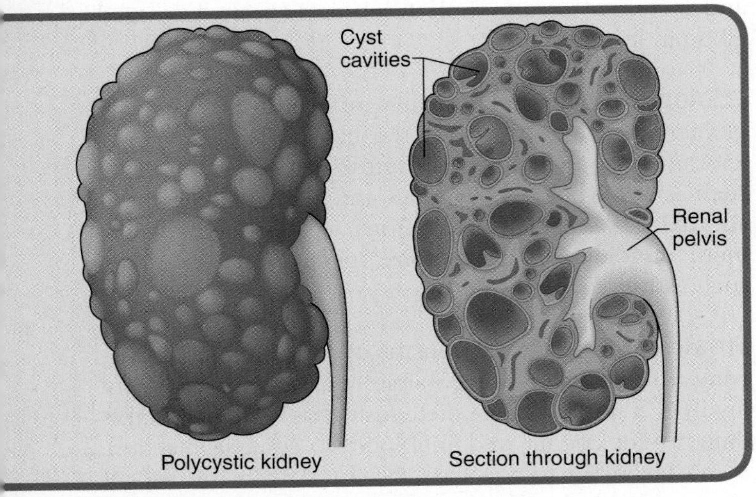

Figure 33–15: Polycystic disease. *Delmar/Cengage Learning.*

Pyelonephritis (Pie-lo-ne-fri′-tis)

Description—This is one of the most common kidney infections.

Signs and symptoms—Symptoms associated with pyelonephritis include fever, urgency, dysuria, back pain, burning during urination, nocturia, and hematuria. The urine may have an ammoniacal or fishy odor and is usually cloudy in appearance. Other common symptoms include chills, lack of appetite, flank pain, and fatigue. The symptoms generally develop rapidly and may subside within a few days. However, a residual bacterial infection may recur at a later time.

Etiology—Acute pyelonephritis is caused by bacteria that normally inhabit the intestines. The bacteria typically spread from the bladder up the ureters and into the kidney pelvis, causing the development of colonies of bacteria within 24 to 48 hours. **Pyelonephritis** may also result from urinary stasis; the inability to empty the bladder completely; or urinary obstruction caused by strictures, tumors, or enlarged prostate in males.

Diagnosis is confirmed by urinalysis, which shows sediment containing bacteria leukocytes and possibly a few red blood cells. Culture reveals a significant population of bacteria. Specific gravity is below normal because of the temporary inability to concentrate urine.

Treatment—Treatment consists of antibiotics determined by culture and sensitivity tests. A course of treatment is usually 10 to 14 days even though urine becomes sterile after two to three days.

Reculturing is sometimes done one week after treatment. Structural problems causing urinary stasis, such as strictures, "dropped" bladder (positioned so that it cannot totally empty), or tumors, should be corrected.

Renal Calculi (Re′-nal Kal′-ku-li)

Description—Kidney calculi (stones) are formed from chemicals in the urine, forming crystals that stick together. They may be as small as a grain of sand or as large as a golf ball. Small stones pass out of the kidney with the urine. Some that are larger become caught in a ureter, where they cause severe pain. Still others may pass into the bladder where they continue to enlarge. They will again cause pain if they wash into the urethra and become lodged.

Kidney stones affect primarily young to middle-aged adults, with men being affected four times as often as women. The condition tends to recur.

Signs and symptoms—

- Severe pain, starting suddenly in the kidneys or lower abdomen and moving to the groin area. It may last for minutes or hours, alternating with periods of relief.

- Nausea and vomiting
- Burning, frequency, urgency
- Chills, fever, and weakness, probably from infection
- Cloudy or foul-smelling urine
- Blood in the urine
- Blocked urine flow

Diagnosis is made based on symptoms, X-rays (such as KUB or IVP), CAT scan, or ultrasound. Once size and location are determined, then an appropriate course of action can be selected. About 90% can be passed without requiring special treatment or surgery. Often, increasing fluids, may assist in stone passage. Some medications like tamsulosin (Flomax) can help stones in the ureter to pass without surgery. However, calcium-containing stones, the most common type, cannot be dissolved.

Etiology—The causes of calculi formation are not always clear; however, certain factors seem to contribute to their development:

- Drinking too little fluid
- Chronic UTIs
- Blockage of the urinary tract
- Prolonged limited activity
- Misuse of certain medications
- Certain genetic and metabolic diseases
- Specific foods in certain susceptible people

Treatment—The simplest treatment is chosen first. Many stones, if in the bladder or ureters, can be removed endoscopically either directly or following fracture of the stone with laser or shock waves. Stones in the kidney may be removed by a scope, inserted through the side of the body and directly into the kidney. This allows removal of the stone when it is visualized or fracture of the stone with instruments passed under direct vision.

Another method of stone removal is called extracorporeal (outside the body) shock-wave **lithotripsy** (ESWL). Shock waves (high-energy pressure waves) similar to sonic booms generated by aircraft are produced outside the body by an electrical spark. There are two types of lithotripsy. One utilizes a tank of warm water with the patient positioned in a hydraulic chair (Figure 33–16A). The chair is positioned so that the stone is in the area where the shock waves can be focused. The waves travel through the water and into the body without damaging the tissues because all tissue is about 80% water.

A newer type of lithotripsy positions the patient in a supine position on a special table. The spark generating device with its cushion of water is positioned behind the kidney (note the red circular area in Figure 33–16B). Using fluoroscopy, the stone is located and the device is centered on target. The procedure is performed using the attached computer (Figure 33–16C).

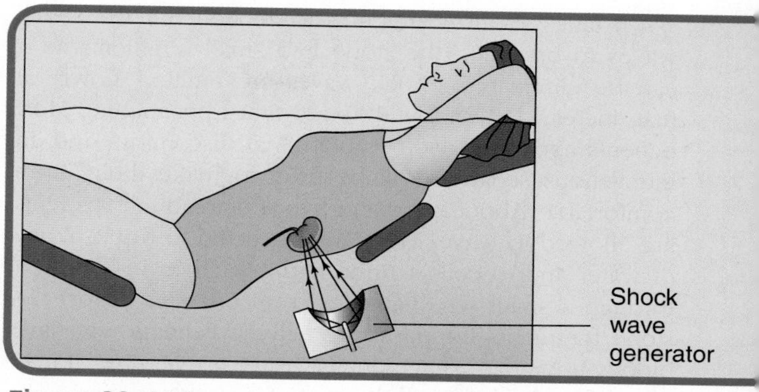

Figure 33–16A: Lithotripsy procedure *Delmar/Cengage Learning.*

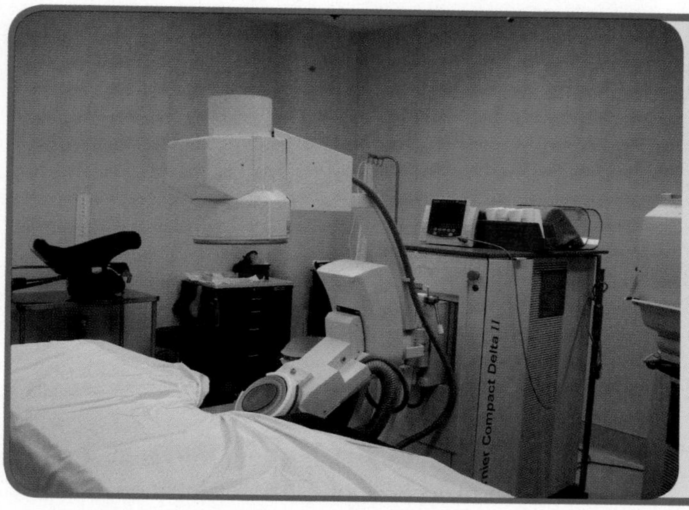

Figure 33–16B: Lithotripsy table. *Courtesy of Barbara A. Wise.*

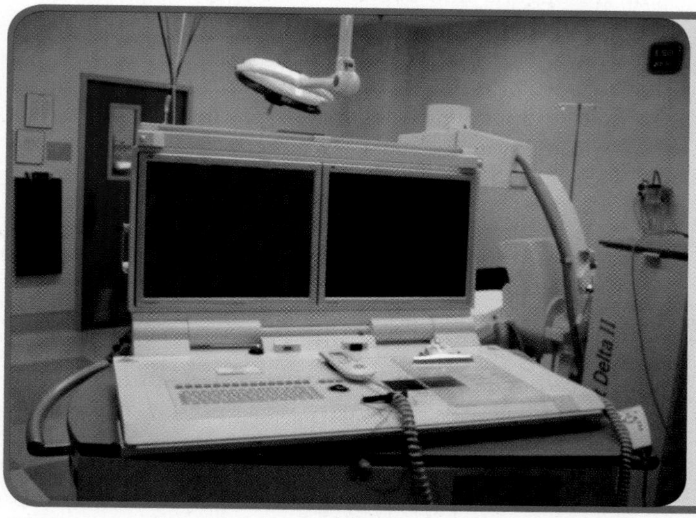

Figure 33–16C: Lithotripsy computer. *Courtesy of Barbara A. Wise.*

It takes about 45 minutes to an hour for the shock waves to break up the stone into small fragments so it can be eliminated. Shock waves are emitted slowly at first, increasing to about 100–120 times per minute. Most patients experience some abdominal discomfort, and an intravenous sedation will be used to make them more comfortable. About an hour or two after treatment, patients are allowed to leave. They are instructed to drink plenty of water and to collect urine in a container and strain it through a small screening device in order to collect the stone fragments for possible analysis. Patients will have bloody urine that will gradually decrease over time. It may take a few weeks for all the stone fragments to pass.

Not all patients with kidney stones qualify for ESWL. Usually, the stone must be no more than 4 cm in diameter and be located within the kidney or ureter. (The lithotripsy device can also be used to break up gallstones lodged in the cystic or common bile ducts). With the water tank method, people over 6 feet 6 inches tall or weighing over 300 pounds may not qualify because of their size. Also, if there is little or no kidney function or an uncontrolled urinary infection, ESWL is not a good choice.

Rarely, if no other method can be used, the stone will be removed by surgical incision into the kidney. This is considered the final choice to solve the problem because of the risks involved with any major surgical procedure and the length of recovery time required.

Renal Failure

Acute Renal Failure

Description—A critical illness, **acute renal failure** results in the sudden cessation of kidney function. Effective medical treatment usually can overcome the problem. If not, however, it will progress to uremia and death.

Signs and symptoms—Symptoms initially apparent are oliguria and azotemia (nitrogenous products of protein metabolism in the blood). Without filtration, the waste products and excess solutes quickly collect in the blood, resulting in severe electrolyte imbalance, acidosis, and uremia, which interfere with the function of the other body systems. A vast number of other symptoms develop, listed here by body system and in ascending order within the system:

- *Gastrointestinal:* anorexia, nausea, vomiting, hematemesis (bloody vomitus)
- *Nervous:* headache, drowsiness, confusion, convulsion, coma
- *Integumentary:* dryness of the skin, pruritus, pallor, uremic frost (powdery white crystals of urea on the skin)
- *Circulatory:* hypotension initially, then hypertension, cardiac rhythm irregularities, CHF, edema, anemia, pulmonary edema
- *Respiratory:* Kussmaul's respirations (fast, deep respirations, over 20 per minute and usually sounding labored, resembling sighs)

Fever and chills, indicators of infection, are an expected complication.

Diagnosis of renal failure is confirmed by blood test findings of greatly elevated quantities of urea, nitrogen, and creatinine and urine samples with casts, protein, and altered specific gravity. Additional verification with diagnostic examinations, such as KUB, IVP, ultrasound, and retrograde pyelography, may be indicated.

Etiology—Renal failure may be caused by an obstruction, inadequate circulation, or damage to the nephrons. Failure caused by bilateral obstruction is usually associated with calculi, blood clots, tumors, strictures, or an enlarged prostate. Inadequate blood flow results from low blood pressure and low volume in the arteries, which eliminates the force required for the kidney to filter water and solutes from the blood. This can result from shock, embolism, hemorrhage, loss of fluid caused by burns, congestive heart failure, and arrhythmias. Nephron damage, which may cause failure, can result from acute glomerulonephritis, sickle cell anemia, bilateral renal vein thrombosis, acute pyelonephritis, renal myeloma (tumor), or toxic substances, like medications.

Treatment—Treatment consists of a high-calorie diet that is low in protein, sodium, and potassium. Fluids are controlled. Dialysis may be required.

Chronic Renal Failure

Description—This is an end result of the progressive loss of kidney function.

Signs and symptoms—Symptoms do not develop significantly enough to warrant investigation until almost 75% of glomerular function is gone. The remaining normal nephrons gradually deteriorate, causing symptoms of renal failure and other system involvement. Signs and symptoms initially are related to an imbalance of sodium and potassium and an accumulation of nitrogen from protein metabolism; these may include hypotension, dry mouth, listlessness, fatigue, and nausea. Later, the patient will begin experiencing mental dullness and confusion. Symptoms increase as more nephrons fail.

Additional system involvement is similar to that described with acute failure, but a few specific differences do occur with the slower progressive course.

Infertility and amenorrhea (lack of menses) in women, impotence in men, and impaired carbohydrate metabolism also result from improper endocrine action. The skeletal system develops a mineral imbalance that results in bone pain because of parathyroid hormone imbalance. This in turn allows the minerals to be withdrawn from the bones, causing fractures. Calcifications develop in the brain, eyes, joints, myocardium, and blood vessels. Children with chronic failure show stunted growth patterns because of endocrine abnormalities.

Diagnosis is made in the same manner as for acute renal failure.

Etiology—**Chronic renal failure** can be the result of many preexisting conditions, such as chronic glomerular disease; chronic infections; obstructions; stones; and endocrine diseases, such as diabetes, vascular diseases, hypertension, and chronic overdose of toxic agents.

Treatment—Treatment is almost exclusively dependent on dialysis to correct the chemical imbalance. Other treatment is required for the complications developed in the other body systems. Long-term dialysis requires specific physical and psychologic therapy. Patients must be meticulous in their personal care. The skin must be clean, and lotions should be applied to combat dryness and itching. Good oral hygiene is a must to alleviate bad breath and counteract excessive dryness and bad taste. Diet is extremely critical and requires individual adjustments in relation to dialysis. Daily records of intake and output aid in determining fluid status. If urine is not being excreted, fluid builds up within the body's tissues. Dialysis removes this fluid, causing the patient to express feelings of being "wrung out."

Stricture (Strik′-chur)

Description—This is a narrowing of a passageway that interferes with the movement of substances through its interior. For example, the **stricture** of a ureter interferes with the flow of urine to the bladder. A more common stricture occurs in the urethra, particularly in males.

Signs and symptoms—Symptoms of urethral stricture, such as a small urine stream and prolonged urination time, are indicative of a decreased passageway. Stricture of a ureter may not be evident until distention occurs because of the buildup of pressure or until kidney stones develop from urinary stasis. Complete stricture of a ureter will destroy the function of the affected kidney.

Etiology—It may be caused by a congenital abnormality or, in either sex, may be the result of scarring following infection or surgery.

Treatment—Urethral stricture in adult men can be treated with dilation of the stricture using increasingly larger dilators to open up the narrowed passageway. If this fails, the stricture is cut through a cystoscope using a knife or laser beam. In some instances, the urethral stricture is excised through an open surgical procedure. Urethral strictures are rather rare in children and are treated in a similar way as adults. In children, surgery is used to remove the area of narrowing.

Uremia (U-re′-me-a)

Description—Literally translated, this term means that the products normally found in the urine are instead in the blood.

Signs and symtoms—Blood analysis shows excess protein by-products because urinary disease prevents their excretion in the urine. It is a toxic condition, leading to coma and death if not treated. End-stage uremia may cause "uremic frost," the presence of crystals from the excretion of urine products through the skin.

Etiology—It can be the end result of many acute and chronic kidney diseases. Any condition that renders the kidney unable to regulate the chemical composition of the blood by excretion of waste products causes the wastes to accumulate, slowly building to a toxic level. When renal failure exists, **uremia** is inevitable.

Treatment—Dialysis is the only substitute for kidney function, except for surgical transplantation of another kidney.

AGE-RELATED BODY CHARACTERISTICS

Incontinence seems to occur at both ends of life. Of course, infants and toddlers must learn to control the urinary sphincter to stay dry and urinate only when appropriate. Unfortunately, as we age, especially women, bladder sphincters are not always capable of controlling urine and we experience stress incontinence with sneezing, coughing, laughing, and exercise. Sphincter control is also inadequate when the bladder is too full. The physical affects of childbirth and obesity may also cause incontinence. Men frequently experience some dribbling due to prostate involvement or following prostate surgery. With advanced age, urinary incontinence is very common as control of body functions becomes more difficult.

System Interaction Associated with Disease Conditions

The urinary system, particularly the kidneys, are so important to the welfare of the body that a great number of symptoms from other systems develop when this system fails. In fact, without kidney function, the patient will die. Fortunately, modern medicine and the use of artificial methods of removing the waste products from the body can prolong life for quite some time. The system interaction and the symptoms exhibited in two disease conditons are shown in Table 33–1.

TABLE 33–1 System Interaction Associated with Disease Conditions

Disease	Systems Involved	Pathology Present
Chronic glomerular nephritis	Urinary	Proteinuria, hematuria, uremia, renal failure
	Circulatory	Hypertension, anemia, congestive heart failure
	Digestive	Nausea, vomiting
Renal Failure	Urinary	Elevated urea, nitrogen and creatinine in urine
	Digestive	Anorexia, nausea, vomiting, hematemesis
	Nervous	Headache, confusion, convulsion, coma
	Circulatory	Hypotension followed by hypertension, cardiac rhythm irregularities, CHF, edema, anemia
	Respiratory	Kussmaul's respiration, pulmonary edema

CHAPTER SUMMARY

- The urinary system performs three main functions: excretion, secretion, and elimination.
- The kidneys remove waste products from the blood to the ureters into the bladder for storage until eliminated through the urethra.
- Kidneys are located retroperitoneally on each side of the spinal column.
- The kidney has a concave boarder notch called the hilum. Internally, there is an outer layer, the cortex, and an inner layer called the medulla.
- The medulla contains renal pyramids that empty into calyces.
- Nephrons are the microscopic units of the kidney. The have a Bowman's capsule, which contains a cluster of capillaries called a glomerulus.
- Filtration results from blood from the glomerulus entering into a single efferent arteriole, which raises the blood pressure and forces fluid into the Bowman's capsule.
- Reabsorption causes 99% of the fluid to re-enter the bloodstream.
- Secretion moves substances directly from the peritubular capillaries into the distal and collecting tubules.
- Urinary output is in relation to the volume of blood and the amount of solutes in the filtrate.
- The ureters extend from the kidney to the urinary bladder. Urine is moved through the ureters by peristalsis.
- The urinary bladder is composed of muscular tissue to expand and contract. The inability to expel urine is called retention.
- The urethra drains the urinary bladder through the urinary meatus. Inability to control urine passage is called incontinence.
- Dialysis is a mechanical process to remove waste products normally removed by the kidneys, from the blood. This is called hemodialysis.
- A hemodialysis site can be an arteriovenous fistula, an arteriovenous vein graft, or a Permacath.
- Peritoneal dialysis used the patient's own abdomen to filter wastes. Methods are CAPD, CCPD, and NIPD.
- Kidney transplant involves finding a match for the greatest chance of success.
- Diagnostic examinations include noninvasive procedures of routine specimens, clean catch, and 24-hour urine test. An X-ray of plain film and ultrasound are also diagnostic.
- Invasive procedures of IVP, cystourethroscopy, catheterization of the kidneys, biopsy calculi removal, and retrograde ureteropyelography are other diagnostic procedures.
- Diseases and disorders discussed were cystitis, acute glomerulonephritis, chronic glomerulonephritis, incontinence, nephritic syndrome, polycystic kidney disease, pyelonephritis, renal calculi, lithotripsy procedures, renal failure, chronic renal failure, stricture, and uremia.

STUDY TOOLS

Workbook	Activities for Chapter 33
Premium Website	
MEDIA LINK	View this **Media Link** for Chapter 33: • Urine formation
StudyWARE	Activities and Quizzes on the **StudyWARE™ Software** for Chapter 33
	Audio Library of medical terms
	Online access to the **Critical Thinking Challenge 2.0**
CourseMate	Activities and Quizzes for Chapter 33
WebTutor	Activities and Quizzes for Chapter 33

CHECK YOUR KNOWLEDGE

1. Which of the following diagnostic procedures is not noninvasive?
   a. Catheterization
   b. Ultrasound
   c. KUB series
   d. Fluoroscopy
2. A clean catch specimen is not:
   a. a sterile specimen.
   b. caught in midstream.
   c. collected by the patient.
   d. obtained after careful cleaning.
3. An intravenous pyelography:
   a. requires catheterization.
   b. is an X-ray study with contrast media.
   c. is a noninvasive procedure.
   d. allows visualization of the bladder interior.
4. Which of the following terms does not refer to a type of incontinence?
   a. Stress
   b. Overflow
   c. Urge
   d. Pressure
5. Polycystic kidney disease is characterized by:
   a. large number of protein molecules in the urine.
   b. fluid-filled structures within the kidney tissue.
   c. a history of a systemic infection.
   d. rapidly developing symptoms.
6. Which of the following is the basic cause of renal calculi?
   a. Drinking hard water
   b. A habit of delaying passing urine
   c. Getting too much calcium in the diet
   d. Crystals formed from chemicals in the urine
7. Acute renal failure may result in all the following except:
   a. uremia.
   b. death.
   c. sudden kidney failure.
   d. progressive loss of kidney function.
8. A long term treatment for uremia is:
   a. a kidney transplant.
   b. antibiotics.
   c. radiation.
   d. blood transfusions.
9. Which of the following is not a type of incontinence?
   a. Retention
   b. Stress
   c. Overflow
   d. Urge
10. Hemodialysis can be achieved through all the following except:
    a. arteriovenous fistula.
    b. indwelling urinary cetheter.
    c. synthetic graft.
    d. Permacath.

WEB LINKS

National Kidney and Urologic Diseases Clearinghouse: http://kidney.niddk.nih.gov/

National Kidney Foundation: http://kidney.org/

MedlinePlus, information about Lithotripsy: www.nlm.nih.gov/medlineplus/ency/article/007113.htm

Chapter 34 The Endocrine System

OBJECTIVES

In this chapter, you will learn the following:

KB KNOWLEDGE BASE

1. Spell and define, using the glossary at the back of the text, all the Words to Know in this chapter.
2. Differentiate between endocrine and exocrine glands and give an example of each.
3. Give five examples of body functions affected by hormones.
4. Name and locate the nine glands discussed in the chapter.
5. Describe the functions of the pituitary, thyroid, parathyroid, adrenal, pancreas, and thymus glands.
6. Describe the hormones and functions of the gonads.
7. Explain the hormone secretion abnormalities that cause gigantism, dwarfism, acromegaly, goiter, tetany, diabetes, cretinism, Cushing's syndrome, and myxedema.
8. List the symptoms of diabetic coma and insulin shock.
9. Identify the diagnostic examinations used to confirm diabetes, thyroid function, pregnancy, and Cushing's syndrome.
10. Describe briefly the symptoms, characteristics, and usual course of action of endocrine disorders presented in the chapter.
11. Discuss the effects of diabetes upon a person as he or she ages.
12. Identify the body systems involved with diabetes and Graves' disease.

WORDS TO KNOW

acromegaly
adrenal
adrenaline
adrenocorticotropic hormone (ACTH)
aldosterone
cretinism
Cushing's syndrome
diabetes mellitus
dwarfism
endocrine
epinephrine
estrogen
exocrine
exophthalmos
gigantism
glucohemoglobin
glycosuria
goiter
gonad
gonadotropic hormone
hyperglycemia
hyperthyroidism
hypoglycemia
hypothyroidism
insulin
islets of Langerhans
luteinizing
mineralocorticoid
myxedema
ovary
parathyroid
pineal body
pituitary
progesterone
puberty
testes
testosterone
tetany
thymus
thyroid
thyroidectomy

THE ENDOCRINE SYSTEM

The **endocrine** system is a group of glands that secrete substances directly into the bloodstream. Endocrine glands are ductless; in other words, their secretions do not drain into the body by way of a duct but are secreted and enter into the capillaries of the circulatory system (Figure 34–1A). Glands secreting substances through ducts are **exocrine** glands (Figure 34–1B). The pancreas secretes pancreatic juices by way of a duct into the duodenum, so it is an exocrine gland. However, the pancreas also secretes insulin directly into the capillaries, which also makes it an endocrine gland.

The secretions from endocrine glands are called **hormones**. A hormone is a complex chemical that influences actions at distant sites and controls body functions. Hormones are chemical messengers that cause changes. Examples of body functions affected by hormones are growth and development, metabolism, the composition of the blood and bones, sexual maturity, and the function of all endocrine glands.

Nine glands or groups of glands will be discussed: the **pituitary**, **thyroid**, **parathyroids**, pancreas (introduced in Chapter 32), **adrenals**, **ovaries**, **testes**, **thymus**, and the **pineal body** (Figure 34–2). Each gland performs a specific function. The hyperactivity or hypoactivity of the gland causes changes in the body, often altering its appearance, always altering its function, even to the point of death in specific hormonal crises. Hormones either increase or decrease glandular function to maintain homeostasis.

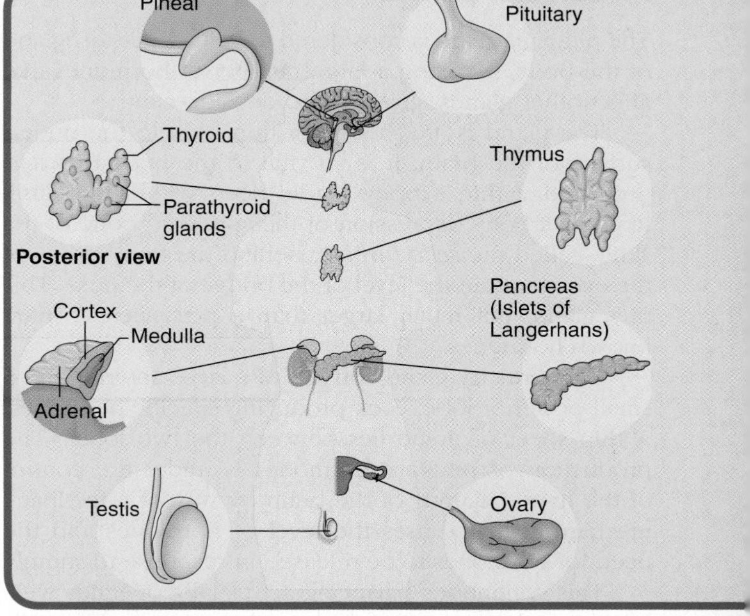

Figure 34–2: The glands of the endocrine system. *Delmar/Cengage Learning.*

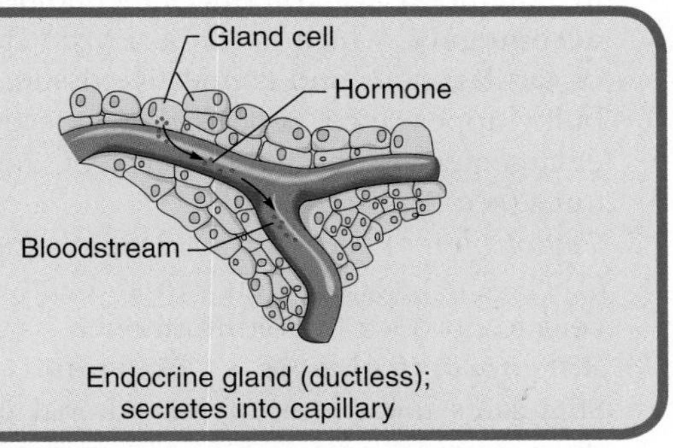

Figure 34–1A: Endocrine gland cells secrete hormones into a capillary. *Delmar/Cengage Learning.*

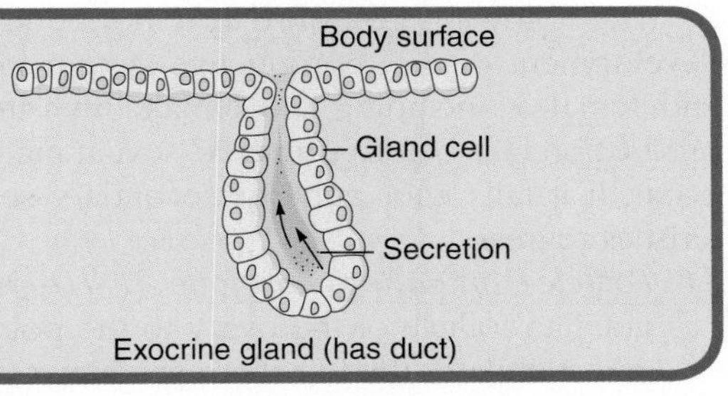

Figure 34–1B: Exocrine gland cells secrete substances directly into a duct. *Delmar/Cengage Learning.*

It is important to know that there are hormones secreted from nontraditional endocrine glands. For example, adipose (fat) cells secrete polypeptides that influence appetite and energy metabolism. Leptin is an example of such a hormone that may be used clinically to influence caloric intake and obesity. Also, gastrointestinal hormones are secreted by intestinal cells and have various actions, such as slowing gastric emptying, affecting insulin resistance in diabetes, and inhibiting the secretion of other hormones. Some of these hormones, such as amylin-like products, dipeptidyl peptidase-4 inhibitors, and somatostatin, have recently become available to treat endocrine disorders.

There are many diseases and disorders that develop from either too little or too much hormone influence. Some effects begin in early childhood, others after years of absence or excess of secretions. Fortunately, with appropriate health care, these abnormal conditions are usually discovered early and treated appropriately. In developing nations or when religious beliefs prohibit medical intervention, conditions that develop from too little or too much hormone influence may still be observable.

MEDIA LINK

Go to the Premium Website and watch the animation, "The Endocrine System," for this chapter.

PITUITARY GLAND

The pituitary gland is considered to be the "master" gland of the body, secreting a large number of hormones that affect other glands, growth, and development.

The gland is attached by a thin stalk to the undersurface of the brain. It is so vital to the body that it is protected within a bony cradle deep within the skull. It sits in a bony depression of the sphenoid bone of the skull, called the *sella turcica,* behind the bony orbits of the eyes at about the level of the bridge of the nose. This tiny gland, not much larger than a pea, secretes nine known hormones.

The pituitary gland consists of a large anterior and a small posterior lobe, each producing specific hormones. A thin sheet of tissue lies between the two lobes. The production of pituitary hormones is under the control of the hypothalamus of the brain by way of a feedback mechanism that senses the level of hormones and the need for hormones to be released in response to stimuli.

This continuous balancing act usually operates well. It is a complex process of the hypothalamus sensing levels of circulating hormones. If the level is too low, a chemical message is sent to the pituitary, which in turn secretes a hormone message to the particular gland to produce the hormone that will raise the level. After enough is produced, the hypothalamus senses the level is sufficient and sends the pituitary another message to reduce the production. The pituitary sends a hormone message to the appropriate gland, and the secretion is slowed. Later you will discover what happens when the hormones are either deficient or excessive because of some abnormality.

Anterior Lobe

The hormones of the anterior lobe of the pituitary are as follows:

1. *Growth hormone (GH)*—Essential for normal growth of the body's tissues, affects the length of long bones and therefore height. Insufficient production during childhood results in **dwarfism**, or short stature, whereas overproduction produces **gigantism**. Figure 34–3 is a modern illustration from a 100-year-old photo showing three different sizes of men: a giant, an average-sized man, and a dwarf. The photograph was demonstrating the effects of growth hormone. The average-sized man was probably about 5 feet, 8 inches tall, and perhaps the "giant" was about 7 feet tall. At that time he would have been considered very unusual. Today, many men reach and surpass this height, as evidenced by collegiate and professional basketball players. Not only men but women have grown taller as well. There are many females reaching 6 feet in height, and some are even taller (again, this can be seen among female basketball players).

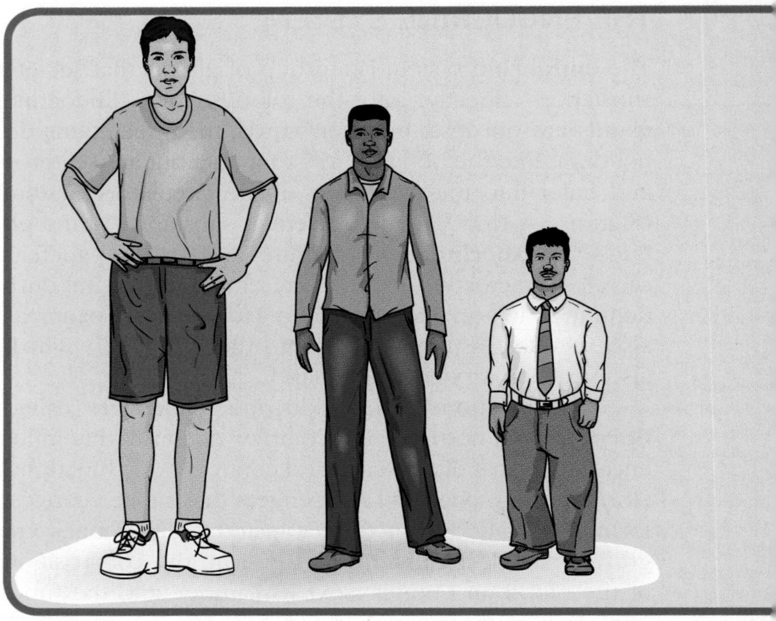

Figure 34–3: The effect of growth hormone: a giant, an average-sized person, and a dwarf. *Delmar/Cengage Learning.*

   What was once considered excessively tall may not be so today.

   However, overproduction of growth hormone beyond maturity is another thing. Overproduction in adulthood will produce a condition known as **acromegaly**, which is characterized by overgrowth of cartilagenous and connective tissue resulting in a bulky appearance, protrusion of the eyebrow area, enlargement of the hands and feet, and coarse features (see Figure 34–4).
2. *Thyrotropin,* the thyroid-stimulating hormone (TSH)—Increases the growth and activity of thyroid cells to produce thyroid hormone.
3. ***Adrenocorticotropic** hormone (ACTH)*—Stimulates the cortex of the adrenal gland to produce steroids.
4. *Melanocyte-stimulating hormone (MSH)*—Increases skin pigmentation.
5. *Prolactin (PR)*—Responsible for breast development and the production of milk.

The following **gonadotropic** hormones control the development of the reproductive system in both males and females, including the female menstrual cycle. If production fails before **puberty**, sexual maturity will not occur. If it fails after puberty, secondary sexual characteristics regress.

6. *Follicle-stimulating hormone (FSH)*—Enlarges the graafian follicle of the ovary to the point of rupture and stimulates the follicle to produce estrogen in the female. FSH stimulates the production of sperm in the male.

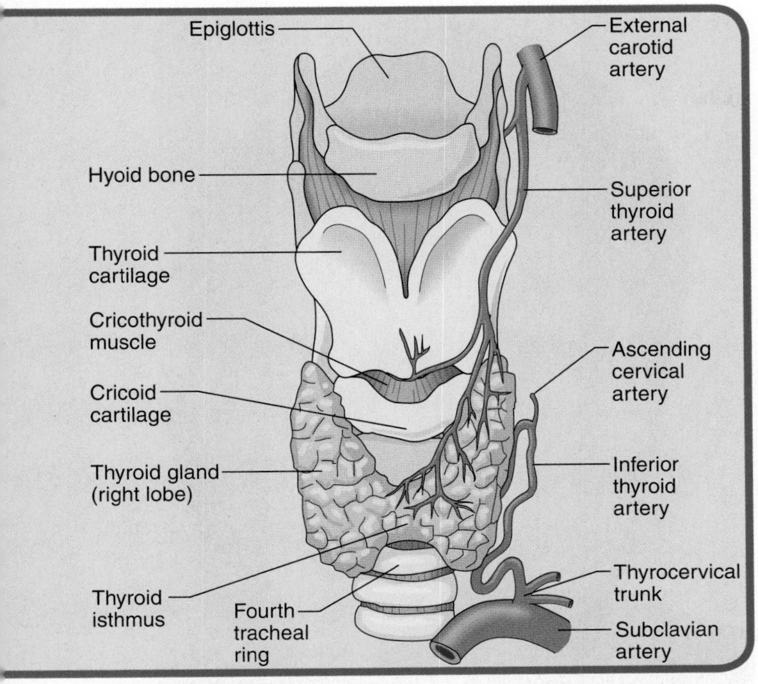

Figure 34–4: The thyroid gland. *Delmar/Cengage Learning.*

7. ***Luteinizing** hormone (LH)*—In the female causes the ruptured ovarian follicle to become a corpus luteum that in turn secretes the hormone progesterone. LH in the male stimulates the interstitial cells in the testes to produce testosterone.

Posterior Lobe

The hormones of the posterior lobe of the pituitary are as follows:

1. *Oxytocin*—Stimulates the contractions of the uterus, especially during childbirth; it also is responsible for the flow of milk from the breast.
2. *Vasopressin, or the antidiuretic hormone (ADH)*—Acts on the kidney tubule cells to concentrate urine and conserve water within the body. It also stimulates the smooth muscles of blood vessels to constrict.

THYROID GLAND

The thyroid gland has two lobes, one on each side of the larynx, with a connecting central section called the isthmus (Figure 34–4). It is located in front of the upper portion of the trachea in the lower part of the neck. The gland is encased in a capsule of connective tissue.

The thyroid gland produces three hormones: thyroxine (T_4), triiodothyronine (T_3), and calcitonin. Calcitonin causes reduction in the level of calcium in the blood. It is synthesized in C cells, which are nonfollicular cells located in the thyroid gland in humans. Calcitonin inhibits the bone cells from releasing calcium, therefore reducing serum calcium. The other two hormones strongly affect metabolism, which influences both the physical and mental activity necessary for normal growth and development. When thyroid activity is below normal, it is called **hypothyroidism**, indicating a decrease in the basal metabolic rate. An overactive thyroid is called **hyperthyroidism** and indicates an increased metabolic rate.

The thyroid gland requires iodine to form the thyroid hormones. Iodine is obtained by eating vegetables grown in soil containing iodine or by eating seafood. Lack of the element causes the thyroid gland to enlarge. When the pituitary receives information from the hypothalamus that the level of thyroid hormones is too low, it secretes TSH to stimulate the thyroid cells and eventually enlarges the entire gland. An enlarged thyroid gland is commonly known as a **goiter**.

The control of hormone release and inhibition by negative feedback is characterized in the relationship between the thyroid and the pituitary gland. When the hypothalamus senses thyroid hormone concentrations are too low, it secretes a releasing factor that travels to the anterior pituitary cells. This thyrotropin-releasing factor stimulates thyrotropin (TSH), which in turn causes the thyroid gland to synthesize and secrete thyroid hormones. As stated, if excessive secretion continues, a goiter may develop. Normally, as these hormones increase in the blood, they negatively "feed back" signals to the hypothalamus to reduce the releasing factor, resulting in the pituitary reducing TSH secretion, and in turn thyroid hormones. This finely tuned system is operative in the healthy state to maintain thyroid levels at the appropriate levels for regulating metabolism and other functions.

A person who has hypothyroidism feels cold and fatigued, has a low pulse rate, often has a subnormal temperature, and may be overweight due to decreased metabolism. The patient with hyperthyroidism is nervous, restless, and irritable, with heart rate above normal and elevated systolic blood pressure. The patient may lose weight despite a good appetite. Occasionally, the eyes protrude dramatically in a condition called **exophthalmos.**

The man in Figures 34–5A and 34–5B had been diagnosed with an enlarged thyroid gland and hyperthyroidism in 1980 and initially treated with propylthiouracil. In May 2001 he felt pressure in his eye and noticed a change in his vision and the bulging of his eye. He was diagnosed with exopthalmos, but only in one eye, an uncommon finding (see Figure 34–5A). By June, he was experiencing increased pressure and having severe pain. The pressure was compressing the optic nerve and would have destroyed his vision. He had his first surgery, an orbital decompression, in June. In this procedure, pieces of the bony orbit are removed to allow for drainage of the fluid

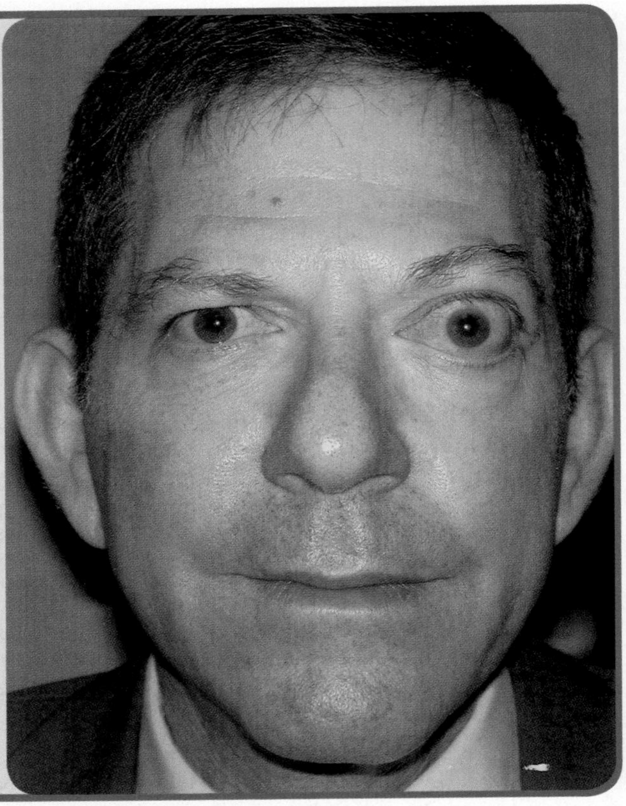

Figure 34–5A: Male with uncommon unilateral exopthalmos. *Courtesy of Barbara A. Wise.*

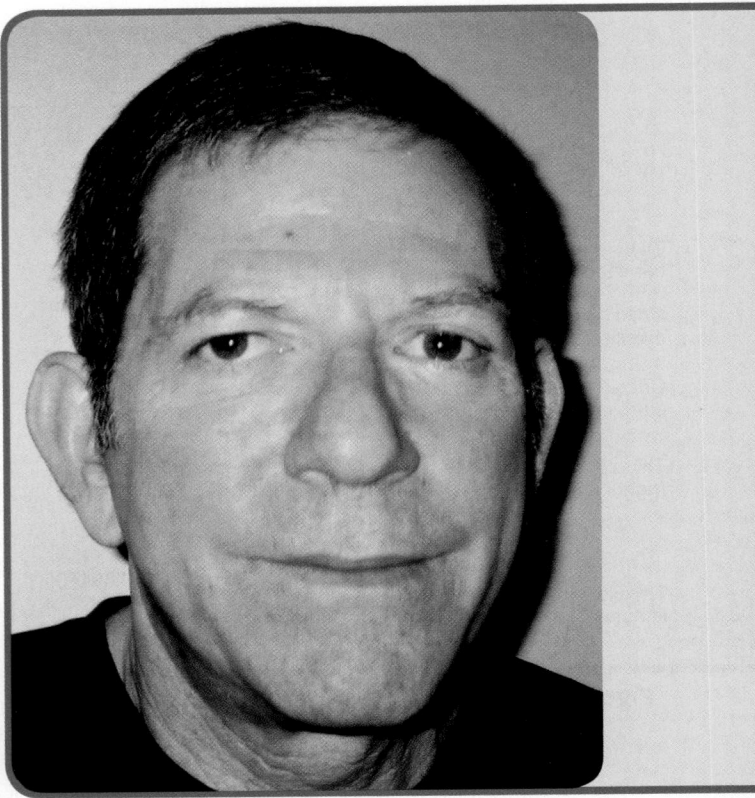

Figure 34–5B: Male with uncommon unilateral exopthalmos, after surgery. *Courtesy of Barbara A. Wise.*

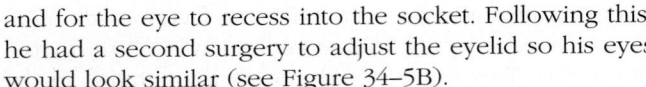

and for the eye to recess into the socket. Following this, he had a second surgery to adjust the eyelid so his eyes would look similar (see Figure 34–5B).

Hyperthyroidism may be treated by removing part or all of the gland or limiting its function by radioactive iodine or antithyroid drugs. The surgical removal of the thyroid is called a **thyroidectomy**. Treatment of hypothyroidism is relatively simple: the thyroid hormone is taken orally as a supplement.

A thyrotoxic crisis or thyroid storm is the extreme clinical development of hyperthyroidism. It produces a greatly accelerated metabolism, severe nervous system malfunction, overheating, and heart failure. The situation is precipitated by stress in an hyperthyroid person, or infection and can be fatal. Antithyroid drugs propylthiouracil or tapazole are used to treat the condition.

PARATHYROID GLANDS

The parathyroid glands, usually two pairs, are embedded on the posterior surface of the thyroid gland. Their number and size vary greatly, but normally they resemble grains of wheat. The parathyroids are responsible for regulating the calcium content of the blood. The hormone parathormone cooperates with vitamin D to balance the level of calcium in the blood by stimulating the bones to release stored calcium and phosphate into the circulation, as well as increasing intestinal absorption.

Hyperparathyroidism results in increased levels of calcium in the blood, which causes lethargy and the excretion of large quantities of calcium salts in the urine, leading to the formation of kidney stones. The condition leads progressively to decalcification of the bones and is usually associated with a tumor of one of the glands. Decalcified bones are prone to pathologic fracture.

Hypoparathyroidism is dramatically demonstrated by a condition known as **tetany**, an uncontrollable twitching and spasm of the muscles of the body. This results from hyperirritability of the nervous system in response to the lowered concentration of calcium in the blood. The condition is treated by the addition of calcium. Hypoparathyroidism occurs following damage to or accidental removal of the parathyroids during a thyroidectomy. Inherited hypoparathyroidism is a rare cause of the disorder.

ADRENAL GLANDS (SUPRARENAL)

The adrenal glands sit atop each kidney, hence the additional name *suprarenal*. Each gland is contained in a fibrous capsule and is composed of two parts, each of which acts separately. The outer glandular tissue is called the *cortex,* and the inner tissue is referred to as the *medulla*.

The principal hormone of the medulla is **adrenaline**, also called **epinephrine**. Another hormone, norepinephrine, has a similar action on the body. Together they are considered to be the "flight-or-fight" hormones because of their effects in emergency situations. The hormones cause an increase in the heart rate, blood pressure, and flow of blood and a decrease in intestinal activity. The adrenal medulla is considered to be nonessential to life.

The cortex of the adrenal gland, however, is essential to life. The cortex produces steroid hormones in three categories: **mineralocorticoids**, glucocorticoids, and sex steroids. The mineralocorticoids, of which **aldosterone** is the principal one, control electrolyte balances through regulating the reabsorption of sodium in the kidney tubules and the excretion of potassium. The glucocorticoids affect the metabolism of protein, fat, and glucose. They stimulate the breakdown of body proteins to amino acids, many of which can be converted to glucose in the liver, thereby increasing blood sugar levels. This process is called gluconeogenesis. They also decrease inflammation by the immune system. ACTH stimulates glucocortocoids to increase in response to stress.

The sex steroids govern certain sexual characteristics, especially those that are male oriented. These steroids are referred to as *androgens.* Excessive secretions cause the virilization and development of masculine secondary sex characteristics in the female and immature male. A mature female's voice will deepen, body hair increases, menstruation will become irregular, and infertility will result.

Androgen excess in the fetus or newborn (e.g., gene mutations causing congenital hyperplasia) may result in abnormalities, particularly of the external genitalia. Clitoral enlargement and pseudohermaphroditism (genitalia with likeness to the male) may be seen. Low-dose glucocorticoid drugs can be given to mothers with certain known genetic conditions. Adults also may benefit from the same medication as well as estrogens or spironolactone. Androgen deficient states of the adrenal usually do not need treatment if testicular function in males is normal.

PANCREAS

The pancreas is a dual-function organ. It has an exocrine function, producing pancreatic juices excreted by way of the pancreatic duct into the duodenum to become part of the digestive juices. It is also an endocrine gland. The hormone *insulin* is secreted by the B cells of the **islets of Langerhans**, often called beta cells (Figure 34–6). There are four cell types located in the pancreas. The alpha cells make up about 25% of the islet cells. Glucagon stimulates new glucose formation by the liver and aids in the breakdown of glycogen to glucose. Thus, its secretion results in a rise in glucose levels. The beta cells are 60% to 80% of the islets and contain the major hormone of the pancreas, **insulin**. Insulin is necessary for the metabolism of carbohydrates. With reduced islet function, the level of blood sugar rises to an abnormal amount, which is referred to as **hyperglycemia**. Conversely, an abnormally low level of blood sugar is known as **hypoglycemia**. When excess glucose is present in the blood, it is excreted in the urine, a finding known as **glycosuria**. Hyperglycemia and glycosuria are the two outstanding characteristics of **diabetes mellitus**.

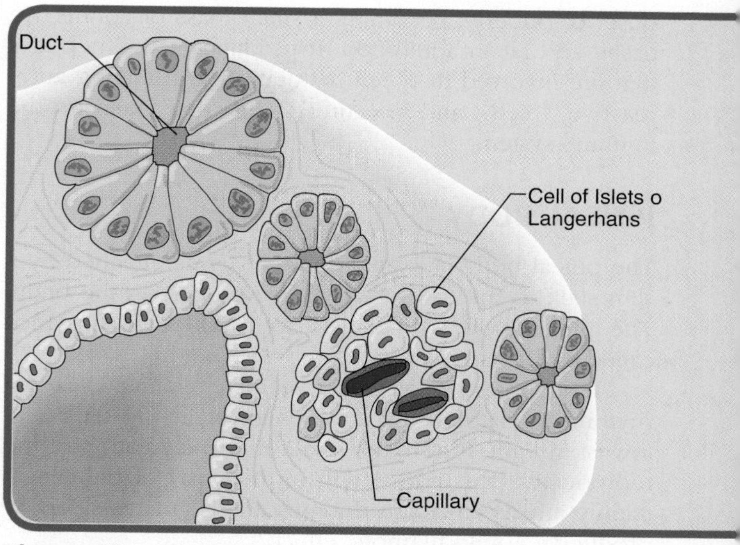

Figure 34–6: Pancreatic structure. *Delmar/Cengage Learning.*

Type 1 diabetes, also known as juvenile diabetes, is an autoimmune disease that eventually results in severe insulin deficiency. These individuals require insulin replacement to survive. Type 2 diabetics have insulin resistance and are usually overweight. Almost 90% of diabetics are type 2, and their numbers are increasing dramatically due to lifestyles that are associated with inactivity and eating excessive calories. Insulin is also required for the appropriate metabolism of fat and protein.

The other two cell types in islets are delta cells, which contain somatostatin, and pancreatic polypeptide-containing cells, which influence intestinal function.

THYMUS GLAND

The thymus gland is a two-lobed structure located under the sternum. It is composed primarily of lymphoid tissue and is enclosed in a fibrous capsule. The thymus is fairly large during childhood but begins to disappear with the onset of puberty, becoming a small mass of connective tissue and fat in adulthood. It produces active peptides that are involved in T cell maturation, eliminating autoreactive T cells, and selecting T cells that make up the immune system.

PINEAL BODY

The pineal body is a small mass of tissue attached by a slim stalk to the roof of the third ventricle in the brain. The pineal body is believed to produce a substance called melatonin.

This substance plays a role in regulating circadian rhythms. Melatonin levels are highest in the dark and lowest in light. It also has a role in the regulation of the reproductive axis and timing of the onset of puberty. It mainly affects circadian rhythms and regulates sleep by producing a mild hypnotic effect.

GONADS (TESTES AND OVARIES)

The ovaries in the female and the testes in the male are called the **gonads**, or sex glands. The ovaries are located in the pelvic cavity, one on each side of the uterus. The testes are located outside the body of the male, suspended in the scrotum. Both gonads secrete hormones that control the development of secondary sex characteristics.

In the female, the ovaries secrete **estrogen**, which reacts on the lining of the uterus, promotes growth and development of the primary and secondary sex organs, and maintains them throughout adult life. Estrogen also affects the release of other hormones from the pituitary. Another hormone, **progesterone**, is also secreted by the ovaries. It affects the uterine lining and the development of the secretory portion of the breasts. It aids in maintaining pregnancy.

In the male, the testes produce a hormone known as **testosterone**. This hormone develops the primary male sexual characteristics and the secondary characteristics of a deep voice, muscular development, and body hair distribution. It facilitates maturation of sperm cells.

The gonads are the organs of fertility and reproduction in both sexes. The maturity of the organs and the proper balance of hormonal secretions create the desire for and ability to engage in sexual activity.

Hypogonadism in males and females may be treated with replacement hormones. Estrogen and progesterone drugs can produce the appropriate sexual characteristics in the female and also alleviate certain symptoms in mature women, for example "hot flashes." Testosterone products such as injections or skin-absorbed testosterone in a patch or cream (Androgel) replaces the hormone in males.

See Table 34–1 for a summary of the glands and their functions.

TABLE 34–1 Endocrine Glands

Gland	Location	Hormone	Principal Effects
Pituitary Anterior lobe	Undersurface of the brain in the sella turcica of the skull	Growth hormone (GH)	Normal growth of body tissues
		Thyroid-stimulating hormone (TSH) (Thyrotropin)	Stimulates growth and activity of thyroid cells to produce and secrete thyroid hormone
		Adrenocorticotropic hormone (ACTH)	Stimulates the cortex of the adrenal gland and the secretion of cortisol
		Melanocyte-stimulating hormone (MSH)	Increases skin pigmentation
		Follicle-stimulating hormone (FSH)	Stimulates the maturity of the graafian follicle to rupture and to produce estrogen in the female. In the male, it stimulates the development of the testes and the production of sperm.
		Luteinizing hormone (LH)	Causes the development of the corpus luteum, which then secretes progesterone in the female. In the male, it stimulates the interstitial cells of the testes to produce testosterone.
		Prolactin (PR)	Develops breast tissue and stimulates secretion of milk from mammary glands

TABLE 34–1 *(Continued)*

Gland	Location	Hormone	Principal Effects
Posterior lobe		Oxytocin	Stimulates contraction of uterus, especially during childbirth; causes ejection of milk from mammary glands
		Vasopressin or antidiuretic hormone (ADH)	Acts on cells of kidney tubules to concentrate urine and conserve fluid in the body; also acts to constrict blood vessels
Thyroid	Lower portion of the anterior neck	Thyroxine (T_4) and triiodothyronine (T_3)	Increase metabolism; influence both physical and mental activity; promote normal growth and development
		Thyrocalcitonin	Causes calcium to be stored in bones; reduces blood level of calcium
Parathyroid	Posterior surface of thyroid gland	Parathormone	Regulates exchange of calcium between the bones and blood and increases blood calcium
Adrenal Medulla Cortex	Superior surface of each kidney	Adrenaline (epinephrine)	Increases heart rate, blood pressure, and flow of blood; decreases intestinal activity
		Aldosterone (mineral corticoid)	Controls electrolyte balances by regulating the reabsorption of sodium and the excretion of potassium
		Glucocorticoids	Affect the metabolism of protein, fat, and glucose, thereby increasing blood sugar; also decrease inflammation
		Sex hormones (androgens)	Govern sex characteristics, especially those that are masculine
Pancreas	Behind the stomach	Insulin	Essential to the metabolism of carbohydrates; reduces the blood sugar level
		Glucagon	Stimulates the liver to release glycogen and convert it to glucose to increase blood sugar levels
Thymus	Under the sternum	Several peptides	React upon lymphoid tissue to produce T lymphocyte cells to regulate immunity
Pineal Body	Third ventricle in the brain	Melatonin	Influences onset of puberty and circadian rhythms
Ovaries	Female pelvis	Estrogen	Promotes growth of primary and secondary sexual characteristics
		Progesterone	Develops excretory portion of mammary glands; aids in maintaining pregnancy
Testes	Male scrotum	Testosterone	Develops primary and secondary sexual characteristics; stimulates maturation of sperm

INTERRELATIONSHIP OF THE GLANDS

As stated previously, hormonal secretion is regulated by a feedback mechanism. When the hormone is present or the substance produced by the effect of that hormone on another gland or organ is present, further secretion is affected. For example, the parathyroids increase secretion of parathormone to raise the serum calcium level, taking calcium primarily from the bones. When the serum level rises, a negative feedback message is signaled, and the secretion of parathormone is decreased. A more complicated feedback was described earlier in the control of TSH and the interaction of the hypothalamus, pituitary, and thyroid glands.

In the next unit, the interrelationship of the pituitary and the ovary will be discussed to explain how this complex balance prepares the female for pregnancy.

DIAGNOSTIC EXAMINATIONS

Many diagnostic tests can be performed on blood and urine that either measure the amount of specific hormones present in the body or measure the effectiveness of their function. A few of the more common tests are:

- *Blood sugar*, frequently measured after fasting (fasting blood sugar, FBS)—To assess the function of the pancreas, including insulin effects
- *T_3, TSH, and T_4*—To measure the level of the thyroid hormones
- *Urine human chorionic gonadotropin (HCG)* (pregnancy test)—To measure the presence of a hormone secreted by the placental cells
- *Glucose tolerance*—To measure the body's ability to process a large dose of glucose. Multiple blood samples are taken at specific intervals following ingestion of the glucose mixture.
- ***Glucohemoglobin*** *or Hemoglobin A1c* (Hgb A1c)—A simple blood test that measures how well the glucose level has been controlled over the previous four to six weeks. The glucose attaches to the hemoglobin of the red blood cells (RBC). A1c is the stable molecule formed when sugar and hemoglobin bind together in the RBC in a process called glycosylation. A1c can be measured. An elevated finding indicates poor glucose control. Measuring A1c reveals a truer picture of blood sugar level control than conventional glucose measurement. If the diabetic patient has not been conforming to diet, except in anticipation of an office visit, the cells will reveal that they have picked up excess sugar. Recently, a Hgb A1c of 6.5% or more is a criterion for diagnosis of diabetes.

There are also specific tests measuring hormone levels in the blood to aid in confirming diagnoses, such as:

- *ACTH, FSH, growth hormone LH, and TSH*—When acromegaly or dwarfism is suspected
- *FSH, LH, estrogen, and testosterone*—When sex organs fail to develop properly
- *ACTH, cortisol*—When Cushing's syndrome (chronic excessive glucocorticoids) is suspected
- *PTH*—When hypoparathyroidism or hyperparathyroidism is suspected
- *Prolactin*—When a common tumor of the pituitary gland is present.

Scanning Tests

The thyroid gland is probably the one most frequently scanned.

- *Radioactive iodine uptake test*—An oral dose of radioactive iodine is given to the patient. After intervals of 6 and 24 hours, an external detector (scintillation counter) measures the amount of the original dose that is present in the gland. Thyroid function can be determined by the gland's ability to absorb and retain iodine.
- *Thyroid scan*—The thyroid gland is viewed by a scintiscanner camera following either an oral or IV dose of a radioactive iodine. The scan is indicated by discovery of a palpable nodule or mass, enlarged thyroid gland, or asymmetrical goiter. The camera is capable of photographing the isotopes, which identify the size of the gland, position, and uniformity of absorption. A nodule with poor or no uptake capability shows as a "cold spot," suggesting a possible malignancy. A "hot spot" indicates a hyperfunctioning nodule, possibly a toxic nodular goiter. A total gland picture that shows little uptake is indicative of hypothyroidism; an enlarged gland showing uniformly increased uptake is indicative of hyperthyroidism.
- *Ultrasound*—Valuable in assessing thyroid size and nodules.

DISEASES AND DISORDERS

Acromegaly (Akro-meg′-a-le)

Description—This is an uncommon hormonal disorder that occurs when the pituitary gland produces excess growth hormone during adulthood, resulting in the characteristic changes of overgrowth of connective tissue. The occurrence of acromegaly is about 6 in every 100,000 adults.

Signs and symptoms—The symptoms develop gradually. There is enlargement of the hands, feet, and prominent facial features such as protruding lower jaw and brow, enlarged nose, thickened lips, and teeth that tend to separate. Patients may also complain of headaches and loss of peripheral vision due to an enlarging pituitary tumor.

Etiology—This condition results from the excessive production of growth hormone and is almost always due to a pituitary tumor. An MRI or CT scan can determine the location and size of the tumor.

Treatment—A surgical procedure known as transsphenoidal resection is the treatment of choice. The surgeon goes through the nose and sphenoid sinus to extract the tumor through a scope, unless the tumor is too large. Medications such as Sandostatin and bromocriptine can be used occasionally to decrease the growth hormone secretion. Radiation may also be necessary to destroy any remaining tumor cells.

The man in Figure 34–7 was diagnosed in 1970 when he was in his twenties. His original complaints were a

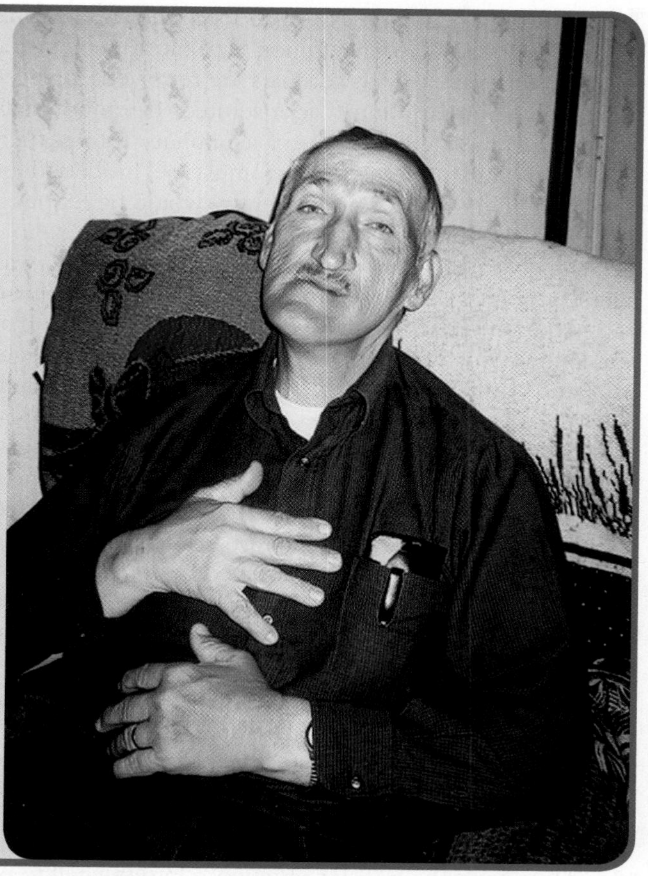

Figure 34–7: Male with acromegaly. *Courtesy of Barbara A. Wise.*

change in his facial appearance, enlarging hands, no energy, headaches, and vision sensitivity to sun or snow. He later developed color blindness. He also noticed his skin became oily, and he perspired excessively. A pituitary tumor was discovered and later resected, but a small portion was apparently missed. He had continuing elevated hormone levels and after three years received radiation therapy. After surgery and radiation, he noticed a significant change in the size of his hands, reducing by four ring sizes. He has recently developed severe arthritis in his back, hands, and lower extremities, but he attempts to walk two to three miles a day despite the discomfort and fatigue. He takes prednisone and synthroid medication daily. The main characteristics of acromegaly are evident in the photo.

Addison's Disease

Description—This condition results from a deficiency of adrenal hormones from the cortex of the adrenal gland. This causes significant metabolic changes that can result in serious illness and even death.

Signs and symptoms—Patients gradually develop a pigmented appearance of the skin due to excessive ACTH and melanocyte-stimulating hormone secretion from the pituitary due to low adrenal hormone concentrations in the blood. Weakness, low blood pressure, tiredness, and salt craving are prominent symptoms. The lack of cortisol (a glucocortocoid) and aldosterone (a mineralocorticoid) impairs normal metabolism of proteins and carbohydrates. Electrolyte disturbances, namely a low serum sodium level and high serum potassium, also occur.

Etiology—The most common cause of adrenal insufficiency is autoimmune destruction of the cells producing the hormones. Other causes include infections such as tuberculosis, histoplasmosis, and meningococcemia; hemorrhage into the adrenal glands; and metastasis of malignant tumors.

Treatment—Hormone replacement therapy with hydrocortisone or prednisone and the mineralocorticoid fludrocortisone results in a positive outcome. Lifetime treatment is needed, and larger doses are given in stressful situations such as infections or surgery.

Cretinism (Kre′-tin-izm)

Description—This is an endocrine disorder of the thyroid gland that has physical and mental ramifications.

Signs and symptoms—**Cretinism** is characterized by lack of mental and physical growth, resulting in mental retardation and a characteristic dwarflike appearance.

The male in Figure 34–8 has cretinism. He was not diagnosed in time to prevent the features of a large, short tongue and coarse facial characteristics. Note his small sloping shoulders and low-set ears.

Etiology—This condition results from a serious lack of the thyroid hormone thyroxine beginning in the early stages of life.

Treatment—If thyroid replacement is initiated early enough, normal development may be achieved, but once cretinism has developed, total normal development is not possible. An infant born without thyroid hormones of its own must be treated within a few weeks to prevent irreversible mental retardation.

Cushing's Syndrome (Koosh′-ings)

Description—This is an endocrine disorder of the adrenal glands that has physical and physiologic effects.

Signs and symptoms—Symptoms include hypertension, obesity, weakness of the muscles, and a tendency to develop bruises. Typical characteristics result from the rapid deposit of body fat: a deposit of fat between the shoulders, referred to as "buffalo hump," and a rounded

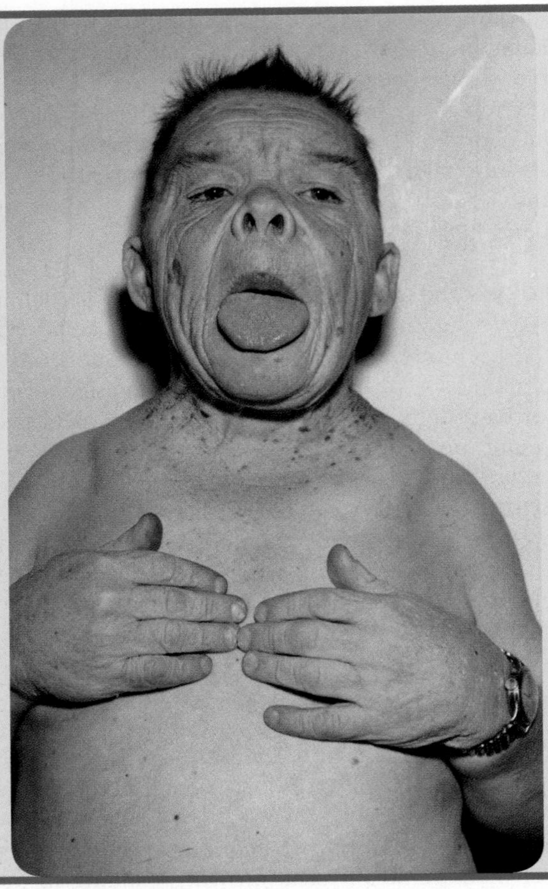

Figure 34–8: Adult male with Cretinism. *Courtesy of Manuel Tzagournis, MD, Endocrinologist; Professor Emeritus, The Ohio State University.*

face referred to as "moon face." Purple streaks called striae (stretch marks) develop in the skin. The trunk becomes obese, yet the arms and legs are slender.

The excess amount of glucocorticoids, increase the breakdown of body proteins to amino acids, many of them being able to be converted to glucose. The process is called gluconeogenesis. The excessive amount however, leads to hyperglycemia, which worsens control of diabetes or produces new "steroid diabetes." The kidney is affected by the hormone imbalance and excretes excessive amounts of potassium, which results in hypokalemia. The lack of potassium results in muscular weakness. Muscle mass slowly wastes away. The decreasing amount of bone structure results in pathologic fractures.

Etiology—This disorder is characterized by a group of symptoms that result from the hypersecretion of glucocorticoids from the adrenal cortex caused by excess ACTH production. **Cushing's syndrome** may also be directly related to a tumor of the cortex of the adrenal gland or long-term steroid treatment for a variety of diseases.

Treatment—Treatment is related to the underlying cause. If there is an adrenal tumor, then the adrenal gland must be removed. If both adrenals are removed, replacement steroid therapy must be instituted. If the adrenals are being stimulated because of a pituitary tumor, then the pituitary gland or adenoma must be irradiated or removed. Afterward hormone therapy would be required to replace the pituitary's secretions.

The woman in Figures 34–9A and 34-9B was diagnosed with Cushing's disease in 2003. She is a nurse and experienced difficulty convincing physicians that "something was wrong with her." Her 45-pound weight gain and "buffalo hump" were dismissed as too much food and not enough exercise. She also had a blood pressure of 176/100, acne, excessive perspiration, weakness, and was growing facial hair. At her insistence, diagnostic and radiologic tests were performed; they indicated excess ACTH and the presence of a microadenoma of the pituitary. The tumor was removed by transphenoidal resection and proved to be benign. As you can see, 18 months after surgery, her appearance had returned to normal, and her other symptoms had subsided.

Diabetes Mellitus (Dia-be′-tez Mell′-i-tus)

Description—A chronic disease of insulin deficiency or resistance, diabetes mellitus interferes with the metabolism of carbohydrates, proteins, and fats. Insulin in the blood facilitates the transfer of glucose into the cell to be used for energy or stored as glycogen. It also stimulates the formation of proteins and free fatty acid storage. Without sufficient insulin being secreted by the pancreas, the body's tissues do not have access to essential nutrients for fuel or storage.

Diabetes mellitus affects an estimated 8% of the United States population or over 25 million people. The prevalence of diabetes has increased greatly in the past decade, and more children and teenagers are being diagnosed with both Type 1 (insulin requiring) and Type 2 diabetes. The reasons are multifactorial, but increasing numbers of obese individuals and inactivity are common risk factors. There are many long-term effects of diabetes. Diabetes is a leading cause of new cases of blindness, end-stage kidney disease, neuropathy, and lower limb amputation in the United States. It develops more often in people who are older than 40 and have a family history of diabetes, or are of African American, Hispanic, or Native American descent. It more than doubles the risk for stroke and heart disease. The disease also interferes with resistance to organisms, which may result in skin and bladder infections. Diabetic retinopathy results from microvascular changes in the retina of the eye, especially in poorly controlled diabetics. In patients who have had diabetes for 20 or more years, 80% develop retinopathy.

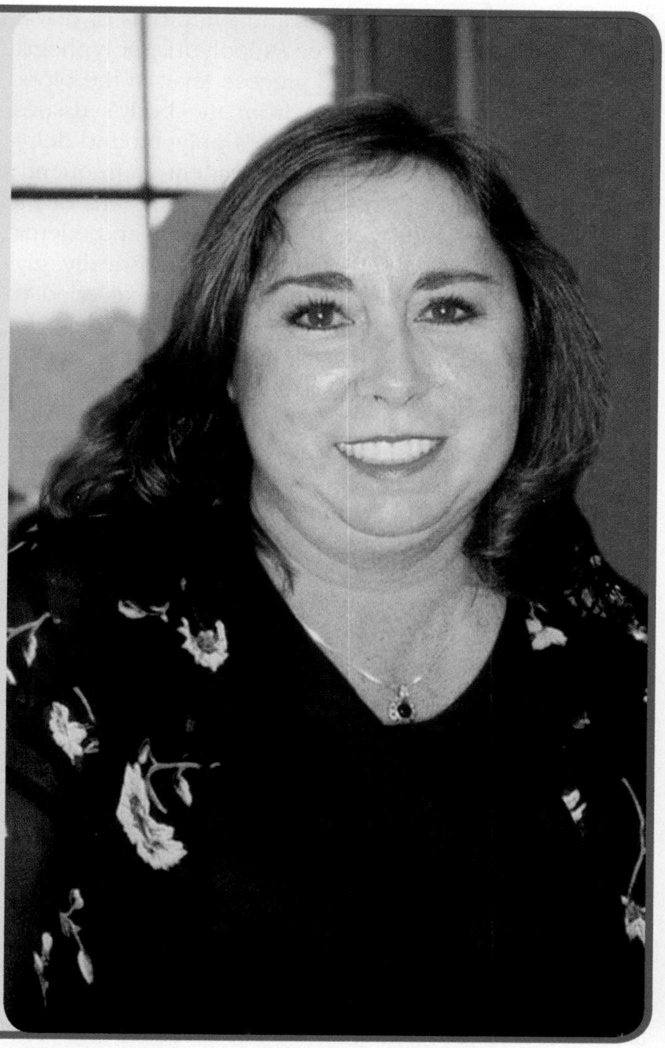

Figure 34–9A: Female with Cushing's disease. *Courtesy of Barbara A. Wise.*

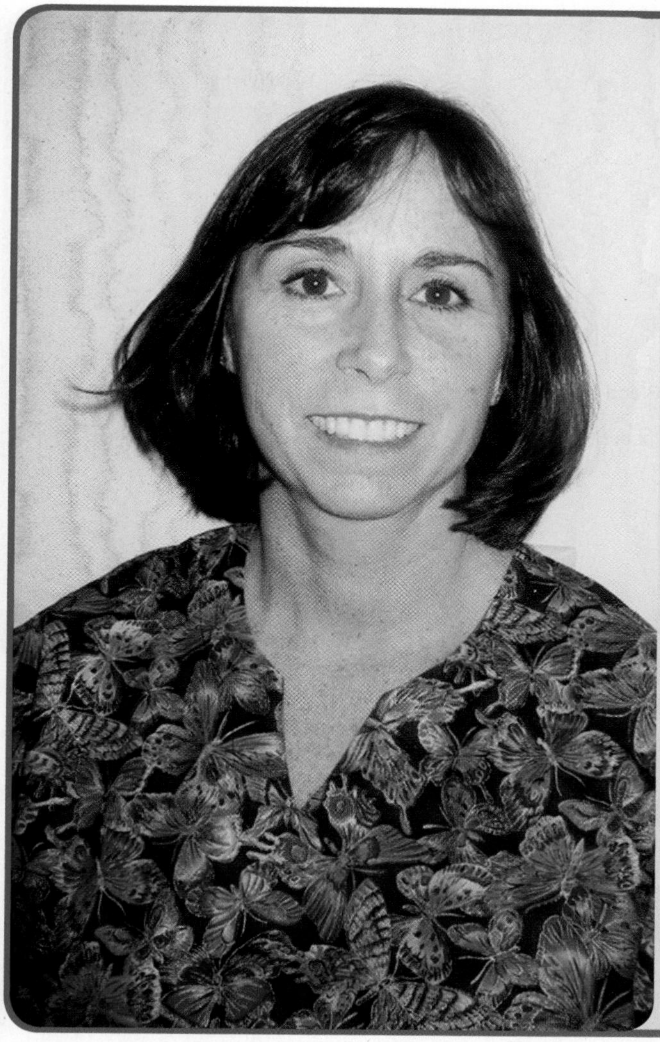

Figure 34–9B: Female with Cushing's disease, after surgery. *Courtesy of Barbara A. Wise.*

How Insulin Works

Insulin is the hormone made in the pancreas and released into the bloodstream as glucose rises. It helps sugar to enter the body's cells, where it is used as fuel for the cell's activities (Figure 34–10). When the sugar level rises, the pancreas secretes more insulin so that the larger amount of sugar can move out of the blood and into the cells. When the sugar level falls too low, insulin secretion is greatly reduced and the hormone glucagon is released. This causes the liver to release stored glycogen into the blood.

To completely understand the role of insulin, we need to consider a basic fact of life. All living organisms are programmed to withstand cycles of feast and famine and have developed ways of storing energy for lean times. In humans and most animals, it is insulin that allows us to store glucose, protein, and fat in the liver, fat, and muscle cells until it is needed. Our bodies are programmed to store glucose and fat that produce excess weight and obesity when excessive calories are consumed, which leads to diabetes and numerous other illnesses. In the United States, obesity is at alarming incidence rates not only for adults but also for children. There is much concern about the future health of our population.

There are two forms of diabetes: Type 1 DM, or insulin-dependent diabetes mellitus, and Type 2 DM, noninsulin-dependent diabetes mellitus, often called adult-onset form. Type 1 DM tends to afflict children and young people, and insulin replacement is necessary for survival. Refer to the boxed information Diabetes Mellitus (Type 1 DM) that summarizes the etiology, signs and symptoms, and treatment as they relate to children.

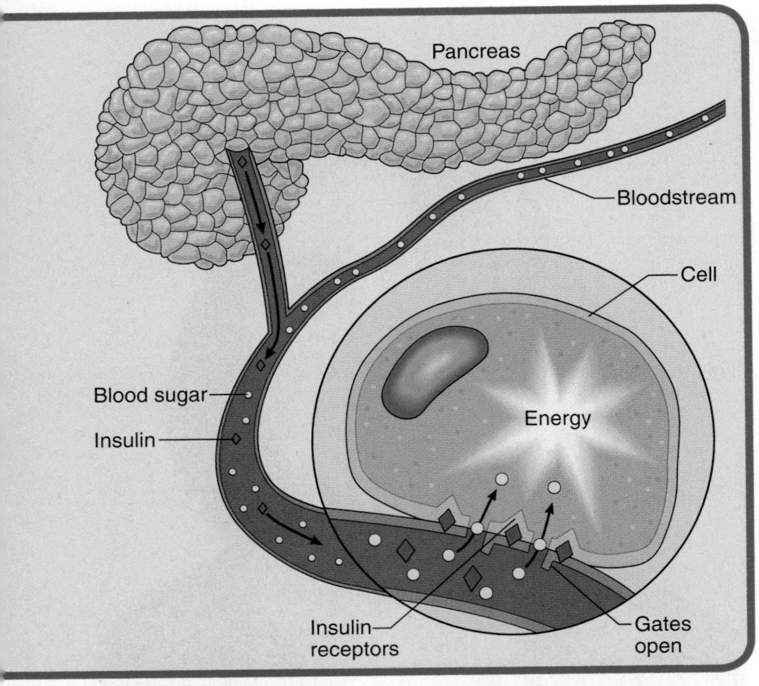

Figure 34–10: How insulin works. Insulin is excreted by the pancreas into the blood. It circulates to an insulin receptor on the membrane of a cell. When it binds to the receptor, a signal is sent, and the gates in the cell wall open, allowing blood sugar to enter the cell to be converted to energy. *Delmar/Cengage Learning.*

Diabetes Mellitus (Type 1 DM)

Etiology—Type 1 diabetes can be considered a genetic disease. It is an autoimmune disorder that attacks the cells of the pancreas known as the islets of Langerhans.

Signs and symptoms—The diagnosis of diabetes in childhood is usually straightforward. The parents report an increased thirst, increased urination, and weight loss. The child will appear to be dehydrated and may have a sweet odor to the breath from the ketones (a by-product of fatty acids). A urinalysis will generally reveal a large amount of ketones and is positive for glucose.

Treatment—A child with newly diagnosed Type 1 DM will be admitted to the hospital for stabilization and treatment. Insulin injections or intravenous insulin are required for initial management. During hospitalization, the parents, caregivers, and the child (if of appropriate age) are taught to administer the insulin injections. Commonly, several types of insulin (short-acting, intermediate, and long-acting) will be used to control the elevated blood sugar and complications with childhood diabetes.

Signs and symptoms—Signs and symptoms of diabetes include fatigue and the three *P*s; polyuria, polyphegia, and polydipsea. The elevated glucose level in the blood causes fluid to be withdrawn from the body's tissues. The excess fluid in the blood causes polyuria and dehydration of the cells. The diabetic patient is frequently thirsty and has dry mucous membranes. The lens of the eye becomes affected by the hyperglycemia and edema, which results in visual difficulties. Characteristically, glycosuria is present when the threshold is exceeded to reabsorb glucose (about 180 mg per dL); the excess glucose spills over into urine. This wasting of sugar causes the weight loss and hunger of the Type 1 DM patient.

Etiology—Type 2 DM is the most common form, usually due to insulin resistance. This is a complex problem arising from the reduced effectiveness of insulin to facilitate glucose entering the cell. The blood sugar level rises, and the liver produces more sugar and often releases lipoproteins full of triglycerides that may decrease HDL cholesterol. Insulin resistance can also result from genetics, aging, and some medications, but being overweight and lack of exercise are the main nongenetic factors. About 90% of all newly diagnosed diabetics are overweight. Some of the hormones secreted by fat cells, for example resistin, interfere with insulin action. The role of fat cells is being studied specifically because obesity is so often associated with the disease.

In addition to resistance, other factors exist. The pancreas compensates by secreting more insulin. Eventually, the insulin-producing cells can no longer keep up, and glucose increases in the blood. Over time, this high level of sugar damages blood vessels, nerves, and other body tissues. It also causes a vicious cycle of increasing resistance and further exhausts the pancreas.

Treatment—Treatment begins with a strict diet, planned to meet the nutritional needs of the individual patient and to control the blood sugar level. Diet can have a significant impact on controlling blood sugar and diabetes. Losing as little as 10 pounds will reduce blood sugar levels. A recent study determined that a high-fiber diet lowered blood sugar levels by 10%, a reduction similar to the effect of some medications. Exercise may be the most important intervention. It not only increases glucose metabolism, but it also increases insulin sensitivity, which causes fat and muscle cells to better respond to insulin. Diet and exercise can have a significant effect in preventing diabetes, but as a treatment, they can only go so far. In most people, the problem of insulin production and insulin resistance tend to worsen in time despite weight loss, diet, and exercise. When diet alone is inadequate, insulin injections or the use of oral hypoglycemic drugs are indicated. Injections may be necessary initially once a day, using a long-acting insulin; when control is more difficult, a short-acting insulin, injected before meals, may be needed. Diabetic patients are taught to evaluate their glucose level by performing a finger stick for blood analysis. The amount of insulin injected is based on the findings. Hypoglycemic drugs are taken orally to aid in the metabolism of sugar. Oral therapy is adequate only for Type 2 DM patients.

The drugs used today address insulin resistance and secretion to reduce blood sugar levels. Physicians are using more drugs and using them more aggressively. Drugs can be categorized according to their actions (see the following).

Increasing Insulin Supplies

1. *Sulfonylureas* stimulate beta cells to release more insulin. This works for a while but then may become ineffective. These drugs can work too well, causing hypoglycemia that can be dangerous for older patients because it causes fainting, falls, and fractures.
2. *Rapid-acting insulin stimulators* are similar to sulfonylureas but faster. They are of short duration and are less apt to cause hypoglycemia. Two drugs in this class are Prandin and Starlix.
3. *Antidiabetic drugs,* relatively recently approved are available. The dipeptidyl peptidase-4 inhibitors, Onglyza (saxagliptin) and Januvia (sitagliptin), increase the presence of gut hormones, which are advantageous for insulin secretion and decrease glucagon levels. In 2008, colesevelam was approved as a glucose, lowering agent. It is an old drug used for a number of years to lower cholesterol.
4. *Injection of insulin* subcutaneously is the ultimate method of overriding pancreatic dysfunction. Type 1 diabetics who lack insulin are dependent on injections. Patients with Type 2 diabetes often can control their disease with diet, exercise, and medications, but if that fails, insulin is the most potent and effective therapy. They usually require higher doses because of the need to overcome resistance. A form of insulin that can be inhaled is being developed. Initial trials have yielded promising results.

Lowering Blood Sugar by Other Means

1. *Alpha-glucosidase inhibitors* block the action of a digestive enzyme that breaks down carbohydrates into smaller sugars. The effect is to moderate blood sugar surges after a meal. These drugs are weaker than some others but very safe.
2. *Biguanides* work to lower sugar levels by blocking the release of glucose by the liver. The only drug currently approved is Glucophage, and it works well in overweight people because it does not cause weight gain or risk of hypoglycemia.
3. *Thiazolidinediones* (TZD) reduces insulin resistance by modulating activity of nuclear transcription factors. They show promise in improving the lipid profiles and other metabolic factors.

Multi-Drug Approach

More physicians are using a multi-drug approach to management. Previously, they would do one thing at a time: diet and exercise, then drug after drug until ineffective, and then insulin. By using drug combinations, lower doses of each are effective, and therefore fewer side effects occur. This approach better addresses the new view of diabetes as a syndrome instead of a simple disease of high blood sugar.

A common drug combination is metformin and sulfonylurea. Clinical trial with metformin-TZD combination showed improved effectiveness in control of blood sugar, insulin sensitivity, and islet cell function. When insulin becomes necessary, combining it with oral medications may mean a lower dose of insulin is needed.

Future Treatments

It is hoped that the human genome project will reveal new information on diabetes and its treatment, but researchers realize this will take some time to determine. Some researchers are focusing on preventing the complications associated with diabetes, such as atherosclerosis; others focus on therapies directed at fat cells. Pancreatic and islet transplantations show encouraging promise.

A study also revealed that the simple action of taking an aspirin a day is a very effective health strategy for diabetics and would help those with cardiovascular disease. Controlling blood pressure and lowering LDL are crucial even if there is no evidence of coronary disease.

Maintaining Health

The glucose level of the blood can be affected by circumstances other than food or insulin. For example, the diabetic requires either less insulin or more food when engaging in a high level of physical activity. Adjustments are also required with illness. A patient who has diarrhea or vomiting may require less insulin. Pregnancy, the use of contraceptives, a fever, and periods of stress all influence the diabetic's need for supplemental insulin or oral hypoglycemic therapy.

Specific symptoms indicate whether the blood sugar is too high or too low. A diabetic must be aware of her physical condition at all times. Should the blood sugar level become significantly low, she may enter into insulin shock; if it goes very high, there is a possibility of a diabetic coma. Both situations require urgent attention. When patients sense impending shock, they will drink orange juice or eat a piece of candy immediately. A patient going into coma needs an urgent blood sugar measurement and injections of insulin. Figure 34–11 illustrates the contrasting symptoms of

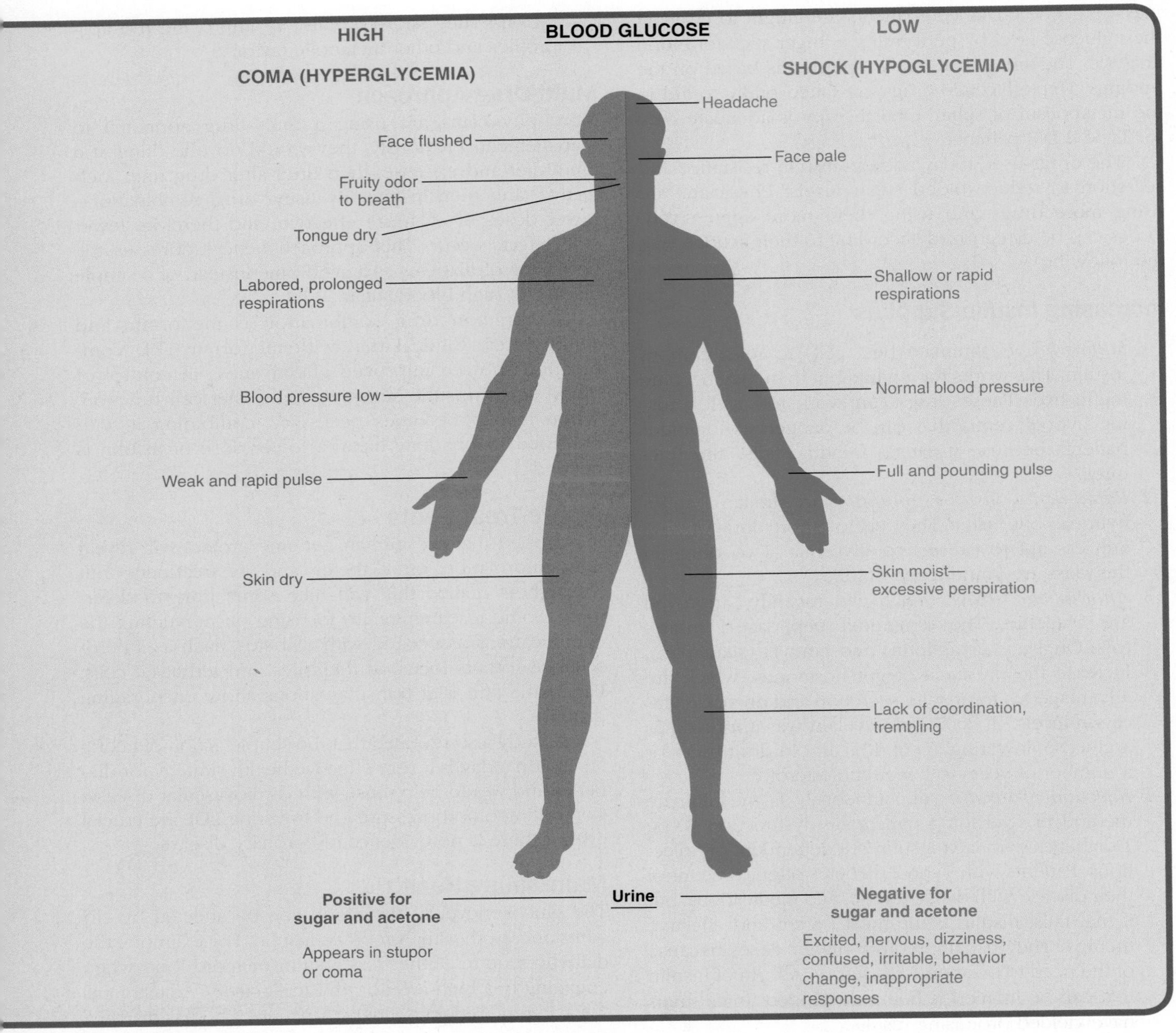

Figure 34–11: Diabetic coma (hyperglycemia) versus insulin shock (hypoglycemia). *Delmar/Cengage Learning.*

shock and coma. Become familiar with the signs and be prepared to act.

Diabetic patients must be encouraged to maintain their optimal level of health. They must guard against injury, especially to the lower extremities, because of difficulty healing. They must use extreme caution when cutting toenails and must not try to remove corns or calluses themselves. Diabetics frequently suffer amputations as a result of infection from an injury that would not heal or from the loss of peripheral circulation, which causes tissue ischemia.

Patients should be encouraged to visit an ophthalmologist at least yearly to detect the possibility of retinal changes. The physician must be alert to signs of cardiovascular complications and urinary tract involvement. Cerebral vascular disease, coronary artery disease, and renal failure resulting from vascular deterioration in the kidney are common.

Graves' Disease

Description—This condition is the most common form of hyperthyroidism.

Signs and symptoms—The thyroid gland enlarges and the patient becomes nervous; has an intolerance to heat; loses weight; sweats; and may have diarrhea, tremors, and palpitations. The increased thyroxine may also cause difficulty in concentrating because of the accelerated cerebral functioning. Mood swings and emotional instability may occur. The cardiovascular system is also affected in the form of tachycardia, increased cardiac output, cardiomegaly, and possibly atrial fibrillation (especially in the elderly). The patient may experience dyspnea and an array of musculoskeletal symptoms ranging from weakness and fatigue to localized or generalized paralysis. The dominant feature of exophthalmos may also be present. The woman in Figure 34–12A was diagnosed with Graves' disease in her early 20s. She experienced weak pelvic muscles, dissociation of thoughts, rapid heart rate, and an intolerance to heat. She also had the traditional exopthalmos and an enlarged thyroid gland. (Enlargement is noticeable in the photo). She was treated with propylthiouracil for one year, and the thyroid gland was later ablated with radioactive iodine. After about six years, she had bilateral orbital decompression to allow fluid to drain from behind the eyes, which permitted them to recess into the bony sockets (Figure 34–12B).

The patient may become seriously ill if the hyperthyroidism escalates into a thyroid storm. The symptoms persist and others develop, such as hypertension, extreme irritability, vomiting, high fever, delirium, and eventually coma.

Etiology—Graves' disease results from an increase in the production of thyroxine that may be caused by a genetic susceptibility to autoimmune factors. The production of autoantibodies arise from a defect in suppressor T lymphocyte function that allows other T cells to make autoantibodies.

Treatment—A common treatment is the use of antithyroid drugs that block the formation of thyroid hormone. Some patients are candidates for an oral dose of radioactive iodine that concentrates in the thyroid, destroying some cells and reducing the size of the thyroid gland. In addition, a portion or all of the gland can be removed surgically to reduce or eliminate the hormone.

In addition to propylthiouracil, methimazole is used to block the release and synthesis of thyroid hormone.

Myxedema (Miks-e-de′-ma) (Hypothyroidism)

Description—This endocrine disorder of the thyroid gland is associated with too little thyroid hormone.

Signs and symptoms—Clinically, **myxedema's** characteristics are in relation to the degree of hypothyroidism.

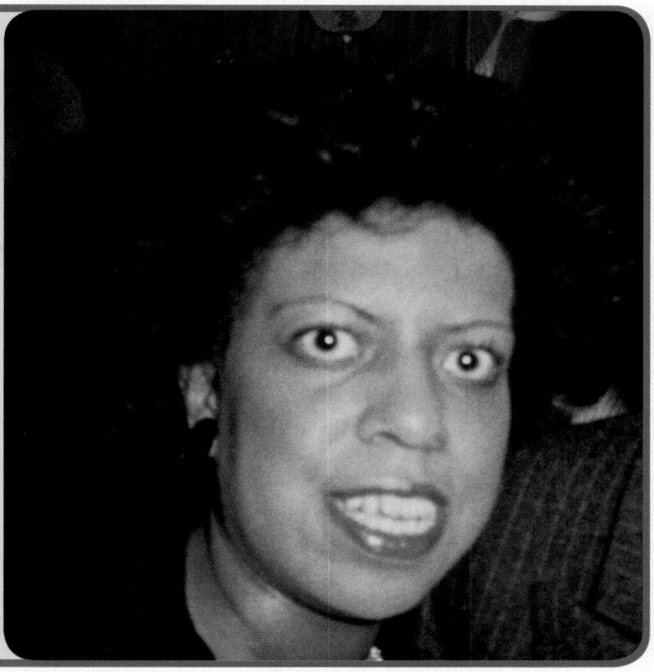

Figure 34–12A: Female with Graves' disease. *Courtesy of Barbara A. Wise.*

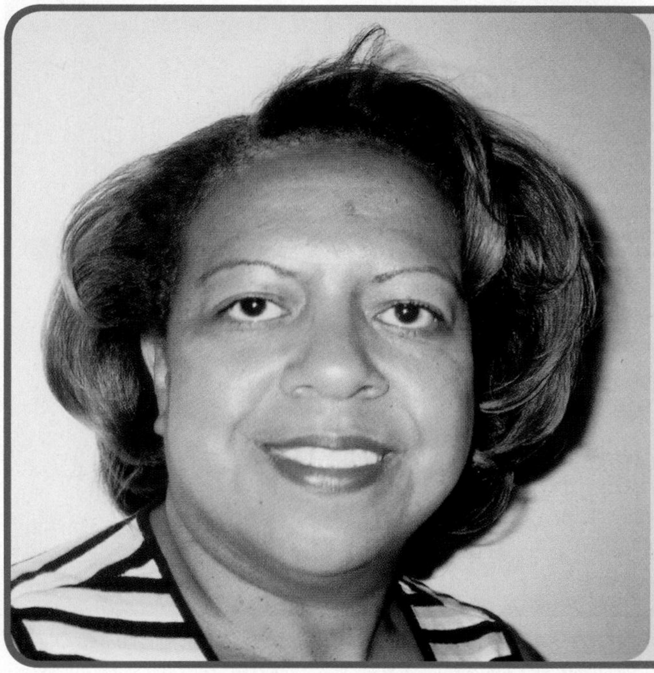

Figure 34–12B: Female with Graves' disease, after treatment and surgery. *Courtesy of Barbara A. Wise.*

If it is mild, the patient will probably complain of forgetfulness, dry skin, and an intolerance for cold. With more severe myxedema, the decreased metabolism causes a marked intolerance for cold and weight gain. Motor function and reflex actions are slowed. The voice becomes low and husky. A characteristic yellowish discoloration of the skin, called *carotenemia,* results from reduction in the conversion of carotene to vitamin A. Levels of cholesterol are increased and may also produce atherosclerosis. Because cardiac function is depressed, the myocardium becomes enlarged and weak. Protein and certain electrolytes accumulate in the tissue spaces, causing edema. Myxedema patients have a characteristic drowsy appearance, with puffiness about the eyes. There is a marked degree of fatigue and weakness. The temperature, pulse, respiration, and blood pressure are all below normal. Figure 34–13 shows a female with mild hair loss, puffy and drooping eyelids, and the puffy face characteristics of myxedema.

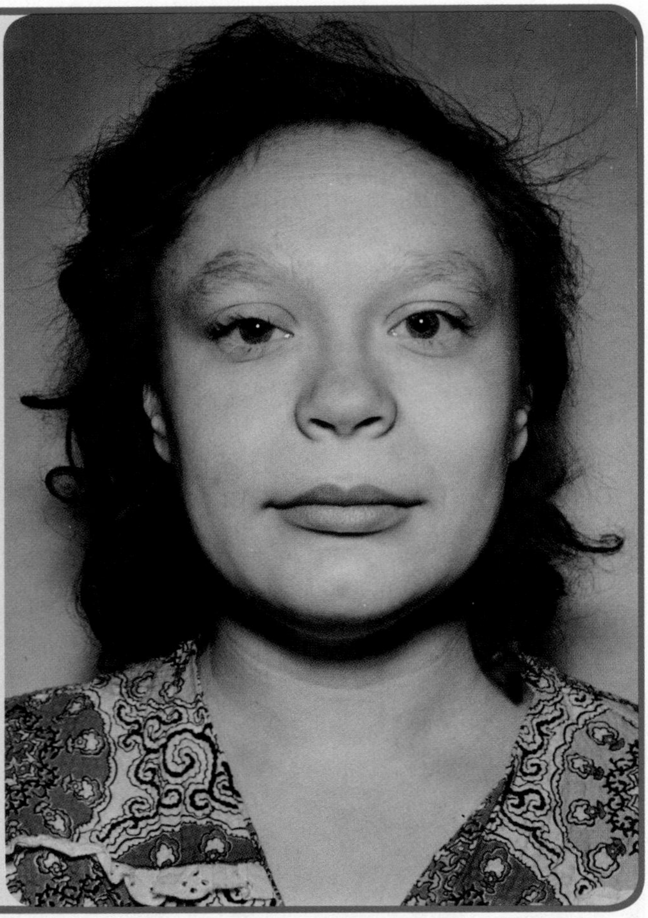

Figure 34–13: Female with myxedema. *Courtesy of Manuel Tzagournis, MD, Endocrinologist; Professor Emeritus, The Ohio State University.*

Etiology—This condition is caused by a hyposecretion of the thyroid gland. It varies in significance in relation to the amount of secretion. Hashimoto's thyroiditis is a common cause of goiter and hypothyroidism.

Treatment—Treatment consists primarily of thyroid hormone replacement to a level necessary to maintain normal balance. Levothyroxine sodium (Synthroid) or Liothyronine sodium (Cytomel) are examples of replacement drugs.

Hormonal Balance

Diagnosing, treating, and maintaining hormonal balance in patients with endocrine gland malfunctions is a challenging endeavor because of the hormone interactions. For example, what may appear to be a simple overproduction by the thyroid may actually be a pituitary malfunction, a failed hypothalamus, or an inhibitor that did not cause the pituitary to stop secreting a thyroid stimulant. Many possibilities must be considered to explain the symptoms presented by a patient with endocrine dysfunction.

AGE-RELATED BODY CHARACTERISTICS

Type 1 DM and Type 2 DM have similar characteristics of increased thirst, urination, and weight loss. As the disease progresses, long-term effects become evident. The vision may become affected due to changes in the lens; blindness may occur from retinopathy, neuropathy, end-stage kidney disease, and often infection that does not respond to treatment and leads to amputation. There is an increased risk of stroke and heart disease. This disease requires a life-long commitment to dietary guidelines and monitoring of glucose levels in addition to healthful practices to maintain an optimal level of health.

System Interaction Associated with Disease Conditions

The endocrine system is especially interconnected due to the interaction of the hormones excreted by the nine organs. The hormones circulate throughout the body and have effects on many body organs and structures. Table 34–2 summarizes the systems involved in two examples of endocrine disorders.

TABLE 34–2 System Interaction Associated with Disease Conditions

DISEASE	SYSTEMS INVOLVED	PATHOLOGY PRESENT
Diabetes	Endocrine	Insulin deficiency, destruction of insulin-producing cells of the pancreas
	Urinary	Glycosuria, polyuria, UTI, kidney disease
	Circulatory	Heart disease, stroke, elevated triglycerides
	Senses	Retinopathy, lens changes
	Integumentary	Skin infection, ulcers
	Nervous	Peripheral neuropathy
Graves' disease	Endocrine	Thyroid enlargement
	Circulatory	Palpitations, tachycardia, cardiomegaly
	Muscular	Weak muscles, fatigue, paralysis
	Nervous	Nervousness, tremors, mood swings, difficulty in concentration
	Senses	Exopthalmos

CHAPTER SUMMARY

- The endocrine system consists of nine glands that are either exocrine or endocrine in their function.
- The glands are pineal, thyroid, pituitary, thymus, parathyroids, adrenal, pancreas, testis, and ovaries.
- Pituitary gland is the master gland of the body. The gland has two lobes that produce nine hormones.
- The thyroid gland has two lobes and produces three hormones. Hyperthyroidism or hypothyroidism refer to increased or decreased thyroid activity. An enlarged thyroid gland is called a goiter.
- Exopthalmos is a symptom of hyperthyroidism.
- A thyroid storm or a thyrotoxic crisis is an extreme development of hyperthyroidism.
- Parathyroid glands are embedded on the surface of the thyroid and secrete parathormone.
- Adrenal glands sit atop each kidney. The glands have a cortex and medulla portion and secrete five hormones. The sex steroids, androgens, govern sexual characteristics.
- The pancreas is a dual-function organ with both exocrine and endocrine functions. The islets of Langerhans secrete the hormone insulin necessary for the metabolism of carbohydrates.
- The thymus gland is present during childhood but begins to disappear with puberty.
- The pineal body is attached by a slim stalk to the roof of the third ventricle in the brain and is believed to produce melatonin.
- The gonads are the testes in the male and the ovaries in the female. The testes produce testosterone and the ovaries produce estrogen and progesterone.
- Diagnostic examinations include blood sugar, T_3, TSH, and T_4, human chorionic gonadotropin, glucose tolerance, hemoglobin A1c. Hormone levels in the blood can also be measured such as ACTH, FSH, LH, TSH, FSH, LH, ACTH, and PTH.
- Various scanning tests can be performed to measure function as well as ultrasound to assess size and nodules.
- Diseases of the system include: acromegaly, Addison's disease, cretinism, Cushing's syndrome, Diabetes mellitus (Type 1 and 2), Graves' disease, and Myxedema.
- Blood sugar can be lowered with insulin, sulfonylureas, and other means.
- Diabetes causes changes in the body as the disease progresses.
- Many body systems interact with diabetes and Graves' disease.

STUDY TOOLS

Workbook	Activities for Chapter 34
Premium Website	
MEDIA LINK	View this **Media Link** for Chapter 34: • The Endocrine system
StudyWARE	Activities and Quizzes on the **StudyWARE™ Software** for Chapter 34
	Audio Library of medical terms
	Online access to the **Critical Thinking Challenge 2.0**
CourseMate	Activities and Quizzes for Chapter 34
WebTutor	Activities and Quizzes for Chapter 34

CHECK YOUR KNOWLEDGE

1. An endocrine gland:
   a. secretes substances into the bloodstream.
   b. secretes substances into a duct.
   c. secretes substances into the lymph vessels.
   d. secretes substances into the stomach.
2. All of these statements are true except:
   a. insulin is secreted by the islets of Langerhans.
   b. hyperglycemia refers to too much insulin.
   c. insulin is an endocrine secretion from the pancreas.
   d. insulin is necessary to metabolize carbohydrates.
3. Which of the following statements is not true?
   a. Type I diabetes is called juvenile diabetes
   b. Type 2 diabetes develops from insulin resistance
   c. Type 1 diabetes is an autoimmune disease
   d. Hypoglycemia is the main symptom of diabetes
4. The following statements about the thymus gland are true except:
   a. it gets smaller as we age.
   b. it causes certain T cells to mature.
   c. it is located in the brain.
   d. it produces peptides.
5. Progesterone is a hormone secreted by the:
   a. ovaries.
   b. testes.
   c. pituitary gland.
   d. pineal gland.
6. A test that measures glucose levels of four to six weeks is:
   a. glucose tolerance.
   b. human chorionic gonadotropin.
   c. fasting blood sugar.
   d. hemoglobin A1c.
7. A moon face and a buffalo hump are symptoms of:
   a. Addison's disease.
   b. Graves' disease.
   c. Myxedema.
   d. Cushing's syndrome.
8. Enlarged thyroid, nervousness, and weight loss are symptoms of:
   a. Addison's disease.
   b. Graves' disease.
   c. Myxedema.
   d. Cushing's disease.
9. The following are symptoms of hypoglycemia except:
   a. nervousness.
   b. paleness.
   c. full bounding pulse.
   d. dry skin.
10. Escalated hyperthyroidism may develop into:
    a. cardiomegaly.
    b. generalized paralysis.
    c. exophthalmus.
    d. a thyroid storm.
11. Diabetes causes:
    a. obesity.
    b. hyperglycemia.
    c. hypoglycemia.
    d. urinary retention.

WEB LINKS

CDC's Diabetes Public Health Resource: www.cdc.gov/diabetes

National Diabetes Information Clearinghouse: diabetes.niddk.nih.gov

AllThyroid.org: www.allthyroid.org

Chapter

35 The Reproductive System

OBJECTIVES

In this chapter, you will learn the following:

KB KNOWLEDGE BASE

1. Spell and define, using the glossary at the back of the text, all the Words to Know in this chapter.
2. Differentiate between sexual and asexual reproduction.
3. Describe the differentiation of reproductive organs.
4. Explain how sperm are able to fertilize an egg.
5. Describe male prenatal development.
6. Name the male sex organs and describe their location and function.
7. Explain how pituitary hormones affect the functions of the testes.
8. Identify the male secondary sex characteristics.
9. Trace the pathway of sperm from production to expulsion.
10. Name the components of semen.
11. Describe four diseases and disorders of the male reproductive system.
12. Name the female sex organs and describe their location and function.
13. Explain the interaction of pituitary hormones with the ovaries and other organs.
14. Identify the female secondary sex characteristics.
15. Describe the maturation and release of an ovum.
16. Compare the internal and external sexual organs of the male and female.
17. Describe the phases of the menstrual cycle and the purpose of menstruation.
18. Explain how fertilization occurs.
19. Describe the events occurring during each trimester of pregnancy as they relate to the woman and the embryo or fetus.
20. Describe the events that occur in the three stages of labor.
21. List the reasons for practicing contraception.
22. Identify the contraceptive methods, stating their relative effectiveness.
23. Describe the diagnostic tests of the female reproductive system.
24. Describe the diseases or disorders of the female reproductive system.
25. Identify the characteristics of the sexually transmitted diseases.
26. Relate how the female body changes in relation to fertility.
27. Discuss the system relationships with premenstrual syndrome.

WORDS TO KNOW

ablation
abortion
alpha-fetoprotein screening (AFP)
amniocentesis
amniotic
anteflexed
anteverted
areola
Bartholin's glands
benign hypertrophy
bulbourethral glands
cervix
cesarean
chlamydia
circumcision
clitoris
coitus
colposcopy
conceive
conception
contraception
contraction
corpus luteum
cryptorchidism
dilation and curettage
dysmenorrhea
dysplasia
ectopic
effacement
ejaculation
ejaculatory duct
embryo
endometrium
epididymis
episiotomy

erectile
erectile dysfunction
fallopian tubes
fertilization
fetus
fibroid
foreskin
gamete
genital herpes
genitalia
gonorrhea
graafian follicle
gynecology
hydrocele
hymen
hysterectomy
hysteroscopy
impotence
inguinal canal
inguinal hernia
interventional hysterosal-pingography
labia majora
labia minora
ligation
mammary glands
mammogram
mastectomy
menarche
menopause
menorrhagia
menstruation
moniliasis
mons pubis
myometrium
nonspecific urethritis
os
ovulation
ovum
Papanicolaou (Pap) smear
penis
perineum
phimosis
placenta
pregnancy
prolapse
prostate
prostatectomy
rectocele
reproductive
retroflexed
retroverted
salpingo-oophorectomy
scrotum
semen
sperm
spermatozoan
syphilis
transurethral
trichomoniasis
trimester
uterus
vagina
vaginitis
vas deferens
vasectomy
vulva
womb
zygote

The **reproductive** system consists of the organs that are capable of accomplishing reproduction, the creation of a new individual. All living organisms reproduce, some very simply by an asexual method or without the need of sexual contact. An example of asexual reproduction is one of the simplest forms of life, a single cell. In binary fusion, a cell divides into two cells by simple cleavage. In mitosis, a single cell rearranges its chromatin into chromosomes and then divides into two cells (the method by which human cells reproduce). Both methods require that the "parents" become the "children"; therefore, both parent and child cannot exist at the same time.

Sexual methods of reproduction are found in multi-celled forms of life, including humans. The methods may vary but certain characteristics are common to all. In each species, there are sexes, namely a male and a female. Each sex has special sex glands, or gonads, that produce sex cells (**gametes**). In humans, the union of the male gamete (a **spermatozoan**) with the female gamete (an **ovum**) forms a new one-celled structure called a **zygote**. The zygote then undergoes mitosis repeatedly to form a new individual.

In Chapter 23, the cell was described as having 46 chromosomes, or 23 pairs. Each chromosome has a partner of the same shape and size. One pair of chromosomes are the sex chromosomes. In the female, both chromosomes in the pair are X chromosomes, but in the male, one is an X and one is a Y. When the gonads produce the ovum and spermatozoan cells, the number of chromosomes is reduced to 23 (one half). When the two cells unite as fertilization occurs, the new cell, a zygote, will again have 46 chromosomes. If the spermatozoan carries an X chromosome, the embryo will develop female characteristics. If it carries a Y chromosome, the embryo will develop as a male.

The reproductive organs are the only organs in the human body that differ between the male and female, yet there is still a significant similarity. This likeness results from the fact that male and female organs develop from the same group of embryonic cells. For approximately two months, the embryo develops without sexual identity. Then the influence of the X or Y chromosome begins to make a differentiation.

DIFFERENTIATION OF REPRODUCTIVE ORGANS

The gonads of the embryo begin to evolve into the sexual organs of the female at about the 10th or 11th week of pregnancy or gestation. The ovaries of the embryo develop high in its abdomen from the same type of tissue as the testes. However, the testes evolve from the medulla of the gonad, whereas the ovaries develop from the cortex. Figure 35–1 illustrates how the undifferentiated external **genitalia** develop into fully differentiated structures. In the male, the tubercle becomes the glans **penis**, the folds become the penile shaft, and the swelling develops into the **scrotum**. In the female, the tubercle becomes the **clitoris**, the folds the **labia minora**, and the swelling the **labia majora**.

Internally, there is also a similarity of structures. The embryonic müllerian ducts degenerate, and the wolffian ducts become the **epididymis**, **vas deferens**, and **ejaculatory duct** in the male. In the female, the wolffian ducts degenerate, and the müllerian ducts develop into the **fallopian tubes**, the **uterus**, and the upper portion of the **vagina**. It is believed that the presence of the testes in the male is the differentiating factor in the development. Without the androgens (male hormones) from the testes, a female develops. With the androgens,

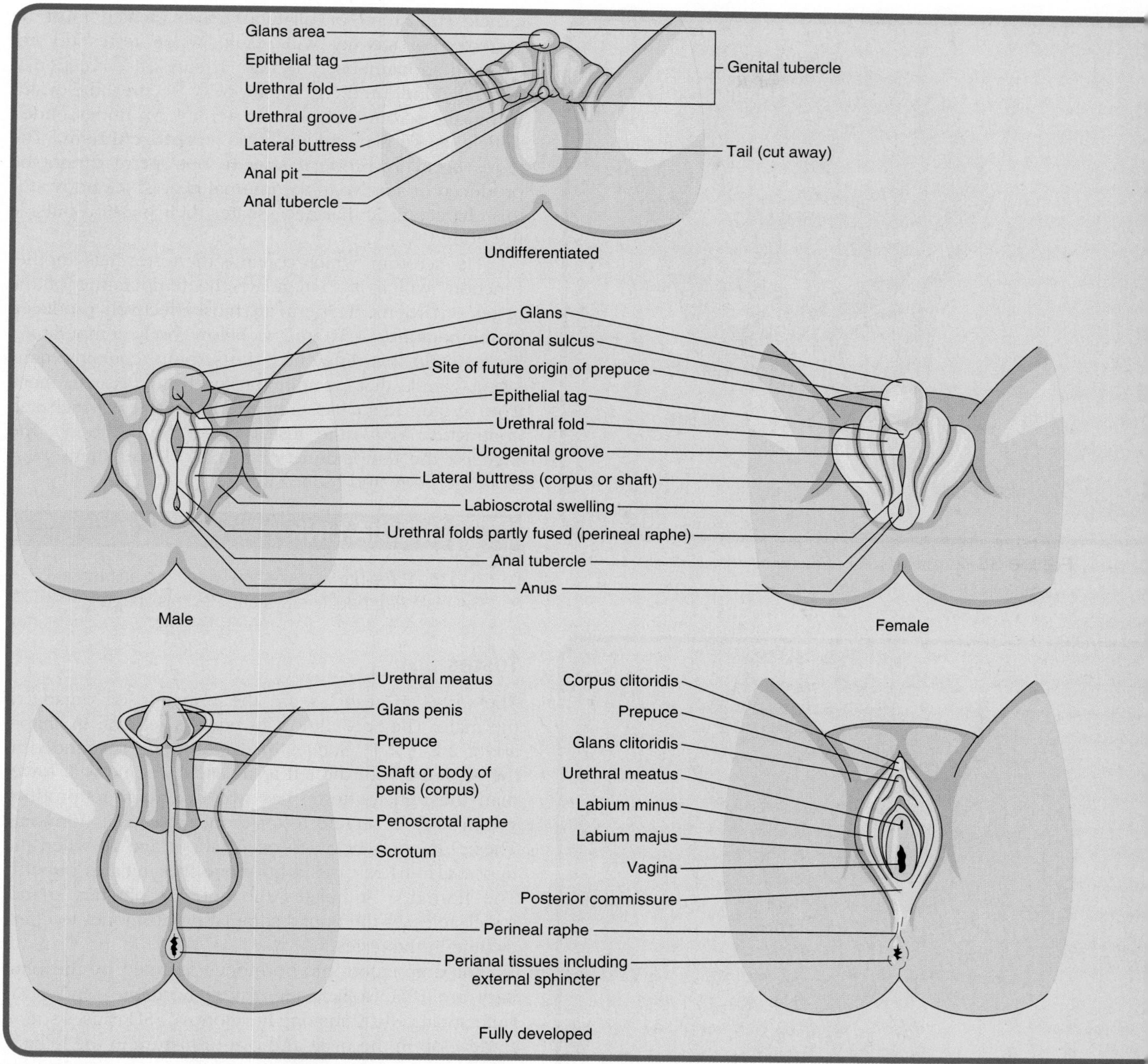

Figure 35–1: Sexual differentiation before birth. *Delmar/Cengage Learning.*

a male develops. Another substance called the müllerian inhibitor works in partnership with the androgens to produce the sex differentiation.

MALE REPRODUCTIVE ORGANS

When the zygote contains a Y chromosome, a male child will develop. About the 7th or 8th week of pregnancy, the testes begin to develop within the abdominal cavity at about the level of the ileum of the pelvis bone. The sex of the fetus is evident by about the 4th month.

During the 8th and 9th months of pregnancy, the testes move from the abdomen through the **inguinal canal** into the external pouch called the scrotum (Figure 35–2). After the testes pass, the canal closes to prevent the descent of other structures into the scrotum or the return of the testes into the abdomen. When a loop of small intestine descends through the canal

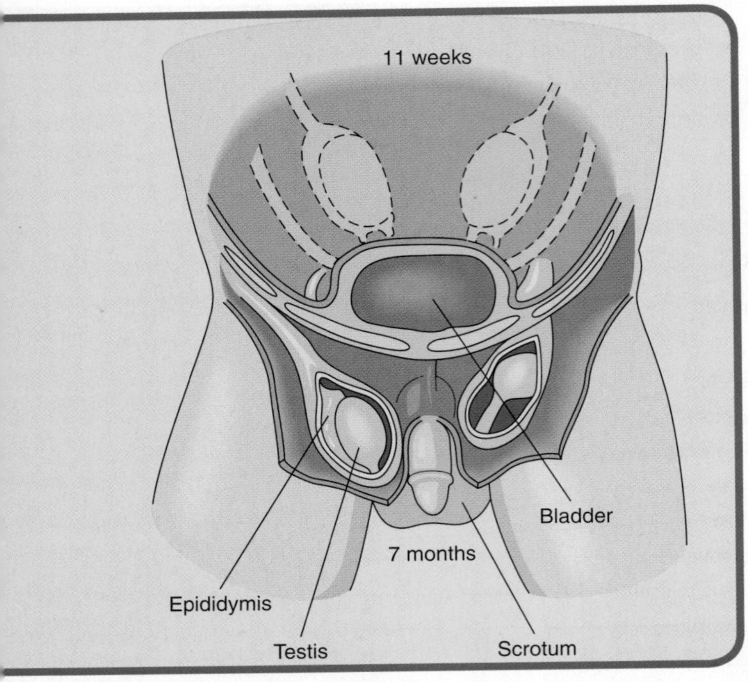

Figure 35–2: The descent of the testes. *Delmar/Cengage Learning.*

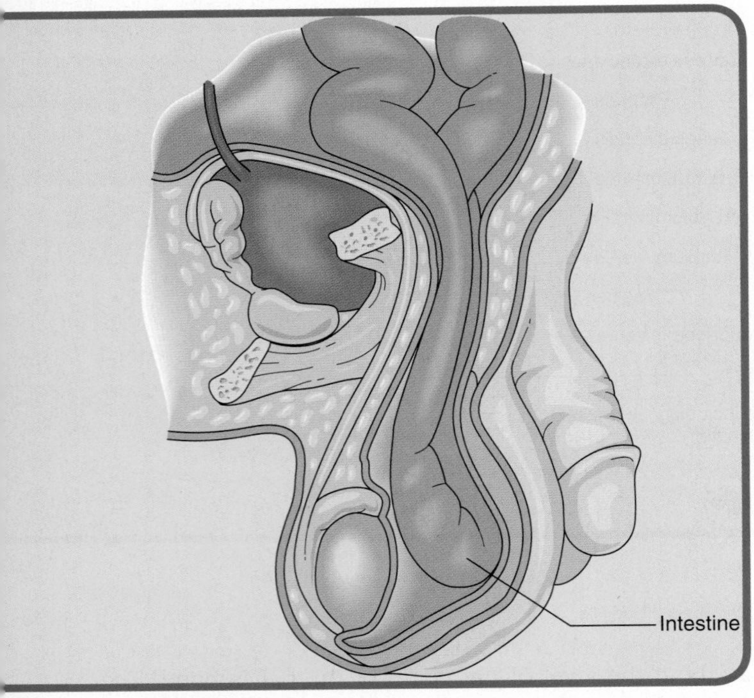

Figure 35–3: Inguinal hernia. *Delmar/Cengage Learning.*

because of improper closure or later in life because of relaxed inguinal structures, it is known as an **inguinal hernia** (Figure 35–3).

If the testes fail to descend or if they return to the abdomen, a condition known as undescended testicle (unilateral or bilateral) exists, which must be corrected or sterility will result. When testes do not descend spontaneously by age 1, surgical correction is generally indicated. An orchiopexy secures the testes within the scrotum to prevent sterility. An undescended testicle is known medically as **cryptorchidism**. The testes normally produce **sperm**, but sperm cannot be produced or survive in the internal heat of the body. It is this characteristic that necessitates their location outside the body.

The scrotum, which contains the testes, has another function, which is to regulate the temperature of the testes' environment. Sperm are most effectively produced at temperatures 1.5° to 2°C below body temperature. To maintain this difference, the scrotum contains many sweat glands that perspire profusely to dissipate heat. The scrotum also has cremasteric muscles, which can contract to draw the testes closer to the body and increase the temperature or relax to lower them away from the body and reduce it.

MEDIA LINK

Go to the Premium Website and watch the animation, "The Male Reproductive System," for this chapter.

Testes

The testes or testicles are the primary sex organs of the male. They are almost of equal size, oval in shape, about 2 × 1 × 1½ inches in size, and are suspended in the scrotum, with the left testis usually somewhat lower than the right. A testis has two functions: to produce sperm and to secrete testosterone, the male hormone. These functions begin to occur about age 10 when the hypothalamus releases a hormone that initiates puberty. The hormone stimulates the anterior pituitary gland, which releases the gonad-stimulating hormones to effect change in the testes.

Male gonadotropic hormones secreted by the pituitary are FSH (follicle-stimulating hormone) and ICSH (interstitial cell-stimulating hormones). FSH causes sperm to develop in the male and ova to mature in the female, a very similar function.

Sperm Production

Sperm develop and mature in microscopic tubes in the testes known as *seminiferous tubules* (Figure 35–4). FSH stimulates the production of sperm in the cells that line the tubules. There are about 300 sections of coiled tubules that, if uncoiled, are estimated to extend over a mile. As the sperm develop, they are released into the tubules to start their journey from the testes. Sperm formation in an adult male requires about 74 days to maturity. The function normally begins to develop at about age 12, and the first mature sperm are ejaculated at about age 14.

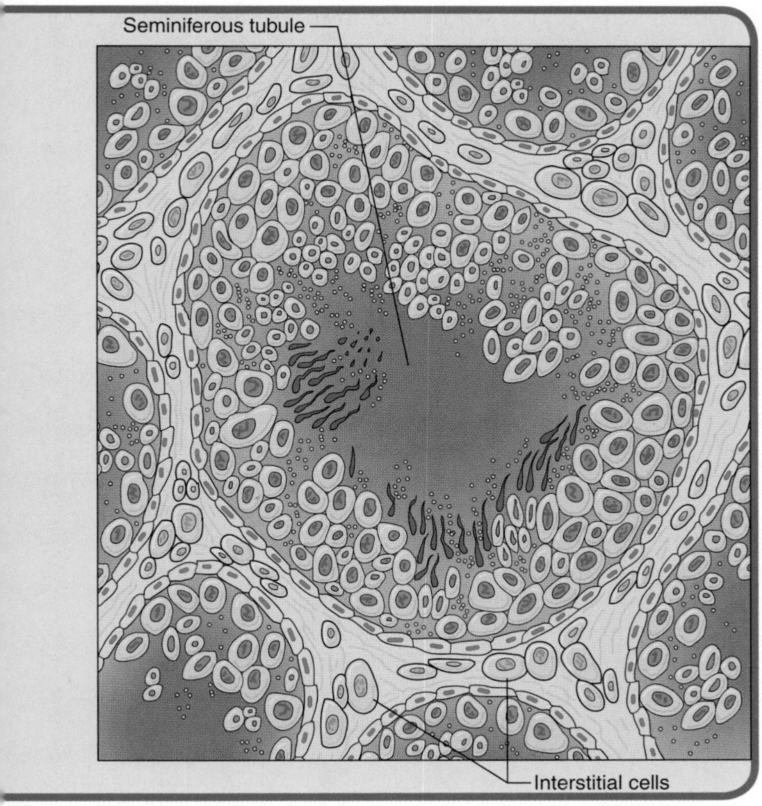

Figure 35–4: The production of sperm in the seminiferous tubules and the secretion of testosterone by the interstitial cells. *Delmar/Cengage Learning.*

Testosterone

As sperm are developing, ICSH is causing the interstitial cells in the network of structures around the tubules to secrete testosterone. Testosterone aids in the maturing of sperm and causes many changes in the male body as it circulates in the bloodstream. These changes are referred to as the development of secondary sex characteristics (Figure 35–5).

In the male, secondary sex characteristics are:

1. Longer and heavier bone structure
2. Larger muscles
3. Deep voice
4. Growth of body hair
5. Development of the genitalia (external sex organs)
6. Increased metabolism
7. Sexual desire

Epididymis, Vas Deferens, and Seminal Vesicles

The epididymis is a coiled structure about 20 feet in length. It is shaped like a half-moon and sits with its head on top of the testes with its tail extending down the side to join the vas deferens (Figure 35–6).

After sperm are produced in the tubules, they pass into the epididymis, where a small number are stored. The sperm mature in the epididymis for about 18 hours. The fluid secreted by the epididymis adds to the volume of ejaculant.

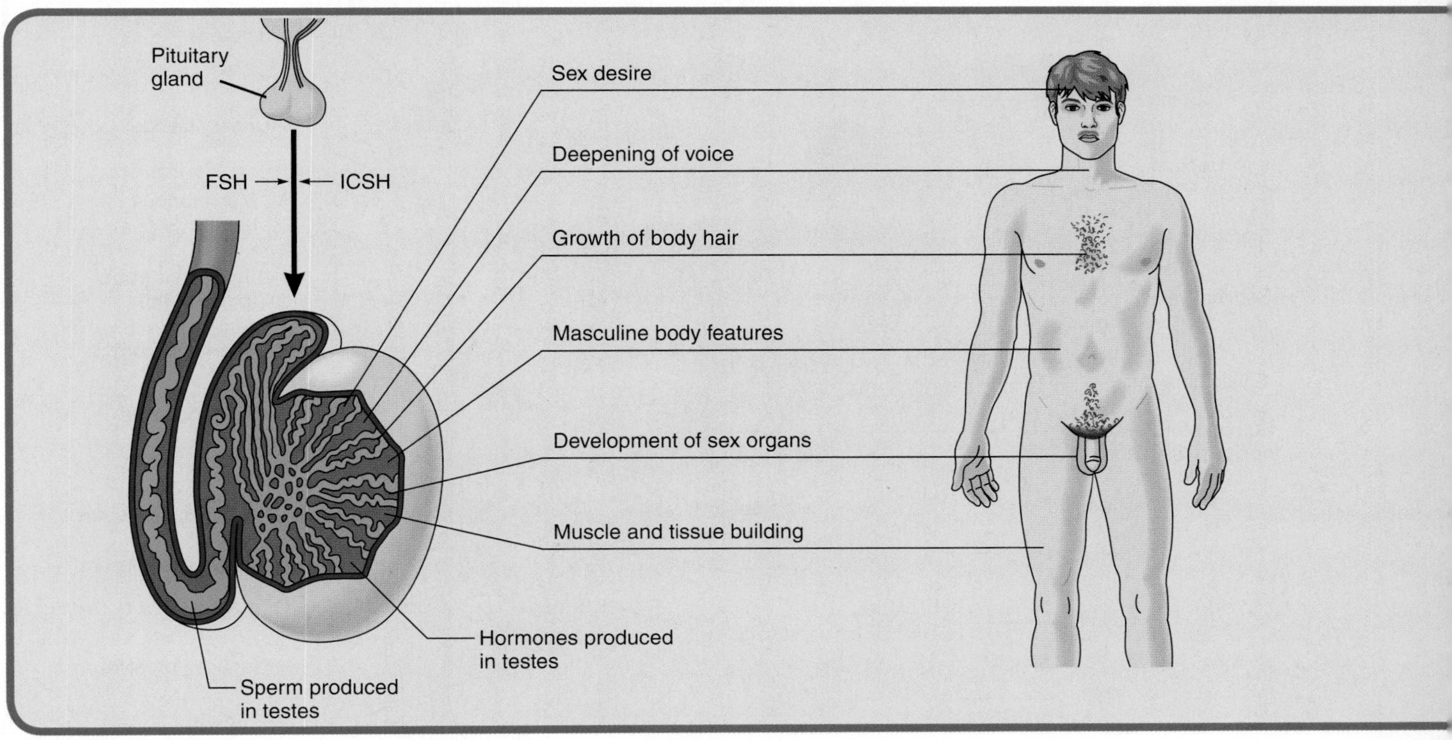

Figure 35–5: Secondary sex characteristics of the male. *Delmar/Cengage Learning.*

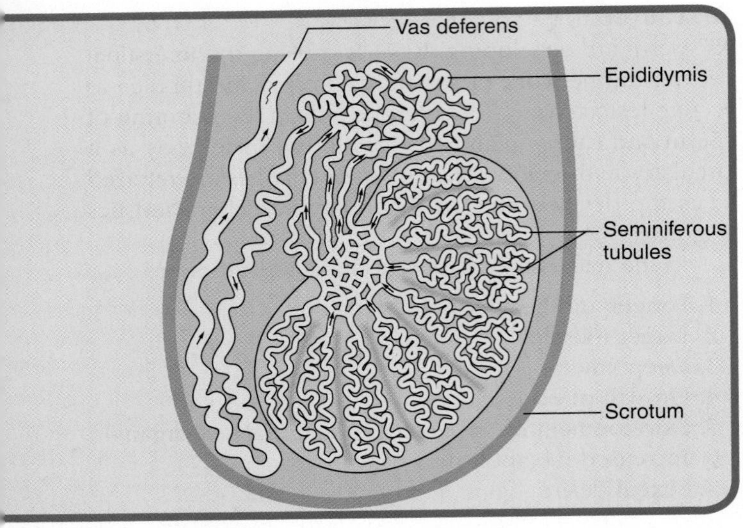

Figure 35–6: Seminiferous tubules, epididymis, and vas deferens. *Delmar/Cengage Learning.*

The vas deferens serves as the passageway for sperm to exit the epididymis. On each side, one vas deferens joins one epididymis, extending upward for about 45 cm through an inguinal canal to the base of the urinary bladder. Each vas joins with a duct from a seminal vesicle to form a common ejaculatory duct (Figure 35–7).

The seminal vesicles are a pair of convoluted tubes lying posterior to the bladder. They also empty into the ejaculatory duct. The vesicles secrete a fluid that contains fructose, a simple sugar, which provides nutrition for the sperm. The fluid makes up a major portion of the ejaculant. The ejaculatory duct is a short straight tube that passes through the **prostate** gland to join the urethra.

Prostate Gland, Bulbourethral Glands, and Urethra

The prostate gland is a donut-like pyramidal structure with the urethra extending through its center (see Figure 35–7). The gland is positioned just beneath the bladder. It produces secretions that are drained through tiny tubules into the prostatic section of the urethra. The fluid secreted is alkaline in nature. Its addition to the ejaculant stimulates sperm motility and preserves sperm life by neutralizing the acidity of the vagina. The prostate is surrounded by muscular tissue that contracts during ejaculation to empty the **semen** (ejaculant fluids and sperm) into the urethra to be propelled from the body.

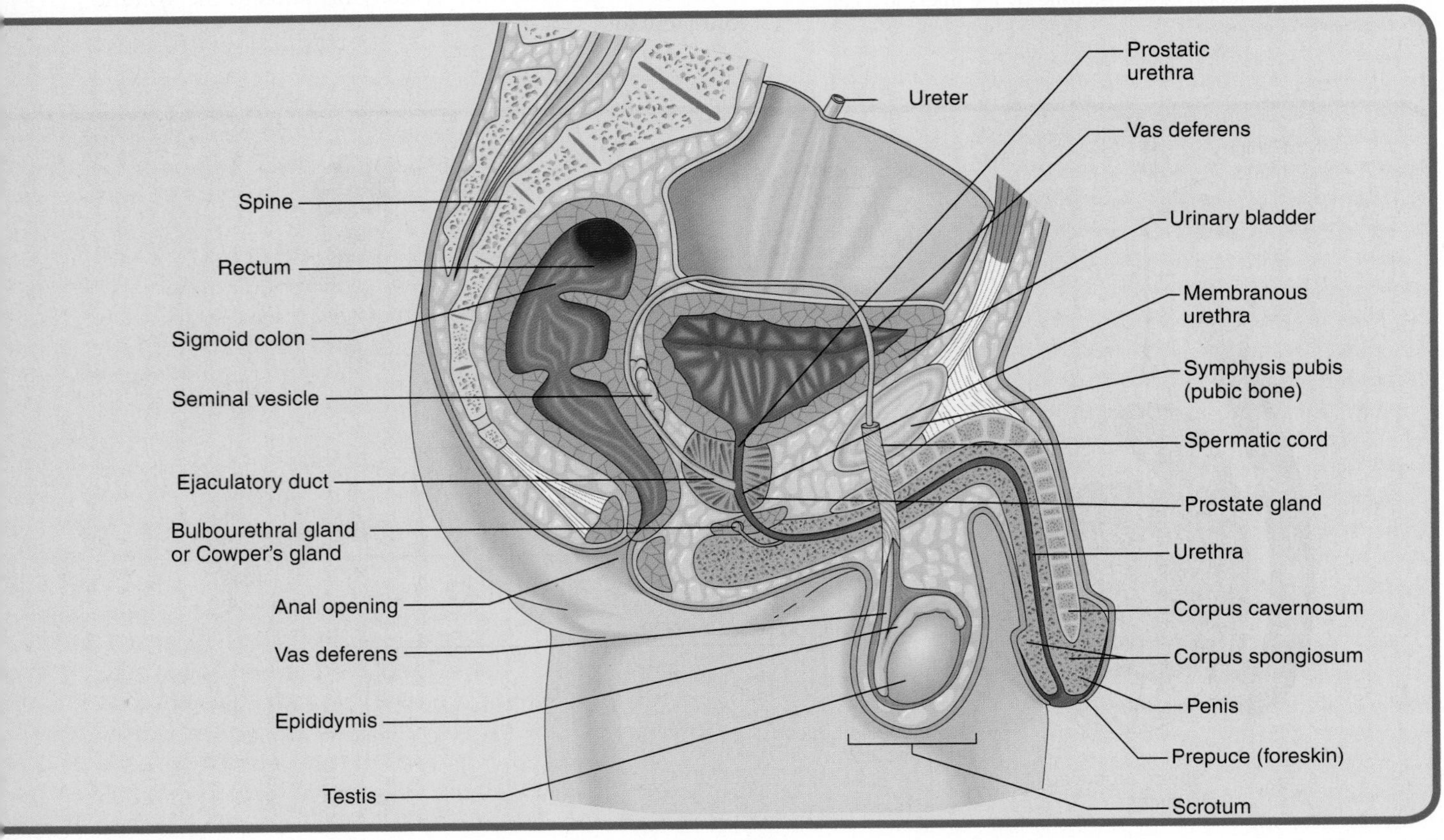

Figure 35–7: The organs and ducts of the male reproductive system. *Delmar/Cengage Learning.*

The **bulbourethral glands** lie beneath the prostate and empty their contents into the urethra. The fluid the glands secrete aids in the movement of sperm and makes the normally acidic male urethra alkaline just prior to **ejaculation**. The secretions may serve as a lubricant for intercourse. Bulbourethral glands are sometimes called Cowper's glands.

Semen

The combined secretions from all the glands and ducts along with the sperm are called the seminal fluid or semen. Approximately 3.5 mL of total fluid are expelled per orgasm (series of rhythmic muscular contractions). Semen is composed of:

- Fluids from the testes and epididymis containing about 350 million sperm (5%)
- Fluid secreted by the seminal vesicles (30%)
- Fluid secreted by the prostate gland (60%)
- Fluid secreted by the bulbourethral glands (5%)

Penis

The penis consists of three columns of **erectile** tissue. Two are called the corpora cavernosa. A third column, the corpus spongiosum, contains the urethra. It is surrounded by a layer of subcutaneous tissue and covered with skin. The distal end of the penis enlarges to form the glans penis. A circular fold of skin that extends down over the glans is called the prepuce or **foreskin**. A number of small glands in the foreskin secrete a waxy, odoriferous substance called smegma onto the glans. A **circumcision** (surgical removal of the foreskin) may be performed on a male infant to prevent accumulation of the smegma, thereby avoiding bothersome infections later in life. It also has been observed that circumcised men have a lower incidence of cancer of the penis and that women married to circumcised men have a lower incidence of cancer of the cervix. Circumcision is indicated to correct **phimosis**, a narrowed opening of the foreskin, which prohibits its retraction over the glans. Phimosis contributes to the accumulation of smegma. Many men feel that sexual sensations are heightened when the glans is not covered or restricted by the foreskin. The urethra extends down the length of the penis, opening at the urinary meatus of the glans. The urethra serves two purposes, to empty urine from the urinary bladder and to expel semen.

Erection and Ejaculation

Successful intercourse is dependent on the two cavernosa columns of erectile tissue in the penis. When a male is sexually aroused, nerve impulses cause the erectile tissue to engorge with blood, which makes the erectile tissue increase in size and become firm. Blood entering the dilated arteries squeezes the veins against the penile structures, prohibiting venous return.

After stimulation of the glans results in maximum stimulation of the seminal vesicles, impulses are sent to the ejaculatory center and orgasm occurs. Orgasm is the result of muscular contractions from the vas deferens, seminal vesicles, ejaculatory ducts, and prostate gland. Secretions produced and stored in these structures, along with the sperm, are forcefully expelled through the urethra, after which the engorgement gradually subsides.

Vasectomy

Vasectomy is a simple surgical procedure to prohibit the ejaculation of sperm and effect sterilization of the male. It has become a popular means of birth control. The procedure involves making a small incision in each side of the scrotum. The vas deferens, on each side, is grasped and a loop is withdrawn through the incision. The physician ties the duct in two places and removes a piece of the duct between the ties. The ends are placed back into the scrotum, and the small incision is closed with sutures. The procedure can be performed in the physician's office under local anesthesia or in a hospital outpatient clinic. It is a much simpler means of sterilization than the surgery required to perform a similar procedure on a female.

A vasectomy does not interfere with the function of the testes or with sexual ability. Sperm are still produced in the testes but, because their exit is blocked, they remain in the testes and epididymis until they die and are reabsorbed into the body. Testosterone, the male hormone produced by the testes, gains access to the body by way of the veins in the scrotum. Vasectomy will have no effect on testosterone levels. Most men report as much or more sexual activity after as before their vasectomy. The only negative aspect is that the procedure is likely to be irreversible. Recently, success at restoring fertility has been achieved by surgical reconnection in one out of five attempts. However, the patient may have developed autoantibodies toward his own sperm and may no longer be fertile.

DIAGNOSTIC EXAMS AND TESTS OF THE MALE REPRODUCTIVE SYSTEM

- *Chromosomal analysis*—Tests to determine genetic defects, such as Klinefelter's syndrome, that cause abnormal growth and development of sexual characteristics and chromosome basis for hypogonadism.
- *Digital rectal examination*—A common manual examination involving insertion of a gloved finger into the rectum to palpate the prostate gland for size, density, and nodules or tumors.

- *Hormonal studies*—Measurement of pituitary hormones, such as interstitial-cell stimulating hormone that causes development of testes and sperm production or adrenal cortex androgens that govern sex characteristics and testosterone levels of the testes, to diagnose conditions like hypogonadism, early or delayed sexual development, and infertility.
- *Prostatic specific antigen (PSA)*—A blood test used to measure the amount of antigen present when there is prostate hypertrophy. An elevated amount may be indicative of cancer.
- *Semen analysis*—Analysis of semen and the sperm to determine the volume of semen; the number, maturity, and motility of sperm; the presence of abnormal or immature sperm; and other characteristics. Approximately 40% to 50% of fertility problems are attributed to the male when couples fail to achieve pregnancy.
- *Testicular biopsy*—Examination of testicular tissue to determine unexplained oligospermia, the absence or great decrease in the amount of sperm, when diagnosing infertility.
- *Testicular self-examination*—The American Cancer Society recommends that men perform routine testicular self-examination (TSE) as a means of early identification of testicular cancer. The cancer tends to occur primarily in men from 20 to 40 years old, but it is the most common site of cancer in men 29 to 35 years of age. The Society recommends monthly TSE beginning at 15 years of age.

DISEASES AND DISORDERS OF THE MALE REPRODUCTIVE SYSTEM

Epididymitis (Epi-didi-mi′-tis)

Description—This is an infection of the epididymis and is an uncommon infection of the male reproductive tract. It may spread to the testicle, causing *orchitis* (inflammation of the testicle).

Signs and symptoms—The primary symptom is intense pain with swelling in the scrotum. Other symptoms include fever, malaise, and a characteristic waddle when walking.

Etiology—The causative organism is usually a coliform bacteria from the intestinal tract and generally follows urinary or prostatic infections. Other causes include trauma, gonorrhea, or syphilis.

Treatment—Treatment may consist of bed rest, elevation of the scrotum on towel rolls, and ice to relieve pain and swelling. A broad-spectrum (inclusive) antibiotic and pain medication are indicated. Therapy must be initiated immediately, especially if there is bilateral involvement, because of the risk of sterility.

Erectile Dysfunction (Impotence)

Description—This is an inability to have or sustain an erection to complete intercourse. Because of the negative connotation of the word "**impotence**," physicians and sex therapists use the term *erectile dysfunction* to identify the occurrence.

Signs and symptoms—Primary **erectile dysfunction** refers to the patient who has never had an erection. Secondary dysfunction refers to the patient who is currently unable to sustain erection but has had intercourse in the past. Transient periods of inability are not considered a dysfunction and probably occur in half the adult male population. The incidence of erectile dysfunction increases with age.

Etiology—Organic factors cause most dysfunction and may result from a chronic illness such as diabetes, renal failure, or cardiopulmonary disease. Spinal cord trauma, the effects of alcohol, or the results of certain drug therapy may also cause organic dysfunction. About 30% may be psychogenic in origin. The usual causes are anxiety, fear of failure, depression, parental rejection, and previous traumatic sexual experiences. Dysfunction may result from stress. Interpersonal factors such as insufficient knowledge of sexual function or lack of communication with a partner may also cause difficulty.

Treatment—Treatment may include sexual therapy to reduce the anxiety and usually involves both partners. The type of therapy chosen depends on the specific cause of the dysfunction. Most often it involves improving communication, reevaluating attitudes toward sex, restricting sexual activity, and encouraging attention to the physical sensations of touching. Many men may benefit from the use of a medication such as Viagra. It can be beneficial for men following prostatectomy where nerves involved in the erection process may be damaged or severed. It is also helpful for men with diabetes or those taking hypertensive medications. It is primarily a trial process to determine whether it will be effective. The medication must be taken one hour prior to intercourse for it to be effective. The drug is contraindicated for patients with severe heart problems or those using nitroglycerin products. Additional methods of medicating may be developed, such as a nasal form to be inhaled or a topical ointment and methods with a shortened period to effectiveness. Patients with organic dysfunction may need to develop alternative means of sexual expression. Some patients may benefit from learning to inject one or a combination of drugs into the spongy erectile bodies of the penis. These drugs stimulate a normal erection. Some may use a vacuum device, which pulls blood into the spongy bodies to effect a firm erection. Others may be candidates for the placement of a prosthesis, a device that is implanted into the spongy bodies. There are two basic types of prostheses: a semi-rigid and an inflatable style. The semi-rigid prosthesis will give a constant state of firmness with flexibility at the base so that the penis can be held against the body with underclothing. The inflatable prosthesis can be made erect for intercourse and can be deflated when the man is not engaged in sexual activity.

Hydrocele (Hi′-dro-sel)

Description—The presence of an excessive amount of fluid within structures around the testes is called a **hydrocele**.

Signs and symptoms—Enlargement of the scrotum.

Etiology—It may occur following injury or inflammation or may develop as a result of the aging process. It usually is caused by excess production of normal body fluid, lack of reabsorption, or blockage of the circulatory process.

Treatment—Surgical correction is indicated with continued enlargement and discomfort.

Prostatic Hypertrophy (Pros-tat′-ik Hi-per′-tro-fe)

Description—This enlargement of the prostate gland is common in men over age 50. In **benign** (nonmalignant) **hypertrophy**, the prostate may enlarge sufficiently to constrict the urethra, making it difficult to empty the bladder. Surgery may be indicated to remove the obstructive tissue. A malignant prostate, one of the most common forms of cancer found in men, is a different disease.

Signs and symptoms—Symptoms of hypertrophy vary with the extent of involvement. Usually, the initial symptoms are reduced force and size of urinary stream, difficulty in starting a stream, dribbling, a feeling of incomplete voiding, nocturia (having to void at night), and frequent urination. As the hypertrophy increases, symptoms become more pronounced, and eventually hematuria and retention may develop. Diagnosis of hypertrophy can be confirmed by a digital examination to palpate the prostate through the rectal wall (Figure 35–8).

Etiology—It may be caused by a change in hormonal activity.

Treatment—Treatment of benign hypertrophy of the prostate will be conservative until the gland squeezes the urethra and interferes with voiding. Medications like tamsulosin (Flomax) have altered management of hypertrophy. This medication improves the force of urine and the ability to empty the bladder. Other medications like finasteride (Proscar) help shrink the size of the prostate. This occurs slowly; about six to nine months with the maximum effect taking about 18 months. The alternative to medical therapy is a more permanent surgical solution to effectively relieve urinary retention and other symptoms.

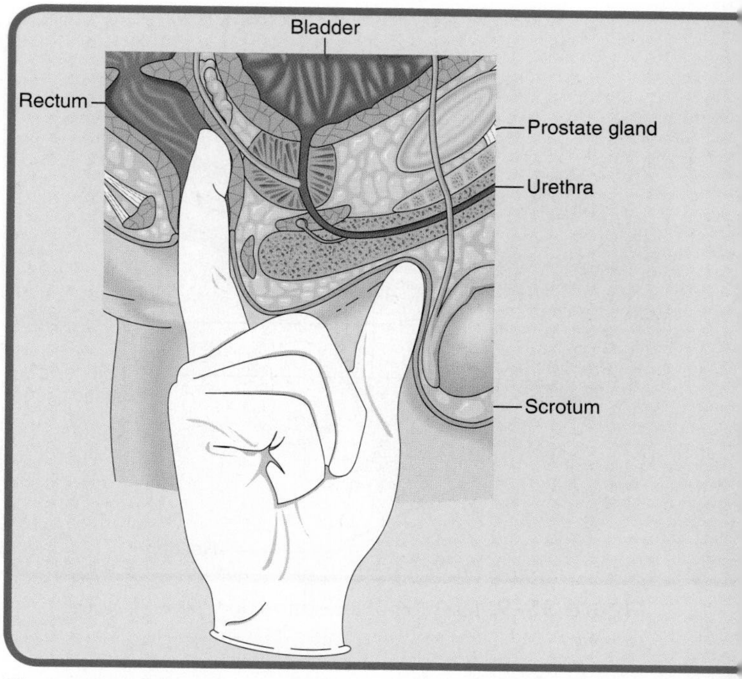

Figure 35–8: Digital examination of the prostate gland. *Delmar/Cengage Learning.*

A **prostatectomy** (removal of the prostate) can be performed by different methods. An open or robotic prostatectomy is indicated with a large prostate or with a contained malignancy. An incision is made in the skin above the pubic bone and below the umbilicus. The prostate is exposed as it lies below the bladder and above the penis. The benign tumor of the prostate is removed when no cancer is expected. When cancer is expected, the entire prostate gland and tumor is removed. A robotic prostectomy involves using a surgeon-controlled robot to remove the prostate. This is performed after the abdomen has been filled with CO_2 (pneumoperitoneum). The benefit of robotic surgery is less blood loss and better visualization of the prostate. Another common method is the **transurethral** prostatectomy (TURP). In this procedure, a resectoscope is inserted into the urethra, and the prostate is approached through an incision in the wall of the urethra (Figure 35–9). A wire loop with electric current removes a segment of the gland, thereby interrupting the integrity of the prostate and prohibiting its

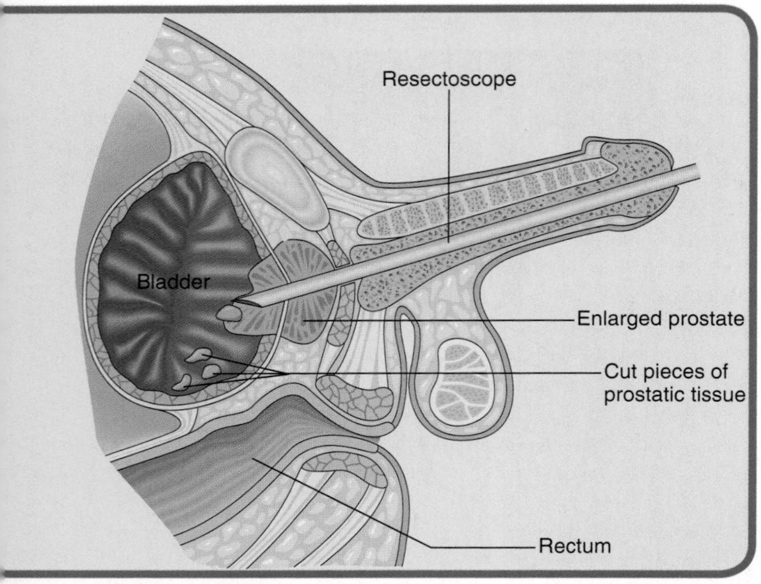

Figure 35–9: Insertion of a resectoscope. *Delmar/Cengage Learning.*

constricting action. Another surgical procedure involves the use of laser energy, which can be directed to either vaporize the prostate tissue or to incise the tissue and remove it in pieces.

When there is a malignancy in the prostate, it may cause no symptoms, or the patient may have urinary obstructive symptoms similar to those seen with benign hypertrophy. Cancer may be identified on a rectal examination as a hardened area and may be palpated, or the suspicion of a malignancy may be raised when the patient's prostatic specific antigen (PSA) blood test is abnormal. PSA is a compound that is made only by cells in the prostate, and malignant cells cause this to rise more quickly than is normally seen with an enlarging prostate or with aging.

The incidence of prostate cancer appears to show a family tendency and to be more prevalent in the black race. All men over 50 years should have a rectal examination and a PSA blood test yearly, but those with a family history or who are black should begin annual testing at 40 years.

Treatment of prostatic cancer—Treatment is determined by clinical assessment, expected life span, the stage of the disease, and tolerance for the therapy. Radiation, a prostatectomy, an orchidectomy (removal of testes to stop hormone production), and oral doses of female estrogen are used alone or in combinations, according to the stage of the involvement, to arrest and control the malignancy. Favorable results are obtained from high doses of radiation. Not only does the cancer go into remission, but the associated metastatic skeletal pain, if present, is also relieved.

With the screening for prostate cancer that is now occurring, many younger, sexually active men are being found with prostate cancer, so treatment offers a chance to cure many individuals, and it is anticipated that survival rates will be greatly improved. Unfortunately, the curative treatments available—cryotherapy, radiotherapy, or radical prostatectomy—all have side effects that are disturbing, but they can be overcome. These include incontinence, erectile dysfunction, cystitis, and proctitis (rectal inflammation). If the cancer has spread outside the prostate, making it incurable, it can be controlled by medications or orchidectomy. The cancer can be put into remission for a significant time.

New methods of prevention and treatment are being continuously developed. The National Cancer Institute, through a study called the Prostate Cancer Prevention Trial (PCPT), determined that the drug finasteride (Proscar) can prevent prostate cancer in men ages 55 and older.

There are other treatments being used. Cryosurgery (freezing) uses liquid nitrogen to kill cancer cells. It appears to be a good alternative to radiation and is less invasive than traditional surgery. But it still poses risks, including impotence and leakage of urine from the bladder or stool from the rectum.

Other treatments include biologic therapy (also called immunotherapy), high-intensity focused ultrasound, proton beam radiation therapy, as well as a number of clinical trials.

FEMALE REPRODUCTIVE ORGANS

Because the similarity in function of the male and female reproductive organs is another indication of their common origin, a comparison will be made, when appropriate, as each organ or structure is presented. The order of presentation will be, as with the male, from the formation of the sex cell to its exit from the body.

MEDIA LINK

Go to the Premium Website and watch the animation, "The Female Reproductive System," for this chapter.

Ovaries

The embryonic gonadal tissue that is to become the ovaries begins to develop about the 10th or 11th week of pregnancy. The ovaries of the fetus develop high in the abdominal cavity near each kidney but descend to the pelvis as the time for delivery nears. Ovaries are small, almond-shaped glands measuring about 1½ × 1 × ¼ to ½ inch (Figure 35–10). They are supported by the ligaments, which attach to the uterus and tubes to ensure their position near the fimbriated (fringelike projections) ends of the fallopian tubes. These two organs play a significant role in the life of every female. They have two main roles: to produce the sex cell and the ovum and to secrete hormones. These functions parallel the role of the testes in the male.

It is estimated that at birth the ovary has between 200,000 and 400,000 primary **graafian follicles** (podlike structures), which contain immature ova. Many follicles never mature and degenerate by puberty. During the reproductive life of a female, about 375 will develop and mature, releasing an ovum. By age 50, most of them have disappeared.

The ovaries are the primary sex organs of the female. When the female is around age 8, the pituitary gland begins to send hormonal messages that puberty is approaching. Within a few years, the messages get stronger, and the pituitary hormone causes the ovaries to begin releasing estrogen into the blood. Estrogen affects the development of the sex organs, such as the fallopian tubes, the uterus or **womb**, and the vagina, causing them to increase in size and maturity.

Estrogen also produces secondary sex characteristics, which alter the shape and appearance of the female body (Figure 35–11). In the female, secondary sex characteristics are:

1. Broadening of the pelvis, making the outlet broad and oval (to permit childbirth) (The male pelvic outlet is oblong and narrow.)
2. The epiphysis (growth plate) becomes bone and growth ceases. In the absence of estrogen, females continue to grow, becoming several inches taller than normal.
3. Development of softer and smoother skin
4. Development of pubic hair in a flat upper border pattern
5. Deposits of fat in the breasts and development of the duct system
6. Deposits of fat in the buttocks and thighs
7. Sexual desire

In addition to physical changes, two physiological functions begin to occur, namely **ovulation** and **menstruation**. The initial menstrual period is known as the menarche. Ova are produced in the germinal epithelium layer of the ovary (Figure 35–12). There, a "nest" of cells undergo change, with some cells forming a wall around a liquid-filled cavity. Other cells join to thicken one area of the wall. This structure is known as a primary follicle. One of the inner cells will become

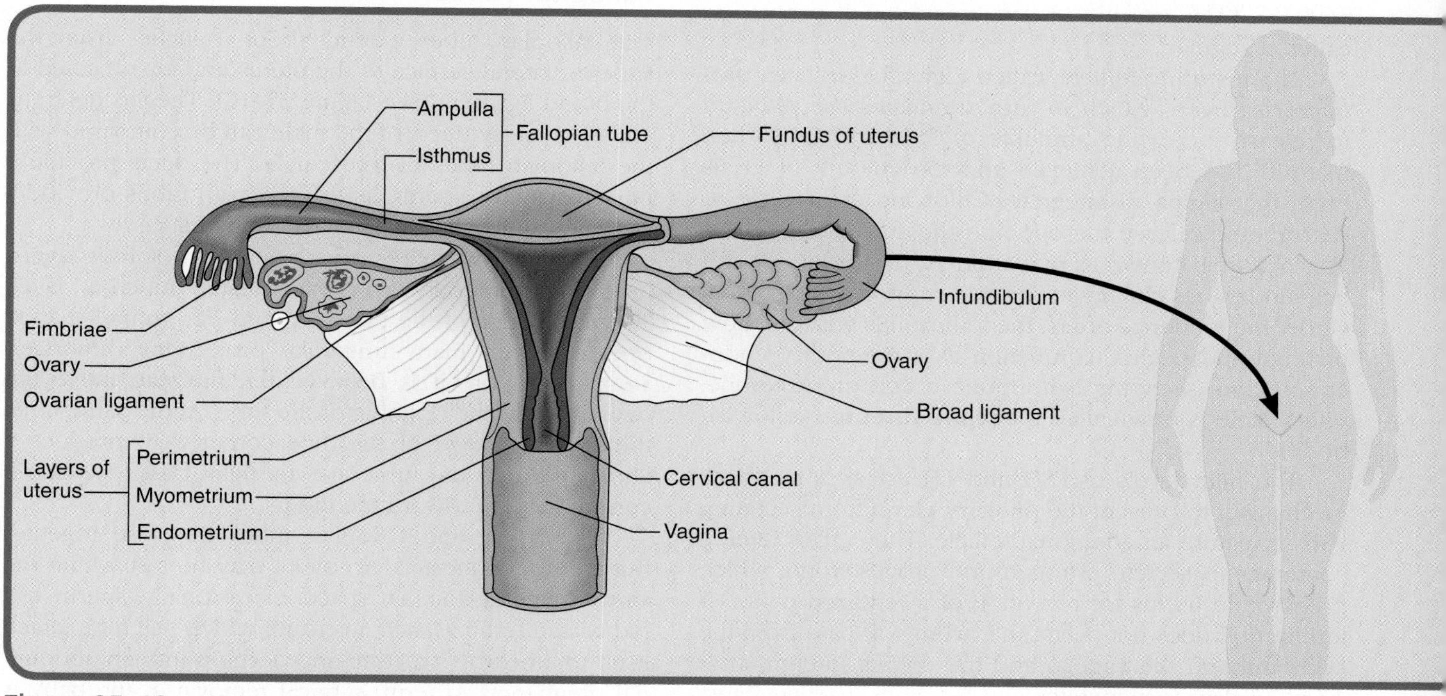

Figure 35–10: Female internal reproductive organs. *Delmar/Cengage Learning.*

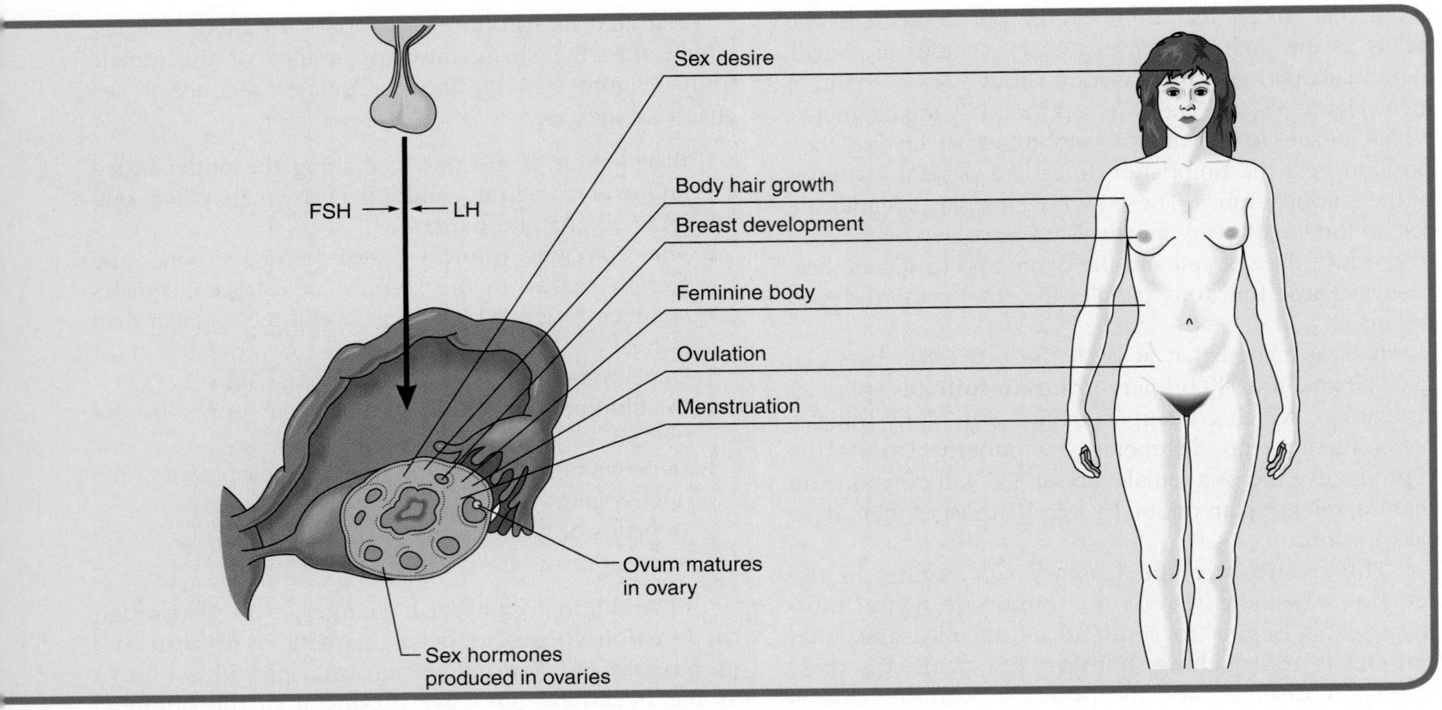

Figure 35–11: Secondary sex characteristics of the female. *Delmar/Cengage Learning.*

the ovum. Under the continued influence of FSH and LH from the pituitary, the follicle and ovum mature. Additional fluid collects within the follicle, and it begins to resemble a blister. The follicle moves toward the surface of the ovary and develops a small protrusion called a stigma.

The maturing follicle, called a graafian follicle, produces estrogen, which in turn stimulates the pituitary to release increasing amounts of FSH and LH. When maturity has been achieved and the amount of LH is high, the stigma disintegrates, allowing the follicle to rupture and release the egg into the surrounding area. This action is known as ovulation. At this point, the follicle undergoes change to provide support to the ovum. Under the influence of LH, the follicle fills with a yellow material and begins to function as a temporary endocrine gland, secreting a hormone called progesterone. The follicle is now called a **corpus luteum** (yellowish body).

The high levels of FSH and LH act as a feedback mechanism to prevent the pituitary gland from secreting FSH to mature an additional follicle. The corpus luteum continues to secrete estrogen and progesterone, which prepare the uterus for reception of a fertilized ovum. If fertilization does not occur, the ovum will pass from the body through the vagina, and the corpus luteum, after 10 or 12 days, degenerates and becomes inactive, causing a sharp decline in the hormonal level. This decline stimulates the pituitary to again begin releasing FSH and LH, and the cycle starts again.

Fallopian Tubes

The fallopian tubes extend about 4 inches from the superior lateral surface of the uterus and are attached to the broad ligament (see Figure 35–10). The vas deferens and ejaculatory ducts of the male can be compared with the fallopian tubes of the female. The ducts provide a passageway for sperm, as the fallopian tubes provide a passageway for the ovum to reach the uterus.

The fallopian tubes are constructed of four layers, including a muscle layer and ciliated mucosal layer. The distal ends of the tubes expand into funnel-shaped openings with many fingerlike projections (fimbriae). Upon ovulation, it is believed the fimbriae move the ovum toward the opening of the tube. At the same time, the muscular layer of the tube contracts to produce a vacuum within the tube, and the cilia beat to create a current moving toward the uterus.

The ovary and fallopian tubes lie close together but are not connected. An ovum may be lost within the surrounding abdominal space. Occasionally, sperm will locate and fertilize such an ovum, which will then attach itself to a nearby structure and develop into an abdominal pregnancy. At term, surgical removal of the baby is necessary because no outlet for delivery exists.

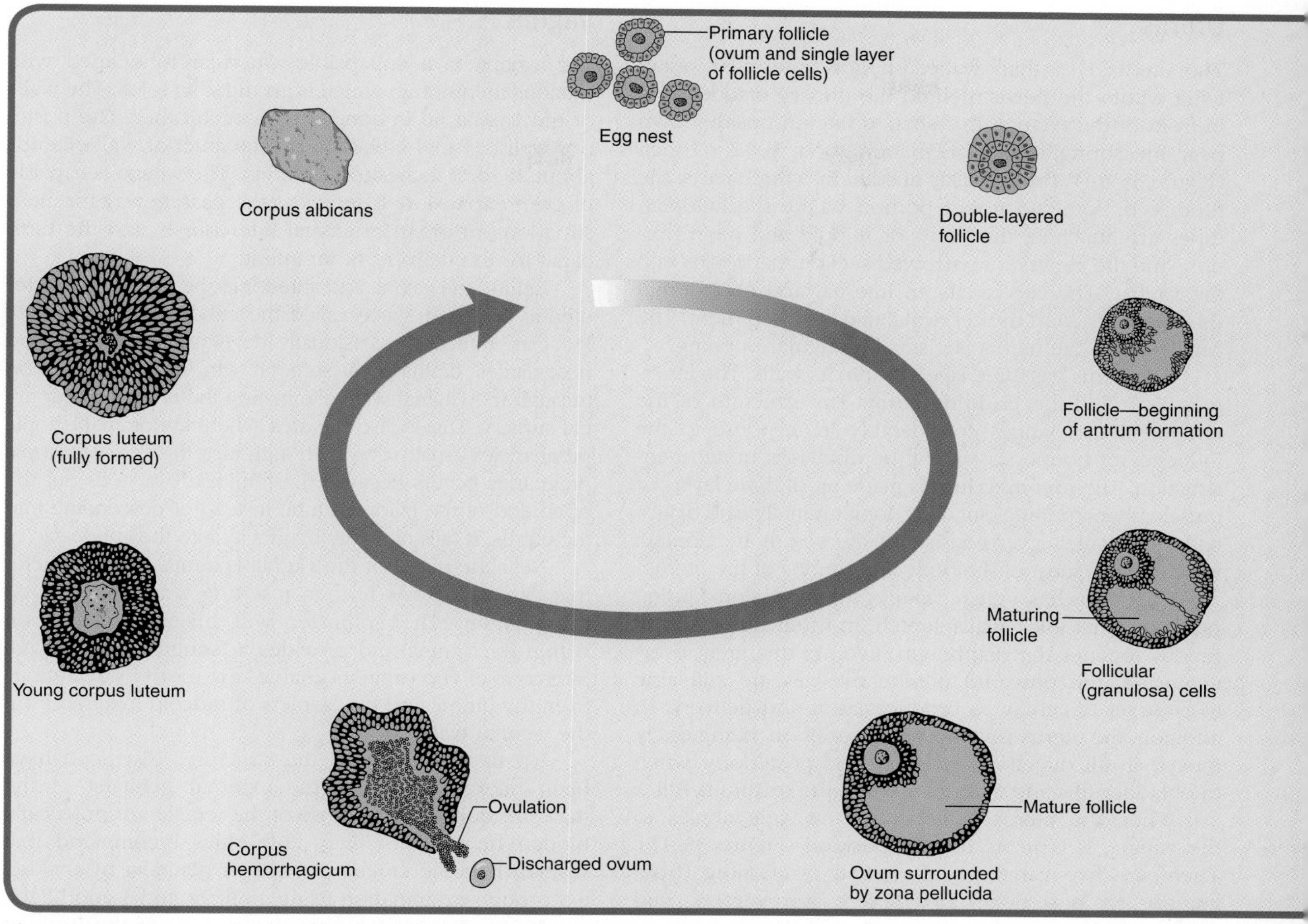

Figure 35–12: The lifecycle of an ovarian follicle and the ovum. *Delmar/Cengage Learning.*

Normally, **conception (fertilization)** takes place in the outer third of the fallopian tube (Figure 35–13). Upon union, the two cells begin to multiply. The corpus luteum causes secretions to be released from glands within the mucosa of the tubes. The secretions provide nutrition for the new zygote, which must now move into the uterus within three to seven days for implantation and development. However, the opening of the tube narrows in the isthmus section to about 1 mm in diameter near the entrance to the uterus. If the zygote is unusually large or slow, or if there is any constriction of the tube, the zygote may not be able to pass through the opening, and an **ectopic** (abnormal location) tubal pregnancy develops. Because there is no space for growth, pain and discomfort will develop within a few weeks. Surgical removal of the embryo is imperative to prevent rupture of the tube.

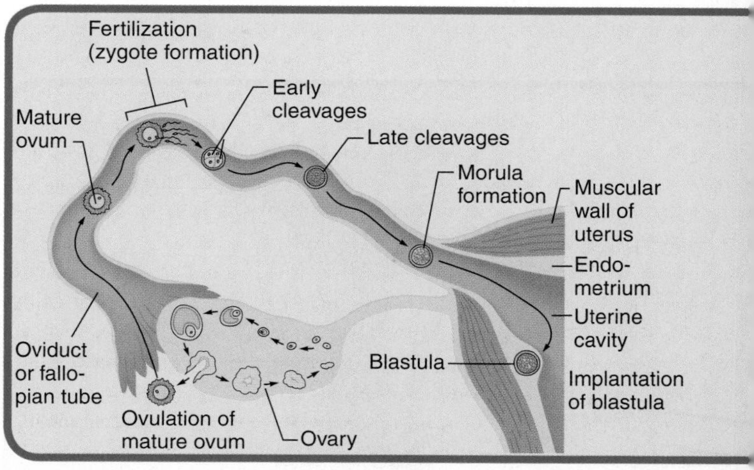

Figure 35–13: Pathway of ovum to fertilization and blastula phase implantation in the uterus. *Delmar/Cengage Learning.*

Uterus

The uterus is a thick-walled, hollow, muscular organ lying within the pelvis, behind the urinary bladder, and in front of the rectum. It is shaped like an upside-down pear, measuring, before pregnancy, about 3 × 2 × 1 inch (Figure 35–14). The uterus is divided into three parts: the fundus, or rounded upper portion where the fallopian tubes are attached; the body, or middle and main portion; and the **cervix**, or narrowed section that opens into the vagina. The cervix has an internal and an external **os** (opening), with the cervical canal between them. The cavity within the uterus is a small triangular opening.

The uterus has three layers within its walls. The innermost is called the **endometrium**. The structure of the endometrium changes considerably in response to the influence of hormones, as will be discussed under menstruation. The **myometrium** is made up of three layers of muscle fibers running circularly, longitudinally, and diagonally. The outer layer consists of the serous membrane, which covers most of the body and fundus of the uterus.

The uterus has a great capacity for expansion. During pregnancy, its thick walls stretch and thin out until the fundus touches the diaphragm. Even at this great overextension, the powerful uterine muscles are still able to contract forcefully to produce labor and delivery. In addition, the uterus is flexible in its position, being easily moved in all directions. It is pressed posteriorly when the bladder fills and anteriorly when the rectum is full.

When the uterus is horizontal, at right angles to the vagina, it is in its normal position (Figure 35–15). There are five variances of normal positioning (from anterior to posterior): **anteflexed**, **anteverted**, mid position, **retroverted**, and **retroflexed**. The uterus may also **prolapse**, or drop downward into the vagina. If these positions cause discomfort or interfere with adjoining structures, a device called a pessary can be inserted into the vagina to support the uterus.

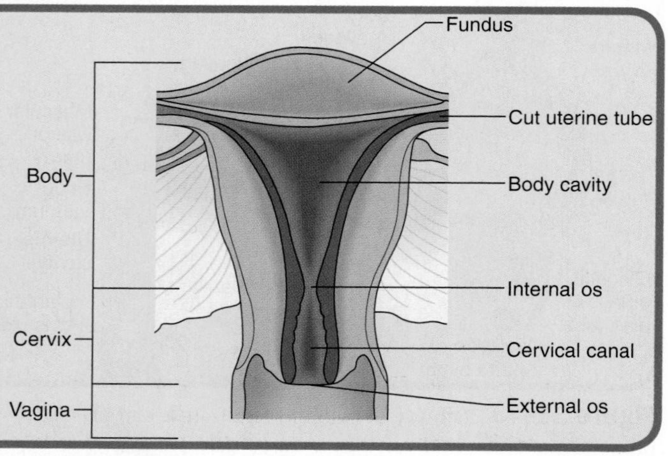

Figure 35–14: The uterus. *Delmar/Cengage Learning.*

Vagina

The vagina is a collapsible muscular tube lined with mucous membrane, which is arranged in folds. The walls of the vagina lie in contact with each other. The posterior wall is 3 to 4 inches long. The anterior wall extends about $2\frac{1}{2}$ or 3 inches to the cervix. The vagina is capable of great expansion. It serves as the passageway for menstruation, an organ of sexual intercourse, and the birth canal for the delivery of an infant.

Behind the vagina and anterior to the rectum is a rectouterine pouch, a space called the cul-de-sac or pouch of Douglas. Infection occasionally develops in this area and necessitates draining. A surgeon can make an incision through the vaginal wall, eliminating the need for abdominal surgery. This is also the area where abdominal ectopic pregnancies usually occur. Though rare, this type of ectopic pregnancy occurs because the fertilized ova goes out the open end of the fallopian tube instead of descending into the uterus. It falls naturally by gravity into the cul-de-sac.

Near the outlet of the vagina is a muscular sphincter that can be detected when inserting tampons or upon examination. The sphincter will maintain a tampon within the vagina and provides a "snugness" for sexual intercourse. The vaginal canal is kept moist by secretions from the uterus and by droplets of mucoid material from the vaginal walls.

Up to this point, all the structures discussed have been internal. Whereas the external genitalia of the male are quite visible, those of the female are practically hidden from sight. Many authorities recommend that women become familiar with their genitalia by making a thorough examination using a mirror and a good light.

The vagina opens onto the surface of the body at the **perineum**, posterior to the urinary meatus and anterior to the anus (Figure 35–16). The external opening is partially covered by folds of mucous membrane called the **hymen**, which border the edges prior to intercourse. Occasionally, the hymen is thicker than normal or covers the entire opening (imperforate hymen). The tissue must be removed prior to menstruation when imperforate. It occasionally requires surgical removal (hymenectomy) to permit intercourse when the narrowing tissue cannot be stretched naturally.

Vulva

The **vulva** is the area of the female external sexual structures. The large pad of fat that is covered with coarse hair on the mature female and overlies the symphysis pubis is known as the **mons pubis**. The labia majora (large lips) are a pair of rounded folds of skin on each side of the vulva and are continuous with the mons pubis. The labia are covered with hair on the exterior surface but with pigmented smooth skin on the inner surface. The labia are composed mainly of fat and numerous glands.

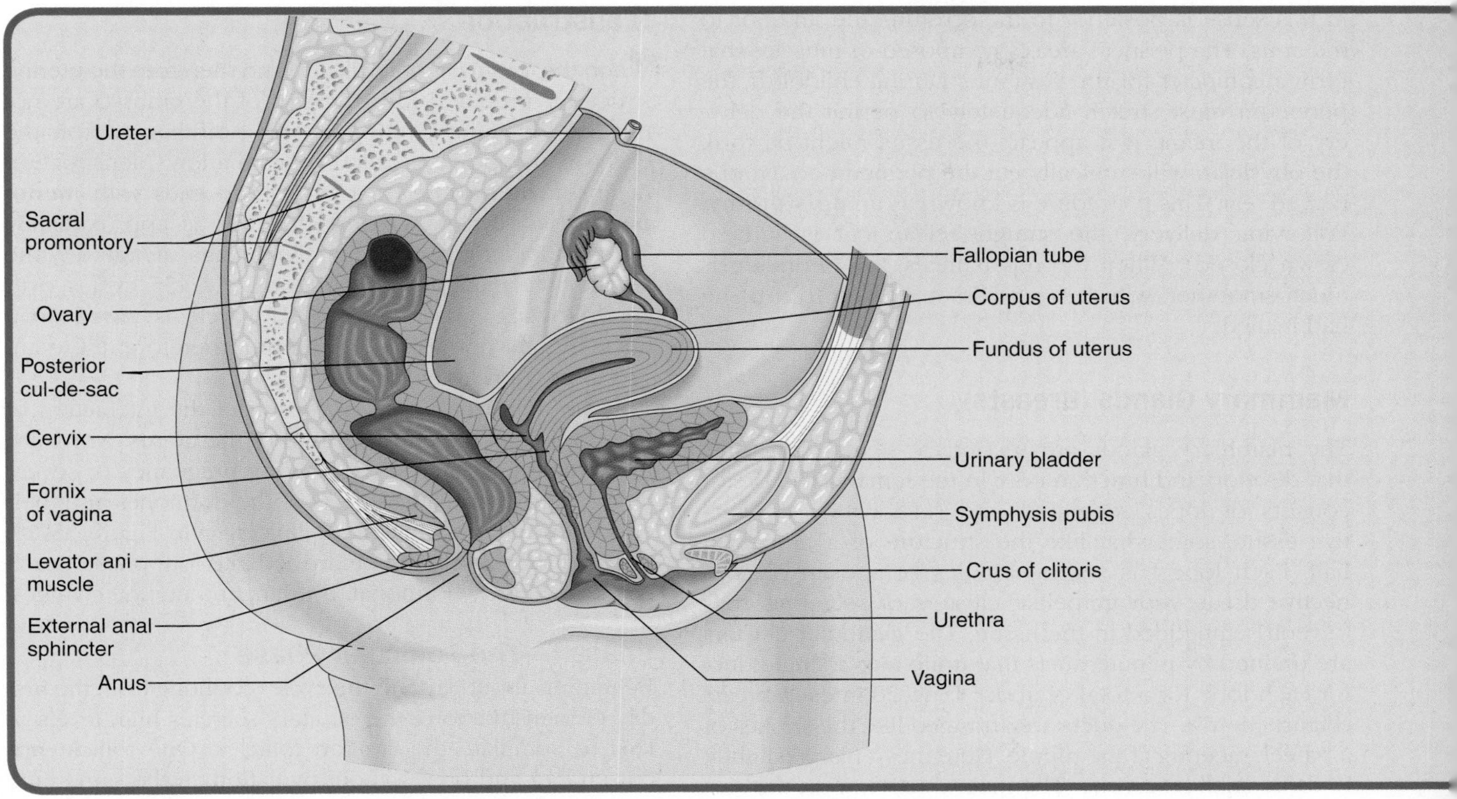

Figure 35–15: Female internal reproductive organs with uterus in normal position. *Delmar/Cengage Learning.*

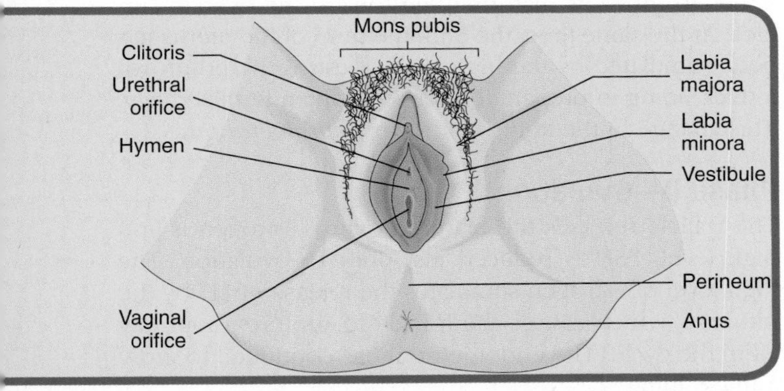

Figure 35–16: Female external genitalia. *Delmar/Cengage Learning.*

The labia majora develop in the female from the same embryonic tissue that becomes the scrotum in the male.

The labia minora (small lips) lie within the labia majora and come together anteriorly in the midline continuous with the prepuce, which covers the glans of the clitoris. The labia minora are covered with mucous membrane that is continuous with the lining of the vagina. The female labia minora develop from the same embryonic tissue as the male penile shaft.

The term vestibule is used to denote that portion of the vulva that lies inside the labia minora and posterior to the clitoris. It contains the opening to the urethra and the vagina. The ducts to the vestibular glands (**Bartholin's glands**) open at the base of the labia minora. They secrete a fluid that serves as a lubricant for coitus (intercourse). Posteriorly, the labia minora are connected by a thin piece of tissue called the fourchette, which is just posterior to the vaginal opening. The fourchette is destroyed by the birth of the first child.

Clitoris

The clitoris is a rounded mass composed of two small columns of erectile tissue. The clitoris develops in the female similarly to the glans and penis of the male, except that the urethra does not descend through its interior. The clitoris and the glans penis are very sensitive and provide for heightening of sexual excitement. The clitoris becomes enlarged and engorged with blood and is involved in the orgasmic response to sexual arousal.

Perineum

The perineum is identified in two different manners. Some physicians consider the entire pelvic floor as the perineum and apply the term to both male and female. But in **gynecology** (the study of female diseases), the perineum refers to the area posterior to the vaginal introitus and anterior to the anus. In the male, the perineum in this sense is posterior to the scrotum and anterior to the anus. The perineal area is composed of muscles that form a sphincter for the vestibule. During childbirth, the perineum must stretch adequately to permit the delivery of the infant. If it appears the tissue might be torn, the physician will surgically cut the perineum to avoid a ragged tear. This procedure is known as an **episiotomy**. Following delivery, the straight, clean cut is sutured (sewn closed). When the repair heals, the perineum is much smoother, with less scar tissue, than if torn tissue had healed.

Mammary Glands (Breasts)

The mammary glands are secondary sexual structures that develop and function only in the female. The breast consists of lobes separated into sections by connective tissue, somewhat like the structure of a grapefruit half. Each lobe has several lobules composed of connective tissue with grapelike clusters of secreting cells (alveoli) embedded in the tissue. The glandular clusters are drained by minute ducts that unite into a single duct for each lobe for a total of about 15 to 20 in each breast (Figure 35–17). The ducts are arranged like the spokes of a wheel, meeting at the nipple. Here they enlarge slightly to form small reservoirs. The main ducts exit on the surface of the nipple through tiny openings.

Fatty tissue is deposited around the surface of the gland, between the lobes and beneath the skin. A darkened area called the **areola** surrounds the nipple. The color of the areola varies from pink in light blonds and redheads to brown in brunettes. A pink areola will turn brown early in pregnancy and regress somewhat after delivery but will not return to pink. About three days after delivery, the glands begin to secrete milk, resulting from hormonal stimulation from the pituitary. The hormone prolactin stimulates the production of milk, whereas oxytocin causes it to be ejected in response to the infant's sucking.

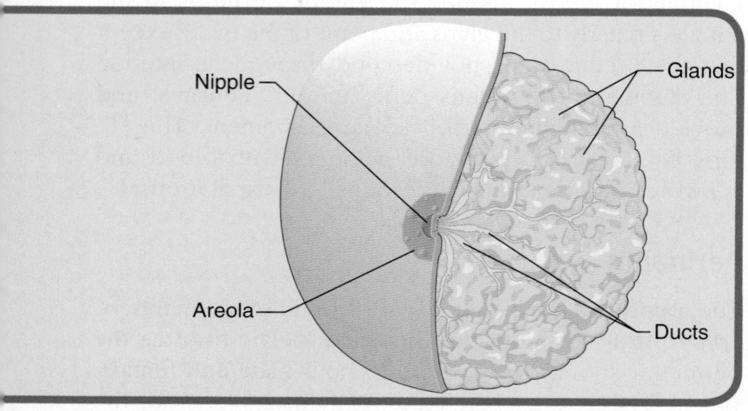

Figure 35–17: The structure of the breast. *Delmar/Cengage Learning.*

Menstruation

When the ovum is not fertilized, and therefore the uterine structures prepared for reception of the embryo are not needed, the lining deteriorates and is discharged from the body in the process called menstruation. Menstruation begins at **menarche** (first cycle) and ends with **menopause** (last cycle). A complete cycle is approximately 28 days in length. If menarche occurs at age 13, the female will experience approximately 455 cycles over the following 35 years. A 28-day cycle is based on a lunar month, not a calendar month; therefore, there are 13 cycles (lunar months) per year.

The menstrual cycle is a result of the interaction of hormones and the endometrium of the uterus. Normally, menstruation is interrupted only by pregnancy or severe illness. The interrelated effects of the hormones and their effects on the sex organs are illustrated in Figure 35–18. The menstrual cycle can be divided into four phases, each characterized by hormonal, ovarian, and uterine changes.

Phase I—The Follicular Phase

Beginning about day 5 in the cycle (counting from the first day of menstruation), the pituitary secretes high levels of FSH to stimulate the ovarian follicles. One follicle ripens an egg and brings about ovulation, at the same time secreting estrogen. About day 10, the pituitary begins to secrete LH in large amounts to react on the follicle. As the estrogen increases, the FSH slows down. The follicle continues to move its maturing egg toward the ovarian surface. At the same time, the endometrium of the uterus has been stimulated by the high level of estrogen and grown a thick lining in preparation for receiving a fertilized egg. This change in the lining is known as *proliferation*.

Phase II—Ovulation

The follicle releases the matured ovum. Estrogen is at a high level; FSH is reduced just prior to ovulation. The high level of estrogen stimulates the release of LH by the pituitary, which causes the follicle to rupture about day 14 in the cycle. The endometrium has continued to grow a thick lining.

Phase III—The Luteal Phase

After the egg is released, the empty follicle undergoes a rapid change caused by the influence of LH. It becomes a glandular mass of cells called the corpus luteum and begins to release progesterone and estrogen. The progesterone reacts on the glands in the endometrium to begin secreting a nourishing substance for the egg. The corpus luteum continues to secrete progesterone for about 12 days until approximately day 26 of the cycle. As the level of progesterone rises, LH is inhibited and the LH level falls. When LH drops, the corpus luteum degenerates, causing the levels of progesterone and estrogen to decline sharply.

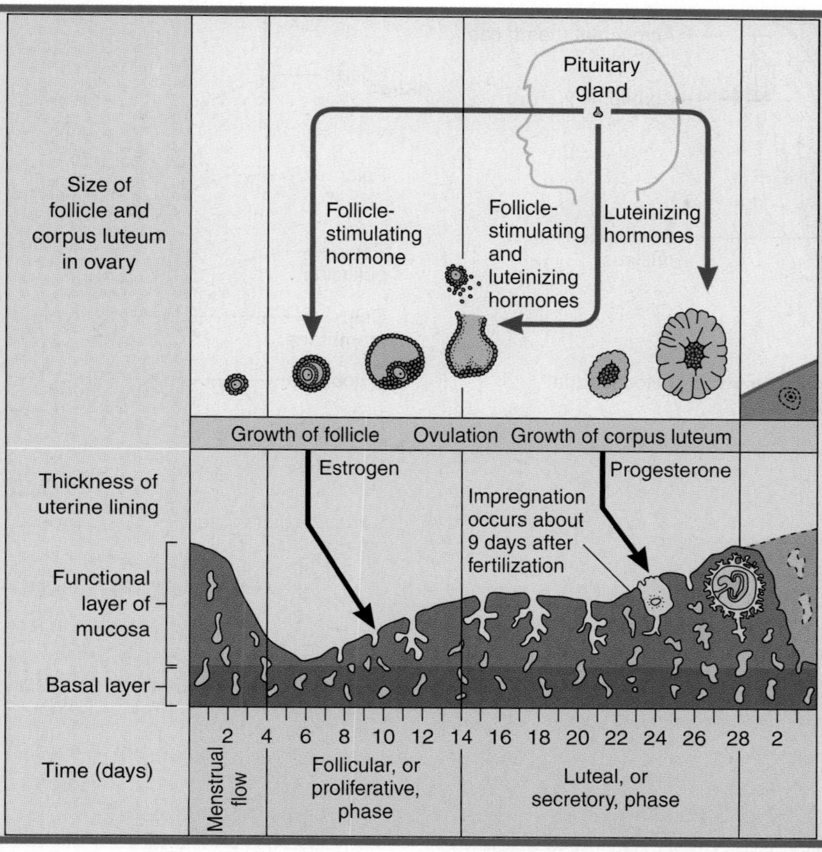

Figure 35–18: Menstrual cycle illustrating the levels of pituitary and ovarian hormones, ovarian cycle, and endometrial changes. *Delmar/Cengage Learning.*

Phase IV—Menstruation

With hormonal support gone, the lining buildup in the uterus begins to slough off (shed), causing menstruation from days 1 to 5. The excess endometrium and a small amount of blood pass out through the cervix. Estrogen and progesterone levels are low, but the FSH level is rising to start the next cycle, preparing the uterine lining and the next ovum for the opportunity of pregnancy.

FERTILIZATION

The miracle of reproduction begins with fertilization. In the process of sexual intercourse, sperm at the rate of about 360 million per ejaculation are deposited into the female vagina. From here the microscopic sperm begin an incredible journey toward a single female ovum, which will normally be in the outer one third of one of the fallopian tubes. The ovum must be fertilized within 24 hours after expulsion from the ovary, or fertilization will have to be postponed until the next ovum is ready in approximately one month.

The sperm travel at a rate of about 1 to 5 millimeters per minute; their course seems to be in a straight line but in a random direction. Studies on humans are difficult to do, but some research has been conducted. In one study, it was found that sperm deposited in the vagina of a woman just prior to surgery had migrated through the fallopian tubes 30 minutes later. This finding could not be explained based on sperm motility alone. It is hypothesized (suggested) that intercourse or artificial insemination causes the release of a hormonal substance that increases uterine contractions, propelling sperm toward their destination.

The ovum is considerably larger than the sperm, yet it is still only about $^{1}/_{125}$ of an inch in diameter (Figure 35–19). When the sperm reach the egg, they surround its outer surface, attempting to enter. Only the strongest sperm are able to survive the acidity of the vaginal secretions to attack the protective corona radiata that surrounds the ovum. In repeated attacks, the sperm release an enzyme called hyaluronidase, which gradually breaks down the ovum's protection. Eventually, an exposed area of membrane will allow one spermatozoan to penetrate the ovum. The head and middle of the sperm enter the ovum while the tail drops off outside. Immediately, the membrane becomes sealed against additional sperm. The nucleus of the sperm moves to combine with the ovum nucleus, and a zygote is formed. At this time, the traits, which are inherited, and the sex of the new individual are determined and cannot be

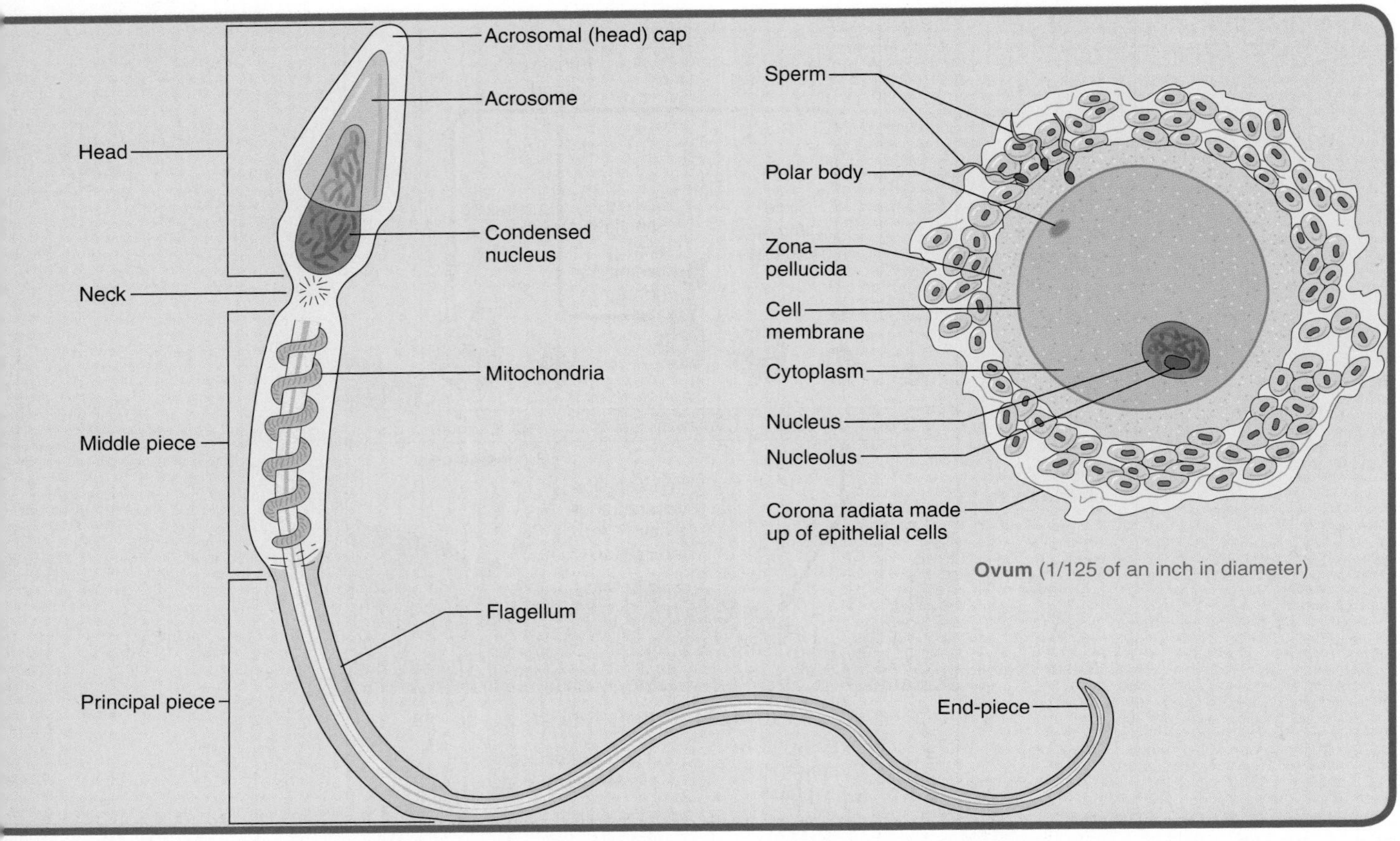

Figure 35–19: Sperm and ovum. (*Note:* Actual size comparison of sperm entering ovum.) *Delmar/Cengage Learning.*

altered. The father has determined the sex, but the other characteristics are contributed by both parents. At this point, conception has occurred.

Following fertilization, the zygote begins the journey to the well-prepared uterus, arriving about six days after ovulation. There it implants itself in the thick wall, and a change in the menstrual cycle begins. At this point, phase III is at about day 20. The endometrium is at its peak. The levels of estrogen and progesterone are high. LH and FSH are low because of the feedback of adequate amounts of hormones; this prevents stimulation of new follicle maturity. The secretions from the fallopian tubes and the uterine glands provide nutrition for the embryo.

The high level of progesterone inhibits the myometrium from contracting; therefore, the embryo cannot be expelled. Progesterone also stimulates development of the ducts of the **mammary glands** (breasts). These effects must be continued to maintain the implantation. If the corpus luteum fails, so does the production of progesterone. Therefore, the developing **placenta** (afterbirth) secretes a hormone, human chorionic gonadotropin (hCG), which maintains the corpus luteum during the early stages of pregnancy. This is the hormone that is detectable on urine pregnancy tests. As the embryo develops, the placenta begins to secrete progesterone and estrogen, and the corpus luteum degenerates and disappears.

The placenta maintains its high level of hormone output throughout pregnancy. When the time for delivery nears, the placenta decreases production of progesterone, which allows the myometrium to begin contracting, and labor begins. With progesterone diminished, the release of prolactin from the pituitary can occur. Prolactin stimulates the mammary glands to produce, for the first few days, *colostrum,* a thin nutritious liquid, and later, milk. The continued production of milk depends on stimulation from the regular sucking of the infant or the removal of milk by pumping.

PREGNANCY

About 36 hours after fertilization occurs, the zygote begins to grow from its one-cell beginning. It is almost beyond comprehension to realize that everything necessary to the formation of a new life, the bones, muscles, blood vessels, the brain, all the organs, and the skin and hair are all contained in one microscopic cell. In addition, the life-support system of the placenta and umbilical cord and the protective membranes and **amniotic** fluid also develop from this single cell. By about day 6, the small cluster of cells firmly implant within the uterine wall, and it enters the embryonic period (8 weeks) of development when most of the major organ systems are formed at an amazing speed. The group of cells arrange themselves into three layers from which the various organs are formed. One layer, the *ectoderm,* becomes the nervous system, skin, hair, and parts of the eye. The *endoderm* layer becomes the digestive and respiratory systems. The skeletal, muscular, connective tissue, reproductive, and circulatory systems develop from the *mesoderm* layer.

The **embryo** develops from the head down, which explains why, in Figure 35–20, the head is so large compared with the rest of the body. By the end of the 10th week of **pregnancy**, all systems are completed, even to nails on the fingers. Many of the organs begin limited function by the 7th week. After 8 weeks, the embryo is called a **fetus**. By week 12, the sex can be determined, and the fetus is about 4 inches long and weighs about two thirds of an ounce. This marks the end of the first **trimester** or one third of the total pregnancy period.

It is obvious the fetus has a lot of growing to do, and it does so rapidly. By week 20, movement can be felt and the heartbeat is detectable with a fetascope. By now, the pregnancy is about half way through. A fetus must be carried past the next several weeks to survive. If born in week 23, a little past 5 months, it will weigh less than 2 pounds and has a 1 in 10,000 chance of surviving.

By the 20th week, the fetus opens its eyes, and by week 24, it can hear sounds from inside the uterus. The movements are very vigorous by now, and there are periods of sleep and wakefulness as the second trimester ends.

During the last trimester, the fetus adds greatly to its size. By the end of the 7th month, it has assumed a head-down position and if born would have over a 50% chance of survival. The odds increase to about 95% at 8 months when weight reaches 5 pounds, to 99% at full-term 9 months with average weight being 7½ pounds and a length of 20 inches.

The pregnant woman also undergoes body changes during pregnancy. Initially, the first sign is a missed menstrual period. This is a time of joy for couples who have been trying to **conceive** but may be less than welcome to others. Another early sign is breast tenderness caused by the stimulation of hormones. Some women will expe-

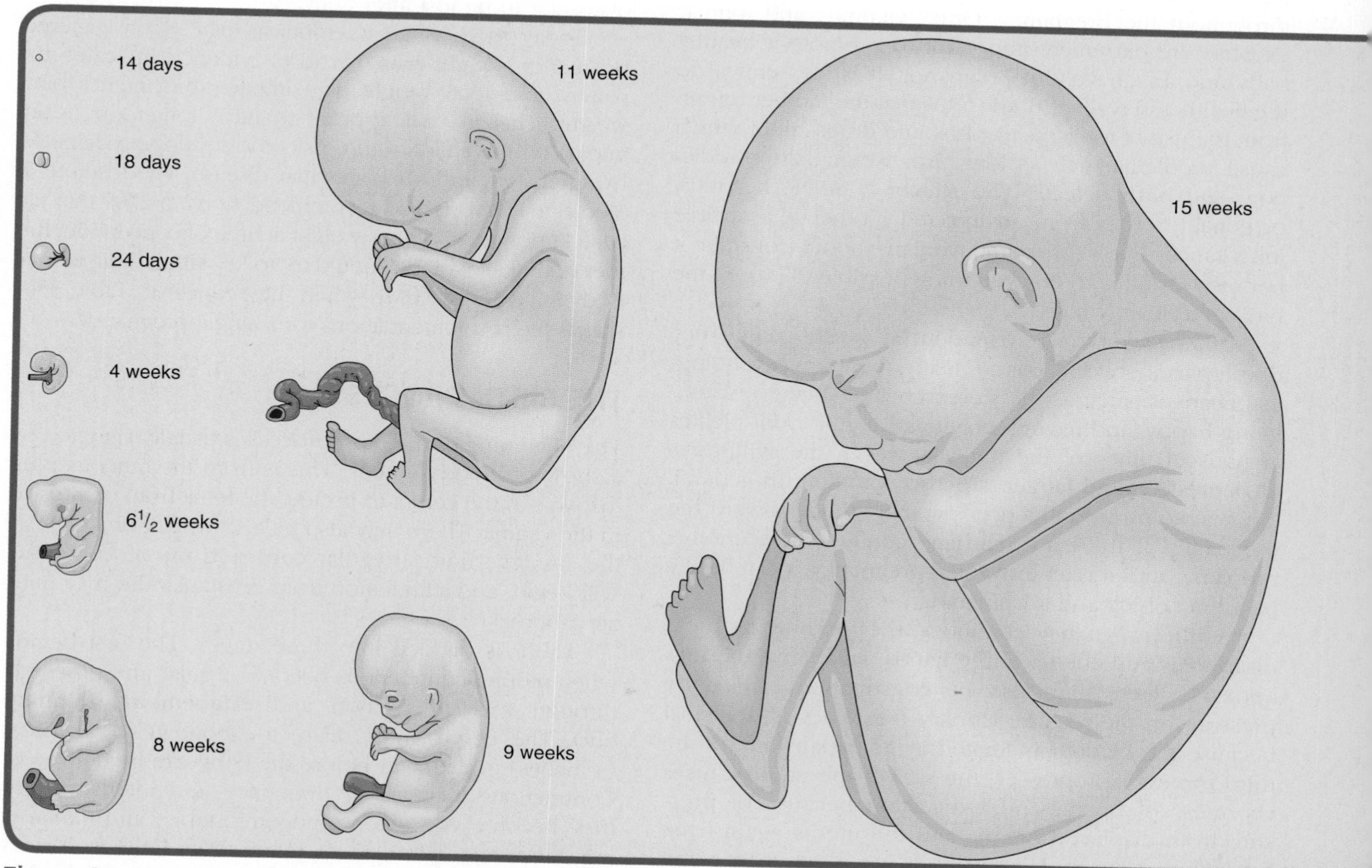

Figure 35–20: Changes in the body size of the embryo and fetus during development in the uterus (all figures natural size). *Delmar/Cengage Learning.*

rience "morning sickness," especially for the first six to eight weeks. Usually, there is more frequent urination, fatigue, and the need for additional sleep. By the 8th to 10th week, pregnancy can be detected by manual pelvic examination and the bluish hue of the formerly pale pink cervix. This change is called "Chadwick's sign." Once pregnancy is confirmed, the woman is usually interested in the expected delivery date. It is calculated using Nagele's rule, which states: Take the first day of the last menstrual period, subtract 3 months, and add 7 days, plus a year. For example, if the first day of the last period was September 1, 2013, the expected day of delivery would be June 8, 2014. Remember, this is only the "expected" date. Babies have a habit of being born when they are "ready." On a percentage basis, 39% are born within five days of the projected date and another 55% are within 10 days. The rest obviously are either early or late.

It is important to confirm pregnancy early so that good prenatal care is started. Proper nutrition, such as 1 mg of folic acid daily, is recommended three months prior to conception to decrease the risk of neural tube defects of the fetus. If a woman has a history of a previous child with a neural tube defect, she should increase the dose to 4 mg daily prior to conception and continue throughout the pregnancy. Other vitamins and regular exercise are extremely important to promote a healthy baby and an uneventful pregnancy. It is also critical to the health and welfare of the fetus that the mother refrain from the use of tobacco, alcohol, and drugs, all of which cause problems such as low birth weight, drug addiction, and birth defects. The effects of AIDS, hepatitis, or genital herpes from an infected mother is a terrible inheritance. Every pregnant woman should consider it her responsibility to do everything possible to ensure the birth of a healthy baby.

Other symptoms experienced with pregnancy develop as the weeks pass. Usually, there are psychological changes, such as the stereotypes of "being radiant," being happy, and having "cravings" (e.g., for dill pickles at unusual times of the day). However, the symptoms of depression and fatigue are also common. In general, the symptoms are influenced by the attitude toward the pregnancy. If there are marriage conflicts or economic problems, or if it is an unwanted pregnancy, it can hardly be a time of joy and anticipation.

As the pregnancy continues, the morning sickness disappears and edema of the hands, face, feet, and legs appears. There may also be constipation caused by pressure on the rectum. Urinary frequency is universal because the bladder is limited in its expansion. As the third trimester progresses, the size of the uterus causes shortness of breath and indigestion because of pressure from displaced organs and the uterus against the lungs and stomach. Hemorrhoids are a common result of constipation and pressure on the blood vessels of the rectum.

TABLE 35–1 IOM Recommendations for Weight Gain During Pregnancy

BMI at Conception	Weight Status	Permissible Weight Gain
BMI 18.5 kg/m2	underweight	28 to 40 lbs.
BMI 18.5 to 24.9 kg/m2	normal weight	25 to 35 lbs.
BMI 25.0 to 29.9 kg/m2	overweight	15 to 25 lbs.
BMI 30.0 kg/m2	obese	11 to 20 lbs.

Weight gain continues throughout pregnancy. Most physicians prefer to establish a set amount of permissible gain. The total weight of the baby (7–8 pounds), placenta (1½ pounds), enlarged uterus (2 pounds), enlarged breasts (1–3 pounds), and additional fat and water (about 6–8 pounds) add up to about 18 pounds, so 20 pounds is sometimes the recommended amount of gain. Excess weight causes complications such as hypertension, increased stress on the heart, and the problem of weight to be lost after delivery.

Today there is great emphasis placed on maternal pregnancy weight gain because evidence indicates the pattern and total weight gain impacts the infant's birth weight. This in turn appears to have long-term health impact on the child's future risks for developing diabetes, hypertension, and cardiovascular disease. The Institute of Medicine (IOM) issued recommendations in 2009 that are based upon the mother's weight at time of conception, further stating all women should try to be within their normal Body Mass Index (BMI) when they conceive. Table 35–1 shows the recommendations for a single pregnancy.

THE BIRTH PROCESS

The beginning of the birth process is usually signaled by a show of bloody mucus. This is from the mucous plug that was in the cervix to protect the fetus from organisms in the vagina. There may also be a slow leak or a gush of the amniotic fluid. Irregular **contractions** of the uterus will begin, and stimulation from prostaglandin may initiate labor.

Labor is divided into three stages. The first begins when uterine contractions become regular and proceeds through cervical dilation and **effacement** (thinning out). The cervix must dilate to about 10 centimeters (4 inches) in diameter before the baby can be delivered. Contractions increase in frequency and intensity until they become very strong, uncomfortable, and exhausting. First stage labor varies between as little as 2 to as long as 24 hours; 12 to 15 hours is average for a first pregnancy.

The second stage of labor begins with complete dilation and the entrance of the head (or another part) into the vagina. Continued contractions and bearing down by the woman push the baby through the vagina until it is visible at the entrance; this is known as *crowning* (if it is a head presentation). Strong contractions and pushing force the head through the vaginal opening, then the baby rotates to the side so the shoulders can be delivered. The rest is easily passed, and the second stage is completed.

The baby is suctioned to remove mucus from its mouth and nose, and crying begins to inflate the lungs. The baby's body function changes dramatically. For the first time, it must breathe on its own to take in oxygen and begin to circulate its own blood. It changes from a bluish color to a healthy skin tone within several minutes. As soon as the baby's condition is satisfactory, the umbilical cord is clamped, tied, and cut.

To help assess a newborn's condition, a universally accepted evaluation technique called the Apgar scoring system is used. Observation of the newborn is made at 1 and 5 minutes following delivery. The ratings are entered on a chart and the scores totaled. A score of 10 is considered the best possible condition. A score of 7 to 9 is considered adequate, and no treatment is required. A score of 4 to 6 indicates close observation, and some intervention, such as suctioning, is necessary. A score below 4 requires immediate intervention and continued evaluation. Table 35–2 is an example of the Apgar scoring system.

The third stage of labor begins with the detachment of the placenta from the uterine wall, and the *afterbirth* (placenta and its membranes) are expelled. Usually, a few more contractions are required to accomplish this stage. After it has emptied, the muscles of the uterus maintain a level of contraction to close off open blood vessels and control bleeding.

In some cases, such as inadequate pelvic outlet, breech presentation (other than head), large baby, ineffective labor, or the development of a serious complication, the baby may need to be removed by **cesarean** section. This involves cutting through the abdomen and into the uterus to remove the baby and the afterbirth. About 30% of all deliveries are cesarean. Pregnancy following a cesarean section may undergo a trial of labor if certain factors are considered. It is commonly called vaginal birth after cesarean (VBAC) and is successful in 60% to 80% of cases. One main concern is the type of *uterine* incision that was made. This may not be the same as that on the surface of the abdomen. If a transverse uterine incision has been made, across the lower, thinner part of the uterus (Figure 35–21), it is the least likely to result in complications in a subsequent vaginal delivery. The low vertical incision is an up and down cut in the lower, thinner area of the uterus, and risks are not well documented. The classic, a high vertical incision in the upper part of the uterus, is not as frequently done now because this type of incision requires that women have repeated cesareans because of the risk of uterine rupture during labor.

INFERTILITY

Infertility refers to the inability to become pregnant after one year of sexual intercourse without the use of birth control. It affects one in seven couples in the United States. One cause for infertility may be the delay in childbearing until after age 30. Infertility can be traced to the woman in about one third of the cases, to the man in another third, and to both in the last third. For the woman, the problem is usually a blocked fallopian tube, damaged ovaries, or abnormally developed tubes. Many times, it is the absence or infrequency of ovulation. In the male, it is usually abnormally developed testicles, a

TABLE 35–2 Apgar Scoring System

Sign	0	1	2	Rating 1 min	Rating 5 min
Heart rate	Not detectable	Below 100	Over 100		
Respiratory effort	Absent	Slow, irregular	Good, crying		
Muscle tone	Flaccid	Some flexion	Active motion of extremities		
Reflex irritability (response to flick on sole)	No response	Grimace, slow motion	Cry		
Color	Blue, pale	Body pink, extremities blue	Completely pink		
			TOTAL		

Scoring system developed by Dr. Virginia Apgar

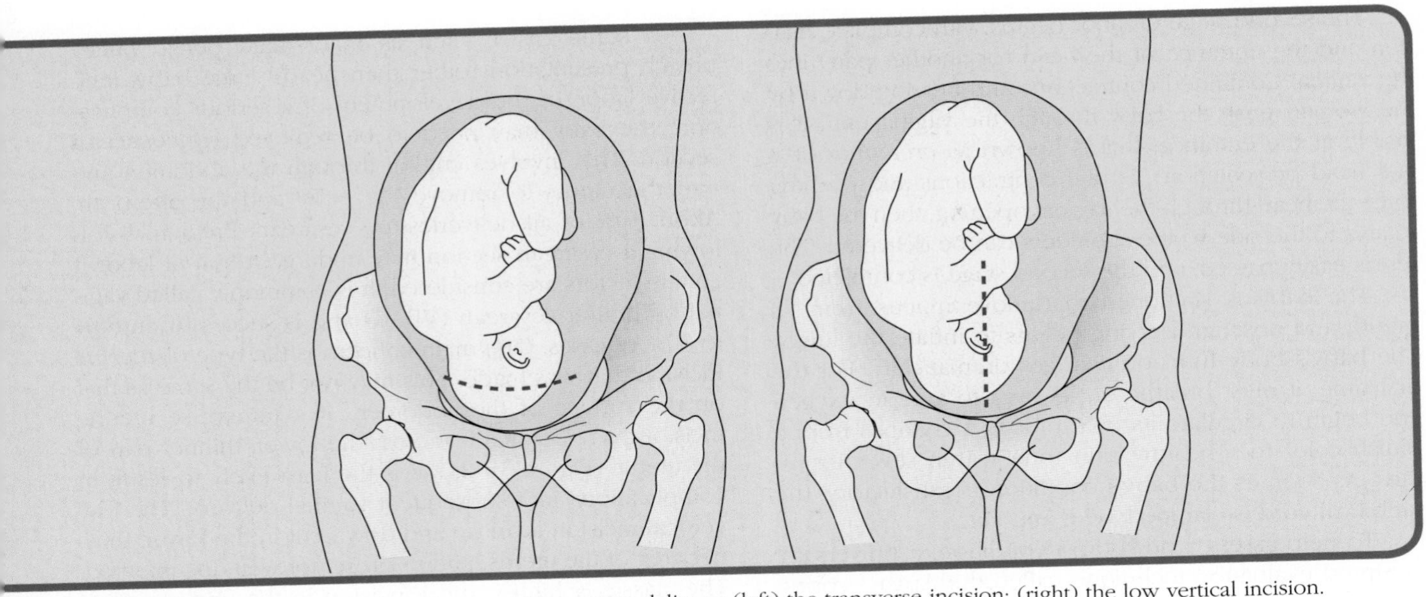

Figure 35–21: The types of incision used in cesarean delivery: (left) the transverse incision; (right) the low vertical incision.
Delmar/Cengage Learning.

low sperm count, or low motility. Sexually transmitted diseases (STDs) account for a large percentage of infertility by silently damaging the fallopian tubes and ovaries. It is very important that young men and women understand the importance of practicing safe sex by using condoms and decreasing the number of sexual partners.

Treatment consists of medications to stimulate egg or sperm production or surgery to repair damaged organs or abnormalities. Other actions such as determining ovulation, intercourse on alternating fertile days (to collect sperm), and the use of boxer shorts for men (this reduces the body heat transferred to the testicles by tight briefs) are indicated. When this is unsuccessful, other methods can be used, such as:

- *Artificial insemination*—The semen is spun down to concentrate the sperm, which are withdrawn and injected into the uterus through a catheter in the cervix. The specimen can be from the women's spouse or another male donor.
- *In vitro fertilization*—The eggs are retrieved through a needle inserted into the ovaries, fertilized with sperm in a laboratory, and placed into the uterus.
- *Gamete intrafallopian transfer (GIFT)*—This involves injection of egg(s) mixed with sperm directly into the fallopian tube(s) so that fertilization can occur.
- *Intracytoplasmic sperm injection (ICSI)*—This is a microsurgical procedure involving the direct injection of a single sperm into an egg cell. This procedure is done in instances where only a very few sperm cells are produced or where those sperm cells are incapable of entering an egg on their own. ICSI is also used in those cases where sperm has to be recovered directly from the testes because of blockage of the normal route of sperm cells.
- *Zygote intrafallopian transfer (ZIFT)*—This is a combination of *in vitro* fertilization and gamete intrafallopian transfer. Eggs are fertilized in the test tube, and the resulting embryos are transferred to the fallopian tube by laparoscopy. ZIFT is infrequently used.

Procedures to produce pregnancy are proceeded by medications that increase the maturation of eggs to increase the odds of fertilization. Due to these processes, multiple fertilzations and embryos can occur, resulting in multiple births.

CONTRACEPTION

The authors acknowledge that some religious and ethnic groups oppose birth control, and this text does not ignore that issue; however, this subject matter is presented factually, from a clinical viewpoint, as information required for practice as a medical assistant. As the word implies, **contraception** is literally "against" conception. Several reasons may be given to avoid pregnancy:

- Avoid health risks to the woman. A woman in poor health may not survive a pregnancy.
- Spacing pregnancies. Some women are very fertile and conceive every year or less. The infant death rate is reported to be 50% higher at one-year intervals than at two or more years.
- Avoid having babies with birth defects. Some women have chromosome defects or are genetic disease carriers (or married to carriers) and choose not to risk pregnancy.
- Delay pregnancy early in marriage to allow a time for adjustment to avoid additional stress in the new relationship and establish a strong marriage.

- Limiting family size. It is sometimes a personal decision and other times a reality of limited resources.
- Avoid pregnancy among unmarried couples. Single parenthood is difficult.
- Permit the woman to develop a successful career with planned pregnancies to integrate motherhood.
- Curbing population growth. The concern over worldwide food supply and supportive environment prompts some to promote contraception.

Several methods to prevent conception and their relative percentage of effectiveness are listed in Table 35–3. Selection is usually made by the woman in consultation with her doctor. The cost, ease of use, degree of effectiveness, and likelihood of side effects must be taken into consideration when selecting a method.

Pregnancy Termination

Abortion (A-bor′-shun) (Miscarriage)

Description—This is the spontaneous (unforced) elective or induced (therapeutic) loss of a pregnancy of less than 20 weeks' gestation.

Signs and symptoms—Symptoms of spontaneous abortion are a pink or brownish discharge for several days followed by uterine cramping and increasing vaginal bleeding. When contractions are sufficient, the cervix dilates and the fetus is expelled. A complete abortion includes expulsion of the fetus, placenta, and membranes, resulting in the end of cramping and minimal bleeding because the uterus contracts to close off the blood vessels. An incomplete abortion results from the retention of some or all of the placenta.

Etiology—A spontaneous **abortion** usually results from one of three factors: (1) *fetal:* defective implantation or development of the embryo (most common cause); (2) *placental:* premature separation or abnormal implantation of the placenta; or (3) *maternal:* endometrial rejection, infection, malnutrition, trauma, drug reaction, endocrine difficulties, or blood group incompatibility. Spontaneous abortions occur in about 30% of all first pregnancies and up to 15% of all pregnancies.

TABLE 35–3 Different Methods of Preventing Conception

% Effective	Method	Description/Comments
100%	Abstinence	Refraining from sexual intercourse; absolutely most effective.
100%	Sterilization	Tubal **ligation** (cutting of the fallopian tubes) is done in the female. The cut ends can be sewn back in opposite directions or cauterized. The surgical procedure is done through a laparoscope inserted into the abdomen. The procedure is considered permanent. A vasectomy is done in the male, with the ends being sewn in opposite directions. The surgery is performed through a small incision at the base of the scrotum. Vasectomies are usually not reversible; however, in some instances, reconstructive surgery has been successful, especially in cases of shorter duration; sperm production is usually significantly decreased in time. Usually, a second marriage and the desire for another child prompt the attempt. The method is relatively expensive initially.
99%	Depo medroxyprogesterone acetate (DMPA) suspension	This is an intramuscular injection that is given quarterly and provides protection for three months. The injection is given during the first five days of a normal menstrual period and provides contraceptive effects immediately. It is contraindicated if there is a possibility of being pregnant, a history of blood clots in the legs or lungs, known or suspected breast cancer, a liver tumor, or unexplained vaginal bleeding. Some side effects may occur, such as nervousness, dizziness, stomach discomfort, headaches, or fatigue. It may reduce the amount of minerals stored in bones, which could contribute to the development of osteoporosis. The most common side effect is irregular or unpredictable menstrual periods. Some women will stop having periods until 6 to 18 months after stopping the injections. A new warning was issued in 2005 that Depo-Provera should not be used more than two consecutive years due to possible bone loss from estrogen suppression.

(continues)

TABLE 35–3 *(Continued)*

% Effective	Method	Description/Comments
95%–99%	Birth control pills	Many different kinds are available. They are a combination of hormones that prevent ovulation; no ovum means no pregnancy. Failure occurs when pills are not taken as prescribed. Side effects can be prohibitive for some women. They are available only by prescription and require regular visits to a physician. Cost is a factor to consider. Examples are Loestrin, Ortho-novum, and Tri-Norinyl.
99%	Contraceptive patch	The contraceptive patch contains hormones similar to those in birth control pills. The patch is just as effective as the pill (99% when used correctly). It is paper thin and as soft as the skin. The patch is changed weekly for three weeks, then left off for the 4th week, when a menstrual period will occur. The side effects and warnings are the same as with oral contraceptives. The patch does not protect against sexually transmitted diseases.
99%	Contraceptive ring	The contraceptive ring is a comfortable, flexible ring about 2 inches in diameter that is inserted into the vagina once per month. The ring will release a low level of hormones to prevent conception. The ring is removed after three weeks so a menstrual period can occur. A new ring is inserted for the next three weeks. The ring is also 99% effective, the same as oral contraceptives, and carries the same risk factors and warnings.
93%–99%	Intrauterine device (IUD)	The intrauterine device is a small piece of plastic or coiled material inserted into the uterus to prevent implantation of a fertilized egg, presumably by providing irritation to the endometrium. Failure can occur if the device is expelled and during the first few months after being inserted. Initial insertion costs and the cost of removal are involved. IUDs are only recommended for women who have had children and who are in monogamous relationships because there is an increased risk of uterine infection with this device. Side effects include increase in menstrual cramping and possible increase in vaginal discharge throughout the month. IUDs are available in two types: one is paraguard copper and is effective for up to 10 years. Another, Nirena, contains progesterone and comes in a five-year form.
90%–99%	Diaphragm	A thin piece of dome-shaped rubber with a firm ring, which is inserted into the vagina to cover the cervix and provide a barrier to sperm. It is most effective when used in combination with a contraceptive cream placed into the dome before inserting. Failure usually results from improper insertion; a defect in the rubber, such as a hole; failure to insert before any penile penetration; or failure to maintain in place at least six hours following intercourse. There is an initial cost to examine and fit and purchase. There are side effects. It requires cleaning and inspection after each use.
85%–97%	Condom	A thin sheath of rubber or latex that fits over an erect penis to catch the semen. A properly used condom is very effective. It must be unrolled onto an erect penis *before* any penetration occurs. It is important to leave about ½ inch of free air space at the tip (unless the condom is constructed with a tip) to catch the semen; otherwise, the force of the ejaculant may burst the condom. It must also remain in place throughout intercourse. After ejaculation has occurred, care must be taken to withdraw with the condom in place. It may require grasping with the fingers. This is the only contraceptive that also provides a level of protection against sexually transmitted diseases. It is relatively inexpensive, easy to use, and readily available. Remember, only a latex condom is also effective against the AIDS virus.

% Effective	Method	Description/Comments
75%–97%	Female condom (Figure 35-22)	This is a latex pouch suspended from an inner ring that fits over the cervix. The pouch extends to the outside and has an external ring that holds the opening outside the vagina. The condom provides a barrier for protection against sexually transmitted diseases and contraception. A new condom must be used with each intercourse. Care must be taken to ensure that the penis enters inside the pouch and that the pouch remains in the proper position throughout intercourse.
70%–75%	Spermicides	Contraceptive foams, jellies, sponges, and creams with *sperm-killing* ingredients, inserted by applicator deep into the vagina before intercourse. It must remain for at least six to eight hours afterward. Each application is good for only one act of intercourse. They should not be relied on alone as an effective contraceptive. Combined with a diaphragm or condom, they are effective. They have few side effects (some report allergic reactions), are easily used, and are readily available. They must not be confused with lubricants such as KY jelly or Lubafax, which contain *no* spermicide.
70%–80%	Withdrawal	This method has been practiced since biblical times. It simply requires that the penis be withdrawn and ejaculation occur outside the vagina. It is not very effective because some sperm are deposited in the vagina before ejaculation occurs. In addition, the man may not be able to withdraw in time. It requires a lot of concentration to control. It is also not advised because it may lead to a sexual dysfunction if practiced for a prolonged time.
65%–85%	Rhythm	The practice of abstinence during an eight–day period from days 10 to 17 of the menstrual cycle when conception is theoretically possible. The method works fairly well for women who are extremely regular in their cycles and couples who can practice strong self-control. However, it requires a careful assessment of at least six months of cycles to establish ovulation days. If cycles vary in length, the period of abstinence must be increased to cover the longest possible time.
Unknown	Douching	Absolutely not effective. It only takes several minutes for sperm to enter the cervix. Douching, in fact, may even assist sperm toward the cervix, thereby increasing the odds of conception.

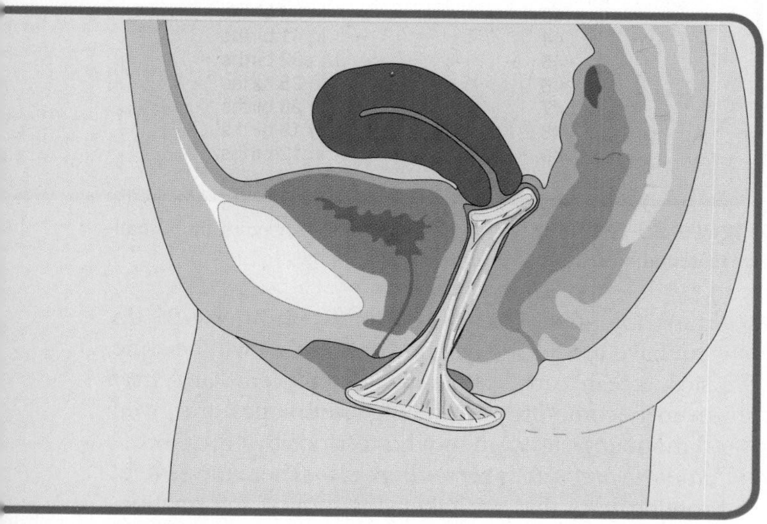

Figure 35–22: Female condom placement. The pouch should not be twisted, and the outer ring must be outside the vagina. *Delmar/Cengage Learning.*

Treatment—If the placenta (or a portion) adheres to the uterine wall, bleeding will persist, necessitating a D & C (**dilation and curettage**) to scrape out the retained placenta and permit the uterus to close off the blood vessels.

A therapeutic abortion is one performed to preserve the mother's mental or physical health in such instances as rape; unplanned pregnancy; or an existing medical condition, such as cardiac or kidney disease.

Diagnostic and Screening Tests in Pregnancy

- ***Alpha-fetoprotein screening (AFP)***—This is a blood test taken at about the 15th to 18th week of pregnancy to aid in the detection of birth defects. It can also indicate the presence of multiple births. If the blood level is too high, additional tests will be performed to rule out neural tube defects. These are instances when there is a failure of the brain and skull to develop or there is an opening in the spine, exposing the spinal cord—a condition known as spina bifida. When the blood level is too low, Down syndrome is suspected. The tests are not 100% accurate but serve as a screening device detecting about 85% of open neural tube defects and about 75% of fetuses with Down syndrome in women under 35 years of age. When positive results are obtained, another blood sample, an ultrasound, and an amniocentesis are indicated. Remember that a negative test does NOT guarantee a baby free of birth defects but only that it is unlikely that there is neural tube defect or Down syndrome.

- *Amniocentesis*—Down syndrome is caused by a chromosomal error (see Chapter 23). This occurs in 1 of every 1,000 live births. A test known as an **amniocentesis** can be done on women who apparently are at risk. Amniotic fluid is withdrawn from the amniotic sac in which the fetus is growing (Figure 35–23). Cells from the skin of the fetus can be grown in a culture and examined for chromosomal abnormalities and neural tube defects. The test is usually done between 13 and 16 weeks, and ultrasound is used to visualize the fetus and amniotic fluid. Amniocentesis is 100% accurate in findings, but it is not without risk. A miscarriage rate of 1 in 200 to 1 in 300 is associated with the procedure. The incidence of Down syndrome correlates to the age of the mother. In her 20s, a woman has only a 1 in 2,500 chance of having a Down syndrome child. That incidence increases dramatically as the woman ages. By age 45, the risk increases to 1 in every 40 births. Figure 35–24 shows the frequency of Down syndrome in relationship to age from 30 to 49 years.
- *Chorionic villi sampling (CVS)*—A procedure similar to amniocentesis but done by removing cells from the chorionic villi. This procedure is not as common as amniocentesis and is associated with more complications. Like amniocentesis, this is 100% accurate for chromosomal testing.
- *Gestational diabetes screening*—This test is done between 24 and 28 weeks of pregnancy by drawing a blood sample after drinking a loading dose of glucose. Gestational diabetes only affects pregnant women. It is absent after delivery.
- *Group B streptococcus (GBS)*—GBS is one of the many bacteria that do not usually cause serious illness. It may be in the digestive, urinary, or reproductive tract, but it is most common in the vagina and rectum. Infected persons who show no symptoms are said to be colonized and usually do not pose any danger to their own health and may not be treated. However, when there is a pregnancy, 1 to 2 out of every 100 babies will be infected. Vaginal cultures are used to test during 35 to 37 weeks of pregnancy. This type of bacteria is found in up to 40% of pregnant women. It can be passed on to the fetus during pregnancy, to the baby during delivery, or to the baby after birth. Most babies who get GBS do not have any problems; however, a few will become sick. It can cause major health problems and may even become life threatening. Antibiotics are given during labor to women who test positive for GBS.
- *Routine pregnancy screening tests*—There are several routine tests that are taken for routine information, such as blood typing, antibody screenings, sexually transmitted disease screening, and urine cultures.

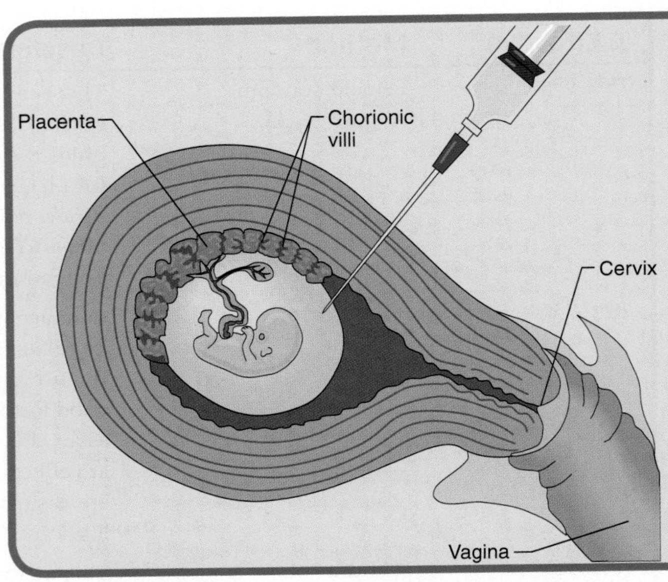

Figure 35–23: Amniocentesis. *Delmar/Cengage Learning.*

DOWN SYNDROME AND MATERNAL AGE

Maternal Age	Frequency of Down Syndrome
30	1 in 885 births
31	1 in 826 births
32	1 in 725 births
33	1 in 592 births
34	1 in 465 births
35	1 in 365 births
36	1 in 287 births
37	1 in 225 births
38	1 in 176 births
39	1 in 139 births
40	1 in 109 births
41	1 in 85 births
42	1 in 67 births
43	1 in 53 births
44	1 in 41 births
45	1 in 32 births
46	1 in 25 births
47	1 in 20 births
48	1 in 16 births
49	1 in 12 births

Figure 35–24: Risk of giving birth to a Down syndrome infant by maternal age. *Delmar/Cengage Learning.*

OBSTERICAL HISTORY

Date	Hospital	Sex	Length of Gestation	Type Delivery	Birth Weight	Anesthesia	Complications

MEDICAL HISTORY

Surgery ______

Medications ______

Alcohol ______

Tobacco ______ Caffeine ______

Drug Abuse ______

Toxoplasmosis exposure: ❑ Yes ❑ No ❑ Advised

Varicella history: ❑ Yes ❑ No ❑ Unknown

Drug allergies (Type Reaction) ______

Latex allergy: ❑ Yes ❑ No

Transfusion (? Reaction) ______

Hospitalizations ______

Recent BC (?) ❑ Yes ❑ No

FAMILY HISTORY

Diabetes ______

Hypertension ______

Multiple Births ______

Genetic Diseases ______

Mental Retardation ______

Birth Defects ______

Signature ______ **R.N. Date** ______

DHYSICIAL EXAM (✓ = Normal) Height ______

HEENT ______

Thyroid ______

Breasts ______

Heart ______

Lungs ______

Abdomen ______

Extremities ______

Pelvic:

Ext. Genitalia ______

Vagina ______

Cervix ______

Uterus ______

Adnexa ______

Capacity ______

Signature ______ **M.D. Date** ______

MEDICAL ILLNESSES (Circle)

HBP DM Thyroid Heart Lungs GI Kidneys

UTI STD Anemia Neurologic Psych Genital Herpes

Specify ______

LABORATORY

Date	Lab	Result
	Blood Type/Rh	
	H/H	______ g/dl ______ %
	RPR	Non reactive / Reactive
	Hb Sag	Negative / Positive
	Rubella	Immune / Non-immune
	Urine Culture & Sensitivity	No Growth / ______
	HIV	Non-reactive / Reactive
	Varicella IgG	Immune / Non-immune
	Sickle Cell Screen	Negative / Positive
	Antibody Screen	Negative / Positive
	GC	Negative / Positive
	Chlamydia	Negative / Positive
	Pap	Normal /Abnormal ______
	MSAFP	Normal /Abnormal ______
	Glucose Challenge	______ mg/dl
	3 hr GTT	______ F ______ 1h ______ 2h ______ 3h
	Rh Immune Globulin (28wk)	
	GBBS	Not Present / Present
	GC	Negative / Positive
	Chlamydia	Negative / Positive

D T 0 1 5 5

Outpatient Clinic
Antepartum Record Part 3

BL 173-1-02 (recorder-PS)

NAME

DOB

MR #

FAN #

Figure 35–25: Sample antepartum form with routine pregnancy screening tests. *Delmar/Cengage Learning.*

Figure 35–25 is an example of an outpatient clinic form used to record obstetrical information that is obtained on all new patients. Note the laboratory section, which lists various routine screening tests performed to assure the patient's health status.

DIAGNOSTIC TESTS OF THE FEMALE REPRODUCTIVE SYSTEM

- ***Colposcopy***—An examination and biopsy of the cervix using a colposcope. It is done to rule out cancer when there are abnormal Pap smear results. Often, cell structure may be temporarily altered by antibiotics, yeast infections, and other reasons, which might give a false positive Pap smear. The cervix is cleansed with a solution of acetic acid and the scope introduced. The cervix can then be viewed through the colposcope, which magnifies the mucosa and makes cellular structure visible. In most cases, biopsies are taken from the abnormal sites. A Pap smear is a screening test, whereas colposcopy is used to obtain a definitive diagnosis.
- ***Hysteroscopy***—A hysteroscope is inserted vaginally into the uterus. It is connected to a monitor that permits viewing of the endometrium. By using instruments through the scope, it is possible to biopsy suspicious areas and remove polyps and fibroids. It is even possible to take photographs or make a videotape for documentation of findings (Figure 35–26). When the hysteroscope is used with a laparoscope, it is possible to increase the visual field and facilitate the performance of surgical procedures. In the Figure 35–26, the use of both scopes permits visualizing both the inside and outside of the uterus at the same time.
- ***Mammogram***—An X-ray of the breast for the detection of malignancy. A mammogram is indicated whenever there are palpable breast masses, breast pain, or nipple discharge. The film can also help differentiate between benign breast disease or breast malignancy. The American College of Radiologists recommends a single baseline mammogram for all women between ages 35 and 40. All women older than 40 should have an annual mammogram. Women at risk require earlier and more frequent examinations. Risk-related factors are fibrocystic disease; history of breast, uterine, ovarian, colorectal, or salivary gland cancer; and a family history of breast malignancy.
- *Maturation index*—A means of determining hormonal level by examining the percentage of certain types of cells in scrapings taken from the lateral vaginal walls.
- ***Papanicolaou (Pap) smear*** (test)—A routine examination done on secretions removed from the cervix and upper vagina to determine the presence of cancerous cells.

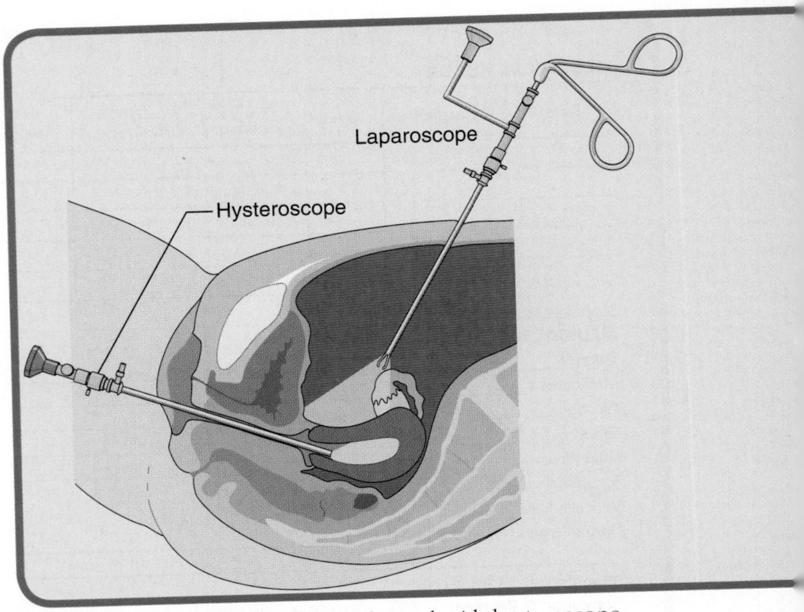

Figure 35–26: Laparoscopy performed with hysteroscope.
Delmar/Cengage Learning.

- *Pregnancy test*—Conducted on a first-voided morning urine specimen to determine presence of the hormone human chorionic gonadotropin (HCG), which is produced by the developing placenta at the onset of pregnancy.
- *Ultrasonography*—A test for malignancy. A transducer is used to focus a beam of high-frequency sound waves through the skin into the breast. Sound waves bounce back echos, which are displayed on a computer screen for diagnosis. Ultrasound can detect tumors less than ¼ inch in diameter and can distinguish between cysts and solid tumors.
- *Ultrasonography* is also used to observe the fetus *in utero*. It can help determine the status of pregnancy, confirm the expected date of delivery, and identify the gender, if desired.

Ultrasonography is also useful to diagnose cysts, fibroids, pelvic masses, and pelvic pain such as with extopic pregnancy.

DISEASES AND DISORDERS OF THE FEMALE REPRODUCTIVE SYSTEM

Cervical Erosion (Ser′-vi-kal E-ro′shun)

Description—This is an ulceration of the epithelium on a portion of the cervix.

Signs and symptoms—The area bleeds easily when touched during examination and may cause intermenstrual bleeding.

Etiology—It results from chronic cervicitis.

Treatment—Erosion is treated locally by cauterization (burning) to destroy the abnormal tissue growth. Cauterizing agents used can be chemical, such as silver nitrate sticks, or electrical, such as electrocautery. The treatment is administered through a vaginal speculum and produces immediate cramping, which subsides quickly. Vaginal discharge will increase for a few days as the tissue sloughs off.

Cervicitis (Ser-vi-si′-tis)

Description—This is inflammation of the cervix.

Signs and symptoms—Often, the only symptoms are a purulent, foul-smelling vaginal discharge and a tenderness of the cervix.

Etiology—It is caused by an invading organism, usually chalmydic staphylococcus or streptococcus. Herpes simplex II is a possible cause. A large percentage of patients in whom the cervicitis is associated with pelvic inflammatory disease are infected with the gonorrhea bacteria.

Treatment—Treatment is usually an antibiotic appropriate for the causative organism.

Cystic (Fibrocystic) Breast Disease (Fibro-sis′-tik)

Description—This is the presence of multiple lumps within the breast tissue. The lumps may be fibrous tumors that have degenerated or cysts (sacs) containing fluid.

Signs and symptoms—They may occur singularly or in multiple clusters. Fibrous tumors are either round or lobular. They are usually firm, well-defined (with definite borders), freely movable, and painless. Cysts are also round, soft to firm, elastic, well-defined, movable, and often tender. Neither type is attached to underlying tissues or to the skin to cause signs of retraction.

Etiology—There is probably no specific "cause" of this disorder. It is not a "disease" as such but rather a condition of normal breast tissue that has just "developed." It tends to occur with aging.

Treatment—Treatment may include needle aspiration of cystic fluid. Often, the cyst will not refill. Women with fibrocystic disease are believed to be at greater risk of developing a malignancy in one of the masses.

Many women naturally have "lumpy" breasts and should not be classified as having a "disease." Young women often have dense breast tissue that feels lumpy all over. This is just a condition of being fibrocystic. Often breasts become fibrocystic as a woman ages. Only professional examination and mammography can accurately diagnose a fibrocystic condition.

Cystocele (Sis′-to-sel)

Description—This is the bulging of the anterior wall of the vagina by the bladder pushing into the vaginal canal, sometimes into the introitus.

Signs and symptoms—It can be demonstrated by asking the patient to bear down or strain as the vaginal opening is observed.

Etiology—Cystocele appears in older women because of poor musculature from aging and the effects of childbearing. Other predisposing factors are obesity, lifting of heavy objects, instrument deliveries, and chronic coughing. The displacement of the bladder contributes to improper emptying, which results in cystitis, frequency (because some urine is always in the bladder), urgency, and incontinence, particularly stress incontinence as a result of coughing, sneezing, or laughing.

Treatment—If it causes discomfort or continual urinary problems, it may be necessary to surgically reposition the bladder and repair the vaginal wall.

A non-surgical option may be appropriate. It involves the use of a pessary, which can be cup-shaped, donut-shaped, an inflated hollow ring, or other shapes that can be inserted into the vagina to support the uterus. The devise puts pressure against the vaginal wall to push against the cystocele.

Dysmenorrhea (Dis-men-o-re′-a)

Description—This is the lower abdominal and pelvic pain associated with menstruation common among young females. It tends to decrease with maturity, particularly after pregnancy. **Dysmenorrhea** in women in their late 20s or early 30s may be a symptom of an organic disease, such as cervical stenosis, pelvic congestion, or endometriosis.

Signs and symptoms—Dysmenorrhea typically begins 12 to 14 hours before the onset of menses and lasts between 24 to 48 hours. It may be associated with headache, nausea, vomiting, fatigue, and diarrhea. Occasionally, pain may be felt in the back and upper legs.

Etiology—It is unrelated to any identifiable cause. However, certain contributing factors are known, such as hormonal imbalances and psychogenic factors. The discomfort probably results from increased secretion of the hormone prostaglandin, which intensifies uterine contractions. Dysmenorrhea is also present with other conditions, such as endometriosis, cervical stenosis, uterine leiomyomas (tumor in the muscle tissue), incorrect uterine positioning, and PID (pelvic inflammatory disease).

Treatment—Treatment consists of analgesics; heat; drugs to decrease uterine contractions; and the use of hormonal therapy, such as oral contraceptives, to suppress ovulation. When discomfort has an organic cause, the underlying condition must be corrected.

Endometriosis (En-do-me-tre-o′-sis)

Description—The presence of endometrial tissue outside the uterus is most commonly found in the pelvic area, affecting the ovaries, ligaments, and peritoneal tissues.

Signs and symptoms—The condition is characterized by dysmenorrhea, with constant pain in the lower abdomen, pelvis, vagina, and back beginning about a week before menses and lasting two to three days after onset. The degree of pain depends on the location of the endometrial tissue. Other symptoms include excessive, profuse menses when ovarian; hematuria when located in the bladder; rectal bleeding when located in the colon; and nausea, vomiting, and abdominal cramps when located in the small intestine.

Etiology—The cause of endometriosis is unknown, but it is believed to be the result of the following:

- Recent surgery that opened the uterus
- Endometrial fragments expelled through the fallopian tubes at menstruation
- Alteration in the epithelium by inflammation or hormones that changes it to endometrium

Treatment—Treatment consists of conservative methods in younger women, such as analgesics, nonsteroidal anti-inflammatory drugs, and oral contraceptives. Oral contraceptives are the current treatment of choice for long-term therapy because of the action of ovulation suppression. Other injectable medications such as Lupron Depot is used for six-month therapy. It works by decreasing estrogen and progesterone normally produced by the ovaries. This is mainly used after the diagnosis of endometriosis has been determined, although some physicians are now using Lupron Depot prior to surgery for treatment. After the six-month therapy, menstrual cycles will return to normal. When ovarian masses exist, they may be surgically removed. In women who no longer desire children, the treatment of choice is **hysterectomy** (removal of the uterus) and bilateral **salpingo-oophorectomy** (removal of both fallopian tubes and ovaries). The condition is not life-threatening, but pain and anemia must be controlled. Because the disease may cause sterility, childbearing should be accomplished as soon as convenient. Endometriosis generally subsides with menopause if surgery is ruled out.

Fibroids (Fi′-broydz)

Description—**Fibroids** are known technically as uterine leiomyomas or myomas; they are a common benign, smooth tumor formed of muscle cells, not fibrous tissue as suggested by the name. Usually, fibroids do not occur singly and are located most often in the body of the uterus.

Signs and symptoms—The primary symptom associated with leiomyomas is **menorrhagia** (excessive menstruation). Other characteristics are pain, a feeling of heaviness in the abdomen if the mass is large, discomfort from pressure against other organs, possible urinary frequency or constipation, and an irregular enlargement of the uterus. When a leiomyoma is attached to the lining by a stalk and is suspended within the uterine cavity, pain is caused by the uterus contracting in an attempt to expel the mass. The patient is frequently anemic because of excessive bleeding. The diagnosis is usually confirmed by a D & C, showing cells from leiomyoma in the scrapings from the endometrium.

Etiology—The cause of leiomyomas is unknown, but it is believed they are cells that have grown into a tumor, probably stimulated by estrogen and the growth hormone, because following menopause they usually shrink in size.

Treatment—Treatment depends on several factors, such as the patient's age, general health, and desire for children; the size of the tumors; and the severity of the symptoms. Lupron Depot is used to treat uterine fibroids for one to three months prior to surgery. The medication shrinks the fibroids, therefore minimizing bleeding with surgery. Small masses can be surgically removed (myomectomy), but a complete hysterectomy is indicated with greater involvement. The ovaries are left intact if possible to maintain hormone levels naturally. Uterine leiomyomas occur in about 20% to 30% of all women older than age 35, with leiomyosarcoma (malignancy) developing in only about 0.1% of patients.

A newer procedure, embolization of the uterine artery, can also treat leiomyomas. A small catheter is passed through the femoral into the uterine artery. A small device is implanted in the appropriate artery to stop the flow of blood. Without blood the uterine mass shrinks and symptoms disappear.

Hysterectomy (His-ter-ek′-to-me)

Description—This is the surgical removal of the uterus. It is one of the most common procedures performed on female patients. It is not usually done on an elective or request basis but as a solution to a problem, such as endometriosis, leiomyomas, uterine rupture, or malignancy. A hysterectomy can be performed in different ways, depending on the situation. Figure 35–27 illustrates the extent of surgery. Removing the uterus through an abdominal incision is called an abdominal hysterectomy. When the uterus is positioned appropriately, it can be removed through the vagina, called a vaginal hysterectomy.

Endometrial **ablation** is used in cases of excessive bleeding from the buildup of endometrium or benign fibroid. A pen-sized instrument called a resectoscope is inserted into the uterus through the cervix. The procedure removes the lining by electrical cautery, using a loop or rollerball attached to the end of the scope. It requires about 20 minutes to perform, is relatively painless, avoids surgery, takes only a few days' recovery time, and is a fraction of the cost of a hysterectomy. In contrast, a hysterectomy is major surgery, requiring well over an hour to perform and approximately six weeks to recover. The ablation is probably an alternative for 20% to 50% of the annual 600,000 hysterectomies done mainly to stop uncontrollable bleeding. The procedure almost always results in sterilization, which of course would also happen with a hysterectomy. There is a slight chance of perforating the uterine wall, which may then lead to a hysterectomy.

Ovarian Cyst

Description—This is a sac of fluid or semisolid material on an ovary; it is usually nonmalignant, small, and produces no symptoms. Common cysts include follicular and lutein types that occur in the follicle or the corpus luteum. They can occur any time between puberty and menopause, including during pregnancy.

Signs and symptoms—An ovarian cyst may cause an acute abdomen (a sudden condition, probably requiring surgical treatment) if the ovary is twisted by the cystic mass or the cyst ruptures. Large or multiple cysts may cause pelvic discomfort, lower-back pain, and abnormal uterine bleeding. Symptoms vary according to the type of cyst. Other possible symptoms are acute abdominal pain similar to appendicitis, massive intraperitoneal hemorrhage, and delayed menses followed by prolonged or irregular bleeding.

Etiology—Follicular cysts develop as a result of an overdistended follicle that fails to close off properly. They secrete excessive amounts of estrogen in response to the FSH hormone. Granular lutein cysts are enlargements of the ovaries caused by excessive accumulation of blood during the bleeding phase of the menstrual cycle. Another form of lutein cyst is usually found bilaterally and contains clear, straw-colored liquid.

Treatment—Follicular cysts generally require no treatment because they spontaneously disappear within 60 days. Oral contraceptives or progesterone for five days reestablishes the hormonal cycle and induces ovulation. Treatment may also include drugs to induce ovulation or surgery to remove a portion of the ovary if drug therapy fails. Treatment generally consists of observation if the cyst is known to be nonmalignant. Signs of cyst rupture, such as increasing abdominal pain, distention, rigidity, fever, tachypnea, hypotension, and symptoms of intraperitoneal hemorrhage, are carefully watched. Occasionally, a cyst becomes so large that it causes discomfort, which may require surgery.

PMS (Premenstrual Syndrome)

Description—This combination of characteristics appears from seven to 14 days before menstruation and usually subsides with the onset. It is estimated that the syndrome occurs in 30% to 50% of women, particularly between the ages of 25 and 40.

Signs and symptoms—Symptoms include any or a combination of the following:

- Behavioral changes, such as nervousness, irritability, fatigue, and depression
- Neurologic changes, including headache, dizziness, numbness of extremities, and fainting
- Respiratory changes, including increase in colds, exacerbation (aggravation or increase) of allergic rhinitis, and asthma

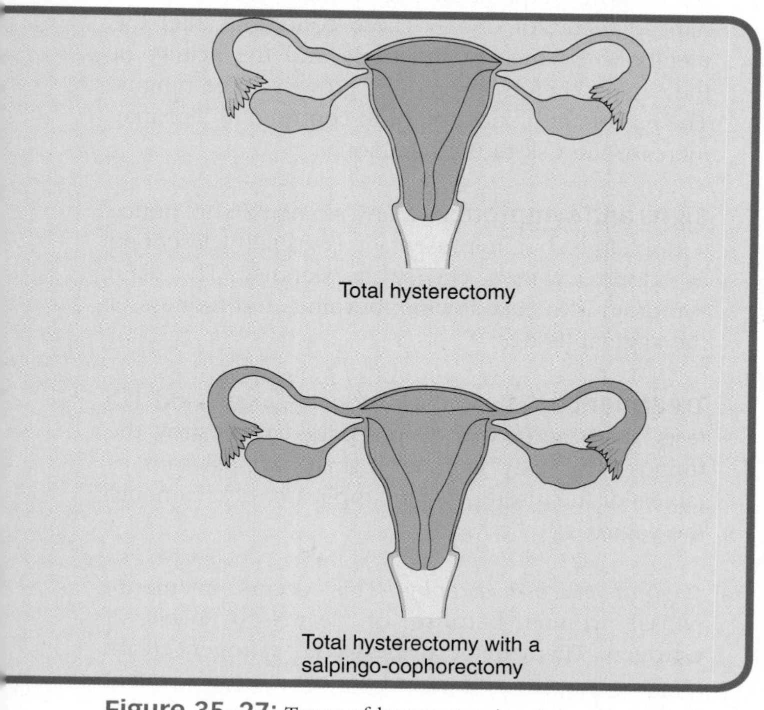

Figure 35–27: Types of hysterectomies. *Delmar/Cengage Learning.*

- Gastrointestinal changes, such as constipation, diarrhea, abdominal bloating, and change in appetite
- General symptoms of backache, palpitations, temporary weight gain, increase in acne, or breast tenderness and enlargement

Etiology—The cause of premenstrual tension is unknown. For some reason, intravascular fluid enters the body tissues and results in secretion of an antidiuretic hormone. This causes fluid retention with characteristic bloating. The tissue edema results in headaches and alterations in mood because of central nervous system changes.

Treatment—Treatment basically is symptomatic. Medication can be used to help relieve emotional symptoms and the physical manifestations.

Polyp (Pol′-ip)

Description—This is a growth with a slender stem attachment usually arising from the mucous membranes.

Signs and symptoms—Polyps of the cervix can often be visualized protruding from the external cervical os. They are red, soft, and rather fragile. If only the tip can be seen, it cannot be differentiated from a polyp of the endometrium.

Etiology—It probably results from the unrestrained cell growth of the epithelium.

Treatment—Depending on the location, size, and attachment, removal may be a simple office procedure or an outpatient surgical procedure. Protruding polyps can be chemically cauterized in the office. The procedure causes some immediate discomfort, primarily cramping, but soon subsides.

Rectocele (Rek′-to-sel)

Description—This is bulging of the posterior vaginal wall, by the rectum, into the vagina.

Signs and symptoms—Inspection of the introitus may disclose a posterior mass, or it may be demonstrable on requesting the patient to bear down. It is most common in postmenopausal women.

Etiology—Contributing factors are believed to be pregnancies, prolonged labor, instrument deliveries, obesity, chronic coughing, and lifting of heavy objects. A **rectocele** of advanced degree may cause difficulty in emptying the rectum.

Treatment—If severe, surgical intervention to repair the vaginal wall and support the rectum can be performed. The nonsurgical option using a pessary may be appropriate. The inserted device puts pressure against the posterior vaginal wall to push against the rectocele.

Vaginitis (Vaj-in-i′-tis)

Description—This is an inflammation of the vaginal mucosa. There are several causes of **vaginitis**, with varying symptoms and treatment.

1. *Allergic reaction*—This usually happens as a result of douche solutions (especially those that are scented), spermicidal materials, deodorant-treated tampons, or other materials inserted into the vagina. This can be treated easily by discontinuing the causative agent.
2. *Bacterial vaginitis (vaginosis)*—This was formerly called gardnerella or nonspecific vaginitis. It is a complex condition that is not understood well at present. The cause of this infection is thought to be an overgrowth of several different types of organisms. The predominant symptom is an increase in vaginal discharge, often with an unpleasant "fishy" odor. Redness and itching are rare; however, because bacterial vaginitis can occur with other types of infections, other symptoms may be present. Treatment involves oral antibiotics or an antibiotic vaginal cream therapy.
3. *Candidiasis*—Also called fungus, yeast infection, or **moniliasis**, this is the most common type of vaginal infection that causes irritation symptoms.

   Etiology—It is caused by a fungus like yeast that requires glucose for growth. It can affect any woman but is more frequent among women who are pregnant, diabetic, or obese. These conditions alter the metabolic balance of the body and the acidity of the vagina, thereby promoting growth of the fungus. The use of antibiotics and birth control pills also may increase the risk of the infection.

   Signs and symptoms—Many women do not notice a discharge, but if present, it is usually described as odorless with a "cheesy" appearance. The main symptom is intense itching, burning, and redness of the vaginal tissues.

   Treatment—With confirmation by exam and lab tests, medication will be prescribed to destroy the fungus. This may include vaginal suppositories or tablets or the insertion of an applicator of cream into the vagina.

4. *Vaginal mucosa atrophy*—This occurs in menopausal women because of decreased levels of estrogen. This can be treated with estrogen cream inserted into the vagina or by estrogen replacement therapy.

MALIGNANCY OF THE FEMALE REPRODUCTIVE ORGANS

Breast

Description—This is the most common malignancy among females and the number two cause of death. It occurs most often in women older than age 35.

Breast cancer is more common in the upper outer quadrant and in the left breast. It spreads through the lymphatic and circulatory system to the lungs, liver, bone, adrenal glands, kidneys, and brain. Cancer may be classified according to its location and cellular type as adenocarcinoma (from the epithelium) or Paget's disease (cancer of the nipple). In addition, most cancers are classified according to stages to identify the amount of tumor, node, and extent of metastasis.

Signs and symptoms—Specific warning signals that may indicate breast cancer are:

- A lump or mass in the breast tissue
- Change in breast size or shape
- Change in appearance of the skin
- Change in skin temperature (a warm, hot, or pink area)
- Drainage or discharge from a non-nursing woman or discharge produced by manipulation
- Change in the nipple, such as itching, burning, erosion, or retraction

Pain should be investigated but is not usually an early symptom.

Diagnosis is most often made by mammography, ultrasonography, and surgical biopsy. A new technique called Elastography may someday be the diagnostic method of choice, replacing the biopsy. The test uses ultrasound waves and compression to diagnose cancer. The breast lump that is a benign tumor is soft and will compress, whereas a malignant tumor is stiff and holds its shape. In preliminary studies, the technique has been nearly 100% accurate in differentiating between benign and malignant tumors. There are major advantages in that a surgical procedure is eliminated, the test is relatively inexpensive, and it can provide results in a matter of minutes. This greatly reduces the anxiety of waiting several days for a diagnosis while a tissue sample is prepared and a microscopic examination is performed.

The best and most reliable means of detecting breast cancer early is mammography. Numerous studies have shown that early detection saves lives and increases treatment options. The 2010 American Cancer Society estimates for new cases of breast cancer in women was 207,090 with an additional 1,970 cases in men. A total of 40,230 deaths were estimated.

Etiology—The cause is not known, but estrogen is believed to be in some way responsible. Predisposing factors include a family history of breast cancer, long menstrual cycles, early menarche or late menopause, first pregnancy after age 30, obesity, and drinking alcoholic beverages. There is also a correlation with diet, especially fat intake.

Treatment—The type of surgical treatment selected for breast cancer takes into consideration, first of all, the stage, the woman's age, the medical circumstances, and the patient's preferences. Physicians have become more aware of the woman's fears, attitudes, and feelings about the disfigurement of her body and will, if possible, choose the least radical method of surgery.

A lumpectomy (removal of the tumor only) can be done on a small mass when there is no evidence of lymph node involvement. The next step would be a lumpectomy and removal of axillary lymph nodes but not the breast itself. With additional breast involvement but no node enlargement, a simple **mastectomy** would remove just the breast and no underlying muscles. A modified radical mastectomy removes the breast and axillary nodes. A radical mastectomy removes the breast, axillary lymph node, and muscles from the chest wall. Radical mastectomies are seldom performed because of the lack of statistical data to verify their additional survival benefit. Treatment of ductal carcinoma *in situ* includes local excision, radiation, and tamoxifen.

Recent advances have been achieved in mastectomy surgery. Reconstruction of a breast mound can be provided for most patients. A prosthesis may be implanted after underlying tissues are excised with the skin and breast surface structures being maintained. The approach is determined by the extent of involvement. A mastectomy is disfiguring surgery that alters the patient's body image drastically, because it can affect a woman's opinion of her sexuality and her relationship with her sexual partner. Numerous volunteer support groups and other services are available to assist with the problems of adjustment.

Surgical treatment is usually combined with chemotherapy and/or radiation in an attempt to destroy cells within other structures of the body. Hormone therapy involves the use of androgens, or an antiestrogen, depending on the hormone-receptive nature of the tumor. Tamoxifen is an antiestrogen drug that is used not only to treat cancer but also to help prevent its initial occurrence in certain women or recurrence following treatment. Another type of drug, a Selective Estrogen Receptor Modulator, called Evista, is used for women at high risk of invasive breast cancer.

The five-year survival rate for localized breast cancer is 97% today. If it has spread regionally, the rate drops to 77%, and with distant metastases, the rate is only 21%. After five years, the rate of survival continues to decline, with the best survival being among women with early-stage disease.

Figure 35–28 shows the chest wall of a female who has had a double mastectomy. Twenty-three years ago,

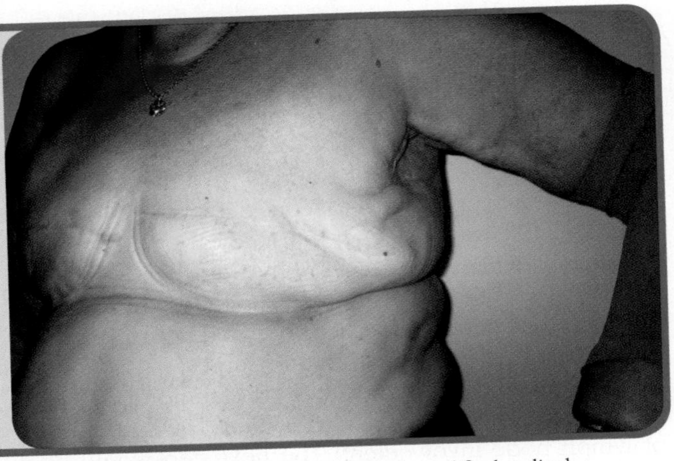

Figure 35–28: Female with bilateral modified radical mastectomy (Note the deep scar in the axilla from lymph node removal.) *Courtesy of Barbara A. Wise.*

when she was in her late 40s, she was diagnosed with breast cancer and had a modified radical mastectomy. Four years later she had a recurrence in the other breast and had another modified procedure. She is truly a cancer survivor. She has been without disease in any other area since her last mastectomy. She had a very supportive husband and with his help she elected to not have reconstructive surgery. She wears prostheses in her brassiere, and no one is aware she has had surgery. Her only remaining problem comes from lymphedema in one arm due to the removal of many lymph nodes.

Inflammatory Breast Cancer

This is an uncommon type of breast cancer, but it is so aggressive that it bears mention. Its symptoms are not what we have been told to observe. The cancer cells block the lymph vessels in the skin of the breast, causing the breast to become red, swollen, and warm. It may also appear bruised or purple, and appear like an orange peel. There may be no lump to be felt and may not be visible with a mammogram. There may be pain and a discharge leaking from the nipple. Diagnosis requires biopsy of the tissue and usually axillary lymph nodes to determine spread.

Inflammatory breast cancer grows and spreads rapidly. Treatment usually involves local treatment to remove the breast and surrounding area followed by radiation. Systemic treatment with chemotherapy and hormonal and even biologic (immune-system stimulation) therapy may also be used prior to surgery to control the disease and swelling within the breast, as well as afterward to destroy cells throughout the body.

Prognosis is guarded; because its progress is rapid and the symptoms are unfamiliar, the disease is often diagnosed late. Researchers are working on effective treatments, and clinical trials are in progress. The National Cancer Institute provides information on its Website or toll-free at 1-800-4-CANCER.

Cervical

Description—This is a cancer of the cervix of the uterus. An estimated 12,200 cases of cervical cancer were expected in 2010 with a death rate of 4,210. The Pap screening has reduced the incidence steadily over the past decades. The Pap test is a simple procedure involving a sampling of cells from the cervix that are easily obtained and examined under a microscope.

Signs and symptoms—It produces no symptoms until the cancer cells penetrate through the membranes and begin to travel through the lymphatic vessels or spread directly to nearby structures. The earliest symptoms are abnormal vaginal bleeding, persistent discharge, and pain and bleeding after intercourse. Cervical cancer can be detected very early by a Pap smear before any clinical evidence is observable. For this reason, the American Cancer Society recommends that all adult women have their first PAP test at age 21 and every year thereafter or every two years with the liquid-based test. At age 30, if there have been three successive normal tests, then you can go two to three years between tests unless certain conditions such as HIV or a weak immune system are present. Over age 30, you may choose every three years with either PAP or the HPV DNA test. After age 70, if three or more successive normal tests and no abnormal test in the past 10 years, then you can choose to stop testing. Pap tests after a total hysterectomy are not necessary unless surgery was performed due to cervical cancer. The Pap test is not a reliable diagnostic tool for uterine cancer, only cervical. Women at risk require more frequent evaluation.

Etiology—Specific causes are unknown, but certain factors are contributory, such as early age intercourse, multiple sexual partners, multiple pregnancies, herpes simplex virus II human papillomavirus (HPV), and other bacterial or viral venereal diseases.

Treatment—A variety of treatments, surgery, radiation, and chemotherapy, are used depending upon the stage of cancer. More common, especially in younger women, are precancerous cells called **dysplasia**, which are detected by Pap smear or colposcopy. For these preinvasive lesions, cryotherapy is used to freeze the area, or a procedure called LEEP (loop electrical excision procedure) uses electric current to excise tissue with intense heat. Other methods use laser ablation or localized surgery.

With invasive cancers, surgery, radiation, or both and chemotherapy may be used. The survival rate for patients with preinvasive lesions is nearly 100%. Even invasive cervical cancer survival is at 92% for five years when discovered early.

In 2006, research identified the HPV virus as the cause of 70% of cervical cancers, and a preventive vaccine was developed. The government issued a policy stating all sexually active females should receive the vaccine. It was recommended that girls even as young as 9 to 10 years old be given the three-injection immunization to establish their protection before sexual activity began.

Ovarian

Description—Ovarian cancer is one of the most common causes of cancer deaths among American women. It accounts for 3% of all cancers among women and ranks second among gynecologic cancers. An estimated 21,880 new cases were expected in 2010 with an estimated 13,850 deaths—more than from any other cancer of the female reproductive system. Prognosis varies with the stage and type of tumor, but only about 25% of patients survive for five years. One type, primary epithelial, accounts for about 90% of the cases. Another form strikes children. It is more prevalent in higher socioeconomic women between the ages of 40 and 65 and in single women. Ovarian cancer spreads rapidly by local extension and occasionally through the blood or lymphatics. The most common metastasis is through the diaphragm into the chest cavity. Because of its location, early diagnosis is difficult.

Signs and symptoms—Symptoms are confined to vague abdominal discomfort and mild gastrointestinal disturbances. With progression, urinary frequency, constipation, pelvic discomfort, and distention develop. Symptoms may be confused with appendicitis. Diagnosis requires careful evaluation, complete history, surgical exploration, and lab studies on tissue samples.

Etiology—Risk factors for ovarian cancer increase with age and peak during the 80s. Women who have never had children, who have had breast cancer, or who have a family history of breast or ovarian cancer are at increased risk. Other genetic factors like *BRCA1* and *BRCA2*, a type of hereditary colon cancer, and living in an industrialized country increase the incidence.

Treatment—Treatment generally involves aggressive surgery to remove all reproductive organs, affected lymph nodes, the omentum (the apron of tissue covering the organs), and the appendix. Chemotherapy may be beneficial in early stages, to extend the survival time. Recent therapy is resulting in prolonged remissions in some patients.

Uterine

Description—Uterine cancer is the most common gynecologic malignancy, usually affecting postmenopausal women between ages 50 and 60. Estimates for 2010 were 43,470 cases of uterine body cancer, usually of the endometrium, with an expected death rate of 7,950. The incidence is higher among white women, but the death rate is higher among black women.

Signs and symptoms—The first signs of uterine cancer are uterine enlargement and unusual premenopausal or any postmenopausal bleeding. It may begin as blood-streaked watery discharge but changes gradually to more bloody drainage. Ultrasound evaluation of the endometrial stripe (thickness) can be diagnostic. If the endometrium is not within normal limits, then the more invasive tests must be done. The most reliable diagnostic test is biopsy, with a follow-up D & C if the biopsy is negative.

Etiology—The prime risk factor that may lead to the most common form of uterine cancer is a high cumulative exposure to estrogen. This can be from hormone replacement therapy, tamoxifen, early menarche, late menopause, never having children, or a history of failure to ovulate. Other factors include infertility, diabetes, gallbladder disease, hypertension, and obesity. A familial tendency, a history of uterine polyps or hyperplasia of the endometrium, and the normal process of aging are also factors.

Treatment—Surgery is the treatment of choice, removing all reproductive organs. Radiation, either by an implanted internal device or externally administered, is indicated before surgery if the tumor is poorly defined. Chemotherapy and hormonal therapy with progesterone may be used. Both cervical and uterine cancers are rated by stages from 0 to IV, with 0 being suspicious and IV-b indicating metastasis to distant organs. The one-year survival rate for endometrial cancer is 92%, and the five-year rate is between 64% and 69%, depending on whether it is discovered early or in a regional stage.

Vaginal

Description—Pertains to the vagina. Vaginal cancer is far less common, occurring primarily in women in their early to mid-50s. It occurs most often in the upper third of the vagina and, like cervical cancer, begins in the epithelial layer, then deepens. It spreads very slowly.

Signs and symptoms—Symptoms include vaginal discharge and bleeding, with an ulcerated, usually firm, lesion of the vagina. Diagnosis is made by the presence of abnormal vaginal cells on a Pap smear. Any visible lesion is biopsied. Involvement of the cervix must be ruled out. Lesions of the vagina are often difficult to visualize because of its physical structure and the presence of the vaginal speculum blades, which obstruct the view.

Etiology—Vaginal cancer appears to be caused by the same factors that contribute to uterine malignancy.

Treatment—Treatment of early stages may be confined to the area alone. Surgery or radiation varies according to the involvement. With extensive disease, surgical exenteration (removal of all pelvic organs) may be required, with construction of a colostomy and an ileal conduit (ureter emptying into the ileum). Radiation is the preferred treatment for vaginal cancer.

Vulva

Description—Pertains to the area of the external genitalia. Cancer of the vulva accounts for 5% of gynecologic malignancies. It occurs usually among older women, most often in their mid-60s, but can occur at any age, even in infancy. Early diagnosis and treatment greatly enhance survival. A five-year survival rate is possible in 85% of patients without lymph node involvement and 75% when removed nodes are positive.

Signs and symptoms—Symptoms often begin with pruritus, bleeding, and a small surface ulcer that becomes infected and painful. Diagnosis is tentatively made from abnormal cells on a Pap smear and the typical clinical findings. Firm diagnosis requires biopsy of the suspected lesion.

Etiology—Risk factors related to vulvular cancer are chronic pruritus of the vulva with friction, swelling, and dryness and the presence of vulval diseases, including venereal diseases. Also, pigmented moles that are constantly irritated by clothing and perineal pads tend to be predisposing. Other systemic conditions, such as obesity, hypertension, diabetes, and absence of childbirth, present risks.

Treatment—Treatment consists of surgery, which varies with the extent of involvement. Small, confined lesions without lymph node involvement are treated by simple vulvectomy, perhaps on only one side. With node involvement in advanced stages a radical vulvectomy is required. This involves the vulva and superficial and deep inguinal lymph nodes. With adjoining tissue metastasis, it may be necessary to excise the urethra, vagina, and rectum, leaving an open perineal wound requiring two to three months to fill in and heal. If surgery is prohibited, radiation may be used to make the patient more comfortable.

SEXUALLY TRANSMITTED DISEASES (STDS)

AIDS—Acquired Immune Deficiency Syndrome

Refer to Chapter 31 for an in-depth look at this disease.

Chlamydia (Kla-mid′-e-a)

Description—This is one of the most frequent sexually transmitted diseases (STDs) in North America, affecting between 3 and 10 million people each year. Approximately 10% of all college students are infected. It is probably present in half of patients with pelvic inflammatory disease (PID).

Signs and symptoms—Symptoms do not easily lead to diagnosis. Men may experience burning on urination and have a mucoid discharge from the penis. They are often misdiagnosed as having gonorrhea. Women experience a vaginal discharge mimicking gonorrhea and have frequent painful urination associated with urinary tract infections. Sometimes **chlamydia** does not cause any visible signs. If there are visible signs, they will be noticeable within one to three weeks after having sexual contact with an infected person.

Etiology—This disease is caused by a specialized bacterium that lives as an intracellular parasite. There are two types of bacteria, both of which are pathogenic to humans. One strain causes a type of pneumonia. The other, *Chlamydia trachomatis,* lives in the conjunctiva of the eye and the epithelium of the urethra and cervix.

Treatment—If chlamydia is misdiagnosed, penicillin (for gonorrhea) or a medication for urinary infection may be given, and the chlamydia remains unaffected. Proper treatment requires repeated doses of tetracycline or erythromycin for at least a week to destroy the organism. If left untreated, or mistreated, it usually has no lasting effect on men, but they carry the organism and infect their sexual partners. In women, the bacteria will travel up the reproductive tract, causing inflammation of the fallopian tubes and eventual scarring. The scarring can interfere with pregnancy by causing tubal implantation of the fertilized ova because of the narrowed opening. Complete blockage may also occur, which prevents conception.

The disease, if contracted during pregnancy, will be transmitted to the baby during birth. The infant may develop conjunctivitis or pneumonia. Some evidence suggests that the infection may cause an increase in premature and still births. Two recently developed tests, which are inexpensive and quick to perform, accurately diagnose the disease. Because of its widespread incidence, many physicians routinely treat patients with symptoms and evidence of PID or gonorrhea even without positive chlamydia test results because of the risk of sterility.

Gonorrhea (Gon-or-re′-a)

Description—This is a common venereal disease. The usual sites are the vagina, penis, rectum, mouth, and throat. Because the organism dies almost immediately on exposure to air, it can be spread only by direct sexual contact.

Signs and symptoms—Symptoms vary between the male and female. Men notice burning, itching, or pain on urination; a sore throat with gland involvement;

discharge from the anus; or penile drainage that begins as a clear, watery fluid but changes to a thick, milky consistency. Women are usually asymptomatic, but they often develop an inflammation with a greenish-yellow discharge from the cervix. Other common symptoms are similar to those experienced by men, including sore throat, anal discharge, and swollen glands. Women may also develop lower abdominal pain, especially if fallopian tubes and other structures become involved (see PID). Diagnosis can usually be made on visual inspection, but confirmation depends on a microscopic examination of the discharge or a positive culture of the gonococcus organism from the discharge. Treatment is necessary; gonorrhea will not go away by itself.

Etiology—An infection caused by gonococcus bacteria is known as **gonorrhea**. The organism is fragile and can survive only in a moist, dark, and warm area within the body.

Treatment—Large doses of penicillin or tetracycline are required to destroy the organism. A follow-up examination after treatment is important, because strains of the gonococcus organism have become so resistant to the drugs that one course may not be sufficient. Untreated or undertreated gonorrhea can continue to spread, causing much damage. Men may develop chronic urethritis, long-term urinary tract inflammation, and sterility. Women may develop PID, which damages the reproductive organs and results in sterility.

Women who are infected with gonorrhea when giving birth pose a grave danger to the newborn. The gonococcus organism can infect the delicate tissues of the newborn's eyes and cause permanent blindness. Because of this possibility, all newborns routinely receive erythromycin solution in their eyes as part of immediate afterbirth care.

Gonorrhea can be controlled and prevented with proper education, treatment, and common sense. Knowledge of a partner's sexual frequency and use of protection with others—*before* engaging in sexual activity—can prevent a person from becoming infected in the first place. Since the advent of the contraceptive pill and the IUD, the use of condoms, diaphragms, and foams has diminished. These chemical and mechanical barriers, especially the condom, deterred the spread of the disease. The condom is encouraged as a deterrent to the spread of all sexually transmitted diseases.

Herpes (Her′-pez)

Description—Genital herpes is an acute, inflammatory disease of the genitalia. It is one of the most common recurring disorders of the genitalia. Prognosis varies according to the age of the patient, the strength of the immune system, and the infection site. Primary genital herpes is usually self-limiting but may cause painful local or systemic disease. For people with weak immune systems, newborns, and others with widespread disease, genital herpes is often severe, with complications and a high mortality rate. Herpes is passed by direct skin-to-skin contact with your own or someone else's lesions, even 24 hours before they erupt. It is possible to spread your own herpes without being aware of its presence.

Signs and symptoms—Herpes takes from three to seven days to erupt. With **genital herpes**, fluid-filled vesicles appear on the cervix (primary site), labia, vulva, vagina, or perianal skin of the female. The male lesions appear on the glans, foreskin, or penile shaft. Nongenital lesions may cause complications, such as herpetic keratitis of the eye, which may lead to blindness. Vesicles are usually painless at first but may rupture and develop into shallow, painful ulcers with edema, redness, and tender inguinal lymph nodes.

Diagnosis is made by observation and from patient history. Confirmation of herpes simplex II is possible from a culture of the vesicle fluid.

Etiology—The virus causing herpes has two strains: type I and type II. Type I is the typical cold sore on the lip or at the edge of the nose. Type II is the form that appears on the external genitalia, mouth, or anus.

Treatment—Treatment with the usual antiviral medications helps reduce edema and ease discomfort. Antibacterial agents help combat secondary infections. Neither medication will treat the virus, but they will help to speed the healing process of the lesions.

After lesions heal, the virus becomes dormant. It may never recur, but about two thirds of herpes sufferers have additional attacks, some within a few months. Future recurrences decrease in frequency and severity. The best defense is a healthy, well-rested body that can fight the disease organism with its natural defense mechanisms.

Other complications demand attention. Newborns can be infected with herpes during vaginal delivery. Some infants survive, but others develop a brain infection that rapidly leads to death. If a woman has active herpes type II lesions at the time of birth, a cesarean section delivery is indicated. Women with herpes genitalis also have a higher-than-usual rate of spontaneous abortion.

Human Papillomavirus (HPV) (Pap-i-lo′-ma-vi′-rus) Infection

Description—Human papillomavirus is the common name given to a group of related viruses. HPV is one of the most common STDs. One form, genital warts, has been around for centuries. Today, its increase may result from women having more sexual partners and being less likely to rely on condoms for birth control—hence, there is no physical barrier.

Signs and symptoms—There are different types of HPV. One causes the common warts that appear on the fingers and hands and rarely spread to the genitalia. These are unsightly but do not cause any health problems. Other types of HPV found on the genitalia cause condylomas, or genital warts. These are usually found in clusters growing on the external structures and inside the vagina and on the cervix. However, HPV can be present without the visible warts because the virus can cause changes that cannot be seen by the naked eye. Often the virus is discovered by the Pap test. When the Pap is positive, a visual examination and sometimes a colposcope, a magnifying instrument, may be used to examine the vagina, cervix, and vulva. Suspicious areas are usually biopsied for diagnosis and signs of precancerous changes.

Etiology—HPV is a very small virus that needs to infect cells in order to survive. Once inside a cell, the virus directs the cell to make copies of itself and to infect other healthy cells. The infected cells eventually die and are shed with the virus from the body. When shed, the virus can be passed to another person who then becomes infected. It often takes several months and maybe even years for the person to show signs of infection. The virus can be passed during sex and is therefore considered to be a STD.

Treatment—Some signs of infection may go away, but the following treatments may still be advisable:

- Trichloroacetic acid (TCA) and bichloroacetic acid (BCA) are strong chemicals that can be applied to destroy genital warts.
- Podophyllin is an old treatment that can also be applied with care to warts because it can burn surrounding tissue. It should not be used during pregnancy.
- Interferon is a new drug to treat genital warts. It can be injected into the warts or into muscle. It must also be avoided during pregnancy.
- Cryotherapy destroys the lesions by freezing.
- Laser treatment destroys the warts with a high-intensity beam of light.
- Electrosurgery uses electric current to burn away the lesion or shave it with a loop.
- Excisional biopsy cuts away the tissue.
- TCA, cryotherapy, or a laser are used to treat pregnant patients.

Genital warts are difficult to remove, and repeated treatment may be necessary for several weeks or months. Even after visibly gone, they may return at a later time. The major concern with HPV is the increased risk of other major health problems, such as cancer, especially cervical cancer.

Nongonococcal Urethritis (NGU, NSU) (Non-gon-o-kok-al U-re-thri′-tis)

Description—This is a group of infections with similar manifestations that are not linked to a single organism. Sometimes it is also called NSU or **nonspecific urethritis**. In men, it causes urethral inflammation; in women, vaginitis. NGU is transmitted by sexual intercourse. Men can also develop inflammation or allergic reactions from vaginal creams, contraceptive foams, soaps, douching solutions, and deodorants used by their sexual partners.

Signs and symptoms—Symptoms are similar to cystitis: burning on urination, frequency, itching (penile or vaginal), and possibly a thin discharge (penile or vaginal).

Differential diagnosis between NGU and gonorrhea must be made because the symptoms are similar, but the treatment is different. Confirmation is made by absence of the gonococcus from the culture of the discharge.

Etiology—It is usually the result of a bacterial infection. In males, it often results from *Chlamydia trachomatis* infection or from bacteria such as staphylococci, diphtheroids, coliform organism, and *Hemophilus vaginalis*. In females, less is known about nonspecific genitourinary infection. The chlamydia or corynebacterial organisms may also be the cause of infection. The disease often has no obvious cause, but sometimes bacteria or bacteria-like organisms are found in the urethral discharge.

Treatment—Treatment is normally with tetracycline or a similar antibiotic, because NGU does not respond to penicillin therapy. If untreated, it may lead to complications like those associated with gonorrhea. The most serious complication is a scarred urethra, which results in problems with urination. In addition, some strains can cause birth defects in newborns whose mothers have the disease.

Pediculosis Pubis (Pe-dik-u-lo′-sis Pu′-bis) (Pubic Lice)

Description—These are little yellowish-gray insects, about the size of a pinhead. They attach themselves to the moist hair roots in the pubic area of humans and feed on the blood of their host, hopping from person to person during sexual contact. It is possible, however, to get lice from contaminated towels, upholstery, clothing, or bedding, because they can survive for about a day without a supporting host.

Signs and symptoms—The prime symptom is an intense itching that cannot be ignored. They are visible on close inspection.

Etiology—Pediculosis is caused by parasitic forms of lice.

Treatment—Treatment is quite simple with a product called Kwell, which is applied to the infected area. All clothing, bedding, and linens must be washed in very hot water and detergent to destroy the nits (eggs) and lice. Nonwashable items can be dry-cleaned or ironed with a hot iron. Lice eggs can survive for a week, so uncleaned items must be avoided.

Pelvic Inflammatory Disease (PID)

Description—This is any acute or chronic infection of the reproductive tract, including the cervix (cervicitis), uterus (endometritis), fallopian tubes (salpingitis), and ovaries (oophoritis). It can also involve the surrounding tissues. Early treatment is important to prevent reproductive damage, infertility, pulmonary emboli, septicemia (blood poisoning), and death.

Signs and symptoms—Symptoms include purulent vaginal discharge, fever, and malaise (especially if gonorrhea-related). There is lower abdominal pain, with severe pain on manipulation of the cervix and adjoining structures.

Etiology—PID is caused by an infection from aerobic or anaerobic organisms. The gonococcus is the most common aerobic organism. It can rapidly destroy the bacterial barrier of the cervical mucus. With the barrier gone, the bacteria present in the vagina can ascend into the uterus and cause infection. Uterine infection can also develop following insertion of an IUD (intrauterine device), which accidentally introduces contaminated cervical mucus into the uterus. Other factors causing PID are abortion, tubal examinations that test patency by inserting air, pelvic surgery, and infection associated with pregnancy. Organisms can enter from the bloodstream, an abscess, an infected tube, or a ruptured appendix.

Treatment—PID can be treated with antibiotics to prevent progressive involvement. Culture of the drainage to identify the organism is important to be certain the appropriate drug is being used. Improper treatment will result in a chronic disease state. If the causative organism is gonorrhea, chlamydia may also be present and require treatment. Bed rest, analgesics, and IV therapy may be indicated. Pelvic abscesses may develop, which require drainage. If permitted to rupture, they may cause a life-threatening situation.

Syphilis (Sif′-i-lis)

Description—This is a venereal disease that inhabits the warm, moist areas of the genitals and rectum. The organism can be viewed by dark-field microscope examination. **Syphilis** is spread by direct sexual contact during either the primary, secondary, or early latent stages of infection. Prenatal transmission to the fetus across the placental barrier is possible, resulting in an infant with congenital syphilis. If the mother is in the primary or secondary stage, the infant will probably die before or shortly after birth. If syphilis is diagnosed and treated before the 4th month of pregnancy, the fetus will not develop the disease. Therefore, a blood analysis for syphilis is routinely performed as part of early prenatal care.

Signs and symptoms—Symptoms vary according to the stage of involvement. Primary stage syphilis begins with entrance of the organism through the mucous membrane of the genitals as the result of contact with an infected person. After three to four weeks, a lesion called a *chancre* appears at the point of entrance. It is an ulcerlike area with a raised, hard edge that looks painful but is not. In the female, it often appears on the cervix and is therefore hidden from sight, going undetected. It may also develop on the vulva and be visible on examination. In the male, the usual site is the glans or corona (ridge) of the penis. It may develop on the penile shaft or scrotum. The spirochete can also enter the mucous membranes of the mouth or rectum during nongenital intercourse, causing chancres to develop on the lip, tongue, tonsils, or around the anus.

The disease progresses through four stages. The primary stage, chancre, even if untreated, disappears within one to five weeks, giving the infected person a false sense of having healed. Actually, the disease enters an asymptomatic period during which the bacteria circulate through the body in the blood. About one to six months later a secondary stage begins. This stage is characterized by a generalized painless, nonitching rash. It is particularly distinctive because of its appearance on the soles of the feet and palms of the hands. During this stage, the following may occur: hair loss; a sore throat; headache; loss of appetite; nausea; constipation; persistent fever; and pain in the bones, muscles, or joints. These symptoms could be indicative of any number of illnesses. If the disease is diagnosed accurately and treated, it can be cured without permanent effects. Without treatment, the disease again "goes away" in two to six weeks, leading to the belief that nothing is wrong, while, on the contrary, a dangerous stage is approaching.

The third stage is the latent stage, which may last for years. There are no symptoms during this stage, but the organism is at work, burrowing into blood vessels, the spinal cord, the brain, and the bones. After the first year, the disease is no longer infectious except to a fetus. About 50% of those who contract syphilis move into the dangerous late or tertiary stage. This stage is further categorized according to the type of involvement:

benign late (affecting internal organs); cardiovascular late (affecting the heart and major blood vessels); or neurosyphilis (affecting the brain and spinal cord). Cardiovascular forms can lead to death; neurosyphilis is almost always fatal.

Diagnosis is difficult by history alone, and physical examination at certain periods would be negative. However, a definitive blood test has been developed and is used routinely for suspected infection and as a mass screening test by some states for persons seeking a marriage license. The test is known as a VDRL, named for the Venereal Disease Research Laboratory of the United States Public Health Service. Another screening test is the Rapid Plasma Reagin test. Like the VDRL, it also screens for antibodies so is not capable of detecting early infection. The blood tests are fairly accurate, cheap, and easy to perform; however, they do not give accurate results until four to six weeks after initial infection. About 25% of the tests will be false negatives during the primary stage, but they are completely accurate in the secondary phase.

Etiology—Syphilis is caused by the spirochete *Treponema pallidum*.

Treatment—Penicillin is the treatment of choice for syphilis, which is relatively easily destroyed. Because some of the spirochetes may survive, a large initial dose of long-acting penicillin (1.2 million units) is divided into two injections, one in each buttock. Much greater doses are required for latent, late, or congenital syphilis. A follow-up exam should be done to confirm freedom from organisms.

Trichomoniasis (Trik-o-mo-ni′-a-sis)

Description—This is a protozoal infection of the lower genitourinary tract. It occurs in 15% of sexually active females and 10% of sexually active males. **Trichomoniasis** can be passed back and forth between sexual partners; therefore, treatment must involve both persons.

Signs and symptoms—The prime and discriminating symptom is abundant, frothy, white or yellow vaginal discharge, which irritates the vulva and has a characteristic foul odor. There are usually no symptoms in the male, except for urethral itching. Diagnosis is made by placing a drop of the secretion on a slide and identifying the organism by microscope. This confirmation rules out ordinary vaginitis from female hygiene products or the presence of rectal *Escherichia coli* in the vagina.

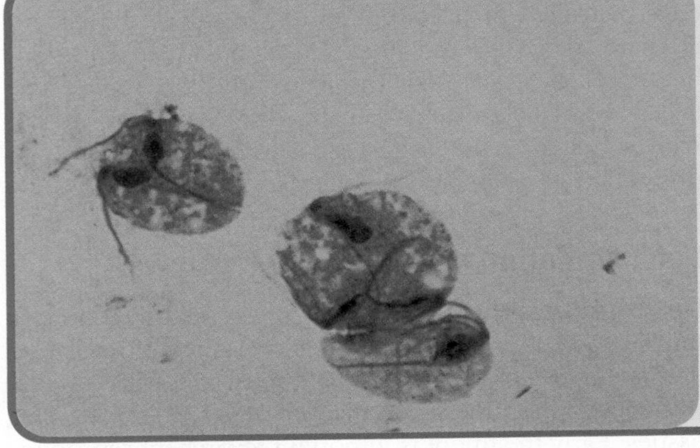

Figure 35–29: *Trichomonas vaginalis. Delmar/Cengage Learning.*

Etiology—It is caused by the single-celled parasitic organism *Trichomonas vaginalis* (Figure 35–29). It is oval in shape, with four hairlike strands protruding from it, which whip back and forth to propel the organism.

Treatment—Treatment of choice is a product called Flagyl, which is taken orally. If left untreated, the female may develop an inflamed cervix and urethra and exhibit abnormal Pap smears. Damaged cells of the cervix may make it more susceptible to cancer. Men develop an infected prostate, testicle, or bladder.

AGE-RELATED BODY CHARACTERISTICS

The female body changes quite drastically throughout life. At about age 10 to 11, the effects of ovarian hormones begin to mature the female and cause the secondary body characteristics to develop. The pelvis broadens, the breasts develop the duct system and gain fat, fat deposits develop on the hips and thighs. The menarche becomes evident with the beginning of menstrual periods.

With maturity, fertility increases and pregnancy may occur. This changes the hormonal influence and results in great body changes including an enlarged uterus and breasts. Again, following delivery, the body is affected by other hormones if the woman chooses to nurse her baby.

As aging occurs, hormonal influence begins to drop significantly. Menstrual periods cease and menopause occurs. Vaginal changes occur, breasts lose their glandular structure, and body shape may change. The possibility of osteoporosis and increased risk of cancer is related to aging.

System Interaction Associatied with Disease Conditions

The reproductive system is very closely related to the endocrine system due to the interaction of the hormones that develop the physical features and regulate the function. With the female in particular, when conception occurs, her whole body must function together to support and deliver a healthy human being. Table 35–4 summarizes the interaction of systems related to two conditions.

TABLE 35–4 System Interaction Associated With Reproductive Conditions

Condition	Systems Involved	Pathology Present
Pregnancy	Reproductive	Enlarged uterus, breasts, cessation of menstruation
	Gastrointestinal	Morning sickness, hemorrhoids
	Circulatory	Edema of hands, face, feet, legs, hypertension
	Urinary	Frequency
	Respiratory	Shortness of breath
Premenstrual Syndrome	Reproductive	Breast tenderness, enlargement
	Respiratory	Increase in colds, asthma, exacerbation of allergic rhinitis
	Nervous	Headache, numbness of extremities, fainting
	Digestive	Constipation, diarrhea, bloating
	Circulatory	Palpitations
	Integumentary	Acne

CHAPTER SUMMARY

- Reproductive system consists of organs capable of accomplishing reproduction
- The male reproductive organs include the testes, penis, prostate gland, bulbourethral glands, epididymis, vas deferens, seminal vesicles
- Diagnostic exams and tests of the male reproductive system: epididymitis, erectile dysfunction, hydrocele, prostatic hypertrophy
- The female reproductive organs include ovaries, fallopian tubes, uterus, vagina, vulva, clitoris, mammary glands.
- Review Table 35-3 for contraception reasons and methods
- Diagnostic and screening tests during pregnancy: alpha-fetoprotein screening, amniocentesis, chorionic villi sampling, gestational diabetes screening, group B streptococcus
- Diagnostic tests of the female reproductive system: colposcopy, hysteroscopy, mammogram, maturation index, Papanicolaou smear, pregnancy tests, ultrasonography
- Diseases and disorders of the female reproductive system: cervical erosion, cervicitis, cystic breast disease, cystocele, dysmemorrhea, endometriosis, fibroids, hysterectomy, ovarian cyst, premenstrual syndrome, polyp, rectocele, and vaginitis
- Malignancy of the female reproductive organs: breasts, inflammatory breast cancer, cervical, ovarian, uterine, vaginal, and vulva
- Sexually transmitted diseases: AIDS, chlamydia, gonorrhea, herpes, human papillomavirus infection, nongonococcal urethritis, pediculosis, pelvic inflammatory disease, syphillis, and trichomoniasis

STUDY TOOLS

Workbook	Activities for Chapter 35
Premium Website	
MEDIA LINK	View these **Media Links** for Chapter 35: • The male reproductive system • The female reproductive system
StudyWARE	Activities and Quizzes on the **StudyWARE™ Software** for Chapter 35
	Audio Library of medical terms
	Online access to the **Critical Thinking Challenge 2.0**
learninglab	Module 16: The Urinary, Endocrine, and Reproductive Systems
CourseMate	Activities and Quizzes for Chapter 35
WebTutor	Activities and Quizzes for Chapter 35

CHECK YOUR KNOWLEDGE

1. Sperm are produced in the:
   a. epididymis.
   b. seminiferous tubules.
   c. vas deferens.
   d. seminal vesicles.
2. The prostate gland is located:
   a. in the testes.
   b. just above the bladder.
   c. in the penis.
   d. just below the bladder.
3. Which of the following is not a treatment for prostate cancer?
   a. Cryosurgery
   b. Radioactive seeds
   c. Female hormones
   d. Prosthesis implant
4. The corpus luteum is a(n):
   a. mature ova.
   b. immature graafian follicle.
   c. primary follicle.
   d. follicle after ovulation occurs.
5. The fallopian tubes are all the following except a:
   a. a passageway for sperm.
   b. a passageway for ova.
   c. attached to the uterus.
   d. attached to the ovaries.
6. Which of the following terms does not refer to a uterine position?
   a. Anteflexed
   b. Retroflexed
   c. Retroverted
   d. Antelapsed
7. The perineum refers to the area:
   a. around the urinary meatus.
   b. within the labia minora.
   c. adjacent to the clitoris.
   d. between the vagina and anus.
8. Menarche means the:
   a. beginning of menses.
   b. end of menses.
   c. highest point in the menstrual cycle.
   d. period of ovulation.
9. Amniocentesis is done to:
   a. determine the sex of the baby.
   b. rule out multiple births.
   c. check for gestational diabetes.
   d. check for chromosomal abnormalities.
10. A colposcope is an instrument used to:
    a. view the cervix.
    b. view the uterus.
    c. evaluate fallopian tubes.
    d. observe the fetus in utero.

WEB LINKS

American Cancer Society, cancer facts and figures: www.cancer.org/Research/CancerFactsFigures /index

National Cancer Institute: www.cancer.gov

CDC, Sexually Transmitted Diseases: www.cdc.gov/std

Section

4

The Back Office

Unit

12

Preparing for Clinical Procedures

When preparing for clinical duties, the medical assistant's responsibilities will vary. An important aspect in the clinical area is ensuring that disease transmission is limited as much as possible. The first goal is protecting the safety of our patients and staff. This can be done in various ways; however, one of the most important things you can do to reduce disease transmission is to wash your hands often and thoroughly. Wearing personal protective equipment; disposing of biohazard items appropriately; and recognizing the proper methodology for the care of instruments and equipment by sanitization, disinfection, and sterilization is essential.

Obtaining the patient's medical history and conducting accurate screening processes is another area in which you, as a medical assistant, need to be confident. When calling patients into the office, you must be able to put the patient at ease and deliver a welcoming setting for the patient. In-person screening requires a professional approach that aids the patient in developing a sense of trust and comfort in disclosing personal information to you. A complete health history is revealing and a great tool to assist in diagnosing conditions.

After the interviewing process is completed, it is usually customary to obtain basic physical measurements, which become the baseline for future comparisons. The patient's height and weight, as well as measurements of blood pressure, pulse, respiration, and temperature, commonly known as vital signs, are routinely obtained.

As the data obtained from the history and measurements is completed, it is documented in the patient's medical record. Because most medical offices are converting from paper charts to electronic files (EHR), it is important to be proficient using either method. With the electronic record system, data is entered at a terminal stationed in the exam room or a on portable system that can be moved from room to room.

Another common responsibility as a medical assistant is to prepare patients for a variety of examinations and procedures performed by the physician. To gain full cooperation, patients need to be informed about what to expect. You must keep in mind that while these procedures and exams are routine for the health care team, they are not for the patient. Part of your duties may include answering questions the patient has regarding the visit. Questions commonly asked may include:

- What exactly is the exam or procedure?
- Why does it need to be done?
- Will it hurt?
- How long will it take?
- When will the results be available?

Even if the physician has already explained all of this to the patient, you may need to review the information and answer questions. In addition to preparing the patient, the medical assistant must also prepare the examination room, including instruments, the table, and supplies. Depending on the provider preference, you might assist with the exam by handing items to the provider or assisting with positioning of the patient.

Certification Connection

	Ch. 36	Ch. 37	Ch. 38	Ch. 39
CMA (AAMA)				
Recognizing and responding to verbal and nonverbal communication		X		
Professional communication and behavior		X	X	X
Patient interviewing techniques		X		
Principles of infection control	X			
Treatment area	X			
Patient preparation and assisting the physician		X	X	X
Patient history interview		X		
Vital signs			X	
Body positions				X
RMA (AMT)				
Patient relations		X	X	X
Patient education				X
Asepsis	X			
Sterilization	X			
Instruments	X			X
Vital signs and mensurations		X	X	
Medical history		X		
Patient positions				X
CMAS (AMT)				
Professionalism		X	X	X
Basic health history interview		X		
Basic charting		X		
Vital signs and measurements			X	
Asepsis in the medical office	X			
Examination preparation		X	X	X

Chapter

36 Infection Control and Medical Asepsis

OBJECTIVES

In this chapter, you will learn the following:

KB KNOWLEDGE BASE

1. Spell and define, using the glossary in the back of the text, all the Words to Know in this chapter.
2. Locate and interpret from the communicable disease chart the means of transmission, incubation time, symptoms, and treatment for a given disease.
3. Describe the infection control cycle and chain of infection links, giving an example of how to break each link.
4. Name five common infectious agents and give an example of each.
5. Explain what direct and indirect contact is.
6. List the five steps in the infectious disease process and give an explanation of each.
7. List the growth requirements of microorganisms and methods of controlling their growth.
8. Explain how used needles, lancets, capillary tubes, glass slides, and other sharp instruments are to be handled.
9. Describe the recommended universal and standard precautions to be taken when you are exposed to human tissue, blood, and body fluids and explain why it is important to follow these precautions.
10. Explain the process for disposal of biohazardous material.
11. List the habits a medical assistant should practice to reduce and prevent disease transmission, including patient education suggestions.
12. Describe the body's defense mechanisms against disease.
13. Define medical asepsis.
14. Explain the importance of proper hand washing and the purpose of wearing gloves and other personal protective equipment (PPE).
15. Explain the preventive measures for health care professionals to protect against the hepatitis B virus.
16. Explain the difference between sanitization, disinfection, and sterilization and the purpose of each.
17. Explain the function of the autoclave and the steps and safety precautions to follow when using the autoclave.
18. Explain the purpose of using sterilization and biological indicators for autoclaving.

S SKILLS

1. Demonstrate the proper procedure for completing an incident exposure report form.
2. Demonstrate proper hand washing.
3. Demonstrate proper removal of non-sterile gloves.
4. Demonstrate application and removal of appropriate personal protective equipment (PPE) when working in potentially infectious situations.
5. Demonstrate sanitization procedures.
6. Demonstrate disinfection procedures.
7. Demonstrate the proper procedure for preparing and wrapping instruments to be autoclaved.
8. Demonstrate the proper procedure for sterilization of instruments by use of an autoclave.

WORDS TO KNOW

aerobe
airborne
anaerobes
asepsis
autoclave
bacteria
biohazardous
bloodborne
Clinical Laboratory Improvement Amendments (CLIA)
coma
communicable
disinfection
droplet infection
exudative
fecal
flora
fomite
fungi
hygiene
incineration
incubation
invasive
malaise
microorganism
morphology
nits
obligate
Occupational Safety and Health Administration (OSHA)
parasites
pathogens
personal protective equipment (PPE)
petechial
pH
protozoa
pruritic
pustular
rickettsiae
resuscitation
sanitization
seizures
serrations
shelf life
spores
Standard Precautions
sterilization
susceptible
vector
vigilant
virulence
viruses
vulnerable

THE INFECTION CYCLE AND DISEASE TRANSMISSION

Infection control is an ongoing aspect of health care for both the patient and the health care provider that is of the utmost importance. As a medical assistant, always be mindful of the necessity of **asepsis** (a state of being free from all pathogenic **microorganisms**) when performing clinical procedures. Although maintaining a completely sterile environment throughout an entire medical facility might not be realistic, the facility must be clean and safe for all who enter.

Table 36–1 lists **communicable** diseases and their means of transmission, **incubation** time, symptoms, and treatment. Becoming familiar with this information will help you serve patients better. Incubation time refers to the time between the initial exposure to the disease-causing microbes and the appearance of the first symptoms or signs of the disease. If a person is **susceptible** to a disease, that person is receptive, or **vulnerable**, to catching it. Generally, the susceptible person is weakened because of a preexisting illness or condition, is overall run down and worn out, or has poor **hygiene** and health habits.

Microorganisms that are the cause of disease are called **pathogens**. They have certain requirements for growth and multiplication. If steps are taken to interrupt and prevent their growth, disease transmission can be reduced. A microorganism's power to produce a disease is know as **virulence**.

It is important to note that not all microorganisms are pathogenic. Some microorganisms are helpful and necessary to normal **flora** in humans and animals because they provide a balance in the body and destroy pathogens. Normal flora is the cohabitation of microorganisms (nonpathogenic and pathogenic in balance) that live in or within an organism to provide a natural immunity against certain infections. Infection occurs when this balance is disturbed.

In the effort to prevent disease transmission, it is helpful to have an idea of what you are trying to prevent. All living organisms have requirements to sustain life and facilitate growth and development. These requirements are:

- *Oxygen.* Microorganisms that need oxygen to grow are called **aerobes**, and those that grow best in the absence of oxygen are called **anaerobes**.
- *pH.* The body has a 6.0 average **pH**, which is an acidic level high enough to protect the body from microorganism invasion. If the pH level is higher, it indicates that microbial growth is present. As bacteria grow and multiply, the pH level becomes higher in alkalinity. A low pH reading, one less than 6, can be the result of ketosis or of not eating for a long period. An environment that is too acidic will not support microbial growth.
- *Temperature (98.6°F).* Microorganisms grow best at the average body temperature (37°C or 98.6°F). The human body has not only a desirable temperature for microbial growth but also darkness and moisture, other growth requirements.
- *Nutrients.*
- *Water.*
- *A host to inhabit.*

darkness

Stages of the Infection Cycle

Study the infection cycle (also known as the "chain of infection") in Figure 36–1 and follow the cycle to see how easily diseases can be transferred from one person to another unless the cycle is broken. Taking care of yourself is extremely important in the scope of disease

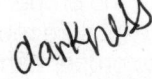

TABLE 36–1 Communicable Diseases

Disease	Means of Transmission	Incubation	Symptoms	Treatment
AIDS (acquired immunodeficiency syndrome)*	Direct contact: sexual, anal, or vaginal intercourse; sharing IV drug needles; infected mother to child (childbirth); blood to blood (from cuts, scrapes, punctures of skin). Indirect contact: blood transfusions	Onset of AIDS following infection with human immunodeficiency virus (HIV) from 6 months to 10+ years	Early—loss of appetite, weight loss, fever, night sweats, skin rashes, diarrhea, fatigue, poor resistance to infections, swollen lymph nodes. Later—cough, fever, shortness of breath, dyspnea, purple blotches on the skin	Research and new developments continue in the search for a cure and a vaccine. The current most commonly used treatments are antiretroviral drugs. (Visit the CDC website for the most up-to-date treatment regimes.)
Chickenpox* (deaths only reportable) (varicella zoster virus)	Direct or indirect contact, droplet, or **airborne** secretion of infected person	2–3 weeks, usually 13–17 days	Crops of **pruritic** vesicular eruptions on the skin, slight fever and headache, **malaise**	Bed rest, topical anti-pruritics
Common cold (upper respiratory infection—URI)	Direct or indirect contact with infected person	12–72 hours (some viruses 2–7 days), usually 24 hours	Slight sore throat, watery eyes, runny nose, sneezing, chills, malaise, low-grade fever	Rest, decongestant, mild analgesics, increased fluid intake
Conjunctivitis (pink eye)	Direct or indirect contact with discharge from eyes or upper respiratory tract of infected person	Viral: 24 hours to days; bacterial: 24–72 hours	Redness of eyes, itching, burning of eyes, matted eyelashes	Antibacterial agents, antibiotics, corticosteroids, depending on causative agent
Head lice (pediculosis)	Direct contact with infested person; indirect contact is rare	1 week (**nits**, or eggs, hatch in 1 week, mature in 2 weeks)	Itching of scalp; presence of small, light-gray lice and nits (eggs) at the base of hairs	Topical use of 1% lindane shampoo, lotion, or cream (7–10 days); comb nits from hair; launder washable items in hot water with hottest drying cycle, dry-clean or seal in plastic bags non-washable items (2 weeks); thoroughly vacuum the environment
Haemophilus influenzae type b Hib (H-flu)* (invasive disease reportable)	Direct and indirect contact and **droplet infection** from respiratory tract	3+ days	URI symptoms, fever, aches, sleepiness, no appetite; as disease progresses, child is irritable and fussy	Antibiotics, increased fluid intake, antipyretics, rest, analgesics

(continues)

TABLE 36–1 (*Continued*)

Disease	Means of Transmission	Incubation	Symptoms	Treatment
Hepatitis A* (acute)	Direct contact or by fecal-contaminated food or water	15–50 days, avg. 25–30 days	Slow onset, fever, malaise, loss of appetite, nausea, vomiting, jaundice, joint pain, dark urine, clay-colored stool	Bed rest, increased fluid intake, proper nourishment (no fats or alcohol)
Hepatitis B* (acute, chronic, and perinatal)	Contact with infectious blood, semen, and other body fluids primarily through birth to an infected mother, sexual contact with an infected person, sharing of contaminated needles, syringes, other injection drug equipment, or needle sticks or other sharp instrument injuries	45–160 days, avg. 120 days	Similar to hepatitis A, but onset is rapid and acute	Acute: Same as hepatitis A. Chronic: regular monitoring for signs of liver disease progression; some patients are treated with antiviral drugs
Hepatitis C* (acute and chronic; formerly non-A, non-B, or NANB)	Contact with blood of an infected person primarily through sharing of contaminated needles, syringes, or other injection drug equipment. Less commonly through sexual contact with an infected person, birth to an infected mother, needle stick or other sharp injuries	14–180 days, avg. 45 days	Same as above	Acute: Antiviral drugs and supportive treatment. Chronic: regular monitoring for signs of liver disease progression; some patients are treated with antiviral drugs
Herpes simplex virus (HSV) (cold sores, fever blisters)	Direct contact with infected person	2–14 days, usually 4–6 days	Painful blisters on lips, which turn pustular and then form crusted scabs; oral lesions are small ulcerated areas	Topical applications of drying medications; antibiotics for secondary infections
H1N1 (Swine Flu)* (associated pediatric mortality)	Direct and indirect contact and by airborne secretions	1–7 days	Fever, cough, sore throat, runny or stuffy nose, body aches, headache, chills, and fatigue. Some people may have vomiting and diarrhea. Can range from an upper respiratory infection to an acute, life-threatening illness.	Bed rest, increased fluid intake, antipyretics, antiviral drugs.

Disease	Means of Transmission	Incubation	Symptoms	Treatment
Impetigo	Direct contact with draining sores	2–10 days	Blister-like lesions (later become crusted), itching	Cleansing of areas with antibacterial soap and water, topical and/or oral antibiotics
Influenza* (associated pediatric mortality)	Direct and indirect contact and by airborne secretions	1–4 days	Sudden onset of fever, chills, headache, sore muscles, malaise (commonly, runny nose, sore throat, and cough)	Bed rest, increased fluid intake, antipyretics
Mesles* (rubeola)	Direct contact by respiratory droplets from an infected person sneezing or coughing	7–18 days	Blotchy rash, fever, cough, runny nose, red watery eyes, malaise, tiny white spots with bluish-white centers found inside the mouth (Koplik's spots)	No treatment; however, measures can be taken to protect individuals exposed to the virus, such as post-exposure vaccination, immune serum globulin, analgesics to relieve the fever, and antibiotics if the person develops a bacterial infection while he or she has the measles
ningitis* (bacterial) *emophilus* and eningococcal	Direct contact and droplet infection from respiratory tract	1–10 days, usually 3–7 days	Sudden onset of fever, intense headache, nausea, vomiting; sometimes **petechial** rash, irritability, sluggishness (possible **seizures** or **coma**)	Antibiotics by intravenous and/or oral administration
eningitis* (viral)	Direct contact, fecal-oral route, and respiratory secretions	Symptoms can appear quickly, or they can take several days to appear, usually after a cold or runny nose, diarrhea, vomiting, or other signs of infection show up.	Symptoms in adults may differ from those in children. Common in infants: Fever, irritability, poor eating, hard to awaken. Common in older children and adults: high fever, severe headache, stiff neck, sensitivity to bright light, sleepiness or trouble waking up, nausea, vomiting, lack of appetite	There is no specific treatment for viral meningitis. Most patients completely recover on their own within 2 weeks. Bed rest, plenty of fluids, and analgesics to relieve fever and headache.

(continues)

TABLE 36–1 *(Continued)*

Disease	Means of Transmission	Incubation	Symptoms	Treatment
MRSA (Methicillin-resistant *Staphylococcus aureus*)	Direct contact or indirect contact. Skin-to-skin contact or shared items, such as towels, razors, and bandages	1–10 days	Skin infections that may look like pimples or boils and can be read, swollen, painful, and full of pus	Antibiotic vancomycin is used to treat resistant germs. In some cases, antibiotics are not necessary, and the superficial abscess can be drained by the physician.
Mumps*	Direct or indirect contact by droplets from the nose or throat of an infected person, usually when they cough or sneeze	12–25 days	Fever, headache, muscle aches, tiredness, loss of appetite, swollen and tender salivary glands under the ears on one or both sides	No specific treatment. Supportive care is needed.
Pertussis* (whooping cough; *Bordetella pertussis*)	Direct contact with discharges from respiratory mucous membranes of infected persons.	7–10 days	Sneezing, runny nose, low-grade fever, and a mild cough. Within two weeks, the cough becomes more severe and is characterized by episodes of many rapid coughs followed by a crowing or high pitched whoop. Thick, clear mucus may be discharged.	Antibiotics such as azithromycin and erythromycin
Pinworms (*Enterobius vermicularis*)	Direct transfer of eggs from anus to mouth; indirect contact with eggs in clothing, bedding	3 weeks–3 months	Anal itching, insomnia, irritability	Anthelmintics, initia scrupulous persona hygiene, shorten fingernails; launder washable items in hottest or boiled water
Pneumonia	Direct and indirect contact	Abrupt onset	High fever, shaking, chills, productive cough	Antibiotics, liquids, rest, antipyretics
Rubella* (German measles)	Direct contact by respiratory droplets from an infected person coughing and sneezing	12–23 days	Rash and fever for 2–3 days	No specific treatment for this disease; patients can take acetaminophen to reduce fever
Scabies	Direct contact or indirect contact with infested clothing/bedding	2–6 weeks	Intense itching of small, raised areas of skin that contain fluid or tiny burrows under the skin, resembling a line—may be anywhere on the body	Topical scabicide, oral antihistamines, and salicylates to reduce itching

Disease	Means of Transmission	Incubation	Symptoms	Treatment
Strep throat	Direct contact	1–3 days	Fever, red and sore throat, pus spots on back of throat, tender and swollen glands of neck	Antibiotics, analgesics, antipyretics, increase fluid intake
Scarlet fever (*scarlatina*) (streptococcal)	Direct or indirect contact	1–7 days	Same as above, plus strawberry tongue, rash on skin and inside mouth, high fever, nausea, and vomiting	Same as above, plus bed rest
VRE (Vancomycin-Resistant Enterococci)	Direct and indirect contact. Person-to-person contact or contact with contaminated surfaces	24 hours	For a skin infection, area may be red and tender. For a urinary tract infection (UTI), possible back pain; a burning sensation when urinating or a need to urinate more often; possible diarrhea, fever, chills; weakness or sick feeling	If no symptoms are present, no treatment is usually needed. Other antibiotics can be used than vancomycin if the VRE infection is in the bladder and a urinary catheter is being used, removal of the catheter can help get rid of the infection

Diseases represented with the (*) must be reported to the National Notifiable Diseases Surveillance System of the CDC, through your local state or county health department. Visit the CDC website at www.cdc.gov/ncphi/disss/nndss/phs/infdis.htm for a comprehensive list of all reportable diseases. Refer also to "Sexually Transmitted Diseases" in Unit 11, Chapter 35.

prevention and protection. You can be instrumental in the interruption of the cycle by being **vigilant** in, and actively making efforts against, the transmission of disease. Breaking the infection cycle helps prevent the spread of disease.

Infectious Agents

Infections occur when a pathogen (infectious agent, the first link in the chain of infection) finds a body (a reservoir or source, the second link) that offers it the conditions necessary for growth. Common infectious agents are microorganisms that are classified as **bacteria**, **viruses**, **fungi**, **parasites**, and **rickettsiae**. Infection control practices such as sanitization, disinfection, and sterilization are methods to break these links in the chain of infection and are discussed later in this chapter.

Bacteria

Bacteria are microorganisms that vary in their **morphology**. Bacteria in the body do not indicate that disease is present; many types are beneficial. However, when it gets into the wrong area of the body such as the bloodstream or becomes overpopulated, it can feed on the body's vital nutrients while releasing toxins, causing problems to the body due to the invasion. These single-celled microorganisms are different from all other organisms because they lack a nucleus and organelles (mitrochondria, chloroplasts, and lysosomes; refer to Chapter 23 to review information about cells). Bacteria reproduce by cell division approximately every 20 minutes. Figure 36–2, A through C, shows the various forms of bacteria. Many species of bacteria are pathogenic to humans and animals. For example, *Escherichia coli* causes urinary tract infections (among other illnesses) in humans; *Bordetella pertussis* causes whooping cough, which is transmitted by droplet infection; and *Vibrio cholerae* causes cholera in humans who ingest contaminated food and water.

Viruses

Viruses, which are the smallest of the microorganisms, may be viewed only by an electron microscope. Figure 36–3 shows a magnified view of a virus. Viruses are classified by the type of DNA or RNA (the type of

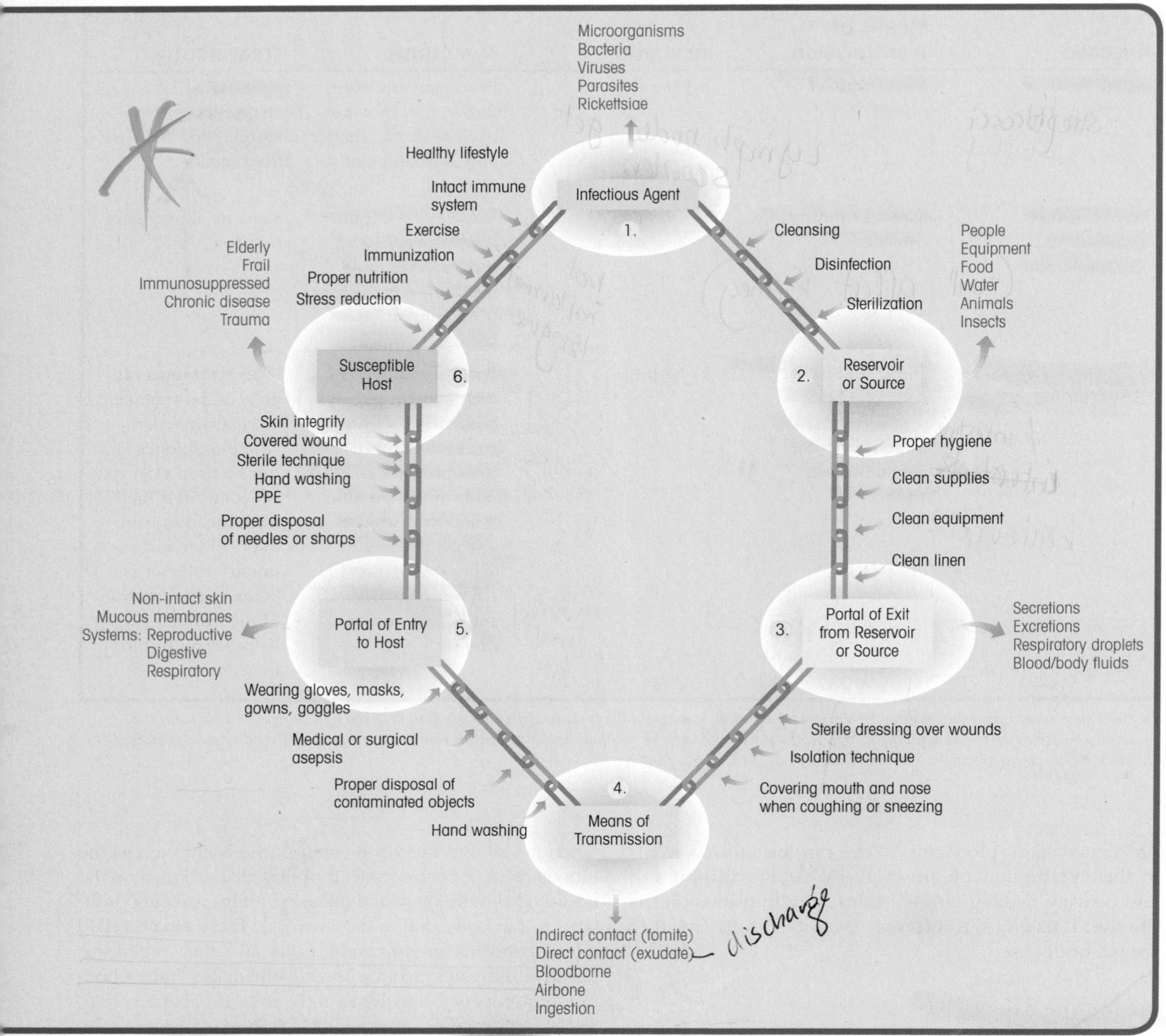

Figure 36–1: The chain of infection. *Delmar/Cengage Learning.*

nucleic acid core) they have or by their clinical properties. Viruses can reproduce themselves only within a host, by attaching itself to a cell and taking over the cell's nucleus. It then uses the hostage cell to self-replicate the virus, often destroying the host cell. Commonly known viruses include HIV/AIDS, herpes, chicken pox, hepatitis, the common cold, and influenza.

Fungi

Fungi are simple parasitic plants that depend on other life forms for a nutritional source. Molds (multicelled) fungi can be found both indoors and outdoors and grow best in warm, damp, and humid conditions. Molds spread and reproduce by spore formation, which is a mode of reproduction in which the organism breaks up into a number of pieces. Mold spores can survive harsh environmental conditions, such as dry conditions, that do not support normal mold growth. Yeasts (single-celled) fungi consist of oval or round cells found in soils and on plant surfaces, in sugary mediums such as flower nectar and fruits, and as mild to dangerous pathogens in humans. The multiplication of yeast cells occurs by

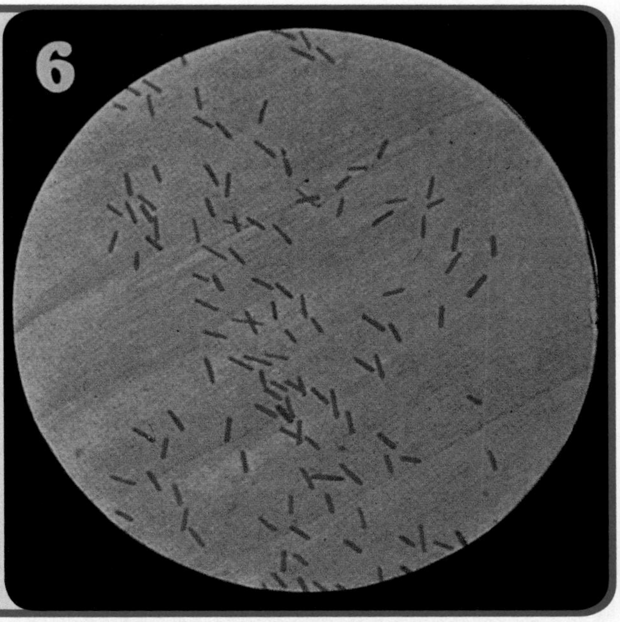

Figure 36–2A: Escherichia coli. *Centers for Disease Control and Prevention.*

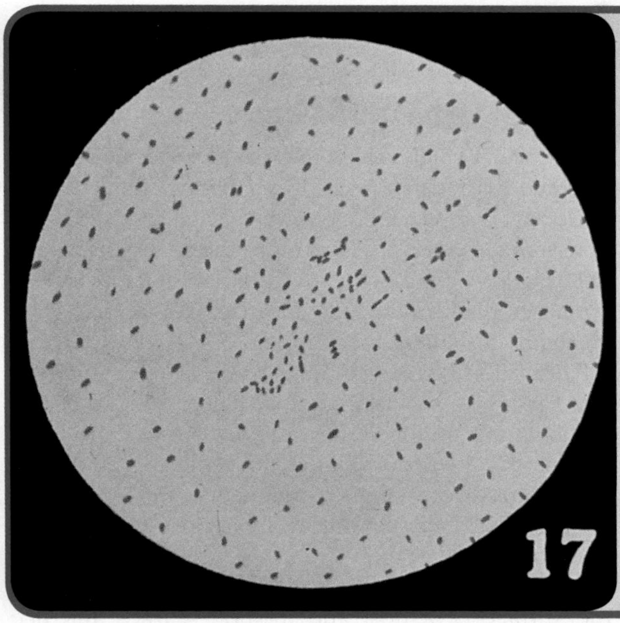

Figure 36–2C: *Vibrio cholerae. Centers for Disease Control and Prevention.*

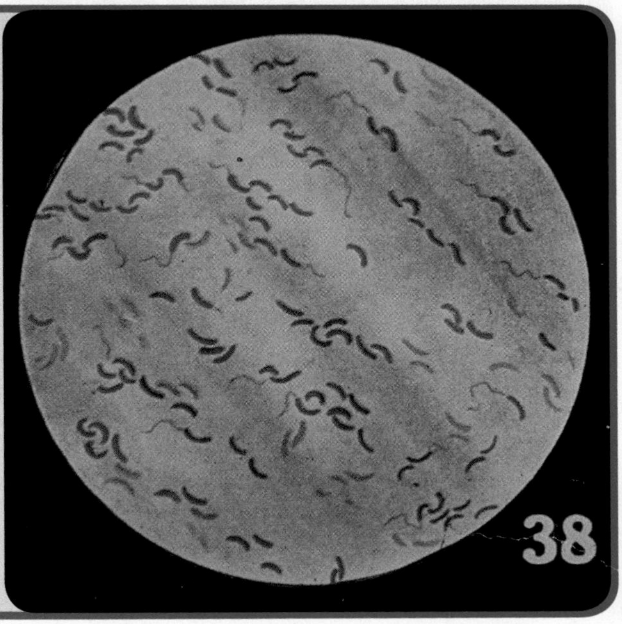

Figure 36–2B: Haemophilus pertussis. *Centers for Disease Control and Prevention.*

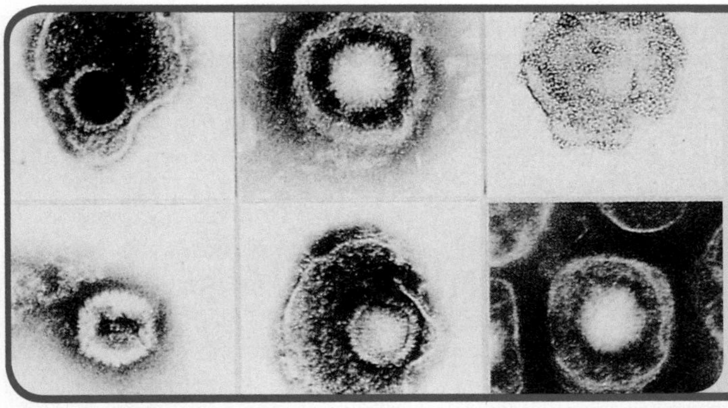

Figure 36–3: Electron micrographs of the various types of *Herpes simplex* virus. *Centers for Disease Control and Prevention.*

a budding process, by the formation of cross walls or fission, and sometimes by a combination of these two processes. Roughly 100 types of fungi are common in humans; approximately only 10 of these are pathogenic. Some examples of pathogenic fungal conditions are histoplasmosis (a lung infection passed on by the droppings of certain birds and bats), *Candida albicans* (yeast infection), and *Tinea pedis* (athlete's foot, see Figure 36–4).

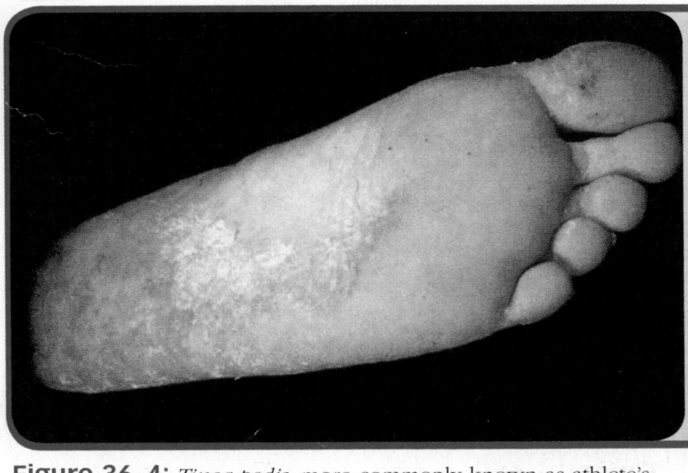

Figure 36–4: *Tinea pedis*, more commonly known as athlete's foot. *Centers for Disease Control and Prevention.*

Parasites

Parasites are organisms that depend on another living organism for nourishment. Parasites are classified as **protozoa**, metazoa, and ectoparasite.

- Protozoa are single-celled internal parasites that have a true nucleus and survive on living matter. Characteristics such as hair-like projections (flagella) and tails determine the classification for these organisms by determining how they move. Common diseases caused by these organisms include malaria, toxoplasmosis, and *Trichomonas vaginalis*. Diarrhea, bowel infection, and inflammation of the brain are some of the symptoms that can be caused by protozoa (Figure 36–5).
- Metazoa are multicellular organisms that cause pinworms, hookworms (Figure 36–6), and tapeworms. Symptoms from these organisms vary but can include diarrhea, itching and rash at site, malaise, and abdominal cramps.
- Ectoparasites, also multicellular parasites, live on the surface of a host and include scabies and lice (Figure 36–7). Intense itching at the site and red, dry, scaly, irritated skin are common symptoms experienced by persons infested by these parasites.

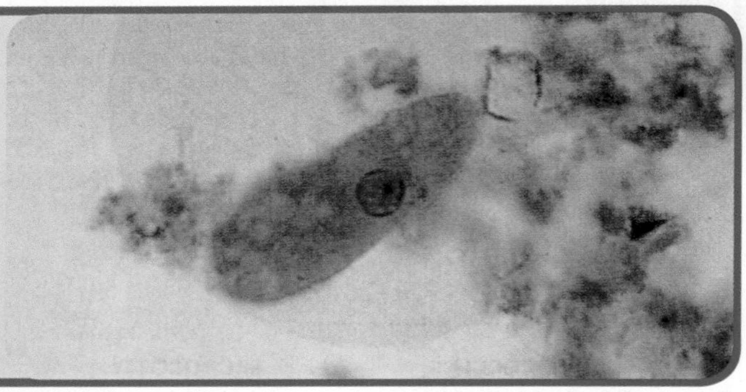

Figure 36–5: Intestinal protozoa *Entamoeba coli*. *Centers for Disease Control and Prevention.*

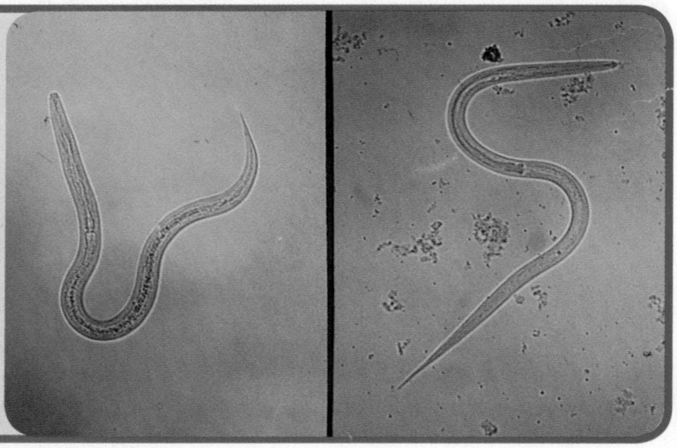

Figure 36–6: Strongyloides—filariform larvae of hookworm and strongyloides. *Centers for Disease Control and Prevention.*

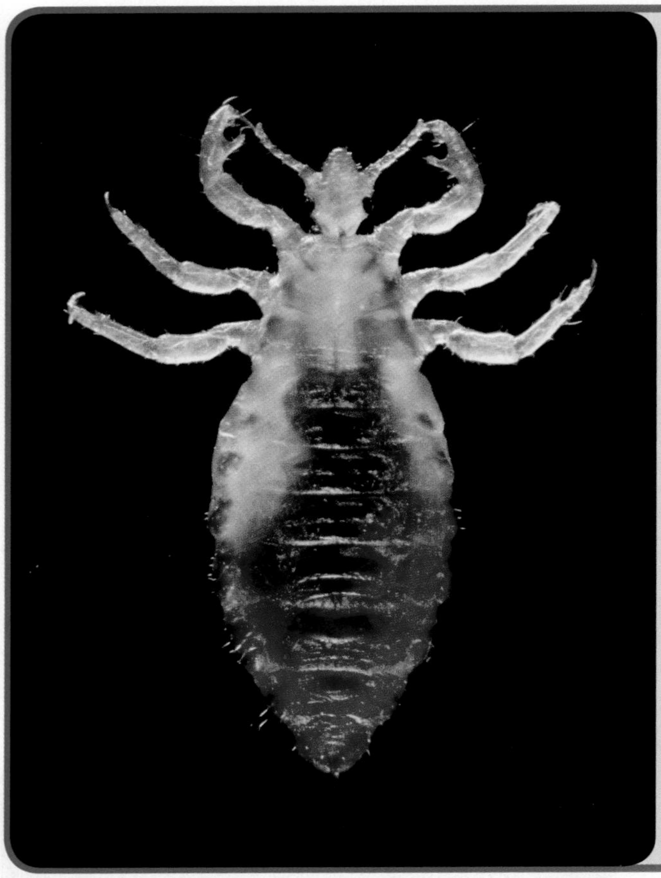

Figure 36–7: Lice. *Centers for Disease Control and Prevention.*

Rickettsiae

Rickettsiae are known as **obligate** parasites because they depend completely on their host for survival. Rickettsiae are larger than viruses and can be seen under conventional microscopes after staining procedures. Most rickettsial pathogens are transmitted by ectoparasites such as fleas, lice, mites, and ticks (Figure 36–8) during blood-feeding or from scarification of infectious feces from these vectors that may be deposited on the skin. Examples of this type of infection include Lyme disease (Figure 36–9), Rocky Mountain spotted fever, and typhus. Different rickettsial infections cause similar symptoms, including fever, severe headache, a characteristic rash, and malaise.

Reservoir or Source

The reservoir is the place where conditions are ripe for replication. This can be a person or object. Sometimes, a human reservoir is called a carrier because the pathogen can survive, grow, and multiply here. Examples include people, equipment, food, water, animals, and insects. Methods to break this link in the chain of infection

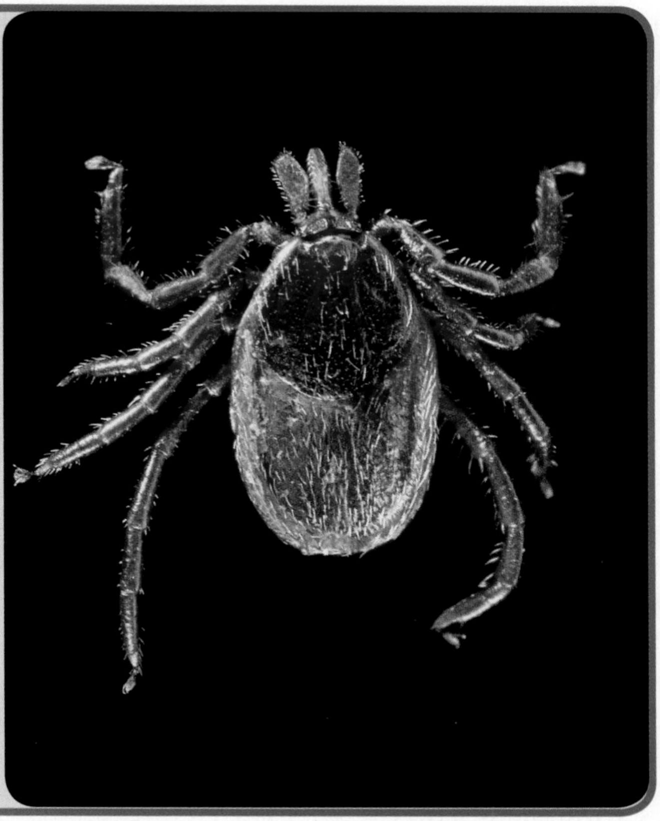

Figure 36–8: Deer tick. *Centers for Disease Control and Prevention.*

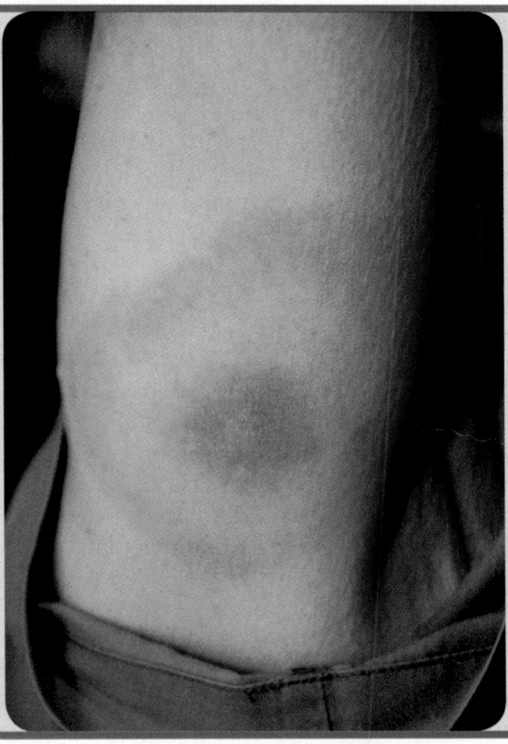

Figure 36–9: Lyme disease rash. *Centers for Disease Control and Prevention.*

include proper hygiene and proper cleaning of supplies, equipment, and linen.

Portal of Exit from Reservoir or Source

The next step in the chain of infection is the portal of exit, how the pathogen departs the reservoir or source to another by way of body openings. The microorganisms leave the reservoir or source through the discharge of body secretions, excretions, respiratory droplets, and blood/body fluids and make either direct or indirect contact with another host. Methods to break this link in the chain include isolation techniques, covering the mouth and nose when coughing or sneezing, and using sterile dressings when applying to wounds.

Means of Transmission

The next step, means of transmission, refers to how the microorganism travels from the reservoir and portal of exit to a susceptible individual. Diseases can be transmitted in different ways, and it is important for you to recognize the ways in which the infectious agent travels to realize and understand the potential danger that an infected person can have.

Direct contact means there is actual contact with the infected person or body fluids, including **blood-borne** transmission, which is acquired when the infected blood enters the susceptible host through blood or body fluids. Direct contact includes eating, drinking, touching, kissing, and sexual intimacy. Indirect contact means that you can contract the disease from inhaling the contaminated air (such as following a cough or sneeze of an infected person), or by handling a **fomite** (such as soiled tissues, piece of equipment, or door knob) that an infected person touched. When a person with a cold coughs or sneezes, the vapor containing the microorganism that is causing the illness can travel up to 3 feet (however, it does not remain suspended in the air for long periods of time). This is known as a droplet infection.

CLINICAL PEARL

When you are around a person who is sick, you should not inhale deeply when you breathe, or you can subject yourself to an even greater risk of contracting the disease.

A similar means of transmission, airborne transmission, involves tiny drops of vapor (moisture) from the person's breath, which, depending on the force of the breath, can carry droplets quite far, possibly projecting them up to 20 feet or more. Ingestion, the consumption of contaminated food or water, and **vector** transmission (transmission by a disease-carrying insect, usually a mosquito or a tick) are additional examples of indirect contact.

Methods to break this link in the chain of infection include hand washing, wearing gloves, masks, gowns, and goggles, medical and surgical asepsis, and proper disposal of contaminated objects.

Portals of Entry

The way the pathogen enters the host is the next link in the chain. Portals of entry include the mouth, nose, throat, ears, eyes, intestinal tract, urinary tract, reproductive tract, or open wounds and breaks in the skin. Methods to break this link include hand washing, wearing **personal protective equipment (PPE)**, using sterile technique, proper disposal of needles or sharps, ensuring skin integrity, and covering wounds.

Susceptible Host

The susceptible host is one who is capable of being infected by the pathogen. The resistance or ability to fight off disease of the host is low, which could be because of poor health, poor nutritional habits, or poor hygiene. Populations that have low resistance and increased susceptibility include the elderly, frail, or immunosuppressive or those with chronic disease, trauma, or both. Methods to break this link include living a healthy lifestyle (exercise, proper nutrition, and stress reduction), maintaining intact immune systems, and immunization.

INFECTIOUS DISEASE PROCESS

After an individual is exposed to a disease-producing pathogen, a series of stages from exposure to recovery from the condition occur. The stages generally occur in order, and each has its own distinctiveness. This can be useful for providing patient education and assisting the physician with the patient's care and treatment.

- *The incubation stage.* This stage is considered the silent stage because often it is not known when the pathogen gains entry into the host and starts replicating. The length of the incubation period depends on the disease; some are very short, whereas others are lengthy. The stage ends when the first signs and symptoms of the disease appear.
- *The prodromal stage.* The first onset of signs and symptoms occur (malaise, runny nose, itchy and dry eyes, and so on). This stage generally lasts about one to two days and is considered to be the time when symptoms show that a disease process is taking place.
- *The acute stage.* The disease reaches its highest point of development (severe aches, chills, vomiting, and so on). The symptoms during this stage can help determine one disease from another.
- *The declining stage.* The symptoms start to subside; the infection is still present, but the patient's health starts to return to normal.
- *The convalescent stage.* The symptoms have all but completely vanished, and the pathogen has been mostly eliminated. The patient begins to regain strength and return to his or her original state of health.

DEFENSE MECHANISMS

The body's immune system has amazing abilities. Immunity is best when the body is in a state of good physical, emotional, and mental condition. Essentially, this means that defense against disease can be maintained most efficiently by practicing the good health habits of proper exercise, adequate rest, good nutrition, and proper hygiene. Exercise is most helpful in resisting disease because it promotes circulation, encourages nutrition, and reduces stress. Following the food pyramid guidelines and developing good eating habits help keep energy levels at a maximum. Getting enough rest according to individual need gives the body time to restore strength and vitality.

The body also has specialized defense mechanisms. The respiratory tract contains hair-like cilia that filter out invading pathogens. Coughing and sneezing are reflexes that rid the body of invaders. Body secretions (such as tears, sweat, urine, and mucus) wash pathogens from the body. These body secretions have a low pH, which discourages bacterial growth. Hydrochloric acid found naturally in the digestive tract has a low pH and discourages growth. Refer to Chapter 31 for more information about the various types of immunity and the immune system.

INFECTION CONTROL AND DISEASE PREVENTION

You can play a useful role in preventing disease transmission and help provide a safe and comfortable environment for staff and patients. For example, when a patient presents with an infectious disease, as a medical assistant, it will be your responsibility to remove the infected individual from the waiting room immediately to prevent others from being infected. Providing patient education is important in breaking the infection cycle. Offer the patient instruction on coughing and sneezing into tissues you provide and show the patient where to deposit the waste. After the patient leaves, it is good practice to follow the patient's steps with a spray disinfectant to help contain the germs. If you do not clean up after the patient carefully (by gloving to pick up used tissues, for example), there is a risk that you and others might contract the same illness. In severe infectious disease cases, it is wise to wear a face mask that covers the mouth and nose. The physician usually suggests this for protection against disease. As you continue reading this chapter, you will learn many more ways to ensure the health and safety of yourself and others.

Universal Precautions

Universal precautions, as defined by the CDC, are a set of precautions designed to prevent transmission of human immunodeficiency virus (HIV), hepatitis B virus (HBV), and other blood-borne pathogens when providing first aid or health care. Under universal precautions, blood and body fluids of all patients are considered potentially infectious for HIV, HBV, and other blood-borne pathogens.

Standard Precautions

In addition to protecting patients from infectious diseases, health care workers are responsible for self-protection. **Standard Precautions** (Figure 36–10) have been recommended by the Centers for Disease Control and Prevention (CDC) since 1987 to provide for the safety and welfare of both health care providers and the public, regarding health care standards.

It recommends using standard blood and body fluid precautions when working with all patients, especially when the infection status of the patient is unknown. Appropriate protection against exposure to blood and body fluids should be routine practice for all health care workers.

Follow these general guidelines for disease prevention and safety:

1. Perform proper hand washing before and after every procedure and before and after gloving. This must become a habit for all health care workers for self-protection from disease transmission. Immediately washing *any* skin surface thoroughly that has been contaminated with any blood or body fluid is vital.
2. Gloves should be worn when in contact (direct or indirect) with blood or any body fluids, mucous membranes, or non-intact skin; in handling items or surfaces soiled with blood or body fluid; and when performing venipuncture or any other surgical procedure. After each patient contact, gloves should be changed and hands washed. If you find that you are allergic to latex gloves, gloves made from other materials are available and can be supplied with or without powder.
3. Bandage all scratches, paper cuts, or any breaks in the skin after hand washing and before gloving for self-protection against possible contamination.
4. Refrain from direct patient care if you have an **exudative** skin condition or laceration (or other contagious disease) until the condition clears up. An appropriate bandage should be worn, and the affected person should follow proper gloving procedures to keep the condition contained.
5. When you are working, never eat, drink, chew gum, smoke, place hands or fingers to the mouth (including nail-biting), or place any item in your mouth (such as a pen or pencil).
6. Wear PPE (protective gloves, masks, face shields, gowns or aprons, and goggles) when splashing of any blood or body fluid is possible while you are working to prevent contact with mucous membranes, blood, or any body fluid of any patient (Figure 36–11A and B).
7. Always recap or close bottles, jars, and tubes immediately after desired amounts are obtained to avoid spills, waste, and accidents.
8. Clean up spills immediately to avoid accidents (Figures 36–12A and B). Spilled blood or any body fluid should be flooded with a liquid germicide or bleach solution with a 1:10 ratio before cleaning up with paper towels (wearing latex or vinyl gloves). Commercial spill kits may also be used to solidify liquids, which makes cleanup easier.
9. Work in a well-lit, properly ventilated, uncluttered, and quiet area for better concentration.
10. Immediately discard all disposable sharp instruments, lancets, syringes, and needles (intact) in proper biohazard, puncture-proof containers (Figure 36–13). *Never* break needles off, handle needles after they are used, or reuse needles. Never put the needle cover between your teeth to remove it when giving an injection.
11. Package broken glass or any sharp, unusable items in a puncture-proof container marked "Caution—Broken glass" to discard in the proper waste receptacle. This protects unsuspecting custodial personnel from injury.
12. Discard *all* hazardous waste in proper containers (Figure 36–14).
13. Place reusable metal instruments in a disinfectant solution after rinsing in cold water in preparation for proper cleaning and sterilization.
14. Use disposable equipment in mouth-to-mouth resuscitation procedures, such as mouthpieces, **resuscitation** bags, or any other ventilation supplies necessary for emergency use.
15. Especially strict adherence to safety precautions should be practiced during pregnancy.

If you or a coworker is sick or feverish, it is wise to refrain from contact with patients. Stay home and take care of yourself until you are well and return to work only after you have been fever-free for at least 24 hours. Working as a cooperative team helps solve these types

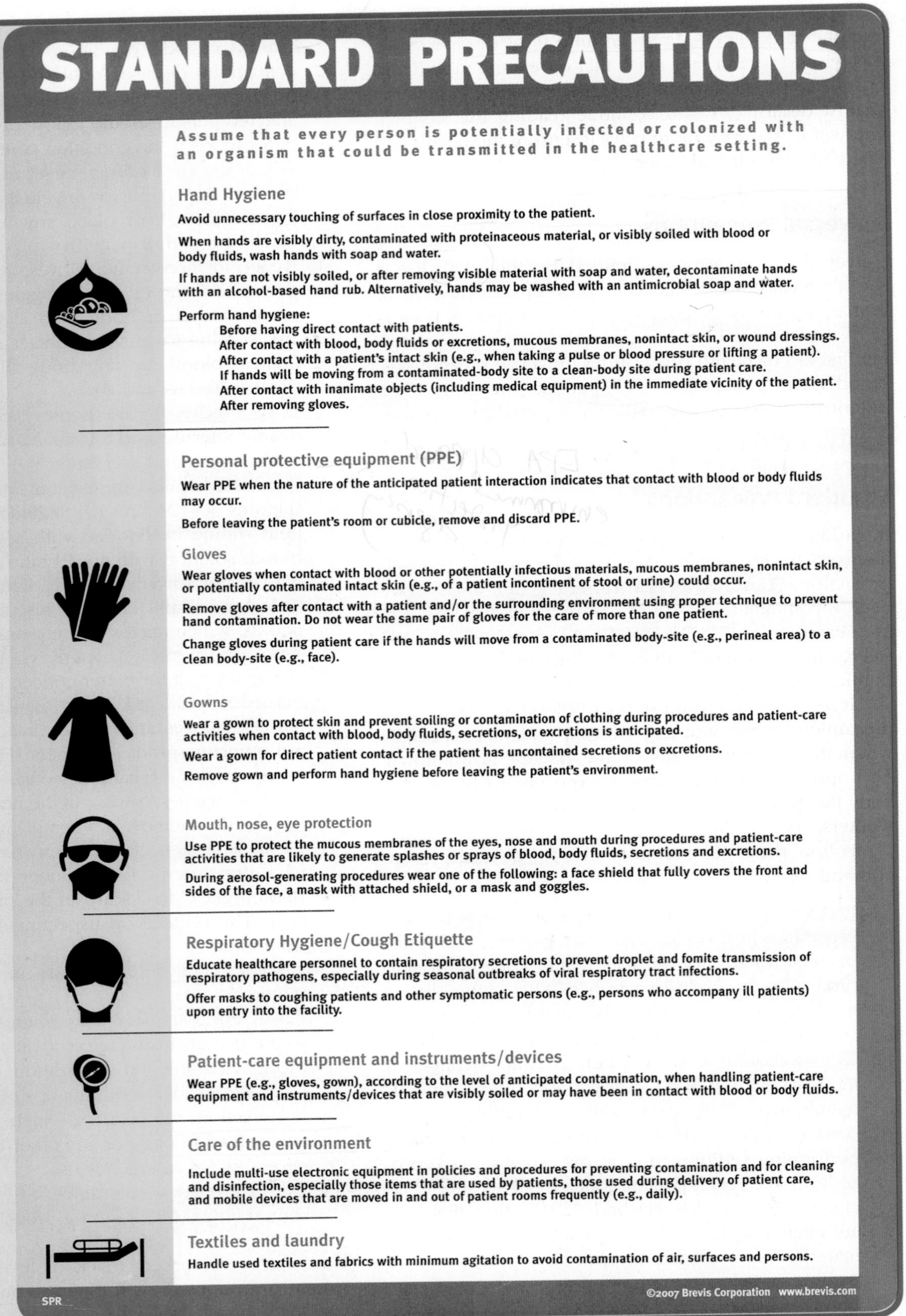

STANDARD PRECAUTIONS

Assume that every person is potentially infected or colonized with an organism that could be transmitted in the healthcare setting.

Hand Hygiene

Avoid unnecessary touching of surfaces in close proximity to the patient.

When hands are visibly dirty, contaminated with proteinaceous material, or visibly soiled with blood or body fluids, wash hands with soap and water.

If hands are not visibly soiled, or after removing visible material with soap and water, decontaminate hands with an alcohol-based hand rub. Alternatively, hands may be washed with an antimicrobial soap and water.

Perform hand hygiene:

- Before having direct contact with patients.
- After contact with blood, body fluids or excretions, mucous membranes, nonintact skin, or wound dressings.
- After contact with a patient's intact skin (e.g., when taking a pulse or blood pressure or lifting a patient).
- If hands will be moving from a contaminated-body site to a clean-body site during patient care.
- After contact with inanimate objects (including medical equipment) in the immediate vicinity of the patient.
- After removing gloves.

Personal protective equipment (PPE)

Wear PPE when the nature of the anticipated patient interaction indicates that contact with blood or body fluids may occur.

Before leaving the patient's room or cubicle, remove and discard PPE.

Gloves

Wear gloves when contact with blood or other potentially infectious materials, mucous membranes, nonintact skin, or potentially contaminated intact skin (e.g., of a patient incontinent of stool or urine) could occur.

Remove gloves after contact with a patient and/or the surrounding environment using proper technique to prevent hand contamination. Do not wear the same pair of gloves for the care of more than one patient.

Change gloves during patient care if the hands will move from a contaminated body-site (e.g., perineal area) to a clean body-site (e.g., face).

Gowns

Wear a gown to protect skin and prevent soiling or contamination of clothing during procedures and patient-care activities when contact with blood, body fluids, secretions, or excretions is anticipated.

Wear a gown for direct patient contact if the patient has uncontained secretions or excretions.

Remove gown and perform hand hygiene before leaving the patient's environment.

Mouth, nose, eye protection

Use PPE to protect the mucous membranes of the eyes, nose and mouth during procedures and patient-care activities that are likely to generate splashes or sprays of blood, body fluids, secretions and excretions.

During aerosol-generating procedures wear one of the following: a face shield that fully covers the front and sides of the face, a mask with attached shield, or a mask and goggles.

Respiratory Hygiene/Cough Etiquette

Educate healthcare personnel to contain respiratory secretions to prevent droplet and fomite transmission of respiratory pathogens, especially during seasonal outbreaks of viral respiratory tract infections.

Offer masks to coughing patients and other symptomatic persons (e.g., persons who accompany ill patients) upon entry into the facility.

Patient-care equipment and instruments/devices

Wear PPE (e.g., gloves, gown), according to the level of anticipated contamination, when handling patient-care equipment and instruments/devices that are visibly soiled or may have been in contact with blood or body fluids.

Care of the environment

Include multi-use electronic equipment in policies and procedures for preventing contamination and for cleaning and disinfection, especially those items that are used by patients, those used during delivery of patient care, and mobile devices that are moved in and out of patient rooms frequently (e.g., daily).

Textiles and laundry

Handle used textiles and fabrics with minimum agitation to avoid contamination of air, surfaces and persons.

SPR

Figure 36–10: A poster such as this one should be posted in the physician's office laboratory to comply with the Standard Precautions and to remind employees of safety precautions. *Courtesy of the Brevis Corp.*

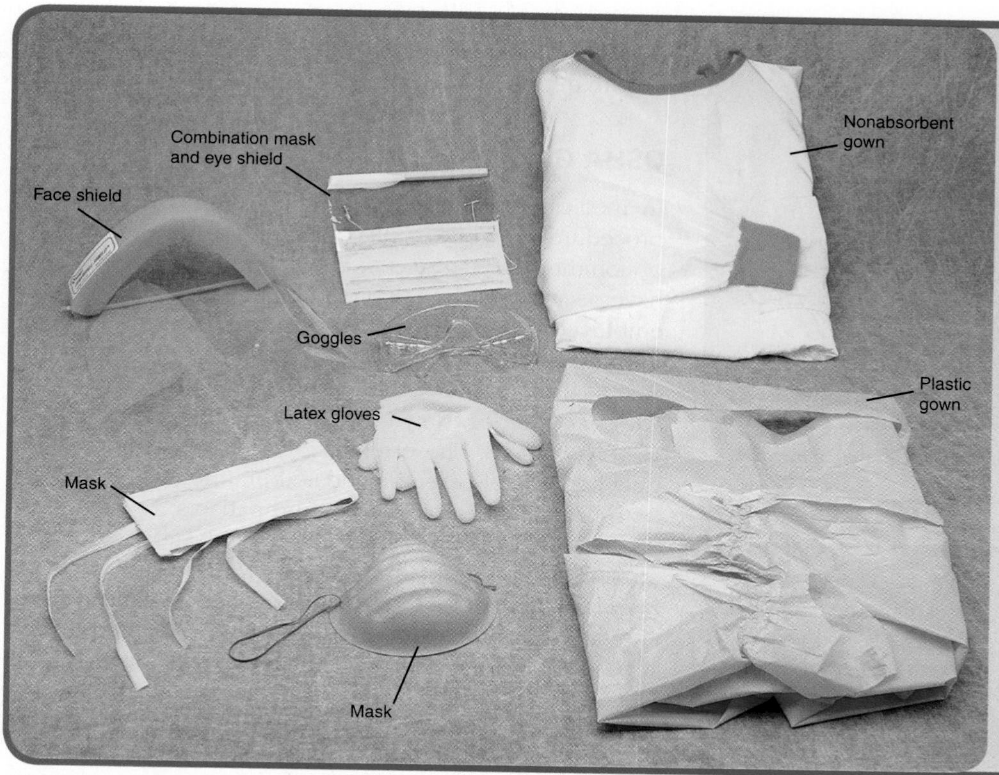

Figure 36–11A: Personal protective equipment (PPE). *Delmar/Cengage Learning.*

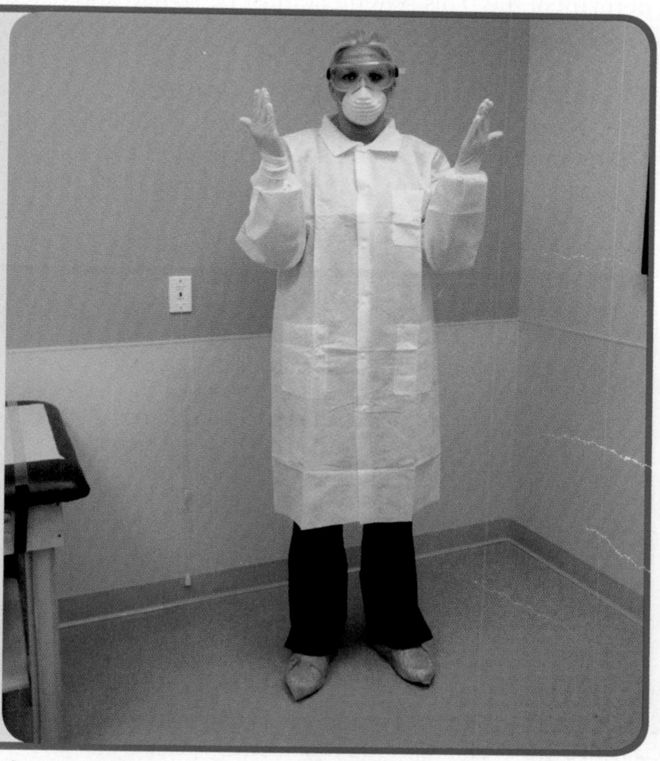

Figure 36–11B: The medical assistant is wearing PPE: goggles, mask, gown, and gloves. *Delmar/Cengage Learning.*

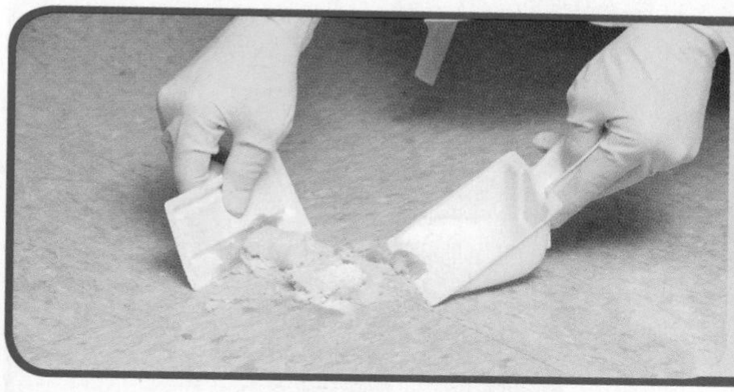

Figure 36–12A: Wear gloves to clean up a spill. *Delmar/Cengage Learning.*

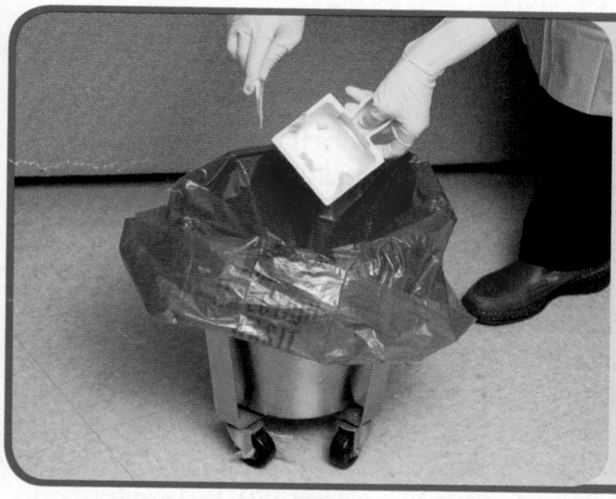

Figure 36–12B: All materials used to clean up the spill are placed in a biohazard waste bag. *Delmar/Cengage Learning.*

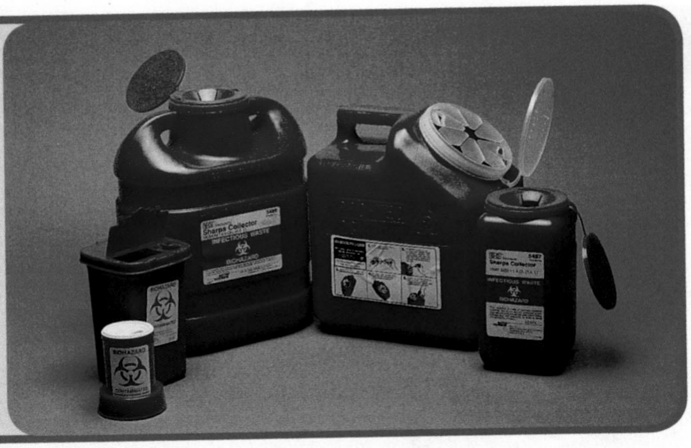

Figure 36–13: Various sizes of sharps containers. *Delmar/Cengage Learning.*

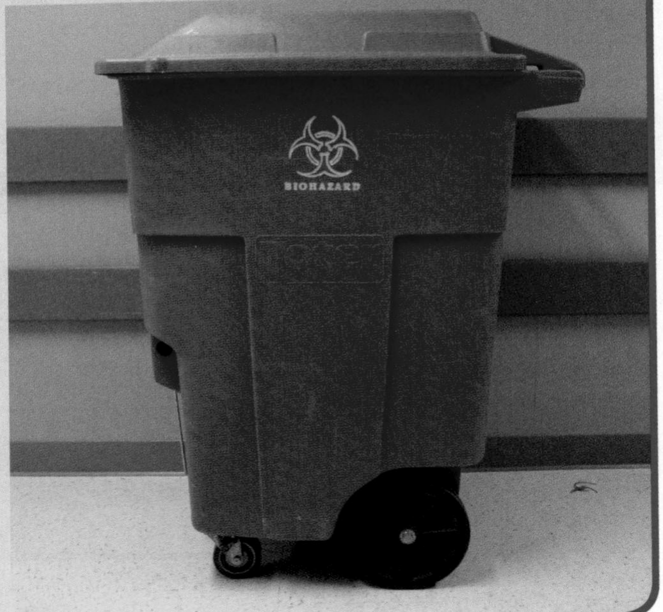

Figure 36–14: Properly dispose of hazardous waste. *Delmar/Cengage Learning.*

of problems, which can and do happen from time to time. Remember that the multiskilled medical assistant is a well-prepared team member who can fill in when other staff members are absent.

Further guidelines are discussed in the next section, regarding mandatory **Occupational Safety and Health Administration (OSHA)** regulations. It is up to each person working in the health care field to be honest and credible about following these guidelines. Remember: Some diseases are dangerous and can be fatal. You have a legal, moral, and ethical responsibility to protect yourself and others from such preventable problems. The best way to do this is to establish a routine and stick to it. It is far better and easier to learn good habits from the start than to break established bad habits.

OSHA Guidelines

In medical care facilities, infection control policies and procedures are put in place to control the transmission of communicable diseases. Regulatory agencies and laws have been established to provide standards for all who are employed with managed care of the public to ensure quality care. Two of the most prominent are the Occupational Safety and Health Administration (OSHA), and the **Clinical Laboratory Improvement Amendments (CLIA)** of 1988. These regulations must be followed not only because of federal mandate but, foremost, to protect both health care professionals and patients.

In each medical office, a posted statement must appear in writing that agrees with compliance of Standard Precautions and other OSHA regulations, as shown in Figure 36–15. Medical offices and employees who do not follow these regulations will be fined by OSHA. Having this statement in clear view provides a constant reminder to all health care personnel to be alert in their duties that they may be exposed to blood or other biohazardous body fluids or infectious waste on a daily basis. Each employee must have this statement explained when he or she is hired and have evidence of this explanation in writing with his or her signature in a permanent file. This statement must be signed and dated by the employer as well.

The Blood-Borne Pathogen Standard

The blood-borne pathogen standard, published by OSHA in 1991, was established to reduce the risk for occupational exposure. As outlined by the CDC, health

Standard Precautions

All employees in this medical practice must follow standard precautions at all times in performing procedures that may expose them to bloodborne pathogens possibly contained in the blood and body fluids from any patient regardless of the patient's health status. All employees must wear protective barriers that are appropriate for the procedure being performed to prevent possible infection. Employees who work with direct patient contact must have HBV vaccine. Any accidental needle sticks, other injuries, or contacts with a potentially infectious body fluid must be reported to the physician at once for treatment and documentation.

Figure 36–15: A statement regarding compliance with Standard Precautions, like this one, should be posted in clear view. *Delmar/Cengage Learning.*

care personnel are at risk for occupational exposure to blood-borne pathogens, including hepatitis B virus (HBV), hepatitis C virus (HCV), and human immunodeficiency virus (HIV). Exposures can occur through needlesticks, cuts from other sharp instruments contaminated with an infected patient's blood, or through contact of the eye, nose, mouth, or skin with a patient's blood. To comply with this standard, employers must have a written exposure control plan to protect workers whose employment puts them at an increased risk of contracting a blood-borne pathogen exposure. Documentation of employee input must be included in the exposure control plan.

In 2001, in response to the Needlestick Safety and Prevention Act, OSHA revised the blood-borne pathogens standard. The revised standard clarifies the need for employers to select safer needle devices and to involve employees in the selection process.

Exposure Control Plan

Employers must update their exposure control plan annually to reflect technological changes that will help eliminate or reduce exposure to blood-borne pathogens. OSHA checks for compliance with this provision during inspections by questioning employees to determine whether and how their input was requested. The plan must include:

- *Engineering controls.* These are devices that isolate or remove the blood-borne pathogen hazard from the workplace. They include sharps disposal containers, self-sheathing needles, and safer medical devices such as sharps with engineered sharps-injury protection and needleless systems.
- *Work practice controls.* These are practices that reduce the likelihood of exposure by changing the way a task is performed. They include appropriate procedures for hand washing, sharps disposing, lab specimen packaging, laundry handling, and contaminated material cleaning.
- *PPE.* Employers must provide PPE such as gloves, gowns, and masks. Employers must clean, repair, and replace this equipment as needed.
- *Hepatitis B vaccinations.* Hepatitis B vaccinations must be available to all employees with occupational exposure to blood-borne pathogens within 10 days of employment, with no cost to the employee. Documentation of the immunization offer must be filed in the employee's record. If the person has already had the vaccine or refuses to be given the vaccine, documentation must be filed in the employee record.
- *Post-exposure follow-up.* Employers must provide post-exposure follow-up to any worker who experiences an exposure incident, at no cost to the worker. This includes conducting laboratory tests; providing confidential medical evaluation; identifying and testing the source individual, if feasible; testing the exposed employee's blood if the worker consents; performing post-exposure prophylaxis; offering counseling; and evaluating reported illnesses. All diagnoses must remain confidential.
- *Labels and signs to communicate hazards.* The standard requires warning labels affixed to containers of regulated waste, refrigerators and freezers, and other containers used to store or transplant blood or other potentially infectious materials. Facilities may use red bags or containers instead of labels (Figure 36–16). Employers also must post signs to identify restricted areas.
- *Information and training to employees.* Employers must ensure that their workers receive regular training that covers the dangers of blood-borne pathogens, preventive practices, and post-exposure procedures. Employers must offer this training on initial assignment and annually thereafter.
- *Documented employee medical and training records.* Medical and training records must be maintained for each employee. The employer also must maintain a log of occupational injuries and illnesses as well as a Sharps Injury Log unless classified as an exempt industry under OSHA's standard on Recording and Reporting Occupational Injuries and Illnesses.

BIOHAZARD LABELS

Containers that hold biohazardous materials must be properly labeled. Biohazardous materials include blood and body fluids as well as garments, gloves, masks, needles, gauze, wipes, aprons, and so on that may be contaminated with blood or other potentially contaminated body fluids. Labels shall be used to identify the presence of an actual or potential biological hazard.

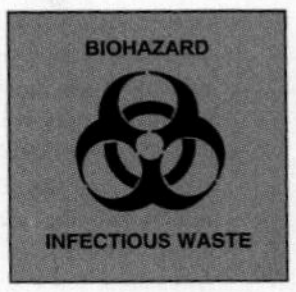

CONSIDERATIONS:

- Labels shall be fluorescent orange or orange-red, with lettering or symbols in a contrasting color.
- Labels should be affixed onto or as close as feasible to the container by adhesive, string, wire, or other method.
- Red bags or red containers may be substituted for labels.
- If blood or control serum is stored in a refrigerator, the refrigerator shall be marked with a biohazard label.
- If blood is stored in a refrigerator for transport or same-day shipment, it does not need to be labeled but should be put in containment bags.

Figure 36–16: Biohazard labels. *Delmar/Cengage Learning.*

Reporting Exposure Incidents Your employer should have in place a system for reporting exposures to evaluate quickly the risk of infection, inform you about the treatments available to help prevent infection, and determine whether infection occurs. The CDC recommends the following steps to be taken immediately following an exposure to blood:

- Wash needlesticks and cuts with soap and water.
- Flush splashes to the nose, mouth, or skin with water.
- Irrigate eyes with clean water, saline, or sterile irrigation.

Additionally, the exposure needs to be reported to the appropriate supervisor or person responsible for managing exposures. The steps required after an incident of exposure are covered in Procedure 36–1. Figure 36-17 shows an example of an incident exposure report form.

Needlesticks and Other Sharps The greatest risk of exposure to blood-borne pathogens occurs when handling contaminated sharps; OSHA estimates approximately 500,000 exposures occur each year. At all times, health care workers must use extreme caution when handling needles, scalpels, and other sharp instruments to avoid self-injury.

To prevent possible self-injury, it is recommended that needles should never be recapped, broken off, or removed from disposable syringes by hand after use. They should be placed carefully in puncture-proof containers after engaging the safety guard over the needle. Always dispose of the entire used needle intact with the syringe to prevent injury. If it becomes necessary to re-cover a needle prior to performing an injection, a one-handed scoop method should be used. (See Chapter 53 for this procedure.)

Many medical devices have been developed to reduce the risk of needlesticks and other sharps injuries. These safer medical devices replace sharps with a non-needle sharp or a needle device used for withdrawing body fluids, accessing a vein or artery, or administering medications or other fluids, with a built-in safety feature or mechanism that effectively reduces the risk of an exposure incident.

Used needles, lancets, capillary tubes, and glass slides should be properly disposed of in a sharps container. These containers are leak-proof and puncture-proof and are usually red in color to identify the contents as biohazard. Some containers are clear or white in color to make it easier to realize when they are full. A biohazardous warning label must be present on all sharps

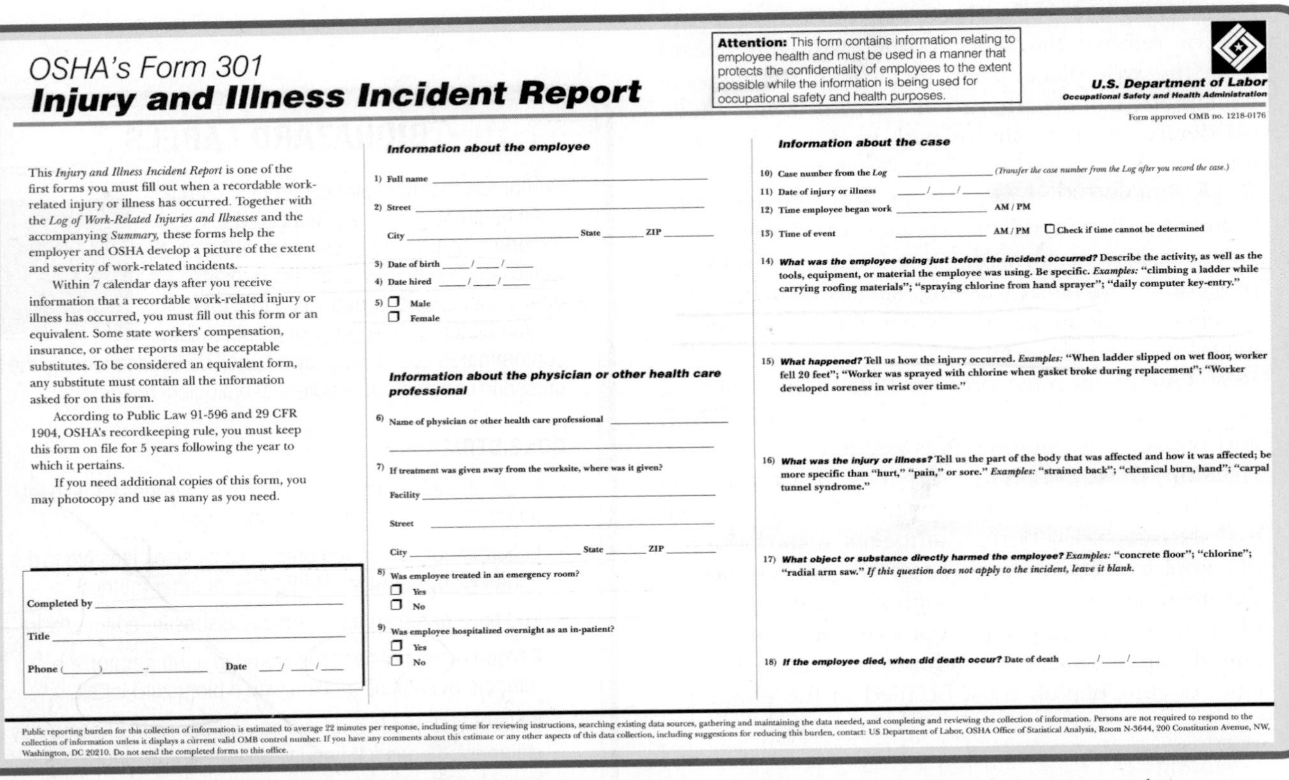

OSHA's Form 301
Injury and Illness Incident Report

Attention: This form contains information relating to employee health and must be used in a manner that protects the confidentiality of employees to the extent possible while the information is being used for occupational safety and health purposes.

U.S. Department of Labor
Occupational Safety and Health Administration

Form approved OMB no. 1218-0176

This *Injury and Illness Incident Report* is one of the first forms you must fill out when a recordable work-related injury or illness has occurred. Together with the *Log of Work-Related Injuries and Illnesses* and the accompanying *Summary*, these forms help the employer and OSHA develop a picture of the extent and severity of work-related incidents.

Within 7 calendar days after you receive information that a recordable work-related injury or illness has occurred, you must fill out this form or an equivalent. Some state workers' compensation, insurance, or other reports may be acceptable substitutes. To be considered an equivalent form, any substitute must contain all the information asked for on this form.

According to Public Law 91-596 and 29 CFR 1904, OSHA's recordkeeping rule, you must keep this form on file for 5 years following the year to which it pertains.

If you need additional copies of this form, you may photocopy and use as many as you need.

Completed by ______
Title ______
Phone (___)___-___ Date __/__/__

Information about the employee

1) Full name ______
2) Street ______
City ______ State ___ ZIP ___
3) Date of birth __/__/__
4) Date hired __/__/__
5) ☐ Male ☐ Female

Information about the physician or other health care professional

6) Name of physician or other health care professional ______
7) If treatment was given away from the worksite, where was it given?
Facility ______
Street ______
City ______ State ___ ZIP ___
8) Was employee treated in an emergency room?
☐ Yes
☐ No
9) Was employee hospitalized overnight as an in-patient?
☐ Yes
☐ No

Information about the case

10) Case number from the *Log* ______ *(Transfer the case number from the Log after you record the case.)*
11) Date of injury or illness __/__/__
12) Time employee began work ______ AM / PM
13) Time of event ______ AM / PM ☐ Check if time cannot be determined
14) ***What was the employee doing just before the incident occurred?*** Describe the activity, as well as the tools, equipment, or material the employee was using. Be specific. *Examples:* "climbing a ladder while carrying roofing materials"; "spraying chlorine from hand sprayer"; "daily computer key-entry."
15) ***What happened?*** Tell us how the injury occurred. *Examples:* "When ladder slipped on wet floor, worker fell 20 feet"; "Worker was sprayed with chlorine when gasket broke during replacement"; "Worker developed soreness in wrist over time."
16) ***What was the injury or illness?*** Tell us the part of the body that was affected and how it was affected; be more specific than "hurt," "pain," or sore." *Examples:* "strained back"; "chemical burn, hand"; "carpal tunnel syndrome."
17) ***What object or substance directly harmed the employee?*** *Examples:* "concrete floor"; "chlorine"; "radial arm saw." *If this question does not apply to the incident, leave it blank.*
18) ***If the employee died, when did death occur?*** Date of death __/__/__

Public reporting burden for this collection of information is estimated to average 22 minutes per response, including time for reviewing instructions, searching existing data sources, gathering and maintaining the data needed, and completing and reviewing the collection of information. Persons are not required to respond to the collection of information unless it displays a current valid OMB control number. If you have any comments about this estimate or any other aspects of this data collection, including suggestions for reducing this burden, contact: US Department of Labor, OSHA Office of Statistical Analysis, Room N-3644, 200 Constitution Avenue, NW, Washington, DC 20210. Do not send the completed forms to this office.

Figure 36–17: OSHA's Injury and Illness incident report. This form can be downloaded and printed from OSHA's website, www.osha.gov/recordkeeping/RKforms.html. *United States Department of Labor, Occupational Safety and Health Administration. www.osha.gov.*

PROCEDURE 36–1 Complete an Incident Report

PURPOSE: To provide documentation required by OSHA in the event an employee becomes injured or is exposed to blood or body fluids. A post-exposure plan must be followed, and an incident report must be filled out.

EQUIPMENT: OSHA's Form 301 (Injury and Illness Incident Report), pen.

S SKILL: Demonstrate the proper procedure for completing an incident exposure report form.

Procedure Steps	Detailed Instructions and/or *Rationales*
1. Report the incident immediately to a supervisor for documentation.	*This helps determine whether a recordable, work-related injury occurred and the proper protocol according to your facility can be followed. In some cases, post-exposure treatment may be needed and should be started as soon as possible after the exposure.*
2. Assemble equipment.	
3. Fill in the demographic information about the employee.	This includes the full name, address, date of birth, date hired, and sex of the employee.
4. Fill in the information about the physician or other health care professional.	This includes the name of the physician or other health care professional, if treatment was given away from the worksite, and where, if the employee was treated in an emergency room, and if the employee was hospitalized overnight as an inpatient.
5. Complete the section regarding information about the case.	This includes the case number from the log, date of injury or illness, time the employee began work and the time of event (check box provided if a time cannot be determined).
6. Fill in what the employee was doing just before the incident occurred.	Describe the activity as well as the tools, equipment, or material the employee was using. Be specific. Examples: "giving a patient an injection," "drawing blood from the patient," and "cleaning a wound."
7. In the space provided, explain what happened.	Describe how the injury occurred. Examples: "Worker was poked with the needle while removing it from the patient's arm"; "Worker was splashed in the eye while irrigating the patient's wound."
8. Explain what the injury or illness was.	Describe what part of the body was affected and how it was affected; be more specific than "hurt, "pain," or "sore." Example: "punctured left hand."
9. Explain what object or substance directly harmed the employee.	Examples: "blood," "body fluid"
10. If the employee died, fill in the section concerned with when the death occurred.	

containers to recognize the hazardous materials that are contained in them. The containers must be sealed and or locked when they are full and disposed of according to EPA regulation as biohazardous waste.

Care must also be taken when handling broken glassware, which might be contaminated. Broken glassware is not to be picked up directly with the hands; instead it should be cleaned up using mechanical means, such as with a brush and dust pan, tongs, or forceps.

Blood Spill Clean Up and Disposal of Hazardous Waste Materials OSHA standards require all contaminated surfaces to be cleaned by a 1:10 bleach solution or an EPA- (Environmental Protection Agency) approved disinfectant. Some contaminants are not visible; therefore, all work areas must be thoroughly disinfected after each use.

All infectious waste must be disposed of by placing each contaminated item in its appropriate hazardous waste container provided by your employer. Any disposable material that has even a trace of human tissue, blood, or other body fluid on it is considered infectious and must be treated with extreme caution. Latex or vinyl gloves must be worn when handling any contaminated item to reduce the possibility of disease transmission, especially the human immunodeficiency virus (HIV), hepatitis B virus (HBV), and hepatitis C virus (HCV).

Regulated Waste and Infectious Laundry According to the blood-borne pathogen standard, any item contaminated with blood, body fluids, or other potentially infectious materials (OPIM) is considered medical or regulated waste. By OSHA standards, regulated waste would contain liquid or semiliquid blood or OPIM that would release blood or OPIM in a liquid or semiliquid state if compressed. Therefore, any contaminated waste that would fall under this category must be disposed of in a red biohazard bag with a biohazard label.

Laundry such as linen, lab coats, and towels can occasionally become contaminated with microorganisms. Although the risk for transmission is minimal, a process must be in place for how to handle the laundry with minimal agitation to prevent contamination into the air as well as of the person handling it. Gloves and other appropriate PPE should be worn during this process. All soiled laundry should be removed and bagged in the area in which it was contaminated and transported to the properly labeled leak-proof biohazard bin to await pickup from the laundry service.

Incineration **Incineration** is a method to completely destroy disposable items by flame. Items that will be treated in this way must be properly bagged for the procedure so that anyone handling the contaminated articles will not be affected.

MEDICAL ASEPSIS

Medical asepsis is a type of infection control that decreases the risk of spreading infection by decreasing the number of pathogenic microorganisms and their spread after they leave the body. Techniques mentioned earlier in this chapter such as practicing standard and universal precautions and using PPE barriers are ways to practice medical asepsis. Other forms of medical asepsis include hand washing, sanitization, and disinfection and sterilization techniques. In addition to practicing medical asepsis in the facility, educating patients should also be part of your daily routine to combat the spread of infection.

Hand Washing

Practicing proper hand washing and developing good habits is essential in infection control and eliminating the potential of contracting diseases. The very best way to prevent the transfer of microorganisms is by regularly washing your hands. This one task alone could help eliminate many diseases before they even begin. Hand washing, according to the CDC standards, should be done vigorously for at least 15 seconds before and after seeing each patient, before and after eating, before and after using the restroom, before and after handling specimens or any soiled or contaminated materials, and after removing gloves. Proper basic hand washing helps remove microorganisms from the skin and from under fingernails. Minimal or no jewelry should be worn because it is impossible to eliminate all pathogens from the crevices of jewelry items.

Hand washing performed before gloving for a surgical procedure, known as a surgical scrub, includes a 2- to 6-minute scrub (or the length of time recommended by the antimicrobial soap manufacturer). Surgical scrubs are covered in more detail in Chapter 49.

CLINICAL PEARL

Lotion may be applied to the hands to prevent dry skin. If you are putting latex gloves on after hand washing, it is important to avoid using lotions that have a petroleum or mineral oil content because they can break down the latex and could intensify a latex allergic reaction. Those who are allergic to latex should use vinyl gloves. To be safe, it is a good practice to use a water-based lotion without perfume.

When a sink is not readily available for hand washing or if hands are not visibly soiled between patients (such as in an area designated for allergy injections or blood pressure readings), a practical way to cleanse the hands is by using an alcohol-based hand-rub preparation. This preparation is a gel or foam applied and spread over the hands in the same manner as you would use soap and water. It dries in approximately one minute. Due to the alcohol in the product, your hands can become dry and chapped; therefore, a supply of hand cream should be readily available. Treating chapped skin with soothing lotions can help prevent a possible infection of the hands.

Learning the correct way to wash the hands thoroughly is outlined in Procedure 36–2. Carefully adhere to each hand-washing step to prevent disease transmission. Even though the hand-washing procedure may seem extensive, it takes only a couple of minutes to complete, and it is done to prevent the spread of disease. Acquiring this important habit is necessary for your well-being and that of others.

PROCEDURE 36–2 Hand Washing for Medical Asepsis

PURPOSE: To reduce pathogens on the hands and wrists, thereby decreasing direct and indirect transmission of infectious microorganisms. Average duration is a vigorous 15-second scrub following each patient contact. (Some facilities might recommend two minutes at the start of your work day, before beginning to work with patients.) Standard precautions recommend proper hand washing to avoid the transfer of microorganisms to other patients, yourself, or the environment.

EQUIPMENT: Sink (preferably with foot-operated controls), antimicrobial soap, nail stick or brush, disposable paper towels, lotion, and a waste receptacle.

S SKILL: Demonstrate proper hand washing.

Procedure Steps	Detailed Instructions and/or *Rationales*
1. Assemble equipment.	
2. Remove all jewelry.	Remove all jewelry, including bracelets and rings. (Wedding rings may be left on but must be scrubbed.) *Jewelry harbors microorganisms.*
3. Use a paper towel to turn on faucet and adjust water temperature to lukewarm (Figure 36–18A).	Stand at the sink and turn faucets on, using a paper towel to avoid direct contact with faucets. Adjust water temperature to moderately warm. Leave water running at desired temperature. *Once the procedure is begun, the faucets cannot be touched because the sink and faucets are considered contaminated.*
4. Discard paper towel.	
5. Wet hands and apply soap, use friction and work into lather, being sure to cover all parts of the hands, including the wrists (Figures 36–18B and C).	Wet hands and press the soap dispenser with the heel of your hand to obtain approximately 1 teaspoon of soap in the palm of one hand. Work soap into a lather and distribute soap over both palms and backs of hands in circular motions constantly and vigorously for 15 seconds. *Circular motion and friction are more effective.*
6. Rinse well, hands pointed down; be sure not to touch the inside of the sink.	Keep hands lower than forearms. Rinse well, being careful not to touch the inside of the sink or faucets during the procedure. *Removed soil and water flows into sink. The inside of the sink and faucets harbor microorganisms.*

(continues)

(continued)

Procedure Steps	Detailed Instructions and/or *Rationales*
7. If the first hand cleansing of the day, use a nail stick or a nail brush on the nails and cuticles and repeat steps 5 and 6 (Figure 36–18D).	Use the nail brush or stick to dislodge microorganisms around cuticles and under nails.
8. Use paper towels to dry hands with a blotting method from hands to elbows discarding each towel after one use (Figure 36–18E).	Rinse hands thoroughly. Leave water running and reach for sufficient paper towels to dry hands completely.
9. Turn faucet off with a clean paper towel and discard (Figure 36–18F).	*Touching the faucet contaminates clean hands.*
10. Apply lotion.	Hand lotion may be applied to prevent skin from becoming dry and chafed.

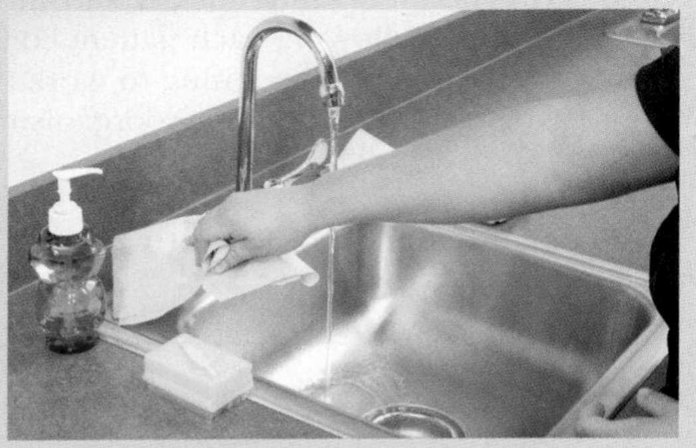

Figure 36–18A: A dry paper towel should be used to turn the faucet on (if not lever-operated). *Delmar/Cengage Learning.*

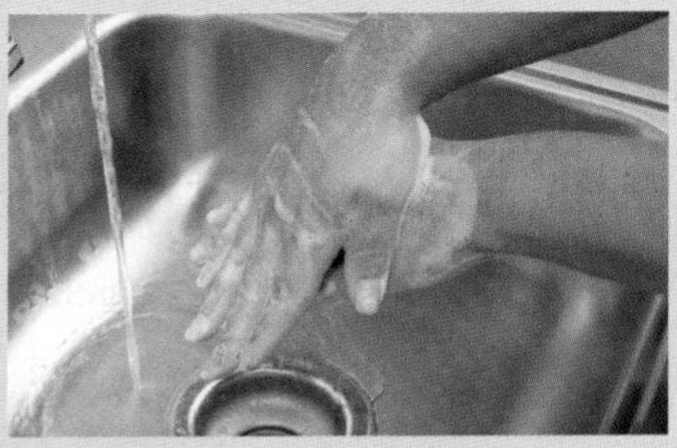

Figure 36–18B: Fingertips should be pointed down while washing hands. Use the palm of one hand to clean the back of the other hand. *Delmar/Cengage Learning.*

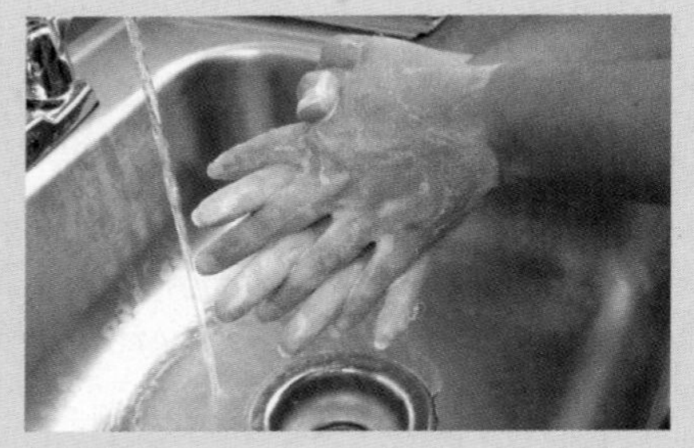

Figure 36–18C: Interlace the fingers to clean between them. *Delmar/Cengage Learning.*

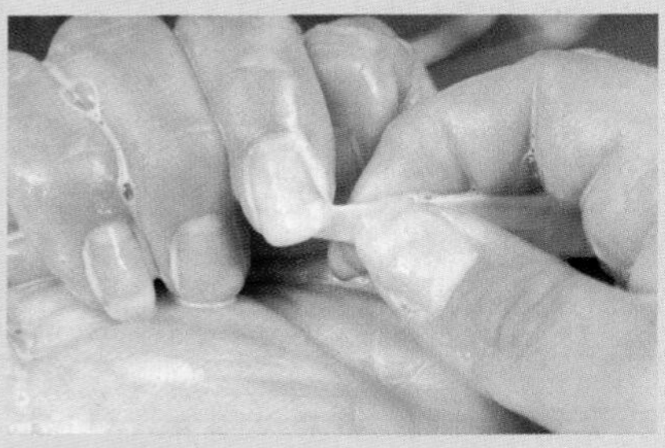

Figure 36–18D: Clean under the fingernails. *Delmar/Cengage Learning.*

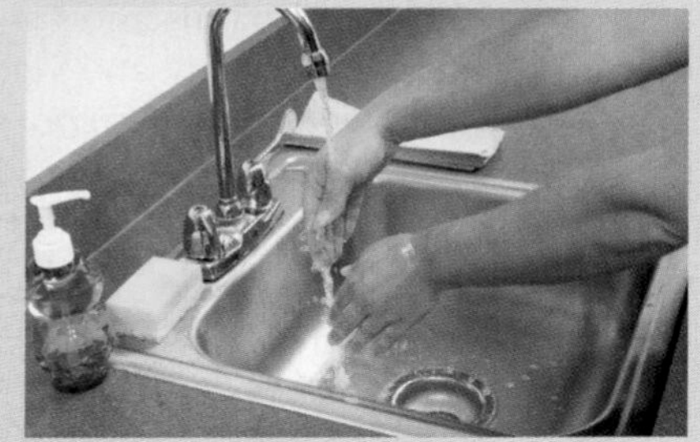

Figure 36–18E: Rinse the hands thoroughly with the fingertips down. *Delmar/Cengage Learning.*

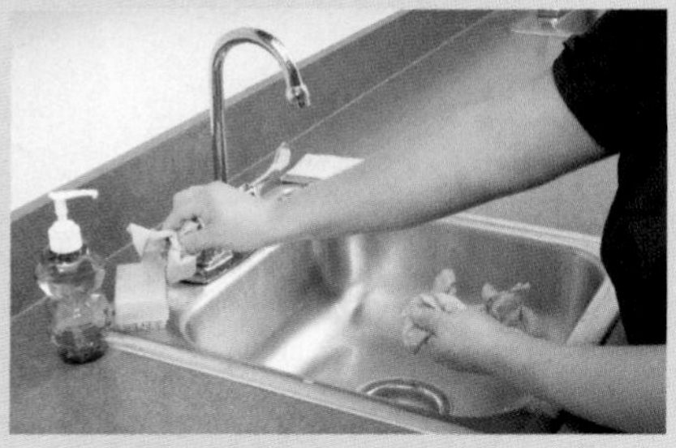

Figure 36–18F: Use paper towels to dry the hands and turn off the faucet (if not lever-operated). *Delmar/Cengage Learning.*

Gloving

Wearing gloves is necessary when cleaning up blood or bodily fluid in the reception area and in the examination or treatment room. Following are three very important reasons latex or vinyl gloves are worn:

1. To provide protection as a barrier and prevent contamination of the hands when touching any blood or body fluid;
2. To reduce the possibility that any pathogens present on your hands will be transferred to another;
3. To diminish the chance of any pathogens being transmitted from you to patients as you go from one patient to another.

Wearing gloves is not a substitute for hand washing. Because gloves can have imperfections, such as small holes or tears, or if gloves are ill-fitting, hand washing is a must before and after wearing them. The risk also exists of becoming contaminated during the removal of soiled gloves. Always remember to protect yourself and follow the proper procedure for removing gloves as outlined in Procedure 36–3.

PROCEDURE 36–3 Remove Non-Sterile Gloves

PURPOSE: To remove and dispose of contaminated gloves without exposing surroundings to contamination.

EQUIPMENT: Biohazard waste container, contaminated gloves, hand-washing equipment.

S SKILL: Demonstrate proper removal of non-sterile gloves.

Procedure Steps	Detailed Instructions and/or *Rationales*
1. Hold hands down and away from the body.	*This helps prevent contaminant exposure.*
2. Grasp the used glove by the palm of the non-dominant hand with the dominant hand and remove it by turning the glove inside out (Figure 36–19A–C).	Take care not to touch bare skin on contaminated glove. *This helps prevent contaminant exposure by keeping the contaminants isolated.*
3. Holding the glove that has been removed in the dominant gloved hand, insert three fingers inside the back of the contaminated glove and turn it inside out over the other (Figures 36–19D–F).	*This keeps the contaminants on the inside of the gloves, preventing contaminant exposure.*
4. Dispose of gloves into biohazard waste container.	*Items exposed with blood or body fluids must be disposed of by placing them in the appropriate biohazard container.*
5. Wash hands thoroughly.	*This is an added precaution to prevent exposure.*

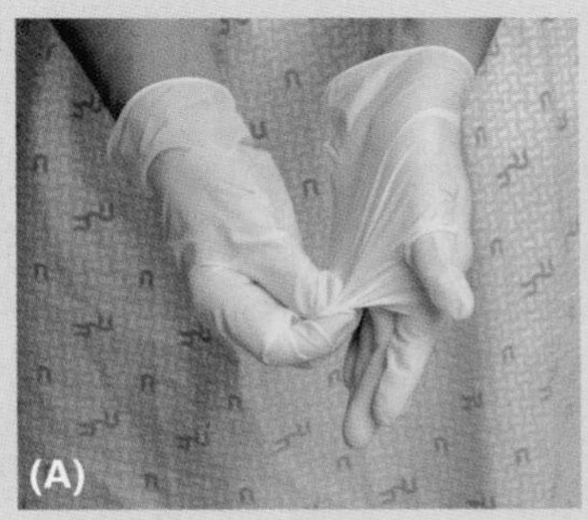

Figure 36–19A: Grasp the palm of the used glove with the right hand. *Delmar/Cengage Learning.*

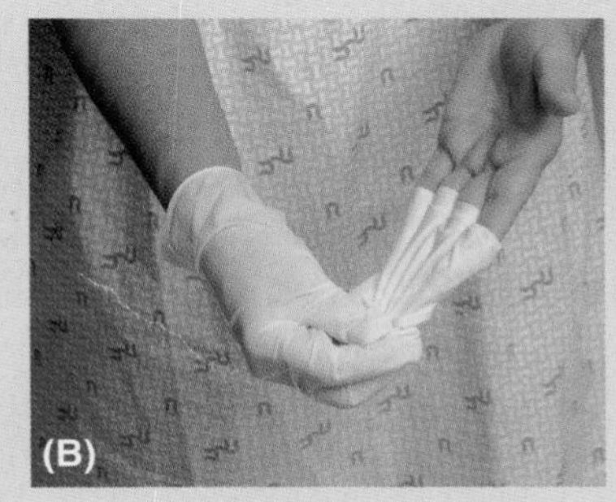

Figure 36–19B: Begin removing the first glove. *Delmar/Cengage Learning.*

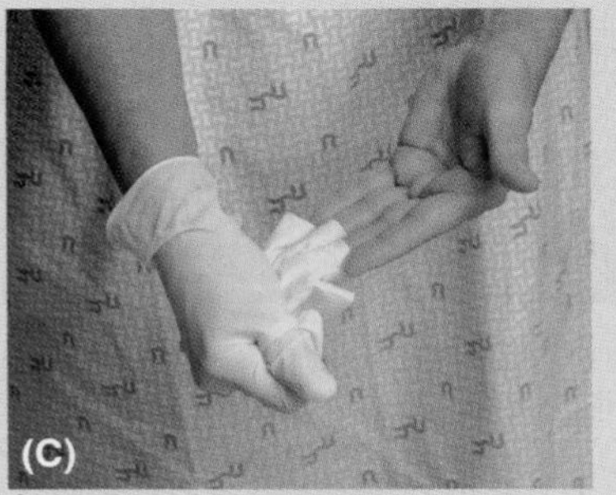

Figure 36–19C: Glove is turned inside out as it is being removed. Take care to not touch bare skin on the contaminated glove. *Delmar/Cengage Learning.*

(continues)

(continued)

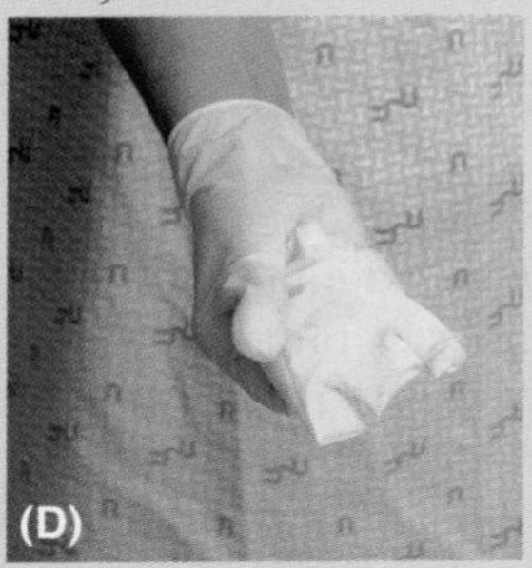

Figure 36–19D: Inverted glove is completely removed into the contaminated glove. *Delmar/Cengage Learning.*

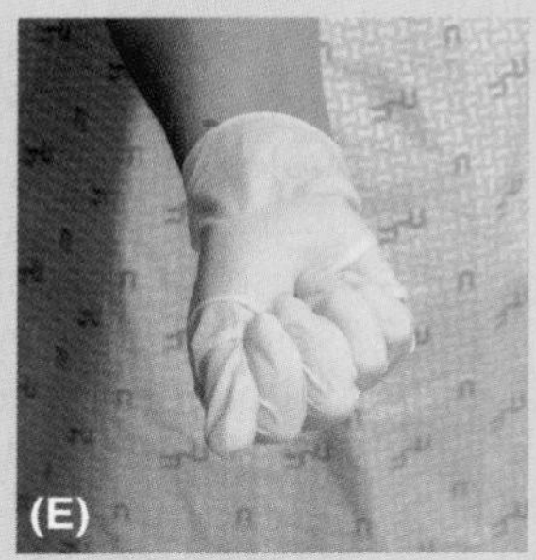

Figure 36–19E: Contain the inverted glove completed in the gloved hand. *Delmar/Cengage Learning.*

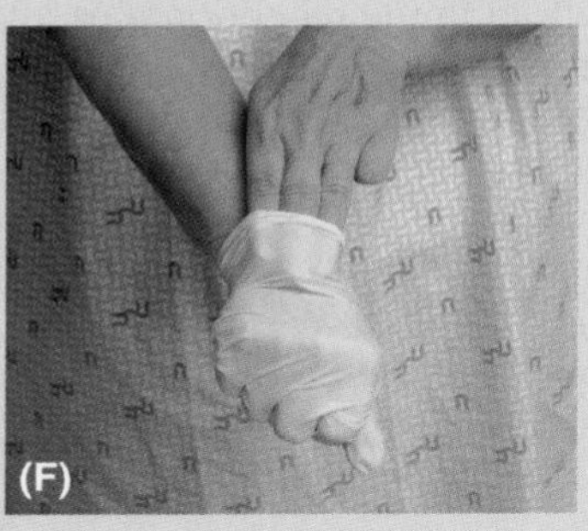

Figure 36–19F: Insert three fingers of the ungloved hand inside the back of the contaminated glove and turn it inside out of the other. *Delmar/Cengage Learning.*

Many of the patients you will serve and possibly some of your coworkers may be highly allergic to latex. Although many health care facilities are phasing out the use of latex and going to a latex-free environment, some products are still in use. Be sure when questioning patients about allergies they may have that latex is included. A practical way to care for patients with this sensitivity is to make one of the examination rooms free of all latex products. When latex-allergic patients are treated in this way, they can be less likely to have an allergic episode when visiting your office.

Applying PPE

Personal protective equipment (PPE) is protective wear required by OSHA and protects health care employees from coming in contact with blood, body fluids, and other potentially infected material. Knowing the appropriate PPE to wear due to the potential exposure is critical for safety. Gloves are generally worn for any direct hand contact exposure. Gowns or lab coats would be worn to protect against any potential splash and sprays or when dealing with large amounts of infectious materials. Safety glasses or face shields should be worn to protect against splashes, sprays, and droplets, and masks against airborne transmission. Refer to Procedure 36–4 for a step-by-step process of choosing, applying, and removing appropriate personal protective equipment.

Sanitization

Processing items and instruments for use in procedures that are **invasive** is a vital responsibility. When handling any of the instruments or articles that need to be sanitized, disinfected, or prepared for sterilization, always wear gloves to protect you from becoming contaminated with any possible lingering microorganisms on the item and the item from any possible contamination from your hands. Whenever you have a cold or the sniffles, wear gloves and a mask to avoid disease transmission. Never sneeze or cough on or over any items you are preparing for any procedure. Always follow standard precautions in performing procedures with patient contact.

PROCEDURE 36–4 Choose, Apply, and Remove Appropriate Personal Protective Equipment (PPE)

PURPOSE: To provide protection from infectious contamination.

EQUIPMENT: Disposable gown, cap, mask, gloves, safety glasses, hand-washing equipment, and biohazard waste receptacle and/or laundry bag.

S SKILL: Demonstrate application and removal of appropriate personal protective equipment (PPE) when working in potentially infectious situations.

Procedure Steps	Detailed Instructions and/or *Rationales*
1. Review provider orders and facility protocols relative to the type of infectious exposure.	*Protocols may vary from facility to facility, depending on the type of exposure.*
2. Choose and place appropriate PPE to be applied in a designated area for application.	*Some facilities have a designated area for applying and removing PPE used for infectious exposures to contain the contaminants.*
3. Remove jewelry, lab coat, and other items not necessary in providing patient care or cleanup process.	*Decreases exposure to microorganisms.*
4. Wash hands, apply safety glasses if necessary, and prepare to apply PPE.	*PPE provides a barrier that prevents the transmission of microorganisms to the medical assistant.*
5. Apply cap if necessary to cover hair and ears completely.	
6. Apply mask if necessary.	Place the top of the mask over the bridge of your nose (top part of the mask has a metal strip) and pinch the metal strip to fit snuggly against nose. Hook straps behind the ears. If using a tie mask, firmly tie the mask at the top and bottom of the back of the head so it covers the nose and mouth entirely. *This protects the mouth and nose from exposures when performing procedures that have the potential for spraying or splashing blood or OPIM.*
7. Apply gown if necessary and tie securely to cover outer garments completely (Figures 36–20A and C).	
8. Apply gloves if necessary and pull over the cuff of the gown to ensure that no skin is exposed.	
9. Enter exposure area and clean up the contaminants following facility protocol.	*Some facilities use specialized kits for cleanup, depending on the type of contaminant.*
10. Dispose of contaminated articles into biohazard bag. If any reusable equipment is involved, transport to appropriate area, following protocol for proper cleaning.	*This prevents transmission and exposure to the contaminant.*
11. Remove contaminated gown (Figures 36–20D and F).	*Untie the gown, pinch a fold in the front of the gown, and pull away from yourself; slide arms out, being careful to turn entire gown inside out and roll into a ball. If disposable, place in biohazard bag; if reusable, place in biohazard laundry bag. By turning the gown inside out, the contaminants remain on the inside, preventing exposure to yourself.*
12. Remove contaminated gloves; place in biohazard bag and wash hands.	
13. Remove safety glasses, mask, and hair covering; dispose of properly. (If they are contaminated, you must reapply new gloves first before removing.)	*This prevents transmission and exposure to the contaminant.*
14. Wash hands.	

(continues)

(continued)

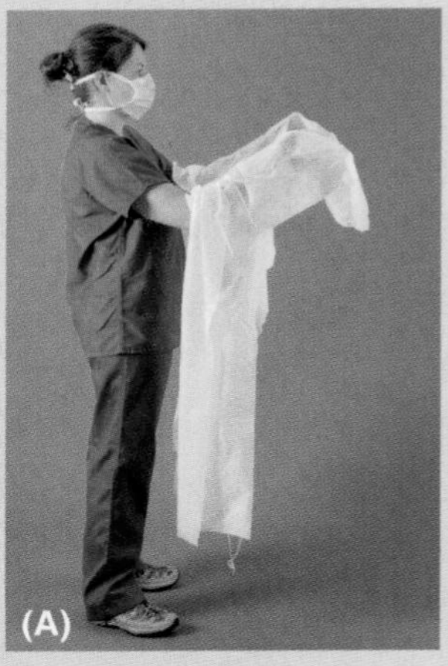

Figure 36–20A: The medical assistant has put on a mask and is applying the gown, pulling on the sleeves. *Delmar/Cengage Learning.*

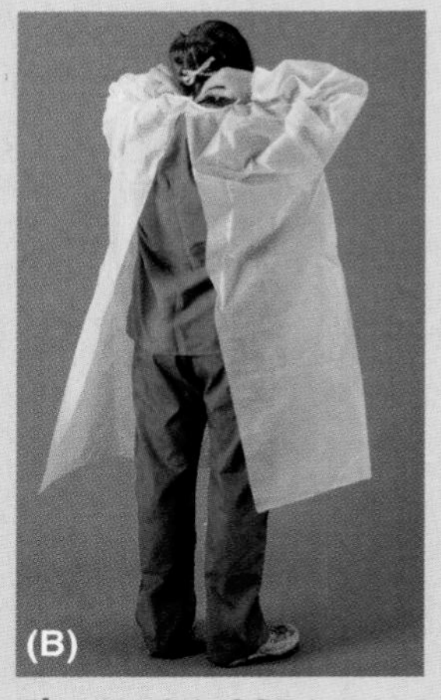

Figure 36–20B: The neck of the gown is secured first. *Delmar/Cengage Learning.*

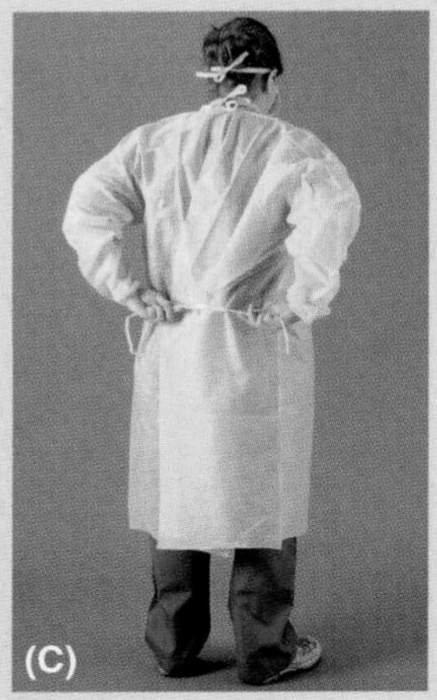

Figure 36–20C: The back of the gown is secured last. *Delmar/Cengage Learning.*

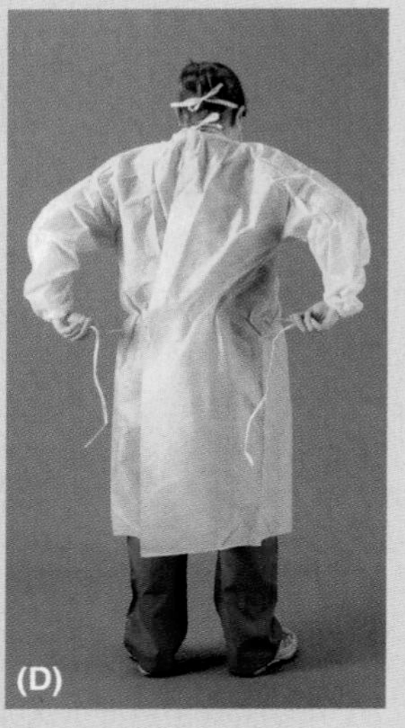

Figure 36–20D: When finished with cleaning of contaminants, the medical assistant removes PPE by untying the gown. *Delmar/Cengage Learning.*

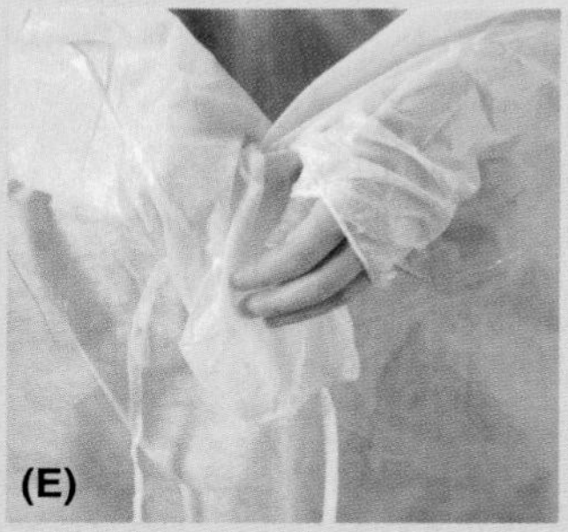

Figure 36–20E: Using the hand covered by the gown, pull down the gown over the other hand. *Delmar/Cengage Learning.*

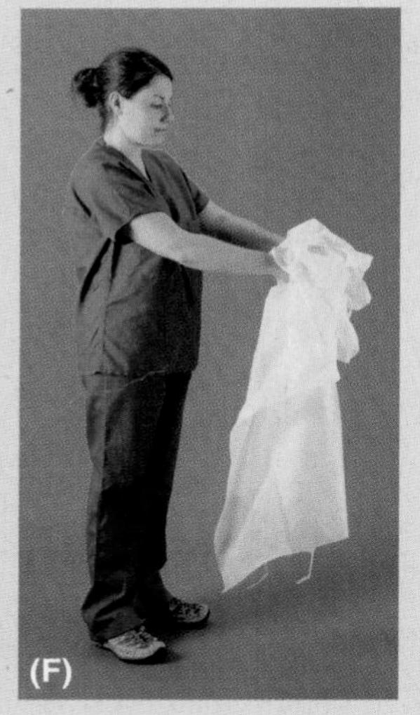

Figure 36–20F: Pinch the gown in the center and pull off the body and roll into a ball with the contaminated side of the gown on the inside. *Delmar/Cengage Learning.*

Sanitization is the process of washing and scrubbing to remove materials such as body tissue, blood, or other body fluids. Wear latex or vinyl gloves, double-gloving as necessary. Additionally, utility gloves are recommended during the process of sanitization of items and equipment to protect your hands from any possibility of contamination and injury from the articles that you handle (Figure 36–21). As you will practice in Procedure 36–5, items should be rinsed in cool water, soaked in a warm detergent solution for about 20 minutes, washed, and scrubbed thoroughly with a brush, being sure to include all **serrations**, grooves, and hinges, rinsed in warm to hot water to remove the detergent, and dried completely. During this process, the gloves also serve to protect your hands from the harshness of repeated contact with soap and water,

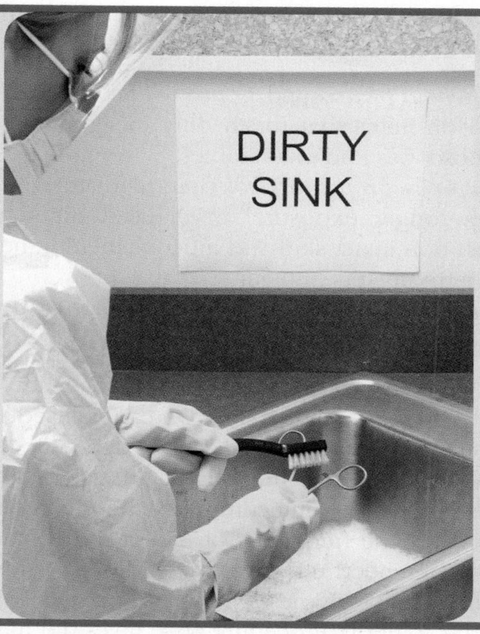

Figure 36–21: Medical assistant sanitizing an instrument. *Delmar/Cengage Learning.*

which can result in chafing and cracking of the skin and possibly lead to infection. Remember to wash your hands before and after gloving and use a soothing hand lotion routinely to help prevent dryness.

Disinfection

Disinfection is a process by which disease-producing microorganisms, or pathogens, are killed; however, disinfectants do not always kill **spores**. Spores are thick-walled, hard capsules formed by some bacteria that allow them to remain dormant until conditions for growth are good (Figure 36–22). When the proper growth conditions are present, the bacteria break out of the capsule, grow, and multiply, starting infection. An example of bacteria that produce spores is *Clostridum tetani*, the cause of tetanus, or lockjaw. The only way to be sure spores are eliminated is to sterilize them.

The term *disinfect* pertains to a chemical or physical means of destroying bacteria. It is sometimes referred to as a germicide or bactericide. Disinfectants are used on objects, not on people, and are used mainly for large

PROCEDURE 36–5 Sanitize Instruments

PURPOSE: To properly clean instruments to remove all tissue and debris.

EQUIPMENT: Sink with running water, sanitizing agent with enzymatic action, soft brush, towels, disposable paper towels, protective plastic apron, heavy-duty gloves, and goggles.

S SKILL: Demonstrate sanitization procedures.

Procedure Steps	Detailed Instructions and/or *Rationales*
1. Apply PPE: Goggles, apron, and heavy-duty gloves.	*This equipment protects you and your clothing from exposure to blood and body fluids through contact, splashing, or punctures.*
2. If instruments need to be transported from one place to another, place the instrument in a container labeled "Biohazard."	*Following standard precautions, keep contaminated items contained to prevent exposure.*
3. Rinse instruments in cool water and place in disinfectant solution.	*This removes any tissue or debris that might dry onto instruments.*
4. Scrub each instrument well with detergent and water (be sure to include inside edges, serrations, grooves, hinges, and all surfaces); scrub under running water.	*This ensures that all debris has been removed prior to sterilization.*
5. Rinse instruments with hot water.	*This removes any residue left behind from the disinfectant solution.*
6. Place instruments on a clean towel and dry thoroughly with disposable paper towels.	*This prevents the instruments from rusting or corroding.*
7. Remove PPE and wash hands.	

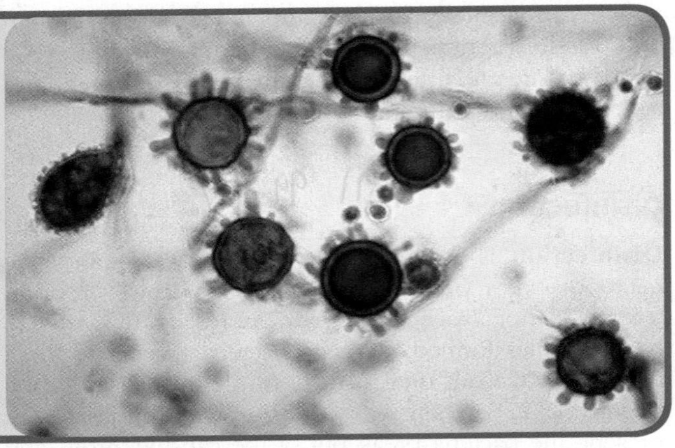

Figure 36–22: This picture shows the tough outer wall of spores, which explains their resistance to disinfectants. *Centers for Disease Control and Prevention.*

instruments, scopes, and heat-sensitive items that can't withstand the autoclaving process. Three levels of disinfecting solutions (low, intermediate, and high) may be used in medical facilities. The level used depends on the item or object being disinfected and its function. Common disinfectants include:

- *Household bleach* and *isopropyl alcohol* (low-level), used on items that touch only intact skin, such as stethoscopes and exam tables
- *Ethyl or isopropyl alcohol* (intermediate when used for a longer exposure time), used on items that touch non-intact skin and mucous membranes, such as thermometers and ear speculas
- *Glutaraldehyde-based formulas* (high), used on endoscopes and laryngoscopes.

Disinfectants that are registered as sterilants with the EPA or cleared for marketing by the FDA can be used as high-level disinfectants or for sterilization, depending on the recommended time per the manufacturer. The chemical solutions used for disinfecting must be changed often, depending on the frequency of use of the container, to ensure the intended effect. Always follow the manufacturer's directions for time of exposure and how often to change the solution. Procedure 36–6 gives the high-level steps to follow to disinfect an endoscope.

PROCEDURE 36–6 Disinfect (Chemical "Cold" Sterilization) Endoscopes

PURPOSE: To sterilize heat-sensitive items such as endoscopes by using appropriate chemical disinfectant (glutaraldehyde-based) solution. (This procedure may also be used for delicate cutting instruments.)

EQUIPMENT: Chemical disinfectant, timer, sterile water, airtight container, heavy-duty gloves, sterile gloves, poly-lined towels, and sterile towels.

S SKILL: Demonstrate disinfection procedures.

Procedure Steps	Detailed Instructions and/or *Rationales*
1. Ensure that the endoscope has been sanitized thoroughly and dried prior to chemical disinfecting (sterilization).	*All debris must be thoroughly removed before sterilization procedure is performed.*
2. Read manufacturer's instructions for preparation of solution.	*Preparation instructions vary depending on the brand of product being used.*
3. Apply PPE.	*Chemical disinfectants are caustic and can be harmful if exposed to the skin.*
4. Prepare solution and pour into a container with an airtight lid, being careful not to splash the chemical (Figure 36–23A).	*If the lid is not airtight, evaporation can occur, causing the product to lose its potency. Splashing can lead to serious injury to the skin and mucous membranes.*
5. Place items into solution and completely submerge (Figure 36–23B).	*Exposed components of the items will not achieve sterility.*
6. Close the lid securely and label the outside of the container with the name of solution, date, and time required according to the manufacturer for sterilization procedure (Figure 36–23C).	*Exposure time must be precise to ensure sterility.*
7. When required processing time is completed, lift lid and remove endoscope, using sterile gloves.	*Item must remain sterile.*

Procedure Steps	Detailed Instructions and/or *Rationales*
8. Rinse scope thoroughly inside and out with sterile water and drain remainder water from scope by holding in an upright position.	*This will remove any chemical that has remained on or inside the scope.*
9. Place scope on sterile poly-lined towels and dry completely, using sterile towels.	*The poly-lined towel acts as a barrier for the sterile scope and prevents contamination while drying.*
10. Place scope in storage container or area until next use.	
11. Remove PPE and dispose of properly.	
12. Wash hands.	

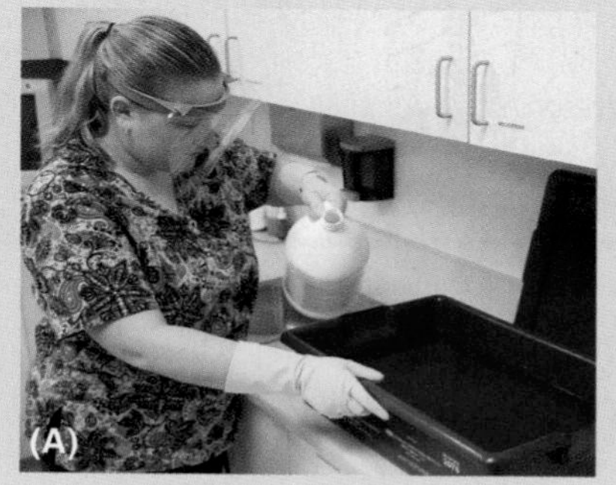

Figure 36–23A: Prepare solution and pour into a container with an airtight lid, being careful not to splash the chemical. *Delmar/Cengage Learning.*

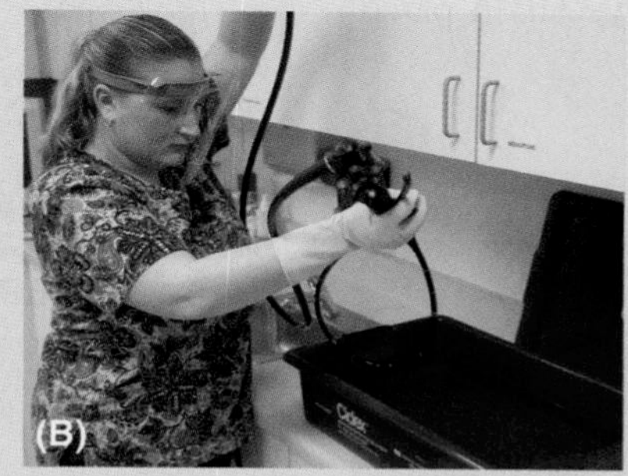

Figure 36–23B: Place items into solution and completely submerge. *Delmar/Cengage Learning.*

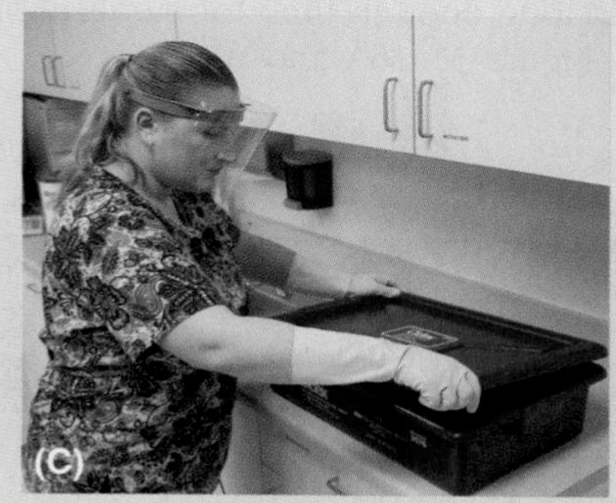

Figure 36–23C: Close the lid securely and label the outside of the container with the name of solution, date, and time required according to the manufacturer for sterilization procedure. *Delmar/Cengage Learning.*

Sterilization

Sterilization is the process that destroys all forms of living organisms. Following the sterilization procedure, which is generally performed by **autoclaving**, the item remains sterile for 30 days if its packaging is kept dry and intact. This period is referred to as **shelf life**.

Many medical practices have an autoclave for sterilization of instruments by steam under pressure, which is a method that guarantees the destruction of spores. After the items are removed from the autoclave, exam and procedure rooms must be restocked. Make sure to place the newly sterilized items in the back of the storage area, behind other previously stored items to ensure that your current stock is up to date and save you time by preventing the need to re-sterilize items. Pay attention to the expiration date on all packages to ensure that the contents are sterile. Do not use any sterile package if it is beyond the expiration date (or more than 30 days from the time it was sterilized). If the package is labeled with just the date, it denotes when it was autoclaved. Autoclaved packages can also be labeled with "expiration date, 3-10-XX," which is the last date you could use the contents and be assured that they are sterile. If the packaging is torn or punctured, has signs of having been wet (watermarks), or is wet, this is an indication that the sterility of the contents has been lost. Microorganisms can enter wrapped or enveloped articles through moisture.

Wrapping Items for Autoclaving

Carefully study and practice the procedure of wrapping items for autoclaving in Procedure 36–7. Articles to be autoclaved must first be sanitized and then wrapped in a double thickness special porous autoclave paper or cloth wrap. Several items may be wrapped together if separated by a gauze square. Items that are up against others during sterilization do not permit the steam to flow properly, and the items do not become sterile. Wrap each package snugly, but not too tight or too loose. If the package is too tight, the steam flow will not be able to get through the package or around each item sufficiently. Packages that are too loose or leave gaps could threaten the sterility of the contents, and they may even come apart.

Envelope packaging is manufactured for some instruments (Figure 36–24), such as scissors, and Figure 36–25 shows a medical assistant inserting an instrument into an envelope type of packaging in preparation for autoclaving. A section on the paper envelope permits recording of the instrument name, the date, and the initials of the person who sterilized it. Sterilization and biological indicators register proper and complete sterilization. Autoclave tape has an indicator stripe that changes color when the proper temperature has been maintained for a long enough time for sterilization to have taken place (Figure 36–26A and B).

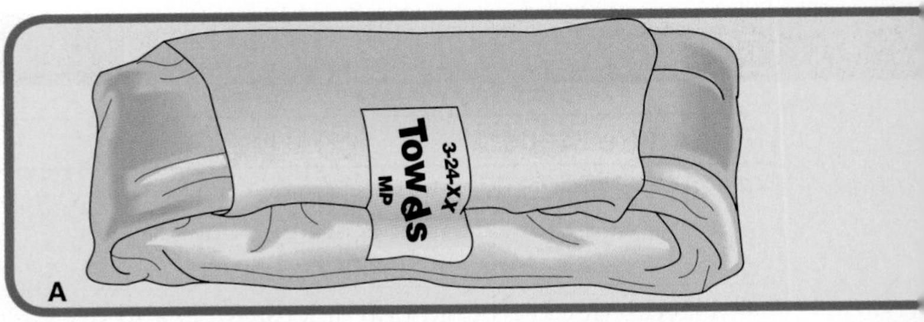

Figure 36–26A: Packaging of towels before autoclaving. *Delmar/Cengage Learning.*

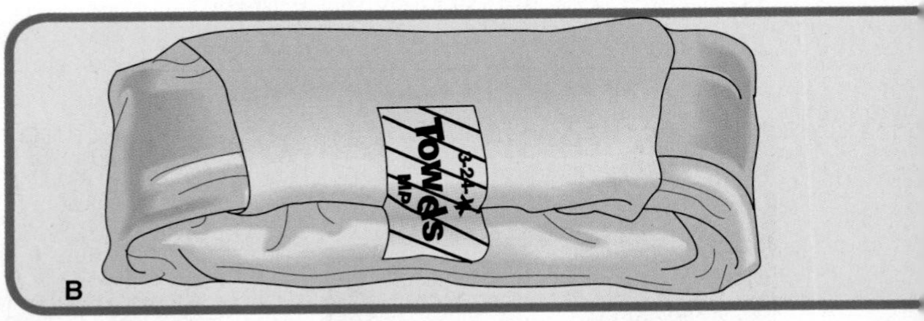

Figure 36–26B: Packaging of towels after autoclaving. *Delmar/Cengage Learning.*

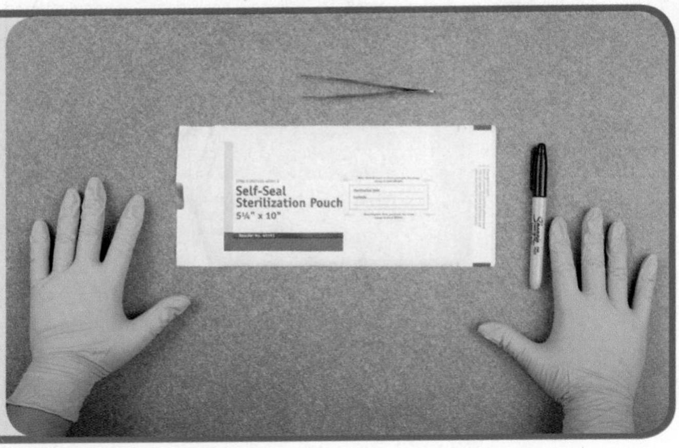

Figure 36–24: Envelope-type packaging for autoclaves. *Delmar/Cengage Learning.*

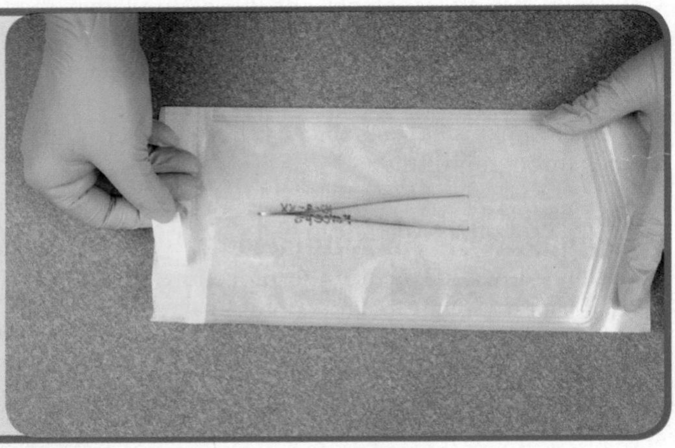

Figure 36–25: Placing a single instrument into the autoclave pouch. *Delmar/Cengage Learning.*

The same principle applies to indicators placed inside the wrapped package. Be aware that gas sterilizers and steam autoclaves require different indicator tapes. There are also envelopes for both types of sterilizers. The manufacturer can inform you of the proper indicator tape to use when you purchase a sterilizer or can tell you which one(s) to use with your present equipment. Biological indicators are used as a quality control method to validate that sterilization has been achieved. A common type is a vial that contains bacterial spores that will be killed when the autoclave is functioning properly. You should also clean the sterilizer routinely according to the manufacturer's recommendations.

Using the Autoclave

The manufacturer's instructions should be followed for the operation and care of the autoclave. Instructions are usually printed either on top of the machine or on a tray that pulls out underneath it. It is important for the desired temperature of the sterilizer to be maintained for the proper time. Temperatures and pressure requirements will vary depending on the type and model of the autoclave as well as on the contents in the load. Following the manufacturer's guidelines ensures that sterility has been achieved. In the process of sterilization, the autoclave exerts approximately 15 to 30 pounds of steam pressure per square inch at a temperature between

121 -250

PROCEDURE 36–7 Wrap Items for Autoclaving

MEDIA LINK: Go to the Premium Website and view the Media Link for this chapter: "Wrap Items for Autoclaving."

PURPOSE: To wrap items to be autoclaved so that they will be protected from contamination after the sterilization process is completed for storage and handling.

EQUIPMENT: Autoclave paper or cloth, disposable plastic sealed pouches, autoclave tape, items to be sterilized or autoclaved, sterilization indicators, gauze, tip protectors, indelible pen.

SKILL: Demonstrate the proper procedure for preparing and wrapping instruments to be autoclaved.

Procedure Steps	Detailed Instructions and/or *Rationales*
1. Wash hands and assemble all necessary items. (Figure 36–27A).	*Some offices may require the use of gloves in performing this procedure. Check your office's policy.*
2. Ensure that items have been sanitized before wrapping for autoclave process.	
3. Check items for flaws and make sure they function properly.	*Instruments must be working properly, and materials must be in usable condition.*
4. Place two squares of autoclave paper adequate in size to wrap item(s) on a clean, flat surface in a diamond shape with one corner of the paper facing toward you; place item(s) as well as a sterilization indicator in the center of the paper (Figure 36–27B).	*Placing a sterilization indicator on the inside of the package ensures sterility of the contents, which is required for quality control.*
5. Place a cotton ball between any hinged instruments and keep all ratchets open during the sterilization process (Figure 36–27B).	All sharp tips on the instruments must be protected with tip protectors or gauze. *Keeping the instruments open ensures that all parts of the instrument are sterilized, and covering the sharp tips prevents the packages from being punctured.*
6. Wrap item(s), using the first square by folding the corner of the paper toward the center and turning a small corner back toward you (Figure 36–27C).	
7. Continue wrapping the items by folding one side toward the center, leaving a small corner toward the back on itself, and then do the same with the other side (Figure 36–27D and E).	
8. Fold the package up from the bottom and secure, folding the last corner back on itself (Figure 36–27F and G).	
9. Wrap the package in the second square of paper using the same technique; be sure there is no opening and seal with autoclave tape. Wrap item(s) snugly (Figure 36–27H).	*Double thickness and complete enclosure prevent exposures to pathogens. The autoclave tape, which is heat sensitive, serves as a sterilization indicator and should be placed over the final tab for ease in opening wrapped packages after autoclaving by taping 1 to 2 inches of tape to the edge of the package.*

(continues)

(continued)

Procedure Steps	Detailed Instructions and/or *Rationales*
10. Label the contents and write the date and your initials on the tape (Figure 36–27I).	*This is required to identify the contents and ensures accountability and responsibility. Sterilized packages are considered sterile for 30 days from the date of sterilization; if you are not sterilizing the packages immediately, wait to adhere a date until the day of processing.*
11. If using a plastic pouch for sterilization, place item into the pouch, seal, and label.	Items suitable for plastic autoclave pouches include but are not limited to forceps, hemostats, needle holders, and towel clamps. Remember that all hinged instruments must be autoclaved open. *The sterilizing process must reach all parts of the instruments.*
12. Place wrapped instruments in the autoclave for sterilizing and return all unused supplies to the proper storage area when finished.	
13. Wash hands.	

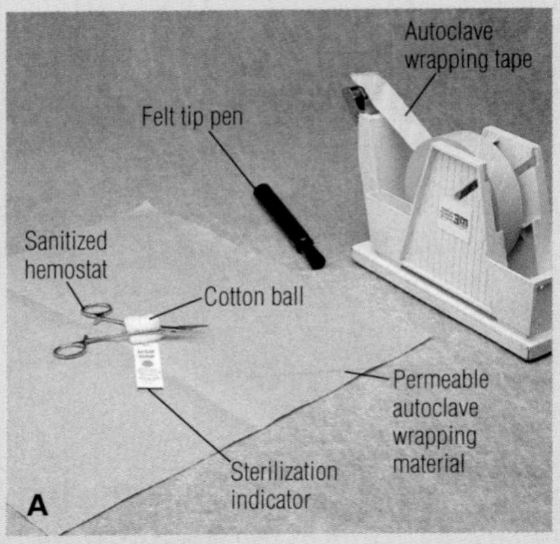

Figure 36–27A: Equipment needed to wrap surgical instruments or equipment for sterilization in an autoclave. *Delmar/Cengage Learning.*

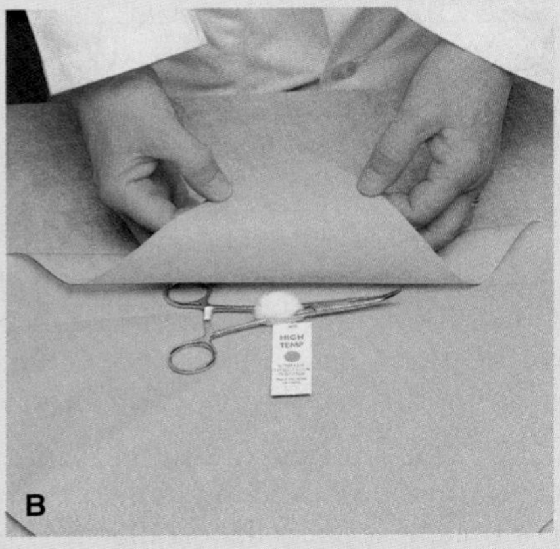

Figure 36–27B: Place a cotton ball between any hinged instruments and keep all ratchets open during the sterilization process. Put a sterilization indicator in with the instruments to be wrapped. *Delmar/Cengage Learning.*

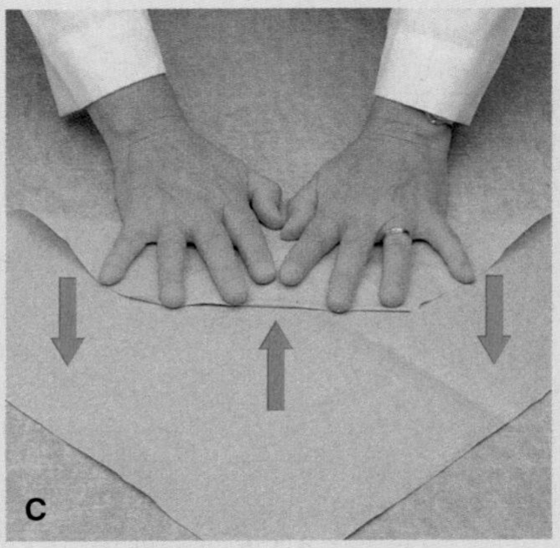

Figure 36–27C: Wrap item(s), using the first square by folding the corner of the paper toward the center and turning a small corner back toward you. *Delmar/Cengage Learning.*

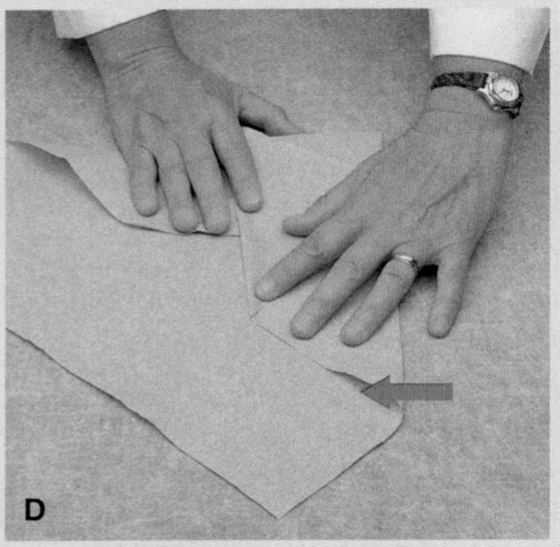

Figure 36–27D: Fold the other side toward center, leaving a small corner turned back on itself. *Delmar/Cengage Learning.*

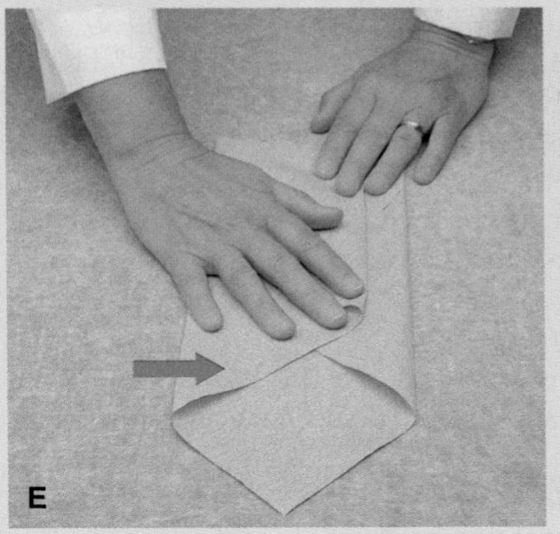

Figure 36–27E: Continue wrapping the items by folding one side toward the center, leaving a small corner toward you back on itself and then do the same with the other side. *Delmar/Cengage Learning.*

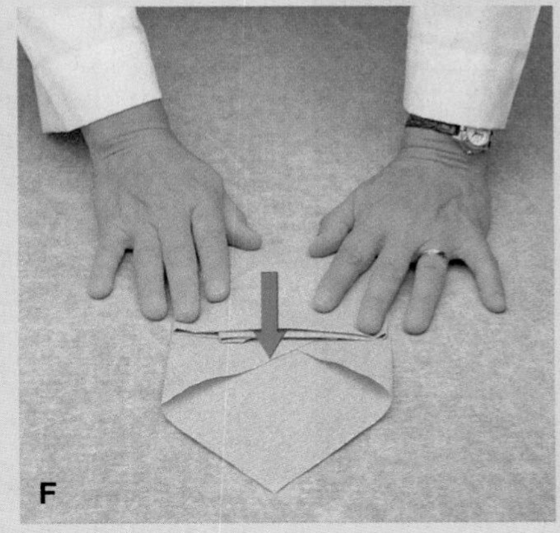

Figure 36–27F: The package is folded up from the bottom, leaving the last corner out. *Delmar/Cengage Learning.*

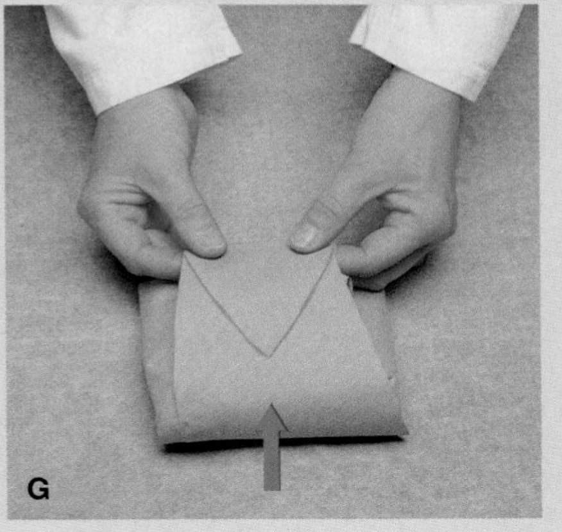

Figure 36–27G: Fold the package up from the bottom and secure, folding the last corner back on itself. *Delmar/Cengage Learning.*

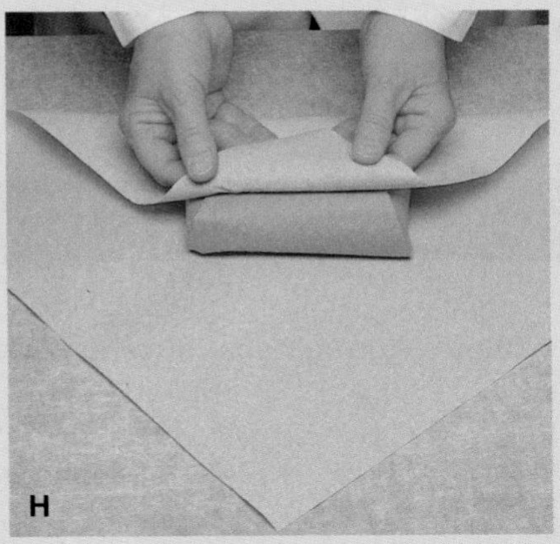

Figure 36–27H: Wrap the package in the second square of paper using the same technique; be sure there is no opening and seal with autoclave tape. Wrap item(s) snugly. *Delmar/Cengage Learning.*

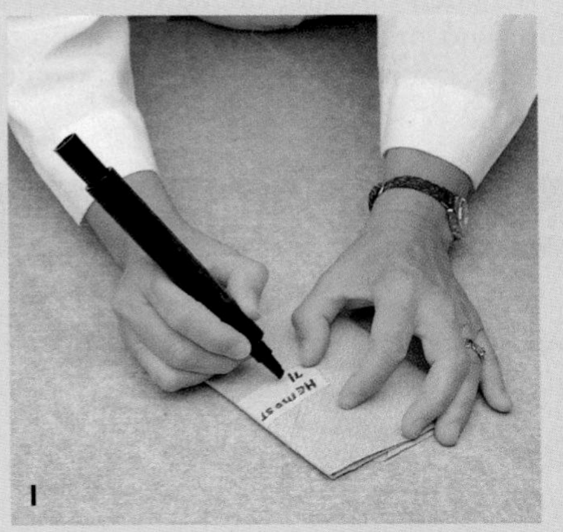

Figure 36–27I: Label the contents and write the date and your initials on the tape. *Delmar/Cengage Learning.*

250-270 121- 132°C

250°F/121° C and 270°F/132°C. The steam flows through the items and destroys all microorganisms and spores (Figures 36–28A, B, and C).

Special care should be taken to avoid touching the autoclave to prevent an accidental burn while sterilization is in progress. It is a good practice to alert the staff

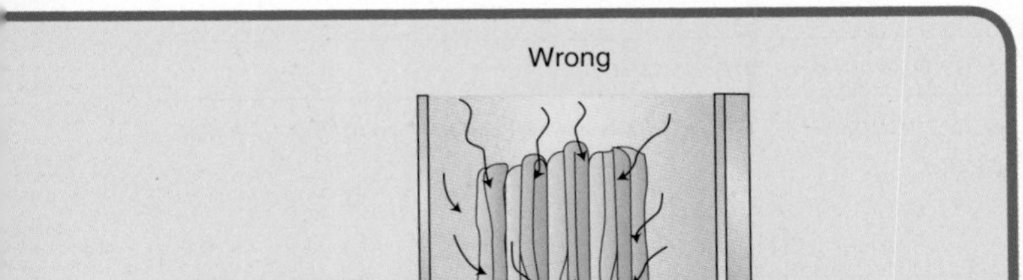

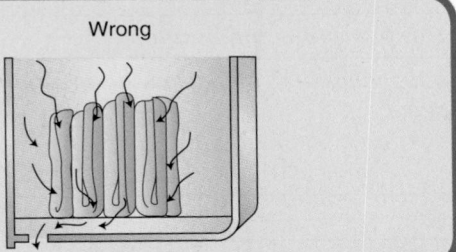

Figure 36–28A: Incorrect method of loading packages. *Delmar/Cengage Learning.*

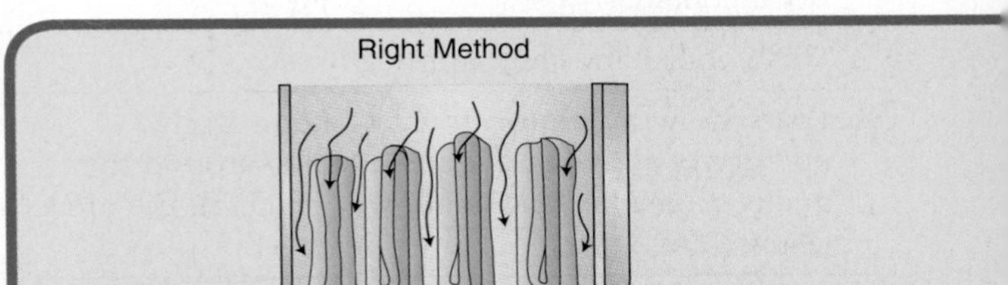

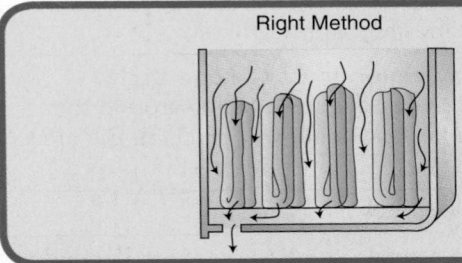

Figure 36–28B: Correct method of loading packages. *Delmar/Cengage Learning.*

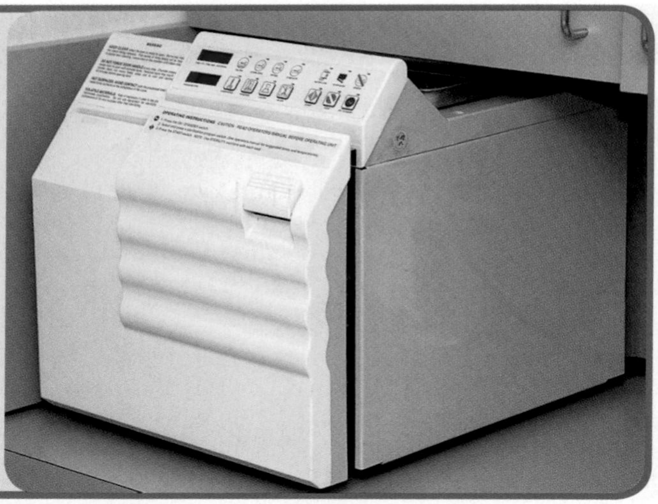

Figure 36–28C: Autoclave. *Delmar/Cengage Learning.*

when the sterilizer is operating so that they will also be cautious. When opening the autoclave door after the temperature and pressure are lowered, step to the side to avoid the possibility of a steam burn to the face and upper body. Use caution with any type of sterilizer. You should leave the items in the autoclave with the door partially opened so that the packages can dry. Allow adequate time for the packaging and contents to cool and dry before handling. If packs are touched before they are thoroughly dry, they are subject to contamination because microorganisms may enter through the wrap by the moisture.

Some offices or medical centers use the autoclaving service of a hospital. In this case, minimum cleaning is all that is necessary because all items are properly sanitized before autoclaving.

Study Procedure 36–8 to learn the basic operational steps for use of an autoclave for sterilization.

Chemical Sterilization

Although the most common method of sterilization is autoclaving, other types of sterilization techniques might need to be used in the medical practice. Because sharp instruments become dull from autoclaving and rubber or vinyl articles are damaged by the intense heat of chemical sterilization, an alternative method for these items is chemical sterilization (refer to Procedure 36–6). In this method, the item is placed in a chemical sterilant (a high-level disinfectant

PROCEDURE 36–8: Perform Autoclave Sterilization

PURPOSE: To sterilize instruments or supplies that will penetrate a patient's skin or come in contact with otherwise sterile areas of a patient's body.

EQUIPMENT: Items properly sanitized and wrapped or sealed in pouches, disposable gloves, protective mitts, sterile transfer forceps

S SKILL: Demonstrate the proper procedure for sterilization of instruments by use of an autoclave.

Procedure Steps	Detailed Instructions and/or *Rationales*
1. Check the water level in the reservoir and add distilled water to the fill line if required.	
2. Any quality control procedures required must be performed with the load to be sterilized and documented.	*This ensures that the autoclave is performing accurately.*
3. Wash your hands and apply gloves.	*This prevents contamination.*
4. Load the wrapped or pouched items in the autoclave, allowing adequate space around the packs to ensure that steam will reach all the areas (Figure 36–29A).	*If the items are compacted, sterilization might not take place.*
5. Remove gloves and wash hands.	
6. Select the appropriate sterilization cycle, depending on the contents loaded, and press the start button.	Follow the manufacturer's guidelines. *Cycles can vary depending on the type and manufacturer of the autoclave.*

Procedure Steps	Detailed Instructions and/or *Rationales*
7. After the cycle has ended, the autoclave will vent on its own. Open the autoclave door to allow the packs to dry before removing them from the autoclave (Figure 36–29B). The door should be ajar only slightly, ¼ to ½ inch.	Check the manufacturer's guidelines regarding opening the door; some models don't require opening during the drying cycle. *Opening the door more than ½ inch causes cold air to enter the autoclave; this can cause excessive condensation in the chamber, preventing the articles from drying completely.*
8. After the drying cycle is completed, wear protective mitts to unload the items, making sure not to unload any packs that are damp (Figure 36–29C).	*Items may still be hot, and the mitts will protect you from getting burned. Organisms can be absorbed through the wet packaging, resulting in contamination.*
9. Check the items to be sure that the stripes on the autoclave tape or indicators on the plastic pouches turned the appropriate color (Figure 36–29D).	*If the stripes or indicators have not changed to the appropriate color, sterilization cannot be guaranteed.*
10. If any individual items have been placed in the autoclave unwrapped, sterile transfer forceps must be used to remove the item and placed in the appropriate storage area (Figure 36–29E).	*This prevents contamination.*
11. Remove the mitts and wash your hands.	

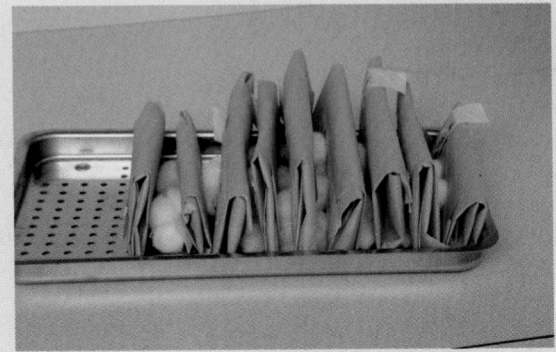

Figure 36–29A: Allow adequate space around the packs to ensure that steam will reach all the areas. *Delmar/Cengage Learning.*

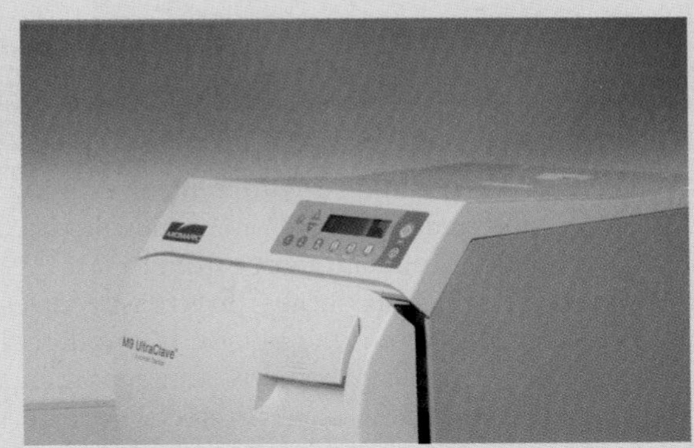

Figure 36–29B: Allow the packs to dry before removing them from the autoclave. *Delmar/Cengage Learning.*

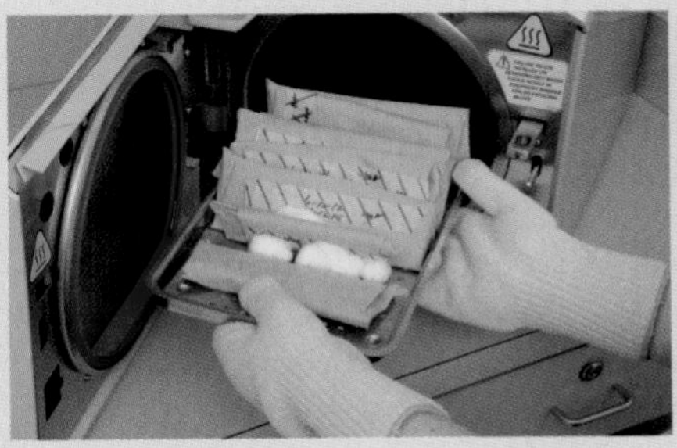

Figure 36–29C: Wear protective mitts to unload the items from the autoclave, making sure not to unload any packs that are damp. *Delmar/Cengage Learning.*

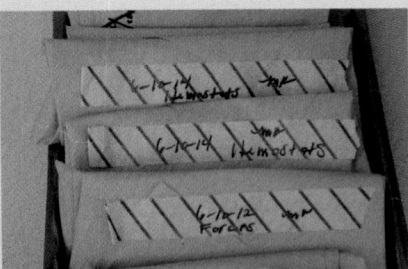

Figure 36–29D: Inspect the items and ensure that the stripes on the autoclave tape or indicators on the plastic pouches have turned the appropriate color. *Delmar/Cengage Learning.*

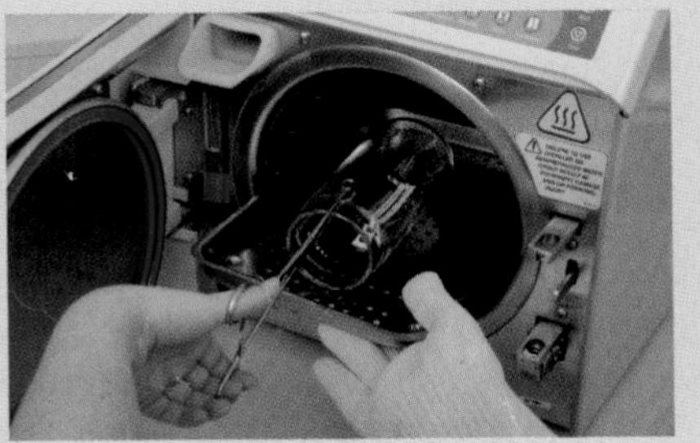

Figure 36–29E: Use sterile transfer forceps to remove items that have been placed in the autoclave unwrapped. *Delmar/Cengage Learning.*

250 → 270
121 → 132

solution) and remains in the solution for an exposure time recommended by the manufacturer to achieve sterility. All instruments must be thoroughly cleaned in a detergent (specifically made for this purpose), brushed, and thoroughly dried before placing them into the sterilant. The hinges and handles of instruments should be kept open to allow all parts to be exposed to the solution. A cover over the sterilant container prevents the evaporation of the solution and keeps the vapor from being inhaled by members of the health care team. This sterilizing solution must completely cover the instruments to be effective. Follow the manufacturer's recommendations regarding sterilant strength, proper disposal, and the frequency of how often the solution must be changed.

Dry Heat Sterilization

Still another method of sterilization is the dry heat oven. Instruments with sharp blades, such as scissors or scalpels, are sometimes sterilized in this way. It is not the most desirable sterilization method for general items because it is time consuming, and spores can still be a threat with this method. The process takes one to two hours at a temperature of 350°F/176.6°C, depending on the article. It is *not* a way to sterilize items made of rubber, which are damaged by the intense heat.

CHAPTER SUMMARY

- It is important to be familiar with transmission means, symptoms, and treatments of communicable diseases and the reporting regulations regarding them.
- The chain of infection shows how easily diseases can be transferred from one person to another. This chain can be broken by a variety of infection control practices such as sanitization, disinfection, and sterilization. Breaking the chain prevents the transmission of contaminants.
- Common infectious agents are microorganisms that are classified as bacteria, viruses, fungi, parasites, and rickettsiae.
- Diseases can be transmitted through direct contact by eating, drinking, touching, kissing, and sexual intimacy or by indirect contact such as inhaling contaminated air or handling items an infected person has had contact with.
- Stages of infection that occur when an individual is exposed to a disease producing pathogen include the incubation, prodromal, acute, declining, and convalescent stages.
- Microorganisms that are the cause of diseases are called pathogens and have certain requirements for growth and multiplication. If steps are taken to interrupt and prevent their growth, disease transmission can be reduced.
- Strict adherence to universal and standard precautions while treating all patients is essential in preventing the spread of infection.
- The greatest risk of exposure to blood-borne pathogens occurs when handling contaminated sharps. Used needles, lancets, capillary tubes, glass slides, and other sharp instruments should be disposed of properly in an appropriately labeled, leak-proof, puncture-proof container.
- The medical assistant's role and responsibilities in maintaining personal safety and well-being of staff and patients can be achieved by assessing their understanding of risk for infection, educating them on steps to eliminate an infection and methods to control the spread of infection.
- Medical asepsis is a type of infection control that decreases the risk of spreading infection by destroying microorganisms after they leave the body. This can be achieved by wearing the appropriate PPE and practicing proper hand washing, sanitization, disinfecting, and sterilizing techniques.
- Acquiring the Hepatitis B vaccination and following standard and universal precautions are preventive measures health care professionals should use to protect against this virus.

- Sanitization is the process of washing and scrubbing to remove materials such as body tissue, blood, or other body contaminants. Disinfection is a process by which disease-producing microorganisms or pathogens (not always their spores) are killed. Sterilization is the process that destroys all forms of living organisms.
- Autoclaves sterilize instruments and other medical supplies by using steam under pressure. Safety must be maintained by wearing proper PPE and following the manufacture's guidelines for use.
- Sterilization and biological indicators are quality control methods used to register proper and complete sterilization of equipment and should be used according to the autoclave manufacturer's guidelines.

STUDY TOOLS

Workbook	Activities for Chapter 36
Premium Website	
MEDIA LINK	View these **Media Links** for Chapter 36: • Wrap Items for Autoclaving
StudyWARE	Activities and Quizzes on the **StudyWARE™ Software** for Chapter 36
	Complete the following **Competency Challenge 2.0** activity: • Tuesday, 8:00 AM, Perform General Clinical Practices
	Audio Library of medical terms
	Online access to the **Critical Thinking Challenge 2.0**
CourseMate	Activities and Quizzes for Chapter 36
WebTutor	Activities and Quizzes for Chapter 36

CHECK YOUR KNOWLEDGE

1. An example of a disease that must be reported to the National Notifiable Diseases Surveillance System of the CDC is:
   a. *herpes simplex* virus.
   b. impetigo.
   c. pediculosis.
   d. meningitis.
2. When the infection cycle is broken:
   a. an individual becomes susceptible.
   b. the spread of disease is prevented.
   c. an individual becomes infected.
   d. disease can be transferred from one person to another.
3. An infectious agent that can be viewed only with an electron microscope and can reproduce itself only within a host is known as:
   a. bacteria.
   b. a virus.
   c. fungi.
   d. a parasite.
4. The stage of infection when the first onset of signs and symptoms of infection occur is the:
   a. incubation stage.
   b. prodromal stage.
   c. acute stage.
   d. convalescent stage.
5. Which of the following organizations established the Blood-Borne Pathogen Standard?
   a. OSHA
   b. CDC
   c. CLIA
   d. EPA
6. Contaminated surfaces must be cleaned with a _____ bleach solution.
   a. 1:100
   b. 100:1
   c. 1:10
   d. 10:1

7. Standard precautions should be used:
   a. only if the infectious status of the patient is unknown.
   b. only if the patient is known to have HIV.
   c. with all patients at all times.
   d. for self-protection rather than for protection of the patient.
8. An exposure control plan should include:
   a. engineering controls.
   b. work practice controls.
   c. PPE.
   d. All of the above
9. Sharps containers should be:
   a. odor-proof.
   b. puncture-proof.
   c. white in color.
   d. red in color.
10. According to CDC standards, vigorous hand washing should be done for at least _____ before and after seeing each patient.
    a. 15 minutes
    b. 30 seconds
    c. 15 seconds
    d. 60 seconds
11. Gloves are worn to:
    a. prevent contamination of the hands when touching blood or body fluids.
    b. increase the possibility of transferring pathogens on your hands to another.
    c. protect hands by reducing the amount of hand washing needed.
    d. all of the above
12. The process that destroys all forms of microorganisms is known as:
    a. disinfection.
    b. sterilization.
    c. sanitization.
    d. Both a and b are correct.
13. Autoclaved items have a shelf life of _____ days if items are kept dried and intact.
    a. 10
    b. 20
    c. 30
    d. 45

WEB LINKS

Centers for Disease Control and Prevention: www.cdc.gov

Occupational Safety & Health Administration: www.osha.gov

RESOURCES

Heller, M., and Veach, L. (2009). *Clinical Medical Assisting: A Professional, Field Smart Approach to the Workplace.* Clifton Park, NY: Delmar, Cengage Learning.

Kennamer, M. (2007). *Basic Infection Control for Health Care Providers* (2nd ed.). Clifton Park, NY: Delmar, Cengage Learning.

Lindh, W., Pooler, M., Tamparo, C., and Dahl, B. (2010). *Delmar's Comprehensive Medical Assisting Administrative and Clinical Competencies* (4th ed.). Clifton Park, NY: Delmar Cengage Learning.

Neighbors, M., and Jones, R. T. (2006). *Human Diseases* (2nd ed.). Clifton Park, NY: Delmar, Cengage Learning.

U.S. Department of Health and Human Services, Centers for Disease Control and Prevention. (2003). *Exposure to Blood: What Healthcare Personnel Need to Know.* Retrieved October 19, 2009, from www.cdc.gov/ncidod/dhqp/pdf/bbp/Exp_to_Blood.pdf.

U.S. Department of Health and Human Services, Centers for Disease Control and Prevention. (2008). *Guideline for Disinfection and Sterilization in Healthcare Facilities, 2008.* Retrieved January 10, 2010, from www.cdc.gov/hicpac/pdf/guidelines/Disinfection_Nov_2008.pdf.

U.S. Department of Labor, Occupational Safety and Health Administration. (2009). *Bloodborne Pathogens and Needlestick Prevention.* Retrieved November 16, 2009, from www.osha.gov/SLTC/bloodbornepathogens/index.html.

Venes, D., (ed.) (2009). *Taber's Cyclopedic Medical Dictionary* (21st ed.). Philadelphia: F. A. Davis.

Chapter 37

The Medical History and Patient Screening

CHAPTER OBJECTIVES

In this chapter, you will learn the following:

KB KNOWLEDGE BASE

1. Spell and define, using the glossary at the back of this text, all the Words to Know in this chapter.
2. Explain the purpose of screening in today's medical office.
3. Describe the process for screening and determining the urgency of a patient's condition.
4. Identify the skills necessary to conduct a patient interview.
5. List the characteristics of the patient's chief complaint and the present illness.
6. Explain the purpose of obtaining a health history.
7. Identify the components of the health history form and their documentation.
8. Compare and contrast the patient's medical, family, and social and occupational histories.
9. Discuss the genogram and explain why it is useful.
10. Explain how the review of systems is obtained and documented.

S SKILLS

1. Perform in-person screening.
2. Obtain and record a patient health history.

B BEHAVIORS

1. Demonstrate professionalism by being courteous and diplomatic; showing respect, empathy, and cultural sensitivity; maintaining privacy and confidentiality; and adapting to change.
2. Apply critical thinking skills in performing patient assessment and care.
3. Use language and verbal skills that enable patients' understanding and appropriate, congruent body language and other nonverbal skills.
4. Apply active listening skills.
5. Demonstrate awareness of the territorial boundaries of the person with whom communicating.
6. Demonstrate recognition of the patient's level of understanding in communications.
7. Analyze communications in providing appropriate responses and feedback.
8. Recognize and protect personal boundaries in communicating with others.
9. Demonstrate sensitivity to patient rights.
10. Use time management and anticipation skills.

WORDS TO KNOW

allergies
biases
chief complaint (CC)
clinical diagnosis
emergent
familial
genogram
interview
objective
over-the-counter (OTC)
patronizing
prioritizing
remedies
screening
subjective
symptoms
triage

hypovolmonic shock

PATIENT SCREENING

Screening is the process of obtaining information from patients to determine who will be the most beneficial to handle their needs. As a medical assistant, one of your responsibilities is to perform both incoming phone call screening (covered in Chapter 9) and in-person screening. Phone screening occurs in some form every time a patient calls into the medical facility, whereas in-person screening occurs in the office every time the patient is seen to identify the **chief complaint (CC)** presented as well as secondary conditions. A more intense form of this process was originated during wartimes and was referred to as **triage**, a concept developed by the military and particularly applicable to trauma and disaster situations. It referred to the sorting and assessment of soldiers' injuries. The French word *triage* means "to sort." After the medics made a decision regarding the seriousness of the wounds, the soldier was taken as soon as possible for treatment. Those in charge of treatment had a clear description of the nature of the wounds from the initial triage.

In addition, triage is a term also used in **prioritizing** the conditions of the injured following a disaster. The injured were separated into groups according to the seriousness of their needs. Usually, they were tagged with a particular color-coded tape or cloth so that the other members of the emergency medical team would know which victims required immediate attention. As discussed more in Unit 18, the rules regarding those who have **emergent** conditions should be given first priority. Conditions that are not life threatening can wait a short time.

Many of the emergent conditions are rarely (if ever) seen initially in the physician's office in metropolitan areas due to the presence of emergency medical services and hospital emergency rooms. The word *screening* has replaced the term *triage* because it is more appropriate for the process used in the medical office.

When conducting the screening process, you must communicate in the most efficient and effective manner for each individual. Patients may be shy or embarrassed by their problems or questions and may not ask and answer direct questions. Therefore, excellent listening skills are vital to understanding what the patient is trying to convey. Be familiar with information about the patient before proceeding with an explanation. This will help determine how to communicate best with each individual.

CLINICAL PEARL

Never assume that a patient already knows the information you are conveying. Sometimes a patient will state that he or she understands something to keep from being embarrassed. If you sense that this is the situation, you should briefly repeat the information to ensure that you are receiving the information accurately.

IN-PERSON SCREENING

In-person screening is the first step taken between the patient and you to make their experience at the office beneficial. Talking to patients one on one and asking questions about their condition requires professional communication skills and the assurance of privacy. Some offices may have a private area specifically for screening (Figure 37–1). Other offices conduct the screening and **interview** in the privacy of the examination room. It is important to remember that all of the data obtained is subject to legal and ethical considerations and must remain confidential. Patients are entitled to certain rights, and these rights must be enforced. (Refer to "Patient Bill of Rights" in Unit 3.) Your ability to obtain and accurately record information received from the patient is crucial. Your goal is to determine why the patient is seeking health care; what he or she sees as the main problem; any other concerns he or she may have; and what, if anything, he or she has done about it.

The purpose of the screening is to help patients focus on their main concern, the CC, and its related **symptoms**. After this is established, it may be necessary to continue the screening to obtain and record other health concerns. For example, a work-in patient whose chief complaint is severe muscle spasms of the back may also express concern because of occasional irregular heartbeats and an increasing need to take antacids for indigestion. These complaints need to be recorded and will probably require an additional visit to address, depending on the severity of the symptoms due to previous patient scheduling.

The patient's initial visit will require varying amounts of questioning depending upon the reason for the visit. Someone requesting a complete physical, but who has no complaints, will not require the in-depth inquiry that someone would who has complaints of intermittent pain, fever, and fatigue for the past two weeks. Face-

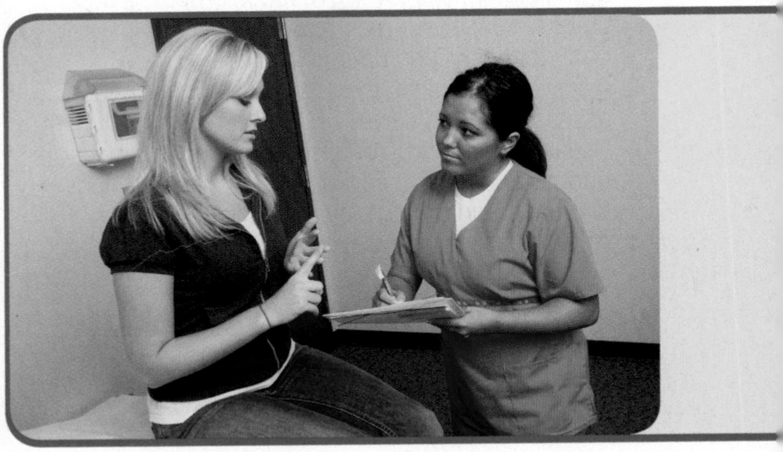

Figure 37–1: A medical assistant and patient are in a private area discussing symptoms and assessing the patient's condition. This is called in-person screening. *Delmar/Cengage Learning.*

to-face screening is also required when patients return for follow-up visits. The line of questioning then is to determine how they have felt since the last office visit. Establishing an accurate database is a very important duty because it is the beginning of the patient's medical record with the physician.

When patients are called into the office, the medical assistant makes the initial personal contact to begin gathering the information that relates to their reason for the office visit. It is important to not appear rushed or as if just performing a routine task. Because this is the patients' first visit, they may be naturally ill at ease and nervous about seeing a new provider, especially if they fear they may have a serious condition. This in-person screening procedure requires a professional approach and is critical to the patient's perception of the practice.

Following the determination of a clear reason the patient is there, it is generally customary on the patient's first visit to obtain an accurate and comprehensive personal and family health history. A complete history is very revealing and a great aid in diagnosing conditions.

CLINICAL PEARL

To follow HIPAA privacy standards, be sure to get the patient's approval to involve another person in the discussion of his or her private health information. Document the permission; without documentation, it is considered "not permitted." For more information about HIPAA, refer to Unit 4.

Factors Influencing Screening

Successfully conducting the first interview with a new patient establishes a favorable relationship among the patient, you, and the practice. Many factors must be considered to make that experience as beneficial as possible. The following gives you some things to remember when you are talking with the patient.

- *Ensure privacy*: Not only in the setting, but also assure the patient that the information you are gathering will be protected within the privacy policy of the office.
- *Be aware of your* **biases**: Our beliefs and behaviors tend to influence how we view others. All patients must be treated with respect without evaluating them based on their race, religion, sexual orientation, cultural or ethnic origin, or socioeconomic or educational status. Take care that your value system does not interfere with what you hear or observe.
- *Establish a non-threatening, relaxed atmosphere*:
  - Greet the patient by name.
  - State your name.
  - Explain what you would like to do.
  - You may say something like this: "Mrs. Green, I am Ginny, Dr. Long's medical assistant. I would like to ask you a few questions about what brought you to the office today. Would you be willing to share this information with me?"
- *Be aware of your own nonverbal messages*: Be attentive and give eye contact so the patient can tell you are interested in who he or she is and what he or she has to say. Do not be overly involved with note taking or watching the time.
- *Be sure the patient understands*: Using medical terminology is not appropriate for most patients. Pay attention to their expressions as you talk. Is there a hearing problem or a lack of understanding? Responses to questions will usually indicate any difficulty. Repeating or restating the question will probably be sufficient. If there is a language barrier, it may be necessary to enlist help from an approved translator. Someone who is hearing or speech impaired will require a person who can sign your questions and speak for them (Figure 37–2).
- *Allow the patient to do most of the talking*: Remember, you are trying to learn about his or her condition and concerns.
- *Listen attentively to what the patient says*: Be an active listener; ask questions to be sure you understand what was said. You can repeat what you think the patient stated to see whether he or she agrees.
- *Nonverbal communication*: Watch the patient's body language; does it agree with what he or she is saying? This may take some experience. For example, if the patient does not look at you when answering personal questions, is it because of embarrassment or is he or she not being truthful? For example, a married

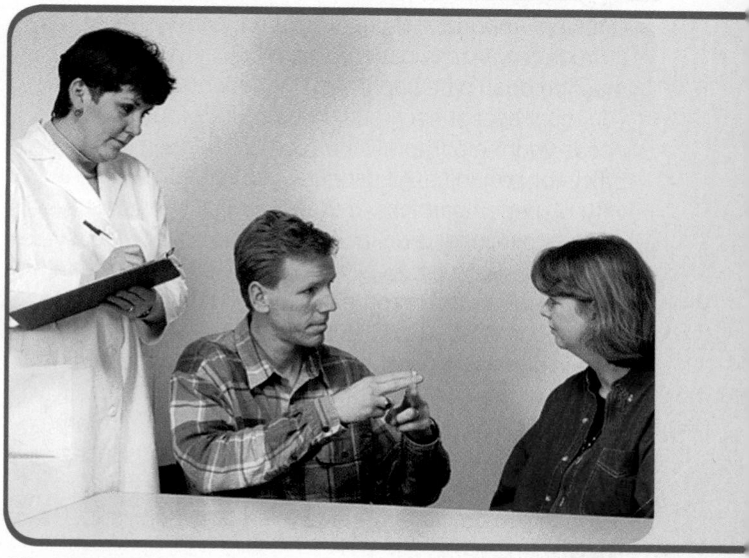

Figure 37–2: A person who can sign may be needed to assist with the patient interview. *Delmar/Cengage Learning.*

person seeking care because of a sexually transmitted disease acquired from an affair may be reluctant to tell anyone other than the provider. Additionally, it may be none of these but rather due to a cultural difference.

- *Use open-ended questions*: These ask for more than a yes or no answer and provide the opportunity for additional information. Asking, "How would you describe your pain?" will get you more information than asking, "Do you have pain now?"
- *Focus on the interview*: Do not allow the conversation to go off course.
- *Conclude the screening portion of the interview with a summary*: State to the patient what has been identified and recorded as the chief complaint and any additional concerns in decreasing order of importance. With the patient's agreement, record the CC and other data.

Conducting the In-Person Screening

What is done by the medical assistant during the in-person screening will be determined by the employing provider. Some providers prefer the medical assistant to do only the chief complaint, and the providers conduct the in-depth interview so they have the advantage of getting the information personally. Other providers want all preliminary questioning done by the medical assistant so they can review it briefly and begin their examination. Detailed information is provided later in the chapter regarding the health history form, the components, and what information is obtained in each section.

CLINICAL PEARL

One very important aspect of patient care is your attitude toward the patient. The medical assistant must be open when approaching patients. This means you must accept each patient as an individual who needs your help. There is no room in the medical office for prejudice. All patients should be treated with respect regardless of their financial status, race, religion, age, or station in life. Remember, your job is to provide assistance. Calling patients by pet names or terms of endearment (e.g., Honey, Hon, and Dear) may be taken as **patronizing**, especially if your attitude is questionable. It is more respectful to patients if you call them by their titles (i.e., Mr. or Ms.) or their full names. The patient will let you know if a first-name basis is all right with him or her. If the patient senses any negative feelings on your part, he or she will be less likely to pay attention to your instructions and suggestions.

Developing the Chief Complaint

After introducing yourself to the new patient, establishing a comfortable environment, and requesting the patient's assistance, it is time to start the interview. Begin by asking what brought the patient to the office today, the CC. Record the CC in the patient's own words on the chart or electronic medical record (EMR) and then add other descriptive information given by the patient. By asking the patient to describe certain characteristics regarding the symptoms, you can ensure that the chief complaint is documented thoroughly. The following are examples of aspects to have the patient consider:

- *Location:* Where is the symptom located?
- *Radiation:* What area does the symptom cover?
- *Quality:* Describe the characteristic of the symptom, for instance, "dull ache," "throbbing," "tingling," and so on.
- *Severity:* Describe the pain associated with the symptom. (A pain scale such as the one in Figure 37–3 can be used.)
- *Associated symptoms:* Describe other minor symptoms in addition to the CC.
- *Aggravating factors:* Describe what makes symptoms worse.
- *Alleviating factors:* Describe what makes the symptoms better.
- *Setting and timing:* Describe when the symptoms started and what the patient was doing at the time.

When the patient has identified all the complaints and together you have determined the specifics of the symptoms, you can summarize the results of your screening. Read to the patient what you have written on the chart or entered into the EMR and ask whether there is anything else to add. The finished statement may read something like this:

8/6/XX 11:30 am	CC: "I have a pain in my stomach." RLQ, Pain level 4, intermittent × 3 days, nausea, no vomiting or diarrhea. Some relief by lying down. G. Jenks, RMA(AMT)

Procedure 37–1 provides a generic guide for in-person screening of a patient.

After obtaining this initial information, you are ready to proceed with interviewing and reviewing the patient's health history. Completing both these tasks establishes a good basis for not only diagnosing and treating the patient's current condition but also understanding the patient's and the family's past health conditions, which might have some bearing on the present.

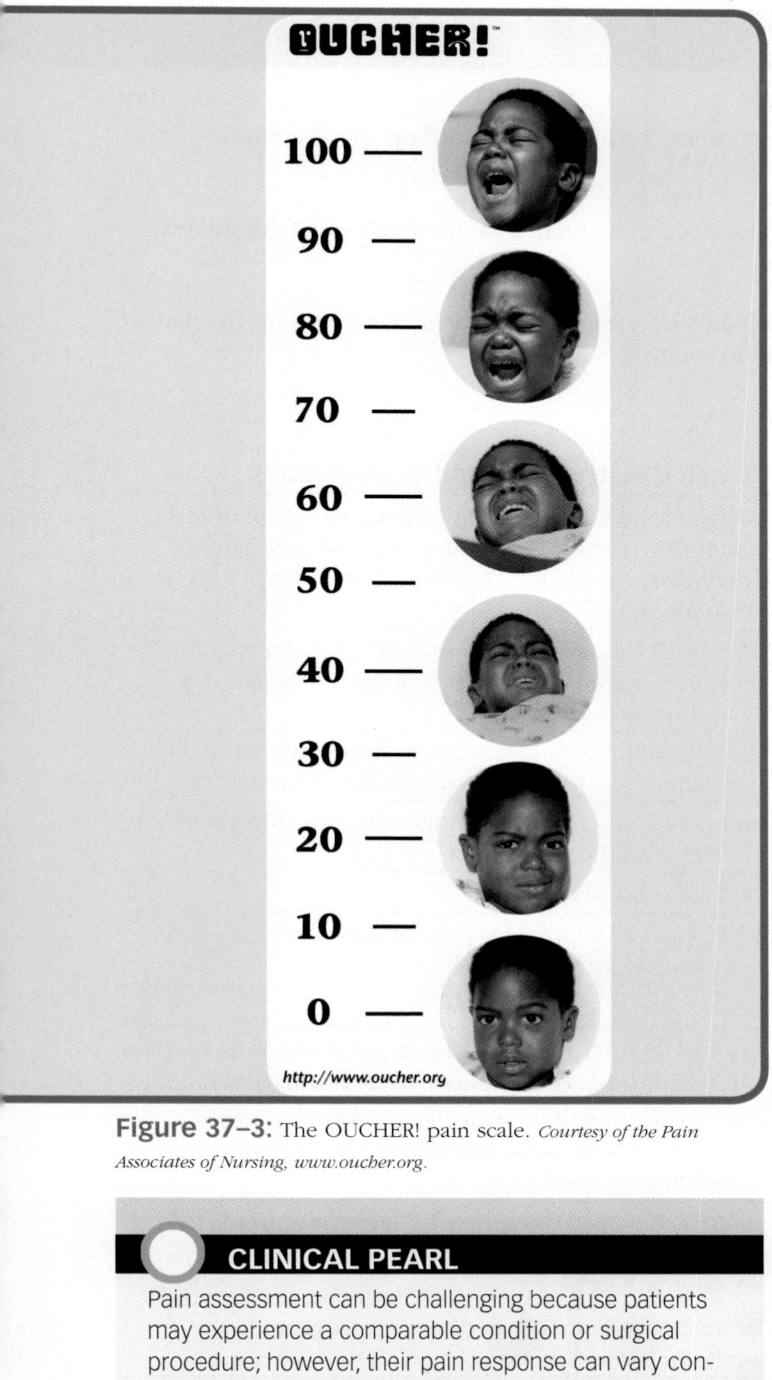

Figure 37–3: The OUCHER! pain scale. *Courtesy of the Pain Associates of Nursing, www.oucher.org.*

CLINICAL PEARL

Pain assessment can be challenging because patients may experience a comparable condition or surgical procedure; however, their pain response can vary considerably. Individuals of every age and culture experience pain, and many practitioners consider pain a fifth vital sign. Because pain is **subjective**, it is whatever the experiencing person says it is and exists whenever the experiencing person says it does. Today, health care providers are more perceptive to pain and recognize that unrelieved pain can have both physiological and psychological effects on patients. Constant pain can slow recovery, create hassles for patients and their families, and increase the cost of care.

THE HEALTH HISTORY

A patient's health history is a comprehensive medical history that includes information about the patient and the patient's family. Information incorporated in the history includes previous illnesses, medications, allergies, and surgical history. The health history is the basis for all treatment given by the provider and is a guide for future treatment of the patient. The history is helpful for patients and providers when patients are seen by a provider who is not their primary provider or when referred to a specialist. This information gives them useful information about past and present health concerns and saves them time from not having to collect that data again. In addition to providing the patient comprehensive health information for the provider, health histories can also provide statistical data to research companies and the health department as well as insurance data.

The health history is acquired when the patient is new to the facility. In general, before extensive care is provided to new patients, a complete physical exam is performed and a complete and thorough medical history is obtained so the providers have a good idea of the patient's current and past health status as well as any family conditions that might factor into the patient's health. All patients are asked to complete a health history form at their initial visit to a provider's office. Some are mailed prior to the appointment, depending on the provider's preference, and others are completed in the office prior to the provider's examination. The standard paper health history form can vary, depending on the type of practice, from short and concise to fairly comprehensive (Figure 37–4). Notice at the end of the comprehensive form a statement regarding errors or omissions. The absence of pertinent information could result in a misdiagnosis, a consequence that this form addresses.

As part of your duties as a medical assistant, you may need to assist in the completion of the history. Refer to Procedure 37–2 to help you practice interviewing a patient. With a copy of a history form or the one included in the workbook, proceed through the form, asking clarifying questions and recording patient information. Include any significant additional remarks in your notes on the patient's chart. If you have access to a computer with office practice software, proceed through the form and enter the patient's responses directly into the EMR.

The patient might need help with some unfamiliar medical terms and some confusing questions. Language, literacy, cultural, and other barriers can prevent completion. Assist these patients with respect and without judgment. Some providers may wish to interview and complete the form themselves as a means to gain insight into the patient's condition. You will need to be familiar with the individual provider's preference.

PROCEDURE 37–1 Perform In-Person Screening

MEDIA LINK: View the video for this chapter, "Developing a Chief Complaint," on the Premium Website.

PURPOSE: To conduct an in-person screening to identify and accurately record the patient's chief complaint (CC) and related symptoms in the patient's medical record.

EQUIPMENT: Patient's chart or computer with appropriate software, pen, any supplies or equipment needed to set up the room according to the reason for the patient being seen.

S **SKILL:** Perform In-Person Screening

Procedure Steps	Detailed Instructions and/or *Rationales*
B 1. ***Select a private location for the interview.***	*Talking to patients one on one and asking questions about their personal condition requires professional communication skills and the assurance of privacy and confidentiality.*
2. Review any completed office forms, including the HIPAA authorization agreement.	*This saves time and helps the medical assistant identify why the patient is there and determine whether any assistance is needed.*
B 3. ***Call the patient by name from the reception room.***	The general rule is to use the patient's full name unless the patient has requested something different.
B 4. ***Take the patient to the interview area and make the patient comfortable.***	Sitting face to face to begin the interview allows for eye contact with the patient.
5. Restate the patient's name and introduce yourself.	*This helps build rapport.*
B 6. ***Explain what you will be doing and request participation.***	*This shows respect for the patient and provides helpful information for the provider.*
7. Ask what brings the person to the office today.	
8. Use questioning to focus on the CC, its characteristics, and any related symptoms.	*Certain characteristics should be obtained for a complete understanding of why the patient is being seen.*
9. Identify and record any secondary concerns.	*Due to the allotted time for the appointment, these might need to be addressed at a future appointment, depending on the severity.*
10. Ask the patient whether he or she is taking any medications.	*Be sure to include prescription, over-the-counter (OTC), and herbal supplements. Include the dosages and reason for taking them.*
11. Ask the patient whether he or she has any allergies.	Be sure to include all medications, food, and environmental allergies.
12. Reconfirm the CC, symptoms, and any other concerns with the patient.	*This clarifies that the information you obtained is accurate.*
13. Record the CC statement and related information on the chart or EMR.	Concise documentation is essential in providing an accurate account of the patient's visit. *Documentation identifies the person responsible for providing the screening.*
B 14. ***Set up the room according to the patient's complaint, demonstrating time management and anticipation skills.***	*This enhances the patient's visit by saving time for the provider, making the visit more efficient.*

Procedure Steps	Detailed Instructions and/or *Rationales*
B 15. ***Dismiss yourself in a professional manner and indicate to the patient the approximate wait time.***	*This is provided as a courtesy to the patient so he or she can anticipate the wait time.*
16. Notify the provider that the patient is ready to be seen.	

Charting Example

8/6/XX 11:30 am	CC, "I have a pain in my stomach." RLQ, pain level 6, intermittent, ×3 days, nausea, no vomiting or diarrhea. Some relief from lying down. Patient not on any medications at this time. Patient has NKDA. G. Jenks, RMA(AMT)

With electronic health records (EHR) software becoming more abundant in the medical office, another common way to collect the history data is electronically. Some facilities enter the data obtained from the paper copy or scan the paper copy the patient fills out into the system. Other systems allow the patient to fill out the forms ahead of time via a patient portal, either in the comfort of his or her home with access to a computer or by a kiosk inside of the facility prior to the appointment. Most of the electronic versions of the health history forms have drop-down lists within the system, making it quicker and easier for the patient to fill in the information. These systems are also easier to update if changes need to be made rather than having the patient fill out an annual paper form. Figure 37–5 shows a screen shot of a completed patient medical history (PMH) form from an EHR program. Whichever technique is used, it may be your responsibility as a medical assistant to review the history with the patient to be certain that all of the data collected is accurate. Before calling the patient in for the in-person screening, if the patient has completed the form ahead of time, you should obtain the form from the receptionist and review its contents.

Reviewing the Patient's Health History

As mentioned earlier, even if the patient has completed the form in its entirety, you must still review all the information for omission and clarity. For instance, if a patient checks "hazardous substances" under occupational concerns, it would be important to identify what those substances are. Another question might arise about who is a "blood relative." You must be thoroughly familiar with the form used by your employer and be prepared to answer any questions. In the sample form in Figure 37–4, notice that not only the patient but also the person reviewing the form must sign and date the document. The validity of this baseline document can become very important later in the patient's course of treatment.

EHR - Electronic Medical Record
EMR - Electronic Health record

CLINICAL PEARL

Note that if the form is not completed, the patient may have a language barrier or reading problem. If this is the case, the patient may be very sensitive about his or her inability to read and write. It may be necessary for you to ask the questions and help complete the form for such a patient. Use tact when asking whether a patient needs assistance with the form.

Sections of the Health History

Most medical facilities have a standard health history form, or electronic template if using EHR, that will be used for all patients. A four-page history form developed for an oncology practice is included in the workbook to provide you with an interview experience. Regardless of the specific form used, some information requests are standard and are elaborated in the next sections.

Chief Complaint

The chief complaint (CC) is why the patient is being seen currently in the office. It should be short and written with precision and conciseness and should contain the subjective and objective data that the patient discusses. Information you receive from patients is subjective, meaning it is based upon symptoms they feel. Subjective symptoms or sensations are those that only the patient can perceive, such as pain, dizziness, itching, or numbness. Information or symptoms that can be observed (that are perceptible to other people), such as swelling, bruising, vital signs, and physical examination findings, are known as **objective** findings. It is important for you to know the difference. These two distinctions become necessary when you proceed with recording information

CONFIDENTIAL HEALTH HISTORY

Name: ______________________ Date: __________

Birthdate: __________ Age: ______ Date of last physical examination: __________

Occupation: ______________________

Reason for visit today: ______________________

MEDICATIONS List all medications you are currently taking	**ALLERGIES** List all allergies

SYMPTOMS Check (✓) symptoms you currently have or have had in the past year.

GENERAL
- ☐ Chills
- ☐ Depression
- ☐ Dizziness
- ☐ Fainting
- ☐ Fever
- ☐ Forgetfulness
- ☐ Headache
- ☐ Loss of sleep
- ☐ Loss of weight
- ☐ Nervousness
- ☐ Numbness
- ☐ Sweats

MUSCLE/JOINT/BONE
Pain, weakness, numbness in:
- ☐ Arms
- ☐ Back
- ☐ Feet
- ☐ Hands
- ☐ Hips
- ☐ Legs
- ☐ Neck
- ☐ Shoulders

GENITO-URINARY
- ☐ Blood in urine
- ☐ Frequent urination
- ☐ Lack of bladder control
- ☐ Painful urination

GASTROINTESTINAL
- ☐ Appetite poor
- ☐ Bloating
- ☐ Bowel changes
- ☐ Constipation
- ☐ Diarrhea
- ☐ Excessive hunger
- ☐ Excessive thirst
- ☐ Gas
- ☐ Hemorrhoids
- ☐ Indigestion
- ☐ Nausea
- ☐ Rectal bleeding
- ☐ Stomach pain
- ☐ Vomiting
- ☐ Vomiting blood

CARDIOVASCULAR
- ☐ Chest pain
- ☐ High blood pressure
- ☐ Irregular heart beat
- ☐ Low blood pressure
- ☐ Poor circulation
- ☐ Rapid heart beat
- ☐ Swelling of ankles
- ☐ Varicose veins

EYE, EAR, NOSE, THROAT
- ☐ Bleeding gums
- ☐ Blurred vision
- ☐ Crossed eyes
- ☐ Difficulty swallowing
- ☐ Double vision
- ☐ Earache
- ☐ Ear discharge
- ☐ Hay fever
- ☐ Hoarseness
- ☐ Loss of hearing
- ☐ Nosebleeds
- ☐ Persistent cough
- ☐ Ringing in ears
- ☐ Sinus problems
- ☐ Vision - Flashes
- ☐ Vision - Halos

SKIN
- ☐ Bruise easily
- ☐ Hives
- ☐ Itching
- ☐ Change in moles
- ☐ Rash
- ☐ Scars
- ☐ Sores that won't heal

MEN only
- ☐ Breast lump
- ☐ Erection difficulties
- ☐ Lump in testicles
- ☐ Penis discharge
- ☐ Sore on penis
- ☐ Other

WOMEN only
- ☐ Abnormal Pap Smear
- ☐ Bleeding between periods
- ☐ Breast lump
- ☐ Extreme menstrual pain
- ☐ Hot flashes
- ☐ Nipple discharge
- ☐ Painful intercourse
- ☐ Vaginal discharge
- ☐ Other

Date of last menstrual period __________

Date of last Pap Smear __________

Have you had a mammogram? __________

Are you pregnant? __________

Number of children __________

MEDICAL HISTORY Check (✓) the medical conditions you have or have had in the past.

- ☐ AIDS
- ☐ Alcoholism
- ☐ Anemia
- ☐ Anorexia
- ☐ Appendicitis
- ☐ Arthritis
- ☐ Asthma
- ☐ Bleeding Disorders
- ☐ Breast Lump
- ☐ Bronchitis
- ☐ Bulimia
- ☐ Cancer
- ☐ Cataracts
- ☐ Chemical Dependency
- ☐ Chicken Pox
- ☐ Diabetes
- ☐ Emphysema
- ☐ Epilepsy
- ☐ Gall Bladder Disease
- ☐ Glaucoma
- ☐ Goiter
- ☐ Gonorrhea
- ☐ Gout
- ☐ Heart Disease
- ☐ Hepatitis
- ☐ Hernia
- ☐ Herpes
- ☐ High Cholesterol
- ☐ HIV Positive
- ☐ Kidney Disease
- ☐ Liver Disease
- ☐ Measles
- ☐ Migraine Headaches
- ☐ Miscarriage
- ☐ Mononucleosis
- ☐ Multiple Sclerosis
- ☐ Mumps
- ☐ Pacemaker
- ☐ Pneumonia
- ☐ Polio
- ☐ Prostate Problem
- ☐ Psychiatric Care
- ☐ Rheumatic Fever
- ☐ Scarlet Fever
- ☐ Stroke
- ☐ Suicide Attempt
- ☐ Thyroid Problems
- ☐ Tonsillitis
- ☐ Tuberculosis
- ☐ Typhoid Fever
- ☐ Ulcers
- ☐ Vaginal Infections
- ☐ Venereal Disease

CONFIDENTIAL HEALTH HISTORY

Figure 37–4: Comprehensive Health History form. *Delmar/Cengage Learning.*

HOSPITALIZATIONS

Year	Hospital	Reason for Hospitalization and Outcome

Have you ever had a blood transfusion? ☐ Yes ☐ No
If yes, please give approximate dates: ______

OCCUPATIONAL CONCERNS Check (✓) if your work exposes you to the following:	HEALTH HABITS Check (✓) which substances you use and indicate how much you use per day/week.
☐ Stress	☐ Caffeine
☐ Hazardous Substances	☐ Tobacco
☐ Heavy Lifting	☐ Drugs
☐ Other	☐ Alcohol

PREGNANCY HISTORY

Year of Birth	Sex of Birth	Complications if any

SERIOUS ILLNESS/INJURIES	DATE	OUTCOME

FAMILY HISTORY Fill in health information about your family.

Relation	Age	State of Health	Age at Death	Cause of Death
Father				
Mother				
Brothers				
Sisters				

Check (✓) if your blood relatives had any of the following

Disease	Relationship to you
☐ Arthritis, Gout	
☐ Asthma, Hay Fever	
☐ Cancer	
☐ Chemical Dependency	
☐ Diabetes	
☐ Heart Disease, Strokes	
☐ High Blood Pressure	
☐ Kidney Disease	
☐ Tuberculosis	
☐ Other	

I certify that the above information is correct to the best of my knowledge. I will not hold my doctor or any members of his/her staff responsible for any errors or ommisions that I may have made in the completion of this form.

______ Signature ______ Date

______ Reviewed By ______ Date

PATIENT EDUCATION

The medical assistant is often involved in patient education, which can include supplying information about diseases and disorders, explaining diagnostic tests, and providing instruction in health care procedures. Recording the patient's health history may identify areas in which educational materials can be helpful. Your office policy may make it appropriate for you to mention these resources. To instruct a patient properly, the medical assistant must know the material. Be prepared to answer any questions from the patient. If you cannot answer one of the patient's questions, tell the patient that you do not know the answer but will ask the physician. Never try to answer a question that you are not prepared to discuss. You could give incorrect information that could harm the patient's well-being. Never give information that is beyond your scope of practice. In teaching a patient about health care and all that is involved in medical well-being, the primary goal of the medical assistant should be good communication. Refer to Chapter 8 for more on patient education and detailed information about instructing patients according to their needs.

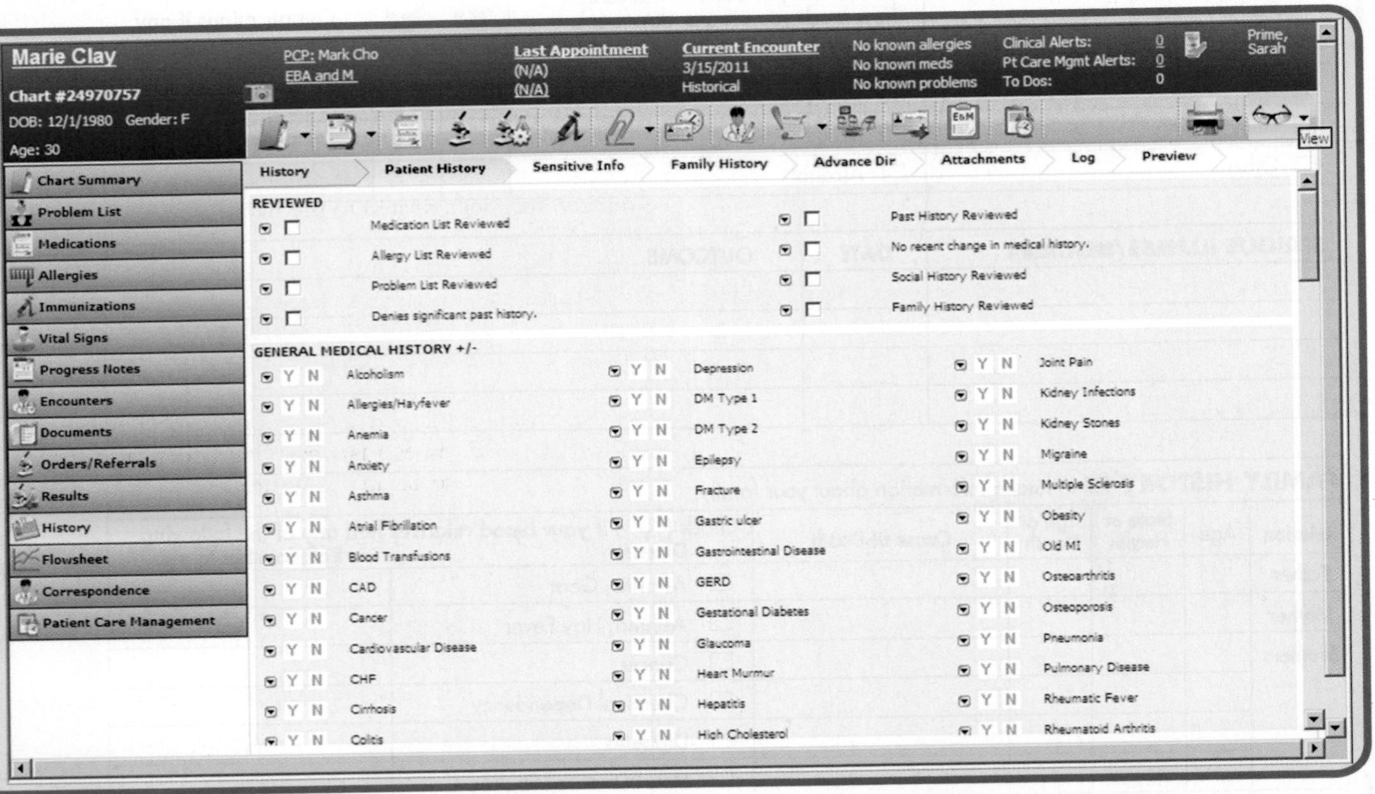

Figure 37–5: Screen shot of a completed patient medical history (PMH) within an EMR health history. *Courtesy of Ingenix CareTracker.*

on the chart. As discussed in Chapter 13, many providers use a method called SOAP (subjective, objective, assessment, and plan) for recording data regarding the patient's office visit. The assessment is made by the provider upon examination, and the plan refers to what course or courses of action will be taken.

Present Illness

The patient will be asked to elaborate on the present illness (PI) or history of present illness (HPI), which will include detailed information about the chief complaint, including when the problem started, concerns on what the patient has done for the condition, and whether any treatment was attempted (such as **over-the-counter [OTC]** medications, vitamins and herbal supplements, or home **remedies**) and, if so, what they were and whether they were effective.

Medical History

The past history (PH) or past medical history (PMH) section identifies all health problems, illnesses, or disorders ever diagnosed and surgeries. In the example, the sections are divided into symptoms during the past year and the history, which refers to present and past *diseases* and *disorders*. Usual childhood diseases (UCHD) are also included in the medical history section, which can help patients remember previous illnesses or symptoms they may have forgotten. Notice some questions are gender specific, and others deal with serious illnesses and hospitalizations. The hospitalization section should include all hospitalizations and any surgeries the patient has had.

If not included in the present illness section, two very important sections within the history list current medications being taken, including dosages and the reason the patient is taking them and a listing of any **allergies** the patient may have. In addition to the health history form, medications and allergies should be discussed with the patient at every visit. Drug reactions and interactions, from both prescribed and OTC medications, can cause significant symptoms. Some offices identify allergies with red ink or separate labels attached to the chart. Always question the patient about any allergies to drugs, including OTC and herbal supplements, food, or environmental factors because true allergic reactions can be very serious, even life-threatening. If the patient indicates he or she does not have any allergies, enter "No known drug allergies" (NKDA) on the form and in the initial charting to indicate the question was addressed and not overlooked.

Family Health History

Most forms also request information about the health status of the immediate family members. These data, in addition to the physical examination, assist the provider with not only the information necessary to arrive at a diagnosis and treatment for the current complaint but also perhaps to forewarn and possibly prevent future conditions that tend to develop within families. The family history (FH) section asks for ages and status of health or age and cause of death for immediate family members. Family members should include siblings, parents, grandparents (maternal and paternal), aunts, uncles, and children. Some forms ask about the incidence of specific diseases among blood relatives and or provide space to add any other conditions.

Providers who treat **familial** disorders and diseases may also use another type of history form called a **genogram**. Figure 37–6 illustrates a family's medical history. Most genograms include at least three generations. This provides visual information to the provider that is helpful in determining the patient's chances of developing a disease that has genetic tendencies.

Social/Occupational History

It is also necessary to determine the patient's personal or lifestyle habits. A patient's lifestyle can have a huge impact on the prevention or creation of certain diseases or conditions. Patients may not want to answer questions pertaining to some of the sensitive subjects in this area and may need to be asked again later by the provider. The excessive use of some prescribed drugs can lead to a dependency the same as with illegal drugs. Alcohol and tobacco are commonly abused substances and may require assistance to control. If any habits are problematic, they may be addressed by the provider. You may be instructed to provide the patient with educational materials related to the problem and to make him or her aware of any community resources or office-sponsored meetings related to the habit.

Work history for the patient is also conducted in this area. Certain occupations may contribute to industrial diseases by exposure to harmful chemicals such as asbestos, coal, and pesticides. Noise level from certain factories can also be problematic. Questioning the patient about the hazardous occupation and how long he or she was employed in that occupation can help in determining illnesses that may have been associated from this or could result in the future.

Additional questioning about the patient's living environment, firearm practices, hobbies, sexual practices, diet, and exercise can also provide insight into his or her health history and give the provider greater detail about the patient's health status and direction.

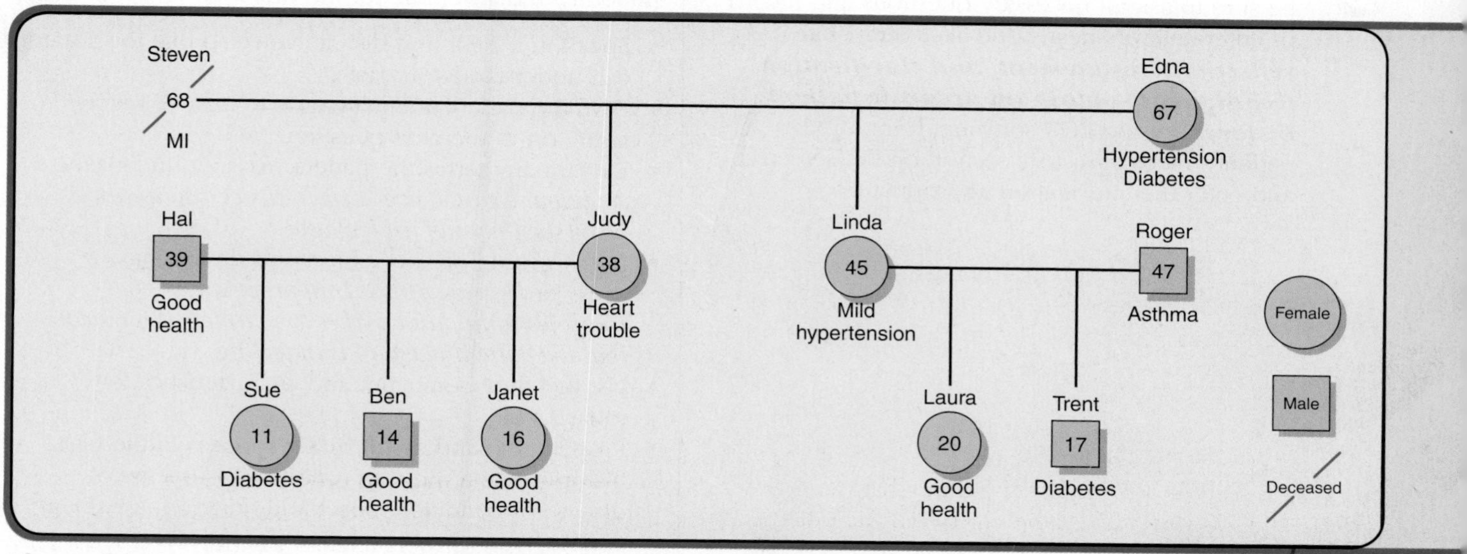

Figure 37–6: Example of a genogram tracing a family's medical history. *Delmar/Cengage Learning.*

no known drug allergies

PROCEDURE 37–2 Obtain and Record a Patient Health History

MEDIA LINK: View the video for this chapter, "Reviewing a Patient's Health History," on the Premium Website.

PURPOSE: To obtain and record a comprehensive health history of a patient, including family, occupational, and social factors; to facilitate the diagnosis and health care plan for the patient.

EQUIPMENT: Health history form, and pen or computer with appropriate software. Using the computer or copies of a medical history form and a pen, obtain and record a medical history by interviewing a person and reviewing the completed form. Allergies are identified or "NKDA" stated. All areas must be addressed and the form signed as appropriate.

S **SKILL:** Obtain and Record a Patient Health History

Procedure Steps	Detailed Instructions and/or *Rationales*
1. If using a paper system, obtain the medical history form and pen.	
B 2. ***Escort the patient to a private area where you can both sit comfortably.***	*Obtaining a history from the patient can be time consuming; you want to ensure the patient's comfort at all times.*
B 3. ***Sit opposite patient.***	*Allows you to establish eye contact.*
B 4. ***Explain the purpose of the health history and inform the patient that all the information obtained is confidential.***	*Helps the patient understand why the information is necessary and allows him or her to be more at ease to discuss sensitive information.*
B 5. If the patient completed the form prior to the visit, review the information with the patient, clarifying information and ensuring no omissions. ***Use reflection, restatement, and clarification techniques to obtain an accurate patient history.***	*Patients may not understand what the questions are asking, omitting some of the data. Reviewing the information also allows them to elaborate on YES answers, saving time for the provider.*
B 6. If you are completing the form with the patient, be sure to ask all necessary questions and record or enter answers neatly and accurately. ***Use reflection, restatement, and clarification techniques to obtain an accurate patient history.*** If using EHR software, bring up the patient's medical history section on the screen and enter the information appropriately.	Following these protocols will make the interview flow smoothly and save time for the provider: • Speak in a clear and distinct voice so that the patient can understand you easily. • Give the patient adequate time to answer before going on to the next question. • Explain any terms the patient may not understand. *A patient cannot give correct answers to inquiries he or she does not understand.* • Avoid getting off the subject and discussing irrelevant topics. *This is inappropriate, unprofessional, and wastes time unless it is obvious that the patient needs to vent feelings.* • List the chief complaint and characteristics for today's visit. • Properly expand on all YES responses in the past history section. Be sure to list concise name of disease or condition, onset and duration, treatment, current status, and resolution if applicable.

Procedure Steps	Detailed Instructions and/or *Rationales*
	• Properly expand on all YES responses in the family and social or occupational sections. • Ensure that all medications (including dosages and reason for taking) and allergies are identified and recorded on the chart as instructed. • Be sure to include all hospitalizations and surgeries on the form.
7. When finished with the form or entering the data, summarize and clarify the information with the patient.	*Helps confirm that the information is concise and accurate.*
B 8. ***Thank the patient and explain the next step in the examination. Ensure that the patient is comfortable and explain whether there will be a wait.***	*This is provided as a courtesy to the patient so he or she can anticipate any wait time that might occur.*
9. Chart a summary of the findings on the patient's chart or EMR. Highlight significant information as instructed.	*Allows the provider to point out any pertinent information easily that needs to be addressed with the patient.*
B 10. Assemble all necessary forms into the patient's chart or templates within EHR software to have them ready for the provider to use during the examination, ***demonstrating time management and anticipation skills.***	

Review of Systems

After the history is completed and appropriate notations are made on the form and on the chart or in the EMR, the patient is weighed and measured and the vital signs are obtained and recorded. This completes the baseline data, and the patient is ready for the provider's examination. With the areas of concern identified, you may have an indication of what type of examination the provider will need to do. According to the office policy, you might begin preparing the patient. This could include partial or complete disrobing and putting on a gown, obtaining a urine specimen, or having the female patient empty her bladder in preparation for a pelvic exam. However, some providers feel it is preferable to meet the patient initially while she is still clothed. They will review the history form and make notations on the chart or in the EMR and conduct a brief screening conversation and then indicate which examination they will be performing.

Whichever procedure is followed, after the history is completed and the baseline measurements and vital signs recorded, express your appreciation to patients for their cooperation and indicate to them what follows next. Be sure to ask whether they have any questions. If there is apt to be a waiting period, try to estimate the time involved and offer reading materials to occupy their time. After the data are accurately recorded on the patient's chart or EMR, it is time for the provider to greet the patient and begin the medical discussion and examination.

The Review of Systems (ROS) is performed by the provider during the physical examination. An orderly and systematic check of each of the body systems is recorded. The ROS can provide information that will be essential in the current diagnostic state of the patient as well as information used as a baseline for subsequent visits. Providers' preference of how the ROS will be performed can vary; however, all the body systems as mentioned in Unit 11 are generally covered.

The provider will document all findings during the ROS, whether positive or negative, on the health history form. If the patient responds positively to an area, the provider will then ask the patient to elaborate. Using the information obtained from the health history, physical exam, ROS, and any laboratory tests completed can help the provider determine a **clinical diagnosis** for the patient. All the sections of the patient's health history must be complete to determine the patient's health condition. With a little experience, you will be able to perform an in-person screening and an interview with confidence.

CHAPTER SUMMARY

- Screening is the process of obtaining information from patients to determine who will be the most beneficial to handle their needs. As a medical assistant, one of your responsibilities is to perform both incoming phone call screening and in-person screening.
- *Triage* is a term used in prioritizing the conditions of the injured following a disaster. The injured are separated into groups according to the seriousness of their needs. Those who have emergent conditions should be given first priority. Conditions that are not life-threatening can wait a short time.
- When conducting the screening process, you must communicate in the most efficient and effective manner for each individual. Patients may be shy or embarrassed by their problems or questions and may not ask or answer direct questions. Therefore, excellent listening skills are vital to understanding what the patient is trying to convey.
- In-person screening is the first step taken between the patient and you to make his or her experience at the office beneficial. Talking to patients one on one and asking questions about their personal condition requires professional communication skills and the assurance of privacy.
- The purpose of the screening is to help patients focus on their main concern, called the chief complaint (CC), and its related symptoms. It should be short and written with precision and conciseness and contain the subjective and objective data that the patient discusses.
- The present illness (PI) or history of present illness (HPI) includes detailed information about the chief complaint, including when the problem started, concerns on about what the patient has done for the condition, whether any over-the-counter (OTC) medications or home remedies were tried, and, if so, what they were and whether they were effective.
- Successfully conducting the first interview with a new patient establishes a favorable relationship among the patient, you, and the practice. Many factors need to be considered to make that experience as beneficial as possible.
- A patient's health history is a comprehensive medical history that includes information about the patient and the patient's family. Information incorporated in the history includes information about previous illnesses, medications, allergies, and surgical history. The health history is the basis for all treatment given by the provider and is used as a guide for future treatment of the patient.
- The past history (PH) or past medical history (PMH) section identifies all surgeries as well as health problems, illnesses, or disorders ever diagnosed.
- Most forms also request information about the health status of the immediate family members. These data, in addition to the physical examination, assist the provider with not only the information necessary to arrive at a diagnosis and treatment for the current complaint but also perhaps to forewarn and possibly prevent future conditions that tend to develop within families.
- It is also necessary to determine the patient's personal or lifestyle habits. A patient's lifestyle can have a huge impact on the prevention or creation of certain diseases or conditions.
- Providers who treat familial disorders and diseases may also use another type of history form called a genogram, which illustrates a family's medical history. Most genograms include at least three generations. This provides visual information to the provider that is helpful in determining the patient's chances of developing a disease that has genetic tendencies.
- The Review of Systems (ROS) is performed by the provider during the physical examination. An orderly and systematic check of each of the body systems is recorded. The ROS can provide information that will be essential in the current diagnostic state of the patient as well as information used as a baseline for subsequent visits.

STUDY TOOLS

Workbook	Activities for Chapter 37
Premium Website	
MEDIA LINK	View the following **Media Link** for this chapter: • Developing the Chief Complaint • Reviewing the Patient's Health History
StudyWARE	Activities and Quizzes on the **StudyWARE™ Software** for Chapter 37
	Audio Library of medical terms
	Online access to **Critical Thinking Challenge 2.0**

CourseMate	Activities and Quizzes for Chapter 37
WebTutor	Activities and Quizzes for Chapter 37

CHECK YOUR KNOWLEDGE

1. The purpose of screening in today's medical office is to:
   a. prioritize the condition of the injured following a disaster.
   b. tag the victims requiring immediate attention.
   c. sort and assess soldiers' injury.
   d. determine who will be the most beneficial to handle the patient's needs.
2. An example of an open-ended question would be:
   a. "How long have you had the pain?"
   b. "Does strenuous activity increase your symptoms?"
   c. "How would you describe your pain?"
   d. "Do you have pain now?"
3. Information collected in the health history includes:
   a. medications.
   b. allergies.
   c. previous illness.
   d. all of the above.
4. When a medical office has the patient fill out the health history form, areas that are incomplete may indicate the following:
   a. laziness
   b. language problem
   c. reading problem
   d. both b and c
5. A genogram determines genetic tendencies and covers how many generations?
   a. Three
   b. Four
   c. Two
   d. Five
6. Questions regarding alcohol and tobacco use would be found under the following section of the health history form:
   a. family health history
   b. review of systems
   c. social or occupational
   d. medical history
7. Where on the health history form is a systematic check of all the body systems recorded?
   a. Medical history
   b. ROS
   c. EHR
   d. Present illness
8. Having the patient elaborate on his or her present illness by asking him or her, "What makes the symptoms better?" would cover the following aspect while the screening the chief complaint.
   a. Aggravating factors
   b. Alleviating factors
   c. Associated symptoms
   d. Severity

WEB LINK

American Medical Association: **www.ama-assn.org**

RESOURCES

Brasin, G.A., & Favreau, C.R. (2010). *The Total Practice Management Workbook: Using e-Medsys*. Clifton Park, NY: Delmar Cengage Learning.

Estes, M. E. Z. (2010). *Health Assessment & Physical Examination* (4th ed.). Clifton Park, NY: Delmar Cengage Learning.

Heller, M., and Veach, L. (2009). *Clinical Medical Assisting: A Professional, Field Smart Approach to the Workplace*. Clifton Park, NY: Delmar Cengage Learning.

Lindh, W., Pooler, M., Tamparo, C., and Dahl, B. (2010). *Delmar's Comprehensive Medical Assisting Administrative and Clinical Competencies* (4th ed.). Clifton Park, NY: Delmar Cengage Learning.

Maki, S. E., and Petterson, B. (2008). *Using the Electronic Health Record in the Health Care Provider Practice*. Clifton Park, NY: Delmar Cengage Learning.

Chapter

38 Body Measurements and Vital Signs

CHAPTER OBJECTIVES

In this chapter, you will learn the following:

KB KNOWLEDGE BASE

1. Spell and define, using the glossary at the back of the text, all the Words to Know in this chapter.
2. Name five types of mensurations.
3. Explain why and when a patient's height and weight is measured.
4. Identify the four vital signs and the body functions they measure.
5. Identify the average normal temperature for aural, axillary, oral, temporal, and rectal measurement.
6. Demonstrate knowledge of basic math calculations by being able to calculate the following: foot and inch measurement conversions, weight and BMI conversions, and Celsius and Fahrenheit temperature conversions.
7. Identify normal pulse rates, describing five factors that affect the rate.
8. Identify and locate five pulse sites and explain the appropriate use of each.
9. Explain indications for apical pulse measurement.
10. Describe normal respiration and explain abnormal breathing patterns.
11. Explain what blood pressure measures.
12. Describe the appropriate equipment for obtaining a blood pressure.
13. Name the two phases of blood pressure; describe the corresponding action that occurs and the relative amount of pressure with each phase.
14. Identify normal and abnormal blood pressure, including factors affecting blood pressure.

S SKILLS

1. Measure and record height and weight.
2. Measure and record oral temperature with an electronic thermometer.
3. Measure and record rectal temperature with an electronic thermometer.
4. Measure and record axillary temperature with an electronic thermometer.
5. Measure and record core body temperature with a tympanic (aural) thermometer.
6. Measure and record temperature with a temporal artery thermometer.
7. Measure and record radial pulse rate and respirations.
8. Measure and record apical pulse rate.
9. Measure and record blood pressure.

B BEHAVIOR

1. Demonstrate professionalism by being courteous and diplomatic; showing respect, empathy, and cultural sensitivity; maintaining privacy and confidentiality; and adapting to change.
2. Use language/verbal skills that enable patients' understanding and appropriate, congruent body language and other nonverbal skills.
3. Apply critical thinking skills in performing patient assessment and care.

WORDS TO KNOW

afebrile
aneroid
antecubital
apex
apical
apnea
arrhythmia
aural
auscultate
axillary
blood pressure
body mass index (BMI)
brachial
bradycardia
bradypnea
carotid
Cheyne-Stokes
diastole
dorsalis pedis
dyspnea
essential
exhale
fatal
febrile
femoral
groin
hyperventilation
idiopathic
infrared
inhale
mensuration
oral
orthostatic
palpate
popliteal
pulse
pulse pressure
pyrogen
radial
rales
rectal
respiration
rhythm
sphygmomanometer
stethoscope
systole
tachycardia
tachypnea
temperature
thermometer
thready
vital signs
volume

BODY MEASUREMENTS

Body measurements are sometimes referred to as **mensuration**, meaning the process of measuring. When used in connection with patient care, it refers to body measurements such as height and weight; length of extremities; and the circumference of head, chest, or abdomen with infants. The initial measurements are usually taken before or after the vital signs are obtained and become the baseline for all measurements that follow. Precise measurements are extremely important with infants and children to ensure that there is proper growth and development. (Refer to Chapter 42 for details about infant and child measurements.) For adults, abnormal changes could indicate the presence of a disease or disorder such as osteoporosis or fluid retention.

Measurements can also provide information concerning treatment. Some diagnostic testing relies on a patient's measurements for correct interpretation. Certain medication dosages are determined by the patient's weight (see Unit 16).

Measurements are obtained at the beginning of the patient's visit, prior to seeing the provider and usually follow the completion of recording the patient history with new patients to complete the initial base information. Any follow-up visit measurement policy will be determined by the provider. Weight may be measured at each visit and height for adults may be monitored only occasionally unless a disease condition warrants more frequent measurement. The measurement performed and the frequency of that measurement will be determined largely by the patient's condition.

Height and Weight Measurements

Measurements are important to patients for many reasons:

- A young adult may be very interested in his height, especially those who wish to play certain sports.
- An elderly patient may be concerned about the loss of height.
- Athletes may have to gain or lose a certain amount of weight to meet regulations or goals.
- People of all ages may be interested in losing excess pounds and achieving a healthier weight range.

Measurement of height and weight are very familiar to patients, and most understand their implications. The accurate measurement of height and weight is best done on a balance beam scale (Figure 38–1). Scales should be balanced frequently and properly maintained to ensure accuracy. The scale should also sit on a firm surface. Figure 38–2 shows an electronic scale. The patient stands on the platform and the weight is displayed in the window of the unit. Many of these electronic scales have the capacity to convert units from pounds to kilograms if needed.

Height

Most of the balance beam scales have a height apparatus attached to them; however, there are also stand-alone devices that can be mounted to a wall. On a balance beam scale, the height bar is calibrated in inches by quarter-inch markings. When the height bar is lowered to touch the patient's head, the extension bar will indicate the height in inches on the calibrated height bar. The height should be measured to the nearest quarter of an inch. Height can be recorded in total inches or

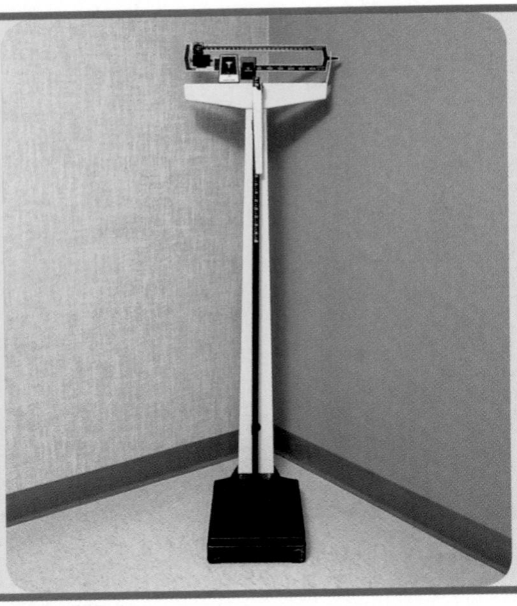

Figure 38–1: The traditional balance beam scales with measuring bar. *Delmar/Cengage Learning.*

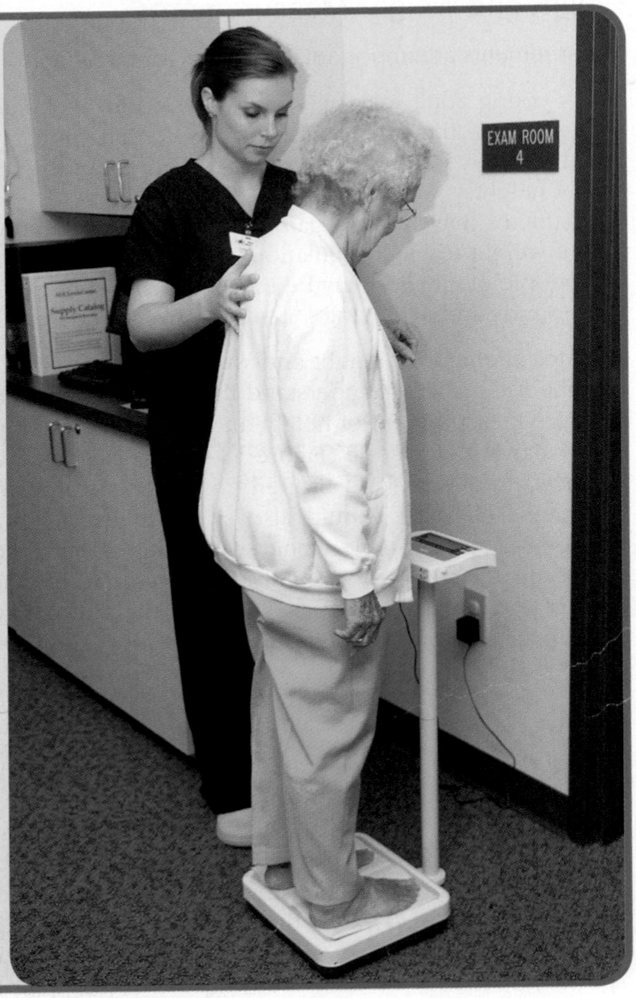

Figure 38–2: An electronic scale. *Delmar/Cengage Learning.*

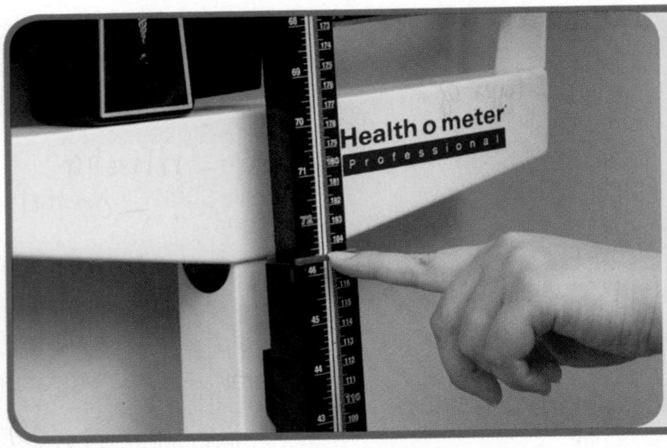

Figure 38–3: The height is read at the movable point on the ruler, where the two sections of the height bar meet. The bars are measured in quarter inches. *Delmar/Cengage Learning.*

converted to feet and inches, obtained by dividing the inches by the number 12 because there are 12 inches in 1 foot. The height bar in Figure 38–3 indicates where the height is read.

Weight

Obtaining the patient's weight by using a balance beam scale requires you to manipulate the two weights on the balance bar until the pointer rests in the middle of the rectangle at the end of the frame. Before an accurate weight can be measured, you must be sure that the scale is calibrated. This is performed by setting both of the weights at zero and making sure that the pointer floats in the middle of the rectangle at the end of the frame. Some scales have a screw at the end that can be adjusted to get the scale to balance. The bottom large weight slides along the balance bar that is calibrated in 50-pound increments. Place the large weight into the groove you estimate closest to the weight of the patient without going over it. The balance beam should indicate an inadequate weight amount by the pointer's position above the center of the rectangle. Move the smaller weight on the top of the balance beam until you have added enough weight for the beam to balance in the center of the rectangle. The top calibration is in full pounds divided into quarters (Figure 38–4). If your large weight estimation was too low, you will need to move that weight to the next higher 50-pound increment and readjust the smaller weight to balance. If you estimated too high, move the large weight one groove lower and then adjust the top. When the beam balances, add the two measurements together and record the patient's weight.

Measuring and Weighing the Patient

After calling the patient into the back office, tell him or her you are going to measure his or her height and weight; instruct the patient to remove his or her shoes.

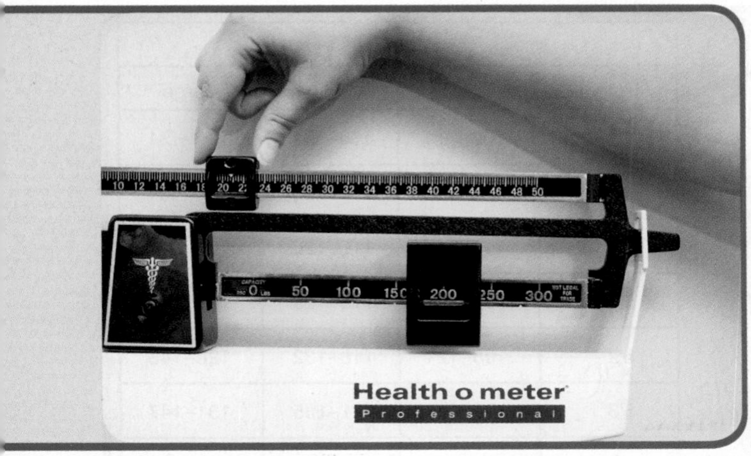

Figure 38–4: The balance bar reads 220¾ pounds. *Delmar/Cengage Learning.*

PATIENT EDUCATION

Patients may be asked to monitor their weight at home when they have certain conditions that can cause fluid retention, such as cardiac or kidney diseases, or for a weight gain or loss program. Remind them to weigh at about the same time each day, since weight varies throughout the day, and to wear clothing of about the same weight. A suggestion to weigh each morning before eating while still in night clothing would provide consistent variables for a more accurate assessment of weight trends.

Remind patients that handbags and items in pockets, such as keys and coin purses, should be put aside. While they are getting ready, check to ensure that the scale is calibrated correctly and reads 0 (zero). If not, make a slight adjustment of the scale as mentioned previously until it does.

Raise the height bar *above* the patient's estimated height and extend the measuring bar. Place a paper towel on the scale base to provide a clean surface. Follow the steps in Procedure 38–1 to obtain the patient's height.

Please note that some providers indicate that the patient should face away from the scale with his or her back to the height bar to ensure that he or she is standing up straight. However, if you are measuring height and weight together, many patients want to face the bar so they can watch you balancing the scale to get their accurate weight. Facing the height bar initially eliminates the need to get off, turn, and get back on or prevents patients from trying to turn around on the narrow scale base, which could result in a fall. It is also more difficult for elderly patients to get on the scale backward. They normally grasp the scale base to aid them when stepping on. Check with your employer to see which technique is used in your office.

While the patient is still on the scale, proceed with Procedure 38–1 to obtain the weight. If there is room to position the scale away from the wall, it is often easier from the other side, where the patient is not in the way. Note that the height bar can remain lowered when you are only measuring the patient's weight. Accurately record your findings on the patient's chart.

CLINICAL PEARL

Most people are very interested in their measurements. Because some may be sensitive about their weight, be careful about any remarks you make. If they are on a weight-gain or weight-loss program and show even a small change, give them praise and encouragement. Some might question what they should weigh for their height. Different weight charts are available, and one should be posted near the scale as a patient education tool. Some charts differentiate by age, whereas others use gender or both. Figure 38–5 is gender-specific and considers relative frame size. These are only guidelines because the composition of the body tissue has an effect on the weight.

Body Mass Index

Another common measurement in the medical office today is the **body mass index (BMI)**. This is a numerical correlation between a patient's height and weight. Many providers prefer the BMI to be calculated by the medical assistant and documented in the patient's record along with the height and weight. There are a number of ways to determine the patient's BMI. You can use the following formula, which is:

- Multiply the patient's weight in pounds by 703.
- Divide this total by the patient's height in inches.
- Divide this total by the patient's height in inches again and then round to the nearest whole number.

EXAMPLE

Calculate the BMI of a patient weighing 140 pounds, and measuring 5'4" (64 inches).

Step 1: 140 × 703 = 98420
Step 2: 98420/64 = 1537.81
Step 3: 1537.81/64 = 24.03

Rounded to the nearest whole number = 24

MEN			
Height	Small	Medium	Large
5'2"	128–134	131–141	138–150
5'3"	130–136	133–143	140–153
5'4"	132–138	135–145	142–156
5'5"	134–140	137–148	144–160
5'6"	136–142	139–151	146–164
5'7"	138–146	142–154	149–168
5'8"	140–148	145–157	152–172
5'9"	142–151	148–160	155–176
5'10"	144–154	151–163	158–180
5'11"	146–157	154–166	161–184
6'0"	149–160	157–170	164–188
6'1"	152–164	160–174	168–192
6'2"	155–168	164–178	172–197
6'3"	158–172	167–182	176–202
6'4"	162–176	171–187	181–207

WOMEN			
Height	Small	Medium	Large
4'10"	102–111	109–121	118–131
4'11"	103–113	111–123	120–134
5'0"	104–115	113–126	122–137
5'1"	106–118	115–129	125–140
5'2"	108–121	118–132	128–143
5'3"	111–124	121–135	131–147
5'4"	114–127	124–138	134–151
5'5"	117–130	127–141	137–155
5'6"	120–133	130–144	140–159
5'7"	123–136	133–147	143–163
5'8"	128–139	138–150	146–167
5'9"	129–142	139–153	149–170
5'10"	132–146	142–156	152–173
5'11"	135–148	145–159	155–176
6'0"	138–151	148–162	158–179

FIGURE 38–5: Chart of desirable weight for men and women. *Delmar/Cengage Learning.*

PROCEDURE 38–1 Measure Height and Weight Using a Balance Beam Scale

PURPOSE: To obtain an accurate measurement of a patient's height and weight.

EQUIPMENT: Balance beam scale with extension measuring bar, paper towel, patient's chart or computer with EHR software, pen.

S SKILL: Measure and record height and weight.

Procedure Steps	Detailed Instructions and/or *Rationales*
1. Wash hands.	
2. Identify the patient and introduce yourself.	*Ensures that you are performing the procedure on the correct patient.*

Procedure Steps	Detailed Instructions and/or *Rationales*
B 3. Explain the procedure, ***using language the patient can understand,*** and instruct the patient to remove shoes and any heavy clothing.	*Ensures understanding, consent, and cooperation from the patient. Accurate measurement cannot be obtained if shoes or heavy clothing are worn.*
4. Place a paper towel on the scale platform (Figure 38–6A).	*Provides a clean surface for the shoeless foot.*
5. Assist patient to the center of the scale (Figure 38–6B).	Make sure the patient is in the center of the platform. Ask the patient to stand still while you adjust the balance and read the weight. Remind the patient not to hold on to the scale. *Holding on to any part of the scale will cause a lighter, inaccurate measurement.*
6. Move the lower weight bar (measured in 50-pound increments) to the estimated number and slowly slide the upper bar until the balance beam point is centered (Figure 38–6C).	You may want to ask the patient for an approximate weight.
7. Read the weight by adding the upper bar measurement to the lower bar measurement. Round to the nearest ¼ pound.	
8. Raise the measuring bar beyond the patient's height and lift the extension (Figure 38–6D).	*Avoids the possibility of striking the patient if the bar is raised after the patient steps on the scale.*
9. Lower measuring bar until firmly resting on top of patient's head (Figure 38–6E).	Measurement of height is from the top of the head, not from the hair.
10. Assist patient off the scale and allow the patient to sit and put on shoes.	Help the patient from the scale and discard the paper towel. Tell the patient to put his or her shoes back on unless ready for a physical exam.
11. Read line where measurement falls. Round to the nearest ¼ inch (Figure 38–6F).	

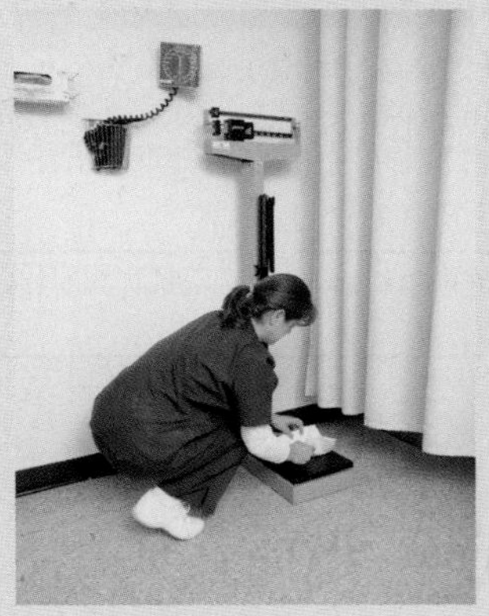

FIGURE 38–6A: Prepare the scale to measure the patient's weight and height by placing a paper towel on the scale platform. *Delmar/Cengage Learning.*

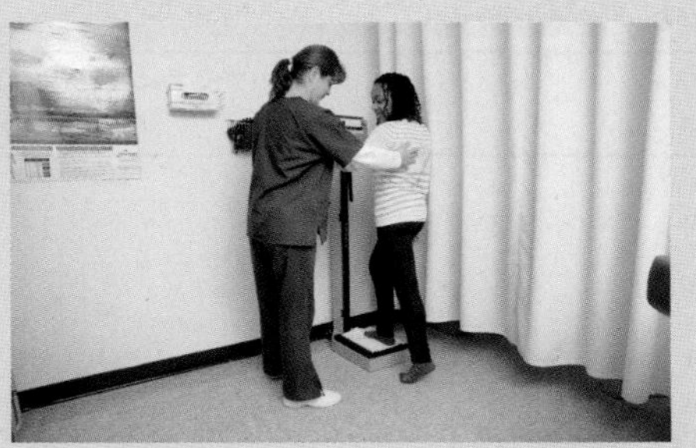

Figure 38–6B: Assist the patient to the center of the scale. *Delmar/Cengage Learning.*

(continues)

(continued)

Procedure Steps	Detailed Instructions and/or *Rationales*
12. Lower measuring bar to its original position and return the weights to zero.	
13. Document in the patient's chart.	Record the weight and height on the patient's chart or in the EMR. Be sure to record whether the patient was wearing street clothing or a gown.

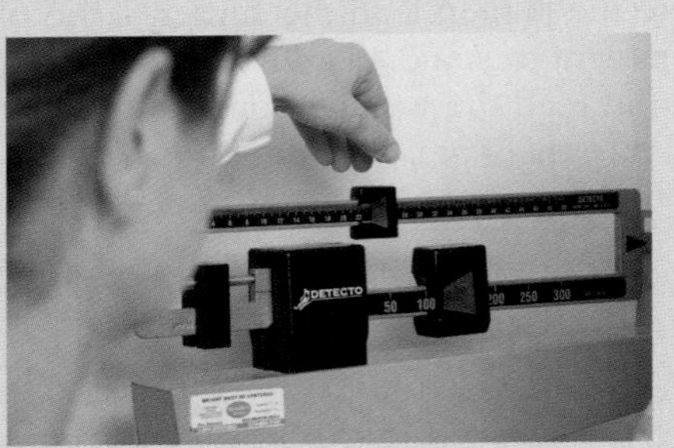

Figure 38–6C: Move the lower weight bar to the estimated number and slowly slide the upper bar until the balance beam point is centered. Read the resulting weight, rounding to the nearest quarter pound. *Delmar/Cengage Learning.*

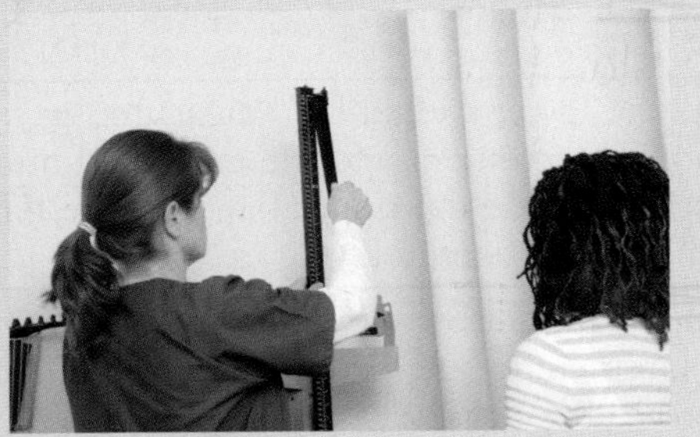

Figure 38–6D: Raise the measuring bar beyond the patient's height and lift the extension. *Delmar/Cengage Learning.*

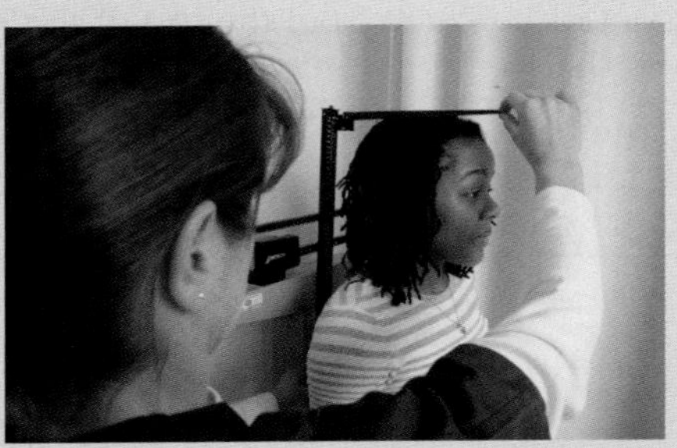

Figure 38–6E: Lower the measuring bar until firmly resting on top of patient's head. Then, assist patient off the scale. *Delmar/Cengage Learning.*

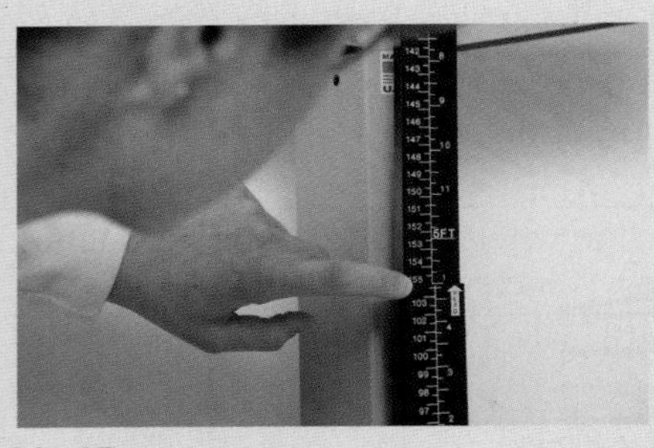

Figure 38–6F: Read the line where the measurement falls, rounding to the nearest quarter inch. *Delmar/Cengage Learning.*

Charting Example

5-12-XX 11:30 am	Wt. 147# (147 lbs) without shoes, in street clothing. Ht. 68". J. Rivera, CMA(AAMA)

Many websites provide a free electronic BMI measurement, and many EHR systems automatically calculate BMI. The National Institutes of Health has published a BMI index chart that is easy to use (Figure 38–7), and many providers prefer to have this chart posted near the scale and in the exam rooms. You can access a copy of this chart on their website at www.nih.gov.

Cardinal Signs

VITAL SIGNS

The term **vital signs** is used by health care personnel to identify the measurement of body functions that are essential to life. The four vital indicators are **temperature**, **pulse**, **respiration**, and **blood pressure**, commonly referred to as TPR and B/P. They indicate

FIGURE 38–7: Body Mass Index table. (Adapted from *Clinical Guidelines on the Identification, Evaluation, and Treatment of Overweight and Obesity in Adults: The Evidence Report*. National Institutes of Health, www.nih.gov.)

Body Mass Index Table

	Normal						Overweight					Obese										Extreme Obesity														
BMI	**19**	**20**	**21**	**22**	**23**	**24**	**25**	**26**	**27**	**28**	**29**	**30**	**31**	**32**	**33**	**34**	**35**	**36**	**37**	**38**	**39**	**40**	**41**	**42**	**43**	**44**	**45**	**46**	**47**	**48**	**49**	**50**	**51**	**52**	**53**	**54**
Height (inches)	**Body Weight (pounds)**																																			
58	91	96	100	105	110	115	119	124	129	134	138	143	148	153	158	162	167	172	177	181	186	191	196	201	205	210	215	220	224	229	234	239	244	248	253	258
59	94	99	104	109	114	119	124	128	133	138	143	148	153	158	163	168	173	178	183	188	193	198	203	208	212	217	222	227	232	237	242	247	252	257	262	267
60	97	102	107	112	118	123	128	133	138	143	148	153	158	163	168	174	179	184	189	194	199	204	209	215	220	225	230	235	240	245	250	255	261	266	271	276
61	100	106	111	116	122	127	132	137	143	148	153	158	164	169	174	180	185	190	195	201	206	211	217	222	227	232	238	243	248	254	259	264	269	275	280	285
62	104	109	115	120	126	131	136	142	147	153	158	164	169	175	180	186	191	196	202	207	213	218	224	229	235	240	246	251	256	262	267	273	278	284	289	295
63	107	113	118	124	130	135	141	146	152	158	163	169	175	180	186	191	197	203	208	214	220	225	231	237	242	248	254	259	265	270	278	282	287	293	299	304
64	110	116	122	128	134	140	145	151	157	163	169	174	180	186	192	197	204	209	215	221	227	232	238	244	250	256	262	267	273	279	285	291	296	302	308	314
65	114	120	126	132	138	144	150	156	162	168	174	180	186	192	198	204	210	216	222	228	234	240	246	252	258	264	270	276	282	288	294	300	306	312	318	324
66	118	124	130	136	142	148	155	161	167	173	179	186	192	198	204	210	216	223	229	235	241	247	253	260	266	272	278	284	291	297	303	309	315	322	328	334
67	121	127	134	140	146	153	159	166	172	178	185	191	198	204	211	217	223	230	236	242	249	255	261	268	274	280	287	293	299	306	312	319	325	331	338	344
68	125	131	138	144	151	158	164	171	177	184	190	197	203	210	216	223	230	236	243	249	256	262	269	276	282	289	295	302	308	315	322	328	335	341	348	354
69	128	135	142	149	155	162	169	176	182	189	196	203	209	216	223	230	236	243	250	257	263	270	277	284	291	297	304	311	318	324	331	338	345	351	358	365
70	132	139	146	153	160	167	174	181	188	195	202	209	216	222	229	236	243	250	257	264	271	278	285	292	299	306	313	320	327	334	341	348	355	362	369	376
71	136	143	150	157	165	172	179	186	193	200	208	215	222	229	236	243	250	257	265	272	279	286	293	301	308	315	322	329	338	343	351	358	365	372	379	386
72	140	147	154	162	169	177	184	191	199	206	213	221	228	235	242	250	258	265	272	279	287	294	302	309	316	324	331	338	346	353	361	368	375	383	390	397
73	144	151	159	166	174	182	189	197	204	212	219	227	235	242	250	257	265	272	280	288	295	302	310	318	325	333	340	348	355	363	371	378	386	393	401	408
74	148	155	163	171	179	186	194	202	210	218	225	233	241	249	256	264	272	280	287	295	303	311	319	326	334	342	350	358	365	373	381	389	396	404	412	420
75	152	160	168	176	184	192	200	208	216	224	232	240	248	256	264	272	279	287	295	303	311	319	327	335	343	351	359	367	375	383	391	399	407	415	423	431
76	156	164	172	180	189	197	205	213	221	230	238	246	254	263	271	279	287	295	304	312	320	328	336	344	353	361	369	377	385	394	402	410	418	426	435	443

Source: Adapted from *Clinical Guidelines on the Identification, Evaluation, and Treatment of Overweight and Obesity in Adults: The Evidence Report.*

temperature — pulse — respiration — BP

the body's ability to control heat; the rate, volume, and rhythm of the heart; the rate and quality of breathing; and the force of the heart and condition of the blood vessels. The vital signs give the provider an assessment of the status of the brain, the autonomic nervous system, the heart, and the lungs. Additionally, it is worth noting here that some providers are also considering pain a fifth vital as discussed in Chapter 37.

The correct measurement of vital signs is extremely important. Proper technique are essential. Findings should be recorded immediately following measurement to avoid a memory error. Always repeat the procedure if you think you might have made a mistake in measuring or recording. Occasionally, you may have a problem measuring a vital sign because a patient's unusual physical condition makes measurement difficult. Inform the provider of your problem and follow the course of action advised. Avoid alarming the patient. *Never* estimate the measurement. The provider's choice of treatment and medication is often based on the findings; therefore, they must be accurate.

Temperature

The temperature of the body indicates the amount of heat produced by the activity of changing food into energy. The body loses heat through perspiration, breathing, and the elimination of body wastes. The balance between heat production and heat loss determines the body's temperature.

Conditions affecting body heat include metabolic rate, time of day, and amount of activity. Body temperature is usually lower in the morning following a period of rest. In the afternoon and evening, body temperature rises because of the heat produced by activity and the metabolism of food. These activities warm the blood that circulates through the body. "Normal" body temperature for an individual is that temperature at which his body systems function most effectively. An *average* normal oral temperature is 37°C (centigrade) or 98.6°F (Fahrenheit), but normal temperatures can vary from 36.5°C to 37.5°C (97.6°F to 99.6°F) (see Table 38–1). A person with a temperature above normal is said to be **febrile** or to have a temperature elevation. A person with a temperature that is normal or subnormal is said to be **afebrile**.

Controlling Body Temperature

The temperature-regulating center in the body is located in the hypothalamus of the brain (Figure 38–8). The action of the hypothalamus can be compared with a thermostat that turns the furnace in your home off and on to keep the room temperature at the set number of degrees. As discussed in Unit 11, the brain, autonomic nervous system, blood vessels, and skin cooperate to regulate temperature through a feedback mechanism from temperature receptors. In the body, the hot and cold peripheral receptors in the skin send messages to the hypothalamus about the environment surrounding the body. Temperature receptors in the spinal cord, abdomen, and other internal structures send messages about the internal body temperature. One section of the hypothalamus also has many heat-sensitive neurons, which increase their output of impulses when temperature rises and decrease their output when it drops. The signals from this section of the hypothalamus merge with those received in another section, along with the internal and skin receptors, to evaluate the situation and send signals to control heat loss or heat production. Therefore, this central center is referred to as the *hypothalamic thermostat.*

The hypothalamic thermostat is very effective. When receptors sense the body is too warm, they send a message to the brain, which in turn acts on the sweat glands of the skin to produce moisture. The moisture evaporates from the skin's surface and cools the body. At the same time, nerve impulses are sent to the surface blood vessels

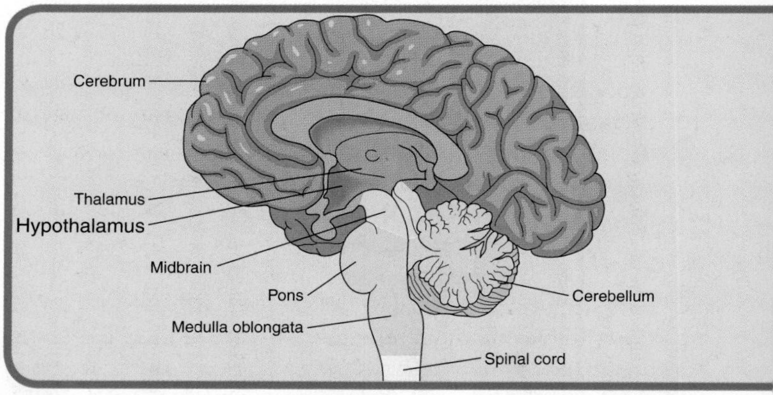

Figure 38–8: The hypothalamus regulates body temperature. *Delmar/Cengage Learning.*

TABLE 38–1 Temperature Variations Considered Normal

	Oral	Axillary	Rectal
Average	98.6°F	97.6°F	99.6°F
Normal temperature	(37°C)	(36.5°C)	(37.5°C)
Range	97.6–99.6°F	96.6–98.6°F	98.6–100.6°F
	(36.5–37.5°C)	(36–37°C)	(37–38.1°C)

to dilate, which brings more blood in contact with the surface of the skin. The blood gives up heat, which cools the blood within the vessels and therefore cools the body.

When the body senses coolness, the opposite activities occur. Surface blood vessels constrict to keep the blood away from the surface of the skin and prevent the loss of heat. Impulses to the sweat glands are stopped when temperature falls below normal, and small papillary muscles around the hair follicles contract, causing goose bumps on the skin. Heat is produced by the activity of the papillary muscles, thereby helping warm the body. In addition, a portion of the hypothalamus becomes active when cold signals are received. Now hypothalamic messages are sent to skeletal muscles throughout the body, causing increased muscle tone that produces heat. When the muscle tone rises above a certain level, shivering results and heat production is raised dramatically. This is evident with an infectious process such as influenza. Microorganisms cause the patient to experience chills and shivering until the temperature rises to warm the body and a fever develops.

During an infectious process, the presence of microorganisms causes **pyrogens** to be secreted, which raise the set point of the hypothalamic thermostat. Pyrogens are toxins from bacteria or a by-product of degenerating tissues. When the set point is higher than normal, the body's heat production and conservation processes are activated. Surface blood vessels constrict, causing the person to feel cold even though the temperature is above normal. No sweat is secreted. Increased white blood cell activity from fighting bacterial invasion also produces heat. Chills and shivering begin and continue until the temperature reaches the higher set point, at which the hypothalamus will continue to operate until the infectious process is reversed. After this occurs, the hypothalamic thermostat is reset to a lower or normal value, and the body's temperature-reduction process results in profuse sweating and hot, red skin from general vasodilation. After this onset reaction, the temperature will begin to fall.

The extent of the infection determines the amount of heat (fever) generated. A mild infection might cause the temperature to rise to 37.7°C (100°F). A moderate infection can elevate the temperature to 38.8°C (102°F). Fevers are categorized by the degree of body heat as slight, moderate, severe, dangerous, or **fatal** (Table 38–2).

TABLE 38–2 Classification of Fevers

	Fahrenheit	Celsius
Slight	99.6°–101.0°	37.5°–38.3°
Moderate	101.0°–102.0°	38.3°–38.8°
Severe	102.0°–104.0°	38.8°–40.0°
Dangerous	104.0°–105.0°	40.0°–40.5
Fatal	over 106.0°	41.1°

PATIENT EDUCATION

Instruct the patient to inform the provider of any significant changes in temperature. Advise the patient at what point an oral temperature should be reported to the provider. Caution the patient that a fever should not be "watched" to see how high it will go. Prolonged high fever can cause seizures, brain damage, and, ultimately, death.

Fatality-associated elevated temperature depends on the extent of time the fever is present. Fevers of short duration well above 41.1°C (106.0°F) have not proved fatal, but immediate measures to reduce body temperature must be administered. Temperatures below normal are called subnormal. Collapse will occur at about 35.5°C (96.0°F), and death follows if temperature goes below 33.8°C (93.0°F) more than briefly.

Thermometer Types and Designs

Body temperature is measured by means of a **thermometer** in scales of Fahrenheit or the metric system equivalent, Celsius. Thermometers are of the following main types: disposable, in the form of plastic strips; battery-operated electronic; self-contained digital; tympanic **infrared**; and temporal artery. The mouth (**oral**), underarm (**axillary**), rectum (**rectal**), ear (**aural** or tympanic membrane), or the temporal area of the forehead may be used to measure body temperature. The large variety of thermometers, each with its own advantages and disadvantages, allows for personal preference in equipment selection for the physician's office. Table 38–3 briefly outlines the main advantages and disadvantages for each type.

Disposable Thermometers

Chemical disposable thermometers can be used by the oral or axillary route (Figure 38–9A and B). When using with the oral route, care must be taken to avoid touching the dot matrix portion, which is placed in the patient's mouth. The dots can be placed up or down. The thermometer must be held under the tongue as far back as possible in the heat pocket, with the tongue pressed against the end and the mouth closed on the stem for the allotted time. The heat in the mouth causes a reaction on the heat-sensitive dots printed on the surface of the plastic strip. The thermometer is then removed and the dots observed for color change. Read the results by counting the number of dots that change color within a degree grouping. The last changed dot on the matrix indicates the correct temperature. Record the temperature and discard the thermometer in a waste container.

TABLE 38–3 Comparison of Thermometer Types

Type	Advantage	Disadvantage
Plastic disposable	Single use avoids cross-contamination, no cleaning, relatively fast	Must protect from heat, somewhat unpleasant for patient, storage and inventory costs
Digital	Quick, signals when registered, easily read, self-contained	Moderate initial cost, plastic cover, and battery expenses
Electronic probe	Quick, signals when registered, easily read, self-contained	Fairly expensive, cumbersome cord, requires recharging, probe cover costs, may cause inaccurate readings if patient bites too hard on probe
Tympanic infrared	Instant results, easily read, core temperature, individualized probe cover, eliminates mucous membrane concerns	Expensive, probe cover costs, replacement battery costs. An improper seal in the ear canal, the presence of cerumen, or an infection of the middle ear can cause inaccurate readings
Temporal artery	Instant results, easily read, as accurate as rectal, noninvasive, no mucous membrane concerns	Expensive, requires probe cover or cleaning when used, requires environmental acclimation, somewhat delicate

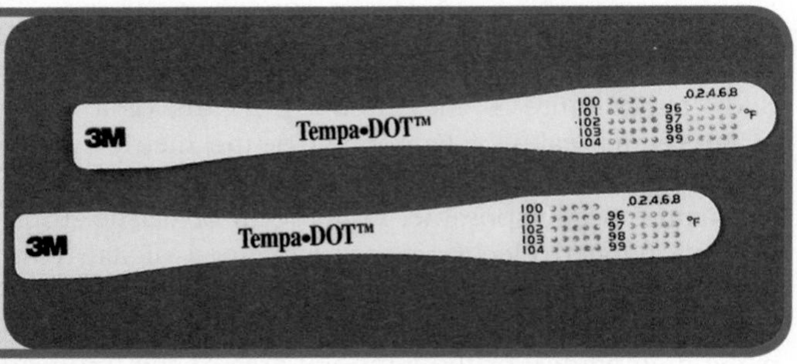

Figure 38–9A: Disposable chemical thermometer. *Delmar/Cengage Learning.*

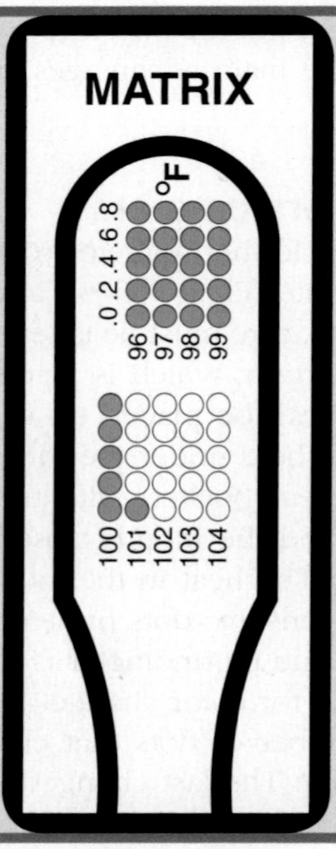

FIGURE 38–9B: The matrix reads 101°F. *Delmar/Cengage Learning.*

When measuring the axillary temperature, the dot matrix portion is placed next to the body, deep in the axillary space, with the handle extending straight down the patient's side. The arm must be held tightly at the side. After time recommended by the manufacturer, remove the thermometer; read and record the temperature.

Electronic Thermometers

The use of electronic thermometers is very common in the medical office. A small, battery-operated unit with a digital read-out window is capable of measuring a temperature within a few seconds (Figure 38–10A). A color-coded probe, blue for oral, red for rectal, is attached by a cord to the battery unit. A disposable cover slips over the probe to provide each patient with an individual barrier for the thermometer. The covered probe is inserted in

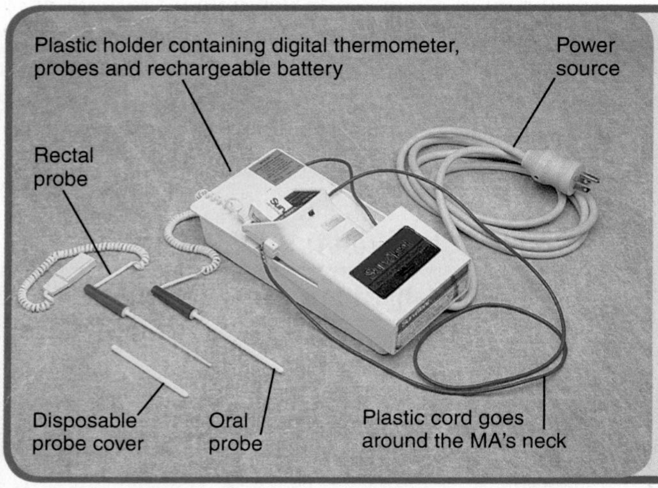

Figure 38–10: Electronic thermometer with labeled parts. *Delmar/Cengage Learning.*

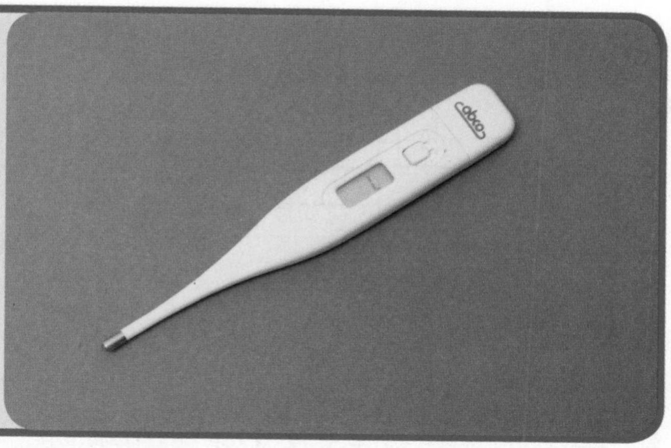

Figure 38–11: Electronic digital thermometer that is excellent for home use. *Delmar/Cengage Learning.*

the patient's mouth. As soon as the temperature level has been reached, the unit will sound a signal and the final reading will appear in the window of the unit. The probe cover is then discarded into a waste container. Refer to Procedure 38–2 for a step-by-step guide on obtaining an oral temperature with this type of thermometer.

Another electronic thermometer that is simple and self-contained is a digital thermometer that is excellent for home use (Figure 38–11). The thermometer registers the temperature in about one to two minutes on an easy-to-read LCD panel that shows the temperature in tenths of degrees. The thermometer can be cleaned with soap and water and sanitized with a disinfectant. Probe covers are available for office or home use. It may be used for oral, axillary, or rectal measurement. Some models have a beeper that sounds when the maximum temperature is reached. This feature is especially appealing to children.

Tympanic Membrane Thermometers

Another method for temperature measurement is the instantaneous tympanic membrane (aural) thermometer (Figure 38–12). The thermometer operates by the principle of measuring the strength of the infrared heat waves generated by the tympanic membrane and digitally displays that temperature in fewer than two seconds. Because the tympanic membrane shares the same blood supply as the hypothalamus, it is believed the auditory canal is an ideal site for obtaining an accurate assessment of the body's core temperature. Studies conducted with temperature-sensing devices placed internally in a large blood vessel have shown strong correlation in results.

Although its greatest asset is the instant result, it is also very easy to use and has become a real benefit to health care professionals in hospital emergency rooms, labor and delivery rooms, and pediatric units because it does not involve contact with mucous membranes and because the site is so easily accessible. Another advantage is that the readings are not affected by hot or cold liquids or smoking, as are oral methods. In addition, the patient does not even need to be conscious. There are a few instances when inaccurate readings can result, including if the probe is not properly sealed in the ear canal, if the beam is not directed toward the eardrum, if cerumen is present, or if there is an infection of the middle ear.

Temporal Artery Thermometers

The latest thermometer to be developed is the temporal scanner or, as it is commonly called, the temporal artery thermometer (TAT) (Figure 38–13). Both home and clinical models are available. The TAT determines body temperature by measuring the temperature of the skin over the temporal artery (TA) of the forehead where the artery is less than 2 mm below the surface of the skin. The probe of the thermometer has a sensor that assesses the infrared heat in the artery. The TAT has another unique feature. If the forehead is not an appropriate site for measurement, temperature can be measured in alternative sites. Temperatures can be taken over the femoral artery or lateral thoracic or axillary areas.

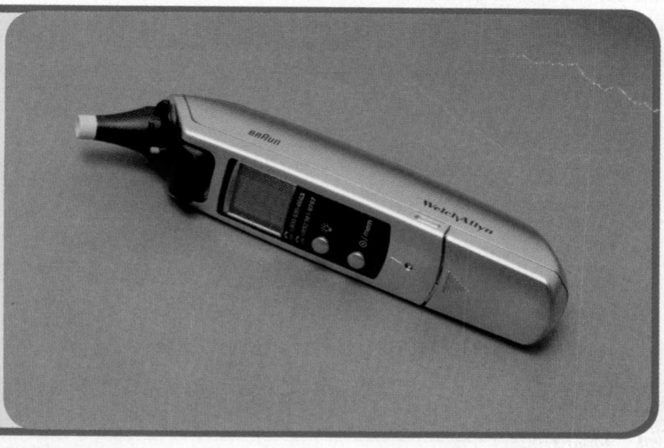

FIGURE 38–12: Tympanic (aural) thermometer. *Delmar/Cengage Learning.*

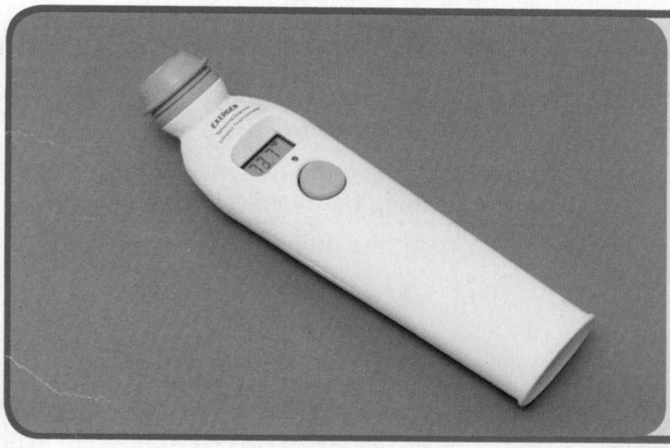

Figure 38–13: Temporal artery thermometer. *Delmar/Cengage Learning.*

It is important for the probe lens and cone to be very clean so the thermometer can register the heat accurately. Follow the manufacturer's instructions for the cleaning process for the specific model you are using. A variety of disposable probe covers, caps, or sheaths can be used instead of cleaning if desired.

Measuring Oral Temperatures

Measuring body temperature by mouth is convenient, quick, fairly accurate, and relatively inexpensive. Refer to Procedure 38–2 for detailed steps for measuring an oral temperature. Remember that oral temperature requires contact with mucous membranes, so a thermometer must either be disposable or require a barrier cover. Some factors also influence the accurate measurement:

- The thermometer must be place sublingually into the heat pocket (Figure 38–14).
- Patients must not have smoked or had anything hot or cold by mouth for at least 15 minutes prior to measuring.
- Patients must be able to maintain the thermometer in place appropriately for the required period of time.

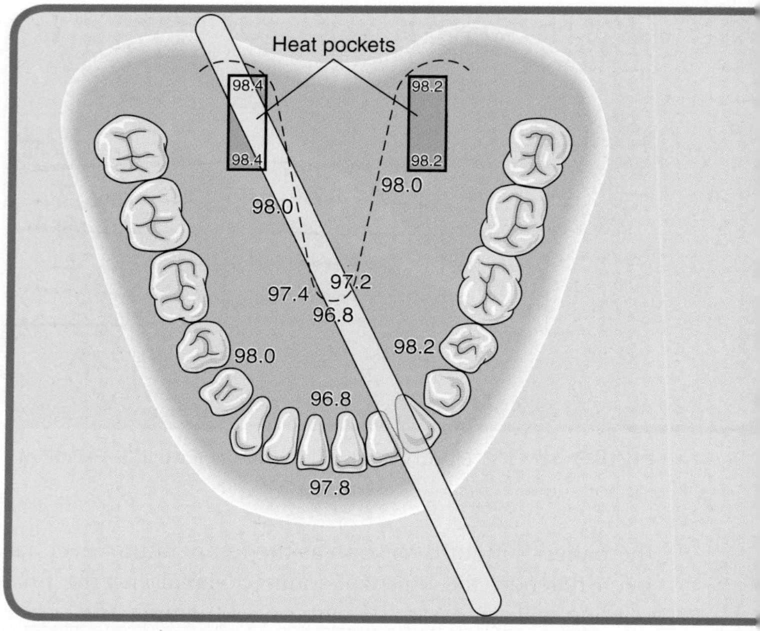

FIGURE 38–14: Placement of an oral thermometer. When taking an oral temperature, place the thermometer under the tongue to the side of the mouth into the heat pockets as shown here.

Courtesy of 3M Healthcare.

PROCEDURE 38–2 Measure and Record Oral Temperature with an Electronic Thermometer

PURPOSE: To determine a patient's oral temperature with an electronic thermometer

EQUIPMENT: Electronic thermometer unit, oral probe, probe cover, waste container, patient chart or EHR, pen

S **SKILL:** Measure and record oral temperature with an electronic thermometer.

Procedure Steps	Detailed Instructions and/or *Rationales*
1. Wash hands; assemble equipment.	
2. Identify the patient and introduce yourself.	*Ensures that you are performing the procedure on the correct patient.*
B 3. Explain the procedure, ***using language the patient can understand.***	*Ensures understanding, consent, and cooperation from the patient.*
4. Ensure that the patient has not smoked or consumed anything hot or cold in past 15 minutes.	*Smoking or consuming hot or cold substances can increase or decrease temperature.*
5. Correctly prepare the thermometer.	a. Be sure the blue probe connector is plugged into the receptacle of the unit base. *The blue probe is used for oral temperatures.* b. Remove probe from the stored position. c. Insert the probe firmly into the probe cover (Figure 38–15A).

Procedure Steps	Detailed Instructions and/or *Rationales*
6. Insert the covered probe into the patient's mouth. Instruct the patient to keep his or her lips pursed around the probe and not to bite down. Maintain the covered probe in position until the unit signals, approximately 10 to 15 seconds (Figure 38–15B).	The probe and connecting cord are rather heavy and cumbersome. It may be necessary to hold the thermometer steady in place. *Early removal results in inaccurate measurement.*
7. Remove the probe from the patient. Do not touch the probe cover.	*Probe is contaminated with patient's saliva.*
8. Read the temperature, noting the temperature.	Temperature is displayed digitally in the window of the unit.
9. Press the eject button to discard the used probe cover into the waste container.	*All materials coming in contact with bodily secretions are deposited in a waste container.*
10. Return the probe to the stored position in the unit and store the unit in the charging stand.	The thermometer display will read zero and shut off. *The unit should remain in the stand so it is fully charged and ready for use.*
11. Wash hands.	
12. Document in the patient's chart.	

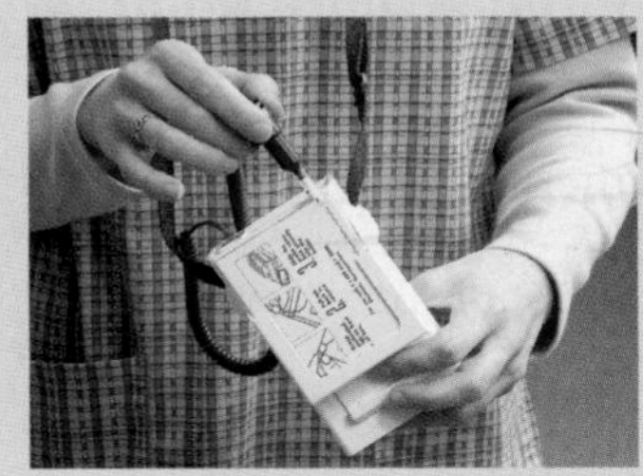

FIGURE 38–15A: Slide the probe into the disposable cover. *Delmar/Cengage Learning.*

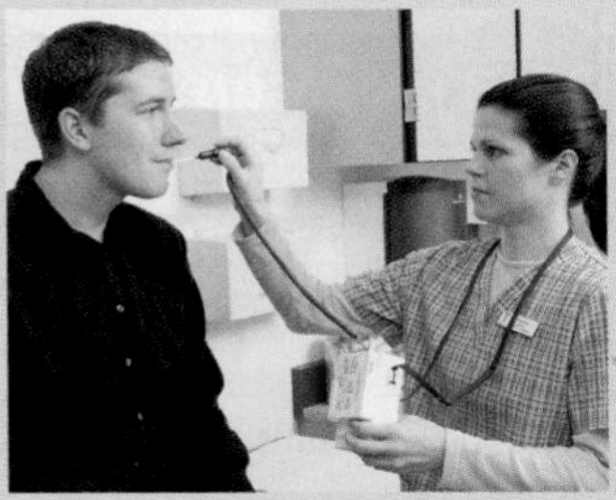

FIGURE 38–15B: The medical assistant holds the probe of the electronic thermometer in the patient's mouth until it signals completion. *Delmar/Cengage Learning.*

Charting Example

5/10/XX 11:30 am	T. 99.8 B. Davis, RMA (AMT)

However, oral temperature measurement is not always the method of choice. Temperature must be measured by an axillary, rectal, tympanic, or temporal method in the following situations:

- Infants and young children
- Patients with respiratory complications that result in mouth breathing or use of supplemental oxygen
- Confused, disoriented, or emotionally unstable patients
- Patients with oral injuries or dental problems such as diseased gums or abscesses
- Patients with recent oral surgery
- Patients with facial paralysis
- Patients with nasal obstruction, sinus congestion, or colds

Measuring Rectal Temperatures

Rectal temperature is a very accurate measurement simply because it is taken internally. Rectal measurement is appropriate with babies and young children who have not yet learned how to keep an oral thermometer in place. Children may complain about having a rectal temperature taken when they think they are "too big." The provider usually has a policy concerning the age limit and recommendations for rectal temperatures, which you must follow.

Electronic thermometers may be used to measure rectal temperature. Gloves must always be worn. Use the rectal (red) probe to take a rectal temperature (refer back to Figure 38–10). Remove the rectal probe from its holder and attach a probe cover. The probe is inserted into the rectum approximately 1 inch for adults and ½ inch for infants and small children. The use of lubricant is optional. After the reading is registered, remove the probe and discard the cover in a waste container.

When measuring the temperature of infants, they may be positioned on the stomach or the back. If positioning on the back, unfasten the diaper to expose the anus. Grasp the ankles securely with one hand, flexing the knees to the abdomen. With the other hand, insert the thermometer into the anal canal. Hold the thermometer securely in place. Maintain your grasp on the ankles so the infant cannot turn over. Be prepared for the procedure to initiate urination or expelling of stool. It would be wise to cover the male infant's penis with a diaper to absorb the urine stream. If positioning prone on a table, be certain to maintain control of the infant or child's position to prevent turning over and causing injury to the rectum from the inserted thermometer probe. Older children can be positioned either on their abdomen or side (lateral or Sims position, Chapter 39), whichever is preferred. Adults would be positioned on their side (lateral or Sims position), generally the left side because the rectum is angled in that direction and draped with a sheet for privacy.

When recording a rectal measurement, place the letter *R* in parentheses following the reading. Normal rectal temperature is 37.5°C or 99.6°F, one full degree above normal oral temperature. Temperature must never be measured rectally if the patient has had recent rectal surgery; it is possible to damage the operative site or perforate newly sutured lines. The rectal route also should not be used in patients with chronic diarrhea. Refer to Procedure 38–3 for detailed steps for measuring a rectal temperature using a digital thermometer.

PROCEDURE 38–3 Measure Rectal Temperature with an Electronic Thermometer

PURPOSE: To determine a patient's rectal temperature using a electronic thermometer

EQUIPMENT: Mannequin (if simulated), electronic thermometer, rectal probe, probe cover, drape (if adult), gloves, lubricant, tissues, waste container, patient chart or EHR, pen

S SKILL: Measure and record rectal temperature with an electronic thermometer.

Procedure Steps	Detailed Instructions and/or *Rationales*
1. Wash hands, assemble equipment, and put on gloves.	*Protects you from microorganism contamination.*
2. Identify the patient and introduce yourself.	*Ensures that you are performing the procedure on the correct patient.*
B 3. Explain the procedure, ***using language the patient can understand,*** and instruct the patient to remove appropriate clothing, assisting as needed.	*Ensures understanding, consent, and cooperation from the patient. Provide privacy when patient is removing clothing.*
B 4. Assist the adult patient onto the examining table, position the patient on his or her side (lateral or Sims position) and cover with a drape, ***displaying sensitivity to patient privacy***.	When performing the procedure on infants or small children, ask the parent or accompanying adult to prepare the child while you prepare the thermometer. Position the infant according to the parent's or physician's preference. Ensure safety during the procedure by maintaining control of the infant's or child's position. (A parent can be instructed to assist you, especially if it comforts the child.)

Procedure Steps	Detailed Instructions and/or *Rationales*
5. Place a small amount of lubricant onto a tissue and place it within reach.	
6. Correctly prepare the thermometer.	a. Place the red probe connector into the receptacle of the unit base. *The red probe is used for rectal temperatures.* b. Remove probe from the stored position. c. Insert the red probe firmly into the probe cover. *Check to make sure it is properly seated.*
7. Apply lubricant to the end of the probe cover.	*This eases the insertion.*
8. Arrange the drape to expose the buttocks, raise the upper buttock to expose the anus, and carefully insert the lubricated thermometer probe into the anal canal approximately 1 inch for adults and ½ inch for infants and children. Hold the thermometer in place until the unit signals.	Angle the probe slightly to ensure contact with mucosa. Do not force the thermometer. Rotating will often facilitate insertion. If opening is not apparent, ask the patient to bear down slightly; this will usually expose the opening.
9. Withdraw the thermometer. Eject the probe cover into the waste container.	*All materials coming into contact with bodily secretions are deposited in a waste container.*
10. Read the thermometer, noting the temperature.	Temperature is displayed digitally in the window of the unit.
11. Replace the probe in the unit and return the thermometer to the charging stand.	The thermometer display will read zero and shut off. *The unit should remain in the stand so it is fully charged and ready for use.*
12. Remove any excess lubricant from the anal area with a tissue.	Wipe from front to back.
13. If the patient is an adult, assist the adult patient from the examining table and instruct him or her to dress. If the patient is a child, ask the parent or accompanying adult to dress an infant or child.	Provide privacy as appropriate for adult patients.
14. Remove and discard gloves in the waste container.	
15. Wash hands.	
16. Document the temperature in the patient's chart, placing an (R) after the finding.	

Charting Example

3-6-XX 11:30 am	T. 100.2 (R) B. Davis, RMA(AMT)

Measuring Axillary Temperatures

Temperature can be measured by placing the electronic or digital thermometer in the axilla (armpit). This method is the least accurate. Axillary measurement is appropriate when oral and rectal temperatures are undesirable or contraindicated. Normal axillary temperature is 36.5°C or 97.6°F, one full degree *below* normal oral temperature. When recording the axillary temperature, place the letters *Ax* in parentheses following the reading.

Some electronic thermometers can change the reading mode to axillary and read the temperature by adding one degree; consult the instructional booklet with your equipment to determine whether your model has this. Apply a probe cover to the probe (unless otherwise indicated, use the oral probe) and insert the tip well into the axillary space with the probe extending down and slightly forward along the patient's side. Press gently into the space to establish good tissue contact. Have the patient lower his or her arm over the probe. Hold the probe in position to maintain good contact. Remove and read after the unit signals completion.

Axillary temperature can also be taken using the digital thermometer. The tip of the thermometer is placed into the axillary space and supported in place. The arm is held tight against the body until the signal is heard. Refer to Procedure 38–4 for detailed steps on measuring an axillary temperature.

Measuring Tympanic (Aural) Temperatures

The normal tympanic (aural) temperature is 99.1 degrees, generally 0.5 degrees higher than the normal oral temperature of 98.6 degrees. Tympanic membrane thermometers are easy, safe, fast to use, and fairly common in many medical offices. You simply remove the thermometer from its charging cradle and apply a disposable sheath. Position the covered plastic tip properly inside the auditory canal by pulling up and back on the ear for adults and down and back for children. Be sure the probe fits snuggly and press the scan button; an infrared beam measures the heat waves. The results are displayed digitally on the screen. A release button ejects the probe cover, and in 10 seconds, another temperature can be taken. The units operate on batteries and will measure approximately 10,000 temperatures before the batteries need to be replaced. Be sure to follow the manufacturer's instructions for the model you are using because each model varies somewhat. Procedure 38–5 provides step-by-step directions for obtaining a temperature by using a tympanic thermometer.

Measuring Temporal Artery Temperatures

Temperature is measured by scanning (gently sliding) the probe of the handheld thermometer across the forehead, halfway between the eyebrow and the hairline, from the midline to the side hairline. As long as the button is depressed and the scanner is moved

PROCEDURE 38–4 Measure Axillary Temperature

PURPOSE: To determine a patient's axillary temperature with an electronic thermometer

EQUIPMENT: Electronic thermometer, probe, probe cover, tissues, waste container, patient chart or EHR, pen

S **SKILL:** Measure and record axillary temperature with an electronic thermometer.

Procedure Steps	Detailed Instructions and/or *Rationales*
1. Wash hands; assemble equipment.	
2. Identify the patient and introduce yourself.	*Ensures that you are performing the procedure on the correct patient.*
B 3. Explain the procedure, ***using language the patient can understand.***	*Ensures understanding, consent, and cooperation from the patient.*
4. Assist the patient, as necessary, to expose the axilla. Pat the axillary space with a tissue to remove perspiration.	Perspiration prevents the probe from coming into direct contact with skin.
5. Correctly prepare the thermometer.	If using an electronic thermometer: a. Be sure the blue probe connector is plugged into the receptacle of the unit base. *The blue probe is used for axillary temperatures.* b. Remove probe from the stored position. c. Insert the probe firmly into the probe cover.

Procedure Steps	Detailed Instructions and/or *Rationales*
6. Insert the covered probe deep in the axillary space.	Position so that it is in direct contact with the top of the axillary space, with the probe extending down and slightly forward.
7. Hold the arm tightly against the body. Maintain the covered probe in position until the thermometer unit signals, approximately 10 to 15 seconds (Figure 38–16).	*Early removal results in inaccurate measurement.*
8. Remove the probe from the patient. (Do not touch the probe cover) and discard the used probe cover into the waste container.	*Probe is contaminated with patient's sweat.* If using an electronic thermometer, press the eject button to discard the probe cover. If using a digital thermometer, a*ll materials coming into contact with bodily secretions are deposited in a waste container.*
9. Read and note the temperature.	Temperature is displayed digitally in the window of the unit.
10. Disinfect thermometer and return the probe to the stored position in the unit. Store the unit in the charging stand.	The thermometer display will read zero and shut off. *The unit should remain in the stand so it is fully charged and ready for use.*
11. Help the patient replace his or her clothing.	
12. Wash hands.	
13. Document the temperature in the patient's chart, placing an (Ax) after the finding.	

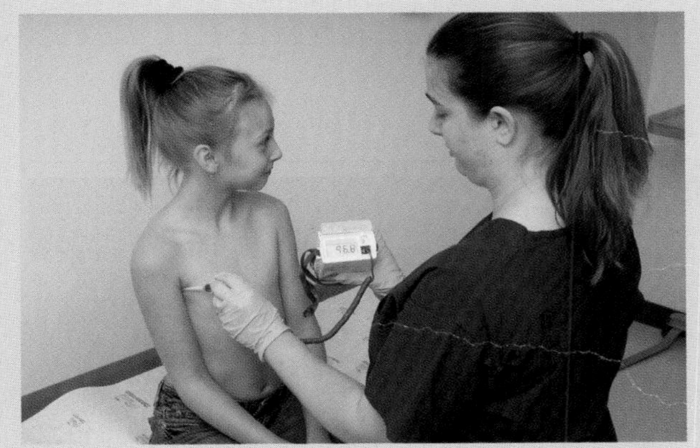

FIGURE 38–16: Measuring axillary temperature with an electronic thermometer. *Delmar/Cengage Learning.*

Charting Example

3-6-XX 11:30 am	T. 97.2 (ax) B. Davis, RMA(AMT)

PROCEDURE 38–5 Measure Core Body Temperature with a Tympanic (Aural) Thermometer

PURPOSE: To determine a patient's core body temperature by using an infrared tympanic thermometer

EQUIPMENT: Tympanic thermometer unit, probe cover, waste container, patient chart or EHR, pen

S **SKILL:** Measure core body temperature with a tympanic (aural) thermometer

Procedure Steps	Detailed Instructions and/or *Rationales*
1. Wash hands; assemble equipment.	
2. Identify the patient and introduce yourself.	*Ensures that you are performing the procedure on the correct patient.*
B 3. Explain the procedure, ***using language the patient can understand.***	*Ensures understanding, consent, and cooperation from the patient.*
4. Correctly prepare the thermometer.	a. Remove the thermometer from the base. b. Attach a disposable probe cover firmly to the ear piece. The display should read "ready."
5. Insert the covered probe into the ear canal, sealing the opening.	Pull up and back on the ear for adults (Figure 38–17 A) and down and back for children (Figure 38–17 B). *Air leaks will occur if the ear canal is not sealed.*
6. Press the scan button to activate the thermometer. Wait until the temperature reading is displayed on the screen.	3 ↓ less baby)
7. Withdraw the thermometer. Observe the display window, noting the temperature.	3 ↑ up for adult
8. Press the release button on the thermometer to eject the probe cover into a waste container and return the thermometer to the base.	
9. Document the temperature in the patient's chart, using (T) or (Tym) to indicate tympanic temperature.	

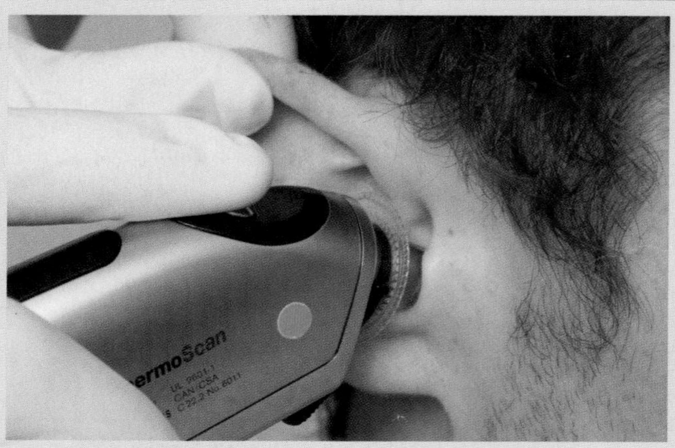

FIGURE 38–17A: For adults, pull up and back on the ear. *Delmar/Cengage Learning.*

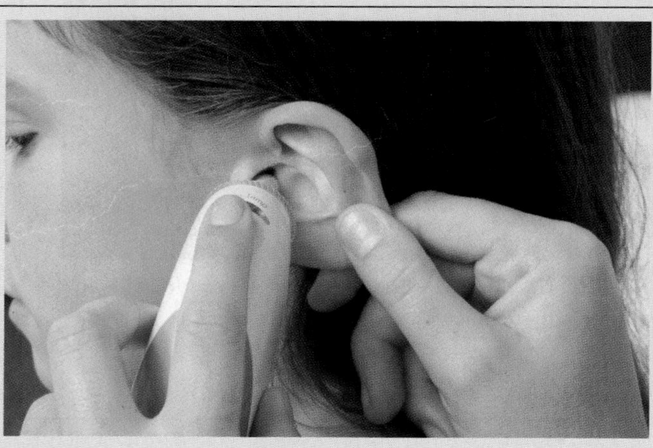

FIGURE 38–17B: For children, pull down and back on the ear. *Delmar/Cengage Learning.*

Charting Example

5/10/XX 11:30 am	T. 100.3 (T or Tym) J. Cook, CMA(AAMA)

slowly, it continually samples and records to measure the highest temperature. Multiple readings can cool the skin, so another immediate measurement may be slightly lower.

Clinical studies have shown TA measurement provides results more closely related to the true internal body temperature measured in a major artery than any other method. The normal TA measurement is equivalent to a rectal temperature; therefore, it is approximately one degree higher than oral measurement. *Note*: When recording on the chart, put (TA) after the temperature to indicate the method used. Measuring temperature by using a TA thermometer has several advantages:

- Appropriate for all ages, infants through elderly
- Convenient, easily accessible, and fast
- Comfortable and safe for the patient
- Proven highly accurate
- No danger from contact with mucous membranes
- Reading is not affected by oral factors such as hot and cold fluids, mouth breathing, oral surgery, or injury.
- Can be sanitized between patients like a stethoscope, with an antiseptic wipe, or clinical models have covers, caps, and sheaths if desired

Temperature of the skin is affected by the temperature of the surroundings. The sensor in the probe performs two processes when temperature is measured. At 1,000 times per second, it reads the infrared heat within the artery and measures the temperature in the immediate environment. The interior software performs calculations to determine the patient's temperature in relation to the surroundings. A few factors, however, affect the accurate measurement:

- Do not glide the probe over burns, open sores, abrasions, or scars.
- The forehead side measured must have been exposed to the environment with no hats, bangs, or bandages to trap heat.
- If there is perspiration on the forehead, measurement will be inaccurate. You must follow TA measurement with placing the probe against the neck behind the earlobe to obtain accurate assessment.
- The TAT must be in the same ambient temperature as the patient. It must be acclimated to the room temperature before it is used if it is moved from a hot to cold area or vice versa (e.g., window ledge exposed to hot sun or in line of air conditioning). Each 10° degree difference can cause a 1° error.
- Some models cannot be used near aerosol products or when oxygen is being administered.

Be sure to follow the manufacturer's guidelines for any additional factors. Procedure 38–6 lists the step-by-step details on how to obtain a temporal artery temperature.

PATIENT EDUCATION

Often, the provider will suggest that a patient should monitor his or her temperature at home. It can be the medical assistant's responsibility to instruct the patient about using a thermometer and how to record the temperature. The provider will name a certain elevated temperature level at which, if reached, the patient should call the office. Many types of less expensive but easy-to-use temperature measuring devices are available for home use in addition to the ones discussed in this unit and are available at most large chain pharmacies and children's stores.

Temperature Conversions

Temperature can be converted from one scale to another by a mathematical calculation:

- To convert from Celsius to Fahrenheit, multiply the degrees by 9/5 and add 32 ($[C \times 9/5] + 32 = F$).
- To change from Fahrenheit to Celsius, subtract 32 and multiply by 5/9 ($[F - 32] \times 5/9 = C$).

PROCEDURE 38–6 Measure Temperature with a Temporal Artery Thermometer

PURPOSE: Measure a patient's temperature with a temporal artery thermometer

EQUIPMENT: Temporal artery thermometer, alcohol wipe or cover, patient chart or EHR, pen

S SKILL: Measure and record temperature with a temporal artery thermometer.

Procedure Steps	Detailed Instructions and/or *Rationales*
1. Wash hands; assemble equipment. Clean the probe with alcohol or attach a cover.	
2. Identify the patient and introduce yourself.	*Ensures that you are performing the procedure on the correct patient.*

(continues)

(continued)

Procedure Steps	Detailed Instructions and/or *Rationales*
B 3. Explain the procedure, ***using language the patient can understand.***	*Ensures understanding, consent, and cooperation from the patient.*
4. Observe the forehead for perspiration and exposure to the environment. Adjust as necessary (e.g., remove hat, hold back hair).	*False readings can occur if the skin is cooled from moisture on the forehead or warmed by a hat or hair covering.*
5. Position the probe at the midline of the forehead.	*Probe must be centered properly over the area for an accurate reading.*
6. Keeping the probe flush on the skin, press, and hold the scan button while slowly sliding the thermometer across the forehead until reaching the hairline (Figure 38–18).	If perspiration is present, continue to hold button, lift probe from forehead, and position on neck behind ear lobe. Note: You will hear clicking, indicating a rise to a higher temperature until the maximum is measured.
7. When scanning is completed, release the button and lift the probe from the forehead or neck. Read the temperature on the display and return the thermometer to storage.	The reading will remain on the display until 15 to 30 seconds after the button is released, depending on the model. To turn off the thermometer immediately, depress and quickly release the button.
8. Document the temperature in the patient's chart, using (TA) to indicate temporal artery temperature.	
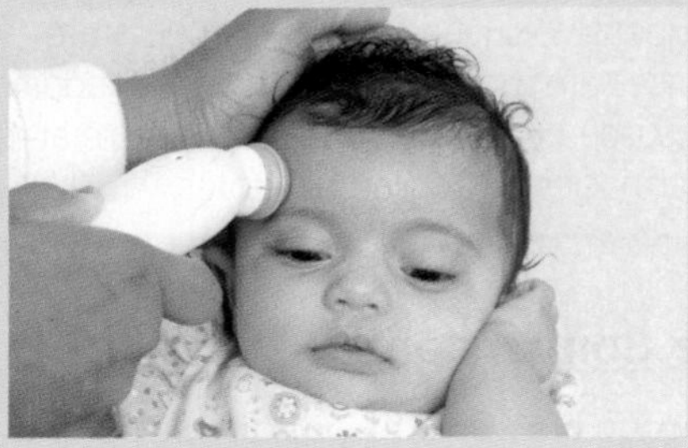 **FIGURE 38–18:** Slide thermometer across forehead. *Delmar/Cengage Learning.*	

Charting Example

5/10/XX 11:30 am	T. 99.5 (TA) B. Davis (RMA)

Another way to convert temperature uses a different mathematical calculation. Some people find this easier to do:

- To convert Celsius to Fahrenheit, the equation is: F = (C × 1.8) + 32.
- To convert Fahrenheit to Celsius, the equation is: C = F – 32/1.8

EXAMPLE

To convert Celsius to Fahrenheit:
37° C × 9/5(333/5) = 66.6 + 32 = 98.6° F
C × F–32/1.8
C = 98.6–32 = 66.6/1.8 = 37

To convert Fahrenheit to Celsius:
98.6° F–32 = 66.6 × 5/9(333/9) = 37° C
F = (C × 1.8) + 32
F = 37 × 1.8 = 66.6 + 32 = 98.6

TABLE 38–4 Temperature Conversion and Comparison

Comparison	Celsius (C)	Fahrenheit (F)
Freezing	0°	32°
Body temperature	37°	98.6°
Pasteurization	63°	145°
Boiling	100°	212°
Sterilizing (autoclave)	121°	250.0°

Table 38–4 compares some common temperatures in Celsius and Fahrenheit.

PULSE

Each time the heart beats, blood is forced into the aorta, temporarily expanding its walls and initiating a wavelike effect. This wave continues through all the body's arteries, causing the alternating expansion and recoil of the arterial walls (Figure 38–19). This effect can be **palpated** (felt) in the arteries that are close to the body surface and that lie over bone or firm structures. When the artery is pressed against the underlying structure, it is possible to feel the rhythmic pulsation, known as the pulse.

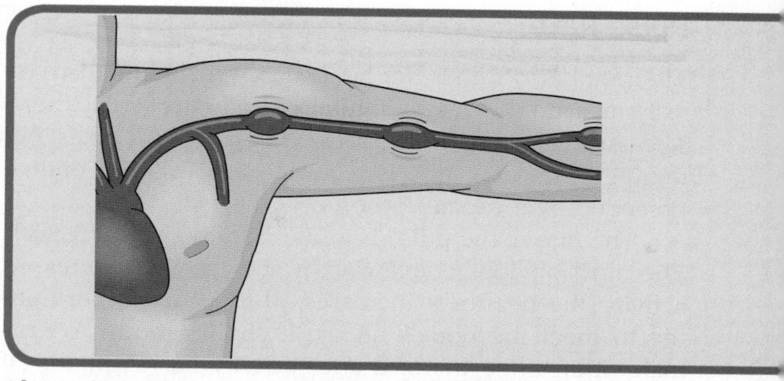

Figure 38–19: Blood pumped from the heart causes a wavelike effect in the arteries. *Delmar/Cengage Learning.*

Pulse Sites

The pulse can be felt in several locations on the body, as shown in Figure 38–20:

- The **radial** pulse is located on the thumb side of the inner surface of the wrist, lying over the radius bone. The radial pulse site is used most frequently when measuring pulse rate.
- The **brachial** artery pulse location is on the inner medial surface of the elbow, at the **antecubital** space (crease of elbow). This site is used to palpate and **auscultate** (listen to) blood pressure.
- The **carotid** pulse can be felt in the carotid artery of the neck when pressure is applied to the area at either side of the trachea. It is the carotid pulse that is palpated during the cardiopulmonary resuscitation (CPR) life-saving maneuver.
- The **femoral** pulse is located midway in the **groin** where the artery begins its descent down the femur.
- The **dorsalis pedis**, on the instep of the foot, and the **popliteal**, at the back ofthe knee, are other sites palpated to evaluate circulation in the lower extremities.

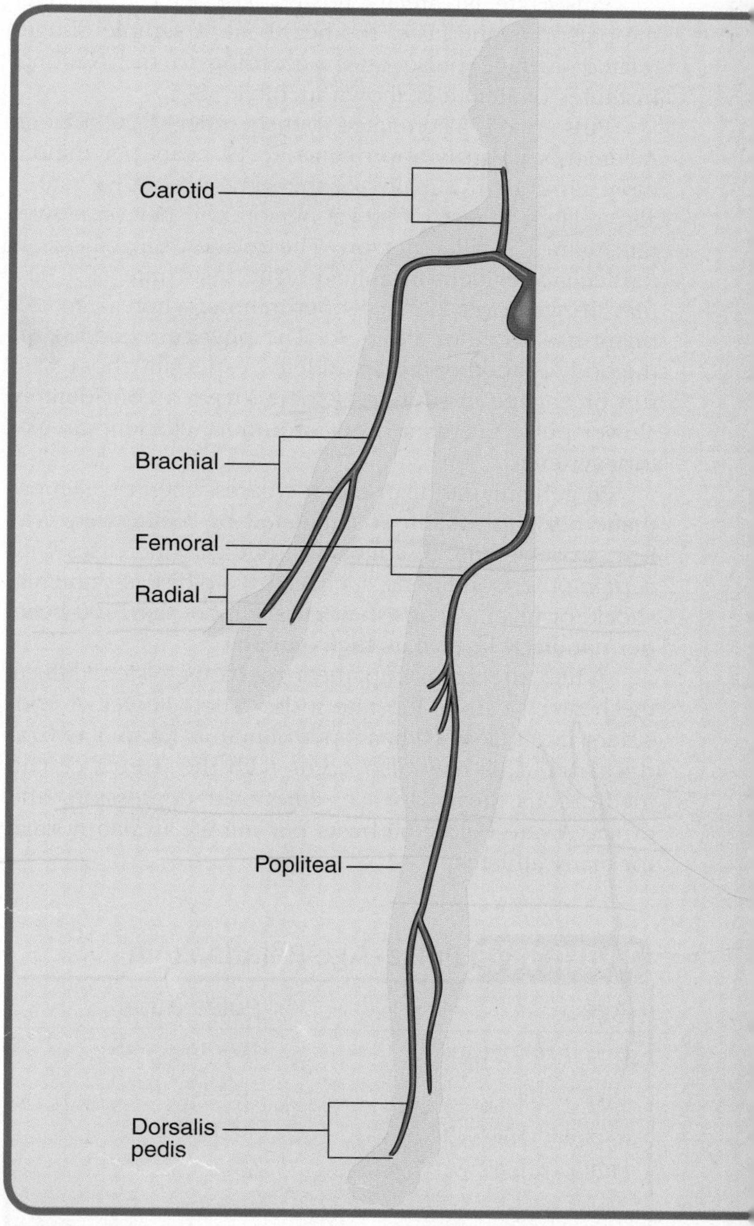

FIGURE 38–20: Pulse sites of the upper and lower extremities and the neck. *Delmar/Cengage Learning.*

Pulse Rate

The number of times the heart beats per minute is typically measured by counting the pulse in the radial artery. The average adult pulse range is 60 to 100 beats per minute. The pulse rate is recorded as beats per minute preceded by a capital *P* (i.e., P. 72).

The rate of the pulse is influenced by several factors. The most obvious is exercise or activity. With increased activity, the heartbeat increases 20 to 30 beats per minute to meet the body's needs. It should return to normal within three minutes after activity has stopped. Of course, the rate of increase will be in proportion to the level of activity.

Pulse rate is directly related to age. The younger the person is, the faster the heartbeat. A sample of age-related average pulse rates according to the National Institutes of Health is shown in Table 38–5.

Pulse rate is also related to the gender of the patient. A female's pulse is approximately 10 beats per minute more rapid than a male's of the same age. Pulse rate is also related to size; a larger person will have a slower rate than a smaller person. The relationship of size is particularly evident in animals. The heart rate of a bird may be well over 200 beats per minute, whereas an elephant has a rate of about 30. The physical condition of the body is another factor. Athletes, especially those who run or engage in strenuous sports, have a considerably slower pulse rate as a result of a more efficient circulatory system.

In general, the heart rate increases when the sympathetic nervous system is stimulated by feelings such as fear, anxiety, pain, or anger. The rate also increases with certain other conditions, such as thyroid disease, anemia, shock, or fever. A consistent rate of more than 100 beats per minute is known as **tachycardia**.

When the parasympathetic nervous system affects the heart, it causes the rate to be much slower. A consistent rate below 60 beats per minute is known as **bradycardia**. This may also occur with the use of certain medications, heart disease, emotional depression, and drugs. A rate below 60 beats per minute is also normal for many athletes.

TABLE 38–5 Pulse–Age Relationship

Age	Pulse Rate
Less than 1 year	100–160
1–10 years	70-120
11–Adult years	60–100
Midlife Adult	60–100
Older adult	50–65

Pulse Characteristics

When measuring pulse rate, two other characteristics must also be observed and recorded. The force or strength of the pulse is referred to as its **volume**. Words to describe this quality are *normal*, *full* or *bounding*, *weak*, and **thready** (scarcely perceivable).

The quality of **rhythm** of the pulse refers to its regularity, or the equal spacing of the beats. The term **arrhythmia** refers to a pulse that lacks a regular rhythm. The pulse can be irregular (without a consistent pattern) or regularly irregular (unequally spaced but consistently the same beating pattern). A pulse can also be intermittent and occasionally skip or insert beats. Often, caffeine or nicotine react on the heart to cause irregularity and increased rate.

Measuring the Radial Pulse

The patient should be completely relaxed and sitting comfortably or lying down when the pulse is measured and evaluated. Ideally, the arm should be well supported, with the wrist near the level of the heart. Place the tips of your fingers at the wrist area, about an inch above the base of the thumb (Figure 38–21). Never use your thumb to measure pulse rate; you might feel and record your own heart rate in your thumb's artery.

An appropriate amount of pressure applied to the artery will permit the pulsations to be felt. Too much pressure will shut off the circulation and therefore eliminate the pulse beat. Too little pressure will not compress the artery sufficiently against the radius. With practice, applying the correct amount of pressure will become routine. The pulse rate may be measured for 30 seconds and multiplied by two; however, if there is any irregularity, the rate should be measured for a full minute. Respirations are often measured at the same time as the

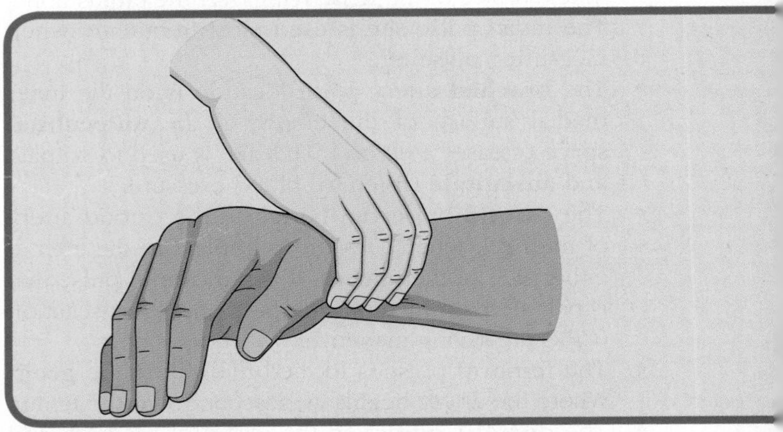

FIGURE 38–21: Measuring the radial pulse. *Delmar/Cengage Learning.*

patient's pulse. After you read the section, "Respiration," later in the chapter, refer to Procedure 38–8 for step-by-step details about how to obtain a radial pulse and respiration rate.

Measuring the Apical Pulse

When measuring heart rate by the radial pulse is not appropriate, it is necessary to listen to the heart at its **apex** with a **stethoscope**. This is a very accurate method of measuring pulse rate. The contraction of the atria and the ventricles will be heard as two closely occurring sounds known as the "lubb dupp"; however, both contraction phases are counted as only one beat. Whenever a pulse rate is measured at a point other than the radial, the location should be noted when recording the rate (e.g., P. 97 [Ap]). Note that an **apical** pulse is counted for a full minute, so it is possible to record an uneven number.

Apical Indications

Apical pulse measurement is indicated for infants and small children because of their normally rapid rate, which is easier to hear and count than to palpate. Patients with heart conditions, especially if being medicated with cardiac drugs, will require apical measurement for greater accuracy. Apical measurement is always indicated if you have difficulty feeling a radial pulse and believe you may be missing beats. Other indications are an excessively rapid or slow rate or a thready or irregular quality.

Locating the Apex

The bottom or lower edge of the heart is known as the apex. This is the point of maximum impulse of the heart against the chest wall. It can be palpated at the left fifth intercostal space in line with the middle of the left clavicle. This spot may be located by pressing the fingertips between the ribs and counting down five spaces on the left chest wall (Figure 38–22 A). Often, the beat at the apex can be felt with the fingertips.

Another, quicker method for estimating the location of the apex is to place the outstretched *left* hand on the chest wall with the tip of the middle finger in the suprasternal notch and the thumb at a 45-degree angle (Figure 38–22 B). The end of the thumb will be approximately over the apex. This is only an approximate measurement because the size of the chest and the hand will vary. For a ready reference point, the apex should be just below the left breast. Again, this is variable, particularly in the female, because of the size and placement of the breast. Refer to Procedure 38–7.

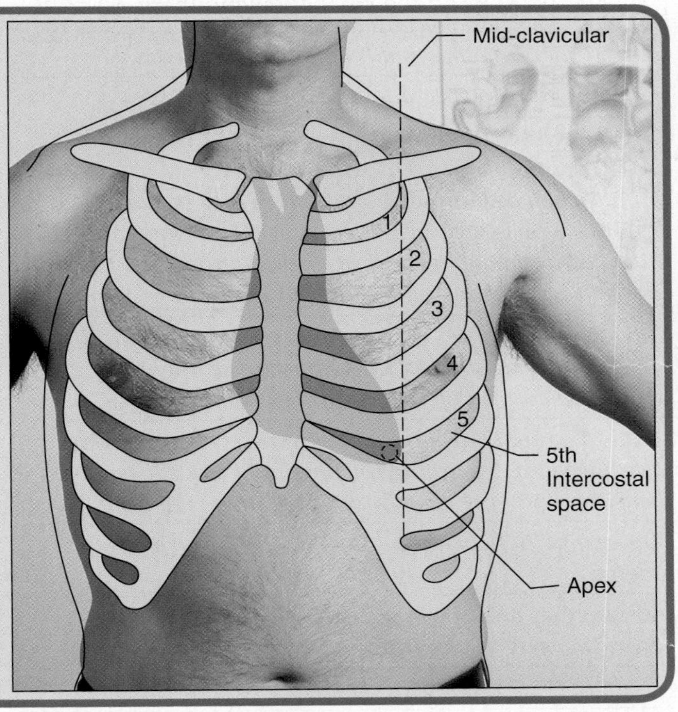

Figure 38–22A: Locate the apical pulse by counting intercostal spaces. *Delmar/Cengage Learning.*

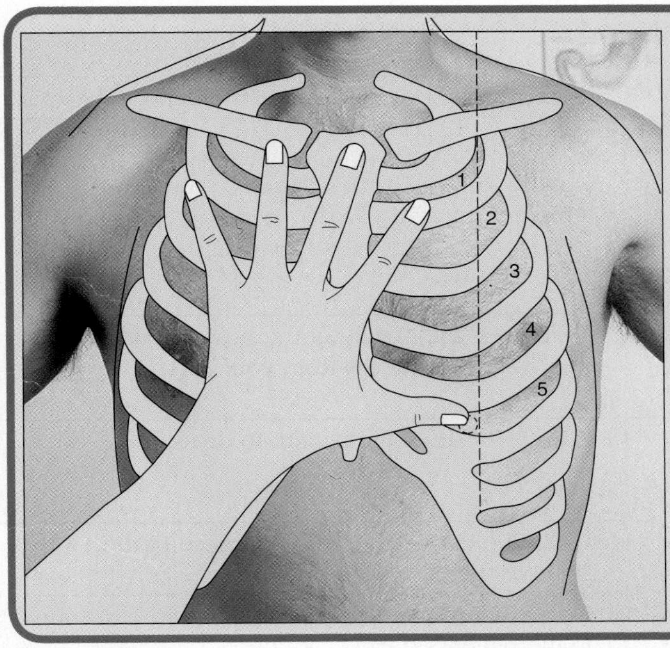

Figure 38–22B: Alternative method for locating the apex of the heart. *Delmar/Cengage Learning.*

PROCEDURE 38–7 Measure the Apical Pulse

MEDIA LINK: View the video for this chapter, "Measure an Apical Pulse," on the Premium Website

PURPOSE: To determine the rate, rhythm, and quality of a patient's apical pulse

EQUIPMENT: Watch with second hand, stethoscope, alcohol wipe, patient chart or EHR, pen

S **SKILL:** Measure and record apical pulse rate.

Procedure Steps	Detailed Instructions and/or *Rationales*
1. Wash hands; assemble equipment. Clean the stethoscope.	Wipe stethoscope earpieces and chest piece with an alcohol pad to *prevent transfer of organisms.*
2. Identify the patient and introduce yourself.	*Ensures that you are performing the procedure on the correct patient.*
B 3. Explain the procedure, ***using language the patient can understand***.	*Ensures understanding, consent, and cooperation from the patient.*
B 4. Uncover the left side of the chest. ***Provide privacy and a gown or drape if indicated***.	*Auscultation must be done directly against the skin surface.*
5. Place the stethoscope earpieces in your ears.	The openings in the tips should be forward, entering the auditory canal.
6. Locate the apex.	Palpate to the left fifth intercostal space at the mid-clavicular line. *Note*: If the chest piece does not have a chill ring, warm it in the palm of one hand while locating the apex. *This also prevents accidental striking against a hard surface and the resulting noise in your ears.*
7. Place the chest piece of the stethoscope at the apex.	
8. Count the beats for a full minute. Note the rate.	Observe wristwatch and begin counting rate when second hand is at 3, 6, 9, or 12. *It is easier to measure* one *minute when beginning at one of these four numbers.* Both pulse phases count as one beat. *Apical rates are indicated when quality or rhythm irregularities are present or possible; therefore, full-minute measurement is essential.*
9. Determine the quality of the heart sounds and remove the earpieces from your ears.	Concentrate on rate, rhythm, and volume. *The quality of the beat is significant in evaluation of the heart action. Be certain of sounds and pattern.*
10. Assist or instruct the patient to dress.	*Unless the physician also wishes to assess heart action. Determine this by asking the physician prior to measurement or if your findings indicate the need.*
11. Clean the earpieces and chest piece of the stethoscope.	*This can be done with an alcohol pad; return it to storage.*
12. Document the rate and quality of the heart sounds in the patient's chart.	Indicate that it is apical measurement. *Immediate recording aids in eliminating errors.*
13. Wash hands.	

Charting Example

5/10/XX 11:30 am	P. 103 (ap), full but irregular with an extra beat every four beats. C. WILLIAMS, CMA(AAMA)

Pulse Oximetry

Many of the electronic blood pressure units, which will be discussed later in the chapter, can check blood pressure, pulse, and oxygen saturation all at the same time and are becoming more and more popular in the medical field. Another device that can be used to obtain a patient's pulse and arterial oxygen saturation in the blood is the pulse oximeter machine, a small, handheld unit with a clip attached that is usually applied to the patient's index finger. The clip uses an infrared light to measure the pulse and oxygen levels. If the pulse is outside of the normal range, it should be taken manually for confirmation. Detailed information along with the procedure on how to perform a pulse oximetry is covered in Chapter 40.

RESPIRATION

One respiration is the combination of total inspiration (breathing in) and total expiration (breathing out). Other frequently used terms are **inhale** and **exhale**. Respirations are usually measured as one part of total vital signs assessment. Because patients can voluntarily control the depth, rate, and regularity of their breathing to some extent, it is important for them to be unaware that the procedure is being done. To accomplish this, it is common practice to observe and measure respiration immediately after assessing the radial pulse, while maintaining your fingers at the radial pulse site.

Quality of Respiration

Respirations should be quiet, effortless, and regularly spaced. Breathing should be through the nose with the mouth closed. Excessively fast and deep breathing, commonly associated with hysteria, is called **hyperventilation**. Difficult or labored breathing is called **dyspnea**. Frequently, dyspnea is accompanied by discomfort and an anxious expression, caused by the fear of being unable to breathe. This patient will use the accessory respiratory muscles of the rib cage, neck, shoulders, and back to assist the breathing process.

The presence of **rales** (noisy breathing) usually indicates constricted bronchial passageways or the collection of fluid or exudate. Rales may be present with pneumonia, bronchitis, asthma, and other pulmonary diseases.

Respirations should be observed for the depth of inhalation. Three words are used to describe this quality: normal, shallow, or deep. Depth of inhalation can be determined by watching the rise and fall of the chest. The rhythm of the respirations must also be assessed. This quality can be described as regular or irregular. Absence of breathing is known as **apnea**. A breathing pattern called **Cheyne-Stokes** occurs with acute brain, heart, or lung damage or disease and with intoxicants. It is characterized by slow, shallow breaths that increase in depth and frequency, followed by a few shallow breaths, and then a period of apnea for 10 to 20 seconds and often longer (Figure 38–23). This type of breathing pattern frequently precedes death.

Respiration Rate

The normal respiration rate for adults is 16 to 20 times per minute. The respiration rate in infants and children has a greater range and fluctuates more during illness, exercise, and emotion than adult rates do. In the newborn, the rate per minute can range from 30 to 60; in early childhood, from 20 to 40; and during late childhood, from 16 to 26. The rate will reach an adult normal range of 16 to 20 by age 16. An abnormally slow rate of respiration is known as **bradypnea**. A faster than normal rate of respiration is known as **tachypnea**.

Counting Respirations

It is necessary to observe the patient carefully while measuring respiration rate. If the patient is lying on the examination table, position the patient's arm across the upper abdominal area, placing your fingers over the radial pulse site. In this position, you can visualize and feel respiration. With the patient in a sitting position, you need to observe more carefully because you count the respirations. Remember, it is also necessary to keep your watch in view as you observe. With a little practice, you will be able to manage both at the same time.

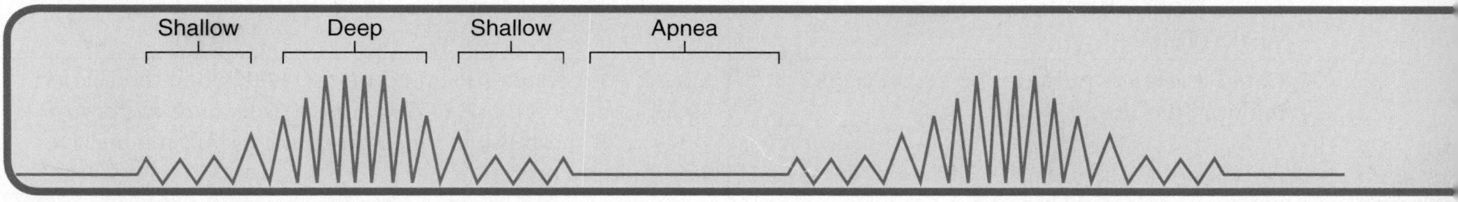

Figure 38–23: Cheyne-Stokes breathing pattern. *Delmar/Cengage Learning.*

When counting respirations as part of the TPR assessment, it is very important to remember the number of heartbeats you have just counted. It may help you to use the following method:

1. Assume the pulse measuring position.
2. Observe, determine the characteristics, and describe to yourself the qualities of both the pulse and the respirations.
3. Count the number of heartbeats during the first 30 seconds of the minute.
4. Repeat the pulse rate to yourself as you count the number of respirations during the second 30 seconds.

(*Note*: You *must* use the word "and" between each respiration so you do not accidentally add counts to the pulse rate.)

For example, if your patient's pulse rate after 30 seconds is 40, repeat this number as you count the respirations: "40 and 1, 40 and 2, 40 and 3," and so on, until the second 30-second period is past. At the end of a minute, you will have counted both rates. Multiply the rates by two and record. Procedure 38–8 gives step-by-step instruction for measuring radial pulse and respirations.

PROCEDURE 38–8 Measure the Radial Pulse and Respirations

PURPOSE: To determine the rate, rhythm, and quality of a patient's radial pulse and the rate, rhythm, sound, and depth of a patient's respirations

EQUIPMENT: Watch with second hand, patient chart or EHR, pen

S SKILL: Measure and record radial pulse rate and respirations.

Procedure Steps	Detailed Instructions and/or *Rationales*
1. Wash hands; assemble equipment.	
2. Identify the patient and introduce yourself.	*Ensures that you are performing the procedure on the correct patient.*
B 3. Explain the procedure, ***using language the patient can understand.***	*Ensures understanding, consent, and cooperation from the patient.* Note: In this procedure, it is preferable to explain only the pulse measurement and not the respirations. If the patient knows you will be counting respirations, control of breathing is possible, resulting in an inaccurate measurement.
4. Determine the patient's recent activity.	*Exertion within the past three to five minutes will cause a temporary increase in pulse and respiration rate.*
5. Position the patient with the wrist supported on a table or lap.	
6. Locate the radial artery on the thumb side of the wrist (Figure 38–24) and observe the quality of the pulse before beginning to count. Determine whether it is regular, strong, weak, or thready.	Do not use your thumb because it has its own pulse. Place the tips of your fingers lightly over the artery. *Concentration on the quality prior to measurement assists in accurate evaluation.*
7. Count a *regular* pulse for 30 seconds and multiply the results by two.	Check your watch. Begin counting beats when the second hand is at 3, 6, 9, or 12. *This makes 30 seconds easier to observe.* If the pulse is irregular, count for full minute. Do not multiply by 2.
8. Assess respiration quality.	Determine depth, rhythm, and sound. *In certain disease conditions, the presence or absence of quality characteristics is a significant finding.*

Procedure Steps	Detailed Instructions and/or *Rationales*
9. Count respirations for 30 seconds and multiply the results by two.	One rise and fall of the chest equals one respiration. Maintain the radial pulse position. Note: If respirations are irregular, count for a full minute and do not multiply results by two.
10. Document the patient's pulse and respiration (including quality characteristics) in the chart.	Record both the pulse and respirations in beats per minute and describe the quality characteristics.
11. Wash hands.	

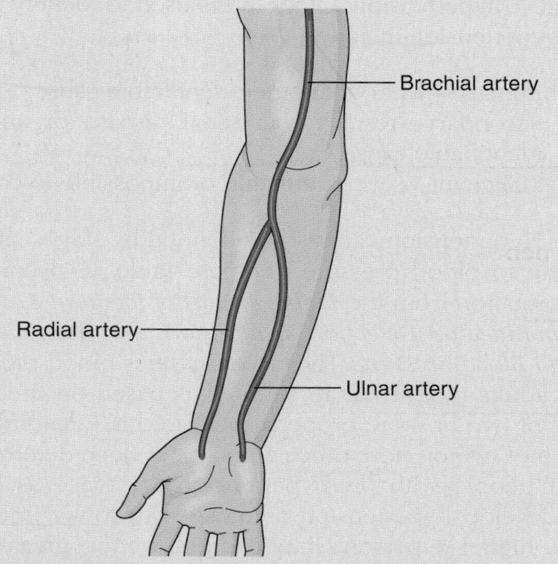

FIGURE 38–24: The radial pulse is measured in the radial artery, on the thumb side of the wrist.
Delmar/Cengage Learning.

Charting Example

5/10/XX 11:30 am	P. 96, weak but regular R. 24, rate and rhythm regular B. Davis RMA (AMT)

BLOOD PRESSURE

Learning to assess blood pressure accurately requires attention to details, careful listening, and correct technique. The term *blood pressure* means the fluctuating pressure the blood exerts against the arterial walls as it alternately contracts and relaxes. The blood pressure reflects the condition of the heart, the amount of blood forced from the heart at contraction, the condition of the arteries, and, to some extent, the volume and viscosity (thickness) of the blood.

Blood pressure is measured in the brachial artery of the arm at the antecubital space (Figure 38–25). It should be measured in both arms, at least initially. There is normally a 5- to 10-mm difference. Subsequent readings should be made on the arm with the higher pressure.

Maintaining Blood Pressure

Two main factors cooperate to maintain a fairly constant blood pressure. The first is the heart or pump, which exerts pressure on the blood. About 100,000 times a

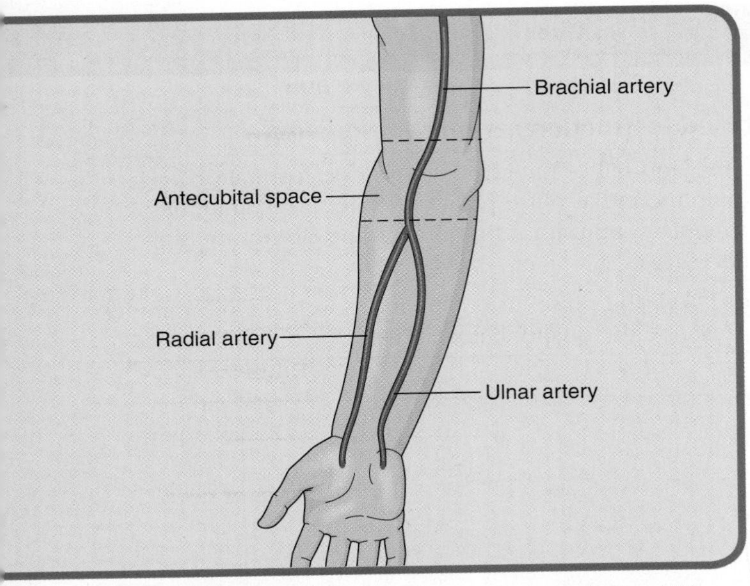

Figure 38–25: Blood pressure is measured in the brachial artery at the antecubital space. *Delmar/Cengage Learning.*

day, the heart contracts, forcing blood into the aorta and throughout the blood vessels of the body. Without a strong, effective pump, the blood will not flow, and the pressure will drop.

The second factor is the brain, which controls, through the autonomic nervous system, the rate of the heart and the size of the opening or caliber of the arteries. When sensors in the arteries detect an increase in arterial pressure, a message is sent to the brain, which in turn directs the arteries to dilate slightly (reducing resistance to the flow of blood) and directs the heart to slow down (reducing the amount of blood being forced out). If the pressure drops too far, the message to the brain results in a slightly increased heart action and constriction of the arteries, which cause the pressure to rise. Both actions are needed to maintain homeostasis.

Blood Pressure Phases

The phases of blood pressure are identical to those of the pulse. A contraction phase, known as **systole**, corresponds to the beat phase of the heart and is the period of greatest pressure. The relaxation phase, known as **diastole**, corresponds to the resting or filling action of the heart and is the period of least pressure.

Normal Blood Pressure

Blood pressure readings are measurements of systolic and diastolic pressure written as a fraction, for example, B/P 120/80, when 120 represents the systolic and 80 represents the diastolic pressure. An adult should have a systolic pressure less than 120 mm Hg and a diastolic pressure less than 80.

Blood pressure readings persistently in the ranges of 140–159 and 90–99 indicate stage 1 *hypertension* (high blood pressure). Hypertension can result from things such as stress, obesity, high salt intake, sedentary lifestyle, and aging. Physical conditions that cause hypertension are kidney disease; thyroid dysfunction; neurological disorders; and vascular conditions (such as atherosclerosis and arteriosclerosis), which make circulation more difficult, therefore requiring a greater pressure to circulate the blood. An elevated pressure without apparent cause is said to be **idiopathic** or **essential** stage 1 hypertension. Other terms used to identify types of hypertension include:

- Primary—without another identifiable cause
- Secondary—results from renal disease or another identifiable cause
- Malignant—severe, difficult, or impossible to control

Hypertension can also be defined by stages as they relate to blood pressure findings. Table 38–6 contains information from the *Eighth Report of the Joint National Committee on Detection, Evaluation, and Treatment of High Blood Pressure*. The table classifies blood pressure for adults older than 18 years. It is based on the average of two or more properly measured B/P readings on each of two or more office visits. It has been determined that people with pre-hypertension are twice as likely to develop hypertension as those with lower findings. The higher a person's blood pressure, the greater the chance for heart attack, heart failure, stroke, and kidney disease.

A blood pressure consistently below 90/60 indicates *hypotension* (low blood pressure), which may be normal for some persons. Hypotension can be present with heart failure, severe burns, dehydration, deep depression, hemorrhage, and shock. A drop in blood pressure can also occur when a patient changes from a sitting to a standing position. This is known as **orthostatic** hypotension and occurs commonly in elderly patients because of decreased circulation efficiency. It often results in dizziness and sometimes syncope. Certain medications can also be the cause of hypotension. Typically, if blood pressure is measured, it will show a drop of at least 20 mm Hg systolic and 10 mm Hg diastolic. Some providers routinely assess orthostatic pressure on all older patients as part of the physical assessment.

Pulse Pressure

Pulse pressure refers to the difference between the systolic and diastolic reading and is an indicator of the tone of the arterial walls. For example, when the

TABLE 38–6 Classification and Management of Blood Pressure for Adults

Blood Pressure Classification	Systolic Blood Pressure (mm Hg)	Diastolic Blood Pressure (mm Hg)	Lifestyle Modification	Initial Drug Therapy: Without Compelling Indication	Initial Drug Therapy: With Compelling Indications
Normal	<120	and <80	Encourage	No antihypertensive drug indicated	Drugs for compelling indications
Pre-hypertension	120–139	or 80–89	Yes	No antihypertensive drug indicated	Drugs for compelling indications; other antihypertensive drugs as needed.
Stage 1 hypertension	140–159	or 90–99	Yes	Thiazide-type diuretics for most; may consider ACEI, ARB, BB, CCB*, or combination	
Stage 2 hypertension	≥160	or ≥ 100	Yes	Two-drug combination for most usually (thiazide-type diuretic and ACEI, ARB, BB, CCB)	

*ACEI, angiotensin-converting enzyme inhibitor; ARB, angiotensin receptor blocker; BB, beta blocker; CCB, calcium-channel blocker.
Source: *Seventh Report of the Joint National Committee on Detection, Evaluation, and Treatment of High Blood Pressure (JNC 7).*

pressure is 120/80, the pulse pressure is 40, which is a normal finding. A pulse pressure over 50 or less than 30 mm Hg may be considered abnormal. A general rule is that the pulse pressure should be approximately a third of the systolic measurement. If less, the patient may have an auscultatory gap (absence of sound), and the pressure may have been incorrectly measured. This disorder is described later.

Equipment Factors

Blood pressure is measured using a stethoscope and a **sphygmomanometer** (Figures 38–26 A and B). It is important for sphygmomanometers be in proper working order, correctly calibrated, and serviced regularly.

Aneroid models must be checked regularly over the entire pressure range. Studies have shown many aneroid sphygmomanometers used in family practice to be faulty. There are two primary areas of failure. The control valves of the cuffs often result in leakage, and a greater problem with accuracy occurs as a result of dial errors because they are rarely calibrated. Faults in aneroid models have to be corrected by service technicians or the manufacturer. The office should have a maintenance policy whereby all sphygmomanometers are on a scheduled service plan.

Blood pressure cuffs are critical to correct measurement. They are available in different sizes to measure blood pressure in neonates (infants), children, adults, obese adults, and adult thighs (Figure 38–27). If the reading is to be accurate, the cuff must be the appropriate size. If it is too small for the upper arm, the reading will be falsely high; if too large, falsely low. To determine the proper size, compare the cuff width to the width of the upper arm. The cuff should be about 20 percent wider than the arm. When a cuff is too small and you do not have access to a wide adult cuff, measure to the width of the forearm. If the cuff is of adequate size, take the blood pressure reading in the forearm by placing the stethoscope over the radial artery.

An electronic sphygmomanometer is totally automatic and facilitates blood pressure measurement by providing a digital readout in the display window (Figure 38–28). It does not require the use of a stethoscope and should eliminate errors from improper technique or hearing

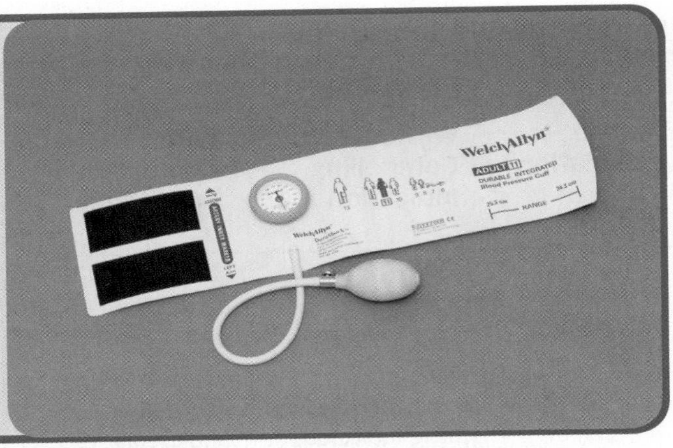

FIGURE 38–26A: Aneroid sphygmomanometer. *Delmar/Cengage Learning.*

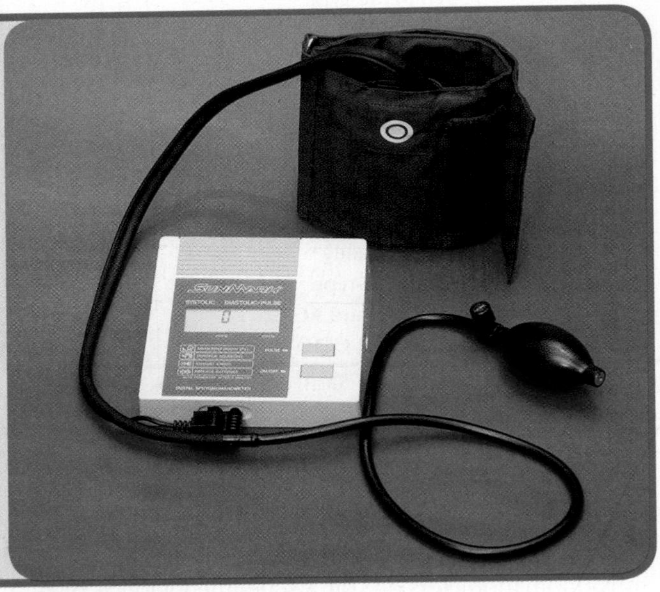

FIGURE 38–26B: Digital sphygmomanometer. *Delmar/Cengage Learning.*

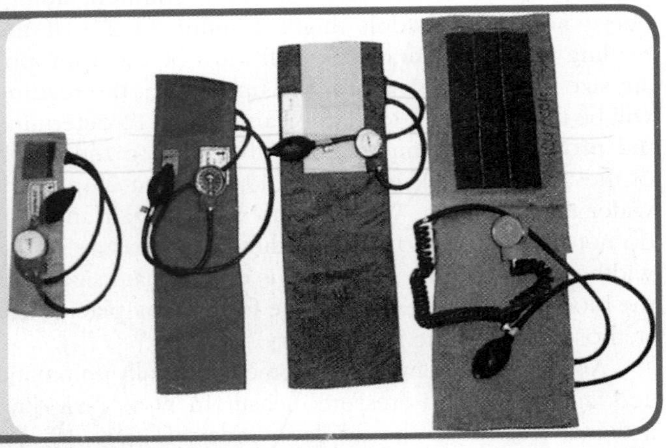

FIGURE 38–27: Blood pressure cuffs in different sizes to fit from the arm of a small child up to an adult thigh. *Delmar/Cengage Learning.*

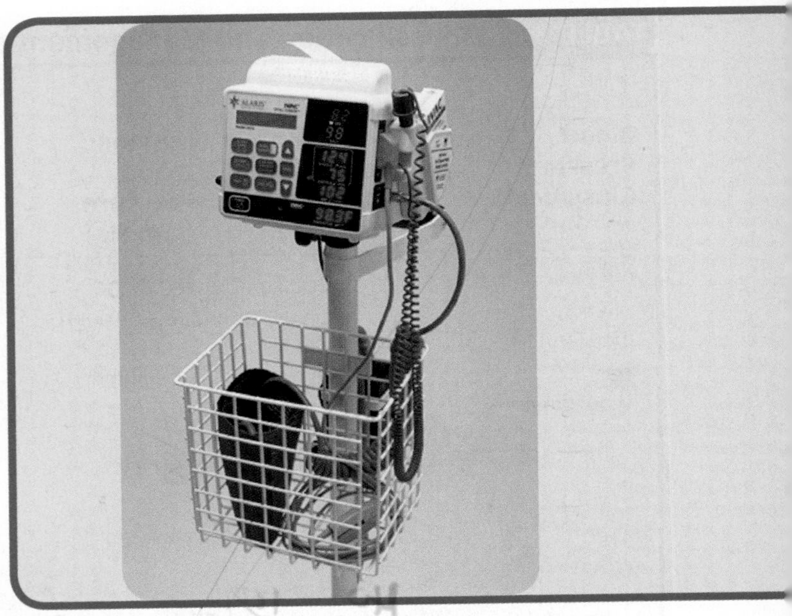

FIGURE 38–28: Electronic sphygmomanometer. *Delmar/Cengage Learning.*

difficulties. After the cuff is applied, the operator presses a button and the cuff automatically inflates, releases pressure slowly, and displays the results. The equipment can also be equipped with a pulse oximeter feature, which measures pulse rate and oxygen saturation when the sensor is attached to the finger. As with any piece of mechanical equipment, if the reading seems unlikely, it should be repeated or checked with another piece of equipment.

Measuring Techniques

Blood pressure readings are critical for the determination of hypertension and for proper medication for managing it; therefore, strict procedure techniques must be followed to ensure the accuracy of the results when using manual equipment.

1. The cuff must be completely deflated when applied.
2. The patient must be comfortable, with the arm slightly flexed at the elbow and the brachial artery on a level with the heart. The arm must be free of a constricting sleeve.
3. The center of the bladder in the cuff must be placed over the brachial artery. Fold the bladder area of the cuff in half to locate the center. Many cuffs have improper artery markings.
4. The manometer must be viewed directly from a distance of not more than 3 feet.
5. A palpatory reading should be taken first to determine proper inflation. This is achieved by placing your fingers on your patient's wrist and slowly opening the valve on the inflation bulb to allow air out at about 5 mm Hg/second. As the brachial artery

CLINICAL PEARL

A study at Duke University, reported in the Harvard Medical School's *Heart Letter*, stated that researchers had taken blood pressure measurements through clothing on 36 volunteers to determine whether readings would be inaccurate. One arm was bare, whereas the other was covered with clothing, either a shirt or a shirt with a light sweater. Simultaneous automated blood pressure measurements revealed that findings through light clothing were within 2 mm Hg of the results on bare skin. It was felt that based on this data, patients visiting a physician for a simple blood pressure reading may not need to change into a gown if the clothing covering the arm is light. This decision, however, needs to be made by the employing physician.

becomes less constricted, blood will begin to flow through. The first beat you feel at the radius is the systolic blood pressure. Afterward, deflate the cuff completely by compressing with your hands before reinflation.

6. A minimum of 15 seconds should elapse between inflations (30 is better) to allow blood pressure to normalize.
7. The cuff should be inflated rapidly to 30 mm Hg above the palpatory reading.

To obtain a baseline reading for new patients, it might be desirable to measure the pressure twice in each arm, once while the patient is sitting and once while lying down. As stated earlier, in certain situations, it may be necessary to obtain orthostatic blood pressure measurement in addition to the general measurement. If this is desired, simply follow the regular sitting or prone measurement by having the patient stand and immediately measure and record the results. Observe the patient for signs of dizziness or syncope.

Blood pressure has two phases, both of which must be determined. When the cuff is properly inflated, the valve must be opened carefully to allow deflation at a rate of 2 to 3 mm Hg per second. Listen for the first sounds of heartbeat and note the reading as the systolic pressure after you have heard at least two consecutive beats. Continue to listen and observe as the cuff is deflated until you hear a sudden change in sound to a softer, muffled tone. Note this reading as the diastolic pressure. Continue to observe the manometer until the sound disappears. Note this reading also, even if 0. To record, for example, you would write: B/P 140/90/70. You should ask the provider for his or her preference about which sound, the change or the absence, you are to record as the diastolic measurement.

Probably the mistake made most often in measuring blood pressure is reinflating the cuff after only partial deflation or too soon after complete deflation. Either error can cause a false reading and will cause difficulty in hearing the sound changes because of venous congestion in the forearm. Procedure 38–9 provides step-by-step details on measuring blood pressure.

PROCEDURE 38–9 Measure Blood Pressure

PURPOSE: To determine a patient's palpatory and auscultatory blood pressure measurements

EQUIPMENT: Stethoscope, aneroid manometer, alcohol wipe, patient chart or EHR, pen

S **SKILL:** Measure and record blood pressure.

Procedure Steps	Detailed Instructions and/or *Rationales*
1. Wash hands; assemble equipment. Clean the earpieces and head of the stethoscope with antiseptic.	*Prevents transfer of organisms.*
2. Identify the patient and introduce yourself.	*Ensures that you are performing the procedure on the correct patient.*
B 3. Explain the procedure, ***using language the patient can understand***.	*Ensures understanding, consent, and cooperation from the patient.*

(continues)

(continued)

Procedure Steps	Detailed Instructions and/or *Rationales*
4. Place the patient in a relaxed and comfortable sitting or lying position. Expose the patient's upper arm well above the elbow, extending the arm with the palm up.	The arm may be either bare or covered with light clothing. Remove the arm from a constricting sleeve. Note: *Arm must be relaxed, on a supporting surface, slightly flexed at the elbow,* with the brachial artery approximately at the level of the heart.
5. With the valve of the inflation bulb open, squeeze all air from the bladder and place it over the brachial artery (Figure 38–29 A). Be sure the aneroid dial is in direct view.	The bottom edge of the cuff should be 1 to 2 inches above the elbow. Wrap the cuff smoothly and snugly around the arm, with the deflated bladder centered over the brachial artery. Be certain the dial can be easily viewed and the end of the cuff does not interfere.
6. With *one hand,* close the valve on the bulb, turning clockwise.	*Do not over-tighten the valve, or it will be hard to open.*
7. Position your other hand to palpate the radial pulse (Figure 38–29 B).	
8. While observing the manometer, rapidly inflate the cuff to 30 mm above the level at which radial pulse disappears.	
9. Open the valve, slowly releasing the air until the radial pulse is detected. Observe the dial reading.	*This provides information for auscultatory measurement. This is palpatory systolic pressure, which may be recorded, for example, as B/P 120 (P).*
10. Deflate the cuff rapidly and completely.	Squeeze the cuff with hands to empty. *All the air must be expressed between inflations to obtain accurate results. Adjust the position if necessary.*
11. Position the earpieces of the stethoscope in your ears.	The openings should be entering the ear canals.
12. Palpate the brachial artery at the medial antecubital space with your fingertips (Figure 38–29 C).	
13. Place the head of the stethoscope directly over the palpated pulse (Figure 38–29 D).	The stethoscope head should not touch the cuff (creates static).
14. Close the valve on the bulb and rapidly inflate the cuff to 30 mm above the palpated systolic pressure.	A minimum of 15–30 seconds must have elapsed since the previous inflation. *This is the minimum time required for the normalizing of blood flow through the artery.*
15. Open the valve, slowly deflating the cuff. Note the reading at which you hear the systolic pressure.	Pressure should drop 2 to 3 mm Hg per second. The reading must be at least two consecutive beats. Remember the systolic measurement.
16. Allow the pressure to lower steadily until you note a change in sound to a softer, more muffled sound. Note this as diastolic pressure (if so instructed).	

Procedure Steps	**Detailed Instructions and/or *Rationales***
17. Continue to release pressure until all sound disappears. Note this point as diastolic pressure (if so instructed).	
18. Remove the stethoscope from your ears and release the remaining air from the cuff.	Squeeze the cuff between your hands. *This removes all the remaining air to make the patient more comfortable and ensures accurate results if re-evaluation is necessary.*
19. Remove the cuff from the patient's arm. Assist the patient with clothing if necessary.	
20. Reevaluate, if indicated, after a minimum of 15 seconds.	
21. Clean the stethoscope. Fold the cuff properly and place it with the manometer and stethoscope in storage.	Use alcohol to disinfect the stethoscope.
22. Wash hands and document the systolic and whichever diastolic reading the provider prefers in the patient's chart.	

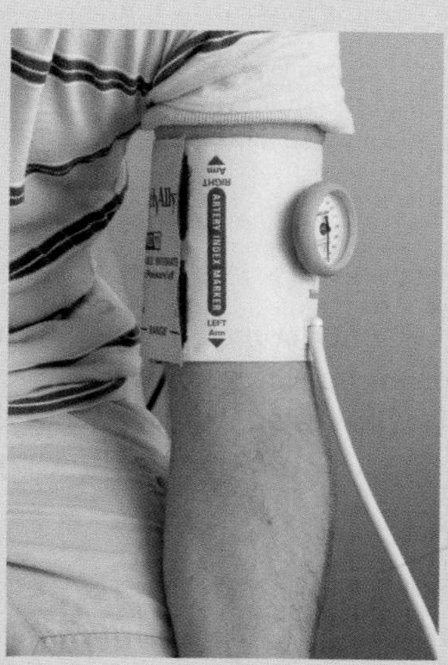

FIGURE 38–29A: Ensure that the patient is comfortable, with the arm slightly flexed at the elbow and the brachial artery on a level with the heart. The arm must be free of a constricting sleeve. With the valve of the inflation bulb open, squeeze all air from the bladder and place it over the brachial artery. *Delmar/Cengage Learning.*

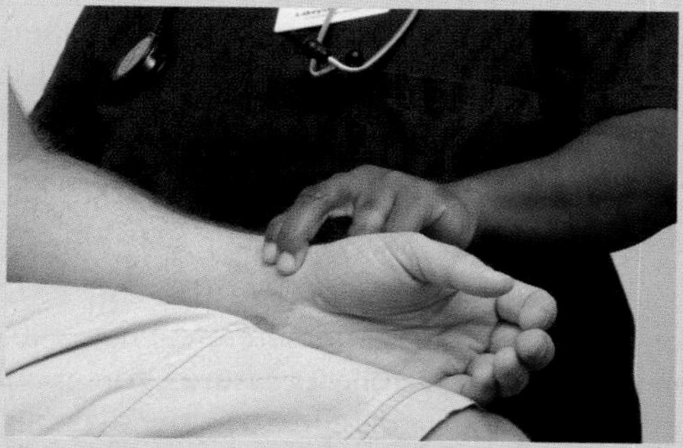

FIGURE 38–29B: With *one hand,* close the valve on the bulb, turning clockwise. Then, position your other hand to palpate the radial pulse. *Delmar/Cengage Learning.*

(continues)

(continued)

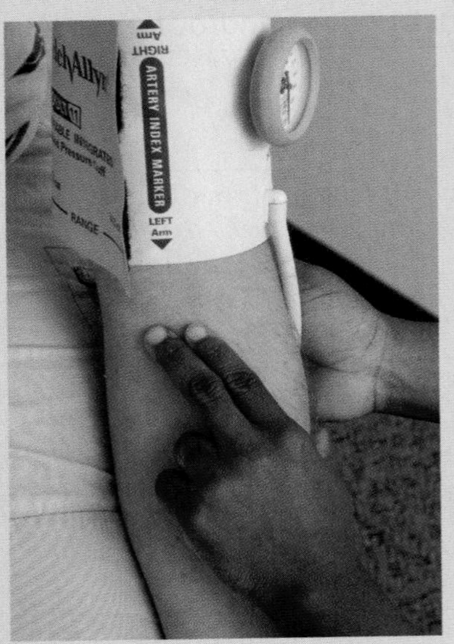

FIGURE 38–29C: Palpate the brachial artery at the medial antecubital space with your fingertips. *Delmar/Cengage Learning.*

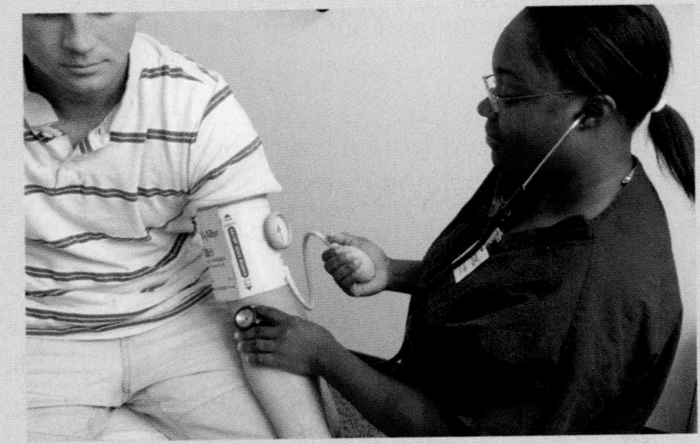

FIGURE 38–29D: Place the head of the stethoscope directly over the palpated pulse. *Delmar/Cengage Learning.*

Charting Example

6-30-XX 11:30 am	B/P 186/94 or B/P 186/94/56. A. Ostroshy, CMA(AAMA)

Auscultatory Gap

In some patients, usually those who are hypertensive, there is a silent interval between systolic and diastolic pressure, called an *auscultatory gap*. If this is not detected, it may lead to serious under-measurement of the systolic pressure. For example, the patient's actual systolic pressure is 200, with a gap from 170 to 140 and a diastolic of 120/110. You inflate the cuff to 170 and hear nothing until the manometer reaches 140, which you presume is the systolic pressure. You would continue deflation and record 120/110 as the diastolic; therefore, you would have a pulse pressure of only 20 or 30 mm Hg. Keeping in mind the normal range for pulse pressure, however, you would view 20/30 as suspicious. Taking one third of 140 would give you about 47. To be certain you had not missed a portion of the pressure, you would remeasure, palpating the systolic and then inflating the cuff 30 mm above. If sounds were still audible at that point, you would wait 15–30 seconds and reinflate it higher *after complete deflation* until you hear the first sounds of systolic pressure. When recording a blood pressure with an auscultatory gap, list your complete findings (e.g., B/P 200/120/110 with the auscultatory gap from 170 to 140).

Blood Pressure in Children

The blood pressure of infants and children is often omitted from the physical examination until the child reaches the age of three or older because it is so difficult to obtain. You must check with the provider for the policy at your specific medical office. Variation in blood pressure caused by anxiety and emotional upset make accurate readings very challenging. Basically, the procedure is the same as with adults; however, providers often prefer to do the measurement last after having established some rapport with the child.

The cuff size is important in measuring a child's pressure. It should be appropriate to the size of the arm.

The inflatable bag must entirely encircle the extremity. The level of systolic pressure gradually rises throughout childhood. Normal pressure for a 6-month-old is 70; at 1 year, it is 95; and it rises to 100 at 6 years. By age 16, the systolic pressure will be 120, the adult average. The diastolic pressure reaches 65 by age 1 and does not change appreciably during childhood.

Measurement of vital signs and body measurements provides essential information regarding the patient's overall condition. Monitoring while treatment and medication are being given for diseases and disorders of these systems is very important. The goal of treatment is to maintain the patient within as normal limits as possible.

CHAPTER SUMMARY

- Body measurements are sometimes referred to as mensuration, meaning the process of measuring. When used in connection with patient care, it refers to body measurements such as height and weight; length of extremities; and the circumference of head, chest, or abdomen with infants.
- Height and weight measurements are important with infants and children to ensure there is proper growth and development. For adults, abnormal changes could indicate the presence of a disease or disorder. Measurements can also provide information regarding treatment, diagnostic testing, and medication dosages.
- The four vital indicators are temperature, pulse, respiration, and blood pressure, commonly referred to as TPR and B/P. They indicate the body's ability to control heat; the rate, volume, and rhythm of the heart; the rate and quality of breathing; and the force of the heart and condition of the blood vessels. Some providers consider pain a fifth vital sign.
- Normal body temperature for an individual is that temperature at which his or her body systems function most effectively. (Refer to Table 38–1 for normal temperature ranges.) All temperature methods have factors that cause inaccuracies; however, the rectal and TA methods are most accurate, and axillary is least accurate.
- The average adult pulse range is 60 to 100 beats per minute. The rate of the pulse is influenced by several factors, including exercise or activity; age; gender; physical condition of the body; and emotions such as fear, anxiety, pain, or anger.
- The radial pulse is used most frequently when measuring pulse rate. The brachial artery is used to palpate and auscultate blood pressure. The carotid pulse is palpated during the CPR life-saving maneuver. The femoral pulse is palpated to evaluate circulation in the lower extremities. Review Figure 38–19 for the locations of these pulse sites.
- Apical pulse measurement is indicated for infants and small children, patients with heart conditions, patients whose radial pulse is difficult to feel or who have an excessively rapid or slow rate or a thready or irregular quality.
- Respirations should be quiet, effortless, and regularly spaced. Abnormalities in respirations can indicate a variety of diseases or disorders.
- The term *blood pressure* means the fluctuating pressure the blood exerts against the arterial walls as the heart alternately contracts and relaxes. The blood pressure reflects the condition of the heart, the amount of blood forced from the heart at contraction, the condition of the arteries, and, to some extent, the volume and viscosity (thickness) of the blood.
- Equipment needed to obtain a blood pressure include a stethoscope; sphygmomanometer; alcohol wipe; blood pressure cuffs available in different sizes to measure blood pressure in neonates (infants), children, adults, obese adults, and adult thighs; or an electronic sphygmomanometer that is totally automatic and facilitates blood pressure measurement by providing a digital readout in the display window.
- An adult should have a systolic pressure less than 120 mm Hg and a diastolic pressure less than 80. Blood pressure readings with a ranges of 140–159 and 90–99 indicate stage 1 hypertension (high blood pressure); above this range indicates stage 2 hypertension.
- Hypertension can result from factors such as stress, obesity, high salt intake, sedentary lifestyle, and aging. Physical conditions that cause hypertension are kidney disease; thyroid dysfunction; neurological disorders; and vascular conditions (such as atherosclerosis and arteriosclerosis).

STUDY TOOLS

Workbook	Activities for Chapter 38
Premium Website	
MEDIA LINK	View this **Media Link** for Chapter 38: • Measure an Apical Pulse
StudyWARE	Activities and Quizzes on the **StudyWARE™ Software** for Chapter 38
	Complete the following **Competency Challenge 2.0** activity: • Tuesday, 9:00 AM, Obtain Vital Signs
	Audio Library of medical terms
	Online access to the **Critical Thinking Challenge 2.0**
CourseMate	Activities and Quizzes for Chapter 38
WebTutor	Activities and Quizzes for Chapter 38

CHECK YOUR KNOWLEDGE

1. The process of measuring body measurements is referred to as:
   a. measuration.
   b. menstruation.
   c. mensuration.
   d. ministration.
2. Although the height bar is usually recorded in inches, you might need to convert into feet and inches by dividing the number of total inches by:
   a. 10.
   b. 12.
   c. 6.
   d. 5.
3. The four vital indicators that measure the body functions essential to life include:
   a. height, weight, temperature, and pulse.
   b. temperature, pulse, respiration, and blood pressure.
   c. temperature, pulse, respiration, and weight.
   d. height, weight, pulse, and blood pressure.
4. When measuring the oral temperature using an electronic thermometer, select the following probe:
   a. green.
   b. red.
   c. blue.
   d. black.
5. The radial pulse can be found:
   a. on the thumb side of the inner surface of the wrist, lying over the radius bone.
   b. on the pinkie side of the inner surface of the wrist, lying over the ulna bone.
   c. on the thumb side of the inner surface of the wrist, lying over the ulna bone.
   d. on the pinkie side of the inner surface of the wrist, lying over the radius bone.
6. Normal respiration rate in adults is:
   a. 16–26 times a minute.
   b. 20–40 times a minute.
   c. 16–20 times a minute.
   d. 30–80 times a minute.
7. The term *systole* refers to:
   a. noisy breathing.
   b. resting phase of the heart.
   c. contraction phase of the heart.
   d. absence of breathing.
8. This type of hypertension is caused by renal disease or another identifiable cause:
   a. primary.
   b. secondary.
   c. tertiary.
   d. malignant.

WEB LINKS

LifeClinic: www.lifeclinic.com

National Institutes of Health: www.nih.gov

RESOURCES

Exergen Corporation. (2005). *Temporal Scanner Reference Manual.* Watertown, MA.

Heller, M., and Veach, L. (2009). *Clinical Medical Assisting: A Professional, Field Smart Approach to the Workplace.* Clifton Park, NY: Delmar, Cengage Learning.

Lindh, W., Pooler, M., Tamparo, C., and Dahl, B. (2010). *Delmar's Comprehensive Medical Assisting Administrative and Clinical Competencies* (4th ed.). Clifton Park, NY: Delmar Cengage Learning.

Rizzo, D. (2010). *Fundamentals of Anatomy and Physiology* (3rd ed.). Clifton Park, NY: Delmar Cengage Learning.

U.S. Department of Health and Human Services. (2003, December). NIH Publication No. 03-5233. Bethesda, MD: National Institutes of Health.

Chapter

39 Preparing for Examinations

OBJECTIVES

In this chapter, you will learn the following:

KB KNOWLEDGE BASE

1. Spell and define, using the glossary at the back of the text, all the Words to Know in this chapter.
2. List the supplies that should be available in an examination room.
3. Explain the steps necessary to prepare for an exam.
4. Explain examination room cleanup and equipment that may need to be disinfected following a patient examination.
5. Name the examination positions and explain the purpose of each.
6. Explain the technique and purpose of draping the patient for each examination position.

S SKILLS

1. Prepare and maintain the examination and treatment areas.
2. Transfer a patient from a wheelchair to the examination table.
3. Transfer a patient from the examination table to a wheelchair.
4. Demonstrate positioning a patient for a variety of examinations.

B BEHAVIOR

1. Demonstrate empathy in communicating with patients, family, and staff.
2. Demonstrate awareness of the territorial boundaries of the person with whom communicating.
3. Apply critical thinking skills in performing patient assessment and care.
4. Use language/verbal skills that enable patients' understanding.

WORDS TO KNOW

anatomical
anterior
dorsal recumbent
dyspnea
fenestrated
Fowler's
horizontal
incompetent
knee-chest
lithotomy
proctological
prone
recumbent
shock
sigmoidoscopy
Sims'
supine
Trendelenburg
dorsal

PREPARING THE ROOM

Preparation and maintenance of the examination room for an exam is the responsibility of the medical assistant. Before every patient encounter in the room, you must ensure that the room is clean, well-organized, and at a comfortable temperature (Figure 39–1). Patients expect to find exam rooms neat and clean. A clean, well-stocked exam room reflects positively on the provider and the staff.

It is important to know how to operate the examination table to ensure a smooth and efficient examination process. The provider might require the patient to assume certain positions during the examination, some of which necessitate changing the table structure. The exam table in Figure 39–2A is limited to changing the angle of the top half, pulling out the leg rest, and extending the hidden stirrups. The power table in Figure 39–2B can be adjusted for the height of the provider as well as for many examination positions. The desired position can be achieved by pressing a button on the programmed hand control or using the optional plug-in foot control.

All surfaces within the room that might be potentially contaminated should be cleaned with a disinfectant between patient examinations. This would include cabinet and table surfaces where used supplies and instruments may be discarded and the examination table that can have soiled table paper. Refer to Chapter 36 for standard precautions that should be followed when cleaning a room and using disinfectants.

After the examination table is cleaned, new table paper at the proper width to appropriately cover the table is pulled down. The paper is supplied in a roll that is inserted on a dowel under the head of the table. The jagged torn edge of the paper is folded and tucked under the seat section of the table for a neat appearance. It is important to check the amount of paper left on the roll periodically. Some tables accommodate two rolls so a replacement one would be available immediately if you ran out; otherwise, you would need to make a trip to the supply cabinet. The table pillow is covered by a disposable cover or towel that is discarded after each use and replaced with a fresh one.

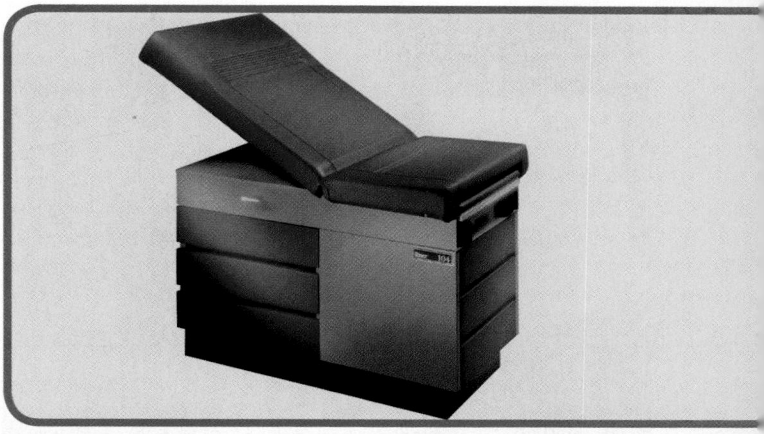

FIGURE 39–2A: A manual medical examination table commonly used in medical offices. *Courtesy of Midmark Corp.*

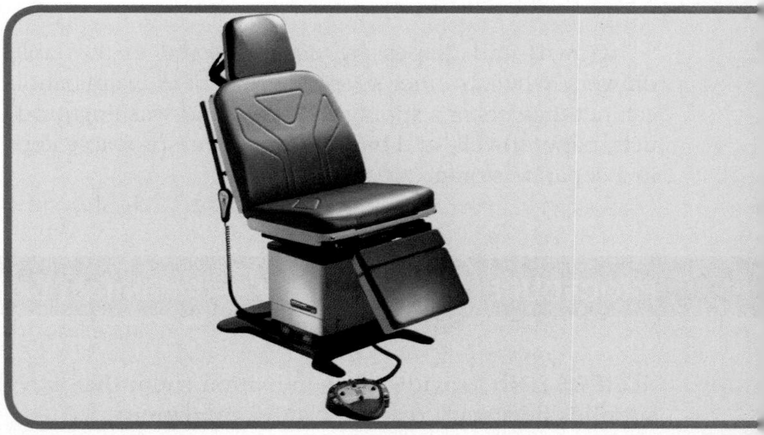

FIGURE 39–2B: A power table that can be adjusted by hand or foot controls. *Courtesy of Midmark Corp.*

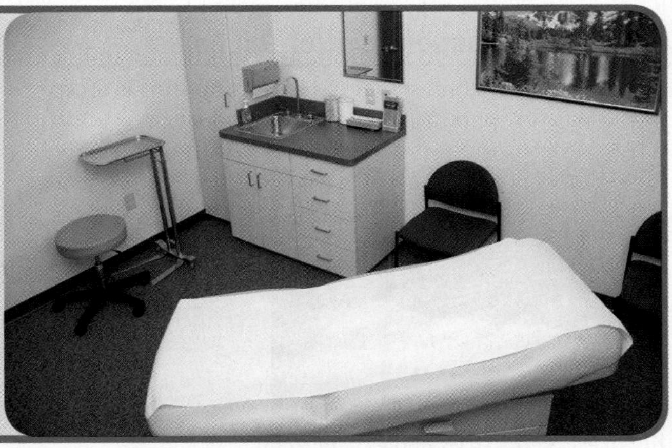

FIGURE 39–1: An example of a clean and well-organized exam room. *Delmar/Cengage Learning.*

Supplies and Equipment

Preparation also includes checking for all the supplies needed within the room, such as:

- A hand-washing product
- Biohazardous waste containers
- Face guards and gloves
- Patient gowns and drapes
- Paper towels, tissues
- A working light source
- Standard examination equipment (tongue blades, speculums, gauze squares, applicators, and so on)

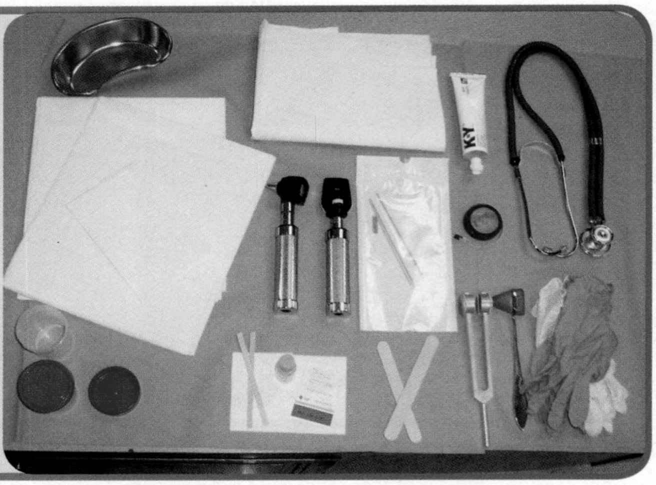

FIGURE 39–3: Standard examination equipment. *Delmar/Cengage Learning.*

Gowns and drapes are usually stored in the table drawers, whereas other supplies are kept in examination cabinet drawers or a supply cabinet. Hand-washing products, paper towels, and biohazard bags are probably kept in a separate storage area.

Table 39–1 Supplies Commonly Used for Patient Examinations

Stethoscope	Penlight
Gloves	Otoscope
Drapes	Ophthalmoscope
Tongue depressor	Lubricant
Percussion hammer	Basin
Tuning fork	Fecal occult blood test
Various specimen collection kits or containers	Tape measure

You may also need to prepare a tray of routine examination instruments used during the physical examination. The items commonly used for patient examinations are shown in Figure 39–3, and listed in Table 39–1. It is important for you to know the name and function of each item so you can anticipate the need and assist the provider if asked.

Procedure 39–1 provides guidelines on how to prepare and maintain an examination room.

PROCEDURE 39–1 Prepare and Maintain Examination and Treatment Areas

PURPOSE: To provide an examination room that is comfortable and clean and has the usual equipment and supplies necessary ready for an examination

EQUIPMENT: Disposable gloves, disinfectant, disposable cloth, exam table, pillow, table paper, patient gowns, drapes, hand-washing liquid, paper towels, gauze squares, examination light, biohazard and regular waste containers, and appropriate supplies and equipment (stethoscope, otoscope, ophthalmoscope, percussion hammer, pin wheel, hemocult supplies, lubricant, pelvic exam supplies, tissues, tape measure).

S SKILL: Prepare and maintain examination and treatment areas

Procedure Steps	Detailed Instructions and/or *Rationales*
1. Assess the room condition, temperature, furniture, and equipment.	Review Figure 39–4, which is an example of a room that is not prepared. 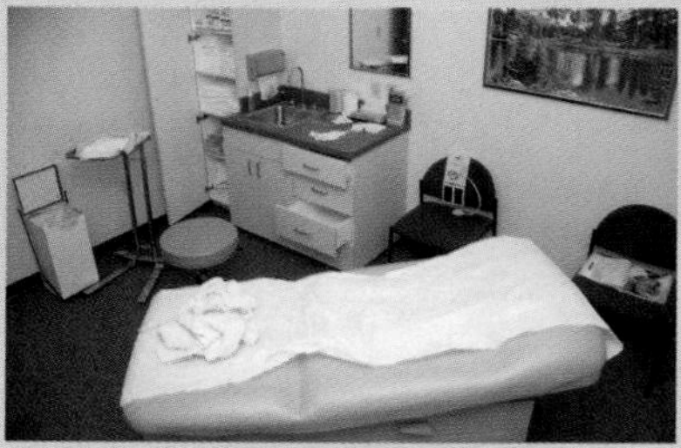 **Figure 39–4:** An example of an exam room that needs to be prepared for the patient. *Delmar/Cengage Learning.*

Procedure Steps	Detailed Instructions and/or *Rationales*
	You want to be sure the room is a comfortable environment for the patient. Check all furniture and equipment to be sure everything is in working order.
2. Wash hands and put on disposable gloves.	
3. Place used supplies and disposable examination equipment in the waste or biohazard container. Check the waste container for space; replace it if the bag is full.	*Depending on the use, supplies and equipment* can *potentially be exposed to microorganisms. Place the used items in the appropriate waste receptacle, depending on exposure, following standard precaution guidelines. Refer to Chapter 36 for guideline information.*
4. Tear the table paper near the top and roll it up with the pillow cover.	Dispose of it in the wastebasket unless contaminated with body fluid, then place it in the biohazard container. Be sure to follow standard precaution guidelines.
5. Wipe permanent examination equipment with disposable cloth or gauze squares and disinfectant.	*Prevents microorganism cross-contamination.*
6. Wipe the examination room table tops with disposable cloth and disinfectant if contaminated from discarded examination supplies. Prepare the exam table for the next patient: a. Pull down clean table paper, fold the ragged edge, and place it under the table seat. b. Place a clean cover on the pillow. c. Check the table paper supply, gowns, and drapes.	Prevents microorganism cross-contamination.
7. Wipe any other equipment contaminated by the provider, such as a stool or exam lamp.	*Prevents microorganism cross-contamination.*
8. Disinfect the examination table and dispose of the cloth in the appropriate container. Remove gloves and dispose and wash hands.	
9. Check the hand-washing dispenser and stock the supply.	
10. Check the paper towel dispenser and supply more if needed.	
11. Check the supplies in the cabinet and the examination table drawers and replace as needed.	*This ensures that all supplies needed by the provider are ready and available, preventing any delay in the patient exam.*
12. Make a final visual check of the room.	

PREPARING AND ASSISTING THE PATIENT

Making sure that patients have a good understanding of what they can expect from the visit and are made to feel as comfortable as possible are the first steps in preparing them for any examination. The medical assistant will probably be the main person with whom the patient interacts prior to the examination. It is important for the patient to feel comfortable in the surroundings and with the anticipated medical exam. Having the patient emotionally prepared goes a long way in helping the provider obtain an accurate assessment of a patient's condition.

> **CLINICAL PEARL**
>
> Some examinations can be embarrassing to a patient, but a clear explanation of each procedure can help relax him or her. You can assist the patient greatly by giving empathy and support and answering any questions he or she may have prior to the exam.

Many times, the provider will want the patient to prep prior to the exam in case laboratory testing is performed. Usually, patients are asked to fast so that specific diagnostic blood tests may be drawn. It can also be more comfortable when other procedures are performed if nothing has been eaten before the examination. In general, the fasting process usually begins at midnight the night before the exam and is indicated as (NPO), meaning "nothing by mouth." The patient needs to understand completely that he or she is to have nothing to eat or drink. Most providers allow the patient to have a small amount of water to take any medications that are prescribed to them or to brush their teeth, but other than that, they must refrain from everything else, including chewing gum or breath mints.

After the initial screening and vitals are taken, instruct the patient to empty his or her bladder. Often, the provider will want to obtain a urine specimen from the patient. If this is the case, provide a specimen container and instruct the patient to collect a sample for you to test. Allowing the patient time to empty his or her bladder will also make the examination process more comfortable.

If gowns and drapes are needed to facilitate examination, ask the patient to disrobe and instruct on how to wear a gown and apply the drape per the provider's preference. Patient gowns and drapes are made of cloth or disposable paper. Depending on the type of exam, the patient may be asked to have the gown either open to the front or open to the back.

After the gown and drapes are applied, ask the patient to have a seat on the examination table. Offer assistance with any of the tasks if the patient needs help. Some patients might need assistance when getting up on the examination table. If the examination table is too high for the patient to get on it comfortably, a foot stool should be provided. Never try to lift a patient who obviously weighs more than you can safely handle; have someone help you. (For more information on proper safety techniques with lifting and moving a patient, refer to the body mechanics section in Chapter 56.) If a patient needs help moving on the table, reach under the arm at the shoulder and help the person move up. You should move with the patient. Additionally, a very ill patient or a small child should never be left alone on a table; a member of the family should be asked to sit with him or her if you must leave the room.

If you are a female medical assistant, you may be asked to remain in the room when a female patient is being examined by a male provider (and vice versa). The rationale is that the patient should feel more relaxed, and the provider is protected from lawsuits that could result from patients claiming the provider acted improperly during the examination.

There may be a period of time before the provider enters the room. If the patient is anxious, this is a good time to reiterate the general format of the exam and answer any questions he or she may have. It can also be an excellent opportunity for patient education. Knowing about the pamphlets and other resources available in your office, you can talk with the patient and supply the material after the exam if the provider indicates. There are patient education boxes within this chapter and throughout the text that can give you some ideas upon which to build conversation and that have general information appropriate for discussion. This skill will become easier after you gain knowledge and experience.

> **PATIENT EDUCATION**
>
> To prevent injuries of the face and head:
>
> - In work and recreational environments, wear protective head gear: hard hat at work (construction sites), helmet for sports (motorcycle riding, football).
> - Wear protective face mask or goggles for sports such as football, hockey, and lacrosse to prevent possible eye injuries.
> - Use ear plugs to protect ears from exposure to loud noises (machinery, band concerts) that can lead to possible damage to auditory nerves resulting in hearing loss.

PATIENT EDUCATION

To protect the skin:

- Keep skin clean and soft by using mild soap and water for bathing and a moisturizing lotion as necessary.
- Discourage sun worship. Encourage remaining covered in the sun or the use of a sun blocker to prevent damage from ultraviolet rays if one must be in the sun for prolonged periods. Do not use tanning beds.
- Wash hands of (chemical) irritants immediately to prevent caustic burns.

PATIENT EDUCATION

To prevent diseases of the respiratory system and other contagious diseases:

- Discourage sharing utensils or drinking out of another person's glass to keep from transmitting viruses and diseases.
- Wash hands after handling items in or from public places (money, doorknobs, and soon).
- Discourage smoking or tobacco use of any kind. (Post antismoking pamphlets or meetings for patients to read.)
- Remind patients of the dangers of drug and alcohol use and abuse. (Display information about Alcoholics Anonymous meetings.)
- Encourage exercise and physical fitness programs with the advice of the provider.
- Promote proper nutrition and weight control by helping patients plan their diets and reminding them to eat well-balanced meals regularly.
- Encourage *safe sex* by providing explicit information to teach patients about the dangers of sexually transmitted diseases, hepatitis, and AIDS.
- Discourage patients from using laxatives and enemas unless specifically ordered by the provider.
- Remind patients about immunizations and encourage compliance.
- Encourage patients to read labels for contents of the products they buy and use for their safety.
- Remind patients to use seat belts.
- Promote regular medical and dental checkups.

WHEELCHAIR TRANSFERS

If a patient comes to your office in a wheelchair, it is important to know how to help that patient from the wheelchair to the examination table and back to the wheelchair. This is not an easy task to do alone if the patient is unable to support his or her own weight. Always enlist help from coworkers to prevent injury to the patient and yourself. Always remember to position the chair and lock the wheels before trying to help the patient move from the chair to the table. To make it easier to assist the patient to stand or walk, a wide-strap called a gait belt should be placed around the patient's waist. The belt provides a way to hold and support the patient while he or she is being transferred in and out of the wheelchair. The belt is grasped in the front to assist the patient to stand from a sitting position and is held in the back if supporting the patient while walking. Procedures 39–2 and 39–3 detail the steps on transferring a patient from a wheelchair to an exam table and vice versa.

PROCEDURE 39–2 Transfer a Patient from a Wheelchair to the Examination Table

PURPOSE: To move a patient safely from a wheelchair to an examination table

EQUIPMENT: Examination table, wheelchair, and gait belt

S SKILL: Transfer a patient from a wheelchair to the examination table.

Procedure Steps	Detailed Instructions and/or *Rationales*
1. Unlock the wheels of the chair and wheel the patient to the examination room.	*Wheelchairs should always be locked in position when sitting still to prevent unexpected movement. This is accomplished by flipping the brake on each wheel.*

(continues)

(continued)

Procedure Steps	Detailed Instructions and/or *Rationales*
2. Position the chair as near as possible to the place you want the patient to sit on the table. Lock the wheels on the chair.	
3. Lower the table to chair level.	Note: If this cannot be done, position a footstool beside the table and determine whether assistance will be needed.
4. Apply the gait belt (Figure 39–5A) and fold the footrests back (Figure 39–5B).	If necessary, assist the patient to move his or her feet.
5. Stand directly in front of the patient with your feet slightly apart.	To give a good base, place one foot forward, between the patient's legs.
6. Bend your knees and have the patient place his or her hands on your shoulders while you place your hands under the gait belt and assist the patient to a standing position.	Pause in this position for a moment before the next step.
7. Maintaining the position of your hands, pivot or side step to a position beside the table (Figure 39–5C).	
8. Place one foot slightly behind you for support and help the patient to a sitting position on the table.	
9. If it is necessary to use a stool, determine the assistance required and enlist the needed help *before* taking the patient from the wheelchair.	
10. While supporting the patient, stabilize the stool by placing your feet on the outside next to the legs and assist the patient to step onto the stool.	Caution: Be certain the patient steps onto the stool squarely to avoid tipping the stool.

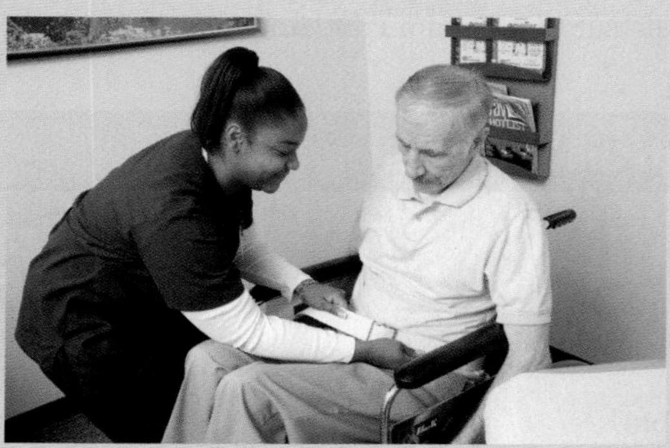

Figure 39–5A: A gait belt makes it easier to support the patient when walking.
Delmar/Cengage Learning.

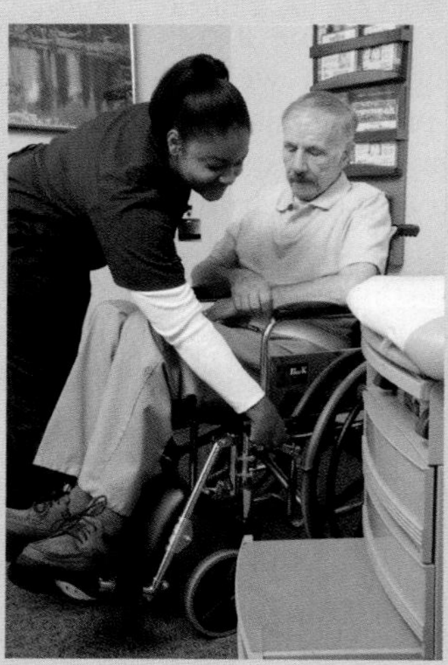

Figure 39–5B: Fold the footrests back.
Delmar/Cengage Learning.

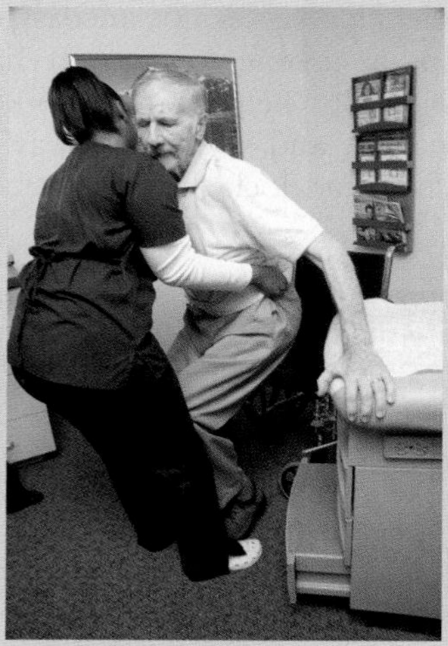

Figure 39–5C: Assisting a patient from a wheelchair.
Delmar/Cengage Learning.

Procedure Steps	Detailed Instructions and/or *Rationales*
11. Assist the patient to sit on the table (Figure 39–5D).	
12. If the patient needs assistance to lie down, place one hand around the patient's back. Help the patient raise his or her legs to the table by placing your free arm under the legs and lifting them as the patient turns.	Note: If the patient needs to remove clothing, get someone to help you. One person balances the patient while the other removes necessary clothing.
13. Place a pillow under the patient's head. Drape the patient appropriately.	*Never leave a very ill or weak patient alone on a table. There is danger of a fall.*
14. Unlock the chair wheels and move the chair out of the way.	Note: If the room is small, it may be necessary to place the chair outside the examination room.

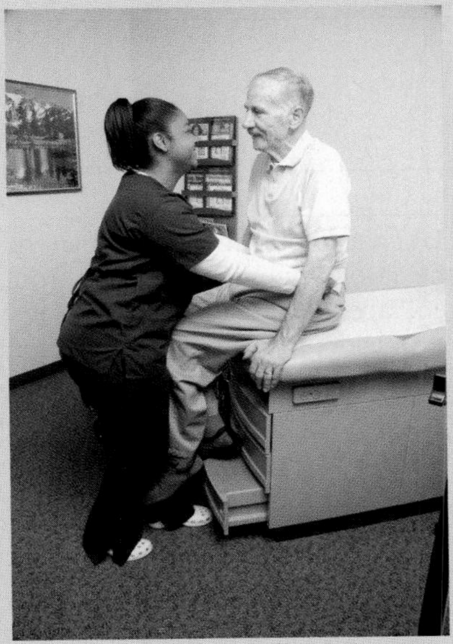

Figure 39–5D: Assist the patient to a comfortable sitting position.
Delmar/Cengage Learning.

PROCEDURE 39–3 Transfer a Patient from an Examination Table to a Wheelchair

MEDIA LINK: View the video clip for this chapter, "Transferring a patient from an exam table to a wheelchair," on the Premium Website.

PURPOSE: To move a patient safely from the examination table to a wheelchair

EQUIPMENT: Wheelchair, gait belt, and examination table

S **SKILL:** Transfer a patient from an examination table to a wheelchair.

Procedure Steps	Detailed Instructions and/or *Rationales*
1. Reposition the chair and lock the wheels.	
2. Assist the patient to a sitting position on the table.	Support the patient's back if necessary. Lift the patient's legs as the patient is turned until his or her feet dangle over the edge of the table.
B 3. Explain the procedure to the patient, ***using language the patient can understand, outlining what you will do and enlisting the patient's help.*** Assist the patient to dress if needed.	
4. Apply a gait belt to the patient.	
5. Move so you are directly in front of the patient. Grasp the patient on the sides below the armpits by placing your hands under the gait belt. Plant your feet a shoulder's width apart and bend your knees. Ask the patient to put his or her hands on your shoulders. Assist the patient to step onto the floor (or have a stepstool in place if the table cannot be lowered to chair height.)	Caution: Take special care to ensure that the patient steps squarely on the stool when getting down from the examining table. Place your feet against the legs of the footstool, on the outside, to maintain its position.
6. Support the patient into a standing position on the stool or floor. (If using a stool, help the patient step down from the stool.) Side step or pivot the patient to a position in front of the chair.	
B 7. Have the patient reach back to the arms of the chair as you help lower the patient into the chair. ***Ensure that the patient is comfortably seated.***	
8. Remove the gait belt from the patient and adjust the footrests.	
9. Unlock the wheels and return the patient to the reception room.	

EXAMINATION POSITIONS

A patient will be asked to assume certain positions to facilitate examination of the body. During a comprehensive physical examination, several of the standard positions may be used. The medical assistant must know their names and be able to assist the patient into each position. The following is a list of examination positions that will be discussed:

- Anatomical
- Sitting
- Horizontal recumbent (supine)
- Dorsal recumbent

- Prone
- Sims'
- Knee-chest
- Trendelenburg
- Fowler's
- Semi-Fowler's
- Lithotomy
- Jackknife or Kraske

Procedure 39–4 has step-by-step instructions for assisting patients to assume most of the examination positions. Performing this procedure will assist you in becoming familiar with their names, the patient's position, and the relationship between the examination and the position. This information, along with mastery of the skills is necessary before you begin to assist the provider to perform a partial or complete physician examination.

PATIENT EDUCATION

It is important to instruct the patient about the need for a specific position for the examination to be performed. This information should be included with the instructions on preparing for the examination. The patient should understand that the provider needs to examine certain parts of the body or perform certain procedures and tests, and the patient must be positioned in the most accessible manner.

The provider may begin the examination by asking the patient to assume the **anatomical** position, which means to stand erect, arms at sides with palms pointed forward. This allows a visual inspection of posture and is usually followed by requests to perform several movements (such as range-of-motion exercises). Next, the patient will be asked to sit at the end of the examination table, with the legs hanging down (sitting position). You should assist the patient as needed. If the patient is shorter in stature, it may be necessary to pull out the step from the bottom of the table or use a small stepping stool. Be careful to be sure the patient does not fall. Once seated on the table, a drape should be placed over the lap and legs for privacy and warmth. Several inspections and examinations are done with the patient in sitting position.

The patient will then be asked to lie down on the table. You will assist the patient to lie back and pull out the leg rest at the bottom of the table to support the patient's legs. A small pillow can be placed under the head for comfort. If a power table is used, and it is in the sitting position, press the appropriate button and reassure the patient as the table levels. Patients often feel like their head is lower than their body after being in an upright position. Readjust the drape as needed.

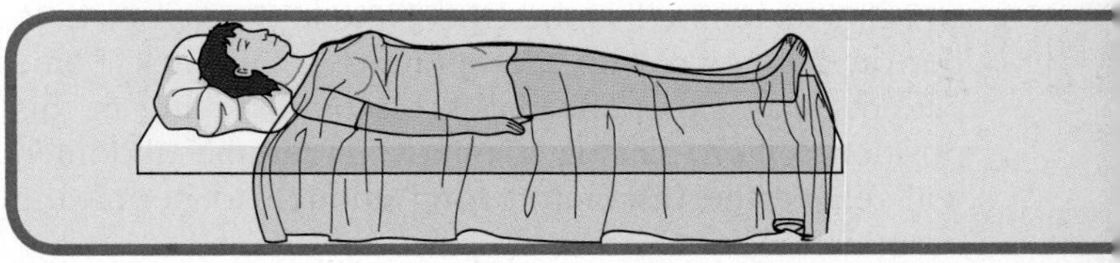

Figure 39–6: Horizontal recumbent or supine position. *Delmar/Cengage Learning.*

The **horizontal** recumbent or **supine** position is used for examination and treatment of the **anterior** portion of the body, including the breasts and abdominal organs (Figure 39–6). The term **recumbent** means lying down. The **dorsal recumbent** position indicates that the knees are bent (Figure 39–7), which allows for relaxation of the abdominal muscles and thus easier examination of the abdominal area. This position may also be used for digital vaginal or rectal examination. The gown is open in the front, and a drape sheet of cloth or paper is used to cover the patient from the neck down.

During a complete physical, the provider may request the patient to turn over so the **dorsal** surface may be examined. This is called the **prone** position (Figure 39–8) and is used to examine the spine and structures of the back. Assist the patient as necessary to turn over, instructing him or her to turn toward you. Watch to be certain the patient does not get too close to the edge when turning and fall off the table. Instruct the patient to lie face down with his or her arms folded to make a place to rest the head. Because the gown was originally put on with the opening in the front, it will be necessary to pull the gown up to expose the back. Reposition the drape from the upper back to the feet to cover the exposed area. When the dorsal surface

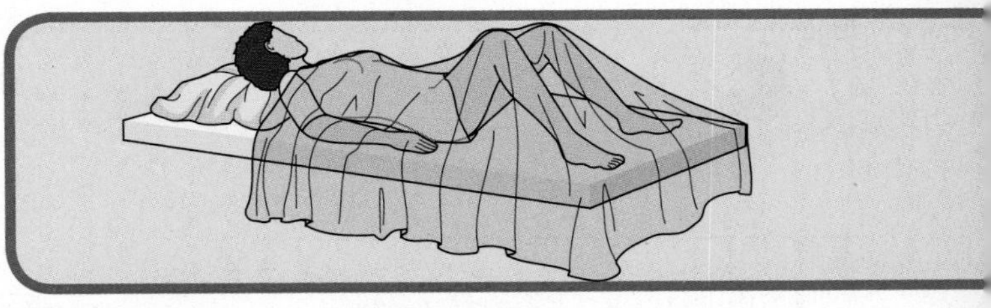

Figure 39–7: Dorsal recumbent position. *Delmar/Cengage Learning.*

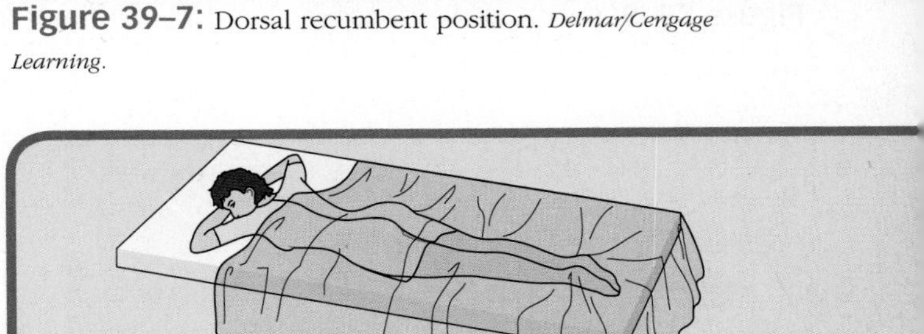

Figure 39–8: Prone position. *Delmar/Cengage Learning.*

is being examined alone, the patient is instructed to put on the gown with the opening in the back. Some patients may experience back discomfort lying in this position. Often placing a pillow under the abdomen will relieve the discomfort long enough to permit the examination.

The **Sims'** position is used in examination and treatment of the rectal area and for enemas, rectal temperature, and instilling rectal medications (Figure 39–9). This position may also be used for perineal and some pelvic examinations. This is also referred to as the lateral recumbent position. The patient is positioned on his or her left side with the left arm extended behind the body and the right arm flexed upward. A pillow under the head adds to the comfort of this position. The left leg may be slightly flexed, but the right leg is sharply flexed upward. The drape should cover at least from the axillary area to below the knees. The drape is raised to permit examination or treatment of the rectal area.

The **knee-chest** position (Figure 39–10) is a difficult position for patients to assume. The chest and knees are placed flat against the table with the knees separated. The arms can be crossed under the head or flexed to each side with the head turned to the side. The buttocks extend upward with the back straight. Patients will need support and assistance in assuming and maintaining this position; therefore, you must remain with the patient while he or she is in this position. The patient should not be placed in the position until the provider is ready to do the examination. If the patient cannot get into the knee-chest position, it can be modified to a knee-elbow position, which is easier to assume and maintain.

The knee-chest position is used for rectal or **proctological** examinations and occasionally for a **sigmoidoscopy** if a proctological table is not available. The position causes the intestinal organs to move toward the chest, thereby somewhat straightening the sigmoid colon to facilitate insertion of instruments. The patient is commonly covered with a fenestrated drape, in which a special opening provides access to the area being examined.

The **Fowler's** position is used for patients with respiratory or cardiovascular problems. The patient who is having **dyspnea** must be in a sitting or semi-sitting position to breathe comfortably. This position is also used to examine the trunk of the body (head, neck, and chest area). The patient may simply sit upright at the foot of the table or be supported by the back of the examination table. When the patient's upper body is at a 90-degree angle to the table, it is known as a Fowler's position (refer to Figure 39–11 B). If the patient is resting against the back of the table and it is lowered to a 45-degree angle, it is known as the semi-Fowler's position (refer to Figure 39–11 A). The patient gown should open in the front, and the drape should cover from the axillary area down to the feet. When the high Fowler's position is used, the drape will naturally fall to cover from the top of the legs to over the feet.

The **lithotomy** position is used for vaginal or rectal examination (Figure 39-12). This position can also be used for examination of the male genital area and for catheterization of a female patient. The primary use of the position is for vaginal examinations of the female patient when a speculum is inserted, as when obtaining Pap smears.

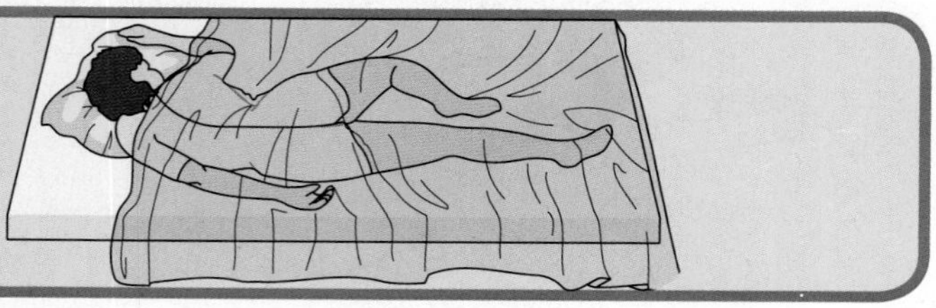

Figure 39–9: Sims' position. *Delmar/Cengage Learning.*

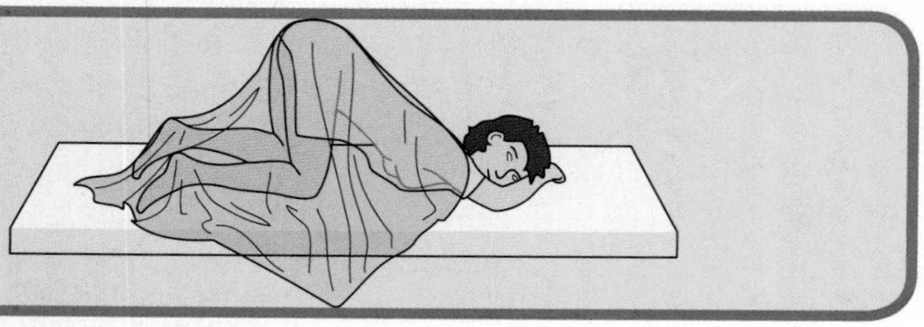

Figure 39–10: Knee-chest position. *Delmar/Cengage Learning.*

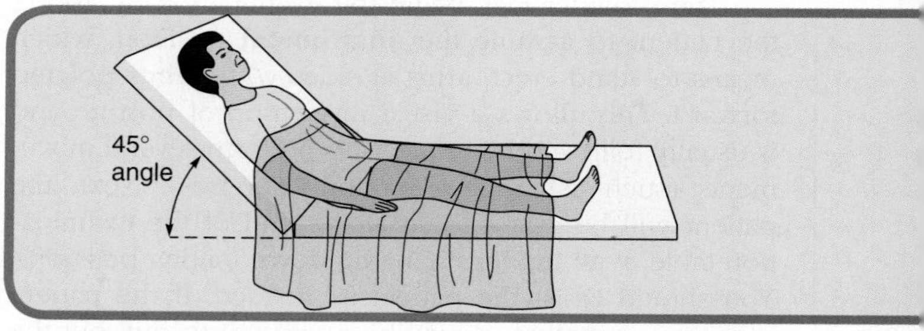

Figure 39–11A: Semi-Fowler's position. *Delmar/Cengage Learning.*

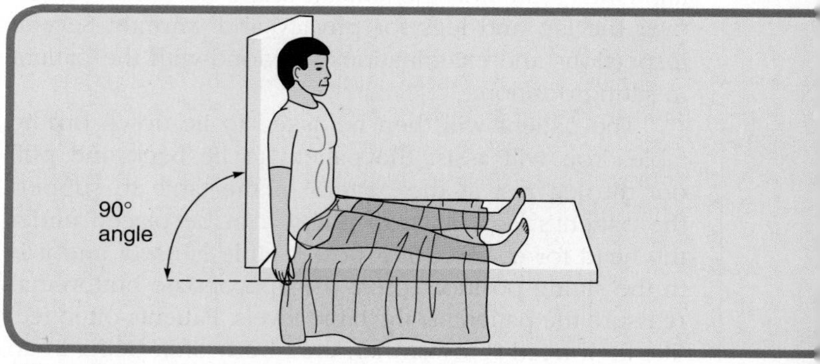

Figure 39–11B: Fowler's position. *Delmar/Cengage Learning.*

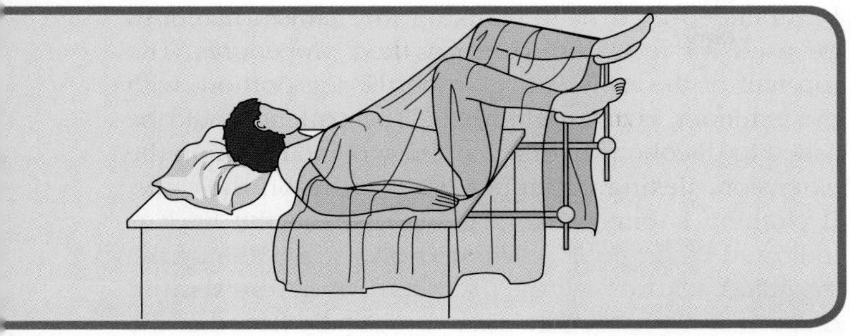

Figure 39–12: Lithotomy position. *Delmar/Cengage Learning.*

Assisting a patient into the lithotomy position requires her first to sit at the end of the table and then lie back. The leg support may be extended temporarily. A drape is placed over the patient from the chest to the feet, usually in the shape of a diamond. Placing the drape with one corner between the legs will make the exam easier in this position. The stirrups are extended from the table and tightened or secured into position. They should be extended far enough to allow the patient to be comfortable to facilitate abdominal relaxation and prevent leg cramps. The legs are flexed, and the heel of each foot is placed in a stirrup. The patient is instructed to slide down so that the hips are at the edge of the table. A pillow under the head will make the patient more comfortable. The arms may be crossed over the abdomen or placed at the sides. You should ensure that the patient is as comfortable as possible and provide support for the anxious patient.

Additional Body Positions

Two additional body positions need mentioning but are used infrequently in most providers' offices: The Trendelenburg and the Jackknife or Kraske. In the **Trendelenburg** or **shock** position, the patient is supine with the feet elevated slightly (Figure 39–13 A). This position may easily be accomplished with a power table. The controls would automatically lower the head of the table while keeping the patient in supine or horizontal recumbent position. With a manual table, the top section can be raised to elevate the thighs and hips, thereby achieving a lower position for the head and a modified Trendelenburg position. The lower legs are bent over the end of the table to maintain the position (Figure 39–13 B). The patient is typically draped from the neck, or the axillary, to the knees. This position would be used if a patient experiences or has symptoms of syncope. Patients may experience difficulty when blood samples are drawn or intravenous therapy is given or with some examinations.

Trendelenburg positioning is frequently used in a critical care facility and by EMS personnel with trauma, hemorrhage, and dangerously low blood pressure. It is also beneficial in certain abdominal and pelvic surgical procedures to

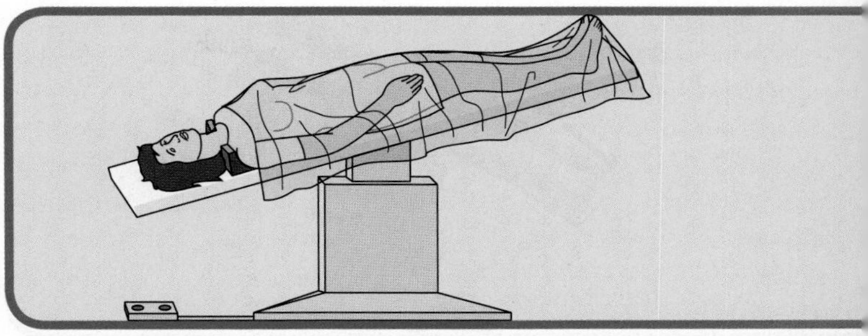

Figure 39–13A: Trendelenburg or shock position with power table. *Delmar/Cengage Learning.*

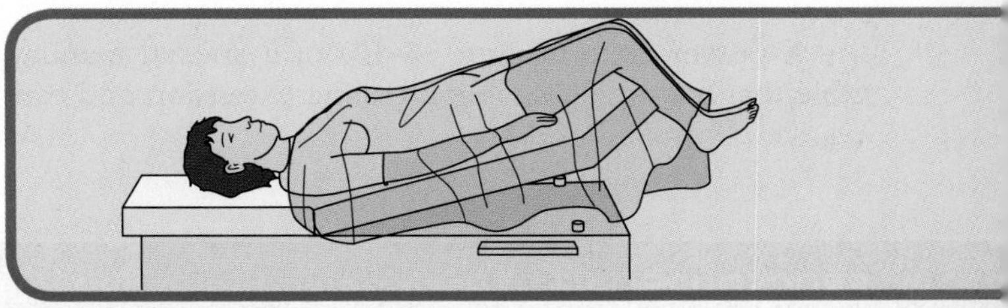

Figure 39–13B: Modified Trendelenburg with manual table. *Delmar/Cengage Learning.*

displace organs upward. The position can also be used as a simple test for **incompetent** valves in persons with varicose veins. After being placed in straight-line Trendelenburg, the patient is asked to stand, and the provider observes whether the veins fill from above or below.

A special table is needed for the jackknife, or Kraske, position to be comfortable. The patient is positioned lying flat on their abdomen. The special table is then raised in the middle with a fold so the hips and pelvic area is lifted and the legs and head remain low (Figure 37-14). This position is especially useful for surgeries related to the rectum, anus and coccyx, as well as examination and treatment of rectal and anal conditions such as thrombosed and internal hemorrhoids. Draping is from the mid-back to the knees.

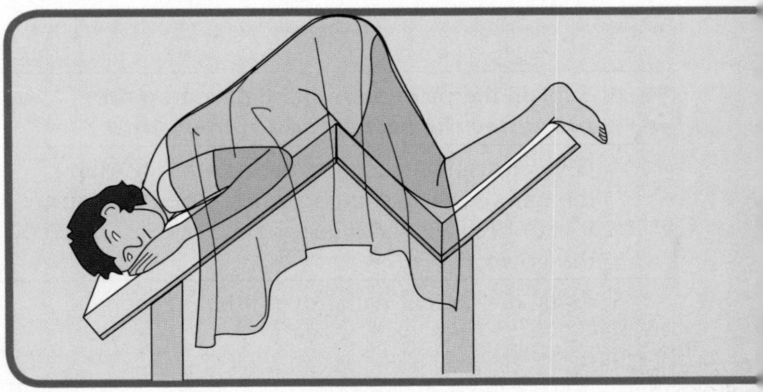

Figure 39–14: Jackknife, or Kraske, position. *Delmar/Cengage Learning.*

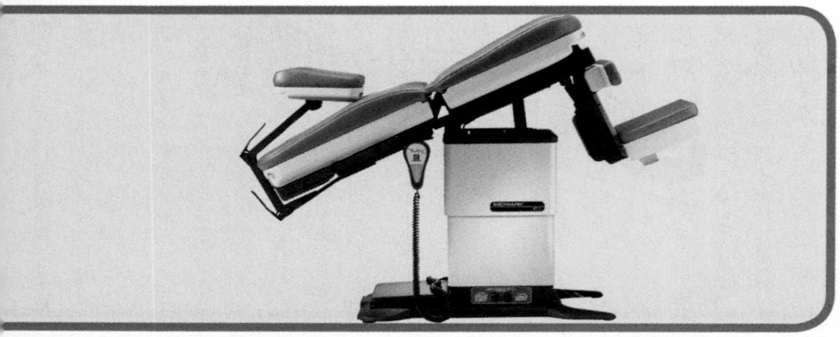

Figure 39–15: The Midmark power table in position for specialty exams. *Courtesy of Midmark Corp.*

A power table (Figure 37–15) or a special manual table that has an attachable kneeling extension and can be upended by a hand-cranking mechanism may also be used for rectal examinations and procedures. The top half of the table is flat, while the leg portion, with the extender, is at a right angle. The patient would be asked to disrobe from the waist down and kneel on the extension, flexing his upper body to lie on the table. If clothing is one piece, a gown open in the back is indicated. A drape is positioned over the patient from the mid-back down past the knees or a **fenestrated** drape may be used. The arms are usually flexed at the side or under the head. The medical assistant operates the controls or cranks the table over until the buttocks are elevated. The head is lower than the body, and the internal abdominal organs move toward the chest. This helps straighten the "S" curve of the sigmoid colon to facilitate sigmoidoscope insertion during a sigmoidoscopy, as discussed in Chapter 39.

PROCEDURE 39–4 Positioning the Patient for an Exam

MEDIA LINK: View the video for this chapter, "Positioning the Patient" on the Premium Website.

PURPOSE: To assist the patient into a variety of positions used in general physical and other examinations

EQUIPMENT: Adjustable examination table, table paper, gown, drape sheet, pillow, disposable pillow cover

S **SKILL:** Demonstrate positioning a patient for a variety of examinations.

Procedure Steps	Detailed Instructions and/or *Rationales*
1. Check the examination room for cleanliness.	Always have clean paper on the table and a clean pillow cover or clean towel over the pillow. *Every precaution must be maintained to prevent any possible cross-contamination of disease.*
2. Identify the patient and introduce yourself.	*Speaking to the patient by name and checking the chart ensures that you are performing the procedure on the correct patient.*
B 3. Explain the procedure to the patient, ***using language the patient can understand.***	
4. Give clear instructions to the patient regarding the amount of clothing to be removed and where it is to be placed and instruct the patient in use of the gown.	*The procedure to be performed dictates whether the front or back should be open.*
5. Assist the patient with gown if help is needed.	*If no help is needed, respect the privacy and modesty of the patient by leaving the room while the patient changes.*

Procedure Steps	Detailed Instructions and/or *Rationales*
6. Assist the patient onto the examination table if help is needed.	
7. Explain to the patient the necessary exam and the position required.	*For some examinations, multiple positions may be needed. Be sure the patient is aware of the position he or she will be assisted into and confirm that he or she is comfortable with this prior to positioning.*
8. Assist the patient into the required position:	A pillow may be used for patient support in any of the positions to aid comfort.
a. Anatomical	Patient stands up straight
b. Sitting	Patient sits at the edge of the examination table, drape on lap covering legs
c. Horizontal recumbent (supine)	Patient lies flat on the back, drape from neck to feet
d. Dorsal recumbent	Patient lies face up, flat on back with knees bent, drape from neck to feet
e. Prone	Patient lies flat, face down, drape from upper back to feet
f. Sims'	Patient lies on left side, leg slightly bent, arm placed behind back, drape from axillary to knees
g. Knee-chest	Patient lies on table face down, supporting body with knees and chest, fenestrated drape used, covering area to be examined
h. Trendelenburg	Patient is in the supine position on a tilted table with head lower than legs
i. Fowler's	Patient lies back on exam table on which head is elevated 90 degrees, drape from waist down
j. Semi-Fowler's	Patient lies back on exam table on which head is elevated 45 degrees, drape from chest down
k. Lithotomy	Patient lies on back with knees bent and feet in the stirrups, drape diamond shape, chest to feet
9. Drape the sheet evenly over the patient but leave loose on all sides.	
10. Assist the patient from the table when the examination is completed.	Patient may be dizzy from the change in position. Allow him or her to sit upright before standing. Clean the room and replace the supplies. *The examination table surface and base must be thoroughly cleaned with disinfecting cleanser at regular intervals and following any contact with body fluids that may contain bloodborne pathogens.*

Now that you have been trained in the skills needed for positioning and draping the patient for physical and other examinations, we will continue in the next unit with the examination process as we proceed through a complete physical examination, OB/GYN exam, and pediatric exam.

CHAPTER SUMMARY

- Supplies used in the preparation of the exam room will vary depending on the provider's preference and the exam being performed; however, common ones include (but are not limited to) hand-washing products; biohazardous and regular waste containers; face guards; gloves; patient gowns; drapes; paper towels; tissues; an examination light source; and standard examination equipment such as tongue blades, speculums, gauze squares, and applicators.
- Preparation and maintenance of the examination room for an exam is also the responsibility of the medical assistant (see Procedure 39–1). Ensure that the room is clean and tidy and at a comfortable temperature.
- Between patient examinations, all surfaces within the room that might be contaminated should be cleaned with a disinfectant between patient examinations. The examination table is cleaned and new table paper and pillow cover is applied. Discard all disposable items into the proper waste receptacle and non-disposables in the laundry bin. Put all reusable supplies in the proper storage area, restock any used items, spray disinfectant or deodorizer if needed.
- Proper transfer techniques for assisting patients from their wheelchair to the exam table and back again is imperative to ensure that injuries don't occur. This is not an easy task to do alone if the patient is unable to support his or her own weight. Always enlist help from coworkers to prevent injury to the patient and yourself.
- Several positions may be incorporated into a patient examination; it may be your responsibility to assist the patient into the various positions appropriate for the provider's examination. Safety and patient comfort must be made a priority in any positioning that occurs. Refer to Procedure 39–4 for a comprehensive list of positions and reasons for their use.
- Draping for the various positions is essential for patient comfort and privacy. Patient gowns and drapes should be positioned so that only the portion of the body being examined is exposed. Positions may frequently change, so be prepared to assist the provider with the changes and keep the patient adequately covered.

STUDY TOOLS

Workbook	Activities for Chapter 39
Premium Website	
MEDIA LINK	View these **Media Links** for Chapter 39: • Transferring a Patient from a Wheelchair • Positioning the Patient
StudyWARE	Activities and Quizzes on the **StudyWARE™ Software** for Chapter 39
	Complete the following Competency Challenge 2.0 activity: • Tuesday, 10:00 AM, Prepare Patients for Exams
	Audio Library of medical terms
	Online access to the **Critical Thinking Challenge 2.0**
learninglab	Module 17: Preparing for Clinical Procedures
CourseMate	Activities and Quizzes for Chapter 39
WebTutor	Activities and Quizzes for Chapter 39

CHECK YOUR KNOWLEDGE

1. The primary use of this position is for vaginal examinations of the female patient when a speculum is inserted, as when obtaining pap smears.
   a. Trendelenburg
   b. Lithotomy
   c. Fowler's
   d. Semi-Fowler's
2. These supplies are usually stored in the table drawers, whereas other supplies are kept in examination cabinet drawers or a supply cabinet.
   a. Tongue depressors
   b. Gauze squares
   c. Gowns and drapes
   d. Applicators
3. The lateral recumbent position is another term that may be used to describe the following position.
   a. Sims'
   b. Lithotomy
   c. Supine
   d. Prone
4. Which position would be used if a patient experiences or has symptoms of syncope?
   a. Prone
   b. Trendelenburg
   c. Sims'
   d. Anatomical
5. The horizontal recumbent or supine position is used for examination and treatment of the _____ portion of the body, including the breasts and abdominal organs.
   a. posterior
   b. superior
   c. inferior
   d. anterior
6. Which position would be used for patients with respiratory or cardiovascular problems?
   a. Fowler's
   b. Prone
   c. Knee-chest
   d. Jackknife

WEB LINKS

Occupational Safety and Health Administration:
www.osha.gov

RESOURCES

Corning Metpath Laboratories. (1996). *Patient Education* [Pamphlet]. Columbus, OH: Author.

Diagnostic tests, nurse's ready reference. (1991). Springhouse, PA: Springhouse Corporation.

Estes, M. E. Z. (2010). *Health Assessment & Physical Examination.* Clifton Park, NY: Delmar Cengage Learning.

Heller, M., and Veach, L. (2009). *Clinical Medical Assisting: A Professional, Field Smart Approach to the Workplace.* Clifton Park, NY: Delmar, Cengage Learning.

Lindh, W., Pooler, M., Tamparo, C., and Dahl, B. (2010). *Delmar's Comprehensive Medical Assisting Administrative and Clinical Competencies* (4th ed.). Clifton Park, NY: Delmar Cengage Learning.

Venes, D. (ed.). (2009). *Taber's Cyclopedic Medical Dictionary* (21st ed.). Philadelphia: F. A. Davis.

Unit

13

Assisting with Examinations

From Chapter 39 you learned that, as a medical assistant, the responsibility of preparing patients for examinations and procedures performed by the providers is mainly yours. In this unit, your role in the patient examination process is stressed. We discuss the preparation of the patient for physical examinations and other procedures and examinations. The performance of several evaluation tests for the eye and ear are discussed as well as your role in assisting with or serving as a scribe for the physical examination. Many of the common specialty examinations and procedures as well as the specific examinations and procedures for assessing the OB/GYN and pediatric patient are also examined.

An important and continuing role for you as a medical assistant is educating the patient in healthful activities and disease or disorder management. Often, opportunities for patient teaching occur before, during, and after the examination process. The medical assistant can make note of these and provide instructional sheets, pamphlets, community resources, and personal instruction following the provider's examination. Many topics are appropriate for discussion within Patient Education boxes throughout this unit.

Certification Connection

	Ch. 40	Ch. 41	Ch. 42
CMA (AAMA)			
Principles of equipment operation	X	X	X
Examinations	X	X	X
Procedures	X	X	X
Patient education	X	X	X
Vision testing	X		
Hearing testing	X		
Respiratory testing	X		
Immunizations			X
RMA (AMT)			
Instruments	X	X	X
Methods of examination	X		
Specialty examinations	X	X	X
Visual acuity	X		
Terminology	X	X	X

Chapter

40 The Physical Exam, Specialty Exams, and Procedures

OBJECTIVES

In this chapter, you will learn the following:

KB KNOWLEDGE BASE

1. Spell and define, using the glossary at the back of the text, all the Words to Know in this chapter.
2. Discuss the reasons a complete physical examination is performed.
3. Explain the role of the medical assistant in the examination process.
4. Discuss patient education as it relates to breast and testicular self-examination and why physical examinations are performed.
5. Name the six examination techniques used by physicians and give examples of each.
6. Discuss the physical examination format for providers and the body systems that are examined.
7. Discuss the examination and specialty procedures routinely performed on patients. (Refer to Table 40–1.)
8. Explain why irrigation of the ear is performed.
9. Describe the audiometric assessment procedures used to assess hearing acuity.
10. Explain why irrigation of the eye is performed.
11. Identify three vision screening tests and explain what they determine.
12. Describe a spirometry test and state the purpose of it.
13. Explain what a peak flow meter measures and why its use may be indicated.
14. Describe pulse oximetry testing and why it is performed.
15. Explain what a flexible sigmoidoscopy can help diagnose.

S SKILLS

1. Prepare a patient for and assist with a routine physical exam.
2. Perform ear irrigation.
3. Perform eye irrigation.
4. Measure distant vision acuity with a Snellen chart.
5. Measure near vision acuity with a Jaeger chart.
6. Determine color vision acuity using Ishihara plates.
7. Perform spirometry testing.
8. Perform peak flow measuring.
9. Perform pulse oximetry testing.
10. Assist with a flexible sigmoidoscopy procedure.

B BEHAVIOR

1. Apply critical thinking skills in performing patient assessment and care.
2. Use language and verbal skills that enable patients' understanding.
3. Demonstrate respect for diversity in approaching patients and families.
4. Demonstrate awareness of the territorial boundaries of the person with whom communicating.

WORDS TO KNOW

acuity
audiometer
auscultation
bimanual
bruit
cerumen
coordination
decibel
digital rectal exam (DRE)
duration
enema
evacuant
fecal
flexible sigmoidoscope
funduscopy
gait
guaiac test paper
heartburn
heart murmur
hernia
inspection
irrigate
Ishihara
Jaeger chart
lavage
laxative
lumen
manipulation
mucosa
obturator
occluder
occult
palpation
peak flow
percussion
peripheral
physical
pitch
polyps
proctoscope
pulse oximetry
resonance
scribe
Snellen chart
spirometer
symmetry
tonometry
turgor
vertex
visceral
vital capacity

THE COMPLETE PHYSICAL EXAMINATION

The primary reason for performing a complete physical examination (CPE) is to determine the general state of health and well-being of the patient. The CPE can be performed for various reasons, such as an insurance examination before issuing a policy, as a requirement with a patient's employment, as a request by a patient, or to assess a patient's state of health. The exam will cover all major organs and systems of the body. The provider's findings enable him or her to establish an opinion about the patient's condition and establish either a tentative or definitive diagnosis when there are abnormal signs and symptoms. Often, laboratory tests or diagnostic procedures are ordered to provide additional information upon which to base the diagnosis. After all data is obtained, the diagnosis is defined and the treatment plan, if indicated, can be established.

The Medical Assistant's Role

As you read in Chapter 39, the medical assistant has many responsibilities in preparing for examinations, including setting up the room and supplies as well as preparing the patient for the exam. During the CPE, you will position the patient, hand examination instruments and supplies to the provider, and provide comfort to the patient as needed. Assisting with the CPE, the general physical exam, history and physical (H and P), physical exam (PE), or just plain **physical** (as it is often termed) is not difficult but is complex in that it is a *set* of procedures. You might also assist with the exam or scribe the findings per the provider.

In many facilities, the medical assistant accompanies the provider in the examination room and records the findings. The term **scribe** is given to the medical assistant who writes what the provider dictates during the exam. To perform this duty well, it is important to have sound knowledge in medical terminology, anatomy, and physiology in addition to good spelling and writing skills. Because the provider bases the diagnosis on these findings, accuracy is vital. Many providers prefer to write their own findings on the progress notes or preprinted physical forms in an outlined order of their choice (see Figure 40–1). Other providers prefer to dictate the findings of an examination into a recorder for transcription later by the medical assistant or medical transcriptionist. With the use of EHR becoming more common, the provider enters findings directly into the software as the examination is conducted (Figure 40–2).

There is no one set format for the examination as long as the provider is consistent, thorough, and complete with each patient. Some providers use the review of systems and physical examination portion of a history and physical examination form (Figure 40–3). In your career as a medical assistant, you might work with providers who may be quite different in their systematic approach to patient examination.

Physical Exam

PLACE PATIENT LABEL HERE

Patient ID #____________________ DATE OF EXAM ___/___/___

❑ New Pt. Well-Woman Exam ❑ New Pt. Problem ❑ Est. Pt. Well-Woman Exam ❑ Est. Pt. Problem

NAME

AGE **DOB** **LMP**

Current MEDS

Current BCM

ALLERGIES

PFSH of ___/___/___ **Reviewed** ❑ No changes ❑ Updated

STI RISKS: Change in partner since last exam? ❑ Yes ❑ No

Are both pt and partner mutually monogamous? ❑ Yes ❑ No

Current partner's STI status: ❑ HSV ❑ HBV ❑ HCV ❑ Unknown

Partners: ❑ Men ❑ Women ❑ Both

❑ Vaginal ❑ Oral ❑ Anal Sex

With partner_________ wks / mos / yrs

EDUCATION [if oral, if written]

❑ Contraceptive options
❑ Method education
❑ Exam/lab findings discussed
❑ Breast health
❑ Problem education
❑ UTI / Cystitis
❑ Anemia / Iron / Diet
❑ Cholesterol management
❑ Infertility
❑ Menopause
❑ HT / ET
❑ Parental involvement
❑ Medications prescribed
____
❑ Initial PT education
❑ Assessment / Plan discussed
❑ STI / HIV education / Safer sex
❑ Vaginitis / Vaginal infection
❑ Partner treatment
❑ Stop smoking
❑ Weight control / Diet / Exercise
❑ Options × 3 (Pregnancy)
❑ Preconception / Folic Acid
❑ Osteoporosis / Calcium
❑ EC offered
❑ Abstinence
❑ HPV vaccine
❑ Other ________________

PATIENT INFORMATION (PI) PROVIDED

PIICs
❑ The Pill
❑ The Ring
❑ The Patch
❑ Special Considerations
❑ HOPE
❑ DMPA
❑ EC
❑ POPs
❑ IUC
❑ IUC with Special Conditions
❑ IUC Use Beyond Recommendations
❑ Misoprostol for GYN Procedures
❑ Barriers
❑ Implants
❑ STI TX without an Exam

PIs Provided in:
❑ English
❑ Other:____________

❑ Treatment of Genital Warts
❑ Treatment of Bartholin's Duct

Cyst or Abscess
❑ PID
❑ Endometrial Biopsy
❑ Services Related to the Menopause

PIs
❑ Herbal Medicine
❑ Instructions for use of the Ring
❑ Instructions for use of the Patch
❑ Pregnancy with an IUC in Place
❑ Condoms and Female Condoms
❑ Sepermicide for Birth Control
❑ Directions for Chlamydia

Treatment of Sex Partners
❑ UTI
❑ Pregnancy Testing, Evaluation & Options Services

S: Reason for Visit / Chief Complaint / History of Present illness

VITAL SIGNS

❑ BP________ ❑ Weight________ ❑ Height ________ ❑ Temp ________

O; Examination / Physical Findings

SYSTEM	WNL	OTHER
GENERAL	❑ No acute distress, grossly WNL	
EYES	❑ Grossly WNL	
ENMT	❑ Grossly WNL	
CV	❑ RRR ❑ Murmurs	
RESP	❑ Clear to auscultation, equal breath sounds	
GI	❑ Abdomen soft / non-tender, no masses ❑ Liver/spleen non-palpable ❑ Rectal exam (req. ≥ age 50) no masses / blood	
GU	❑ Breasts w/no masses/discharge/tenderness ❑ No urethral discharge ❑ No CVAT ❑ Vulva, no lesions, skin intact w/no discoloration ❑ Vagina, normal color, no unusual discharge, no Bartholin enlargement/tenderness ❑ Cervix, no lesions, no contact bleeding ❑ Uterus, NS / NT / mobile / no CMT ❑ AF ❑ AV ❑ RF ❑ RV ❑ Adnexa, non-tender w/no masses	
MUSC.	❑ Back w/no curvature ❑ Extremities full ROM	
SKIN	❑ Intact w/no lesions ❑ Piercing ❑ Tattoo If yes, where ? _____	
ENDO	❑ Thyroid NS / NT / equal bilateral	
LYMPH	❑ No lymphadenopathy neck /axilla / groin	

LAB TESTS DONE

❑ Hct __________

❑ Urine Dip (circle): Glucose Protein Nitrites Leukocytes

❑ Pregnancy Test Pos Neg ❑ Slide Pap ❑ Liquid Based Pap ❑ HSV ❑ GC ❑ CT

❑ HPV ❑ Other: ___________

❑ Wet Mount: KOH Saline WNL + Clue/+ Whiff pH____ +Hyphae +Trich

WBC _____hpf

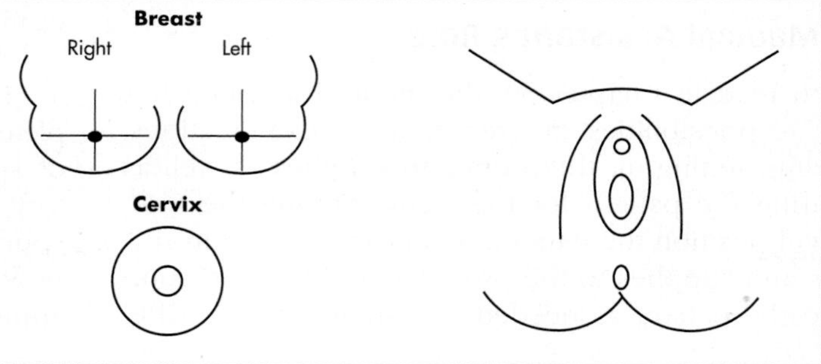

Figure 40–1: Example of a preprinted general physical exam form. *Delmar/Cengage Learning.*

Physical Exam

PLACE PATIENT LABEL HERE

ASSESSMENT

PLAN

Referral provided for ______________________ Referral to ______________________
❑ Explained nature and implication of abnormal findings.
❑ Explained consequences of not receiving additional care.
❑ Explained management option and referral.
❑ Explained responsibility to obtain follow-up care.

Patient demonstrated understanding of education / findings / plan by
❑ Asking appropriate questions / returning
❑ Interpreter / Language Line. Provided by (name/relationship) ______________
❑ Other______________

PRESCRIPTION

❑ DMPA 150 mg IM/Sq q 12 weeks × 5 ❑ Given today
❑ OCs________ Sig: 1 qd × 1 yr # _____ today _____
❑ NuvaRing PV × 3 wks; out for 1 wk. × 1 yr # _____ today
❑ Ortho Evra 1 patch/wk × 3, none for 1 wk. × 1 yr # _____ today
Start: ❑ Sunday p next menses ❑ Day ____ ❑ Today ❑ Continue
❑ IUD ❑ ParaGard ❑ Mirena Date inserted: ________
❑ Implanon Date inserted ________
❑ Condoms #______ requested by client for ❑ contraception/BUM ❑ STD prevention
❑ Other__________

❑ OK for emergency pack of pills if needed
❑ Advanced Rx EC × 1 year ____ today ❑ EC now: ____

INTERVIEWER ______________________ CLINICIAN ______________________

DATE ______________________

Figure 40–1: *(continued)*

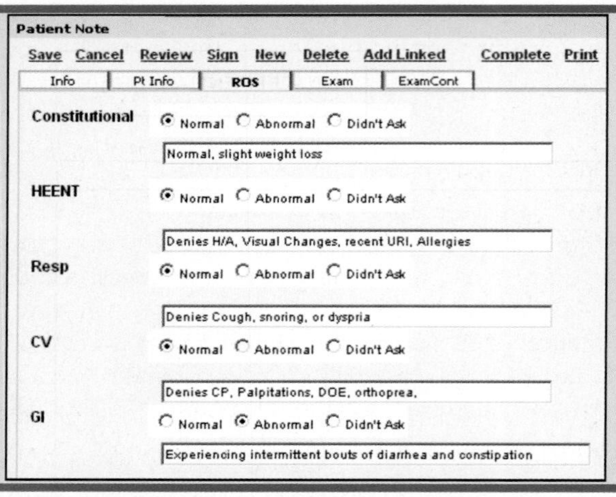
Patient Note

Save Cancel Review Sign New Delete Add Linked Complete Print

Info | Pt Info | ROS | Exam | ExamCont

Constitutional ◉ Normal ○ Abnormal ○ Didn't Ask
Normal, slight weight loss

HEENT ◉ Normal ○ Abnormal ○ Didn't Ask
Denies H/A, Visual Changes, recent URI, Allergies

Resp ◉ Normal ○ Abnormal ○ Didn't Ask
Denies Cough, snoring, or dyspria

CV ◉ Normal ○ Abnormal ○ Didn't Ask
Denies CP, Palpitations, DOE, orthoprea,

GI ○ Normal ◉ Abnormal ○ Didn't Ask
Experiencing intermittent bouts of diarrhea and constipation

Figure 40–2: Part of a physical exam screen in an EHR. *Courtesy of TriMed Technologies, Corp.*

EXAMINATION TECHNIQUES

Providers are skilled in a variety of techniques used to evaluate patients in the examination process. You are expected to have a basic knowledge of these six techniques used to evaluate patients during physical examinations. Each technique provides specific information regarding the condition of the patient's body.

1. **Inspection** is evaluation by the use of sight. This is usually the initial part of the exam, when the provider looks at the patient to observe the skin's color and condition (rashes and discoloration), the general appearance (grooming, apparent state of health, posture), the level of anxiety, and **gait**. Awareness of person, place, and time as well as any visible injuries or deformities are noted.

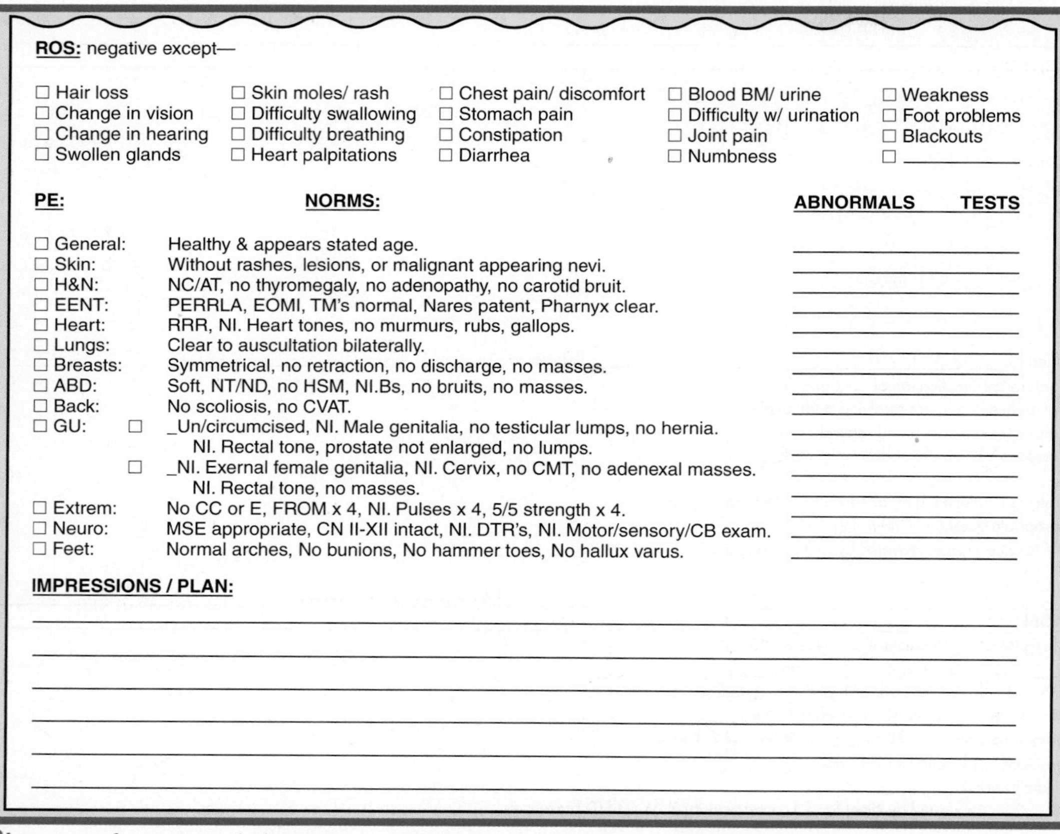
ROS: negative except—

☐ Hair loss ☐ Skin moles/ rash ☐ Chest pain/ discomfort ☐ Blood BM/ urine ☐ Weakness
☐ Change in vision ☐ Difficulty swallowing ☐ Stomach pain ☐ Difficulty w/ urination ☐ Foot problems
☐ Change in hearing ☐ Difficulty breathing ☐ Constipation ☐ Joint pain ☐ Blackouts
☐ Swollen glands ☐ Heart palpitations ☐ Diarrhea ☐ Numbness ☐ ________

PE: NORMS: ABNORMALS TESTS

☐ General: Healthy & appears stated age.
☐ Skin: Without rashes, lesions, or malignant appearing nevi.
☐ H&N: NC/AT, no thyromegaly, no adenopathy, no carotid bruit.
☐ EENT: PERRLA, EOMI, TM's normal, Nares patent, Pharnyx clear.
☐ Heart: RRR, Nl. Heart tones, no murmurs, rubs, gallops.
☐ Lungs: Clear to auscultation bilaterally.
☐ Breasts: Symmetrical, no retraction, no discharge, no masses.
☐ ABD: Soft, NT/ND, no HSM, Nl.Bs, no bruits, no masses.
☐ Back: No scoliosis, no CVAT.
☐ GU: ☐ _Un/circumcised, Nl. Male genitalia, no testicular lumps, no hernia. Nl. Rectal tone, prostate not enlarged, no lumps.
☐ _Nl. Exernal female genitalia, Nl. Cervix, no CMT, no adenexal masses. Nl. Rectal tone, no masses.
☐ Extrem: No CC or E, FROM x 4, Nl. Pulses x 4, 5/5 strength x 4.
☐ Neuro: MSE appropriate, CN II-XII intact, Nl. DTR's, Nl. Motor/sensory/CB exam.
☐ Feet: Normal arches, No bunions, No hammer toes, No hallux varus.

IMPRESSIONS / PLAN:

Figure 40–3: Review of systems and physical examination portion of an H and P form. *Delmar/Cengage Learning.*

2. **Palpation** is evaluation using the sense of touch. The body can be felt using one hand, two hands (**bimanual** as in vaginal and rectal examinations), or one finger only (digitally as in **digital rectal examination [DRE]**). Examination of the breasts is done with the flat surfaces of the fingers of both hands. Palpation can determine skin temperature, size and shape of organs, the position and presence of abnormal structures, and the degree of abdominal rigidity and aortic pulsations.
3. **Percussion** is a means of producing sounds by tapping various parts of the body. The provider listens to the sounds to determine the size, density, and location of underlying **visceral** organs. **Pitch**, quality, **duration**, and **resonance** are terms used by providers when referring to percussion. Direct

percussion is termed *immediate* and is done by striking the finger against the patient's body. The type of percussion most often used is *indirect* or *mediate.* With indirect percussion, the examiner's finger is placed on the area and struck with a finger of the other hand.

4. **Auscultation** is listening to sounds made by the patient's body. Indirect or mediate auscultation is done with the stethoscope to amplify sounds that arise from the lungs, heart, and visceral organs. Sounds heard by this method of examination include **bruits**, murmurs, rales, rhythms, and bowel sounds. Direct or immediate auscultation is done by placing the ear directly over the bare surface area. Auscultation skill is acquired with experience. The provider must be able to determine normal from abnormal sounds. Some, such as the heart valve sounds, last only a fraction of a second and demand concentrated listening.
5. Mensuration, as you learned in Chapter 38, means measurement. In this part of the examination, the patient's chest and extremities are measured and recorded. Usually, a standard flexible tape measure is used. Mensuration includes all the following measurements: height, weight, head, chest, and other parts of the body as appropriate; temperature; pulse; respirations; and blood pressure. All measurements should be recorded in centimeters, inches, or feet; and pounds or kilograms; being consistent is especially necessary in keeping track of the pediatric patient's growth and development or in assessment and evaluation of any patient's change in readings that may contribute to a diagnosis.
6. **Manipulation** is the passive movement of a joint to determine the range of extension and flexion. This evaluation is especially important when patients have had joint injuries or have arthritis. Orthopedic providers evaluate range of motion following surgical procedures such as knee and hip replacements. Insurance companies and state industrial commissions may request evaluation to determine continuation of coverage following trauma injuries and industrial accidents.

PHYSICAL EXAMINATION FORMAT

In reviewing the medical examination form in Figure 40–3, notice that the section immediately following "Review of Systems" has the areas outlined for recording the findings of the complete physical examination. It is concise and requires listing only abnormal findings to conserve time and writing. Additionally, many abbreviations are used (and some may be facility-specific).

The following pages provide an explanation of each of the body areas examined to help you become familiar with what the provider does in each section of the physical examination. Even though H and P and customized physical forms vary in appearance, the contents are basically be the same. The form has small boxes to check to be sure nothing is omitted. Each exam area has conditions to be observed and a line to note any abnormalities. If an additional diagnostic test is needed, it can also be noted after the abnormal finding.

Remember that the very first part of the physical includes measurement, vital signs, and vision screening (covered later in this chapter), which you will have initially completed before the provider's examination. To make the physical examination format easier to read and understand, it is presented in a modified outline format.

1. First, the examination area is listed in the heading.
2. Next [enclosed in brackets] is the patient's position, the examination technique(s), and the equipment or supplies needed. The patient is gowned throughout the examination, positioned, and draped as explained in Chapter 39. The gown will probably be opened in the back and simply raised by you or the provider for examining the chest and abdomen. The drape will also be repositioned throughout the examination to allow inspection and examination of the patient while providing as much coverage as possible.
3. There is a brief description of how the provider may conduct this portion of the examination.
4. Within each examination area are listed characteristics the provider may be observing and, *in italics*, some applicable descriptive terms. Each provider has his or her own style and depth of examination, which may not include all the areas and characteristics mentioned. The following will help you understand the components of a complete physical examination.

General Appearance

[Anatomical, ambulate, or sitting; inspection; no equipment or supplies, just provider observations]

The provider may ask the patient to stand in front of him in the anatomical position while he observes the patient's general appearance. A few questions may be asked to judge speech and appropriate responses. The patient is asked to walk across the room to observe the manner of walking and body movements.

- Appearance—*grooming, state of health, body stature, nourished, appears stated age*
- Awareness—*to person, place, and time; confused; distressed*
- Gait—*manner of walking: shuffle, limp, balance, evidence of stiffness or pain*
- Speech—*slurring, stutter, loss of voice, impediment*
- Hearing—*response to sound, volume of speech*
- Breath—*odors: sweet and fruity with diabetes, acetone with acidosis, oral hygiene*

Diabetes ketoacidosis (DKA) high sugar level

Skin

[Sitting or standing; inspection or palpation; no equipment or supplies, just provider observations]

The provider will inspect anterior and posterior skin surfaces while the patient stands in front of him or her and as he or she progresses through the examination.

- Color—*redness, bruising, birth marks, darker areas*
- Condition—*dry, flaky, soft, calloused fingers or hands, skin cracks,* **turgor** (measured by pinching back of hand and observing the length of time for return to normal; provides estimate of hydration)
- Blemishes—*moles, warts, scars, acne, rashes*
- Lumps—*palpable masses under the skin*
- Nails—*cuticles, groomed, brittle, peeling, grooved, spooning, clubbing, white lines*

Neck

[Sitting; inspection, palpation, auscultation, or manipulation]

The provider observes the patient in a sitting position, palpating and giving instructions for movement to evaluate range of motion.

- Range of motion
- Thyroid gland for *size, nodules, and symmetry*
- Lymph nodes and parotid glands palpated,
- Observation of swallowing,
- Auscultation of carotid arteries (Figure 40–4). (Blockage of the artery causes a sound known as a *bruit.*)

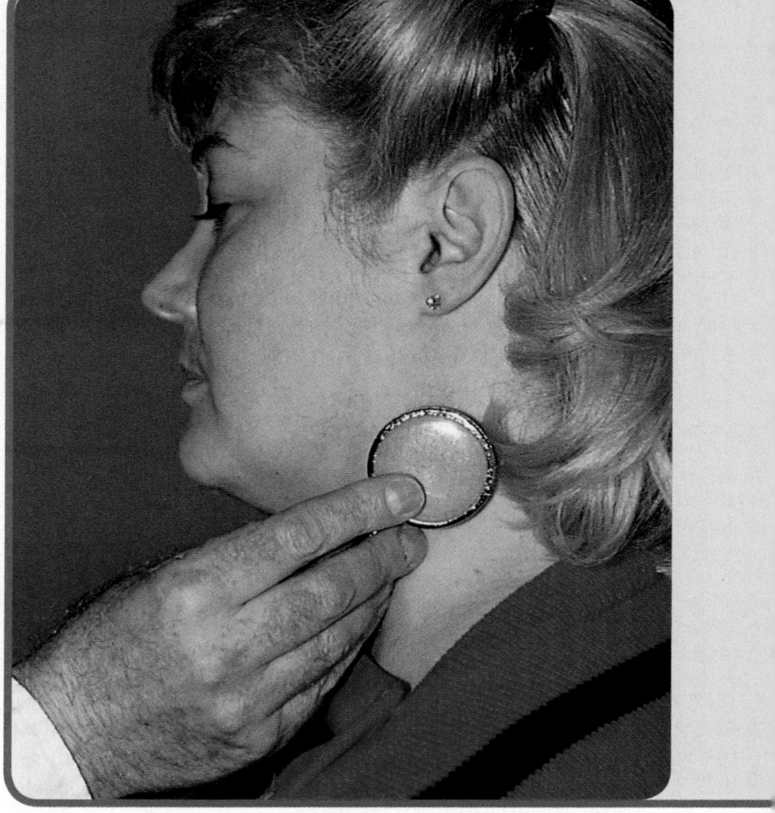

Figure 40–4: The physician auscultates the neck for the sounds made by blood flowing through the carotid artery. *Delmar/Cengage Learning.*

HEENT (Head, Eyes, Ears, Nose, and Throat)

[Sitting; inspection, palpation; ophthalmoscope, otoscope, tuning fork, nasal speculum, tongue depressor, sterile gauze square]

The provider visually observes each area and uses the ophthalmoscope and otoscope to view internal structures. Eye musculature is observed by requesting patient movement. Hearing is evaluated using the tuning fork, and the nasal passages are examined with a speculum. The mouth, throat, and tongue are checked for lesions, and oral hygiene is evaluated.

- Head—**symmetry**, *nodules, hair texture and distribution, scalp*
- Face—*skin condition, presence of facial hair, facial paralysis, eye symmetry*
- Eyes—*observed for protrusion, lashes, symmetry, general condition*

  Vision—*The results of the Snellen, Jaeger, and Ishihara screening procedures previously completed following mensuration are indicated on the form.*

  Pupils (in darkened room with light source)—*These are checked for reaction to light and accommodation (LandA); if equal, it is recorded as PERRLA (pupils equal, round, and respond to light and accommodation).*

  Sclera—*color, clarity, scarring*

  Musculature—*extraocular movements (EOM) are checked for: movement up, down, right, and left while following the provider's finger.*

  Peripheral—*This is side vision while looking straight forward.*

  Internal structures—*Provider views these with an ophthalmoscope: retina, optic disc, blood vessels*

- Ears—*visual and otoscope inspection*

  External—*size, symmetry, lobes, structure*

  Middle—*with otoscope: external auditory canal, cerumen, drainage, tympanic membrane (should be pearly gray), scars from perforations and infection*

  Hearing—*tuning fork to test air, nerve conduction*

- Nose—*visual and nasal speculum inspection*

  Exterior—*structure: straight, curved, bulbous, color*

  Interior—*with nasal speculum and light; checks mucosa, septum, polyps*

- Throat—*inspection with light source*
- Mouth—*with light and tongue depressor, checks inside surface of cheeks and jaw alignment; with gauze to hold tongue, check under tongue and mouth floor, frenulum*

  Tongue—*surface, mobility, depress while patient says "ah" to view tonsils, posterior pharynx*

  Teeth—*oral hygiene, condition of teeth, gums, bite, dentures* (*Note:* If poor oral hygiene, provide patient education and instructional materials following examination and encourage dental visit.)

Chest

[Sitting; inspection or palpation; no equipment or supplies, just provider observations]

The provider observes the seated patient as the chest is palpated for underlying nodes or masses. The chest structure is noted, and the movement in response to breathing is observed.

- Inspection—*for symmetry of sides, shape deformities, intercostal spaces when breathing (retract or bulge), posterior spine alignment, scapula levels*
- Palpation—*lymph nodes, nodules, tenderness* (Figure 40–5)

Heart

[Sitting; auscultation; stethoscope]

The provider auscultates the heart from both anterior and posterior chest wall. The medical assistant and patient must maintain silence during the examination for the provider to hear the heart sounds. Abnormalities may indicate the need for further testing or a cardiologist referral.

- Rate and rhythm—*beats per minute, regularity, volume, premature contractions*
- Sounds—***heart murmurs***

Lungs

[Sitting; auscultation or percussion; stethoscope]

The provider auscultates the lungs on posterior and anterior chest wall. Again, the medical assistant and patient must maintain silence except for the patient's making speech sounds the provider may request. Percussion may be used if fluid, excess air, or a mass is suspected within the chest cavity (Figure 40–6).

- Rate and rhythm—*breaths per minute, regularity, volume, depth*
- Sounds—*posterior auscultation (breathe with open mouth): wheeze, rales, rhonchi, crackling, bronchial constriction; percussion for lung consolidation, hyperinflation, pleural fluid*
- Capacity—*measured by the* **spirometer**; *different tests can be done: forced vital capacity involves forced inhalation followed by quick and complete exhalation to determine the capacity of lungs.* (Review the procedure for performing spirometry later in the chapter).

Breasts

[Sitting or recumbent; inspection or palpation; no equipment or supplies, just provider observations]

The provider inspects and palpates the breasts with the patient in sitting and lying positions. The provider may provide breast self-examination instruction to the patient or defer the responsibility to the medical assistant.

- Inspection—*size, shape, symmetry, position, nipples, dimpling*

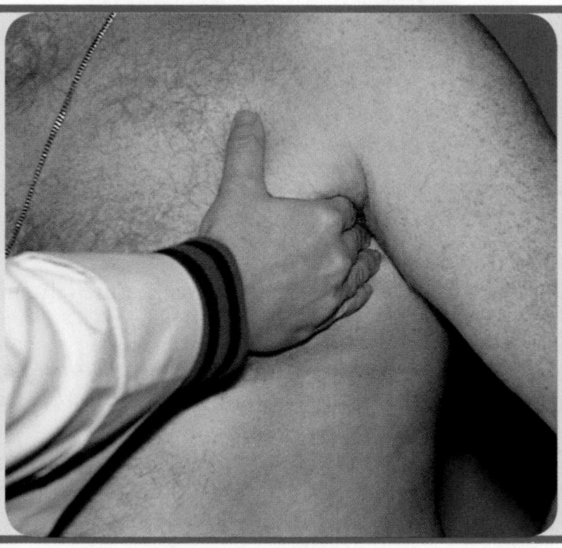

Figure 40–5: Palpation of the patient's axillary region. *Delmar/Cengage Learning.*

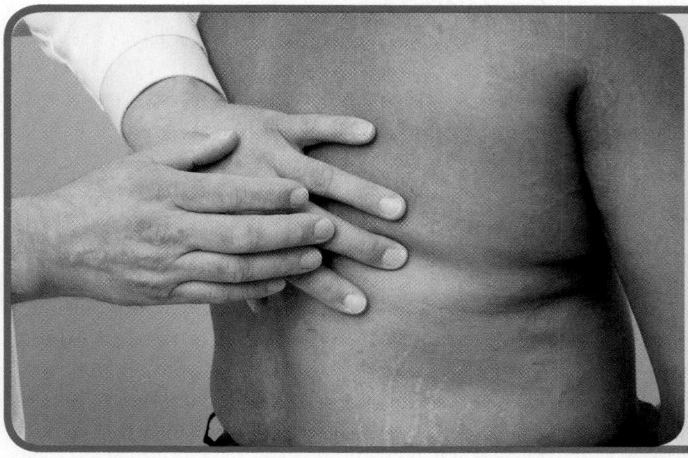

Figure 40–6: Using blunt percussion to examine the base of the lung. *Delmar/Cengage Learning.*

- Palpate—*lumps, nodules, tenderness, mass, in both supine and sitting position*
- Patient education—*Men can also develop breast cancer and should be examined. Instruct the female patient to perform monthly breast self-examination following her menstrual period. Provide visual educational handout. Encourage regular mammograms as appropriate for her age group.*

PATIENT EDUCATION

Breast Self-Examination

Breasts should be examined on a specific day every month, 7 to 10 days following the beginning of a period for women who still menstruate. Learn what your breasts feel like so you can identify a change. Normal changes of breast tissue due to hormonal fluctuations during the cycle could be mistaken for an abnormality.

1. Lie on your back with a pillow or a large folded towel under the same shoulder as the breast you're examining.
2. For the right breast, use the ends of the three middle fingers of the left hand to press the breast tissue against the chest wall to feel for lumps or thickening (Figure 40–7A). Move the fingers in a pattern: Start at the nipple and move around the breast in circles toward the chest wall or move up and down or in a wedge pattern. Use the same pattern each month. Cover the entire breast area.
3. Repeat for the left breast.
4. Stand in front of a mirror (Figure 40–7B). Look at the breasts for symmetry; observe for any area that appears to be attached or falls differently. Observe with arms at sides and with arms raised.
5. Do an extra breast exam while showering. Wet, soapy hands glide over the skin, making feeling the tissue easier.
6. Report any abnormal findings to your physician as soon as possible.

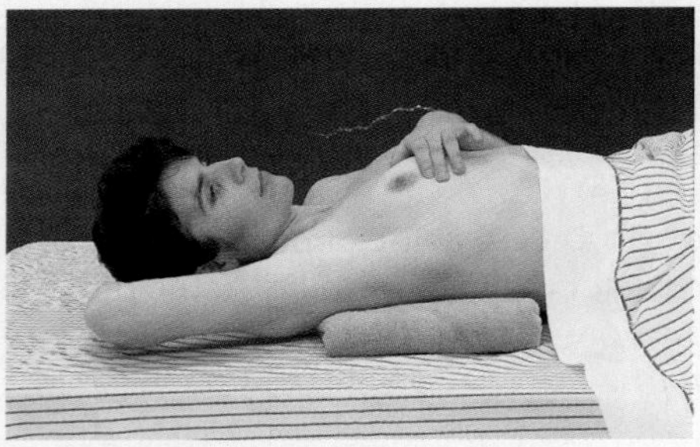

Figure 40–7A: Breast self-exam, lying down. *Delmar/Cengage Learning.*

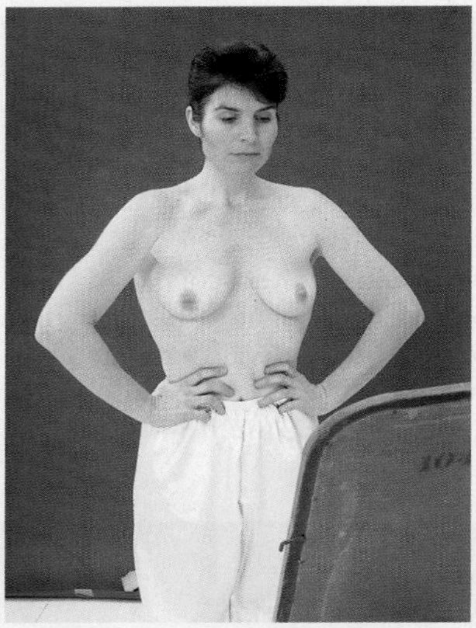

Figure 40–7B: Breast self-exam, in front of mirror. *Delmar/Cengage Learning.*

Abdomen

[Supine or dorsal recumbent; auscultation, inspection, palpation, or percussion; stethoscope]

Refer to Figures 40–8A, B, and C to review the sections of the abdomen and the location of the underlying organs.

The provider stands at the side to inspect, auscultate, palpate, and percuss the abdomen with the patient in the supine and dorsal recumbent positions. A pillow under the patient's head and relaxing the abdominal muscles facilitate deep palpation of the abdominal organs. Auscultating for bowel sounds requires the medical assistant and patient to maintain silence.

- Auscultation—*(should be done first because palpation and percussion can alter bowel sounds); bowel sounds' character and frequency, bruits*
- Inspection—*symmetry, operative scars, protrusions (hernias), umbilicus*
- Palpation—*abdominal aorta pulse, masses,* ***hernias****, tenderness, organs, muscular tension*
- Percussion—*liver, spleen, and stomach size; presence of air*

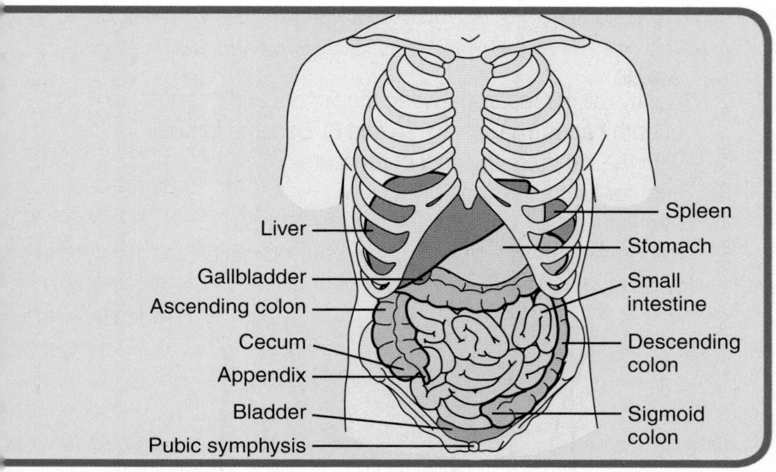

Figure 40–8A: Position of abdominal organs in the nine abdominal regions. *Delmar/Cengage Learning.*

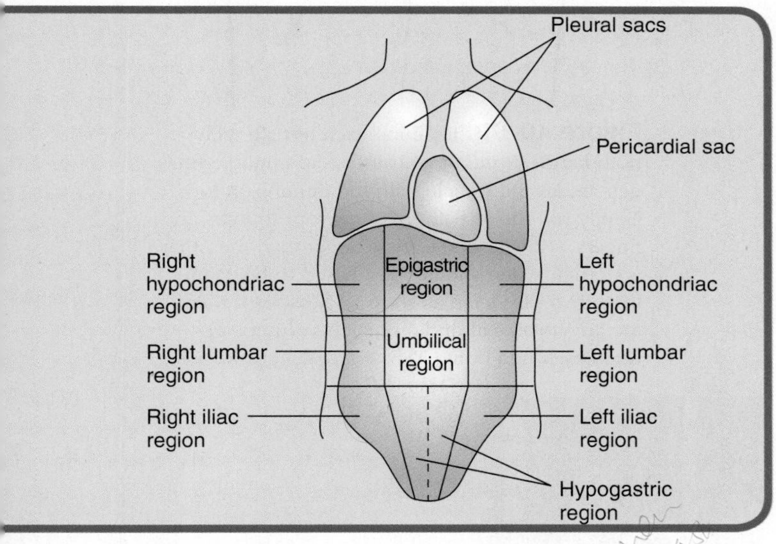

Figure 40–8B: Position of the nine abdominal regions. *Delmar/Cengage Learning.*

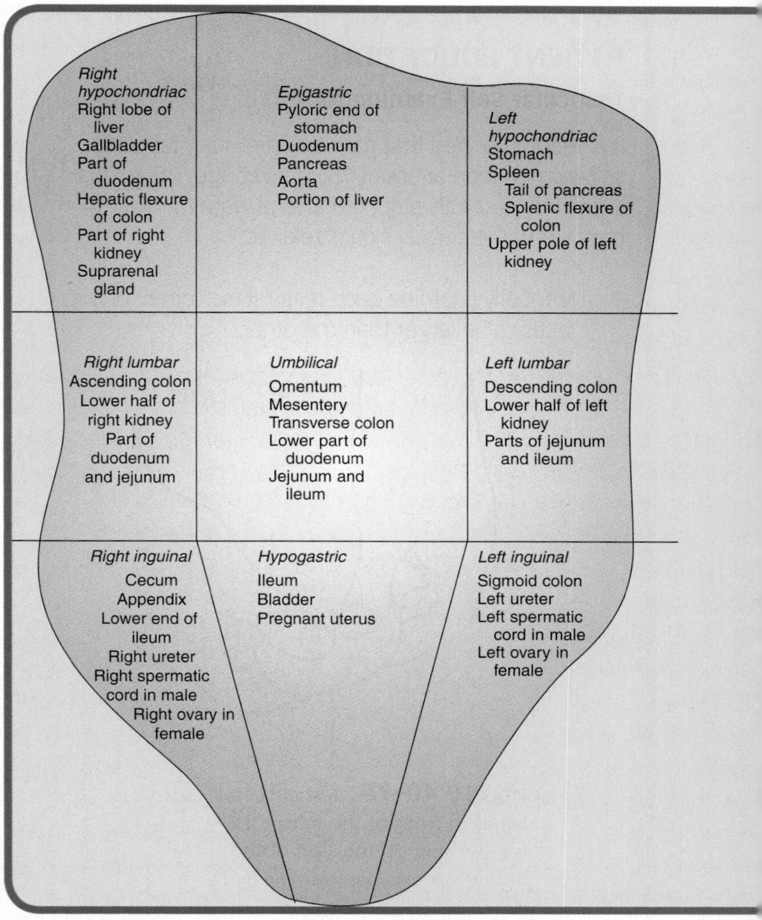

Figure 40–8C: The nine regions of the abdominal cavity with underlying visceral organs. *Delmar/Cengage Learning.*

Back

[Standing; inspection, palpation, or manipulation; no equipment or supplies, just provider observations]

The provider inspects the posterior surface to observe the spine and symmetry of bony prominences. A lateral view will detect excessive anterior and posterior curvatures. The patient may be asked to twist and bend over to evaluate curvatures and flexibility.

- Spine—*straight, concave and convex curvatures, kyphosis, lordosis, scoliosis, manipulation to sides, twist, bend over, front and back, cervical manipulation and head all directions*
- Symmetry—*sides equal, pelvis and scapula even*

Genitourinary and Rectal (Male)

[Standing; inspection or palpation; physician's senses, glove, lubricant, **guaiac test paper** (occult blood test kit), tissues]

The provider wears gloves to inspect the external genitalia of the standing male patient. When the testes are palpated, males past puberty should be instructed in testicular self-examination (TSE). Printed instructions should be provided following the examination. The patient is asked to bear down and cough while the provider checks for hernias in the scrotum and inguinal ring. The patient is then instructed to turn around and bend over the table. The provider inspects the anus and then inserts the gloved and lubricated index finger into the anal canal to evaluate sphincter tone and internal hemorrhoids. The prostate is palpated through the anterior wall of the rectum. A test for **occult** blood is taken from a small amount of stool on the withdrawn index finger placed on the guaiac test paper. Tissues are used to remove the excess lubricant.

- Pubis—*lesions, infestation, distribution of hair*
- Penis—*lesions, scars, deformity, discharge, circumcision, urinary meatus*

PATIENT EDUCATION

Testicular Self-Examination

It is recommended that men begin routine testicular self-examination at about 15 years of age. The testes should be carefully palpated after a warm shower or bath when the scrotal skin is relaxed.

1. Manually examine each testis. It is normal for one testis to be larger than the other.
2. Gently roll the testes between the fingers and thumbs of both hands (Figures 40–9A and B). Become familiar with the structure and feel of the testes.
3. Feel for lumps or nodules.
4. See Figure 40–9C to identify the structures.
5. Report any abnormal findings to your physician as soon as possible.

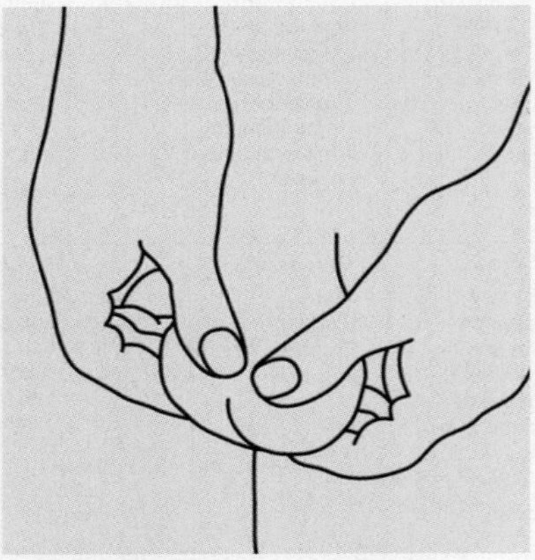

Figure 40–9A: Testicular self-exam. Stand in front of the mirror. Look for swelling on the skin of the scrotum. *Delmar/Cengage Learning.*

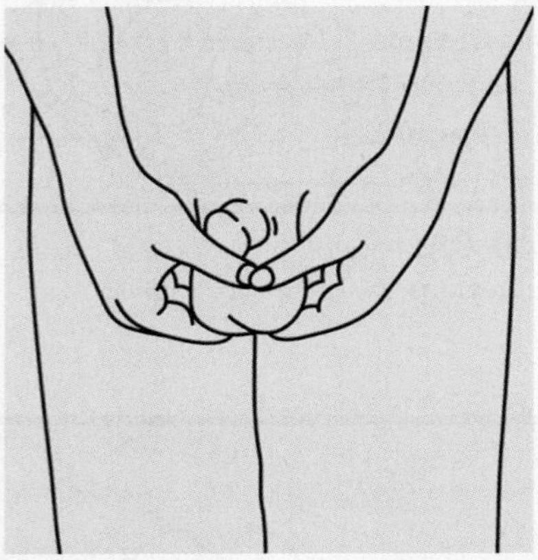

Figure 40–9B: Examine each testicle with both hands. Position your index and middle fingers under the testicle with the thumbs on top. Gently roll the testicle between your thumbs and fingers. (Having one testicle larger than the other is normal.) Men should be advised to be examined by a physician as soon as possible if there are any abnormal findings, such as lumps or nodules, when doing TSE. *Delmar/Cengage Learning.*

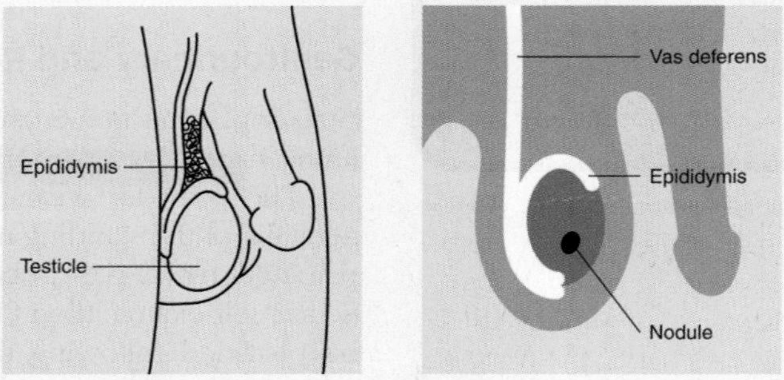

Figure 40–9C: Illustration of testicular structures. *Delmar/Cengage Learning.*

- Scrotum—*symmetry, swelling, varicosities, fluid, masses, presence of hernia*
- Anus—*hemorrhoids, lesions, fissures, prolapse, sphincter tone*
- Prostate—*size, tenderness, nodules*

Genitourinary and Rectal (Female)

[Lithotomy; inspection or palpation; gloves, lubricant, vaginal speculum, examination stool, exam lamp, guaiac paper (occult blood test kit), tissues]

The medical assistant assists the patient into the lithotomy position. The provider puts on gloves or is assisted into gloves by the medical assistant. The provider usually sits on a stool at the foot of the table, with the light coming over his or her shoulder. First the perineal and anal areas are inspected. Then the speculum, which the medical assistant has warmed in running water, has lubricant applied and is inserted into the vagina to view internal structures. A bimanual examination follows. The provider inserts two fingers of the well-lubricated gloved hand into the vagina and examines internal structures by deep palpation with the other hand, and then the index finger is inserted into the anus to examine the anal and rectal area. A test for occult blood is taken from a small amount of stool on the withdrawn index finger placed on the guaiac test paper. Tissues are used to remove the excess lubricant. Additional tissues are offered to remove any residual lubricant. For information on gynecological exams and collecting a Pap test, refer to Chapter 41.

- Pubis—*lesions, infestation, distribution of hair*
- Labia—*edema, redness, cysts, masses, varicosities*
- Vaginal orifice—*hymen, inflammation, bleeding, discharge, lesions*
- Vagina—*discharge, redness, lesions, mass, cervix*

Bimanual examination by palpation:

- Uterus—*size, masses, symmetry, tenderness, position*
- Ovaries—*size, masses, symmetry, tenderness*
- Anus—*Inspection for hemorrhoids, lesions, fissures, prolapse; palpation: sphincter tone, internal hemorrhoids, masses*

Extremities

[Recumbent; mensuration and manipulation; tape measure]

The provider sometimes measures different parts of the body; however, the lower extremities are probably the most frequently measured, especially if the patient complains of back problems. It is very common to find one leg slightly longer than the other, but when the difference is too great, the pelvis and back are out of alignment, and muscles, therefore, might react with spasms.

- Leg—*Medial surface is measured bilaterally from the anterior superior iliac spine to the bony prominence of the tibia at the ankle; legs and ankles are assessed for edema.*
- Feet—*Arches, toes, and toenails are examined, and feet are checked for deformities and bunions.*

All extremity joints are observed for range of motion (refer to Chapter 56) by the provider either requesting the patient to move extremities or by passively flexing, extending, and rotating the arms and legs to evaluate the shoulders, hips, elbows, knees, wrists, and ankles. This can be combined with evaluating muscle strength.

Muscle Strength

Muscle strength is sometimes observed by asking the patient to perform a set of movements that the provider counteracts with resistance. Figure 40–10 shows some examples.

- Fingers—The patient is asked to spread his or her fingers (abduction); then the provider tries to force them together to measures ulnar nerve function.
- Grip—The patient is asked to squeeze the index and middle finger of the provider as the provider tries to remove them to evaluate forearm muscles and condition of the hands.
- Elbow—The patient pushes and pulls against the provider's resistance to check flexion and extension strength of the arms.
- Hip—Flexion of the hip is evaluated by having the patient try to raise his or her leg while the provider pushes down on the thigh.
- Knee—Flexion of the knee is evaluated by having the patient flex the leg with the foot on the table and maintaining the position as the provider tries to straighten the leg.
- Knee—Extension of the knee is evaluated by having the patient try to straighten the leg while the provider holds the leg flexed and exerts pressure at the ankle.
- Ankle—The patient pushes or pulls against the provider's hand to evaluate the plantar flexion and dorsiflexion.

Reflexes

[Sitting or supine; percussion; percussion hammer]

The provider systematically evaluates *involuntary* reflex action at several locations on the body with the patient in a sitting or lying position. The patient is instructed to relax the muscle. The provider positions the extremity so that the muscle is mildly stretched. Then the partially stretched tendon is tapped sharply to stimulate the sensory nerve endings in the muscle to cause a reaction (Figure 40–11). These tests evaluate the condition of the sensory nerve, the *automatic* synapse in the spinal cord, the motor nerve, and the innervated muscle. The biceps, triceps, patellar, Achilles, and plantar reflexes are checked. The plantar reaction is stimulated by stroking the plantar surface with the handle of the hammer or an object such as a key. Note on the physical exam form in Figure 40–4 the neuro area, the examination of CN II–XII, and the motor and sensory nerves.

Other Evaluations

In addition to the many examinations already discussed, the physician may include others such as:

1. *Romberg balance test*—Performed to detect any muscle abnormality. The patient stands with feet together and eyes open; if the balance seems all right, the examiner asks the patient to close the eyes. If there is any muscle abnormality, the patient can possibly fall. Assist by standing close enough to help prevent this from happening.

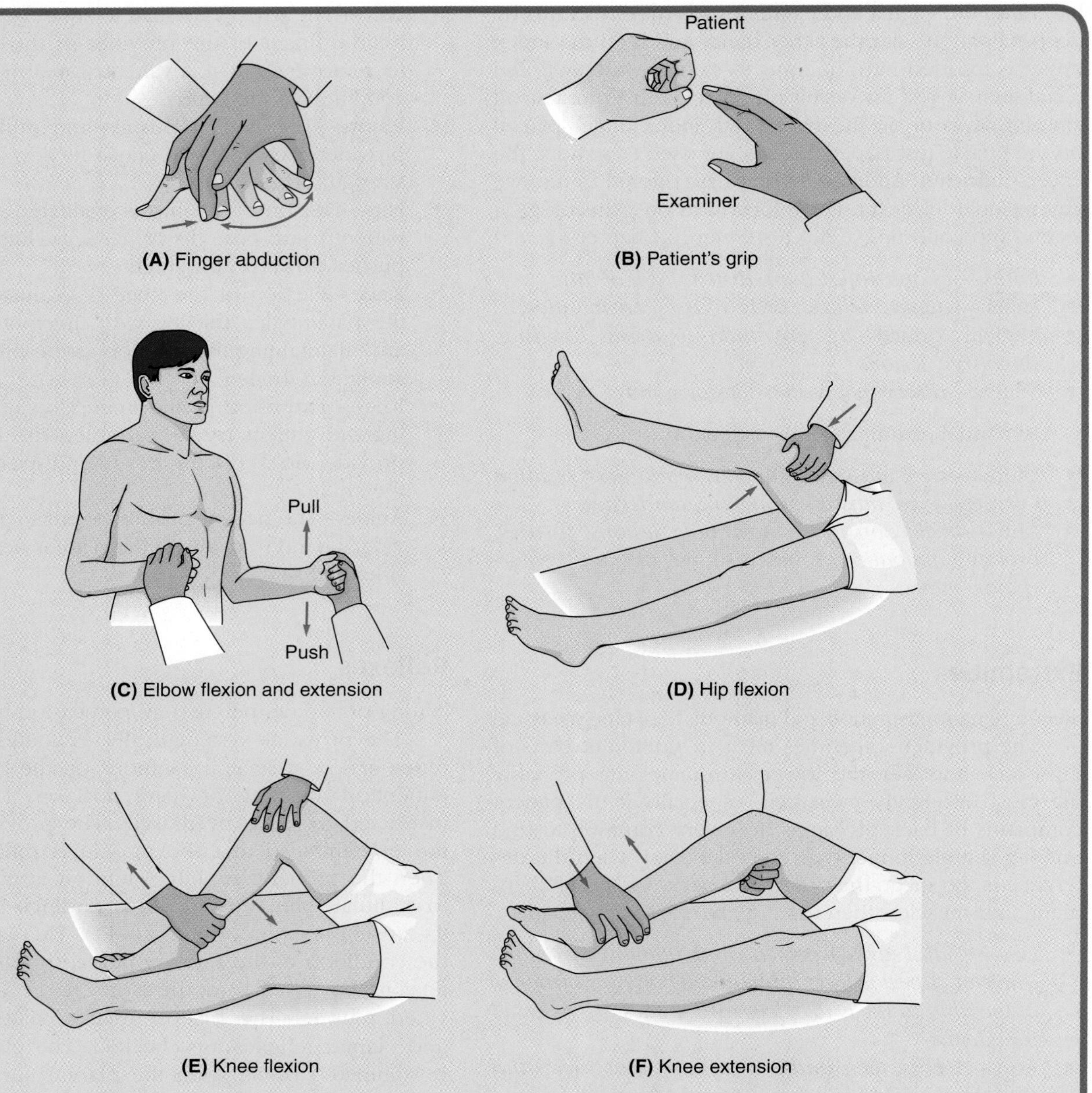

(A) Finger abduction
(B) Patient's grip
(C) Elbow flexion and extension
(D) Hip flexion
(E) Knee flexion
(F) Knee extension
(G) Plantar flexion
(H) Dorsiflexion

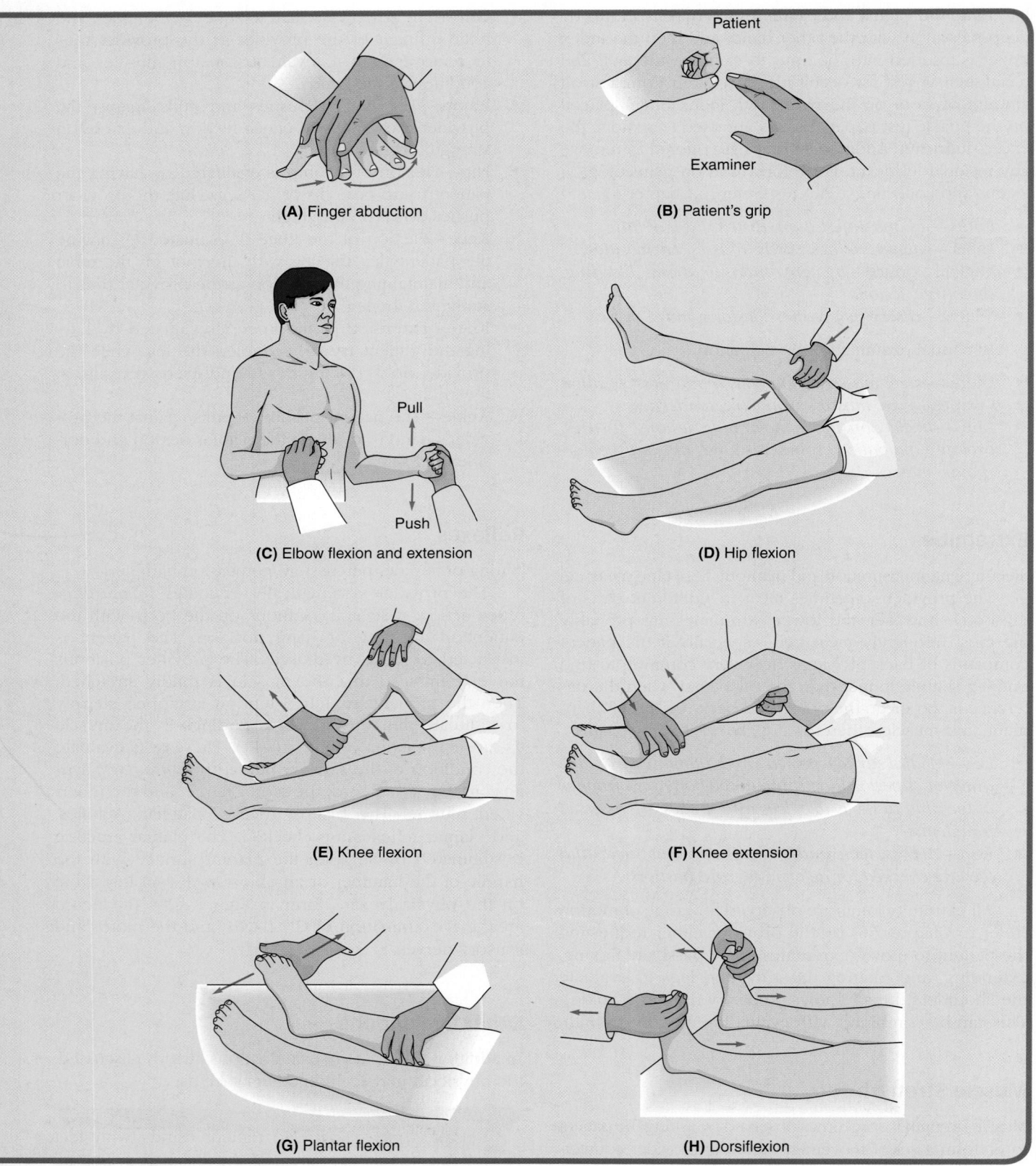

Figure 40–10: Testing muscle strength. *Delmar/Cengage Learning.*

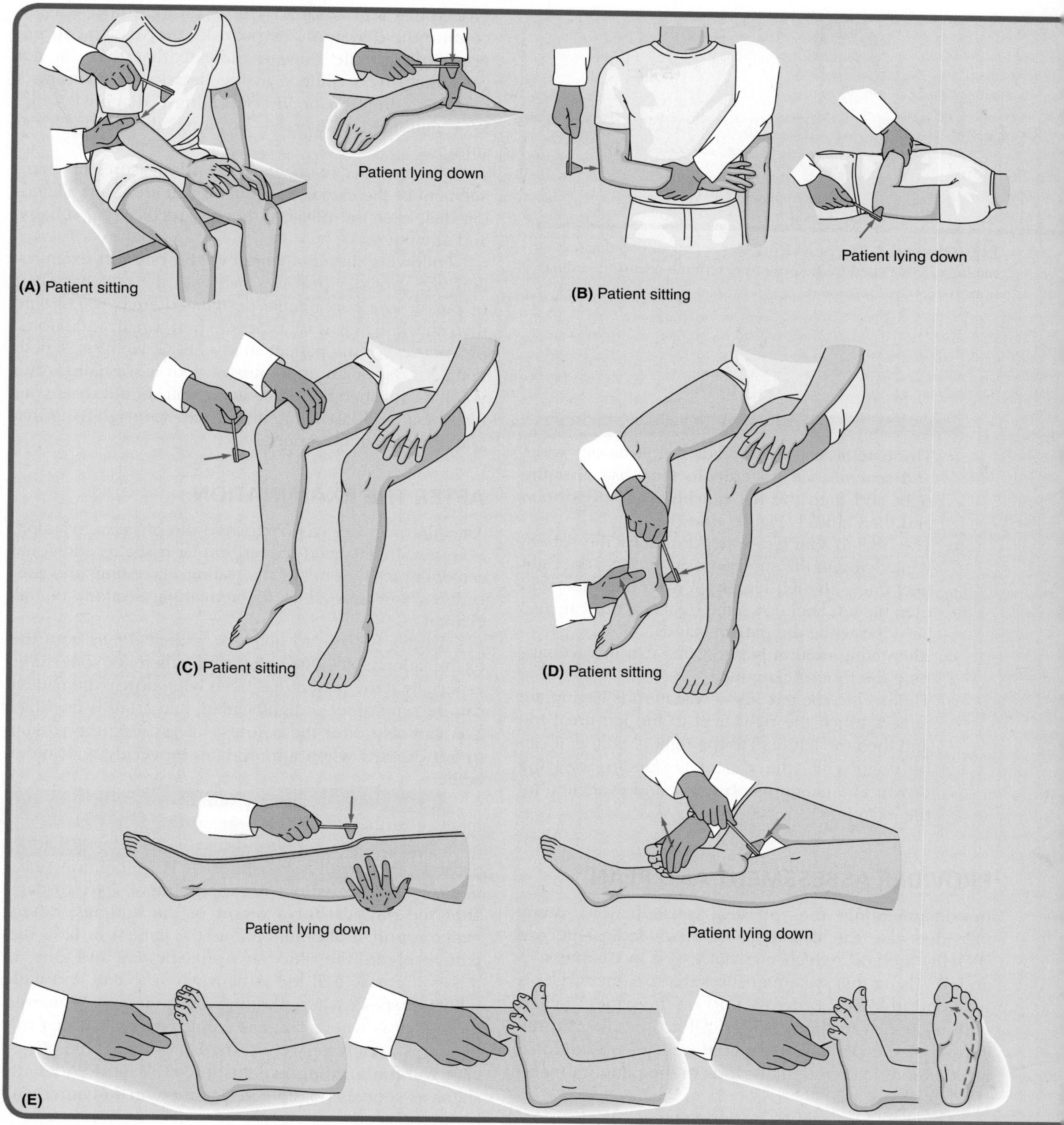

Figure 40–11: A percussion hammer is used to test (A) biceps, (B) triceps, (C) patellar, (D) Achilles, and (E) plantar reflexes. *Delmar/ Cengage Learning.*

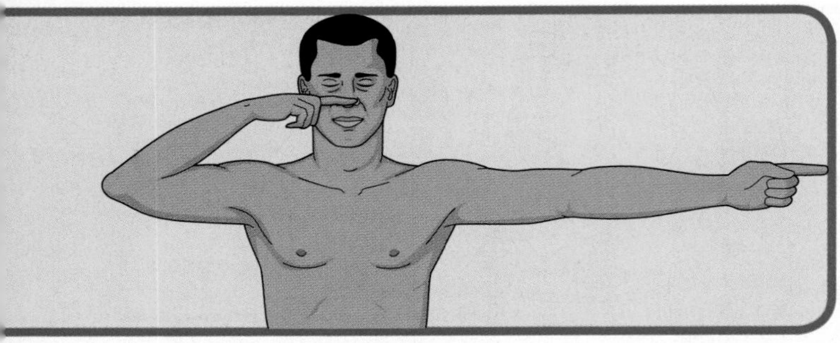

Figure 40–12: The provider observes patient coordination as the finger is touched to the nose to determine normal coordination. *Delmar/Cengage Learning.*

2. Other tests for **coordination**, which can include:
   a. The patient sits up, spreads the arms out wide, and touches the fingertip to the nose, first the right and then the left quickly, with eyes open and then closed (Figure 40–12).
   b. The heel-to-shin test is performed by the patient while lying in the supine position: First, the right heel traces the left leg down from the knee, and then the left heel down the right leg; this can also be done while the patient stands.
   c. Alternating motion is a test that can involve tapping the foot or clapping.
   d. The heel-to-toe test of coordination is having the patient touch the right heel to the left great toe and then the left heel to the right great toe; it can be done while the patient is standing or lying down. The patient is observed and evaluated by the examiner.

PROVIDER ASSESSMENT AND PLAN

In documenting the physical examination, many providers use the Problem Oriented Medical Record (POMR) method, which was discussed in Chapters 13 and 37. Using this system ensures that pertinent data is recorded in logical order (SOAP) on the patient's chart with each visit to the provider. All action taken in the course of the patient's treatment generates additional information that continually adds to the patient's medical record.

The provider makes an *assessment,* or decision, about the patient's condition based on the health history, symptoms, examination findings, and any other procedures and laboratory tests thought necessary to confirm the decision. The provider may use the abbreviation R/O (rule out) to indicate that there is not yet conclusive evidence in the decision concerning a patient's condition or in confirming a diagnosis (e.g., R/O gallbladder disease—awaiting diagnostic X-ray studies).

The provider's *plan* includes *all* measures for management of the care of the patient that are listed, including diet, exercise, physical therapy, medication, surgery, and any others.

Following the completion of the physical examination, the provider provides you with the patient's chart or puts it in a confidential designated area. You should then check the chart for orders to perform any additional procedures for the patient such as ECG, lab tests, scheduling X-rays, or an appointment with a specialist. After you have finished the procedures, you should write your first initial and last name after each one, signifying that you completed the orders.

AFTER THE EXAMINATION

After the provider has completed the physical examination, you might need to perform or assist in additional screening tests. Some of the testing, screening, and procedures are covered in the remaining sections of this chapter.

Always be sure to help the patient down from the examination table. Often after sitting there for some time, especially if the patient has been lying down, the patient can become dizzy or lightheaded, and a fall is possible. You can also offer the courtesy of assisting the patient to get dressed when appropriate, especially with older adults.

Answer any questions about the follow-up appointment or further studies. Let the patient know how long to expect to wait for reports from the lab, radiology, or other diagnostic procedures. It is a common practice to give the patient an appointment 7 to 10 days after the physical for a report of the findings; others mail a report. Still others phone the patient or have the patient phone the office at a specific day and time. If this is the case, tell the patient when to call and with whom to speak when phoning for the report. Whatever the policy is where you are employed, realize that the patient is usually very concerned about what the physician will find. Letting patients know about their health status as soon as possible in a professional manner will be appreciated.

Procedure 40–1 provides step-by-step instruction for assisting with a general physical examination.

PROCEDURE 40–1 Prepare a Patient for and Assist with a Routine Physical Examination

PURPOSE: To have the patient, the room, and the examination equipment prepared for the physician to complete a physical examination as you assist with the process as needed

EQUIPMENT: Gown, drape, stethoscope, ophthalmoscope, otoscope, tongue depressors, sterile gauze squares, tuning fork, nasal speculum, tape measure, percussion hammer, vaginal speculum, guaiac test kit, disposable gloves, lubricant, tissues, towel, Mayo tray, examination stool, exam lamp, regular and biohazardous waste container, patient chart or EMR, and a pen

S **SKILL:** Prepare a patient for and assist with a routine physical exam.

Procedure Steps	Detailed Instructions and/or *Rationales*
1. Prepare the examination room as in Procedure 39–1.	
2. Review the patient's chart for completed history and the physical examination form.	Have a pen ready if you are to scribe for the physician.
3. Wash hands.	
4. Prepare the examination equipment on the Mayo tray in order of use and cover with a towel.	Place the Mayo tray in a convenient location in the room.
5. Pull out the step from the table. Place a gown and drape on the table.	
B 6. Identify the patient, introduce yourself, check the chart, and explain the procedure to the patient, ***using language the patient can understand.***	*Ensures that you have the correct patient. Ask the patient to follow you to the room. Using appropriate language ensures that the patient understands the examination process.*
7. Measure and record vital signs, height, and weight.	If the physical follows the in-person interview and history, the mensuration would have been completed and recorded.
8. Instruct the patient to go to the bathroom to empty the bladder.	Provide a labeled specimen bottle for a urine sample to be tested later.
9. Instruct the patient to remove clothing and place it on a chair, to put on the gown with the opening in back, to sit at the end of the table, and to cover the legs with the drape.	Evaluate ability to undress and to get onto the table unassisted. Assist the patient as needed, especially the elderly, weak, or disabled. Do not leave disoriented, weak, dizzy, or ill patients alone. Request temporary family assistance if you must leave the room.
10. Ensure that the patient is ready and notify the provider.	
11. Assist the provider as needed with the examination. Position and drape the patient, adjust lights, and hand equipment as appropriate for each body system.	• **General appearance and skin inspection—**When instructed, remove the drape, help the patient from the table for inspecting posterior surface and gait evaluation and assist to sit again. • **Neck—**Stand by. • **HEENT—**If provider requests, turn off lights for pupil and ophthalmoscope evaluation. (If physician desires, hand ophthalmoscope, then otoscope, nasal speculum, tongue blade, gauze squares, and tuning fork.)

(continues)

(continued)

Procedure Steps	Detailed Instructions and/or *Rationales*
	• **Chest—**Might need to raise gown • **Heart—**Ensure silence. Might need to raise the gown. Note whether ECG is requested. • **Lungs—**Ensure silence. Might need to raise the gown. Note whether vital capacity is requested. • **Breasts—**Raise gown for sitting exam and then assist the patient to lie back. Expose the breasts and cover with the drape. • **Abdomen—**Raise gown to the breasts and then cover with the drape. Stand away from the side of the table. • **Back—**Provider's preference; may be done while the patient is standing for general inspection. If not, assist the patient to sit and then stand in front of the provider. • **Extremities—**Position the patient in supine position and cover with the drape. Hand tape measure. • **Reflexes—**Position patient in sitting position (most common). Hand percussion hammer. • **Muscle strength—**Begin with sitting patient *and t*hen assist to supine and drape. • **Genitourinary and rectal (female)—**assist the patient into lithotomy position and drape. Assist the provider to glove and then adjust lamp. Warm the speculum; hand when ready. Apply lubricant to a gloved finger. Prepare the guaiac paper.
12. When the exam is completed, allow the patient to relax a moment and then help to sitting position.	
13. Provide tissues to remove excess lubricant and instruct the patient to dress.	
14. Take specimens from the room to the laboratory for testing.	
15. Return to the room, provide patient instructions, and see the patient out.	• Determine whether the patient has any questions. • Provide instructions and schedule any additional procedures requested by the physician. • Provide information for receiving the examination results.
16. Properly clean the room and prepare it for the next patient.	• Put on gloves to wrap up the table paper and dispose of used supplies in appropriate waste containers. • Disinfect table tops, exam lamp, and examination table. • Remove and discard gloves in the appropriate waste container; wash hands.

Procedure Steps	Detailed Instructions and/or *Rationales*
	• Replace used supplies and cover the table and pillow with clean paper.
17. Give the room a visual check for completeness.	

Charting Example

2-14-XX 11:30 am	Patient here for a complete physical today. Refer to physical form for findings. T. EDWARDS, CMA(AAMA)

Patient Follow-up

Patients might ask how often they need to have a physical. Some providers recommend annual physicals for their patients, others every two to three years unless a specific or chronic medical problem exists. *The physical exam schedule in Table 40–1 is meant to serve as a guide. The medical needs of patients will vary, as will physicians' recommendations. You will need to check with the provider who employs you because office policies can vary.*

TABLE 40–1 Physical Examination Frequency

Procedure/Screening	Age
Hearing	Annually 65 years+, or as necessitated by symptoms
Vision	Annually 65 years+, or as necessitated by symptoms
	Tonometry or funduscopy at 40, then every 4 years
Urinalysis	Annually 65 years+, or as necessitated by symptoms
Skin for melanoma	Begin at 40, then annually
Fecal occult blood test Feces	Begin at 50, then annually Guaiac reagent
Males: Digital rectal exam (DRE) and Prostate Specific Antigen (PSA)	Begin at 50, then annually
Sigmoidoscopy (flexible fiber-optic)	Begin at 50, then annually
Colonoscopy	Starting at age 50, every 10 years or as directed by provider
Pulmonary function tests	As needed for high-risk patients (COPD and smokers)
Total blood cholesterol	At age 20, start screening every 5 years or as directed by provider.
Thyroid testing	As needed for symptoms; baseline for females at menopause, then every 2 years
H and P	20–39, every 3 years; then annually after 40
Height and weight	Annually 13–65+, then as directed by provider
Blood pressure	Annually 13–65+, then as directed by provider if higher than 140/90
Males: testicular self-exam	Monthly (13–65+ as needed for symptoms) or as directed by provider
Females: mammogram	Baseline at 40, every 1–2 years, then annually at 50
Breast self-exam	Monthly self performed, 18–39, at least every 3 years; 40+, annually (by provider)
Pap test and pelvic exam	Begin no later than age 21. At least every 1–3 years for sexually active women

EYE AND EAR EXAMINATIONS

In assisting with eye and ear examinations, you may be expected to hand instruments to the provider as needed. Assembling the instruments in the order of use will be most helpful. You will be responsible for making sure that the instruments are clean and in working order.

Most often, wall-mounted otoscope and ophthalmoscope instruments with electrically powered light sources are used in the medical office (Figure 40–13). Otoscopes and ophthalmoscopes should be checked to be sure the light bulbs are providing strong enough light and changed periodically. If these instruments are the handheld portable type, the batteries must also be changed or charged periodically. Cleaning of the scopes after patient use is performed by wiping them down with a gauze pad and disinfectant or disinfectant wipe as discussed in Chapter 39.

You might also be responsible for providing education and assurance to the patient and recording the procedure performed along with documenting the results in the patient's chart or EHR.

Ear Examinations

Most physicians use a disposable plastic ear speculum to prevent disease transmission. If non-disposable specula are used, they must be sanitized after every use with a mild detergent and sterilized so they can be reused safely to examine another patient. (Refer to Chapter 36 for infection control techniques.) If the patient has an infected ear that has a discharge containing blood, a disposable ear speculum is preferred and protective gloves must be worn.

Sometimes it is difficult for the provider to inspect the patient's ear due to a buildup of **cerumen** (earwax) in the ear. Patients sometimes try to remove it by using a cotton-tipped swab, but this often pushes it farther into the ear canal, where it becomes lodged and hardens. This buildup can become very uncomfortable and eventually impair hearing. The ear may require **irrigation** (also known as **lavage**) to remove the excessive wax. The provider will determine whether the ear needs to be irrigated and direct the medical assistant to perform the procedure. Occasionally, it is necessary to instill a softening solution in the ear to soften ear wax before an irrigation procedure can be performed. Refer to Chapter 52 for the procedure for ear medication instillation.

Patients should have impacted cerumen removed to avoid further discomfort or possible injury to the ear. Many offices have adopted Waterpik® or electronic ear irrigators for this purpose because of the gentle flow produced and convenience for irrigation procedures. A bulb, metal, or plastic syringe may also be used to perform the ear irrigation procedure.

After irrigation procedures are performed, even with gentle care, many patients feel a little dizziness. Be sure that patients are completely stable before permitting them to leave. After the ear wax is removed, the provider will be able to visualize the ear canal to determine whether infection or other conditions are occurring. Perform irrigations of the ear following the steps in Procedure 40–2.

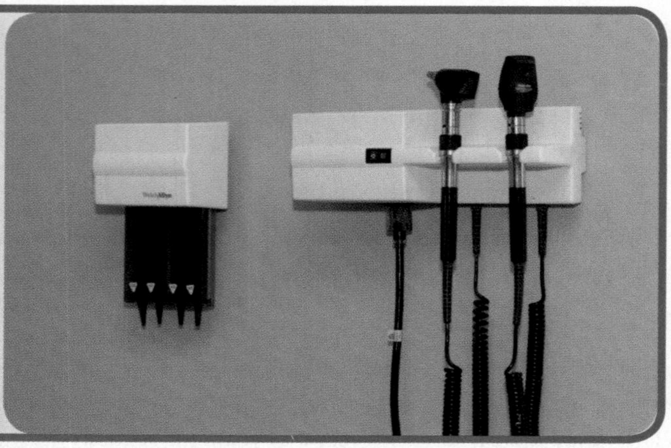

Figure 40–13: Wall-mounted set of scopes. *Delmar/Cengage Learning.*

PATIENT EDUCATION

1. Advise patients not to put anything into their ears to avoid damaging the tympanic membrane. Cerumen is produced to protect and moisten the membrane of the ear canal. Many people feel that they must completely remove this daily with a swab, which often results in it being packed down into the ear canal, where it hardens. Impacted cerumen must be removed by a health care professional.
2. Instruct patients that ear drops and other ear medications should be used only with the advice of their provider. Earache, pain, or discharge should be reported to and examined by the provider as soon as possible.
3. Discuss the possibility of permanent hearing loss with patients who work around extremely loud noise or who listen to audio systems, radios, or TVs with the volume up high. Suggest to these patients to wear protective ear coverings or ear plugs and turn down the volume on audio systems to avoid nerve damage.
4. Urge patients to have regular hearing tests to detect loss of hearing or other related problems. It is recommended this to be done annually, unless otherwise instructed by the provider, if there is a noticeable difference or problem with hearing. If there is a history of ear infections, the patient should have periodic hearing tests.

PROCEDURE 40–2 Irrigate the Ear

PURPOSE: To irrigate the ear canal to remove foreign objects, impacted cerumen, or drainage

EQUIPMENT: Gloves, small basin, ordered lukewarm irrigation solution, towel, ear basin, syringe, gauze squares, otoscope, ear speculum, tissues, patient chart or EMR, and a pen

S **SKILL:** Perform ear irrigation.

Procedure Steps	Detailed Instructions and/or *Rationales*
1. Wash hands. Prepare the solution as ordered and assemble the necessary items for the procedure.	The solution is usually between 99°F and 100°F for patient comfort.
B 2. Identify the patient, introduce yourself, and explain the procedure, ***using language the patient can understand.***	This *ensures* that *you are performing the procedure on the correct patient.*
3. Assist the patient onto the examination table or to a chair.	
4. Put on gloves.	
5. View the affected ear with an otoscope to see where cerumen or the foreign object is located so that the flow of solution can be directed properly.	The flow should be directed upward and to one side. To use the otoscope, place one hand gently against the patient's head, and grasp the auricle with your thumb and index finger, pulling up and back for adults and older children and down and back for infants up to 36 months. Avoid using too much pressure as you insert the speculum into the ear canal.
6. Ask the patient to turn his or her head to the affected side and toward the back. Place a towel over the patient's shoulder to protect his or her clothing.	For pediatric patients, ask a parent to hold the child on his or her lap and assist you during the procedure.
7. Position the ear basin under the ear for the patient to hold to catch the solution.	
8. Use a gauze square to wipe away any particles from the outer ear before proceeding.	child – down & back
9. Fill the syringe with the ordered solution.	
10. With one hand, gently pull the auricle up and back for an adult (or down and back for an infant or small child) (Figure 40–14A–B). With the other hand, place the tip of the syringe into the canal and aim the flow of solution upward so the entire ear canal will be irrigated.	*Pulling the auricle straightens the ear canal.* DO NOT direct the flow of the solution straight into the ear or use force, or the result will be quite painful for the patient and may damage the tympanic membrane.
11. Use gauze squares to wipe the excess solution from the outside of the patient's ear.	
12. Give the patient several gauze squares or tissues and have the patient tilt his or her head to the side to allow drainage of excess solution from the canal.	All material must be removed to inspect the ear canal and tympanic membrane adequately. Patients sometimes feel a little dizzy following this procedure. Allow the patient time to gain balance; assist the patient from the examination table or call the provider to examine.
13. Inspect the ear canal with an otoscope to determine whether the desired results have been obtained. Repeat irrigation if necessary.	

(continues)

(continued)

Procedure Steps	Detailed Instructions and/or *Rationales*
14. Record the procedure on the patient's chart.	Include which ear was irrigated, the solution used, the results of the procedure, and any other important observations.
15. Wash equipment and return it to the proper storage area.	
16. Remove gloves and wash hands.	

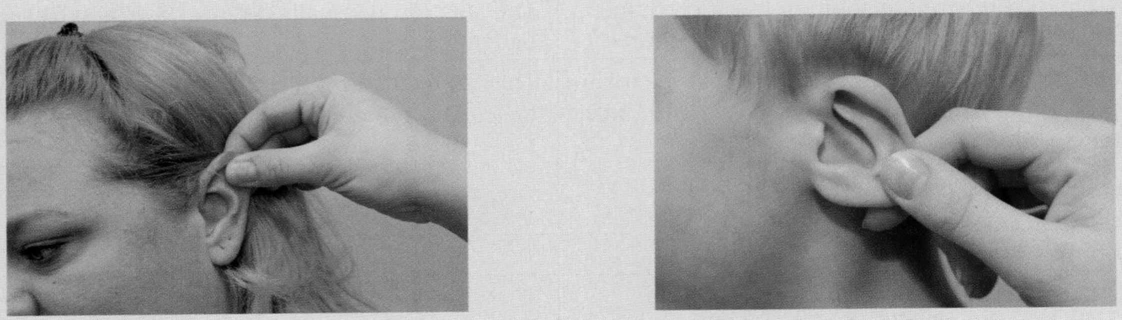

Figure 40–14: (A) Positioning the ear up and back for an adult. (B) Positioning the ear down and back for a child. *Delmar/Cengage Learning.*

Charting Example

5-20-XX 11:30 am	Irrigated pt's right ear with water @ 100°F, per Dr. Long; returned three pieces of cerumen (1.25 cm each). Eardrum is shiny with a pearl-gray color. T. Edwards, CMA(AAMA)

Auditory Acuity

The function of the ear is to enable sound to be perceived. If this process is impaired, hearing loss results. Diseases or conditions of the ear, if not treated, can cause damage to nerves and tissues, which can result in mild to profound deafness.

Sometimes an auditory problem may be as simple as the patient having impacted cerumen, and after irrigation, the person's hearing returns to normal. Other times, further measures are necessary. One of your most important duties is relaying important information observed to the provider about patients. Often, it is a family member who makes the appointment for a patient with an obvious hearing problem. You can watch for any behaviors as you have contact with the patient or when you talk to him or her over the phone.

Common behaviors of patients that indicate the loss of hearing ability are:

- Frequently asking to repeat what was said during conversation.
- Talking in an inappropriately loud voice.
- Not responding when spoken to if out of sight range.
- Not pronouncing words well.
- Responding only when you speak very loudly.

Certain complaints can suggest hearing loss or auditory nerve damage. When patients disclose any of the following symptoms, you should bring it to the attention of the provider for further assessment:

- Ringing in the ears
- Decreased hearing in one ear (or both), sometimes caused by impacted cerumen
- Infection or injury to the ear
- Bleeding or discharge from the ear(s)
- Any unusual noise or feeling inside the ears

These signs and any others that patients tell you should be documented in the chart during in-person screening. Further examination by the provider is necessary to determine the extent of the problem and its treatment.

CLINICAL PEARL

Some patients might try to hide hearing loss if they perceive it to be embarrassing or are afraid they might have to wear a hearing aid or undergo surgery. A patient may try to compensate for the hearing loss by:

- Learning to read lips
- Turning the best ear toward the sound source
- Pretending that he or she heard
- Increasingly turning up the volume on audio equipment
- Standing very close during conversation
- Sometimes withdrawing

If family members of the patient relate this information to you, advise the person to have the patient schedule a time to have a provider examine the ears and have a hearing test. Note the information on the patient's chart and bring it to the provider's attention. The provider will discuss the problem with the patient during the scheduled appointment.

Hearing Assessment

Providers use several audiometric assessment procedures to determine the cause of the patient's hearing loss, some of which are a part of the complete or routine physical examination.

An **audiometer** is an instrument that measures one's hearing; it determines the hearing thresholds of pure tones of frequencies that are normally audible by an individual. Tone frequency refers to the sound vibrations per second; tone intensity refers to the loudness. Some also measure bone and air conduction. The threshold of hearing is the point at which a sound can barely be heard. Figure 40–15 illustrates the **decibels** of common environmental noise levels. The audiometer is cleaned after patient use by wiping the unit down with disinfectant wipes or a disinfectant cleaner and gauze squares.

Audiometric devices are powered by either batteries or electricity. The devices should be checked periodically for proper performance and accuracy. If the batteries need to be changed or if a wire is frayed, it should be taken care of before being used with patients, not only for their safety but to make sure that it works efficiently. Several types of audiometers are available for use in determining hearing acuity. Many are still used that require the operator to turn a dial manually to emit the various frequencies for the patient to hear during the test. Companies that manufacture audiometers offer in-service demonstrations to make sure their equipment is used properly. Operational manuals should be kept with the instrument for handy reference.

The procedure for most audiometers is basically the same. The patient is instructed to place the earphones (marked red for the right ear and blue for the left ear) over the ears. The medical assistant tells the patient how the earphones are to be placed and how to work the

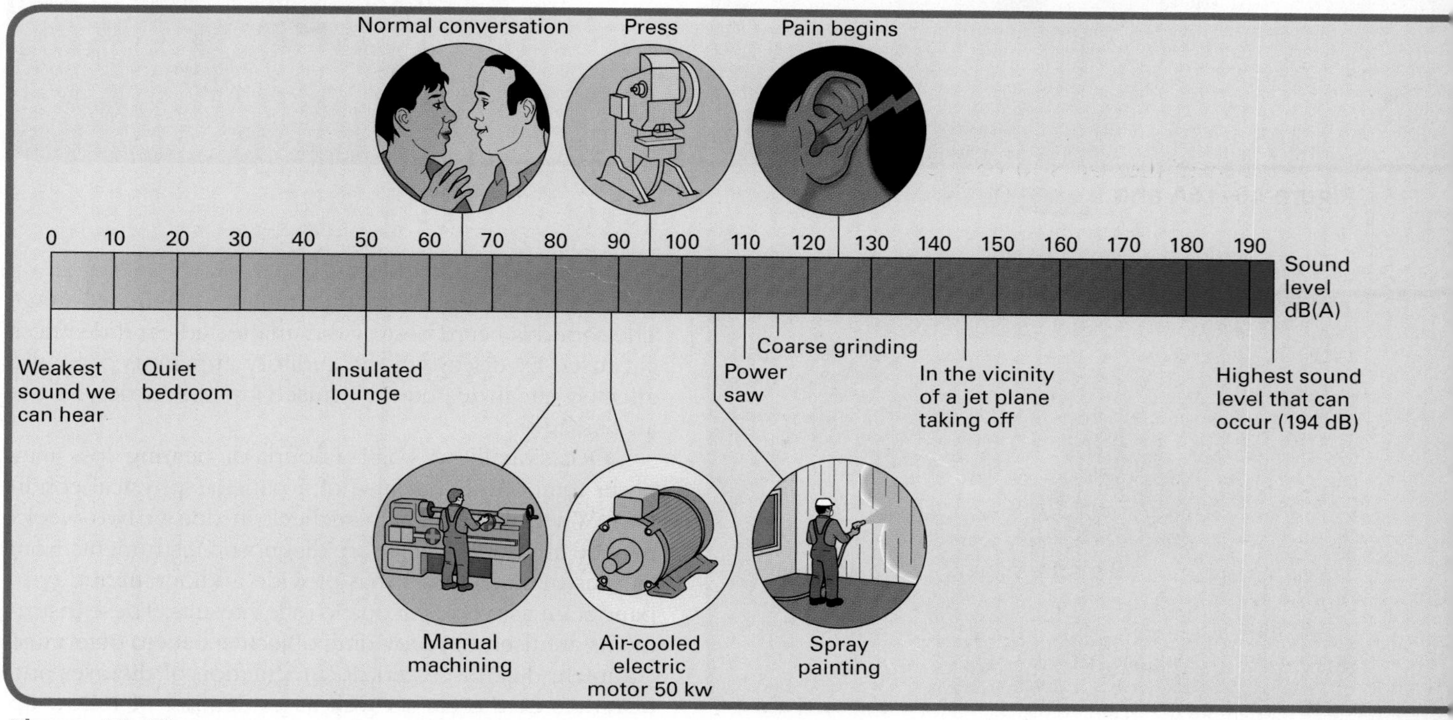

Figure 40–15: Noise levels associated with selected environments and machinery. *Delmar/Cengage Learning.*

control signal. The printer records the results of the hearing test or, if not an automatic machine, you might need to fill out the form manually with the patient's responses. The printout is called an audiogram and is filed in the patient's chart after the provider reads the results of the test and makes an evaluation.

During the procedure, the machine tests one ear at a time. In the ear that is being tested, the machine provides a series of tones. The sound is automatically blocked in the ear that is not being tested. The patient listens and signals (either by raising a finger or by using a handheld control) as the various sounds are heard. The tones range in frequencies from very low to very high with a varied level of decibel intensity. After the right ear has been tested, the machine switches automatically to test the left ear. Report any complaints the patient may have and any unusual behavior before or during the hearing test to the provider and in the patient's chart, along with the results of the test, and place your initials indicating that you have completed the test.

Tympanometry is a procedure that determines the ability of the middle ear to transmit sound waves and is commonly performed on children to diagnose middle ear infections. A probe is inserted into the ear canal to measure the air pressure of the ear canal in relation to the air pressure found in the middle ear.

During the physical examination, the provider will use a tuning fork to test the patient's hearing. A two-pronged metal tuning fork is used, its frequency varying with the size of the instrument. The common tests done are the Rinne and the Weber (Figure 40–16A–C).

In the Rinne test, the examiner strikes the fork and then holds the shank (stem) against the patient's mastoid bone until the patient no longer hears the sound; this is performed to assess nerve or conduction deafness (Figure 40–16A). The prongs of the tuning fork are then placed about 1 inch from the auditory meatus (opening to the ear) and then next to it (Figure 40–16B). In a normal ear, the sound is heard about twice as long by air conduction as by bone conduction. If hearing by bone conduction is greater, the result is spoken of as a negative Rinne.

In the Weber test, the vibrating tuning fork is held against the **vertex** (crown of the head) or against the skull or forehead in the midline (Figure 40–16C). The sound is heard best by the unaffected ear if deafness is caused by disease of the auditory apparatus or by the affected ear if deafness is caused by obstruction of the air passages.

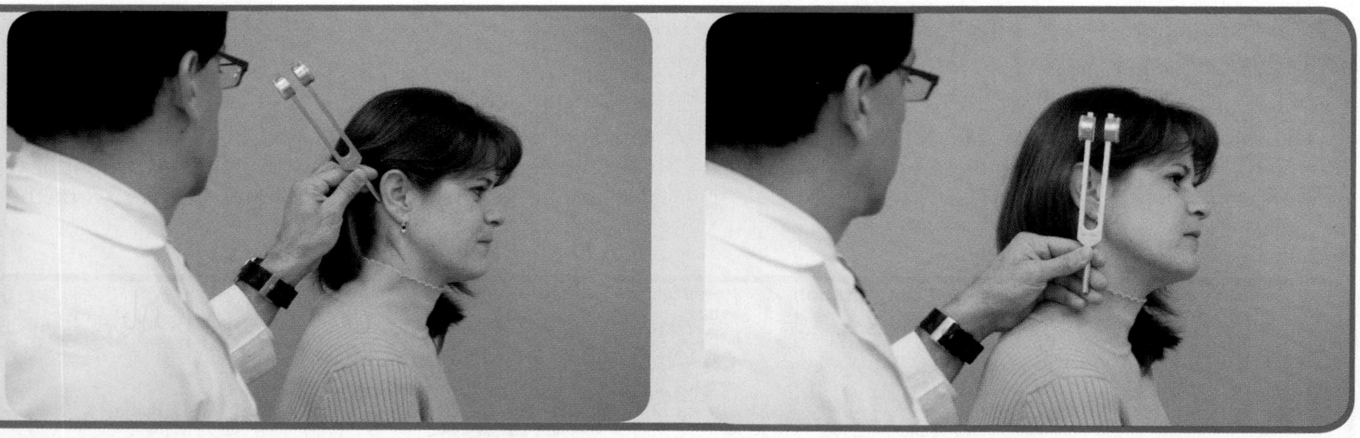

Figure 40–16A and B: Rinne test. *Delmar/Cengage Learning.*

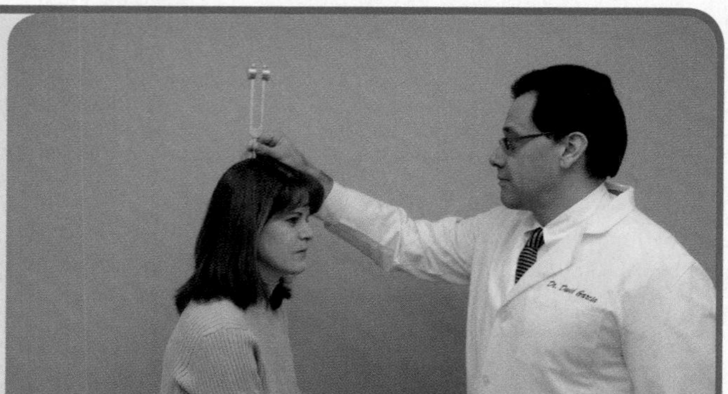

Figure 40–16C: Weber test. *Delmar/Cengage Learning.*

Occasionally, a small amount of hearing loss may occur temporarily because of a patient's physical condition. When this occurs, a recheck in one or two weeks may be advisable. There are diagnostic instruments from various manufacturers that provide audiogram and tympanogram as well as acoustic reflex results. These instruments are useful in providing objective data to determine complete diagnoses and documentation of diseases and disorders of the ear as well as evaluation of follow-up treatment.

Eye Examinations

For examinations of the eye, the provider uses an ophthalmoscope, an instrument used to examine the internal structures of the eye. Visual examinations can be performed if a patient has an eye infection or injury or needs additional screening to check vision acuity or color vision. Often, the screenings are performed prior to the provider's examination so the results can be discussed during the physical exam. The provider will advise you to do this, depending upon his or her preference.

Occasionally, the eye may need to be irrigated if there is inflammation, secretions in the eye due to infection, a chemical contamination, or a foreign particle in the eye. Your role may be to perform the irrigation. Eyes that have come in contact with a chemical are usually flushed with plain water using an eyewash station, whereas other flushing may be performed with a rubber bulb syringe or Waterpik. For these types of irrigations, a sterile saline solution is used.

Patients should be instructed to lie on their side with their face turned to the side of the eye being irrigated. A basin will be placed under the eye to catch the solution. A water-absorbent pad may also be placed under the patient. The eye should be flushed from the inner canthus or corner of the eye to the outer canthus to prevent any debris being removed from reentering the eye. Procedure 40–3 lists the steps on how to perform eye irrigation.

PATIENT EDUCATION

1. While performing procedures involving the eye, the medical assistant may want to remind patients to use eye protection when indicated, such as the use of safety glasses or goggles when working with tools that could cause particles of material to fly into the eye and cause injury.
2. Remind patients to wear protective sunglasses when out in direct sunlight for extended periods.
3. Remind patients to have routine eye examinations, especially when the family medical history includes glaucoma, cataracts, or diabetes. **Tonometry** and **funduscopy** are recommended every four years for patients past 40 years old.
4. Explain to patients that over-the-counter eye drops should be used carefully and only as directed because extended use can cause tissue damage. Used only when necessary and with the advice of the provider.
5. Advise patients not to rub their eyes because further irritation and possibly tissue damage could result. Itching, burning, or watering eyes can be signs of infection. Rubbing the eyes can transmit the infection to others.
6. In the event of a chemical splash in the eye, patients should flush the eye with clear, room temperature water for 20 minutes (nonstop) and seek medical attention immediately.

PROCEDURE 40–3 Irrigate the Eye

PURPOSE: To irrigate the patient's eye(s) to soothe tissues, relieve inflammation, and remove foreign objects and discharge

EQUIPMENT: Gloves, small basin of lukewarm irrigation solution, towel, emesis basin, irrigation syringe or bottle of solution, gauze squares, patient chart or EMR, and a pen

S **SKILL:** Perform eye irrigation.

Procedure Steps	Detailed Instructions and/or *Rationales*
1. Wash hands. Assemble the items needed for the procedure; prepare lukewarm solution.	
B 2. Identify the patient, introduce yourself, and explain the procedure, ***using language that the patient can understand.***	*Ensures that you are performing the procedure on the correct patient.*
B 3. ***Ask the patient which position would be more comfortable, sitting or lying down.*** Drape the patient with a towel to protect clothing.	Assist onto the examination table if desired.

(continues)

(continued)

Procedure Steps	Detailed Instructions and/or *Rationales*
4. Put on gloves.	
5. Ask patient to tilt his or her head back and to the side. Place the emesis basin against the head. Instruct patient to hold the basin to catch the solution during irrigation (Figure 40–17).	Placing several tissues, gauze squares, or a towel between the face and the basin will help prevent the patient from getting wet during the procedure. You might have to hold the basin yourself.
6. Gently wipe eye with gauze square from the inner to outer canthus to remove any particles before proceeding with irrigation.	
7. Fill syringe with ordered solution.	
8. Hold the affected eye open with the thumb and index finger and slowly release the solution over the eye gently and steadily.	This must be done from inner canthus to outer canthus *to prevent any solution from entering the other eye, which may not be affected, and for ease of catching solution.*
9. When irrigation is completed, use gauze squares or tissues to blot the area dry.	
10. Record the procedure in the patient's chart.	Record the type of solution that was used, which eye was irrigated, results, and any other important information you may have observed while performing the procedure.
11. Wash the items and return them to the proper storage area.	
12. Remove gloves and wash hands.	Deposit gloves in an appropriate container based upon the conditions under which irrigation was performed.

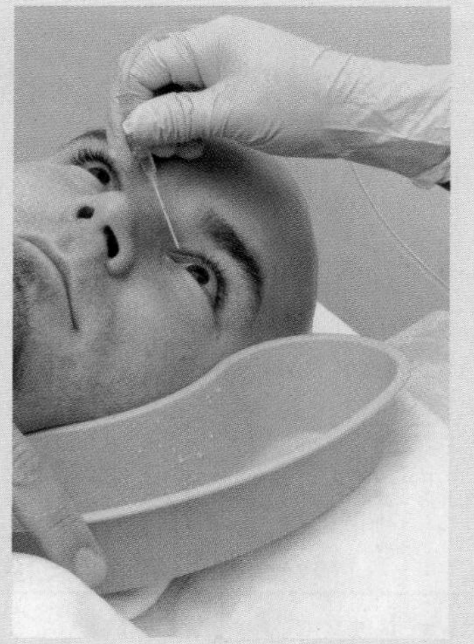

Figure 40–17: Irrigating the eye. *Delmar/Cengage Learning.*

Charting Example

3-30-XX 11:30 am	Right eye irrigated w/ H_2O to remove sand, per Dr. White; tolerated well. pt. states, "eyes less scratchy." T. EDWARDS, CMA(AAMA)

Visual Acuity

Measuring visual **acuity** is a diagnostic screening procedure most often done by the medical assistant on the patient's initial visit, prior to the physical examination. It should be performed in a well-lighted area with no interruptions. Observation of the patient for any conditions or behaviors that may indicate visual disturbances is an essential part of the overall examination.

The following are examples of what to look for when performing visual acuity tests:

- Tilting the head to the side or forward
- Blinking or watering of the eyes
- Frowning or puckering of the face
- Closing of one eye when testing both eyes
- Any sign of straining to see

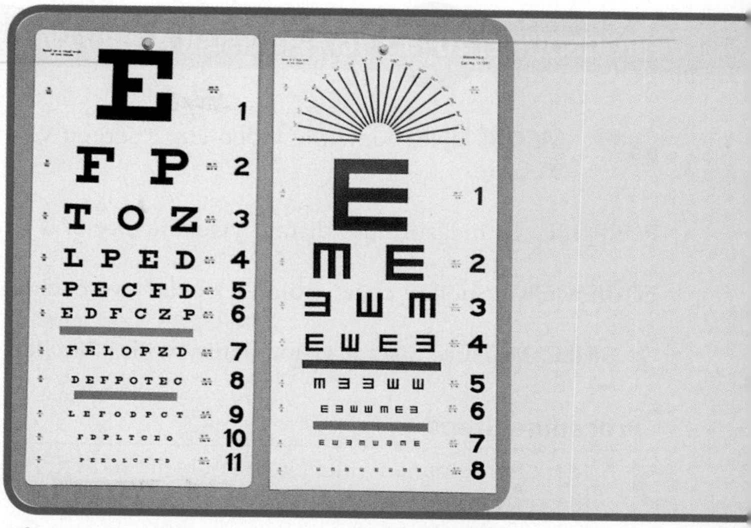

Figure 40–18: Snellen visual acuity screening charts. *Delmar/Cengage Learning.*

The most common screening device for *distance* vision is a **Snellen chart**, which shows at what distance the chart can be read by the patient. The regular chart has letters arranged in rows from largest to smallest. Those who might have difficulty with reading or are non-English speakers should be tested with the chart or cards of the letter *E* arranged in different directions. The patients are directed to use their hand, particularly the three middle fingers to show the direction the E is facing. Figure 40–18 shows two Snellen vision screening charts, which are made to standard specifications. These charts are hung on the wall with a mark 20 feet away to show where the patient should stand or sit to read the chart. The chart should be at the patient's eye level. The patient covers one eye with an **occluder** so each eye may be tested individually.

Distance visual acuity is written as a fraction. The numerator is the number of feet, or the distance from the chart; the denominator is the numbered line the patient can read. If one's distant visual acuity results are 20/100, it means that the person stood 20 feet from the chart and read the line that should be read at 100 feet. One who has 20/10 acuity can see at 20 feet what should be seen at a distance of 10 feet. A finding of 20/20 is average. Patients should be screened with and without their corrective lenses and the results recorded as such on their charts. Note that if visual acuity is 20/200 or less in the better eye with corrective lenses, the patient is considered legally blind.

Common complaints that can indicate vision problems are listed in Table 40–2. These complaints pertain to both children and adults. Perform Procedure 40–4 to measure distance vision.

TABLE 40–2 Possible Indications of Visual Disturbance

During Activities That Require Reading	Conditions	Behaviors	Complaints
1. Exhibits difficulty with near or distance vision	1. Redness of the eye(s) or eyelid(s)	1. Looks cross-eyed	1. Blurriness of vision
2. Avoids reading, writing, and related activities	2. Sties or crusting or swelling of eyelid(s)	2. Rubbing eyes frequently	2. Nausea
	3. Poor eye coordination	3. Confuses letters (e.g., *a* and *c*, *f* and *t*, *m* and *n*)	3. Headaches often
	4. Watering or discharge	4. Turns head or leans forward to see better	4. Dizziness
	5. Accident or injury to the eye	5. Blinks continually	5. Eyes sensitive to light
		6. Irritable at attempting close work	6. Feels like something in the eye(s)

PROCEDURE 40–4 Screen Visual Acuity with a Snellen Chart

MEDIA LINK: View the video clip, "Screen Visual Acuity," on the Premium Website.

PURPOSE: To measure the distant visual acuity of a patient

EQUIPMENT: Snellen chart, pointer, ocular eye occluder, patient chart or EMR, and a pen

S **SKILL:** Measure distant vision acuity with a Snellen chart.

Procedure Steps	Detailed Instructions and/or *Rationales*
B 1. Identify the patient, introduce yourself, and explain the procedure, ***using language that the patient can understand.***	*Ensures* that *you are performing the procedure on the correct patient.* The patient is to read each line from the chart as you point to it with a pointer. Tell the patient to keep both eyes open when covering one eye. This prevents squinting and blurring.
2. Ask the patient to read the chart with both eyes (OU) first, standing 20 feet from the chart.	The chart should be at the patient's eye level. Follow office policy in giving the test. Asking patients to read only certain lines of the chart may be less time consuming (e.g., "Begin at line 6.").
3. To test acuity of the right eye, have the patient cover the left eye with an occluder.	If patient wears corrective lenses, the procedure should be performed first wearing lenses and then without and recorded as such.
4. Record the smallest line the patient can read without making a mistake.	Some physicians allow up to two errors on the smallest line read. Record any observations of individual accommodations made to read chart, such as squinting or turning the head.
5. Have the patient cover his or her right eye and test acuity of the left, following the same procedure.	
6. Record the number of the smallest line the patient can read.	

Charting Example

2-14-XX 11:30 am	Snellen findings: Vision screening per Dr. White, right eye 25/30, left eye 20/40, no squinting observed. T. EDWARDS, CMA(AAMA)

The **Jaeger chart** is a common method of screening for **near** vision acuity. The screening procedure should be conducted in a well-lighted room without interruptions. The patient should be tested with and without wearing corrective lenses, and each eye is tested separately for a complete assessment to be made by the provider. The chart used for this procedure is a card held by the patient between 14 and 16 inches from the eye (measure with a yardstick, a meterstick, or a tape measure for accuracy). This is the distance at which one with normal vision is able to read printed material (a magazine) or work on something that requires close attention (sewing). The Jaeger screening test consists of reading material that has ascending sizes of type ranging from 0.37 mm to 2.5 mm (Figure 40–19). The test contains excerpts from a manuscript sectioned into short paragraphs, none of which are the same. Observe the patient for any difficulty (e.g., holding the

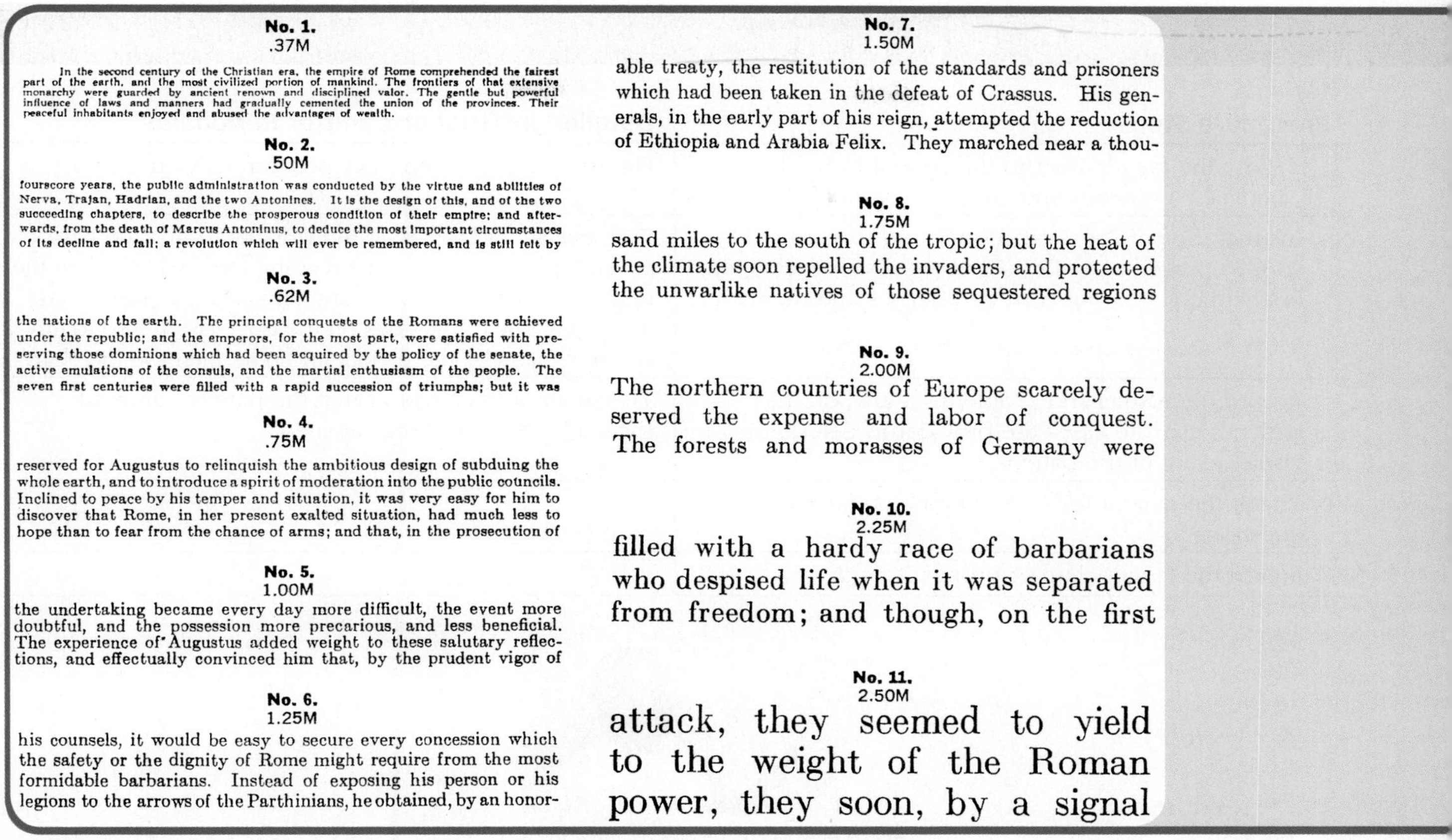

No. 1.
.37M

In the second century of the Christian era, the empire of Rome comprehended the fairest part of the earth, and the most civilized portion of mankind. The frontiers of that extensive monarchy were guarded by ancient renown and disciplined valor. The gentle but powerful influence of laws and manners had gradually cemented the union of the provinces. Their peaceful inhabitants enjoyed and abused the advantages of wealth.

No. 2.
.50M

fourscore years, the public administration was conducted by the virtue and abilities of Nerva, Trajan, Hadrian, and the two Antonines. It is the design of this, and of the two succeeding chapters, to describe the prosperous condition of their empire; and afterwards, from the death of Marcus Antoninus, to deduce the most important circumstances of its decline and fall; a revolution which will ever be remembered, and is still felt by

No. 3.
.62M

the nations of the earth. The principal conquests of the Romans were achieved under the republic; and the emperors, for the most part, were satisfied with preserving those dominions which had been acquired by the policy of the senate, the active emulations of the consuls, and the martial enthusiasm of the people. The seven first centuries were filled with a rapid succession of triumphs; but it was

No. 4.
.75M

reserved for Augustus to relinquish the ambitious design of subduing the whole earth, and to introduce a spirit of moderation into the public councils. Inclined to peace by his temper and situation, it was very easy for him to discover that Rome, in her present exalted situation, had much less to hope than to fear from the chance of arms; and that, in the prosecution of

No. 5.
1.00M

the undertaking became every day more difficult, the event more doubtful, and the possession more precarious, and less beneficial. The experience of Augustus added weight to these salutary reflections, and effectually convinced him that, by the prudent vigor of

No. 6.
1.25M

his counsels, it would be easy to secure every concession which the safety or the dignity of Rome might require from the most formidable barbarians. Instead of exposing his person or his legions to the arrows of the Parthinians, he obtained, by an honor-

No. 7.
1.50M

able treaty, the restitution of the standards and prisoners which had been taken in the defeat of Crassus. His generals, in the early part of his reign, attempted the reduction of Ethiopia and Arabia Felix. They marched near a thou-

No. 8.
1.75M

sand miles to the south of the tropic; but the heat of the climate soon repelled the invaders, and protected the unwarlike natives of those sequestered regions

No. 9.
2.00M

The northern countries of Europe scarcely deserved the expense and labor of conquest. The forests and morasses of Germany were

No. 10.
2.25M

filled with a hardy race of barbarians who despised life when it was separated from freedom; and though, on the first

No. 11.
2.50M

attack, they seemed to yield to the weight of the Roman power, they soon, by a signal

Figure 40–19: Example of a Jaeger chart. *Delmar/Cengage Learning.*

chart right in front of the face, squinting, or blinking) while trying to read the card. You then record the section number that the patient can read easily. Refer to Procedure 40–5.

Electronic devices that screen both near and distance visual acuity are also available. Some products are capable of fully automating the screening process and generating a final results report.

PROCEDURE 40–5 Screen Visual Acuity with the Jaeger System

PURPOSE: To determine near distance visual acuity of a patient by using the Jaeger system

EQUIPMENT: Jaeger near vision acuity chart, patient chart or EMR, and a pen

S SKILL: Measure near vision acuity with a Jaeger chart.

Procedure Steps	Detailed Instructions and/or *Rationales*
B 1. Identify the patient, introduce yourself, and explain the procedure, ***using language that the patient can understand.***	*Ensures that you are performing the procedure on the correct patient.*
2. Have the patient sit up straight but comfortably in a well-lighted area.	

(continues)

(continued)

Procedure Steps	Detailed Instructions and/or *Rationales*
3. Hand the Jaeger chart to the patient to hold, between 14 inches and 16 inches from the eyes.	Figure 40–20 shows proper positioning of the card.
4. Instruct the patient to read (out loud to you) the various paragraphs of the card with both eyes open, first without wearing corrective lenses and then with.	Each eye should be tested individually having the person cover the left eye first while reading the card and then the right. Observe carefully for any difficulty the patient has in reading any of the lines on the card. Listen also to any remarks made by the patient and note them on the chart.
5. Record the results and problems, if any, on the patient's chart to assist the provider in determining the visual acuity of the patient.	The smallest line of print that the patient can read should be recorded and initialed.
6. Thank the patient for cooperation and answer any questions.	
7. Return the Jaeger chart to proper storage.	

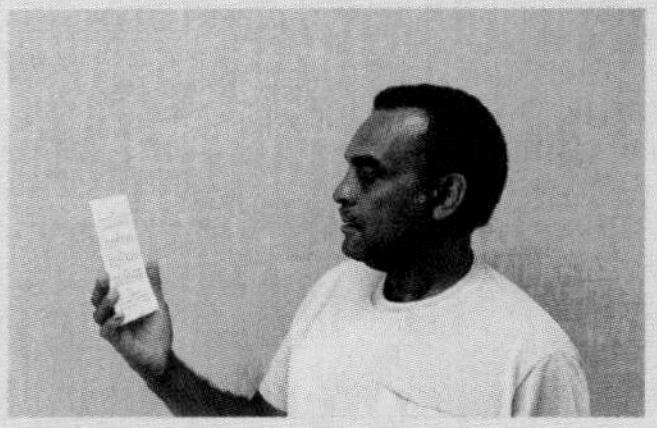

Figure 40–20: Proper distance for near visual acuity screening. *Delmar/Cengage Learning.*

Charting Example

8-17-XX 11:30 am	Screened vision w/Jaeger per Dr. White; read No 3 (62M) both eyes w/corrective lenses; No 11 (2.5) right eye (squinting); No 10 (2.2) left eye. T. EDWARDS, CMA(AAMA)

Color vision acuity means that one can accurately recognize colors. The inability to perceive colors of the spectrum distinctly is commonly termed *color blindness* or the technically correct and preferred term, *color deficient.* This is caused by changes that happen in the pigments of the cones in the retina of the eyes as they react to red, green, and blue light wavelengths.

There are two primary types of color deficiency: daltonism and achromatic vision. Daltonism, which is the most common, is a hereditary visual disorder in which the person cannot tell the difference between red and green. Achromatic vision is total color blindness (the person cannot recognize any color at all) and is very rare. These people see everything in white, gray, and black. The probable cause for this condition is defective cones in the retina or complete absence of them.

Several other conditions involve one's inability or weakness in distinguishing certain colors. In deuteranopia, a person has trouble telling any difference between varying shades of green and of bluish reds and neutral shades. Protanopia is partial color blindness. These people have trouble with the perception of reds, and sometimes yellows and greens are confused. This condition is often referred to as red blindness. Tritanopia, which is the rarest, means that the person cannot distinguish blue color.

Although electronic devices are available for screening color vision, the most common method for screening patients for defects in distinguishing color vision acuity is with an **Ishihara** color plates book. A sample of the series of multicolored charts in the test book is shown in Figure 40–21. In these pictures of the color plates, a person with normal color vision acuity can see a pink-red number 8 against a blue-green background and a blue-green number 5 against a pink-red background.

Patients may be asked to trace the patterns of color with a cotton swab as you observe them. Instruct the patients not to use their fingers for the tracing because the oil on their skin can discolor the plates. There are letters

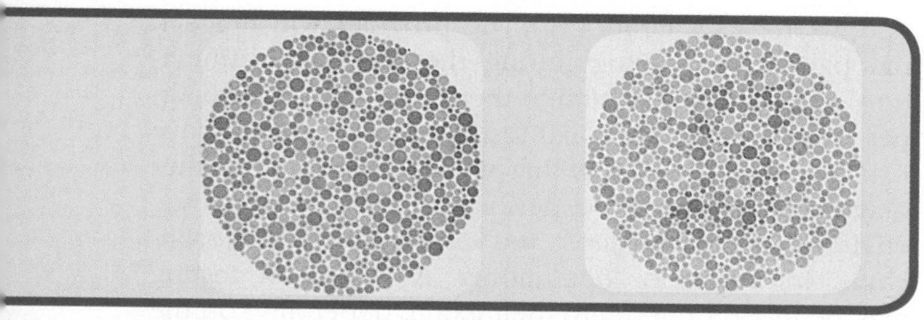

Figure 40–21: Sample of Ishihara color plates. *Delmar/Cengage Learning.*

and numbers (and curved lines and shapes for nonreaders) that are one color within another. When administering this procedure, make sure that the room is well-lit, preferably with natural daylight (not direct sunlight), so that the patient is able to follow your instructions without straining to see. Whatever method of color vision assessment is used where you are employed, it is vital for you to be accurate in reporting the results. You need to have your own eyes tested first to determine whether they have normal color vision before administering the test to patients. Perform Procedure 40–6 to measure color vision acuity.

Patients with thyroid conditions should be routinely screened for color vision acuity during scheduled visits. The procedure should include testing with both eyes first and then each eye separately to see whether there is any difference in the perception of color in either eye. The eye not used should be covered with an occluder and not held shut. Grave's disease patients especially need frequent assessment of their color vision acuity changes. The color vision test results may lead to earlier diagnosis and treatment of Grave's ophthalmopathy.

PROCEDURE 40–6 Determine Color Vision Acuity by the Ishihara Method

MEDIA LINK: View the video, "Color Vision Acuity," for this chapter on the Premium Website.

PURPOSE: To determine color vision acuity of a patient by using the Ishihara method

EQUIPMENT: Ishihara book, proper lighting, occluder, patient chart or EMR, and a pen

S SKILL: Determine color vision acuity by using Ishihara plates.

Procedure Steps	Detailed Instructions and/or *Rationales*
1. Obtain the chart from the back of the book.	Before administering this screening test, you should be tested.
B 2. Identify the patient, introduce yourself, and explain the procedure, ***using language that the patient can understand.***	*Ensures that you are performing the procedure on the correct patient.*
3. Ask the patient first to read the plates with both eyes.	If the patient wears corrective lenses, perform the testing with the patient wearing them and be sure to document it in the patient's chart.
4. Have the patient cover the left eye to test the right eye and then cover the right to test the left.	Make sure to note any difficulty or complaint of the patient during the screening process.
5. Compare answers given with those on chart. Record those frames the patient misses and write down what the patient reports so that the degree of color deficiency may be determined by the provider.	
6. Document results in the patient's chart.	

Charting Example

9-24-XX 11:30 am	*Color vision screening per Dr. White; Ishihara color plates—accurately read.* T. EDWARDS, CMA(AAMA)

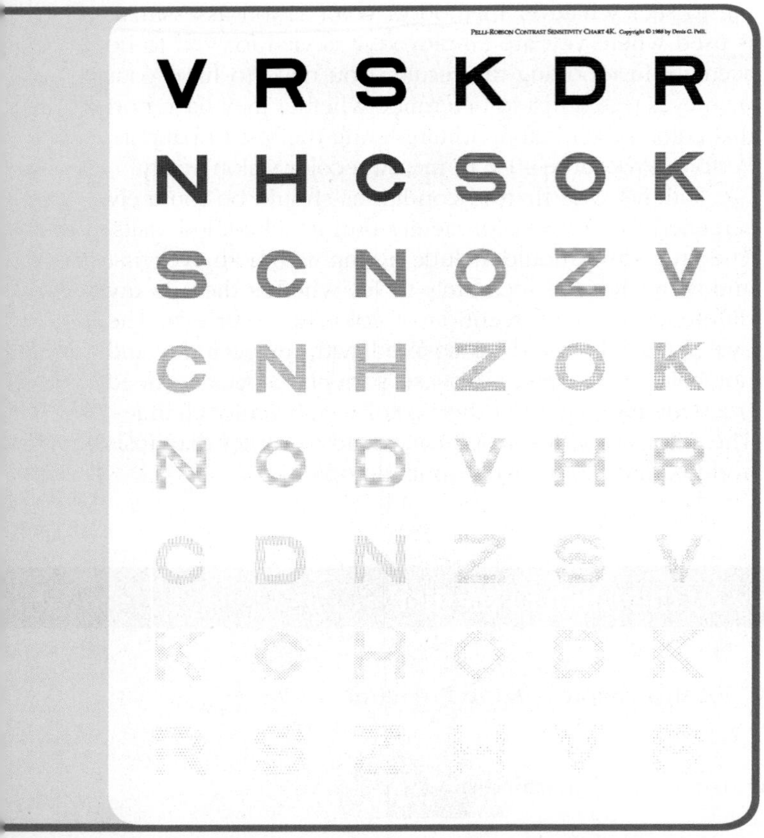

Figure 40–22: Pelli–Robson contrast sensitivity chart. *Courtesy of Dr. Denis Pelli, NYU.*

Contrast Sensitivity Screening

The Pelli–Robson *contrast sensitivity* chart measures contrast sensitivity by determining the faintest contrast an observer can see (Figure 40–22). Clinical evidence shows that contrast sensitivity is affected by all the major eye diseases—diabetic retinopathy, macular degeneration, glaucoma, and cataract. Therefore, measuring contrast sensitivity provides a sensitive screening test for eye disease to provide earlier diagnosis and treatment.

Another contrast sensitivity screening method is the CSV-1000, developed by Vectorvision. All patients can be tested with this method, but it is especially useful in screening small children, internationals, and people who are illiterate. This test has a series of four groups of circles. In these rows of circles, some are solid gray in color and some have vertical lines. The patient is instructed to look at the first group and tell which circles have lines within them. The last correctly identified circle in each group is charted on a graph. The results of this test are interpreted by the provider.

RESPIRATORY EXAMINATIONS

When the patient arrives for his or her visit, recall that one of the first procedures performed is the monitoring of his or her vital signs, including the respiratory rate. (Refer to Chapter 38.) The provider will recheck the patient's breathing during the physical examination to determine whether there are any abnormalities that warrant additional testing. Many patients have risk factors or infections that would encourage further diagnostic testing to be performed, such as smoking, environmental exposures, and infections such as bronchitis, influenza, or pneumonia. A variety of testing may be incorporated into their exam, depending on the patient's symptoms.

Vital Capacity Tests

Vital capacity is defined as the greatest volume of air that can be expelled during a complete, slow, unforced expiration following a maximum inspiration. Vital capacity should equal inspiratory capacity plus expiratory reserve. Vital capacity is usually reported in both absolute values and statistically derived values based on the age, sex, and height of the patient. The statistical value is reported as a percentage.

The spirometer is an instrument that tests the capacity of the lungs. Many providers prefer to use the handheld spirometer, which comes with vital capacity charts. Vital capacity testing is performed to evaluate patients who are suspected of having pulmonary insufficiency. Vital capacity testing aids in the diagnosis and degree of functional or obstructive abnormalities. It also helps the provider find the cause of dyspnea and evaluate the effectiveness of medication and therapy.

PATIENT EDUCATION

When scheduling patients for vital capacity tests, it is important to advise them to eat lightly and not to smoke for at least six hours before the appointment. Patients should refrain from routine treatment, and medication should not be taken until after the test is completed.

In preparing to perform this diagnostic procedure, instruct the patient regarding the necessary steps and demonstrate the use of the spirometer. Routine procedures, such as height, weight, and vital signs, should have already been taken and recorded in the patient's chart. Showing the patient how to hold the instrument and what is expected will yield a more accurate test result. Disposable mouthpieces are used to prevent disease transmission. Most spirometers are computerized and have a printout of the results within minutes of administering the test. Type in the patient's name, age, height, race, gender, account number, and any other information, if applicable, before you start the test.

Figure 40–23 pictures a medical assistant coaching a patient through the procedure. A clip is placed on the patient's nose to force the expired air out of the lungs directly into the mouthpiece (make sure patient's mouth is sealed around the mouthpiece) and into the spirometer. Instruct the patient to stand up straight and to take in a slow deep breath. Coach the patient to expel all the air from the lungs quickly until it is not possible to exhale any more, within approximately 15 seconds. Give the patient several practice runs before beginning the official test because it is an awkward procedure for most people. Follow each of the expirations with a few seconds of resting for the patient. Watch for signs of stress, dizziness, coughing, or other problems the patient might have during the test. Generally, three to five expirations are tested. The results are analyzed by the computerized instrument, and the diagnostic data are printed for evaluation by the provider. Test results below 80 percent are usually considered abnormal. This spirometry reading is placed in the patient's chart, along with a notation of any symptoms or problems the patient might have had during the test and your initials. Spirometry tests should not be performed when the patient has been diagnosed with angina, acute coronary insufficiency, or recent myocardial infarction. Allow the patient to sit and relax to wait for consultation with the provider. Instruct the patient to resume medication and therapy routine as directed by the provider. Procedure 40–7 provides step-by-step instruction.

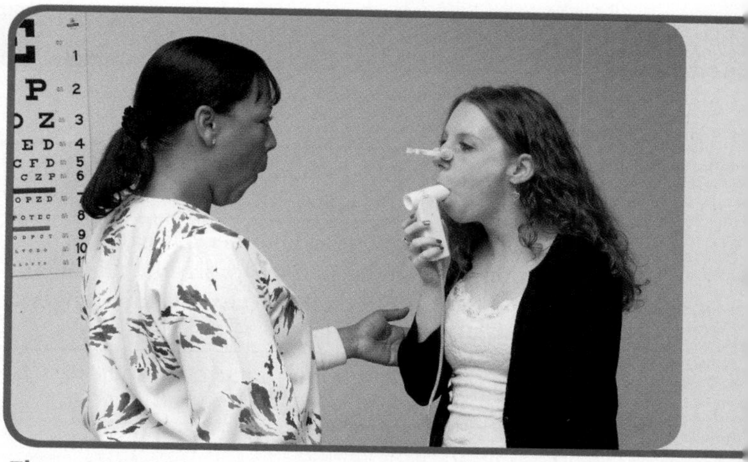

Figure 40–23: The medical assistant coaches the patient during the spirometry test. *Delmar/Cengage Learning.*

PROCEDURE 40–7 Perform Spirometry Testing

PURPOSE: Evaluate patients suspected of having pulmonary insufficiency

EQUIPMENT: Spirometer and disposable mouthpieces, patient chart or EMR, and a pen

S **SKILL:** Perform spirometry testing.

Procedure Steps	Detailed Instructions and/or *Rationales*
1. Obtain the spirometer machine, assemble the necessary equipment and supplies; wash hands.	
B 2. Identify the patient, introduce yourself, and explain the procedure and equipment, ***using language the patient will understand.***	*Ensures that you are performing the procedure on the correct patient.* Let the patient become familiar with the equipment by having the patient breathe into the machine.
B 3. ***Be sure the patient is in a comfortable position and any restrictive clothing (such as a tie or collar) is loosened before initiating the procedure.***	
4. Instruct the patient to sit or stand as straight as possible and not bend at the waist while blowing into the disposable mouthpiece.	

(continues)

(continued)

Procedure Steps	Detailed Instructions and/or *Rationales*
5. Instruct the patient to make a tight seal around the mouthpiece with the lips.	
6. After telling the patient to take deep breaths in (inhalation), coach the patient to breathe all the air out of the lungs until unable to exhale any longer, usually about 15 seconds.	
7. Allow the patient to have a practice run before performing the actual test.	
8. Support the patient during the test and have the patient keep blowing into the mouthpiece until told to stop.	Watch for signs of stress, dizziness, coughing, or other problems during the test.
9. Document the procedure in the patient's chart and place the results in the chart for the provider's review.	

Charting Example

3-30-XX 11:30 am	Spirometry testing performed per Dr. White. Patient tolerated well. T. EDWARDS, CMA(AAMA)

Peak Flow Testing

Peak flow testing measures a patient's ability to exhale. A peak flow meter is a monitoring device that measures the peak expiratory flow rate, that is, the highest speed at which one can forcibly blow air from the lungs after taking in as deep a breath as possible (Figure 40–24). Peak flow testing may be used if a patient had an inconclusive or normal spirometry test but is still presenting with asthma symptoms. It can also be performed to monitor the effectiveness of medications or to determine whether another form of treatment should be tried. Daily peak flow readings can help detect subtle changes in lung function, sometimes even before the patient is aware of them. Patients can benefit from a peak flow meter in several ways: to recognize that asthma may be occurring at night, to improve perception of asthma, to identify factors that worsen asthma and to predict worsening of asthma. Peak flow measurements can change over time, depending on the patient's current medical condition, age, weight, and the time of day it is taken. Procedure 40–8 provides complete steps on how to perform a peak flow measurement on a patient.

Although the predicted "normal" peak flow is determined by height, age, and sex, it is preferable to gauge asthma control by comparing daily peak flow readings with the patient's personal best reading. This is defined as the highest measurement the patient can achieve in the middle of a good day, after using any prescribed inhaled bronchodilators. The patient might need to use a peak flow meter for one or two weeks to arrive at the personal best number. After a personal best peak flow has been established, every effort must be made to maintain values within 80 percent of this number. If the reading falls between 50 percent and 80 percent, the patient will usually need to take a quick action inhaler; if it falls below 50 percent, the patient must seek emergency care. Providers will have guidelines they want their patients to follow.

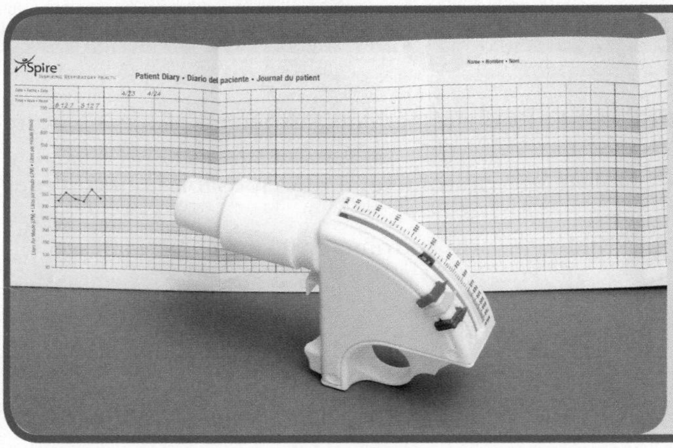

FIGURE 40–24: Peak flow meter with patient diary. *Delmar/Cengage Learning.*

PROCEDURE 40–8 Perform Peak Flow Testing

MEDIA LINK: View the animation, "Peak Flow Testing," for this chapter on the Premium Website.

PURPOSE: Correctly instruct the patient to measure his or her peak expiratory flow rate

EQUIPMENT: Peak flow meter, mouth piece, medical order, waste container, patient chart or EMR, and a pen

S **SKILL:** Instruct the patient to measure his or her peak expiratory flow rate.

Procedure Steps	Detailed Instructions and/or *Rationales*
1. Assemble equipment and supplies; wash hands.	
B 2. Identify the patient, introduce yourself, and explain the procedure and equipment, ***using language the patient will understand.***	*Ensures that you are performing the procedure on the correct patient.*
B 3. ***Be sure the patient is in a comfortable position, and any restrictive clothing (such as a tie or collar) is loosened before initiating the procedure.***	Help the patient to a standing position (if needed).
4. Set the indicator to the bottom (lowest number) of the scale.	
5. Instruct the patient to take in a deep breath, place the meter to mouth, close lips around the mouthpiece, and blow as hard as he or she can.	
6. Write down the number the patient achieved.	
7. Repeat steps 5, 6, and 7 two more times.	
8. Instruct the patient to do a peak flow 2–3 times a day.	Instruct the patient to take readings in the AM, PM, and when he or she is short of breath.
9. Explain to the patient how to establish his or her "Personal Best"; explain the "Three Zone" system and how to record results in his or her peak flow diary.	
10. Dispose of mouthpiece in the waste container.	
11. Document.	

Charting Example

3-30-XX 11:30 am	Patient instructed on how to measure peak expiratory flow, using a peak flow meter, how to obtain personal best, and how to monitor the three zones with their results. T. EDWARDS, CMA(AAMA)

Pulse Oximetry

As discussed in Chapter 38, **pulse oximetry** is a simple, noninvasive test that measures the patient's pulse rate and oxygen saturation (SAT) level in the blood. Many cardiopulmonary conditions could warrant the provider seeking a patient's oxygen saturation level. Common cardiac and pulmonary conditions include heart attacks, congestive heart failure (CHF) and coronary artery disease (CAD), asthma, pneumonia, and respiratory syncytial virus (RSV), a common but serious respiratory virus often seen in infants and children.

Many oximeter models are available; common ones are small, handheld devices with a monitor and a sensor that is clipped onto the patient's finger (Figure 40–25). The sensor has an infrared light in it that transmits through the patient's tissues to a photo detector on the opposite side of the clip. The device measures the amount of light that is absorbed by the hemoglobin, which is then displayed as a percentage on the monitor. Additional attachments can be used in the event of poor circulation, calloused fingers, nail polish, or if the patient is an infant or small child. The attachment can be wrapped around the toe, earlobe, or bridge of the nose and is held in place similar to a bandage. A normal pulse oximeter reading is 95 percent or higher. Refer to Procedure 40–9 for instructions on how to perform a pulse oximeter test.

You may be instructed to schedule patients for further pulmonary function studies to be performed by a pulmonary and thoracic specialist. More sophisticated equipment may be necessary to evaluate a patient's condition.

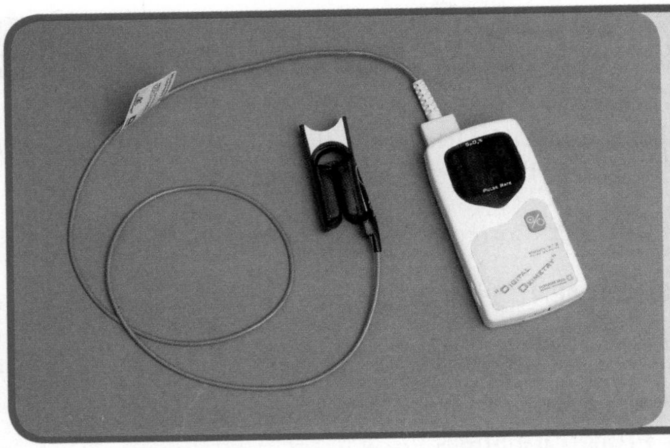

Figure 40–25: Pulse oximeter. *Delmar/Cengage Learning.*

PROCEDURE 40–9 Perform Pulse Oximetry Testing

PURPOSE: To measure a patient's oxygen level in the blood

EQUIPMENT: Pulse oximeter, alcohol wipes, nail polish remover if needed, patient chart or EHR, and a pen

S **SKILL:** Perform pulse oximetry testing.

Procedure Steps	Detailed Instructions and/or *Rationales*
1. Wash hands and assemble equipment.	
B 2. Identify the patient, introduce yourself, and explain the procedure and equipment, ***using language the patient will understand.***	*Ensures that you are performing the procedure on the correct patient.*
3. Select a site for the sensor.	The finger is commonly used. If the patient has poor circulation, use another site such as the bridge of the nose, earlobe, or forehead (you need a special sensor for this).
4. Clean the site with alcohol. Remove nail polish if needed. Wash with soap and water.	
5. Apply sensor, read results.	
6. Note the results (including pulse) according to the manufacturer's instructions. (Take reading after 10 seconds.)	
B 7. ***Apply critical thinking skills in performing patient assessment and care, notifying provider immediately of abnormal results.*** Abnormal results are less than 95%.	
8. Document procedure, site of application, (sensor applied to left index finger), and results.	

Charting Example

3-30-XX 11:30 am	Pulse oximetry sensor applied to L index finger per Dr. White. P 70 SpO2 99%. T. EDWARDS, CMA(AAMA)

PROCTOLOGIC EXAMINATIONS

In the diagnosis of hemorrhoids, fissures, and ulcerations, the provider usually begins investigative procedures by examining the anus and the interior of the rectum with a **proctoscope**. The proctoscope permits viewing of the anal canal and lower rectal area when sigmoidoscopy is not necessary; for example, the provider may view the intestinal **mucosa** following a normal bowel movement. Figure 40–26 shows a tray setup for a basic rectal exam.

Some of the instruments used in these procedures are shown in Figure 40–27A through C. The rectal speculum (A) allows viewing of the anal canal and rectum, the biopsy forceps (B) permit removing a tissue sample for examination, and the snare (C) is used to detach polyps or other pendulous growths from the mucosa to be examined. All instruments and items that come in contact with a body cavity must be free from microorganisms. The medical assistant is generally responsible for this task. Some instruments can be disinfected and then autoclaved. Delicate instruments and those with plastic or rubber parts will require processing in a germicidal solution. (Refer to Chapter 36.)

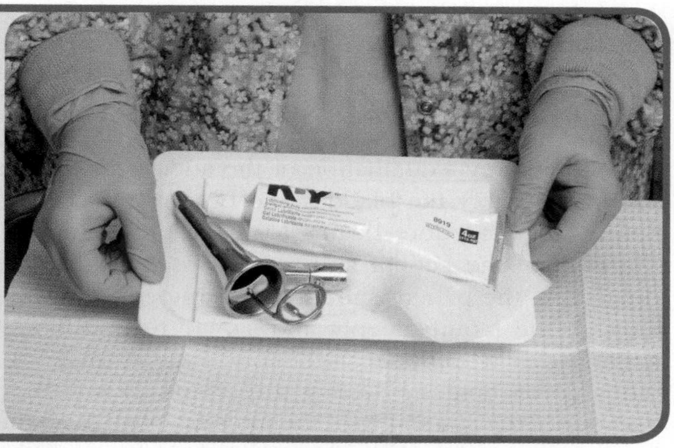

Figure 40–26: Tray setup for a rectal exam. *Delmar/Cengage Learning.*

Proper positioning of patients during the exam is important for both the provider's viewing of the rectum and sigmoid colon and for the patient's comfort. Proctology tables (refer to Figure 39–9) are designed especially for this procedure. They provide support of the patient's chest and head with the arm resting against the headboard as the table is tilted to the knee-chest position. Those who cannot tolerate this position are assisted into a Sims' position for the exam. You should ask about the provider's preference in patient position because there are variations.

Patient Instructions and Preparation

Patients may be instructed to eat a light diet containing plenty of clear liquids and avoiding dairy products for 24 hours before the exam and to have a plain cleansing **enema** the morning of, or two hours before, the exam. Other providers may wish patients to use **laxatives** the day before and an enema the night before and the morning of the exam.

Some exams require the use of **evacuants** by the patient before the exam; if this is the case, instructions should be made clear to the patient before the appointment is scheduled. Helping him or her choose a convenient appointment time and explaining the reasons for the preparations they must undergo will usually be appreciated.

For the patient's convenience, make sure that you use an examination room that is close to the restroom if an enema is administered. The enema is a simple procedure, one that patients can do at home when advised by the provider. Your patience and understanding are needed here because most patients are embarrassed to have this done.

Occasionally, even when the patient follows the list of instructions, the enema solution is not retained long enough for it to work. Encourage the patient to hold the contents of the enema longer and perhaps explain that the longer the contents are held, the more successful

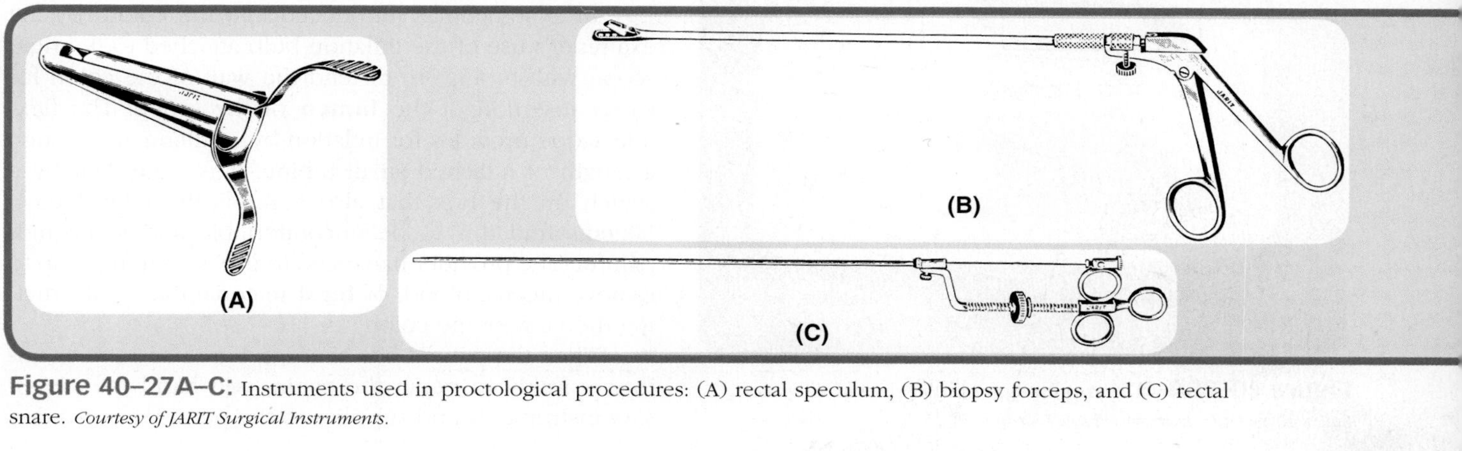

Figure 40–27A–C: Instruments used in proctological procedures: (A) rectal speculum, (B) biopsy forceps, and (C) rectal snare. *Courtesy of JARIT Surgical Instruments.*

the results will be. Often, encouraging deep breathing and placing a couple of tissues over the anal opening and applying gentle pressure will aid in retaining the fluid. Otherwise, it may have to be repeated or the exam rescheduled.

Sigmoidoscopy

Sigmoidoscopy is a diagnostic examination of the interior of the sigmoid colon. It is a useful aid in the diagnosis of cancer of the colon, ulcerations, **polyps**, tumors, bleeding, and other lower intestinal disorders. The sigmoidoscope is an instrument with a light source and a magnifying lens, which permits viewing the mucous membranes of the sigmoid colon. Many providers use a **flexible sigmoidoscope** (Figure 40–28), although metal and plastic (disposable) scopes are still occasionally used. The flexible sigmoidoscope can be inserted much farther into the colon with less discomfort. This instrument makes it possible to view more of the interior of the colon.

When using the metal or plastic type, an **obturator** (a tool with a solid, rounded end) is inserted into the sigmoidoscope. The tip of the obturator and scope are lubricated and carefully inserted into the rectum and sigmoid. Then the obturator is removed so that the S shape of the colon can be seen. Patients find this an uncomfortable and unpleasant procedure.

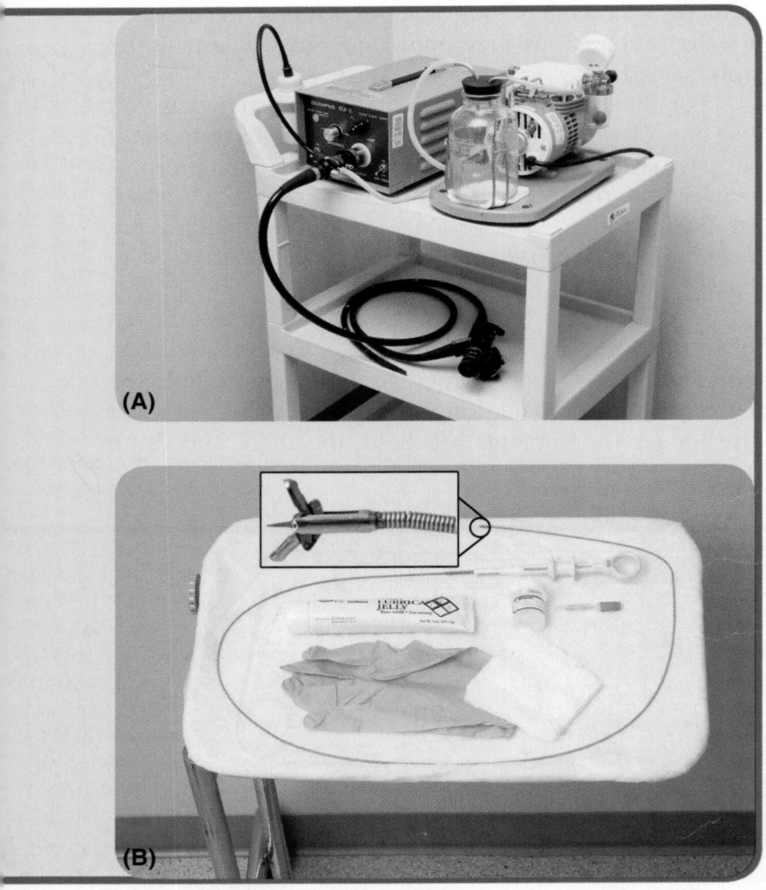

Figure 40–28A–B: Setup for sigmoidoscopy with flexible sigmoidoscope. *Delmar/Cengage Learning.*

PATIENT EDUCATION

The medical assistant often instructs the patient in how to prepare for the sigmoidoscopy and explains how the test is performed. For successful examination, proper preparation is essential. In addition to having the patient restrict dairy products, raw fruits and vegetables, and grains and cereals from his or her diet, encourage the patient to drink plenty of clear liquids and eat lightly the day before the scheduled appointment for the sigmoid colon exam.

Manufactured preps are used to clean the colon and, usually, an enema should be self-administered at home approximately two hours before the exam. Providers may vary the instructions according to the patient's condition, so it is best to ask before proceeding with instructions. If patients are not completely informed about preparations and the exam is attempted with unsatisfactory results, it will have to be repeated. It is best to give patients both oral and written instructions.

As with any examination of the abdomen, ask the patient to empty the bladder and evacuate the bowel before the procedure begins to make the exam easier for both the patient and the provider. During the procedure, the patient should be instructed to breathe through the mouth deeply and slowly relax abdominal muscles to reduce discomfort. Patients may feel the urge to defecate during any colon examination because of the stretching of the intestinal wall from the instrument passing through and air being introduced with it. The procedure should last only a minute or two, especially if patients have followed preparation instructions.

Air is sometimes introduced into the colon (by the examiner's use of the inflation bulb attached to the rigid scope with tubing) to distend the wall of the colon for easier insertion of the **lumen** of the scope. The flexible scope provides for inflation by instilling air through a length of attached small tubing. It is controlled by a switch on the box that also controls the light source. Patients find this to be uncomfortable and sometimes painful. The provider may need to use a suction pump to remove mucus, blood, or **fecal** material that is obstructing the view of the colon.

When the patient has been prepared and the examiner is ready to begin the exam, you hand the necessary instruments and supplies to the provider as needed and provide support to the patient. During the sigmoidoscopy, the provider might want to take a biopsy of questionable tissue from the sigmoid colon to aid in confirming the diagnosis. A biopsy lab request form must be completed and accompany any tissue sent to the lab. Containers for biopsy specimens have a preservative solution to preserve the tissue until the analysis is done.

Remember to advise patients to report any problems, such as bleeding, discharge, swelling, or any other unusual discomfort, following any proctologic procedure.

The examinations discussed in this chapter are by no means the only ones performed in medical offices and clinics. You will learn many others as you gain experience and knowledge in assisting.

PATIENT EDUCATION

When patients come in for rectal or sigmoidoscopy examinations, here are a few informative topics you might discuss with them:

1. Laxatives and enemas should be used only at the direction of the provider.
2. Constipation may be avoided or relieved by including fresh fruits and vegetables and cereals and grains in the diet, drinking plenty of liquids (water), and getting regular exercise.
3. If patients have any of the following symptoms persistently, consulting the provider is strongly advised because it could mean that a disease or an abnormal condition is present: **heartburn** or indigestion; nausea, vomiting, or both; constipation or diarrhea; excessive gas or bloating; or feces that is tarry (black) or other than a normal brown color.
4. Inform patients over age 40 that they should routinely test their stool for blood every two years for detection of cancer of the colon or more often if advised by the provider. Patients over age 50 should test annually.

PROCEDURE 40–10 Assist with a Flexible Sigmoidoscopy

PURPOSE: To assist in examination of the sigmoid colon

EQUIPMENT: Gloves; water-soluble lubricant; gauze squares; flexible sigmoidoscope; long cotton-tipped swabs; drape sheet (fenestrated optional); suction machine (container with room temperature water); tissues; if ordered by physician: biopsy forceps, specimen container for transport to lab; lab request form; patient chart or EMR; and a pen

S **SKILL:** Assist with a flexible sigmoidoscopy procedure.

Procedure Steps	Detailed Instructions and/or *Rationales*
B 1. Identify patient, introduce yourself, and explain the procedure, ***using language that the patient understands.***	*Ensures that you are performing the procedure on the correct patient.* Ask the patient to empty the bladder and bowel.
2. Assemble all needed items on a Mayo tray near the end of the examination table.	If a biopsy is scheduled, complete the lab request form and label the specimen container.
3. Plug in cord of light source to make sure it works properly; then turn it off.	*If left on, it will be uncomfortably warm for the patient and can cause a burn.*
B 4. ***Instruct the patient to disrobe from the waist down and let you know when he or she is ready. Assist the patient to sit at the end of the table and cover him or her with the drape sheet for privacy.***	
5. Wash hands and put on gloves.	

(continues)

(continued)

Procedure Steps	Detailed Instructions and/or *Rationales*
6. Just before the provider is ready to begin the exam, assist the patient into a knee-chest or Sims' position, whichever the provider prefers.	Many providers have an examining table that permits the patient to kneel on a pad and then be placed in a proctological position to facilitate the procedure.
7. Assist the provider by applying about two tablespoons of lubricant on gauze square for the tip of the gloved fingers.	The provider makes a digital examination of the anus and rectum prior to insertion of the endoscope.
8. As the provider finishes the digital exam, plug the sigmoidoscope into the light source. Secure the air-inflation tubing and have it ready to hand to the provider; activate the switches for air inflation and light.	
9. As the provider inserts the sigmoidoscope, be ready to hand items as needed.	Have the suction machine plugged in and suction tip secured. *Often, fecal material or unexpelled enema fluid is present and must be removed before adequate viewing can be accomplished.*
10. Be prepared to rinse the suction tip in water if it becomes clogged.	Flexible scopes aspirate through the attached tubing when suction is activated.
11. If biopsy is indicated, hand biopsy forceps to the provider and have a specimen container open so the provider can place tissue in it. Place the cap on the container securely.	
12. Use tissues to clean lubricant and waste from the patient's anal area and discard it into the waste container.	
13. Place a small pad or dressing over the anal area in case of light bleeding.	
14. Assist the patient to resting prone position (or return table to starting position).	
B 15. ***Assist the patient to a sitting position, allowing time for balance to return before helping him or her down from the table. Instruct the patient to dress.***	
16. Wear gloves to clean the exam table and instruments. The scope and suction tip should be cleaned with detergent and water and placed in a disinfectant to be sterilized.	Follow the manufacturer's instructions for cleaning, disinfecting, and sterilization.
17. Remove gloves and wash hands.	
18. Attach a label and the completed requisition form to the specimen container. Place the specimen container in the area for laboratory pickup.	
19. Restock the room and return the instruments to storage.	
20. Document the procedure on the patient's chart.	

Charting Example

4/19/XX 11:30 am	Flexible sigmoidoscopy exam tolerated well by patient; biopsy of lesion on anterior wall at 10 inches. Pad placed over anal area in case of light bleeding. Specimen sent to lab. Follow-up when results received. T. EDWARDS, CMA(AAMA)

CHAPTER SUMMARY

- The primary reason for performing a complete physical examination (CPE) is to determine the general state of health and well-being of the patient. The CPE can be performed for various reasons such as an insurance examination before issuing a policy, as a requirement with a patient's employment, as a request by a patient, or to assess a patient's state of health.
- Your role in the physical examination process in addition to preparing the room is to provide assistance and instruction to the patient, assist the provider by anticipating the provider's needs during the exam, handing him or her instruments, positioning and draping the patient, and performing as a scribe if needed.
- You may be expected to provide patient education on a variety of topics. When you know about the pamphlets and other resources available in your office, you can talk with the patient and indicate that you will supply the material after the exam if the provider concurs with the necessity of it.
- The provider uses six examination methods while performing a physical examination. They are inspection, palpation, percussion, auscultation, mensuration, and manipulation.
- The physical examination is performed by the provider. Within each examination area are characteristics the provider may be observing and some applicable descriptive terms. Providers have their own style and depth of examination, which may not include all the areas and characteristics mentioned. You must be aware of the various examination components and the significance of each.
- Patients may ask how often they need to have a physical or a checkup, as they call it. You may use Table 40–1 as a guide in giving advice to adult patients about examination and specialty procedures routinely performed on patients.
- Sometimes it is difficult for the provider to inspect the patient's ear due to a buildup of cerumen (earwax) in the ear. This buildup can become very uncomfortable and eventually impair hearing. The ear may require irrigation (also known as lavage) to remove the excessive wax.
- Providers use several audiometric assessment procedures to determine the cause of the patient's hearing loss: Audiometry is a procedure that measures one's hearing; tympanometry is a procedure that determines the ability of the middle ear to transmit sound waves and is commonly performed on children to diagnose middle ear infections; and a two-pronged metal tuning fork, its frequency varying with the size of the instrument, tests nerve or conduction deafness.
- Occasionally, the eye might need to be irrigated if there is inflammation, secretions in the eye due to infection, a chemical contamination, or a foreign particle in the eye.
- Measuring visual acuity is a diagnostic screening procedure most often done by the medical assistant. Common vision screening tests include the Snellen chart, which measures *distance* vision; the Jaeger system, which screens for *near* vision acuity; and the Ishihara color plates book, which screens patients for defects in distinguishing *color vision* acuity.
- The spirometer is an instrument that tests the capacity of the lungs. Vital capacity testing aids in the diagnosis and degree of functional or obstructive abnormalities. It also helps the provider find the cause of dyspnea and evaluate the effectiveness of medication and therapy.
- Peak flow testing measures a patient's ability to exhale. A peak flow meter is a monitoring device that measures your peak expiratory flow rate, the highest speed that you can forcibly blow air from your lungs after taking in as deep a breath as possible. Peak flow testing can be used if a patient had an inconclusive or normal spirometry test or to monitor the effectiveness of medications.
- Pulse oximetry is a noninvasive test that measures the patient's pulse rate and oxygen saturation (SAT) in the blood. It is a simple test that is performed in many clinical facilities to determine a patient's oxygen status.
- Flexible sigmoidoscopy is a diagnostic examination of the interior of the sigmoid colon. It is a useful aid in the diagnosis of ulcerations, polyps, tumors, bleeding, cancer of the colon, and other lower intestinal disorders.

STUDY TOOLS

Workbook	Activities for Chapter 40
Premium Website **MEDIA LINK**	View these **Media Links** for Chapter 40: • Screen Visual Acuity • Screen Color Vision Acuity • Peak Flow Testing

StudyWARE	Activities and Quizzes on the **StudyWARE™ Software** for Chapter 40
	Complete the following **Competency Challenge 2.0** activities: • Tuesday, 11:00 AM, Prepare and Assist with Procedures, Treatments, and Minor Office Surgeries • Wednesday, 1:00 PM, Perform Respiratory Testing • Thursday, 3:00 PM, Provide Patient Instructions
	Audio Library of medical terms
	Online access to the **Critical Thinking Challenge 2.0**
CourseMate	Activities and Quizzes for Chapter 40
WebTutor	Activities and Quizzes for Chapter 40

CHECK YOUR KNOWLEDGE

1. The following examination technique uses a means of producing sounds by tapping various parts of the body.
   a. Inspection
   b. Palpation
   c. Percussion
   d. Manipulation
2. Which examination technique must be used to detect sounds, including bruits, murmurs, rales, rhythms, and bowel sounds?
   a. Auscultation
   b. Inspection
   c. Mensuration
   d. Percussion
3. The Rinne and Weber tests are performed by using the following piece of equipment.
   a. Ophthalmoscope
   b. Otoscope
   c. Audiometer
   d. Tuning fork
4. The breast examination is best done on the ______ days following the menstrual cycle of menstruating women.
   a. 21–28
   b. 7–10
   c. 5–10
   d. 7–14
5. At what age should men begin a routine testicular self-examination?
   a. 12
   b. 15
   c. 16
   d. 18
6. What is the name of the chart used most commonly for screening distance vision?
   a. Jaeger
   b. Snellen
   c. Ishihara
   d. Pelli-Robson
7. Which of the following devices are used to measure the capacity of the lungs?
   a. Spirometer
   b. Peak flow
   c. Tuning fork
   d. Both a and b
8. In the diagnosis of ulcerations, polyps, tumors, bleeding, cancer of the colon, and other lower intestinal disorders, the examination of the interior of the sigmoid colon can be done using a:
   a. proctoscope.
   b. rectal speculum.
   c. rectal snare.
   d. sigmoidoscope.

WEB LINKS

Centers for Disease Control and Prevention: www.cdc.gov/nip

Hearing Loss Web: www.hearinglossweb.com

RESOURCES

Estes, M. E. Z. (2010). *Health Assessment & Physical Examination* (3rd ed.). Clifton Park, NY: Delmar Cengage Learning.

Heller, M., and Veach, L. (2009). *Clinical Medical Assisting: A Professional, Field Smart Approach to the Workplace*. Clifton Park, NY: Delmar, Cengage Learning.

Lindh, W., Pooler, M., Tamparo, C., and Dahl, B. (2010). *Delmar's Comprehensive Medical Assisting Administrative and Clinical Competencies* (4th ed.). Clifton Park, NY: Delmar Cengage Learning.

Venes, D. (ed.). (2009). *Taber's Cyclopedic Medical Dictionary* (21st ed.). Philadelphia: F. A. Davis.

Chapter 41

OB/GYN EXAMINATIONS

OBJECTIVES

In this chapter, you will learn the following:

KB KNOWLEDGE BASE

1. Spell and define, using the glossary at the back of the text, all the Words to Know in this chapter.
2. Differentiate between gynecology and obstetrics.
3. Identify five reasons the liquid-based Pap test is preferred.
4. Interpret the American Cancer Society (ACS) guidelines for frequency of Pap tests.
5. Identify four specific ACS patient preparation instructions for more accurate Pap results.
6. Stress why breast self-examination is necessary even when the provider performs an annual exam.
7. Give two reasons the medical assistant should accompany the provider when a pelvic exam is performed.
8. List the three main Pap test reporting categories.
9. Identify three processes or procedures done to confirm a diagnosis of pregnancy.
10. List five general responsibilities of the medical assistant in prenatal care.
11. Explain how to determine the estimated due date using Naegele's rule.
12. List seven assessment responsibilities of the MA before the provider performs the prenatal examination.

S SKILLS

1. Prepare a patient for and assist with a gynecological exam and Pap test.

B BEHAVIOR

1. Apply critical thinking skills in performing patient assessment and care.
2. Use language and verbal skills that enable patients' understanding.
3. Apply active listening skills.
4. Use appropriate body language and other nonverbal skills in communicating with patients' family and staff.
5. Demonstrate awareness of the territorial boundaries of the person with whom communicating.
6. Demonstrate recognition of the patient's level of understanding in communications.
7. Recognize and protect personal boundaries in communicating with others.
8. Explain the rationale for performance of procedure to the patient.
9. Show awareness of patients' concerns regarding their perceptions of the procedure being performed.

WORDS TO KNOW

atypical
cervical
cytology
douche
endocervical
exfoliated
fundus
gestation
Lamaze
Naegele's rule
Papanicolaou
pregnancy
prenatal
ThinPrep
trimester
vaginitis

GYNECOLOGICAL EXAM

In assisting with the complete physical exam (CPE, discussed in Chapter 40), the examination of the vagina and genitalia was described as part of the total exam; however, a Pap test is not necessarily done at that time. Women may schedule appointments with their general or family practitioners for a Pap test or might prefer to see a gynecologist for this type of examination. The OB/GYN (obstetrics/gynecology) practice focuses on the female reproductive system. (Refer to Chapter 35 for a complete discussion of the anatomy and physiology of this system.) Obstetrics focuses on pregnancy and childbirth, whereas the gynecology practice addresses diseases and disorders of the female reproductive system. When a patient calls a general or family practice for an appointment, be sure to make a distinction between a physical exam and a gynecological exam with a Pap test so that the appropriate amount of time is allotted and proper instructions are given. Remember that the CPE is a review of systems (ROS) of the total body, and the gynecologic exam is of the female reproductive organs only.

PATIENT EDUCATION

Remind the patient at the time she schedules the appointment for a Pap test that she should not **douche** or engage in sexual intercourse for 48 hours before the examination. Because the specimen analysis could be misinterpreted during the menstrual flow, the patient should be advised to schedule the test about five days after her period.

THE PAP TEST

The **Papanicolaou** (Pap) technique is a cytological screening test to detect cancer of the cervix. This method of detection was developed by an American physician, George N. Papanicolaou, in 1883. This simple smear technique used samples taken from the vagina, the cervix, and the endocervix to look for **atypical cytology**. The samples were smeared onto slides and then sprayed with a fixative or placed in an alcohol solution and sent to a lab. Studies have shown that the technique produced many inadequate specimens, sometimes requiring repeating the procedure. Up to two thirds of the false negative reports were caused by the limitations of the sampling technique and the slide preparation. Often, cells on the slide were piled up so those underneath could not be seen. Additionally, **cervical** cells were hidden by pus cells from infection, yeast cells, bacteria, and increased mucus. Therefore, precancerous cells were not visible, and the results were incorrectly reported negative. Furthermore, if the slide was not treated immediately after the smear was done, the cells dried out and became distorted, leading to possible reading errors.

In May 1996, after 50 years of conventional Pap testing, the U.S. Food and Drug Administration (FDA) approved a new, liquid-based method known by the brand names of **ThinPrep** and AutoCyte. This improved technique involves collecting the sample with a plastic **endocervical** "broom" and immediately placing it into a bottle of preservative solution (Figure 41–1). The broom is swished 10 times in the solution to remove the collected cells. The solution prevents the cells from drying out and significantly reduces the presence of mucus, bacteria, yeast, and pus cells on the slide prepared from the diluted cell samples in the solution.

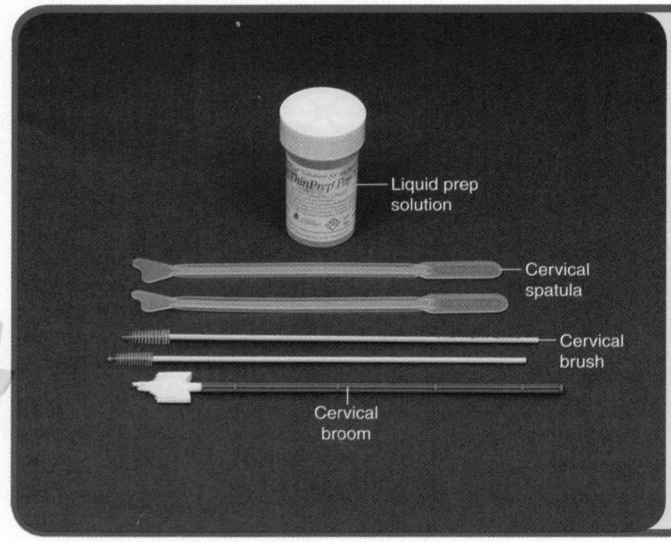

Figure 41–1: Liquid prep solution with cervical spatula, brush, and broom. *Delmar/Cengage Learning.*

This technique slightly improves the detection of cancers but greatly improves the detection of precancers. This method also provides the ability to do additional studies from the same sample, such as tests for the presence of HPV, chlamydia, and gonorrhea.

The AutoPap Primary Screening System has been approved by the FDA for use in screening smears before a provider or technologist analyzes them. Anything identified as abnormal would still be examined by a technologist. Additionally, these computerized instruments will retest Pap samples interpreted as normal by technologists, with the intent to detect abnormal cells that are missed by humans.

Female patients usually have the Pap test done routinely either as part of the CPE with their family doctor or by their gynecologist. Patients who have complaints of severe menstrual pain or discomfort, unusual vaginal discharge, or lower abdominal pain (or any other problems) may have a Pap smear taken during the pelvic examination to rule out gynecological problems.

The American Cancer Society recommends the following guidelines for early detection of cervical cancer:

- All women should begin screening tests about three years after they begin having vaginal intercourse but no later than 21 years old. Screening should be done every year with a regular Pap test or every two years with a liquid-based Pap test.
- At age 30, women with three normal Pap tests in a row may have a screening every two to three years with either test method. Women with risk factors such as diethylstilbestrol exposure before birth; HIV infection; or a weakened immune system due to organ transplant, chemotherapy, or chronic steroid use should continue with annual testing.
- An option for women older than 30 is screening every three years plus the HPV DNA test. Human papillomavirus (HPV) is a known risk factor for developing cervical cancer because it can cause normal cells on the cervix to become abnormal. The virus causes changes in cervical cells that can be observed from the Pap test. At least 50 percent of sexually active people will have HPV at some time in their lives, according to the Centers for Disease Control and Prevention (CDC). For more information about HPV, visit www.cdc.gov/hpv.
- Women 70 or older who have had at least three normal Pap tests in a row and no abnormal findings in the past 10 years may choose to stop cervical cancer screening. Women with the risk factors named previously should continue as long as they are in good health.
- Women who have had a total hysterectomy (cervix and uterus removed) may choose to stop screening unless surgery was performed as a treatment for precancerous cells or cervical cancer. Women who have had a hysterectomy without removal of the cervix should still follow the guidelines.

Women should be especially conscientious in scheduling Pap tests if they have a family history of uterine or cervical cancer. You should check with your provider employer for his or her preference and advise patients accordingly.

Patient Preparation for the Pap Test

When the patient is scheduled for a Pap test, she must be given clear instructions to follow in preparation for the test. The following are recommended by the American Cancer Society for accurate results:

- Do not use tampons, birth control foams, jellies, or other vaginal creams for 48 hours before the test. (They alter the cervical and vaginal environment.)
- Do not douche for 48 hours prior to the test. (Douching could wash away **exfoliated** cancer cells and cause the test to be falsely reported as negative.)
- Do not have sexual intercourse for 48 hours before the test. (This adds extra cells and fluid to the environment, making reading more difficult.)
- Try to schedule the Pap test at least five days after the menstrual period. Avoid scheduling during the period. (Red blood cells make the test more difficult to read.)

The Medical Assistant's Role in Gynecological Exams

Prior to bringing the patient into the examination room for the pelvic exam and Pap, the medical assistant should make the necessary preparations. As with any procedure or patient contact, wash your hands before you begin. The exam table should have a clean, protective covering. Place a gown and drape sheet on the end of the table for the patient (either cloth or disposable paper).

Prepare the Mayo tray with the instruments and supplies the provider will need to perform the pelvic exam and obtain the Pap test (Figure 41–2). Speculums can be reusable or disposable. Place the tray in a convenient location near the end of the exam table. Cover the equipment with a towel to help allay the patient's anxiety from seeing the equipment. To aid in the inspection part of the pelvic exam, an exam lamp should also be placed within reach of the examiner's stool at the end of the table. (Most lamps are expandable and attached to the wall.)

Call the patient from the reception room to prepare her for the exam. Instruct her to go to the bathroom to empty her bladder before the test. If a specimen is to be

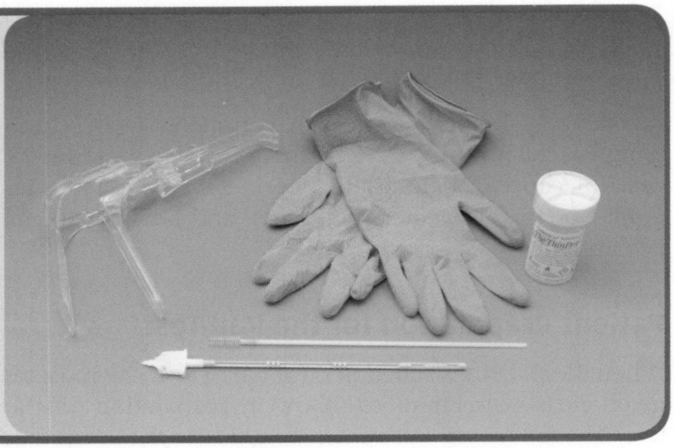

Figure 41–2: Equipment for a Pap smear.
Delmar/Cengage Learning.

obtained, instruct her in the method of collection. A pelvic examination is uncomfortable for the patient if the bladder is full, besides making the examination difficult for the provider to perform.

CLINICAL PEARL

Pelvic examinations that have to be delayed while the patient goes to the bathroom disrupt the schedule and should be avoided. Certainly there are exceptions; some patients may have trouble with bladder control or some other condition that requires frequent trips to the bathroom. Help these patients feel at ease because they will most likely feel embarrassed.

When the patient comes back to the examination room, try to determine her level of anxiety regarding the examination. Take time to explain the procedure, letting her know what to expect, especially if it is her first time having a pelvic exam. *Never* assume that a patient knows about a procedure. Some patients are both afraid and embarrassed to ask questions because they believe they should already know about procedures. Try to make patients feel comfortable and at ease to help them relax for the exam. Complete the cytology request form (see Figure 41–3), making sure that you ask the patient all necessary questions. Many of the questions that are asked when taking a complete GYN history will be needed for the requisition form. They should include:

- Age at onset of menstrual cycle
- Gravida (how many pregnancies the patient has had)
- Para (how many live births the patient has had)
- Abortions: How many? Were they spontaneous or elective?
- Date of last menstrual period (LMP) (you need to record the day it started)
- Regularity and duration of cycles
- Date of last Pap smear, result, and if any abnormal Pap smear results or biopsies in the past
- Contraception method used
- Hormone replacement therapy (HRT) if patient is taking any
- Date of last mammogram if had one
- Any GYN surgeries and dates
- Past and present sexual activity
- Any abnormal discharge or pain

After the patient is questioned and you fill in the required information on the requisition form, label the ThinPrep collection bottle and place it on the stand. Some requisition forms come with prenumbered stickers you can attach to specimens. This helps eliminate errors from mismatching requisitions to specimens. You can then instruct the patient to undress completely, tell her where to put her belongings, explain how to put on the exam gown with the opening in the front, and offer your assistance if needed. Allow the patient privacy for several minutes to change and then knock before entering to see whether the patient is ready.

Enter the room when the patient lets you know she is ready. Pull out the footstep at the end of the exam table and help her step up onto the exam table and sit at the end. Place the drape sheet over the top of her legs for privacy and warmth. Remember to push the footstep back in after the patient has been seated to avoid injury to you or the provider.

Alert the provider that the patient is ready to be examined. Most providers prefer the medical assistant to accompany them into the exam room, not only to assist with the procedure, but also for legal and safety reasons as discussed in Chapter 39.

Because of the importance of early detection of breast cancer, providers include the breast exam during the patient's annual appointment for the Pap test and pelvic exam. Patients should be reminded to do a breast self-examination each month following their menstrual period (see the Patient Education box in Chapter 40, page 870). Giving them a pamphlet of instructions to take with them for this procedure is recommended (Figure 41–4). Explain to the patient that the exam conducted by the provider with the annual Pap test is important but insufficient in detecting abnormal breast tissue between visits to the provider. Most women discover a lump or mass in their breasts themselves and report it to the provider. This leads to early detection and treatment, which greatly increases the survival rate.

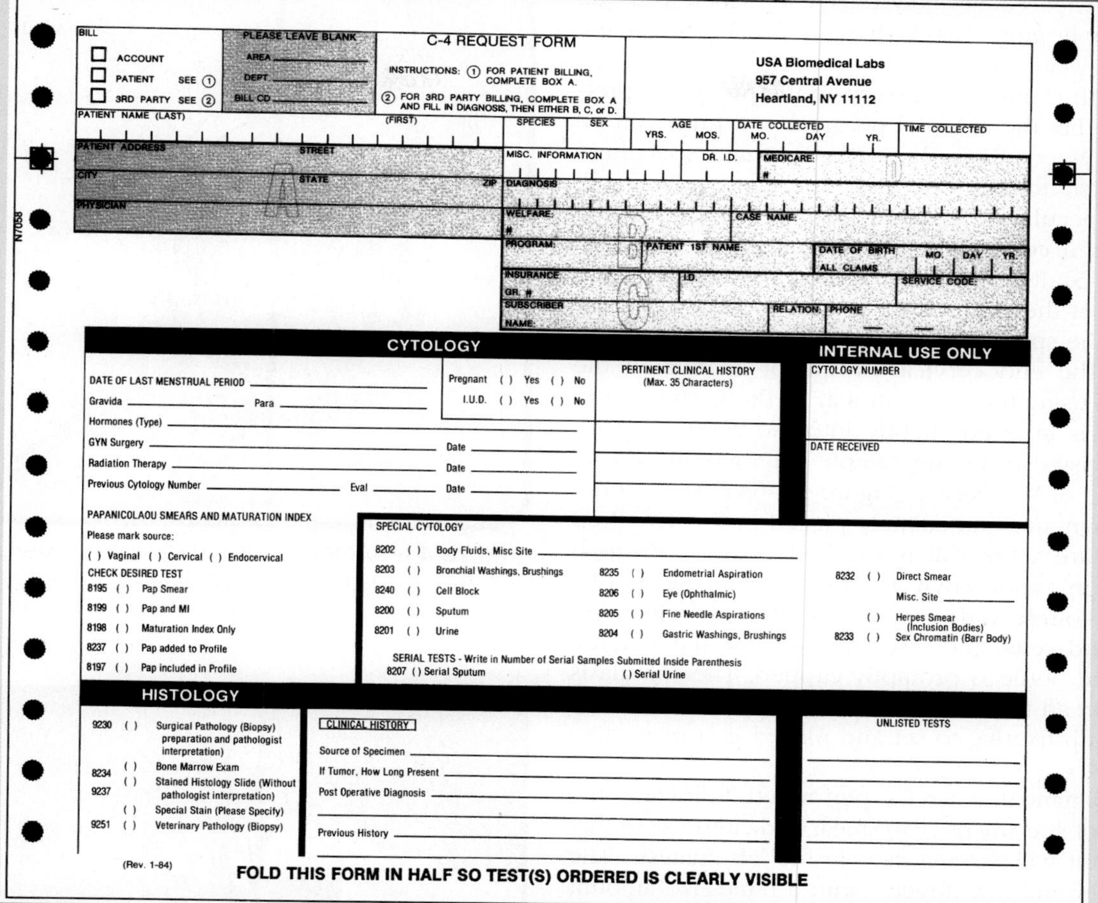

BILL
☐ ACCOUNT
☐ PATIENT SEE ①
☐ 3RD PARTY SEE ②

PLEASE LEAVE BLANK
AREA
DEPT
BILL CD

C-4 REQUEST FORM
INSTRUCTIONS: ① FOR PATIENT BILLING, COMPLETE BOX A.
② FOR 3RD PARTY BILLING, COMPLETE BOX A AND FILL IN DIAGNOSIS, THEN EITHER B, C, or D.

USA Biomedical Labs
957 Central Avenue
Heartland, NY 11112

PATIENT NAME (LAST) (FIRST) SPECIES SEX AGE YRS. MOS. DATE COLLECTED MO. DAY YR. TIME COLLECTED
PATIENT ADDRESS STREET
CITY STATE ZIP
PHYSICIAN
MISC. INFORMATION DR. I.D. MEDICARE: #
DIAGNOSIS
WELFARE: # CASE NAME:
PROGRAM: PATIENT 1ST NAME: DATE OF BIRTH MO. DAY YR. ALL CLAIMS
INSURANCE GR. # I.D. SERVICE CODE:
SUBSCRIBER NAME: RELATION PHONE

N7058

CYTOLOGY

DATE OF LAST MENSTRUAL PERIOD
Gravida Para
Hormones (Type)
GYN Surgery Date
Radiation Therapy Date
Previous Cytology Number Eval Date

Pregnant ( ) Yes ( ) No
I.U.D. ( ) Yes ( ) No

PERTINENT CLINICAL HISTORY (Max. 35 Characters)

INTERNAL USE ONLY
CYTOLOGY NUMBER
DATE RECEIVED

PAPANICOLAOU SMEARS AND MATURATION INDEX
Please mark source:
( ) Vaginal ( ) Cervical ( ) Endocervical
CHECK DESIRED TEST
8195 ( ) Pap Smear
8199 ( ) Pap and MI
8198 ( ) Maturation Index Only
8237 ( ) Pap added to Profile
8197 ( ) Pap included in Profile

SPECIAL CYTOLOGY
8202 ( ) Body Fluids, Misc Site
8203 ( ) Bronchial Washings, Brushings
8240 ( ) Cell Block
8200 ( ) Sputum
8201 ( ) Urine
8235 ( ) Endometrial Aspiration
8206 ( ) Eye (Ophthalmic)
8205 ( ) Fine Needle Aspirations
8204 ( ) Gastric Washings, Brushings
8232 ( ) Direct Smear
Misc. Site
( ) Herpes Smear (Inclusion Bodies)
8233 ( ) Sex Chromatin (Barr Body)

SERIAL TESTS - Write in Number of Serial Samples Submitted Inside Parenthesis
8207 ( ) Serial Sputum ( ) Serial Urine

HISTOLOGY

9230 ( ) Surgical Pathology (Biopsy) preparation and pathologist interpretation)
8234 ( ) Bone Marrow Exam
9237 ( ) Stained Histology Slide (Without pathologist interpretation)
( ) Special Stain (Please Specify)
9251 ( ) Veterinary Pathology (Biopsy)

CLINICAL HISTORY
Source of Specimen
If Tumor, How Long Present
Post Operative Diagnosis
Previous History

UNLISTED TESTS

(Rev. 1-84)
FOLD THIS FORM IN HALF SO TEST(S) ORDERED IS CLEARLY VISIBLE

Figure 41–3: Cytology requisition form. *Delmar/Cengage Learning.*

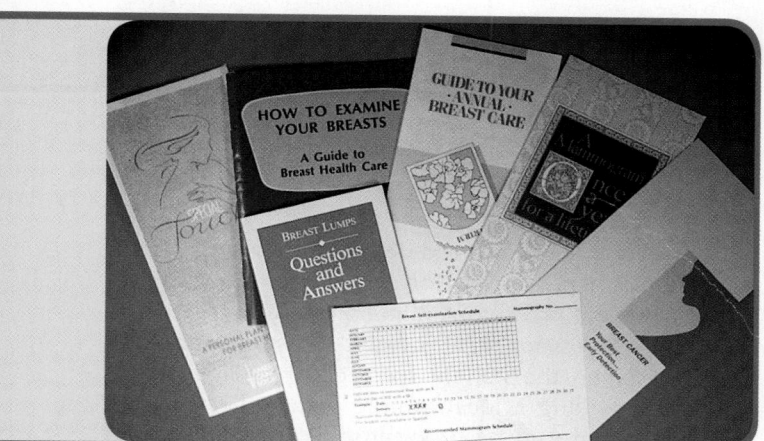

Figure 41–4: Breast self-examination (BSE) pamphlets and schedule. *Delmar/Cengage Learning.*

Conducting the Examination

The provider usually listens to the heart and lungs and does a brief general check of the patient first. Then the patient's gown is lowered to the waist while the patient is still sitting up for the inspection part of the breast exam and palpation for lumps and masses. When this part is completed, you will pull the table extension out to support the patient's lower legs and feet and help the patient lie down. This assists the provider in further palpation for any abnormalities of the breast tissue. (Often, a towel is placed over the chest to provide a sense of privacy for the patient.) Next, the provider will inspect and palpate the abdominal and pelvic areas. Remind patients to breathe slowly through the mouth to help relax abdominal muscles during the exam.

The next step is for you to help the patient into the lithotomy position. Assist her in getting her feet in the stirrups, adjusting them as necessary, and place the drape sheet over her knees. Ask her to scoot down to the end of the table until the buttocks are just at the edge. Be careful in assisting patients into positions because the exam tables are usually rather narrow, and there *is* the possibility of a patient falling *off* the table. The exam lamp should be adjusted at the end of the table and the stool positioned comfortably for the provider. You will need to apply gloves as well as supply a pair for the provider to wear.

Adjust the lamp if necessary, to the provider's preference, so that the external perineal structures can be observed. When ready, hand the warmed speculum, handles first, to the provider. Some providers may want the speculum ran under warm water to facilitate insertion and comfort for the patient. After insertion (Figure 41–5), it might be necessary to adjust the light again so that the cervix can be seen clearly within the blades of the speculum.

Hand the endocervical broom or spatula to the provider if using the conventional method. The broom or spatula is inserted slightly into the cervical opening and twisted to obtain sample cells within and on the surface of the cervix (Figure 41–6A). The broom is withdrawn and immediately placed in the ThinPrep bottle (Figure 41–6B). It is swished 10 times through the solution, withdrawn to the top of the bottle, tapped a couple times to knock off any remaining solution and cells, and discarded on the Mayo stand. The labeled bottle is promptly capped. The spatula is used to spread the cells on a glass slide which is then sprayed with fixative to set and placed in a protective cover.

The bimanual exam is performed following the collection of specimens (Pap smear and cultures) so that the lubricant will not interfere in the lab analysis. The examiner inserts two fingers (with a dime-size amount of water-soluble lubricant) into the vagina and palpates the pelvic area with the other hand (Figure 41–7). The provider then places one finger into the vagina and the other in the rectum simultaneously checking for any abnormalities of the pelvic organs and rectum. You should hand the doctor a clean glove and lubricant to prevent cross-contamination between the vaginal and rectal tissues for this exam. The provider might want to screen the patient for rectal bleeding at this time by providing a fecal sample obtained during the bimanual exam to a fecal occult test card as discussed in Chapter 40.

Alternately, instead of assisting, the medical assistant may be asked to write or scribe the findings of this examination while the provider conducts the exam. Regardless of your tasks, you can be a valuable assistant to both provider and patient.

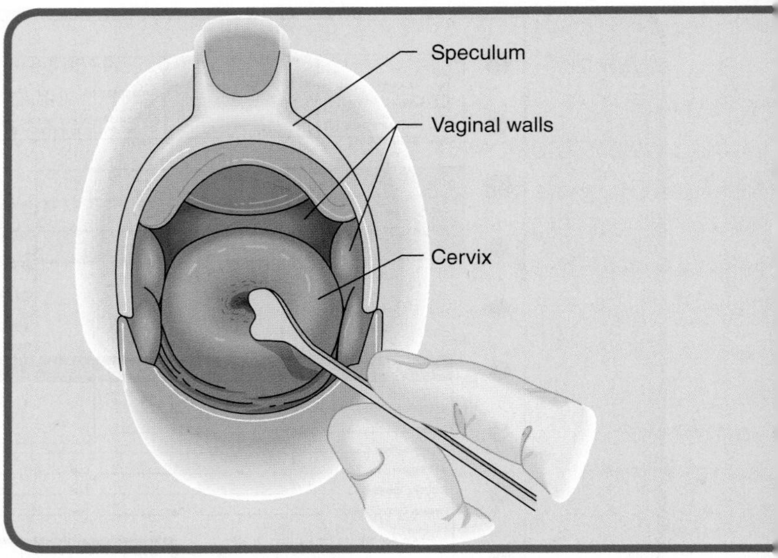

Figure 41–6A: The cervix is scraped with a spatula to obtain cells for a Pap test. *Delmar/Cengage Learning.*

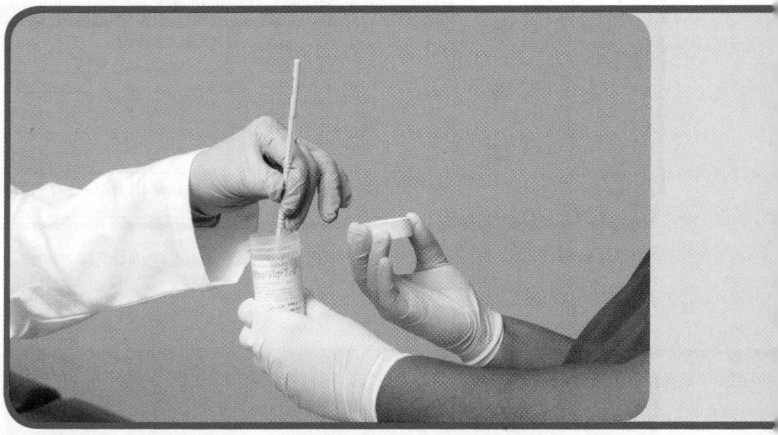

Figure 41–6B: The provider swishes the broom in the ThinPrep bottle. *Delmar/Cengage Learning.*

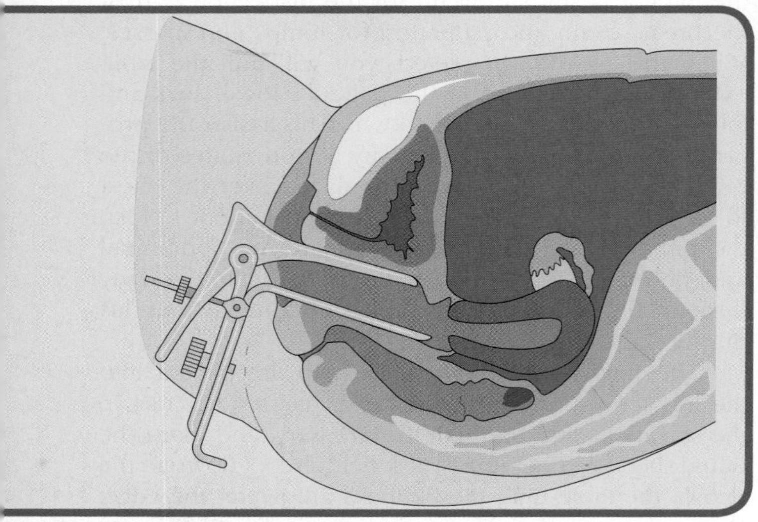

Figure 41–5: Lateral view of vaginal speculum in place for inspection and for obtaining specimens. *Delmar/Cengage Learning.*

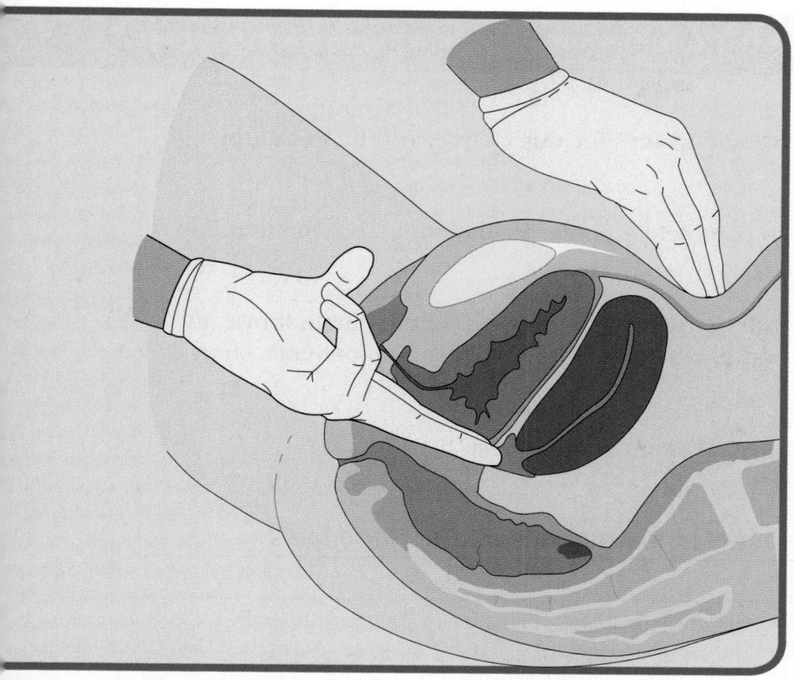

Figure 41–7: Bimanual pelvic exam. *Delmar/Cengage Learning.*

After the Examination

When the exam has been completed, push the stirrups and the extension of the table in and assist the patient to sit up. After lying down for the exam, the patient may feel faint or dizzy; if she attempts to stand up too quickly, she can fall. After she has let you know that she has regained her balance, help her down from the table and offer tissues to the patient to wipe away any residual lubricant. Discard the used tissues in a waste container. Ask her to get dressed and offer assistance to the patient if needed.

Remember to advise her when to expect to receive the results of the Pap test and other reports in the mail or when she should call to find out the results. Giving these instructions will decidedly reduce unnecessary phone calls to the office. If the provider requests a return appointment for the patient, politely assist her in scheduling it or direct her to the administrative area. As time permits, you may discuss patient education topics either before or after the exam as appropriate to the age and needs of the patient.

Return to the examination room to clean up the exam area. Wear gloves to protect yourself from disease transmission. Discard all disposables in appropriate waste containers, remove gloves, and wash hands. Restock the supplies as necessary, making the room ready for the next patient to be seen. Place the labeled specimen(s) and attached requisition form in the proper area for pickup by the lab representative.

Follow the steps in Procedure 41–1 to assist the provider with a gynecological examination and a ThinPrep Pap test.

PATIENT EDUCATION

Here are a few informative topics you might want to discuss with female patients coming in for Pap tests:

1. Explain to patients that they should *not* douche routinely because it washes away natural protective vaginal secretions that aid in the resistance of possible invading microorganisms. Douching should be done only with the provider's orders.
2. Patients who are sexually active and not in a committed, monogamous relationship should be instructed to use condoms when engaging in sexual intercourse for protection against both sexually transmitted diseases and unwanted pregnancies.
3. Educate all females to perform breast self-examination at home routinely after their menstrual period. (Refer to Chapter 40.) Pamphlets for distribution can be obtained from the American Cancer Society to help patients with the procedure.
4. Remind all female patients over age 40 to schedule a routine mammography for early detection of breast cancer.
5. Explain to female patients that any of the following symptoms could mean that infection or disease is present and that they should call for an appointment: foul vaginal odor; vaginal discharge that is other than clear; unusual bleeding; vaginal itching or soreness; or any other **vaginitis**, pain, or discomfort.
6. Advise female patients to refrain from using perfumed toilet articles such as soaps or bubble baths, vaginal sprays, tampons, toilet tissue, or feminine napkins because they may be irritating to the delicate vaginal tissues. Chronic irritation can lead to infection.

PROCEDURE 41–1 Prepare the Patient for and Assist with a Gynecological Exam and Pap Test

MEDIA LINK: View the video, "Assist with a Gynecologic Exam," for this chapter on the Premium Website.

PURPOSE: To prepare the patient and assist the provider to complete a pelvic examination and obtain a Pap test to determine a patient's gynecological health

EQUIPMENT: Mayo tray, two cloth or paper towels, three pairs of disposable gloves, water-soluble lubricant, vaginal speculum, tissues, endocervical broom, ThinPrep bottle, label, laboratory requisition, patient's chart or EMR, and pen

S **SKILL:** Prepare the patient for and assist with a gynecological exam and Pap test.

Procedure Steps	Detailed Instructions and/or *Rationales*
1. Wash hands.	
2. Prepare the room and equipment.	• Place a towel on the Mayo tray, assemble all necessary equipment, and cover. • Place the requisition form on a nearby table. • Place the gown and drape on the exam table.
3. Call the patient from the reception room; introduce yourself and identify the patient.	*Ensures that you have the correct patient.*
4. Instruct the patient to go to the bathroom to empty the bladder.	Provide instructions and a specimen container if a urine specimen is needed.
B 5. Explain the procedure, ***using language the patient can understand; answer any questions, making the patient feel at ease about the procedure to be performed.***	
6. Obtain the necessary information to complete the cytology requisition form.	
7. Attach a label to the ThinPrep bottle and place it on the Mayo tray.	
B 8. Instruct the patient to remove all clothing and put on the examination gown with the opening in front. ***Leave the room to allow for privacy unless assistance is needed.***	Show her where to put her clothing.
9. When the patient is gowned, enter the room and pull out the step from the end of the table. Ask the patient sit on the table. Cover the patient's legs with the drape. Push in the table step.	Provide assistance as needed. The step is small, and the patient may step off the edge when trying to turn around to sit down.
B 10. Notify the provider that the patient is ready. ***If the patient is apprehensive, provide reassurance and support. Answer any questions she may have.***	
11. Accompany the provider into the room and apply critical thinking skills to provide assistance as needed. Be sure to use proper body mechanics when positioning the patient.	

Procedure Steps	Detailed Instructions and/or *Rationales*
12. Position the patient in a sitting position for basic assessment and initial breast examination. Be sure to show awareness to any patient concerns regarding the procedure.	
13. Assist the patient to a supine position for a continued breast exam.	Put the pillow under her head. Uncover her chest, and cover her breasts with the towel covering the Mayo tray if desired.
14. When the breast exam is completed, assist the patient to cover her chest with the gown and drape and prepare for the pelvic exam.	*For modesty and patient comfort.*
15. Assist the patient into a lithotomy position, helping her place her feet into the stirrups, and adjust as needed.	Push in the table extension.
16. Place the drape over the patient from the chest to the feet. Push the drape down between her legs until it touches the table. Instruct the patient to slide her buttocks down to the end of the table.	*The patient's buttocks must be at the end of the table so that the vaginal speculum can be inserted without the handle hitting the table.*
17. The provider will take his or her position on the exam stool at the end of the table. Remove the cover from the Mayo tray if not previously done. Hand gloves to the provider.	
18. Adjust the lamp so that the light facilitates inspection of the perineal and anal areas.	
19. Put on gloves and run warm water over the speculum.	
20. Hand the speculum, handle first, to the provider.	
21. Hand the endocervical broom, handle first, to the provider.	
22. Open the labeled specimen bottle and be ready to accept the endocervical broom.	Hold the bottle securely while physician swishes the broom, or take the handle of the broom and swish thoroughly in the solution 10 times. Withdraw it from bottle, tap it against the bottle edge to dislodge any cells and excess fluid, and place it on the Mayo tray. Cap the bottle securely and place it on the Mayo tray.
23. The provider will stand to perform the bimanual pelvic and rectal exam. Apply lubricant to the gloved index and middle fingers of the examining hand.	
24. When the provider has finished the exam, have the patient push back up the table, help her get her feet out of the stirrups, and push the stirrups in.	
25. Assist the patient to sit up. Pull out the table step. When the patient's sense of balance has returned, assist her down from the table.	
26. Hand tissues to the patient to remove any residual lubricant.	
27. Instruct the patient to dress. Provide assistance as needed. Remove gloves and wash hands.	

(continues)

(continued)

Procedure Steps	Detailed Instructions and/or *Rationales*
28. Advise the patient when results will be available and schedule a follow-up appointment if indicated.	
29. Provide any patient teaching information pamphlets that are appropriate and dismiss the patient. Record exam, Pap test, and any teaching in the chart.	
30. Apply gloves; properly clean and disinfect the room and all instruments and restock supplies.	• Discard all disposable items in the appropriate waste container. Wrap up the table paper and towels and discard. • If a metal speculum was used, place it in cool water, then wash, wrap, and autoclave. • Disinfect table surfaces and the exam room furniture. • Restock supplies. Pull down fresh table paper on the exam table.
31. Place the labeled specimen bottle with the attached requisition in the lab pickup area.	
32. Pull down fresh table paper on the exam table.	
33. Remove gloves and wash hands.	

Charting Example

8/28/XX 2:30 PM	Annual pelvic exam and ThinPrep Pap test performed. See patient history/physical form. G. Talbert, RMA(AMT)

Reporting Pap Test Results

The system most widely used to describe Pap test findings is the Bethesda System. It was developed in 1988 and revised in 1991 and 2001. There are three general categories:

1. Negative for intraepithelial lesion or malignancy *(Means there are no signs of cancer or precancerous changes. Other findings may be reported, such as yeast, herpes, Trichomonas, or cellular changes caused by irritation or infection.)*
2. Epithelial cell abnormalities *(Means the cells of the lining layer of the cervix show changes that might be cancer or a precancerous condition. The cells are divided into (a) atypical squamous cells, (b) low-grade squamous intraepithelial lesions (SILs), (c) high-grade SILs, and (4) squamous cell carcinoma. These findings require repeat Pap tests and other interventions such as colposcopy (examining the cervix with a magnifying lens instrument) and biopsy.*
3. Other malignant neoplasms *(Means there is likely an invasive squamous cell cancer. Additional diagnostic tests will be performed, followed by radiation, chemotherapy, or radical surgery.)*

Figure 41–8 lists and defines some terms used in the cytology reports of Pap tests.

atypical—not typical
CIN—cervical intraepithelial neoplasia
CIS—carcinoma in situ
condyloma—a lesion caused by human papillomavirus
dysplasia—precancerous lesion
epithelial—pertaining to epithelium
epithelium—cellular tissue that covers the surface of a body or that lines a body cavity
glandular—the cell making up the epithelium of a body cavity
HPV—human papillomavirus
lesion—a change in the tissue cells or a wound
malignant—a lesion that spreads out of the epithelium into underlying tissues
reactive changes—changes in cells caused by their reaction to infectious agents or a foreign body
reparative changes—changes in cells as they divide rapidly in an attempt to repair damaged tissue
SIL—squamous intraepithelial lesion (that lies within the squamous epithelium)
squamous—a type of cell that makes up the epithelium, the purpose of which is to protect underlying tissues

Figure 41–8: Terms and abbreviations used in cytology/Pap test reports. *Delmar/Cengage Learning.*

OTHER GYNECOLOGICAL PROCEDURES

Other procedures can be performed to make decisions regarding the condition of the uterus and cervix. Figures 41–9A through D show gynecological instruments used in some of these procedures. The uterine sound Figure 41–9A is inserted into the uterus to explore the cavity and measure the depth. Note it is graduated in inches or centimeters. The curettes (Figure 41–9B and C) are used to scrape the lining of the uterus for a specimen and to remove growths or remnants of an abortion. The biopsy forceps (Figure 41–9D) permits taking a small piece of tissue for diagnostic examination. These instruments are most often used when performing surgical procedures.

OBSTETRICS PATIENTS

When patients suspect that they are pregnant, their visit to the doctor is to confirm pregnancy. Usually, the patient has missed one or two menstrual periods. Because home pregnancy tests are convenient and accessible, many women have already tested their urine at home prior to coming into the office. However, even after having performed the home test, they still may not be certain of the results. The diagnosis is made by the provider only after the patient has been given a complete evaluation. This is generally done by (1) interviewing the patient and obtaining a complete **prenatal** health assessment and history; (2) doing a complete physical examination; (3) ordering laboratory tests such as urinalysis and pregnancy tests, blood tests, and cultures; and (4) performing any other diagnostic test indicated by the patient's condition.

The same principles apply in assisting with obstetrics patients as apply in assisting with the complete physical examination. Documentation of the prenatal history, vitals, and any past or current medical conditions of the patient must be complete and efficient. This enables the providers to give quality care to their patients. Refer to Chapter 35 for review of the anatomy and physiology of the reproductive system and information regarding **pregnancy**, labor, and childbirth. You need to be familiar with the terminology when discussing issues with patients.

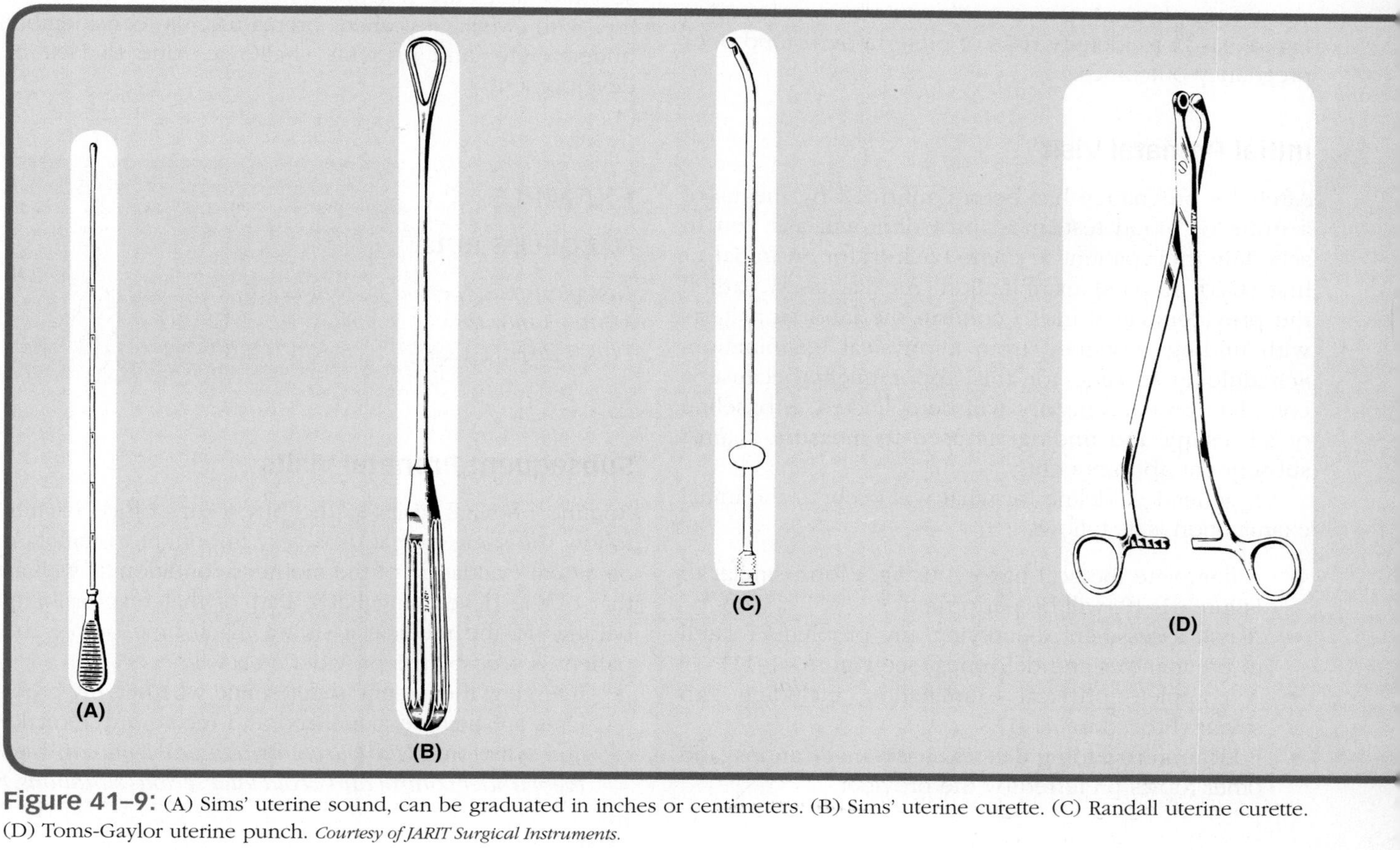

Figure 41–9: (A) Sims' uterine sound, can be graduated in inches or centimeters. (B) Sims' uterine curette. (C) Randall uterine curette. (D) Toms-Gaylor uterine punch. *Courtesy of JARIT Surgical Instruments.*

The Medical Assistant's Role in Obstetrical Exams

In addition to assisting the provider with all the examinations, your role in prenatal evaluation and care of patients is to instill the importance of keeping regular appointments; encourage patients to eat a sensible, well-balanced diet; alert the doctor of any problems or concerns; and provide patient education materials with explanations. Follow your office policy regarding prenatal and childbirth classes to provide information about times and places of such programs as **Lamaze** classes.

A prenatal medical history form (Figure 41–10) and a risk assessment form (Figure 41–11) are used to assess the health status of pregnant women and is generally filled out at the patient's initial visit after the pregnancy has been confirmed. Subsequent findings during prenatal visits are recorded on the spaces provided on the bottom half of the form or on progress notes. Careful attention should be given to sections regarding (1) medications, drugs, alcohol, and smoking (consumption and use); (2) preexisting risk factors; and (3) past menstrual and obstetrical health history.

The effects on the fetus are well documented from certain medications, smoking, and alcohol as well as from illicit drug use. Risks are also associated with certain systemic disease conditions, sexually transmitted diseases, age, physical stature, and mental factors. Examine Figure 41–11 to identify risks of preterm births and poor pregnancy outcomes.

Initial Prenatal Visit

After the pregnancy has been confirmed by means of a urine or blood test, most providers will ask you to schedule their patient to come back in for an initial or first (OB) prenatal examination. As discussed earlier, the provider will want to confirm the laboratory tests with findings obtained from a physical examination. Schedule extra time for this appointment because a complete prenatal history will be collected. A baseline of all testing and findings is used to measure against subsequent appointments.

A general guideline for what will occur at the initial examination is as follows:

- A complete medical history, using a form similar to Figure 41–10, will be performed
- A risk assessment identifying any problems related to pregnancies and deliveries (see Figure 41–11)
- A complete physical examination, including Pap smear (Procedure 41–1)
- Education regarding diet, exercise, medications, and other topics preferred by the provider
- Laboratory testing, which usually includes a prenatal profile to check the patient's blood type and RH factor; HIV, hepatitis, and VDRL screening; complete blood count to check the iron level and screen for infection; urinalysis and cultures to check for chlamydia and gonorrhea (refer to Unit 14 for descriptions on laboratory testing)
- An estimation of the date of confinement or date of delivery
- The provider's request for the patient to return in one month for the next prenatal visit

Estimating the Date of Delivery

Probably the question of most interest to the expectant couple is when the baby will be born. This is known medically as the estimated day or date of delivery (EDD) or the estimated date of confinement (EDC). This can be determined, with a fair amount of accuracy, by using a formula known as **Naegele's rule**. The method was devised by Franz Naegele, a German obstetrician, in the early eighteenth century. The period of gestation (conception to birth) is determined by using the first day of the last menstrual period (LMP), subtracting three months, and then adding seven days plus one year.

A normal pregnancy can range from 37 to 41 weeks, so exact dates are not possible. An infant born before the 37th week is called premature, is considerably underweight, and presents challenges due to lack of development.

EXAMPLE

NAEGELE'S RULE

Last menstrual period	August 10, 2012
Minus 3 months	May 10, 2012
Plus 7 days, 1 year	May 17, 2013

Subsequent Prenatal Visits

Routine prenatal visits to the physician's office usually follow the same format. It is very important to maintain continual evaluation of the mother's condition as well as that of the developing baby. Part of that responsibility belongs to the medical assistant. Each time before the patient is seen by the provider, you will:

- Interview the patient to determine whether any problems are being experienced and record any remarks and symptoms. (*Early treatment of problems can keep them under control and avoid later serious situations.)*

PLEASE USE BALL POINT PEN

NAME ______ SEND TOP (WHITE) COPY TO DEL. ROOM TERM ______
ADDRESS ______ LMP ______ LIFE ______ EDC ______
PHONE ______ RELIGION ______ NURSING ______ PEDIATRICIAN ______
AGE ______ GR ______ PARA ______ AB ______ ANESTHESIA ______
BLOOD TYPE ______ RH ______ SEROLOGY ______ REFERRING M.D. ______
HUSB. BL. TYPE ______ RH ______ GENOTYPE ______ PRENATAL PREPARATION ______
HUSBAND IN DELIVERY ROOM? ______
RUBELLA TITER ______
MENSTRUAL CYCLE ______
PAP SMEAR ______ G.C. CULTURE ______

PP AR SE T G.		DATE	WHERE CONFINED	WEEKS GESTATION	LENGTH OF LABOR	INFANT WT.	COMPLICATIONS
	1						
	2						
	3						
	4						

HISTORY AND PHYSICAL

CHILDHOOD ______ HT. ______ NORMAL WT. ______ NORMAL B.P. ______
FAMILY ______ HEENT ______
TRAUMATIC ______ HEART & LUNGS ______
ADULT ______ BACK & BREASTS ______
BLOOD TRANSFUSIONS ______ ABDOMEN ______
ALLERGIES ______ SKIN & EXTREMITIES ______
SURGERY ______ PELVIC CAPACITY ______
COMMENTS: ______
MEDICATIONS ______
RH TITERS DATES: ______

PERIODIC VISITS		DATE	WEIGHT	BP	URINE	FHT	FUNDUS	PELVIC	COMMENTS
	1								
	2								
	3								
	4								
	5								
	6								
	7								
	8								
	9								
	10								
	11								
	12								
	13								
	14								

DELIVERY ROOM - TERM SIGNATURE: M.D.

Figure 41–10: Prenatal health history form. *Delmar/Cengage Learning.*

- Request her first morning urine specimen, which she brought with her, or have her give you one now. (*Some complications of pregnancy can be identified by urine tests.*)
- Obtain a blood sample if needed: Some providers monitor the patient's iron level by checking the hemoglobin routinely. Also, screening tests for alpha-fetoprotein (AFP), a test to check for neural tube defects, may be performed at 15–18 weeks, and gestational diabetes, known as a glucose tolerance test, is performed during weeks 24–28 of gestation.
- Measure the patient's weight and record the findings. (*Weight reflects the mother's nutrition and the related health of the fetus. Excess as well as insufficient weight gain is undesirable. Excess gain could indicate fluid retention.*)
- Measure and record her vital signs. (*Monitoring blood pressure is extremely important. Hypertension is indicative of complications.*)

PRENATAL RISK ASSESSMENT FORM

Please print or type:

Patient Name	Case Number	ADC Number	E.D.D. month / day / year
Physician Name	Physician Telephone		

Please check all that apply:

AT RISK OF PRETERM BIRTH

ABSOLUTE FACTORS *(one factor puts patient at risk)*

OBSTETRICAL HISTORY

- ❑ 1. PRETERM DELIVERY
- ❑ 2. DES EXPOSURE
- ❑ 3. CONE BIOPSY
- ❑ 4. SECOND TRIMESTER ABORTION
- ❑ 5. 1st TRIMESTER SPONTANEOUS ABORTIONS, more than 2

CURRENT PREGNANCY

- ❑ 6. UTERINE ANOMALY OR FIBROIDS
- ❑ 7. MULTIPLE GESTATION
- ❑ 8. ABDOMINAL SURGERY
- ❑ 9. CERVIX DILATED, more than 1.5 cm before 29 weeks
- ❑ 10. CERVIX EFFACED, less than 1 cm before 29 weeks
- ❑ 11. IRRITABLE UTERUS, more than 6 contractions per hr. confirmed
- ❑ 12. POLYHYDRAMNIOS
- ❑ 13. BLEEDING, if significant after 12 weeks
- ❑ 14. PYELONEPHRITIS
- ❑ 15. PRETERM LABOR
- ❑ 16. SMOKING, more than 10 cigarettes per day
- ❑ 17. PROM, confirmed

❑ YES ❑ NO At least ONE of the above conditions has been checked. Patient is at risk of preterm birth.

AT RISK OF POOR PREGNANCY OUTCOME

ABSOLUTE FACTORS *(one factor puts patient at risk)*

OBSTETRICAL HISTORY

- ❑ 18. INFANT DEATH, stillborn, neonatal, post neonatal
- ❑ 19. CONGENITAL ANOMALY, major
- ❑ 20. LOW BIRTH WEIGHT, less than 2500g.
- ❑ 21. ECLAMPSIA or severe preeclampsia
- ❑ 22. INCOMPETENT CERVIX

CURRENT PREGNANCY

- ❑ 23. HEART DISEASE, class III or IV
- ❑ 24. DIABETES, insulin dependent
- ❑ 25. SICKLE CELL ANEMIA or other hemoglobinopathy
- ❑ 26. MALIGNANCY or leukemia
- ❑ 27. THYROID DISEASE, confirmed
- ❑ 28. EPILEPSY or on anticonvulsant
- ❑ 29. HEPATITIS or chronic liver disease
- ❑ 30. ASTHMA, on medication
- ❑ 31. TUBERCULOSIS, active
- ❑ 32. PNEUMONIA
- ❑ 33. HYPERTENSION, on medication
- ❑ 34. DEEP VENOUS THROMBOSIS
- ❑ 35. PLACENTA PREVIA, 3rd trimester
- ❑ 36. OLIGOHYDRAMNIOS
- ❑ 37. ECLAMPSIA or preeclampsia
- ❑ 38. ALLOIMMUNIZATION associated with fetal disease
- ❑ 39. RUBELLA EXPOSURE with rising titer
- ❑ 40. POSITIVE SEROLOGY
- ❑ 41. ACTIVE HERPES or positive culture, 3rd trimester
- ❑ 42. PRIMIGRAVIDA, less than 17 years or more than 35 years
- ❑ 43. FAMILIAL GENETIC DISORDER, confirmed
- ❑ 44. PSYCHOSIS
- ❑ 45. MENTAL RETARDATION
- ❑ 46. DRUG OR ALCOHOL ABUSE
- ❑ 47. OTHER ______________________

❑ YES ❑ NO At least ONE of the above conditions has been checked. Patient is at risk of poor pregnancy outcome.

RELATIVE FACTORS *(two factors put patient at risk)*

- ❑ 48. PRIOR C-SECTION
- ❑ 49. PRENATAL CARE NON-COMPLIANCE, most recent pregnancy
- ❑ 50. GRAND MULTIPARA, more than 5 of 20 weeks or more
- ❑ 51. RECENT DELIVERY, less than 1 yr.
- ❑ 52. LATE INITIAL VISIT, after 14 weeks of pregnancy
- ❑ 53. MISSED PRENATAL APPOINTMENTS, 2 consecutive
- ❑ 54. AGE, less than 17 years or more than 35 years
- ❑ 55. Height, less than 5 ft.
- ❑ 56. OBESITY, more than 20% weight for height
- ❑ 57. UNDERWEIGHT, more than 10% weight for height
- ❑ 58. WEIGHT LOSS, continuing after 14 weeks
- ❑ 59. ANEMIA, less than 10 Hgb, or less than 30% Hct.
- ❑ 60. GONORRHEA, positive culture
- ❑ 61. DIABETES, gestational, diet controlled
- ❑ 62. CHRONIC BRONCHITIS
- ❑ 63. TRAUMA, requiring hospitalization
- ❑ 64. ILLITERACY or language barrier
- ❑ 65. DOMESTIC VIOLENCE
- ❑ 66. OTHER ______________________

❑ YES ❑ NO At least TWO of the above conditions have been checked. Patient is at risk of poor pregnancy outcome.

Physician's Signature	Date

Figure 41–11: Prenatal risk assessment form. *Delmar/Cengage Learning.*

- Check the chart to be sure all lab reports from tests ordered since the last visit are in the chart. Also check that any other studies or referral letters are included.
- If the provider will be performing an examination, prepare the patient by having her remove her clothes from the waist down, unless the breasts are also to be examined, and put on a gown with the opening in the front. (Providers have different preferences for how often they will do an exam; be sure to check with your provider for specifics.)
- Assist the patient onto the examination table and have her sit at the end. (Provide a drape for her lap and legs if an exam is being performed.)
- Notify the provider that the patient is ready for the examination.

After the provider reviews any returned reports and your chart notes, the patient's current general condition is discussed, and the reported problems or findings are further explored. Then it is time to proceed with the examination or additional testing if desired or needed.

- Assist the patient into supine position for the prenatal examination.
- Provide assistance to the provider as appropriate for the **trimester** (three-month period) of the patient's **gestation** (nine [ten lunar] months or 38 to 42 weeks).
- A fetoscope (special stethoscope) or a Doppler fetal pulse monitor and gel are applied to the abdomen to determine the developing fetus's heart rate.
- The provider may palpate the abdomen to evaluate fundic height as a means of estimating the duration of the pregnancy. If it is not as expected, it could be an indication of multiple fetuses, excess amniotic fluid, poor development of the fetus, or even fetal death.
- A flexible centimeter tape is used to measure the height of the **fundus** (top of the uterus) from the symphysis pubis to evaluate the growth of the fetus after approximately the third month.
- Upon completion of the examination, assist the patient to a sitting position and instruct her to dress.
- Record the appropriate information such as fundic height, fetal heart rate, procedures performed, and other pertinent patient or provider observations and remarks.
- Ultrasonography may be performed the first trimester to confirm pregnancy and later to monitor its progress (Figure 41–12). One of the most exciting times for the expectant parents is when the physician or technician locates the fetus by using ultrasound technology. The equipment is capable of displaying the image on the screen and printing out the baby's first "picture" for the proud parents to show to family and friends.

Patient Care

After the provider has completed the examination and talked with the patient, offer to answer any questions the patient might have. Encourage the patient to make her next appointment before leaving the facility. Figure 41–13 illustrates the frequency of office visits for a normal pregnancy. Persons experiencing difficulties or at high risk require more frequent evaluation. Give support and assistance by reminding her to call if she has any questions or problems.

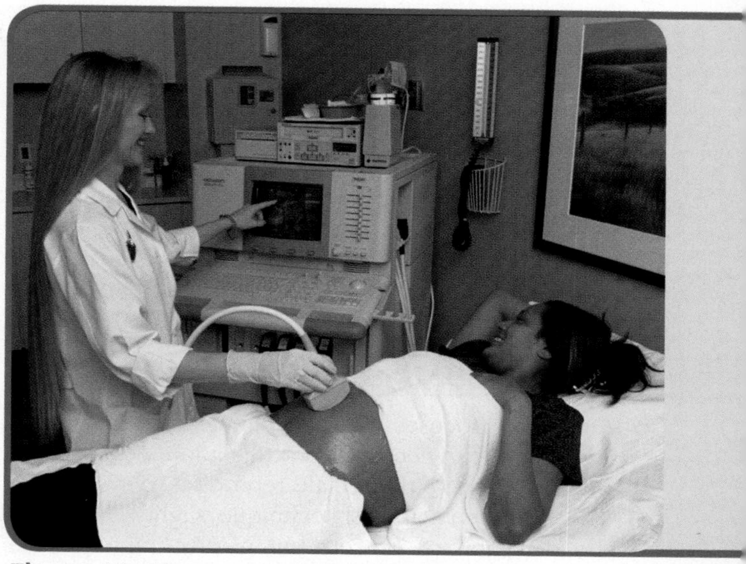

Figure 41–12: An ultrasound being performed.
Delmar/Cengage Learning.

PATIENT EDUCATION

It is very important for prenatal patients to receive regular, systematic evaluation. You must stress the importance of keeping scheduled appointments so the mother and baby can be monitored closely.

The medical assistant should return to the exam room to clean up the area. Wear gloves to protect yourself from disease transmission. Discard all disposables in appropriate waste containers, remove gloves and dispose of them properly, and wash hands. Restock supplies as necessary, making the exam room ready for the next patient. Place any specimens in the area for pickup by the lab representative.

GENERAL SCHEDULE FOR PRENATAL OR OBSTETRICAL APPOINTMENTS

FIRST AND SECOND TRIMESTER:
Monthly or every four weeks through the 28th week.

THIRD TRIMESTER:
Every two weeks in the 30th–36th weeks. Every week in the 36th+ week up to delivery.

Figure 41–13: Prenatal appointment schedule.
Delmar/Cengage Learning.

> **CLINICAL PEARL**
>
> Especially in an OB/GYN practice, the possibility exists of patients who might be bleeding or who have an infection that can be transmitted by body fluids and therefore could be a threat to others.

To be of further assistance to both provider and patient, you might want to check all patients' charts to make sure that findings are documented in a neat and legible manner and signed by the provider. Remember, records are legal documents and may be requested at any time by insurance providers to verify the diagnosis and coding, leading to more efficient and expedient payment.

CHAPTER SUMMARY

- Obstetrics focuses on pregnancy and childbirth, whereas the gynecology practice addresses diseases and disorders of the female reproductive system.
- The ThinPrep Pap test technique slightly improves the detection of cancers but greatly improves the detection of precancers. This method also enables additional studies from the same sample, such as tests for the presence of HPV, chlamydia, and gonorrhea.
- The ACS recommends that all women should begin Pap screening tests about three years after they begin having vaginal intercourse but no later than 21 years old. Screening should be done every year with a regular Pap test or every two years with a liquid-based Pap test. At age 30, women with three normal Pap tests in a row may have a screening every two to three years with either test method. Women with risk should continue with annual testing or follow provider's recommendations.
- The ACS has recommendations in place for women to follow to assist in making their Pap results more accurate.
- Breast self-exams need to be performed by the patient monthly. Although the breast exam conducted by the provider with the annual Pap test is important, it is insufficient in detecting abnormal breast tissue between visits to the provider. Most women discover a lump or mass in their breasts themselves and report it to the provider. This leads to early detection and treatment, which greatly increases the survival rate.
- Most providers prefer the medical assistant (or nurse) to accompany them into the exam room, not only to assist with the procedure, but also to verify their behavior in case of patient accusations.
- Three main reporting categories for Pap smears are: negative for intraepithelial lesion or malignancy; epithelial cell abnormalities; and other malignant neoplasms.
- To confirm pregnancy, the diagnosis is made only after the patient has been given a complete evaluation by (1) interviewing the patient and obtaining a complete prenatal health assessment and history; (2) doing a complete physical examination; (3) ordering laboratory tests, such as urinalysis and pregnancy tests, blood tests, and cultures; and (4) performing any other diagnostic test indicated by the patient's condition.
- In addition to assisting the provider with all the examinations, your role in prenatal evaluation and care of patients is to instill the importance of keeping regular appointments; encourage patients to eat a sensible, well-balanced diet; alert the doctor of any problems or concerns; and provide patient education materials with explanations.
- Naegele's rule is determined by using the first day of the last menstrual period (LMP), subtracting three months, and then adding seven days plus one year.
- Your role in assessing the patient prior to her prenatal appointment can include: interviewing the patient to determine whether any problems are being experienced; requesting lab and urine specimens; measuring the patient's weight and recording the findings; measuring and recording her vital signs; checking the chart to be sure all lab reports from tests ordered since the last visit are in the chart; preparing the patient if the provider will be doing an examination; and notifying the provider that the patient is ready for the examination.

STUDY TOOLS

Workbook	Activities for Chapter 41
Premium Website MEDIA LINK	View this **Media Link** for Chapter 41: • Assist with a Gynecologic Exam

StudyWARE	Activities and Quizzes on the **StudyWARE™ Software** for Chapter 41
	Audio Library of medical terms
	Online access to the **Critical Thinking Challenge 2.0**
CourseMate	Activities and Quizzes for Chapter 41
WebTutor	Activities and Quizzes for Chapter 41

CHECK YOUR KNOWLEDGE

1. Over what age is it recommended that women start routine yearly mammograms?
   a. 21
   b. 30
   c. 40
   d. 50
2. All women should begin screening tests about three years after they begin having vaginal intercourse but no later than ______ years old.
   a. 16
   b. 21
   c. 18
   d. 40
3. The system most widely used to describe Pap test findings is the Bethesda System, which reports the test results by using _______ general categories:
   a. three
   b. two
   c. four
   d. six
4. Which of the following gynecological instruments are inserted into the uterus to explore the cavity and measure the depth of the uterus?
   a. Sims' uterine curette
   b. Randall uterine curette
   c. Toms-Gaylor uterine punch
   d. Sims' uterine sound
5. During the 24th to 28th week of gestation, the following blood test is obtained from the mother:
   a. Alpha-fetoprotein (AFP)
   b. Glucose tolerance test
   c. HIV
   d. Hepatitis
6. Using Naegele's rule, the period of gestation (conception to birth) is determined by using the:
   a. first day of the last menstrual period (LMP), subtracting three months, and then adding seven days plus one year.
   b. last day of the last menstrual period (LMP), subtracting three months, and then adding seven days plus one year.
   c. first day of the last menstrual period (LMP), subtracting nine months, and then adding seven days plus one year.
   d. last day of the last menstrual period (LMP), subtracting three months, and then adding seven days plus one year.

WEB LINKS

American Cancer Society: www.cancer.org

RESOURCES

Estes, M. E. Z. (2010). *Health Assessment & Physical Examination* (3rd ed.). Clifton Park, NY: Delmar Cengage Learning.

Heller, M., and Veach, L. (2009). *Clinical Medical Assisting: A Professional, Field Smart Approach to the Workplace*. Clifton Park, NY: Delmar, Cengage Learning.

Lindh, W., Pooler, M., Tamparo, C., and Dahl, B. (2010). *Delmar's Comprehensive Medical Assisting Administrative and Clinical Competencies* (4th ed.). Clifton Park, NY: Delmar Cengage Learning.

Venes, D., (ed.). (2009). *Taber's Cyclopedic Medical Dictionary* (21st ed.). Philadelphia: F. A. Davis.

Chapter 42 Pediatric Examinations

OBJECTIVES

In this chapter, you will learn the following:

KB KNOWLEDGE BASE

1. Spell and define, using the glossary at the back of the text, all the Words to Know in this chapter.
2. Interpret from the AAP's Recommendations for Preventive Pediatric Health Care chart for frequency and types of recommended screenings and procedures for pediatric patients.
3. Explain the Early and Periodic Screening, Diagnostic, and Treatment (EPSDT) program.
4. Identify and discuss developmental stages of life.
5. Identify gross motor activities that are appropriate for 6-month-, 1-year-, and 18-month-old children using childhood growth and development tables.
6. Explain how to plot height and weight measurements on a National Center for Health Statistics growth chart.
7. Explain the difference between a well-child and sick-child visit.
8. List five responsibilities of the medical assistant when assisting with pediatric examinations.
9. Explain the difference between neglect and abuse, citing five examples of each.
10. Identify immunizations given to 2- and 12-month-old children according to the Childhood and Adolescent Immunization Schedule.
11. Identify two charts used to perform pediatric vision acuity and explain how each is used.

S SKILLS

1. Measure length, weight, and head and chest circumference measurements of an infant and child.
2. Plot pediatric patients' measurements on a growth chart.
3. Perform pediatric vision acuity screening.

B BEHAVIOR

1. Apply critical thinking skills in performing patient assessment and care.
2. Explain the rationale for performance of procedure to the patient.
3. Show awareness of patients' concerns regarding their perceptions of the procedure being performed.

WORDS TO KNOW

Apgar
attachment
bonding
caregiver
child abuse
child neglect
chronologic
circumference
development
failure to thrive (FTT)
immunization
intercede
lethargic
listlessness
malnutrition
pediatric
percentile
preventive
vaccination information statement (VIS)

PEDIATRICS

Pediatrics is a specialty of medicine that cares for children from birth until essentially adulthood. The initial pediatrician's examination will often be done in the hospital a few hours after birth, but the state of health of the newborn actually began many months before with the prenatal care of the mother. Some practices limit care at 16 years of age, whereas others may continue until patients reach 18 years of age or high school graduation.

Almost immediately after birth, the infant is evaluated by the **Apgar** scoring system, which is an indication of the newborn's well-being (described in Chapter 35). This score, from 0–10, determines the infant's first individual experience with medical care. A score of 10 is considered the best possible condition; a score below 4 requires immediate intervention and continued evaluation.

With many hospital discharges occurring between 24 and 48 hours after birth, infants begin their journey through the pediatrician's office at approximately one to two weeks of age. At this visit, the height and weight are measured, diet and eating concerns discussed, and any lab tests such as PKU and bilirubin screenings or other procedures deemed necessary are performed. By 2 months, infants return for another examination and evaluation and begin the **immunization** schedule. Infants continue on with the immunization schedule if they have already started immunizations in the hospital.

After that, infants continue to be examined at 2- to 3-month intervals throughout the first 18 months, and immunizations should be completed. Children continue to be examined on a yearly basis to monitor their development toward maturity. The American Academy of Pediatrics (AAP) has established Recommendations for Preventive Pediatric Health Care, a chart that outlines the types and frequency of examinations to provide **preventive** care for normally developing, healthy children. Go to the AAP's Website at www.aap.org and search for "Recommendations for Preventive Pediatric Health Care" to view and download the most up-to-date, comprehensive chart. If health or development problems occur, a more frequent schedule will be necessary.

Another program that requires regular health maintenance exams and careful documentation of examination findings is the Early and Periodic Screening, Diagnosis, and Treatment (EPSDT) program, Medicaid's comprehensive and preventive child health program. This is for eligible Medicaid patients who are between birth and 21 years of age. This program requires regular routine health maintenance checkups to detect and treat medical problems before they become serious or beyond treatment stages. The parent or primary **caregiver** must accompany the child at each visit.

The program includes the following screening services:

- Comprehensive health and developmental history (assessment of both physical and mental health development)
- Comprehensive unclothed physical exam
- Appropriate immunizations
- Laboratory tests
- Lead toxicity screening
- Health education
- Vision services
- Dental services
- Hearing services
- Other necessary health care (states must provide other necessary health care, diagnosis services, treatment, and other measures to correct problems discovered by the aforementioned screening services.)

PEDIATRIC GROWTH AND DEVELOPMENT

Pediatric patients are examined much more frequently than adults and must be monitored carefully because of their rapid growth and **development**, especially in the first year. Growth refers to the changes in height and weight that can be measured as the infant begins to mature. Development refers to an infant's ability to control his or her body and use verbal and mental skills. These areas of assessment, as well as the apparent intellectual and social development of the developing child, are closely observed and compared with acceptable national standards. This comparison determines whether the child is at the appropriate level of development as compared to the **chronologic** age. Children will vary in individual development, but when characteristics are beyond acceptable levels, intervention will be initiated to identify the reason.

A great deal of physical, mental, and social development occurs within a relatively short period of 2 years. The ability to sit, stand, and walk; hold and use toys and utensils; and progress from babbling sounds to words all unfold over that time period. Children develop their own personality and exhibit a degree of independence (Figure 42–1). Table 42–1 highlights growth and development during infancy and toddlerhood. The table shows the age at which the average child should be able to perform the activities listed.

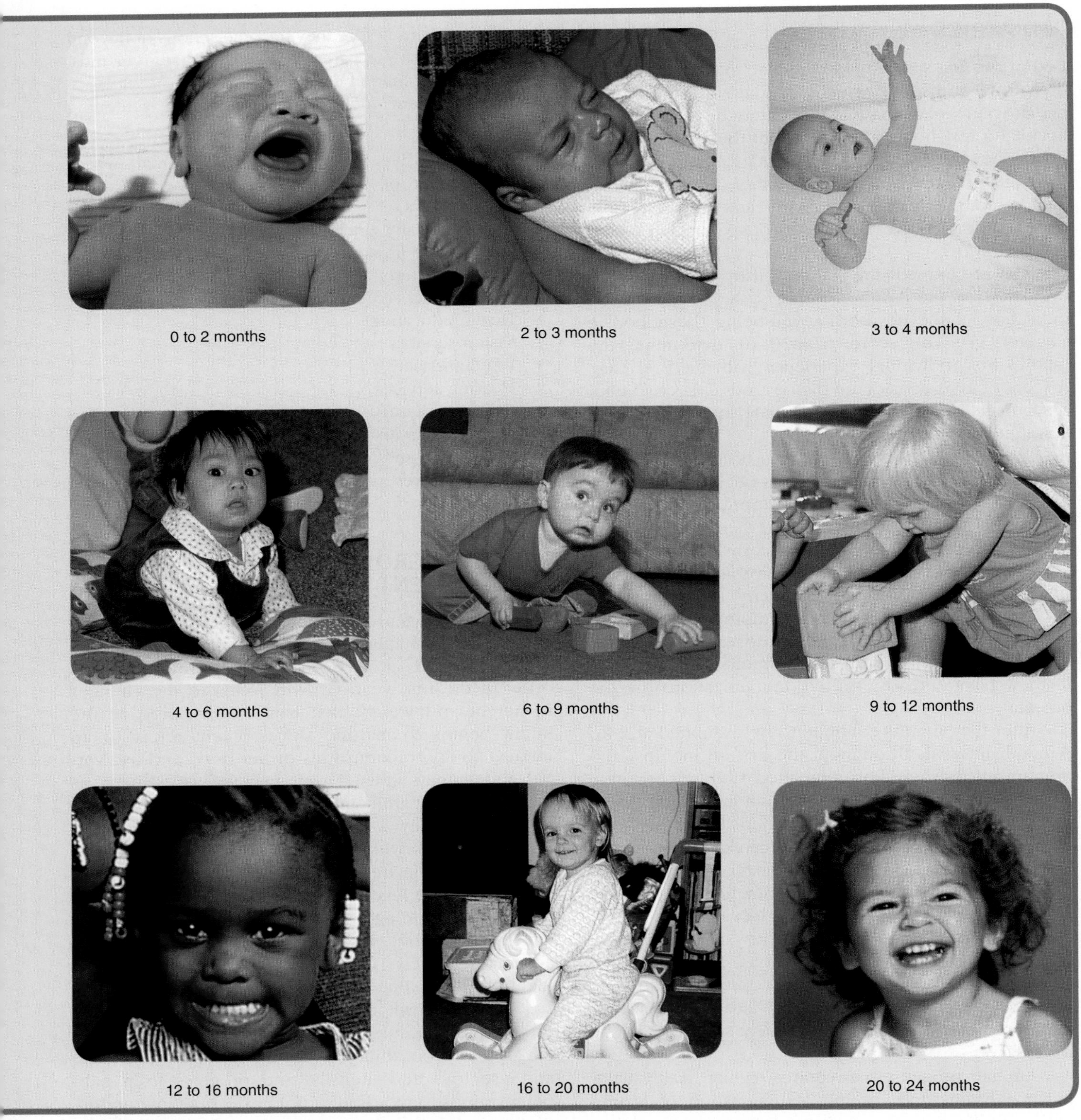

Figure 42–1: Growth and development stages of infants and toddlers. *Delmar/Cengage Learning.*

TABLE 42–1 Growth and Development from Newborn to 30 Months

Age	Gross Motor	Fine Motor	Language	Sensory
Birth to 1 month	• Assumes tonic neck posture • When prone, lifts and turns head	• Holds hands in fist • Draws arms and legs to body	• Cries	• Comforts with holding and touch • Looks at faces • Follows objects when in line of vision • Alert to high-pitched voices • Smiles
2 to 4 months	• Can raise head and shoulders when prone to 45–90 degrees; supports self on forearms • Rolls from back to side	• Hands mostly open • Looks at and plays with fingers • Grasps and tries to reach objects	• Vocalizes when talked to; coos, babbles • Laughs aloud • Squeals	• Smiles • Follows objects 180 degrees • Turns head when hears voices or sounds
4 to 6 months	• Turns from stomach to back and then back to stomach • When pulled to sitting, almost no head lag • By 6 months, can sit on floor with hands forward for support	• Can hold feet and put in mouth • Can hold bottle • Can grasp rattle and other small objects • Puts objects in mouth	• Squeals	• Watches a falling object • Responds to sounds
6 to 8 months	• Puts full weight on legs when held in standing position • Can sit without support • Bounces when held in a standing position	• Transfers objects from one hand to the other • Can feed self a cookie • Can bang two objects together	• Babbles vowel-like sounds, "ooh" or "aah" • Imitation of speech sounds ("mama," "dada") begins • Laughs aloud	• Responds by looking and smiling • Recognizes own name
8 to 10 months	• Crawls on all fours or uses arms to pull body along floor • Can pull self to sitting • Can pull self to standing	• Beginning to use thumb-finger grasp • Dominant hand use • Has good hand-mouth coordination	• Responds to verbal commands • May say one word in addition to "mama" and "dada"	• Recognizes sounds

(continues)

TABLE 42–1 *(Continued)*

Age	Gross Motor	Fine Motor	Language	Sensory
10 to 12 months	• Can sit down from standing • Walks around room holding onto objects • Can stand alone	• Picks up and drops objects • Can put small objects into toys or containers through holes • Turns many pages in a book at one time • Picks up small objects	• Understands "no" and other simple commands • Learns one or two other words • Imitates speech sounds • Speaks gibberish	• Follows fast-moving objects • Indicates wants • Likes to play imitative games such as patty cake and peek-a-boo
12 to 15 months	• Can walk alone well • Can crawl up stairs	• Can feed self with cup and spoon • Puts raisins into a bottle • May hold crayon or pencil and scribble • Builds a tower of two cubes	• Says four to six words	• Binocular vision developed
18 months	• Runs, falling often • Can jump in place • Can walk up stairs holding on • Plays with push and pull toys	• Can build a tower of three to four cubes • Can use a spoon	• Says 10 or more words • Points to objects or body parts when asked	• Visual acuity 20/40
24 months	• Can walk up and down stairs • Can kick a ball • Can ride a tricycle	• Can draw a circle • Tries to dress self	• Talks a lot • Approximately 300-word vocabulary • Understands commands • Knows first name, refers to self • Verbalizes toilet needs	
30 months	• Throws a ball • Jumps with both feet • Can stand on one foot for a few minutes	• Can build a tower of eight blocks • Can use crayons • Learning to use scissors	• Knows first and last name • Knows the name of one color • Can sing • Expresses needs • Uses pronouns appropriately	

PEDIATRIC MEASUREMENTS

Precise measurements of the pediatric patient are essential for monitoring the growth and development of the child. In addition to monitoring normal physical development, the provider may use growth patterns and developments to assist in diagnosing diseases. Routine measurements that are obtained at every well-child visit include height or recumbent length, weight, and **circumference** of the head and chest.

Measuring Height

Measuring the height of a baby from infancy to 36 months by recumbent length is recommended as the most accurate method of measurement. The baby should be placed on a pediatric scale with built-in height measurement apparatus or on an infant height measurement chart board with the placement of the baby's head at the headboard. If necessary, someone holds the head in position while you stretch the legs out straight. (Infants tend to flex their legs.) You then slide the footboard up to the infants' heels and measure from the vertex of the head to the heel of the baby. Refer to Figure 42–2 and Procedure 42–1 regarding how to place the baby on the exam table for measuring the recumbent length.

It is also possible to measure the recumbent length of an infant without a measuring scale or chart. Place the infant lying on an examination surface that is covered with paper and make a mark on the paper at the top of the infant's head. (Enlist the parent or another medical assistant to help position the infant.) With the parent holding the infant in position, straighten out one leg and mark on the paper at the bottom of the heel. Ask the parent to pick up the infant. Using a flexible tape or ruled measuring device, measure the distance between your two markings on the paper to obtain the recumbent length of the infant. Whether you are using a table that has a headboard, a measuring scale, or a portable measuring chart (shown in Figure 42–2), follow the directions for that particular device in your facility.

When the child reaches 3 years of age (36 months), he or she generally is old enough to cooperate, and you can begin to measure the height and weight on a regular balance beam scale, following the same procedure as an adult patient (refer to Procedure 38–1). The child's shoes should be removed and the measuring bar placed on the top (vertex) of the child's head to get an accurate measurement (Figure 42–3). The child must stand still in the center of the platform until the height measurement is obtained. To reduce the amount of time the child is in place on the platform of the scales, look at the chart and see what the measurement was at the last exam so that you can have an idea where the measurement will be.

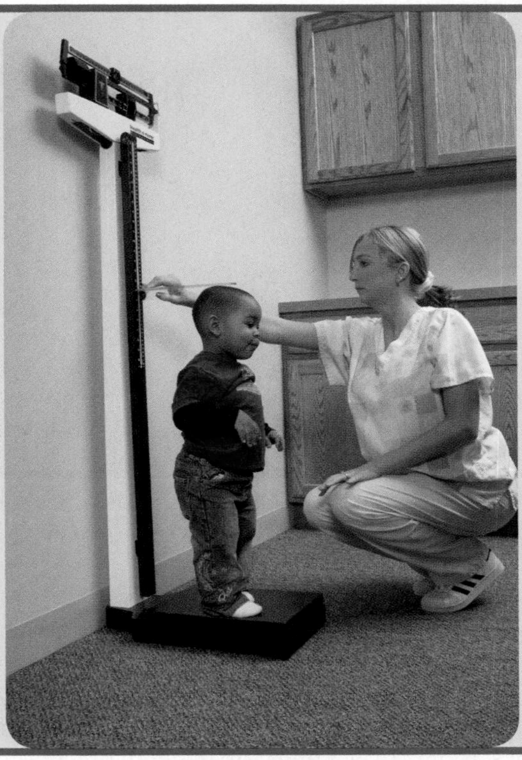

Figure 42–3: Measuring the child's height on a regular balance beam scale, placing the measuring bar at the vertex of the patient's head. *Delmar/Cengage Learning.*

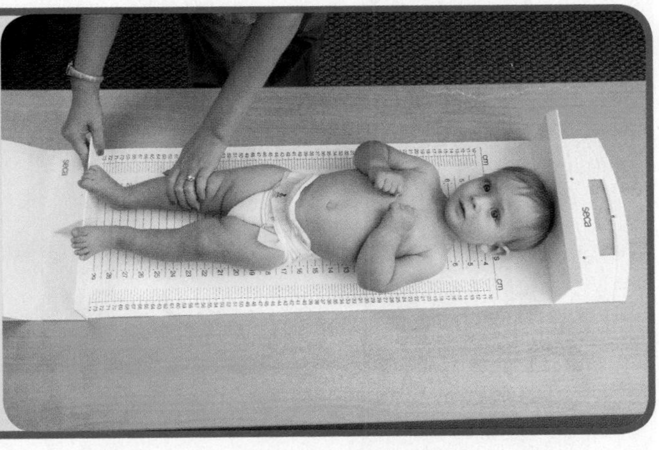

Figure 42–2: Measuring recumbent length of an infant, measuring from the vertex of the child's head to the heel. *Delmar/Cengage Learning.*

Weighing the Pediatric Patient

It is customary to weigh infants unclothed for greater accuracy. Remember, a wet diaper can weigh several ounces, which would lead to an inaccurate measurement of the infant's true weight. Because you cannot control an infant's elimination, a disposable, waterproof pad should be placed on the scale, and a dry diaper can be placed over the genital area in case urination occurs. It is possible to adjust the weight to accommodate for the pad and diaper if the infant's weight is of great concern. Simply place it on the scale and adjust the balance weight to zero *before* the infant is placed on the scale. If an infant gains or loses weight too quickly, it could be a signal of a disease or disorder and should be brought to the provider's attention. It is also important to ask the

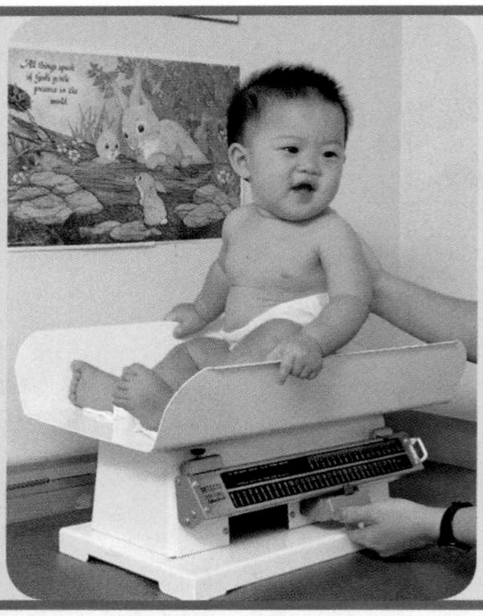

Figure 42–4: A baby weighed in sitting position; place your hand close to the child for safety. *Delmar/Cengage Learning.*

caregiver about the feeding schedule and appetite of the infant or child.

In some offices and clinics, the pediatric scale is kept on a stainless steel cart and simply wheeled to the patient's room. In a family or general practice office, the facility may have a pediatric room where all infants and children are examined. In a pediatric office, every patient room may have an infant scale, or the scale may be kept in a specific location where all infants and children are examined. Figures 42–4 and 42–5 show the proper positioning of the baby on the scales. Follow Procedure 42–1 to weigh an infant or baby up to 36 months or 38 pounds.

As the infant grows into the toddler stage and on to a preschooler and passes the weight limit of the infant scale, the weight can be measured on the regular balance beam scale used for older children and adults. (Refer to Procedure 38–1.) Often, the provider asks for the weight to be taken with the child unclothed except for the underwear. This is a good time for you to provide a gown for the patient, as mentioned earlier, for while he or she waits for the provider. Remember that children have feelings and may be embarrassed without their clothes.

Head Circumference

The head circumference is measured by placing a flexible tape measure around the infant's or child's head. You want the tape measure to go around the back part of the skull that protrudes out the farthest and around in front on the forehead. It is often necessary to ask for assistance in keeping the child from pulling on the tape while you are measuring the head. Place the tape under the head if the patient is lying down, about an inch above the ears, and around to the forehead. To get an accurate measurement, you should take the measurement more than once. This measurement should be performed and recorded routinely at each office visit until the child is 36 months of age. This is important for

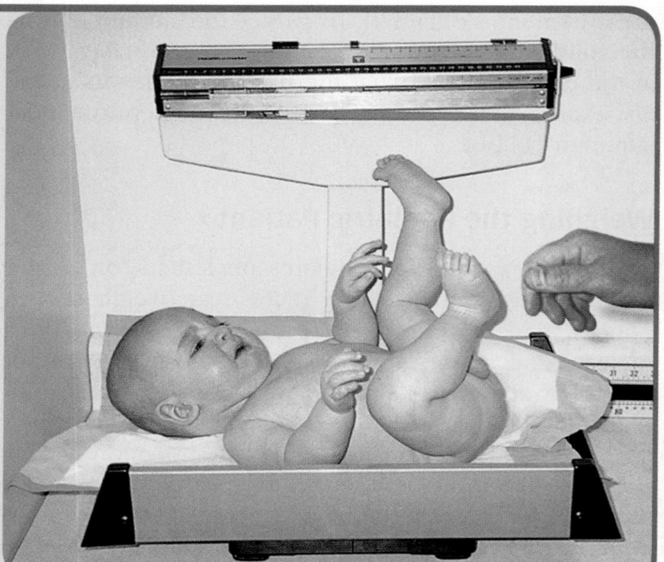

Figure 42–5: Infants too young to sit are weighed lying down; place your hand close to the child for safety. *Delmar/Cengage Learning.*

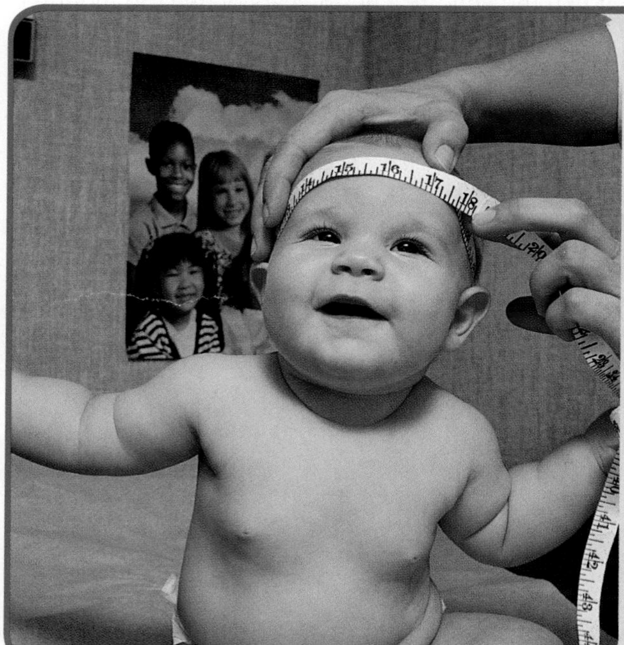

Figure 42–6: Measuring the head circumference of an infant. *Delmar/Cengage Learning.*

alerting the provider of abnormal development. Refer to Figure 42–6 to see the correct placement of the measuring tape. Procedure 42–1 will help you perform this measurement.

Chest Circumference

The chest circumference is measured by placing the flexible measuring tape around the child's chest just above the nipples (Figure 42–7). Often, it is difficult to keep the baby from moving. As said before, ask for assistance from the caregiver or another medical assistant. Place the measuring tape under the child and bring it around the baby's back to the chest to meet the zero mark. This measurement is not required on the growth graph but should be recorded on the chart. Refer to Procedure 42–1 for measuring an infant's chest circumference.

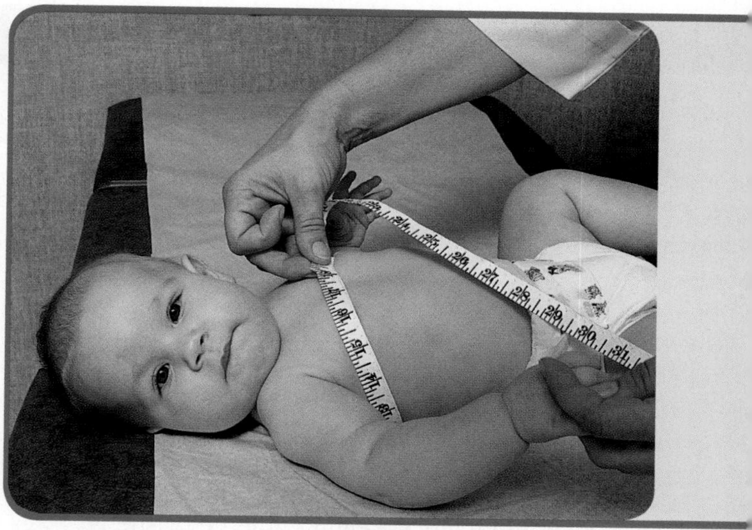

Figure 42–7: Measuring the chest circumference of an infant. *Delmar/Cengage Learning.*

PROCEDURE 42–1 Measure Length, Weight, and Head and Chest Circumference of an Infant or Child

PURPOSE: To obtain an accurate measurement of an infant or child's length, weight, and head and chest circumference

EQUIPMENT: Exam table with table paper, portable measurement chart board, measuring tape, patient's chart with growth chart or EMR; parents' record booklet, pediatric scale, and pen

S SKILL: Measure length, weight, and head and chest circumference of an infant or child

Procedure Steps	Detailed Instructions and/or *Rationales*
Measure Weight	
B 1. Introduce yourself, identify the patient, and explain the procedure to the parent or caregiver, ***using language that the parent or caregiver will understand.*** Wash hands.	
2. Ask the parent to undress the infant or child, including diaper.	*This alleviates the infant's apprehension and conserves your time.*
3. Place both weights to the left of the scale to check the balance.	
4. Place a water absorbent pad on the scale; reset scale to zero if necessary.	*To avoid disease transmission and decrease shock from the cold metal for the infant. This will decrease the chance that the infant will move because of being uncomfortable or afraid.*

(continues)

(continued)

Procedure Steps	Detailed Instructions and/or *Rationales*
B 5. Gently place the infant on his or her back on the scale; ***place your hand slightly above the child to ensure safety.***	The age of the baby may determine how the child is placed on the scales. Small infants will be easier to weigh lying down; those who can sit up on their own will most likely be more cooperative sitting on the scales. In either case, the safety of the baby is primary.
6. Place the bottom weight to the highest measurement that will not cause the balance bar to drop to the bottom edge.	
7. Slowly move upper weight until the balance bar rests in the center of the indicator. Read the infant's weight while he or she is lying still.	
8. Return both weights to their resting position to the extreme left.	
9. Gently remove infant and assist parent to apply diaper.	
10. Discard the used absorbent pad.	
Measuring Length	
B 1. Explain the procedure to the parent or caregiver, ***using language that the parent or caregiver will understand.***	
2. Gently place infant on his or her back on the portable measurement chart board with the top of the infant's head flush to the top of the board. Keep the legs straight and slide the footboard up so it is flush with the infant's heels.	There can be discrepancies with measurement of newborns because they are so used to the fetal position that it is difficult to straighten the legs.
3. Gently remove the infant. Measure the distance the between the headboard and the footboard. Read the length in inches to the nearest ¼, ½, or ¾ inch.	
Measuring Head Circumference	
B 1. Explain the procedure to the parent or caregiver, ***using language that the parent or caregiver will understand.***	
2. Place measuring tape snug around the forehead at the widest part.	Pull the tape snugly to compress any hair.
3. Read measurement to the nearest ¼, ½, or ¾ inch.	
Measuring Chest Circumference	
B 1. Explain the procedure to the parent or caregiver, ***using language that the parent or caregiver will understand.***	

Procedure Steps	Detailed Instructions and/or *Rationales*
2. Use one thumb to hold the tape measure at the zero mark against the infant's chest at the midsternal area and around the nipples.	The infant or child may lie down on the examination table or be held by a parent or guardian for the procedure. Children of 2 or 3 years and older may sit or stand on their own if they will cooperate and remain still for the procedure. Accurate measurement cannot be achieved if the child is crying. The measurement should be taken when the child is breathing normally, not with forced inspiration or expiration.
3. Read measurement to the nearest ¼, ½, or ¾ inch.	
4. Document the measurements in the patient's medical record and growth chart.	No chest measurements are included on the growth chart. The next section, and Procedure 42–2, details the steps in plotting measurements on growth charts.

Charting Example

5-12-XX 11:30 am	Wt. 16 lbs 9 oz, Ht. 26 in., head circumference 16 ¼ inches., Chest circumference 64 cm. G. Jenks, CMA(AAMA)

GROWTH CHARTS

All babies grow at different rates. The growth and development of the child is recorded in the patient's chart, in the caregiver's record booklet (if he or she has one), and on growth charts from the National Center for Health Statistics (NCHS), a division within the Centers for Disease Control and Prevention (CDC). These charts can be downloaded from the CDC's Website at www.cdc.gov/growthcharts and allow providers to see at a glance the child's growth and development pattern. The growth chart shows the normal growth of infants and children up to 20 years of age. The provider can then compare the child's measurements in relation to the **percentile**, that of other children the same age. (This percentile is to the far right of the graph; see Figure 42–8A.) The percentiles are calculated by plotting the child's measurements on the graph paper and locating the percentile it falls into by following the line it is plotted on to the outside of the paper where the percentiles are listed. The curved-line section closest to the top of the page, is where the height, length, and stature are recorded. The curved-line section below that is for plotting the weight of children. If the percentile of the height and weight of the child combined is wanted, the back section of the chart contains an area in which you draw an imaginary line from the child's weight to the height and plot it. You can then follow the line up the curved graph to the percentile on the right. If the measurements of a baby or child fall above or below the normal height or weight areas and the family history does not warrant it, further examination and diagnostic testing is usually scheduled.

If using an EMR system for documentation, the growth chart will display the height and weight information that you enter into the system through either the physical examination and vitals section or onto the growth chart itself, depending on the system. The record will then show the data points of the infant or child in comparison to other infants and children of that same age. The EHR provides a screen shot of this graphical data for the provider to use to monitor the child's physical development as is done with the paper chart documentation.

The growth charts become a permanent record of the child's development and are to be filed in the patient's chart. At each subsequent visit, the child's growth should be recorded. These growth graphs aid in the diagnosis of growth abnormalities, nutritional disorders, and diseases of children from birth to 20 years of age. Of course, hereditary factors also influence growth patterns, hence the importance of having a complete family health history in the medical record.

Refer to Figures 42–8A through D to see the growth graphs for boys and girls. Two graphs record growth patterns of infant males and females from birth to 36 months, and two record growth patterns record growth patterns of boys and girls from 2 to 20 years of age.

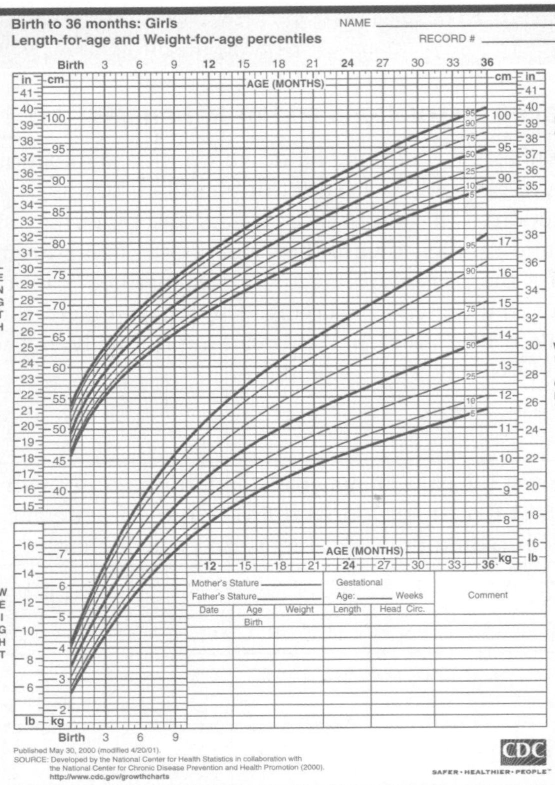

Figure 42–8A: Growth graph for height and weight, girls 0–36 months. *Courtesy of the Centers for Disease Control and Prevention.*

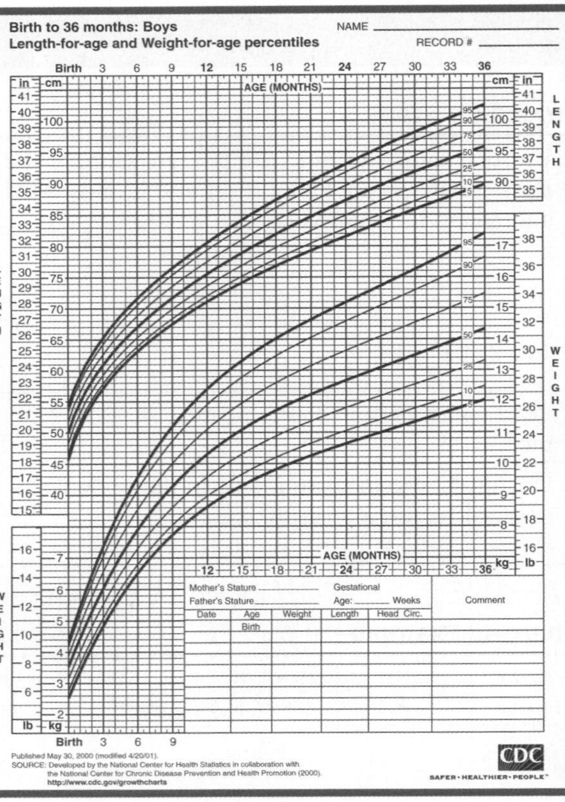

Figure 42–8B: Growth graph for height and weight, boys 0–36 months. *Courtesy of the Centers for Disease Control and Prevention.*

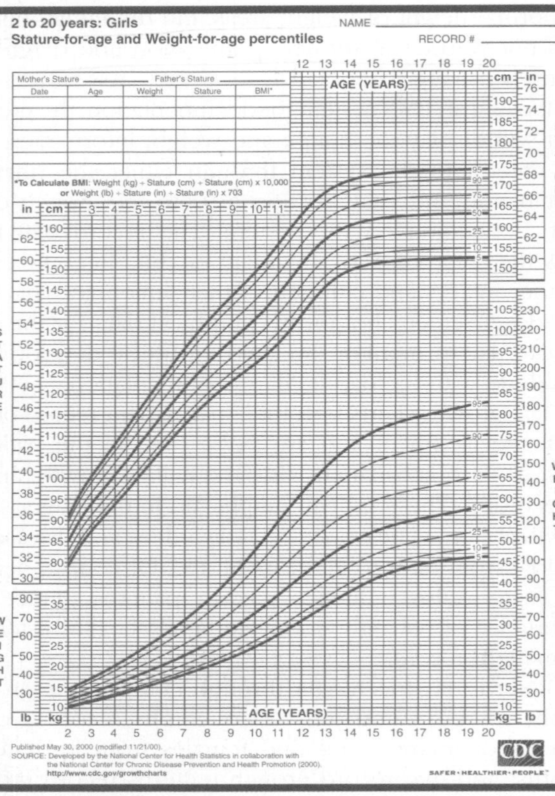

Figure 42–8C: Growth graph for height and weight, girls 2–20 years. *Courtesy of the Centers for Disease Control and Prevention.*

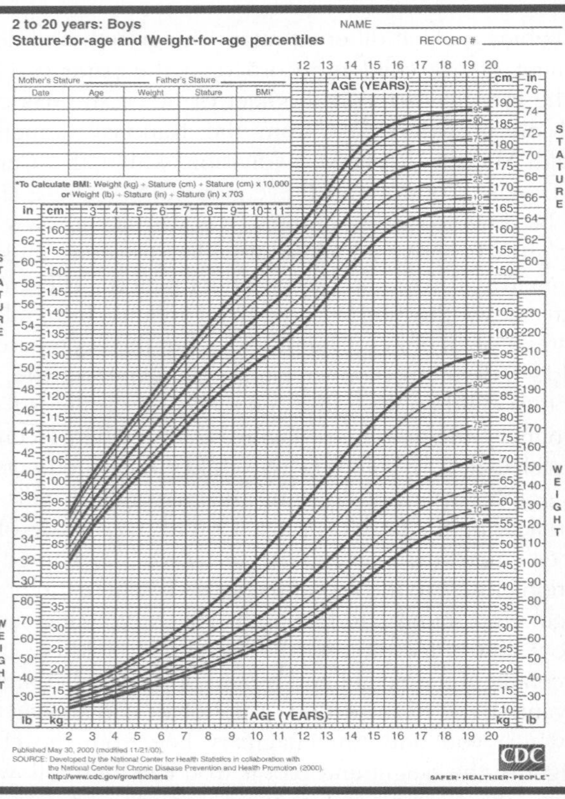

Figure 42–8D: Growth graph for height and weight, boys 2–20 years. *Courtesy of the Centers for Disease Control and Prevention.*

This information is printed across the top and bottom of the graph. Each of the squares across the page represents one month for the birth to 36-month graph and one year for the 2- to 20-year graph. Be sure you use the appropriate chart for the patient because the normal development and growth patterns are different for males and females. On the front of each of the graphs is a ruled section to record the date; age; length, height, and stature; and weight of the child at each appointment. The line for comments is for you to record a brief chief complaint that the caregiver (or the child, if old enough to speak) tells you. By looking at the line provided for the comments, you can see it is vital for you to print small and neatly so that it can be read easily. The complaint or problem should also be neatly recorded on the chart.

After the measurements of height, weight, and head circumference have been obtained, they are plotted on the graph where the age and the measurement intersect. To record the height measurement, simply follow the age line (vertically) to the child's length measurement (horizontally) on the left, follow the horizontal line to the point at which the two intersect, and place a dot there with your pen. For recording the weight of the infant or child, stay on the vertical (age) line and look to the right side of the graph if over 16 pounds or on the left if under. Following the horizontal line from right to left, you then place a dot at the intersection of the weight and age lines. The recumbent length of the child is recorded in inches or centimeters and the weight in either pounds or kilograms. Be consistent when measuring the child to avoid confusion.

Procedure 42–2 describes how to plot measurements on a growth chart.

PROCEDURE 42–2 Plot Data on a Growth Chart

PURPOSE: To record the growth and development of a patient accurately on a growth chart

EQUIPMENT: Patient's chart and growth chart; pen or EHR

S SKILL: Plot pediatric patient's measurements on a growth chart.

Procedure Steps	Detailed Instructions and/or *Rationales*
1. Obtain measurement data from the patient's chart.	This should include the patient's weight, height, and head circumference.
2. Locate the patient's age on the growth chart.	This runs across the top and bottom of the growth chart.
3. Locate the patient's height on the growth chart.	Depending on the child's length, you will find this on the left or right margin of the chart.
4. Locate the patient's weight on the growth chart.	Depending on the child's weight, you will find this on the left or right margin of the chart.
5. Find where the age on the horizontal line and child's height or length on the vertical line intersect and plot the measurement by making a dot on the chart.	You can then follow the curved line that you plotted on up to the right where it ends to read the percentile.
6. Do the same for the child's weight.	
7. On the back side of the chart, find the graph for the head circumference. This is plotted the same way.	
8. Fill in the box chart on the growth chart with the date, patient's age, weight, height, and head circumference.	This allows the provider to see the development at a glance.
9. Some providers want you to connect the dots of the measurements over time with a thin line. You can also determine the child's percentile by following the line on which the measurement is plotted to the side of the paper where the percentiles are indicated.	Refer to Figure 42–9 for a sample of a completed growth chart.

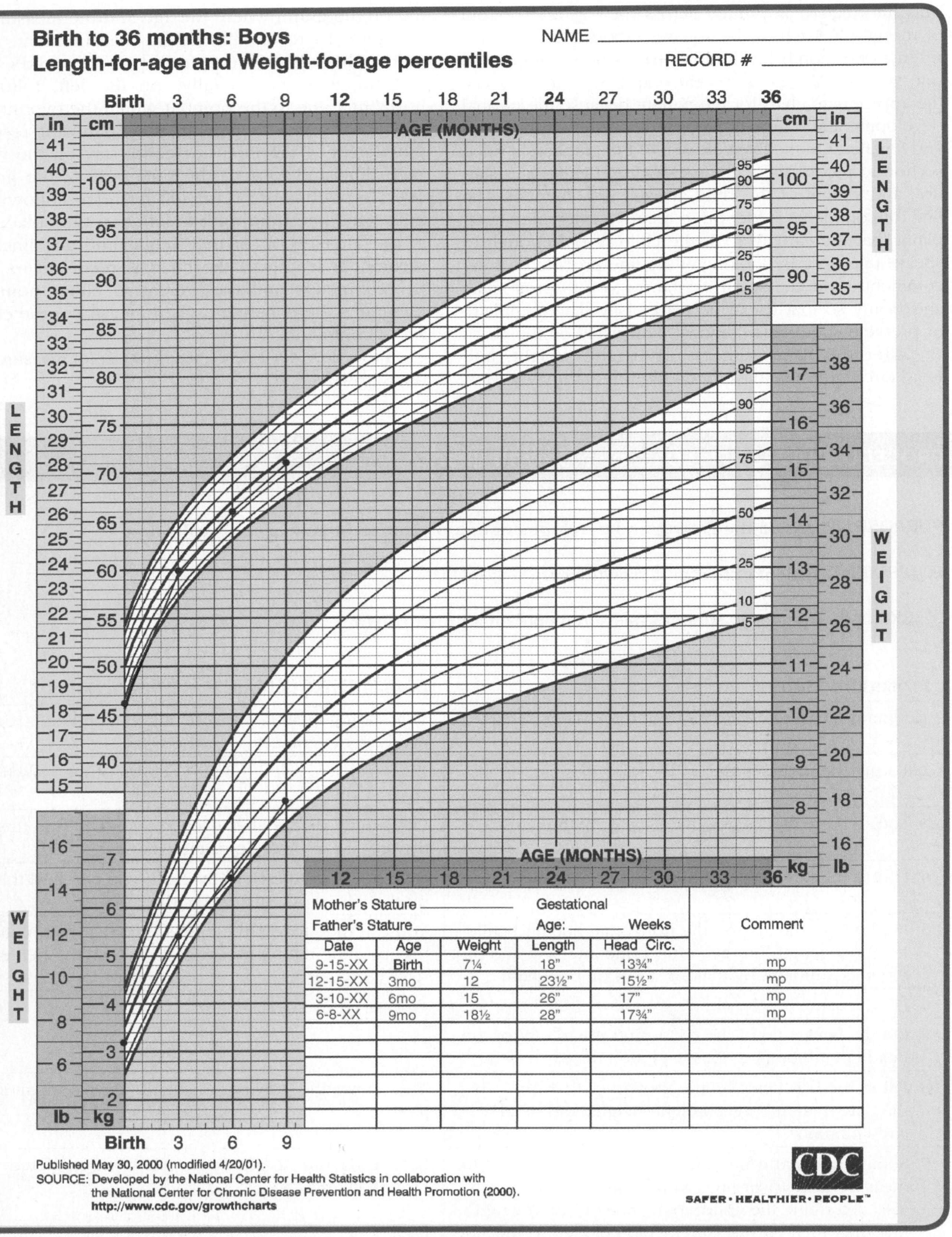

Date	Age	Weight	Length	Head Circ.	Comment
9-15-XX	Birth	7¼	18"	13¾"	mp
12-15-XX	3mo	12	23½"	15½"	mp
3-10-XX	6mo	15	26"	17"	mp
6-8-XX	9mo	18½	28"	17¾"	mp

Figure 42–9: Completed growth chart. *Courtesy of the Centers for Disease Control and Prevention.*

brain, heart, lungs, ht & wt is developing regularly

Failure to Thrive

An infant or young child who is below the third percentile on standardized growth charts is said to have a **failure to thrive (FTT)**. The cause may be from a physical problem (such as an unrepaired cleft palate or a disease condition) or associated with a poor physical and emotional environment. Normally, when a baby is born, a great deal of examining, touching, cuddling, and expressions of love are directed toward it. The infant is known to respond to this behavior, and this parent-child relationship is called **attachment** and **bonding**. When this does not occur, the baby lacks emotional support. Often, care is not provided on a consistent basis. If food is offered, the baby might be too **lethargic** to eat. Parents might lack knowledge about infant care, have anxiety about being a parent, or just be unconcerned. Parental illness, drug abuse, an unwanted or ill infant, and other factors can cause difficulty. With irregular and often absent care, the infant will show physical, emotional, and social delays in development.

When conducting the interview and performing the procedures prior to the provider's examination, the medical assistant has an opportunity to observe the parental behavior as well as the baby's condition. Some symptoms of an FTT baby are **listlessness** and avoidance of eye contact. Additionally, the infant will not seem concerned about you, a stranger, and there might be no cooing or crying. Older infants may not be interested in toys or playing. Parents may exhibit a lack of concern, not ask questions, and express negative comments about the baby. Inform the provider of any behaviors you observe that seem different to you so that awareness can be established and further examined.

WELL-CHILD OR SICK-CHILD VISITS

When a parent calls for an appointment, it should be determined whether the visit is for a routine well-child examination or the child has symptoms of an illness. Specific well-child hours are usually set aside in each day's schedule to care for the routine examinations and procedures (as identified on the Recommendations for Preventive Pediatric Health Care chart). However, when a child is ill, most pediatricians will attempt to see the child within a few hours of a parent's call. Parents can usually phone the pediatrician's office at all hours of the day or night and someone who is on call will respond. Some practices use an answering device or service to receive parental messages and then respond to those accordingly. Practices may also set aside early office hours to see children who have become ill overnight. Check with your employer for the guidelines at your facility.

The Pediatric Office Environment

When young patients come in to see the provider, your attitude may be the deciding factor in their cooperation during the visit. Greeting them with a smile and speaking to them on their developmental level will help gain their trust and cooperation.

CLINICAL PEARL

Patients of all ages are much more cooperative when they feel welcome. Some children may be fearful of health care providers or the medical office, due to prior traumatic experiences in emergency care centers because of serious illness or injury, or even because of an immunization. Some parents may even contribute to this fear by using threats of medical care and shots when disciplining children. If you take time, showing interest and patience, you can establish a rapport with the patients and help eliminate this potential problem.

The play area in the reception area helps the children feel welcome and provides a comfortable environment. A variety of safe, durable, washable, and educational toys should be provided. Toys that have many or tiny parts are not appropriate because they can be a potential choking hazard or create an unsafe walkway if left out, causing others to fall and possibly be hurt. Keeping the toys clean and contained in one area will be one of your duties.

CLINICAL PEARL

Often, a child will find an interesting toy while waiting to be called in to the examination room. The child's cooperation will be greater if the patient is permitted to bring the toy back to the exam room, which helps you gain compliance in performing any necessary procedures in preparation for the provider's examination. When the child is finished with the toy, ensure that it is sanitized properly before returning it to the play area for other children.

Ideally, the play area should be used only for well children who are waiting for annual physical examinations or other well visits, checkups, allergy injections, or immunizations. Every attempt should be made to provide for the separation of well and sick children in the office, including providing separate reception areas. When an ill child is brought to the office, the administrative medical assistant should be notified and accommodations made to take the sick child back into an examination or other private area immediately. At the very least, a separate area with its own toys should be set aside so that the office play area and toys are not available to the sick child.

CLINICAL PEARL

Children (and patients of any age) becoming sick and vomiting is a concern in any medical facility. The administrative medical assistant should keep a disposable emesis basin near the front desk for this potential situation. You should also keep a commercial preparation accessible for use in cleaning up this type of waste. Gloves, paper towels, facial tissues, and biohazardous plastic waste bags should also be easily accessible. A covered waste receptacle lined with a biohazardous plastic bag for disposal of contaminated items should be available.

There can be occasions when a parent or caregiver brings a seriously ill or injured child into the facility unannounced. You must act quickly to provide immediate care to the patient and protect others from the possible transmission of the disease.

Medical Assistant Responsibilities

As a medical assistant, you will have certain routine responsibilities to perform with each pediatric examination. Generally, you will:

- Assist in gathering data.
- Document information.
- Perform screening tests within your skill and ability level.
- Assist the patient.
- Assist the provider.
- Provide patient education.

Some providers require all patients from age 2 to 100 years to have vital signs taken and recorded at every visit regardless of the reason for the appointment. Others feel it is necessary only periodically or when indicated by symptoms. Check with your employer for his or her preferences. Accuracy in the documentation of each of these components is essential to quality care for these young patients. You also should afford time with parents or caregivers and children to provide patient education as appropriate to the child's age and developmental stage.

When you are assisting with the examination of a child, a very important responsibility is relaying information to the provider from the parent or caregiver and from the provider to the patient and parent or caregiver. Your careful observation of the child and the parent or caregiver–child relationship could be critical information to the provider in the care and treatment of the child. Make note of any unusual observations and advise the provider before the child is seen.

Child Neglect and Abuse

One area of awareness concerns the suspicion of **child neglect** or **child abuse**. Neglect refers to the lack of or withholding of care. Abuse refers to inflicting emotional, physical, or sexual injury. The federal Child Abuse Prevention and Treatment Act states that all threats or acts that might cause physical or mental harm to a child *must be* reported. This refers to suspicion of neglect of care as well as of abuse. Anyone, whether a teacher, neighbor, social worker, family member, or health care worker, is obligated to report neglect or abuse to the proper authorities. The law protects the person who makes the report under a confidentiality provision. It should be mentioned that although parents are responsible for their child's care, that responsibility is often given to other caregivers such as grandparents, babysitters, or boyfriends or girlfriends of the single parent. This act applies to all caregivers.

As a medical assistant, be aware of neglect and abuse symptoms, some of which are not too obvious. During your interview and performance of routine procedures, you might feel there is a possibility of inadequate care. Alert the provider of your suspicions before the examination because they must be evaluated by the provider. It is beyond your scope of practice as an MA to determine whether neglect or abuse is occurring; only the provider can make such a diagnosis and will contact the appropriate authorities. The appropriate authorities to whom the provider should make a report in your community should be identified in the office manual. Table 42–2 lists some of the more obvious examples of neglect and abuse for your information.

Establishing Rapport

Cooperation with youngsters is generally obtained by explaining, in a calm, simple manner appropriate to their stage of development, what you and the provider are going to do and why. If you sense behavior that is not cooperative, you must ask the parent or caregiver to **intercede**. A child who is uncooperative for a necessary procedure has to be restrained safely by you and the parent or another health care worker. Doing what has to be done as quickly as possible is the best way to handle the situation.

Young children are often amused with items that are not ordinary toys during an examination, such as a plastic drinking cup or tongue depressor (with supervision, of course). Giving children non-sharp instruments

TABLE 42–2 Symptoms of Neglect and Abuse

Neglect	Abuse
Excessive length of time before seeking medical attention for illness or injury	Discoloration or bruises on the back, buttocks, or any other area
Apparent **malnutrition**	Evidence of burns in unusual places
Obvious lack of dental care	Internal abdominal pain
Immunizations neglected or incomplete	Dislocation of joints, such as shoulder and wrist
Poor personal hygiene	Frequent injuries requiring medical attention
Inadequate clothing for season or size; unclean	An X-ray of current injury showing evidence of untreated previous fractures
Developmental delay	Suspicious story about the injury; difference between description by child and parent or caregiver
Parental comments indicating lack of concern or not wanting child	Reports by the child of sexual or physical abuse

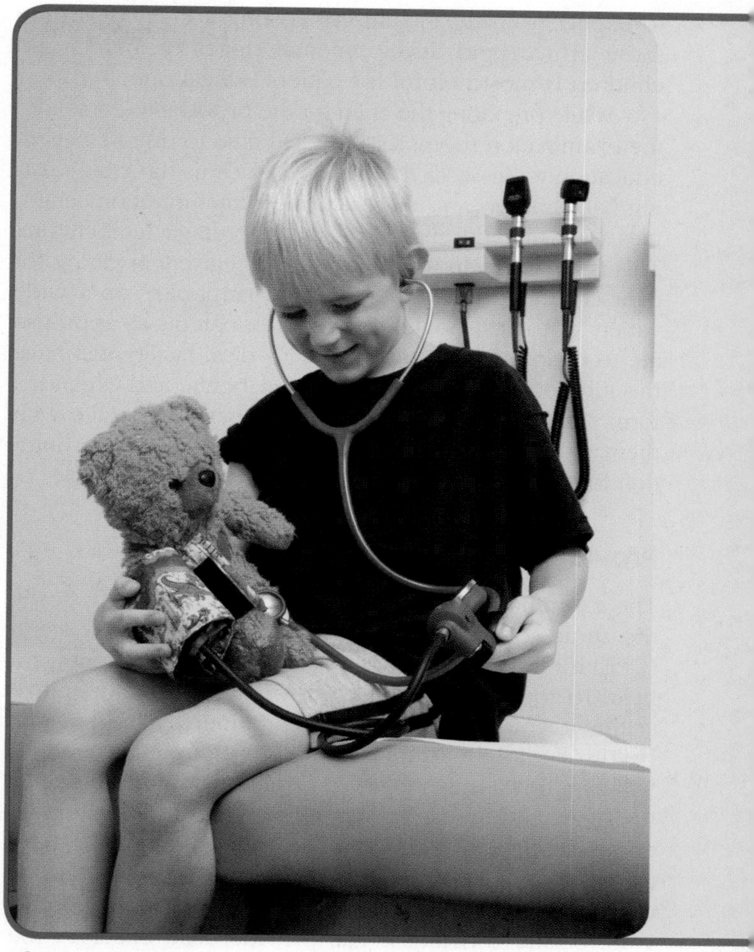

Figure 42–10: The child is allowed to become familiar with the blood pressure instruments the provider will use to examine him. *Delmar/Cengage Learning.*

such as a percussion hammer, stethoscope, or penlight to examine can help them overcome fear of their use by the doctor during the exam (Figure 42–10). Be sure to clean these items properly when the examination is completed.

Pediatric patients should be regarded as individuals and given the kindness and respect you give all patients. Be sure to provide a gown for them; many practices have specific gowns for pediatric patients with child-friendly prints on them. Young children are often embarrassed and chilled sitting on the examination table in their underwear, awaiting the doctor. This is an easy way to help them feel more comfortable and keep them warm, and they like the special treatment.

Another common practice to help little ones feel special is to provide them with bandages in colorful prints or cartoon characters for their minor cuts and abrasions or for injection sites following immunizations. Most health care providers in medical facilities that treat pediatric patients offer a small token reward such as stickers, balloons, or trinkets after their treatment or exam is completed. (Ask the parent or caregiver for approval first.) This gives the child positive reinforcement and helps establish and keep a good rapport between the medical team and the child.

MEDIA LINK

View the video, "Communicating with Pediatric Patients," for this chapter on the Premium Website.

Examination Preparation

The initial part of the pediatric checkup and examination is the preparation of the baby or child. Remember to establish a good rapport with the child and the caregiver by being friendly and relaxed. Ask the caregiver about the child and how everything has been regarding the child's behavior and health as well as whether there are any problems or questions. Many caregivers or parents are unaware of developmental stages and what to expect from their children. Posting a chart regarding these growth and developmental stages of infants and children is most helpful for patient education.

While preparing the child for the provider to come into the examination room, it is an ideal time to discuss patient education topics with the caregiver such as the child's eating habits, sleep and daily activities, immunization schedules, toilet training, and taking and recording a temperature. This is a great help to parents and caregivers in caring for their children. Printed booklets and pamphlets on a wide variety of topics should be offered to parents as appropriate to their children's ages. Your medical facility will have this kind of information in a more elaborate and expanded form. Patient education materials for patients to take with them about specific topics, such as sleep disturbances, nutrition for toddlers, and toilet training, should be available.

Provider Examination

The examination of a pediatric patient follows basically the same format of the comprehensive physical exam (CPE) for adults. The provider examines the patient from head to toe. Because little ones may be uncooperative at times, you should assist the provider by holding the child still until the exam is completed. Often the provider will ask the caregiver to hold the baby while listening to the heart and lungs. The provider will ask the caregiver about the baby's eating and sleeping schedule and how the development is progressing (e.g., at 2 to 3 months, is the baby playing with his or her own hands? at 6 months, is he or she crawling?). The provider also observes the parent or caregiver relationship. Part of the examination of toddlers and children is to observe their gait by placing the child across the room and observing him or her from behind as he or she walks to the caregiver.

IMMUNIZATIONS

As part of the pediatric exam and AAP's Recommended Preventive Pediatric Health Care chart, babies and children receive their immunizations. You are required to have the proper immunizations ready for the provider to administer, or you may be asked to administer them yourself (office policies and providers differ regarding this procedure). You are required to record this information on the patient's immunization record in his or her chart and in the booklet that parents or caregivers keep.

Documentation of shot records is law, so recording them accurately is mandatory. The Immunization Action Coalition (IAC) provides excellent resources on its Website, www.immunize.org, including blank Vaccine Administration Records for Children and Teens and examples of how to document on them. Completed examples of these forms are shown in Figures 42–11A to B.

Make sure, before the immunizations are given, that you give the caregiver or parent the **vaccination information statement(s) (VIS)**, which provides detailed information about the immunization(s), including possible side effects in printed form for him or her to keep (Figure 42–12). A VIS for every immunization can be downloaded from the Centers for Disease Control and Prevention (CDC) Website at www.cdc.gov/vaccines/pubs/vis/default.htm. VISs in different languages can be found on the IAC Website at www.immunize.org.

> **CLINICAL PEARL**
>
> Go to www.immunize.org/handouts/ to search and download other educational handouts and resources from the IAC.

Allow parents or caregivers the time to read the sheets and ask questions. The parent or caregiver should sign for consent after he or she has read it or you have explained the information to him or her. Instruct the caregiver to contact the doctor immediately if a serious reaction should occur from the immunization. If the child has a fever the day of the scheduled appointment, the provider will check the child before giving any immunizations. Be sure to have the provider outline exactly what needs to be done as a routine so you will be efficient in getting pediatric patients ready for the provider to examine. Many practices post an immunization schedule near the immunizations to be used as a reference guide. The CDC releases annual Recommended Childhood and Adolescent Immunization Schedules for children in the United States. It is approved by the AAP and the American Academy of Family Physicians. Figures 42–13A and B show the schedule for the year 201X. In Chapter 53, you will learn more about immunizations and how to prepare the injections.

VISION SCREENING

Vision and hearing screenings are also identified on the AAP Recommended Preventive Pediatric Health Care chart. On the chart, notice that for the first 36 months, vision screening is considered to be subjective or evaluated by history. At age 3, the child is old enough to identify items on a vision screening chart and can be evaluated more easily.

Unless the vision is considerably impaired, deficiencies might not be too obvious. Usually, the parent or caregiver will indicate that the child either holds books too closely to the face or rubs the eyes frequently. Other observations can include excessive blinking, looking cross-eyed, or turning and tilting the head forward to see well. The subspecialty area of pediatric ophthalmology can evaluate the vision of very small children and should be consulted if indicated. However, the routine screening can be done in general at pediatric offices by using the modified Snellen charts as discussed in Chapter 40.

Vaccine Administration Record for Children and Teens

(Page 1 of 2)

Patient name: *Emily Jacobs*

Birthdate: *6/2/2005*

Chart number: ______

Before administering any vaccines, give copies of all pertinent Vaccine Information Statements (VISs) to the child's parent or legal representative and make sure he/she understands the risks and benefits of the vaccine(s). Always provide or update the patient's personal recor d card.

Vaccine	Type of Vaccine[1]	Date given (mo/day/yr)	Funding Source (F,S,P)[2]	Site[3]	Vaccine		Vaccine Information Statement (VIS)		Vaccinator[5] (signature or initials & title)
					Lot #	Mfr.	Date on VIS[4]	Date given[4]	
Hepatitis B[6] (e.g., HepB, Hib-HepB, DTaP-HepB-IPV) Give IM.[7]	HepB	6/2/2005	F	RT	0651M	MRK	7/11/01	6/2/05	JTA
	Pediarix	8/2/2005	F	RT	635A1	GSK	7/11/01	8/2/05	DCP
	Pediarix	10/2/2005	F	RT	712A2	GSK	7/11/01	10/2/05	DCP
	Pediarix	12/2/2005	F	RT	712A2	GSK	7/11/01	12/2/05	DLW
Diphtheria, Tetanus, Pertussis[6] (e.g., DTaP, DTaP/Hib, DTaP-HepB-IPV, DT, DTaP-IPV/Hib, Tdap, DTaP-IPV, Td) Give IM.[7]	Pediarix	8/2/2005	F	RT	635A2	GSK	7/30/01	8/2/05	DCP
	Pediarix	10/2/2005	F	RT	712A2	GSK	7/30/01	10/2/05	DCP
	Pediarix	12/2/2005	F	RT	712A2	GSK	7/30/01	12/2/05	DLW
	DTaP-Hib	9/2/2006	F	RA	P0897AA	SPI	7/30/01	9/2/06	RLV
	DTaP	8/2/2010	F	RA	326-912	SPI	5/17/07	8/2/10	JTA
***Haemophilus influenzae* type b**[6] (e.g., Hib, Hib-HepB, DTaP-IPV/Hib, DTaP/Hib) Give IM.[7]	Hib	8/2/2005	F	LT	UA744AA	SPI	12/16/98	8/2/05	DCP
	Hib	10/2/2005	F	LT	UA744AA	SPI	12/16/98	10/2/05	DCP
	Hib	12/2/2005	F	LT	UA744AA	SPI	12/16/98	12/2/05	DLW
	DTaP-Hib	9/2/2006	F	RA	7172AA	SPI	12/16/98	9/2/06	RLV
Polio[6] (e.g., IPV, DTaP-HepB-IPV, DTaP-IPV/Hib, DTaP-IPV) Give IPV SC or IM.[7] Give all others IM.[7]	Pediarix	8/2/2005	F	RT	635A2	GSK	1/1/00	8/2/05	DCP
	Pediarix	10/2/2005	F	RT	712A2	GSK	1/1/00	10/2/05	DCP
	Pediarix	12/2/2005	F	RT	712A2	GSK	1/1/00	12/2/05	DLW
	IPV	8/2/2010	F	RA	U4569-8	SPI	1/1/00	8/2/10	DCP
Pneumococcal (e.g., PCV7, PCV13, conjugate; PPSV23, polysaccharide) Give PCV IM.[7] Give PPSV SC or IM.[7]	PCV7	8/2/2005	F	LT	489-835	WYE	9/30/02	8/2/05	DCP
	PCV7	10/2/2005	F	RT	489-835	WYE	9/30/02	10/2/05	DCP
	PCV7	12/2/2005	F	LT	489-835	WYE	9/30/02	12/2/05	DLW
	PCV7	9/2/2006	F	LA	501-245	WYE	9/30/02	9/2/06	RLV
	PCV13	8/2/2010	F	LA	E44433	PFI	12/9/08	8/2/10	DCP
Rotavirus (RV1, RV5) Give orally (po).									

DTaP-HepB-IPV (Pediarix)

DTaP-Hib (TriHIBit): 2 lot #s, 2 different VISs

Pediarix: 3 different VIS dates

See page 2 to record measles-mumps-rubella, varicella, hepatitis A, meningococcal, HPV, influenza, and other vaccines (e.g., tra vel vaccines).

How to Complete This Record

1. Record the generic abbreviation (e.g., Tdap) or the trade name for each vaccine (see table at right).
2. Record the funding source of the vaccine given as either F (federal), S (state), or P (private).
3. Record the site where vaccine was administered as either RA (right arm), LA (left arm), RT (right thigh), LT (left thigh), or IN (intranasal).
4. Record the publication date of each VIS as well as the date the VIS is given to the patient.
5. To meet the space constraints of this form and federal requirements for documentation, a healthcare setting may want to keep a reference list of vaccinators that includes their initials and titles.
6. For combination vaccines, fill in a row for each antigen in the combination.
7. IM is the abbreviation for intramuscular; SC is the abbreviation for subcutaneous.

Abbreviation	Trade Name & Manufacturer
DTaP	Daptacel (sanofi); Infanrix (GlaxoSmithKline [GSK]); Tripedia (sanofi pasteur)
DT (pediatric)	Generic (sanofi pasteur)
DTaP-HepB-IPV	Pediarix (GSK)
DTaP/Hib	TriHIBit (sanofi pasteur)
DTaP-IPV/Hib	Pentacel (sanofi pasteur)
DTaP-IPV	Kinrix (GSK)
HepB	Engerix-B (GSK); Recombivax HB (Merck)
HepA-HepB	Twinrix (GSK); can be given to teens age 18 and older
Hib	ActHIB (sanofi pasteur); Hiberix (GSK); PedvaxHIB (Merck)
Hib-HepB	Comvax (Merck)
IPV	Ipol (sanofi pasteur)
PCV13	Prevnar 13 (Pfizer)
PPSV23	Pneumovax 23 (Merck)
RV1	Rotarix (GSK)
RV5	RotaTeq (Merck)
Tdap	Adacel (sanofi pasteur); Boostrix (GSK)
Td	Decavac (sanofi pasteur), Generic (MA Biological Labs)

Technical content reviewed by the Centers for Disease Control and Prevention, August 2010.

www.immunize.org/catg.d/p2022.pdf • Item #P2022 (8/10)

FIGURE 42–11A: Vaccine Administration Records for Children and Teens, completed for a child. *Acquired from www.immunize.org/catg.d/p2022.pdf on 1/3/2010. We thank the Immunization Action Coalition.* (*continues*)

(Page 2 of 2)

Vaccine Administration Record for Children and Teens

Patient name: *Jessica Ashley*

Birthdate: *10/15/1991*

Chart number: ____________

Before administering any vaccines, give copies of all pertinent Vaccine Information Statements (VISs) to the child's parent or legal representative and make sure he/she understands the risks and benefits of the vaccine(s). Always provide or update the patient's personal recor d card.

Vaccine	Type of Vaccine[1]	Date given (mo/day/yr)	Funding Source (F,S,P)[2]	Site[3]	Vaccine		Vaccine Information Statement (VIS)		Vaccinator[5] (signature or initials & title)
					Lot #	Mfr.	Date on VIS[4]	Date given[4]	
Measles, Mumps, Rubella[6] (e.g., MMR, MMRV) Give SC.[7]	MMR	1/15/1993	P	RA	0857M	MRK	10/15/91	1/15/93	DLW
	MMR	10/15/2003	P	LA	0946M	MRK	1/15/03	10/15/03	PWS
Varicella[6] (e.g., VAR, MMRV) Give SC.[7]	VAR	10/15/2003	P	LA	0799M	MRK	12/16/98	10/15/03	PWS
	VAR	10/15/2007	P	LA	0689M	MRK	1/10/07	10/15/07	JTA
Hepatitis A (HepA) Give IM.[7]									
Meningococcal (e.g., MCV4; MPSV4) Give MCV4 IM[7] and MPSV4 SC.[7]	MCV4	6/12/2010	P	LA	28011	NOV	1//28/08	6/12/10	MAT
Human papillomavirus (e.g., HPV2, HPV4) Give IM.[7]	HPV2	12/12/2009	P	LA	0331Z	GSK	2/2/07	12/12/09	TAA
	Cervarix	2/13/2010	P	LA	0331Z	GSK	2/2/07	2/13/10	PWS
	Garadasil	6/12/2010	P	LA	0637F	MRK	2/2/07	6/12/10	DLW
Influenza (e.g., TIV, inactivated; LAIV, live attenuated) Give TIV IM.[7] Give LAIV IN.[7]	FluMist	10/15/2007	P	IN	500491P	MED	10/4/07	10/15/07	MAT
	TIV	10/12/2008	P	RA	878771P	NOV	7/24/08	10/12/08	JTA
	Fluzone	10/2/2009	P	RA	U100461	SPI	8/11/09	10/2/09	DLW
	H1N1	12/7/2009	P	LA	1009224P	NOV	10/2/09	12/7/09	MAT
Other									

When recording the type of vaccine, use the generic abbreviation, tradename, or both. By recording the manufacturer, you will always be able to determine the brand of vaccine given.

See page 1 to record hepatitis B, diphtheria, tetanus, pertussis, *Haemophilus influenzae* type b, polio, pneumococcal, and rotavirus vaccines.

How to Complete this Record

1. Record the generic abbreviation (e.g., Tdap) or the trade name for each vaccine (see table at right).
2. Record the funding source of the vaccine given as either F (federal), S (state), or P (private).
3. Record the site where vaccine was administered as either RA (right arm), LA (left arm), RT (right thigh), LT (left thigh), or IN (intranasal).
4. Record the publication date of each VIS as well as the date the VIS is given to the patient.
5. To meet the space constraints of this form and federal requirements for documentation, a healthcare setting may want to keep a reference list of vaccinators that includes their initials and titles.
6. For combination vaccines, fill in a row for each antigen in the combination.
7. IM is the abbreviation for intramuscular; SC is the abbreviation for subcutaneous; IN is the abbreviation for intranasal.

Abbreviation	Trade Name & Manufacturer
MMR	MMRII (Merck)
VAR	Varivax (Merck)
MMRV	ProQuad (Merck)
HepA	Havrix (GlaxoSmithKline [GSK]); Vaqta (Merck)
HepA-HepB	Twinrix (GSK)
HPV2	Cervarix (GSK)
HPV4	Gardasil (Merck)
LAIV (Live attenuated influenza vaccine]	FluMist (MedImmune)
TIV (Trivalent inactivated influenza vaccine)	Afluria (CSL Biotherapies); Agriflu (Novartis); Fluarix (GSK); FluLaval (GSK); Fluvirin (Novartis); Fluzone (sanofi)
MCV4	Menactra (sanofi pasteur); Menveo (Novartis)
MPSV4	Menomune (sanofi pasteur)

FIGURE 42–11B: *(continued)*

YOUR BABY'S FIRST VACCINES
WHAT YOU NEED TO KNOW

Babies get six vaccines between birth and 6 months of age.

These vaccines protect your baby from 8 serious diseases (see the next page).

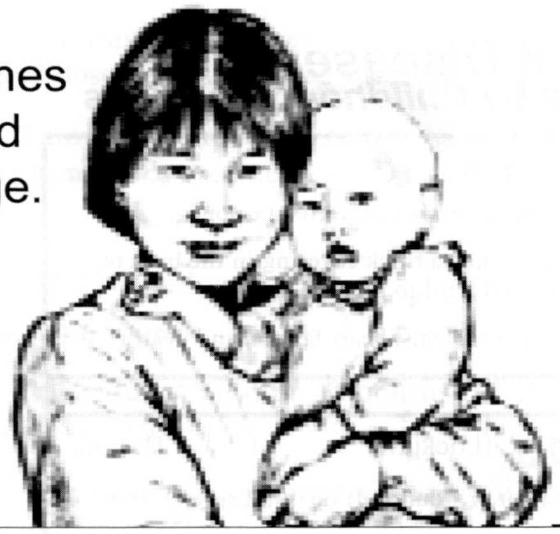

Your baby will get vaccines today that prevent these diseases:

☐ Hepatitis B ☐ Polio ☐ Pneumococcal Disease
☐ Diphtheria, Tetanus & Pertussis ☐ Rotavirus ☐ Hib

(Provider: Check appropriate boxes)

These vaccines may be given separately, or some might be given together in the same shot (for example, Hepatitis B and Hib can be given together, and so can DTaP, Polio, and Hepatitis B). These "combination vaccines" are as safe and effective as the individual vaccines, and mean fewer shots for your baby.

These vaccines may all be given at the same visit. Getting several vaccines at the same time will not harm your baby.

This *Vaccine Information Statement* (VIS) tells you about the benefits and risks of these vaccines. It also contains information about reporting an adverse reaction, the National Vaccine Injury Compensation Program, and how to get more information about childhood diseases and vaccines.

Please read this VIS before your child gets his or her immunizations, and take it home with you afterward. Ask your doctor, nurse, or other healthcare provider if you have questions.

Individual Vaccine Information Statements are also available for these vaccines.
Many Vaccine Information Statements are available in Spanish and other languages. See www.immunize.org/vis

DEPARTMENT OF HEALTH AND HUMAN SERVICES
CENTERS FOR DISEASE CONTROL AND PREVENTION

Vaccine Information Statement
(Interim)
42 U.S.C. § 300aa-26
9/18/2008

FIGURE 42–12: Example of a vaccine information statement. *Courtesy of the Centers for Disease Control and Prevention.* (continues)

have mild, temporary diarrhea or vomiting. This happens within the first week after getting a dose of vaccine. Rotavirus vaccine does not appear to cause any serious side effects.

FIGURE 42–13A: Recommended immunization schedule 0–6 yrs. *Courtesy of the Centers for Disease Control and Prevention.*

Precautions

If your child is sick on the date vaccinations are scheduled, your provider *may* want to put them off until she recovers. A child with a mild cold or a low fever can usually be vaccinated that day. But for a more serious illness, it may be better to wait.

Some children should **not get certain vaccines.** Talk with your provider if your child had a serious reaction after a previous dose of a vaccine, or has any life-threatening allergies. (These reactions and allergies are rare.)

- If your child had any of these reactions to a previous dose of DTaP:
  - A brain or nervous system disease within 7 days
  - Non-stop crying for 3 or more hours
  - A seizure or collapse
  - A fever over 105°F

  Talk to your provider before getting **DTaP Vaccine.**

- If your child has:
  - A life-threatening allergy to the antibiotics neomycin, streptomycin, or polymyxin B

  Talk to your provider before getting **Polio Vaccine.**

- If your child has:
  - A life-threatening allergy to yeast

  Talk to your provider before getting **Hepatitis B Vaccine.**

- If your child has:
  - A weakened immune system
  - Ongoing digestive problems
  - Recently gotten a blood transfusion or other blood product
  - Ever had intussusception (an uncommon type of intestinal obstruction)

  Talk to your provider before getting **Rotavirus Vaccine.**

What if my child has a moderate or severe reaction?

What should I look for?

Look for any unusual condition, such as a serious allergic reaction, high fever, weakness, or unusual behavior.

Serious allergic reactions are extremely rare with any vaccine. If one were to happen, it would most likely come within a few minutes to a few hours after the shot.

Signs of a serious allergic reaction can include:

- difficulty breathing	- weakness	- hives
- hoarseness or wheezing	- dizziness	- paleness
- swelling of the throat	- fast heart beat	

What should I do?

Call a doctor, or get the child to a doctor right away.

Tell your doctor what happened, the date and time it happened, and when the shot was given.

Ask your healthcare provider to report the reaction by filing a Vaccine Adverse Event Reporting System (VAERS) form. Or you can file this report yourself through the VAERS website at **www.vaers.hhs.gov**, or by calling **1-800-822-7967**.

VAERS does not provide medical advice.

The National Vaccine Injury Compensation Program

A federal program exists to help pay for the care of anyone who has a serious reaction to a vaccine.

For information about the National Vaccine Injury Compensation Program, call **1-800-338-2382** or visit their website at **www.hrsa.gov/vaccinecompensation.**

For More Information

Ask your healthcare provider. They can show you the vaccine package insert or suggest other sources of information.

Call your local or state health department.

Contact the Centers for Disease Control and Prevention (CDC) at **1-800-232-4636 (1-800-CDC-INFO).**

Visit CDC websites at **www.cdc.gov/vaccines** and **www.cdc.gov/ncidod/diseases/hepatitis.**

FIGURE 42–13B: Recommended immunization schedule 7–18 yrs. *Courtesy of the Centers for Disease Control and Prevention.*

The Snellen big E chart (Figure 42–14A) requires the child to indicate with his or her fingers which way the E is facing. The Es become smaller and less bold as the acuity gets more difficult. Results are recorded on the last line correctly identified, the same as with adults on the regular screening chart. The kindergarten version of the chart (Figure 42–14B) uses various shapes and symbols in descending size to evaluate vision. When using either of these, review the charts up close with the child to be sure they know what they are supposed to do and that they can name the symbols. This determines whether the child is actually having trouble seeing the chart or simply does not know what to call the letter or symbol you are pointing to.

Most preschoolers have a short attention span, so you might need some assistance from the parent or caregiver, who can help by restating your instructions and maintaining the child's position. He or she can also monitor the covering of one eye as you proceed through the test. Watch the child for signs of visual difficulty such as tilting the head and frowning or straining to see as he or she reads the chart. Procedure 42–3 provides instruction to screen a child's vision.

CLINICAL PEARL

You can make the screening fun by taking your turn first. This also helps the child to understand what he or she is to do. Remember to praise the child during the screening to encourage cooperation.

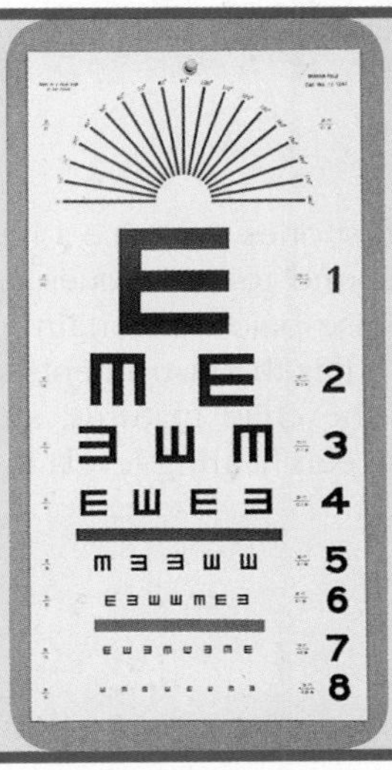

FIGURE 42–14A: Snellen E chart. *Delmar/Cengage Learning.*

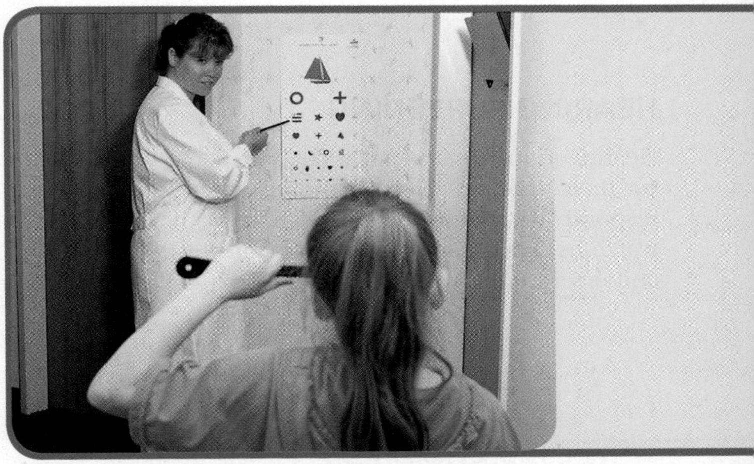

FIGURE 42–14B: Kindergarten chart. *Delmar/Cengage Learning.*

PROCEDURE 42–3 Screen Pediatric Visual Acuity with a Modified Snellen Chart

PURPOSE: To measure distant visual acuity of a child

EQUIPMENT: Modified Snellen chart, pointer, eye occluder, patient's chart or EMR, and pen

S SKILL: Perform pediatric vision acuity screening.

Procedure Steps	Detailed Instructions and/or *Rationales*
1. Identify the patient and introduce yourself.	*Ensures that you are performing the procedure on the correct patient.*
B 2. Explain the procedure to the patient, ***using language that is appropriate for the patient.***	
3. Ask the patient to read the chart with both eyes at a distance of 20 feet from the chart.	
4. Have the patient cover the left eye with the occluder to test the acuity of the right eye.	

(continues)

(continued)

Procedure Steps	Detailed Instructions and/or *Rationales*
5. Record the smallest line the patient reads without making a mistake.	Some providers allow up to two errors on the smallest line read.
6. Have the patient cover the right eye with the occluder to test the acuity of the left eye.	
7. Record the smallest line read.	

Charting Example

4/17/XX 11:30 am	Vision screening with kindergarten screening chart per Dr. White, findings R eye 20/35, L eye 20/40; appeared to understand chart. Noticed some squinting during screening. G. Jenks, CMA(AAMA)

HEARING SCREENING

Hearing in infants and small children is usually observed by their reaction to surrounding sounds. Infants will respond by turning their head toward the ticking of a watch held near their ear. Older infants respond to verbal and environmental sounds. The parents or caregiver will probably be the first ones to notice a hearing deficit. The child will not respond to voice cues and will not react to surrounding noise below a certain intensity. Again, a pediatric specialist has the instruments and skills to evaluate hearing. As the child matures, an audiometer test can be given to screen hearing levels more accurately.

CHAPTER SUMMARY

- The American Academy of Pediatrics (AAP) has established Recommendations for Preventive Pediatric Health Care, a chart that outlines the types and frequency of screening examinations and procedures. It can be downloaded from the AAP website at www.aap.org.
- Table 42–1 highlights growth and development during infancy and toddlerhood. The table shows the age at which the average child should be able to perform the activities listed.
- Pediatric growth measurements are documented on the patient's chart and on a growth chart. This chart gives the provider an ongoing quick-glance reference to the child's growth and development and is used to determine any abnormal patterns.
- Medicaid's comprehensive and preventive child health program, known as the Early and Periodic Screening, Diagnosis, and Treatment (EPSDT) program, is a program that requires regular health maintenance exams and careful documentation of examination findings for Medicaid patients who are between birth and 21 years of age.
- When a parent calls for an appointment, determine whether the visit is for a routine well-child examination or whether the child has symptoms of an illness. Specific well-child hours are usually set aside in each day's schedule.
- As a medical assistant, you have certain routine responsibilities to perform with each pediatric examination. Generally, you will assist in gathering data, document information, perform screening tests within your skill and ability level, assist the patient, assist the provider, and provide patient education.
- Child neglect refers to the lack of or withholding of care; child abuse refers to inflicting emotional, physical, or sexual injury. Examples are provided in Table 42–2.
- The CDC releases annual Recommended Childhood and Adolescent Immunization Schedules for children. You can download the latest schedule from the CDC Website at www.cdc.gov.
- To screen for visual acuity, alternate versions of the Snellen chart are used, the Snellen big E chart and the kindergarten shapes and symbols chart.

STUDY TOOLS

Workbook	Activities for Chapter 42
Premium Website	
MEDIA LINK	View this **Media Link** for Chapter 42: • Communicating with Pediatric Patients
StudyWARE	Activities and Quizzes on the **StudyWARE™ Software** for Chapter 42
	Audio Library of medical terms
	Online access to the **Critical Thinking Challenge 2.0**
learninglab	Module 18: Assisting with Clinical Procedures
CourseMate	Activities and Quizzes for Chapter 42
WebTutor	Activities and Quizzes for Chapter 42

CHECK YOUR KNOWLEDGE

1. At what age will the infant begin the immunization schedule?
   a. 1 day
   b. 2 months
   c. 6 weeks
   d. 1 year
2. An infant or young child who is below the __________ percentile on standardized growth charts is said to be failing to thrive.
   a. third
   b. fifth
   c. seventh
   d. tenth
3. Which of the following persons are obligated to report neglect or abuse to the proper authorities?
   a. Family members
   b. Health care workers
   c. Neighbors
   d. All of the above
4. Up until what age would you record the head circumference measurement?
   a. 12 months
   b. 24 months
   c. 36 months
   d. 48 months
5. Which measurement is taken and recorded in the patient's record but not on the growth chart?
   a. Head circumference
   b. Chest circumference
   c. Height
   d. Weight
6. The kindergarten version of the Snellen chart uses:
   a. signs and symbols.
   b. the capital letter *E*.
   c. letters.
   d. numbers.
7. When using the growth chart, each month is represented by a:
   a. dot.
   b. square.
   c. line.
   d. circle.

WEB LINKS

American Academy of Pediatrics: www.aap.org

Centers for Disease Control and Prevention: www.cdc.gov

Immunization Action Coalition: www.immunize.org

RESOURCES

Estes, M. E. Z. (2010). *Health Assessment & Physical Examination* (3rd ed.). Clifton Park, NY: Delmar Cengage Learning.

Heller, M., and Veach, L. (2009). *Clinical Medical Assisting: A Professional, Field Smart Approach to the Workplace.* Clifton Park, NY: Delmar, Cengage Learning.

Lindh, W., Pooler, M., Tamparo, C., and Dahl, B. (2010). *Delmar's Comprehensive Medical Assisting Administrative and Clinical Competencies* (4th ed.). Clifton Park, NY: Delmar Cengage Learning.

Venes, D. (ed.). (2009). *Taber's Cyclopedic Medical Dictionary* (21st ed.). Philadelphia: F. A. Davis.

Unit

14

Laboratory Procedures

Patient and health care provider safety is at the forefront of collection of specimens. Prevention of disease is of utmost importance in preparing for these clinical tasks. A medical assistant must be alert and conscientious in the performance of his or her duties to ensure the prevention of disease transmission. The medical assistant must also remember to practice standard precautions with each patient as he or she collects and handles patient specimens.

In addition to following safety precautions, the medical assistant should check with his or her family physician to ensure that he or she does not have any updates due within his or her own immunizations because staying up to date with immunizations is critical for the medical assistant. Because medical assistants work directly with patients and the potential to be exposed to blood or other body fluids, it is important for them to have been administered the series of three HBV (hepatitis B virus) injections. After the medical assistant has received this vaccination series, a permanent record should be kept within the employee file. However, if a medical assistant is hired in a new position in which the employer states that it is not necessary for him or her to receive the vaccination, the employer must sign a waiver stating so and such a waiver should be kept within the employee file.

All guidelines should be noted regarding safe and efficient practice of procedures in the physician's office laboratory (POL) and in dealing with patients. The medical assistant must pay attention to proper fit of protective barriers such as gowns and gloves. Even though these small items seem trivial, gloves that are too small can tear; a gown that is too large can catch on something and rip, resulting in a safety risk for the medical assistant and patient and a possible exposure to potentially infectious materials.

The medical assistant must be careful not to touch items with gloves on that would normally be touched without gloves on. Such items include light switches, door handles, drawer handles, phones, charts, and other equipment. He or she must develop a habit of completing one task at a time. For example, complete the procedure that requires gloves and other personal protective equipment (PPE) and then record the results after the protective barriers have been removed. If a medical assistant touches an item that does not require gloves with contaminated gloves on, he or she is contaminating everything that is touched and is putting others at risk to be exposed to biohazardous residue.

Certification Connection

	Ch. 43	Ch. 44	Ch. 45	Ch. 46
CMA (AAMA)				
Legislation: Occupational Safety and Health Act (OSHA), Clinical Laboratory Improvement Act (CLIA '88)		X		
Safety regulations: Occupational Safety and Health Act (OSHA)	X	X	X	X
Standard precautions	X	X	X	X
Principles of equipment operation: microscope		X		
Patient preparation and assisting the physician	X		X	X
Collecting and processing specimens; diagnostic testing	X		X	X
RMA (AMT)				
Understand the application of the Clinical Laboratory Improvement Amendments of 1988 (CLIA '88)		X		
Employ procedures in compliance with Occupational Safety and Health Administration (OSHA) guidelines and regulations	X	X	X	X
Clinical Laboratory Improvement Amendments of 1988 (CLIA '88)		X		
Laboratory procedures	X	X	X	X

Chapter

43 Blood Specimen Collection

OBJECTIVES

In this chapter, you will learn the following:

KB KNOWLEDGE BASE

1. Spell and define, using the glossary at the back of the text, all the Words to Know in this chapter.
2. State the purpose of wearing gloves when performing capillary blood collection procedures.
3. Explain the reasons for performing capillary blood collection in the medical office.
4. Explain how to obtain serum from whole blood.
5. List the different colors used to code blood specimen tubes.
6. List the correct order of draw for blood specimen tubes.
7. Identify by the colors of the tubes what additives are contained in the tubes.

S SKILLS

1. Perform capillary blood collection procedures for obtaining specimens.
2. Perform a venipuncture, using a syringe and needle.
3. Perform a venipuncture, using a vacuum tube and multiple-sample needle and adapter.
4. Perform a venipuncture, using the butterfly syringe method.

B BEHAVIORS

1. Use language and verbal skills that enable patients' understanding of the procedure being performed.
2. Explain the rationale for performance of a procedure to a patient.
3. Show awareness of patients' concerns regarding their perceptions of the procedure being performed.
4. Display sensitivity to patient rights and feelings in collecting specimens.

WORDS TO KNOW

centrifuge
diffuse
elasticity
gauge
hematoma
hemolysis
heparin
lancet
meniscus
oxygenate
phlebotomy
plasma
puncture
serum
sterile
tourniquet
venipuncture
venous

Wipe off the first drop of blood

CAPILLARY BLOOD COLLECTION

Capillary blood tests are frequently performed in the medical office or clinic because of the small amount of blood required, usually one to a few drops. Because most patients are extremely apprehensive, you must develop skill not only in performing the procedures but in conveying reassurance to the patient. When capillary **puncture** procedures, also referred to as finger sticks, are done correctly, the patient should feel minimal discomfort. Displaying confidence in carrying out the procedures competently ensures patient safety and comfort.

Capillaries are minute blood vessels that convey blood from the arterioles to the venules. At this level, blood and oxygen **diffuse** to the tissues, and products of metabolic activity enter the bloodstream. For this reason, capillary blood is an ideal sample for many screening tests that require a very small amount of blood.

Capillary blood is just under the surface of the skin. The most practical sites to use are the ring and great finger, rarely the earlobe, and, in infants, the lateral sides of the heel (Figure 43–1A and 43–1B). Skin punctures should be made across fingerprints, not parallel to them (Figure 43–2).

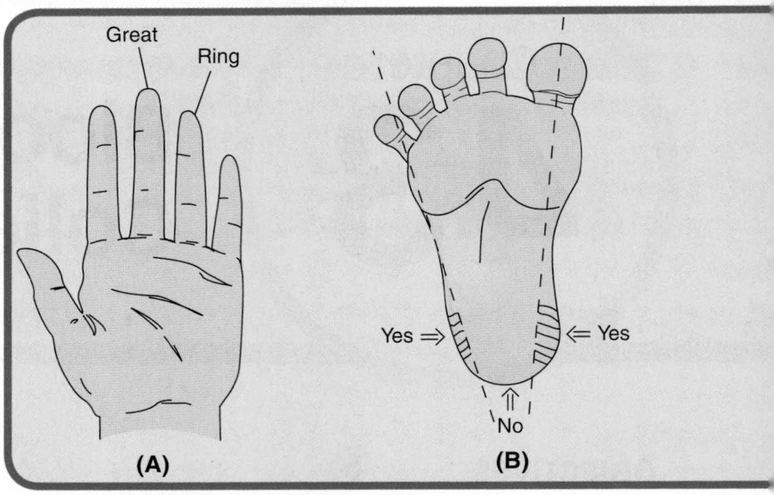

Figure 43–1: (A) Sites for finger capillary punctures. (B) Sites for heel sticks on infants for capillary collection. *Delmar/Cengage Learning.*

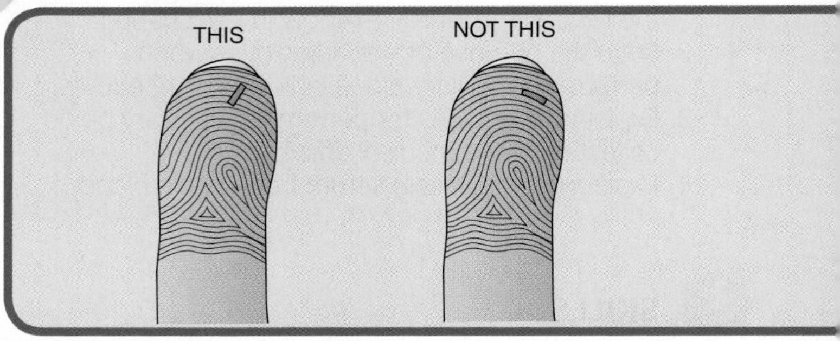

Figure 43–2: Correct and incorrect capillary punctures (finger sticks). A correct puncture must go across fingerprints. *Delmar/Cengage Learning.*

Performing a Capillary Puncture

The **sterile lancet** is widely used for simple blood tests that require capillary blood. You might be given the duty of instructing patients in the use of one of the skin puncturing devices shown in Figure 43–3. Patients who use this technique daily should simply wash the puncture site thoroughly with soap and water. Alcohol tends to break down the skin if used for extended periods. Patients should be provided with a sharps container to keep at home to dispose of the lancets after use. Encourage them to dispose of the three-fourths-full container appropriately. Refer to Procedure 43–1 for steps in performing a capillary puncture.

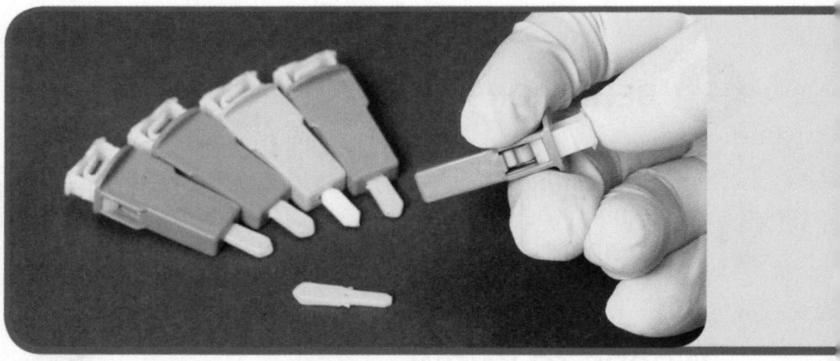

Figure 43–3: Picture of different lancets that are available for various purposes. *Delmar/Cengage Learning.*

CLINICAL PEARL

Most patients, especially youngsters, are apprehensive about having blood taken. The medical assistant must calmly explain to each patient that screening tests, such as a hemoglobin or a blood glucose, are performed with a small amount of blood taken from the finger, earlobe, or infant's heel. Let the patient know ahead of time what you are going to do to gain cooperation. You should tell the patient that there will be a little pain or discomfort during the initial skin puncture, but it will not last long. Reassure the patient that this procedure is short-lived and necessary for the physician to aid in making a diagnosis or evaluating the condition.

VENOUS BLOOD COLLECTION

When more than a few drops of blood are required to perform tests, a **venous** collection of blood is performed. **Venipuncture**, also called **phlebotomy**, is the surgical puncture of a vein. A phlebotomist is a person trained to perform this procedure.

Site Selection

The area of choice for venipuncture is most often the inner arm at the bend of the elbow (Figure 43–5). The veins in this area are the median basilic and the median cephalic (commonly referred to as antecubital) veins. A means of promoting better palpation and sometimes visual position of the veins is a tourniquet.

Applying the Tourniquet

Tourniquets are available in many materials. Soft, flat bands made of latex, or latex-free rubber, are probably the most popular and economical. Some medical facilities use a tourniquet only once and then discard it with the gloves removed after drawing blood samples. It comes in widths of 1 to 2 inches and can be cut into

PROCEDURE 43–1 Puncture Skin with a Sterile Lancet

PURPOSE: Puncture skin with a sterile lancet to obtain a few drops of capillary blood for screening tests

EQUIPMENT: Latex or vinyl gloves; sterile lancet; alcohol; cotton balls; sharps container; flat, stable surface

S SKILL: Perform a capillary puncture.

Procedure Steps	Detailed Instructions and/or *Rationales*
1. Identify the patient.	*Speaking to the patient by name and checking the chart ensures that you are performing the procedure on the correct patient.*
B 2. Explain the procedure to the patient, ***including the rationale for performing the procedure, using language and verbal skills the patient can understand. Show awareness of patients' concerns regarding their perceptions of the capillary puncture by answering any questions the patient might have and assisting the patient into a comfortable position before you proceed.***	
3. Inspect the patient's fingers (or other puncture site) and select the most desirable site.	The main sites are the ring or great finger, earlobe, or infant's lateral areas of heel. Some patients have a preference for a particular site. Do not use areas that are bruised, calloused, or injured.
4. Wash hands, put on gloves, and assemble the needed items on the flat surface.	
5. Wipe the desired site with an alcohol-saturated cotton ball and let dry (Figure 43–4A).	*Do not blow on the skin to expedite drying—you can contaminate the skin with microorganisms in the exhaled air.*
6. Take the sterile lancet out of the package without contaminating the point.	*Another must be used if the point is touched.*
7. Hold the patient's finger (or other site) securely between your thumb and great finger. In your other hand hold the lancet, pointed downward, with your thumb and index or great finger. Puncture the site quickly with a firm, steady, down-and-up motion to approximately a 2-mm depth (Figure 43–4B).	Control entry and exit of lancet in same path to avoid ripping skin. To obtain a better blood sample, puncture across fingerprints, not parallel to them.
8. Discard the first drop of blood by blotting it away with a dry gauze square.	*The first drop can contain traces of alcohol or tissue fluid that would dilute the sample and make the test inaccurate.*

(continues)

(continued)

Procedure Steps	Detailed Instructions and/or *Rationales*
9. Keep applying gentle pressure on either side of the puncture site until the necessary amount of blood has been obtained.	*Too much pressure will cause tissue fluid to mix with blood, resulting in a diluted sample and incorrect test results.*
10. Wipe the site with a cotton ball and ask the patient to hold it gently for a minute or two.	Check the site to be sure the bleeding has stopped. Determine whether the patient is allergic to adhesive before applying a bandage to the puncture site. (Use a gauze square and hypoallergenic tape if patient is allergic.)
11. Remove gloves, wash hands, and discard used items in the proper receptacle (Figure 43–4C).	A solution of approximately $\frac{1}{4}$ cup bleach per gallon of tap water (a 1:100 dilution of common household bleach) should be made fresh daily and kept readily available for cleanup of accidental spills of blood or body fluids.
12. Record the procedure on the patient's chart.	

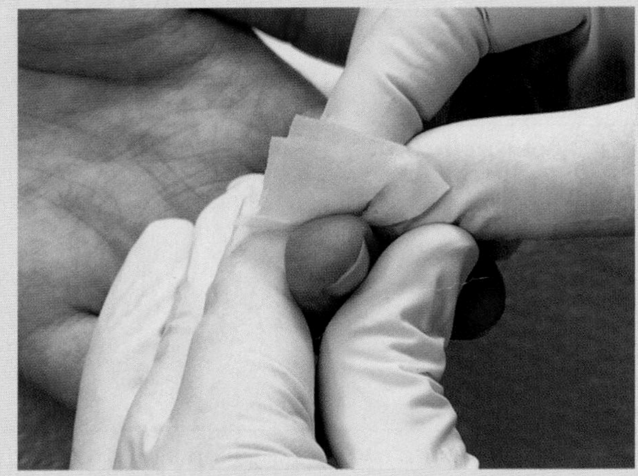

Figure 43–4A: Wipe the desired site with an alcohol-saturated cotton ball and let dry. *Delmar/Cengage Learning.*

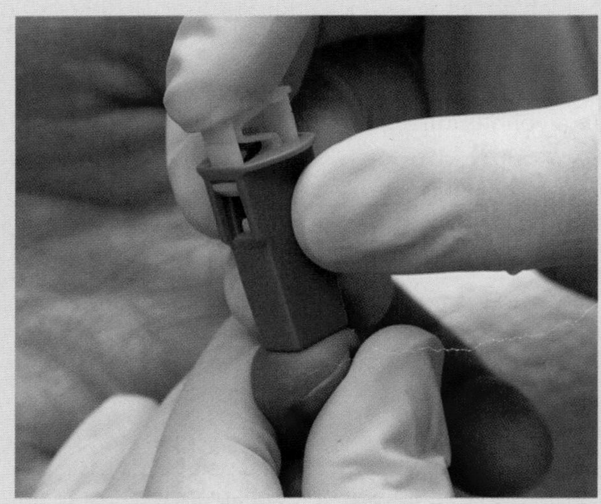

Figure 43–4B: Puncture the site quickly with a firm, steady, down-and-up motion to approximately a 2-mm depth. *Delmar/Cengage Learning.*

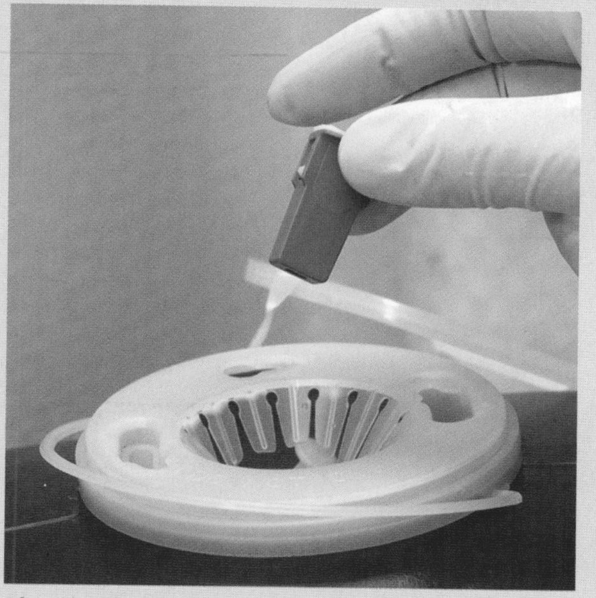

Figure 43–4C: When the procedure is complete, remove gloves, wash hands, and discard used items in the proper receptacle. *Delmar/Cengage Learning.*

Charting Example

8-5-XX 10:20 am	*Rt. ring finger punctured, filled two microhematocrit tubes with capillary blood; Hct 37%; Hgb 12.4. J. Watkins, CMA (AAMA)*

40–60

Can use blood pressure cuff for older people for blood draw

any length desired, usually from 12 to 16 inches. If the hair on the patient's arm is especially thick, it might be wise to apply the tourniquet over the patient's sleeve. This keeps the tourniquet from pinching and pulling the hair, and the patient most likely will be more cooperative for your thoughtfulness. Tourniquets are easily washed with a detergent solution and quickly cleaned with alcohol and a cotton ball. Tourniquets that are worn or permanently visibly soiled (even after washing) should be discarded. Velcro tourniquets are cloth strips, approximately 1½ to 2 inches wide. They are not so easily cleaned and cannot be used on patients with larger than average arms. Wiping the Velcro tourniquets off with alcohol helps prevent most staining problems.

Before applying the tourniquet, it is a good idea to check both arms of the patient or simply ask the patient which arm is better for this procedure. Many patients have had the procedure performed and know that one arm is better. Some patients will have a preferred arm because of their work or planned activities.

The tourniquet is placed on the patient's upper arm, about 3 inches above the elbow (Figure 43–6A through D).

(2–4")

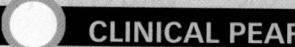

CLINICAL PEARL

In patients whose blood is very difficult to draw, try using a blood pressure cuff as a tourniquet. Be careful not to inflate it too tightly on the patient's arm, or you can cut off the circulation completely and cause unnecessary discomfort to the patient. Be sure the cuff size is appropriate for the size of the arm. Care also must be taken to avoid getting blood on the cuff. It must be discarded (or sanitized and sterilized before reuse) if it does become contaminated.

Bring the ends of the tourniquet up evenly and cross them. Switch so that you are holding an end in each hand comfortably. Stretch the end in your right hand to apply gentle pressure over the area of the arm while you hold the other end against the patient's arm. Tuck any excess stretched end under the section that is held against the arm so there is nothing in the way of the puncture site.

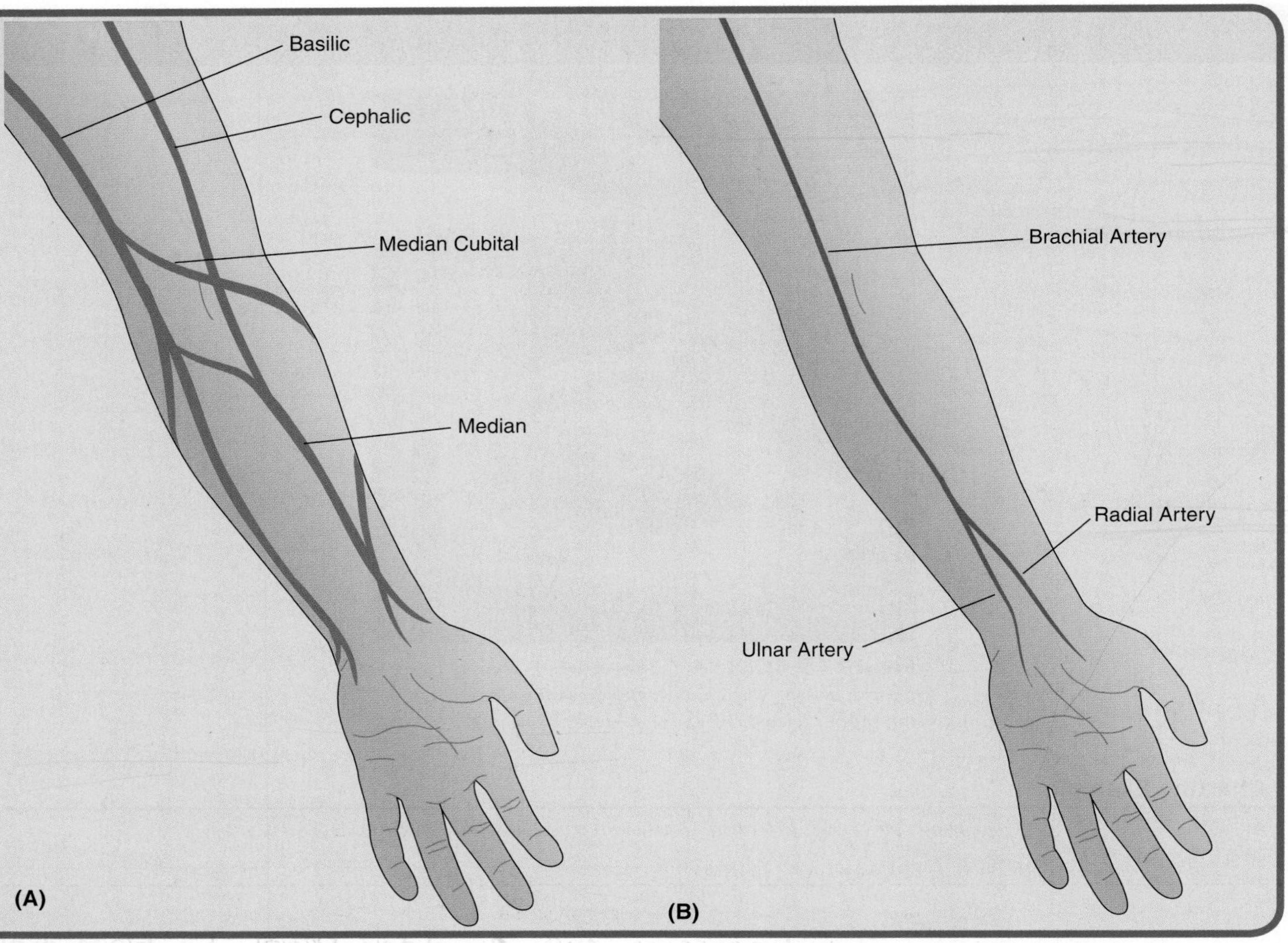

Figure 43–5: (A) Veins of the arm (in blue); the most popular area of choice is the inner arm at the bend of the elbow. (B) Arteries of the arm (in red); do NOT draw from these. *Delmar/Cengage Learning.*

When you draw blood for culture, use betadin (no alcohol swab)

Preparing the Site

Use a cotton ball saturated with alcohol or a presaturated alcohol pad to swab the entire area. The alcohol helps make the skin more sensitive to your touch and disinfects the area. Slowly move your fingertip across the patient's arm at the bend of the elbow. Veins have **elasticity** and give somewhat when depressed. Feeling the subtle spring-back movement helps you find a suitable vein for the procedure. You should ask the patient to clench the fist only if the vein does not stand out. The pressure of the clenched fist can interfere with some chemistry tests. A few gentle taps to the antecubital area with two of your fingers also help the vein stand out for better view and access. Another method to encourage blood flow in patients whose blood is difficult to draw is to place a warm compress on the antecubital area for a few minutes before you begin the procedure to help make the veins stand out to the touch if not to the sight.

Do not leave on patient longer than 1 minute

CLINICAL PEARL

- Explain to the patient that there will be minimal pain or discomfort, similar to how as it feels when you stick yourself with a pin accidentally. Normally, this slight pain lasts only momentarily.
- Explain to the patient that relaxing helps speed up the procedure. Occasionally, there is some bruising at the venipuncture site, but this does not last long. Even if the patient has had previous venipunctures, explain the procedure and answer questions. The patient will feel more relaxed if you display confidence in your ability.
- If the patient expresses concern about contracting an infection from the needle puncture, reassure the patient that the needle is sterile, is used once, and then is discarded.
- If the patient has questions concerning the diagnosis, it is wise for the medical assistant to refer the patient to the physician.

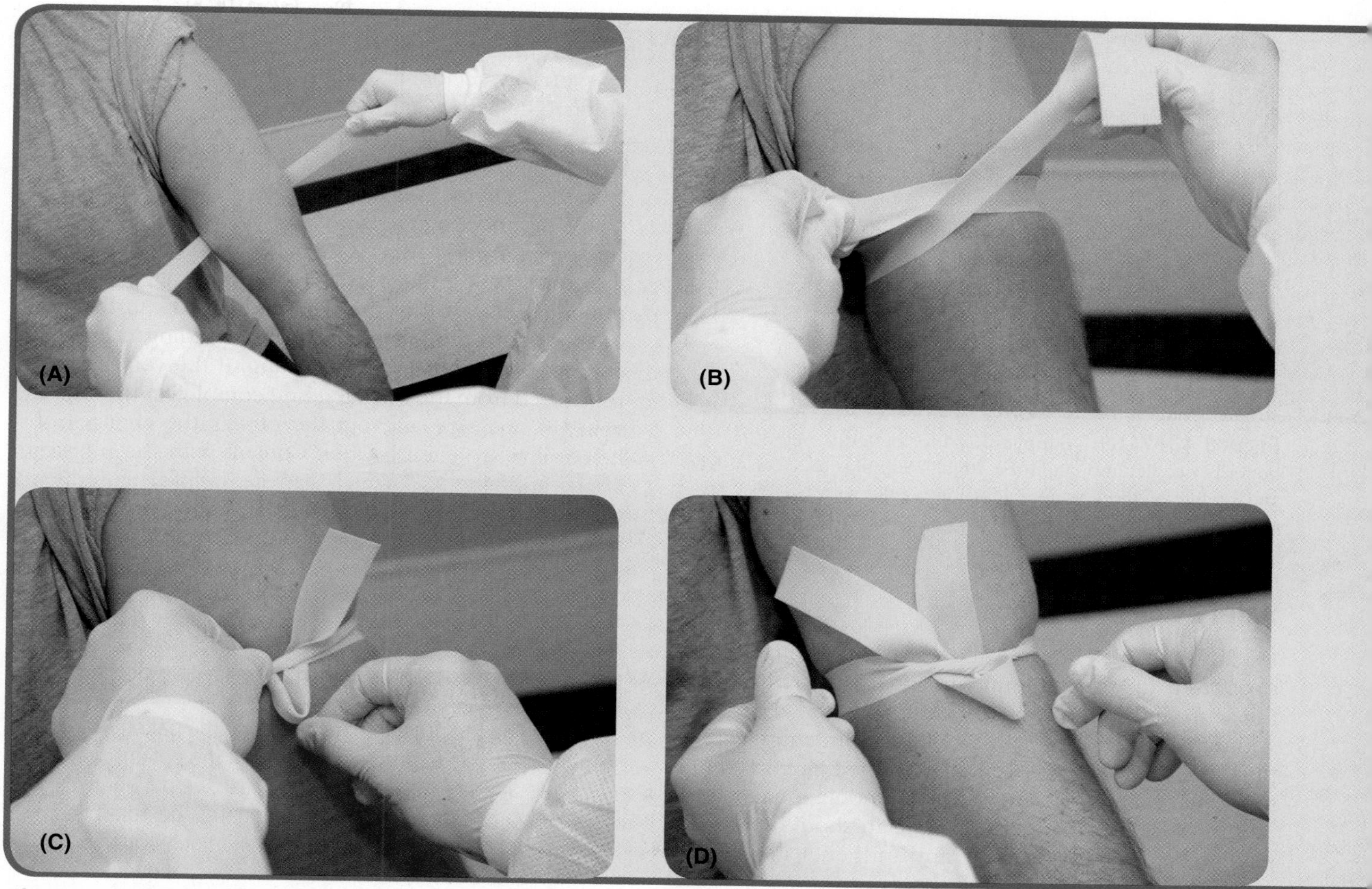

Figure 43–6A-D: (A) Wrap the tourniquet around the patient's arm at no more than 3 inches above the venipuncture site. (B) Grab tourniquet close to the patient's arm, stretch the tourniquet tight, and cross the ends. (C) As you hold ends tight, tuck one portion of the tourniquet under the other. (D) Check that the tourniquet is secure and that the ends are pointed upward.
Delmar/Cengage Learning.

genetic
hemophilia - blood does not clot.

Venipuncture Methods

There are several methods of performing the venipuncture procedure: the syringe and sterile needle method, the vacuum tube method, and the butterfly needle method. Sterile technique must be used because a foreign object is introduced directly into the vein.

A 21- to 23-**gauge** needle is generally used. The gauge must be large enough to allow blood to flow through the needle without causing **hemolysis** (breakdown of blood cells).

Needle and Syringe Method

The needle and syringe method is often used when very small veins are involved because it is less damaging to the tissues than the vacuum method. The size of the syringe varies according to the amount of blood needed. Usually, a 10- to 20-mL syringe is used when drawing several tubes, each 5 to 15 mL. (Refer to Procedure 43–2.)

vaco container - 21g

Vacuum Method

The vacuum method is probably the most popular because it is so convenient. Blood specimens enter directly into the tubes for the desired tests rather than having to be transferred. It is vital to use the correct tubes, however. (Refer to Procedure 43–3.)

Butterfly Needle Method

Some patients are extremely difficult to obtain blood from; in these cases, it might be necessary to draw the sample from a vein on the back of the hand using a smaller gauge needle. These veins are small, and the procedure is painful for these patients. A method that can be used in this type of situation is called the butterfly needle method (Figure 43–7). The tourniquet should be applied just above the wrist in this case. A skilled phlebotomist can perform this procedure successfully alone. (Refer to Procedure 43–4.)

23 gauge (more fine than 21g)

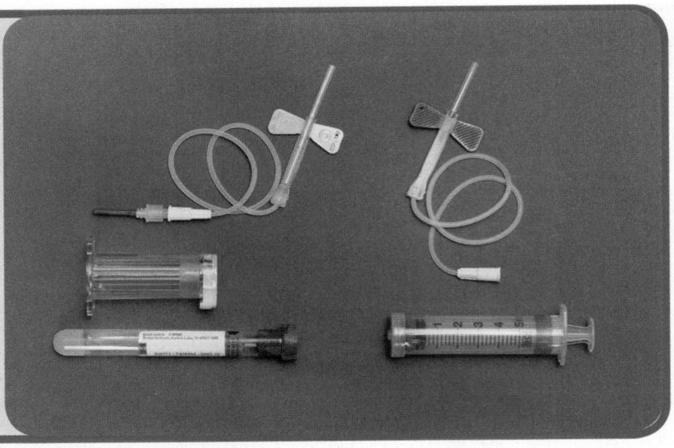

Figure 43–7: Left—Supplies used for butterfly method: butterfly needle, hub, and tube. Right—Supplies used for needle and syringe method: winged infusion needle with Luer-Lok adapter and Luer-Lok syringe. *Delmar/Cengage Learning.*

Safety Considerations

Usually, the patient is seated in a chair with the arm supported for the venipuncture procedure. If a patient faints from this position, first remove the tourniquet, withdraw the needle, and hold a bandage over the puncture site. Then the patient must be helped carefully to the floor. Spirits of ammonia (ammonia inhalant) can help revive the patient. The physician should check the patient before you proceed any further. Patients who say they feel faint should put their head down between their knees. Usually, this helps within a few minutes, and the procedure can be accomplished with no further interruptions. Often, following a complete physical examination, the patient might still be lying on the examination table. This makes an ideal work area for the medical assistant, and the position for the patient is most comfortable. In case the patient feels faint, there is no worry of accidental falling when the patient is lying down. The law regarding who performs venipuncture varies from state to state. Usually, the health care provider is aware of it and will not ask you to perform the procedure unless it is lawful.

Venipuncture must always be done carefully to avoid causing a **hematoma** (collection of blood just under the skin). When the needle is inserted into the vein, it punctures the wall of the vein and blood can then leak out into surrounding tissues. This bleeding causes discoloration and sometimes swelling. If the vein has been punctured from the needle going completely through the vein (in one side and out the other), the chances of a hematoma are even greater. Consult with the physician about applying ice, which can be helpful in reducing discomfort and swelling. Gentle pressure applied immediately on withdrawing the needle will help prevent this problem.

CLINICAL PEARL

Explaining the procedure and making the patient comfortable is of great importance. If the patient shows any signs of apprehension, ask the patient to lie down and try to relax. This eliminates the possibility of a patient falling as the result of fainting during the procedure. Some patients experience a queasy (nauseated) feeling, so it is a good idea to keep an emesis basin nearby. Displaying competency and efficiency in carrying out the procedure will gain the patient's confidence and cooperation.

PROCEDURE 43–2 Obtain Venous Blood with a Sterile Needle and Syringe

PURPOSE: To obtain venous blood specimens with a sterile needle and syringe when the amount needed is more than a few drops

EQUIPMENT: Sterile needle (19–23 G, 1 to 1 $\frac{1}{2}$ inches in length), 10–20 mL syringe for specimen tubes, laboratory specimen packaging materials, pen, patient's chart, alcohol, latex or vinyl gloves, cotton balls, tourniquet, lab request form (labeled appropriately with the vacuum blood specimen tubes that were ordered), gauze squares, adhesive bandage, spirits of ammonia, emesis basin, biohazard waste container (should be within reach), and sharps container

S SKILL: Perform a venipuncture, using the needle and syringe method.

Procedure Steps	Detailed Instructions and/or *Rationales*
1. Identify the patient by using two identifiers.	*Speaking to the patient by name and checking the chart ensures that you are performing the procedure on the correct patient.*

Procedure Steps	Detailed Instructions and/or *Rationales*
2. Assemble all needed items on a flat, stable surface next to the patient. Wash hands. Put on gloves.	
3. Secure a needle onto a syringe by holding the needle guard in one hand and turning the syringe barrel clockwise. Push in the plunger of the syringe all the way to release any air from the barrel.	It is a good practice to pull back one half to one third of the way and then push forward to push out all the air. This makes it easier to start pulling back when you are in the vein. It is also less traumatic to the patient.
B 4. Explain the procedure to the patient, ***including the rationale for performing the procedure, using language and verbal skills the patient can understand. Show awareness of patients' concerns regarding their perceptions of the venipuncture procedure by answering any questions the patient might have and assisting the patient into a comfortable position before you proceed.*** After consulting the patient, select a vein that can be palpated.	Ask the patient to lie down if there is any sign of apprehension. Most often, the patient will be sitting down with one arm extended and supported on the arm rest of the chair or on a table. *Providing a comfortable position relaxes the patient and elicits better cooperation.* Ask the patient whether there is a preferred venipuncture site. If the patient has no preference, visually check both arms and select a vein that can be palpated (felt) easily with your fingertip after application of alcohol. Ask a patient who is eating or chewing gum to remove the contents from his mouth before you begin, *to eliminate any possibility of the patient choking if he or she faints or becomes ill during the procedure.*
5. Apply a tourniquet to the patient's upper arm, about 3 inches above the bend in the elbow (Figure 43–13A).	*The tourniquet slows down blood flow, increasing volume within the vein and thereby aiding palpation and visualization of the blood vessel.* Proceed quickly because a tourniquet should not be left on longer than one minute. A tourniquet applied too tightly prevents blood flow, and the patient will be most uncomfortable.
6. Clean the site lightly with an alcohol-saturated cotton ball and let it air dry (Figure 43–13B).	*Blowing on the site to dry it contaminates the tissue.*
7. Ask the patient to clench the fist only if the vein does not stand out.	
8. Take off the needle guard and, with the bevel of the needle up, insert the needle tip into the vein with a quick and steady motion, following the path of the vein at approximately a 15-degree angle.	Holding the skin at the site to stretch it slightly will help keep the vein from moving during the puncture. The needle should be inserted no more than $\frac{1}{4}$ to $\frac{1}{2}$ inch, or it can pass through the vein. *This helps maintain the position of the vein.*
9. Hold the barrel of the syringe in one hand and, with the other hand, pull the plunger back slowly and steadily until the barrel is filled with the amount of blood needed to fill the specimen tubes (Figures 43–13C and D). As you observe the blood flow into the syringe, ask the patient to open the fist slowly; release the tourniquet (Figure 43–13E).	Release the tourniquet by quickly pulling up on the end of the portion that is tucked in.

(continues)

(continued)

Procedure Steps	Detailed Instructions and/or *Rationales*
10. Pull the needle out in the same path as it was inserted and place a gauze square or cotton ball over the site as the needle is withdrawn. Have the patient apply gentle pressure and slightly elevate the arm (Figure 43–13F and G). Activate the needle safety device and discard the needle into a sharps container (Figure 43–13H).	
11. Attach a blood transfer device to the syringe and allow the blood to transfer using the tube's vacuum (Figure 43–13I and J). Do not depress the plunger of the syringe. Fill the tubes with blood from the syringe according to the correct order of draw. Blood smears should be made at this time if needed.	Forcing blood into tubes causes hemolysis. Vacuum tubes fill easily because the vacuum draws in blood. Specimen tubes must be filled quickly because clotting will begin within minutes in the syringe and needle. Before filling the tubes containing powdered additives, you should tap the tubes gently to allow any of the contents that might have collected around the top to fall to the bottom of the tube. Check with the laboratory manual regarding the required amount of blood for tests ordered by the provider that contain additives. Test results can be false or inaccurate if there is a ratio imbalance of blood and additive.
12. Immediately invert tubes, and stand red stoppered tubes vertically to clot. In tubes that contain an anticoagulant, use a figure-eight motion to mix the blood gently.	*Do not shake blood, or hemolysis will occur.*
13. Deposit the entire syringe and blood transfer device intact in the sharps biohazard waste container (Figure 43–13K). Label all required specimen tubes and complete a lab request form. The completed lab request form is usually placed in one side of the lab-provided biobag and the specimens in the other, protected (sealed and leak-proof), side to be sent to a reference lab for analysis.	*Keep the labeled specimen tubes near the centrifuge so that serum-only transfer tubes may be added when completed.*
B 14. ***Attend to the patient's needs and comfort;*** once it is determined that a patient doesn't have an allergy to adhesives, apply a bandage over the puncture site (Figure 43–13L).	
15. Discard disposables in the proper receptacles. Remove gloves, wash hands, and return items to the proper storage area.	
16. Record the procedure in the log book and on the patient's chart and initial.	Refer to the charting example.

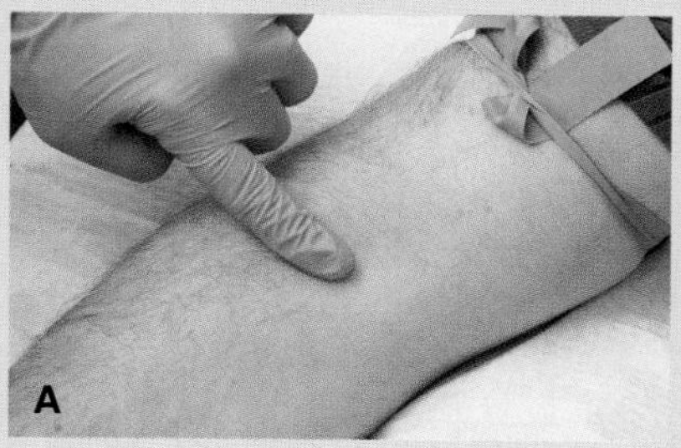

Figure 43–13A: Venipuncture by syringe and needle method series. Apply a tourniquet to the patient's upper arm. *Delmar/Cengage Learning.*

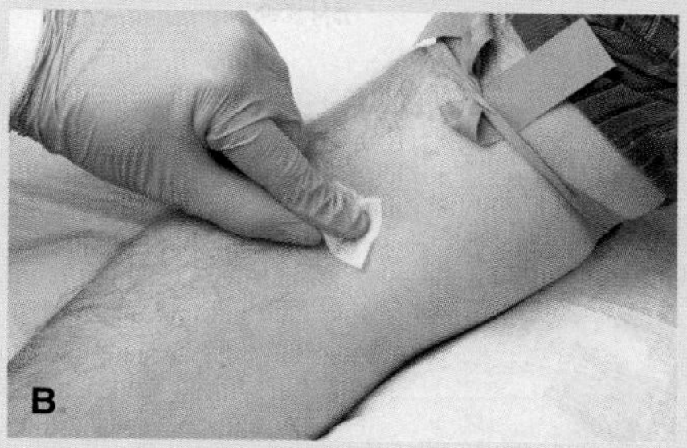

Figure 43–13B: Clean the site and let it air dry. *Delmar/Cengage Learning.*

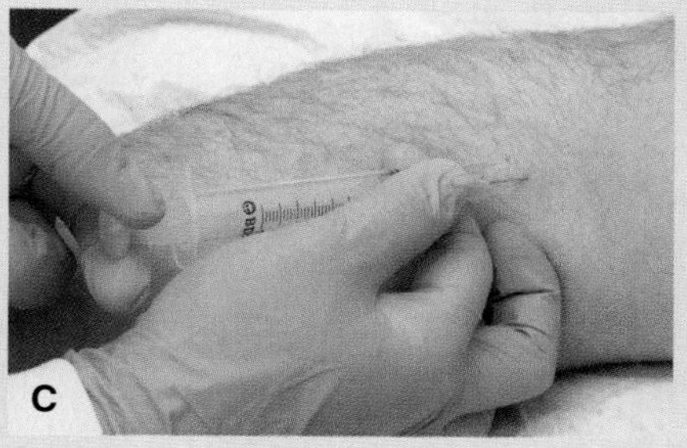

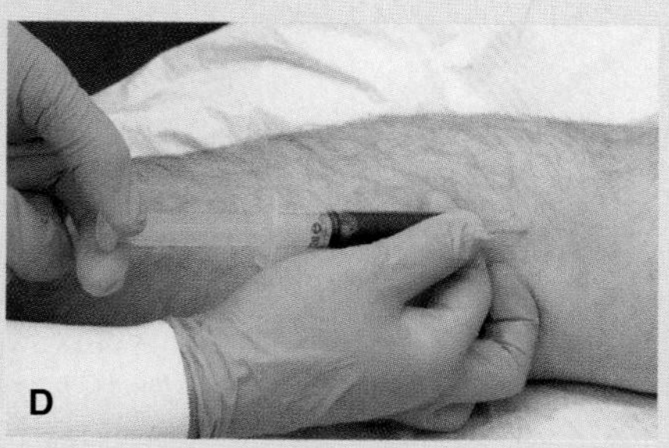

Figure 43–13C and D: Insert the needle tip into the vein with a quick and steady motion; holding the barrel of the syringe in one hand, pull the plunger back slowly with the other hand. *Delmar/Cengage Learning.*

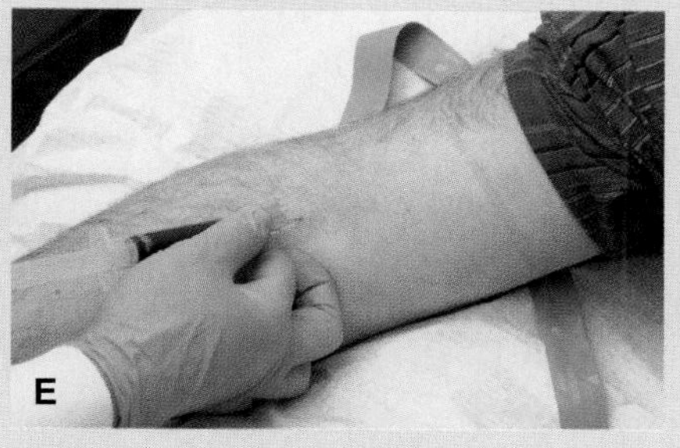

Figure 43–13E: Ask the patient to open the fist slowly, and then release the tourniquet. *Delmar/Cengage Learning.*

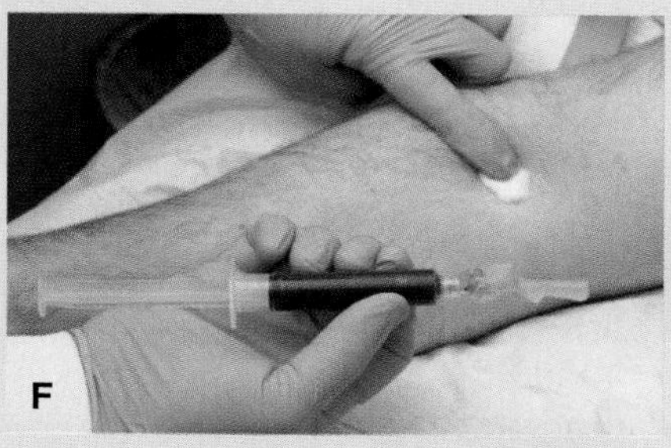

Figure 43–13F: Apply a gauze square or cotton ball over the site after the needle is withdrawn. *Delmar/Cengage Learning.*

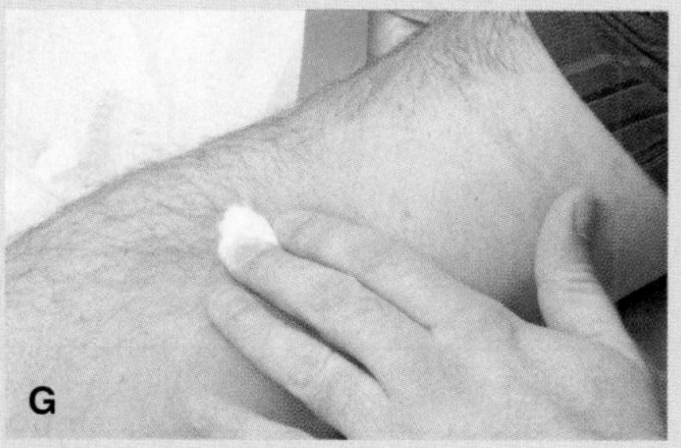

Figure 43–13G: Have the patient apply gentle pressure and slightly elevate the arm. *Delmar/Cengage Learning.*

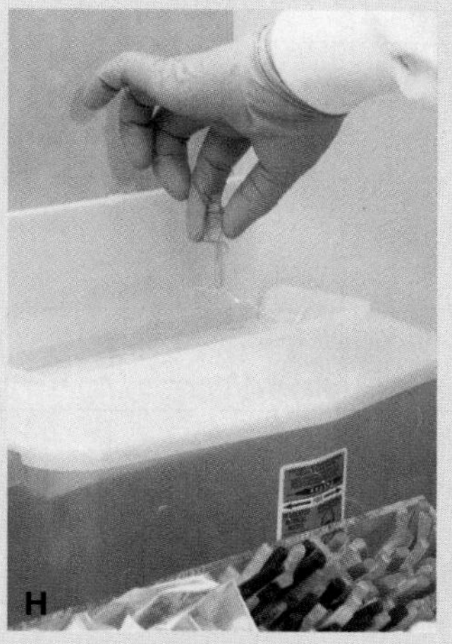

Figure 43–13H: Discard the needle (with safety device activated) into a sharps container. *Delmar/Cengage Learning.*

(continues)

(continued)

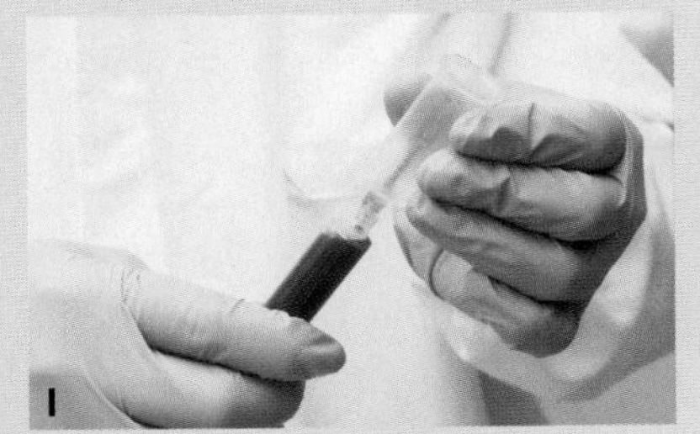

Figure 43–13I: Attach a blood transfer device to the syringe. *Delmar/Cengage Learning.*

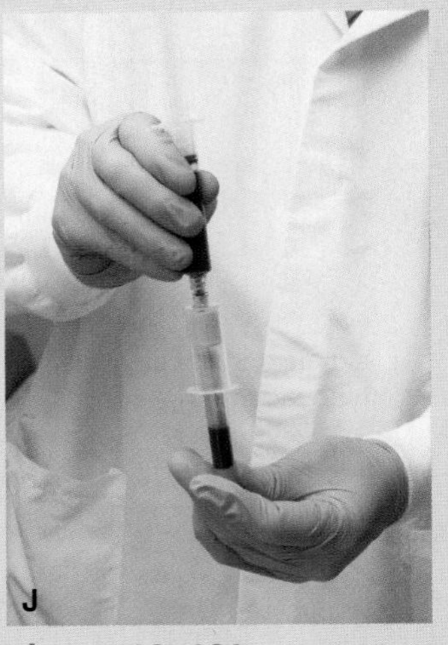

Figure 43–13J: Allow the blood to transfer using the tube's vacuum; do not depress the plunger of the syringe. Fill the tubes with blood from the syringe according to the correct order of draw. *Delmar/Cengage Learning.*

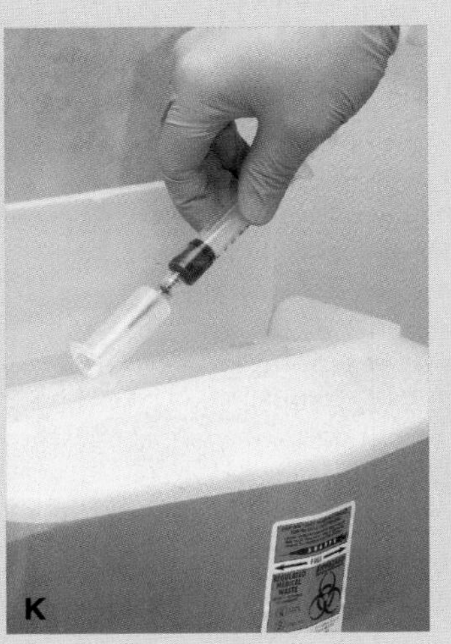

Figure 43–13K: Deposit the entire syringe and blood transfer device intact into a sharps container. *Delmar/Cengage Learning.*

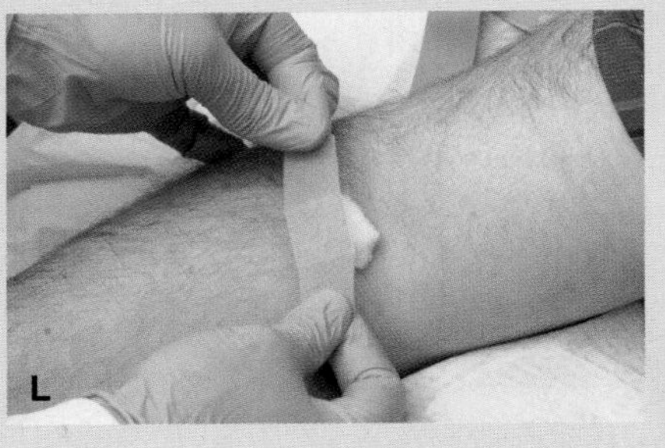

Figure 43–13L: Apply a bandage over the puncture site. *Delmar/Cengage Learning.*

Charting Example

4-18-XX 3:15 PM	One CBC tube drawn from Mr. Mitchell's L arm; packaged for reference lab pickup. J. Watkins, CMA(AAMA)

Log Book Example

Date	Patient's Name	Number	Test	Sent	Result	Filed by
4-18-XX	Bernie L. Mitchell DOB 7-19-61	7843	CBC	4-18-XX		

PROCEDURE 43–3 Obtain Venous Blood with a Vacuum Tube

PURPOSE: To obtain venous blood specimens with a vacuum tube when the amount needed is more than a few drops

EQUIPMENT: Multiple sample sterile needles (19–23 G, 1 to 1 $\frac{1}{2}$ inch in length), plastic adapter (a shielded blood needle adapter is recommended for safety), labeled specimen tubes (vacuum), alcohol, latex or vinyl gloves, sharps container, cotton balls, gauze squares, tourniquet, lab request forms, pen, patient's chart, bandages, biohazard waste container, and laboratory specimen packaging material

S **SKILL:** Perform a venipuncture, using the vacuum tube method.

Procedure Steps	Detailed Instructions and/or *Rationales*
1. Identify the patient by using two identifiers.	*Speaking to the patient by name and checking the chart ensures that you are performing the procedure on the correct patient.*
2. Assemble all needed items on a flat, stable surface next to the patient. For needle assembly, secure a needle onto the adapter by screwing the grooved end of the needle into the grooved tip of the adapter, holding the needle guard, and turning the adapter in a clockwise motion. Set aside. Wash hands. Put on gloves.	
B 3. Explain the procedure to the patient, ***including the rationale for performing the procedure, using language and verbal skills the patient can understand. Show awareness of patients' concerns regarding their perception of the procedure by answering any questions the patient might have and assist the patient into a comfortable position before you proceed.*** After consulting the patient, select a vein that can be palpated.	Ask the patient to lie down if there is any sign of apprehension. Generally, the patient will be sitting down with the arm extended and supported on the arm rest of chair or on a table. *Providing a comfortable position helps relax the patient and elicits better cooperation.* Ask the patient whether there is a preferred venipuncture site. If the patient has no preference, visually check both arms and select a vein that can be palpated (felt) easily with your fingertip after application of alcohol. Ask a patient who is eating or chewing gum to remove the contents from his mouth before you begin, *to eliminate any possibility of the patient choking if he or she faints or becomes ill during the procedure.*
4. Apply a tourniquet to the patient's upper arm, about 3 inches above the bend in the elbow (Figure 43–14A).	*The tourniquet slows down blood flow, increasing volume within the vein and thereby aiding palpation and visualization of the blood vessel.*
5. Clean the site with a lightly alcohol-saturated cotton ball and let it air dry (Figure 43–14B).	*Blowing on the site to dry it contaminates the skin.*
6. Ask the patient to clench the fist only if the vein does not stand out.	*This pressure of the clenched fist can interfere with some chemistry tests.*
7. Take off the needle guard and, with the bevel of the needle up, insert the tip of the needle into the vein with a quick and steady motion, following the path of the vein at approximately a 15-degree angle (Figure 43–14C).	Holding the skin at the site to stretch it slightly helps keep the vein from moving during the puncture. The needle should be inserted no more than $\frac{1}{4}$ to $\frac{1}{2}$ inch, or it can pass through the vein. *This helps maintain the position of the vein.*

(continues)

(continued)

Procedure Steps	Detailed Instructions and/or *Rationales*
8. Hold the adapter with one hand and, with the other hand, place your index and great fingers on either side of the protruding edges of the adapter. Push the vacuum tube completely into the adapter with your thumb, allowing the needle to puncture the stopper (Figure 43–14D). Blood will flow into the tube by vacuum force if the other end of the needle is in the vein properly. As you observe blood flow into the tube, ask the patient to open the fist slowly and then release the tourniquet. When the tube is filled, pull it out of the adapter by holding it between your thumb and great finger and pushing against the adapter with your index finger (Figure 43–14E).	Release the tourniquet by quickly pulling up on the end of the portion that is tucked in.
9. Fill the required number of tubes for the tests ordered by the provider according to the correct order of draw (Figure 43–14F). Blood smears should be made at this time if needed.	Before filling the tubes containing powdered additives, tap the tubes gently *to allow any of the contents that might have collected around the rubber stopper to fall to the bottom of the tube.* Check with the laboratory manual regarding the required amount of blood for tests ordered by the provider that contain additives. *Test results can be false or inaccurate if there is a ratio imbalance of blood and additive.*
10. Pull the needle out in the path by which it was inserted and place a gauze square over the site as the needle is withdrawn. Have the patient apply gentle pressure and slightly elevate the arm. Activate the needle safety device and discard entire adapter and needle into a sharps container (Figure 43–14G).	If a blood smear is needed for a differential, turn the CBC (lavender) tube (if still attached to adapter) upside down and gently press tube down to release a drop of blood onto the glass slide. Make blood smear (or as many as have been ordered), label the frosted end with a pencil, air-dry quickly, and send with other specimens. If using a blood analyzer system, place the lavender stopper tube in the closed vial to run the test.
11. Immediately invert tubes, and stand red stoppered tubes vertically to clot. In tubes that contain an anticoagulant, use a figure-eight motion to mix the blood gently.	*Do not shake blood or hemolysis will occur.*
12. Label all required specimen tubes and complete a lab request form (Figure 40–14H).	*Keep the labeled specimen tubes near the centrifuge so that serum-only transfer tubes can be added when completed.*
B 13. ***Attend to the patient's needs and comfort;*** once it is determined that the patient does not have an allergy to adhesives, apply a bandage over the puncture site (Figure 43–14I).	
14. Discard disposables in the proper receptacle. Remove gloves, wash hands, and return items to the proper storage area.	
15. Record the procedure in the log book and on the patient's chart and initial.	Refer to the charting example and log book example.

Procedure Steps	Detailed Instructions and/or *Rationales*
16. Place labeled specimen tubes with the lab request form securely in the appropriate specimen container for safe transport to the lab. The completed lab request form is usually placed in one side of the lab-provided biobag and the specimens in the other, protected (sealed and leak-proof), side to be sent to a reference lab for analysis.	

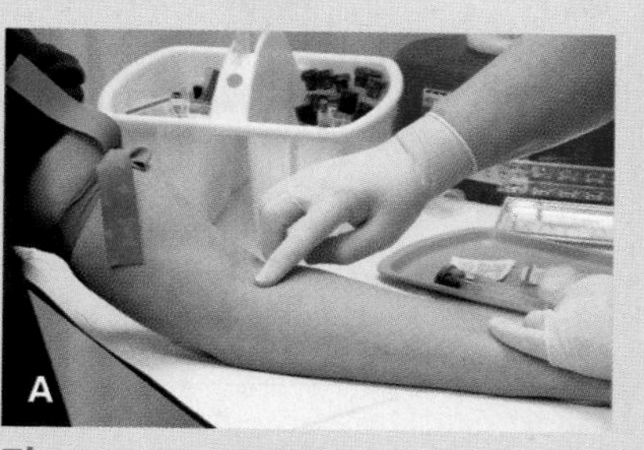

Figure 43–14A: Venipuncture by vacuum tube method series. Apply a tourniquet to the patient's upper arm. *Delmar/Cengage Learning.*

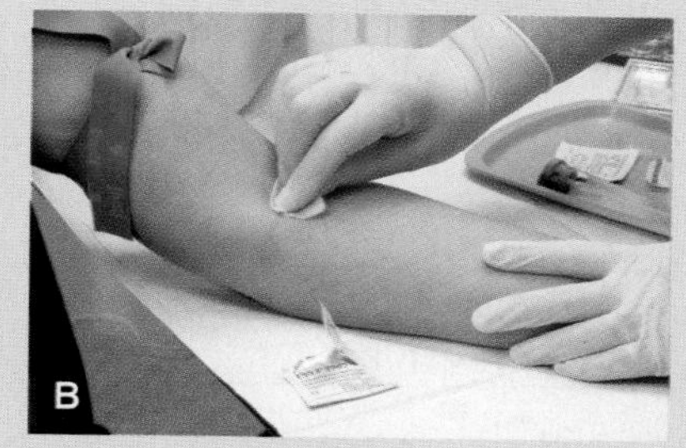

Figure 43–14B: Clean the site and let it air dry. *Delmar/Cengage Learning.*

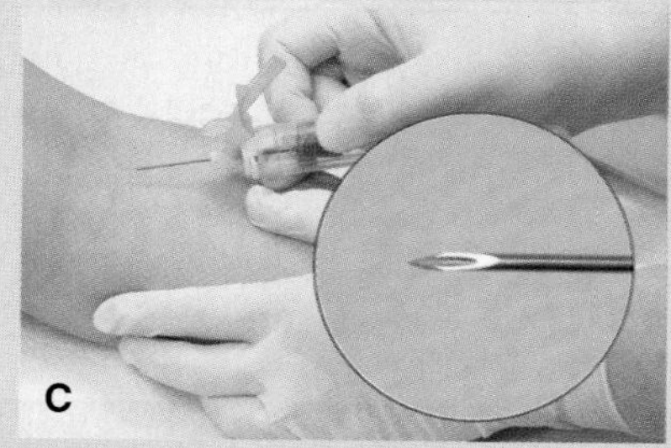

Figure 43–14C: Insert the needle tip into the vein with a quick and steady motion. *Delmar/Cengage Learning.*

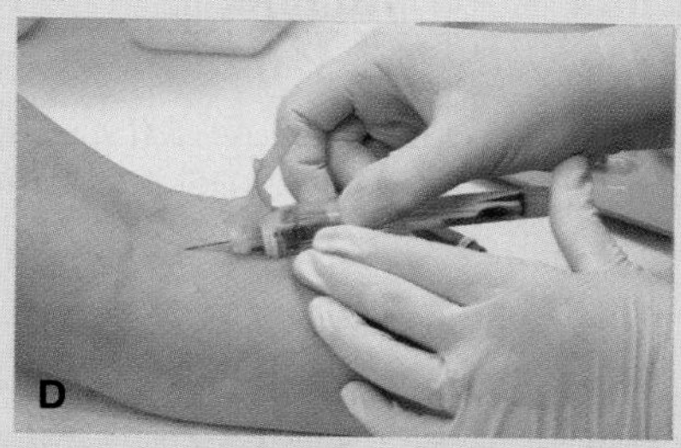

Figure 43–14D: Push the vacuum tube completely into the adapter with your thumb, allowing the needle to puncture the stopper. *Delmar/Cengage Learning.*

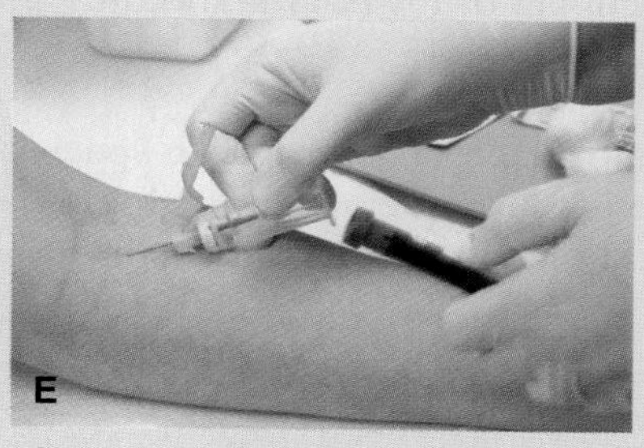

Figure 43–14E: As you observe blood flow into the tube, ask the patient to open the fist slowly, and then release the tourniquet. When the tube is filled, remove it from the adapter. *Delmar/Cengage Learning.*

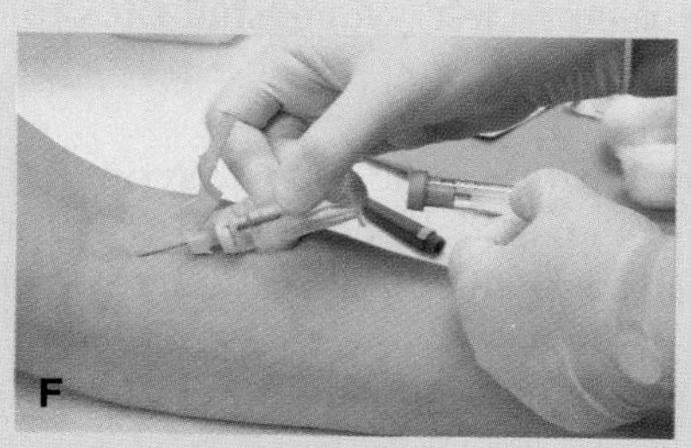

Figure 43–14F: Fill the required number of tubes according to the correct order of draw. When the last tube has been filled, smoothly remove the needle. Place a gauze square or cotton ball over the site; have the patient apply gentle pressure and slightly elevate the arm. *Delmar/Cengage Learning.*

(continues)

(continued)

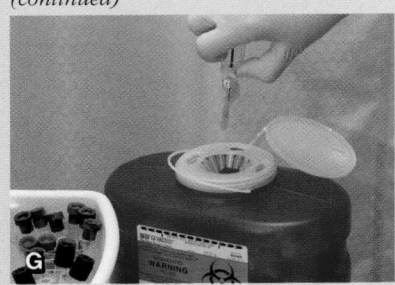

Figure 43–14G: Activate the needle safety device and discard into a sharps container. *Delmar/Cengage Learning.*

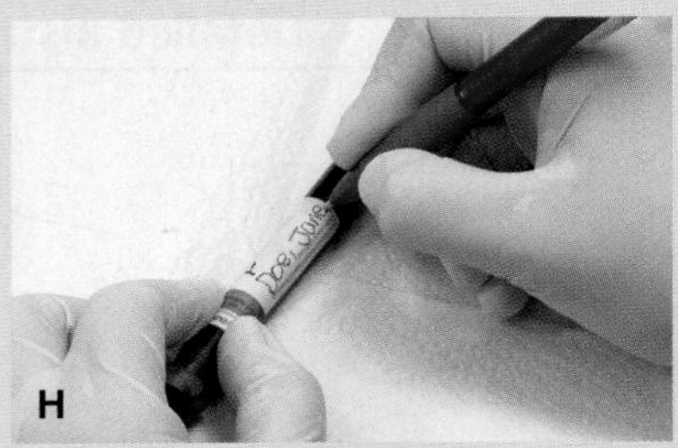

Figure 43–14H: Label all tubes and complete a lab request form. *Delmar/Cengage Learning.*

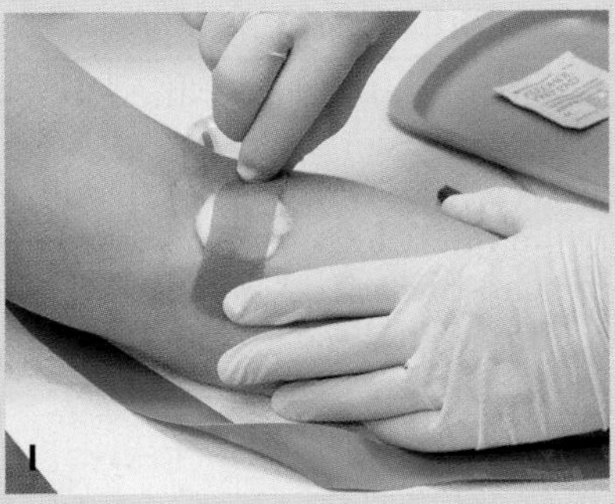

Figure 43–14I: Place a bandage over the puncture site. *Delmar/Cengage Learning.*

Charting Example

4-18-XX 11:15 am	One CBC tube drawn from Mr. Mitchell's L arm; packaged for reference lab pickup. R. Ropitzky, RMA(AMT)

Log Book Example

Date	Patient's Name	Number	Test	Sent	Results	Filed by
4-18-XX	Bernie L. Mitchell DOB 7-19-61	7843	CBC	4-18-XX		

PROCEDURE 43–4 Obtain Venous Blood with the Butterfly Needle Method

PURPOSE: To obtain venous blood specimens from infants, children, or patients with veins that are difficult to draw (veins not easily seen or felt). Suggested sites to obtain blood are the antecubital or lower arm and the back of the hand.

EQUIPMENT: Sterile butterfly needle (22 G), syringe (or vacuum tubes and needle adaptor), appropriate specimen tubes, pen, patient's chart, lab request form, spirits of ammonia, emesis basin, tourniquet, latex or vinyl gloves, alcohol prep, cotton balls or gauze squares, bandage, Mayo tray table, and biohazard sharps container

S SKILL: Perform a venipuncture, using the butterfly needle method.

Procedure Steps	Detailed Instructions and/or *Rationales*
1. Identify the patient by using two identifiers.	*Speaking to the patient by name and checking the chart ensures that you are performing the procedure on the correct patient.*

Procedure Steps	Detailed Instructions and/or *Rationales*
2. Assemble all needed items on a flat, stable surface next to the patient. For needle assembly, secure a needle onto the adapter by screwing the grooved end of the needle into the grooved tip of the adapter, holding the needle guard, and turning the adapter in a clockwise motion. Push any air out of syringe before using it to draw a blood specimen Set aside. Wash hands. Put on gloves.	
B 3. Explain the procedure to the patient, ***including the rationale for performing the procedure, using language and verbal skills the patient can understand. Show awareness of patients' concerns regarding their perceptions of the venipuncture procedure by answering any questions the patient might have and assisting the patient into a comfortable position before you proceed.*** After consulting the patient, select a vein that can be palpated.	
4. Apply the tourniquet to the patient's arm, about 3 inches above the needle insertion site (Figure 43–15A).	
5. Clean the site lightly with an alcohol-saturated cotton ball and let it air dry (Figure 43–15B).	
6. Ask the patient to make a fist and hold it until you say to release it.	
7. Remove the needle guard and quickly insert the butterfly needle into the vein (Figure 43–15C).	
8. Pull back on the plunger of the syringe slowly until an adequate amount of blood is obtained (Figure 43–15D) and then ask the patient to release the fist.	
9. Release the tourniquet and withdraw the needle quickly.	
10. Apply gentle pressure over the site with cotton or gauze and ask the patient to hold the arm slightly up for a few minutes (Figure 43–15E).	*Holding the arm up can help prevent a hematoma.*
11. Retract the needle or activate the safety lock on the needle and then place the used needle and all other contaminated supplies in a biohazard sharps container (Figure 43–15F–G).	

(continues)

(continued)

Procedure Steps	Detailed Instructions and/or *Rationales*
12. Attach a blood transfer device to the syringe and allow the blood to transfer using the tube's vacuum. Do not depress the plunger of the syringe. Fill the tubes with blood from the syringe according to the correct order of draw. Blood smears should be made at this time if needed.	Forcing blood into tubes causes hemolysis. Vacuum tubes fill easily because the vacuum draws in blood. Specimen tubes must be filled quickly because clotting begins within minutes in the syringe and needle. Before filling the tubes containing powdered additives, tap the tubes gently to allow any of the contents that might have collected around the top to fall to the bottom of the tube. Check with the laboratory manual regarding the required amount of blood for tests ordered by the provider that contain additives. Test results can be false or inaccurate if there is a ratio imbalance of blood and additive.
13. Stand red-stoppered tubes vertically to clot so that serum can be drawn after centrifugation. In tubes that contain an anticoagulant, use a figure-eight motion to mix the blood gently.	*Do not shake blood or hemolysis will occur.*
14. Deposit the entire syringe and blood transfer device intact in the sharps biohazard waste container. Label all required specimen tubes and complete a lab request form. The completed lab request form is usually placed in one side of the lab-provided biobag and the specimens in the other, protected (sealed and leak-proof), side to be sent to a reference lab for analysis.	
B 15. ***Attend to the patient's needs and comfort;*** once it is determined that the patient does not have an allergy to adhesives, apply a bandage to the site (Figure 43–15H).	Ask whether the patient has an allergy to adhesive.
16. Place specimens in the appropriate lab transport container.	
17. Remove gloves and discard them in a biohazard container or bag. Wash hands and return items to the proper storage area.	
18. Record the procedure in the log book and on the patient's chart and initial.	

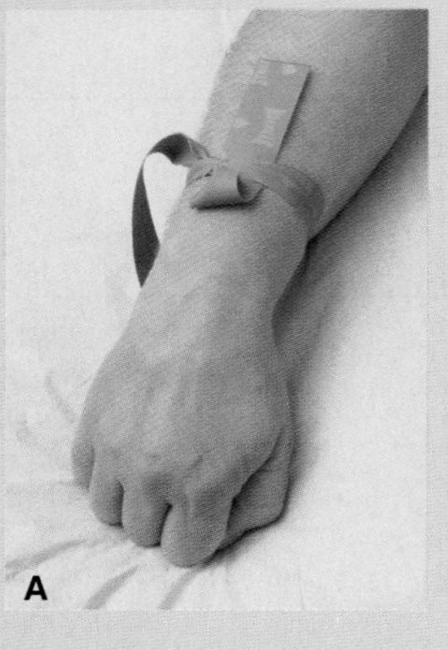

Figure 43–15A: Venipuncture by butterfly method series. Apply a tourniquet about 3 inches above the insertion site. *Delmar/Cengage Learning.*

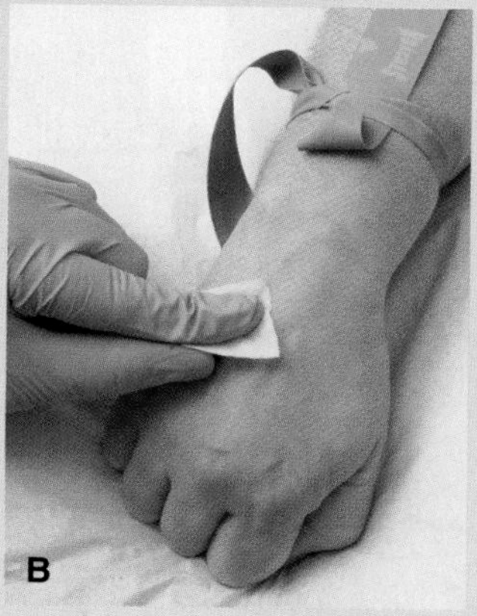

Figure 43–15B: Clean the site and let it air dry. *Delmar/Cengage Learning.*

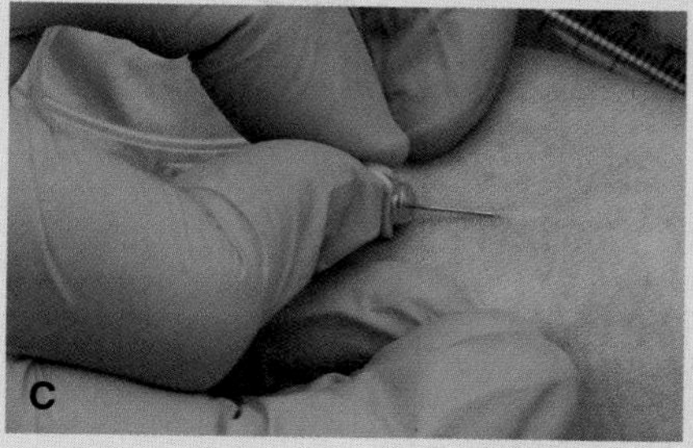

Figure 43–15C: Insert the needle tip into the vein with a quick and steady motion. *Delmar/Cengage Learning.*

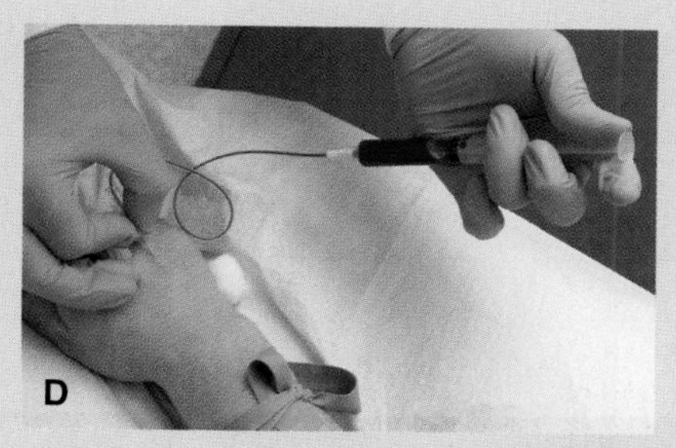

Figure 43–15D: Pull back on the plunger of the syringe slowly until an adequate amount of blood is obtained. *Delmar/Cengage Learning.*

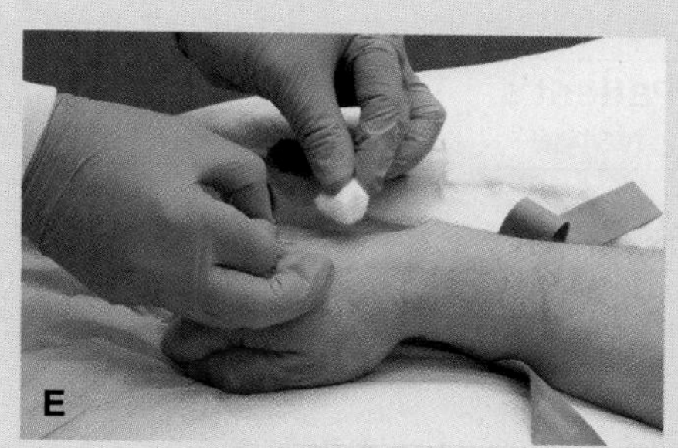

Figure 43–15E: Release the tourniquet, withdraw the needle quickly, and apply gentle pressure over the site with cotton or gauze. *Delmar/Cengage Learning.*

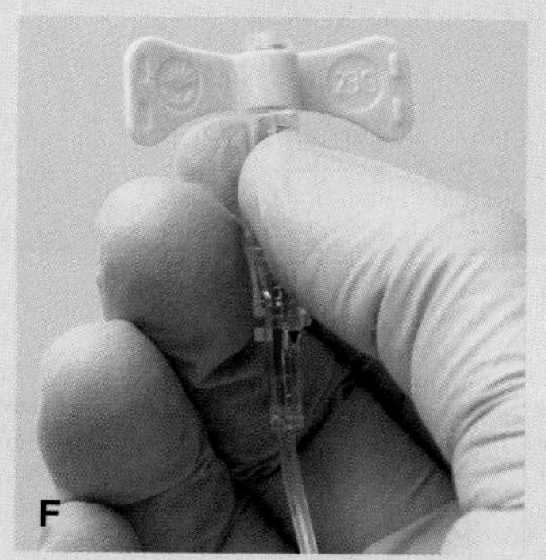

Figure 43–15F: Retract the needle or activate the safety lock on the needle. *Delmar/Cengage Learning.*

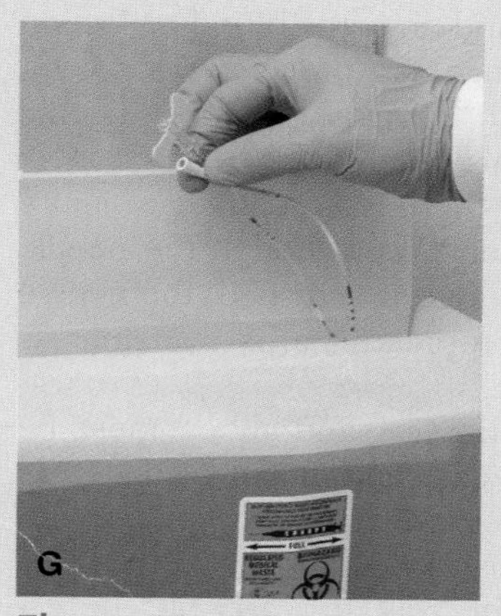

Figure 43–15G: Dispose of needle in a sharps container. *Delmar/Cengage Learning.*

(continues)

(continued)

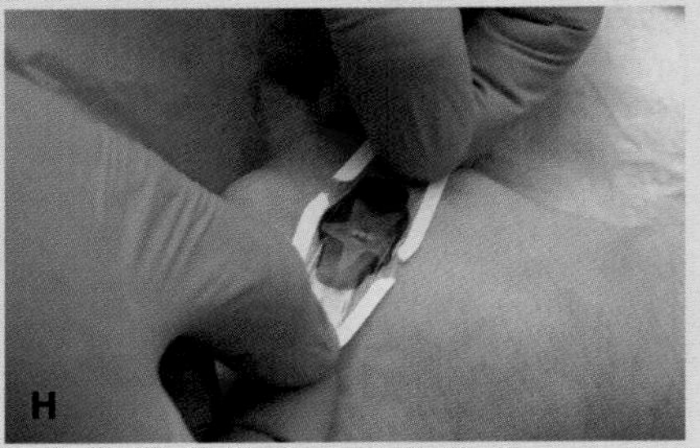

Figure 43–15H: Place a bandage over the puncture site. *Delmar/Cengage Learning.*

Charting Example

4-18-XX 11:15 am	One CBC tube drawn from Mr. Mitchell's L arm; packaged for reference lab pickup. R.Ropitzky, RMA(AMT)

Log Book Example

Date	Patient's Name	Number	Test	Sent	Results	Filed by
4-18-XX	Bernie L. Mitchell DOB 7-19-01	7843	CBC	4-18-XX		

Equipment and Supplies Used in Venipuncture

Figures 43–8A and 43–8B shows the BD Eclipse Blood Collection needle with a safety device on it. The design protects users from accidental needle injury, thereby reducing possible disease transmission.

This safety device is found on many blood collection needles and does not change the procedure for venipuncture. After its use, push the guard over the needle until you hear a click. At this point, the needle is safely covered and locked so that there is no danger of injury to the phlebotomist or patient. Even though the needle is covered and the safety device is activated, the needle must be placed in the appropriate sharps container as soon as possible.

All blood collection supplies and tubes must be checked for the expiration date and, if out of date, not used. This is in compliance with quality control and quality assurance regulations.

A tray is a convenient way to carry all necessary items for venipuncture procedures. It should be stocked with lab request forms, specimen tubes, cotton balls, alcohol dispenser, syringes, sterile needles, sharps container, latex or vinyl gloves, tourniquet, frosted-end slides, adapter for vacuum tube method, pen and pencil, gauze squares, spirits of ammonia,

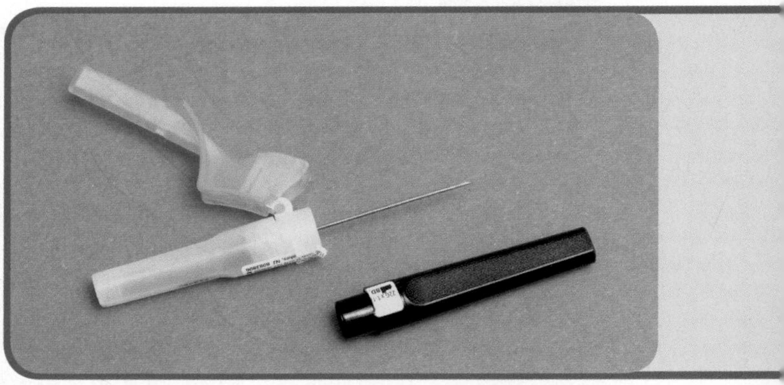

Figure 43–8A: BD Eclipse Blood Collection needle with cap off. *Delmar/Cengage Learning.*

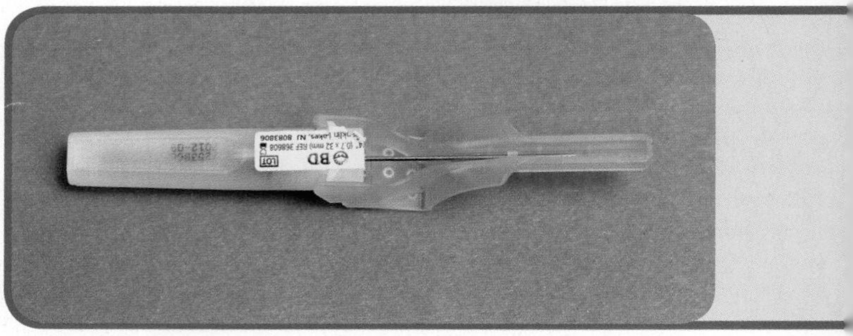

Figure 43–8B: BD Eclipse Blood Collection needle with safety device activated. *Delmar/Cengage Learning.*

and bandages. This handy carrier may be set next to the patient. It should be restocked daily during routine checking of supplies.

Blood Collection Tubes

Blood collection tubes are color coded for the various departments in the lab. Red-stoppered tubes come in sizes ranging from 3 to 15 mL. They are used to collect whole blood that is allowed to clot so that the **serum** can be drawn off by centrifugation. The serum can be drawn out by a disposable pipette and deposited into a transfer tube, which is labeled for the particular test to be done. There are other methods to transfer serum easily from the centrifuged tube. The most efficient way is to use the red/black stoppered tube, which has a gel in the bottom. During centrifugation, the gel liquefies and travels to the center of the tube, separating the red cells from the serum. You can then pour the serum carefully into a transfer tube and label for analysis. Another method is to place a slender, rubber-tipped tube down carefully into the centrifuged tube (pushing the tube down forcefully will result in hemolysis) just to the **meniscus** of the packed red blood cells. The screened, filtered opening at the rubber end of the inner tube allows the serum to fill the tube, leaving the red blood cells at the bottom. Then, pour off the serum into a transfer tube and label for analysis.

Lavender-stoppered tubes contain ethylene diamine tetracetic acid additive (EDTA) and are generally called CBC tubes. They are usually 5 or 10 mL in size and are also used to collect whole blood specimens.

Gray-stoppered tubes are used in blood glucose tests and are usually 5 mL. They contain oxalate.

Blue-stoppered tubes must be completely full because of the large amount of citrate. These tubes are most often the 5-mL size and are used for testing prothrombin times. For accurate test results, the test should be performed within two hours from the time it is drawn.

The green-stoppered tubes generally are 5-mL tubes that contain **heparin** and are used to determine several chemical constituents.

The blood specimen vacuum tubes used for pediatric patients are the same as the tubes used for adults except for the sizes, which are between 2 mL and 3 mL. Tests drawn in the blue tubes should be performed within two hours for accurate results or centrifuge. Freeze the plasma until testing can be performed.

Order of Draw

When several blood specimens are ordered, they should be drawn into the color-coded stoppered tubes in the following order: yellow (for blood cultures), blue, red or red/black (red-gray), green or blue or blue/black, lavender, and gray (Figure 43–9). The red or red/black tubes do not contain additives and should be drawn first in multiple sample draws to prevent possible contamination from the additives in the other tubes (Figure 43–10). In cases that require only one blue stoppered tube, a 5-mL red-stoppered tube should be drawn first and discarded to prevent thromboplastin from the site of the draw from interfering with the results of coagulation testing.

Blood in specimen tubes that contain an anticoagulant must be mixed immediately in a figure-eight motion 8 to 10 times. Gentle mixing prevents hemolysis. The tubes with red stoppers must be allowed to stand vertically and undisturbed for at least 15 to 30 minutes to allow clotting to occur. They must then be properly balanced in a centrifuge and spun for varying lengths of time, depending on the centrifuge speed. The serum, which is a clear, light-yellow liquid, is then carefully drawn off with a pipette (usually disposable ones provided by the laboratory) or by using one of the methods discussed earlier.

DOCUMENTING BLOOD COLLECTION

A log book must be kept of all specimens collected and sent for analysis. The log book must contain the following information:

1. Date collected
2. Patient's full name, DOB, Social Security number, or records number
3. Date sent to lab
4. Test requested
5. Date results received
6. Test results—may not be kept in specimen log book unless the test is being performed in house. Generally, a copy is filed in the patient's chart and a copy in the lab file in order of the date collected.

A lab request form, such as the one in Figure 43–11, must be completed and sent with the specimens and listed in the log book.

Often, specimens are picked up by couriers for delivery to out-of-town or out-of-state laboratories for analysis. The federal government requires specimens to be shipped or transported in securely closed, watertight containers. Blood tubes should be enclosed in a second durable watertight container. The doubly secured specimens are then placed in a shipping container with a label stating it is biohazardous. It is then ready for safe transport to the reference laboratory. A second label should read, "In case of breakage, send to this address: Centers for Disease Control and Prevention, Attention: Biohazards Control Office, 1600 Clifton Road, Atlanta, GA 30333."

BD Vacutainer® Order of Draw for Multiple Tube Collections

Designed for Your Safety

Reflects change in NCCLS recommended Order of Draw (NCCLS H3-A5, Vol 23, No 32, 8.10.2)

Closure Color	Collection Tube	Mix by Inverting
	BD Vacutainer® Blood Collection Tubes *(glass or plastic)*	
	• Blood Cultures - SPS	8 to 10 times
	• Citrate Tube*	3 to 4 times
or	• BD Vacutainer® SST™ Gel Separator Tube	5 times
	• Serum Tube *(glass or plastic)*	5 times (plastic) none (glass)
	• Heparin Tube	8 to 10 times
or	• BD Vacutainer® PST™ Gel Separator Tube With Heparin	8 to 10 times
or	• EDTA Tube	8 to 10 times
	• Fluoride (glucose) Tube	8 to 10 times

* When using a winged blood collection set for venipuncture and a coagulation (citrate) tube is the first specimen tube to be drawn, a discard tube should be drawn first. The discard tube must be used to fill the blood collection set tubing's "dead space" with blood but the discard tube does not need to be completely filled. This important step will ensure maintenance of the proper blood-to-additive ratio of the blood specimen. The discard tube should be a nonadditive or coagulation tube.

Note: Always follow your facility's protocol for order of draw

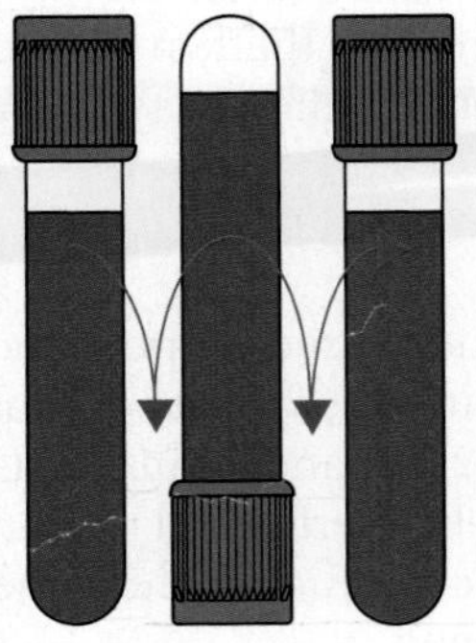

= 1 inversion

BD Global Technical Services
1.800.631.0174

BD Customer Service
1.888.237.2762
www.bd.com/vacutainer

Handle all biologic samples and blood collection "sharps" (lancets, needles, luer adapters and blood collection sets) according to the policies and procedures of your facility. Obtain appropriate medical attention in the event of any exposure to biologic samples (for example, through a puncture injury) since they may transmit viral hepatitis, HIV (AIDS), or other infectious diseases. Utilize any built-in used needle protector if the blood collection device provides one. BD does not recommend reshielding used needles, but the policies and procedures of your facility may differ and must always be followed. Discard any blood collection "sharps" in biohazard containers approved for their disposal.

BD Diagnostics
Preanalytical Systems
1 Becton Drive
Franklin Lakes, NJ 07417
www.bd.com/vacutainer

Figure 43–9: BD Vacutainer® Order of Draw for Multiple Collections wall chart. *Courtesy and © Becton, Dickinson and Company.*

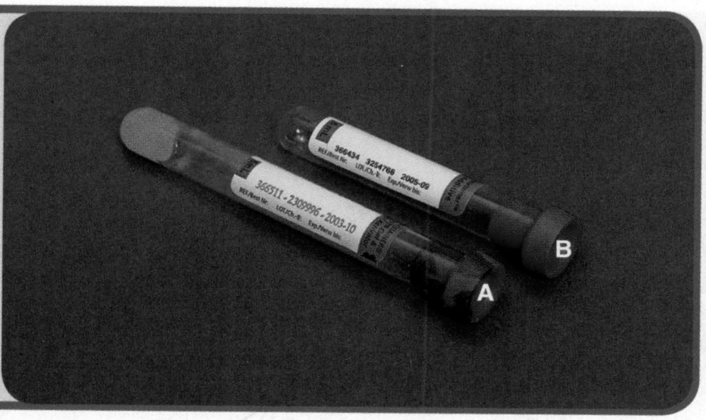

Figure 43–10: Standard vacuum tubes. (A) Red gray-top tube that contains clot activators and thixotrophic gel. (B) Plain red-top tube that contains no anticoagulant or additives. *Delmar/Cengage Learning.*

PROCESSING SPECIMENS FOR TRANSPORT

When processing specimens for transport by a reference laboratory, you will be provided with a laboratory manual that specifies the collection procedure for accurate specimen reporting. A piece of equipment that is essential to processing specimens is a **centrifuge**, an instrument that rotates at variable rates of speed to separate components of the blood (Figure 43–12).

For serum specimens, blood in the evacuated tube must be allowed to clot for 15 to 30 minutes prior to being loaded in the centrifuge. Serum is then extracted from the specimen and sent for testing in a properly labeled tube with a laboratory requisition form. **Plasma** specimens result from an anticoagulant present in the vacuum tube; care must be taken when removing the specimen from the centrifuge to prevent mixing the cells and the plasma together. It is also imperative to load the centrifuge properly; a centrifuge must be properly balanced to function as intended. An improperly loaded centrifuge can vibrate and literally walk off a countertop, resulting in instrument damage and possible injury to workers. If you have never used a centrifuge, be sure to have someone demonstrate the proper balancing procedure for loading tubes for centrifugation to prevent this accident from occurring.

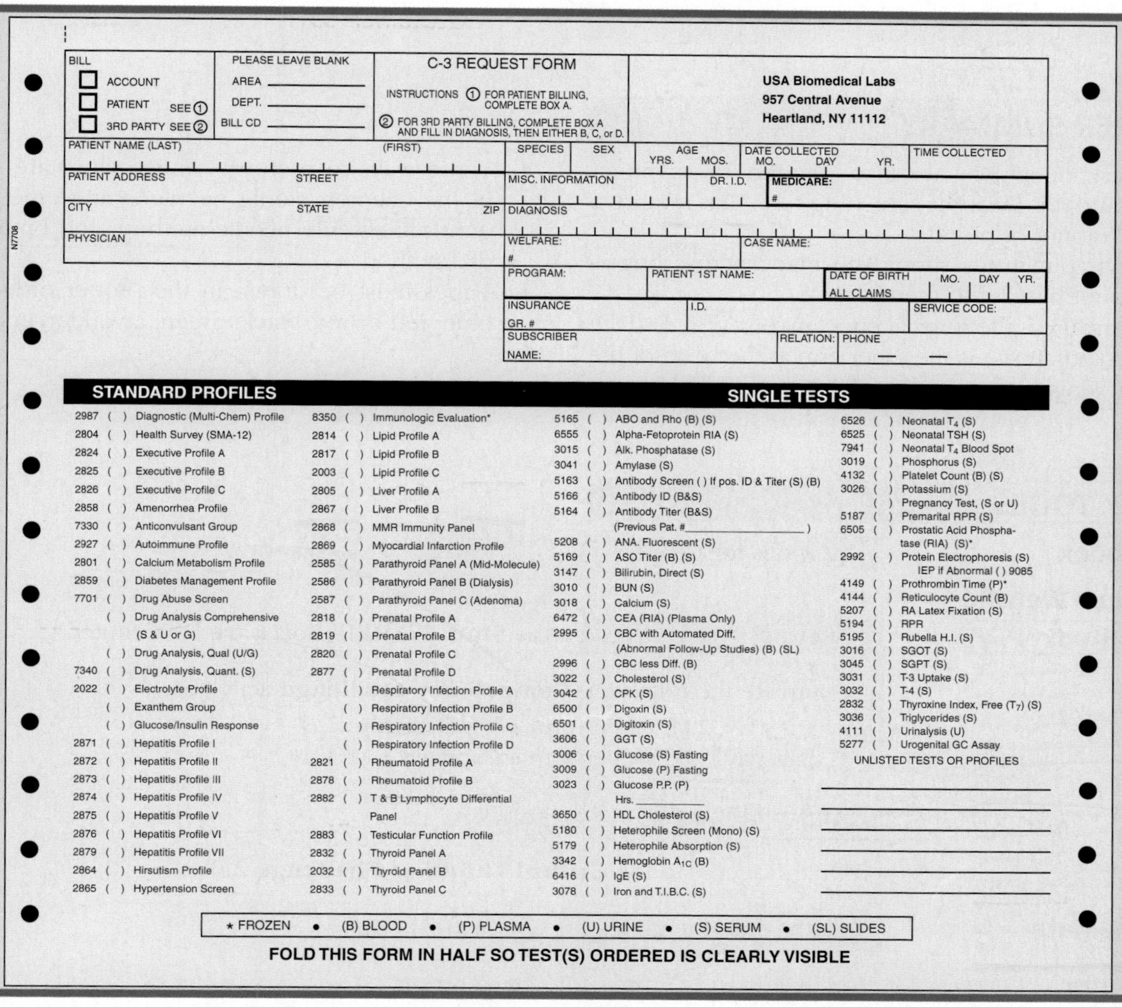

N7708

BILL
☐ ACCOUNT
☐ PATIENT SEE ①
☐ 3RD PARTY SEE ②

PLEASE LEAVE BLANK
AREA ______
DEPT. ______
BILL CD ______

C-3 REQUEST FORM
INSTRUCTIONS ① FOR PATIENT BILLING, COMPLETE BOX A.
② FOR 3RD PARTY BILLING, COMPLETE BOX A AND FILL IN DIAGNOSIS, THEN EITHER B, C, or D.

USA Biomedical Labs
957 Central Avenue
Heartland, NY 11112

PATIENT NAME (LAST) (FIRST) | SPECIES | SEX | AGE YRS. MOS. | DATE COLLECTED MO. DAY YR. | TIME COLLECTED
PATIENT ADDRESS STREET | MISC. INFORMATION | DR. I.D. | **MEDICARE:** #
CITY STATE ZIP | DIAGNOSIS
PHYSICIAN | WELFARE: # | CASE NAME:
PROGRAM: | PATIENT 1ST NAME: | DATE OF BIRTH ALL CLAIMS MO. DAY YR.
INSURANCE GR. # | I.D. | SERVICE CODE:
SUBSCRIBER NAME: | RELATION: | PHONE

STANDARD PROFILES

2987 ( ) Diagnostic (Multi-Chem) Profile
2804 ( ) Health Survey (SMA-12)
2824 ( ) Executive Profile A
2825 ( ) Executive Profile B
2826 ( ) Executive Profile C
2858 ( ) Amenorrhea Profile
7330 ( ) Anticonvulsant Group
2927 ( ) Autoimmune Profile
2801 ( ) Calcium Metabolism Profile
2859 ( ) Diabetes Management Profile
7701 ( ) Drug Abuse Screen
( ) Drug Analysis Comprehensive (S & U or G)
( ) Drug Analysis, Qual (U/G)
7340 ( ) Drug Analysis, Quant. (S)
2022 ( ) Electrolyte Profile
( ) Exanthem Group
( ) Glucose/Insulin Response
2871 ( ) Hepatitis Profile I
2872 ( ) Hepatitis Profile II
2873 ( ) Hepatitis Profile III
2874 ( ) Hepatitis Profile IV
2875 ( ) Hepatitis Profile V
2876 ( ) Hepatitis Profile VI
2879 ( ) Hepatitis Profile VII
2864 ( ) Hirsutism Profile
2865 ( ) Hypertension Screen
8350 ( ) Immunologic Evaluation*
2814 ( ) Lipid Profile A
2817 ( ) Lipid Profile B
2003 ( ) Lipid Profile C
2805 ( ) Liver Profile A
2867 ( ) Liver Profile B
2868 ( ) MMR Immunity Panel
2869 ( ) Myocardial Infarction Profile
2585 ( ) Parathyroid Panel A (Mid-Molecule)
2586 ( ) Parathyroid Panel B (Dialysis)
2587 ( ) Parathyroid Panel C (Adenoma)
2818 ( ) Prenatal Profile A
2819 ( ) Prenatal Profile B
2820 ( ) Prenatal Profile C
2877 ( ) Prenatal Profile D
( ) Respiratory Infection Profile A
( ) Respiratory Infection Profile B
( ) Respiratory Infection Profile C
( ) Respiratory Infection Profile D
2821 ( ) Rheumatoid Profile A
2878 ( ) Rheumatoid Profile B
2882 ( ) T & B Lymphocyte Differential Panel
2883 ( ) Testicular Function Profile
2832 ( ) Thyroid Panel A
2032 ( ) Thyroid Panel B
2833 ( ) Thyroid Panel C

SINGLE TESTS

5165 ( ) ABO and Rho (B) (S)
6555 ( ) Alpha-Fetoprotein RIA (S)
3015 ( ) Alk. Phosphatase (S)
3041 ( ) Amylase (S)
5163 ( ) Antibody Screen ( ) If pos. ID & Titer (S) (B)
5166 ( ) Antibody ID (B&S)
5164 ( ) Antibody Titer (B&S) (Previous Pat. #______)
5208 ( ) ANA. Fluorescent (S)
5169 ( ) ASO Titer (B) (S)
3147 ( ) Bilirubin, Direct (S)
3010 ( ) BUN (S)
3018 ( ) Calcium (S)
6472 ( ) CEA (RIA) (Plasma Only)
2995 ( ) CBC with Automated Diff. (Abnormal Follow-Up Studies) (B) (SL)
2996 ( ) CBC less Diff. (B)
3022 ( ) Cholesterol (S)
3042 ( ) CPK (S)
6500 ( ) Digoxin (S)
6501 ( ) Digitoxin (S)
3606 ( ) GGT (S)
3006 ( ) Glucose (S) Fasting
3009 ( ) Glucose (P) Fasting
3023 ( ) Glucose P.P. (P) Hrs. ______
3650 ( ) HDL Cholesterol (S)
5180 ( ) Heterophile Screen (Mono) (S)
5179 ( ) Heterophile Absorption (S)
3342 ( ) Hemoglobin A_{1C} (B)
6416 ( ) IgE (S)
3078 ( ) Iron and T.I.B.C. (S)
6526 ( ) Neonatal T_4 (S)
6525 ( ) Neonatal TSH (S)
7941 ( ) Neonatal T_4 Blood Spot
3019 ( ) Phosphorus (S)
4132 ( ) Platelet Count (B) (S)
3026 ( ) Potassium (S)
( ) Pregnancy Test, (S or U)
5187 ( ) Premarital RPR (S)
6505 ( ) Prostatic Acid Phosphatase (RIA) (S)*
2992 ( ) Protein Electrophoresis (S) IEP if Abnormal ( ) 9085
4149 ( ) Prothrombin Time (P)*
4144 ( ) Reticulocyte Count (B)
5207 ( ) RA Latex Fixation (S)
5194 ( ) RPR
5195 ( ) Rubella H.I. (S)
3016 ( ) SGOT (S)
3045 ( ) SGPT (S)
3031 ( ) T-3 Uptake (S)
3032 ( ) T-4 (S)
2832 ( ) Thyroxine Index, Free (T_7) (S)
3036 ( ) Triglycerides (S)
4111 ( ) Urinalysis (U)
5277 ( ) Urogenital GC Assay

UNLISTED TESTS OR PROFILES

★ FROZEN • (B) BLOOD • (P) PLASMA • (U) URINE • (S) SERUM • (SL) SLIDES

FOLD THIS FORM IN HALF SO TEST(S) ORDERED IS CLEARLY VISIBLE

Figure 43–11: A laboratory requisition form for diagnostic tests. *Delmar/Cengage Learning.*

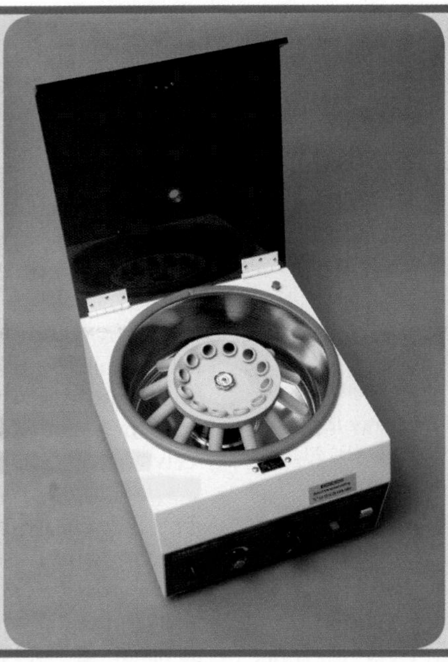

Figure 43–12: Centrifuge. *Delmar/Cengage Learning.*

CHAPTER SUMMARY

- Capillary punctures are also referred to as finger sticks and are ideal for screening tests that require a small amount of blood.
- Capillary punctures should be made across fingerprints, not parallel to them.
- Venipuncture is the surgical puncture of a vein, and the most common site is the inner arm at the bend of the elbow. Venipuncture is also referred to as phlebotomy.
- Three ways to perform venipuncture are described in the chapter: sterile needle/syringe method, vacuum tube/sterile needle method, and butterfly needle method.
- Tubes must be drawn in the proper order: Yellow, blue, red or red/black, green, lavender, and gray.

STUDY TOOLS

Workbook	Activities for Chapter 43
Premium Website StudyWARE	Activities and Quizzes on the **StudyWARE™ Software** for Chapter 43
	Complete the following **Competency Challenge** activities: • Tuesday, 2:00 PM Perform a Venipuncture • Tuesday, 3:00 PM Perform a Capillary Puncture
	Audio Library of medical terms
	Online access to the **Critical Thinking Challenge 2.0**
CourseMate	Activities and Quizzes for Chapter 43
WebTutor	Activities and Quizzes for Chapter 43

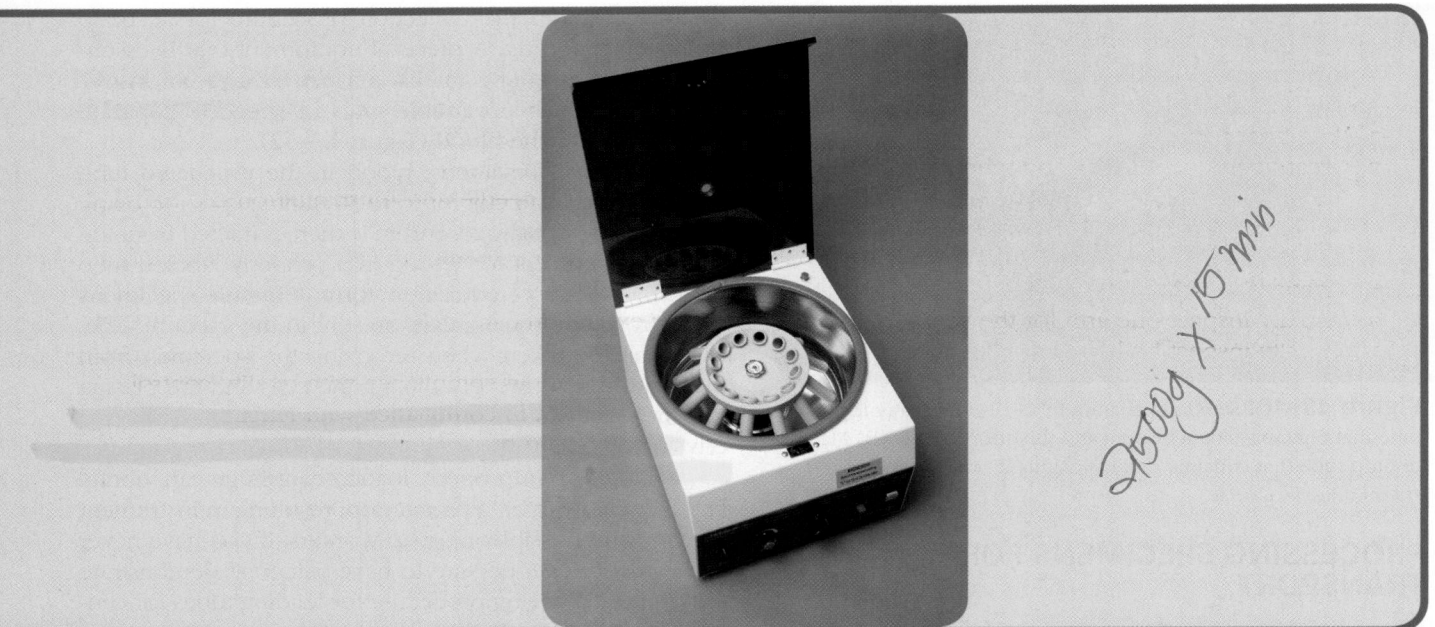

CHECK YOUR KNOWLEDGE

1. Which are the most ideal areas for capillary puncture on the hand?
   a. Ring finger and great finger
   b. Great finger, ring finger, and thumb
   c. Pinky finger, thumb, and great finger
   d. Any of the five fingers
2. What should you do prior to applying a tourniquet to a patient's arm?
   a. Visually inspect one arm for the vein
   b. Visually inspect both arms for the vein
   c. Ask the patient which site is preferred or best site
   d. Both b and c
3. To prepare the site for venipuncture, you should clean the site with alcohol and then do the following.
   a. Fan the site to dry the alcohol
   b. Have patient blow on the site to dry
   c. Blow on the site to dry
   d. None of the above
4. What is the first step for an MA to do if a patient faints when he or she is performing venipuncture?
   a. Remove the needle
   b. Remove the tourniquet
   c. Keep the needle and tourniquet on the arm and call for help
   d. None of the above
5. Why must an MA check all blood collection supplies for expiration date?
   a. To remain in compliance with quality assurance
   b. To remain in compliance with quality control
   c. To remain in compliance with HIPAA
   d. Both a and b

WEB LINKS

BD Medical Supplies (Becton, Dickinson, and Company): www.bd.com

Center for Phlebotomy Education: www.phlebotomy.com

Clinical Laboratory Standards Institute: www.clsi.org

Chapter 44

The Physician's Office Laboratory

OBJECTIVES

In this chapter, you will learn the following:

KB KNOWLEDGE BASE

1. Spell and define, using the glossary at the back of the text, all the Words to Know in this chapter.
2. Identify and describe the three laboratory classifications of testing under the Clinical Laboratory Improvement Amendments of 1988 (CLIA '88).
3. List and describe the regulatory bodies that govern the physician's office laboratory (POL).
4. List and describe the laboratory practices that yield quality assurance in the POL.
5. Define the terms *quality assurance* and *quality control*.
6. Describe guidelines for a well-managed and efficient POL.
7. Discuss safety precautions that should be taken when working in the POL.
8. Explain the general purpose of the microscope in a medical office.
9. Identify the parts of the microscope and the purpose of each.
10. Describe the proper way to adjust and focus the objectives and state their magnification powers.
11. Explain how to maintain the microscope properly.

S SKILLS

1. Properly use a microscope.

WORDS TO KNOW

binocular
compensate
condenser
control
high-power field (hpf)
low-power field (lpf)
magnify
minute
monocular
objectives
ocular
physician's office laboratory (POL)
provider-performed microscopy procedures (PPMP)
proficient
quality assurance (QA)
quality control (QC)
stage
waived

LABORATORY CLASSIFICATION AND REGULATION

The **physician's office laboratory (POL)** falls under many regulatory bodies. The complexity of the laboratory tests performed determines the classification of the POL and the body under which it will be regulated.

The three laboratory classifications under the Clinical Laboratory Improvement Amendments of 1988 (CLIA) are **waived**; moderately complex, including the subcategory of **provider-performed microscopy procedures (PPMP)**; and highly complex. The Centers for Medicare and Medicaid Services (CMS) regulate all laboratory testing performed on humans (except for clinical trials and basic research) through CLIA.

Other bodies that provide regulation inspections of a POL are CLIA, administered by the Centers for Medicare and Medicaid Services (CMS), and the Occupational Safety and Health Administration (OSHA). Private agencies also issue accreditation and state licensing for approved operation of the POL. The laboratory can be operated under a provisional certificate, which is issued until the Department of Health and Human Services (HHS) inspects the facility. Unannounced inspections of laboratory facilities can be made at any time. If OSHA, a separate entity from CMS, finds a POL in noncompliance of regulations during a visit, a monetary fine per item and per employee is applied.

All state and federal health and safety regulations and laws apply to the POL according to the three lab categorizations. It is important to stay abreast of current regulations applicable to the facility in which you are employed.

Categories of Testing

A certificate of waiver allows only those tests to be performed in a POL that are on the list of waived tests. The *waived* status is granted according to the difficulty in performing the diagnostic tests. Waived tests that can be performed in a medical office following package insert directions are basically those that have been manufactured for patient home testing and cleared by the Food and Drug Administration (FDA). The thought behind this category of tests is that the tests employ methodology that is so simple and accurate that an error in completion of the test or in the interpretation of the results would do no harm to the patient. Due to technology, this category of testing changes frequently, so consulting the Centers for Disease Control and Prevention (CDC) Website for governmental regulations is advisable (www.cdc.gov/dls/waivedtests). Generally speaking, nonautomated tests such as visual color comparison tests fall into the waived category.

> **CLINICAL PEARL**
>
> You can search for tests on the Food and Drug Administration's CLIA database at www.accessdata.fda.gov/scripts/cdrh/cfdocs/cfCLIA/search.cfm.

The application for the certificate of waiver is obtained from the CMS when the facility registers with this organization. Laboratory tests on the certificate of waiver list may be billed to Medicare and Medicaid for reimbursement. The certification must be renewed every two years for a published fee, and all tests performed by the medical assistant in the POL must be restricted to this list. CMS does not stipulate any specific staff requirements or proficiency tests, although it is stipulated that the laboratory must follow good laboratory practices, including quality assurance and quality control.

Moderately complex laboratory tests must be performed under more stringent regulations and with a more expanded requirement of personnel. For instance, CLIA mandates that the office must have a personnel director such as a physician who oversees the non-waived laboratory; testing personnel who are responsible for processing the specimens, monitoring the testing process for reliability, and reporting the results; a technical consultant who oversees all the testing performed in the facility; and a clinical consultant with a minimum of a doctoral degree. An error in the testing or reporting of tests in this category could endanger a patient's life—thus the additional requirements for patient safety.

Provider-performed microscopy procedures (PPMP) have several criteria for allowing testing to be performed by trained individuals other than laboratory personnel such as physicians, mid-level practitioners under the supervision of a physician or a dentist. The primary instrument, as you should be able to identify from the category of testing, is the microscope, limited to bright-field or phase-contrast microscopy.

Highly complex laboratory tests go beyond the preceding requirements in that the testing personnel must have very specific and specialized training to perform those tests. Testing of this nature would not typically be performed in a POL and is usually found in hospital laboratory settings and reference laboratories.

Quality Assurance

Regulatory bodies periodically inspect laboratories and medical offices to ensure quality assurance and quality control. **Quality assurance (QA)** in the health care field refers to all evaluative services and the results compared with accepted standards.

In the POL, no matter what the classification, the following practices must be followed to ensure reliable and accurate data and to ensure quality health care to the patients being served.

Quality assurance involves proper:

1. Patient identification.
2. Patient preparation and specimen collection.
3. Specimen processing and transportation.
4. Instrumental and technical performance.
5. Safety.
6. In-service training and education of all health care personnel.

All laboratories are required to follow quality assurance programs. The purposes of quality assurance programs are to evaluate the quality and effectiveness of health care according to accepted standards and to ensure accuracy and validity in testing procedures. When required, POLs must also participate in proficiency testing programs for the procedures they perform; additionally, strict records of quality control results, temperature readings, and maintenance logs are required.

Quality Control

Quality control (QC) is a process that assesses testing procedures, reagents, and technique of the person performing the tests. It is defined as a process that validates final test results and determines any variations. Quality control feeds directly into quality assurance in the laboratory setting because before any patient tests are performed and reported, the instruments and reagents are first tested with the QC material, with the results compared against standard results for these manufactured products. Results from the QC that do not fall within the prescribed parameters must be investigated and rectified to protect patients from receiving erroneous lab results and subsequent treatment.

Every laboratory, including the physician's office laboratory, is required by law to have a carefully performed, documented, and ongoing quality control program in place. This program assures both the physician and the patient that test results are accurate and is designed to discover and eliminate error.

The quality control program is designed to monitor all aspects of laboratory activity, including specimen collection and processing and the actual testing and reporting of results. It not only monitors the test procedure itself but also monitors reagents used in testing, the instruments, and personnel technique in performing tests.

Thorough and accurate records must be maintained on all equipment used to test patient samples. Temperatures must be checked daily and recorded in a log book on any refrigerators or freezers that store reagents and patient samples and incubators used for cultures. Automated equipment must be maintained according to the manufacturer's recommendations.

Each test kit used comes with a **control**, which is a sample with a known value range to be tested along with the patient specimen. The value range of the control can be a range of numbers or simply a positive or negative result. Controls are tested at specific intervals, usually according to manufacturer's directions. For example, a positive and negative control may be performed with each patient sample when using test kits, such as rapid strep and pregnancy tests (refer to the manufactures guidelines). Urine reagent strips should be checked daily and each time a new bottle is opened. Manufacturer's directions should be followed when performing control samples on all automated analyzers.

Carefully maintained records showing consistent and accurate control sample results ensure that test conditions, procedures, and results are accurate.

POL GUIDELINES

Guidelines for a well-managed and efficient POL include:

1. Following current state and federal regulations and keeping them on file.
2. Making sure files of correspondences and all other documents regarding the lab are up to date and accessible.
3. Maintaining all material safety data sheets (MSDS) regarding all chemicals, reagents, and solutions (such as isopropyl alcohol, disinfectants, and even correction fluid) in a notebook that is readily accessible to all employees.
4. Have a biohazard communications manual that includes:
   - A chemical hygiene plan (the employer's plan) to prevent employees from being exposed to dangerous chemicals.
   - A biohazard safety section that includes universal precaution techniques that conform to OSHA and CLIA regulations.
5. Retaining copies of all biohazard box or bag pickups per state regulation.
6. Keeping a log of all accidents and what was done for the person (i.e., who used the eye wash station and for what reason). The designated person enters this data on the OSHA log.
7. Placing all sharps, including intact needles and syringes (do not recap), into the biohazard sharps container.
8. Keeping long hair tied back securely and wearing only a minimum amount of jewelry.
9. Keeping a 10 percent bleach solution (made fresh daily) ready for cleanup of infectious wastes.

10. Recording all performed lab work in a log with the date, time, name of test, who performed it, the results, when it was sent to the reference lab, and when the results were received.
11. Clearly posting standard precautions for employees as a safety reminder.
12. Providing adequate lighting in all work areas.
13. Having a properly maintained fire extinguisher readily available and the directions for use clearly posted with it.
14. Keeping hallways and walking paths free of clutter.
15. Having fire and evacuation routes clearly posted.

SAFETY IN THE POL

The safety of all patients and health care providers is foremost regarding the collection of specimens. As you learned in previous chapters, prevention of disease is of vital importance in preparation for these clinical tasks. You must be alert and conscientious in the performance of your duties to avoid disease transmission. Remember to practice standard precautions, including proper hand washing, with each patient when you collect or handle a specimen. Hand washing is critical in preventing cross-contamination between patients, patients and health care workers, specimens and patients, and specimens and health care workers.

Credibility of each individual is challenged in compliance of standards and guidelines set by regulatory bodies. In most situations, you are the only one who will know if you did or did not follow standard precautions and quality assurance recommendations. You must keep your mind on your work and pay attention to detail to protect yourself and others from possible contamination. You must also focus on accuracy and efficiency of the procedures and charting of information. Expedient and efficient work practices do not mean that you should hurry and make patients feel the brunt of it. Using a methodical and a steady pace will help you in accomplishing a great deal of work in a reasonable amount of time.

Wearing Protective Barriers

Selecting and wearing appropriate personal protective equipment (PPE) is essential in infection control and contributing to a safe work environment. When collecting specimens from patients, the basic recommended PPE includes gloves, face shields, fluid-resistant lab coats, and respirators for airborne pathogens. Pay attention to proper fit when wearing protective barriers. If a gown is too large or too small, the purpose of the gown will be defeated. Latex or vinyl gloves should also fit snugly but not too tight or too loose. These simple problems can seem trivial points but could pose a problem situation and a safety risk. Gloves that are too small will most likely tear. Loose clothing or gloves could catch on something and be ripped or snagged, which could present a possible exposure to potentially infectious materials.

When working with specimens and recording information, you must be careful not to touch items that you would normally touch without gloves, such as light switches, door and drawer handles and pulls, phones, charts, and equipment. Develop the habit of completing one task at a time when possible. Complete the procedure that requires gloving and other personal protective equipment (PPE) and then record the results after you have removed the protective barriers. For example, if you are assisting with a sigmoidoscopy wearing PPE, complete the assisting, clean up, remove the contaminated barriers, and then perform the charting of the procedure. If you write in the patient's chart with the contaminated gloves still on, you will be contaminating everything you touch and possibly exposing others to biohazardous residue.

Appropriate Attire

Appropriate attire is a necessity as a medical assistant at all times. A reminder about jewelry and hairstyles must be discussed here for safety reasons. Excessive jewelry is not only inappropriate but could present a dangerous situation; for example, it could get caught on a piece of equipment or harbor pathogens in the crevices of the metal. When you are dealing with babies for their check-ups and often when they are ill, they can be tempted to pull at dangling earrings, necklaces, and bracelets. This is a danger for many reasons: The jewelry could break, which could result in an injury to both you and the child; the pathogens that are on the jewelry could be transmitted to you or the child; or you could transmit the microorganisms from one patient to another. Remember that you cannot see microorganisms without a microscope, but they are everywhere.

Another safety consideration is how you wear your hair. Both male and female medical assistants who have long hair must keep their hair worn back and secured because of a chance that a patient could grab your hair. Hair jewelry and ribbons should be conservative and, if worn, cleaned periodically to reduce the possibility of disease transmission. These seem to be remote possibilities but could actually happen, and it takes only one exposure to transmit diseases that are opportunistic. Remember: The health status of the patients is unknown in most cases. A patient can be susceptible and become infected with a microbe from the medical facility during a routine office call.

Keeping Immunizations Up to Date

When working in the medical field with patients, it makes good sense to be protected from every possible disease. Check with your family physician and find out whether you need any updating on your own immunizations. Staying current with immunizations is essential. For those who have respiratory conditions, having protection against pneumonia and influenza is also generally recommended.

If you are going to be working directly with patients and there is a risk of coming in contact with blood or other body fluids, you should receive the series of three HBV (hepatitis B virus) injections. The permanent record of this vaccine should be kept in your employee file. If you are hired in a new position in which you supposedly will not be in contact with patients and you have not received the HBV and your new employer states that it is not necessary for you to have the vaccine, the employer must sign a waiver regarding this. This signed document should also be kept in your employee file.

In addition, some individuals are allergic to the contents of the culture media of certain vaccines. If you are allergic, this should be documented also in your employee file. Refer to Figure 44-1 for an example statement to decline the administration of the HBV immunization.

THE MICROSCOPE

The microscope is an essential piece of equipment in the laboratory. It is used to examine and identify **minute** objects that cannot be seen with the naked eye.

The part of the microscope that supports the eyepiece is called the arm. Figure 44-2 shows the labeled parts of a **binocular** microscope. The proper way to carry the microscope is by grasping the arm with one hand and placing the other hand under the base, holding it at waist level. To secure a microscope while transporting it, the electrical cord for the light source should be loosely wrapped and secured with a twist tie or a rubber band. Wrapping the cord too tightly can cause the enclosed wires to break and lead to a short that could cause an electrical fire. The cord of the microscope should be kept loosely wrapped and out of the work area when not in use. It should always be unplugged by grasping the plug, never by pulling the cord. As when using any electrical appliance, all surrounding surfaces and hands should be dry. Wet hands or floors can lead to electric shock.

Parts of the Microscope

A binocular microscope has two eyepieces. The **monocular** microscope has only one eyepiece or ocular lens. The eyepiece or **ocular** lens is in the upper part of the tube of the microscope. The eyepiece contains a lens to **magnify** what is being seen.

The body tube leads to the revolving nosepiece. Attached to the revolving nosepiece are three (sometimes four) small lenses called **objectives**, each of which has a different magnifying power. The shortest has the lowest power. It is called the **low-power field (lpf)**. On most microscopes, it will magnify the object to be viewed 10 times or make it 10× larger than when viewed by the naked eye. The low-power field is the lens that

Wise Family Clinic
1234 Sunnyvale Road
Sunnyville, USA 98765
Phone: 555-444-1212
Fax: 555-444-2121

HEPATITIS B VACCINE DECLINATION DOCUMENT

I understand that due to my occupational exposure to blood or other potentially infectious body fluids and materials, I may be at risk of acquiring hepatitis B virus (HBV) infection. Through my employer, I have been offered the opportunity to be vaccinated with the hepatitis B vaccine at no expense to myself. I, however, decline the hepatitis B vaccination at this time. In declining this vaccination, I understand that I will continue to be at risk of acquiring hepatitis B, which is a serious disease. I also understand that if I continue to have occupational exposure to blood or other potentially infectious body fluids and materials and want to be vaccinated with the hepatitis B vaccination, I will be eligible to receive the vaccination series at no charge to me.

Employee Signature

Social Security Number

Witness Signature

Date

Figure 44–1: Example of an HBV declination document. *Delmar/Cengage Learning.*

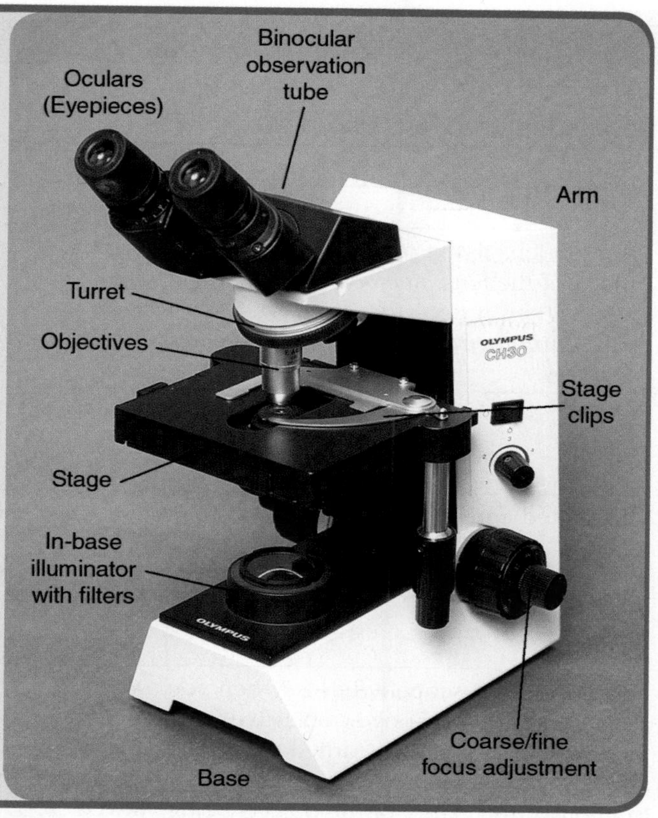

Figure 44–2: Binocular microscope with parts labeled. *Delmar/Cengage Learning.*

scans the field of interest and focuses in on the specimen. To position each objective, you simply rotate the nosepiece until you hear a click.

For greater detail in viewing the specimen, turn the nosepiece to the next longer objective, the **high-power field (hpf)**. It will magnify the object approximately 40 times, or 40×. The longest objective is the oil-immersion objective. This high-power lens, when used with oil, magnifies objects about 100 times, or 100×. Using the fine-focus dial brings the specimen into good definition.

The **stage** of the microscope has two clips that hold the specimen slide to be viewed. Just underneath the stage is a substage where a **condenser** is held that regulates the amount of light directed on the magnified specimen. It has a shutter or diaphragm to control the amount of light desired. The substage may be raised or lowered in focusing on the specimen.

A supply of lens paper should be kept nearby to clean the lenses after each use. Makeup, oil, secretions from the eyes, and dust can make it difficult to see through the lens, besides being a possible means of transmitting disease among office personnel. Because several individuals in a medical office might use the microscope, it is advised to wipe the eyepieces with a disinfectant after each use to avoid the transmission of diseases. Eyeglasses are not necessary when performing microscopic work because the microscope can be focused to **compensate** for all visual defects except astigmatism.

It takes time and patience to learn how to operate the microscope. The supervision of an experienced operator is essential to becoming **proficient** in its use and care. Refer to Procedure 44–1.

Care of the Microscope

Microscopes are fine and expensive technical instruments that must be handled with great respect. The operation and care manual should be kept handy for reference because each microscope is slightly different. The amount of routine maintenance required varies with the amount of use. Each POL must keep a maintenance log of all equipment. Routine inspection and maintenance should be recorded in this maintenance log with information regarding what was done, when it was done, and the agency that did the required labor to fix it. All maintenance forms or documents should be kept on file.

PROCEDURE 44–1 Use a Microscope

PURPOSE: To gain skill in the use of the microscope. Provided with all necessary equipment and supplies, demonstrate the use of the microscope following the steps in the procedure with the instructor observing each step.

EQUIPMENT: Microscope, electrical outlet for light source of microscope, specimen on disposable glass slide with frosted end, cover glass (used usually for wet specimens only), lens cleaning tissues, latex or vinyl gloves

S SKILL: Use a microscope properly.

(continues)

(continued)

Procedure Steps	Detailed Instructions and/or *Rationales*
1. Wash hands and put on latex or vinyl gloves.	
2. Assemble the necessary equipment.	
3. Clean the ocular lens with lens cleaning tissues.	Use only lens tissue paper to prevent damaging the surface of the lens. *Removal of makeup, oil, and eye secretions is necessary to ensure clear viewing and eliminate transmission of disease among office personnel.*
4. Plug the microscope light source into an electrical outlet and turn on the light switch at the front base of the microscope.	
5. Place the specimen slide on the stage with the frosted end up between the clips and secure it over the opening of the stage.	The frosted end is used for labeling the specimen in pencil.
6. Watch carefully as you raise the substage so that it does not come in direct contact with the slide.	
7. Turn the revolving nosepiece to low-power objective (10×) and begin to focus the coarse-adjustment dial until a wide shaft can be seen.	Regarding microscope lighting: When you switch from a lower- to a higher-power objective (or vice versa), the light will need to be turned up. The light source should be kept at a fairly low level for each objective to improve the clarity of the objects being viewed. Too much light can have a bleaching or glaring effect, and the object might not be seen at all or at least not be seen well.
8. When the outline of the specimen is in view, turn the fine-adjustment dial until the specimen can be seen in detail.	
9. Adjust the substage diaphragm level or adjust the mirror to obtain proper lighting.	
10. If sharper detail is needed, carefully turn the revolving nosepiece to the intermediate-power objective and adjust the fine-focus dial.	
11. When using the oil-immersion lens objective, oil should be used very sparingly.	A disposable cover slide should be used, and the lens must be cleaned after each use. Adjustment must be made for the amount of light needed by adjusting the diaphragm lever under the stage.
12. When the specimen has been identified, turn off the light and return all items to the proper storage area. The microscope stage should be cleaned and recorded in the maintenance log.	Results of the actual examination should be read and recorded in the laboratory test log by the physician. The medical assistant is responsible for assisting with the preparation of the specimen for microscopic examination unless otherwise instructed by the physician.
13. Remove gloves and wash hands.	

CHAPTER SUMMARY

- The three laboratory classifications of testing under the Clinical Laboratory Improvement Amendments of 1988 (CLIA '88) are waived, moderately complex, and highly complex.
- In addition to CLIA '88, other bodies that provide regulation inspections of a POL are the Centers for Medicare and Medicaid Services (CMS), the Occupational Safety and Health Administration (OSHA), private agencies, and the Department of Health and Human Services (HHS). All state and federal health and safety regulations and laws apply to the POL according to the three lab categorizations.
- All laboratories are required to follow quality assurance programs. The purposes of quality assurance programs are to evaluate the quality and effectiveness of health care according to accepted standards and to ensure accuracy and validity in testing procedures.
- Quality assurance involves proper (1) patient identification; (2) patient preparation and specimen collection; (3) specimen processing and transportation; (4) instrumental and technical performance; (5) safety; and (6) in-service training and education of all health care personnel.
- Every laboratory, including the physician office laboratory, is required by law to have a carefully performed, documented, and ongoing quality control program in place. Quality control is a process that assesses testing procedures, reagents, and technique of the person performing the tests.
- There are many guidelines to running an efficient and well-managed POL. Always remember to practice standard precautions with each patient when you collect or handle a specimen.
- Pay attention to proper fit when wearing protective barriers. Also be careful not to touch items that you would normally touch without gloves. Excessive jewelry and long hair not pulled back are not only inappropriate when working as a medical assistant but could also present a dangerous situation.
- In addition to following safety precautions, check with your family physician and find out whether you need any updating on your own immunizations. Staying current with immunizations is essential.
- The microscope is an essential piece of equipment in the laboratory, which takes time and patience to learn to use properly.

STUDY TOOLS

Workbook	Activities for Chapter 44
Premium Website	
StudyWARE	Activities and Quizzes on the **StudyWARE™ Software** for Chapter 44
	Audio Library of medical terms
	Online access to the **Critical Thinking Challenge 2.0**
CourseMate	Activities and Quizzes for Chapter 44
WebTutor	Activities and Quizzes for Chapter 44

CHECK YOUR KNOWLEDGE

1. The *waived* status is granted according to what?
   a. The tests cleared by the DFA
   b. That the tests are manufactured for clinical use only
   c. The difficulty in performing the diagnostic tests and whether they can be performed in a medical office following package insert directions
   d. The amount of time it takes to perform the diagnostic tests
2. Which of the following properly describes inspections of laboratory facilities?
   a. May be made unannounced at any time
   b. A monetary fine per item may be assessed on the clinic if a violation is found
   c. A monetary fine per employee is applied if a violation is found
   d. All of the above

3. Why should the operation and care manual for the microscope be kept?
   a. It does not need to be kept
   b. Only one needs to be kept because all microscopes are the same
   c. It needs to be kept because it is a HIPAA standard
   d. It needs to be kept because all microscopes are slightly different
4. How many injections are involved with the hepatitis B vaccine?
   a. 2
   b. 3
   c. 4
   d. None of the above
5. High-power field, without oil submersion, magnifies objects by:
   a. 40 times.
   b. 50 times.
   c. 75 times.
   d. 20 times.
6. Low-power field magnifies objects by:
   a. 5 times.
   b. 10 times.
   c. 15 times.
   d. 20 times.

WEB LINKS

Occupational Safety & Health Administration: www.osha.gov

Centers for Disease Control and Prevention: www.cdc.gov

Clinical Laboratory Improvement Amendments: wwwn.cdc.gov/clia/default.aspx

FDA's CLIA database: www.accessdata.fda.gov/scripts/cdrh/cfdocs/cfClia/Search.cfm

Chapter 45 Diagnostic Testing

OBJECTIVES

In this chapter, you will learn the following:

KB KNOWLEDGE BASE

1. Spell and define, using the glossary at the back of the text, all the Words to Know in this chapter.
2. Differentiate between normal and abnormal results for common diagnostic tests performed in the POL.
3. Identify panic values for diagnostic test results.
4. Describe how the erythrocyte sedimentation rate is useful in diagnoses.
5. Explain the purpose of the glucose tolerance test (GTT).
6. Define and describe the indications for the hemoglobin A1C test.
7. Identify common immunology tests ordered by health care providers and how they are used in diagnoses.
8. Describe scratch, patch, and intradermal skin tests and state their purpose.
9. Describe patient education concerning allergies and treatment.
10. Explain the need for collecting a PKU test and describe the proper collection procedure for the specimen.
11. Differentiate between a properly collected and improperly collected PKU blood specimen.

S SKILLS

1. Perform a hemoglobin test on a blood specimen and document the quality control(s) for the test.
2. Perform a hematocrit test on a blood specimen.
3. Perform an erythrocyte sedimentation rate (ESR).
4. Perform a glucose test on a blood specimen and document the quality control(s) for the test.
5. Perform a hemoglobin A1C screening on a blood sample.
6. Perform an infectious mononucleosis screening on a blood sample.
7. Review a laboratory report for blood studies and make notations about whether the results are normal, abnormal, or panic value and follow up.

B BEHAVIORS

1. Display sensitivity to patients' rights and feelings in collecting specimens.
2. Explain the rationale for performance of a procedure to the patient.
3. Show awareness of patients' concerns regarding their perceptions of the procedure being performed.

WORDS TO KNOW

adrenalin
adverse
allergy
allosteric protein
anaphylactic
anemia
antibody
antigen
cholesterol
complete blood count (CBC)
contact dermatitis

pale skin
SOB
tiredness

desensitizing
eosinophil
epinephrine
extract
gestational diabetes
glucose
glycohemoglobin
glycosylation
histamine
hypersensitive
immune
immunology
immunoassays
infectious mononucleosis
interpreted
ketone (acetone)
metabolism
microhematocrit
morphology
panic value
percentage
phenylalanine
phenylketonuria (PKU)
polycythemia
RAST
reagent
systemic
venom
WBC differential
wheal

QUALITY CONTROL AND QUALITY ASSURANCE

Very important to the integrity of diagnostic test results is for you to perform the quality controls at the beginning of each day and log the results prior to reporting any patient results. Also, if you have to open a new bottle of reagent strips during the day, you might need to calibrate the instrument, change the code to agree with what is printed on the bottle, and repeat the quality controls. This helps ensure that both the meter and the reagents are working properly so that you do not provide inaccurate results.

With strict regulations regarding quality control and quality assurance, you are required to keep a log book to record all specimens and the results of the tests performed. The log should include:

1. Date.
2. Patient's name.
3. Test performed.
4. Results of the test.
5. Your initials.
6. Any kit, reagent strip, or **reagent** lot numbers and expiration dates.
7. Quality control results.

HEMATOLOGY TESTING

Recall information you learned on the circulatory system and the blood. Remember that:

- The red blood cells are filled with hemoglobin, making their primary function delivering oxygen to the cells and picking up carbon dioxide to be exhaled.
- The chief function of the white blood cells is to protect the body against invaders such as bacteria and viruses. The granulocytes engulf bacteria and debris, as do the monocytes. The lymphocytes produce antibodies against specific antigens, usually viruses.
- The platelets, with other clotting factors, stop bleeding when an injury occurs.

There are several automated hematology instruments on the market that are relatively inexpensive and easy to operate. These instruments have the capability of measuring:

- Total red blood cell count.
- Total white blood cell count.
- Total platelet count.
- Hemoglobin.

CLINICAL PEARL

Many patients can be frightened or confused about some of the laboratory procedures requested by the health care provider to aid in diagnosis. You might perform some of these in the office or clinic setting or send the patient to the lab for tests. If you send patients elsewhere, make sure you give accurate directions on how to get there.

Each test or procedure must be explained clearly and concisely to relieve patients' anxiety. Use language that patients understand. Most people have little or no knowledge of medical terminology.

Certain lab tests require preparation by patients prior to arrival (e.g., fasting or taking or omitting certain medications). Be sure to instruct patients in these preparations and have clear, concise, written instructions available. Do not presume that patients know all about a procedure even if they have had the test before. Often, new techniques require additional or different instructions for preparation. Medical technology is constantly changing. It is important for all health care personnel (including medical assistants) to keep abreast of new developments in medicine. Inform patients that some procedures can cause temporary discomfort and tell them how it may be relieved.

Give patients enough time to look over the printed instruction sheet or pamphlet and make certain you answer all of their questions thoroughly before they leave.

- Hematocrit.
- Total granulocyte count.
- Total lymphocyte and monocyte count.
- Percentage of granulocytes.
- Percentage of lymphocytes and monocytes.
- Red blood cell indices.

Hemoglobin

Hemoglobin and hematocrit screening tests require a small amount of blood, most often capillary blood. Hemoglobin (Hgb or Hb) is an **allosteric protein** found in erythrocytes, which transports molecular oxygen in the blood to the cells of the body. The red blood cells circulate to deposit the oxygen and carry away carbon dioxide as a waste product. One quick and easy method for measuring a patient's hemoglobin is the use of a hemoglobinometer (Figure 45–1A). Older technologies made this procedure a more tedious process, but today, instrumentation has advanced to the point that a drop of blood is applied to a card, and in a short period of time (usually less than one minute), a result is displayed (Figure 45–1B). Refer to Procedure 45–1 for performing this important screening test.

Because hemoglobin is essential to oxygen circulation in the body, it is important for you to be familiar with the normal ranges for hemoglobin for males and females in case you need to contact the health care provider immediately. **Anemia** is the medical term given when a patient's circulating erythrocytes are deficient. The normal range of hemoglobin for males is 14 to 18 g/dL; for females, the range is 12 to 16 g/dL. When a patient's hemoglobin falls below 10 g/dL, the patient can experience shortness of breath and tiredness and have a pale appearance to his or her skin. It is generally accepted that a hemoglobin result of less than 5 g/dL is not compatible with life; it is doubtful you would come across a result such as this in the ambulatory health care setting.

However, when taking results by phone from other laboratory facilities, a report of a very low hemoglobin could be reported, so you should be aware that this result would be considered a **panic value**. A panic value always requires immediate intervention by the health care provider. Although most attention is given when a patient's hemoglobin is low, another condition, **polycythemia**, needs to be considered in patient screening. When a patient experiences polycythemia, the bone marrow is producing too many red blood cells, and the patient most likely will experience weakness and fatigue. Other symptoms include redness of the skin, pain in the extremities, and what appears to be bruising. When a patient has profound anemia, a blood transfusion might be indicated to increase the circulating red blood cells; a patient with polycythemia might need to have a unit of blood withdrawn to provide relief of the symptoms.

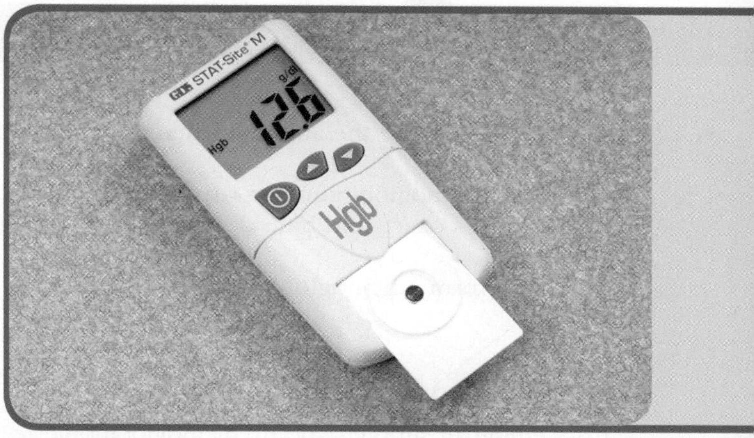

Figure 45–1B: Results from performing a hemoglobin test on capillary blood. *Delmar/Cengage Learning.*

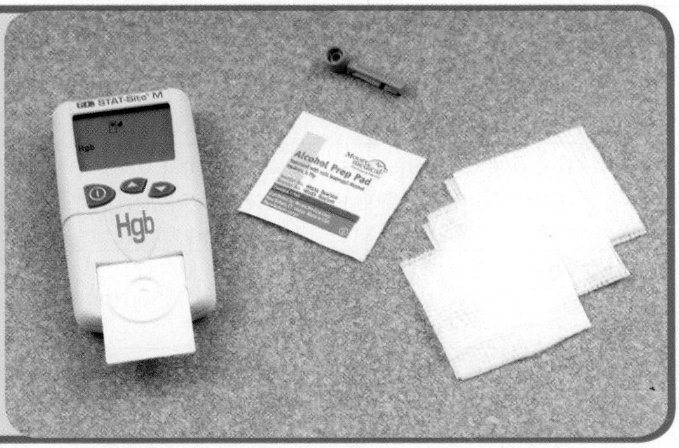

Figure 45–1A: A handheld hemoglobinometer that is commonly found in the physician office laboratory. *Delmar/Cengage Learning.*

Hematocrit

The hematocrit (Hct) is another hematology test, not used as commonly now as it was in recent years, that screens patients for anemia. Very small glass or plastic tubes are used for the testing procedure (Figure 45–2A); the hematocrit performed in this manner is referred to as a **microhematocrit**. Either capillary blood or venous blood may be used for this test. Most of the tubes are marked approximately three fourths of the way up the tube to prevent overfilling of the tube; the tubes are designed to draw by capillary action so that no additional equipment is needed for aspirating the blood into the tubes. After the tubes are filled, a small amount of clay sealant closes one end of the tube so the blood

PROCEDURE 45–1 Determine Hemoglobin Using a Hemoglobinometer

PURPOSE: To measure the amount of hemoglobin (Hbg or Hb) in the circulating blood

EQUIPMENT: Hemoglobinometer, reagent card, sterile lancet, cotton balls or gauze, alcohol, gloves, work surface, patient's chart, and blue or black pen or electronic medical record

S **SKILL:** Perform a hemoglobin determination.

Procedure Steps	Detailed Instructions and/or *Rationales*
1. Assemble all supplies and the hemoglobinometer; place them on a secure work surface.	
B 2. Identify the patient. Explain the procedure to the patient, ***including the rationale for performing the procedure, using language and verbal skills the patient can understand. Show awareness of patients' concerns regarding their perceptions of the procedure by answering any questions the patient might have and assisting the patient into a comfortable position before you proceed.***	*Speaking to the patient by name as well as checking the chart ensures that you are performing the proper procedure on the correct patient.*
3. Wash hands and don gloves.	
4. Perform a capillary puncture.	Follow the desired capillary puncture procedure as outlined in Procedure 43–1.
5. Place a large, beaded drop of blood on the reagent card while making sure the instrument is on. Wipe the patient's finger with a cotton ball or dry gauze and have the patient apply pressure to the site of the puncture.	
6. After the instrument displays the results, chart this in the patient's medical record.	The results should be expressed as [the number] g/dL.
7. Dispose of the lancet in the biohazard sharps containers. Dispose of the remaining soiled articles in the biohazard trash container.	
B 8. ***Take care of the patient's needs*** once it is determined that the patient does not have an allergy to adhesives, and put a bandage over puncture site.	
9. Record the results, as well as the quality control sample results, in the log book.	Refer to the package insert to ascertain that the controls are within the prescribed range set by the manufacturer.

Charting Example

10/9/XX 11:30 am	Capillary puncture of Lt. middle finger performed for Hbg. Results: 14.3 g/dL. Roger Wong, CMA(AAMA)

Log Book Example

Date	Patient's Name	Test	Results	Performed by
10/9/XX	Melody C. Jones	Hbg	14.3 g/dL	RW
10/9/XX	High control	Hbg	19.8 g/dL	RW
10/9/XX	Low control	Hbg	7.6 g/dL	RW

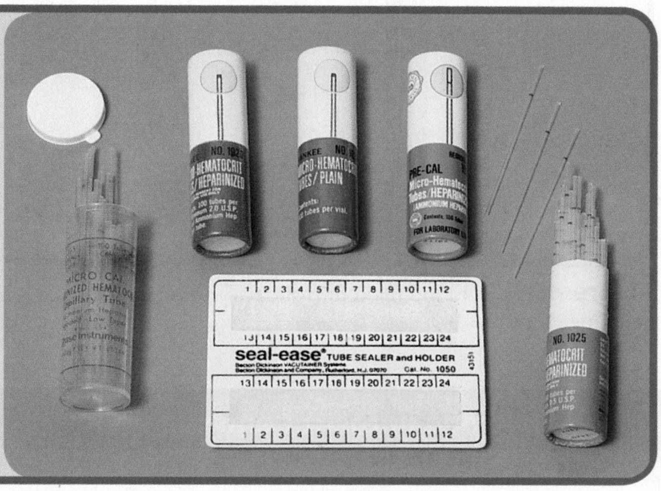

Figure 45–2A: Sample of microhematocrit (capillary blood) tubes with clay sealant. *Delmar/Cengage Learning.*

Red tube - heparinised

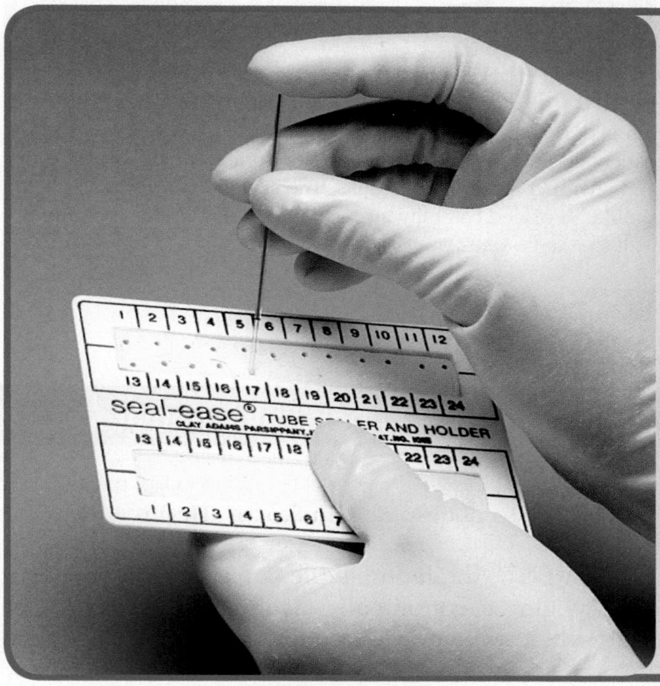

Figure 45–2B: Before placing the glass tube that is filled to the line with capillary blood in the microhematocrit centrifuge, carefully push the glass tube into the clay to seal one end. *Delmar/Cengage Learning.*

does not leak out during the centrifugation process (Figure 45–2B). Be sure that you have adequately sealed the tube prior to centrifuging, or the blood can be spun out of the tube, resulting in no measurement of the hematocrit value. Microhematocrits should always be collected in duplicate with the results between the two readings averaged for the result.

The tubes are then placed in a microhematocrit centrifuge, commonly called a *microfuge*, as seen in Figure 45–3. The tubes are centrifuged at a very high speed for a relatively short period of time, usually not more than five minutes; the process of centrifuging separates the cell components, with the erythrocytes going to the bottom of the tube because they are heaviest and the plasma migrating to the top. In the middle of the tube is a very thin layer known as the *buffy coat* that contains the leukocytes and platelets (Figure 45–4).

The hematocrit is always expressed as a **percentage** of the total blood volume, and what you are measuring and recording is the percentage of packed red blood cells in the microhematocrit tube as compared with the rest of the blood sample. The normal hematocrit range for adult males is 40 percent to 54 percent; the adult female range is 37 percent to 47 percent. (Refer to Procedure 45–2).

Hematocrits are read by looking down onto the tube against the values chart within the centrifuge. Refer to Figure 45–5 for a closer look into the centrifuge to understand how the measurement is read. After the tubes have been centrifuged, the readings are performed by placing the sealed end of the tube against the padding or gasket, making certain that where the clay ends is at the 0 point of the reader. Read the hematocrit at the bottom end of the meniscus, although with most microhematocrit tubes, the meniscus is not obvious. Use of a magnifying lens to

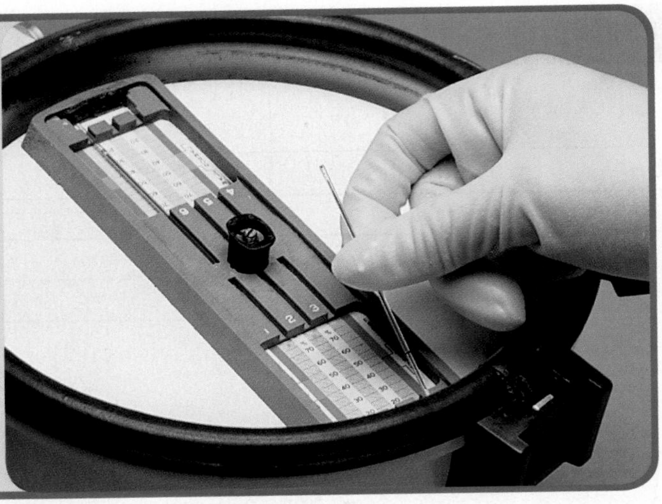

Figure 45–3: Up to six microhematocrit tubes can be centrifuged at once in grooved slots. Make sure to write down the patient's name and corresponding slot number to avoid confusion and incorrect reporting of results. The sealed end of the tube should be placed carefully against the padding of the centrifuge wall. *Delmar/Cengage Learning.*

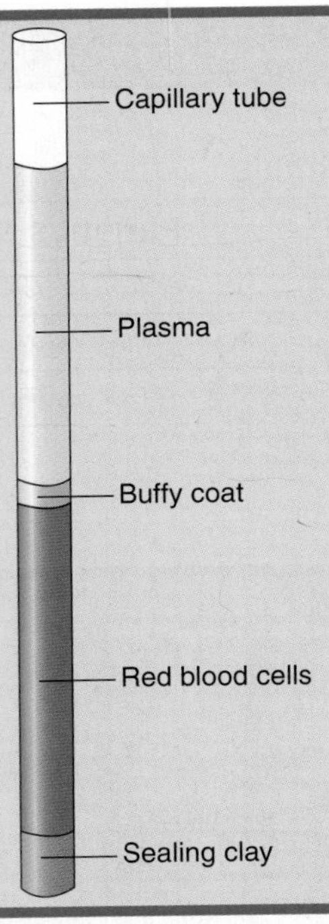

Figure 45–4: A blood-filled microhematocrit tube after centrifugation. *Delmar/Cengage Learning.*

PROCEDURE 45–2 Determine Hematocrit (Hct) Using a Microhematocrit Centrifuge

PURPOSE: To determine hematocrit (Hct) readings using the microhematocrit centrifuge

EQUIPMENT: Autolet or sterile lancet, microhematocrit tubes, sealing clay, microhematocrit centrifuge, latex or vinyl gloves, cotton balls, alcohol, patient's chart, pen (if hemoglobin is done by this procedure, conversion chart will also be needed to determine Hb), and Table 45–1

S **SKILL:** Determine hematocrit (Hct) readings by using the microhematocrit centrifuge.

Procedure Steps	Detailed Instructions and/or *Rationales*
1. Assemble the needed items on a Mayo table. Check to see that the centrifuge is plugged into the electrical outlet.	
B 2. Identify the patient. Explain the procedure to the patient, ***including the rationale for performing the procedure, using language and verbal skills the patient can understand. Show awareness of patients' concerns regarding their perceptions of the procedure by answering any questions the patient might have and assisting the patient into a comfortable position before you proceed.***	*Speaking to the patient by name as well as checking the chart ensures that you are performing the proper procedure on the correct patient.*
3. Wash hands and don gloves.	

Procedure Steps	Detailed Instructions and/or *Rationales*
4. Perform a capillary puncture.	Follow the desired capillary puncture procedure as outlined in Procedure 43–1.
5. Hold the microhematocrit tube as you would hold a pencil or pen, horizontally with the opening next to the drop of blood that appears at the puncture site. Hold the tip of a gloved finger over the Hct tube to keep blood from flowing out. Obtain as many tubes as ordered.	*Holding the tube horizontally slightly tilted downward assists the flow of blood to enter the tube by capillary action until it reaches the fill line or three quarter point.* Avoid bubbles in the capillary tube(s). Usually one or two tubes are ordered.
6. Wipe the outside end of the glass tube with a gauze square while still holding it horizontally. Carefully seal *only one end* of the tube by placing it into the clay and turning it until the entire end is solid clay. You may leave the tube standing up in the tray until you are finished tending to the needs of the patient.	Note: When sealing one end of the tube, do not apply too much pressure or the glass tube will break. Only a very small amount of clay is needed.
7. Have the patient hold a dry gauze square on the puncture site. Make sure bleeding has stopped; offer the patient a bandage.	
8. Secure the sealed end of the tube against the rubber padding in the centrifuge (clay end of tube is always toward you). Balance the centrifuge with another tube opposite it.	If two or more patients' tubes are placed in the centrifuge at the same time, make sure that you note the numbers of the spaces to avoid a mix-up. *Accurate identification is essential to assigning results to the proper patients.*
9. Close the inside cover carefully over the tubes and lock it into place by turning the dial clockwise. Then close and lock the outside cover. Listen for it to click into place.	
10. Turn the timer switch to 3 to 5 minutes. It will automatically turn off. Wait until the centrifuge has completely stopped spinning and unlock both covers.	Most timing switches indicate that you turn past the desired time and then back to the time you want set. *Opening a centrifuge before it stops spinning is very dangerous—centrifugal force pulls objects such as hair, jewelry, or loose sleeves of lab coats into it.*
11. Accurately read the results.	Read the results by placing the bottom line of packed RBCs (up to buffy coat but not including it) against the calibrated chart in the centrifuge where the tube is resting. There is usually a magnifying glass attached to the centrifuge to assist in reading Hct accurately. Keep the cover of the centrifuge closed when not in use.
12. Discard used items in the proper waste receptacles, remove gloves, and wash hands.	
13. Record the reading in the patient's chart and on the log sheet.	The results should be expressed as a percentage.
14. Return items to the proper storage areas.	

Charting Example

4-21-XX	Finger stick of L ring finger for capillary blood for Hct—reading is 47%. S. Davis, RMA(AMT)

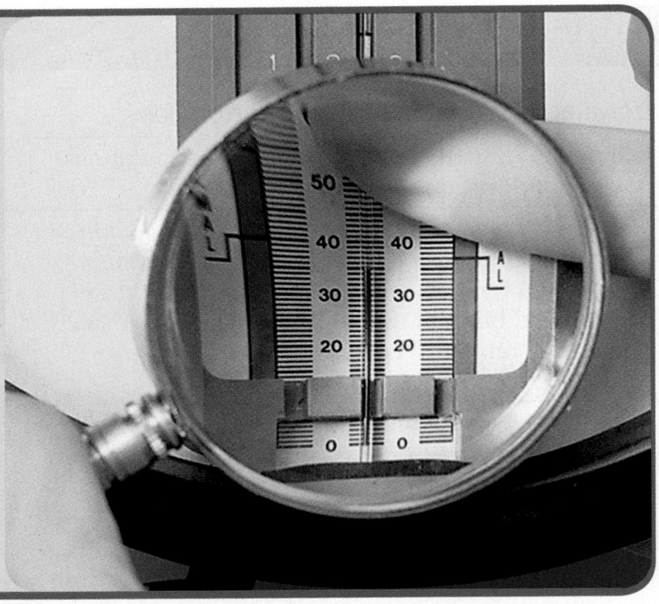

Figure 45–5: A hematocrit reading can be obtained by looking down onto the tube against the values chart within the centrifuge. The reading is obtained after centrifugation by placing the sealed end against the padding and reading the hematocrit at the bottom of the meniscus. The reading in the photo is 35 percent.
Delmar/Cengage Learning.

read the hematocrit is advised for accuracy in reporting the results (Figure 45–5). There are also microhematocrit readers that are not built within the centrifuge, but these are more complicated to use. Remember to measure both tubes and average the results for reporting. You can also roughly calculate what the hemoglobin for that patient might be by dividing the hematocrit value by 3; for example, a patient with a hematocrit value of 45 percent would have a hemoglobin of approximately 15 g/dL. Conversely, you could take the hemoglobin value for a patient and multiply it by 3 for an estimate of the hematocrit value—for example, a hemoglobin of 12 g/dL should yield a result of 36 percent plus or minus 3 percent (refer to Table 45–1).

Complete Blood Count

Many factors go into interpreting results from what is commonly known as the **complete blood count**, or **CBC**, one of the more common tests ordered in health care providers' offices. When a health care provider looks at the total red blood cell count, the hemoglobin, hematocrit, and indices are also considered for the big picture. Although the total white blood cell count is reviewed, the ratios or percentages of the granulocytes to the lymphocytes or monocytes is considered because

TABLE 45–1 Approximate Relationship between Hematocrit and Red Blood Cell Count and Hemoglobin in Adults

For Red Blood Cells of Normal Size—To Be Used for Checking Purposes Only*		
Hematocrit %	**Red Blood Cell Count (× 1 million per millimeter of blood)**	**Hemoglobin (in grams per 100 mL)**
30	3.4	9.8
31	3.6	10.4
32	3.7	10.7
33	3.8	11.0
34	3.9	11.3
35	4.0	11.6
36	4.1	11.9
37	4.3	12.4
38	4.4	12.8
39	4.5	13.1
40	4.6	13.3
41	4.7	13.6
42	4.8	13.9
43	4.9	14.2
44	5.1	14.8
45	5.2	15.1
46	5.3	15.4
47	5.4	15.7
48	5.5	16.0

Hematocrit %	Red Blood Cell Count (× 1 million per millimeter of blood)	Hemoglobin (in grams per 100 mL)
49	5.6	16.2
50	5.7	16.5
51	5.9	17.1
52	6.0	17.4
53	6.1	17.7
54	6.2	18.0
55	6.3	18.3
56	6.4	18.6
57	6.6	19.1
58	6.7	19.4
59	6.8	19.7
60	6.9	20.1
61	7.0	20.3
NORMAL HEMATOCRITS	NORMAL RED BLOOD CELL COUNTS	NORMAL HEMOGLOBINS
Men:	Men:	Men:
Range	Range	Range
40–54%	4,600,000–6,200,000	14.0–18.0 grams
Aver. 47%	Aver. 5,400,000	Aver. 15.8 grams
Women:	Women:	Women:
Range	Range	Range
37–47%	4,200,000–5,400,000	11.5–16.0 grams
Aver. 42%	Aver. 4,800,000	Aver. 13.9 grams

**The relationship shown between hematocrit and red blood cell count is based on normal cells (which have an average mean corpuscular volume of 0.87). The relationship between hemoglobin and red blood cell count is based on normal cells (with a mean corpuscular hemoglobin of 29). These relationships do not hold true in cases of microcytic or macrocytic anemias, which probably will not be more than 5% to 10% of blood examined by clinical laboratories and blood banks.*

these cells protect the body in different ways. Generally speaking, consider the following when reviewing a CBC.

- The normal total red blood cell count for an adult male is 4.5 to 6.0 million per millimeter. A decrease in the total number of red blood cells constitutes a type of anemia.
- The normal total red blood cell count for an adult female is 4.0 to 5.5 million per millimeter. A decrease in the total number of red blood cells constitutes a type of anemia.
- The normal total platelet count for males and females is 150,000 to 400,000 per millimeter.
- The normal total white blood cell count for males and females is 3,500 to 11,000 per millimeter. When the WBC count is elevated, it indicates a disease process of some type, whether it is an infection or a precursor to leukemia. When the WBC is decreased, the patient could be immunocompromised due to HIV or AIDS infection or current cancer therapy in the form of chemotherapy or radiation treatments. When the WBC count is decreased, the patient is more prone to opportunistic infections because immunity is compromised.
- The granulocyte ratio should be larger than the lymphocyte/monocyte ratio. The normal percentage range for granulocytes is 50 percent to 70 percent with the lymphocyte/monocyte percentage generally in the 20 percent to 40 percent range.

The WBC Differential

The **WBC differential** is a count performed on 100 white blood cells and differentiates the various types seen in that representative sample. The numbers of neutrophils, eosinophils, basophils, monocytes, and lymphocytes are counted and, during this screening, the technician reviews the slide for abnormalities of the red blood cells such as in size and shape, referred to as **morphology**. Often, premature white or red blood cells are seen on the differential slide that indicate disease processes such as leukemia.

CLINICAL PEARL

Medical assistants are not trained to perform these counts, but it is useful for you to have an idea of what such a report entails.

Refer to Figure 45–6 for an illustration of how cells become mature and how they appear upon maturity. Table 45–2 provides a specific description of the function of each of the cells counted in a WBC differential. For the differential count to be performed, a slide must be prepared and stained for examination under the microscope. Many laboratories use an automated slide preparer as well as an automated staining apparatus. Because the cells cannot be differentiated into their categories without staining, laboratories use either the Wright's stain or the Giemsa stain prior to reviewing the slides under the oil immersion lens of the microscope.

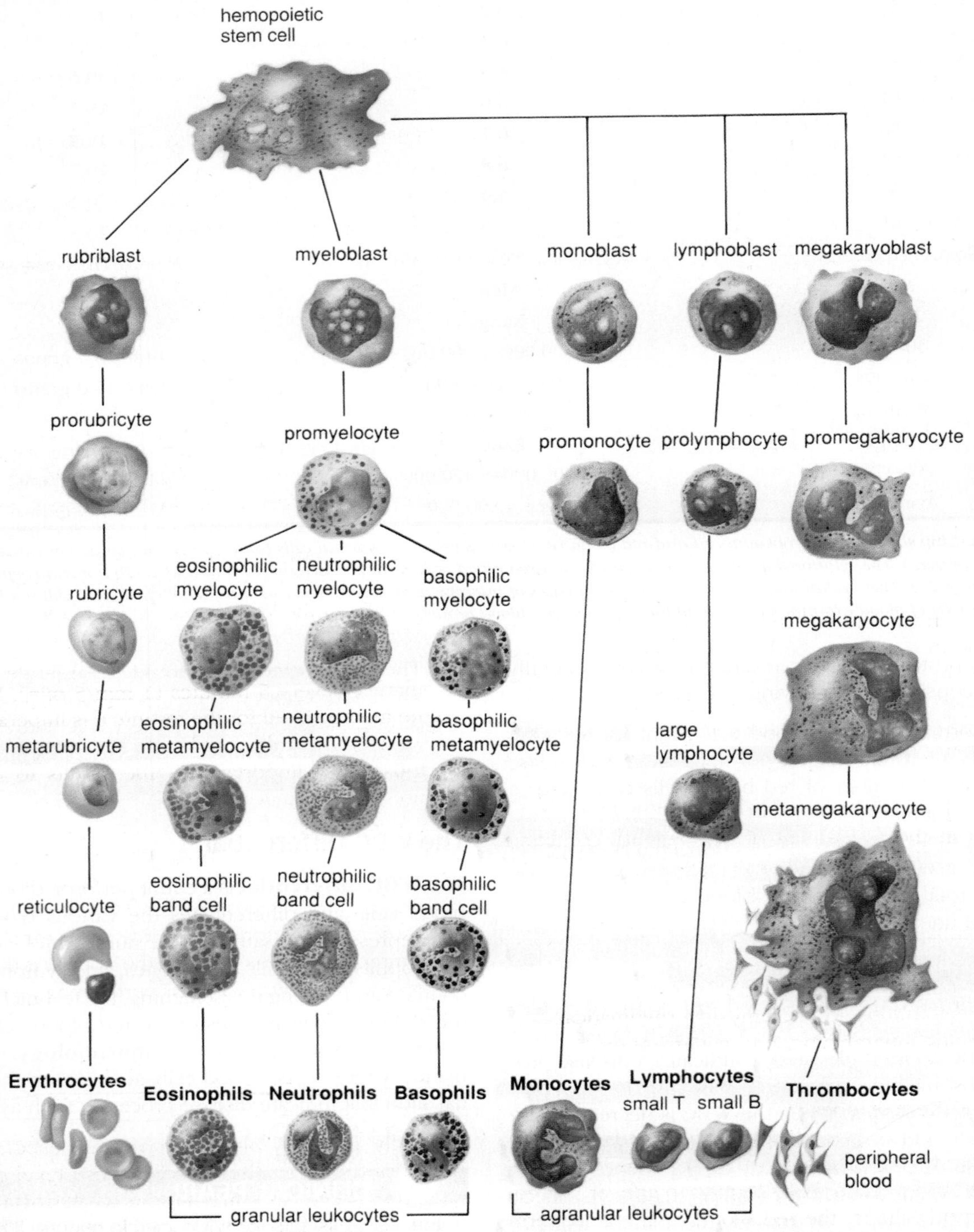

Figure 45–6: Chart of blood cells and platelets from stem cell to maturity. *Delmar/Cengage Learning.*

TABLE 45–2 Categories of White Blood Cells and Their Functions

White Cell Type	Percent in Normal WBC	Function
Granulocytes		
Neutrophils		Phagocytosis and killing of bacteria; release of pyrogen that produces fever
Segmented	56 ± 10	
Band	3 ± 2	
Eosinophils	2.7 ± 2	Phagocytosis of antigen-antibody complexes; killing of parasites
Basophils	0.3 ± 1	Release of chemical mediators of immediate hypersensitivity
Lymphocytes	34 ± 10	
B lymphocytes		Humoral immunity; production of specific antibodies against viruses, bacteria, and other proteins
T lymphocytes		Cell-mediated immunity, including delayed hypersensitivity and graft rejection; regulation of immune response
Monocytes	4 ± 3	Phagocytosis of microorganisms and cell debris; cooperation in immune response

Erythrocyte Sedimentation Rate

The erythrocyte **sedimentation** rate is also known as the ESR or the sed rate. It is the rate at which red blood cells settle in a calibrated tube within a given time, ranging from one to two hours, depending on the method used. This test is not a true diagnostic test but, instead, gives the health care provider an idea of how much inflammation is occurring in a patient's body in response to a disease condition. The basis of the test is that certain proteins in the blood become altered in disease processes that in turn allow the red blood cells to stick together and thus become heavier, settling at a higher rate of speed than would normally occur.

Some of the indications in which the ESR would be helpful in the assessment of the patient's condition include:

- Acute infections.
- Acute inflammatory processes.
- Chronic infections.
- Rheumatoid arthritis or autoimmune disorders.
- Temporal arteritis and polymyalgia rheumatica.
- Monitoring inflammatory and malignant diseases.

There are also conditions in which there is inflammation, but the ESR does not increase. An example of one of these conditions is *sickle cell anemia*; the red blood cells are not shaped in their normal biconcave disk shape but are abnormally formed to appear curved. Because of this shape, the red blood cells cannot form the *rouleaux* pattern in which the cells stack upon one another, thus resulting in a low ESR value. Another example is *polycythemia vera* or *secondary polycythemia*, in which the body produces too many cells, leaving little plasma for the red blood cells to fall through within the designated period of time for the test.

The two most common methods used for performance of the ESR are the Westergren (modified Westergren) and the Wintrobe methods. Figure 45–7A–C show the waived ESR test. The normal rate at which red blood cells fall is 1 millimeter every 5 minutes (1 mm/5 min). Depending on the method used for the testing, it is imperative, when recording the results, to denote the method of testing. It is also very important for the results to be read at precisely the time at which the test is timed for conclusion. Reading the test before the designated time can yield a false negative result, and reading the test after the designated time could yield a false positive result. Commonly, female patients have higher ESR rate readings than males; a normal ESR rate value for a female is 0 to 20 mm/hr, whereas for men the normal is 0 to 10 mm/hr. Review Procedure 45–3 for performing an erythrocyte sedimentation rate.

GLUCOSE TESTING

Typically, capillary blood samples are used in medical practices to screen the blood glucose level of diabetic patients. These tests are simple to perform and relatively painless and provide quick results. This type of testing uses a handheld meter with specially designed

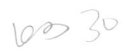

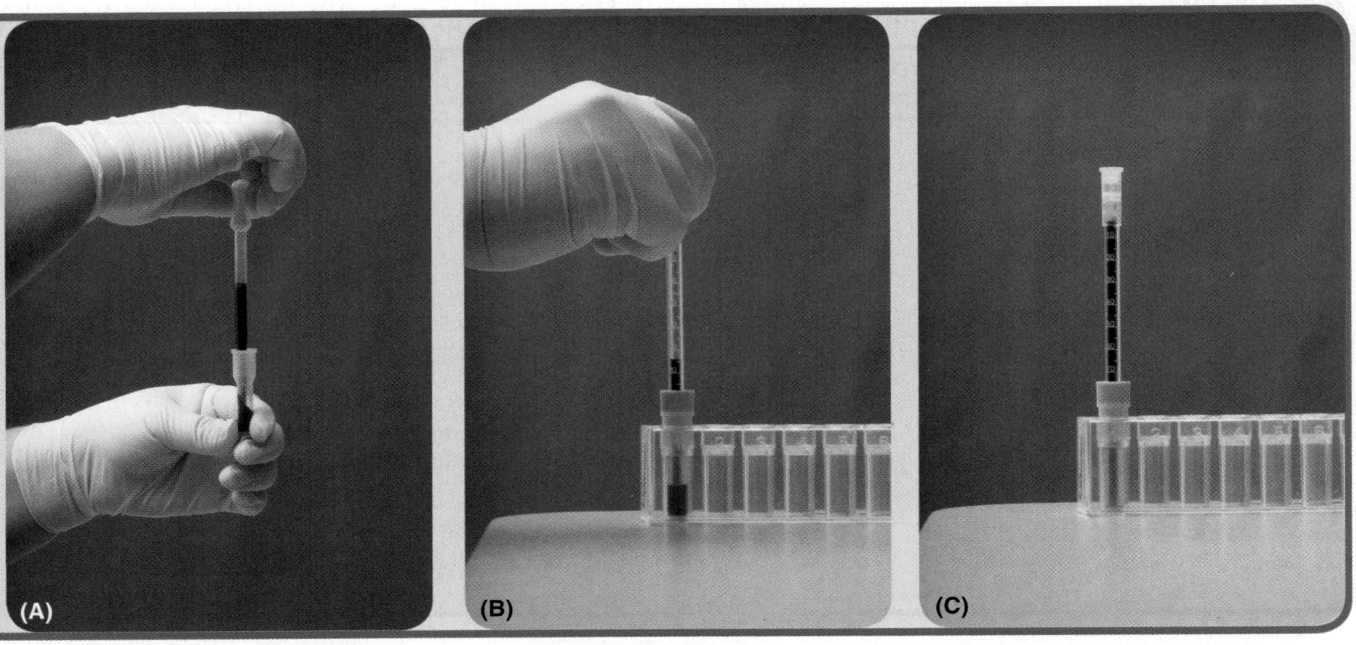

Figure 45–7: (A) Remove the stopper on the prefilled vial and fill to the indicated line with blood. Replace stopper and invert several times to mix. (B) Insert the pipette through the stopper and push down until the pipette touches the bottom of the vial. The pipette will autozero the blood, and any excess will flow into the closed reservoir compartment. (C) Let the pipette stand for one hour and then read the numeric results of the ESR. *Delmar/Cengage Learning.*

PROCEDURE 45–3 Perform an Erythrocyte Sedimentation Rate (ESR)

MEDIA LINK: View the video for this chapter, "Perform an ESR," on the Premium Website.

PURPOSE: To measure the rate of fall of red blood cells within a prescribed time

EQUIPMENT: Goggles or face shield, gloves, prefilled vial, calibrated sed rate pipette, EDTA tube with patient's blood, sed rate stand, flat work surface, timer, patient's chart or laboratory report form, and blue or black pen or electronic medical record

S SKILL: Perform an erythrocyte sedimentation rate (ESR).

Procedure Steps	Detailed Instructions and/or *Rationales*
1. Assemble all supplies at the flat work surface.	
2. Don gloves and goggles or face shield before uncapping the EDTA sample.	
3. Remove the stopper on the prefilled vial; fill to the indicated line with blood. Replace the stopper on the prefilled vial and invert several times to mix.	
4. Insert the pipette through the pierceable stopper, pushing down in a twisting motion until the pipette touches the bottom of the prefilled vial.	

Procedure Steps	Detailed Instructions and/or *Rationales*
5. Set the timer.	Set the timer for exactly one hour if performing the Wintrobe method of testing; two hours if performing the Westergren method.
6. After the appropriate time, read the numeric results of the test, using the designation of mm/hr after the numeric reading.	
7. Dispose of the testing materials in a biohazard waste container.	

reagent strips to which the blood sample is directly applied. Many types of meters, known as *glucometers* or glucose meters (Figure 45–8), are available that give reliable results.

Many patients perform this testing at home to assist them in monitoring their blood sugars in case insulin adjustment is needed. Some of the meters use a blood sample so small that instead of puncturing the finger, the patient punctures the forearm to obtain the specimen, and technology has accelerated to make these instruments much more common and affordable for home use.

Procedure 45–4 provides general instructions for performance of a blood sugar test. Remember, many types of meters are on the market, so you must check the manufacturer's instructions prior to testing.

Glucose Tolerance Test

The reported normal fasting blood glucose range varies; however, if you learn that 70 to 126 mg/dL is an average range for a fasting specimen, you will be able to determine the correct range on an examination.

When a patient has a consistently high fasting blood sugar (FBS), the next test usually ordered is the *glucose tolerance test*, or GTT. There are basically two reasons for this test to be ordered: diagnosis of diabetes mellitus or hypoglycemia. This test determines the patient's ability

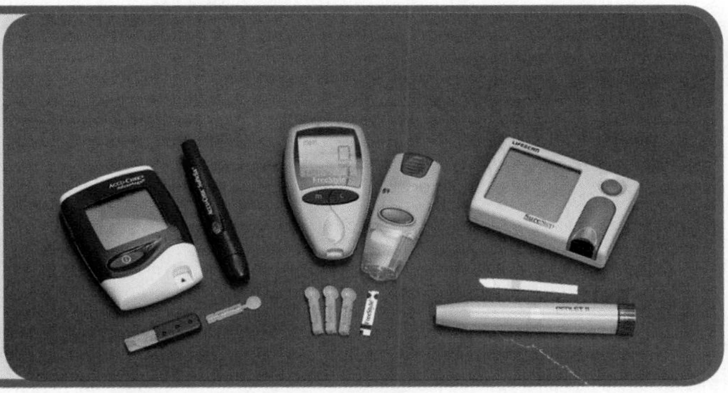

Figure 45–8: A variety of handheld glucometers available for home or clinic use. *Delmar/Cengage Learning.*

CLINICAL PEARL

As you converse with the patient, be sure to inquire about medications (both prescription and OTC), any home remedy he or she has taken, and his or her diet and record all information on the patient's chart. Most diabetics are encouraged to keep a record (or diary) of their daily routine of medicines, blood glucose readings, nutritional intake, and exercise, especially if one's condition has been unruly. Reporting this information to the physician is valuable in assessing the patient's condition and plan of treatment because some substances can affect the accuracy of some blood glucose monitors.

PROCEDURE 45–4 Screen Blood Sugar (Glucose) Level

MEDIA LINK: View the video for this chapter, "Perform Glucose Testing," on the Premium Website.

PURPOSE: To determine the sugar (glucose) level in the blood

EQUIPMENT: Sterile lancet, reagent strips, bottle (for color chart), glucometer, latex or vinyl gloves, cotton balls, alcohol, gauze squares, watch or clock, and facial tissue

S SKILL: Perform a glucose test on a blood specimen and document the quality control(s) for the test.

Procedure Steps	Detailed Instructions and/or *Rationales*
1. Assemble all needed items on a Mayo table or comparable flat, steady surface.	If a glucometer is to be used, make sure it has been turned on for the required time and has been calibrated for accuracy. (Follow instruction manual.)
B 2. Identify the patient. Explain the procedure to the patient, ***including the rationale for performing the procedure, using language and verbal skills the patient can understand. Show awareness of patients' concerns regarding their perceptions of the procedure by answering any questions the patient might have and assisting the patient into a comfortable position before you proceed.***	*Speaking to the patient by name and checking the chart ensures that you are performing the procedure on the correct patient.* If the test is to be for a fasting blood sugar level, be certain the patient has not had anything by mouth for the past 8 to 12 hours.
3. Wash hands and don gloves.	
4. Perform a capillary puncture.	Follow the desired capillary puncture procedure as outlined in Procedure 43–1. You should perform a capillary puncture for a glucose reagent strip from an FBS sample unless otherwise ordered by the health care provider.
5. Open the reagent strip bottle and take one of the plastic strips out without touching the chemically treated pads. Reclose the bottle.	*Touching the reagent strip pad can alter the results.*
6. Apply a large drop of blood from the patient's finger so that the pad is completely covered.	
7. Begin timing *immediately* for *exactly* the amount of time specified by the manufacturer.	
8. Give the patient a dry gauze square to hold over the puncture site after wiping it with an alcohol-saturated cotton ball. Offer a bandage.	
9. Wait for the instrument to display the results. The number displayed is the blood glucose level. Record the result in the patient's chart.	For example: 98 mg/dL of blood, initial.
10. Discard all used items in the proper receptacle, remove gloves, and wash hands.	
11. Record in the log book the lot number and the expiration date of the reagent test strips.	

Charting Example

6-12-XX 3:30 PM	Finger stick of L great finger for capillary blood for FBS—reading is 98 mg/dL of blood. S. Davis, RMA(AMT)

Log Book Example

Date	Patient's Name	Test	Results	Obtained by
6-12-XX	Mark J. Stanford	FBS	98 mg/dL	S. Davis, RMA(AMT)
glucose reagent strips Lot #875913-42 Exp 9/30/XX				

CLINICAL PEARL

Remember what the term *fasting* means—that the patient has had nothing to eat or drink for at least 12 hours prior to having the test drawn. Patients frequently ask about the term *fasting*; it should be emphasized that they should not eat mints, chew gum, drink coffee or juices, or smoke. However, some providers permit their patients to sip a small amount of water to take their medications. Always be sure to ask the patient whether he or she has adhered to the requirement prior to taking the sample.

to metabolize a glucose (carbohydrate) load within a prescribed amount of time. Figure 45–9 displays various types of readings and their indications.

If you are administering this test, check with the health care provider and policy and procedure manual to see whether urine specimens are to be collected with the blood samples; this used to be common practice, but the stress of the test and the timing has led many providers to believe that the urine tests do not have to be collected. Before you begin the test, it is essential to collect the fasting specimen. If the patient's fasting blood sugar is 150 mg/dL or above, do not administer the glucose load to the patient. Immediately inform the provider of the results and await further instructions; administering the glucose load could be very dangerous to the patient when the blood sugar is already this high. Timing for the collection of subsequent samples is critical; usually, 30 minutes after the glucose load has been ingested, a blood sample is collected. Following that

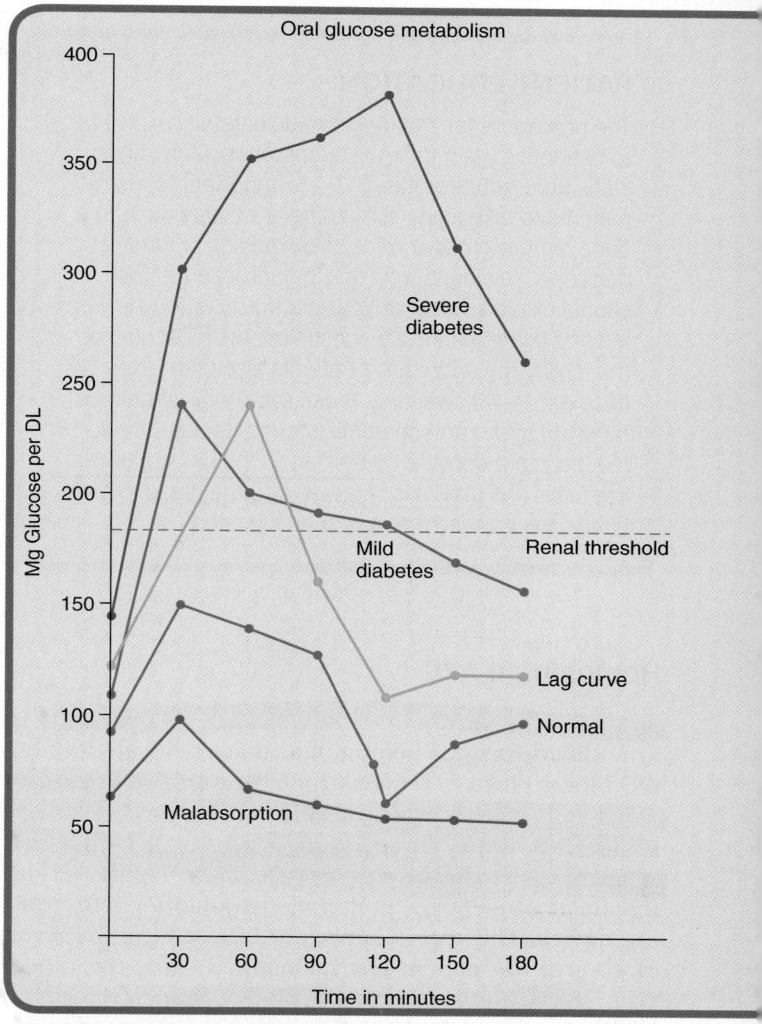

Figure 45–9: Graph of three-hour glucose metabolism. *Delmar/Cengage Learning.*

initial collection, another will be collected 30 minutes later and then once every 60 minutes for the duration of the test. If the patient becomes nauseated and vomits, the test must be discontinued and the provider informed.

A GTT is performed on many pregnant women to determine whether they have **gestational diabetes**. This test may be ordered at any time during pregnancy when there are symptoms that might be associated with diabetes such as extreme thirst, visual difficulties, fatigue, weight loss, dehydration, and a high glucose reading. Women who have miscarried or have delivered very large babies are most at risk for having gestational diabetes. If the patient is a known diabetic, regular home glucose screenings will be ordered by the provider; in addition, frequent office exams and in-office glucose screening will be used to monitor the patient's condition to help prevent complications during the pregnancy.

PATIENT EDUCATION

The procedure for a GTT should be carefully explained to patients to gain their full cooperation. Many physicians order a three-hour GTT. It is important to instruct patients to take along something to occupy their time (for example, crossword puzzles, reading or writing materials, sewing) during this long procedure. They should also be told about the possibility of feeling weakness or fainting during the test. Patients must stay at the facility the entire time. Patients also often experience excessive sweating. These symptoms should be reported to the person administering the test. These reactions are considered normal as the blood glucose level falls and insulin is secreted into the blood in reaction to the glucose that has been ingested.

Hemoglobin A1C

Glycohemoglobin, or hemoglobin A1C (HbA1c), is a modified form of hemoglobin that is elevated when the blood glucose remains high. A capillary puncture helps determine how the diabetic patient has been controlling the blood sugar during the past two or three months since the last office visit. See Figure 45–10 for an example of a common hemoglobin A1C testing device. This test is important in assessing the level of control the patient has maintained since the office visit. Hemoglobin A1C is the stable molecule formed when sugar and hemoglobin bond, a process known as **glycosylation**. Very commonly, the provider will request a random blood sugar level with the HbA1C to assess fully the patient's compliance with the diabetic regimen. Follow the steps in Procedure 45–5 to perform a hemoglobin A1C screening.

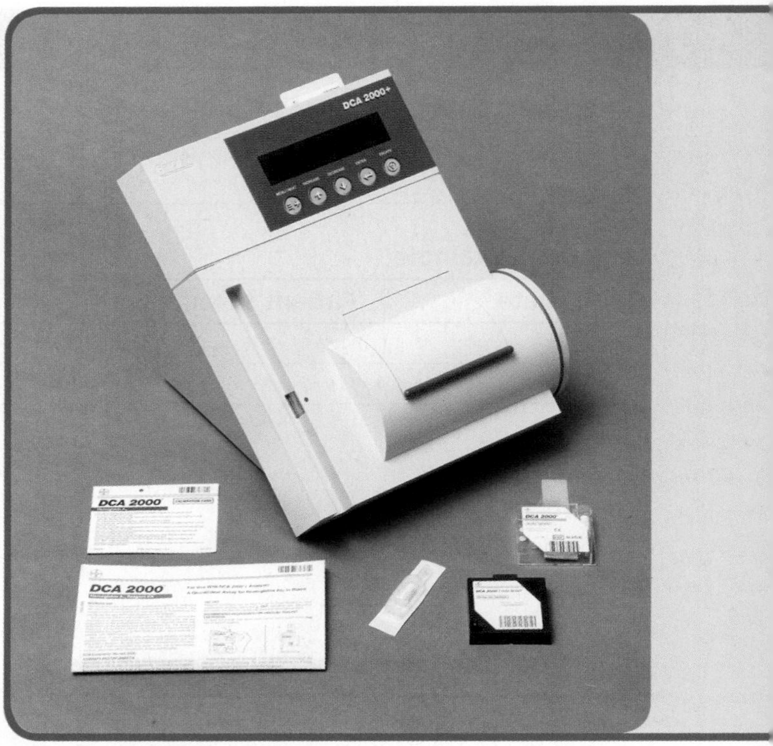

Figure 45–10: The DCS 2000 is a common hemoglobin A1C testing unit found in the POL. *Delmar/Cengage Learning.*

CHOLESTEROL TESTING

Cholesterol is a steroid normally found in the body; however, when cholesterol levels are over 200 mg/dL (hypercholesterolemia), this can cause *atherosclerosis* or *arteriosclerosis*, a hardening of the arteries. Also, if cholesterol levels stay elevated for an extended period of time, *plaque* can build up on the inside of the arteries, narrowing the size of the artery and not allowing blood to flow through normally. You have probably heard of *angioplasty*, a surgical procedure by which a cardiac surgeon goes into an affected artery or arteries with special instruments and removes the plaque by inflating a small balloon on the tip of the scope and dragging it along the arterial walls. Several CLIA-waived tests are available on the market for screening cholesterol levels in the POL; one is a card that does not provide a specific number for the cholesterol level but a range. Instruments are also available that use the same technology as many of the glucometers for testing and provide a specific number for the cholesterol level.

PROCEDURE 45–5 Perform Hemoglobin A1C (Glycosylated Hemoglobin) Screening

PURPOSE: Evaluate diabetic patients' overall compliance with diet regimen for management of blood glucose levels

EQUIPMENT: Sterile lancet, disposable gloves, other personal protective equipment (PPE) per laboratory policies, alcohol wipe, clean gauze or cotton balls, testing instrument, reagents, black or blue pen, biohazard waste container, and sharps container

S SKILL: Perform a hemoglobin A1C screening on a blood sample.

Procedure Steps	Detailed Instructions and/or *Rationales*
1. Assemble the necessary equipment and supplies.	
B 2. Identify the patient. Explain the procedure to the patient, ***including the rationale for performing the procedure, using language and verbal skills the patient can understand. Show awareness of patients' concerns regarding their perceptions of the procedure by answering any questions the patient might have and assisting the patient into a comfortable position before you proceed.***	*Speaking to the patient by name as well as checking the chart ensures that you are performing the proper procedure on the correct patient.*
3. Wash hands, don gloves and other PPE as required.	
4. Perform the capillary puncture and collect the blood sample per the manufacturer's directions for the instrument.	Follow the desired capillary puncture procedure as outlined in Procedure 43–1.
5. Record the results of the test on the patient's chart and flow sheet.	
6. Check the patient's finger for excessive bleeding and provide clean gauze or a cotton ball, instructing the patient to apply pressure to the site. Offer a bandage.	
7. Dispose of contaminated sharps in the sharps container and other contaminated materials in the biohazard waste container.	
8. Remove gloves and wash hands.	

Charting Example

Lafferty, Jerry B. ID# 143896LA 07/27/XX	0855	Hemoglobin A1C	5%	Brooke Bourne, RMA(AMT)

Cholesterol tests should be collected as a fasting specimen, so patients should be instructed to refrain from eating or drinking anything for 12 to 16 hours prior to the test. The cholesterol numbers considered ideal vary, ranging from 180 to 200 mg/dL. Your health care provider will establish the ideal level for the particular office and patients. Procedure 45–6 provides steps to perform a cholesterol screening.

PROCEDURE 45–6 Perform a Cholesterol Screening

PURPOSE: Screen a cholesterol level for hypercholesterolemia.

EQUIPMENT: Sterile lancet, disposable gloves, other personal protective equipment (PPE) per laboratory policies, alcohol wipe, clean gauze or cotton balls, testing instrument (if indicated—some tests are done without an instrument), reagents, black or blue pen, biohazard waste container, and sharps container

S **SKILL:** Perform a cholesterol screening on a blood sample.

Procedure Steps	Detailed Instructions and/or *Rationales*
1. Assemble the necessary equipment and supplies.	
B 2. Identify the patient. Explain the procedure to the patient, ***including the rationale for performing the procedure, using language and verbal skills the patient can understand. Show awareness of patients' concerns regarding their perceptions of the procedure by answering any questions the patient might have and assisting the patient into a comfortable position before you proceed.***	*Speaking to the patient by name as well as checking the chart ensures that you are performing the proper procedure on the correct patient.*
3. Wash hands, don gloves and other PPE as required.	
4. Perform the capillary puncture and collect the blood sample per the manufacturer's directions for the instrument or the reagent card.	Follow the desired capillary puncture procedure as outlined in Procedure 43–1.
5. Record the results of the test on the patient's chart.	
6. Check the patient's finger for excessive bleeding and provide clean gauze or a cotton ball, instructing the patient to apply pressure to the site. Offer a bandage.	
7. Dispose of contaminated sharps in the sharps container and other contaminated materials in the biohazard waste container.	
8. Remove gloves and wash hands.	

Charting Example

Bennett, Anna ID# 145709 1/7/XX	1050	Fasting cholesterol	156 mg/dL	Mary Adams, CMA(AAMA)

IMMUNOLOGY

Immunology is the study of the body's ability to prevent and fight off infection. Although this sounds like a very detailed science, and indeed it is, tests have been developed that can be performed at the waived level to diagnose common diseases and illnesses. **Immunoassays** are the diagnostic tests that use techniques for measuring the amount of antigens and antibodies present relative to a specific illness.

Mononucleosis Testing

Infectious mononucleosis is an illness caused by the Epstein Barr virus (EBV); you might have heard it referred to as the kissing disease or mono. This virus can be transmitted in other ways, but all transmissions involve contact with saliva. It is considered an extremely contagious disease, and it is most commonly found in individuals between the ages of 10 and 25 years. EBV is related to the herpes virus and can be spread for a period of up to six months after initial contact and infection. The symptoms are similar to those of the flu, and the infection can affect the lymph nodes, throat, salivary glands, liver, and spleen; bed rest, good nutrition, and plenty of fluids are indicated for treatment of the viral infection. The presence of the virus remains throughout a patient's life, although the symptoms associated with mononucleosis usually do not recur. Testing for infection and subsequent antibody production is performed by a monotest, a type of immunoassay that detects the presence or absence of the antibodies to EBV for diagnosis. Procedure 45–7 describes steps for performing an infectious mononucleosis screening.

Allergy Testing

Allergy tests are another type of immunology testing found in certain offices such as otorhinolaryngologists' (ENT) offices or allergy specialists. Basically, three types of direct allergy tests are performed.

- *Skin prick test.* The allergen (the substance to which the patient is suspected to be allergic) is applied directly to the patient's skin and scratched or pricked into the epidermis. The areas of application are observed for reaction from antibodies, usually as a reddening of the area with itching.
- *Intradermal injections.* This test is more sensitive than the skin prick test. A small amount of

PROCEDURE 45–7 Perform a Screening for Infectious Mononucleosis

PURPOSE: To determine the presence (or absence) of antibodies to the Epstein-Barr virus (EBV)

EQUIPMENT: Sterile lancet, disposable gloves, other personal protective equipment (PPE) per laboratory policies, alcohol wipe, clean gauze or cotton balls, quality control materials, reagents, black or blue pen, biohazard waste container, and sharps container

S **SKILL:** Perform an infectious mononucleosis screening on a blood sample.

Procedure Steps	Detailed Instructions and/or *Rationales*
1. Assemble the necessary equipment and supplies.	
B 2. Identify the patient. Explain the procedure to the patient, ***including the rationale for performing the procedure, using language and verbal skills the patient can understand. Show awareness of patients' concerns regarding their perceptions of the procedure by answering any questions the patient might have and assisting the patient into a comfortable position before you proceed.***	*Speaking to the patient by name as well as checking the chart ensures that you are performing the proper procedure on the correct patient.*
3. Wash hands, don gloves and other PPE as required.	
4. Perform the capillary puncture and collect the blood sample per the manufacturer's directions.	Follow the desired capillary puncture procedure as outlined in Procedure 43–1.

(*continues*)

(continued)

Procedure Steps	Detailed Instructions and/or *Rationales*
5. Perform quality control testing on two additional cards, one negative and one positive, while performing testing on the patient's sample.	Control samples must be run only once per day or anytime a new box of reagents has been opened.
6. Record the results of the quality control analyses in the quality control log; do not report patient results if quality control results are not in the acceptable range.	
7. Record the results of the test on the patient's chart.	
8. Check the patient's finger for excessive bleeding and provide clean gauze or a cotton ball, instructing the patient to apply pressure to the site. Offer a bandage.	
9. Dispose of contaminated sharps in the sharps container and other contaminated materials in the biohazard waste container.	
10. Remove gloves and wash hands.	

Charting Example

Thomas, Ronald ID# TH0932 1-07 9/12/XX	1448	Monotest	Positive	Kristina Frye, CCMA

Quality Control Log

Date	Control Level	Control Lot #	Expiration Date	Reagent Lot #	Expiration Date	Results	Initials
09/12/XX	Positive	40589J	02/28/11	32159	04/25/09	Positive	dlr
09/12/XX	Negative	40593J	02/28/11	32159	04/25/09	Negative	dlr

the allergen is injected between the epidermis and dermis with an observation of the area for a reaction. Usually, reactions occur immediately, although patients can be instructed to return 24 to 72 hours later for delayed responses to the allergen.

- *Skin patch test.* An allergen-soaked pad is placed on the surface of skin for 24 to 72 hours to observe for a reaction.

In certain cases, the *radioallergosorbent test* (RAST) is indicated because some individuals cannot tolerate the skin tests; this test determines the presence of immunoglobulins (IgE among others) present in greater amounts in those with allergies. This test is not as specific as the specific allergen applications.

The provider determines the diagnosis by evaluating the results of the tests along with the patient's medical history, physical exam, and other laboratory tests. The medical assistant might assist the provider in performing these tests or might perform them by order of the provider. Tests should always be performed under the direct supervision of the provider.

The tests involve introducing an **antigen** directly into the patient's skin to induce a reaction. If the reaction is negative (normal), there will be no change in the appearance of the skin following testing. A normal **immune** reaction occurs in the body when an antigen and **antibody** unite and the foreign substance is excreted by the body.

A positive allergic reaction to a test is shown by a raised area on the skin, much like a mosquito bite, called a **wheal** (hive). This is caused by interaction of the antigen and antibody, which releases **histamine** and is termed a **hypersensitive** reaction. Histamine is naturally produced by the body to attach itself to certain cells to cause dilation of blood vessels and contraction of smooth muscles. Most cells release histamine during allergic reactions. As part of the normal inflammatory response of the body, histamine protects tissue against injury (the scratch test), and it is why redness and a wheal are produced. The inflammatory response of the body is specific in that it is the whole body's defense against infection, chemicals, or other physical factors.

Besides histamine, researchers are finding other chemicals released during the allergic response. Many people have allergies to a variety of substances, including certain foods, pollens, dust, drugs (medications), chemicals, **venom** of stinging insects, animal dander, molds, pollutants, and other allergens. There are also some that are not so well known. It is very important to realize that cockroaches and their egg casing and fecal matter are major sources of allergens in large cities. The extermination of these roaches is of concern because the chemicals used to eliminate them can cause serious problems for those who have allergies and respiratory diseases. Asthma patients are most sensitive to these sprays and other methods of getting rid of the roaches. The allergen remains even after the roaches are killed. Thorough cleaning is necessary to rid the home of the allergen as much as possible after extermination has been completed. Advising patients of the risks is extremely important.

Certain irritants can make allergies worse. These irritants can be caused by smoke, paint fumes, perfumes, insect sprays, gasoline, cleaning materials, and personal grooming products (hair sprays, soaps, lotions, and so on). Sensitivity to these irritants is most likely in those who have allergies. The best advice for such patients is to avoid being around these substances. Reaction to these substances ranges from slight to severe. Severe reactions can be life threatening. A life-threatening reaction must be counteracted with an injection of **adrenalin** immediately to prevent **anaphylactic** shock. Symptoms of anaphylactic shock initially include intense anxiety, weakness, sweating, and shortness of breath. These can be followed by hypotension, shock, arrhythmia, respiratory congestion, laryngeal edema, nausea, and diarrhea.

For example, those who have known allergies to the venom of stinging insects or to certain foods that produce intense life-threatening allergic reactions are instructed to carry an anaphylactic shock kit with them at all times. The kit contains a self-injecting dose of adrenalin for emergency use. Instruct patients with food allergies to read the contents (ingredients) on all labels of foods and over-the-counter medications to avoid adverse reactions. Also explain that herbal remedies, when combined with prescribed medications and foods, can produce health risks and that the patient should always check with his or her pharmacist before taking any combinations of over-the-counter medicines and prescriptions from the provider. It is also a good practice to advise patients to ask the server or the dinner host about the contents of some foods on restaurant menus such as soups, breads, and desserts. Some of these foods can contain ingredients that result in an allergic reaction for those who are sensitive to these substances. You might also want to inform these patients, if they do not already wear them, to get a medic alert bracelet or necklace. These are very helpful if a medical emergency occurs; the medic alert tag informs others of their condition if they are not able to speak or if they are found unconscious.

Treatment for many allergy patients consists of an allergy immunotherapy program. Over a considerable period, which can be indefinite, this therapy gradually provides immunization against the substance to which the person is allergic. Increasing amounts of the allergen are injected as long as the patient can tolerate each dose. Treatment generally takes a few years. It is usually effective in reducing symptoms of most allergies. Often, patients bring their serum from the allergy specialist to the family doctor's office or clinic for administration. All allergy serum should be refrigerated unless otherwise specified. These **desensitizing** injections of allergy serum (which patients refer to as allergy shots) should always be administered under the direct supervision of a provider because anaphylactic shock can occur within seconds. Following any injection, the patient must be observed for 20 minutes for possible reaction. Any reaction or unusual symptom must be reported to the provider and noted on the patient's chart and on the schedule sheet accompanying the allergy serum. An example of this schedule is shown in Figure 45–11.

Because patients generally continue this therapy once a week (or even more frequently) over a few years, it is vital to rotate the injection sites frequently. A practical method of keeping a record of where the allergy serum is injected each time is by alternating arms and numbering the injection sites. This pattern allows up to 18 injection sites, and then it can be repeated. This can help prevent tissue damage from recurring frequent injections of the same area. Keep track of the pattern on the schedule that comes with the allergy serum, or in the patient's chart, by recording which arm, the number of the injection site, and, of course, the date and your initials.

Company's Name
(maker of serum)

Physician's Name/Allergist
Address and Phone Number

Patient's Name
Account Number

Lot Number of Serum
Expiration Date

INSTRUCTIONS FOR ADMINISTRATION

—Preparations should always be made for physician to treat anaphylaxis should it occur.
—Patients who are being treated with beta-blocker medications should not be given allergy serum.
—Use 27G 1/2-inch needle.
—Administer 3/8 to 1/2 inch into subcutaneous tissue between deltoid and biceps muscle (but not into the muscle).
—Aspirate plunger of syringe to ensure needle is not in a blood vessel.
—Reschedule patient for injection if he or she is feverish or is wheezing.
—Observe patient for possible reaction for 20 minutes following injection.
—Administer cold packs on site if local redness, itching, or wheal develops—alert physician for administration of antihistamine PRN.
—If a systemic or general reaction occurs, such as hives, sneezing, or wheezing, alert physician for dosage and administration of epinephrine (subcutaneous).
—Contact allergist for rescheduling instructions if systemic reaction occurs.

SCHEDULE

Administer allergy serum injections every ______________ days. If no adverse reaction occurs, resume scheduled dose. If adverse local reaction occurs, resume schedule with the last well-tolerated dose. Proceed with the following schedule until maximum dose is reached and well-tolerated. Then repeat maximum dose tolerated until vial is empty.

Dose	Date Administered	Adverse Reaction
0.10 mL	Month/day/year	Type of reaction,
0.15 mL	Initials of one who	if any (note the
0.20 mL	administered the	severity and
0.30 mL	injection	symptoms of
0.40 mL	and which arm	the patient)
0.50 mL	was injected	
*0.50 mL	Rt or L	

*Reorder before last dose is administered. Allow 2 weeks for delivery.

Figure 45–11: Example of schedule and instructions for allergy serum injections. *Delmar/Cengage Learning.*

Allergy injections are administered to patients who have demonstrated a reaction to one or more allergens. One method of testing is administration of an intradermal injection; a minute amount of allergen is introduced just below the epidermis of the skin, and the site is observed for a reaction. A positive reaction to the allergen is the appearance of a wheal.

The size of the wheal is **interpreted** by the provider after a timed 20- to 30-minute period. Wheals are measured in centimeters by using a tape measure or by comparison (Figure 45–12). A trained skin tester may observe the reaction and make an interpretation by inspection alone.

Extracts of substances that are commonly the cause of allergy in patients are manufactured in applicator bottles. These should be refrigerated and the expiration date noted for accurate test results. Many of the skin testing extracts vary in strength from one company to another. Because specific allergens can also differ geographically, skin tests are sometimes unreliable. New methods are being researched, and skin testing might one day become an obsolete procedure.

Scratch Test and Skin Prick Test

Desirable sites for the scratch test and skin prick test are the arms and the back, depending on the number of tests to be performed and, in some cases, the preference of the patient. Small children are easier to restrain if they are lying face down while the test is being administered. The area to be tested should be comfortably accessible to both patient and provider or assistant. The patient must stay in the same position for at least 20 minutes, so comfort is essential for compliance.

The tests should be numbered in a pattern with washable ink on the surface of the skin. Explain to the patient that there is some discomfort when

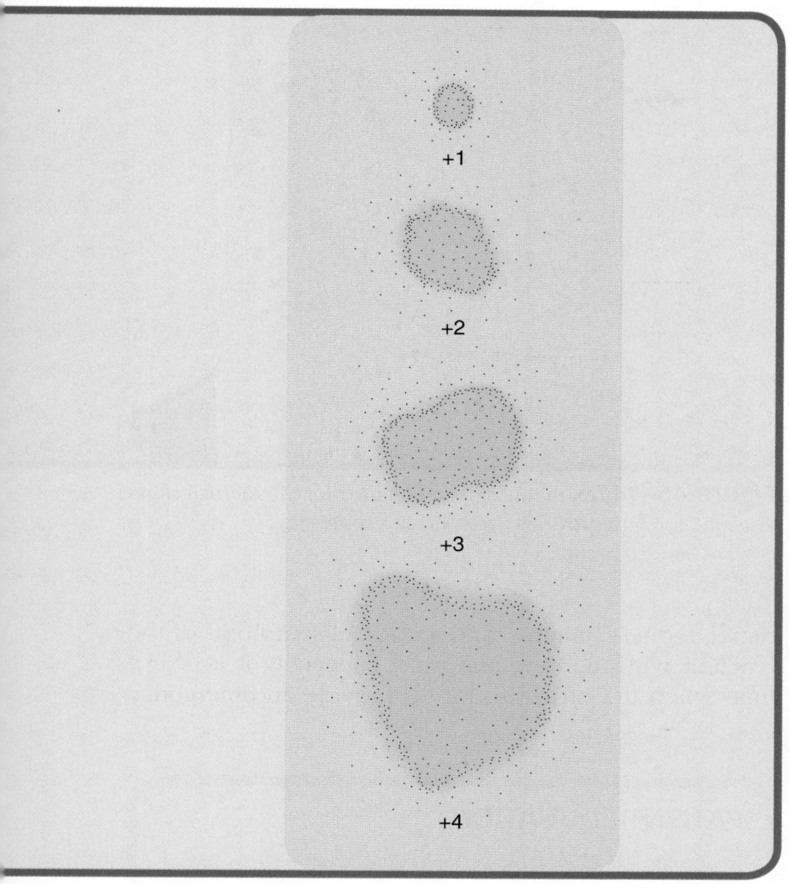

Figure 45–12: Sizes of wheals from +1 to +4 in reaction to scratch testing of allergens. *Delmar/Cengage Learning.*

administering either the scratch test or the intradermal test, but it does not last long. Instruct the patient to inform you of any itching, redness, or swelling at the site of injection. Advise the patient to avoid scratching the area to allow for accurate interpretation following the prescribed timing of the test(s). Several extracts might be applied to the patient's skin in rows from evenly spaced applicators that have been dipped into various bottles of allergen substances. The applicator provides a small drop of the substance on the skin in preparation for the scratch test. Figure 45–13A shows a medical assistant applying seven extracts on the patient's skin. Usually, the skin is prepared with alcohol and allowed to air dry. Alcohol can also be used to remove the ink after the test is completed. A sterile needle or lancet tears the surface of the skin in a scratch of about ⅛ inch or less to allow a drop of the antigen to enter the epidermis (Figure 45–13B). Some test materials are packaged in sealed glass capillary tubes, the contents of which are shaken onto the skin after the tube is snapped. Only a small drop should be used. Otherwise, antigens might run together, rendering the test results inaccurate. The scratches should be from 1½ to 2 inches apart, allowing possible reactions to spread without interfering with each other. A nonallergenic plain base fluid control is used for comparison in interpreting the results.

Reactions usually occur within the first 20 minutes. (Itching at the test site can be relieved by application of cold or ice packs after the test site has been evaluated by the provider. Look at the examples in Figure 45–13C of graduated sizes of reactions to allergy testing.) Many providers wish to recheck the test sites in 24 hours for delayed reactions. If the provider's interpretation of the

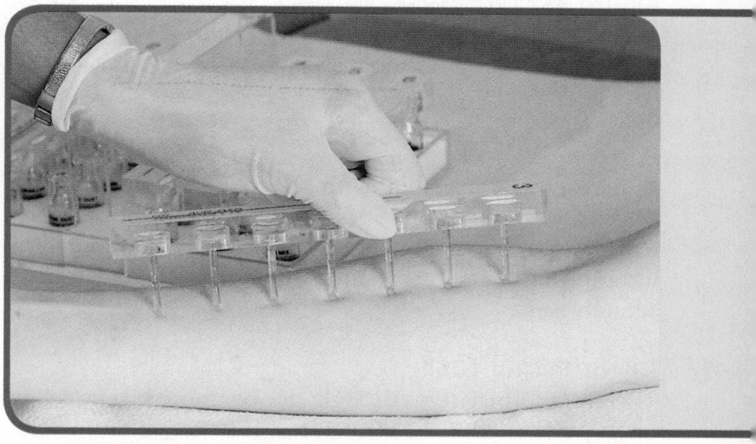

Figure 45–13A: An example of how a multiple applicator is used to place allergy extracts on the skin. *Delmar/Cengage Learning.*

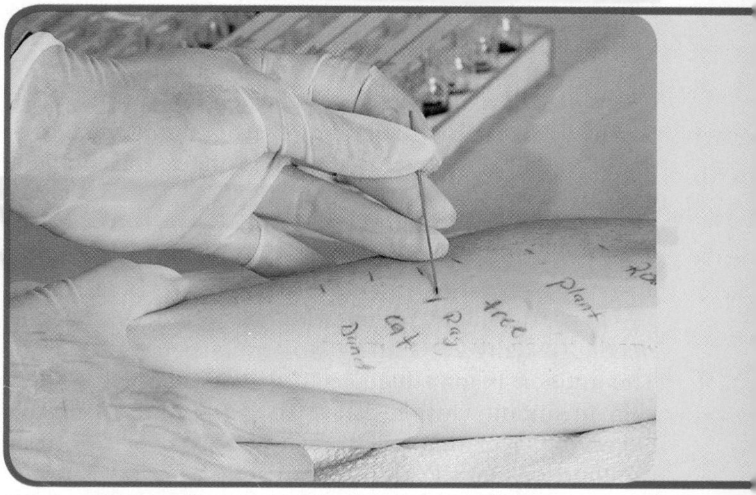

Figure 45–13B: After extracts are placed on the skin, each is labeled with ink for identification. To allow the extract to enter the epidermis, the medical assistant uses a sterile fine-point needle or lance to scratch the surface of the skin. *Delmar/Cengage Learning.*

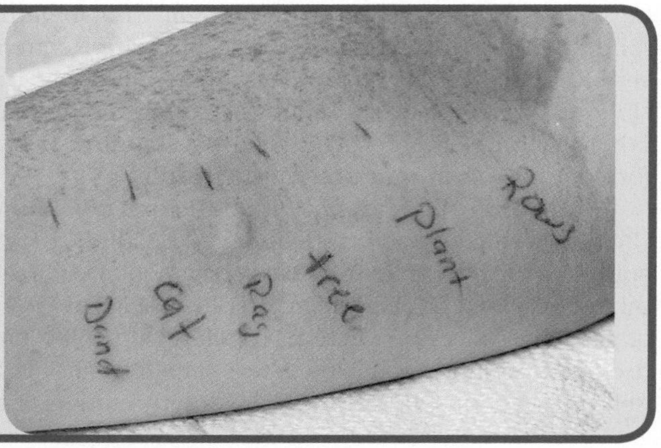

Figure 45–13C: The test needs to be timed for 20 minutes. After the allotted time is completed, the reaction must be observed and recorded on the patient's chart. A + 3 reaction to ragweed is pictured. *Delmar/Cengage Learning.*

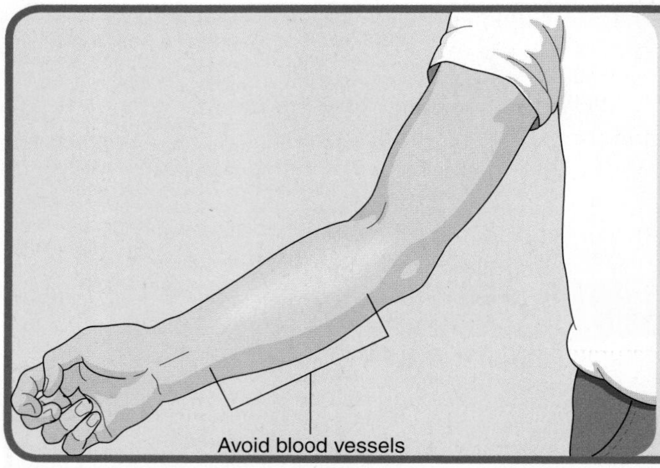

Figure 45–14: As the most common area for intradermal skin tests, the forearm provides up to 14 sites for testing. *Delmar/Cengage Learning.*

skin tests is consistent with the patient's history and physical examination findings, more advanced studies are not necessary. It is not advisable to perform intradermal tests on patients who have had positive scratch tests.

Intradermal Test

The intradermal test, thought to be more accurate, is often performed if the scratch test is negative or unclear. Although the solutions used for intradermal tests are about 100 times more dilute than those used for scratch tests, they are still potentially dangerous. Severe reactions can occur, however, with either method. Generally, the diluted solutions prevent **systemic** reactions. Intradermal test sites are performed at spaced intervals on the forearm (Figure 45–14) or scapular area. In the event of a severe **adverse** reaction, a tourniquet can be applied proximal to the site when the arm is used. Serum or vaccine is sometimes used in intradermal testing. If the initial test is negative, it is often repeated with a stronger solution. Usually, the reaction time is 15 to 30 minutes. **Epinephrine** should be administered about an inch above the site by order of the provider if severe reaction occurs.

In performing an intradermal test, a fine-gauge needle (usually 26 G and $\frac{3}{8}$ to $\frac{5}{8}$ inches long) is used. The antigen is introduced into the dermal layer of the skin in minute dosages of 0.01 to 0.02 mL by sterile technique. The area will appear as a small blister from the fluid raising the skin. The reaction period is up to 30 minutes, and the interpretation of the results is the same as in the scratch tests. Some antigens such as fungi and bacteria produce delayed reactions 24 to 48 hours after administration. Be sure to impress upon the patient the importance of comparing the reaction to something well known (e.g., size of welt [size of a dime], redness, itching) and record all symptoms of the reaction with the date and time, especially if it is at a time when the office is closed. Provide an emergency

PATIENT EDUCATION

During the allergy patient's visit, especially if he or she is recently diagnosed as such, advice concerning the condition and the prevention of further problems is well received. The following are a few suggestions for discussion with patients who have allergies.

1. Urge patients to follow the allergy serum desensitizing schedule closely to help build up immunity to the substance to which they are allergic.
2. Advise them to avoid what they are allergic to if at all possible.
3. Instruct patients to read all labels carefully (household products, clothing, consumable products, and so on) to identify possible allergens.
4. Urge them to develop and practice good health habits such as following a sensible, well-balanced diet, proper rest, and exercise. They should also be encouraged to wash their hands frequently with soap and warm water for 20 seconds (approximately the length of time it takes to sing the Happy Birthday song at a traditional pace) and teach their families to do so.
5. Advise them to take only prescribed medication and to avoid OTC medications unless advised by the provider.
6. If patients have a known severe reaction to a particular substance, remind them to carry their kit with them at all times.

phone number or instructions to call EMS (911 where applicable) in case a severe or life-threatening reaction occurs.

Providers sometimes use intradermal tests to determine medication sensitivity or immunization needs. Follow the procedure for intradermal injections in Chapter 54.

Patch Test

The patch test is performed to determine the cause of **contact dermatitis**. A patch consisting of a gauze square saturated with the suspected allergy-causing substance is placed on the surface of the skin and secured with nonallergenic tape. The arm is the usual site of choice for convenience. The results are read after a 24-hour period and then repeated after a 48-hour period. A control is necessary and should be placed on the arm near the patch if the substance of the patch test is not a known skin irritant. Redness or swelling of the area indicates a reaction, and its interpretation is based on grading as for scratch and intradermal tests.

RAST Testing

The radioallergosorbent test (**RAST**) is a blood test that can be done with a skin test or instead of one. Individual allergens or allergen groups can be identified by the measurement of serum antibodies. (An example of an allergen group could be a food panel.) The antibody tested is immunoglobulin E (IgE), which can be produced in response to exposure to certain allergens; many times, the IgE levels are found to be higher in individuals with allergies or asthma. The RAST test is useful for those patients who cannot have the skin tests because they are taking certain medications such as some antidepressants.

Nasal Smear

A helpful aid for years in the diagnosis of allergies has been a smear done with nasal secretions to observe the **eosinophil** count. If there are many and they are clumped together, that is a strong indication of allergy. This is a simple means of screening for an allergy and is usually the first step in the testing program.

Testing for HIV

Another type of immunology testing includes testing for human immunodeficiency virus (HIV), which can result in acquired immunodeficiency syndrome (AIDS), a tragic disease in which the body can no longer fight off any type of infection. The first stages of the infection mimic the flu or mononucleosis with fatigue, slight fever, aching, lymph node swelling (lymphedema) and tenderness, and weight loss. Rapid tests are available for home use that detect the antibody to HIV; the results are generally available in 30 minutes. The standard screening tests are *enzyme immunoassays* (EIA), which take approximately a week to report the results. Depending on the office in which you are assigned for your externship or employed, you might be drawing blood specimens for this screening. Always remember to follow policy and procedure for collection and follow standard precautions—treat all patients as if they are or could be infected with HIV or hepatitis to protect yourself and others.

PKU TESTING

A screening test done with capillary blood from an infant's heel is the **phenylketonuria** (PKU). Phenylketonuria is a congenital disease caused by a defect in the **metabolism** of the **phenylalanine** amino acid. This unmetabolized protein accumulates in the bloodstream and can prevent the brain from developing normally. If this condition goes undetected and untreated, the result is mental retardation. This screening is required in all states and Canadian provinces, most commonly by the blood test but occasionally with a urine specimen. The blood test requires a few drops of the infant's blood to be soaked through the outlined circles (from the back of the card) of the treated paper attached to a health department's requisition (Figure 45–15A–B). The requisition is a multipart form that must be completed accurately and fully; usually, the parents bring the form with them when they return with the infant for the testing. Upon completion of the requisition form and collection of the specimen, the form and the PKU testing card is to be mailed to the state health department for processing. Most often, this test is done in a hospital or larger clinic facility setting, but you might be requested to perform this test in a pediatrician's office.

TESTING OUTSIDE THE POL

Typically, when a series of related tests are ordered for outside testing, the tests will be compiled into a panel or a profile. For instance, a liver panel would include enzymes and chemistries related to liver function and dysfunction: LDH, alkaline phosphatase, AST, ALT, and total **bilirubin** may be included in such a panel or profile. Another example of a profile would be a kidney function test that might include electrolytes (sodium, potassium, chloride, carbon dioxide), BUN (blood urea nitrogen), and creatinine.

Many times when individual tests are ordered on a laboratory requisition form, the reference or testing laboratory will combine them into a profile for better reimbursement by insurance providers.

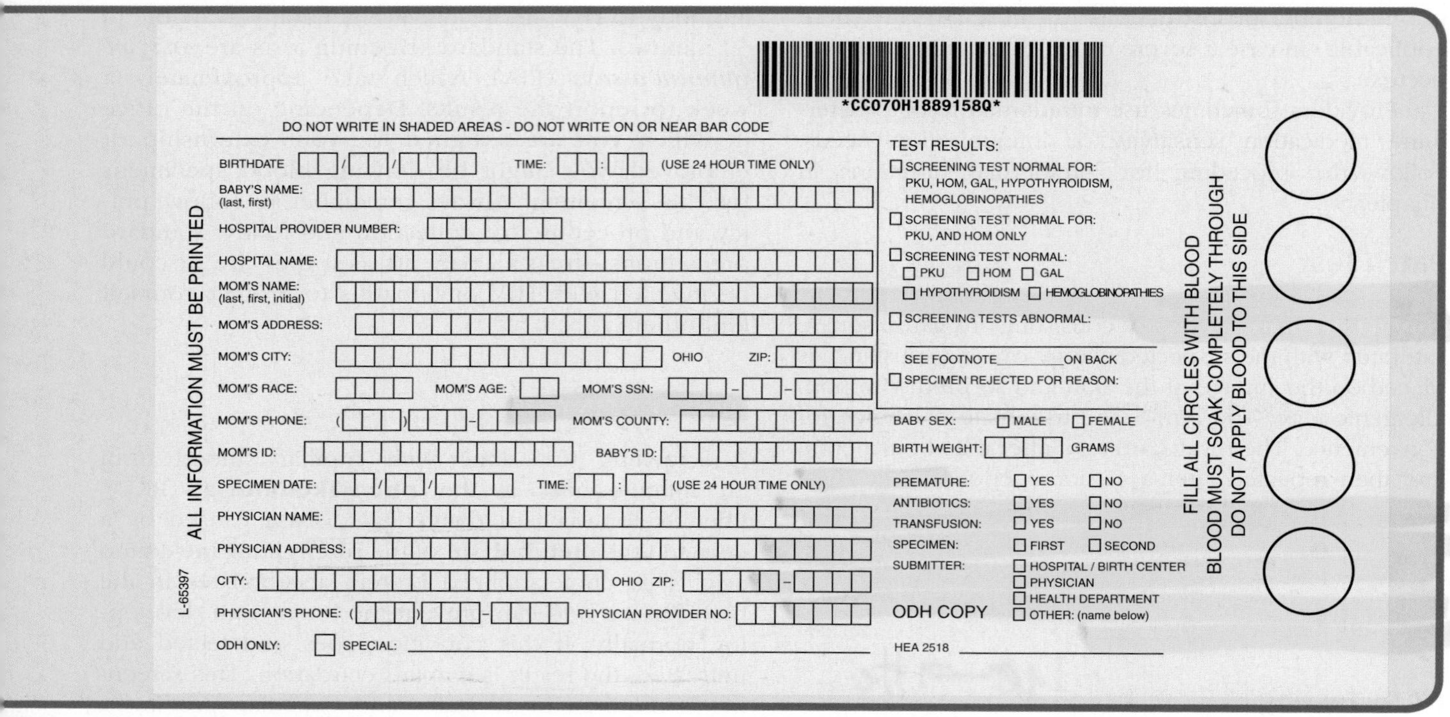
CC070H1889158Q

DO NOT WRITE IN SHADED AREAS - DO NOT WRITE ON OR NEAR BAR CODE

ALL INFORMATION MUST BE PRINTED

BIRTHDATE __/__/____ TIME: __:__ (USE 24 HOUR TIME ONLY)
BABY'S NAME: (last, first)
HOSPITAL PROVIDER NUMBER:
HOSPITAL NAME:
MOM'S NAME: (last, first, initial)
MOM'S ADDRESS:
MOM'S CITY: OHIO ZIP:
MOM'S RACE: MOM'S AGE: MOM'S SSN: ___-__-____
MOM'S PHONE: (___)___-____ MOM'S COUNTY:
MOM'S ID: BABY'S ID:
SPECIMEN DATE: __/__/____ TIME: __:__ (USE 24 HOUR TIME ONLY)
PHYSICIAN NAME:
PHYSICIAN ADDRESS:
CITY: OHIO ZIP: _____-____
PHYSICIAN'S PHONE: (___)___-____ PHYSICIAN PROVIDER NO:
ODH ONLY: ☐ SPECIAL:

L-65397

TEST RESULTS:
☐ SCREENING TEST NORMAL FOR: PKU, HOM, GAL, HYPOTHYROIDISM, HEMOGLOBINOPATHIES
☐ SCREENING TEST NORMAL FOR: PKU, AND HOM ONLY
☐ SCREENING TEST NORMAL: ☐ PKU ☐ HOM ☐ GAL ☐ HYPOTHYROIDISM ☐ HEMOGLOBINOPATHIES
☐ SCREENING TESTS ABNORMAL:
SEE FOOTNOTE ______ ON BACK
☐ SPECIMEN REJECTED FOR REASON:

BABY SEX: ☐ MALE ☐ FEMALE
BIRTH WEIGHT: GRAMS
PREMATURE: ☐ YES ☐ NO
ANTIBIOTICS: ☐ YES ☐ NO
TRANSFUSION: ☐ YES ☐ NO
SPECIMEN: ☐ FIRST ☐ SECOND
SUBMITTER: ☐ HOSPITAL / BIRTH CENTER ☐ PHYSICIAN ☐ HEALTH DEPARTMENT ☐ OTHER: (name below)
ODH COPY
HEA 2518

FILL ALL CIRCLES WITH BLOOD
BLOOD MUST SOAK COMPLETELY THROUGH
DO NOT APPLY BLOOD TO THIS SIDE

Figure 45–15A: Sample of a PKU testing form. *Delmar/Cengage Learning.*

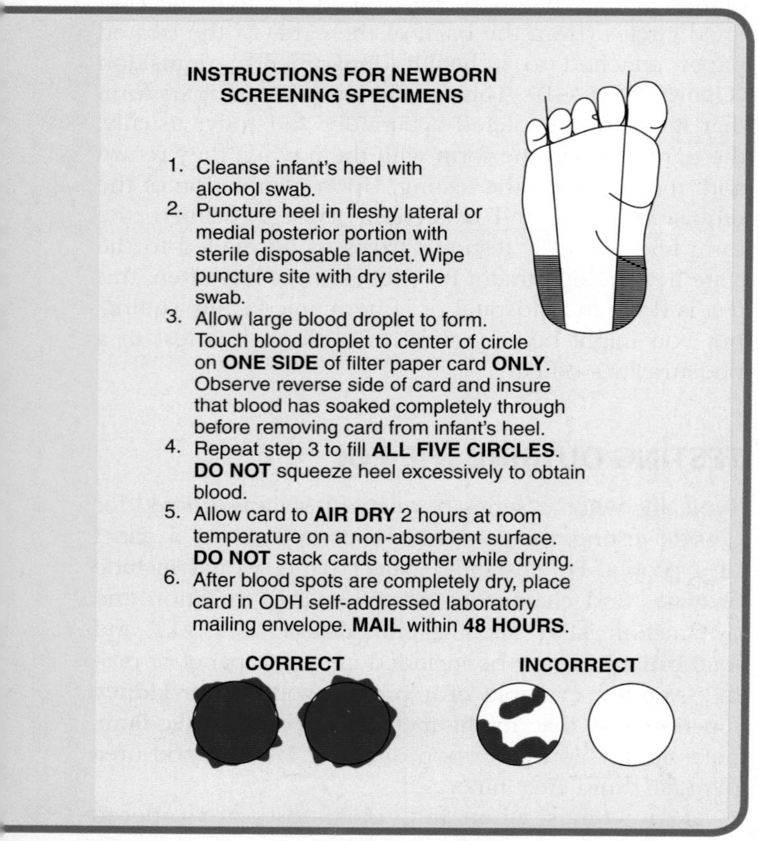
INSTRUCTIONS FOR NEWBORN SCREENING SPECIMENS

1. Cleanse infant's heel with alcohol swab.
2. Puncture heel in fleshy lateral or medial posterior portion with sterile disposable lancet. Wipe puncture site with dry sterile swab.
3. Allow large blood droplet to form. Touch blood droplet to center of circle on **ONE SIDE** of filter paper card **ONLY**. Observe reverse side of card and insure that blood has soaked completely through before removing card from infant's heel.
4. Repeat step 3 to fill **ALL FIVE CIRCLES**. **DO NOT** squeeze heel excessively to obtain blood.
5. Allow card to **AIR DRY** 2 hours at room temperature on a non-absorbent surface. **DO NOT** stack cards together while drying.
6. After blood spots are completely dry, place card in ODH self-addressed laboratory mailing envelope. **MAIL** within **48 HOURS**.

Figure 45–15B: Instructions for completion of information and examples of properly and improperly completed slides. *Delmar/Cengage Learning.*

Figure 45–16 is an example of a typical laboratory requisition form for outside testing. Panels are usually less expensive than the individual tests based on how insurance companies reimburse for health care. Health insurance carriers constantly change their methods for reimbursement, so it is vital to stay abreast of insurance developments when completing the requisitions for maximum reimbursement.

Although many tests are not performed in the health care provider's office, it might be your responsibility to screen the test results as they are returned to the provider's office in hard copy, over the Internet, or on the telephone. Most laboratory reports will come with flagged results for abnormalities, but you should have an idea of what a **panic value** is as well as how to follow up on the results as the provider instructs. Refer to Table 45–4 for commonly ordered tests, their indications, and normal value ranges. Procedure 45–8 reviews screening and following up test results.

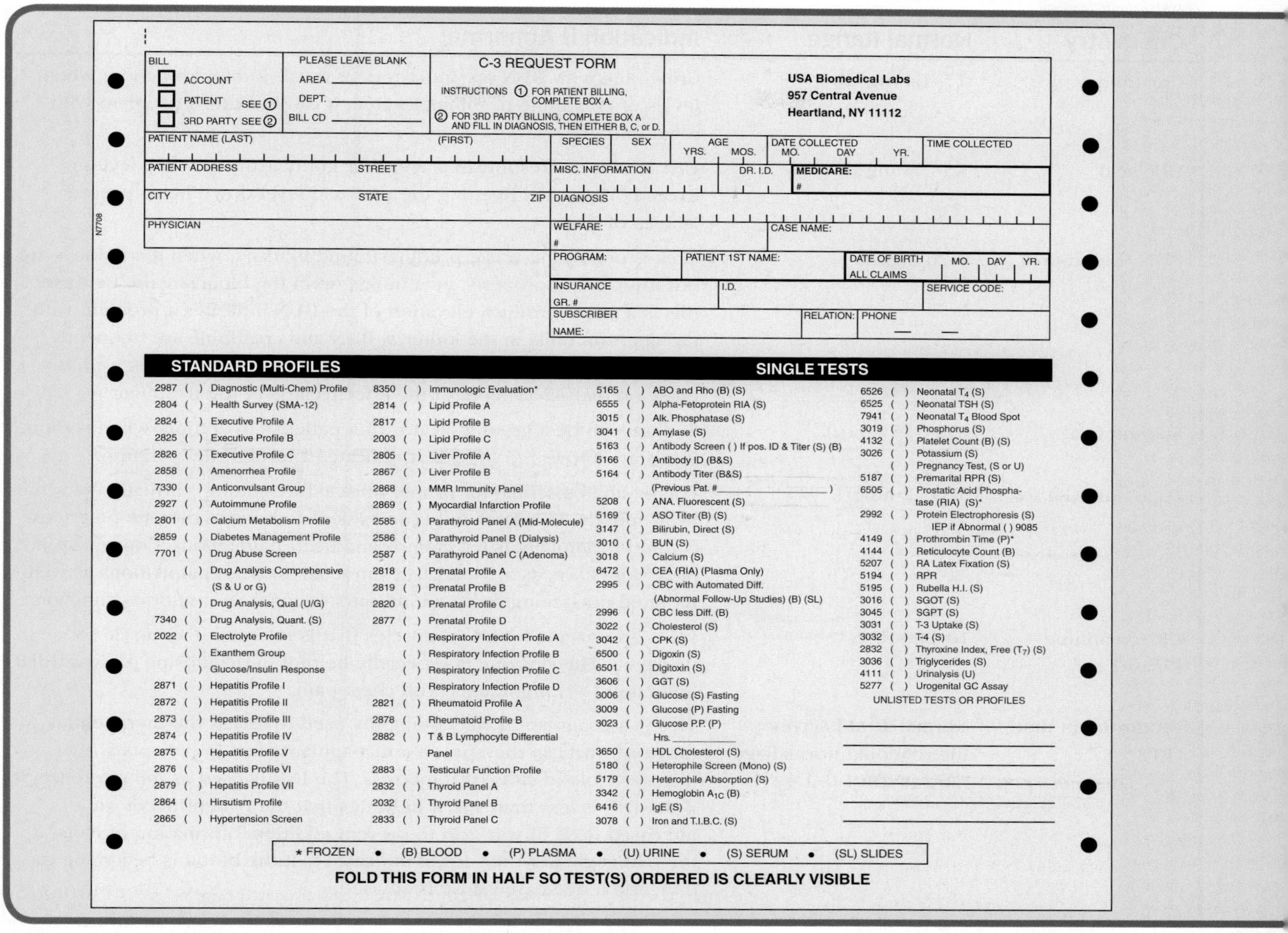

N7708

BILL
☐ ACCOUNT
☐ PATIENT SEE ①
☐ 3RD PARTY SEE ②

PLEASE LEAVE BLANK
AREA
DEPT.
BILL CD

C-3 REQUEST FORM
INSTRUCTIONS ① FOR PATIENT BILLING, COMPLETE BOX A.
② FOR 3RD PARTY BILLING, COMPLETE BOX A AND FILL IN DIAGNOSIS, THEN EITHER B, C, or D.

USA Biomedical Labs
957 Central Avenue
Heartland, NY 11112

PATIENT NAME (LAST) (FIRST) | SPECIES | SEX | AGE YRS. MOS. | DATE COLLECTED MO. DAY YR. | TIME COLLECTED
PATIENT ADDRESS STREET | MISC. INFORMATION | DR. I.D. | MEDICARE: #
CITY STATE ZIP | DIAGNOSIS
PHYSICIAN | WELFARE: # | CASE NAME:
PROGRAM: | PATIENT 1ST NAME: | DATE OF BIRTH ALL CLAIMS MO. DAY YR.
INSURANCE GR. # | I.D. | SERVICE CODE:
SUBSCRIBER NAME: | RELATION: | PHONE

STANDARD PROFILES

2987 ( ) Diagnostic (Multi-Chem) Profile
2804 ( ) Health Survey (SMA-12)
2824 ( ) Executive Profile A
2825 ( ) Executive Profile B
2826 ( ) Executive Profile C
2858 ( ) Amenorrhea Profile
7330 ( ) Anticonvulsant Group
2927 ( ) Autoimmune Profile
2801 ( ) Calcium Metabolism Profile
2859 ( ) Diabetes Management Profile
7701 ( ) Drug Abuse Screen
( ) Drug Analysis Comprehensive (S & U or G)
( ) Drug Analysis, Qual (U/G)
7340 ( ) Drug Analysis, Quant. (S)
2022 ( ) Electrolyte Profile
( ) Exanthem Group
( ) Glucose/Insulin Response
2871 ( ) Hepatitis Profile I
2872 ( ) Hepatitis Profile II
2873 ( ) Hepatitis Profile III
2874 ( ) Hepatitis Profile IV
2875 ( ) Hepatitis Profile V
2876 ( ) Hepatitis Profile VI
2879 ( ) Hepatitis Profile VII
2864 ( ) Hirsutism Profile
2865 ( ) Hypertension Screen
8350 ( ) Immunologic Evaluation*
2814 ( ) Lipid Profile A
2817 ( ) Lipid Profile B
2003 ( ) Lipid Profile C
2805 ( ) Liver Profile A
2867 ( ) Liver Profile B
2868 ( ) MMR Immunity Panel
2869 ( ) Myocardial Infarction Profile
2585 ( ) Parathyroid Panel A (Mid-Molecule)
2586 ( ) Parathyroid Panel B (Dialysis)
2587 ( ) Parathyroid Panel C (Adenoma)
2818 ( ) Prenatal Profile A
2819 ( ) Prenatal Profile B
2820 ( ) Prenatal Profile C
2877 ( ) Prenatal Profile D
( ) Respiratory Infection Profile A
( ) Respiratory Infection Profile B
( ) Respiratory Infection Profile C
( ) Respiratory Infection Profile D
2821 ( ) Rheumatoid Profile A
2878 ( ) Rheumatoid Profile B
2882 ( ) T & B Lymphocyte Differential Panel
2883 ( ) Testicular Function Profile
2832 ( ) Thyroid Panel A
2032 ( ) Thyroid Panel B
2833 ( ) Thyroid Panel C

SINGLE TESTS

5165 ( ) ABO and Rho (B) (S)
6555 ( ) Alpha-Fetoprotein RIA (S)
3015 ( ) Alk. Phosphatase (S)
3041 ( ) Amylase (S)
5163 ( ) Antibody Screen ( ) If pos. ID & Titer (S) (B)
5166 ( ) Antibody ID (B&S)
5164 ( ) Antibody Titer (B&S) (Previous Pat. #______)
5208 ( ) ANA. Fluorescent (S)
5169 ( ) ASO Titer (B) (S)
3147 ( ) Bilirubin, Direct (S)
3010 ( ) BUN (S)
3018 ( ) Calcium (S)
6472 ( ) CEA (RIA) (Plasma Only)
2995 ( ) CBC with Automated Diff. (Abnormal Follow-Up Studies) (B) (SL)
2996 ( ) CBC less Diff. (B)
3022 ( ) Cholesterol (S)
3042 ( ) CPK (S)
6500 ( ) Digoxin (S)
6501 ( ) Digitoxin (S)
3606 ( ) GGT (S)
3006 ( ) Glucose (S) Fasting
3009 ( ) Glucose (P) Fasting
3023 ( ) Glucose P.P. (P) Hrs.____
3650 ( ) HDL Cholesterol (S)
5180 ( ) Heterophile Screen (Mono) (S)
5179 ( ) Heterophile Absorption (S)
3342 ( ) Hemoglobin A_{1C} (B)
6416 ( ) IgE (S)
3078 ( ) Iron and T.I.B.C. (S)
6526 ( ) Neonatal T_4 (S)
6525 ( ) Neonatal TSH (S)
7941 ( ) Neonatal T_4 Blood Spot
3019 ( ) Phosphorus (S)
4132 ( ) Platelet Count (B) (S)
3026 ( ) Potassium (S)
( ) Pregnancy Test, (S or U)
5187 ( ) Premarital RPR (S)
6505 ( ) Prostatic Acid Phosphatase (RIA) (S)*
2992 ( ) Protein Electrophoresis (S) IEP if Abnormal ( ) 9085
4149 ( ) Prothrombin Time (P)*
4144 ( ) Reticulocyte Count (B)
5207 ( ) RA Latex Fixation (S)
5194 ( ) RPR
5195 ( ) Rubella H.I. (S)
3016 ( ) SGOT (S)
3045 ( ) SGPT (S)
3031 ( ) T-3 Uptake (S)
3032 ( ) T-4 (S)
2832 ( ) Thyroxine Index, Free (T_7) (S)
3036 ( ) Triglycerides (S)
4111 ( ) Urinalysis (U)
5277 ( ) Urogenital GC Assay

UNLISTED TESTS OR PROFILES

* FROZEN • (B) BLOOD • (P) PLASMA • (U) URINE • (S) SERUM • (SL) SLIDES

FOLD THIS FORM IN HALF SO TEST(S) ORDERED IS CLEARLY VISIBLE

Figure 45–16: Sample of a laboratory request form. *Delmar/Cengage Learning.*

TABLE 45–4 Normal Values of Commonly Performed Laboratory Tests and Their Indications

Chemistry	Normal Range	Indication if Abnormal
Total cholesterol	130–200 mg/dL (fasting)	Atherosclerosis, arteriosclerosis
HDL cholesterol	>45 mg/dL (fasting)	This is the good cholesterol; when levels are less than 45 mg/dL, the patient is more apt to have deposits of plaque in the arteries. The function of this type of cholesterol is to transport the bad cholesterol out of the vessels and to the liver.
LDL cholesterol	<100 mg/dL (fasting)	This is the bad cholesterol, primarily responsible for depositing plaque on the interior of arterial walls. If the LDL cholesterol cannot be controlled through diet, medication can help lower it as well as the total cholesterol.
Triglycerides	40–150 mg/dL (fasting)	This is a lipid but is not as structurally complex as cholesterol molecules. High levels of triglycerides can contribute to heart disease and hardening of the arteries. Lipid panels usually consist of the total cholesterol, HDL cholesterol, LDL cholesterol, and triglycerides.

(continues)

TABLE 45–4 *(Continued)*

Chemistry	Normal Range	Indication if Abnormal
Creatinine	0.7–1.4 mg/dL	Creatinine with BUN are indicators of renal (kidney) function; when levels of creatinine become elevated, it can indicate a problem with renal function.
Uric acid	3.5–7.5 mg/dL	Uric acid is the responsible agent for gouty arthritis when levels exceed 7.5 mg/dL. Keeping the uric acid level down helps prevent attacks of gout.
BUN (blood urea nitrogen)	8–20 mg/dL	Urea is one of the waste products found in urine; when the kidneys are not functioning properly, urea builds up in the bloodstream. Because this is a waste product, elevation of the BUN indicates a problem with the nephron units in the kidneys. BUN and creatinine are frequently ordered tests for those patients who have renal problems as well as those on dialysis to monitor the effectiveness of the treatment.
Sodium (Na)	132–145 mEq/L	Sodium can be a good indicator of a patient's hydration; when sodium levels are above 145 mEq/L, it indicates a level of dehydration.
Potassium (K)	3.5–5.2 mEq/L	Potassium is essential for proper muscle functioning, particularly for the heart muscle. If potassium becomes depleted due to diuretics, the most common complaint is leg cramps and heart palpitations. Conversely, if potassium exceeds 5.2 mEq/L, it can result in heart palpitations as well. Elevated potassium is also an indicator of renal disease or dysfunction.
CK (creatinine kinase)	10–200 IU/L	CK is an enzyme found in muscles that is released if a muscle is damaged. This enzyme is especially helpful in diagnosing a myocardial infarction (MI) in patients with chest pain.
Prothrombin time (PT)	Normal 10–13 seconds International normalized ratio (INR): 1.0–1.4	This is a coagulation test commonly used to assess the therapeutic range of warfarin therapy, an anticoagulant used in patients with a history of blood clots (thrombosis). The INR is used as the reference; if the INR is less than 1.0, it indicates that the patient needs an increased dose of warfarin to prevent additional formation of clots. If the INR is greater than 1.4, it indicates that the blood is becoming too thin, and a decreased dose is advised.

PROCEDURE 45–8 Screen and Follow Up Blood Test Results

PURPOSE: Screen and follow up lab results for normal, abnormal, and panic values to relay information to the health care provider

EQUIPMENT: Scenarios of simulated lab reports for examination and analysis and reference materials supplied by the instructor (e.g., Internet, laboratory reference manuals, textbook, and so on).

S SKILL: Review a laboratory report for blood studies and make notations about whether the results are normal, abnormal, or panic value and follow up.

Procedure Steps	Detailed Instructions and/or *Rationales*
1. Screen the test results to determine whether they are normal, abnormal, or panic value.	
2. Screen the test results to determine whether laboratory reports are missing any key elements.	

Procedure Steps	Detailed Instructions and/or *Rationales*
3. Identify panic values, the disease state that might be a result of them, or the disease state that might be caused if left untreated.	
4. Identify the appropriate action for panic values with the health care provider.	
5. Identify the appropriate action for abnormal values with the health care provider.	
6. Identify the appropriate action for normal values with the health care provider.	
7. Accurately chart action taken in the patient's medical record.	

Charting Example

Amick, Deborah Ann ID# 27456123 08/03/XX	1802	Spoke with patient regarding low Hgb level per Dr.'s instructions. Phoned Rx into pharmacy for her to start immediately. Return 4 weeks for repeat hgb check. Laura Treolo, RMA(AMT)

CHAPTER SUMMARY

- It is important for the medical assistant to perform the quality controls at the beginning of each day and log the results prior to reporting any patient results to preserve the integrity of the test results.
- Always instruct patients in preparation for testing and have clear, concise, written instructions available. *Do not* presume that patients know all about a procedure even if they have had the test before.
- The erythrocyte sedimentation rate is also known as the ESR or the sed rate.
- Many types of glucometers are on the market; make sure always to check the manufacturer's instructions prior to testing.
- Fasting means that the patient has had nothing to eat or drink for at least 12 hours prior to having specific testing drawn. Emphasize that he or she should not eat mints, chew gum, drink coffee or juices, or smoke.
- Always remember to follow policy and procedure for proper collection and follow standard precautions—treat all patients as if they are or could be infected with HIV or hepatitis to protect yourself and others.
- Panic values require immediate intervention by health care providers.

STUDY TOOLS

Workbook	Activities for Chapter 45
Premium Website MEDIA LINK	View these **Media Links** for Chapter 45: • Perform an ESR • Perform Glucose Testing
StudyWARE	Activities and Quizzes on the **StudyWARE™ Software** for Chapter 45

(continues)

	Complete the following **Competency Challenge 2.0** activities: • Wednesday, 8:00 AM: Perform Hematology Testing • Wednesday, 9:00 AM: Perform Chemistry Testing • Wednesday, 10:00 AM: Perform Immunology Testing
	Audio Library of medical terms
	Online access to the **Critical Thinking Challenge 2.0**
CourseMate	Activities and Quizzes for Chapter 45
WebTutor	Activities and Quizzes for Chapter 45

CHECK YOUR KNOWLEDGE

1. The medical assistant will be responsible for quality control and assurance. All the following are required components to be recorded in the log book *except*:
   a. patient's name.
   b. results of the test.
   c. doctor's initials.
   d. test performed.
2. Hemoglobin is an allosteric protein found in:
   a. monocytes.
   b. erythrocytes.
   c. lymphocytes.
   d. granulocytes.
3. Hemoglobin is responsible for transporting __________ to cells of the body.
   a. oxygen
   b. carbon dioxide
   c. iron
   d. vitamins and nutrients
4. Hematocrit is never expressed as a percentage.
   a. True
   b. False
5. If a patient has a rheumatoid arthritis, the provider will order which of the following tests to monitor inflammation?
   a. Hemoglobin
   b. CBC
   c. ESR
   d. Hemoglobin A1C
6. The forearm provides 14 prime sites for intradermal testing.
   a. True
   b. False
7. Which of the following are indicators of renal function?
   a. Triglycerides
   b. CK with PT
   c. Na with uric acid
   d. BUN with creatinine

WEB LINKS

MedlinePlus Laboratory Tests: www.nlm.nih.gov/medlineplus/laboratorytests.html

WedMD Phenylketonuria (PKU) Test: www.webmd.com/parenting/baby/phenylketonuria-pku-test

Chapter

46 Specimen Collection and Processing

OBJECTIVES

In this chapter, you will learn the following:

KB KNOWLEDGE BASE

1. Spell and define, using the glossary at the back of the text, all the Words to Know in this chapter.
2. Identify different types of urine specimens and why they are ordered for testing.
3. Explain the procedure for collecting urine specimens for substance analysis and the chain-of-custody procedure.
4. Define the three components of the routine urinalysis.
5. Understand various collection techniques for fecal specimens.
6. Identify tests that require sputum specimens and properly instruct a patient on collecting a specimen.
7. Explain the need for bacterial specimen collection.
8. Identify various types of microbiologic collection techniques and diagnostic tests that would be ordered on such specimens.
9. Differentiate between culture and sensitivity.
10. Explain the proper procedure for performing the gram's stain and identify each of the components of the stain.
11. Differentiate between Gram-positive and Gram-negative reactions on a Gram's stain.
12. Identify the basic morphologic shapes for various types of microorganisms.
13. Differentiate between some common Gram-positive and Gram-negative descriptions for bacterial identification.
14. Describe various media for cultures; differentiate between primary media, selective media, and enrichment media.
15. Describe how to label specimens properly.

S SKILLS

1. Instruct a male and a female patient on the proper procedure for obtaining a midstream, clean-catch urine specimen.
2. Perform a pregnancy test and document the quality controls for the test.
3. Perform the chemical examination of a urinalysis.
4. Prepare a urine specimen for microscopic examination.
5. Review a laboratory report and make notations about whether the results are normal, abnormal, or panic value and follow up.
6. Instruct a patient on the proper procedure for collecting a fecal specimen for occult blood screening.
7. Perform occult blood testing.
8. Instruct a patient on collecting a sputum specimen.
9. Obtain a wound culture.
10. Obtain a throat culture.
11. Test a throat swab for group A strep with a rapid diagnostic test and interpret the results.
12. Appropriately document information regarding specimens on the patient's chart.

B BEHAVIORS

1. Display sensitivity to patient rights and feelings in collecting specimens.
2. Explain the rationale for performance of a procedure to the patient.
3. Show awareness of patients' concerns regarding their perceptions of the procedure being performed.

WORDS TO KNOW

agar
bilirubin
catheterization
chemical
culture
exudate
glucose
Gram-negative
Gram-positive
guaiac
hematuria
hemolysis
human chorionic gonadotropin (hCG)
in vivo
ketone (acetone)
nitrite
physical
protein (albumin)
sensitivity
specific gravity
sputum
stability
supernatant
urinalysis
urobilinogen

COLLECTING URINE SPECIMENS

Urine specimens are usually collected in plastic disposable containers, either non-sterile or sterile, depending on the type of specimen indicated for testing (Figure 46–1). The following should be noted on the container: patient's name, date of collection, time of collection, and tests to be performed on the specimen. Ideally, any testing should be performed within one hour of collection to prevent decomposition of the specimen due to bacterial overgrowth and cellular breakdown. If the specimen cannot be tested within the one-hour time frame, the specimen must be refrigerated to preserve its integrity; just as important is that when testing is to be performed on the refrigerated specimen, the specimen must be allowed to return to room temperature and must be stirred well prior to any analysis, whether it is physical, chemical, or microscopic.

First Morning Urine Sample

The first morning urine sample is the best for testing because it is the most concentrated specimen because the urine has been in the bladder overnight. Most often, however, health care providers order random specimens that most patients have little difficulty in providing; *random* means the specimen is not scheduled and requires no advance preparation.

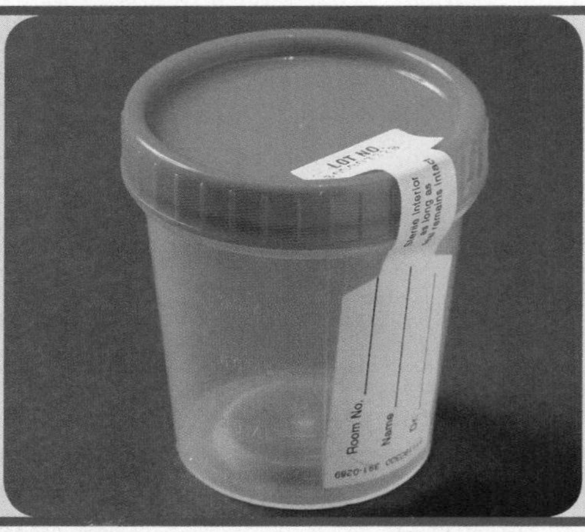

Figure 46–1: Urine collection cup. *Delmar/Cengage Learning.*

Midstream Clean-Catch Specimen

Many providers prefer the specimens to be collected as midstream clean-catch specimens, and for this type of specimen, you must be able to provide adequate instructions for compliance.

PATIENT EDUCATION

Patients should be instructed to use the provided antiseptic wipes to cleanse the genital area from front to back in a single motion and discard, and repeat with a second wipe whether they are male or female. Women need to be instructed to spread the labia gently during the cleansing and during the collection of the specimen. In the case of the male patient, instructions must be provided to those who are not circumcised that the foreskin must be retracted prior to the area being cleansed. If the male is circumcised, the antiseptic wipes are to be used as previously described, in a single front-to-back motion and discarded.

After this step of the procedure, the patient should be instructed to:

- Not touch the inside of the sterile specimen container nor the inside of the lid.
- Void partially into the commode and stop.
- Collect the middle portion of the specimen in the cup and stop (usually about three ounces).
- Finish voiding into the commode.
- Replace the lid on the container, wipe any residual urine from the outside of the container, and either return the container to you or place it in a designated spot.

The partial voiding before collection of the specimen clears the urethra of contaminants such as bacteria, mucus, cells, or other debris that could adversely affect the results. This step helps provide a more sterile specimen so that if a culture of the urine is indicated, the specimen is less likely to be contaminated. Refer to Procedure 46–1.

PROCEDURE 46–1 Instruct a Patient on the Collection of a Clean-Catch, Midstream Urine Specimen

MEDIA LINK: View the video for this chapter, "Clean-Catch Midstream Urine Specimen," on the Premium Website.

PURPOSE: Prepare a written brochure for instructing both a male and a female patient in the collection of a clean-catch, midstream urine specimen. Use the brochure to instruct the patient in the collection of the specimen and give the container to the patient for collecting the specimen.

EQUIPMENT: Computer, printer, paper, sterile container, antiseptic wipes, disposable gloves, pen, and label for container

SKILL: To instruct a male or female patient in the proper collection of a clean-catch, midstream urine specimen to prevent contamination of the urine sample.

Procedure Steps	Detailed Instructions and/or *Rationales*
1. Prepare printed brochures for instructing male and female patients in the proper collection of urine specimens.	The evaluator should review the brochures for accuracy in instruction, grammar, spelling, and punctuation prior to giving to the patient.
2. Assemble supplies to provide to the patient.	
3. Identify the patient and instruct him or her for the collection as outlined in the brochure, ***including the rationale for performing the procedure, using language and verbal skills the patient can understand. Answer any questions the patient might have prior to the collection.***	
4. Provide the patient with the labeled sterile cup and antiseptic wipes. Direct the patient to the restroom.	The sterile cup should be labeled with the patient's name, identification number, the date, and the time.
5. Properly collect the specimen from the patient upon exit from the restroom.	Observe standard precautions in handling the specimen.

24-Hour Urine Specimen

On occasion, a 24-hour urine specimen is ordered. A written laboratory order is given to the patient, and either you or a laboratory technician will be responsible for providing the instructions for collection to the patient. It is essential to provide instructions the patient can understand for proper collection of this specimen, and printed instruction sheets are most helpful for this. The patient is provided with a container in which to collect the sequential specimens over the 24-hour period; it is up to you to check the lab manual to see whether a preservative must be added to the container or special instructions provided. In some cases, the patient simply needs to refrigerate the specimen the entire length of the 24 hours prior to submitting the specimen to the laboratory for testing. A difficult concept for patients to grasp is the timing of the specimen; the patient begins the timing of the 24-hour period at the first void of urine on the first day, although this specimen is not collected as part of the total specimen.

Following this void (the time of which the patient must document), the patient collects all urine specimens and places those in the collection container until the 24-hour period is over. Any specimen voided after the 24 hours is over should *not* be collected; as soon as convenient for the patient, the container should be returned to the laboratory or hospital for testing. Depending on the test being performed, the health care provider might receive results in as little as a day, or results might take several days before being reported.

Pediatric Urine Specimens

Pediatric urine specimens are another type of specimen collection that can be encountered in pediatrician or family practice offices. Special urine collection bags fit over

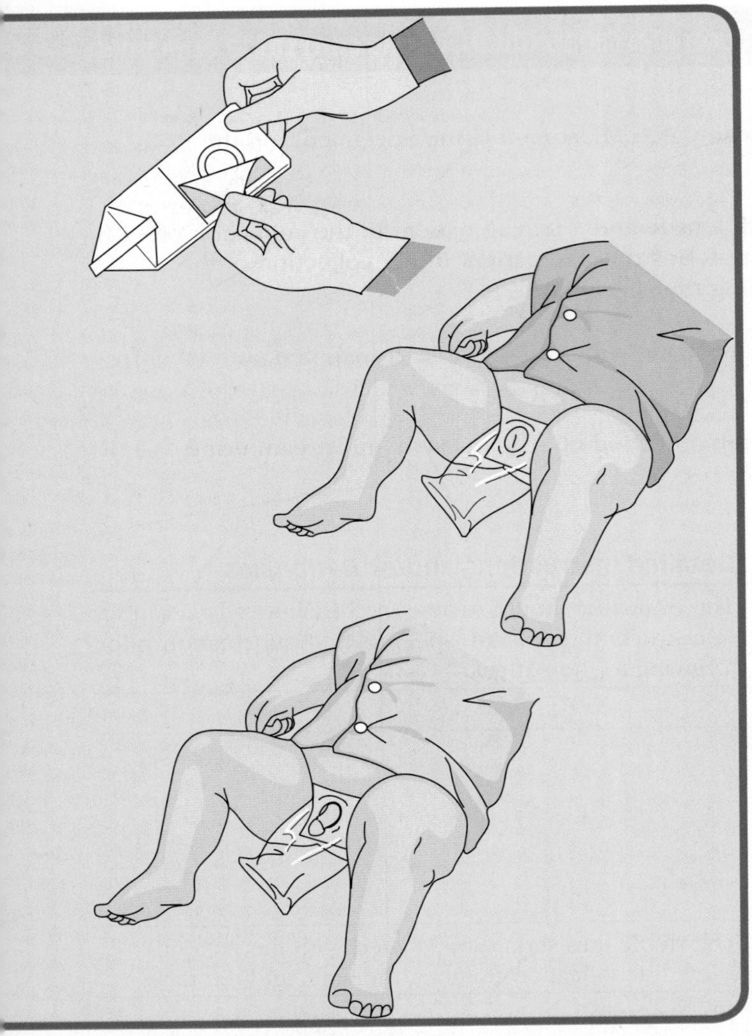

Figure 46–2: Example of a pediatric urine collection unit in the proper position. *Delmar/Cengage Learning.*

the genital area of the baby and are secured with adhesive (Figure 46–2). The infant's skin should be washed and dried thoroughly, usually by the parent, prior to the bag being affixed to the skin; otherwise, the bag will not remain in place for the collection of the specimen. After the pediatric bag is returned to the office, it is necessary to transfer the contents to a container. The parents must provide the baby's name as well as date and time of collection before processing; parents should also be advised that if the specimen cannot be returned to the facility prior to one hour following collection, the specimen should be refrigerated to protect its integrity and accuracy of results.

Urinary Catheterization

Catheterization is a specialized type of urine collection that is indicated in the following instances:

- A sterile specimen is indicated for testing.
- The patient is unable to void.
- Medication must be instilled in the bladder.

When catheterization is ordered, the procedure includes the introduction of a sterile plastic tube into the bladder; catheters can be straight, which means they are used only on a short-term basis, or in-dwelling when they remain for a longer period of time (e.g., Foley catheters). This procedure is not performed routinely in most offices, although you might encounter it in urology offices and even sometimes in obstetrics and gynecology offices. Generally, the urologist performs the catheterization. Many times, a culture and sensitivity (discussed later in the chapter) will be ordered on the specimen because an infection might be causing the patient's inability to void. If you are in an office where catheterization is performed often, your primary role will probably be one of assisting the health care provider. Remember that catheterization is a *sterile* technique, and contamination of any part of the catheterization kit is unacceptable. Severe bladder infections can occur with compromise of the sterile technique required for this procedure.

Collection of Specimens for Substance Abuse Analysis and Chain of Custody

The purpose of this test is to detect the presence of illegal or illicit drugs or chemical substances and might prevent a person from obtaining or retaining a job. Most commonly, urine specimens are collected for this testing; if alcohol abuse is detected, it is most often tested by blood testing, although breath tests are commonly employed.

It is essential for the procedure to be explained to the patient in its entirety before you ask him or her to sign the consent and release form for testing of this sort. Often, this type of collection is performed by the medical assistant, so it is important to understand the implications of this procedure.

Patients should be informed that all drugs that have been consumed within the 30 days prior to testing are likely to be revealed by the test, even including over-the-counter (OTC) medications. Explain that concealing information is inadvisable because the testing procedure is very sensitive; advise patients that a section of the form allows the patient to list all substances consumed in the past month. Ask the patient to be as accurate and honest as possible when completing this form to be fair to him or her in interpretation of the results.

After you explain the procedure to the patient, before you proceed with collection of the specimen, you must have the patient to sign the *chain-of-custody* form that further informs the patient regarding the reason for the test. After the patient signs the chain-of-custody form, it releases you to collect the specimen, prepare it for transport to the testing facility, and release the results to the agency requesting the testing.

Although different testing facilities have different requirements, the following are usually followed for collection:

- Prior to the patient entering the bathroom facility, either bluing is added to the toilet or the handle for flushing is taped down.
- If you are the same sex as the patient, you might be required to be present in the bathroom facility for monitoring purposes.
- The temperature of the specimen is immediately checked following collection and recorded with the patient observing you.
- The lid of the container is taped closed, and the patient is asked to initial as verification that this is his or her specimen and that he or she has observed you closing the specimen.
- Most often, after specimen collection, the patient again signs or initials the form to indicate that he or she has seen his or her specimen processed.

Figure 46–3 displays a sample chain-of-custody form. Persons who require Department of Transportation (DOT) physicals have this type of testing on a routine or random basis, and you will find this type of testing often in pre-employment screening.

After the specimen has been collected, verified as valid by you, and initialed by the patient and signatures have been obtained for the chain-of-custody form, the form accompanies the specimen to the testing facility. It is important to press down hard when completing the form for all carbon copies to be legible. Copies of the form are then routed as follows:

- Medical review officer
- Laboratory (testing facility)
- Patient
- Collector
- Employer

Pregnancy Testing

Pregnancy tests are performed to measure the amount of **human chorionic gonadotropin (hCG)** in the blood or urine. Occasionally, testing is ordered for hCG in the diagnosis of certain tumors, such as germ cell tumors originating in the ovaries or male testes, because hCG or a similar substance might be produced by these tumors. Normally, hCG is produced by the placenta during pregnancy, which helps maintain the pregnancy and normal development of the fetus. Levels of hCG show a steady increase in the first 14 to 16 weeks following fertilization.

Home pregnancy tests and screening tests in most POLs are performed on a urine specimen, ideally a first morning specimen, because that specimen is the most concentrated. Although the quantity of hCG cannot be determined, the test will indicate whether hCG levels have exceeded the non-pregnant levels. Simple urine tests commonly employ either a plus (+) mark or two lines that are similar to an equals (=) sign upon completion of a positive test. A single line (–) indicates the patient is not pregnant or that the level of hCG is undetectable (Figure 46–4). When obtaining a specimen from a patient in the provider's office, ask when the last menstrual period (LMP) occurred and document this on the patient's chart. See Procedure 46–2.

The blood test is a more accurate test than the urine test, provides a quantitative result that indicates how long the woman has been pregnant, and gives an idea of when the fetus is due for delivery. This test also is tracked to make sure the fetus is developing at a normal rate for those women who have had problem pregnancies or miscarriages in the past and can be used to assist in the determination of ectopic pregnancies.

URINALYSIS

Urinalysis is probably the most frequently performed test in the medical office. Examination of the urine consists of the major areas of testing: **physical**, **chemical**, and microscopic (Figure 46–5).

Physical Urinalysis

Included in the physical testing of the specimen are the following.

- Color
- Clarity
- Volume (in certain specimens)
- Odor (although not reported on lab report form)
- Specific gravity

Color and Clarity

Standard color descriptions include yellow, straw, dark straw, light straw, light yellow, and dark yellow; occasionally, colors will be described as red (blood), brown (old blood), orange (pyridium), green (jaundice), and blue (certain medications). The clarity of a specimen refers to how clear it is; therefore, standard clarity descriptions include clear, slightly hazy, hazy, cloudy, and turbid. The most accurate way to describe color and clarity is to decant (pour) the specimen into a clear tube so that the opaqueness of the collection container does not adversely affect your analysis of these properties. If you can easily read print through the tube containing the specimen, the description would be clear; a few particles floating around in the specimen would be slightly hazy. If the print is fuzzy, the specimen would be described as hazy, and if you cannot see the print at all, the specimen will be described as cloudy or turbid, with turbid being the worst description.

USA LABS
ID#

Referred by

Health Care Provider
Address
Phone

DO NOT WRITE IN THIS AREA

CHAIN OF CUSTODY

STEP 1 — TO BE COMPLETED BY EMPLOYER/COLLECTOR.
DONOR IDENTIFICATION—PLEASE PRINT

LAST NAME ____________________

FIRST NAME ____________________ M.I.

SOC. SEC. NO. ______ — ______ — ______

EMPLOYEE NO. ____________________

DONOR I.D. VERIFIED ☐ PHOTO I.D. ☐ EMPLOYER REPRESENTATIVE

____
SIGNATURE OF EMPLOYER REP.

REASON FOR TEST (CHECK ONE)
☐ (1) PRE-EMPLOYMENT ☐ (2) POST ACCIDENT ☐ (3) RANDOM
☐ (4) PERIODIC ☐ (5) REASONABLE SUSPICION/CAUSE
☐ (6) RETURN TO DUTY
☐ (99) OTHER (SPECIFY)

TESTS REQUESTED: TOTAL TESTS ORDERED ☐

SPECIMEN ☐ Urine ☐ Blood (SUBMIT ONLY ONE SPECIMEN WITH EACH REQUISITION)

STEP 2—COLLECTOR, FOR URINE SPECIMENS, READ TEMPERATURE WITHIN FOUR MINUTES OF COLLECTION.
CHECK THE BOX IF TEMPERATURE IS WITHIN THE SPECIFIED RANGE ☐ 90°–100°F / 32°–38°C
OR RECORD ACTUAL TEMPERATURE HERE: ____________

STEP 3—TO BE COMPLETED BY COLLECTOR. COLLECTION SITE

COLLECTION DATE ____________ TIME ____________ ☐ AM PM

ADDRESS ____________________

REMARKS ____________________

CITY STATE ZIP

( )
PHONE

I certify that the specimen identified on this form is the specimen presented to me by the employee identified in Step 1 above, and was collected, labeled and sealed in the donor's presence.

COLLECTOR'S NAME PRINT (FIRST, M.I., LAST) SIGNATUE OF COLLECTOR

STEP 4—TO BE INITIATED BY THE DONOR AND COMPLETED AS NECESSARY THEREAFTER.

PURPOSE OF CHANGE	RELEASED BY SIGNATURE	RECEIVED BY SIGNATURE	DATE
A. PROVIDE SPECIMEN FOR TESTING			
B. SHIPMENT TO LABORATORY			
C.			

COMMENTS:

Self-stick identification
Labels for sealing specimen:
(123) (123) (123) (123)

SPECIMEN PACKAGE INTEGRITY WAS ☐ACCEPTABLE ☐ UNACCEPTABLE WHEN RECEIVED IN LAB.

RECEIVER'S INITIALS

FOR OFFICE USE

Figure 46–3: Sample chain-of-custody form. *Delmar/Cengage Learning.*

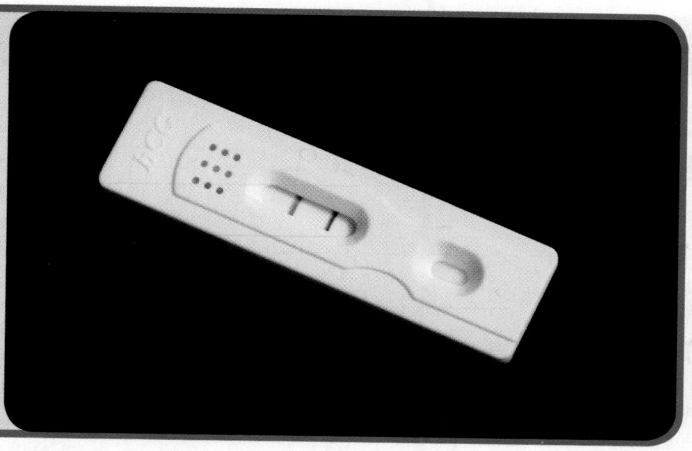

Figure 46–4: Positive pregnancy test result showing the double line resembling an equal sign "=". © *Anthony Jay D. Villalon/ www.Shutterstock.com.*

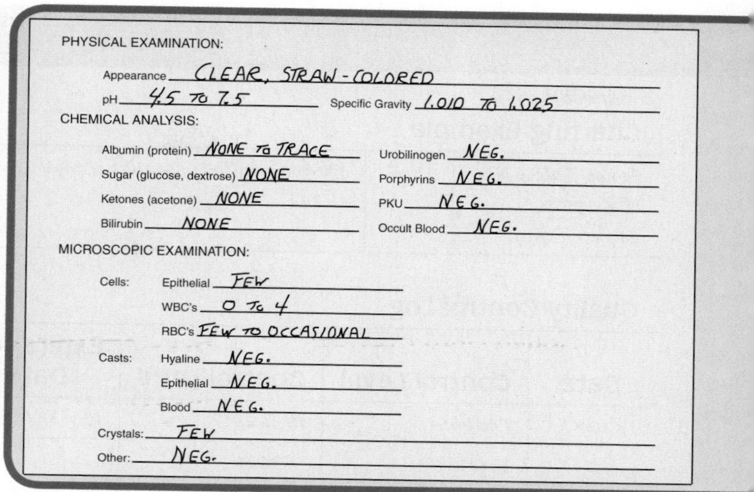

PHYSICAL EXAMINATION:

Appearance CLEAR, STRAW-COLORED

pH 4.5 TO 7.5 Specific Gravity 1.010 TO 1.025

CHEMICAL ANALYSIS:

Albumin (protein) NONE TO TRACE Urobilinogen NEG.

Sugar (glucose, dextrose) NONE Porphyrins NEG.

Ketones (acetone) NONE PKU NEG.

Bilirubin NONE Occult Blood NEG.

MICROSCOPIC EXAMINATION:

Cells: Epithelial FEW

WBC's 0 TO 4

RBC's FEW TO OCCASIONAL

Casts: Hyaline NEG.

Epithelial NEG.

Blood NEG.

Crystals: FEW

Other: NEG.

Figure 46–5: Lab report form showing normal values for a routine urinalysis in the physical, chemical, and microscopic examinations and analyses. *Delmar/Cengage Learning.*

PROCEDURE 46–2 Perform Screening for Pregnancy

PURPOSE: Perform a pregnancy screening on a urine sample to determine the presence (or absence) of human chorionic gonadotropin (hCG)

EQUIPMENT: Disposable gloves, other personal protective equipment (PPE) per laboratory policies, urine specimen, quality control materials, reagents, black or blue pen, and biohazard waste container

S SKILL: Perform a pregnancy test and document the quality controls for the test.

Procedure Steps	Detailed Instructions and/or *Rationales*
1. Assemble the necessary equipment and supplies.	
2. Wash hands and don disposable gloves and other PPE as required.	
3. Perform quality control testing on two reagent cards, one negative and one positive.	Control samples must be run only once per day or any time a new box of reagents has been opened.
4. Record the results of the quality control analyses in the quality control log; do not report patient results if quality control results are not in the acceptable range.	
5. Prepare the reagent for patient testing and process it according to the manufacturer's directions.	
6. Record the results of the test on the patient's health record.	
7. Dispose of contaminated waste in the biohazard waste container.	
8. Remove gloves and wash hands.	

(continues)

(continued)

Charting Example

Jones, Sally Mae ID# 098762 01/10/XX	1347	pregnancy test, negative. Bryan Riffe, CMA(AAMA)

Quality Control Log

Date	Control Level	Control Lot #	Expiration Date	Reagent Lot #	Expiration Date	Results	Initials
1/10/XX	positive	15962V	12/31/09	454590	6/7/10	positive	jva
1/10/XX	negative	15963V	12/31/09	454590	6/7/10	negative	jva

Volume

Twenty-four hour urine specimens must have the volume assessed, although only a representative sample is submitted to the laboratory for testing; it is unnecessary to assess the volume of a routine urine specimen for testing.

Odor

The odor of a specimen can provide you with insight about what abnormal condition the patient might have. For instance, if you notice a very strong ammonia-like smell, it probably indicates a urinary tract infection (UTI) from the presence of bacteria. A mousy or musty odor is associated with phenylketonuria, while a fruity smell is linked to diabetes from the presence of ketones. Although you do not record the odor of a specimen on the report form, these particular odors are helpful in confirming findings as you perform the testing. Keep in mind that certain foods, garlic in particular, can emit a strong odor that does not indicate a pathologic condition.

Specific Gravity

distilled water has no SG

Specific gravity, defined as the weight of substances dissolved in a substance as compared with those found in distilled water, once were assessed as a physical process, either by a urinometer or a refractometer. However, the chemical reagent strips now include this parameter, so offices no longer assess the specific gravity as a physical property but rather as a chemical property. You should keep in mind that the specific gravity of water is 1.000 to 1.003, and the normal range of the specific gravity of urine is 1.005 to 1.030, with most urine results falling in the 1.015 number. The more dilute the specimen (the more water and less dissolved substances in the specimen), the lower the specific gravity will be. Conversely, more substances in the specimen with less water results in a higher specific gravity. Remember you are comparing the specimen with distilled water, a substance that should not have anything dissolved in it and is considered relatively pure and without any solutes.

Chemical Urinalysis

Urine specimens should be analyzed as soon as possible after collection; if more than an hour has transpired and the specimen has been refrigerated, be sure to allow the specimen to return to room temperature and gently mix it before testing because constituents settle to the bottom. Also, because specimens with bilirubin can become degraded from exposure to light, it is important for all specimens to be collected in an opaque container so analysis does not yield false negative results.

Reagent strips are convenient, relatively inexpensive, reliable, and quick and serve to reveal the presence of abnormal substances in the urine as well as assess other numerical values such as pH, urobilinogen, and specific gravity. The reagent strips provide both qualitative and quantitative assessments. Qualitatively, the strips reveal the presence of an abnormal result, and quantitatively, they determine how much of a substance is actually present in the specimen. The specially treated pads on the reagent strip are designed so that the specific pad reacts chemically with the urine to produce a color change. After the color change, the strip is compared with known values on the bottle for reporting (Figures 46–6A and B).

These reagent strips can be used in a manual method in which the person performing the test views the strip and reports the color change as a result at the appropriate time, or instruments are available that read and print out the results when the strip is inserted in the instrument (Figure 46–7). The instruments must be checked daily with quality control and trends that show the instrument might need calibration, cleaning, or new reagent strips.

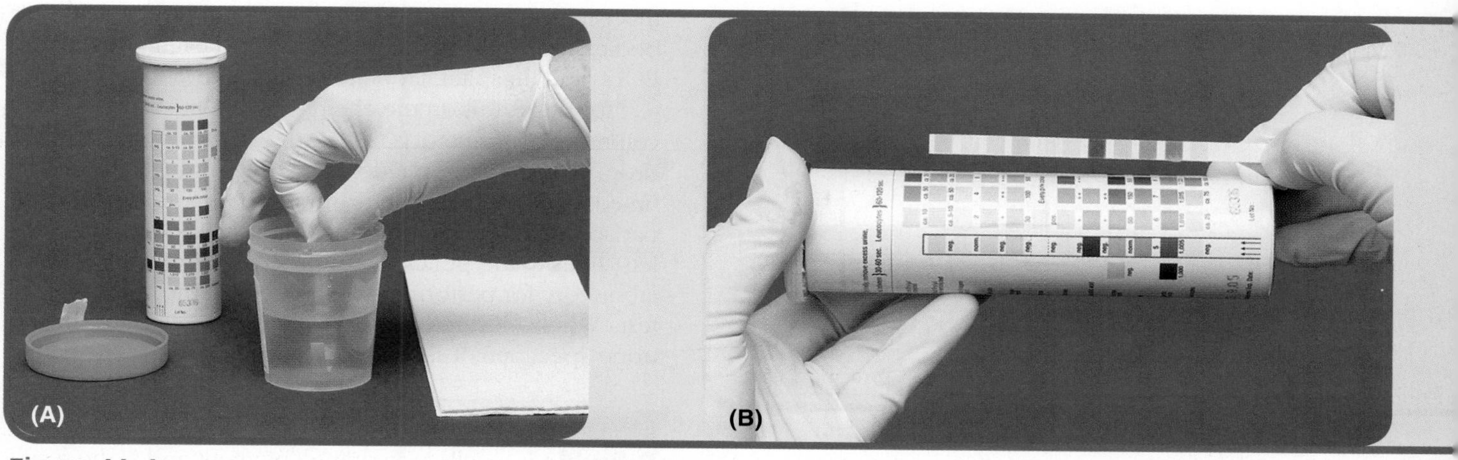

Figure 46–6: (A) The reagent strip is immersed in the urine. (B) The reagent strip is compared with the color chart of known values on the bottle. *Delmar/Cengage Learning.*

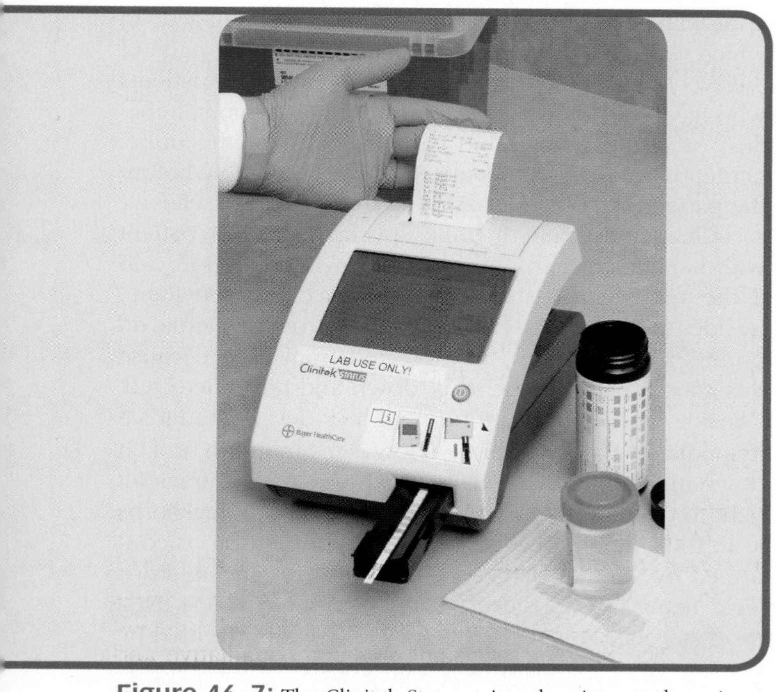

Figure 46–7: The Clinitek Status urine chemistry analyzer is a commonly used machine in the POL. *Delmar/Cengage Learning.*

These results must be recorded in a log each time they are checked as part of the quality assurance program. The following indicates some or all the analytes that can be checked either manually or with the use of an instrument: glucose, protein, ketone, bilirubin, urobilinogen, blood, nitrate, pH, leukocyte esterase, and specific gravity.

Fresh urine specimens should be used, and, when testing manually, it is imperative for exact timing of each of the analytes to be employed. You should have adequate lighting for reading the color changes on the strips as well as color vision to differentiate color changes on the pads. If no change is apparent after the pads have been dipped in the specimen and the appropriate time has elapsed, the result is reported as negative. However, remember that specific gravity, pH, and urobilinogen always have number designations associated with them; for the other pads not related to specific gravity, pH, and urobilinogen that change, you must compare the pads to the strip bottle and consult with your supervisor or policy and procedure manual to see how abnormal results are reported.

Proper handling of the reagent strips includes protecting them from light, capping them tightly after a strip has been removed, and protecting them from exposure to moisture. Unless manufacturers' instructions state otherwise, reagent strips should be stored at room temperature, not in the refrigerator. Be certain to check the expiration date on the bottle; when testing patient specimens, it is unacceptable procedure to use expired strips for reporting results. Additionally, many reagent strip bottles indicate that they should not be used 60 days after the bottle is opened; it is imperative for the person opening the strips to record that date, and the date must be monitored. Using the strips after 60 days exceeds the open vial **stability**, which can affect the accuracy of the testing.

Many companies manufacture urine test strips and many manufacture the strips to be used with instruments to read the results. Many of the instruments provide standardized readings of reflectance photometry with a printout for the patient's record.

Urine can be analyzed for any of several chemical characteristics, as the following sections discuss.

pH

The normal pH for urine is 5.0 to 7.0; remember the pH scale: Anything less than 7.0 is acid in nature, 7.0 is neutral, and readings above 7.0 are alkaline. Urine should be slightly acidic to combat bacteria because bacteria do not like acidic environments; therefore, the majority of urine specimens should be in the 5.0 to 6.5 range (Figure 46–8).

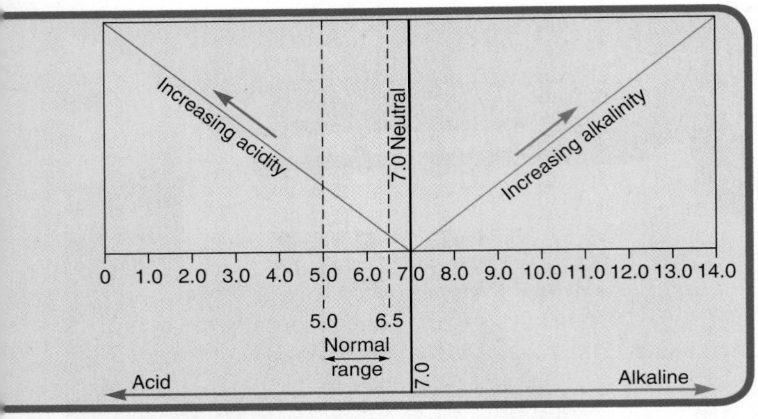

Figure 46–8: Scale of pH for urine. *Delmar/Cengage Learning.*

Protein

Protein (albumin) is a substance that should not normally be found in urine specimens; one of the functions of the tubules in the nephrons of the kidneys is to reabsorb the protein for the body. In cases of kidney disease or infection, protein can be found in the specimen; depending on the circumstances, this can be a very important indicator of kidney disease or failure. Most laboratories require a *confirmatory* test be performed so that a result is not reported erroneously; in this case, the confirmatory test is the sulfosalicylic acid (SSA) test. The SSA test *precipitates* albumin (a protein) in a measurable visual state for reporting purposes; if the SSA is negative, this confirmatory test overrides the results of the reagent test. If the confirmatory test shows the presence of albumin, consult the practice's policy and procedure manual for reporting the results. Protein can be found in specimens of renal failure as well as in specimens in which urinary tract infection (UTI) is found. (Bacteria are protein-based, thus resulting in the increased levels of protein.) Also, increased protein levels can be found in cases of blood in the urine from injury, infection, or menstruation because red blood cells are composed of protein. Thus, there are many causes of protein presence in the urine, and it is up to you to be discriminating in reporting the results and their follow up.

Ketone

Ketone (acetone) bodies are not normally present in urine specimens; ketonuria indicates that fat has been broken down and metabolized in the digestive tract. Urine specimens with ketone bodies present are described as having a fruity odor, something you might notice when you uncap the specimen for testing. Ketones can be found in the following conditions: uncontrolled diabetes mellitus; diet high in fat; starvation (anorexia); and wasting of the body from other disease conditions. Patients who are restricted in their caloric intake for weight loss can have ketone bodies in their urine, but this is a desirable presence because it indicates that their bodies are burning fats, resulting in weight loss. Many POLs and hospital laboratories require a confirmatory test for this result on the chemical reagent strip; the most common confirmatory test is the Acetest®, in which a drop of urine is applied directly to a tablet, the test is timed, and the results are reported according to comparison with a color chart included with the reagent tablets. Follow the policies and procedures of the office or laboratory for performing and reporting the confirmatory test. When elevated levels of ketones are found in the urine specimen, it is termed *ketonuria*.

Bilirubin

Bilirubin is a yellow to orange pigment and is the result of the liver's degradation of hemoglobin. Part of the liver's function within the circulatory system is to recycle red blood cells by removing them from circulation after approximately 120 days (unless they are damaged, in which case they are removed sooner) and using parts of these cells to build new blood cells. However, in patients who have liver damage or disease such as tumors, hepatitis, or cirrhosis, bilirubin can be found in the urine. Often, bilirubin can be detected in a urine sample before the patient exhibits traits such as jaundice and ascites.

Characteristically, a urine specimen from a patient with hepatitis has an orange to greenish coloration, and if the specimen is shaken, it will have a green foam. Besides taking care to protect yourself from this virus, *all* urine specimens must be protected from light because this causes bilirubin to break down and go undetected. Consider babies who are born with or develop jaundice immediately following birth—how is the bilirubin broken down in the infant? The baby is exposed to an ultraviolet light to degrade the bilirubin so that the body reabsorbs it. In most laboratories, the presence of bilirubin is confirmed by another diagnostic test because reagent strips yield many false positives. The most common test used for confirmation is the Ictotest®; the test is performed by placing 10 drops of urine on an absorbent mat, applying a tablet to the top of the pad, adding two drops of water, and timing the test to report the results. If the mat shows a bluish to purple color, the results are positive; if the mat shows a pink to red color, no bilirubin is in the specimen, and these results override the results of the reagent strip.

Urobilinogen

Urobilinogen is a normal by-product of hemoglobin degradation that occurs in the intestines by normal intestinal flora (bacteria). The chemical reaction that occurs in the intestines by the normal flora is what gives stools their normal brown color. Urobilinogen is excreted through the intestines, and most laboratories require that, when reporting, a number is reported with the units expressed in *Ehrlich* units. When urobilinogen is found in the urine in high levels, it often indicates that the liver or gallbladder are dysfunctional as well as being indicative of spleen and heart problems.

Hematuria

Hematuria is the presence of red blood cells or hemoglobin in the urine. Hemoglobin is not normally found in urine specimens except in cases of women who are menstruating. When screening urine specimens, three types of reactions with the reagent strip yield a positive result: the presence of red blood cells; the presence of hemoglobin; and the presence of myoglobin, a globin released in cases of extensive muscle injury. If the reagent strip detects any of these substances as a positive result, the confirmation of results is done by a microscopic examination of the specimen. Even then, there could be a positive blood result but no red blood cells seen in the urine because the tested substance is hemoglobin released from the red blood cells; also, if myoglobin is present from muscle injury, nothing will be seen on microscopic examination. This is why microscopic examinations are designated for those specifically trained to make these types of distinctions.

Nitrite

Nitrite is present in urine samples that have increased numbers of microorganisms, namely bacteria. Normally, urine is considered a sterile fluid excreted from the body; however, in cases in which bacteria have invaded, nitrates are reduced to nitrites **in vivo**. Urine specimens that have a high number of bacteria will have a characteristic smell of ammonia; remember that urine specimens left out at room temperature for longer than an hour encourage bacterial growth, so it is imperative to refrigerate a urine specimen that cannot be tested within an hour to prevent this overgrowth of bacteria from occurring and giving a false positive result. As bacteria change nitrate to nitrite, these microorganisms also ingest glucose and cellular elements and excrete protein, all of which could be misinterpreted in diagnosing and treating the patient. Confirmation of bacteria in the urine, *bacteriuria*, is achieved by microscopic examination as well as by culture and sensitivity, discussed later in this chapter.

Leukocyte Esterase

Leukocyte esterase is commonly checked with other analytes on the reagent strip. This test detects esterase, an enzyme released by white blood cells when significant numbers of these cells are present in a fluid. When a health care provider reviews symptoms of the patient as well as the results of the chemical analysis, particularly if nitrites are positive also, a diagnosis of a urinary tract infection may be made. Confirmation of the presence of white blood cells (leukocytes) is done by microscopic examination. *Pyuria* is the term used when white blood cells are found in the urine specimen in increased numbers.

Glucose

Glucose is a substance that is not normally found in urine samples. The reagent strip that tests for the presence of glucose is specific to that sugar specifically; bear in mind that other sugars exist and can be excreted by the body, such as fructose (fruit sugar), lactose (milk sugar), and galactose (also a milk sugar). Glucose in a urine specimen indicates that the *renal threshold* has been exceeded.

> **CLINICAL PEARL**
>
> Recall in Chapter 33, on the urinary system, that the nephrons are responsible for reabsorbing glucose (sugar) because this is the body's major nutrient.

When the glucose level in the blood is greater than the nephrons can reabsorb, the result is for glucose to spill over into the urine, a condition known as *glycosuria* or *glucosuria*. Different patients will have different renal thresholds; some might have low thresholds in which glucosuria results if the blood sugar exceeds 130 mg/dL. In other patients, the renal threshold can be as high as 200 mg/dL before glucose can be detected in the urine. Normally, the renal threshold is established at 180 mg/dL, meaning that if the blood glucose level exceeds 180 mg/dL, the overage of glucose will be secreted in the urine. At one time, it was common practice for diabetic patients to check their urine specimens for glucose; however, this practice is no longer commonly used for controlling diabetes. Also, remember that technologic advances with home blood glucose meters make it very easy and relatively painless for patients to check their blood sugars, thus providing more accurate results and interpretation of their results. The only confirmatory test for the presence of urine glucose is checking the blood glucose due to variances in renal thresholds.

Specific Gravity

Specific gravity is a complex concept for many people to grasp. When specific gravity was first measured as part of urinalysis, it was considered a physical examination because the measurement was made with a refractometer or a urinometer. However, with scientific advances, reagent strips now measure this. Specific gravity indicates how concentrated or how dilute a specimen is. Remember how specific gravity is based—distilled water provides the basis. Distilled water should have no particles dissolved in it; it should be pure. The specific gravity of distilled water is 1.000 + 0.003. (Memorize this value for certification and registration exams.) Because urine should have some dissolved substances in it, the specific gravity of urine will be higher than the value established for distilled water. Values for the specific gravity of urine range from 1.005 to 1.030, with most specimens falling in the range of 1.010 to 1.025. The higher the specific gravity reading, the more dissolved substances are present, and the lower the reading, the fewer dissolved substances are present, with more fluid. This can be very important in patients with dehydration as well as for those patients suspected of having diabetes insipidus, a condition in which large amounts of very dilute urine are excreted by the body. A good indicator of specific gravity can be the color of the urine: If the specimen is a very light yellow or straw, chances are that the specific gravity will be low. Conversely, if the specimen has more of a medium straw to darker straw or yellow color, it probably will have more dissolved substances and a higher specific gravity. Review the steps of Procedure 46–3 for chemical testing of urine specimens by using a reagent strip.

PROCEDURE 46–3 Test Urine with Reagent Strips

PURPOSE: To detect pH, protein, glucose, ketones, blood, bilirubin, urobilinogen, leukocytes, and specific gravity in urine

EQUIPMENT: Multistix® 10 SG reagent strips, fresh urine specimen, disposable gloves, watch or other timepiece, tongue depressor, patient's chart, pen, and adequate lighting to read color chart on reagent bottle. (For accurate test results, use strips before the expiration date on the bottle.)

S SKILL: Perform the physical and chemical parts of a urinalysis.

Procedure Steps	Detailed Instructions and/or *Rationales*
1. Assemble the necessary equipment and supplies.	
2. Wash hands and don disposable gloves and other PPE as required.	
3. Stir the urine with a tongue depressor to distribute solutes evenly throughout the specimen.	
4. Remove the cap from the bottle and take out one reagent strip without touching the test paper end. Place the cap securely back on bottle.	Study times are given on the bottle for reading each test section.
5. Dip the test paper end of the reagent strip into the urine specimen. With the reagent side of the strip down, pull it across the inside of the specimen container opening to remove excess urine.	*If the strip is too saturated, treated test paper chemicals will run together and make results inaccurate.*
6. Begin timing tests immediately. kidney problem / proteinuria infection, kidney stone, menses	The following scale is in the same order as the reagents on the strip and on the color chart on the bottle when properly aligned and observed from left to right: 2 minutes—leukocytes infection 60 seconds—nitrite — UTI 60 seconds—urobilinogen — liver 60 seconds—protein (albumin) acidity — 60 seconds—pH 50 seconds—blood hematuria 45 seconds—specific gravity [ ] conc. 40 seconds—ketone ketonuria (fasting) 30 seconds—bilirubin (liver) 30 seconds—glucose (quantitative) glucosuria 10 seconds—glucose (qualitative)

Procedure Steps	Detailed Instructions and/or *Rationales*
7. Place the bottle on its side and hold it at the bottom with your left hand. Place the reagent strip next to the color chart on the bottle.	Hold the bottom of the bottle in your left hand. Hold the reagent strip in your right hand with your thumb and index finger and line it up with the color chart on the bottle.
8. Read the test results from the bottom to the top in order of shorter to longer timings.	Proper timing is essential for accurate results. Read the results by comparing the color of the reacted reagent strips with the color chart on the bottle.
9. Discard the used reagent strip, gloves, and other disposables in the proper receptacle. Wash hands. Return reagent strips to the proper storage area.	
10. Record the results as indicated for each section on the patient's chart and in the log book.	

Charting Example

7-17-XX 11:00 am	Clean-catch urine specimen from Marcene Mitchell tested with Clinitek 50 shows clear yellow urine positive for leukocytes, all other tests negative. J. Watkins, CMA(AAMA)

Log Book Example

Date	Patient's Name	Number	Test	Sent	Results	Filed by
7-17-XX	Marcene Mitchell BD 8-8-63	7539	UA Clinitek	7-17-XX	large amount of leukocytes	J. Watkins, CMA

Microscopic Examination of Urine

According to CLIA '88, medical assistants may not read or interpret results of microscopic urine sediments; however, preparation of the urine specimen may be requested of the medical assistant for another to view the slide and report the results. Refer to Procedure 46–4 for proper preparation of urine sediment for microscopic analysis.

PROCEDURE 46–4 Obtain Urine Sediment for Microscopic Examination

PURPOSE: To obtain urine sediment to determine microscopic contents of urine

EQUIPMENT: Fresh urine specimen, disposable latex or vinyl gloves, two centrifuge tubes, centrifuge, frosted-end glass slides with cover glass, tapered pipette, patient's chart, pen, pencil, tongue depressor, microscope with light source, urine sediment chart, timer or timepiece, and sharps container

S SKILL: Prepare a urine specimen for microscopic examination of urine sediment.

Procedure Steps	Detailed Instructions and/or *Rationales*
1. Wash hands, put on gloves, and assemble all the needed items on a cleared counter surface near the centrifuge.	

(continues)

(continued)

Procedure Steps	Detailed Instructions and/or *Rationales*
2. Stir the urine specimen with tongue depressor and pour equal amounts (approximately 10 mL) into each of two test tubes or use plain water in one of the test tubes.	Remember that equal weight is required for proper operation of the centrifuge.
3. To balance the centrifuge, place the centrifuge tubes on opposite sides. Urine should be spun at 1,500 revolutions per minute for 3 to 5 minutes.	Set the timer or write down the start time.
4. When the centrifuge has completely stopped, lift out the tube containing the urine specimen and carefully pour off the urine (**supernatant**).	
5. There will still be a few drops of urine in the bottom of the test tube with the sediment. Gently tap the bottom of the tube on the counter or against your palm to mix the urine and sediment together.	Make sure that all sediment is thoroughly mixed.
6. Obtain a drop or two of urine sediment with a tapered pipette and place it on a clean frosted-end glass slide or calibrated slide for urine sediment.	
7. Place a cover slip over the specimen, allow it to settle, and place it on the microscope stage. If using a calibrated slide, this step is omitted.	Unless you are highly experienced in this area, the health care provider will perform provider-performed microscopy procedures. Consult with your employer about the office policy in this matter before proceeding with the examination.

You should be familiar with some of the microscopic findings and are required to be reported in the sediment of a urine specimen; some of these elements require immediate attention for pathologic conditions. Figure 46–9 displays common microscopic elements found and reported in urine sediment. Usually, red and white blood cells are reported in increments of five; bacteria and epithelial cells are quantitated as rare, few, moderate, or many or slight, 1+, 2+, 3+, 4+; mucus is identified as slight, moderate, or much.

Remember that each laboratory has its own reporting system, so familiarize yourself with each lab. Table 46–1 includes guidelines for normal values. Procedure 46–5 reviews screening and following up test results.

COLLECTING FECAL SPECIMENS

It is not unusual to find that fecal specimens are hard for patients to collect properly, and it can be difficult for you to instruct proper collection of these specimens. Fecal specimens can provide a great deal of diagnostic insight into a patient's condition, and it is essential to instruct the patient properly on collection of the specimen. Stool (fecal) specimens may be ordered to check for occult (hidden) blood, ova and parasites, or bacterial or viral infections. There is also a collection for pinworm screening in which ordinary office transparent tape is affixed to a tongue depressor (sticky side out) and used while a child is asleep to check for eggs being laid outside the rectum during the nighttime hours.

Normal practice is for patients to be instructed to obtain a stool specimen at home and bring it to the laboratory for testing. Depending on the type of testing being performed, refrigeration might or might not be required. Testing for occult blood is discussed in a subsequent section because the instructions to the patient are more detailed than for other specimens. Fecal specimens are not considered sterile, so a patient may collect the specimen in a clean container. It used to be customary practice for the patient to bring only a small amount of the specimen for testing; however, in testing for bacterial or viral infections and ova and parasites, the entire specimen should be collected and transported for testing. The patient should be advised not to contaminate the stool specimen with urine because constituents of urine destroy microorganisms in the stool specimen; this can present a challenge for many female patients.

Laboratory personnel observe the specimen for abnormalities such as obvious discoloration, pus, or other such things and test those areas specifically. It is

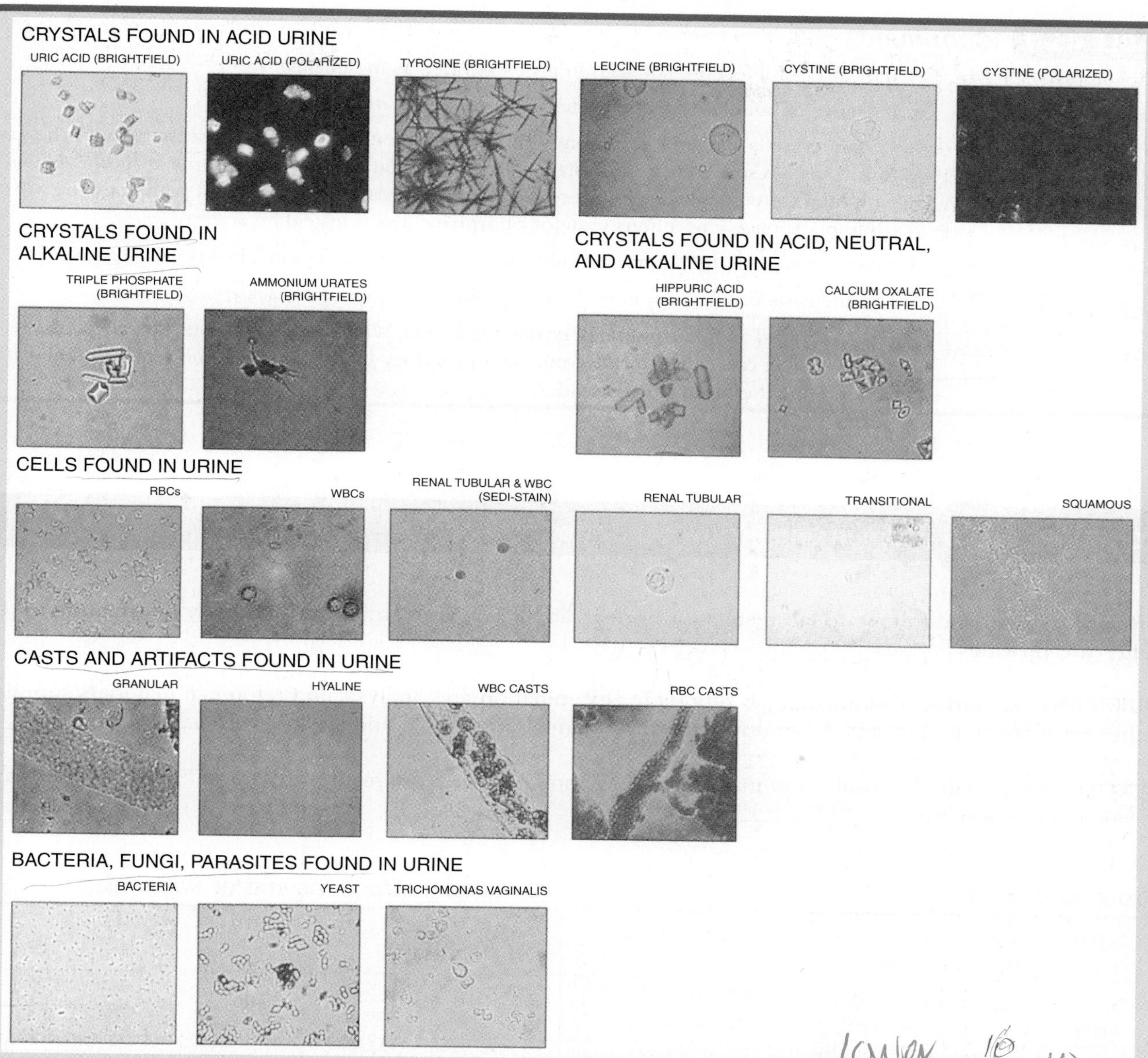

Figure 46–9: Crystals, cells, and casts found in urine sediment. *Courtesy of Bayer Diagnostics.*

lower 10 40
high power 100 400
oil emulsion 1000

TABLE 46–1 Normal Values

WBCs	• Females, 10 to 20/hpf • Males, 0 to 10/hpf
RBCs	• Females, 5 to 10/hpf (unless on menstrual period) • Males 0
Epithelial cells	• Few to moderate (not seen as often in male patients)
Bacteria	• None to slight (remember urine is considered a sterile body fluid)
Mucus	• Slight
Spermatozoa	• Indicative of pathologic state in men • Should not be reported in females except in rape cases and then only under legal authority because it could be perceived as an invasion of privacy

(continues)

TABLE 46–1 (*Continued*)

Trichomonas	• Indicative of infection, not seen in males as often as in females
Yeast	• Presence of budding yeast indicates infection with *Candida albicans*
Crystals	• Certain crystals can appear in urine specimens without indication of disease because they are formed as a result of diet. For instance, calcium oxalate crystals might appear in individuals with high caffeine intake. Other crystals identified in specimens without pathology include triple phosphate, amorphous urate or phosphate, and uric acid. • Crystals that indicate disease include cholesterol, tyrosine, cystine, leukocine, and sulfa
Casts	• Hyaline casts can be seen in specimens without indication of disease • Casts reported as finely granular, coarsely granular, WBC casts, RBC casts, mixed cell casts, waxy, or fatty casts are indicative of a serious kidney (renal) problem and require immediate attention by the health care provider

PROCEDURE 46–5 Screen and Follow Up Urine Test Results

PURPOSE: Screen and follow up lab results for normal, abnormal, and panic values to relay information to the health care provider

EQUIPMENT: Scenarios of simulated lab reports for examination and analysis and reference materials supplied by the instructor (e.g., Internet, laboratory reference manuals, textbook, and so on).

S SKILL: Review lab test results and make notations about whether the results are normal, abnormal, or panic value and follow up.

Procedure Steps	Detailed Instructions and/or *Rationales*
1. Screen the test results to determine whether they are normal, abnormal, or panic value.	
2. Screen the test results to determine whether laboratory reports are missing any key elements.	
3. Identify panic values, the disease state that might be a result of them, or the disease state that might be caused if left untreated.	
4. Identify the appropriate action for panic values with the health care provider.	
5. Identify the appropriate action for the abnormal values with the health care provider.	
6. Identify the appropriate action for the normal values with the health care provider.	
7. Accurately chart action taken in the patient's medical record.	

Charting Example

Denson, Anita ID# DEN0345678 06/07/XX	1725	Called patient to inform her that her urinalysis results were normal. Judy Adams, CCMA

not unusual for a health care provider to order fecal specimens in sequences of three consecutive specimens; that is, for three consecutive days that a patient has a bowel movement, the specimen should be collected.

CLINICAL PEARL

Many patients misinterpret these directions, so use caution when instructing patients for this collection. Patients might not void on consecutive days and, if this is the case, they simply collect the specimens on the three days they have had a bowel movement. For instance, if a patient has a bowel movement on Monday, Thursday, and Saturday, this is three consecutive days for that particular patient. On the other hand, if a patient has more than one bowel movement per day, only one specimen should be collected for that given day.

Refer to Procedure 46–6 as well as Figure 46–10 for an example of a collection container.

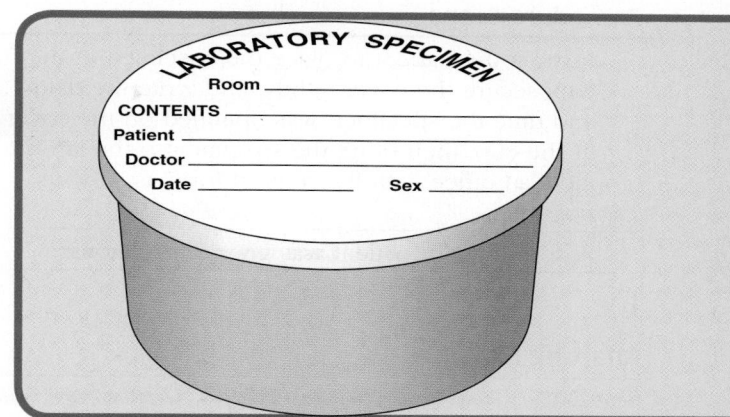

Figure 46–10: Laboratory stool specimen container with identification lid. *Delmar/Cengage Learning.*

PROCEDURE 46–6 Instruct a Patient to Collect a Stool Specimen

PURPOSE: To instruct patients to obtain an adequate stool specimen for laboratory analysis

EQUIPMENT: Specimen container with lid, lab request form, pen, patient's chart, label, rubber band, printed instructions (optional), tongue depressors, and note pad

S SKILL: Instruct a patient on the proper procedure for collecting a fecal specimen for occult blood screening.

Procedure Steps	Detailed Instructions and/or *Rationales*
1. Assemble the items next to the patient.	
2. Write identifying information on the request form and label (usually on the cover) and affix the label to specimen cup.	
B 3. Identify the patient and explain the provider's orders, ***including the rationale for performing the procedure, using language and verbal skills the patient can understand. Show awareness of patients' concerns regarding their perceptions of the procedure by answering any questions the patient might have.*** Give printed instructions or write out if necessary.	*Speaking to the patient by name and checking the chart ensures that you are performing the procedure on the correct patient.*
4. Instruct the patient to obtain a small amount of stool (about 3 or 4 tablespoons) from the next bowel movement, within next few days. Explain that nothing else should be placed in the cup besides stool (no tissue paper, urine, and so on).	Patients may defecate onto a paper plate and obtain a small specimen from the plate, which is then discarded. Or, they may use a tongue depressor to obtain the specimen from the toilet bowl.

(continues)

(continued)

Procedure Steps	Detailed Instructions and/or *Rationales*
5. Instruct the patient to place the specimen in the cup, secure the cover tightly, and write the date and time the specimen was obtained on the cover of the cup; then bring the specimen to the lab or medical office with the request form as soon as possible.	To prevent bacterial growth, the specimen should be refrigerated if it cannot be received by the lab within two hours.
6. Record that the patient was given instructions.	

Charting Example

5-30-XX 2:00 PM	Verbal and printed instructions to collect stool specimen given to patient. J. Watkins, CMA (AAMA)

Occult Blood Specimens

Occult blood specimens from stools are common screening tools for early detection of the possibility of colon cancer, particularly in those patients older than 50 years. These tests are based on the **guaiac** reagent that turns blue when oxidized in the presence of blood. The test might detect bleeding in the digestive tract that is invisible to the naked eye but is enough to follow up with other diagnostic testing such as colonoscopy. When the patient collects the specimen at home, he or she should be instructed to collect only a very small amount for the test. A tongue depressor or disposable stick is used to collect a minute amount to be applied to the reagent packet; usually, there are two areas upon which the specimen should be applied, and these windows should come from different parts of the fecal specimen. If the specimen is returned to the office, you might have the responsibility of applying the specimen to the appropriate areas of the reagent slide and processing it by applying the color developer for observation of either the blue (positive) or brown-green (negative) reaction. Be certain to observe the control area to ascertain that the control reactions are correct prior to reporting any patient results. Refer to Figure 46–11 for instructions regarding collection of the specimen and interpretation of results.

This test is also indicated in patients with a personal or family history of colorectal cancer, rectal polyps, or ulcerative colitis. Remember that bleeding hemorrhoids can also give a positive result for occult blood, although this condition is not serious besides being uncomfortable for the patient. The test was designed to help detect hidden, invisible (occult) blood in the stool early enough to take corrective measures to avoid the spread of cancer. Cancer of the colon is one of the leading cancer killers in the country, so it makes sense to check fecal specimens periodically to protect patients' health. The test is painless to complete, and the results are quick; it is advisable for the patient to collect a minimum of three consecutive specimens in the event that bleeding is present on one day but perhaps not on others. It is common practice for many providers to perform this test while examining patients; therefore, it might be your responsibility to develop the test after the provider has collected the specimen by digital swab. If the patient is provided with slides to take home and mail in at a later time, special envelopes that protect the mail carriers are provided. There are many types of slide tests for this type of analysis. Procedure 46–7 explains the proper method for developing and interpreting an occult blood slide.

COLLECTING SPUTUM SPECIMENS

Sputum specimens are indicated for diagnostic analysis when a patient has an unresolved cough with mucus production. Although the upper respiratory tract is not considered sterile, the lower respiratory tract is, and when infection occurs in the lower respiratory tract, it can be serious for the patient. Instructing patients in the proper collection of a sputum specimen can be difficult because it is vital for a specimen representative of the lower respiratory tract to be obtained for the diagnostic testing. (Refer to Procedure 46–8.)

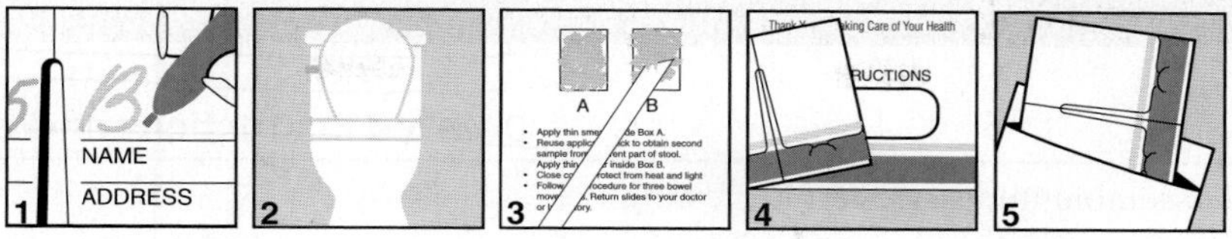

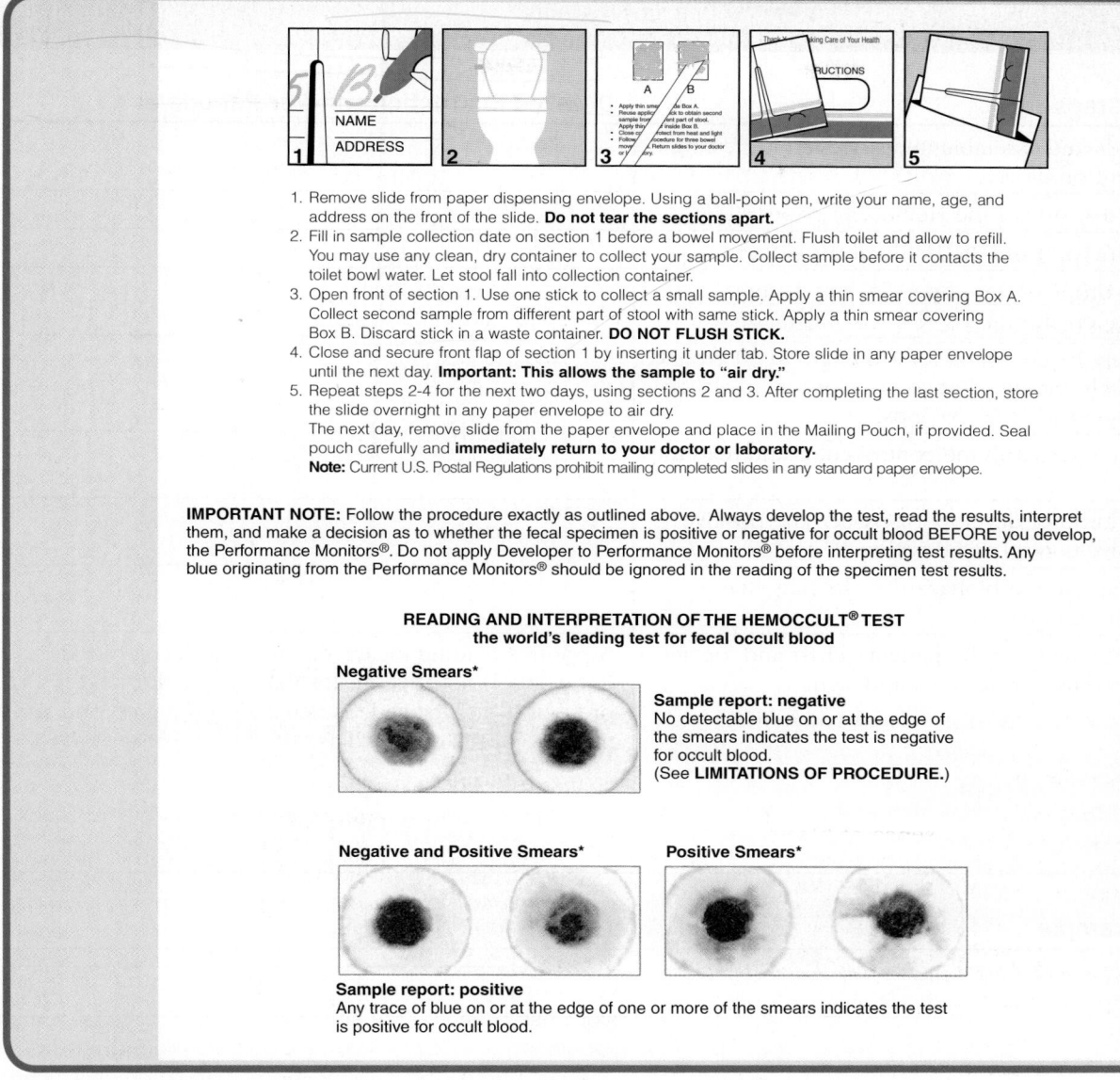

1. Remove slide from paper dispensing envelope. Using a ball-point pen, write your name, age, and address on the front of the slide. **Do not tear the sections apart.**
2. Fill in sample collection date on section 1 before a bowel movement. Flush toilet and allow to refill. You may use any clean, dry container to collect your sample. Collect sample before it contacts the toilet bowl water. Let stool fall into collection container.
3. Open front of section 1. Use one stick to collect a small sample. Apply a thin smear covering Box A. Collect second sample from different part of stool with same stick. Apply a thin smear covering Box B. Discard stick in a waste container. **DO NOT FLUSH STICK.**
4. Close and secure front flap of section 1 by inserting it under tab. Store slide in any paper envelope until the next day. **Important: This allows the sample to "air dry."**
5. Repeat steps 2-4 for the next two days, using sections 2 and 3. After completing the last section, store the slide overnight in any paper envelope to air dry.
   The next day, remove slide from the paper envelope and place in the Mailing Pouch, if provided. Seal pouch carefully and **immediately return to your doctor or laboratory.**
   Note: Current U.S. Postal Regulations prohibit mailing completed slides in any standard paper envelope.

IMPORTANT NOTE: Follow the procedure exactly as outlined above. Always develop the test, read the results, interpret them, and make a decision as to whether the fecal specimen is positive or negative for occult blood BEFORE you develop, the Performance Monitors®. Do not apply Developer to Performance Monitors® before interpreting test results. Any blue originating from the Performance Monitors® should be ignored in the reading of the specimen test results.

READING AND INTERPRETATION OF THE HEMOCCULT® TEST
the world's leading test for fecal occult blood

Negative Smears*

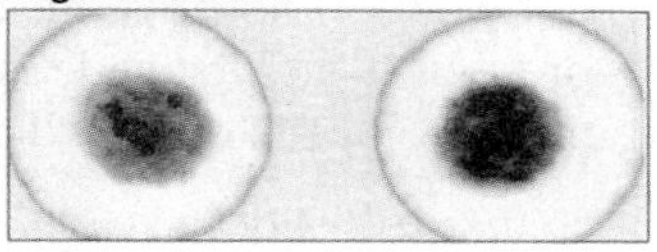

Sample report: negative
No detectable blue on or at the edge of the smears indicates the test is negative for occult blood.
(See **LIMITATIONS OF PROCEDURE.**)

Negative and Positive Smears*

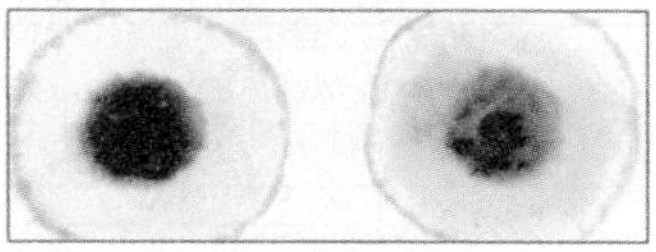

Positive Smears*

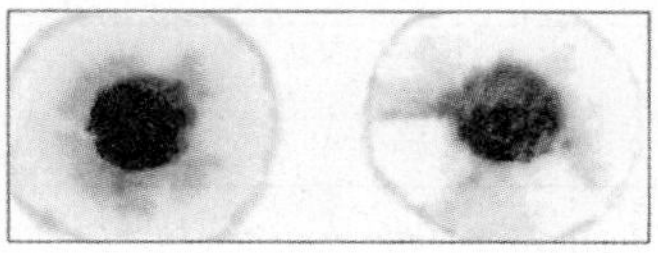

Sample report: positive
Any trace of blue on or at the edge of one or more of the smears indicates the test is positive for occult blood.

Figure 46–11: Hemoccult® test. *Courtesy of Beckman Coulter, Inc.*

PROCEDURE 46–7 Perform an Occult Blood Test

MEDIA LINK: View the video for this chapter, "Perform an Occult Blood Test," on the Premium Website.

PURPOSE: To determine the presence of occult blood in the stool

EQUIPMENT: Hemoccult® slides prepared by patient, developer, timer or timepiece, patient's chart, pen, biohazard bag, and latex or vinyl gloves

SKILL: Perform an occult blood test.

(continues)

(continued)

Procedure Steps	Detailed Instructions and/or *Rationales*
1. Wash hands and assemble items needed for testing on counter. Put on gloves.	
2. Open the test side of the Hemoccult paper slide.	
3. Remove the cap from the bottle of developer.	
4. Place two drops of developer on each section of the reagent paper slide: A, B.	
5. Immediately begin timing for 1 minute. At 30 seconds, watch closely for any change of color that might be developing. Read at 60 seconds.	
6. Compare the test with the control color and read the results.	
7. Place one drop of developer between the positive and negative control. Read within 10 seconds.	
8. Discard the test in a biohazard waste bag. Remove gloves and wash hands.	
9. Record test results on the patient's chart and log sheet as either positive or negative and sign.	A positive reading means that there is occult blood in the stool. Negative means that no occult blood is present. If the first slide is negative and the second and third are positive, record as: Hemoccult slides: 1. neg. 2. pos. 3. pos.

Charting Example

7-24-XX 9:30 am	Hemoccult slides: 1. neg. 2. pos. 3. pos. J. Watkins, CMA(AAMA)

PATIENT EDUCATION

When instructing a patient on collecting a sputum specimen, provide the following directions.

- The first morning specimen is the best specimen for testing; the most productive cough with the most concentrated specimen occurs upon waking.
- Rinse the mouth with water and expel the water. This action washes the superficial cells from the oral (mouth) cavity. Saliva and mucus from the mouth and nasal passages are *not* the desired secretions for the analysis and can interfere with the test results, yielding false positive for infection.
- Uncap the sterile container without touching the inside of the container or the lid.
- Cough deeply from down deep in the lungs and expel the specimen into the cup. The container should not be more than half full.
- Securely recap the container, indicate the date and time of the collection of the specimen, and store the container according to which specimen testing has been ordered.

PROCEDURE 46–8 Instruct a Patient to Collect a Sputum Specimen

PURPOSE: To instruct a patient in the collection of an adequate sputum specimen for laboratory analysis

EQUIPMENT: Sputum specimen container and lid, label, pen, patient's chart, label request form, note pad, rubber band, and printed instruction sheet (optional)

S SKILL: Instruct a patient in the collection of a sputum specimen for analysis.

Procedure Steps	Detailed Instructions and/or *Rationales*
1. Assemble the items next to the patient.	
2. Write the patient's name on a specimen cup label and complete the lab request form.	
B 3. Identify the patient and explain the provider's orders. Identify the patient and explain the procedure, ***including the rationale for performing the procedure, using language and verbal skills the patient can understand. Show awareness of patients' concerns regarding their perceptions of the procedure by answering any questions the patient might have.*** Give printed instructions or write them out if you feel the patient has a difficult time understanding you.	
4. Instruct the patient to remove the lid from the sterile specimen container and to expel secretions from a first morning coughing episode into the center of the cup, being careful not to touch the inside of the cup. The container should not be more than half full.	
5. Instruct the patient not to allow saliva, tears, sweat, mucus from the nose or mouth, or any other substance to enter the cup.	Secretions must be coughed up (expectorated) from the lower respiratory tract (lungs, bronchial tubes, and trachea), or the test will not be acceptable.
6. When secretions have been obtained and the cup sealed with its cover, the patient should write the time and date that it was obtained on the label and the lab request form and bring them to the lab or medical office as soon as possible.	If the patient cannot bring the specimen in within two hours after collection, it should be refrigerated.
7. Secure the completed lab request form to the specimen container with a rubber band or tape. Send it to the lab.	If the patient prepares the specimen at home, show the patient how to do this.
8. Record that instruction was given to the patient in sputum collecting.	

Charting Example

5-30-XX 4:30 PM	*Verbal and printed instructions for collection of sputum specimen given to Jaren. Judy Adams, CCMA*

Occasionally, the health care provider will induce coughing in a patient to produce the specimen; however, this is rarely done. More commonly, if a provider needs a more specific sample, the patient is scheduled for an outpatient procedure for a bronchial washing or brushing to obtain a lower respiratory tract specimen. Emphasize to the patient how important it is to follow the directions provided to obtain an accurate diagnosis.

Sputum specimens are used to diagnose several conditions, including cancer, viral infections, bacterial infections, fungal infections, and tuberculosis. Each of these conditions is different from the others, and different testing is used for the diagnoses. Tuberculosis is a unique type of bacterial infection most commonly found in the lungs with extremely contagious implications. Bacterial cultures are discussed later in this unit. Cancer is detected in the sputum specimen through the use of the Papanicolaou stain, the same stain used for the detection of cancer of the cervix in women. The sputum specimen is processed, centrifuged, and applied to a microscopic slide, then stained and examined by either a cytologist or pathologist to confirm or refute the presence of cancerous cells.

COLLECTING BACTERIAL SPECIMENS

Although it is typical for us to think of bacteria as being the primary cause of infections, several types of microorganisms can and do cause infections in susceptible individuals. Bacteria, viruses, and fungi can all be extracted from specimens for identification, leading to a decision about which medication can eliminate the infection from the patient (Figure 46–12).

BILL
- ☐ ACCOUNT
- ☐ PATIENT SEE ①
- ☐ 3RD PARTY SEE ②

PLEASE LEAVE BLANK
AREA ______
DEPT. ______
BILL CD ______

C-5 REQUEST FORM
INSTRUCTIONS ① FOR PATIENT BILLING, COMPLETE BOX A.
② FOR 3RD PARTY BILLING, COMPLETE BOX A AND FILL IN DIAGNOSIS, THEN EITHER B, C, or D.

USA Biomedical Labs
957 Central Avenue
Heartland, NY 11112

PATIENT NAME (LAST) (FIRST) | SPECIES | SEX | AGE YRS. MOS. | DATE COLLECTED MO. DAY YR. | TIME COLLECTED

PATIENT ADDRESS STREET | MISC. INFORMATION | DR. I.D. | **MEDICARE:** #

CITY STATE ZIP | DIAGNOSIS

N5961

PHYSICIAN | WELFARE: # | CASE NAME:

PROGRAM: | PATIENT 1ST NAME: | DATE OF BIRTH ALL CLAIMS MO. DAY YR.

INSURANCE GR. # | I.D. | SERVICE CODE:

SUBSCRIBER NAME: | RELATION: | PHONE

VIROLOGY

VIRUS ISOLATION

9325 ( ) GENERAL VIRUS
9326 ( ) INFLUENZA VIRUS
9327 ( ) HERPES SIMPLEX VIRUS
9328 ( ) CYTOMEGALOVIRUS

9329 ( ) CHLAMYDIA CULTURE
9330 ( ) ROTAVIRUS ANTIGEN SCREEN
9332 ( ) C DIFFICILE TOXIN SCREEN

CLINICAL INFORMATION

VIRUS SUSPECTED
SOURCE OF SPECIMEN ______
DATE COLLECTED ______
IS PATIENT PREGNANT YES ___ NO ___
PATIENT SYMPTOMS ______
EPIDEMIOLOGIC FACTORS ______
SIMILAR ILLNESS IN FAMILY ______
LOCAL EPIDEMICS ______
RECENT TRAVEL ______
ANIMAL CONTACT ______
IMMUNIZATION (SPECIFY TYPE AND DATE OF LAST DOSE)
POLIO ______ INFLUENZA ______ OTHER ___
MISCELLANEOUS INFORMATION

MICROBIOLOGY

SOURCE OF SPECIMEN ______

9219 ( ) ACID FAST CULTURE & SMEAR
9220 ( ) ACID FAST SMEAR ONLY
9245 ( ) ANAEROBIC CULTURE
9209 ( ) BETA STREP (A), FA
9214 ( ) BLOOD CULTURE
9226 ( ) FECES, FAT & MUSCLE FIBER
9225 ( ) FECES, OCCULT BLOOD
9309 ( ) FECES, OVA & PARASITES
9221 ( ) FUNGUS CULTURE
9204 ( ) FUNGUS, ID. COMPLETE
9222 ( ) FUNGUS, KOH PREP
9232 ( ) GENERAL CULTURE
9215 ( ) GONOCOCCUS CULTURE
9218 ( ) GRAM STAIN ONLY
9207 ( ) LEGIONELLA CULTURE
9228 ( ) PINWORM EXAM
9241 ( ) POST VASECTORY EXAM

9233 ( ) SALMONELLA & SHIGELLA SCREEN
9203 ( ) SPUTUM CULTURE
9227 ( ) STOOL, COMPREHENSIVE
9208 ( ) STREP SCREEN, THROAT
9202 ( ) UPPER RESPIRATORY TRACT CULTURE
9212 ( ) URINE, COMPREHENSIVE CULTURE
9213 ( ) URINE, SCREEN CULTURE
9234 ( ) UROGENITAL CULTURE

UNLISTED TESTS

ADDITIONAL CLINICAL INFORMATION

SENSITIVITIES ARE PERFORMED AS PART OF THE ROUTINE CULTURE AT NO ADDITIONAL CHARGE WHERE ORGANISMS ARE CONSIDERED PATHOGENIC. SENSITIVITIES ARE NOT PERFORMED ON NORMAL FLORA, ALPHA STREPTOCOCCUS, PNEUMOCOCCUS OR BETA STREPTOCOCCUS ROUTINELY.

FOLD THIS FORM IN HALF SO TEST(S) ORDERED IS CLEARLY VISIBLE

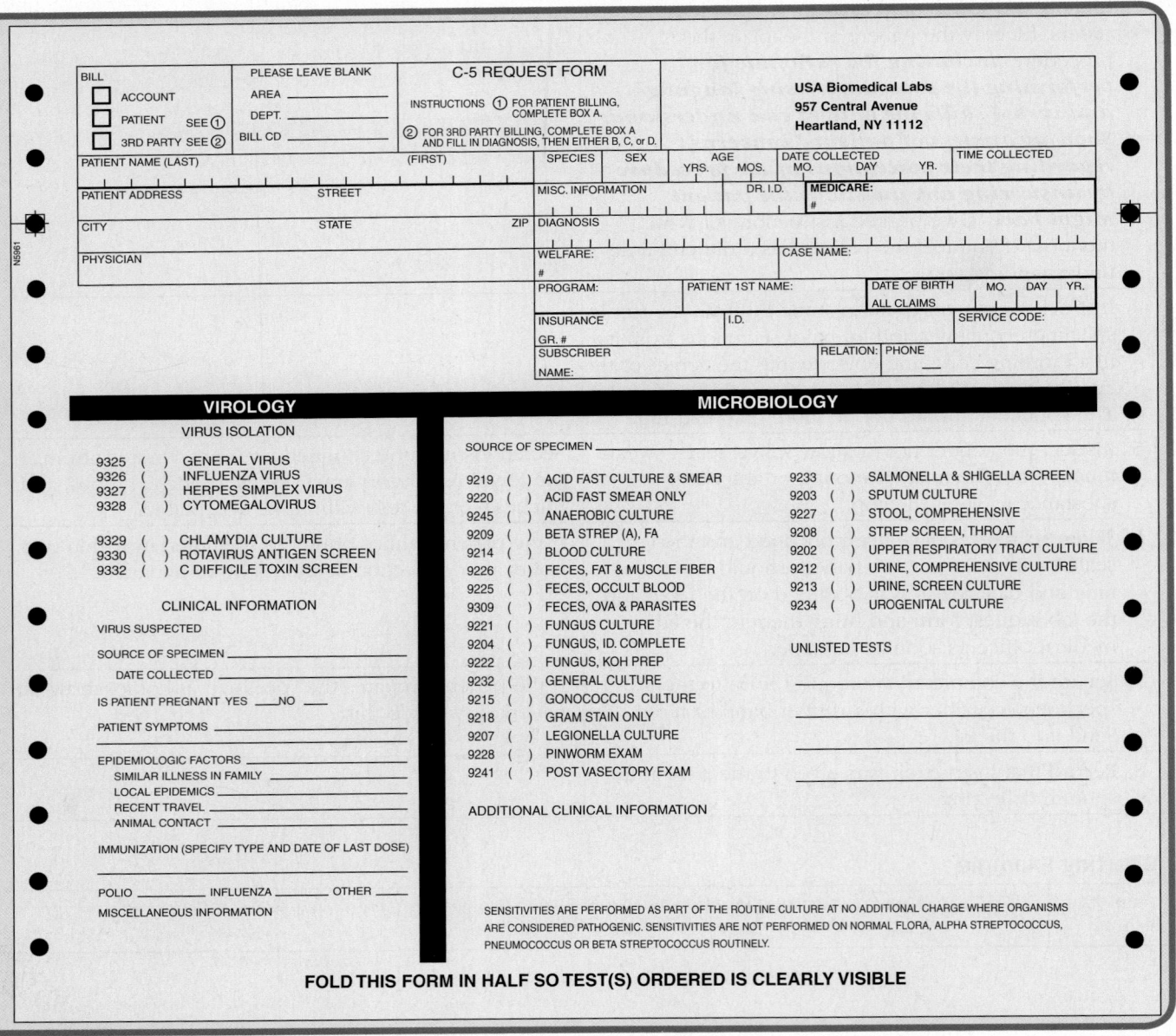

Figure 46–12: Example of a laboratory requisition form for a study to determine different types of microorganisms. *Delmar/Cengage Learning.*

Most commonly, a **culture** is obtained from a patient from the part of the body that appears to be infected. Cultures are performed by a qualified individual by swabbing a sample of the **exudate** (drainage) from the throat, mouth, ear, eye, nose, vagina, anus, or infected wounds (Procedure 46–9). The cultures are collected in a specialized container usually referred to as a *culturette*; the culturette is a sterile swab with a soft tip that is brushed against the infected area and replaced in the sleeve of the collection device (Figures 46–13A and B). The ampule in the culturette must be crushed after collection; it keeps the specimen moist and nourished until the specimen can be processed. In cases of the rapid group A strep test, a sterile swab, *not* cotton-tipped, is used for collection of the specimen and immediately processed; this is discussed later in this unit. Keep in mind that culturing is the means of *isolating* a disease-causing microorganism, a process that takes longer than a bacteriologic smear.

Throat Cultures

In most practices and clinics, throat swabs are obtained from patients complaining of sore throats, fever, swollen glands, and cough. Common practice in the past was to obtain the culture to send to the laboratory for the traditional performance of the culture, isolation of the microorganism, and susceptibility testing. However, now, many rapid group A strep kits are available that provide results of the swab in just a few minutes' time, so waiting 24 to 48 hours is no longer necessary. Some health care providers order a traditional throat culture if the group A strep test returns negative because this test is specific for only this group of strep; keep in mind that there are more groups of strep than just group A. Whether you are collecting a throat swab from a patient for the rapid test or routine culture, remember that you should swab the peritonsillar area in the back of the oral cavity, taking care not to touch the swab to the lips, cheeks, gums, teeth, or tongue. Inform your patient that there might some momentary discomfort while obtaining the specimen and be certain to have the patient to open his or her mouth wide with the head tilted back for better visualization and access to the oral cavity. If obtaining a specimen from a small child, it is easier for you and less traumatic for the child if the parent or guardian holds the child in the lap. Refer to Procedure 46–10 for the proper collection of a throat culture and to Procedure 46–11 for performance of a rapid group A strep test.

Blood Culture

A specialized type of culture is a *blood culture*; blood is drawn from the patient, usually directly into a particular formulated broth in a vacuum bottle. Blood is considered a sterile fluid, and when a blood culture is positive for infection, this indicates a systemic infection, a very important finding that requires immediate attention. Of the utmost importance in collecting such a specimen is protection of the sterile environment; there are specific procedures for collecting the specimen, from the preparation of the patient's skin to placement of the collected specimen into a microbiologic incubator designed for such specimens.

Culture and Sensitivity

Usually when a health care provider orders a test for analysis for detection of a microorganism, the order calls for a culture and **sensitivity**. For a sensitivity to be performed, an organism must be present. The first step of this type of order is the collection of the specimen and inoculation of special media, or **agar**, to encourage the growth of microorganisms present in the specimen.

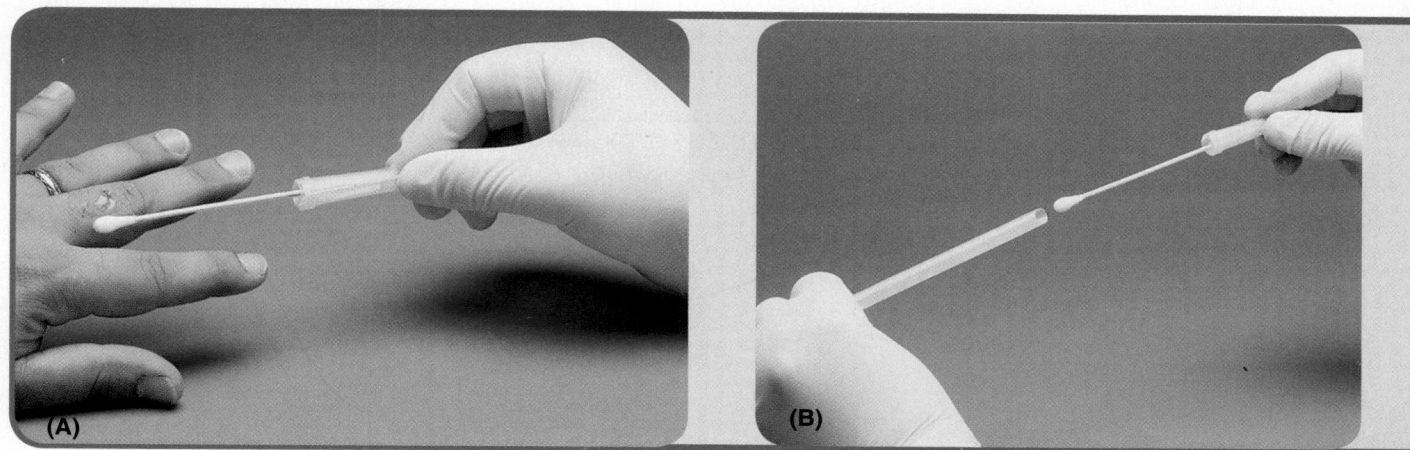

Figure 46–13: (A) Use of a culturette to obtain a wound culture. (B) After the specimen is collected, the swab should be placed into the protective sheath. *Delmar/Cengage Learning.*

PROCEDURE 46–9 Perform a Wound Collection for Microbiologic Testing

PURPOSE: Obtain a wound culture from a patient, using sterile technique

EQUIPMENT: Sterile culturette, gloves, other personal protective equipment as required by the collection procedure, pen, and simulated patient chart

S **SKILL:** Obtain a wound culture from a patient, using sterile technique that protects the integrity of the specimen.

Procedure Steps	Detailed Instructions and/or *Rationales*
1. Assemble necessary supplies for collection of the specimen and ascertain that the culturette is not expired.	
B 2. Identify the patient and explain the procedure, ***including the rationale for performing the procedure, using language and verbal skills the patient can understand. Show awareness of patients' concerns about the procedure by answering any questions the patient might have and assisting the patient into a comfortable position before you proceed.***	
3. Verify the health care provider's order.	
4. Remove the sterile swab from the sleeve.	
5. Collect an adequate specimen without touching any other area except for the exudate and gently rolling the swab in the affected area.	
6. Reinsert the sterile swab in the sleeve and break the ampule.	
7. Record the patient information on the culturette (not the wrapper); if required, complete a lab requisition form for an outside laboratory.	
8. Correctly document the procedure in the patient's medical record.	

Charting Example

Burress, Donald ID# 222558-07 05/15/XX	0830	Infected appendectomy surgical site (LLQ) swabbed per provider's orders; C&S sent to Ace Reference Laboratories for processing. Joni Purcell, RMA(AMT)

PROCEDURE 46–10 Obtain a Throat Culture

PURPOSE: To isolate a disease-causing organism to determine effective treatment of the patient

EQUIPMENT: Sterile swabs, sterile tongue depressor, disposable gloves, pen, patient's chart, penlight (optional), and wax crayon or label

S SKILL: Perform the procedure for obtaining a throat culture.

Procedure Steps	Detailed Instructions and/or *Rationales*
1. Assemble the needed items near the identified patient. Label the culture plate and complete a request form if required. Wash hands and put on gloves.	
B 2. Identify the patient and explain the procedure, ***including the rationale for performing the procedure, using language and verbal skills the patient can understand. Show awareness of patients' concerns about the procedure by answering any questions the patient might have and assisting the patient into a comfortable position before you proceed.***	*Speaking to the patient by name and checking the chart ensures that you are performing the procedure on the correct patient.*
3. Open a sterile swab and ask the patient to open the mouth as wide as possible.	
4. Depress the tongue with a sterile tongue depressor held in one hand. Hold the sterile swab in the other. Ask the patient to say "ah" to assist depression of the tongue. Quickly insert the swab into the back of the throat and roll over at least two areas, touching areas with obvious exudate.	*Asking the patient to say "ah" also prevents the patient from feeling a gag reflex by diverting attention.*
B 5. Remove the swab and depressor from the patient's mouth. ***Attend to the patient's needs and offer tissues.***	*Tearing can result from the procedure.*
6. Place the swab in the container for transportation to the lab. Tape the request form securely.	
7. Discard all disposable items in the proper receptacle. Remove gloves and wash hands.	
8. Record the procedure on the patient's chart and initial.	

Charting Example

5/4/XX 11:50 am	Throat culture obtained and sent to reference laboratory. E. O'Nan, RMA (AMT)

PROCEDURE 46–11 Perform a Rapid Strep Screening Test for Group A Strep

PURPOSE: To screen a patient specimen for the presence of group A strep

EQUIPMENT: Gloves, sterile throat swab, tongue blade, commercial test kit for group A strep with positive and negative controls, patient's chart or laboratory report form, biohazard container

S **SKILL:** Test a throat swab for group A strep with a rapid diagnostic test and interpret the results.

Procedure Steps	Detailed Instructions and/or *Rationales*
1. Assemble supplies.	
B 2. Identify the patient and explain the procedure, ***including the rationale for performing the procedure, using language and verbal skills the patient can understand. Show awareness of patients' concerns about the procedure by answering any questions the patient might have and assisting the patient into a comfortable position before you proceed.***	
3. Wash your hands and don gloves.	
4. Using the tongue blade to keep the tongue out of the way, insert the sterile swab into the back of the oral cavity to collect the specimen from the peritonsillar crypts.	Do not touch the swab to the lips, gums, cheeks, teeth, or tongue.
5. Label the reagent chamber for the test with the patient's name.	
6. Following the manufacturer's instructions exactly, perform the test on the patient's specimen.	
7. Perform the positive and negative controls, recording the results in the laboratory log record, knowing what action must be taken if the results of the quality control are not within the manufacturer's prescribed range.	
8. Dispose of waste in a biohazard waste container.	
9. Properly complete the lab report form or accurately enter the results on the patient's chart.	

Charting Example

7/6/XX 1435	Group A Strep positive. J. Hart, CMA(AAMA)

Quality Control Log

Date	Control Level	Control Lot #	Exp. Date	Reagent Lot #	Exp. Date	Results	Initials
7/6/XX	Positive	14567	9/12/2015	19865	12/10/2010	Positive	JH
7/6/XX	Negative	14568	9/12/2015	19865	12/10/2010	Negative	JH

If after 48 hours no growth is observed by the microbiologist, a sensitivity will not need to be performed. However, when growth of a microorganism is identified in a specimen, the next step of the procedure is for the microbiologist to test the organism against different types of antibiotics for sensitivity to the antibiotics. If an organism is sensitive to an antibiotic, growth of that organism is prohibited; conversely, if an organism is resistant to an antibiotic, that organism will grow up to the antibiotic with no inhibition.

Some POLs still perform testing in this manner for primarily urine specimens; however, the latest methodology employs *minimum inhibitory concentration* (MIC), a specialized test performed only in a microbiology lab, that not only identifies the microorganisms but also identifies the most appropriate antibiotic to be used as well as the lowest dose that is effective in combating the infection. Most instruments can also identify the cost of the indicated medications for the health care provider for making the decision in prescribing the most appropriate medication. This saves on health care costs when the least expensive medication indicated for use as well as the dose is identified for the patient.

Culture Media

Media come in petri dishes, tubes, and broths, to name a few. Depending on the type of specimen, a multitude of media may encourage the growth of the organism for health providers to prescribe the most appropriate medication for the infection.

Primary media encourage the growth of all microorganisms; typically, tryptic soy agar with 5 percent sheep blood is a primary medium. Blood agar is used for the colony count for urine specimens, and the plate is streaked in a distinctive fashion. As a rule, greater than 100,000 colonies indicates a urinary tract infection (UTI), particularly if the organism is identified as Gram negative. A *selective* medium is an agar that discourages the growth of certain organisms; examples of selective media include EMB (eosin-methylene-blue) and MacConkey, which are formulated to encourage only the growth of Gram-negative organisms and inhibit the growth of any Gram-positive organisms.

Selective media are commonly used for urine specimens to control the growth of Gram-positive organisms and encourage the growth of Gram-negative ones; Gram-negative organisms are found in the intestinal tract and are commonly a source of infection in the urinary tract due to improper wiping of the anus. Another commonly used selective medium is the Thayer-Martin plate, which isolates gonorrhea from vaginal or penile excretions. Enrichment medium is an agar that has additional nutrients to encourage the growth of more *fastidious* organisms, such as a "chocolate" agar, named so from the color of the medium in the petri dish. Throat cultures are usually inoculated to blood agar and chocolate agar; if strep is present in the specimen, the blood agar will show **hemolysis**, which assists the microbiologist in determining the strain of *Streptococci*. Stool specimens are planted on several types of agar plates to isolate a pathogenic organism; remember that stool is not considered sterile, so extra steps must be taken to isolate a disease-causing organism in this type of sample.

Some of the more common pathogens found in stool specimens are *Shigella*, *Salmonella*, and *Campylobacter*, all of which produce intense gastrointestinal symptoms such as intense diarrhea and are considered extremely contagious if hands are not adequately washed. Often, an infection will break out in a day care center and spread quickly because the young children do not wash their hands properly. To control such an outbreak, it is important for everyone involved to be instructed in proper hand-washing technique to control the spread of the pathogen.

If culturing for tuberculosis, the media used are commonly referred to as an L-J (Lowenstein-Jensen) slant, a medium that is a sea-green color. Tuberculosis is a slow grower, so these slants are maintained for a minimum of four weeks to observe for growth on the slants. If growth is observed, the slant is sent to a state health laboratory for confirmation of the results. Even slower growers are fungi; the agar plates are maintained for up to eight weeks, and, to prevent the agar from drying out during this lengthy time, *parafilm* is used to seal the plates.

Although it is doubtful that a medical assistant would inoculate the media with a collected specimen, you should know what is involved because you could be hired as a specimen processor. The basic steps for inoculation of a plate follow.

- Check the patient's identification on the swab as well as the type of culture ordered.
- Collect the appropriate agar for inoculation.
- Label the agar with the patient's name, identification number, the source of the specimen, the date and time of inoculation, and your initials. This identification is placed on the bottom side of the petri dish with a marker, wax pencil, crayon, or adhesive label.

- Remove the swab from the culturette and gently roll it on approximately one fourth of the plates. After inoculation, dispose of the culturette in the biohazard waste container.
- Most commonly in microbiology labs, a disposable plastic loop is used for *streaking* the plates, although some labs use a fine-wire loop that must be *flamed* between inoculations. (Refer to Figure 46–14B for an idea of a properly streaked plate.) The idea is to isolate the organism for identification so that as the plate is turned, smaller amounts of the original specimen are streaked out by the fourth turn of the plate. There is a definite art to proper inoculation of plates.
- After the plates have been streaked, place them in an incubator. Usually, incubators are maintained at 37°C/98.6°F (normal body temperature); however, depending on the microorganism suspected, incubators may also be set at 25°C/77°F (fungal isolation and identification) and 42°C/107.6°F (*Campylobacter*). Recall also that there are anaerobic microorganisms that grow better with increased carbon dioxide (CO_2) and decreased oxygen, so there are special packages for incubating these types of organisms. Temperatures are monitored and recorded on a daily basis as part of the quality control and quality assurance for the lab.

CLINICAL PEARL

This would end your part of the processing; from here, a specially trained microbiologist is responsible for looking at the plates at 24 and 48 hours for the presence of a pathogenic microorganism, isolation identification of that organism, and drugs that inhibit the growth or kill the organism.

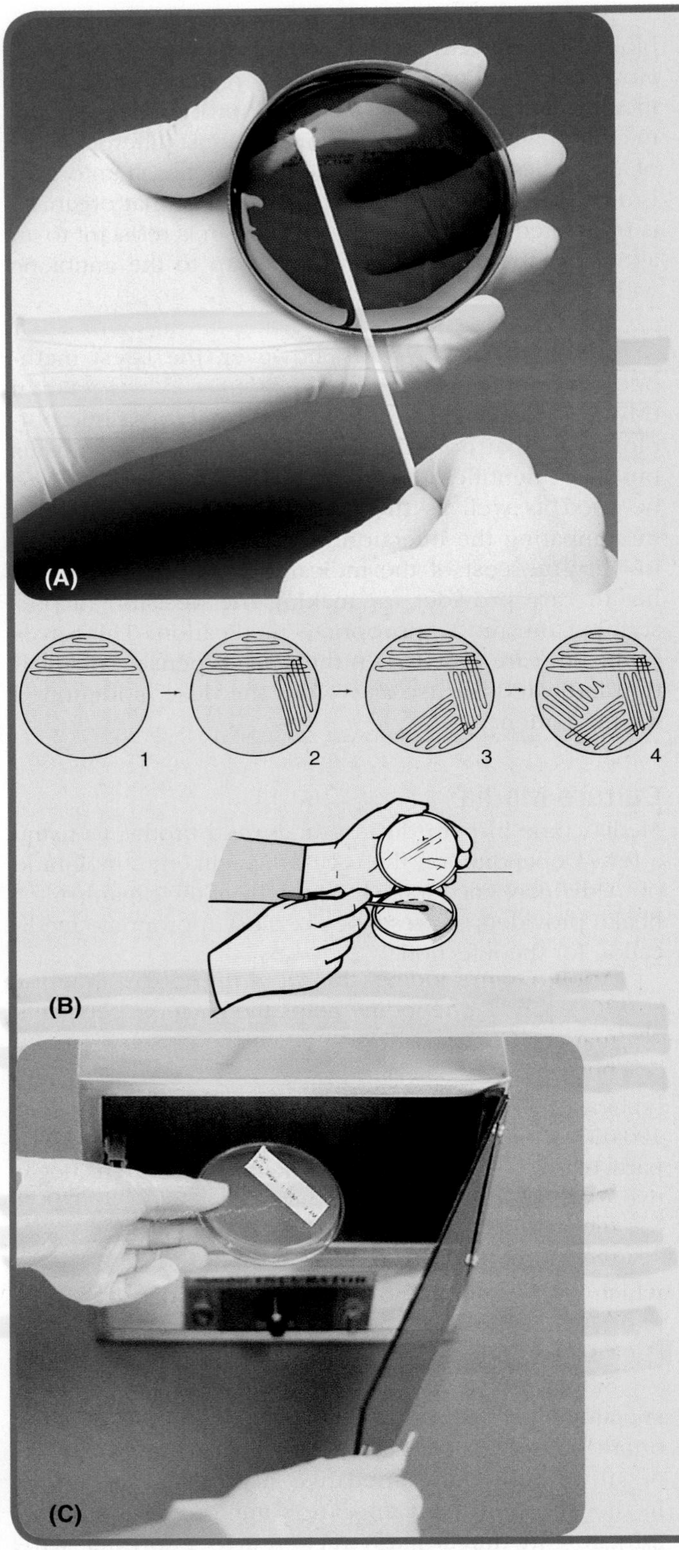

Figure 46–14: (A) The culture plate should be smeared with the specimen from a swab. (B) Pattern for streaking an agar plate. The plate is turned to aid in isolating the microorganism. (C) Place the culture plate in the incubator with the agar side up. Ensure that the label is placed on the agar side for proper identification of the specimen. *Delmar/Cengage Learning.*

Refer to Figures 46–14A–C for proper inoculation of an agar plate.

Gram Staining and Microbiologic Smears

CLINICAL PEARL

As a medical assistant, you probably will not perform either Gram staining or preparation of microbiologic smears; however, it is important to understand the reasons for this type of testing and indications of various results because this is a content area on medical assisting certification examinations.

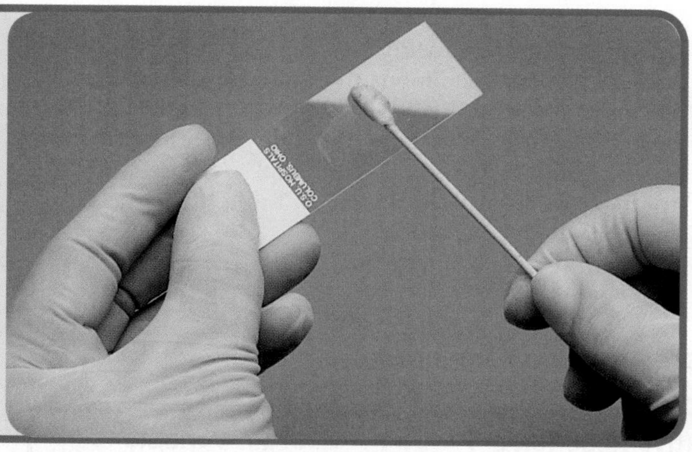

Figure 46–15: The proper method for applying a specimen to a slide for bacteriologic staining. *Delmar/Cengage Learning.*

Hans Christian Gram, a Danish scientist, developed the staining technique in 1884 for identification of various microorganisms that caused pneumonia. With this technique, you should be familiar with several distinctive steps and elements of the stain.

- Apply the specimen to the microscopic slide and affix the necessary, required identification (Figure 46–15).
- Heat-fix the slide by placing it on a slide warmer for the facility's prescribed amount of time.
- First, apply the *primary dye*, which is the crystal violet (purple-colored dye). Usually, this stain is left on the slide for 30 seconds.
- Wash the slide with distilled water.
- Apply Gram's iodine, the *mordant*, to the slide for 30 seconds. The iodine helps the bacterial cell walls that are Gram positive to retain the crystal violet or purple part of the stain.
- Flood the slide with distilled water.
- Apply ethanol or acetone, which is the *decolorizer*. This ensures that a microorganism does not retain the crystal violet to give a false positive result. Flood the slide with the decolorizer until you no longer see the purple color but be careful not to rinse too long.
- Flood the slide with distilled water.
- Apply safranin (red stain) to the slide for 30 seconds.
- Flood the slide with distilled water.
- Drain the slide and blot with bibulous paper; a qualified individual will examine the sample microscopically to interpret the results of the staining procedure.

If the microorganisms on the slide are identified as **Gram positive**, the color of those organisms will be dark blue to violet because the bacterial cell walls retained the crystal violet color even after the decolorizer was applied. If the microorganisms are **Gram negative**, their color characteristics will be red or pink; these organisms do not have the same cell wall characteristics and thus will absorb the counterstain (safranin) in their cell walls. Characteristically, Gram-negative microorganisms have a more dangerous connotation than Gram-positive organisms.

Morphologic Shapes

Also significant when taking certification examinations is a basic understanding of the description of the shape of the organisms. There are three basic morphologic shapes when describing bacteria: *coccus*, *bacillus*, and *spiral*. Coccus-shaped organisms are very round; the Latin term *coccus* means "berry-shaped." Bacillus-shaped organisms are rod-shaped. (Think of a fat hyphen; this is how they appear under the microscope.) Spiral-shaped organisms, also referred to as *spirochetes*, are corkscrew-shaped. Figure 46–16 illustrates these shapes.

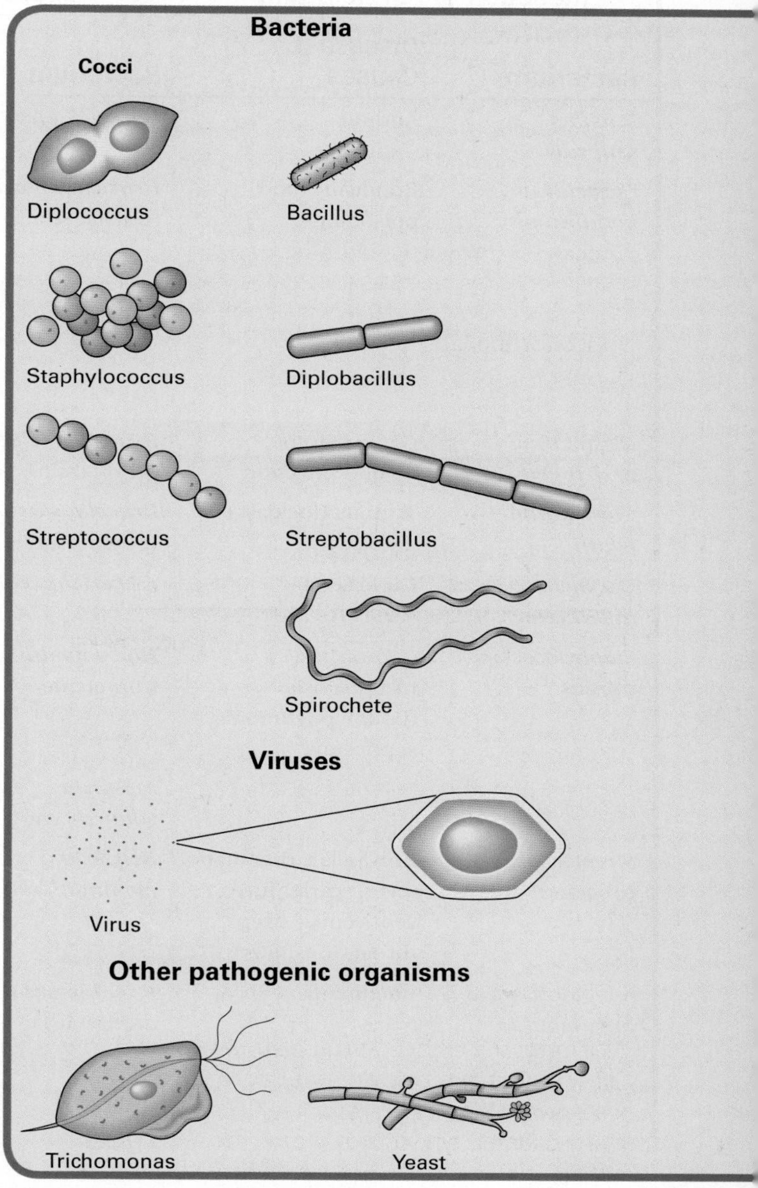

Figure 46–16: Pathogenic microorganisms. *Delmar/Cengage Learning.*

Gram negative - E.coli, salmonella / Shigella

Make a note of the following shapes:

- Gram-positive cocci in clusters: *Staphylococci*
- Gram-positive cocci in chains: *Streptococci*
- Gram-negative cocci in pairs (diplococci): *Neiserria gonorroeae*
- Gram-negative bacilli (rods): *Escherichia coli*

Remember that the bacteriologic smear is not definitive for diagnosing the type of microorganism present in the specimen; the staining characteristics are helpful for the health care provider to get an early start on treating the infection, but the identification of the microorganism is the final definite step for appropriate treatment. Refer to Table 46–2 for stain-

TABLE 46–2 Some Important Pathogenic Bacteria and Their Reaction to the Gram Stain

Gram-Positive Reaction (+) (Reaction of Purple Stain)		Gram-Negative Reaction (−) (Loss of Purple Stain)		Gram-Variable Reaction (+/−)	
Bacterium	**Disease It Causes**	**Bacterium**	**Disease It Causes**	**Bacterium**	**Disease It Causes**
Bacillus anthracis	Anthrax	*Bordetella pertussis*	Whooping cough	*Mycobacterium leprae*	Leprosy
Clostridium botulinum	Botulism (food poisoning)	*Brucella abortus* (bovine strain)	Flu-like symptoms (acute form); fevers, arthritis, neurologic symptoms (undulant form); chronic fatigue syndrome, depression, arthritis (chronic form)	*Mycobacterium tuberculosis*	Tuberculosis
Clostridium perfringens	Gas gangrene, wound infection	*Brucella melitensis* (goat strain)			
Clostridium tetani	Tetanus (lockjaw)	*Brucella suis* (porcine strain)			
Corynebacterium diphtheriae	Diphtheria	*Escherichia coli*	Urinary infections		
Staphylococcus aureus	Carbuncles, furunculosis (boils), pneumonia, septicemia	*Haemophilus influenzae*	Meningitis, pneumonia		
		Neisseria gonorrhoeae	Gonorrhea		
Streptococcus pyogenes	Erysipelas, rheumatic fever, scarlet fever, septicemia, strep throat, tonsillitis	*Neisseria meningitidis*	Nasopharyngitis, meningitis		
Streptococcus pneumoniae	Pneumonia	*Pseudomonas aeruginosa*	Respiratory and urogenital infections		
		Rickettsia rickettsii	Rocky mountain spotted fever		

Gram-Positive Reaction (+) (Reaction of Purple Stain)		Gram-Negative Reaction (−) (Loss of Purple Stain)		Gram-Variable Reaction (+/−)	
Bacterium	**Disease It Causes**	**Bacterium**	**Disease It Causes**	**Bacterium**	**Disease It Causes**
		Salmonella paratyphi	Food poisoning, paratyphoid fever		
		Salmonella typhi	Typhoid fever		
		Shigella dysenteriae	Dysentery		
		Treponema pallidum	Syphilis		
		Vibrio cholerae	Cholera		
		Yersinia pestis	Plague		

ing characteristics of certain bacteria and the diseases they cause.

A different type of stain is used when a patient is suspected of having tuberculosis, a very contagious airborne disease. The stain is called an *acid-fast* stain; tuberculosis will not appear definitively on the Gram stain, so the acid-fast stain must be used. If microorganisms stain pinkish to red, the possibility is good that the patient has a type of *Mycobacterium*, but until the culture is completed, it cannot be known whether it is tuberculosis or another type of *Mycobacterium* infection.

CHAPTER SUMMARY

- Patient's name, date of collection, time of collection, and the tests(s) to be performed must be noted on a urine specimen container.
- The first morning urine sample is the best for testing because it is most concentrated from being held in the bladder overnight.
- Catheterization is a specialized type of urine collection that is used when a sterile specimen is indicated for testing, the patient is unable to void, or medication must be instilled into the bladder.
- In collection of specimens for substance abuse analysis, it is important to inform the patient that all drugs consumed within the 30 days prior to testing are likely to be revealed by the test.
- Pregnancy tests are performed to measure the amount of human chorionic gonadotropin (hCG) in the blood or urine.
- The urinalysis is the most frequently performed test in the medical office and consists of physical, chemical, and microscopic testing of the urine.
- It is essential for the medical assistant to explain properly how to collect stool specimens because they can provide a great deal of diagnostic insight into the patient's condition.
- When a culture is obtained within the doctor's office, it can be sent out for a culture and sensitivity test.

STUDY TOOLS

Workbook	Activities for Chapter 46
Premium Website	
MEDIA LINK	View these **Media Links** for Chapter 46: • Clean-Catch Midstream Urine Specimen • Perform an Occult Blood Test
StudyWARE	Activities and Quizzes on the **StudyWARE™ Software** for Chapter 46
	Complete the following **Competency Challenge 2.0** activities: • Wednesday, 11:00 AM: Perform Microbiology Testing • Wednesday, 2:00 PM: Instruct in Urine Specimen Collection and Perform Urinalysis • Wednesday, 3:00 PM: Instruct in Fecal Specimen Collection
	Audio Library of medical terms
	Online access to the **Critical Thinking Challenge 2.0**
learninglab	Module 19: Laboratory Procedures
CourseMate	Activities and Quizzes for Chapter 46
WebTutor	Activities and Quizzes for Chapter 46

CHECK YOUR KNOWLEDGE

1. Using the word *random* to describe a urine specimen means what?
   a. The provider has ordered a specimen that is collected in the morning.
   b. They provider has ordered a specimen without specifying the time of collection.
   c. The provider has ordered a specimen collected at bedtime.
   d. The provider has ordered a specimen to be collected at lunchtime.
2. There are special urine collection bags that fit over the genital area of an adult and are secured with adhesive.
   a. True
   b. False
3. All the following are portions of physical urinalysis testing *except*:
   a. color.
   b. clarity.
   c. glucose.
   d. specific gravity.
4. Which of the following components could be found in a patient's urine specimen when the patient has a urinary tract infection?
   a. Protein
   b. Nitrite
   c. Leukocytes
   d. All the above
5. Which of the following is the normal value range for specific gravity?
   a. 1.015–1.025
   b. 1.005–1.020
   c. 1.010–1.025
   d. 1.005–1.030
6. Medical assistants are not allowed to read or interpret results of microscopic urine sediments according to OSHA.
   a. True
   b. False

7. Which color does the guaiac reagent turn when oxidized in the presence of blood?
   a. Purple
   b. Black
   c. Blue
   d. Yellow
8. Exudate is another word for:
   a. drainage.
   b. sputum.
   c. pus.
   d. blood.
9. When did Hans Christian Gram develop the staining technique?
   a. 1883
   b. 1884
   c. 1885
   d. 1886
10. Which disease does the bacterium *Bordetella pertussis* cause?
    a. Tuberculosis
    b. Anthrax
    c. Leprosy
    d. Whooping cough

WEB LINK

Clinical Laboratory Improvement Amendments (CLIA): www.cms.gov/CLIA/

Common Laboratory Values: www.globalrph.com/labs.htm

Mayo Clinic – Urinalysis: www.mayoclinic.com/health/urinalysis/MY00488

Unit

15

Cardiology and Radiology Procedures

Cardiology and radiology procedures are discussed in this unit. The medical assistant has a multiple role in these diagnostic areas. You will be responsible for instructing and preparing patients for procedures, tests, and X-rays. In some cases, you will either carry out the tests or procedures or assist the health care provider. After completion, you will alert the provider of the results and, on the order of the provider, notify the patient. You might even be responsible for filing the report of results in the patient's chart.

Often, as part of the complete physical examination, the provider might order certain tests or other procedures (e.g., ECG, chest X-ray, or mammography). If these diagnostic tests are performed on-site, the results can often be determined while the patient is still present. If referrals must be made for diagnostic tests and procedures, patients might be asked to return within a week to 10 days for a final report of the findings. This gives the medical assistant and the provider time to gather reports in the patient's chart to screen and follow up. You might want to advise patients to bring a list of concerns so they will not forget to ask necessary questions. This practice can reduce the number of phone consultations.

Certification Connection

	Ch. 47	Ch. 48
CMA (AAMA)		
Anatomy and physiology: Systems, including structure, function, related conditions and diseases, and their interrelationship	X	
Principles of equipment operation: electrocardiograph	X	
Patient preparation and assisting the provider	X	X
Electrocardiography (EKG/ECG)	X	
Medical imaging		X
RMA (AMT)		
Anatomy and physiology (cardiovascular)	X	
Standard, 12-lead electrocardiogram	X	
Mounting techniques	X	
Other electrocardiographic procedures	X	

Chapter

47 Cardiology Procedures

OBJECTIVES

In this chapter, you will learn the following:

KB KNOWLEDGE BASE

1. Spell and define, using the glossary at the back of the text, all the Words to Know in this chapter.
2. Describe the electrical conduction system of the heart.
3. Explain the reasons for performing an ECG.
4. Discuss the equipment and supplies needed to perform an ECG.
5. Identify the 12 leads and describe which area of the heart each represents.
6. Explain the purpose of standardization for an ECG.
7. Define *artifacts* and list their causes on an ECG.
8. Discuss cardiac arrhythmias and your role in identifying them.
9. State the purpose of a Holter monitor and explain the procedure to a patient.
10. Discuss why cardiac stress testing is performed.
11. Explain echocardiography.
12. State the purpose of a defibrillator.

S SKILLS

1. Obtain a standard 12-lead ECG.
2. Demonstrate the procedure for proper hookup of a Holter monitor.

B BEHAVIOR

1. Apply critical thinking skills in performing patient assessment and care.
2. Use language and verbal skills that enable patients' understanding.

WORDS TO KNOW

amplifier
arrhythmia
artifacts
atrial depolarization
augmented
cardiology
countershock
current
defibrillator
echocardiography
echoes
electrocardiogram
electrocardiograph
electrode
galvanometer
Holter monitor
impulse
interference
intermittent
interpretive
interval
limbs
mechanical
multichannel
precordial
Purkinje
reliable
repolarization
sedentary
segment
simultaneous
somatic
standardization
stylus
trace
voltage

ELECTROCARDIOGRAM

In family and general practice, internal medicine, and **cardiology**, a procedure frequently used in the diagnosis of heart disease and dysfunction is the **electrocardiogram** (referred to as an ECG or EKG for short; in this chapter, it will be abbreviated as ECG for consistency). All muscle movement produces electrical impulses, and the ECG is a recording of the electrical impulses of the heart muscle. This procedure is noninvasive, painless, and safe, and patients should be told so to eliminate apprehension. Chapter 30 covered the anatomy and physiology of the heart, common cardiovascular tests, and diseases and disorders of the circulatory system. Having an understanding of the circulatory system is essential to performing cardiac testing accurately.

Electrical Impulses of the Heart

The heart is a four-chambered pump that produces a tiny electrical current by muscular contraction. Electricity in the heart is produced by a chemical exchange at the cellular level and muscle contraction. An electrical impulse originates in the modified myocardial tissue of the sinoatrial (SA) node, also known as the sinus node or pacemaker of the heart, causing the atria to contract. This contraction is the beginning of **atrial depolarization**, which is the first part of the cardiac cycle. The first impulse as recorded on the graph paper is termed the P wave. The impulse continues through the heart tissue to the atrioventricular (AV) node, to the bundle of His, and spreads to the **Purkinje** fibers. These fibers cause the muscles of the ventricles to contract and produce the QRS complex of waves on the ECG paper. The T wave on the graph paper follows, representing the **repolarization** of the ventricles, or the time of recovery before another contraction. This is considered a normal ECG cycle (Figure 47-1).

Reasons for Performing an ECG

The ECG can detect damage from previous heart attacks, enlargement of the heart muscle, disturbances in the rhythm, and other abnormal conditions.

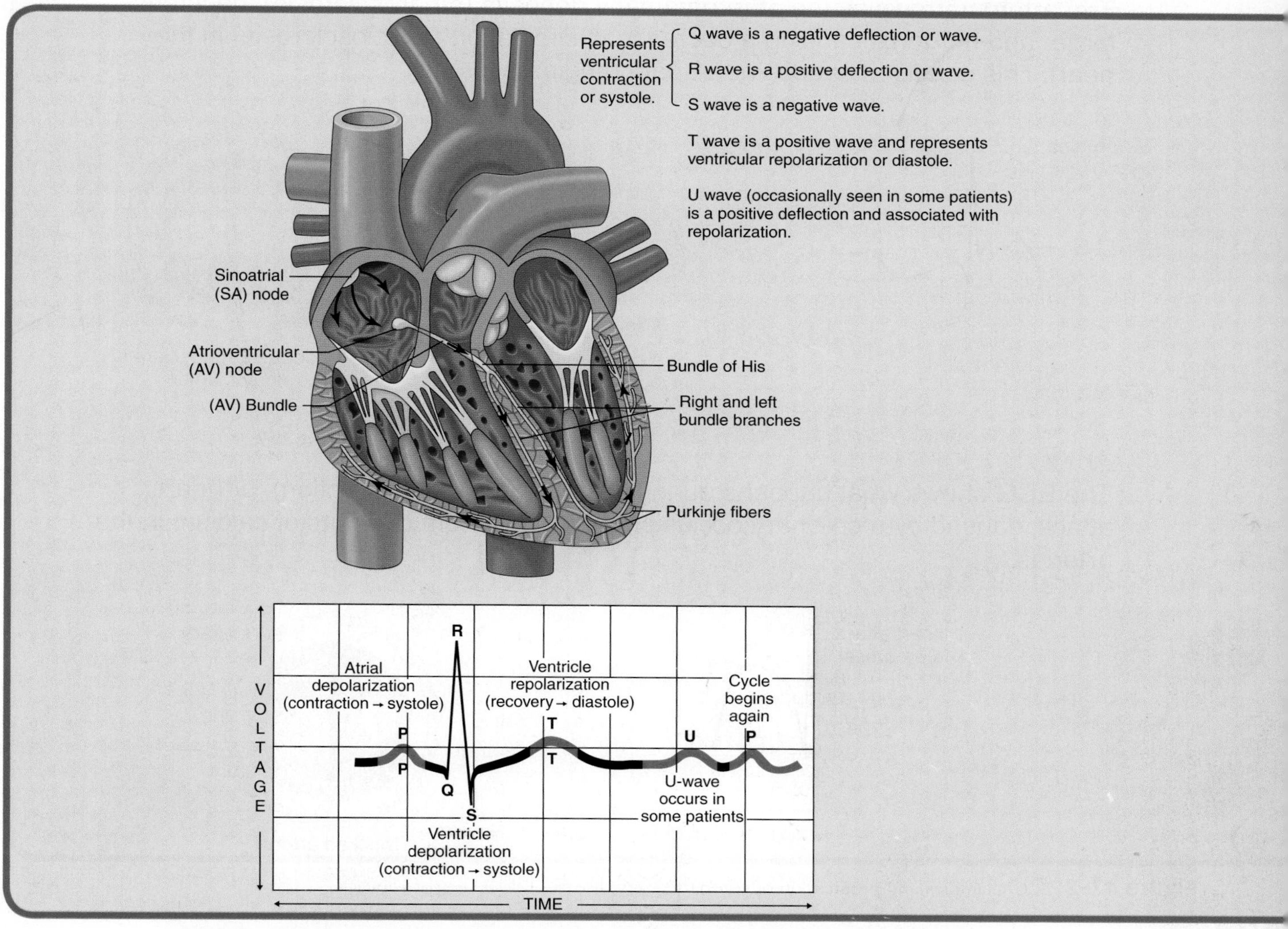

Figure 47–1: Conduction of the heart and ECG graphic representation of the cardiac cycle. *Delmar/Cengage Learning.*

Three examples of the heart's electrical activity and progression of coronary artery disease are shown in Figure 47–2. This might give you a better understanding of what happens during normal beating of the heart and when it is in crisis. As you can see, the changes in the normal pattern can aid the provider in detecting many heart conditions as well as predict the potential for future heart conditions such as a heart attack. Before the provider can confirm a diagnosis, an examination that considers the patient's symptoms, medical history, and other diagnostic tests are necessary. It is usually recommended for patients between

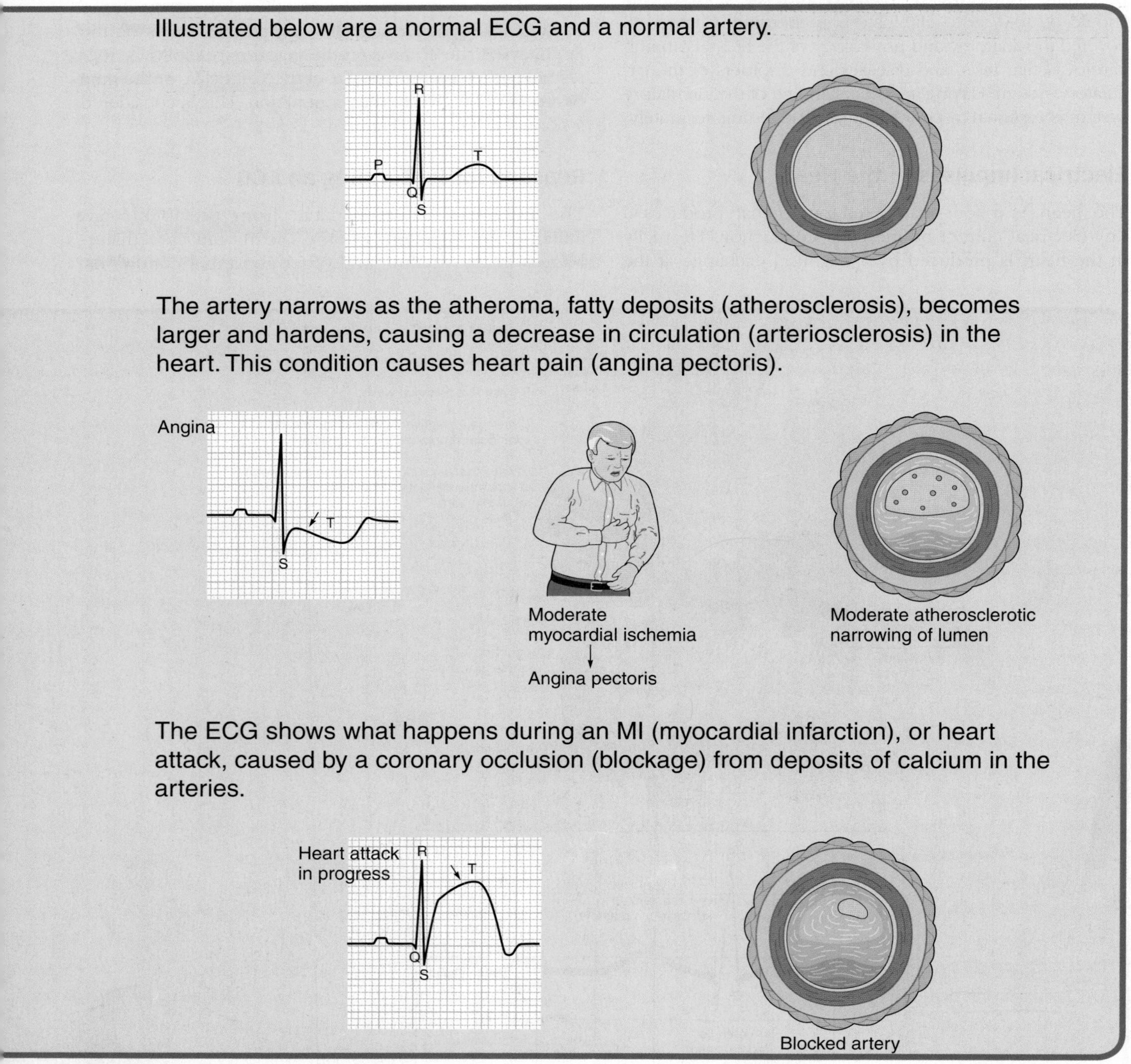
Illustrated below are a normal ECG and a normal artery.
R
P
T
Q
S
The artery narrows as the atheroma, fatty deposits (atherosclerosis), becomes larger and hardens, causing a decrease in circulation (arteriosclerosis) in the heart. This condition causes heart pain (angina pectoris).
Angina
T
S
Moderate myocardial ischemia
Angina pectoris
Moderate atherosclerotic narrowing of lumen
The ECG shows what happens during an MI (myocardial infarction), or heart attack, caused by a coronary occlusion (blockage) from deposits of calcium in the arteries.
Heart attack in progress
R
T
Q
S
Blocked artery

Figure 47–2: ECG examples and progression of coronary artery disease. *Delmar/Cengage Learning.*

the ages of 40 to 45 to establish a base reading. Providers can then refer to this ECG in the event of later problems. Most often, an ECG is performed along with the routine annual physical examination every 5 to 10 years after a baseline normal reading has been established. Some providers prefer to have a tracing more often, even annually, for patients who have a history of hypertension, smoking, obesity, a high serum cholesterol level, or a family history of heart disease. Another factor in heart problems providers consider is a **sedentary** lifestyle, which is usually accompanied by obesity.

ELECTROCARDIOGRAPH MACHINES

The ECG recording is obtained by operating the **electrocardiograph** machine. Many types of electrocardiographs are available for use in the medical field today. The ones shown in Figure 47–3A–B are **multichannel**, 12-lead instruments, which record the electrical activity of the heart simultaneously from 12 views.

Computerized electrocardiographs have **simultaneous** 12-lead, **interpretive** analysis. Data is not only printed out but also stored in memory. The ECG **tracing** is generated in about one minute on a single 8" × 10" sheet of ECG paper, and no time is involved in mounting. A manual mode provides additional leads such as the rhythm strip of lead II. These machines are relatively lightweight and can be moved easily if necessary.

There are also older models, which measure only one lead and one view of the heart at a time, known as single-channel electrocardiographs. The older, single-channel model electrocardiographs produce a strip reading that has to be mounted onto permanent folders for filing. Regardless of which model is used, it is important to understand the operation of the machine you are operating. Each machine comes with an operating manual, step-by-step instructions, maintenance, and troubleshooting for the unit.

Through a process of electrical transmission, the ECG machine traces **impulses** of the heart onto a specially coated, heat-sensitive paper to create a permanent record of its activity. ECGs can also be recorded digitally directly into the patient's EHR and can be sent to a specialist by fax or through the EHR if warranted. To accomplish this, **electrodes** are placed on the patient's **limbs** and chest and pick up the electrical **current** produced by the contractions of the heart. The tiny impulses are transmitted to the electrocardiograph by metal tips (or clips) on the patient cables (wires) that are attached to the

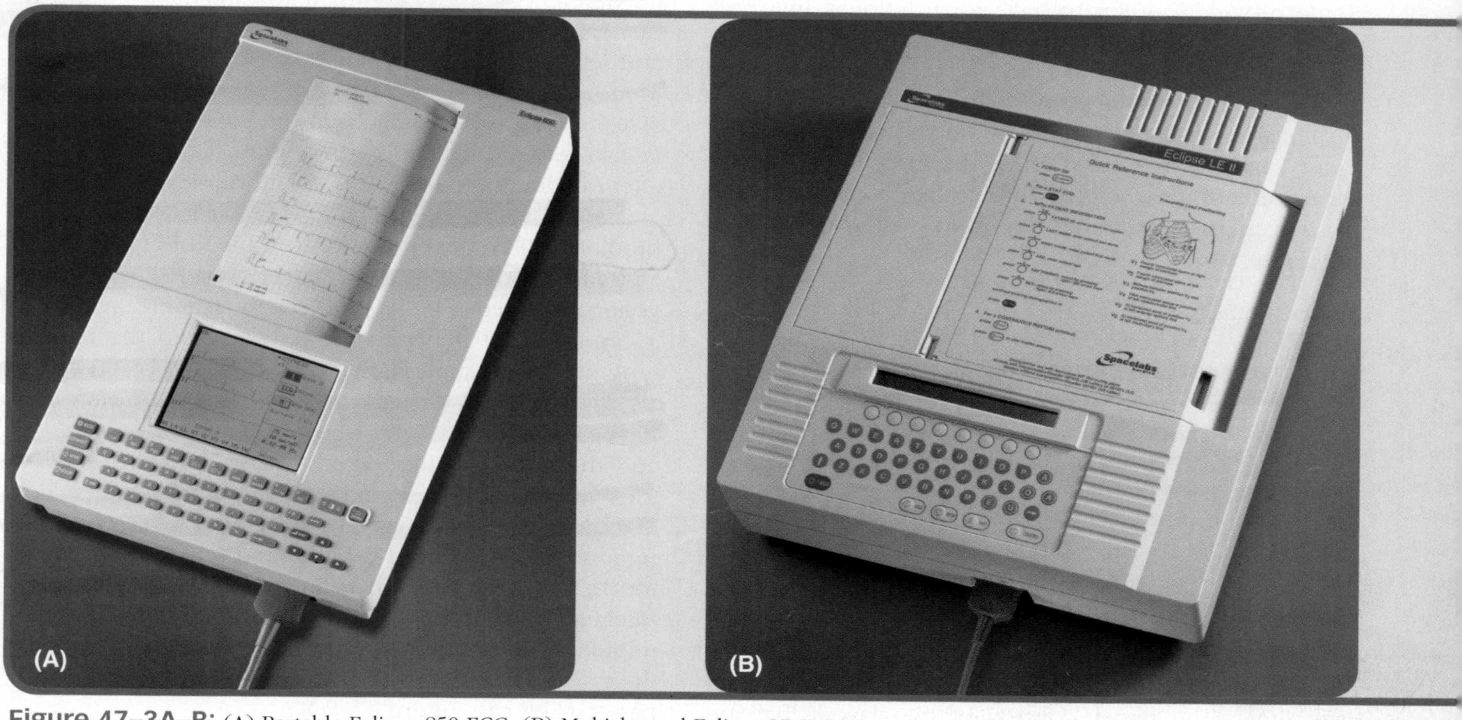

Figure 47–3A–B: (A) Portable Eclipse 850 ECG. (B) Multichannel Eclipse LE II ECG. *Courtesy of Spacelabs Medical, Inc.*

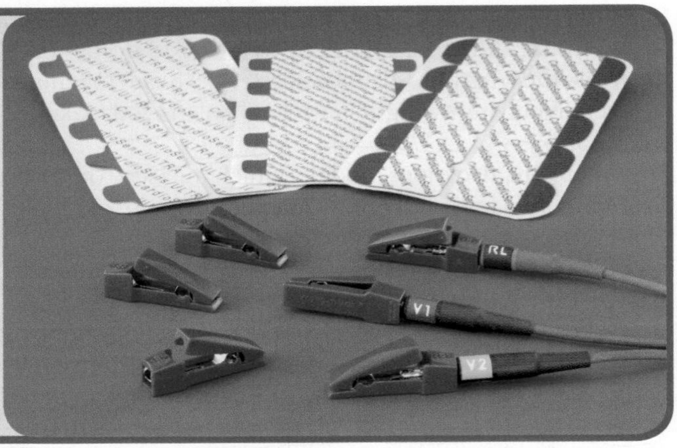

Figure 47–4: Disposable sensors, clips, and electrodes.
Courtesy of Spacelabs Medical, Inc.

electrodes (Figure 47–4). The current enters the electrocardiograph through the wires to reach the **amplifier**, which enlarges the impulses. They are transformed into **mechanical** motion by the **galvanometer**. The **stylus**, a heated, pen-like instrument, produces a printed representation on the ECG paper. As the heated stylus moves against the tracing paper, the impulses given off by the heart are recorded.

The ECG is interpreted by a provider, usually the one ordering the procedure. Newer models have interpretive capability to perform basic interpretations of the tracings, although a provider will still review them. Some providers prefer to have a cardiologist interpret the ECG and submit the results in the form of a written report. ECGs can be faxed, scanned, and emailed or sent by EHR to the cardiologist to be read with the results sent back the same way or phoned to the provider. The provider interpreting the ECG compares the measurement, rate, and rhythm; duration of the electrical waves; **intervals**; and **segments** with known normal ECG readings.

CLINICAL PEARL

As with any faxed document, you must be sure to follow HIPAA guidelines to ensure that the fax reaches the intended recipient.

Electrocardiograph Paper

Electrocardiograph paper comes in either a roll (for single-channel machines) or a pad (for multichannel machines). The paper consists of two layers that are heat- and pressure-sensitive and marked with light and dark dots and lines that form squares. The vertical axis of the paper records the voltage, and the horizontal axis measures time.

The paper moves through the machine at a rate of 25 mm per second. Each small square, or square area defined by dots, measures 1 mm by 1 mm and represents 0.04 second. Each large square measures 5 mm by 5 mm and represents 0.2 second. The distance across five large squares represents 1.0 second. Review Figure 47–5. The tracing paper should be handled carefully to protect it from being accidentally marked. Dot matrix paper makes tracings easy to read and copy because they are clear and legible and standardized to make the reading process universal for all providers.

Electrocardiograph Leads

The routine ECG consists of 12 leads, or recordings of the electrical activity of the heart from different angles. Most electrocardiographs have an automatic lead marker to identify each of the 12 standard leads (Figure 47–6). The first three leads are called standard or bipolar leads and are labeled with Roman numerals I, II, and III. They are termed bipolar because they monitor two electrodes. These leads are obtained by placing limb electrodes on the fleshy part of the upper outer arms and the inner lower calves. Lead I records the electrical voltage difference between the right arm and left arm. Lead II records the difference between the right arm and the left leg. Lead III records the **voltage** difference between the left arm and left leg (Figure 47–7). Many providers request you to run an additional two-foot-long strip of lead II only to assess for any abnormalities in the patient's rhythm; this is also referred to as a rhythm strip. If this is the case, after obtaining the ECG, you would run lead II alone.

The **augmented** leads, also known as standard or bipolar, are the next three in the 12-lead ECG. They are aVR, aVL, and aVF. aVR is the recording of the heart's voltage difference between the right arm electrode and a central point between the left arm and the left leg (augmented voltage right arm). aVL is the recording of the heart's voltage difference between the left arm electrode and a central point between the right arm and the left leg (augmented voltage left arm). aVF is the recording of the heart's voltage difference between the left leg electrode and a central point between the right arm and left arm (augmented voltage left leg or foot). The term *augmented* means "to become larger." Because these three leads are produced by such small impulses, the amplifier of the ECG machine augments their size sufficiently for recording them on the graph paper. (Refer to Figure 47–8.)

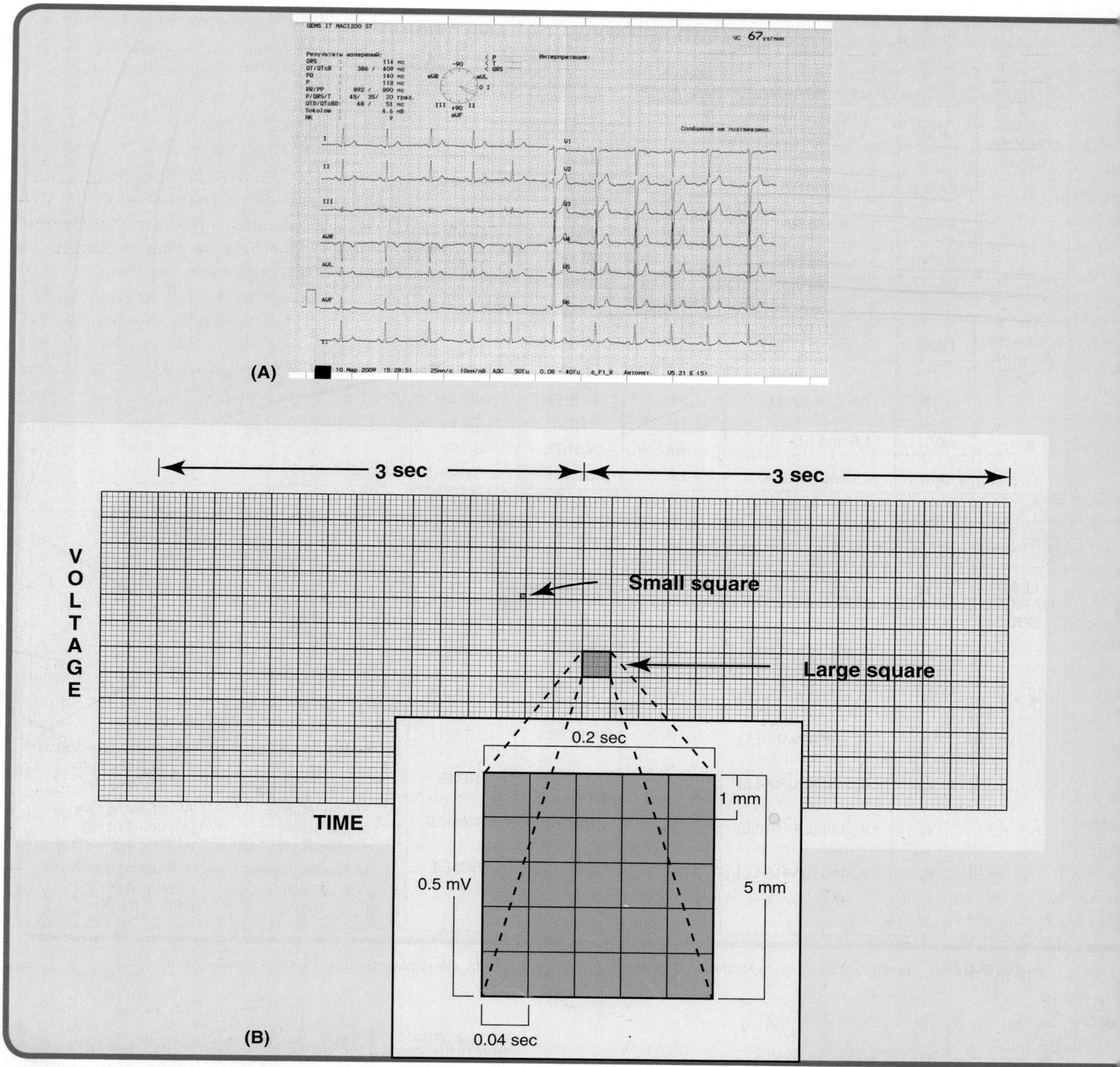

Figure 47–5A–B: (A) ECG tracing. *Courtesy of Shutterstock. Used under license from Shutterstock.com* (B) ECG graph paper illustrating the size of the squares used to measure time and voltage of heartbeats. *Delmar/Cengage Learning.*

The six standard chest or **precordial** leads are unipolar leads and are obtained by affixing the electrodes to the anatomical positions shown in Figure 47–6. Each precordial lead monitors one electrode and a point within the heart. The leads are labeled with a letter and a number that are known as V_1–V_6. Table 47–1 includes the anatomical positioning of the chest or precordial leads.

LEAD ARRANGEMENT AND CODING

STANDARD LIMB LEADS

LEAD MARKING CODE	LEAD	ELECTRODES CONNECTED	COLOR CODE		
				BODY	INSERT
•	LEAD 1	LA and RA	RL	GREEN	GREEN
	LEAD 2	LL and RA	LL	RED	RED
			RA	WHITE	GRAY
	LEAD 3	LL and LA	LA	BLACK	GRAY

AUGMENTED LIMB LEADS

LEAD MARKING CODE	LEAD	ELECTRODES CONNECTED	COLOR CODE		
				BODY	INSERT
• •	aVR	RA and (LA-LL)	RL	GREEN	GREEN
	aVL	LA and (RA-LL)	LL	RED	RED
			RA	WHITE	GRAY
	aVF	LL and (RA-LA)	LA	BLACK	GRAY

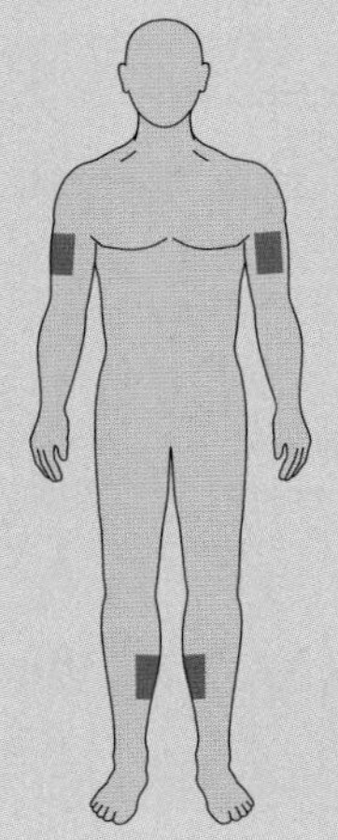

CHEST LEADS

LEAD MARKING CODE	LEAD	ELECTRODES CONNECTED	COLOR CODE		
				BODY	INSERT
• • •	V_1	V_1 and (LA-RA-LL)	V_1	BROWN	RED
	V_2	V_2 and (LA-RA-LL)	V_2	BROWN	YELLOW
	V_3	V_3 and (LA-RA-LL)	V_3	BROWN	GREEN
• • • •	V_4	V_4 and (LA-RA-LL)	V_4	BROWN	BLUE
	V_5	V_5 and (LA-RA-LL)	V_5	BROWN	ORANGE
	V_6	V_6 and (LA-RA-LL)	V_6	BROWN	VIOLET

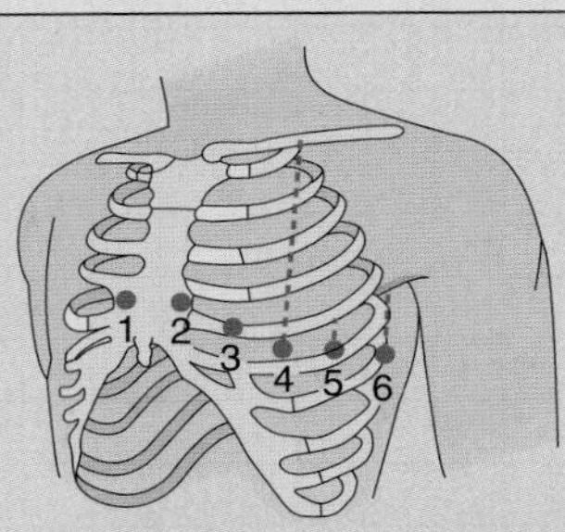

V_1 Fourth intercostal space at right margin of sternum

V_2 Fourth intercostal space at left margin of sternum

V_3 Midway between position 2 and position 4

V_4 Fifth intercostal space at junction of left midclavicular line

V_5 At horizontal level of position 4 at left anterior axillary line

V_6 At horizontal level of position 4 at left midaxillary line

Figure 47–6: International marking codes and diagram with arm, leg, and chest placement. *Courtesy of Spacelabs Medical, Inc.*

PERFORMING THE ECG

The ECG is an important procedure, and every detail must be performed perfectly to ensure accurate results. You will be responsible for preparing the room and equipment prior to administering the ECG. ECG tracings are sensitive to other electrical equipment, so you must ensure that all other equipment in the room, such as exam tables and lamps, is turned off or unplugged because it could cause electrical interference.

Ensure that the ECG machine has been inspected and calibrated and that it is safe for use. Turn the machine on to let the stylus warm up and be sure if using the battery mode for operation that it is currently charged. (Not all models have this availability and must be plugged in.) Look over the lead wires and cables to make sure there are no cracks or damage and check to be sure the clips are attached correctly and are in proper working order. Check the paper in the machine to be sure that it will not run out and restock any materials that will be needed, such as electrodes, alcohol wipes, and disposable razors (in case shaving is necessary). Be sure drapes, gowns, and blankets are available for the patient.

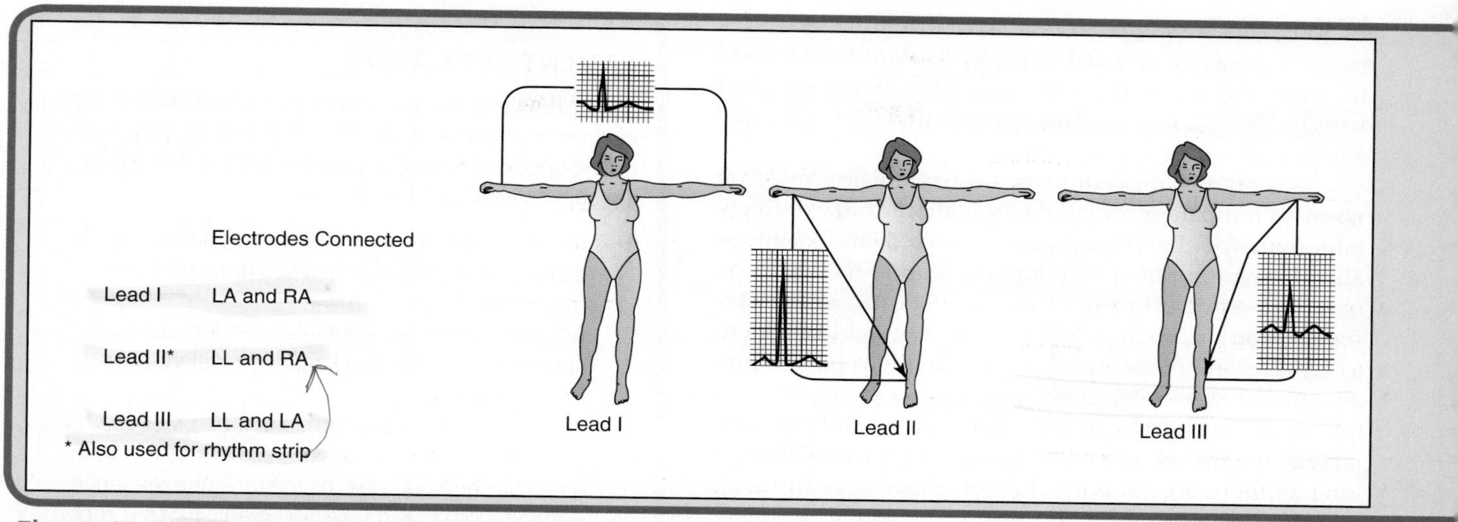

Figure 47–7: Standard limb or bipolar leads. *Delmar/Cengage Learning.*

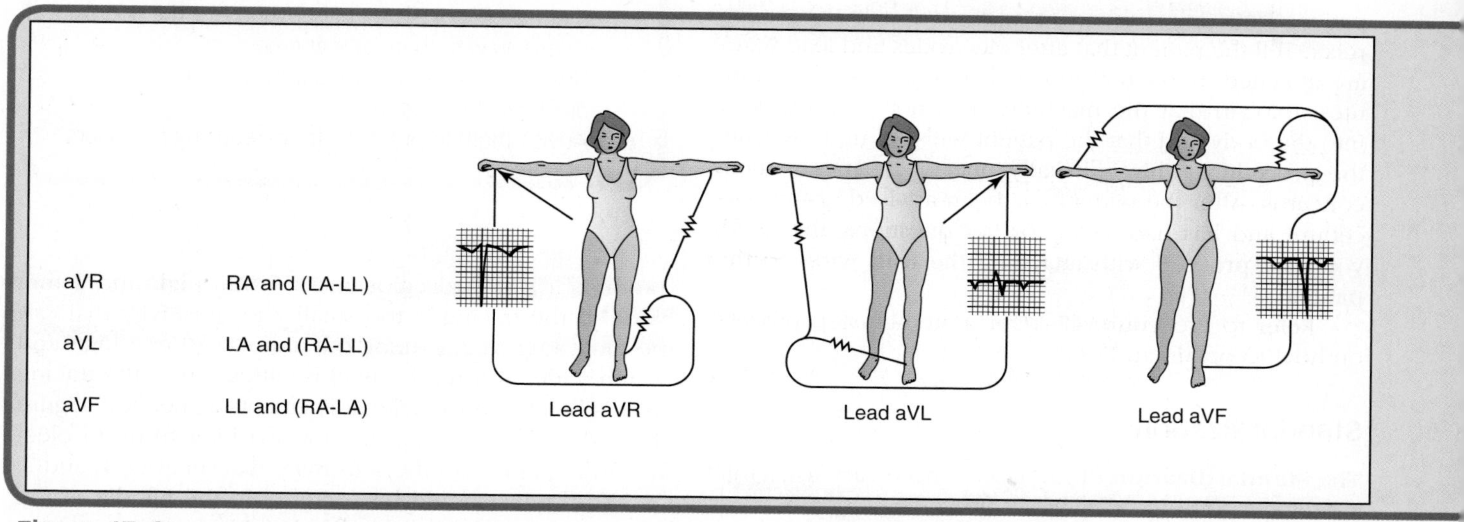

Figure 47–8: Augmented limb leads. *Delmar/Cengage Learning.*

TABLE 47–1 Anatomical Positioning of the Chest or Precordial Leads

Lead	Position placement
V_1	Fourth intercostal space at right margin of sternum
V_2	Fourth intercostal space at left margin of sternum
V_4	Fifth intercostal space on left midclavicular line
V_3	Midway between V_2 and V_4 (V_3 is placed after V_4)
V_5	Horizontal to V_4 at left anterior axillary line
V_6	Horizontal to V_4 at midaxillary line

Preparing the Patient

The room should be quiet and private and the temperature at a comfortable level for the patient, who must disrobe and put a gown on so it opens to the front or will be covered with a drape. Because electrodes must be placed on the patient's arms, legs, and chest, interference can occur if the patient is particularly hairy and must be shaved. Always obtain the patient's permission prior to performing this function.

Lotions, oils, and creams can also cause the electrodes to come loose or not attach properly. You might need to wipe the areas the electrodes are being applied to with an alcohol pad to ensure that the adhesive sticks well.

As with any procedure, a full explanation must be given to the patient to gain cooperation. It is extremely important for the patient to be relaxed and comfortable during the ECG procedure for a good tracing to be obtained; any movement by the patient can cause **interference** on the tracing. Additionally, instruct the patient to remove any metal items he or she might be wearing and his or her cell phone from any pockets because this could cause electrical interference as well. Female patients might ask to wear a sports bra for modesty. As long as there are no wire clips or underwires in them, and they do not get in the way of attaching the electrodes properly, this is generally all right. You can help with this by answering any questions and reassuring the patient. Your calm, efficient manner will help the patient relax. Tell the patient that after electrodes and lead wires are attached, the actual test will only take several minutes. Explain that the machine does not put electricity into the body and that the patient will feel nothing from the procedure. This is usually one of a patient's main concerns. After the patient has been advised of the procedure and has had all his or her questions answered, you may proceed with attaching the lead wires to the patient.

Refer to Procedure 47–1 for a step-by-step process on how to obtain an ECG.

PATIENT EDUCATION

During the time you spend with patients in performing electrocardiographic instruction and testing, you have ample opportunity to give patients some of the following suggestions for a healthy heart:

1. Remind them to eat a low-fat, low-cholesterol diet and keep their salt and sodium intake at a minimum.
2. Advise them to get proper rest, perform provider-approved exercise, and keep their weight at an acceptable level.
3. Instruct cardiac patients to take their prescribed medication regularly and immediately to report to the provider any problems they might experience. Remind them not to take OTC medications without the permission of the provider.
4. Remind them to keep their scheduled appointments and make a list of questions for the doctor to review with them at that time.
5. Urge them not to use tobacco and to avoid alcoholic beverages.
6. Advise them to practice stress-reducing behaviors.

Standardization

The **standardization** of the ECG is necessary to enable a provider to judge deviations from the standard. Most machines used today perform automatic standardization. The usual standardization mark is 2 mm wide and 10 mm high. The sensitivity setting should be set at 1. The standardization mark should be indicated in the front of each lead to provide a **reliable** reading. If the tracing is too large, the sensitivity dial should be turned down to ½ to produce a standardization mark 5 mm high and 2 mm wide. If the tracing is too small, the sensitivity dial can be turned up to 2, making the impulse 20 mm high and 2 mm wide. You must pay close attention to the tracing as it is being run to make adjustments as needed. Figure 47–9 shows the standardization marking from an electrocardiograph with the sensitivity dial set at ½, 1, and 2.

The stylus should be centered in the middle of the paper. The baseline allows you to observe the centering and make adjustments as necessary. The temperature of the stylus can be adjusted to control the thickness of the line.

As mentioned, the tracing paper is normally run at a speed of 25 mm per second. If the ECG cycles are too

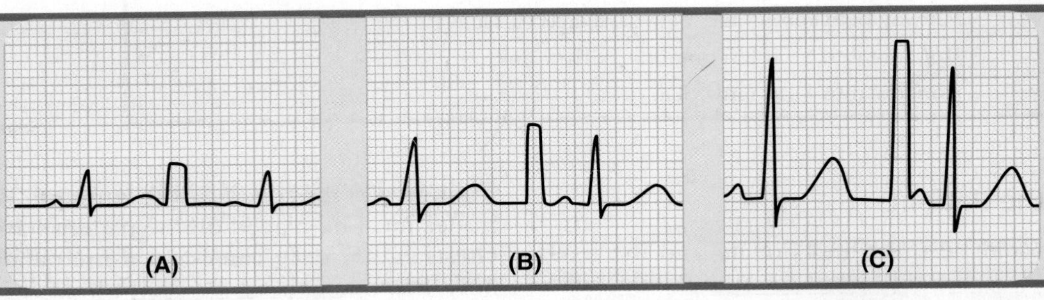

Figure 47–9: Standardization markings with sensitivity dial set on (A) ½, (B) 1, and (C) 2. *Delmar/Cengage Learning.*

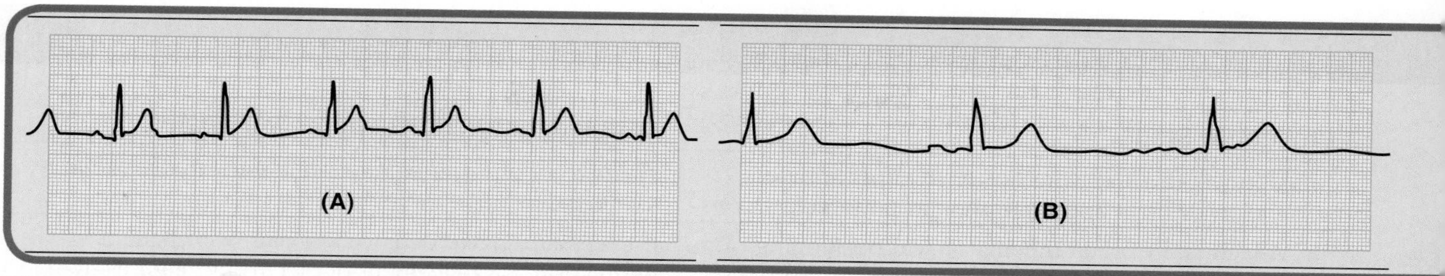

Figure 47–10: (A) Lead run at 25 mm/sec and (B) lead run at 50 mm/sec. *Delmar/Cengage Learning.*

close together, the speed can be changed to 50 mm per second (Figure 47–10). This adjustment should be noted in pen on the tracing.

Any obvious abnormality should be brought to the provider's attention immediately if the patient is experiencing pain or discomfort at the time it is observed.

PROCEDURE 47–1 Obtain a Standard 12-Lead Electrocardiogram

MEDIA LINK: View the video, "Applying Chest Electrodes," for this chapter on the Premium Website.

PURPOSE: Obtain a graphic representation of the electrical activity of the patient's heart

EQUIPMENT: Electrocardiograph; ECG paper; disposable, pre-gelled adhesive electrodes as appropriate for use with patient cable of ECG machine; patient cable and lead wires with clips to attach to electrodes; exam table; pillow; drape sheet or patient gown; gauze squares; alcohol pads; patient's chart or EHR; pen; and disposable razor

S **SKILL:** Obtain a standard 12-lead ECG.

Procedure Steps	Detailed Instructions and/or *Rationales*
1. Prepare the ECG machine and other equipment.	Plug in the ECG machine. Be sure no other electrical equipment is plugged in that might cause electrical interference. Check the cable wires and clips to be sure they are in proper working order. Turn the machine on.
2. Wash hands and assemble other equipment.	
B 3. Introduce yourself, identify the patient, and explain the procedure, ***using language the patient can understand.***	
4. Ask the patient to disrobe from the waist up and remove clothing from the lower legs.	Provide privacy and show the patient where to put belongings.
B 5. ***Assist the patient onto the treatment table and cover the patient with a drape sheet.***	Ask the patient to lie down. Pull out the leg rest. Adjust a pillow under the patient's head for comfort.
6. Place the arm electrodes on the fleshy outer area of the upper arm, with the connectors pointing down. Leg electrodes should be placed on the fleshy inner area of the lower leg near the calf, with connectors pointing up.	*This placement of electrodes reduces tension on the electrodes.* If skin has lotion, oil, or cream on it, use a gauze square or alcohol pad to remove to promote better contact of the electrodes. You might also need to shave the area, with the patient's permission, if there is excess hair.

(continues)

(continued)

Procedure Steps	Detailed Instructions and/or *Rationales*
7. Connect the lead wire tips to the appropriate electrodes by clipping to the tab on the electrodes.	*The power cord and patient cable must not be allowed to touch.*
8. Attach and explain the anatomical positioning of all six disposable adhesive chest electrodes, V_1 through V_6.	If necessary, shave dense chest hair, with patient's permission, for placement of electrodes. Figures 47–11 A through C show male and female patients with electrodes properly placed for a 12-lead ECG. ***Note:*** Performing an ECG on a female patient who has larger breasts might present a problem when attaching the leads. Because the left breast can extend down over the location of the 3rd, 4th, and 5th leads, it might be necessary to elevate the breast tissue before they can be correctly applied. You should elevate the breast using the back of the hand instead of touching the breast with your fingers (shown in Figure 47–11 D).
B 9. ***Cover patient with the drape.***	*To provide for minimum exposure and for warmth while the ECG is obtained.*
10. Enter patient information.	*Follow the manufacture's instructions for proper entering of patient information. Machines allow for various information to be entered; be sure to check with your provider about his or her preference of what data to enter.*
11. Remind the patient not to move and press the Auto button.	*The machine will automatically record and standardize the tracing.*
12. Tear the tracing off from the machine.	
13. Alert the provider of any complaints or unusual findings. With provider approval, remove the lead wires from the limb electrodes. Remove the electrodes from the patient.	*Clean sites with alcohol pad if necessary.*
14. Assist the patient to a sitting position and then down from the table when ready.	*Assist the patient in dressing if necessary.*
15. Change the table paper and pillow cover and discard used disposables.	
16. Wash hands.	
17. Place the tracing in the patient's chart for the provider to interpret.	
18. Document.	Record the appropriate entry on the patient's chart.

Charting Example

4/17/XX 11:30 am	12-Lead ECG obtained. Patient experienced shortness of breath while lying flat. G. JENKS, CMA(AAMA)

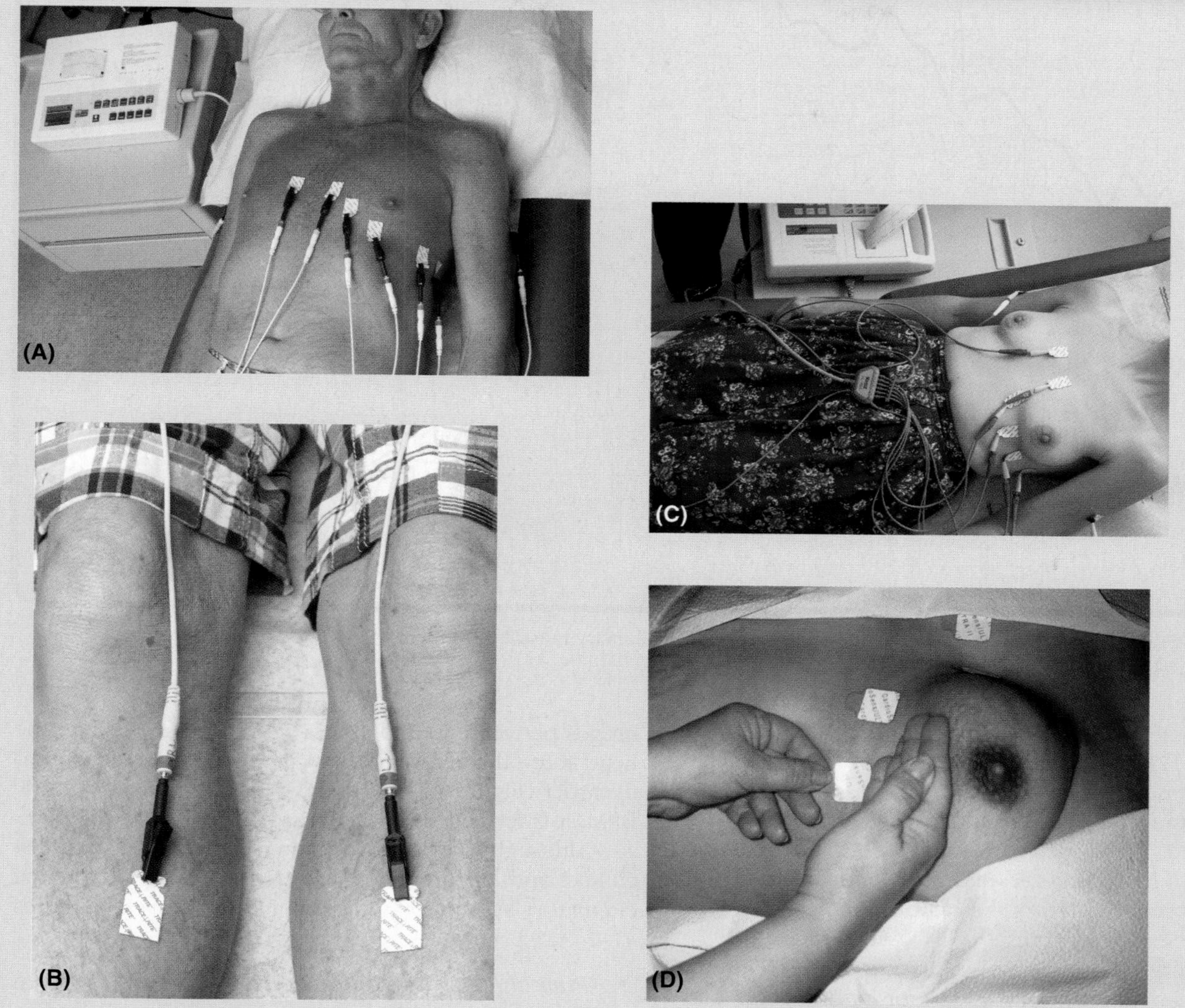

Figure 47–11A–D: A male patient with electrodes placed properly for a standard 12-lead ECG. (B) Lead wires attached to the patient's legs. (C) A female patient with electrodes placed properly for a standard 12-lead ECG. (D) When placing electrodes for a standard 12-lead ECG on a female with a larger breast, elevate the breast using the back of the hand. *A–C Delmar Cengage Learning; D Courtesy of Barbara A. Wise.*

Artifacts

After the ECG is obtained, look over the tracing to determine whether there are any artifacts. This should be done prior to disconnecting the patient. You should be able to recognize any artifacts and identify the source of the interference. Artifacts can occur for a variety of reasons, but if one is found, the interference should be corrected, and a new ECG should be run.

Shivering from nervousness or cold or patients with various neurological conditions such as Parkinson's disease can produce muscle voltage artifacts. This additional activity is called **somatic** tremor. Arm electrodes should be placed close to the shoulders of the upper outer arms to decrease the possibility of muscle voltage **artifacts** and arrhythmias (Figure 47–12A).

AC (alternating current) interference is caused by electrical activity. The latest models of electrocardiographs have sensitive filtering devices that eliminate most of the interference; however, all power cords should be kept away from the patient, and the patient table should be away from the wall to eliminate the possibility of interference from electrical wiring within the wall. The patient must be properly connected

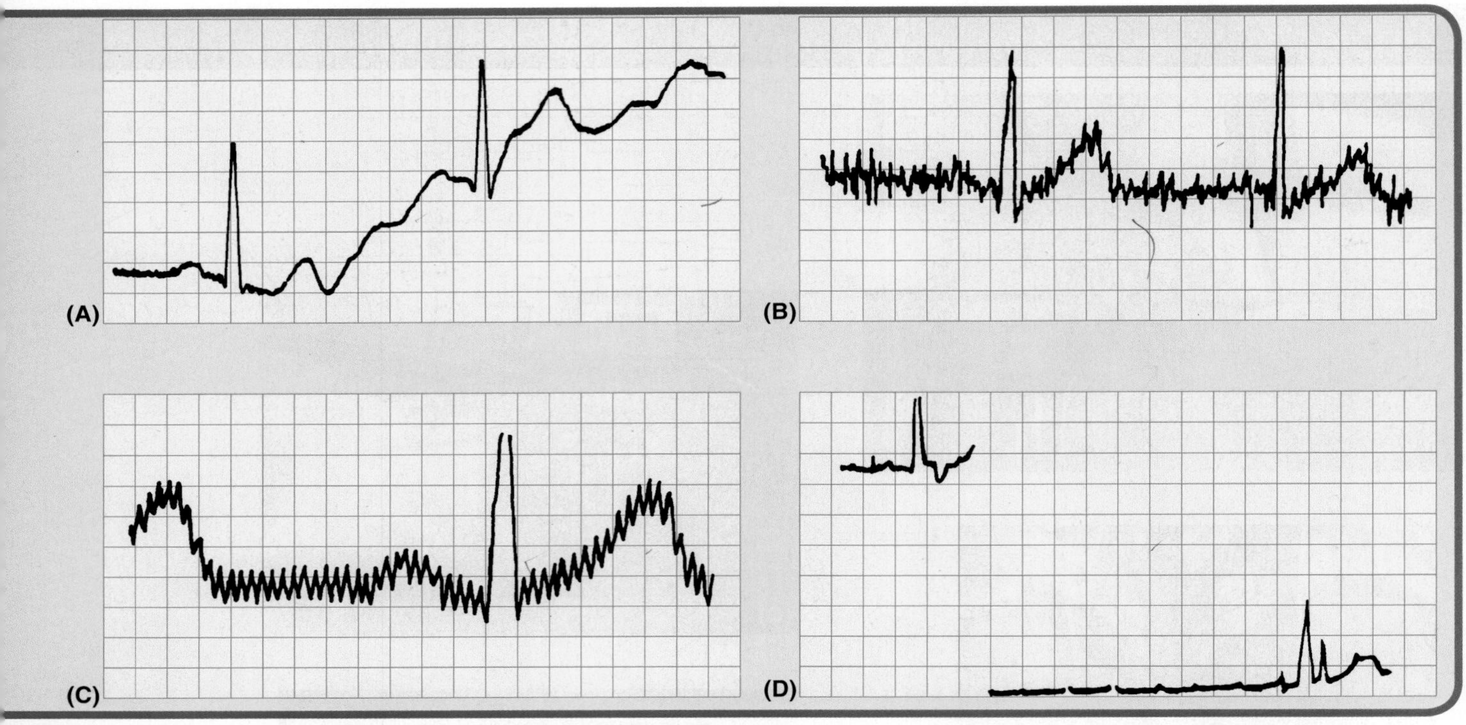

Figure 47–12A–D: (A) Wandering baseline. (B) Somatic tremor or involuntary muscle movement. (C) AC (alternating current). (D) Interrupted baseline. *Courtesy of Quinton Cardiology.*

with the electrodes and properly grounded (see Figure 47–12B). Using good technique also reduces AC interference.

Wandering baseline can be caused by improperly applied electrodes or improperly cleaned skin (Figure 47–12C). Oils, creams, and lotions should be removed from the patient's skin with alcohol, or the conduction of electrical impulses will be impaired.

Interrupted baseline is caused by an electrode becoming separated from the wire or by a broken lead wire (Figure 47–12D). Be sure that the electrode is securely attached to the wire and follow the manufacturer's instructions for repairing the broken wire if needed.

Cardiac Arrhythmias

Irregularities in the hearts rhythm are known as **arrhythmias.** Not all arrhythmias are dangerous or will cause problems; however, for those that are, it is vital for providers to be able to detect them on an ECG. Although it is beyond your scope of practice to interpret ECGs, you should be able to recognize what arrhythmias look like so you can alert the provider, and proper care can be given to the patient. You've learned that with a normal ECG, the P wave, QRS complex, and T wave continually repeat their patterns. When this happens without any abnormalities, the patient is said to be in normal sinus rhythm. When an abnormality in the beat, rate, or rhythm occurs, that is when an arrhythmia is considered. As learned in Chapter 38, a patient's normal heart rate ranges between 60 and 100 beats per minute. When the heart rate falls below 60 BPM, it is known as sinus bradycardia (Figure 47–13A), and when it rises above 100 BPM, it is termed sinus tachycardia (Figure 47–13B).

Although a few of the common arrhythmias are discussed and pictured here, refer to Chapter 30 on the circulatory system for additional information (see Figures 47–14A–F).

- *Premature atrial contractions (PACs):* Can be seen in healthy individuals and people who smoke or use stimulants such as caffeine. Can indicate a serious cardiac problem. On the ECG, they are indicated by a cardiac cycle that occurs before the next cycle is due, with the P waves shaped differently than on a normal ECG (Figure 47–14A).
- *Paroxysmal atrial tachycardia (PAT):* Can be seen in both healthy individuals as well as in those with cardiac disease. It is an episode during which the heart rate ranges from 160 to 250 BPM and lasts momentarily. Patients often describe it as a flutter in the heart (Figure 47–14B).
- *Atrial fibrillation (A-Fib):* Although relatively rare in healthy individuals, it still can be seen in both healthy individuals and those with cardiac disease. It causes rapid multiple electrical signals that fire from areas in the atria other than the SA node. The heart rate can range from 400 to 500 BPM. Some causes are myocardial infarction, hypertension, mitral valve diseases, heart failure, thyroid disorders, pulmonary

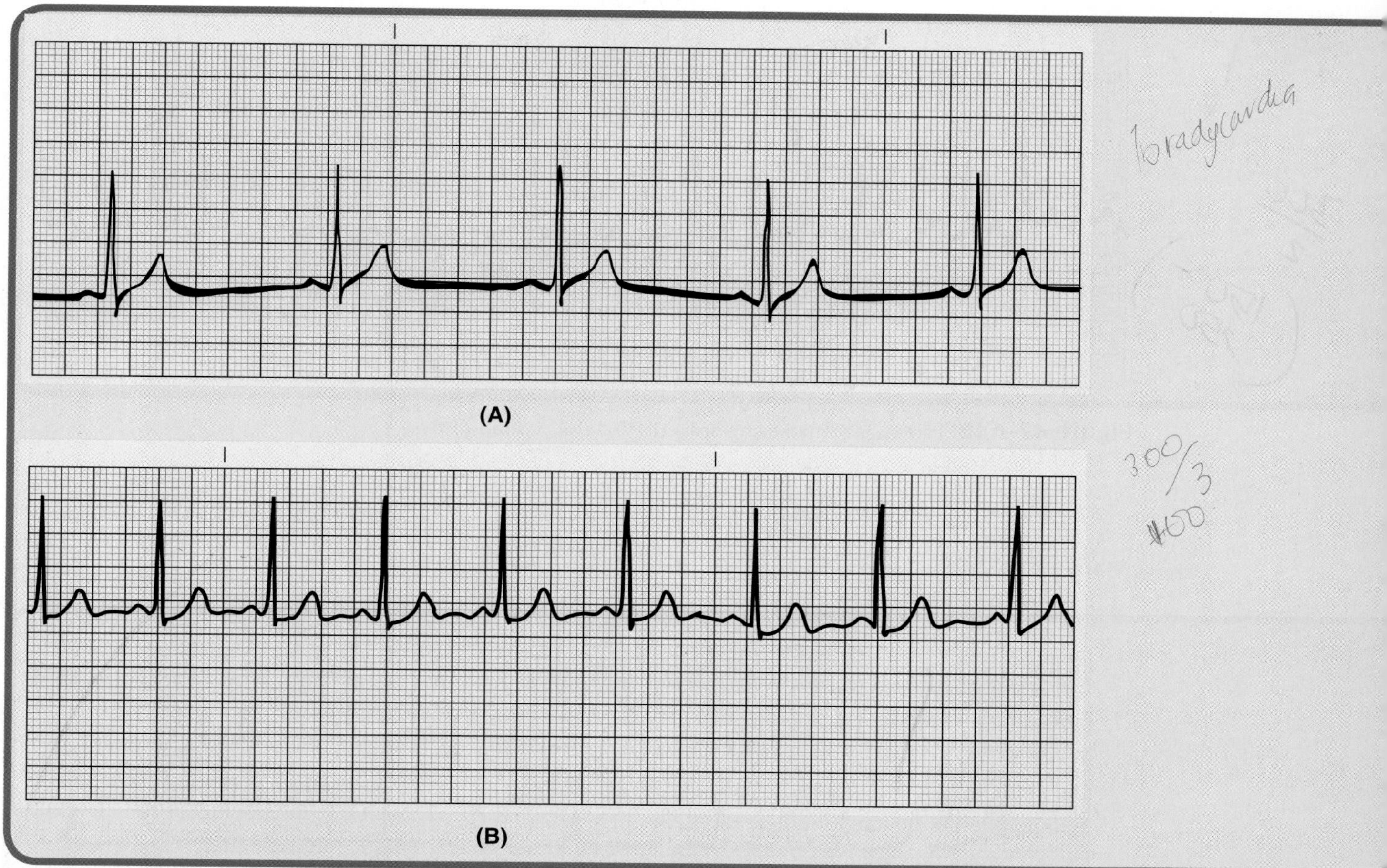

Figure 47–13A–B: (A) A heart rate less than 60 BPM is known as sinus bradycardia; (B) a heart rate above 100 BPM is known as tachycardia. *Delmar/Cengage Learning.*

emboli, and excessive alcohol consumption. On the ECG, it looks like small, irregular complexes that are hard to interpret because the P waves can't be identified (Figure 47–14C).

- *Premature ventricular contractions (PVCs):* Can be seen in healthy individuals who use tobacco and other stimulants as well as in patients with hypertension, coronary artery disease, and lung disease. Other causes include myocardial infarction, electrolyte imbalances, lack of oxygen, and certain medications. They are indicated on the ECG by a beat that occurs early in the cycle and is followed by a pause before the next cycle occurs (Figure 47–14D).

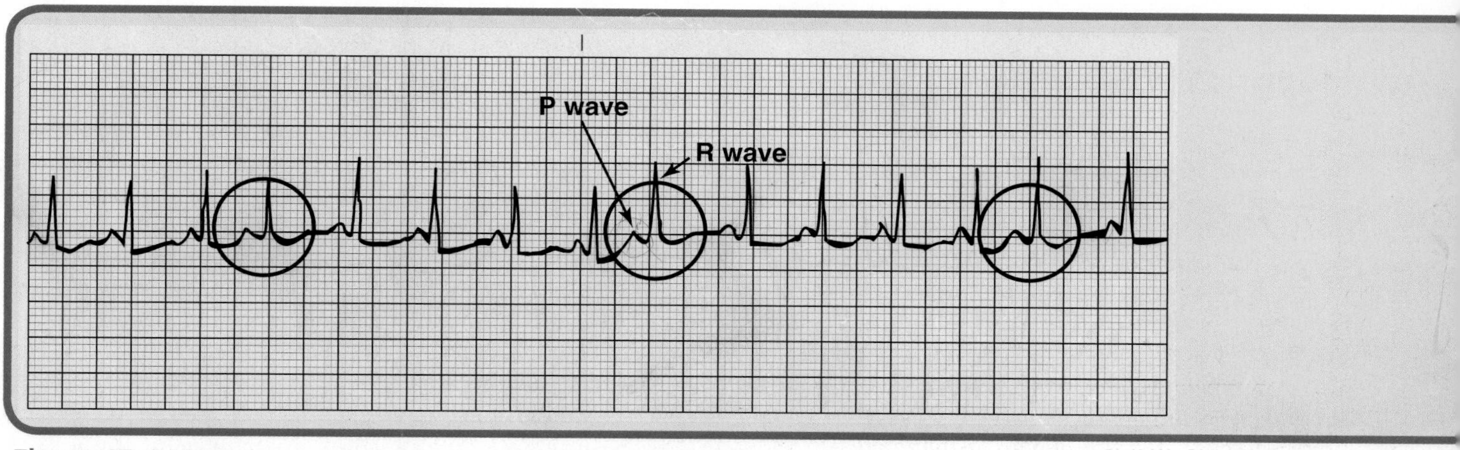

Figure 47–14A: Premature atrial contractions (PAC). *Delmar/Cengage Learning.*

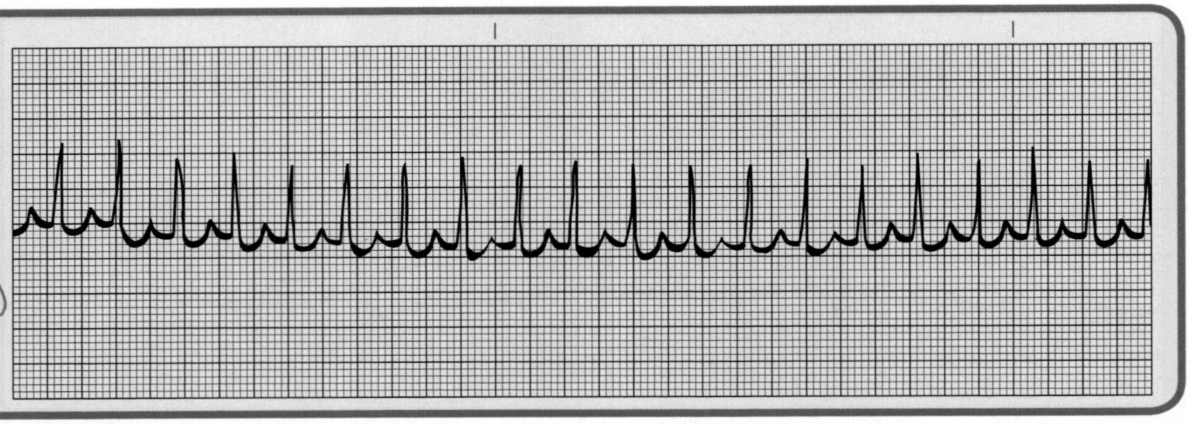

Figure 47–14B: Paroxysmal atrial tachycardia (PAT). *Delmar/Cengage Learning.*

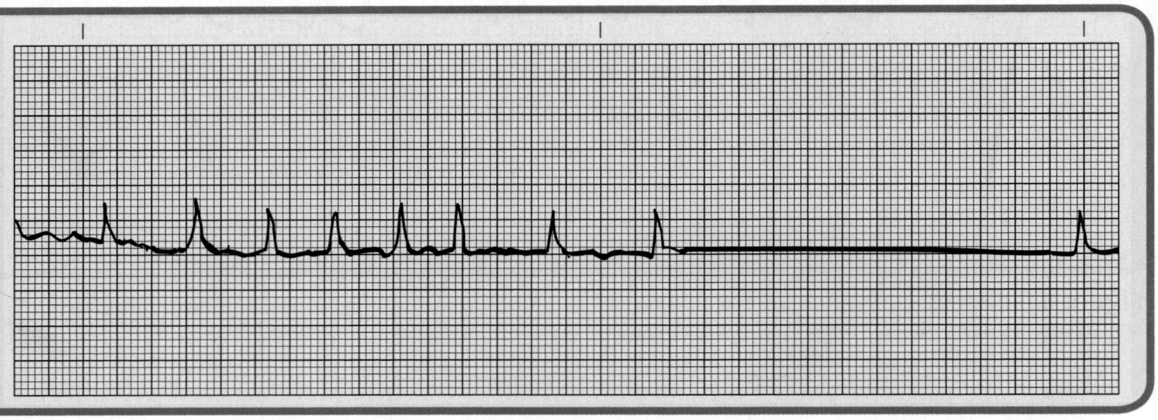

Figure 47–14C: Atrial fibrillation with a sinus pause. *Delmar/Cengage Learning.*

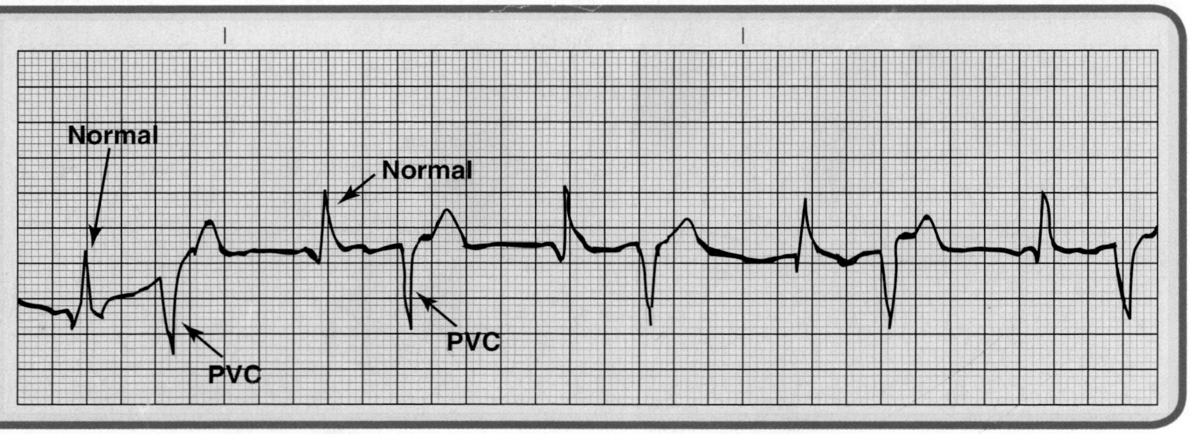

Figure 47–14D: Premature ventricular contractions (PVC). *Delmar/Cengage Learning.*

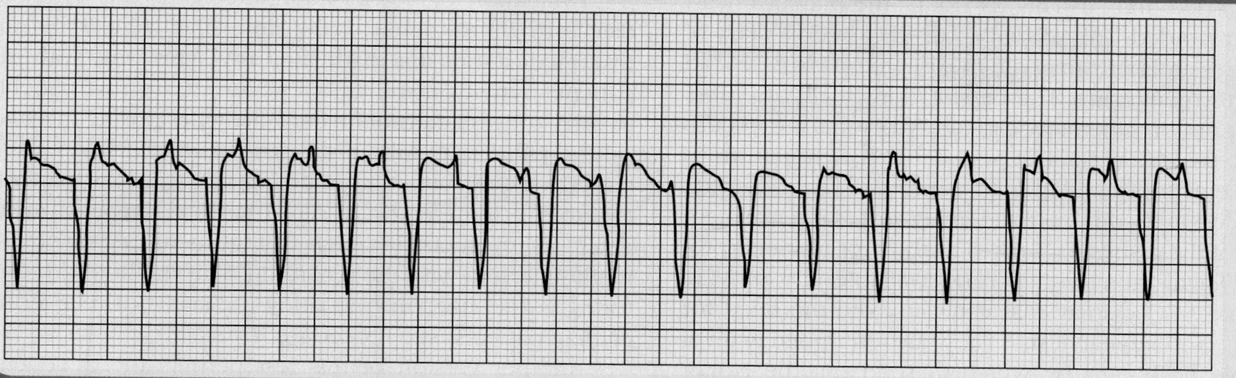

Figure 47–14E: Ventricular tachycardia. *Delmar/Cengage Learning.*

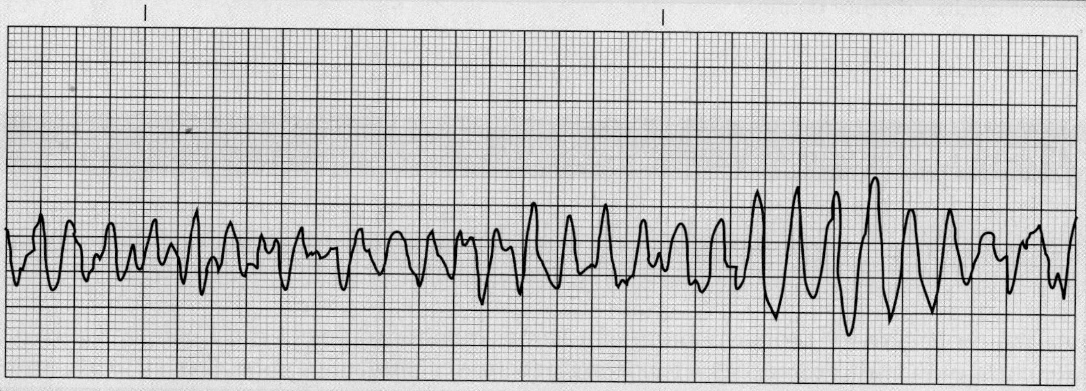

Figure 47–14F: Ventricular fibrillation. *Delmar/Cengage Learning.*

- *Ventricular tachycardia:* This is seen in patients with cardiac disease. It often occurs when a patient is having a myocardial infarction. This is a life-threatening condition. On the ECG, it is identified by three or more PVCs occurring at a rate of 150 to 250 BPM. There are no P waves, and the QRS complexes are imprecise (Figure 47–14E).
- *Ventricular fibrillation (V-Fib):* This is seen in patients with cardiac disease or those who are experiencing a myocardial infarction. The ventricles appear to tremor, and there is no cardiac output. Some providers refer to this jagged rhythm as a sawtooth rhythm. This is a life-threatening condition that appears on the ECG as an erratic, jagged rhythm (Figure 47–14F).

HOLTER MONITOR

Patients who have routine normal ECGs but still have **intermittent** or irregular chest pain or discomfort are often tested over a period of 24 hours or more by a device known as a **Holter monitor** (Figure 47–15). This method of recording the electrical activities of a patient's heart for a time is also referred to as an ambulatory (walking), or 24-hour, ECG.

The ECG electrodes are attached to the patient's chest wall. A portable cassette recorder (monitor) is attached to a belt worn around the patient's waist. During

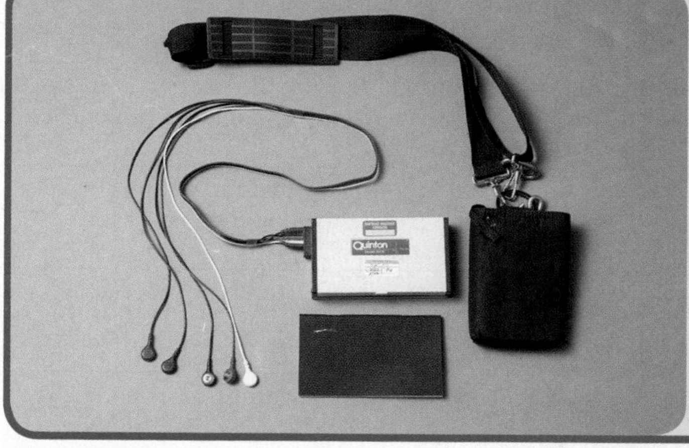

Figure 47–15: Holter monitor and supplies. *Delmar/Cengage Learning.*

the prescribed time, usually 24 hours, the patient's heart action is recorded. The patient is asked to keep a diary of all activities and note any pain or discomfort experienced during this monitoring. The patient is instructed to press the event button when any cardiac symptoms are experienced. At the end of the test period, the patient returns to have the electrodes and monitor removed. The cassette is then placed in a computerized analyzer for a permanent printout of the results (or sent to a laboratory for interpretation). Digital monitors are now available and provide a real-time ECG display that can eliminate the need for test jacks and repeat tests. They are equipped with a removable flash card by which to send out the Holter recording immediately with no wait time to download previous patient results. Special software is required for the devices that provide quick turnaround time and can capture even the smallest of cardiac rhythm changes.

Evaluation of the 24-hour tracing reveals any cardiac arrhythmias, chest pain, and effectiveness of cardiac medications and correlates any symptoms with the patient's activity at the time it occurred. Instruct patients to carry on with all routine daily activities during this test. Advise patients to take a sponge bath rather than a tub bath or shower while conducting this test. Ask patients to avoid using electric blankets or being around metal detectors, magnets, and high-voltage areas because these might interfere with the recording. This method of monitoring is also used in evaluating the status of recovering cardiac patients; see Procedure 47–2.

Another version of this test permits the patient to activate the recording device only when experiencing symptoms. This patient-activated monitor can be worn for several days.

PROCEDURE 47–2 Holter Monitoring

MEDIA LINK: View the video, "Patient Instructions for Holter Monitor," for this chapter on the Premium Website.

PURPOSE: Demonstrate the procedure for proper hookup of a Holter monitor to detect chest pain and cardiac arrhythmias, to evaluate chest pain and cardiac status following pacemaker implantation or after an acute myocardial infarction, and to determine correlation of symptoms and activity

EQUIPMENT: Holter monitor, disposable razor, alcohol wipes, disposable adhesive electrodes, blank magnetic tape or flash memory card, diary for patient, belt or shoulder strap for recorder, patient's chart or EHR, and pen

S **SKILL:** Demonstrate the procedure for proper hookup of a Holter monitor

Procedure Steps	Detailed Instructions and/or *Rationales*
1. Wash hands and assemble the equipment and supplies.	Test the Holter monitor for proper working order and replace the batteries if indicated. *Batteries must function for the entire test period.* Insert a blank tape or flash card in the monitor.
B 2. Introduce yourself, identify the patient, and explain the procedure, ***using language the patient can understand.***	*Adherence to the patient guidelines helps ensure an accurate tracing.*
3. Ask the patient to remove clothing from the waist up. Assist the patient to sit at the end of the examination table.	
4. Use the razor to remove chest hair if necessary.	*A smooth area provides optimal skin contact.* Rinse and dry the electrode sites and clean them with alcohol swabs.
5. Rub each site vigorously with gauze square and apply the electrodes and lead wires carefully, making sure there is good skin contact.	

Procedure Steps	Detailed Instructions and/or *Rationales*
6. Place the belt around the patient's waist or drape around the patient's shoulder and advise the patient about proper care of the recorder and precautions.	Assist the patient in dressing to help avoid disturbing the wires and electrodes.
7. Instruct the patient to go about his or her routine daily activities but to be sure to note in the diary any symptoms or problems experienced. (Include the time it occurred and how long it lasted.)	Remind the patient not to take a tub bath or shower during the 24-hour period. *Accurate reporting and recording is essential for correct interpretation of findings when compared with activity taking place when symptoms occurred.*
8. Give the patient the diary to take for completion and arrange a return appointment time.	See Figure 47–16.
9. Document in patient's chart. Record the date and time the monitor began on the patient's chart and in the patient's diary and initial.	
10. When the patient comes in for the appointment the next day, assist in disrobing. Remove the electrodes and wires; clean the electrode sites and remove the memory card or cassette from the recorder.	
11. Document.	Document that the patient returned with equipment, place the diary in the patient's chart for evaluation by the provider, and initial.

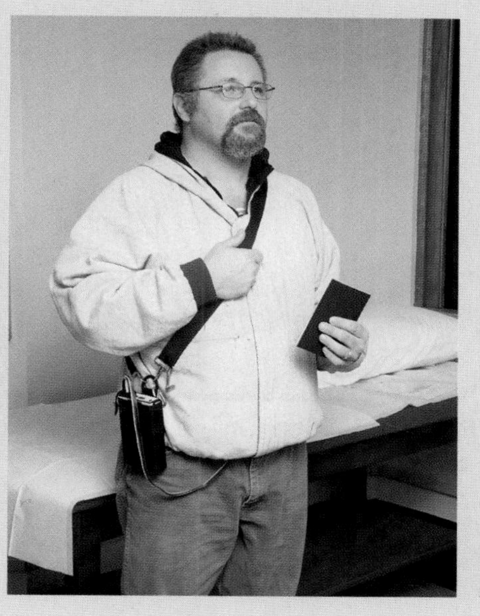

Figure 47–16: Correct placement of the Holter monitor on a patient. *Delmar/Cengage Learning.*

Charting Example

4/17/XX 11:30 am	Holter monitor applied. Patient given complete written and verbal instructions. Patient given activity diary and date and time noted. Appointment visit scheduled for patient to return to have monitor removed tomorrow at 11:30 am G. Jenks, CMA (AAMA)
4/18/XX 11:30 am	Holter monitor electrodes removed from patient. Cassette removed and given to provider for computer analyses. Patient activity diary placed in patient's chart for provider review. G. Jenks, CMA (AAMA)

STRESS TESTS

ECG stress tests are done by some providers on a routine basis for patients with a high risk of developing heart disease. They are more often done in a limited manner for patients interested in starting a strenuous exercise program or those who continue to have chest pain even after a routine ECG has been read as normal. The stress test ECG is done while a patient is exercising on a treadmill under careful supervision. Figure 47–17 shows a provider reading the computerized readout of a stress test in progress. The medical assistant monitors the patient's blood pressure while he or she exercises on the treadmill. The purpose of this test is to detect the unknown cause of a patient's heart trouble.

ECHOCARDIOGRAPHY

Echocardiography is a noninvasive diagnostic tool that tests the structure and function of the heart through the use of sound waves, or **echoes** reflected through the heart. The sound waves are projected through the chest wall into the heart and are reflected back through a mechanical device. A transducer (similar to a microphone) sends and receives these sound waves and records them on paper or video. Measurements are calculated to determine abnormalities within the heart.

OTHER CARDIOVASCULAR EQUIPMENT

Many medical offices, clinics, and emergency centers are equipped with a **defibrillator** (Figure 47–18). These units are designed to provide **countershock** by a trained individual to convert cardiac arrhythmias into regular sinus rhythm. More on defibrillation is covered in Chapter 54. Part of your routine duties might be to check this machine, along with other equipment and supplies, to ensure that they are in proper working order and that everything is ready in case of a cardiac emergency. Employers offer in-service training periodically to all employees in assisting with emergency procedures. All employees should have current cardiopulmonary resuscitation (CPR) certification. Refer to Chapter 54 for more on cardiac emergencies and CPR.

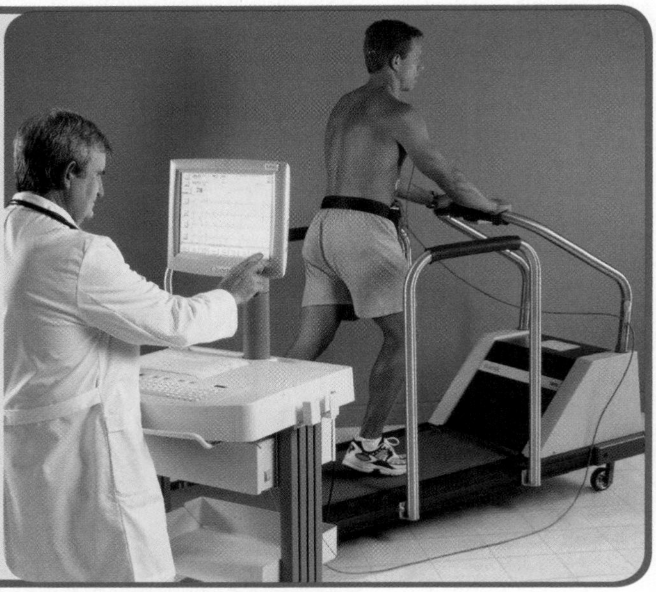

Figure 47–17: The Quest exercise stress system. *Courtesy of Quinton Cardiology.*

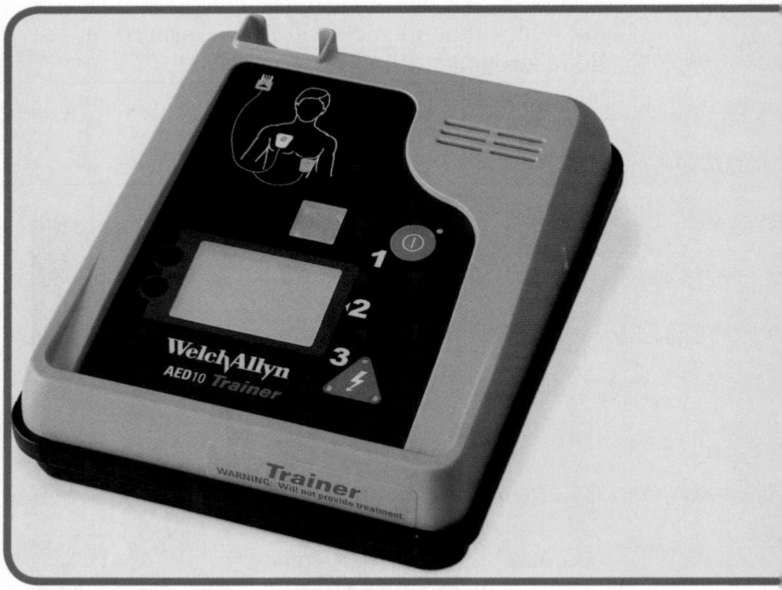

Figure 47–18: Portable AED. *Courtesy of Welch-Allyn.*

CHAPTER SUMMARY

- Many types of electrocardiographs are available for use in the medical field today. Multichannel, 12-lead instruments can record the electrical activity of the heart simultaneously from 12 views; single-channel instruments measure only one lead and one view of the heart at a time. Computerized electrocardiographs offer simultaneous 12-lead interpretive analysis.
- The heart is a four-chambered pump that produces a tiny electrical current by muscular contraction. An electrical impulse originates in the modified myocardial tissue of the sinoatrial (SA) node, also known as the sinus node or pacemaker of the heart, causing the atria to contract. This contraction is the beginning of atrial depolarization, which is the first part

of the cardiac cycle. The impulse continues through the heart tissue to the atrioventricular (AV) node, to the bundle of His, and spreads to the Purkinje fibers. The heart then recovers, representing the repolarization of the ventricles before another contraction. This is considered a normal ECG cycle.

- The ECG can detect damage from previous heart attacks, enlargement of the heart muscle, disturbances in the rhythm, and other abnormal conditions.
- Each machine comes with an operating manual, many with a DVD as well, providing step-by-step instructions, maintenance information, and troubleshooting tips for the unit. Look over the lead wires and cables to make sure there are no cracks or damage; check to be sure the clips are attached correctly and are in proper working order; check the paper in the machine to be sure you will not run out, and restock any materials that will be needed such as electrodes, alcohol wipes, and disposable razors (in case shaving is necessary).
- The standardization of the ECG is necessary to enable a provider to judge deviations from the standard. Most machines used today perform automatic standardization. The usual standardization mark is 2 mm wide and 10 mm high.
- During the time you spend with patients in performing electrocardiographic testing and its instruction, you will have ample opportunity to provide patients with education regarding diet, exercise, rest, and living a healthy lifestyle.
- The routine ECG consists of 12 leads, or recordings, of the electrical activity of the heart from different angles. The first three leads are called standard or bipolar leads and are labeled with Roman numerals I, II, and III. Lead I records the electrical voltage difference between the right arm and left arm. Lead II records the difference between the right arm and the left leg. Lead III records the voltage difference between the left arm and left leg. The augmented leads are also known as, aVR, aVL, and aVF. aVR is the recording of the heart's voltage difference between the right arm electrode and a central point between the left arm and the left leg. aVL is the recording of the heart's voltage difference between the left arm electrode and a central point between the right arm and the left leg. aVF is the recording of the heart's voltage difference between the left leg electrode and a central point between the right arm and left arm. The six standard chest or precordial leads are unipolar leads; each precordial lead monitors one electrode and a point within the heart. The leads are labeled with a letter and a number, V_1 to V_6.
- Many artifacts can occur during the ECG tracing and cause interference. They are known as somatic interference, AC interference, wandering baselines, and interrupted baselines. You must understand the causes and be able to eliminate them.
- You must be able to recognize abnormal heart rhythms such as premature atrial and ventricular contractions, atrial and ventricular fibrillation, and paroxysmal atrial and ventricular tachycardia and alert the provider of these rhythms.
- Patients who have routine normal ECGs but still have intermittent or irregular chest pain or discomfort are often tested over a period of 24 hours or more by a device known as a Holter monitor. The ECG electrodes are attached to the patient's chest wall. A portable cassette recorder (monitor) is attached to a belt worn around the patient's waist; the patient's heart action is recorded. The patient is asked to keep a diary of all activities and note any pain or discomfort experienced during this monitoring. The patient is instructed to press the event button when any cardiac symptoms are experienced.
- ECG stress tests are performed by some providers on a routine basis for patients with a high risk of developing heart disease and are more often done in a limited manner for patients interested in starting a strenuous exercise program or those who continue to have chest pain even after a routine ECG has been read as normal.
- Echocardiography is a noninvasive diagnostic tool that tests the structure and function of the heart through the use of sound waves, or echoes reflected through the heart.
- Many medical offices, clinics, and emergency centers are equipped with a defibrillator. These units are designed to provide countershock by a trained individual to convert cardiac arrhythmias into regular sinus rhythm.

STUDY TOOLS

Workbook	Activities for Chapter 47
Premium Website MEDIA LINK	View this **Media Links** for Chapter 47 • Applying Chest Electrode • Patient Instructions for Holter Monitor

StudyWARE	Activities and Quizzes on the **StudyWARE™ Software** for Chapter 47
	Complete the following **Competency Challenge 2.0** activity: • Tuesday, 1:00 PM, Perform an Electrocardiogram
	Audio Library of medical terms
	Online access to **Critical Thinking Challenge 2.0**
CourseMate	Activities and Quizzes for Chapter 47
WebTutor	Activities and Quizzes for Chapter 47

CHECK YOUR KNOWLEDGE

1. A heated pen-like instrument that produces a printed representation on the ECG paper is known as a/an:
   a. galvanometer.
   b. stylus.
   c. amplifier.
   d. electrode.
2. Each large square on the ECG paper measures 5 mm by 5 mm and represents ____ seconds.
   a. 0.2
   b. 0.04
   c. 0.1
   d. 1.0
3. Which of the following wave(s) on the graph paper represents the repolarization of the ventricles or the time of recovery before another contraction?
   a. P
   b. QRS
   c. ST
   d. T
4. What can you do with the sensitivity dial if the ECG tracing is too small?
   a. Turn down to 1
   b. Turn down to 1/2
   c. Turn up to 5
   d. Turn up to 2
5. The routine ECG consists of how many leads?
   a. 12
   b. 10
   c. 6
   d. 4
6. The augmented leads are also known as:
   a. leads I, II and III.
   b. chest leads.
   c. aVL, aVR, aVF.
   d. precordial leads.
7. What kind of interference is caused by improperly applied electrodes?
   a. Somatic tremor
   b. Wandering baseline
   c. Interrupted baseline
   d. AC interference
8. The following is a diagnostic tool that tests the structure and function of the heart through the use of sound waves reflected through the heart.
   a. Defibrillator
   b. Holter monitor
   c. Echocardiography
   d. Treadmill

WEB LINKS

American Heart Association: www.heart.org

National Institutes of Health: www.nih.gov

U.S. National Library of Medicine: www.nlm.nih.gov

RESOURCES

Estes, M. E. Z. (2010). *Health Assessment & Physical Examination*. Clifton Park, NY: Delmar Cengage Learning.

Heller, M., and Veach, L. (2009). *Clinical Medical Assisting: A Professional, Field Smart Approach to the Workplace*. Clifton Park, NY: Delmar, Cengage Learning.

Lindh, W., Pooler, M., Tamparo, C., and Dahl, B. (2010). *Delmar's Comprehensive Medical Assisting Administrative and Clinical Competencies* (4th ed.). Clifton Park, NY: Delmar Cengage Learning.

Chapter

48 Radiology Procedures

OBJECTIVES

In this chapter, you will learn the following:

KB KNOWLEDGE BASE

1. Spell and define, using the glossary at the back of the text, all the Words to Know in this chapter.
2. Define radiologic testing and explain your role in radiographic procedures.
3. Define X-rays.
4. Explain the methods and importance of using safety precautions in radiographic procedures.
5. Explain why pregnant women should not have X-rays.
6. Instruct patients in diet and preparation for radiologic studies.
7. Compare and contrast the types of radiologic procedures used to diagnose patients.
8. Describe sonography and ultrasound and state the purpose of them.
9. Explain patient preparation for ultrasound procedures.
10. Explain what magnetic resonance imaging (MRI) is and list the contraindications.
11. Describe patient education concerning the procedures discussed in this chapter.

WORDS TO KNOW

brachytherapy
cholecystogram
claustrophobia
compression
computerized transverse axial tomography (CTAT)
conjunction
contrast media
cystoscopy
diagnostic
distends
dosimeter
electromagnetic radiation
electromagnetic
electron
enema
evacuants
flatus
fluoroscope
implants
intravenous pyelogram (IVP)
iodine
KUB (kidneys, ureters, bladder)
lesion
magnetic resonance imaging
mammography
maturity
noninvasive
planes
radioactive
radiograph
radiologist
radiopaque
residual barium
retrograde pyelogram
roentgen rays
sonogram
teletherapy
therapeutic radiation
transducer

after mammogram, a biopsy is ordered.

mammogram - screening

RADIOLOGIC STUDIES

Radiologic testing is an important tool providers use for screening, diagnostic procedures, and therapeutic uses. It has a significant role in the diagnosis and monitoring of many diseases and injuries. As a medical assistant, your role might be to assist the radiology technologist at your facility or, depending on the practices in your state, you might be allowed to take certain X-rays and operate the equipment yourself if you obtain the appropriate licenses. Another area in radiology you will be involved with is scheduling patients for radiology procedures and testing at outside facilities. Many patients have routine screenings for mammograms and chest X-rays, whereas others are performed as a **diagnostic** tool to rule out or confirm a diagnosis. No matter what your role is, you must be familiar with the field of radiology and have a general understanding of the various procedures, screenings, and therapies you might be involved with.

Safety

Any person working in a facility that performs radiologic tests can be at risk for excessive radiation exposure. Therefore, standard safety precautions must be followed to ensure protection for yourself and patients from radiation exposure. All staff working in the radiology department or taking **radiographs** must wear a radiation exposure badge known as a **dosimeter** or film badge (Figure 48–1). This dosimeter has a sensitized piece of film in it that monitors the amount of radiation you are exposed to. Each worker has a maximum permissible dose (MPD) he or she is allowed to be exposed to. The limitations are determined by the age of the worker. The badges are sent in to the monitoring company they were purchased from and measured for exposure, and a report is sent back to the facility. Film badges generally are good for up to a month, whereas dosimeters can last up to three months. In addition, protecting yourself with a lead shield any time you might be exposed is crucial. Wall shields made of lead generally protect the worker while taking the radiograph, and both lead aprons and gloves are available for assisting (Figure 48–2). If you are pregnant or think you might be pregnant, you must discuss the risks with your providers and follow your facility protocols regarding pregnancy and radiation exposure.

All radiology departments have safety signs prominently displayed in several areas of their facility that tell female patients to inform the radiology technologist or radiologist provider whether they are pregnant or if they possibly could be pregnant. Radiation and X-rays are contraindicated in pregnant women; they can be damaging to an unborn child, especially in the first three months of pregnancy (first trimester), sometimes before the patient is even aware she is pregnant. Many X-ray examinations, such as imaging the arms, legs, head and chest, don't involve exposing your reproductive organs or unborn baby to the direct X-ray beam. In these cases, lead shielding can block any scattered radiation. However, X-ray examinations of your abdominal area, such as the stomach, lower back, pelvis, and kidneys, are more of a concern because they expose the developing fetus to the direct X-ray beam. There has been disagreement about the exact amount of risk to the unborn child from the

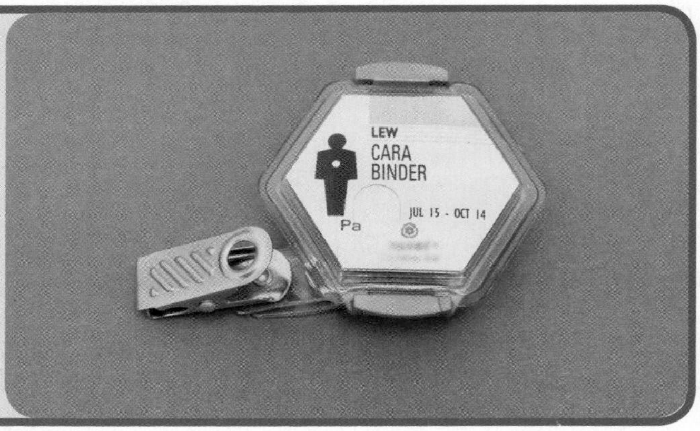

Figure 48–1: A film badge worn by personnel working with X-rays. *Delmar/Cengage Learning.*

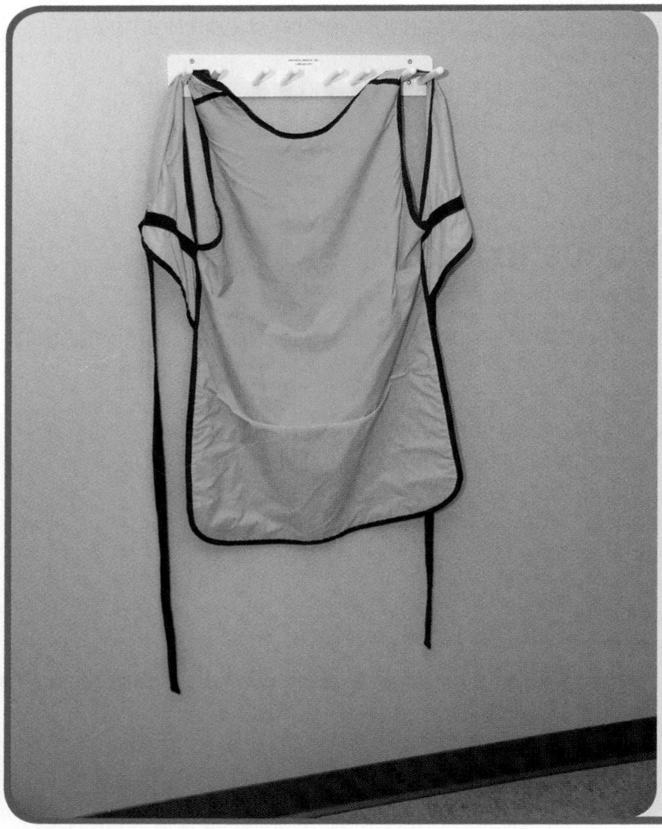

Figure 48–2: An example of a lead apron. *Delmar/Cengage Learning.*

radiation from X-ray examinations, but it's believed to be small. Yet, even small risks should not be taken if they're unnecessary. Any pregnant patient must be informed to discuss the risks with her provider and make a decision based on whether the risk of having the X-ray is less of a danger than not having one at all.

Before scheduling any female patient whose age indicates that she is within the childbearing years, you must always ask if she could be pregnant. During screening, always ask females for the date of the first day of menstrual flow of their last menstrual period (LMP) and document this in their chart to help prevent any misunderstanding concerning a possible pregnancy. Other diagnostic exams can be performed that are safe for the fetus during this time as necessary.

CLINICAL PEARL

Informing patients of risks and safety precautions might be your responsibility. Advising the patient to discuss with her provider questions she might have regarding a radiology procedure can set her mind at ease about the procedure. Inform the patient that the evolution of radiology has come a long way, and much lower doses of radiation are now being used in many of the procedures ordered.

PATIENT EDUCATION

With any radiological procedure, assure the patient that the studies are done in a controlled environment. Always provide clear and concise oral *and* written instructions for examinations that require advance preparation. Be sure the patient understands the necessary preparations. Answer all questions. Emphasize the importance of being on time for the radiologic appointment to avoid unnecessary delays because some examinations are very long. If the patient is not familiar with the facility at which the X-ray studies are scheduled, give specific instructions (and a map) of how to get there and where to park. Patients appreciate this courtesy. Often, this information is printed on the appointment or information sheet the facility provides to medical offices and clinics for referral appointments.

X-rays and Radiation Therapy

Radiologic studies are made by the use of X-rays (**roentgen rays**), which are high-energy **electromagnetic radiation** produced by the collision of a beam of **electrons** with a metal target in an X-ray tube. The roentgen ray or X-ray was discovered in 1895 by Wilhelm Konrad Roentgen (1845–1923). An X-ray photograph is taken of the requested part of the patient's body, and a permanent film picture is made. In addition, some electronic medical records systems now allow results and reports to upload directly on the provider's desktop and to the patient's electronic chart. Results and reports from outside organizations may also be imported through scanning and importing features.

When the provider orders an X-ray of the chest (Figure 48–3), the patient is asked to hold still in the positions shown in Figure 48–4 so that a permanent film (upon inspiration of breath) can be taken. The provider might request to view the films, but usually it is a **radiologist** who determines the final evaluation of the films. If a radiologist is not onsite to read the films, the films are sent out to the radiologist contracted with your facility to be read, and a report of the radiologic studies is sent to the primary provider.

Another type of radiology, known as **therapeutic radiation** or radiation therapy, is used in the treatment of cancer by preventing cellular reproduction. Two main types of this therapy are **teletherapy**, which allows deep penetration for deep tumors and is performed on an outpatient basis, and **brachytherapy**, by which radioactive implants

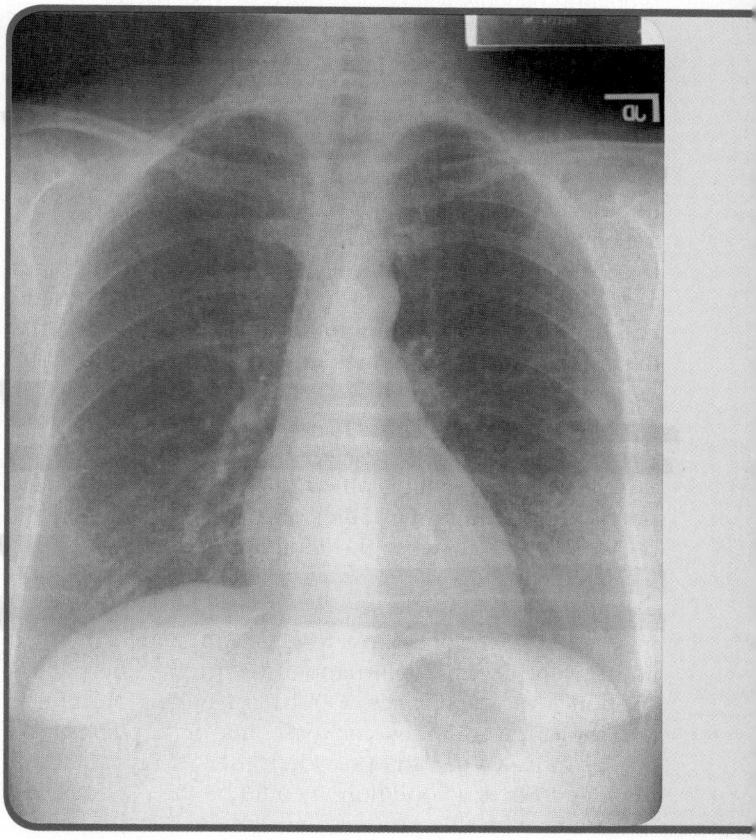

Figure 48–3: Chest X-ray: anterior posterior (AP) view of the chest. *Delmar/Cengage Learning.*

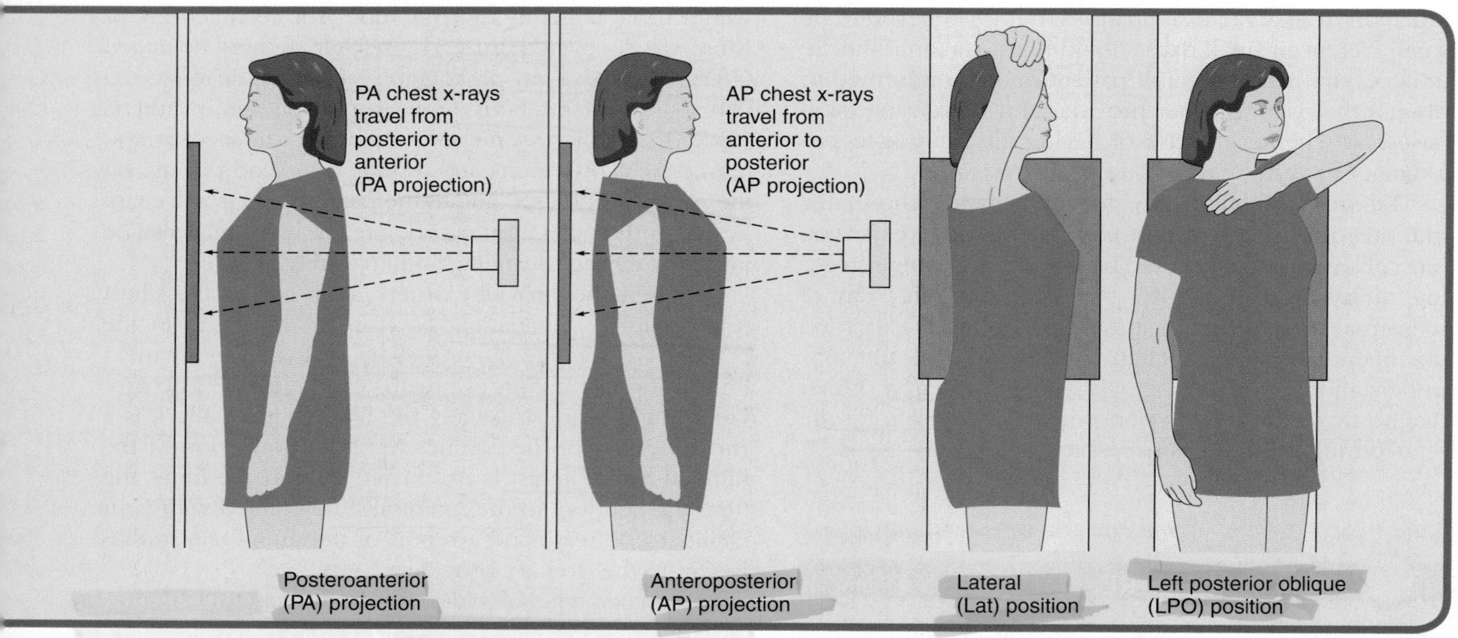

Figure 48–4: Radiographic projection positions to obtain different views of the chest. *Delmar/Cengage Learning.*

prostate cancer / cervical cancer

are placed by the radiologist close to or into the cancerous tissue. Some of the most commonly ordered radiologic studies for which you might be responsible in scheduling and preparing patients will be addressed in this chapter.

Preparing Patients for X-rays

Depending on the radiology study, the patient might be required to follow a preparation prior to the film being taken. It is very important to review the preparation instructions for various radiologic studies when you schedule the patient's appointment because techniques and preparations can vary from one facility to another and are subject to change with technology. For example, bone studies do not require preparation and are performed to aid in the diagnosis of tumors, fractures, and other disorders and diseases. Chest X-rays also do not normally need advance preparation. Make sure the patient understands all instructions clearly to avoid misunderstandings and time delays.

Patients can exhibit a fear of what is going to happen to them during the radiology procedures and might be worried about what the radiologist might find. It is important to show genuine caring and compassion to patients who are in pain and discomfort. When they are in your care and it is apparent that they are confused and unsure of what will happen next, offer the patient support and reassurance. Often, just talking to him or her for a few minutes can ease his or her fears and uncertainties. When the provider orders X-rays to aid in the diagnosis of a condition, it could be the patient's first encounter with this process, so ask whether the patient has ever had an X-ray before. If you can give the patient an idea of what to expect and describe what it is like, you can decrease the stress and anxiety of the patient.

> **CLINICAL PEARL**
>
> Children especially can be apprehensive about what is going to happen to them. You can explain to a child that having X-rays taken is just like having pictures taken with a camera; the X-ray machine is really a great big metal camera taking a picture of the inside of their body. Explain that you have to be very still when having an X-ray taken just like when you have a photograph taken so that the picture does not get blurred and out of focus. The child will be more cooperative when given an explanation of what to expect.

Explain that a big lead apron will be put over the patient to protect the reproductive organs from the X-rays. Visual aids are helpful to show patients what radiologic equipment looks like. The X-ray the provider has ordered will determine the extent of what patient education is indicated. Often, the explanation will be quite simple because the patient already knows there is an obvious problem, such as an injury. For example, Figure 48–5 shows a severe fracture of the femur.

RADIOLOGIC PROCEDURES

The provider can order a variety of radiological imaging tests to assist him or her with the diagnosis of a condition or injury. Many of these procedures show how a specific anatomic structure appears, and some require the patient to follow special preparation or require a contrast agent or **contrast media**. By adding a contrast agent,

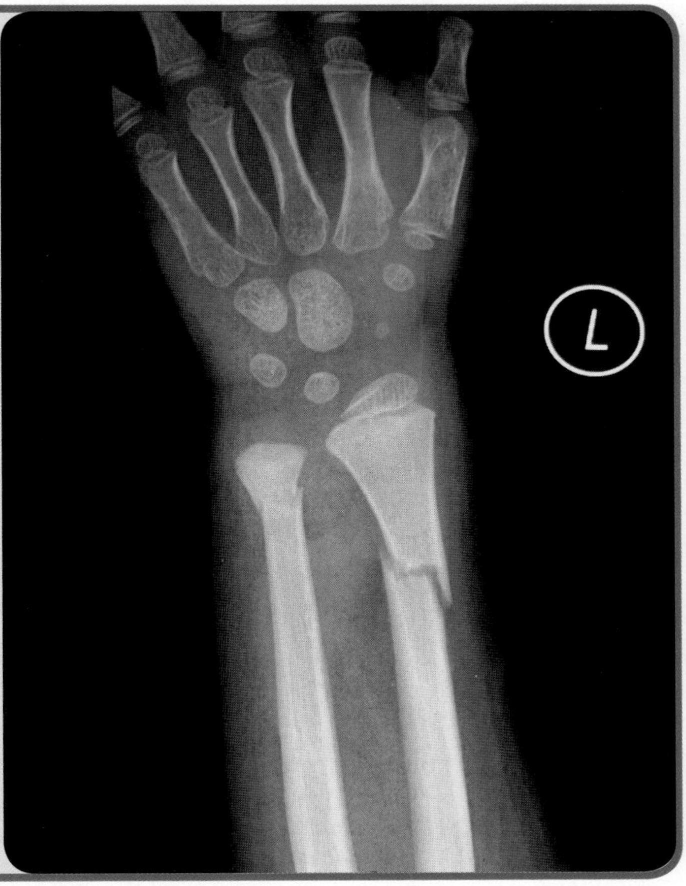

Figure 48–5: X-ray showing severe fracture of the wrist. *Courtesy of Shutterstock. Used under license from Shutterstock.com.*

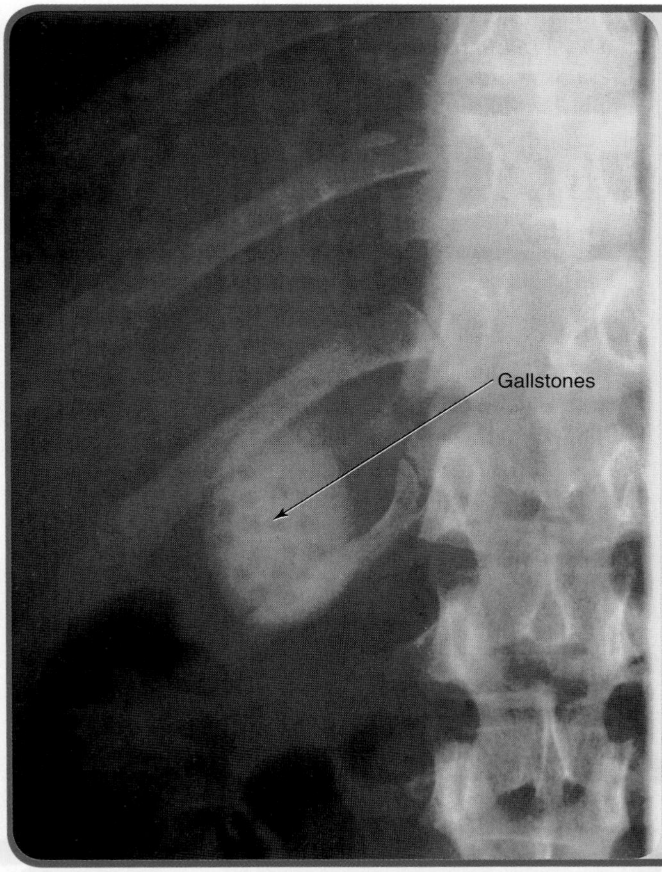

Figure 48–6: Gallbladder X-ray showing gallstones. *Delmar/Cengage Learning.*

the density of the structure being assessed changes and the visualization is improved.

Gallbladder Imaging

The gallbladder stores bile produced in the liver to break down fat in the digestive process. When the gallbladder malfunctions, the patient experiences abdominal discomfort (nausea) and pain. The **cholecystogram** enables the provider to diagnose the cause of the patient's distress. The oral cholecystogram is also referred to as a gallbladder series and a double-dose gallbladder. Refer to Figure 48–6, which shows gallstones present on the permanent film of the cholecystogram.

In preparation for this study of the gallbladder, the patient must follow a prescribed diet and take prescribed medications (a contrast medium) to make the gallbladder visible on the X-ray film. Generally, the patient is advised to avoid drinking alcoholic and carbonated beverages the day before the exam because these drinks can produce **flatus** (gas). Unless otherwise specified by the provider, remind patients to take their regularly prescribed medications.

The abdominal ultrasound, an imaging technique, is now being used by some in place of the cholecystogram. Ultrasound, or sonography, is a process of using sound waves with a frequency of over 20,000 vibrations per second to produce images of the internal structures of the body. An image (**sonogram**) is produced when continuous sound waves are projected toward the desired area to measure and record the reflected image. The abdominal ultrasound includes the gallbladder, pancreas, liver, and other visceral organs. The preparation for the gallbladder or abdominal ultrasound is minimal in comparison

PATIENT EDUCATION

The usual preparation for a cholecystogram is to eat a high-fat meal (eggs, butter, milk, or fatty meats) at noon the day before the test. That evening, a low-fat meal of fresh fruits and vegetables, lean meat (broiled), toast, bread, jelly, and coffee or tea should be consumed. Two hours after the low-fat meal, the contrast medium should be taken. Nothing else should be consumed until after the test. The contrast medium is usually in pill form with directions to swallow all six tablets, one at a time, with a minimum amount of water until all are consumed. As mentioned, the patient is instructed to eat or drink nothing until after the cholecystogram is performed.

with the cholecystogram. The preparation for the sonogram is much easier for the patient because it requires preparation only on the same day as the appointment. You should still advise patients regarding their diet and what to expect during the visit to the radiology facility. Sonograms as discussed in more detail later in the chapter are very useful in aiding in the diagnosis of gallstones, tumors, heart defects, and fetal abnormalities.

PATIENT EDUCATION

This procedure requires a 12-hour fast for a morning appointment. This generally means that the patient should have nothing to eat or drink past midnight the night before the scheduled ultrasound and no breakfast the morning of the appointment. Some radiology facilities offer afternoon appointments for abdominal ultrasounds. To prepare for this, the patient is instructed to have a fat-free liquid breakfast before 9:00 AM the day of the appointment with nothing to eat or drink until after the ultrasound.

Upper GI Series—Barium Swallow

For an upper GI series study, the patient must drink the contrast medium during the examination while the radiologist observes the flow of the substance directly by means of a **fluoroscope**. The contrast medium is a milkshake-like drink that contains a substance called barium. It is usually flavored to increase palatability. Radiologic films are taken for a permanent record of the upper digestive tract. During the study, the patient is positioned so that different angles of the digestive organs can be seen. (Figure 48–7). If needed, further enhancement of the different structures can be obtained by having air as well as barium in the stomach. This can be done by using crystals similar to Alka-Seltzer combined with a small amount of water to add air to the stomach. This is called double contrast. Next a thickened barium mixture is ingested by mouth. Then to further examine the esophagus and duodenal bulb, a thin barium mixture is given to the patient. This allows for better images. Permanent radiographs are taken periodically during the procedure.

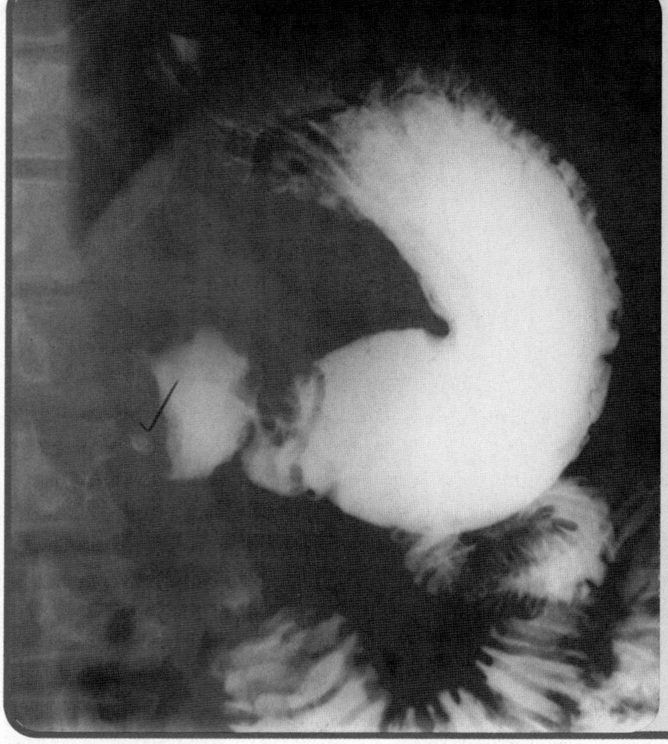

Figure 48–7: An X-ray of the stomach after the ingestion of barium. *Delmar/Cengage Learning.*

PATIENT EDUCATION

Upper GI preparation requires the patient to eat a light evening meal of only clear liquids. The patient should have nothing to eat or drink from midnight until after the X-ray series the next day. The provider will advise whether there are any medication restrictions. Generally, patients can continue taking oral medications. Dairy products, carbonated beverages, and alcohol are not permitted. The digestive tract should be clear of all foods to avoid blockage of or shadows on the anatomical structures to be observed.

Constipation can result from the barium, and patients should be advised to drink plenty of clear liquids to help relieve it. You should also mention that their stool might appear lighter-colored than usual from the white barium and that this is not a cause for concern. Laxatives are ordered only by the provider. Patients should phone the medical office if any problem arises.

Lower GI Series—Barium Enema

Patients who are scheduled for a lower GI series study should follow the preparation listed in Table 48–1 very strictly. Stress the avoidance of milk and all dairy products for better visualization of the colon (Figure 48-7).

CLINICAL PEARL

In an all-liquid diet, the patient may have any of the following: coffee, tea, carbonated beverages, clear gelatin desserts, strained fruit juice, bouillon, clear broths, tomato juice. Do not drink milk of any kind.

Table 48–1 Preparation for Barium Enema

1. Beginning the morning of the day before the examination, change to an all-liquid diet (see Clinical Pearl box on previous page). Do not take any more solid food until after the examination.
2. At 12:30 PM, or half an hour after lunch on the day before the examination, drink entire contents of a bottle of citrate of magnesia (10 oz).
3. At 1:00 PM, drink one glass of fluid.
4. At 3:00 PM, take two Dulcolax tablets with a large glass of water.
5. At 4:00 PM, drink one large glass of fluid.
6. At 5:00 PM, or as close as possible, have a liquid dinner.
7. At 6:00 PM, drink one large glass of fluid.
8. Bedtime, drink one large glass of fluid.
9. You may have one cup of coffee, tea, or water on the morning of the examination.

Be sure to explain the importance of adequate preparation for these studies. Improper preparation could result in the need to repeat the tests. In this examination, barium sulfate is used as the contrast medium. It is introduced into the colon by an **enema** tube, and the radiologist observes the flow into the lower bowel. After barium is introduced into the large intestine, several permanent radiographs are performed. Many providers order a barium enema with air-contrast. Most of the barium is emptied from the colon and air is introduced. This procedure **distends** the barium-filled colon with air to make the structures more visible by fluoroscopy. This is called a double contrast study. This study is helpful in diagnosing diseases of the colon, tumors, and **lesions**.

The barium enema procedure generally takes several minutes and produces discomfort and some pain. Patients should be told to breathe through the mouth slowly and deeply to help relax the abdominal muscles. A strong urge to defecate is normal, and patients often cannot resist the urge. After several films have been taken and the study of the lower bowel is completed, the patient is allowed to use the toilet.

Table 48–2 Preparation for Intravenous Pyelogram (IVP)

1. All-liquid diet.
2. Day prior to the examination, take three Dulcolax 5 mg tablets from 2 to 4 PM
3. Drink only one glass of liquid on the morning of the exam.

Intravenous Pyelogram

In studies of the genitourinary system, the **intravenous pyelogram (IVP)** requires the patient to prepare with laxatives, enemas, and fasting (see Table 48–2). The IVP consists of an intravenous injection of **iodine**, the contrast medium, to define the structures of the urinary system.

PATIENT EDUCATION

Caution: *Patients who have a known iodine allergy should alert the radiology department personnel so that a non-iodine preparation may be used in their X-ray studies. Patients who are suspected of having an allergy to iodine should have iodine-sensitive tests prior to the examination to determine the possibility of an allergic reaction by order of the provider. This information should be obtained during the medical history interview and documented accurately. Allergies should be recorded so that attention is brought to this vital information.*

A **retrograde pyelogram** is a study of the urinary tract done by inserting a sterile catheter into the urinary meatus, through the bladder, and up into the ureters. The **radiopaque** contrast medium then flows upward into the kidneys. This diagnostic test is usually done in **conjunction** with **cystoscopy**. A voiding cystogram might be ordered in conjunction with an IVP; if so, the contrast medium is injected into the bladder by catheter, and no special patient preparation is needed.

PATIENT EDUCATION

Patients must prepare for a barium enema by following instructions precisely, usually beginning the day before the appointment. The instructions generally include using **evacuants** such as laxatives and enemas to clear the bowel of fecal matter and gas. The patient should eat lightly, avoid dairy products, and drink plenty of clear liquids to encourage more comfortable evacuation. Patients should have nothing to eat or drink past midnight the night before the X-ray. On the day of the appointment, the patient should have an enema two hours before the scheduled appointment. Patients should be encouraged to drink plenty of liquids for the next few days to help evacuate the **residual barium** sulfate in the lower colon.

KUB

The **KUB (kidneys, ureters, bladder)** is an X-ray of the patient's abdomen, sometimes termed *flat plate of abdomen* (Figure 48–8). This requires no patient preparation and is used in the diagnosis of urinary system diseases and disorders. It can also be useful in determining the position of an intrauterine device (IUD) or in locating foreign bodies in the digestive tract. In some cases, surgery is indicated to remove an object that might block the normal digestive flow, but many small objects are easily passed with solid foods, especially in young children whose internal structures are more flexible. The provider ultimately makes this decision in patient care.

Mammography

Mammography aids in the diagnosis of breast masses, some of which can be as small as 1 cm in size or less. Women who practice self-examinations regularly each month and find lumps in breast tissue early have a much better cure rate if a malignancy is found. Breast self-examination (see Chapter 40) and regular examinations by the provider should be strongly reinforced to female patients in addition to their scheduled mammography. The American Cancer Society recommends a baseline mammography at the age of 40 for all women. After age 40, women are urged to have a mammography every one to two years.

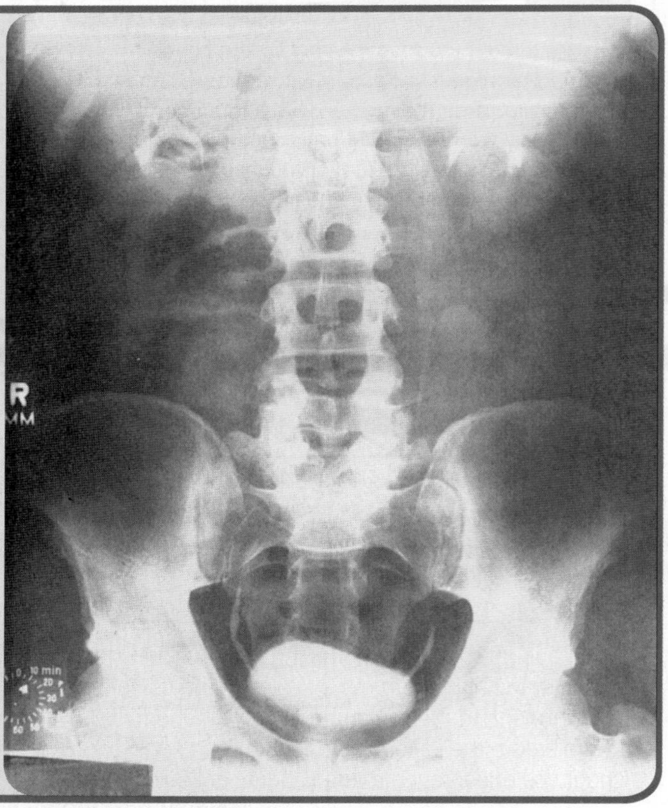

Figure 48–8: Radiologic X-ray of the kidneys, ureters, and bladder (KUB). *Delmar/Cengage Learning.*

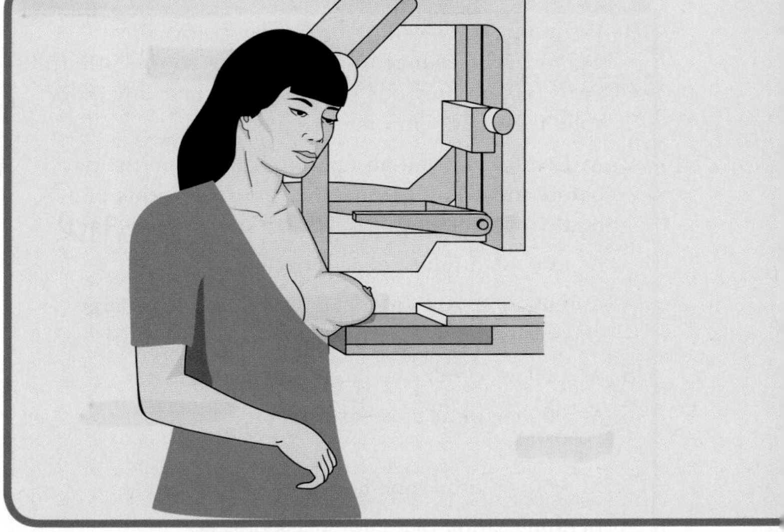

Figure 48–9: Breasts are compressed by plates during mammography to produce a clearer image of the mammary structures. *Delmar/Cengage Learning.*

Remind patients again of the importance of breast self-examinations on a continuing basis. The mammography is not a substitute for this important means of detection. If at any time a lump is found, patients should be advised to see the provider immediately for examination. The mammography procedure requires the patient to move into various positions so that different angles of the breast tissue may be X-rayed (Figure 48–9). The X-ray pictures are called mammograms. **Compression** of the breasts during this procedure requires less radiation to be used. It also allows a much clearer picture to be taken of the breast tissue. Patients are usually advised to wear slacks or a skirt for ease in preparation for the procedure (see Table 48–3) because the patient must undress to the waist for the examination. The only preparation required is for the patient to wash the chest and underarms and

Table 48–3 Instructions for Mammography Preparation

1. Be sure to notify personnel if you are pregnant.
2. Please shower or bathe as close to your appointment as possible.
3. Do not use deodorants, powders, or perfumes on the breast or underarm areas.
4. You must undress at the waist, so wear an easily removable top such as a blouse.

rinse and dry thoroughly. No deodorants, perfumes, or powders are to be used on the day of the mammography because the film on the skin from these substances could interfere with the radiograph.

PATIENT EDUCATION

Because this procedure is often very uncomfortable and even sometimes painful for many women, some suggestions might be helpful in reducing the discomfort:

- Schedule the mammography during the first week following the patient's menstrual cycle because the breasts must be compressed firmly during the procedure to obtain a satisfactory image for diagnostic purposes, and during this time, the patient would experience less discomfort.
- Advise patients to omit caffeine from their diets for 7 to 10 days prior to this examination to reduce the possible effects of swelling and soreness that caffeine often produces.
- After the procedure, some areas of the breasts might become temporarily discolored. However, it does not damage the breast tissue and should not be alarming.
- At the advice of the provider, a mild analgesic may be taken to relieve any discomfort or aching the patient might experience.

Explaining these details to patients and requesting their cooperation with the radiology technician during this procedure is helpful in obtaining a quality mammogram for diagnostic study by the provider. It is also important to let patients know when the results will be available so that they will not worry unnecessarily.

CLINICAL PEARL

It is very important to realize that in some cultures and religions, women are to keep themselves covered at all times when they are in public and in the presence of men. A breast examination and mammography would be especially problematic for the patient unless a female provider or technologist conducted the exam or the mammography. Be sure you explain to the patient or ask an interpreter to explain the preparation, examination, and the imaging to prepare the patient for this experience. Relieving anxiety about this matter helps the patient understand and not be afraid of what to expect.

CT Scans

Rapid scanning of single-tissue **planes** is performed by a process that generates images of the tissue in slices about 1 cm thick. Figure 48–10 illustrates how different parts of the body are sectioned for the image. This method of

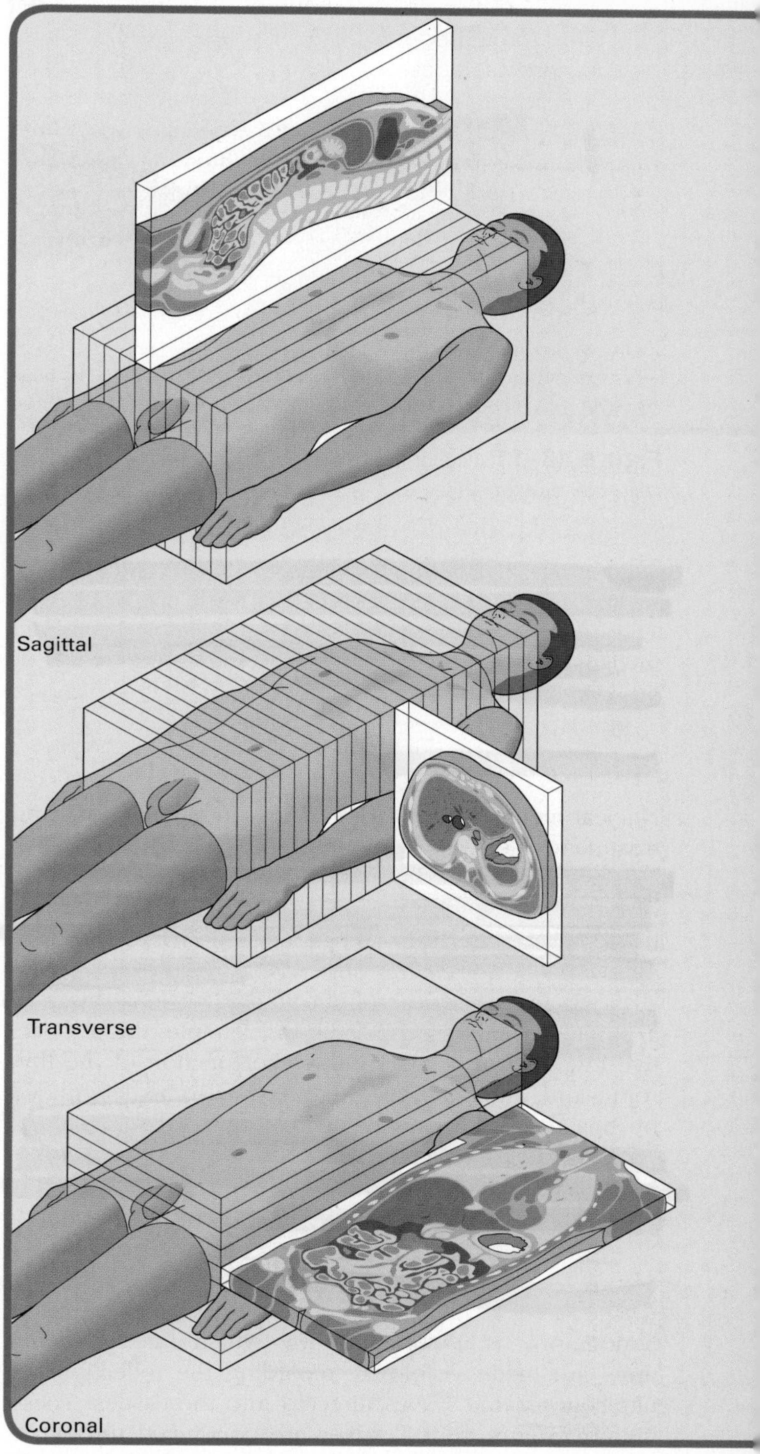

Figure 48–10: Computed tomography provides a three-dimensional view of the internal structures of the body. *Delmar/Cengage Learning.*

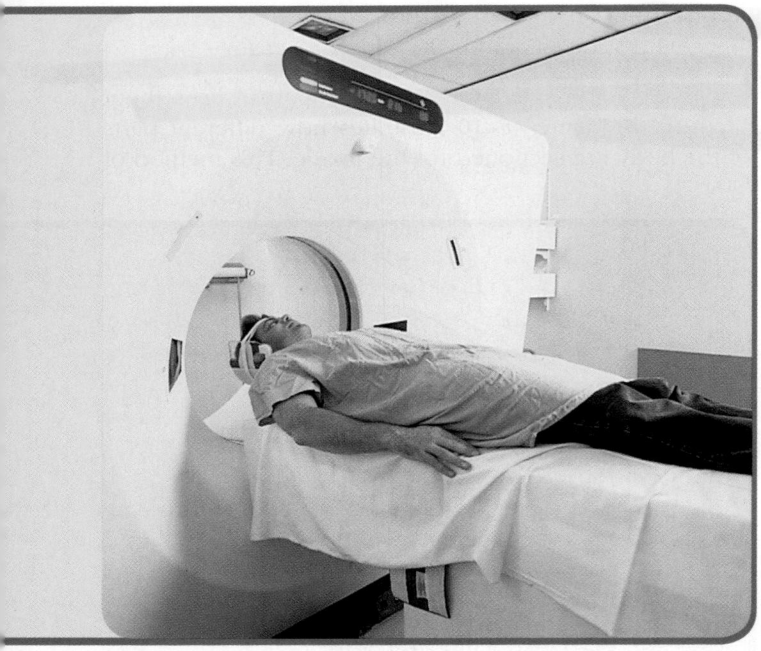

Figure 48–11: Patient in position for a CT scan.
Delmar/Cengage Learning.

radiology is called computed tomography (CT) scan or **computerized transverse axial tomography (CTAT)**. These procedures can be performed in seconds and aid in diagnosis of diseases and disorders of the breast or other internal organs (Figure 48–11).

Nuclear Medicine

Nuclear medicine uses radionuclides in the diagnosis and treatment of disease. Almost any organ of the body can be viewed and recorded by having the patient ingest, or be injected with, radioactive material. Uptake studies refer to procedures in which patients ingest a **radioactive** substance under careful supervision and return within 24 hours to have the amount of radioactive substance in a particular organ measured. For example, the radioactive thyroid uptake determines the function of the thyroid gland. Tumors of the thyroid can also be determined by this method. In female patients, pregnancy should be determined prior to the radioactive thyroid uptake because it is seriously damaging to the fetus, especially within the first trimester of pregnancy.

SONOGRAPHIC STUDIES

Sonography is a technique by which internal structures are made visible by recording the reflections of ultrasonic sound waves directed into the tissues. These high-frequency sound waves are conducted through a **transducer** (a handheld instrument resembling a microphone). While the transducer is held against the body area to be tested, it sends sound waves through the skin to various organs. As the sound waves are sent back, the transducer picks them up and changes them into electrical energy. This energy is transmitted into an image on a monitor or printed out on paper in wavy lines. The picture formed on the screen represents a cross section of the organ. Photos of these images are taken for permanent records. The provider interprets these images to aid in the diagnosis and treatment of the patient. Ultrasound technology does not use radiation, so it is considered to be very safe. Sonograms are not useful in viewing the lungs because sound waves are not created by structures containing air.

The abdominal ultrasound procedure is an accurate and painless diagnostic tool. It involves lying on an examination table for 45 to 60 minutes. A gel or lotion is used to produce better sound wave conduction and to allow the transducer to glide more easily across the skin. Ultrasonography is useful in examination of the abdominopelvic cavity to locate aneurysms of the aorta and other blood vessel abnormalities. The size and shape of internal organs can also be determined with ultrasound. It can be valuable in the identification of cysts and tumors of the eye and in the detection of pelvic masses and obstructions of the urinary tract.

> **PATIENT EDUCATION**
>
> When scheduling patients for studies such as an abdominal ultrasound, give them a few important instructions. Patients should avoid eating foods that produce gas and drink plenty of fluids (specific amounts are required for certain tests) as shown in Table 48–4. Check with the radiology facility regarding what the patient may drink. Some facilities allow other liquids besides water. Alcoholic beverages are not permitted. Additionally, instruct the patient *not* to void following drinking the water (or other liquids).

Table 48–4 Preparation for Ultrasound Procedure

Abdominal ultrasound	Take nothing by mouth after midnight. No breakfast on the morning of the examination.
Pelvic ultrasound	Drink 24–30 ounces of fluid one hour before examination. Do not urinate after drinking the liquid.
Fetal ultrasound	Drink 24–30 ounces of fluid one hour before examination. Do not urinate after drinking the liquid.

In addition to abdominal ultrasound examinations, you might be required to give patients necessary information about pelvic and fetal ultrasound procedures. In the procedure for a pelvic ultrasound, a vaginal probe is used to aid in visualizing internal structures. This is known as an *invasive ultrasound* and shows the ovaries and uterus in great detail. It is helpful for patients to be aware of this before it is done so that they will be prepared. In obstetrics and gynecology, where the radiation of X-ray examination is avoided, ultrasound is useful in the diagnosis of multiple pregnancies and in determining the size, **maturity**, and position of the fetus. Patient preparation can vary, but usually the patient is instructed to drink a large amount of water, up to a quart to distend the bladder, help push the uterus into place, and increase the conduction of the sound waves.

Besides being a diagnostic procedure, ultrasound is used in the treatment of diseased or injured muscle tissue. Sound waves vibrate into the tissues, producing heat, which helps relieve inflammation and pain. It also increases circulation, which speeds up healing of injured muscle tissues. Another common use of ultrasound is in dentistry. Sound vibrations make it possible for tartar to be painlessly removed from the teeth.

MAGNETIC RESONANCE IMAGING (MRI)

Another technique to view the structures inside the human body is called **magnetic resonance imaging** (MRI). This method allows providers to examine a particular area of the body without exposing the patient to X-rays or surgery. This **noninvasive** procedure, which can range from 30 to 60 minutes, requires the patient to lie on a padded table that is moved into a tunnel-like structure (Figure 48–12). Some patients experience **claustrophobia** when a closed MRI is used; this can be handled by counseling or the use of a sedative administered by a provider before the procedure is begun. Open MRIs are now available for claustrophobic or obese patients; however, the image quality may not be as clear or accurate as the traditional MRI.

No advance patient preparation is required for this examination. The MRI procedure becomes an *invasive* procedure only when an intravenous contrast media is administered to the patient under certain conditions. This *contrast enhanced* technique is performed during the last series of images of the examination to detect certain pathologies. The patient may resume normal activity following the procedure. There are no known harmful effects to the patient from this imaging technique.

The magnetic resonance machine scans all planes of a body structure to produce an image processed by a computer without moving the patient. Radio signals are sent from the scanner that are influenced by strong magnetic fields to which the body responds. Figure 48–13 shows an image of the lumbar spine in the sagittal plane. Note the herniated disc and the clarity of the image. The MRI has reduced a great number of diagnostic exploratory surgeries. It is most useful in diagnosing brain and nervous system disorders, cardiovascular disease, cancer, and diseases of the visceral organs. Magnetic resonance imaging can be performed for particular areas of the body such as the hip, shoulder, or neck. This specific imaging of small areas takes less time, approximately a half hour. Explain the time requirement to the patient as a courtesy. The patient can plan transportation better if the time of the appointment and the length of

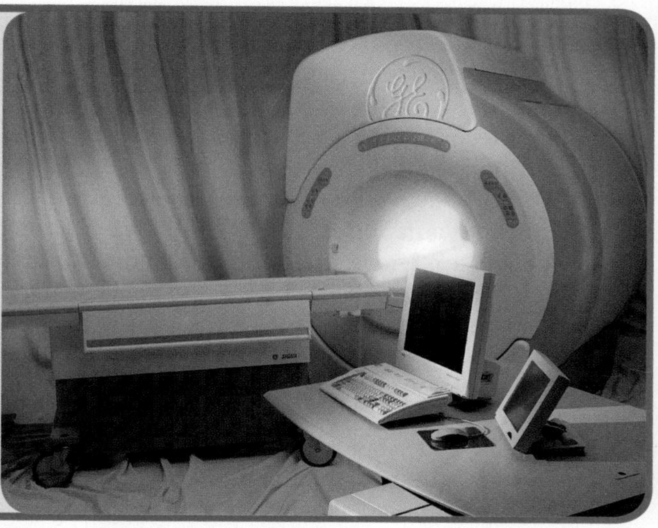

Figure 48–12: Magnetic resonance imaging (MRI).
Courtesy of GE Medical Systems.

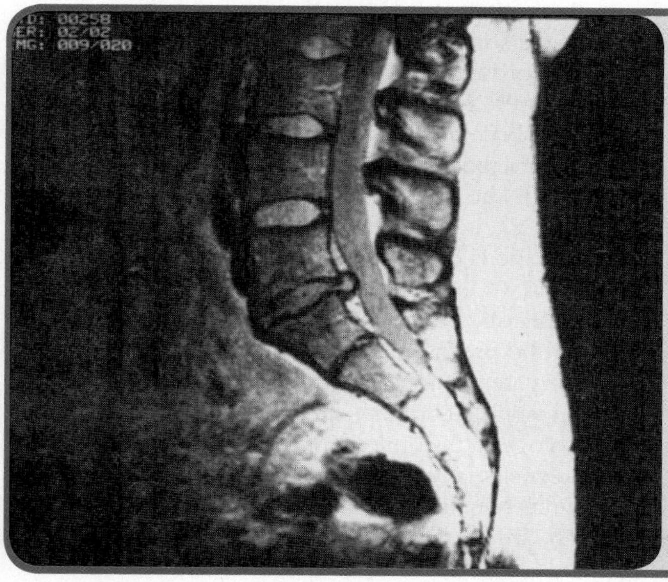

Figure 48–13: MRI showing a herniated disc.
Courtesy of GE Medical Systems.

vasopresser - norepinephrine

time the test takes is known. MRI also helps monitor the effectiveness of treatment. Because the MRI uses a strong **electromagnetic** field, it is extremely important for any metal objects to be removed before the procedure is performed. The technician will request the patient to remove all metallic objects, including jewelry, hairpins, and nonpermanent dentures before being placed in the tunnel for the MRI. Patients should be interviewed thoroughly regarding their health history. Inform patients that at the facility where the MRI will be performed, they will generally be asked to sign a consent form prior to the procedure. Female patients should refrain from even wearing mascara, since tiny metallic flakes can be present in it. During the procedure, these minute pieces of metal can become hot and burn the patient.

During the process, mention that the patient might hear many repetitive noises that sound like clanging and banging, humming, and whirring—this is just the sound of the electromagnetic field. Patients are usually given headphones and are allowed to listen to a radio station or are given ear plugs to help to drown out some of the noise. There are no sensations of pain and no known side effects. The patient must be still and relax for the test to be completed properly. The technician observes the patient during the entire time. Patients may speak to the technician by the use of a microphone inside the tunnel.

The MRI procedure is contraindicated in patients who have pacemakers, have metallic **implants**, are in the first trimester of pregnancy, are severely claustrophobic, or are obese.

CHAPTER SUMMARY

- Radiologic testing is an important tool providers use for screening, diagnostic procedures, and therapeutic purposes. Your role might be to assist the radiology technologist at your facility or to schedule patients for radiology procedures and testing at outside facilities; depending on the practices in your state, you might be allowed to take certain X-rays and operate the equipment yourself.
- Radiologic studies are made with X-rays (roentgen rays), which are high-energy electromagnetic radiation produced by the collision of a beam of electrons with a metal target in an X-ray tube.
- Any person working in a facility that performs radiologic tests can be at risk for excessive radiation exposure. You must institute safety measures to protect both you and the patients.
- X-rays can be damaging to an unborn child, especially in the first three months of pregnancy (first trimester), sometimes before the patient is even aware she is pregnant. Before scheduling any female patient whose age indicates that she is within the childbearing years, you must always ask whether she could be pregnant.
- Dietary restrictions, special preps, contrast agents, and fasting techniques are required for many of the radiology procedures. By adding a contrast agent, the density of the structure being assessed changes, and the visualization is improved. Be sure to explain the requirements to the patient so he or she understands clearly.
- The provider might order a variety of radiological imaging tests to assist him or her with the diagnosis of a condition or injury. Common procedures include bone studies; chest, abdomen, and pelvic studies; KUB; sonograms; CTs and MRIs.
- Sonograms are records obtained by ultrasonic scanning. Ultrasound technology does not use radiation, so it is considered to be very safe. Ultrasonography is a technique by which internal structures are made visible by recording the reflections of ultrasonic sound waves directed into the tissues.
- When scheduling patients for ultrasound studies, advise them about the preparation for the exam. Patient preparation varies, depending on the exam, but avoiding foods that produce gas and drinking plenty of fluids (specific amounts are required for certain tests) are generally the rule. Check with the radiology facility regarding what the patient preparation will be.
- Another technique to view the structures inside the human body is called magnetic resonance imaging (MRI). This method allows providers to examine a particular area of the body without exposing the patient to X-rays or surgery. Contraindications include claustrophobia, obesity, pacemakers, and metal implants.
- When educating the patient, always provide clear and concise oral *and* written instructions for examinations that require advance preparation. Be sure the patient understands the necessary preparations. Answer all questions. Emphasize the importance of being on time for the radiologic appointment to avoid unnecessary delays because some examinations are very long.

STUDY TOOLS

Workbook	Activities for Chapter 48
Premium Website StudyWARE	Activities and Quizzes on the **StudyWARE™ Software** for Chapter 48 **Audio Library** of medical terms Online access to the **Critical Thinking Challenge 2.0**
learning**lab**	Module 20: Cardiology and Radiology Procedures
CourseMate	Activities and Quizzes for Chapter 48
WebTutor	Activities and Quizzes for Chapter 48

CHECK YOUR KNOWLEDGE

1. In this type of therapeutic radiation, radioactive implants are placed by the radiologist close to or into the cancerous tissue.
   a. Teletherapy
   b. Brachytherapy
   c. Physical therapy
   d. None of the above
2. A dosimeter can last up to:
   a. 1 month.
   b. 2 months.
   c. 3 months.
   d. 6 months.
3. Sonograms can be very useful in diagnosing:
   a. gallstones.
   b. tumors.
   c. heart defects.
   d. all the above.
4. Which of the following studies does not require special preparation?
   a. Chest X-ray
   b. Cholecystogram
   c. Upper GI
   d. Barium enema
5. This method of radiology generates images of the tissue in slices about 1 cm thick.
   a. CT scan
   b. MRI
   c. Mammogram
   d. Sonogram

WEB LINKS

National Institutes of Health: www.nih.gov

U.S. National Library of Medicine: www.nlm.nih.gov

RESOURCES

Carlton, R., and Adler, A. (2006). *Principles of Radiographic Imaging* (4th ed.). Clifton Park, NY: Delmar Cengage Learning.

Campeau, F. E., and Fleitz, J. (2010). *Limited Radiography* (3rd ed.). Clifton Park, NY: Delmar Cengage Learning.

Estes, M. E. Z. (2010). *Health Assessment & Physical Examination*. Clifton Park, NY: Delmar Cengage Learning.

Heller, M., and Veach, L. (2009). *Clinical Medical Assisting: A Professional, Field Smart Approach to the Workplace*. Clifton Park, NY: Delmar, Cengage Learning.

Lazo, D. (2005). *Fundamentals of Sectional Anatomy: An Imaging Approach*. Clifton Park, NY: Delmar Cengage Learning.

Lindh, W., Pooler, M., Tamparo, C., and Dahl, B. (2010). *Delmar's Comprehensive Medical Assisting Administrative and Clinical Competencies* (4th ed.). Clifton Park, NY: Delmar Cengage Learning.

Unit

16

Minor Surgical Procedures

As a clinical medical assistant, you might assist with a variety of sterile procedures, including minor office surgery. Maintaining surgical asepsis is vital to prevent the transmission of diseases *before*, *during*, and *following* any of the invasive procedures performed in the medical office or clinic. In compliance with Standard Precautions, proper barriers such as gloves, gown, and face mask or shield must be worn to protect the health care staff from possible contamination while performing these procedures. All disposable waste must be placed in a plastic biohazard bag or in a sharps container and discarded properly to prevent disease transmission.

The medical assistant must have a good working knowledge of the care and function of basic instruments used in the medical office to perform minor surgical procedures. Setup for various procedures can vary slightly according to the provider's preference. However, aseptic technique is always the same for any invasive procedure. Basic information for assisting the provider and preparing the patient is covered in this unit, along with a description of the specialized instruments used in the performance of minor office surgery.

Certification Connection

	Ch. 49	Ch. 50
CMA (AAMA)		
Principles of asepsis	X	
Surgical asepsis	X	X
Preparing/maintaining treatment areas	X	X
Patient preparation and assisting the physician—Procedures	X	X
Instruction for procedure preparation	X	X
Processing specimen		X
Cultures—Wounds		X
RMA (AMT)		
Identify and understand the application of disclosure laws and regulations	X	
Identify and apply proper written and verbal communication to instruct patients in pre- and postoperative care	X	X
Understand and use proper documentation of patient encounters and instruction		X
Know and understand terminology associated with asepsis	X	
Surgical asepsis	X	X
Instruments	X	
Surgical supplies	X	X
Surgical procedures	X	X

Chapter

49 Preparing for Surgery

OBJECTIVES

In this chapter, you will learn the following:

KB KNOWLEDGE BASE

1. Spell and define, using the glossary at the back of the text, all the Words to Know in this chapter.
2. Explain scheduling and preoperative and postoperative instructions for patients for minor office surgery.
3. Discuss the different parts of surgical instruments.
4. Describe the proper care of surgical instruments.
5. List the function of all instruments discussed in this chapter.
6. Discuss the importance of maintaining the sterile field.
7. Explain the importance of obtaining the consent form for the surgical procedure.
8. Explain the importance of proper skin preparation before an invasive procedure.
9. Differentiate between the methods of sterilization.

S SKILLS

1. Set up a sterile tray.
2. Open packages on a sterile tray.
3. Perform hand washing for surgical asepsis.
4. Apply sterile gloves.
5. Prepare skin for a minor surgical procedure.

WORDS TO KNOW

antiseptic
aseptic technique
contamination
fenestrated
forceps
hemostat
microbial
microorganism
needle holder
preoperative (preop)
postoperative (postop)
ratchet
retractor
scrub
serrations
speculum
strikethrough
surgical asepsis

SCHEDULING MINOR OFFICE SURGERY

Many minor surgical procedures are now performed in the medical office, clinic, and ambulatory care center. It is usually the medical assistant's duty to schedule the surgery, educate the patient about **preoperative (preop)** and **postoperative (postop)** care, prepare the room and equipment for the surgery, and assist the physician as needed.

Many providers prefer to perform minor surgical procedures at the beginning of the day's schedule. Some might require patients to fast for a certain amount of time before the procedure. (Fasting lessens the possibility of nausea and vomiting, which some patients can experience during and following any type of surgery.)

You might be asked to schedule an appointment for a patient to have a surgical procedure as an outpatient at a large ambulatory care center or hospital. Be sure to check with the person who makes the appointment regarding the preparation for the patient. When you write the appointment date and time for the patient, make certain the patient has directions to the facility. The assistant in the hospital or surgeon's office generally phones the patient the day before the surgery to confirm the appointment.

Be sure to cover all points listed in the patient education box when scheduling a patient for a minor surgical procedure.

PATIENT EDUCATION

When scheduling, advise patient of the:

1. Surgical procedure, by providing printed education materials.
2. Approximate length of time for procedure.
3. Appropriate clothing to wear at appointment.
4. Amount of time to fast as instructed by provider if applicable.
5. Arrangements necessary for someone to accompany the patient and drive him or her home if necessary.
6. Anticipated time off work or arranging for home care.

When patient arrives for the appointment:

1. Ascertain whether the patient has any allergies to any medications, including topical preparations, latex products, and adhesive tapes.
2. Provide written instructions regarding the surgical procedure and follow-up care.
3. Ensure that the patient has signed a surgical consent form.
4. Answer any questions concerning procedure.

Be sure the patient understands the procedure and the instructions regarding preoperative and postoperative care. Most medical facilities have printed instructions for patients. Remember that some patients you see cannot read or might not speak English. You must explain as well as you can verbally and observe the patient's reactions to your instructions. Printed instructions in other languages and the services of an interpreter should be made available to the patient. This eliminates any misunderstandings, and patients feel more at ease knowing they can refer to it. Patients should be advised of the appropriate clothing to be worn on the day of the surgery. Loose-fitting clothing, clothing easy to put on and take off, and clothing appropriate for the anatomical area of surgery should be suggested. It is a good practice to phone the patient the day prior to the appointment, not only to reassure the patient and answer any questions but to confirm the appointment.

PREPARING THE ROOM

Prior to the scheduled surgery, get all the necessary surgical instruments and supplies ready. A routine inventory of all supplies and sterile items is vital so that a sterile tray can be set up for any surgical procedure.

Instruments

Each instrument used in the performance of minor surgical procedures has a specific function. Many times, its function can be determined simply by a visual inspection of the instrument. Surgical instruments used in the medical office are very costly and must be carefully maintained for longevity and maximum function. Always follow manufacturer's recommendations for cleaning, sterilization, and storage of all instruments. All surgical instruments must be properly labeled and sterilized. Most of the instruments will already be sterilized (as they should be after each use). Disposable instruments are being used more frequently as a way to control the spread of infection. These instruments are designed to be used one time and then properly discarded.

Instrument Care and Handling

Most instruments should be cared for in the same manner. The following is a list of general rules to follow when cleaning and caring for instruments.

1. Blood, tissue, and other body fluids must not be allowed to dry on an instrument.
2. Instruments should be rinsed and then soaked in a room-temperature solution containing a detergent and a solvent immediately after each use.
3. The detergent in the soaking solution should be of a neutral pH, which will help prevent corrosion of the surfaces of the instrument.

4. The soaking solution should contain a special protein that breaks down blood and body fluids on the surface of the instrument.
5. Instruments should be placed in a plastic container for soaking to prevent damage to their points and cutting edges.
6. Separate delicate instruments from heavier ones to prevent damage.
7. Separate sharp instruments from others when cleaning and storing.
8. All surfaces and crevices must be scrubbed with a brush to remove any foreign material.
9. A careful visual inspection should be conducted during each cleaning to check for any nicks, dullness, or warping of the surfaces.
10. Damaged instruments should not be used and should be either repaired or replaced.

Instrument Components

Each part of an instrument's structure has a specific function. Figures 49–1A through C illustrate the key components of an instrument; an explanation of their function follows.

- *Thumb handle* (Figure 49–1A): A handle similar to that of a tweezer that is squeezed between the thumb and finger.
- *Ring handle* (Figure 49–1B): Designed so that the thumb and finger can be inserted into the rings.
- *Ratchet* (Figure 49–1B): Locking mechanism designed to close in varying degrees to hold the instrument closed, used to clamp tissue and vessels.
- *Serrations* (Figure 49–1C): Little fissures engraved into the surface of the blades of hemostats and forceps designed to prevent slippage and provide a firm grip when clamping a tissue. Instruments can have serrations, cross serrations, or longitudinal serrations.
- *Teeth* (Figure 49–1C): Very sharp projections designed to hold the tissue when grasping. Teeth can be heavy or delicate, and some are classified as non-traumatic.

Instrument Classification

Most instruments are classified according to their function as follows:

- *Cutting and dissecting*: Includes scissors, scalpels, and curettes
- *Clamping and grasping*: Includes **hemostats**, clamps, **forceps**, and **needle holders**
- *Dilating, probing, and visualizing*: Includes **retractors**, scopes, **specula**, probes, and dilators

Table 49–1 lists some common instruments along with their use.

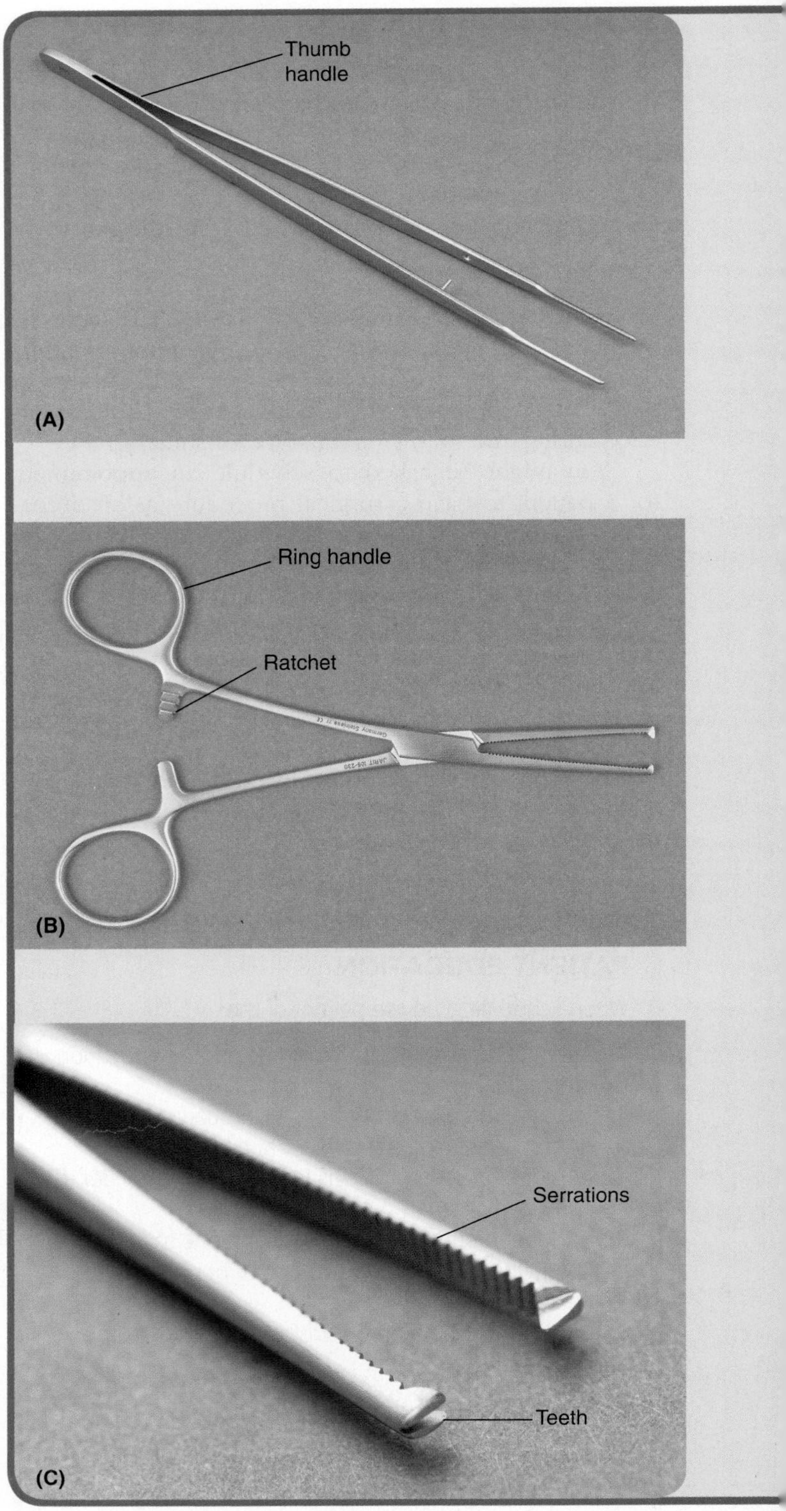

Figure 49–1A–C: Structural features of instruments: (A) Thumb handle. (B) Ring handle and ratchet. (C) Serrations and teeth. *Delmar/Cengage Learning.*

TABLE 49–1 Instruments Used in Minor Office Surgical Procedures

Figure Number	Category: Description	Use
	Cutting and Dissecting	
A	**Operating scissors** $5\frac{1}{2}$" (14 cm), straight, sharp-blunt points	Cut tissue
B	**Operating scissors** $5\frac{1}{2}$" (14 cm), straight, sharp-sharp points	Cut tissue
C	**Lister bandage scissors** $7\frac{1}{4}$" (18.4 cm)	Cut dressings, tape, gauze, bandages
D	**Knife handle #3** 5" (12.7 cm), holds blades 10, 11, 12, 15	
E	**Knife handle #3L** $8\frac{3}{8}$" (21.3 cm), holds blades 10, 11, 12, 15	Accepts blades; used when cutting deeper tissue

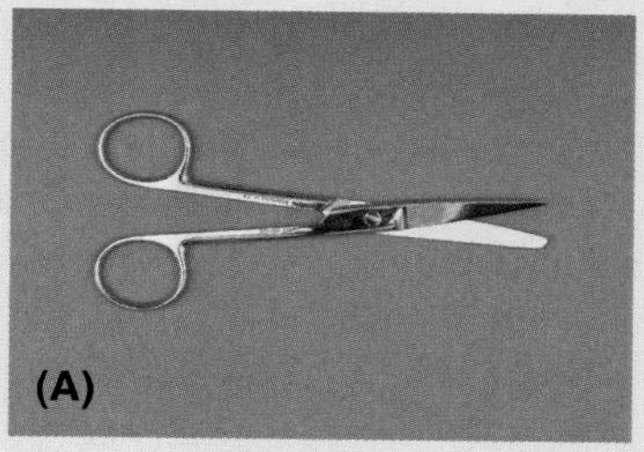
(A)

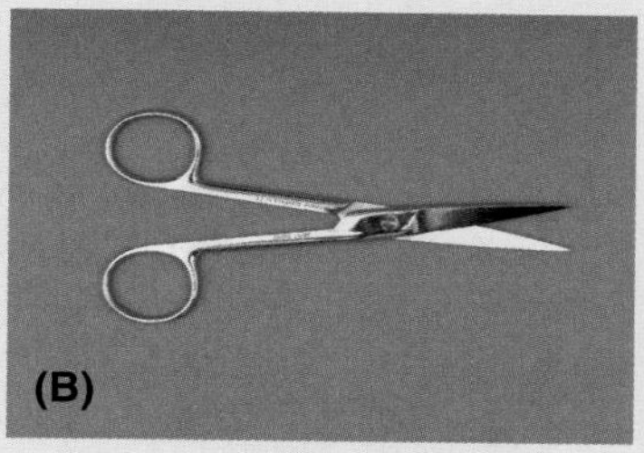
(B)

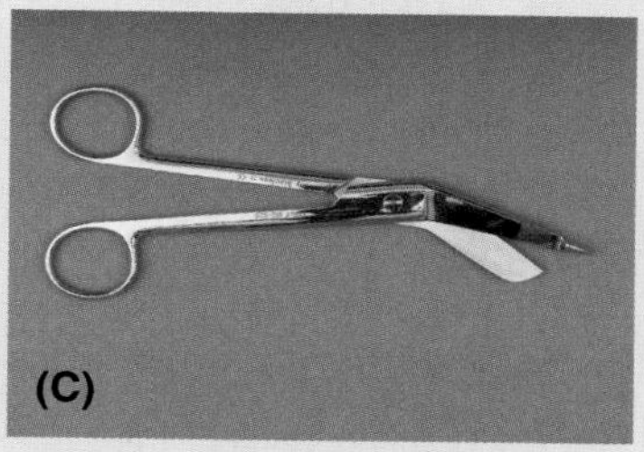
(C)

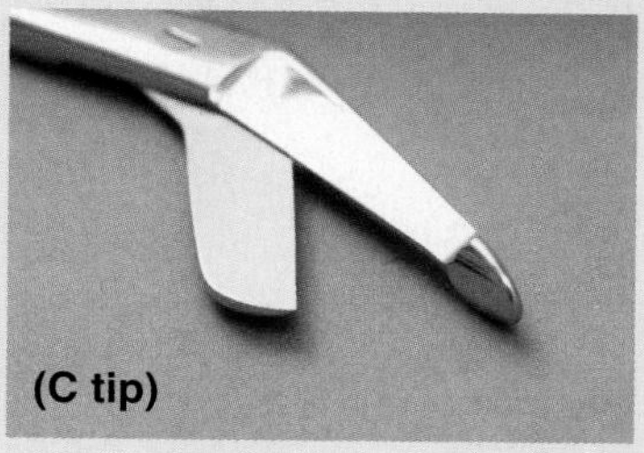
(C tip)

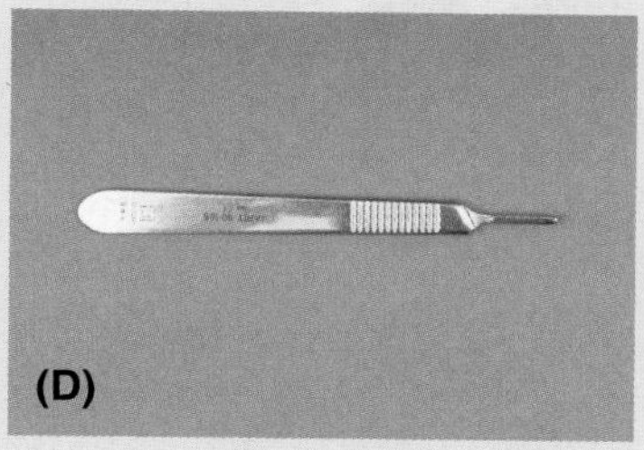
(D)

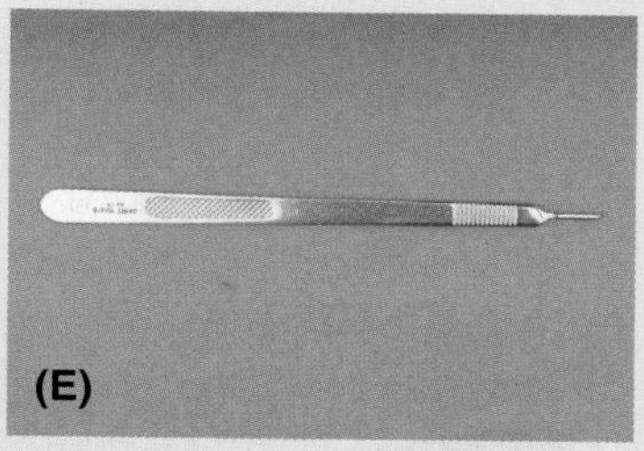
(E)

Figure Number	Category: Description	Use
	Clamping and Grasping	
F	**Dressing or thumb forceps** 6" (15.2 cm), serrated	Pick up dressings, delicate tissue
G	**Adson tissue forceps** $4\frac{3}{4}$" (12.1 cm), serrated	Grasp delicate tissue securely for control during dissection or suturing
H	**Allis tissue forceps** 6" (15.2 cm), 4 × 5 teeth	Grasp tissue securely for control during dissection or suturing
I	**Foerster sponge holding forceps** $9\frac{1}{2}$" (24.1 cm), straight, serrated jaws	Pick up and hold dressings
J	**Hartmann mosquito hemostatic forceps** $3\frac{1}{2}$" (8.9 cm), curved, serrated jaws the entire length of the tip	Grasp tissue to hold, clamp, or pull out of the way
K	**Kelly forceps** $5\frac{1}{2}$" (14 cm), curved, partially serrated jaws	Grasp tissue to hold, clamp, or pull out of the way
L	**Olsen Hegar needle holder** $5\frac{1}{2}$" (14 cm)	Grasp suture needle

(continues)

TABLE 49–1 (*Continued*)

Figure Number	Category: Description	Use
M	**Backhaus towel forceps**	Grasp towels, dressing; hold drape towels in place (use caution—will puncture skin)

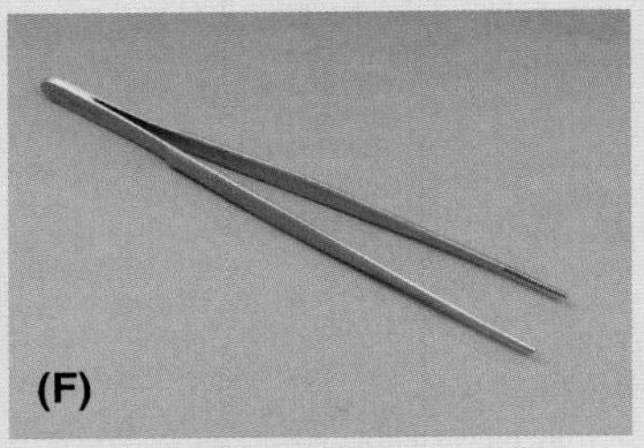

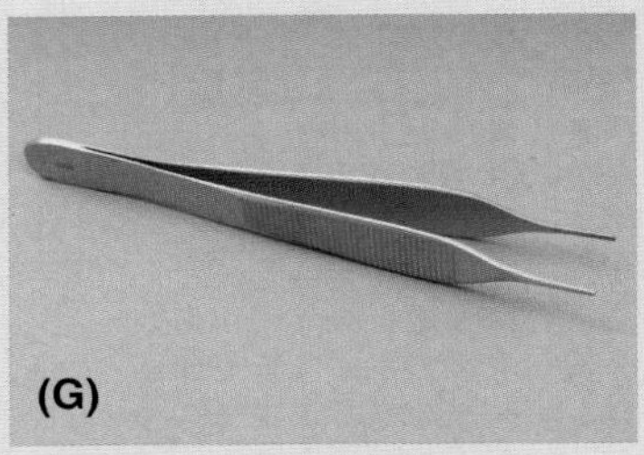

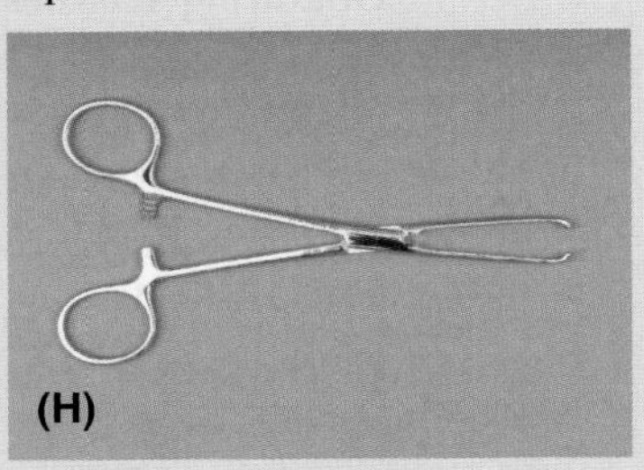

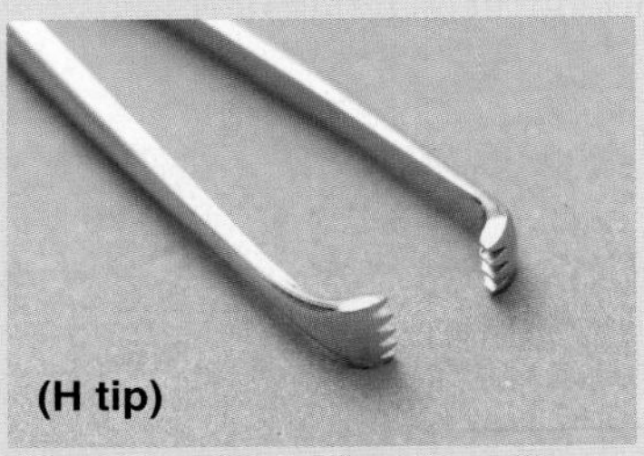

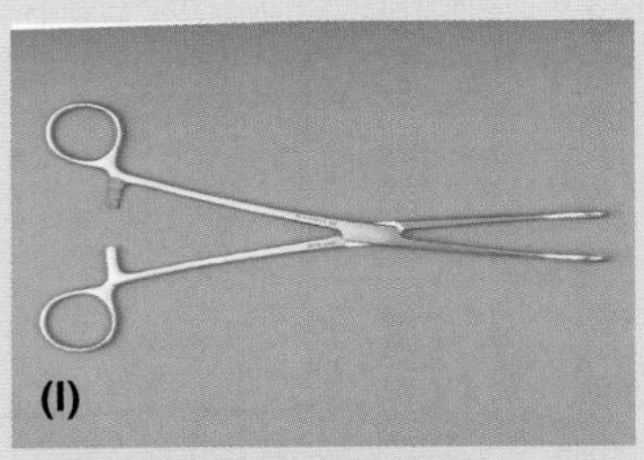

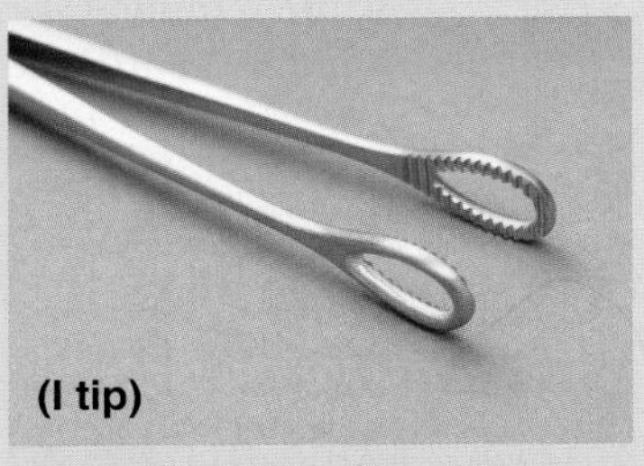

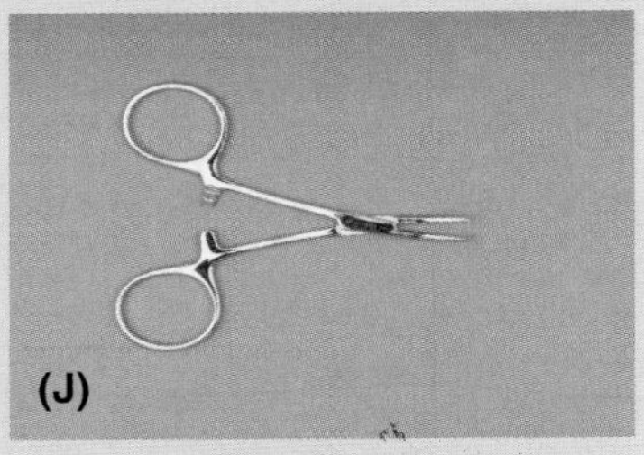

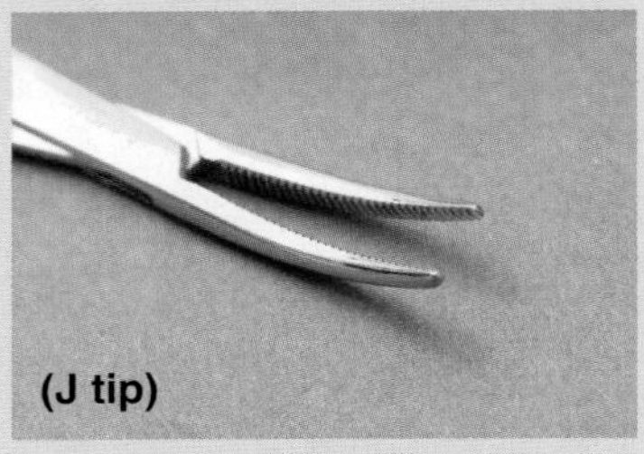

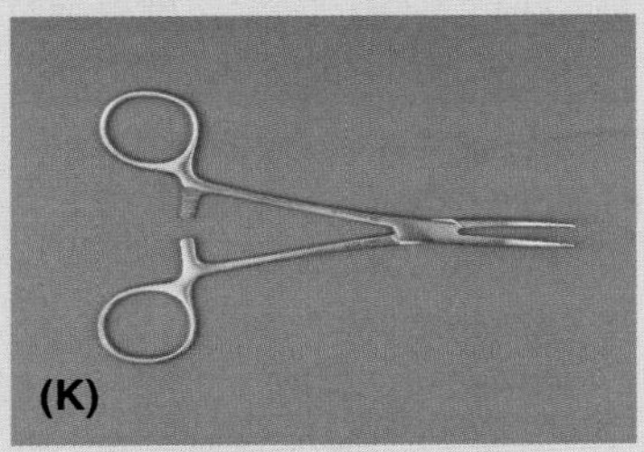

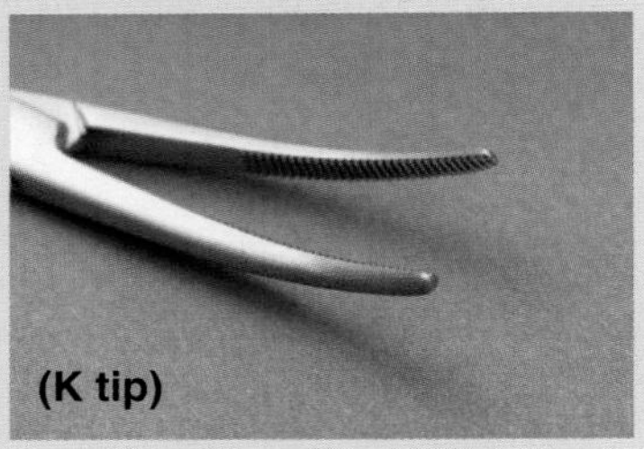

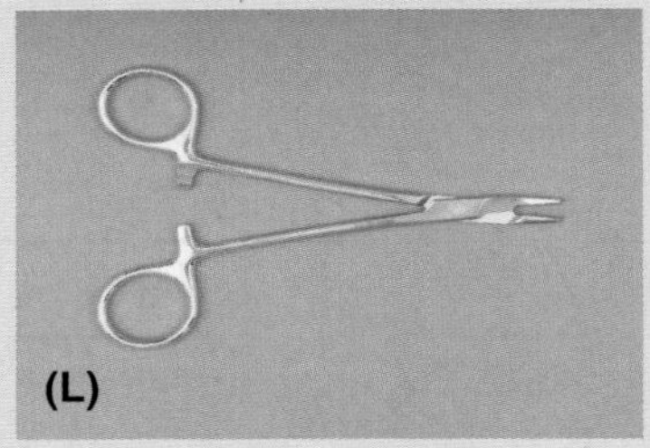

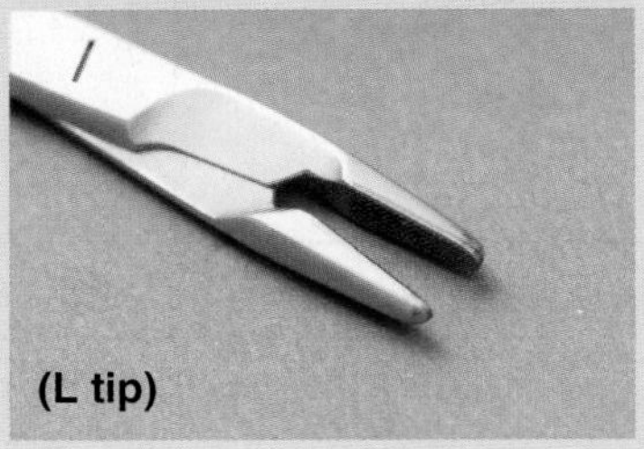

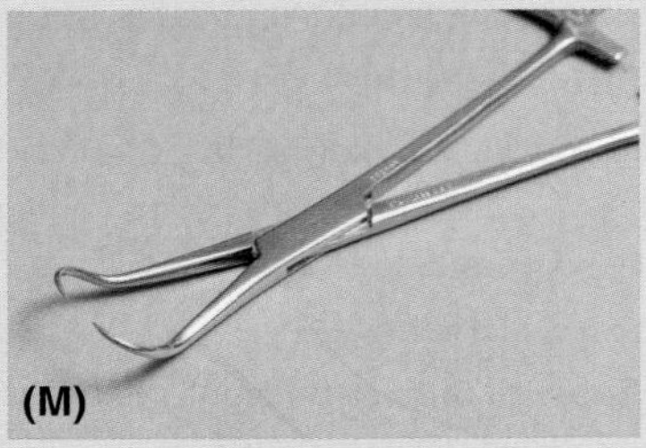

Figure A–X: *Courtesy of Delmar/Cengage Learning.*

Figure Number	Category: Description	Use
	Dilating, Probing, and Visualizing	
N	**Senn retractor** 6¼" (15.9 cm), double-ended, 3 sharp prongs, solid blade	Pull aside tissue to visualize an area better
O	**Ribbon retractor** 1½" (3.8 cm) wide × 13" (33 cm) long 5¼" (13.5 cm)	Pull aside tissue to visualize an area better Grasp suture needle

TABLE 49–1 (*Continued*)

Figure Number	Category: Description	Use
P	**U.S. Army retractor** $\frac{5}{8}$" (1.5 cm) wide × 8-1/4" (21 cm) long	Pull aside tissue to visualize an area better
Q	**Deaver retractor** 1" (2.5 cm) wide × 13" (33 cm) long	Pull aside tissue to visualize an area better
R	**Richardson retractor** $9\frac{1}{2}$", loop handle (1" wide × $1\frac{1}{4}$" deep)	Pull aside tissue to visualize an area better
S	**Flexible probe**	Explore a wound or body cavity
T	**Grooved director** with probe tip and tongue tie	Explore a wound or body cavity
U	**Uterine dilators** Long instrument with calibrations	Measure the depth of the urethra; relieve urethral strictures
V	**Urethral sound** Double-ended smooth rods with rounded tips	Dilate the cervix and gain access to the uterus for examination
W	**Grave's vaginal speculum**	Enlarge vaginal cavity (not shown)
X	**Vienna nasal speculum**	Enlarge nasal cavity (not shown)

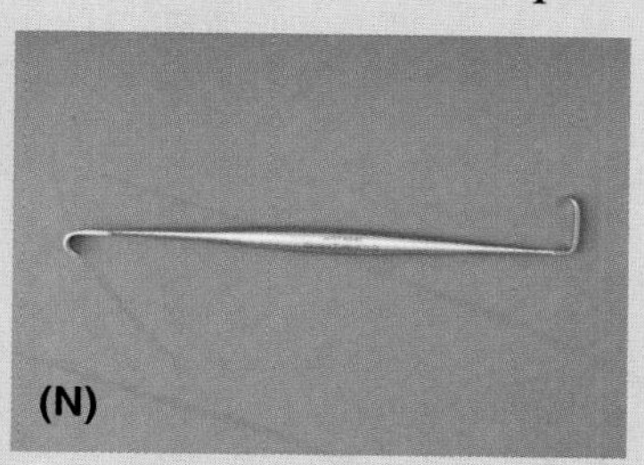
(N)

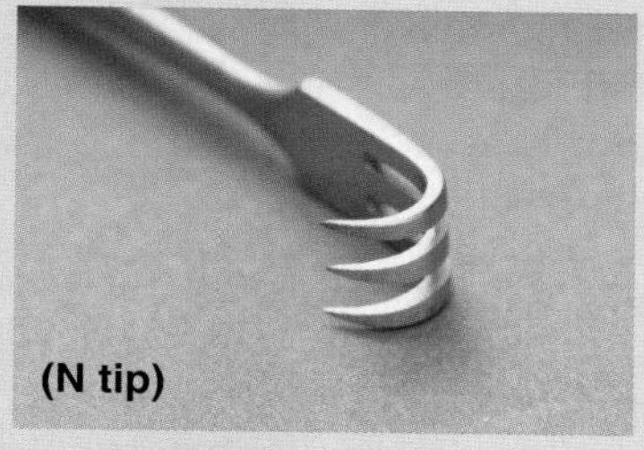
(N tip)

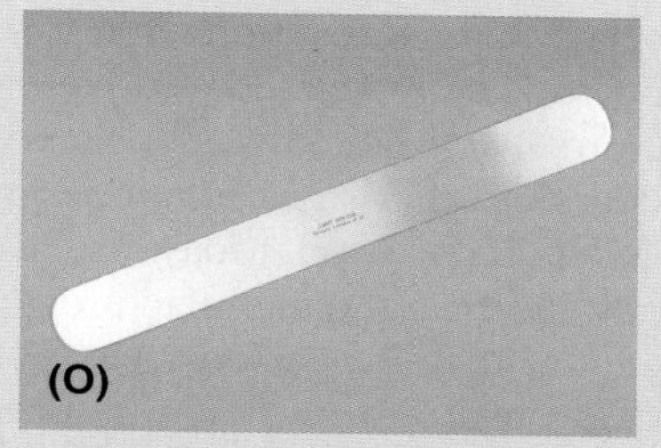
(O)

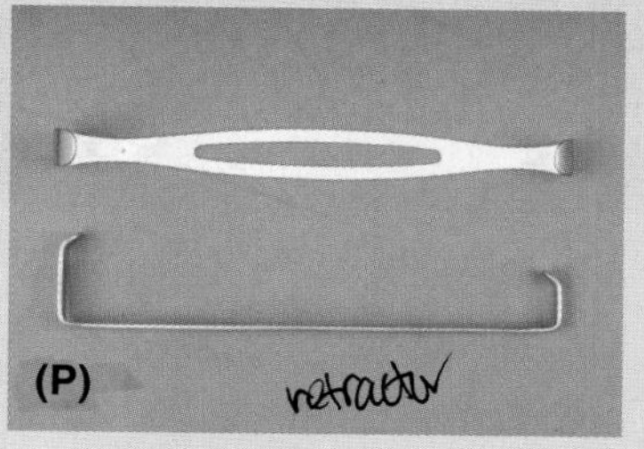
(P)

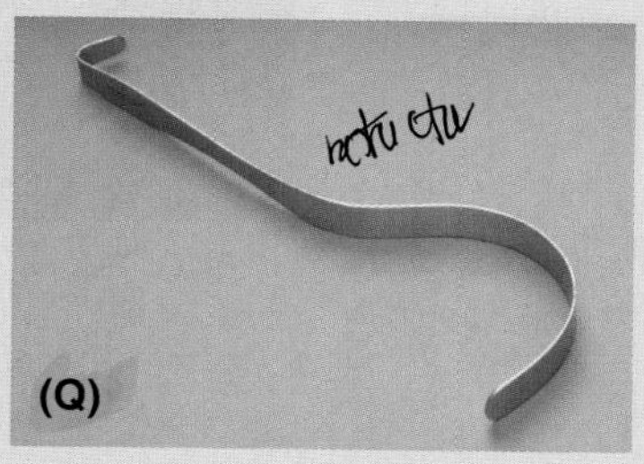
(Q)

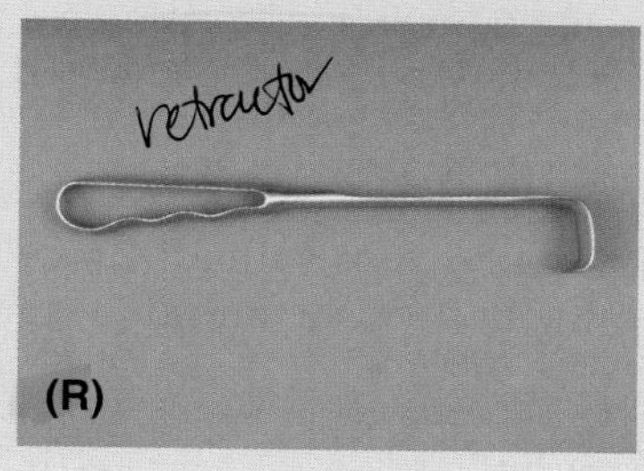
(R)

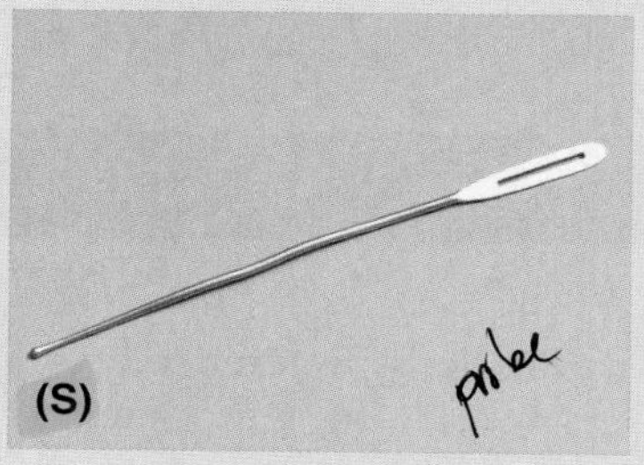
(S)

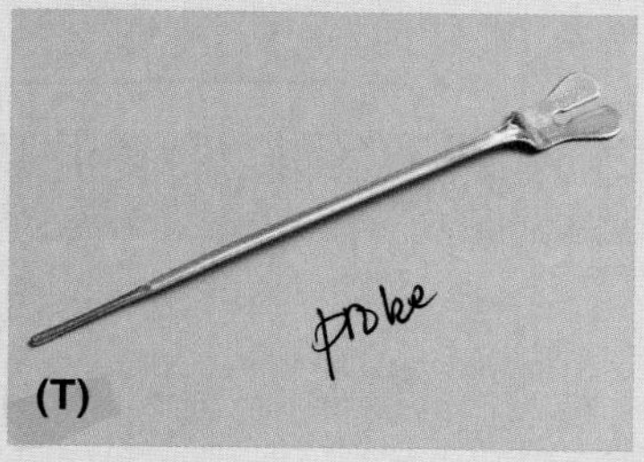
(T)

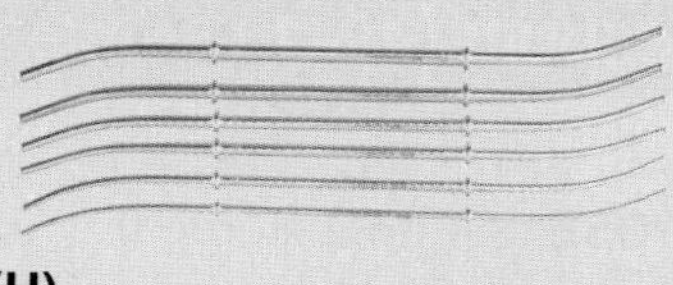
(U)

(V)

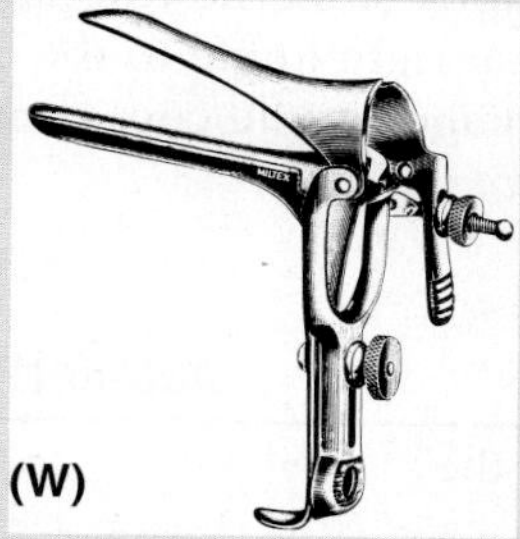
(W)

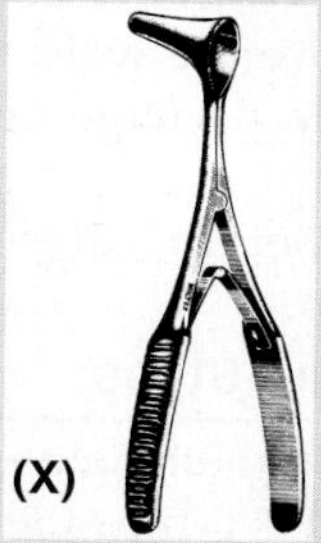
(X)

Supplies

The basic setup for most minor surgical procedures includes the following sterile items:

- Scalpel handle and blades or disposable scalpel
- Hemostats
- Needle holder
- Needles and suture material (absorbable or nonabsorbable)
- Suture scissors
- Thumb forceps
- Probe
- Gauze squares
- Vial of **anesthetic** medication
- Needles and syringes
- Towels
- Bandages

Some of these supplies can be wrapped and sterilized together. All sterile packages must be labeled with the contents, date the package was sterilized, and the signature of the person who prepared and sterilized it. Autoclaved items remain sterile for 30 days if they have been properly processed and have been protected from moisture. Packages should be checked before use for any tears or other signs of tampering to ensure sterility.

Most items used today are disposable and come already sterile in the manufacturer's packaging. You must make sure that the package has not been torn or punctured to ensure sterility. The sterilization of the product is guaranteed only to a certain date marked on the package, and this date must be checked.

Preparing Trays

A variety of minor surgical procedures are performed in the medical office, and each requires several instruments. Proper setup of the surgical tray is a vital part of the surgical process. The medical assistant must become familiar with the provider's preference for particular items and the way they are to be arranged for use. Until you are certain about the details of a particular procedure, you might keep a notebook handy for reference. Many offices keep a card file or computerized listing. Figure 49–2 shows an example of a specific surgical instrument tray setup and supplies commonly used in minor office procedures.

The room where the surgery will take place and the sterile tray should be set up before the patient is escorted to the area to be prepared for the procedure. Procedure 49–1 lists the steps involved in setting up a sterile tray.

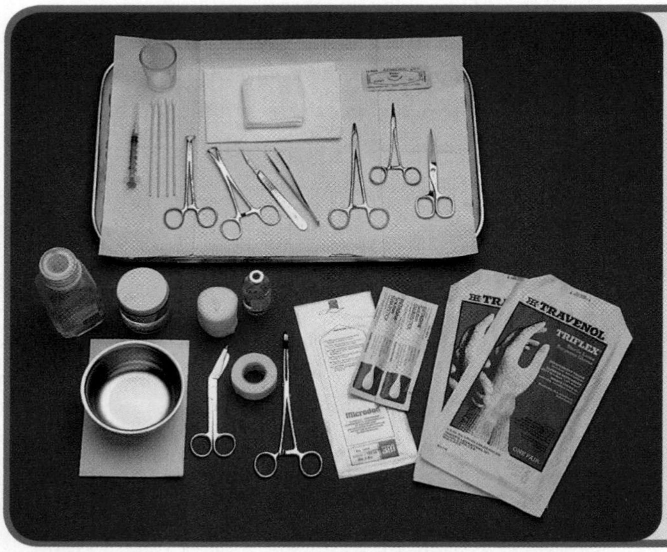

Figure 49–2: An example of a surgical tray setup.
Delmar/Cengage Learning.

PROCEDURE 49–1 Sterile Tray Setup

PURPOSE: Set up a sterile tray for a minor surgical procedure, according to the provider's preference

EQUIPMENT: Disposable sterile poly-lined drapes or sterile towels (two); Mayo instrument tray or stand positioned above the waist with stem to the right, at right angle to the counter; disposable sterile field drapes; peel-apart sterile package or autoclaved sterile package; sterile cup; container of sterile solution

S SKILL: Set up a sterile tray.

Procedure Steps	Detailed Instructions and/or *Rationales*
1. Adjust the height of the Mayo tray so that the stand is at waist level (Figure 49–3A).	

Procedure Steps	Detailed Instructions and/or *Rationales*
2. Clean the Mayo tray, starting from the center and working in a circular pattern (Figure 49–3B).	
3. Place a sterile drape package on a clean, dry surface and open the pack, exposing the sterile drape with the corners facing you (Figure 49–3C).	*You may turn the package to position its contents properly.*
4. Grasp the sterile drape by the corner and lift up enough to unfold but do not touch anything (Figure 49–3D).	*Be sure the drape does not brush up against your uniform or the counter.*
5. Grasp the opposite corner, allow the drape to unfold completely, and place the drape over the Mayo tray (Figure 49–3E). Do not reach over the drape.	*Reaching over the sterile drape will contaminate it.*

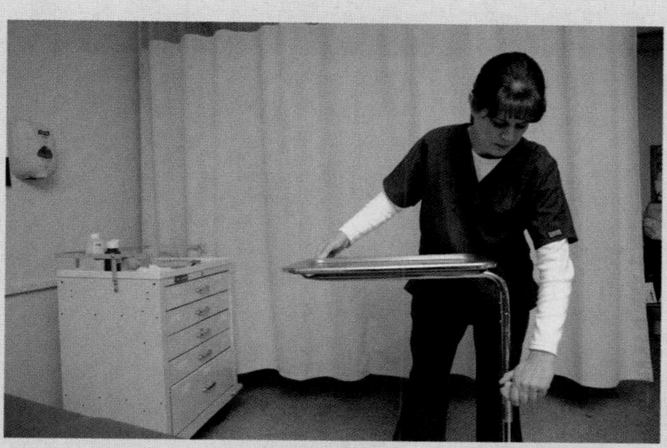

Figure 49–3A: Adjust the Mayo stand to the proper height. *Delmar/Cengage Learning.*

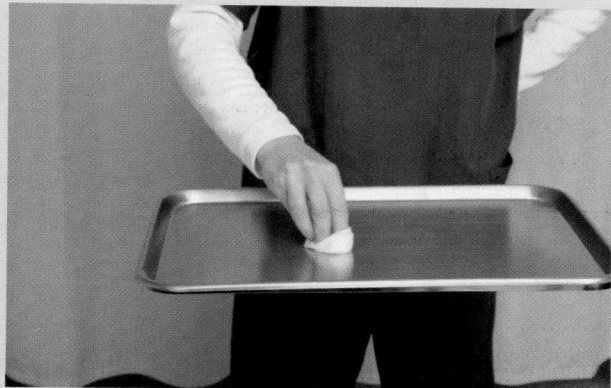

Figure 49–3B: Sanitize and disinfect the tray. *Delmar/Cengage Learning.*

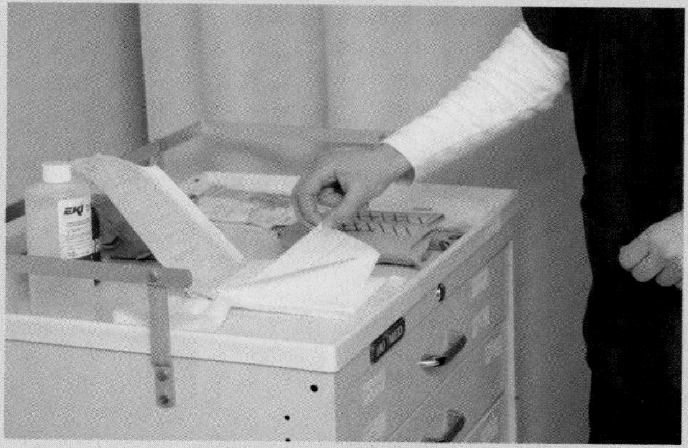

Figure 49–3C: Open the pack to expose the sterile drape with the corners facing toward you. *Delmar/Cengage Learning.*

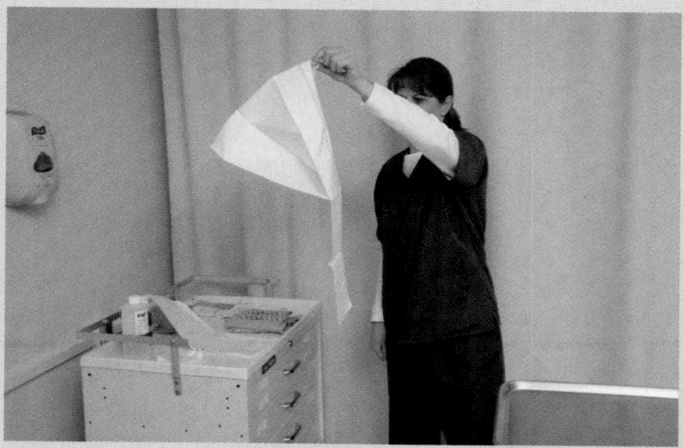

Figure 49–3D: Unfold the drape, without touching or reaching over it. *Delmar/Cengage Learning.*

(continues)

(continued)

Procedure Steps	Detailed Instructions and/or *Rationales*
6. Properly open a fanfolded (Figures 49–3F through J) or prepackaged sterile pack (Figures 49–3K and L) and allow the contents to drop onto the sterile field.	*Never reach over the sterile field because it could become contaminated.*
7. After all supplies have been dropped onto the sterile field, apply sterile gloves or use sterile transfer forceps to arrange the instruments on the field according to the provider preference (Figure 49–3M). Pour any solutions as appropriate (Figure 49–3N).	
8. Place a sterile drape over the field to protect it until the procedure begins (Figure 49–3O).	

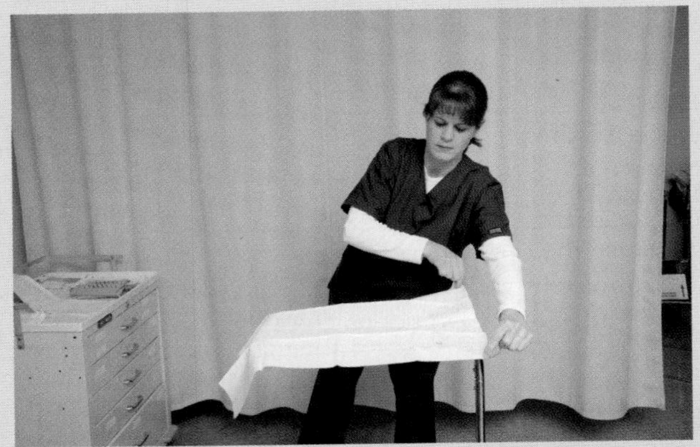

Figure 49–3E: Grasp the opposite corner of the unfolded drape and place the drape over the Mayo tray, without reaching over the drape. *Delmar/Cengage Learning.*

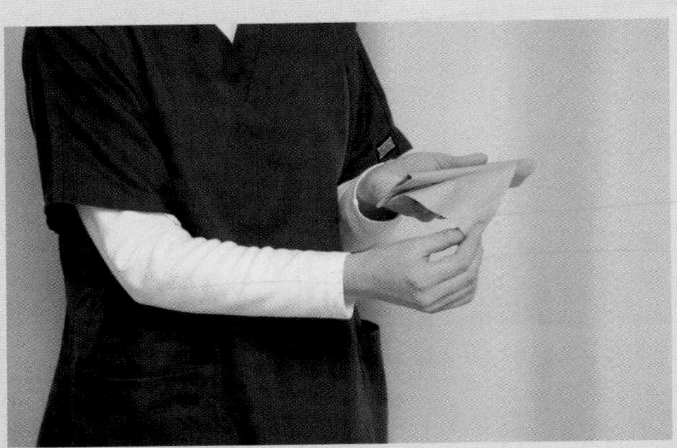

Figure 49–3F: To properly open a fan-folded sterile pack onto the sterile field, begin by grasping the tape on the top flap, and opening the flap away from you. *Delmar/Cengage Learning.*

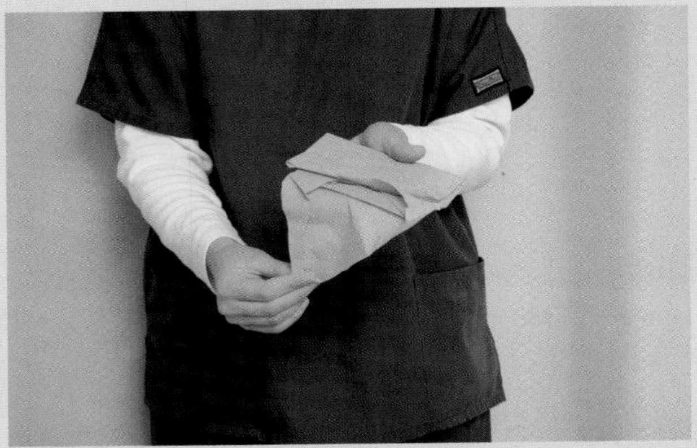

Figure 49–3G: Gently unroll the pack in the palm of your hand, being careful not to touch the inside of the pack. *Delmar/Cengage Learning.*

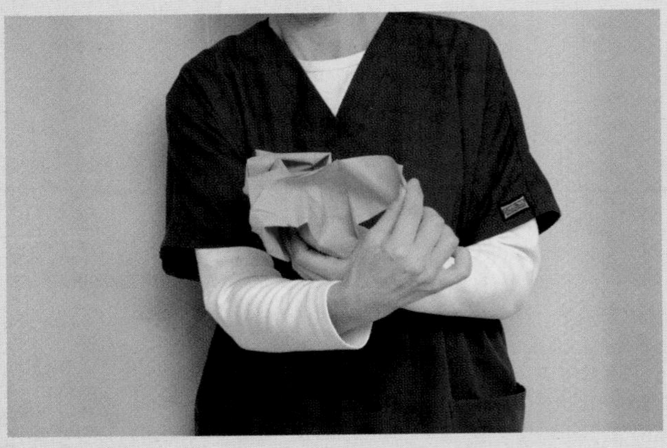

Figure 49–3H: Grasp the tips of the side flaps and unfold them by reaching around the side or under the pack. Do not reach over the pack. *Delmar/Cengage Learning.*

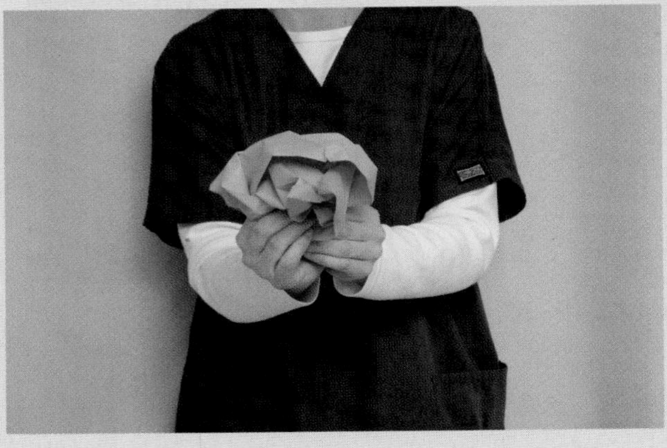

Figure 49–3I: Gather all the flaps together in the palm of your hand so they are back out of the way when the item is dropped onto the field. *Delmar/Cengage Learning.*

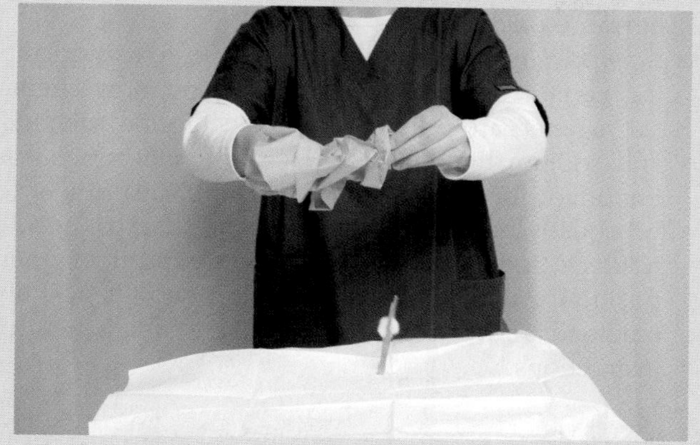

Figure 49–3J: Drop the instrument onto the sterile field. *Delmar/Cengage Learning.*

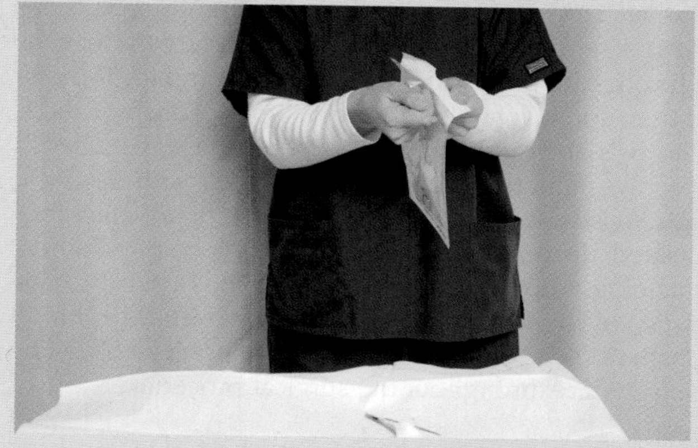

Figure 49–3K: To properly open a sterile peel-apart pack onto the sterile field, begin by grasping the flaps. *Delmar/Cengage Learning.*

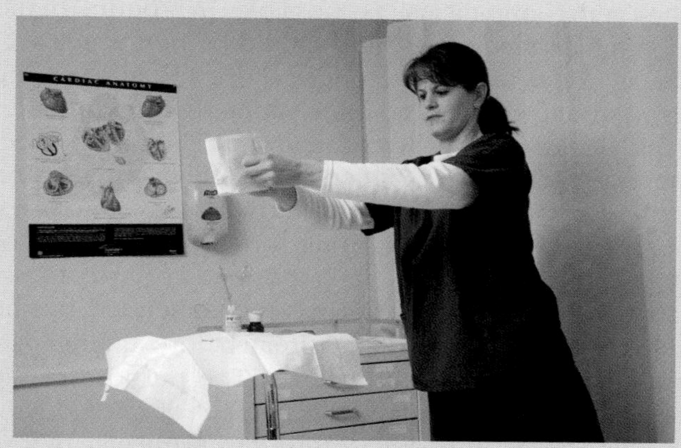

Figure 49–3L: Turn the pack so that the instrument will fall easily onto the sterile field when released. Drop the instrument onto the sterile field. *Delmar/Cengage Learning.*

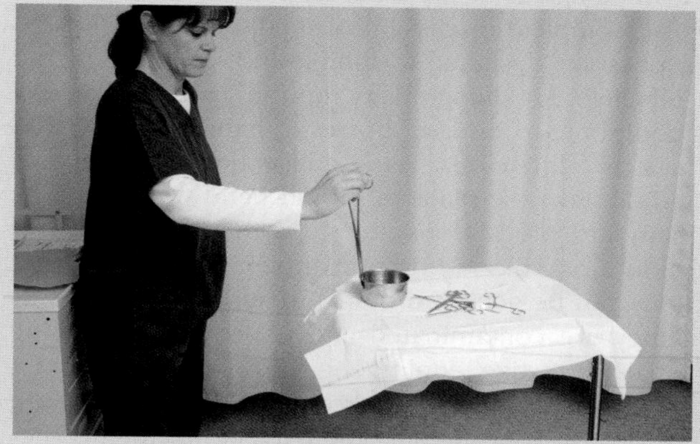

Figure 49–3M: Transfer forceps (or sterile gloves) may be used to arrange the instruments on the tray in the proper order. *Delmar/Cengage Learning.*

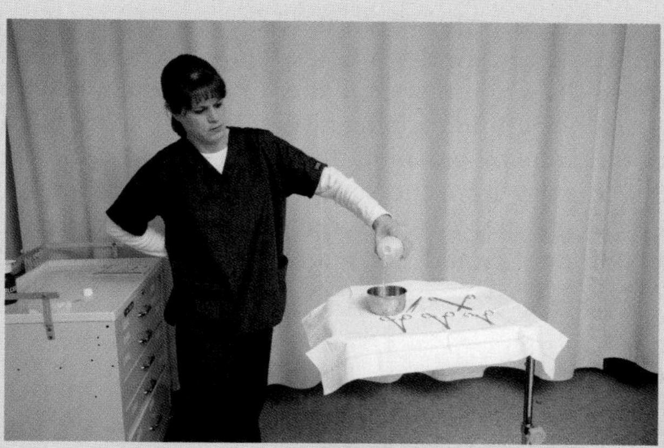

Figure 49–3N: Pour any solutions as appropriate. *Delmar/Cengage Learning.*

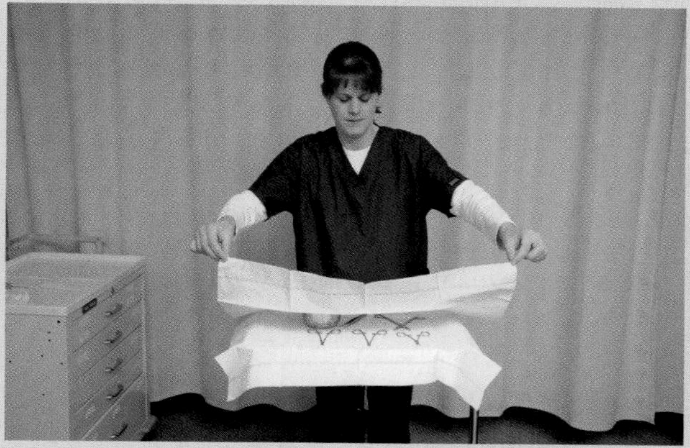

Figure 49–3O: Grasp another sterile drape by the corners and cover the sterile tray until the procedure begins. *Delmar/Cengage Learning.*

SURGICAL ASEPSIS

Asepsis is defined as freedom from disease-causing agents such as microorganisms, viruses, and drug-resistant bacteria. The purpose of asepsis is to protect the patient and health care professional from disease and to stop disease from spreading. There are two types of asepsis, medical asepsis and surgical asepsis. Medical asepsis aims to reduce the number of microbes associated with diseases. **Surgical asepsis** is the total removal of all microbe-associated diseases. Even in minor surgery procedures, maintaining asepsis by aseptic technique is critical to the recovery of the surgical site and to the overall health of the patient. **Aseptic technique** is the process of maintaining sterility throughout the surgical procedure.

Methods of Asepsis

Medical asepsis can be obtained through hand washing or cleaning agents such as antiseptics. (Refer to Chapter 36 for a complete discussion of medical asepsis.) Hand antiseptics are designed to inhibit and kill bacteria and are effective in killing many of the harmful bacteria that contribute to disease; however, hand antiseptics do not destroy all bacteria. Hand antiseptics are useful but should not take the place of proper hand washing.

Standard precautions are steps that reduce risk of infection from blood-borne pathogens. Standard precautions can be achieved by (1) treating all body fluids as if they are contaminated and (2) correctly donning personal protective equipment (PPE) such as gloves, masks, gowns, and eye protection. Employers are responsible for training all employees on standard precautions. Other safety measures include having policies and procedures in place that explain medical asepsis and standard precautions.

Surgical asepsis is obtained through sterilization. Sterilization is defined as the process of destroying all disease-causing microorganisms. Effective sterilization in the office setting is imperative in eliminating inadvertent **contamination** with disease-causing microorganisms. Selecting the type of sterilization depends on the item to be sterilized; many manufacturers suggest the best way to decontaminate and sterilize their instrumentation. Sterilization can occur by autoclave, dry heat, gas, and chemical agents. Steam is the most widely used method of sterilization.

Sterilization Techniques

- *Autoclave:* The autoclave renders sterility by a combination of steam and pressure.
- *Dry heat:* Dry heat sterilization is accomplished by raising the temperature of surgical instrumentation to the designated temperature that renders it sterile.
- *Gas sterilization:* Sterilization by gas occurs with ethylene oxide.
- *Chemical agents:* Chemicals can be used as sterilants for certain surgical instruments. Common chemical agents are glutaraldehyde, chlorine dioxide, and sodium hypochlorite. During sterilization, it is important for all parts of the surgical instrument to be equally exposed to the sterilant. Clamps, needle holders, and scissors should be sterilized in open position. All other instrumentation should be fully emerged and sterilized according to manufacturer instructions.

Scrubbing

Before you put sterile gloves on, you must perform a complete and careful hand washing to remove as many microorganisms as possible. A routine hand washing for medical asepsis should be performed vigorously for at least 15 seconds before and after seeing each patient, before and after eating, before and after using the restroom, before and after handling specimens or any soiled or contaminated materials, and after removing gloves. Skin carries many microbes, and a thorough hand washing for surgical asepsis, or surgical **scrub**, should be performed for two to six minutes (or the length of time recommended by the antimicrobial soap manufacturer) before taking part in any sterile surgical procedure. The purpose of the surgical scrub is to reduce the number of microorganisms and make the skin surgically clean. Just before the surgical scrub, you should put on the appropriate personal protective equipment (PPE). This can include face shield or face mask and eye protectors (goggles). The gown, gloves, and sterile drying towel should be laid out before the surgical scrub is completed. All hand and wrist jewelry must be removed prior to conducting the surgical scrub. Refer to Procedure 49–2 for instructions for performing a surgical scrub. Dry hands and forearms by grasping the sterile towel by the corner and away from the sterile field. When drying, the medical assistant must be careful not to recontaminate the skin and should not retrace any of the skin with the towel.

Gowning

Donning a sterile gown is a must for anyone assisting is surgery. The medical assistant will be required to don a sterile gown when participating in surgery and might also be required to assist the provider in donning sterile attire (Figure 49–4). The procedures for donning a sterile gown are described in Chapter 36.

PROCEDURE 49–2 Hand Washing for Surgical Asepsis

PURPOSE: To reduce the number of microorganisms on the skin and make the skin surgically clean

EQUIPMENT: Personal protective equipment (eye protection, mask), sterile gloves, surgical scrub agent, surgical sink, sterile dry towel

S SKILL: Perform a surgical scrub.

Procedure Steps	Detailed Instructions and/or *Rationales*
1. Don all personal protective equipment needed (eye protection, mask).	
2. Lay out sterile dry towel and gloves.	
3. Remove all hand and wrist jewelry.	*Jewelry harbors microbes.*
4. Open surgical scrub agent and place in sink area.	(If using impregnated scrub sponge)
5. Turn on water by using the automatic sensor or foot and knee controls. Wet hands and forearms, keeping hands pointed upward (during the entire procedure).	Hands should be held away from the body and higher than the elbows at all times during the procedure.
6. Using the nail stick, clean under each nail. Drop the nail stick in the sink and rinse hands.	
7. Wet hands and forearms up to the elbow, starting with the fingers and working down.	
8. Scrub one side (hands and forearms up to the elbow), using the surgical scrub agent, starting from the fingers and working down. Rinse.	Do not go over a section that has already been scrubbed.
9. Scrub the opposite side, using the same steps as in step 8. Drop the scrub brush in the sink. Rinse. The entire rinse should take between two and six minutes.	
10. Turn off the water with the automatic sensor or foot and knee control.	
11. Pick up the sterile dry towel, and, keeping it several inches from your body, start at the fingertips of one side and pat dry all the way up to the elbow. Repeat this procedure with the opposite side of the arm, using the opposite side of the towel. Apply sterile gloves.	Do not rub the towel back and forth. Remember to continue to hold the hands and arms pointed upward.

Gloving

If the provider wishes you to assist directly with the surgical procedure, sterile gloves must be worn. Dressing changes should also be performed wearing sterile gloves to protect both you and the patient. In addition, you might assist with needle biopsies, intrauterine device (IUD) insertions, and lacerations resulting from injuries. All these procedures require sterile techniques. Additional pairs of sterile gloves should be kept nearby during the surgical procedure in case of an accidental tear or puncture. Refer to Procedure 49–4 for instructions on properly putting donning sterile gloves.

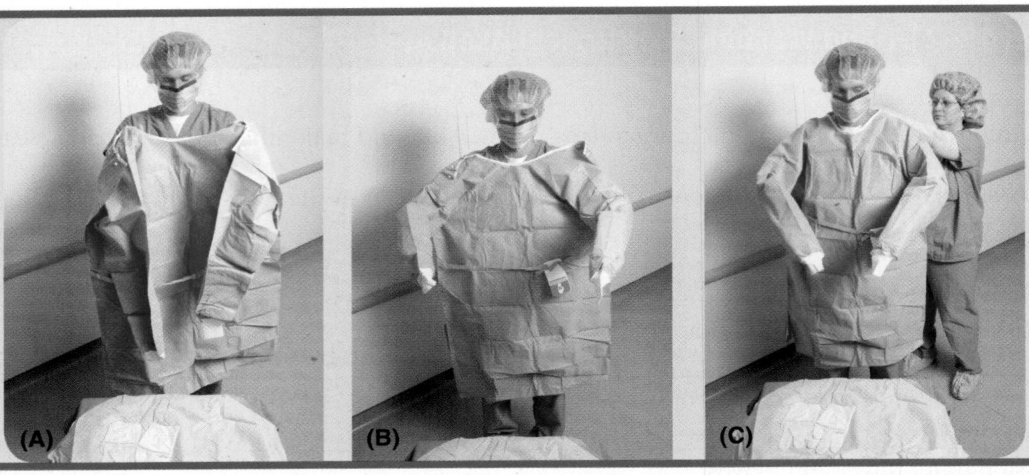

Figure 49–4A–C: Gowning. (A) Grasp gown by the neckline with both hands and allow it to unfold with the inside facing you. (B) Put hands and forearms into the gown without exposing the hands through the cuff. (C) An unsterile team member will assist with gown closure. *Delmar/Cengage Learning.*

PREPARING THE PATIENT FOR MINOR SURGERY

When the patient arrives for surgery, a consent form must be completed. An example is shown in Figure 49–6. Allow the patient time to ask any questions about the procedure and answer them adequately. The patient's signature must be on the consent form, which is filed in the chart or scanned into the patient's electronic medical record (EMR). If the patient is a minor or incompetent, the person authorized to give consent must sign for the patient following an explanation of the procedure and answering any questions. The patient's vital signs should be taken, and any complaints or problems should be recorded on the patient's chart. The patient should then empty the bladder before being positioned and draped for the procedure.

PROCEDURE 49–3 Sterile Gloving

MEDIA LINK: View the video, "Sterile Gloving," for this chapter on the Premium Website.

PURPOSE: Standing in front of a clean, clear counter surface, demonstrate the correct method of putting on sterile gloves

EQUIPMENT: Package of sterile gloves of proper size and biohazard waste bag. To comply with standard precautions, gloves and other protective barriers must be worn if there is any possibility of coming in contact with blood or any body fluids.

S **SKILL:** Apply sterile gloves.

Procedure Steps	Detailed Instructions and/or *Rationales*
1. Remove your wristwatch, rings, and other jewelry from your hands and wrists and perform hand washing for surgical asepsis, following the instructions in Procedure 49–2.	
2. Tear the seal and open the package of sterile gloves as you would open a book (Figure 49–5A). Place it on a clean counter surface with the cuff end toward your body.	Do not touch the inside of the package. *Hands would contaminate the inside of the sterile package.*

Procedure Steps	Detailed Instructions and/or *Rationales*
3. Grasp the glove for your **dominant** hand by the fold of the cuff with the finger and thumb of your nondominant hand (Figure 49–5B). Insert your dominant hand, carefully pulling the glove on with the other hand, keeping the cuff turned back.	Dominant hand is now gloved and sterile.
4. Place gloved fingers under the cuff of the other glove and insert your nondominant hand (Figure 49–5C). Put the glove on by pulling on the inside fold of the cuff (Figure 49–5D–E). Avoid touching the thumb of your dominant hand to the outside cuff of the other glove where it has been contaminated.	
5. Now both hands are gloved and sterile. Place your fingers under the cuffs to smooth the gloves over the wrists and smooth out the fingers for better fit. Check for tears and holes (Figure 49–5F).	*Any break in the integrity of the glove would not maintain sterility.*
6. Keep your hands above waist level. Do not touch anything other than items in the sterile field.	*Contact with any non-sterile object or surface will contaminate gloved hands, requiring removal and re-gloving.*
7. Remove the gloves by pulling the glove off your dominant hand with your thumb and fingers at the palm (Figure 49–5G). Pull the glove off inside-out (Figure 49–5H).	Be careful not to touch the contaminated side of the gloves when removing.
8. Slip your ungloved hand into the inside top cuff of the gloved hand (Figure 49–5I) and slip the glove off inside-out (Figure 49–5J).	
9. Deposit the gloves in a biohazard waste bag if they came in contact with body fluids or other potentially infectious material.	
10. Wash hands.	

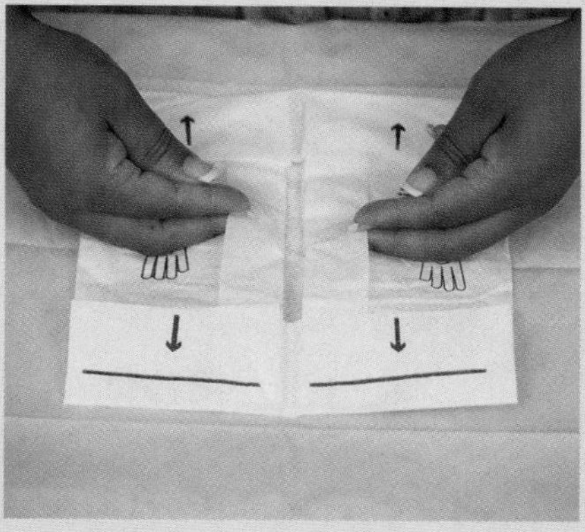

Figure 49–5A: Open the package by pulling on the center paper folds. *Delmar/Cengage Learning.*

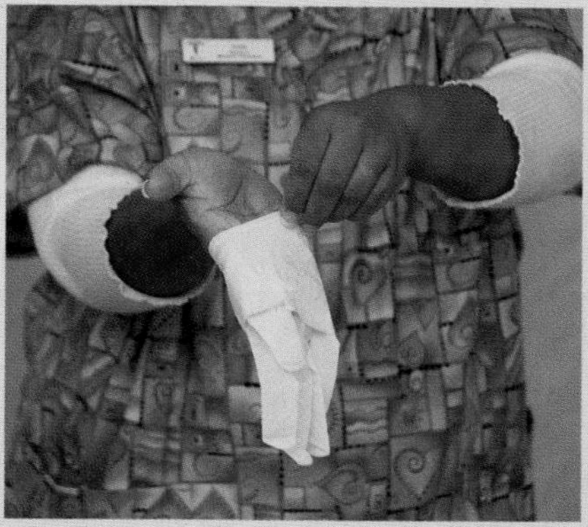

Figure 49–5B: Grasp the fold of the inside cuff of the gloves with the thumb and fingers of your nondominant hand. Insert your dominant hand, carefully pulling the glove on with the other hand, keeping the cuff turned back. *Delmar/Cengage Learning.*

(continues)

(continued)

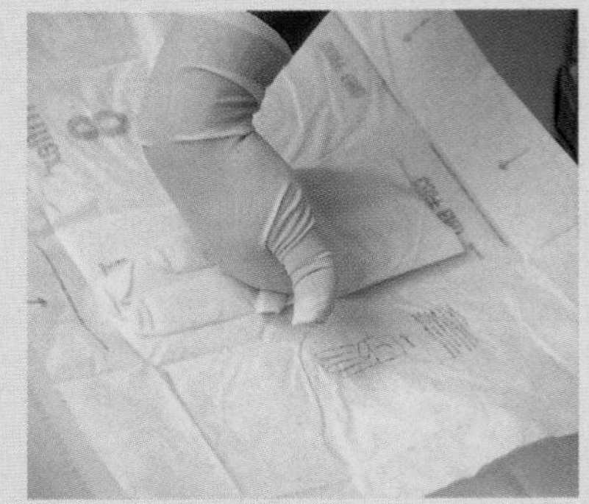

Figure 49–5C: Place gloved fingers under the cuff of the other glove. *Delmar/Cengage Learning.*

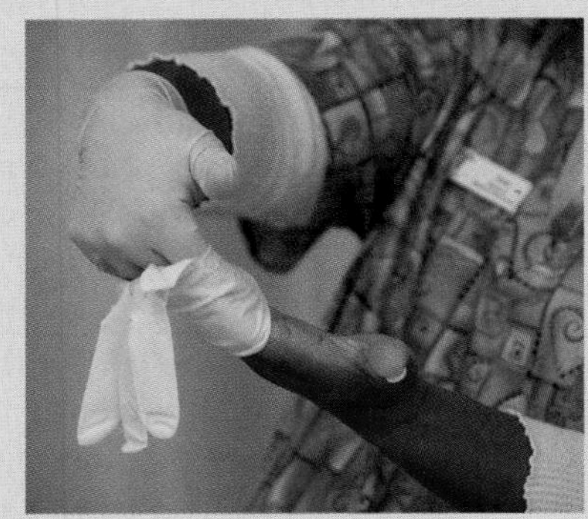

Figure 49–5D: With palm up, insert your nondominant hand. *Delmar/Cengage Learning.*

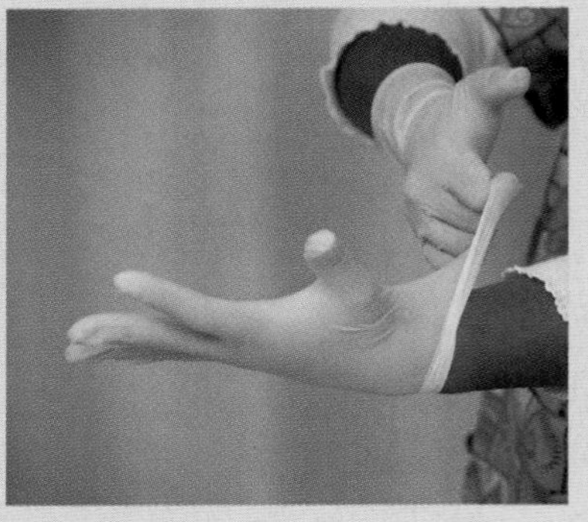

Figure 49–5E: Put on the glove by pulling on the inside fold of the cuff. *Delmar/Cengage Learning.*

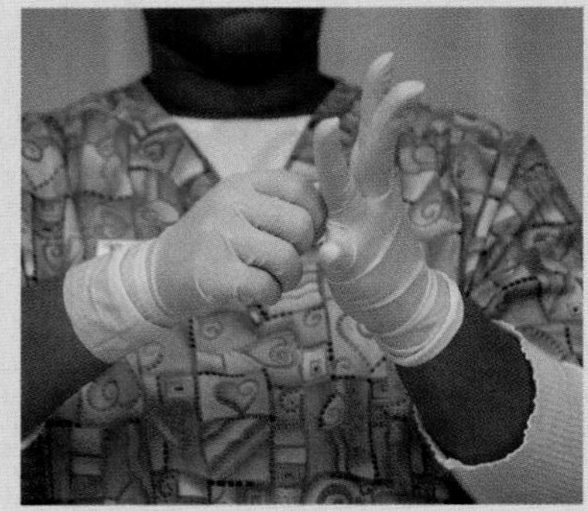

Figure 49–5F: Place your fingers under the cuffs to smooth the gloves over the wrists and smooth out the fingers for better fit. *Delmar/Cengage Learning.*

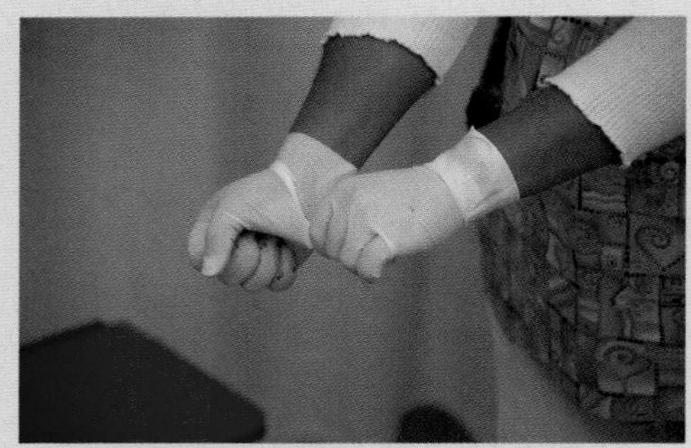

Figure 49–5G: Remove gloves by grasping the gloved palm of the dominant hand. *Delmar/Cengage Learning.*

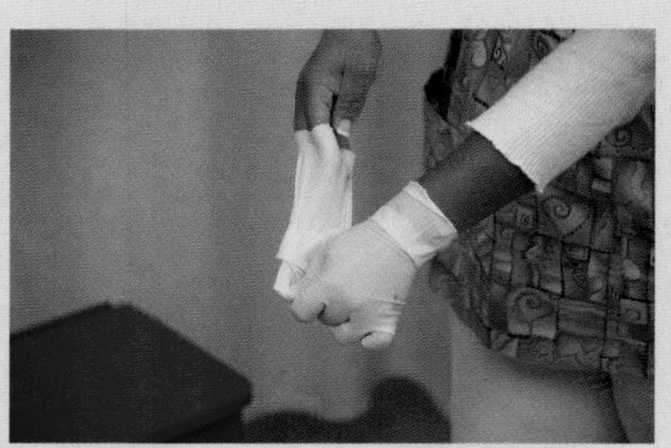

Figure 49–5H: Pull the glove off, turning the glove inside-out as it is being removed. *Delmar/Cengage Learning.*

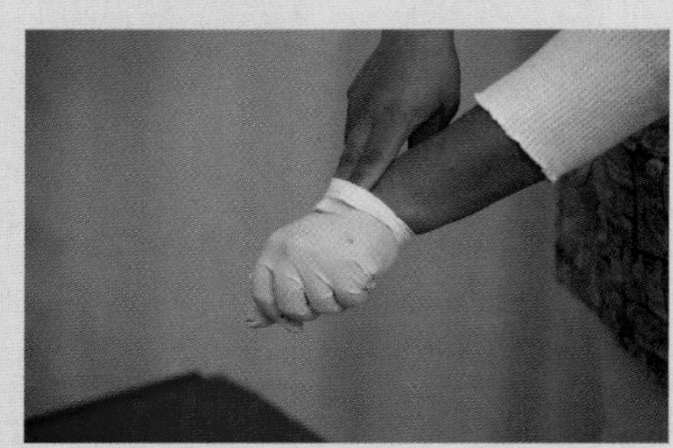

Figure 49–5I: Insert the ungloved hand inside the top cuff of gloved hand. *Delmar/Cengage Learning.*

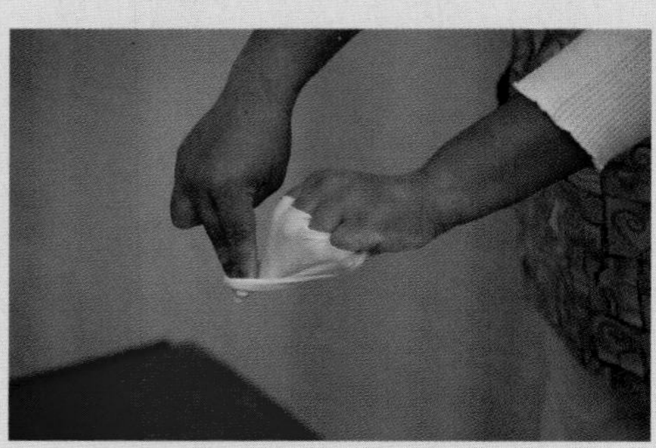

Figure 49–5J: Remove the glove, turning the glove inside-out as it is being removed. *Delmar/Cengage Learning.*

CONSENT TO OPERATE

Date __________ Time __________ AM/PM

1. I authorize the performance upon ______________________
   of the following operation ______________________
   to be performed under the direction of Dr. ______________________
2. The following have been explained to me by Dr. ______________________
   A. The nature of the operation ______________________
   B. The purpose of the operation ______________________
   C. The possible alternative methods of treatment ______________________
   D. The possible consequences of the operation ______________________
   E. The risks involved ______________________
   F. The possibility of complications ______________________
3. I have been advised of the serious nature of the operation and have been advised that if I desire a further and more detailed explanation of any of the foregoing or further information about the possible risks or complications of the above listed operation it will be given to me.
4. I do not request a further and more detailed listing and explanation of any of the items listed in paragraph 2.

Signed ______________________
(Patient or person authorized to consent for patient)

Witness ______________________

Figure 49–6: A sample consent form for surgical procedures. *Delmar/Cengage Learning.*

Positioning the Patient

The patient might need to be positioned in any of a number of numerous positions for in-office surgery procedures. The position of the patient depends on the surgical site and provider preference. All the positions mentioned in Chapter 39 are suitable for minor office surgery. The following positions are the most common:

1. Horizontal recumbant or supine
2. Prone
3. Sims'
4. Fowler's
5. Knee-chest
6. Lithotomy
7. Dorsal recumbent
8. Proctologic

When you touch anything that you are not suppose to touch

Draping

Drapes are an extension of the sterile field and are designed to prevent the spread of bacteria and **strikethrough**. During surgery, drapes provide a surface on which sterile surgical supplies can be placed during surgery. Drapes can be reusable and disposable. Disposable drapes are usually the drapes of choice in a medical office. The type of drape chosen—**fenestrated** or nonfenestrated—will depend on surgical procedure, surgical site, and provider preference (Figure 49–7).

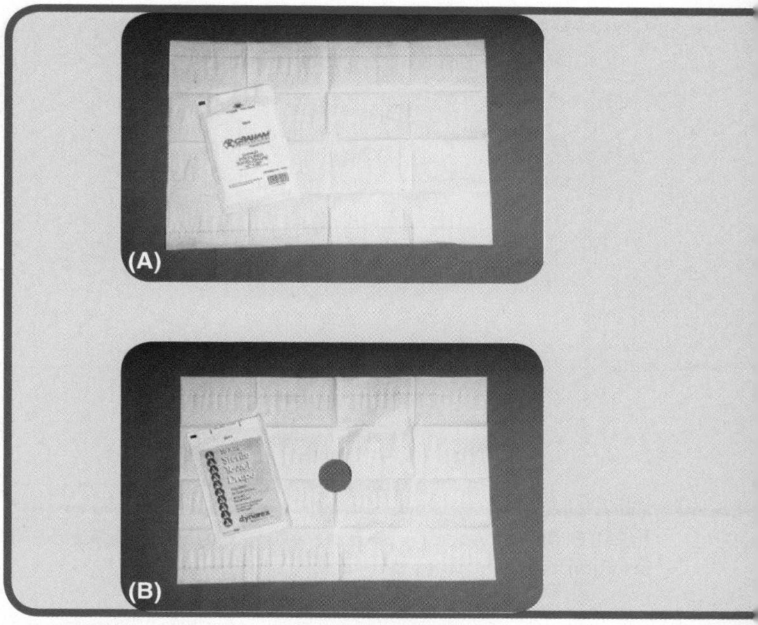

Figure 49–7: (A) Nonfenestrated surgical drapes and (B) Fenestrated surgical drapes. *Delmar/Cengage Learning.*

When draping the patient, the medical assistant must be careful to adhere to aseptic technique; follow these guidelines:

1. Always drape from the sterile to the unsterile.
2. Do not reach across a sterile area to drape.
3. Do not move drapes after they are placed.
4. Do not shake, flip, or fan drapes. Drapes should be unfolded and carefully placed in position.
5. Discard any drapes that become contaminated.

Skin Preparation

Preparation of the area of skin that will be affected by the surgical procedure is called skin prep. Many providers prefer disposable skin-prep kits that contain all the necessary items for this procedure. To protect yourself and the patient from possible disease transmission, you should wear gloves during the skin prep procedure.

Because body hair encourages **microbial** accumulation, it is sometimes shaved. You must be extremely careful to avoid nicking the patient's skin (see Figure 49–8). Microorganisms can enter the body through a break in the skin, and an infection could develop from carelessness. If the skin is nicked, the provider must be notified immediately. Practice in the procedure for this skill is necessary to become proficient.

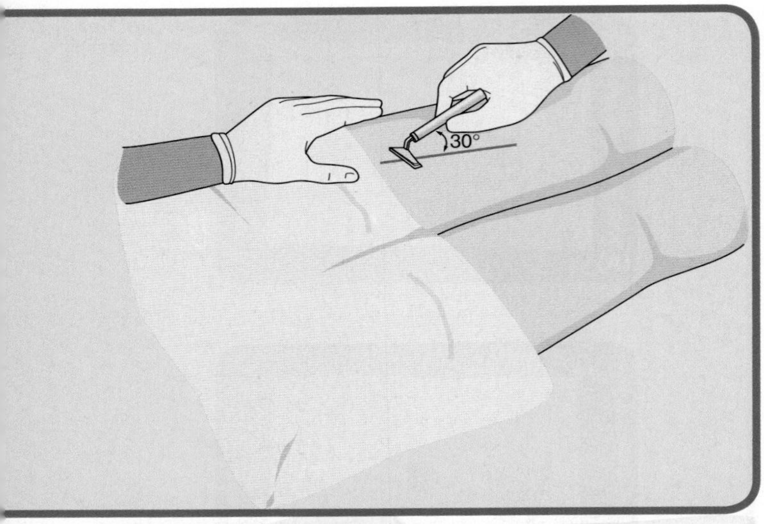

Figure 49–8: Angle for shaving a surgery site (or for suture insertion). *Delmar/Cengage Learning.*

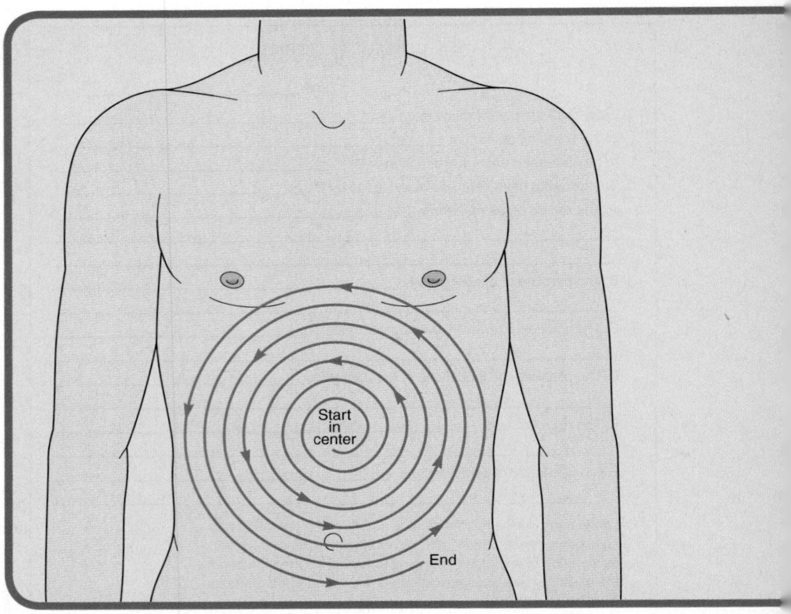

Figure 49–9: Apply all solutions to the skin in this circular pattern. Prepping the skin with an antiseptic solution should begin at the center of the incision site and proceed outward in one continuous circular motion as shown. *Delmar/Cengage Learning.*

The skin cannot be completely sterilized, or the cells would be destroyed, but an **antiseptic** can be used to reduce microbial growth prior to surgery. The antiseptic is applied after the skin has been shaved and properly cleansed. The solution is applied in a circular motion (see Figure 49–9), using care not to contaminate the area during the application.

When assisting with acupuncture procedures, preparation of the skin is simply to use an antiseptic such as alcohol. (If the skin is obviously dirty, wash the area with soap and water and dry it before proceeding.)

Refer to Procedure 49–4 for preparing a patient's skin for minor surgery.

PROCEDURE 49–4 Prepare Skin for Minor Surgery

PURPOSE: Demonstrate each of the steps required in the skin prep procedure. *In the institutional setting, preparing the forearm might be sufficient; moreover, the shaving process can be demonstrated by using a razor with no blade.*

EQUIPMENT: Small basin for soap solution, 4 × 4-inch gauze squares (sponges), disposable razor, scissors, antiseptic soap solution, emesis basin for disposables, gooseneck lamp, sterile drape sheet or towels (or fenestrated drape sheet), latex or vinyl gloves, and skin antiseptic. To comply with standard precautions, gloves and other protective barriers must be worn if there is any possibility of coming in contact with blood or any body fluids.

S SKILLS: Prepare skin for a minor surgical procedure.

Procedure Steps	Detailed Instructions and/or Rationales
1. Assemble all items and wash and glove hands.	
2. Introduce yourself and identify the patient.	*Speaking to the patient by name and checking the chart ensures that you are performing the procedure on the correct patient.*

B 3. Explain the procedure to the patient, ***including the rationale for why the procedure is being performed, using language the patient can understand.*** Ask the patient to remove necessary clothing and explain where the patient should put any belongings. Assist the patient if necessary.	
4. Assist the patient into the proper position on the treatment table and drape with a sheet or light bath blanket as directed by the provider.	
5. If appropriate, apply an absorbent towel underneath area to be shaved to catch water. Adjust the gooseneck lamp to light the area.	
6. Place gauze squares in the soapy solution and use one at a time to soap the area to be shaved. After use, discard each in an emesis basin.	
7. When the skin prep site is covered by scalp hair, beard, or pubic hair, use scissors to clip hair in preparation for shaving. Shave hair by placing the razor against the skin at about a 30-degree angle.	Hold the skin taut for easier shaving. Shave in the direction hair grows. Wipe soap and hair from the razor with a tissue. Swish the razor through soapy water, shake excess water from it, and shave the next area. *Use caution when clipping hair with scissors and in shaving with a razor to avoid both self-injury and harm to the patient.*
8. Remove all soap and hair from the area by wetting a sterile gauze square with sterile water and wiping the area. Dry the area with sterile gauze squares. Remove the absorbent towel if used.	
9. Apply antiseptic solution to the surgery site with a gauze square held by transfer forceps or disposable skin prep kit. Begin application in the center of the site and move outward in a circular motion.	*This pattern of continuous movement ensures total coverage without contamination from untreated areas.*
10. Cover the prepared area with a sterile drape sheet or towel until the provider is ready to begin.	Instruct the patient not to touch the sterile field (either the sterile field of the surgical site or the instrument tray setup).
11. Discard disposable items and return other items to the proper storage area. Remove gloves and wash hands.	
B 12. ***Attend to the patient's comfort. Patients are usually apprehensive about even minor surgical procedures. Reassurance at this time is most important.***	

CHAPTER SUMMARY

- When scheduling minor surgery, advise the patient of the approximate length of time for the procedure, appropriate clothing to wear, fasting instructions, whether someone should accompany the patient and whether the patient should anticipate time off from work or arrange for home care. The patient should be given printed education materials at this time as well.
- Be sure the patient understands the procedure and the instructions regarding preoperative and postoperative care. Provide the patient with printed materials.
- Surgical instruments might have thumb or ring handles, ratchets, serrations, and teeth (see Figure 49–1).
- Most instruments are classified according to their function, including: (1) *cutting and dissecting* (scissors and scalpels), (2) *clamping and grasping* (hemostats, clamps, forceps, and needle holders), and (3) *dilating, probing, and visualizing* (retractors, scopes, specula, probes, and dilators). Review Table 49–1 for a list of common instruments used in minor surgery.
- Proper setup of the surgical tray is a vital part of the surgical process. The room where the surgery will take place and the sterile tray should be set up before the patient is escorted to the area to be prepared for the procedure.
- Surgical asepsis is obtained through sterilization, which is the process of destroying all disease-causing microorganisms. Sterilization can occur by autoclave, dry heat, gas, and chemical agents. Steam is the most widely used method of sterilization.
- Skin carries many microbes, and a thorough surgical scrub should be performed for six minutes before taking part in any sterile surgical procedure.
- It is also important to know how to apply a surgical gown and gloves properly. The medical assistant might also be required to assist the provider in donning sterile attire.
- When the patient arrives for surgery, a consent form must be completed and filed in the patient's chart. Allow the patient time to ask any questions about the procedure and answer them adequately.
- During skin prep, the affected area is cleansed and an antiseptic is applied in a circular motion. The area might also be shaved prior to cleansing if appropriate. To protect yourself and the patient from possible disease transmission, wear gloves during the skin prep procedure.

STUDY TOOLS

Workbook	Activities for Chapter 49
Premium Website	
MEDIA LINK	View this **Media Link** for Chapter 49: • Sterile Gloving
StudyWARE	Activities and Quizzes on the **StudyWARE™ Software** for Chapter 49
	Audio Library of medical terms
	Online access to the **Critical Thinking Challenge 2.0**
CourseMate	Activities and Quizzes for Chapter 49
WebTutor	Activities and Quizzes for Chapter 49

CHECK YOUR KNOWLEDGE

1. A fenestrated sheet is one that has a(n):
   a. fold.
   b. pleat.
   c. stain.
   d. opening.

2. Autoclaved items remain sterile for __________ if they have been properly processed and protected from moisture.
   a. 3 days
   b. 30 days
   c. 3 weeks
   d. 3 months

3. To reduce the possibility of infection from a surgical procedure, skin preparation includes:
   a. cleaning the site with a soapy solution.
   b. shaving the skin.
   c. applying antiseptic solution.
   d. all of the above.
4. Before a surgical procedure can be performed, you must obtain a:
   a. signed consent form.
   b. verbal authorization.
   c. medical history.
   d. medication list.
5. The sterile tray should be set up:
   a. just before the provider enters the room.
   b. prior to the patients entering the room.
   c. 30 minutes before the procedure.
   d. while the patient is gowning.
6. The Mayo stand should be adjusted to:
   a. waist level.
   b. hip level.
   c. be level with the countertop.
   d. be level with the exam table.
7. During skin prep, avoid nicking the skin because this could cause a(n):
   a. rough surface.
   b. infection.
   c. irritation.
   d. redness.

WEB LINKS

Integra Surgical Instruments: www.integra-ls.com/home/medical/isurgical/Miltex, Inc.: www.miltex.com

Chapter

50 Assisting with Minor Surgery

OBJECTIVES

In this chapter, you will learn the following:

KB KNOWLEDGE BASE

1. Spell and define, using the glossary at the back of the text, all the Words to Know in this chapter.
2. Describe the in-office minor surgical procedures discussed in this chapter.
3. Describe the types of anesthetics used in minor surgical procedures performed in the office.
4. List the medical assistant's duties in minor surgery performed in the office.
5. Explain the tray setup for suture removal.
6. Explain the cleanup process following an in-office minor surgery.
7. Describe important information that should be recorded on the patient's chart.

S SKILLS

1. Demonstrate wound collection procedures.
2. Demonstrate the medical assistant's role in assisting with a minor surgical procedure.
3. Demonstrate the medical assistant's role in assisting a provider to apply sutures.
4. Demonstrate suture and staple removal.

B BEHAVIORS

1. Apply principles of aseptic techniques and infection control.
2. Use language and verbal skills that enable patients' understanding.
3. Display sensitivity to patients' rights and feelings in collecting specimens.
4. Explain the rationale for performance of a procedure to the patient.
5. Show awareness of patients' concerns about the procedure being performed.

WORDS TO KNOW

anesthesia
biopsy
coagulate
cryosurgery
electrocautery
excision
exudate
hemophilia
hypoallergenic
incision and drainage (I&D)
suture

SURGICAL PROCEDURES IN THE MEDICAL OFFICE

The medical assistant might have various roles while assisting the provider with minor surgical procedures. He or she must ensure the comfort and safety of the patient and be knowledgeable enough about the procedures to assist during surgery with little or no direction, if required. Maintaining sterile technique, being knowledgeable about the provider's preferences and of the surgery being performed are critical.

Table 50–1 lists some of the common surgical procedures performed in the medical office along with some general information about each.

Outpatient, or ambulatory, surgery in recent years has become more acceptable than ever before for a number of reasons. Anesthesia has been significantly improved and causes fewer side effects in patients following surgical procedures, so patients awaken faster and easier. Also, the required time for many surgeries has decreased due to improved techniques and instruments such as the scopes used in laparoscopic surgeries. For example, an abdominal laparoscopy requires two to three very small incisions for insertion of the scope, suction, and possibly a third instrument. The gallbladder, growths, and tumors can be removed with this advanced technology. Because patients naturally feel more comfortable at home following the same-day surgery, most patients of all ages are sent home to recover and do so more rapidly than when in the hospital. Postsurgical infection rate has also declined in those patients who go home immediately following surgery. All this is highlighted by the reduced cost from the elimination of a hospital stay.

ASSISTING WITH MINOR SURGERY

Some providers prefer to perform minor surgical procedures themselves and have the medical assistant prepare the patient, the room, and the equipment only. However, other providers like to have the medical assistant directly involved in assisting with the procedure, and those providers usually have their own preference of how the instruments are set up and what duties the medical

TABLE 50–1 In-office Minor Surgical Procedures

Procedure	General Description
Laceration repair	Closing a wound or laceration by placing **sutures** or stitches or staples in the skin to hold the edges of the wound together for proper healing.
Sebaceous cyst removal	**Excision** of a small, painless sac containing a build-up of sebum, the secretion from a sebaceous gland.
Incision and drainage (I & D)	Incision into a localized infection, such as an abscess, to drain the **exudate** from the area.
Biopsy	Excision of a small amount of tissue for microscopic examination. Specimen must be preserved in a solution of 10% formalin until transported to the laboratory and prepared for examination.
Needle biopsy	Fluid or tissue cells aspirated through a needle into a syringe for microscopic examination. This specimen must also be properly preserved.
Cryosurgery	Destruction of tissue and skin lesions by using extremely cold temperatures.
Electrocautery	Removal of benign skin lesions, such as warts and skin tags, by use of electric current. This procedure is performed when a biopsy is not required and to control bleeding during a procedure.
Chemical destruction	Tissue destroyed by applying silver nitrate to the area.
Laser surgery	A concentrated laser beam (intense light beam) destroys a target area without harming the surrounding tissue.
Loop electrosurgical excision procedure (LEEP)	A thin, low-voltage, electrified wire loop removes abnormal cervical tissue. A vinegar (acetic acid) or iodine solution can be applied to the cervix prior to the procedure to help make abnormal cells more visible.
Vasectomy	The vas deferens is cut, separated, and then sealed by electrocautery or clamping. This prevents sperm from entering the semen, thus making a man sterile.
Circumcision	The removal of some or all the foreskin (the skin that covers the tip of the penis) from the penis.
Debridement	Excision of lacerated, dead, or contaminated tissue and removal of foreign matter from a wound.

assistant is expected to perform. When assisting with a surgical procedure, it is critical to maintain strict sterile technique. A break in sterile technique or a breach of the sterile field can result in an infection for the patient.

Anesthetics

Most in-office minor surgical procedures are performed under local **anesthesia**, which the provider administers. Local anesthesia causes a loss of sensation in a specific area of the body (the area in which the procedure will be performed) as opposed to general anesthesia, which causes a loss of sensation over the entire body (unconsciousness).

The most common local anesthetic agents are Xylocaine (lidocaine hydrochloride) and Novocain (procaine hydrochloride). The provider is the one to actually inject the anesthetic into the area, but you might be asked to hold the vial while the provider draws up the medication (Figure 50–1). The anesthetic usually begins to numb the area within approximately 5 to 15 minutes and will keep the area anesthetized for up to three hours. Some providers prefer to use an anesthetic with epinephrine additive to help constrict the blood vessels in the area, which prolongs the effect of the anesthetic.

Specimen Collection

In procedures requiring a biopsy for analysis, carefully labeling and handling the specimen is vital. The laboratory provides a formalin solution container for preservation of the tissue specimen. This container is sterile, and the specimen must be placed directly in the solution with sterile transfer forceps. A completed lab request form must accompany the specimen for analysis.

In certain surgical procedures, such as the removal of warts or polyps, an electrocautery device may be used

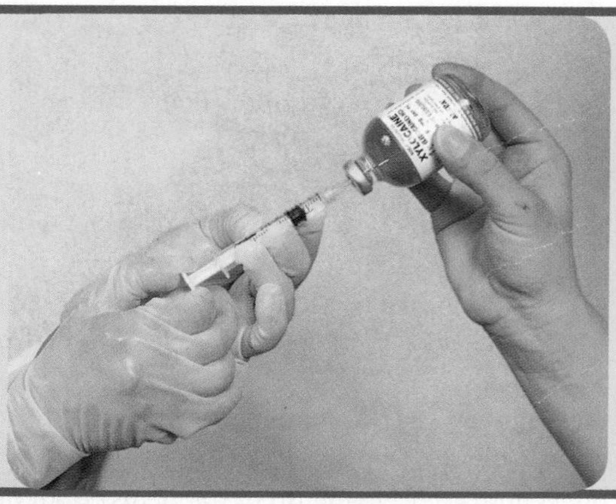

Figure 50–1: Hold the anesthetic solution in a convenient position so the provider can fill the syringe without contamination. *Delmar/Cengage Learning.*

CLINICAL PEARL

A careful medical history must be taken from the patient to determine possible allergic or adverse reactions. Ask about current medications and any over-the-counter, herbal, or diet supplements taken. This helps avoid complications during and after the procedure. If the patient discloses any significant medical history or abnormality, such as **hemophilia** (a serious blood-clotting disease in which the absence of one of the necessary blood-clotting factors prevents blood from coagulating), you should bring it to the provider's attention immediately. This information should be marked in red ink on the patient's chart. Hemophilia is a sex-linked hereditary trait that occurs mostly in males. Patients who have this diagnosis must have surgery of any type *only* at a completely equipped, well-staffed medical-surgical hospital to protect their safety and well-being.

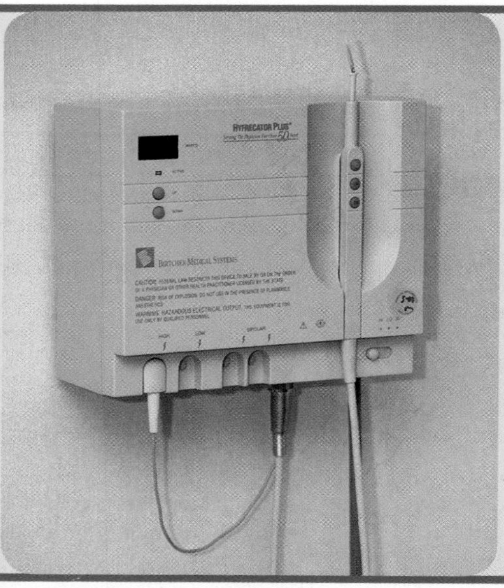

Figure 50–2: An electrocautery unit. *Delmar/Cengage Learning.*

(Figure 50–2). Often, this controls bleeding of the surgical site by electrocoagulation. Controlled high-frequency current is applied by the provider to the surgical area to **coagulate** the blood to close the incision. If the reusable tips are preferred by the provider for surgical procedures, they must be autoclaved to prevent possible cross-contamination. Disposable tips are available.

Another method for removing skin tags, warts, and other skin disorders and growths is by cryosurgery. Often, certain gynecologic treatments and surgical procedures are performed with this instrument. This process uses subfreezing temperature to destroy or remove tissue. Generally, the substances used are solid carbon dioxide or liquid nitrogen. It is sometimes referred to as cold cautery.

Bandaging

Patients will present with skin sensitivities to various materials; the type of bandage the provider orders will vary and should be appropriate for the wound and for the patient's skin. For patients who are very active or who are employed in activities that could further injure or cause the wound to become dirty or wet, the wound should be wrapped in a very thick dressing to cushion and protect it and allow it to heal. Make sure you advise the patient to keep the dressing clean and dry. Remind the patient to place a plastic bag over the extremity to keep it dry during showers or baths. If the wound is on the trunk of the body, taking a shower or bath should be discouraged unless the provider has approved it. Usually, a sponge bath is preferred until the bandage comes off. This is important in minimizing the possibility of infection.

If an infection should occur, you might be asked to obtain a specimen for laboratory analysis and culture. Procedure 50–1 explains wound collection procedures. Simply use a sterile swab and insert the tip into the center of the infected area of the wound. Then transfer the swab with the specimen into the culture medium. Provide patient education regarding care of the site and when to return for a follow-up appointment. In addition, providers advise using an elastic bandage to offer more protection and support of surgical areas of the extremities, especially for pediatric and physically active patients. Application of an ACE wrap increases circulation of the area, which hastens the healing process.

POSTOPERATIVE INSTRUCTIONS

Printed instructions should be given to the patient and explained to both the patient and family members. The patient should, of course, be given the provider's phone number and urged to phone if there are any complications or concerns. You should have a standard set of printed instructions readily available for telephone screening of those outpatient surgery patients who call in with questions or concerns. Any calls that suggest a serious problem or condition should be referred to the provider immediately. Refer to the patient education box regarding what you should caution patients about following any surgery.

PROCEDURE 50–1 Perform Wound Collection

PURPOSE: To collect a wound culture while maintaining sterile technique

EQUIPMENT: Appropriate personal protective equipment as required by procedure, sterile gloves, sterile instrumentation, ampule, and swab

S **SKILL:** Collect a sterile wound culture.

Procedure Steps	Detailed Instructions and/or *Rationales*
1. Assemble all necessary supplies.	
2. Introduce yourself and identify the patient.	The patient can be identified by asking his or her name and date of birth and checking the information in the chart.
3. Verify the provider's orders.	
B 4. ***Explain the procedure and rationale for the procedure to the patient, using language the patient can understand.***	
5. Remove the sterile swab from the container.	
6. Collect a sterile specimen. Roll the sterile swab in the exudate.	The swab should not touch any part of the wound except the exudate.
7. Insert the sterile swab back into the container and crush the ampule.	
8. Record the patient information on the container.	
9. Document the procedure in the patient's chart.	

PATIENT EDUCATION

Usual care of patient:

1. Keep site clean and dry.
2. Place no stress on the area.
3. Drink plenty of fluids.
4. Get proper rest.
5. Eat a sensible, well-balanced diet.
6. Return for follow-up appointment.

Patients should report to the provider any of the following:

1. Unusual pain, burning, or other uncomfortable sensation
2. Swelling, redness, or other discoloration
3. Bleeding or other discharge
4. Fever above 37.7°C (100°F)
5. Nausea and vomiting
6. Any other problem or symptom

Make sure that return appointment visits are confirmed and reminder cards are given to patients before they leave the office. Phoning patients the next day is an excellent way to follow up and reassures them that you and the provider are genuinely concerned about their progress. It will also bring to the provider's attention any problems that could be eliminated early. If patients do have complaints, it is best to have the provider check the problem as soon as possible.

Follow-up visits are essential so that assessment of progress can be made by the provider and sutures or staples can be removed. Specific instructions, such as soaking or applying topical medications, will be given by the provider for certain individual cases. Providers generally instruct patients (or teach you how to instruct patients) about packing or special bandaging procedures such as with ingrown toenail removals. Providers can prescribe an analgesic for minor pain and discomfort the patient might experience following the procedure.

DOCUMENTING SURGICAL PROCEDURES

Like all procedures, surgical procedures are to be documented in the medical record thoroughly and completed immediately. The medical record entry should include:

- *A patient identifier:* The patient's name or patient ID number can be used.
- *Informed consent:* Informed consent should be obtained from the patient before the procedure.
- *The date and time:* The date and time of the procedure should be recorded. The provider might also request the start (time of incision) and stop time of the procedure to be recorded.
- *The reason:* The provider should record in the patient chart the reason for the surgical procedure.
- *The procedure:* The provider or the medical assistant should record the procedure to be done. If the medical assistant records the procedure, it should be rechecked with the provider.
- *Specimen:* Specimen removal should be documented. The medical assistant documents what the specimen is and its source. The medical assistant also labels the specimen container with the patient's name and other patient-identifying information (name, date of birth).
- *Postoperative instructions:* The medical assistant is responsible for ensuring that the patient or his or her caregiver understands the postoperative instructions.

Procedure 50–2 lists the general steps involved when assisting with a minor surgical procedure.

PROCEDURE 50–2 Assist with Minor Surgery

PURPOSE: To demonstrate (insofar as possible) each of the steps required in assisting with minor surgery

EQUIPMENT: Basic sterile setup: needle and syringe; needle holder; appropriate suture, scalpel handle, and blade; thumb forceps; surgical scissors; hemostats; retractor; three or four pairs of latex or vinyl gloves; gauze squares; cotton-tipped applicators; alcohol pad; fenestrated sheet or towels; towel clamps; bandages; bandage scissors; tape; ordered anesthetic; antiseptic (small glass container for antiseptic solution); plastic biohazard sharps container and waste bag (and waste receptacle); patient's chart; pen; histology request form for laboratory analysis if a biopsy is indicated; Mayo tray table; and proper lighting (extra backup sterile setup) *NOTE:* **Some of the equipment might differ according to the procedure performed.**

S **SKILL:** Demonstrate the medical assistant's role in assisting with a minor surgical procedure.

Procedure Steps	Detailed Instructions and/or *Rationales*
1. Wash hands.	
2. Assemble the appropriate equipment and supplies.	Assemble supplies on a counter or table near a Mayo tray. Position the Mayo tray table next to the treatment table and check the condition and expiration dates of sterile items. *If an item is expired or the package shows signs of improper conditions, items might no longer be sterile.*
3. Correctly set up a sterile tray, maintaining sterile technique, and cover it with a sterile drape per office policy.	Refer to Procedure 49–1 for setting up a sterile tray.
4. Introduce yourself and identify the patient.	
B 5. ***Explain the procedure and rationale for the procedure to the patient, using language the patient can understand.*** Ensure that the patient has signed the informed consent form. Advise the patient to empty the bladder. If a biopsy is to be taken, complete a lab request form for histology analysis.	*A signature on the consent form is absolutely essential before any invasive procedure is performed.* *Emptying the bladder ensures the patient's comfort during the procedure. Anxiety often results from the urge to void.*
6. When the patient returns, take vital signs and record.	*Vital signs must be within acceptable limits to proceed with the procedure.*
B 7. Instruct the patient to disrobe as necessary for the procedure and advise where to place any belongings. Assist the patient if needed. ***Allow privacy and ask the patient to let you know when he or she is ready for positioning.***	
B 8. Assist the patient to the treatment table and into the desired position for surgery. Perform a skin prep procedure. ***Give the patient support and understanding and answer any questions at this time.*** Drape the patient appropriately.	Refer to Procedure 49–4 for preparing a patient's skin for minor office surgery.
9. When the provider is ready to begin the procedure, remove the sterile towel from the prepared sterile setup. Assist the provider by handing sterile gloves (if indicated) and assist with drawing up anesthesia as needed.	Use an alcohol prep to wipe the top of the anesthetic vial and hold it for the provider to draw out the amount needed.
10. If you are to assist with the surgical procedure, wash hands and put on sterile gloves. Hand instruments and other sterile items to the provider as needed; mop excessive blood with gauze sponges as needed.	If additional sterile items are needed during the procedure, open the package and hand it to the provider for removal or drop it onto the center of the sterile field.
11. Assist with collecting any specimen as needed by the provider.	If a biopsy is to be performed, take special care to preserve the specimen. Deposit the specimen directly into an open specimen container. Label and attach a completed laboratory requisition when the procedure is completed.
12. Assist with suturing or stapling the incision as needed by the provider.	You might assist the provider in suturing the incision by clipping each individual suture after the provider ties the knot. You should perform any other assistance as directed by the provider during the procedure.
13. When the surgery is completed, assist in (or perform) cleaning and bandaging the surgery site, remove gloves, and wash hands.	If the patient is allergic to adhesive, use **hypoallergenic** tape to secure the bandage.

(continues)

(continued)

Procedure Steps	Detailed Instructions and/or *Rationales*
14. ***Attend to the patient's comfort by helping the patient into a sitting position to regain balance and, when stable, from the table. Assist in dressing if necessary.***	
15. Give the patient postoperative instructions.	Instructions should include education regarding any return visit, care of surgery site, and any other orders from the provider.
16. Document the procedure in the patient's chart.	
17. Put on gloves and clean up the treatment area. Wash hands and restock treatment room.	Clean up treatment table, discard contaminated items in a biohazard waste bag, rinse the instruments with cold water and place in a detergent solution, remove gloves and wash hands, and restock the room.

APPLYING SUTURES

The term *suture* means a type of thread that joins the skin of a wound, either an accidental laceration or a surgical incision, together. A type of suture called catgut is eventually absorbed by the body and does not need to be removed (generally used in major surgeries). It is made from the intestines of sheep. Suture is also made of a material such as silk, nylon, or other manufactured substances that must be removed in a matter of days, depending on the area of the body in which they are inserted. For convenience, most providers prefer to use suture that has a needle already attached. Figures 50–3A and B shows examples of different types of suture materials and needles used in closing wounds.

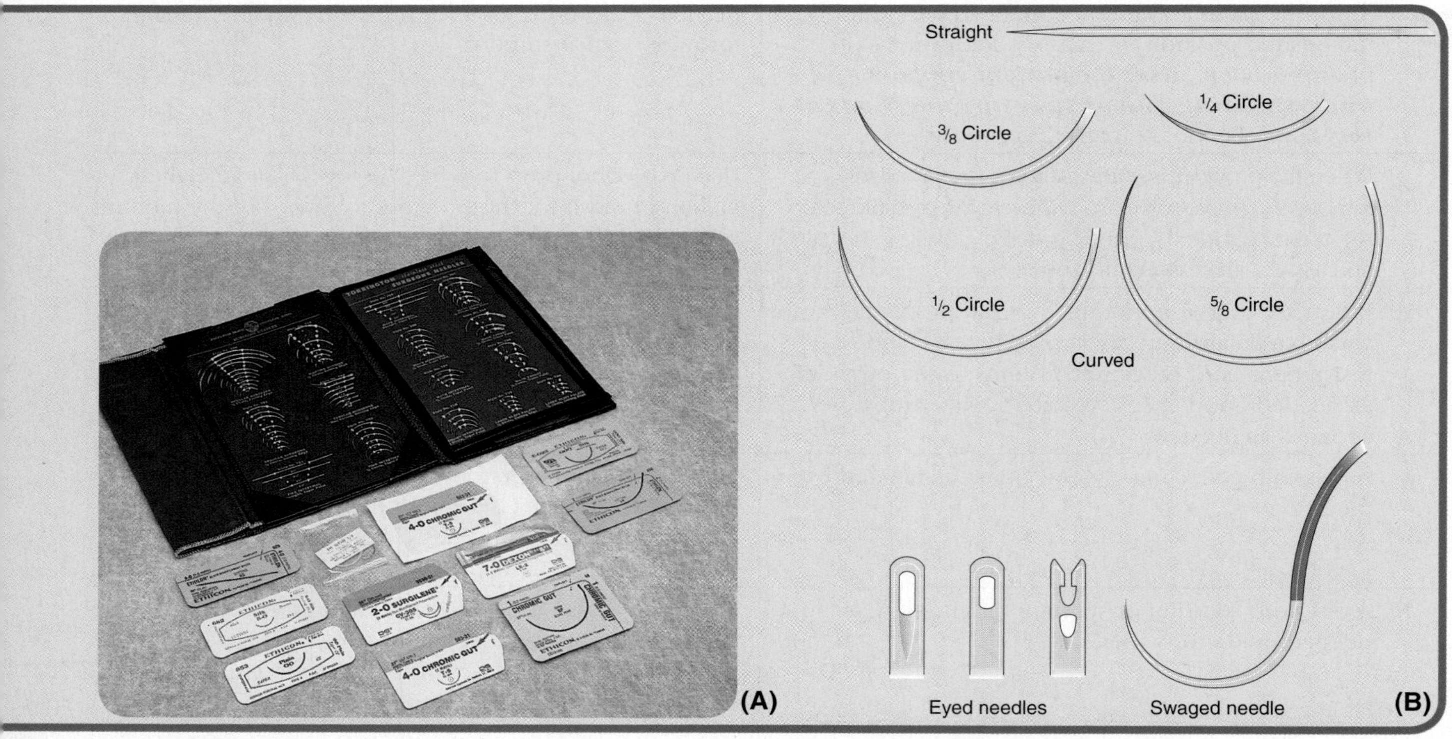

Figure 50–3A–B: (A) A variety of suture packs and curved and straight surgical needles. (B) Various needle shapes used in the insertion of sutures to close wounds. *Delmar/Cengage Learning.*

Most offices have a policy regarding the treatment of lacerations. If the injury is severe and might result in serious blood loss, it is usually treated in the emergency room or trauma center. However, many patients will come to their primary care physician to have a laceration sutured. Working these patients into an already full schedule can present delays for other patients waiting for scheduled appointments. Prepare the patient for the provider and assist as needed. After the suturing is complete, the provider can see other patients while you take care of the laceration patient and clean up the work area.

Your efficiency and expedient preparation of setting up the treatment room will be appreciated by both the provider and the patient in this situation. Follow the steps in Procedure 50–3 for assisting with suturing a laceration. Always make sure that you record the number of sutures (stitches) the provider inserts and the anatomical location. Go over patient education and any additional instructions from the provider before the patient leaves the office. If the patient is given instructions by the provider to redress and bandage the wound at home, show the patient how to do this. Alert patients to call with any questions or concerns.

PROCEDURE 50–3 Assist with Suturing a Laceration

PURPOSE: Demonstrate each of the steps required in the procedure to assist with suturing a laceration while maintaining sterile technique

EQUIPMENT: Items needed for skin prep: alcohol, cotton balls, PPE, biohazard bag, gauze squares, bandages and tape, bandage scissors, antiseptic, ordered anesthetic, tetanus toxoid, patient's chart, pen; sterile items: swabs, needle and syringe, latex or vinyl gloves, fenestrated drape, ordered suture material, gauze squares, hemostats, needle holder, scissors, sharps container

S **SKILL:** Demonstrate the medical assistant's role in assisting a provider to apply sutures.

Procedure Steps	Detailed Instructions and/or *Rationales*
1. Wash hands and assemble all needed items, using sterile technique.	
2. Introduce yourself and identify the patient.	*Speaking to the patient by name and checking the chart ensures that you are performing the procedure on the correct patient.*
B 3. ***Explain the procedure to the patient, using language the patient can understand and explaining the rationale for the procedure.*** Advise the patient to empty the bladder.	*Emptying the bladder ensures the patient's comfort during the procedure. Anxiety often results from the urge to void.*
4. When the patient returns, take and record vital signs.	*Vital signs must be within acceptable limits to proceed with the procedure. The patient might have lost a considerable amount of blood, which could alter vital signs.*
B 5. Ask the patient to remove necessary clothing. Explain where the patient should place any belongings. Assist the patient if needed. ***Allow privacy if needed.***	*The patient might experience weakness and might not feel well enough to be left alone.*
6. Assist the patient into the appropriate position for skin prep of the wound. Proceed with the steps for preparing skin for minor surgery and then drape the patient appropriately.	Refer to Procedure 49–4 for preparing a patient's skin for in-office minor surgery.
7. Put on PPE and sterile gloves. Arrange the instruments and other sterile items in the order the provider will use them. Remove gloves and wash hands.	*Do not reach, cough, sneeze, wave, talk, or cross over the sterile field, or it can become contaminated.* Carefully cover the sterile field with a sterile towel until the provider is ready to begin.

(continues)

(continued)

Procedure Steps	Detailed Instructions and/or *Rationales*
8. When the provider is ready to begin the suturing procedure, remove the sterile towel from the prepared sterile setup. Assist the provider by handing sterile gloves (if indicated) and assist with drawing up anesthesia as needed.	Use an alcohol prep to wipe the top of the anesthetic vial and hold it for the provider to draw out the amount needed.
9. If you assist with the suturing procedure, wash hands and put on sterile gloves. Hand instruments and other sterile items to the provider as needed; mop excessive blood from the wound with sterile gauze as needed.	Assist the provider by clipping each individual suture as directed by the provider.
10. When the wound has been closed with sutures, assist with (or perform) cleaning and bandaging the site per the provider's orders. When bandaging is done, remove and properly dispose of gloves and wash hands.	If cleaning and bandaging the site, you might need to re-glove to keep from soiling the dressing and bandage. *Some individuals are allergic to adhesive; hypoallergenic tape is then preferred.*
11. Administer tetanus toxoid if ordered.	If administered, ensure that this is documented in the patient's chart as part of the entry.
B 12. ***Tend to the patient's needs and comfort. Assist with sitting up, getting dressed, and helping from the treatment table as needed.***	*Allow the patient sufficient time to regain balance before standing alone because dizziness can occur.*
13. Give the patient postoperative instructions.	Instruct the patient in the care of sutures and provide a return appointment for their removal.
14. Document the procedure in the patient's chart.	
15. Put on gloves and clean up the treatment area. Wash hands and restock treatment room.	Clean up the treatment table, discard contaminated items in a biohazard bag and sharps container, rinse the instruments with cold water and place in detergent solution, remove gloves and PPE, and dispose of them in the biohazard bag.

SUTURE AND STAPLE REMOVAL

Patients usually see the family or general practitioner for suture removal following laceration repair from an injury. In many offices, it is the medical assistant's responsibility to remove the sutures. It is vital to check the emergency center's report regarding the number of sutures put in so you can be sure to remove all of them.

Be sure to remove the same number of sutures as were inserted by the primary care physician. Suture that is not removed can become infected, so care in removing all the material is vital. Patients sometimes report that one or two stitches have already come out during a bandage change at home. This should also be noted on the patient's chart. Follow the steps in Procedure 50–4 for suture removal. Removal of staples is performed with a staple extractor as described in the procedure for suture removal. Check the report also for a tetanus booster and record on the patient's chart to bring the immunization record up to date. Before you remove the sutures, check the number of days the provider who put them in recommended as the time to wait before removal. Ask the provider to inspect the healing wound. After the sutures or staples have been removed, providers might order additional closure materials to cover healing incisions or lacerations (Figures 50–4A through D). A support skin closure might be necessary to keep the skin together until the wound is completely healed. The type of supportive closure should be noted on the patient's chart.

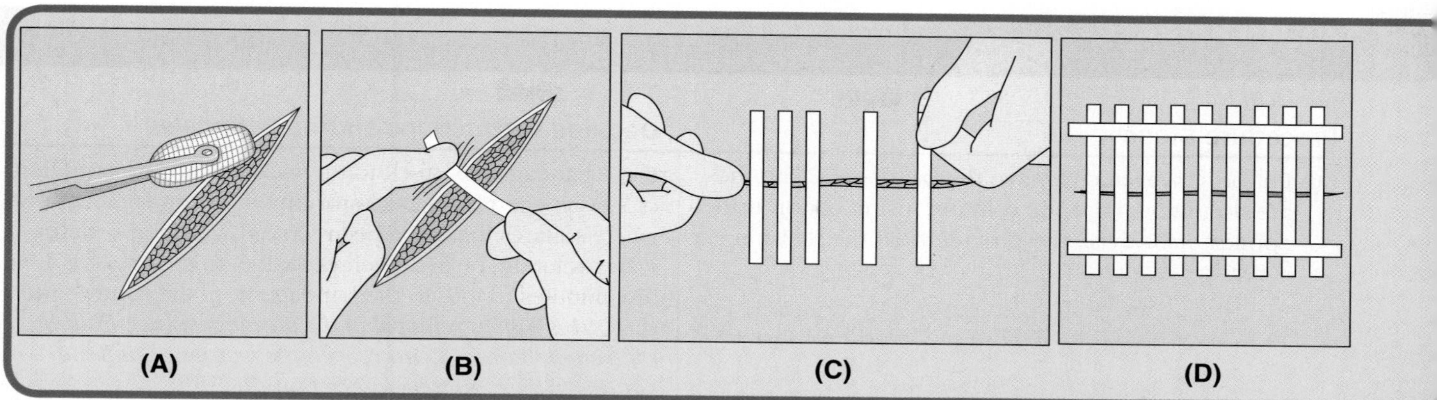

Figures 50–4A–D: (A) Care of an incision or wound with a closure application: Use transfer forceps with sterile gauze to apply antiseptic. (B) Apply Steri-Strip closure to the center of the incision. (C) Apply closures to each side for evenness and then fill in and cover the full wound area. If ordered, apply a topical medication and a sterile bandage. (D) For additional support, closures can also be applied parallel to the incision or wound. *Delmar/Cengage Learning.*

PROCEDURE 50–4 Remove Sutures or Staples

PURPOSE: Demonstrate the steps required to remove sutures (using a mannequin or model as the patient)

EQUIPMENT: Sterile: thumb forceps, suture-removal scissors (or staple extractor), gauze squares, latex or vinyl gloves, cotton-tipped applicators, butterfly or Steri-Strip™ closures; skin care and documentation: antiseptic solution, hydrogen peroxide, tincture of benzoin, basin with warm soapy water, bandages, tape, towels, biohazard waste bag, sharps container, bandage scissors, patient's chart, and pen

S **SKILL:** Remove sutures from a healing laceration or incision.

Procedure Steps	Detailed Instructions and/or *Rationales*
1. Wash hands and assemble all needed items, using sterile technique..	
2. Introduce yourself and identify the patient.	
B 3. ***Explain the procedure and rationale for the procedure, using language the patient can understand,*** and answer any questions. Ask the patient about the healing condition of the incision or laceration, take vital signs, and record them on the patient's chart.	If sutures resulted from a laceration injury, ask appropriate questions regarding where and when injury occurred and when a tetanus booster was administered [file ER report in chart]. Record.
B 4. Ask the patient to remove necessary clothing for inspection of the healing incision. Explain where the patient should place any belongings. Assist the patient if needed. ***Allow privacy if needed.***	
5. Assist the patient to the treatment table and into the required position and drape appropriately.	

(continues)

(continued)

Procedure Steps	Detailed Instructions and/or *Rationales*
6. Put on gloves and remove the bandage. Clean the incision with antiseptic solution, using cotton-tipped applicators. Advise the provider that the incision site is ready.	If the bandage has stuck to the incision (record condition of site on chart [e.g., excessive blood or drainage]), apply gauze squares that have been soaked with soapy warm water solution, or hydrogen peroxide, to the area for a few minutes to loosen the bandage from the sutures and scab. *This makes removal of the bandage easier. Pulling off a stuck bandage can reopen the wound or pull out sutures; either result would be painful.*
7. After the provider orders suture or staple removal, open a sterile package containing the necessary instruments on the Mayo tray and proceed.	*Do not reach, cough, sneeze, wave, talk, or cross over the sterile field, or it can become contaminated.* Carefully cover the sterile field with a sterile towel until the provider is ready to begin.
For Suture Removal:	
8. Grasp the knot of the suture material with thumb forceps and gently but firmly pull up, making just enough space to place the suture removal scissors to clip the suture as close to the skin as possible (Figures 50–5A and B). Pull the suture with the forceps (back) toward the healing incision so that no stress is put on it. Continue until all are removed. Count the number of sutures removed and compare with the number in the patient's chart.	*Pulling the suture away from the site could pull the incision open.* Caution: Do not pull a suture that has been on the surface of the skin (exposed to the outside) through the path of the suture being removed, or infection can develop.

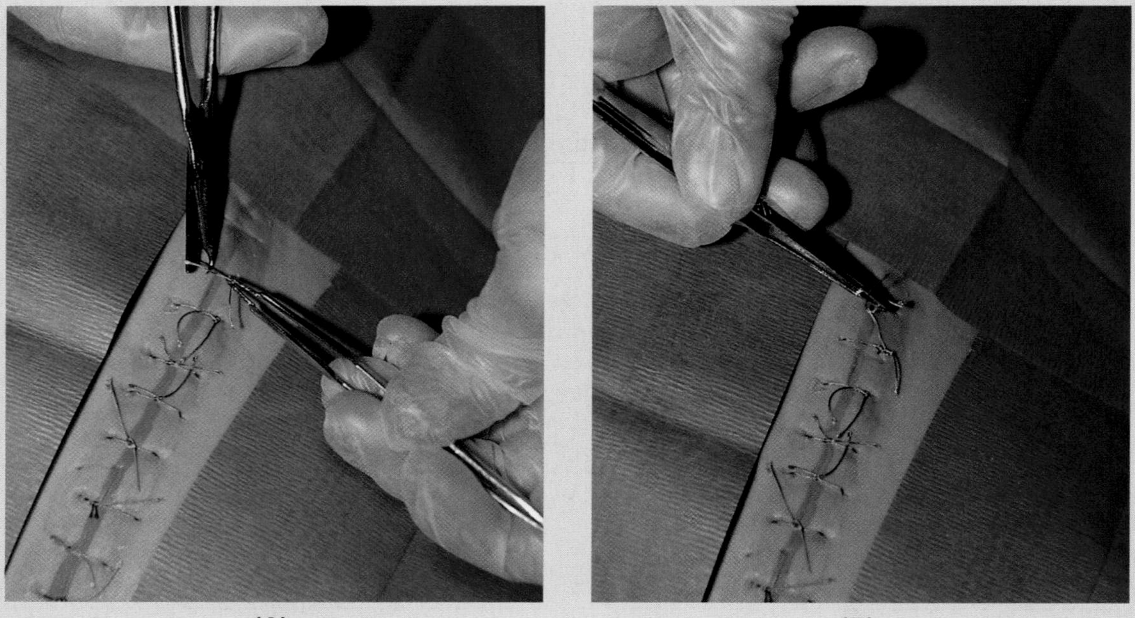

(A) (B)

Figures 50–5A–B: (A) Grasp the suture knot with thumb forceps and place the curved tip of the suture-removal scissors just next to the skin under the suture and clip. (B) Gently pull the suture up and toward the incision with the thumb forceps to remove. (Pulling the suture away from the incision can pull the incision open.) *Delmar/Cengage Learning.*

Procedure Steps	Detailed Instructions and/or *Rationales*
For Skin Staples:	
9. If skin staples are to be removed, place the sterile staple extractor under a staple (one at a time) and squeeze the handles of the extractor completely closed (Figure 50–6). Lift the staple away from the skin and dispose in a sharps container. Continue until all are removed.	Explain to the patient that he or she might feel a tugging sensation.
10. Apply antiseptic solution to the site and allow it to air dry. Apply Steri-Strips or a butterfly closure if necessary for support during the healing process and bandage.	
11. Remove gloves and wash hands.	
12. Give the patient postoperative instructions.	Instruct the patient to keep the bandage clean and dry for 24 to 48 hours or as directed by the provider. Advise the patient to avoid undue stress for the appropriate amount of time for the anatomical area. Schedule a follow-up appointment if ordered by the provider.
13. Document the procedure in the patient's chart.	Document: (1) anatomical area of incision or laceration, (2) condition of site, (3) number of sutures removed, (4) type of antiseptic applied, (5) support closures applied, (6) type of bandage applied, and (7) your signature or credentials. Be sure to include the ER report if sent from the facility where the injury was treated and record the date of the tetanus booster if applicable.
14. Put on gloves and clean up the treatment area. Wash hands and restock treatment room.	Clean up the treatment table, discard contaminated items in a biohazard bag and sharps container, place instruments in detergent solution after rinsing with cool water, remove gloves and PPE, and dispose of them in the biohazard bag.

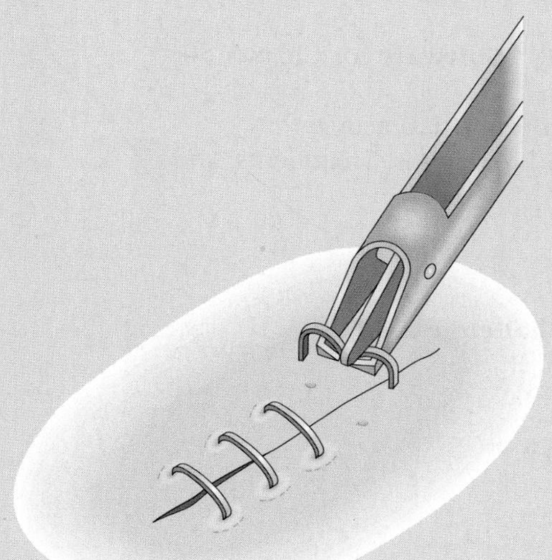

Figure 50–6: Removal of a staple: The staple extractor reforms the staple (clip). Then, the staple is then lifted from the incision. *Delmar/Cengage Learning.*

Advances in skin closures offer a sutureless substance applied to small lacerations. This type of closure is an adhesive material and is used frequently with children who can be frightened and thus uncooperative. A sutureless procedure is much quicker and less traumatic for the child and staff as well. Skin closures give support to the wound and offer the patient more flexibility.

PATIENT EDUCATION

Following suture removal, patients should be advised to:

1. Keep the site dry for at least 24 hours.
2. Cover the area to keep it clean.
3. Apply supportive bandaging as needed.
4. Report any sign of infection immediately to the provider.

CHAPTER SUMMARY

- Medical assistants should have a general knowledge of the procedures performed in their place of employment and be able to assist the provider with little or no direction. Some common procedures include laceration repair, sebaceous cyst removal, incision and drainage, biopsy, needle biopsy, cryosurgery, electrocautery, chemical destruction, laser surgery, loop electrosurgical excision procedure (LEEP), vasectomy, circumcision, and debridement.
- Most procedures are performed under local anesthesia, which the provider administers. The medical assistant might be asked to hold the vial while the provider draws up the anesthesia.
- If a biopsy is taken, careful labeling and handling of the specimen is vital. A completed lab request form must accompany the specimen for analysis.
- After a procedure, printed instructions should be given to the patient and verbally explained to both the patient and family members.
- Complete documentation includes a patient identifier, informed consent, the date and time, the reason, the procedure, any specimen collected, any postoperative instructions given, and the medical assistant's signature and credentials.

STUDY TOOLS

Workbook	Activities for Chapter 50
Premium Website StudyWARE	Activities and Quizzes on the **StudyWARE™ Software** for Chapter 50
	Complete the following **Competency Challenge 2.0** activity: • Tuesday, 11 AM: Prepare and Assist with Procedures, Treatments, and Minor Office Surgeries
	Audio Library of medical terms
	Online access to the **Critical Thinking Challenge 2.0**
learning**lab**	Module 21: Minor Surgical Procedures
CourseMate	Activities and Quizzes for Chapter 50
WebTutor	Activities and Quizzes for Chapter 50

CHECK YOUR KNOWLEDGE

1. Which of the following types of anesthesia is not used in minor surgical procedures performed in the office?
   a. Local
   b. Nerve block
   c. Topical
   d. General
2. The method used to remove skin tags and warts is:
   a. electrocautery.
   b. cryosurgery.
   c. laser surgery.
   d. both a & b.
3. Local anesthesia begins to numb an area in:
   a. 30 minutes.
   b. 5–15 minutes.
   c. 1 hour.
   d. 3 hours.
4. A serious blood-clotting disease in which the absence of one of the necessary blood-clotting factors prevents blood from coagulating is:
   a. coagulitis.
   b. hemophilia.
   c. hemophilitis.
   d. angiocoagulitis.
5. A type of suture that does not need to be removed is called:
   a. silk.
   b. nylon.
   c. catgut.
   d. all of the above.

WEB LINKS

American Association of Medical Assistants (AAMA)
www.aama-ntl.org/

Association of Surgical Technologists (AST)
www.ast.org/

Unit

17

Medication Administration Procedures

Correct and accurate medication administration is the responsibility of all health care workers at every level of care. According to the Agency for Healthcare Research and Quality (AHRQ), medication errors cost the nation approximately $37.6 billion annually—*with $17 billion of those costs being associated with preventable errors*. As many as 44,000 to 98,000 people die in hospitals each year as the result of such errors, making medication errors—even when using the lower end of the range—the eighth leading cause of death in the United States (AHRQ, 2010, retrieved from www.ahrq.gov/qual/errback.htm).

The medical assistant's role in administering medications is an important one and should not be taken lightly. Regardless of the prescriber's credentials, the ultimate responsibility for accurately providing the *right* dose of the *right* medication at the *right* time, to the *right* patient, by the *right* route lies with the person who administers the medication. This cannot be emphasized enough. The *Physician's Desk Reference* (or PDR) with supplementary publications and a nursing drug book are both invaluable office resources. Keeping up to date on and knowing how to use appropriate references help the MA ensure patient safety by correctly administering medications, recognizing adverse reactions, and providing answers to patients' questions about their medications.

Laws vary from state to state regarding to whom and under what conditions medical assistants may administer which types of medications. It is the responsibility of the person administering the medication to know whether he or she is permitted to provide a particular medication and in what setting. It is also the legal responsibility of the prescriber to know to whom he or she may delegate this task. Know your own state laws.

Proficiency with basic math skills is necessary for preparing medications. Aside from the basic function of addition, subtraction, multiplication, and division, the MA should also be able to calculate and convert fractions, decimals, percentages, and ratio proportions.

Certification Connection

	Ch. 51	Ch. 52	Ch. 53	Ch. 54
CMA (AAMA)				
Legislation: Food and Drug Administration (FDA)	X			
Legislation: Drug Enforcement Administration (DEA)	X			
Pharmacology	X			
Preparing and administering oral and parenteral medications		X	X	X
Prescriptions	X	X		
Immunizations	X			X
RMA (AMT)				
Laws, regulations, and acts pertaining to the practice of medicine	X			
Maintain records of biohazardous waste and chemical disposal	X			
Clinical pharmacology: Terminology	X	X	X	X
Parenteral medications	X		X	X
Prescriptions	X		X	
Drugs	X		X	X
CMAS (AMT)				
Pharmacology	X	X	X	X

Chapter 51 Pharmacology Fundamentals

OBJECTIVES

In this chapter, you will learn the following:

KB KNOWLEDGE BASE

1. Spell and define, using the glossary at the back of the text, all the Words to Know in this chapter.
2. Recognize and categorize many of the most commonly used prescription and non-prescription medications, including desired effects, side effects, and adverse reactions.
3. List and identify the most common drug forms.
4. Recognize and describe medical, legal, and ethical concerns regarding medications and appropriate actions to be taken for each.
5. Define *controlled substances* and describe the five schedules in which controlled substances are categorized.
6. Identify the various print and online drug reference sources that are used in the medical office to obtain information on dosages, routes of administration, side effects, and contraindications.
7. Describe proper storage and disposal of medications.

S SKILLS

1. Locate specific information on medications in the PDR.

WORDS TO KNOW

additive effect
administer
allergy
agonist
antagonist
Drug Enforcement Administration (DEA)
Food and Drug Administration (FDA)
indication
generic
intolerance
license
narcotic
over-the-counter (OTC)
pharmaceutical
pharmacology
Physician's Desk Reference (PDR)
prescribe
prescription
side effect
synergistic
tolerance
trade name
vial

DRUG CATEGORIES AND CLASSIFICATIONS

Drugs are divided into different categories or classifications by the chemical type of the active ingredient contained in the drug or by how it is used to treat a disease or symptom. Many classifications of medications produce similar results but do so through different mechanisms of action. For example, in the category of pain relievers, drugs classified as analgesic, anesthetic, and **narcotic** all provide relief from pain. An analgesic drug relieves pain by blocking prostaglandins and providing a longer duration of pain control without significant, if any, decrease in alertness. Narcotics relieve pain by interfering with the central nervous system's recognition of pain impulses, which provides a greater level of pain relief than analgesics but also causes drowsiness and sometimes respiratory depression, with the possibility of developing dependence. Anesthetics block sensation at the nerve ending, being very useful for site-specific, local pain relief but providing a very limited and shorter duration of action. Additionally, a single drug can also provide multiple effects, placing it in several categories.

In addition to many classifications having similar uses and effects, there are often many medications working through different mechanisms of action within each classification. Antihypertensives, for example, control blood pressure through blocking calcium channels, inhibiting conversion of angiotensin 1 into angiotensin 2, relaxing arterial smooth muscle and slowing heart rate. Although the intended result is the same for all, the final effect is achieved through a different chemical action; the best approach must be determined by the prescribing provider. For this reason, among many others, patients should be advised of why they are given a particular medication and that it may not be substituted, changed, or stopped without consulting his or her provider.

Commonly Prescribed Medications

Certain medications will be **prescribed** and **administered** more commonly in certain practices and specialties than in others. The medical assistant should prepare and maintain, in consultation with the prescribing providers, an updated list of these medications tailored to the use of that particular practice and make it readily accessible to all staff. The list should include the usual dosage, possible **side effects**, contraindications, and possible interactions that might be experienced when taken with other commonly used medications or foods.

After becoming familiar with the different categories and classifications of drugs mentioned previously, refer to Table 51–1 to review a list of common classes and examples within each class of medication, which might vary from region to region and practice to practice. You can use this table as a guide to develop one appropriate for the particular specialty your practice serves.

TABLE 51–1 Drug Classifications, Categories, and Examples

Classification	Category Description/Important Characteristics	Action(s)	Examples
Analgesic	These medications provide mild to moderate pain relief without interfering with the patient's level of consciousness; most useful for minor to moderate symptoms of traumatic injury and skeletal muscle aches and pains.	Prostaglandin inhibitors and antagonists, non-steroidal anti-inflammatories (NSAIDs), and COX-2 inhibitors	Advil, naproxen, Celebrex, aspirin, Tylenol
Anesthetic	Medications in this group vary from topical to intravenous to inhaled preparations. Topical agents may be used to facilitate suturing of traumatic lacerations, with effects lasting for a few hours. Produces a lack of feeling. May be local or general, depending on the type and the route of administration. Most of the drug's effects resolve with discontinuation of the drug, but some residual effects can remain for several hours following discontinuation.	Anesthetics interfere with the body's ability to experience pain sensations, blocking conduction of neural impulses or enhancing naturally occurring inhibitory channels	lidocaine HCl (Xylocaine), procaine HCl (Novocaine), Esfluorane

Classification	Category Description/Important Characteristics	Action(s)	Examples
Antacid	Aluminum-containing antacids can cause constipation; those containing magnesium can cause diarrhea; and those containing calcium can increase serum calcium levels and decrease phosphate levels. All these drugs can have significant effects on the metabolism of other medications, which might cause toxicity or prevent absorption.	Neutralize stomach acid by increasing pH	Amphojel, Gelusil, Mylanta, Aludrox, Milk of Magnesia
Antianxiety	Antianxiety drugs relieve anxiety and muscle tension. They are supplied in oral and injectable forms, and some are available for intravenous injection.	Produces a calming effect or increases a patient's feelings of well-being by helping balance certain chemicals in the brain, either enhancing some or decreasing the effects of others	benzodiazepines: diazepam (Valium) and chlordiazepoxide HCl (Librium)
Antiarrhythmic	Cardiac electrical rhythm is maintained through a balance of chemical activity.	These medications control cardiac arrhythmias by altering chemical activity through suppression of extra electrical impulses or blocking the effects of certain chemicals. Actions are divided into four categories: • **Class I** drugs act on sodium channels by slowing conduction in fast-channel tissues that are in the atria and ventricles. • **Class II** drugs are beta blockers, working on the slow-channel tissues of the sinoatrial and atrioventricular nodes. *These drugs are contraindicated in asthmatic patients. • **Class III** drugs interfere with potassium channels to prolong the period in which the next heart beat can occur. These drugs work in slow- and fast-channel tissues to reduce automaticity (the capacity of all cardiac tissues to conduct impulses) without interfering with the conduction velocity (speed of impulse conduction) of impulses that are permitted.	lidocaine HCl (Xylocaine), propranolol HCl (Inderal)

Lecture
arrhythmias – irregular heart beat (without HB)

(continues)

TABLE 51–1 *(Continued)*

Classification	Category Description/Important Characteristics	Action(s)	Examples
		• **Class IV** drugs work by blocking calcium channels, reducing automaticity, conduction velocity, and refractoriness (increasing the period in which the next heart beat can occur).	
Antibiotic	Those at increased risk of developing a secondary bacterial infection may be given antibiotics as a preventive measure. "Broad spectrum" antibiotics may also affect good bacteria that reside in the intestinal tract, causing diarrhea or constipation. Some antibiotics require monitoring of levels to avoid toxicity, especially in patients with liver or kidney disease. Unnecessary use of antibiotics increases the occurrence of antibiotic-resistant bacterial infections, e.g., MRSA (Methicillin-resistant *Staphylococcus aureus*)	Used to cure infections by either killing or injuring bacteria to render them incapable of replication. Antibiotics treat only bacterial infections and have no effects on viral or fungal infections.	penicillins (Pentids, Duracillin, Polycillin, Pipracil, Augmentin), cephalosporins (Keflin, Mandol, Rocephin)
Anticholinergic	Used for stomach and intestinal cramping and reduction of acid secretion	Blocks parasympathetic nerve impulses to slow stomach and intestinal tract activity	atropine, scopolamine, trihexyphenidyl HCl (Artane)
Anticoagulant	Used for patients with a genetic trait that causes them to form clots more readily than others, those with an irregular heart rhythm, patients with artificial heart valve, those at increased risk of heart attack or stroke from clots of any source. Commonly referred to as blood thinners, these medications do not really thin the blood, but they inhibit the action of blood proteins the body uses to form clots in response to injury or inflammation. Coumadin requires careful monitoring; Lovenox does not.	Prevents or delays blood clotting and prevents existing clots from extending or getting larger	heparin sodium, Dicumarol, warfarin sodium (Coumadin), enoxaparin (Lovenox)
Anticonvulsant	Seizures or convulsions are caused by sudden or abnormal amounts of electrical activity in the brain, which can be a result of a chemical imbalance or a traumatic injury.	Prevents or relieves seizures by halting or delaying transmission of excess electrical impulse; prevents skeletal muscles from responding to the impulses.	carbamazepine (Tegretol), phenytoin (Dilantin), ethosuximide (Zarotin)

Classification	Category Description/Important Characteristics	Action(s)	Examples
Antidepressant	An important note on these drugs is that a side effect may be *worsening* depression, especially in the initial treatment phase, so careful monitoring is required. MAOIs interact with a number of foods, including wine and fermented cheeses, which can cause a dangerous and sudden increase in blood pressure.	Prevents or relieves the symptoms of depression by interfering with the brain's ability to receive certain chemicals that affect mood and feelings of well-being	monoamine oxidase (MAO) inhibitors: isocarboxazid (Marplan), phenelzine sulfate (Nardil), amitriptyline HCl (Elavil), imipramine HCl (Tofranil)
Antidiarrheal	Diarrhea can quickly lead to dehydration, especially in the very young and very old. Patients should increase fluid intake while taking these medications to avoid constipation. Caution should be advised when using these drugs in children with infections such as chickenpox or the flu because bismuth-containing medications might contribute to Reye's syndrome.	Prevents or relieves diarrhea by either causing a thickening of the stools, as in psyllium-containing compounds, or by decreasing intestinal spasms	Lomotil, Pepto-Bismol, Kaopectate, Imodium
Antidote	The type and form of an antidote administered depends on the poison or overdose taken; there is no universal antidote. One concern regarding administration of Narcan is for patients who have *accidentally* overdosed on pain medications needed to control the pain of terminal illness. Narcan will remain in the patient's system for several hours and block the effects of narcotic pain medications; it can also induce withdrawal symptoms. The decision to administer an antidote is not based solely on the compound taken but on the consequences of not only the agent ingested but of that agent's sudden reversal.	Counteracts poisons and their effects selectively by binding with the drug or toxin to inhibit further absorption, blocking further effects on target receptor sites or by reversing the actions of the ingested agent	naloxone (Narcan), activated charcoal, atropine
Antiemetic	In controlling nausea and vomiting, the antiemetic chosen is based on the suspected cause of the symptoms as well as underlying medical problems and other medications the patient might be taking. Pregnancy, motion sickness, chemotherapy, migraines, and postoperative nausea are causes of nausea that can require the use of antiemetics.	Prevents or relieves nausea and vomiting by blocking the effects of dopamine, serotonin, or histamine release	Tigan, Dramamine, Phenergan, Reglan, Marinol, Scopolamine

(continues)

TABLE 51–1 *(Continued)*

Classification	Category Description/Important Characteristics	Action(s)	Examples
Antihistamine	Histamine is a protein released by the body in response to allergens. Its release causes an inflammatory response and constriction of smooth muscles, particularly in the airways of asthmatic patients. In a mild reaction, the effects of histamine release will continue to resolve over several hours even after administration of antihistamines. For more severe reactions, other medications can be used in conjunction with the antihistamine to reverse the allergic reaction's effects. Patients who are taking certain medications, such as MAO inhibitors or, drugs that cause drowsiness, and patients with glaucoma or women who are breastfeeding should avoid taking antihistamines.	Antihistamines act by blocking the effects of histamine at the receptor sites. When administered in response to an allergic reaction, antihistamines prevent further activation of the receptor sites that are causing the response but it does not reverse what has already occurred.	Dimetane, Benadryl, Seldane
Antihypertensive	Blood pressure control is essential in patients with hypertension to protect them from kidney damage, heart complications, and stroke. Patients often experience fatigue, sexual side effects, or other symptoms that can interfere with their willingness to continue drug therapy. The MA can help the patient anticipate potential side effects and understand that they might resolve after a period of time on the medication.	Prevents or controls high blood pressure through decreasing heart rate, dilating blood vessels, or reducing circulating fluid volume.	methyldopa (Aldomet), clonidine HCl (Catapres), metoprolol tartrate (Lopressor)
Anti-inflammatory	Pain and swelling may be treated with anti-inflammatory drugs such as aspirin, ibuprofen, or naproxen. They may be used alone, for milder symptoms, or in conjunction with narcotic pain relievers to reduce the amount of narcotics required for adequate relief. Certain anti-inflammatory drugs, NSAIDs (non-steroidal anti-inflammatory drugs), or COX-2 inhibitors have been known to contribute to heart attack and stroke in patients who are at increased risk of developing blood clots. Although useful for acute inflammation, they can delay healing.	Counteracts inflammation by blocking the release of certain chemicals	naproxen (Naprosyn), aspirin, ibuprofen (Advil, Motrin)
Antimanic	Antimanic drugs can help level patients' moods in both directions, not just treat the manic episodes. These patients might need encouragement to continue their medication when they are feeling better.	Used for the treatment of the manic episode of manic-depressive disorder	lithium

Classification	Category Description/Important Characteristics	Action(s)	Examples
Antineoplastic	Although antineoplastic agents are very useful in treating cancers, they have toxic effects on healthy tissues as well and cause a number of unpleasant and sometimes dangerous side effects.	Stops the development, maturation, or spread of a neoplasm or cancer cell	busulfan (Myleran), cyclophosphamide (Cytoxan)
Antiplatelets	Patients who are at increased risk of heart or stroke from blood clots. Antiplatelets do not require the monitor associated with anticoagulants and have less of a bleeding risk. Patients would be advised of increased tendency toward bruising or bleeding.	*Interferes with the stickiness of platelets to help prevent blood clot formation.*	Plavix (clopidogrel), Ticlid (ticlopidine), aspirin
Antipyretic	Febrile seizures in toddlers have not been shown to be predictive of seizures when the child is older.	Reduces fever by acting on the hypothalamus, the heat-regulating part of the brain	aspirin, acetaminophen (Tylenol)
Antitussive	Antitussives can be narcotic or non-narcotic preparations.	Decreases the cough reflex by acting on the central and peripheral nervous systems	codeine, dextromethorphan
Bronchodilator	These medications often make patients feel jittery. Some are used as a "rescue" for acute onset of symptoms, whereas others are used for maintenance and prevention.	Dilates the bronchi by relaxing the smooth muscle that lines the air passages	isoproterenol HCl (Isuprel), albuterol (Proventil)
Contraceptive	Women who are overweight, older than 35 years old, or who smoke are at increased risk of heart attack and stroke from blood clots when taking estrogen-containing oral contraceptives. The morning-after pill is a form of emergency contraception containing progestin if a barrier method fails or there is unintended, unprotected sex (regardless of whether consensual). It is not an abortion pill but works the same three ways as ordinary hormonal birth control methods to prevent pregnancy when taken within 120 hours of intercourse.	Oral contraceptives act by preventing release of an ovum, preventing fertilization of an egg, or inhibiting implantation in the uterus of a fertilized egg. Forms of contraception include condoms, diaphragms, intrauterine devices, sponges, and cervical caps	Enovid-E 21; Ortho-Novum 10/11–21, 10/11–28; Triphasil-21
Decongestant	Because these drugs act through vasoconstriction, patients with heart disease and high blood pressure should not take OTC decongestants without first discussing with their doctor.	Reduces swelling in nasal passages through vasoconstriction to help relieve the pressure sensation in sinuses, improving airflow and making it easier to breathe through the nose	oxymetazoline (Afrin), epinephrine HCl (Adrenalin), phenylephrine HCl (Neo-Synephrine), pseudoephedrine HCl (Sudafed)
Diuretic	Useful either alone or in combination with other drugs to treat hypertension, heart failure, pulmonary edema, edema associated with severe head trauma, and glaucoma	Increases the production of urine and decreases circulating fluid volume by increasing renal blood flow to improve filtration and by decreasing sodium reabsorption	chlorothiazide (Diuril), furosemide (Lasix), Mannitol (Osmitrol)

(continues)

TABLE 51–1 *(Continued)*

Classification	Category Description/Important Characteristics	Action(s)	Examples
Expectorant	Patients should be advised to drink plenty of water when using these medications.	Thins mucus, making it easier to cough it up and clear the airway of secretions	guaifenesin (Robitussin)
Fibrinolytics	Sudden onset (acute) episodes of heart attack or stroke may be caused by a blood clot blocking a critical artery. Used with other anticoagulants, such as Heparin, to prevent smaller clots from forming from the destruction of larger clots.	Clot-buster drugs that dissolve blood clots for emergency treatment of heart attacks and strokes. Destroys existing clots.	TNK, tPA
Hemostatic	May be supplied in an oral form for a genetic clotting deficiency; injectable for surgical bleeding or to reverse the effects of anticoagulant medications; or as a topical dressing containing a hemostatic agent used for external bleeding	Encourages the formation of a blood clot to control or stop bleeding	Humafac, Amicar, vitamin K, alginate dressings
Hypnotic	Patients may develop dependency when using hypnotics for long periods of time. Not to be taken with alcohol or other sedating medications to avoid respiratory depression.	Acts on brain receptors to induce a sense of calm and reduce tension and anxiety	secobarbital (Seconal); chloral hydrate ethchlorvynol (Placidyl), flurazepam (Dalmane), diazepam (Valium)
Hypoglycemic, oral	Many of these drugs may be used alone or in conjunction with insulin. Careful monitoring of liver and kidney function should be observed. Diabetics need to receive adequate dietary and blood glucose monitoring and control teaching.	Lowers blood glucose levels by causing beta cells of the pancreas to release more insulin; acts on the liver to decrease formation of glycogen; decreases absorption of glucose in the intestines; blocks the breakdown of some sugars; prevents the breakdown of GLP-1, a naturally occurring substance that breaks down sugars; and improves use of glucose by tissues, especially skeletal muscles The six types of oral hypoglycemics are sulfonylureas, meglitinides, biguanides, thiazolidinediones, alpha-glucosidase inhibitors, and DPP-4 inhibitors.	(Diabinese), glyburide (Micronase), Amaryl, Glucophage
Insulins	Injectable insulin is given on a routine schedule based on mealtimes to help the body use sugars. In emergencies, the	Insulins lowers blood glucose levels to a normal range by allowing the sugar to cross the	Lantus, Humulin, Novolin

Classification	Category Description/Important Characteristics	Action(s)	Examples
	insulin may be given through an IV. To decrease the number of injections a person receives, some insulins may be combined in one injection, which will be covered later in this unit.	cell membrane to be used for energy. (This is a decidedly oversimplified explanation; much is still not understood about insulin.) There at least 20 types of insulins, which are divided into four basic categories: rapid-acting, regular or short-acting, intermediate, and long-acting insulins. Some patients require more than one type of insulin to control their diabetes.	
Laxative	Lubricants, stimulants, and stool softeners are also effective and may be used in combination for better result. Salts are used for rapid action. Lactulose causes a slower onset of action, is suitable for more prolonged use, and is available only with a prescription. Polyglycol causes water to be retained in stool and is used for short periods of time. Abuse of laxatives is a common issue in anorexic or bulimic patients.	Relieve constipation by absorbing liquid into the intestines to form a soft stool, encourage bowel movements by drawing water into the bowel.	Metamucil powder, Dulcolax
Muscle relaxant	These medications are NOT interchangeable for muscle spasms of different disease processes or injuries.	Muscles spasms are caused by peripheral musculoskeletal problems, such as back or neck pain, and neurological conditions such as multiple sclerosis. The mechanism of action is not well understood. Most appear to act on receptor sites in the central nervous system; a few act directly on striated muscle tissue.	Robaxin, Norflex, Paraflex, Skelaxin, Valium
Sedative/ Tranquilizer	Often considered part of the hypnotics or sedative-hypnotics. Many sedatives are habit-forming or addictive when used improperly. Advise patients to avoid taking sedatives with alcohol because a dangerous decrease in consciousness or breathing can occur.	Produces a calming effect to reduce mental tension and anxiety without causing sleep. They work by suppressing activity in the central nervous system.	amobarbital (Amytal), butabarbital sodium (Buticaps), phenobarbital, zolpidem (Ambien), Haldol, thorazine
Vasodilator	Increases blood supply to tissues, i.e., the heart muscle, to prevent permanent damage and to lower blood pressure. Caution patients beginning a new vasodilator to sit or lie down to avoid an unsafe drop in blood pressure. Use in conjunction with Cialis or Viagra can cause a dangerous and irreversible drop in blood pressure.	Relaxes the smooth muscle inside the vessel walls to cause the inner diameter of the vessel wall to widen, lowering blood pressure and allowing for increased circulation to the area supplied by the vessel	isorbide dinitrate (Isordil), nitroglycerin

(continues)

treatment of Angina Pectoris (Chestpain)
given underneath the tongue
sym – dizziness, headache

TABLE 51–1 *(Continued)*

Classification	Category Description/Important Characteristics	Action(s)	Examples
Vasopressor	Either during or following major surgery, sepsis, or significant blood loss, patients might need chemical blood pressure support in the form of a vasopressor. These are available only in IV form to be used in the hospital setting.	Causes contraction of the smooth muscles that line the walls of blood vessels to increase blood pressure	Neosynephrine, norepinephrine (Levophed)

DRUG ACTIONS

Although many complex and intricate processes are involved in the way different drugs affect the body, we will attempt to provide an easily understandable listing of these actions. Drugs can do many things to help cure disease, but drugs cannot restore lost function of organs that are damaged beyond repair, and it is very important for medical personnel to keep this in mind. Medications can enhance remaining function of a damaged organ or replace hormones and chemicals the body can no longer produce on its own.

Drugs are divided into main groups by types of action on the body: chemotherapeutic, pharmacodynamic, and miscellaneous agents.

Chemotherapeutic Drugs

The chemotherapeutic group includes drugs used to cure a disease caused by an infectious organism or cancer. Chemotherapeutics are used to treat:

- Infections by killing microorganisms or preventing them from reproducing.
- Allergic diseases.
- Metabolic disorders.
- Cancer.
- Toxic diseases as a result of poisoning.
- Mental illness.

Pharmacodynamic Drugs

Pharmacodynamic drugs treat noninfectious processes by acting on different systems in the body to suppress chemicals or hormones being released by the body in excess or to augment chemicals or hormones that are being produced in insufficient amounts. By changing actions that normally occur in the body or interfering with unwanted actions, certain drugs exert their effects by:

- Preventing the action of naturally occurring enzymes or by mimicking the actions of enzymes, as one example of a pharmacodynamic drug. In this way, they can trick the body into either producing more or preventing the production of an enzyme that is causing or worsening a disease process.
- **Agonists** and **antagonists**. Drugs can compete for a certain receptor site to stimulate or prevent the action of that particular receptor. An agonist stimulates a particular action, whereas an antagonist acts to prevent an action or effect on a receptor site. Drugs can also be **synergistic** to each other, meaning that they enhance or multiply the effects of other drugs or have **additive effects**, simply adding each drug's effects to the other.

Nonspecific actions of drugs can be less distinct. They may be used to relieve itching on the skin or reduce stomach acids by changing the pH levels, as examples.

Miscellaneous Agents

Miscellaneous agents include pain relievers.

Drug Effects

The effects of drugs are generally categorized as:

- *Local:* having its effect restricted to the area in which it was administered.
- *Remote:* its effect takes place in areas other than the place of administration.
- *Systemic:* the effect is generalized throughout the body.

Considerations of Drug Action

Several considerations can affect how the body responds to a drug: age, weight, body surface area (BSA), method of administration, **tolerance**, allergies, time, and interaction. Pediatric and geriatric patients and individuals with certain illnesses require a smaller dose than an average adult.

Another consideration is the *rate* at which the body responds to a drug. Medications given by injection reach the bloodstream more rapidly than other routes, whereas transdermal patches deliver small amounts of medication in a sustained, time-release manner. Additionally, when a patient takes a medication for a long time, he or she can develop a tolerance that requires an increase in dosage or a different medicine to obtain a desired effect.

A medication **allergy** may occur at any time in an individual, even if he or she has taken the same medication several times before. Careful attention must be given to the medical history and to the patient's responses during the interview. The MA should note any allergies—whether food, environmental, or drug allergies—in red ink. If a patient phones you to let you know that a new or recently started medication gave him or her a reaction, the MA should describe the reaction and its severity as clearly as possible in the patient's chart.

Occasionally, a patient might experience **intolerance** to a medication and not a true allergic reaction. A medication intolerance (e.g., nausea or upset stomach) should also be charted. Many patients take several medications daily and tend to avoid those that cause them undesirable effects. Helping the patient determine when and how best to take medicines to avoid intolerances or manageable side effects encourages him or her to continue with the prescribed therapy.

DRUG FORMS

Drugs can come in a single form or in a variety of forms (see Table 51–2). The choice of which form to use can depend upon the age of the patient, medical conditions, desired rate of absorption, or inability to tolerate one route or another.

TABLE 51–2 Drug Forms

Capsules	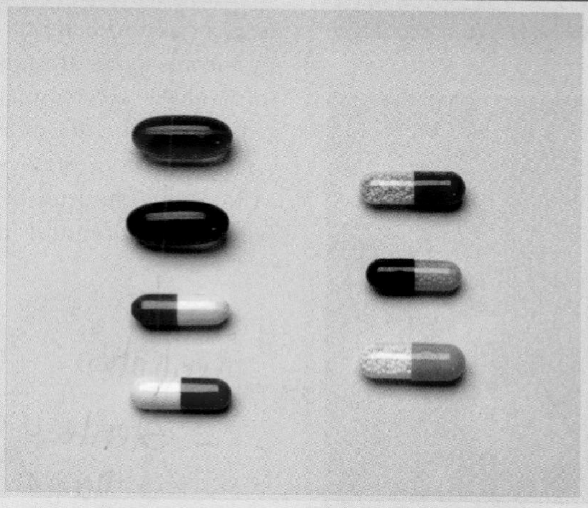 Delmar/Cengage Learning.	Cylinder-shaped enclosure for medication of either a gelatin-coated or time-released coating
Drops	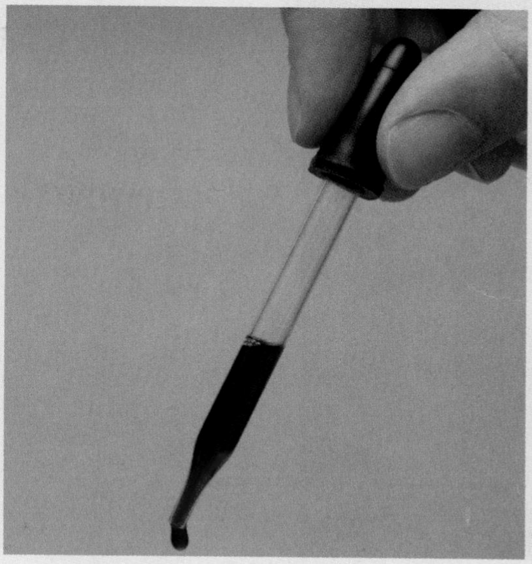 Delmar/Cengage Learning.	Sterile solution that contains medication intended to be delivered directly into the area to be treated, e.g., eyes, ears, nose, and so on

(continues)

TABLE 51–2 *(Continued)*

Inhalants	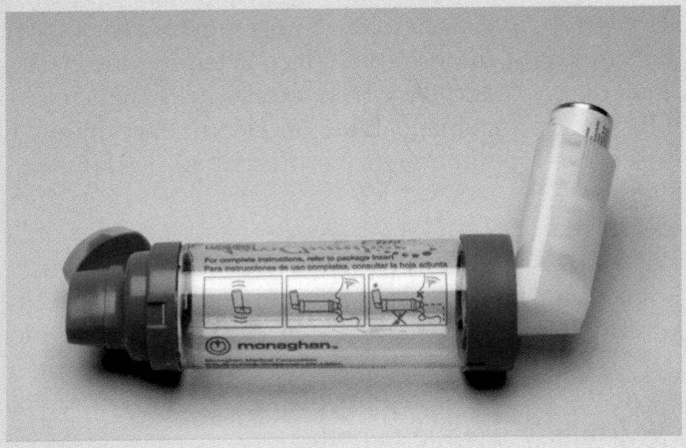 *Delmar/Cengage Learning.*	Medications prepared to be delivered in either a fixed or non-fixed dose to be breathed in through the nose or the mouth. May be oxygen delivery, sprays, or aerosolized medications. MDS – meter dose O_2 – inhaled LPM – liters per min
Liquids	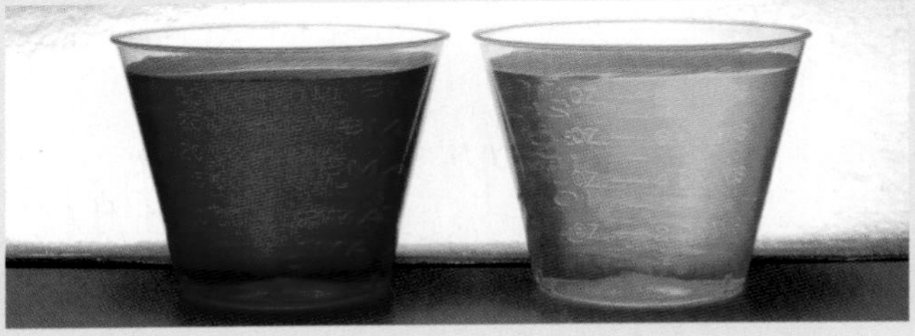 *Delmar/Cengage Learning.* 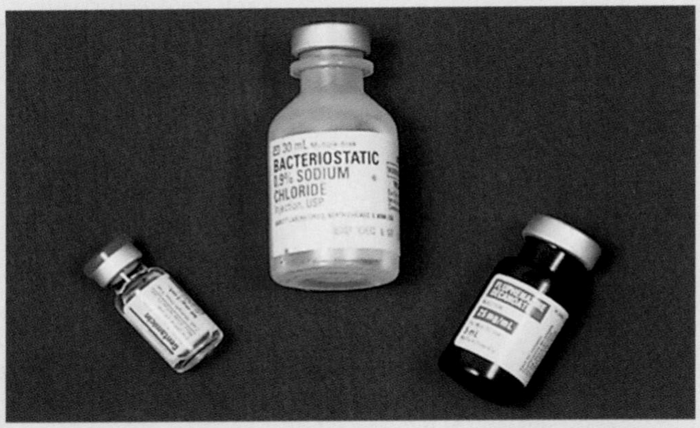 *Delmar/Cengage Learning.* 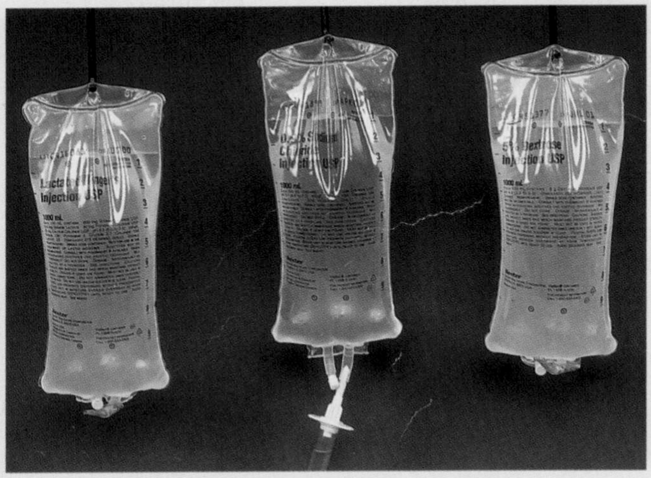 *Delmar/Cengage Learning.*	Medication suspended in alcohol or water. Liquid forms may be prepared for oral, intramuscular, subcutaneous, intravenous, intraarterial, intrathecal, nasogastric, or orogastric delivery as well as for irrigation of body cavities, wounds, or external sites. A less common site of delivery is by intraosseous administration. An implantable device may provide a constant and consistent delivery of a specific dose of medication. Examples of implantable drug delivery include pain medication and insulin pumps. irrigation – sterile water normal water for flashing – oral – injection

Powders

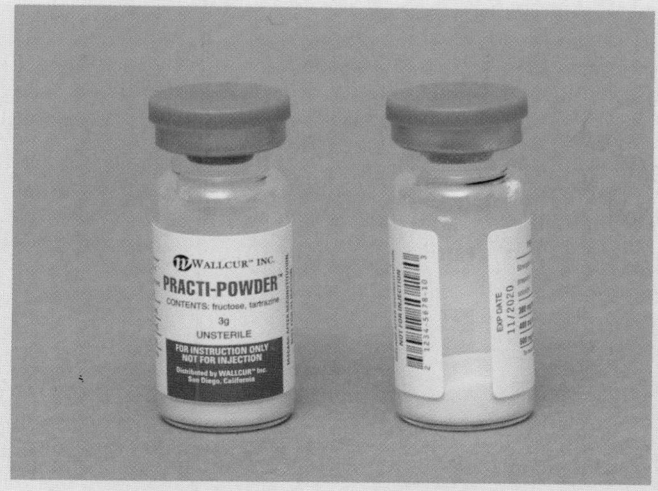

Delmar/Cengage Learning.

Fine particles intended to be dissolved in liquids or foods just prior to being taken.

Skin Preparations

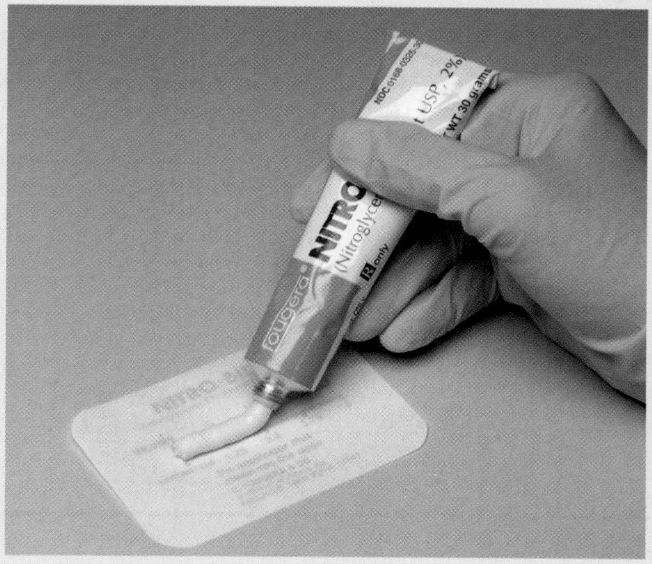

Delmar/Cengage Learning.

Ointments, creams, or lotions that can be applied directly to the skin.

Suppositories

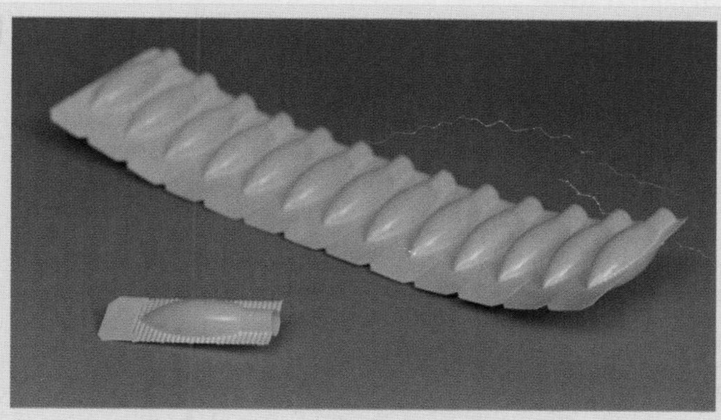

Delmar/Cengage Learning.

Bullet-shaped tablets that melt easily at body temperature for administration through the vagina, urethra, or rectum.

(continues)

TABLE 51–2 *(Continued)*

Tablets	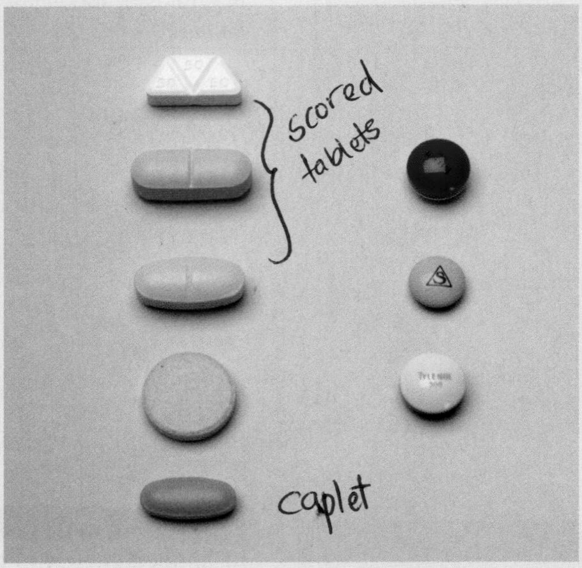 *Delmar/Cengage Learning.*	Medication that is bound together by substances that dissolve in stomach acids; some may have flavorings added to make them more palatable.
Transdermal patches	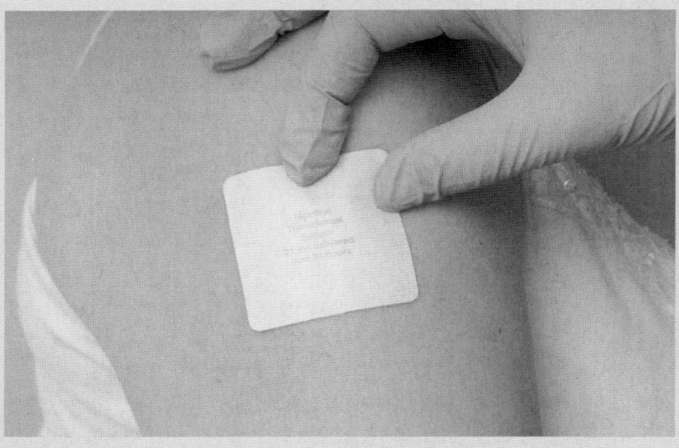 *Delmar/Cengage Learning.*	Adhesive patch with time-released dose of medication to be worn for a specified period of time.

DRUG NAMES

Drugs are identified by four names: **generic** name, **trade name**, chemical name, and official name.

- *Chemical name*: When a drug is first discovered, it is described by its atomic or molecular structure. This name is too complicated for everyday use, so researchers assign a shorthand or abbreviated version of its chemical name for easier discussion.
- *Generic name (also official name)*: When the drug is approved by the **Food and Drug Administration (FDA)**, it is assigned a generic name or official name by the United States Adopted Names (USAN) Council. Generic names are not capitalized.
- *Trade name*: The drug manufacturer assigns a unique name to each drug for marketing. To avoid having more drug names that sound or look alike, which leads to medication errors, the FDA must approve all proposed trade names. Trade names are usually easier to remember than generic names and are capitalized.

Table 51–3 gives some examples of familiar medications.

Newly approved drugs are granted a non-compete status as a trade name drug for seven years, following approval, to give the manufacturer the opportunity to recover development costs, which are often in the millions of dollars. Unless the manufacturer introduces a new **indication** warranting renewal of the non-compete status before the seven-year patent period expires, another company may produce a generic formulation that is usually sold at a lower cost. (An *orphan drug*, one that is the only drug available, approved treatment for a given indication, is the exception to this rule.) Generic drugs contain the same active ingredients as trade name drugs; however, a trade name drug may have a different coating that controls the rate of release in the body or it may have a different type of preservative, which can make a patient intolerant to a generic versus a trade name drug or vice versa.

TABLE 51–3 Generic, Trade, and Chemical Names of Four Common Medications

Generic Name	Trade Name	Chemical Name	Indication
acetaminophen	Tylenol	N-(4-hydroxyphenyl) acetamide	Pain relief, fever reducer
aspirin	Ecotrin	acetylsalicylic acid, 2-(acetyloxy)benzoic acid	Pain relief, fever reducer, decrease platelet adherence
captopril	Capoten	1-[(2S)-3-mercapto-2-methylpropionyl]-L-proline	Hypertension
morphine sulfate	Roxanol	Morphinan-3,6-diol, 7,8-didehydro-4, 5-epoxy-17-methyl-,(5α,6α)-, sul-fate(2:1) (salt), pentahydrate	(Narcotic) pain reliever

Look-Alike, Sound-Alike Drug Names

Beware! Many drugs have similar, sometimes identical-sounding names. Even more confusing, a number of medication names can look alike when handwritten. For this and other reasons, it is important for health care workers to be well versed in the medications most common to his or her particular practice or specialty. According to the *Guidance for Industry* document published by the FDA in February 2010, the FDA updated and reiterated previous recommendations to drug manufacturers to evaluate the proposed names for new drugs to reduce sound-alike names. Table 51–4 provides examples of look-alike or sound-alike drug names.

Prescription Drugs

Prescription drugs are those that may be purchased or given to a patient only with written instructions, known as a **prescription**, from a **licensed** health care provider. For a prescription to be considered valid, it must be issued for a legitimate medical purpose by a licensed practitioner. The FDA is responsible for ensuring that products available for consumption by the public are safe. This includes food, drugs (both prescription and over the counter), and cosmetics. When a drug is developed by a pharmaceutical company, it is evaluated through laboratory and animal testing and then, finally, through a series of controlled clinical trials in humans prior to being approved by the FDA for availability to the general public. The FDA verifies that the data presented regarding the drug's safe use, its ingredients, and what conditions it should be used for are correct and that all these are accurately reflected in its labeling. Sometimes a drug can be recalled, which is actually a voluntary act of the manufacturer on the recommendation of the FDA, not because the drug was unsafe but because its labeling was inaccurate. A drug available for prescription is considered safe by the FDA for use but only so long as its use is determined appropriate and is monitored by a health care provider, therefore requiring a prescription. Many drugs requiring a prescription have serious side effects even when used appropriately. Levels of the drug or other blood tests may need to be performed periodically to ensure that the effects are not more detrimental than the condition the drug is being used to treat.

TABLE 51–4 Look-Alike or Sound-Alike Drug Names

Atarax (antihistamine)	may be confused with …	Ativan (used for anxiety and sedation)
Benylin (cough suppressant)	may be confused with …	Benadryl (antihistamine)
Diovan (treats high blood pressure)	may be confused with …	Zyban (smoking cessation)
enflurane (inhalation anesthesia)	may be confused with …	isoflurane (also inhalation anesthesia but used WITH enflurane)
Lamictal (epilepsy control)	may be confused with …	Lamisil (antifungal treatment)
nelfinavir (antiretroviral used for HIV)	may be confused with …	nevirapine (reverse transcriptase, used for AIDS also but to be used WITH antiretrovirals)
prochlorperazine (anti-nausea, antiemetic)	may be confused with …	trifluoperazine (antipsychotic)

Controlled Substances

A controlled substance is any drug, whether prescription or illegal, that has the potential for abuse or addiction. Controlled substances come under a category of prescription drugs that have an elevated level of restrictions for the public's protection. The 1970 Controlled Substances Act established the **Drug Enforcement Administration (DEA)**, under the Department of Justice, which maintains oversight for legally prescribed and used narcotics drugs and for containment of illegal drugs. This legislation was designed to implement controls on drugs that were commonly abused by society, control prescriptions provided for these drugs, and require prescribers of these medications to be registered with individual DEA numbers.

These drugs are categorized into five schedules, which are regulated under the Controlled Substances Act. The schedules are arranged by most dangerous drugs in Schedule I (illegal substances that are not available for prescription) to least dangerous in Schedule V (see Table 51–5). The drugs in schedules with lower numbers have stricter controls for prescribing and obtaining. There are subcategories within each schedule, and the DEA may alter levels of a drug if there is evidence of increased abuse.

The five schedules include:

- *Schedule I:* These drugs have no recognized medicinal use in the United States, and prescriptions for such drugs are prohibited. Examples include heroin and cocaine.
- *Schedule II:* These drugs must have a written or typed prescription order with the provider's personal signature and DEA registry number and may not be refilled. In an emergency, the doctor may phone in a limited amount of the medication to the pharmacist. However, a written, signed prescription order for the controlled substance must be presented to the pharmacist within 72 hours in compliance with DEA regulations.
- *Schedule III:* Prescriptions may be written or phoned in for these drugs, and they may be refilled five times within six months.
- *Schedule IV:* Prescriptions may be refilled up to five times in six months.
- *Schedule V:* These drugs are subject to state and local regulations. A written prescription for Schedule V medications may not be required.

Each licensed prescriber must display his or her DEA registration certificate at each place of practice where he or she prescribes controlled substances. The registration for prescribers must be renewed every three years. The Website for the DEA's Office of Diversion Control, www.deadiversion.usdoj.gov, contains various forms, both online and mail-in, to apply for and renew DEA registration.

There are strict guidelines not only for prescribing controlled substances but also for their storage in the medical office, which is discussed in the next chapter.

MEDIA LINK

View the video, "DEA and Controlled Substances," for this chapter on the Premium Website.

Storing Controlled Substances

The storage of controlled substances is of particular concern and bears a great deal of not only ethical and professional responsibility but legal oversight as well. Controlled substances and the records of their prescribing and dispensing must be protected from misuse by storing them

TABLE 51–5 Schedules of Controlled Substances

Drug Category	Potential for Abuse (Addiction)	Medical Use	Potential for Dependence	Example
Schedule I	High	Unaccepted; limited to research	High	Heroin, LSD, marijuana, peyote
Schedule II	High	Accepted; tightly restricted	Severe psychic or physical	Amphetamines, morphine
Schedule III	Less than I or II Low to moderate	Acceptable	High psychological	Certain opioids, barbiturates, and some depressants
Schedule IV	Low	Acceptable	Limited physical and psychological	Phenobarbital, propoxyphene
Schedule V	Low	Acceptable	Limited physical and psychological	Small amounts of codeine in cough preparations and analgesics

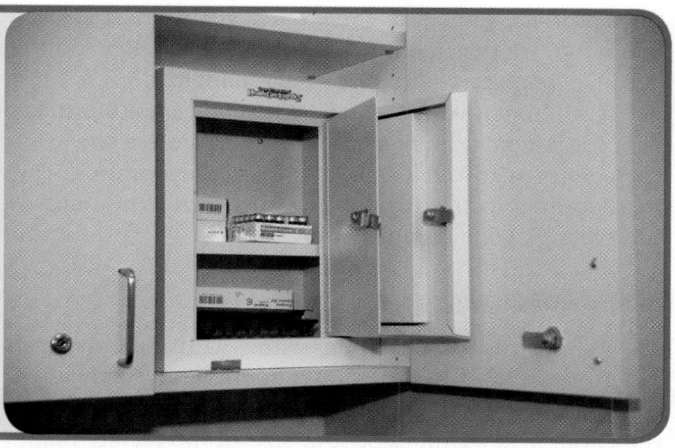

Figure 51–1: Controlled substances must be kept secure in a double-lock system. *Delmar/Cengage Learning.*

under double lock (Figure 51–1). This double-lock system can be a combination of two keys, as to an outer and inner cabinet; the keys are accounted for by each user, whose possession of them is recorded on a daily basis.

Electronic dispensing systems, such as Pyxis®, meet the double-lock criterion by requiring unique user identification and password combinations for an appropriate professional to access controlled substances. To meet these requirements, controlled substances may not be kept in the same compartments or cabinets as uncontrolled **pharmaceuticals** in the office setting. Records of daily counts reconciled by two parties who have legally authorized access to controlled substances must be maintained for DEA review on demand for three years and submitted every two years. Due to an increase in theft and substance abuse, many offices no longer keep controlled substances in the office.

Controlled Substances and the Medical Assistant

The medical assistant must be well informed about the regulations that encompass controlled substances. He or she might be responsible for the following:

- Knowledge of federal and state laws that manage controlled substances, drugs, and pharmaceutical samples
- Keeping a thorough record and inventory of all drugs and samples
- Keeping all drugs, including controlled substances, in a secure location
- Reminding the provider of DEA registration or renewal
- Keeping track of all prescription pads and ensuring their safekeeping in secured areas where only staff may access them
- Properly disposing of expired drugs and keeping a record of their disposal

Nonprescription Drugs

Nonprescription drugs or **over-the-counter (OTC) drugs** are considered safe and effective for use by the general population without requiring a prescription. Many nonprescription drugs have required prescriptions prior to being transitioned to OTC status. Over time, these drugs might have been found to show a low incidence of any serious side effects or may be formulations of prescription drugs in a reduced strength. The FDA still monitors these medications for reports of problems and ensures that the labeling accurately reflects the ingredients and in what conditions they should be used. It should be stressed to patients, however, that improper use of over-the-counter medications can still be harmful *even though these medicines do not require a prescription*.

Vitamins, Herbal Supplements, and Alternative Remedies

The FDA provides little if any oversight regarding vitamins, herbal supplements, and alternative remedies. Many patients choose to take herbal remedies either instead of or in addition to prescription medications. This is an acceptable practice but *only* so long as these herbal remedies are revealed to the patient's provider and recorded accurately in the patient's record. Herbal remedies may be derived from naturally occurring substances that are the same as or similar to the substances found in many prescribed medications. When taking herbal preparations, it is critical not to duplicate the same compound by the use of prescription medications. Just as important, the provider must also be aware of herbal remedies the patient is using that might counteract prescription medications because lack of such knowledge can lead the provider to presume the dose is insufficient or the patient isn't responding to that particular medication, falsely altering the diagnostic process. Toxicity can also develop when a supplement is similar to or mimicking the effects of a prescription medication.

HANDLING MEDICATIONS IN THE MEDICAL OFFICE

The proper storage and preparation of medication is important, not just for the patient's safety but also for the safety of members of the health care team.

Stock Medications

Medication storage involves more than simply putting away packages. Many necessary forms, prescription blanks, and records must be kept. Medications must be rotated according to their expiration dates. They may be stored according to their classification (refer to Table 51–1) or alphabetically, as long as the method used is consistent and known to all who have access to the medications.

The MA might label shelves or have pullout shelves installed to increase efficiency. The medication storage cabinet, closet, or room must be locked and accessed only by a qualified member of the health care team.

Samples

Pharmaceutical companies send their representatives to visit medical facilities on a regular basis. They often provide samples of new or frequently used medications along with information about the cost. Most representatives are more than willing to answer questions from the provider and medical assistant to provide them with the most up-to-date information.

Samples allow the provider to introduce a new medication to a patient to determine whether the patient can tolerate it prior to obtaining a full prescription and allow for an immediate loading dose to be given. When samples are given to patients, the quantity and dosage strength must be recorded on the patient's chart. Maintaining samples is an ongoing task, and they should be stored separately from other medications. The MA may wish to categorize them, just as other medications, but it should be clear that they are samples and not stock medications. Pay careful attention to the product's expiration date and properly discard outdated substances. Check with local regulatory agencies on how to discard expired medications in your area.

Refrigerated Medications

Special attention should to be given to the many medicines that require refrigeration, such as antibiotics and immunizations. Sometimes refrigeration is necessary only after the bottle or **vial** has been opened or after it has been reconstituted; these containers should be clearly labeled with the date and time of opening or reconstitution to determine expiration. The office might maintain medications that must be stored in the freezer, such as the polio vaccine. Also be sure to note whether medications or vaccines that are to be stored under refrigeration actually *arrive* in shipment refrigerated properly by the carrier or packed appropriately by the shipper. For example, if the dry ice is no longer present or the packaging or packing material feels warm, contact the supplier immediately for instructions concerning the safety of the contents for use or to have replacements issued.

Daily temperature logs for both refrigerators and freezers where medications are stored are required to ensure that the necessary temperatures are maintained and your office is in compliance with Material Safety Data Sheet (MSDS) regulations. The appropriate temperature range for each may be determined by your state's laboratory certifying agency or your parent company if your office is part of a larger health care system. A procedure should also be in place concerning what to do in the event of a failure to maintain a prescribed temperature. Check labels, directions, and package inserts to determine the proper method of storage for all products because storage requirements can change.

It is imperative that medications and immunizations kept for patient administration *not be* stored in the same refrigerator with office staff food and medications. This is an unsafe practice for staff members and is contrary to accrediting agency regulations.

Disposing of Drugs

The proper disposal of drugs varies considerably from state to state and is generally influenced by regulations of the FDA and the Environmental Protection Agency (EPA) but also by the type and size of the facility that is disposing of the unused medications. Local communities also have significant variances in the manner of disposal. The best practice is to contact the local municipal government for small practices or to consult with pharmacists in the case of a practice that is part of a larger health care system. Some communities and pharmacy chains have a take-back program by which unused drugs may be returned for disposal. Again, check with the local government agencies, either wastewater treatment departments or trash and recycling services, for guidance.

Controlled substance disposal also varies, and most states require witness of destruction by licensed pharmacists, nurses, and, sometimes, even law enforcement personnel. Your state's drug enforcement authority can provide you more detailed information, but a general listing is available in the *Health Services Industry Study: Management and Disposal of Unused Pharmaceuticals*, published on the EPA's National Service Center for Environmental Publications at www.epa.gov/. As Websites change and are reorganized, use the search term "unused pharmaceuticals" to find links to the most current guidelines. You may also email unusedpharms@epa.gov with specific questions.

A number of drugs are still considered suitable for disposal by flushing down the toilet or sink drain. Based on concerns of news stories in the past few years, flushing certain types of drugs into the local sewage system became a concern. However, a number of scientists and pharmaceutical experts report that more drugs actually enter the sewage and water systems through normal body excretion due to incomplete absorption by the body than through intentional disposal of unused drugs in their manufactured forms. A continuously updated list of drugs suitable or recommended for flushing down the toilet or drain can be found in the article, "Disposal by Flushing of Certain Unused Medicines: What You Should Know," on the FDA's Website. To access, go to www.fda.gov and type the article name in the search bar.

How to Dispose of Unused Medications is a general set of guidelines for consumer disposal of prescription drugs issued by the FDA in conjunction with the Office of National Drug Control Policy (ONDCP) in February 2007. To access, go to www.fda.gov and type

"How to Dispose of Unused Medicine" in the search bar. The guidelines recommend first looking for specific disposal instructions on the label and flushing drugs down the toilet only when the information specifically indicates that it is acceptable to do so. In the absence of specific instructions, drugs may be disposed of in the trash after taking a few precautions:

- They should be removed from the original container and mixed with an undesirable substance to discourage accidental ingestion by humans or animals if found.
- They should be placed in a plastic bag to prevent leakage.
- To protect the patient's identity, the label of any containers should have all personal information scratched off or obliterated in some manner.

PHARMACEUTICAL REFERENCES

So far in this chapter, different types of medications have been discussed as well as the importance of verifying the accuracy of the medication order or prescription. So how does a medical assistant ensure that this information is correct, particularly when new drugs seem to be released almost on a daily basis? Because the medical assistant is legally, ethically, and morally responsible for ensuring that the information is correct to promote patient safety, it is necessary to verify the information personally. A number of references are available that provide the necessary information, both in print and online. Bear in mind that none of these is absolutely comprehensive, so more than one source might need to be referenced, depending on the drug, to find the needed information. By familiarizing yourself ahead of time and learning the organization of different available references, you will be more effective and more efficient in finding the information.

Physician's Desk Reference

The ***Physician's Desk Reference*** (or **PDR**) and *Physician's Desk Reference for Nonprescription Drugs* are valuable resources that should be accessible for easy reference by all members of the health care team. The PDR can be accessed online as well. The purpose of the PDR is to provide accurate, reliable, and current information about most prescribed medications and related products. The MA might need to consult the PDR for the proper spelling, strength, or other information concerning medications that are not given frequently to verify accuracy of a medication order prior to administering medications. Not all medications are included in every edition of the PDR, particularly if they have been in use for a long period of time. For this reason, keeping older editions as well as other supplemental resources is highly recommended, which will be discussed a little later in this chapter. It may be among the MA's assigned duties to ensure that the most current edition of the PDR and quarterly supplements are available in the practice to enable all personnel to stay up to date on the newest FDA-approved pharmaceuticals.

Using the PDR

Learning to use the PDR may seem like a daunting task at first but can be mastered with a systematic approach to understanding its organization. If you are using an older edition of the PDR, the sections are color-coded. Be sure to check the organization of the edition you are using. In the 64th edition of the PDR, PDR–2010, there are six sections to become familiar with:

- **Section 1**: **Manufacturer's Index** (gray pages)–Includes an alphabetic listing of all manufacturers listed in the PDR along with their addresses, phone numbers, and emergency contact information. Also contains a listing of each manufacturer's products and the page number for each product in the PDR. W
- **Section 2**: **Brand and Generic Name Index** (white pages)–Lists the page number of each product by both brand and generic name. P
- **Section 3**: **Product Category Index** (gray pages)–Lists all products by category. Also includes a key to controlled substances categories, key to FDA use-in-pregnancy ratings, U.S. FDA contact numbers, poison control centers listing by states, a section on drugs that can cause photosensitivity, and a listing of drugs that should not be crushed. B
- **Section 4**: **Product Identification Guide** (glossy gray pages)–Displays full-color photo image examples of different forms of the products. This section is organized alphabetically by manufacturer. G
- **Section 5: Product Information Section** (white pages)–Includes an alphabetic listing by manufacturer of products. Section 5 is arranged by manufacturer, and the content is presented for each product in the following sequential format: W
    - *Brand name*: Name assigned by manufacturer.
    - *Description*: Chemical composition of the drug and its origin.
    - *Clinical* ***Pharmacology***: Drug's effects on the body and mechanism of action.
    - *Indications & Usage*: Conditions for which the drug is prescribed.
    - *Contraindications*: Conditions and situations in which the drug should *not* be given.
    - *Warnings*: Potential dangers associated with the drug.
    - *Precautions*: Describes measures to be taken if prescribed in patients with certain conditions (i.e., blood levels or equipment to have available in event of emergency, and so on).
    - *Adverse Reactions*: Side effects or undesirable effects patients might experience when taking the drug.

- *Dosage & Administration*: Usual daily dosage for adults and children with recommended time intervals for dosing. Also includes recommended routes for administration or routes that should *not* be used.
- *How supplied*: Available forms of the drug.

- Following Section 5 is an FDA MedWatch form and Vaccine Adverse Event Reporting Form (VAER).

Note: Older versions of the PDR can contain a sixth section that describes diagnostic product information.

Helpful Guidelines for Using the PDR

1. Find the brand name of the drug in the second section (brand and generic name index) of the PDR. There are two page numbers listed after the manufacturer's name (which is in parentheses). The first page number locates the product identification number, and the second page number is the location of the product information.
2. If only the classification of the drug is known, go to Section 3 to find the drug category.
3. If the desired drug is not listed in the PDR, other reference sources should be consulted until the information is located.

Note: The medical assistant should become familiar with the PDR's contents pages with each new edition to become proficient in assisting the provider with needed information.

Physician's Desk Reference for Nonprescription Drugs

The *Physicians' Desk Reference for Nonprescription Drugs* is a resource that can be of great assistance in identifying over-the-counter (OTC) medicines that patients use for self-medication. The format of this reference book is similar to the PDR for prescription products. Sections on patient education material, support groups, and diagnostic home use products are also included.

CLINICAL PEARL

Pillbox™ is an application currently under development on the NIH (National Institutes of Health) Website that will help health care providers identify a pill by using its physical characteristics. This may be a very helpful tool in cases of accidental poisoning when a sample of the pill is provided but its name is unknown.

PROCEDURE 51–1 Use the PDR to Find Medication Information

PURPOSE: Effectively use a PDR to obtain information on dosages, routes of administration, side effects, and contraindications

EQUIPMENT: PDR

S SKILL: Locate specific information about medications in a PDR

Procedure Steps	Detailed Instructions and/or *Rationales*
1. Obtain name of ordered medication. Determine whether generic or trade name; locate page number.	Locate ordered medication in appropriate section of PDR. *Two page numbers are provided: one for visual identification of medication, the other for prescribing and administration information.*
2. Note appearance of brand-name medication.	Choose page number corresponding to photo of drug and compare drug being given to medication photo if it is an unfamiliar brand-name drug. *May help to prevent giving wrong drug if it does not match photo. Generic medications most likely will not match the photo.*
3. Locate prescribing information. Confirm order matches drug name.	Choose page number that corresponds to prescribing information. Compare to order for dose, route, and any contraindications or precautions to be observed. *To prevent giving incorrect medication, dose, or by wrong route.*
4. Verify accuracy of order and medication	Double-check order **again** and compare to PDR information.

Additional Drug References

Although the PDR is among the most up-to-date and comprehensive references available for verifying medication information, it can be cumbersome to use. Other references designed for everyday practice can be easier to look up most-used information and might also contain older drugs no longer included in the PDR. Although a few of these are discussed in the following text, understand that there are a number of reliable sources. If the MA is unsure of the usefulness or reliability of a particular resource, consider consulting with the provider or other advanced practitioners who work in the office to determine which resource materials might be appropriate for that particular practice.

Product Inserts

Drug information is provided by the manufacturer with medications. When a prescription medication is sent to a pharmacy for dispensing, the product insert is sent along with the original packaging for review by the pharmacist. This information is used for preparation and dispensing purposes and only the required information is printed on the label. OTC medications package inserts are included with every container of medication and contain the information found in the PDR regarding structure, description, indications, side effects, and dosing.

> **CLINICAL PEARL**
>
> When package inserts are received with bulk medication shipments in the office setting, prepare a notebook or file that contains these for easy reference and replace with updated ones as they arrive with new shipments to create your own condensed office PDR.

Professional Drug Handbooks

The medical assistant might also find a nursing drug book an excellent supplementary resource to the PDR because the language and organization is often more readable and more focused on dose, route, side effects, and cautions. A number of companies offer drug handbooks based on different professional perspectives such as that of nursing, provider, or even veterinary. These drug handbooks provide condensed, most frequently used information in an easy-to-find format with an alphabetical index of both trade and generic drug names. Besides being organized by discipline, handbooks can also be organized by specialized areas of medical practice: oncology, emergency, obstetrics and gynecology, pediatrics, and so on. They will include the prescribing information; dosage calculations; and recommended dose ranges, warnings, precautions, and side effects. They do not generally include elaborate chemical structural information. These types of references make an excellent addition to the office library as a supplement to the PDR, and it is often much easier to locate basic information.

Electronic and Online Resources

- **USP-NF** The U.S. Pharmacopeia-National Formulary (USP-NF) is a compilation of standards related to medications, drug substances, medical devices, and vitamins. It is provided in print form, and the online version can be found at www.usp.org/USPNF/. Revisions are issued as supplements as information becomes available. The USP also maintains monographs or structural information on medications and issues reference standards for evaluating drugs and laboratory samples, providing these to laboratories all over the world.
- **PDR.net** provides access to the PDR information online and can be found at www.pdr.net. It requires registration with a DEA or NPI number for access by a provider, advanced practice nurse, provider assistant, or medical student or resident. Separate, less inclusive access may be obtained by patients and other health care workers.
- **Downloadable applications** Many drug information applications are available in downloadable versions that can be readily accessed on handheld devices, providing portable references for medical professionals to use during the course of practice.
- **Online drug Websites** When using an online reference site, you must be very careful to verify its validity. Not all Websites provide accurate information. RxList.com and WebMd® are two helpful Internet drug index resources. Caution in using online Websites for drug referencing cannot be emphasized enough. Wikipedia, for example, is not a reliable resource because it can be changed by input of information from variable and nonvalidated sources.

CHAPTER SUMMARY

- Drugs are divided into different categories or classifications by the chemical type of the active ingredient contained in the drug or by how it is used to treat a disease or symptom.
- Many classifications of medications produce similar results but do so through different mechanisms of action. Additionally, a single drug can also provide multiple effects, placing it in several categories.

- Drugs are divided into groups by types of action on the body: chemotherapeutic, pharmacodynamic, and miscellaneous agents.
- The effects of drugs are generally categorized as: local (effects in the area in which it was administered); remote (effects in areas other than the place of administration); or systemic (generalized throughout the body).
- Drugs can come in a single form or be available in a variety of forms: capsules, drops, inhalants, liquids, powders, skin preparations, suppositories, tablets, and transdermal patches.
- Drugs are identified by four names: generic name, trade name, chemical name, and official name.
- Prescription drugs are those that may be purchased or given to a patient only with written instructions, known as a prescription, from a licensed health care provider. Controlled substances come under a category of prescription drugs that has the potential for abuse or addiction. These drugs are categorized into five schedules, arranged by most dangerous drugs in Schedule I (illegal substances that are not available for prescription) to least dangerous in Schedule V.
- The *Physician's Desk Reference* (or PDR) and *Physician's Desk Reference for Nonprescription Drugs* are valuable resources that should be accessible in the medical office. Additional resources include product inserts, professional drug handbooks, and a variety of electronic and online resources.

STUDY TOOLS

Workbook	Activities for Chapter 51
Premium Website	
MEDIA LINK	View these **Media Links** for Chapter 51 • DEA and Controlled Substances
StudyWARE	Activities and Quizzes on the **StudyWARE™ Software** for Chapter 51
	Audio Library of medical terms
	Online access to **Critical Thinking Challenge 2.0**
CourseMate	Activities and Quizzes for Chapter 51
WebTutor	Activities and Quizzes for Chapter 51

CHECK YOUR KNOWLEDGE

1. Which of the following is one of the main groups that describe actions of drugs?
   a. Inhalation
   b. Pharmacodynamic
   c. Narcotic
   d. Mood altering
2. Drugs can be used to do which of the following EXCEPT:
   a. Restore lost function of an irreparably damaged organ
   b. Enhance remaining function of a damaged organ
   c. Replace hormones no longer being made by the body
   d. Reverse allergic reactions
3. Upon learning that a patient is taking herbal supplements, the MA's most appropriate response is to:
   a. advise the patient to stop taking all herbal supplements at once.
   b. advise the patient to stop taking any prescription medications that interact with the herbal supplements.
   c. record in the patient's chart the herbal supplements, doses, and reasons the patient is taking them and alert the provider.
   d. this is not a concern because herbal supplements are not really medications.

4. Which of the following is correct?
   a. Schedule IV drugs have no legal or medicinal purpose.
   b. Schedule I drugs include street drugs.
   c. Schedule III drugs cannot be refilled.
   d. All schedule drugs require a prescription.
5. Drugs are more likely to enter the sewer and water systems through:
   a. Flushing unused medication down the toilet.
   b. Excesses released from manufacturing plants.
   c. Illegal suppliers disposing of excess inventory.
   d. Natural excretion of drug not completely absorbed by the body.
6. Which of the following best describes a pharmacodynamic drug?
   a. Treatment for allergies
   b. Remedy for metabolic disorders
   c. Cures cancer
   d. Inhibits the action of an enzyme
7. What is required to store controlled substances legally?
   a. DEA license
   b. Current medical credentials of provider prominently displayed
   c. Double-lock system of access
   d. Refrigerator with temperature log
8. Which of the following comments is true?
   a. A medication can fall into only one category.
   b. Over-the-counter medications do not require a prescription but can still be harmful if used incorrectly.
   c. Schedule I drugs require a handwritten prescription.
   d. If a medication allergy does not manifest after the first exposure to a drug, there is no need to be concerned about an allergy in the future.

WEB LINKS

DEA registration applications: www.deadiversion.usdoj.gov/drugreg/reg_apps/index.html

Food and Drug Administration: www.fda.gov

PDR online: www.pdr.net

Pillbox™: http://www. pillbox.nlm.nih.gov/

RxList (online drug information resource): www.RxList.com

U.S. Pharmacopoeia: www.usp.org/USPNF/

RESOURCES

Guidance for Industry Contents of a Complete Submission for the Evaluation of Proprietary Names. (February 2010.) U.S. Department of Health and Human Services, Food and Drug Administration. Retrieved 4/23/2010 from www.fda.gov/downloads/Drugs/GuidanceComplianceRegulatoryInformation/Guidances/UCM075068.pdf.

Pillbox™. National Institutes of Health. Retrieved on 4/24/2010 from http://www. pillbox.nlm.nih.gov/index.html

Chapter 52

Measurement Systems, Basic Mathematics, and Dosage Calculations

OBJECTIVES

In this chapter, you will learn the following:

KB KNOWLEDGE BASE

1. Spell and define, using the glossary in the back of the text, all the Words to Know in this chapter.
2. Identify measurement systems.
3. Define basic units of measurement and equivalents in metric, apothecary, and household systems.
4. Describe the steps in solving basic math computations.
5. Identify both abbreviations and symbols used in calculating medication dosages.

S SKILLS

1. Demonstrate knowledge of basic math computations.
2. Apply mathematical computations to solve equations.
3. Convert among measurement systems.

WORDS TO KNOW

decimal
denominator
dividend
divisor
extremes
fraction
improper fraction
means
metric system
mixed fraction
numerator
percentage
product
proportion
ratio

SYSTEMS OF MEASUREMENT

Because medications can be prescribed in either metric or household measurements, it is important to know equivalents between the two to calculate the dose of the prescribed medication.

MEDIA LINK

Review the "Systems of Measurement" tutorial on the Premium Website to help practice the concepts in this section.

The Metric System

The **metric system** is the primary system of measurement in medicine, based on multiples of 10. There are three basic units:

- gram (g), which measures mass (weight)
- liter (L), which measures volume (liquid)
- meter (m), which measures length (size)

The metric system adds prefixes to the basic units to indicate the value (multiple or submultiple) of the unit. For example, when the prefix "kilo-" is added to the unit "meter," it becomes "kilometer," which has a value of one thousand meters. Table 52–1 lists common prefixes in the metric system, with their values.

Household Measures

Patients at home typically use household measurements such as tablespoon and teaspoon (Figure 52–1). It is important to understand these measurements so you can explain to patients how to take their medications after discharge. The basic units of this system are:

- drop (gtt)
- teaspoon (t or tsp)
- tablespoon (T or tbs)
- ounce (fluid) (fl oz)
- cup
- pint (pt)
- quart (qt)
- ounce (weight) (oz)
- pound (lb)

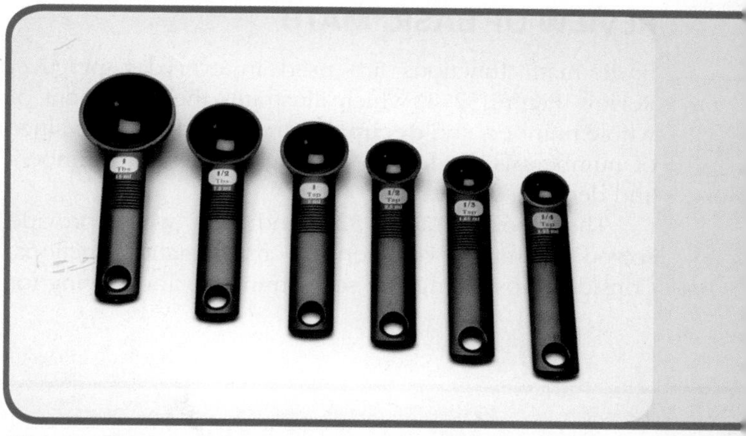

Figure 52–1: Standard measuring spoons. *Delmar/Cengage Learning.*

Table 52–2 shows common household equivalents of these units.

TABLE 52–1 Metric System Prefixes

Prefix	Unit Value	Decimal Value
micro-	1/1000000 of a unit	0.000001
milli-	1/1000 of a unit	0.001
centi-	1/100 of a unit	0.01
deci-	1/10 of a unit	0.1
No prefix (meter, liter, gram)	1 unit	1
deka-	10 units	10
hecto-	100 units	100
kilo-	1000 units	1000

The Apothecary System

The apothecary system was the first system of medication measurement and was developed hundreds of years ago. It consists of several measurements of volume that in the past have been used for prescribing and measuring drugs. Although this system is not commonly used in today's medical office, you should be familiar with the basic units of it, which follow:

- grain (gr)
- quart (qt)
- pint (pt)
- ounce or fluid ounce (oz)
- dram
- minim

TABLE 52–2 Household Equivalents

60 gtt	=	1 t or tsp
3 t or tsp	=	1 T or tbs
2 T or tbs	=	1 fl oz
1 cup	=	8 fl oz
1 pt	=	2 cups
1 qt	=	4 cups (2 pts)
1 lb	=	16 oz

REVIEW OF BASIC MATH

Basic math functions are used in everyday practice. Review Figure 52–2, which illustrates the placement of whole numbers and **decimals**. Knowing the place values of numbers is the key to reading and writing numbers and decimals accurately.

Then look at Tables 52–3 and 52–4, which provide solved examples of everyday mathematic functions. Consider substituting any set of numbers and solving for the answer and then check the solution with a calculator. Practice by solving the sample problems found in the accompanying workbook.

MEDIA LINK

You can also review the "Fractions and Decimals" tutorial on the Premium Website to help practice the concepts presented in this section.

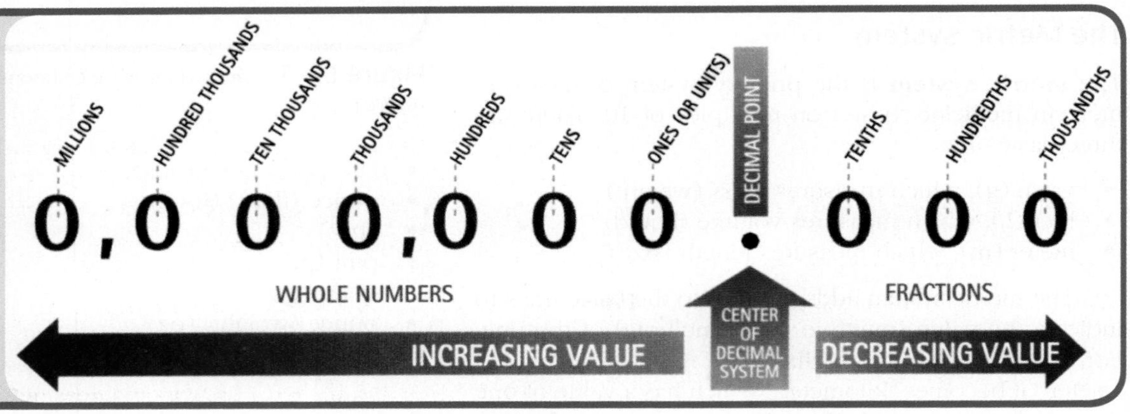

Figure 52–2: Whole numbers and decimals. *Delmar/Cengage Learning.*

TABLE 52–3 Review Examples of Math Problems

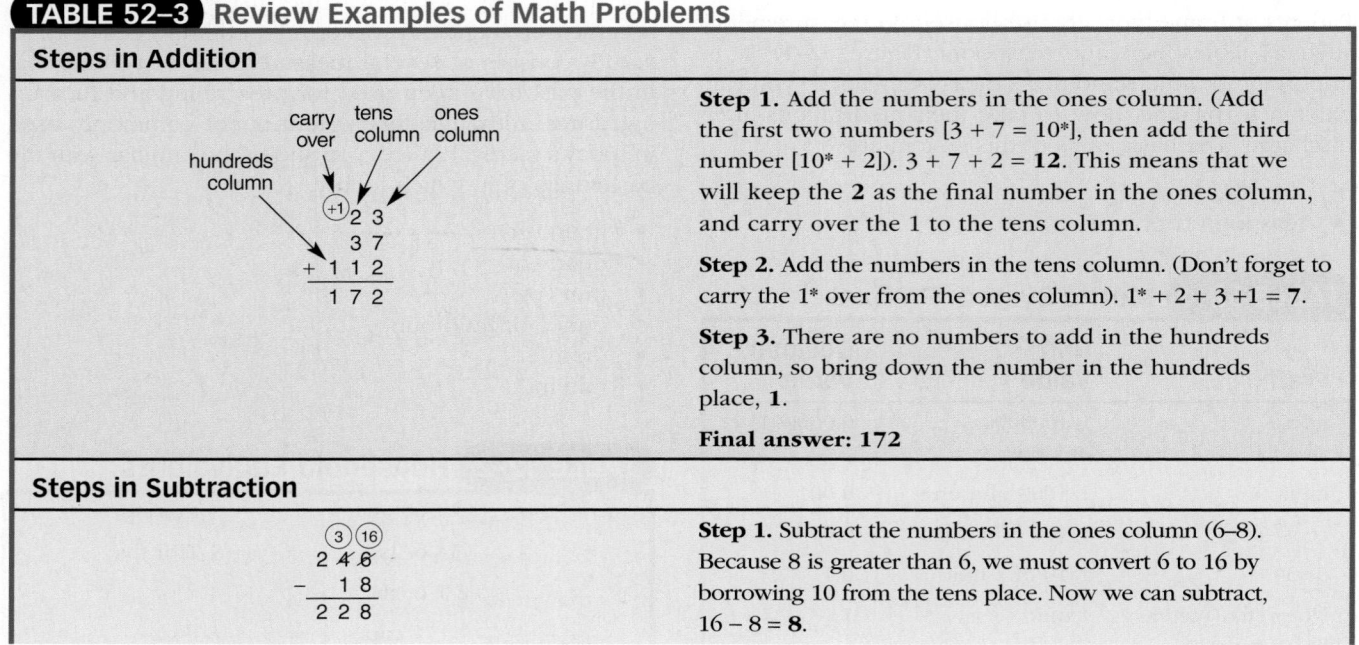

Steps in Addition	
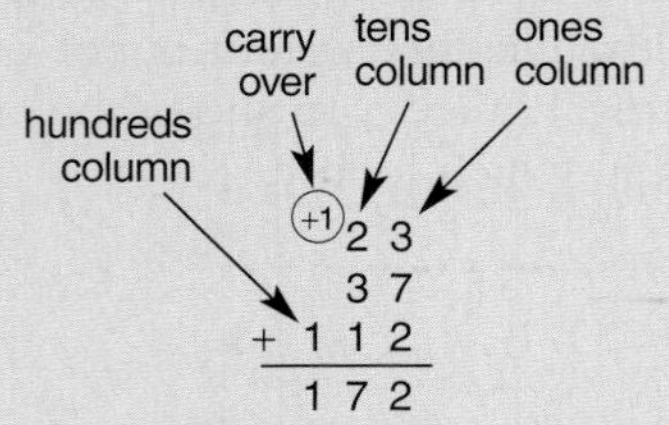	**Step 1.** Add the numbers in the ones column. (Add the first two numbers [3 + 7 = 10*], then add the third number [10* + 2]). 3 + 7 + 2 = **12**. This means that we will keep the **2** as the final number in the ones column, and carry over the 1 to the tens column. **Step 2.** Add the numbers in the tens column. (Don't forget to carry the 1* over from the ones column). 1* + 2 + 3 +1 = **7**. **Step 3.** There are no numbers to add in the hundreds column, so bring down the number in the hundreds place, **1**. **Final answer: 172**
Steps in Subtraction	
(3)(16) 2 ~~4~~ ~~6~~ − 1 8 2 2 8	**Step 1.** Subtract the numbers in the ones column (6–8). Because 8 is greater than 6, we must convert 6 to 16 by borrowing 10 from the tens place. Now we can subtract, 16 – 8 = **8**.

Step 2. Subtract the numbers in the tens column, *remembering* that 4 has been reduced to 3 (because we borrowed for the ones place). So, 3 – 1 = **2**.

Step 3. Subtract the numbers in the hundreds column. 2 – 0 = **2**.

Final answer: 228

Steps in Multiplication

```
 (+2)
  5 1 4
×     5
2 5 7 0
```

Step 1. Multiply 5 by the number in the ones column: 4 × 5 = **20**. Enter the **0** in the ones column and carry over the 2 to be added to the product of the tens column.

Step 2. Multiply 5 by the number in the tens: 5 × **1** = 5*. Now, add the number carried over from the ones column (2): 5* + 2 = **7**.

Step 3. Finally, multiply 5 by the number in the hundreds column: 5 × 5 = 25. Enter that number in the hundreds and thousands columns.

Final answer: 2570

Steps in Division

```
      1 6.5
32 | 5 2 8.0
   - 3 2
     2 0 8
     1 9 2
       1 6 0
       1 6 0
           0
```

Step 1. Read the problem (i.e., 528 divided by 32) and identify the **divisor** and **dividend**. The divisor is the number after "divided by" and goes outside of the bracket (32). The dividend is the number before "divided by" and goes inside the bracket (528).

Step 2. Divide 32 into the first two numbers of the dividend, 52. 32 goes into 52 evenly one time, so put 1 on the top of the bracket, and put 32 (1 × 32) beneath the 52.

Step 3. Subtract 32 from 52. 52 – 32 = 20.

Step 4. Bring down the next digit, 8, making 208.

Step 5. Divide 32 into 208. 32 goes into 208 six times evenly, so put 6 on the top of the bracket and put 192 (6 × 32) beneath the 208.

Step 6. Subtract 192 from 208. 208 – 192 = 16.

Step 7. Add a decimal point and a zero. This does not change the value of the dividend but allows you to continue dividing.

Step 8. Bring the 0 down, making 160.

Step 9. Divide 32 into 160. 32 goes into 160 five times evenly, so put 5 on top of the bracket, and put 160 (5 × 32) beneath the 160.

Step 10. Subtract 160 from 160. 160 – 160 = 0.

Final answer: 16.5

TABLE 52–4 General Rules for Working with Decimals

Adding Decimals

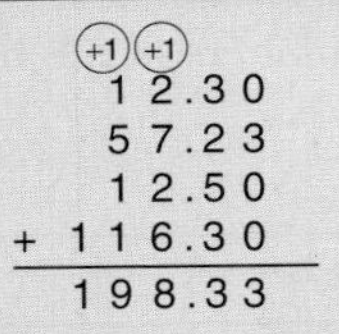

Step 1. Line up the decimal points for each number.

Step 2. Add columns starting on the right. Work from the top down.

Final answer: 198.33

Subtracting Decimals

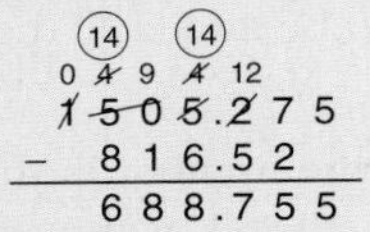

Step 1. Line up the decimal points for each number.

Step 2. Subtract columns starting on the right. Borrow from the number place to the left when needed.

Final answer: 688.755

Multiplying Decimals

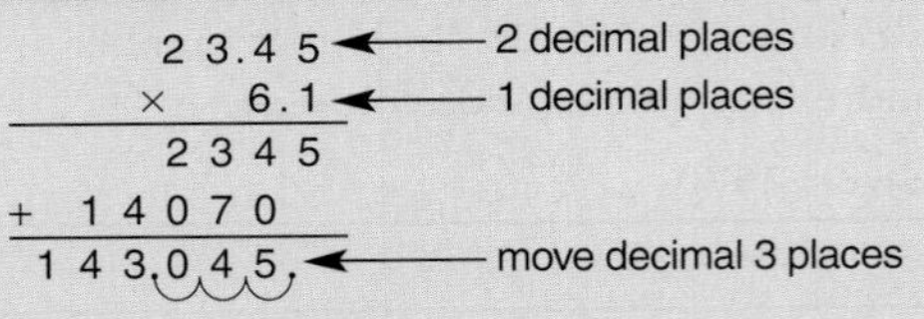

Step 1. Temporarily disregard the decimal points and multiply as you would a whole number.

Step 2. Count the number of decimal places in the numbers being multiplied. In this example, the total number of decimal places is three.

Step 3. In your product, move the decimal point over number of total decimal places.

Final answer: 143.045

Dividing Decimals

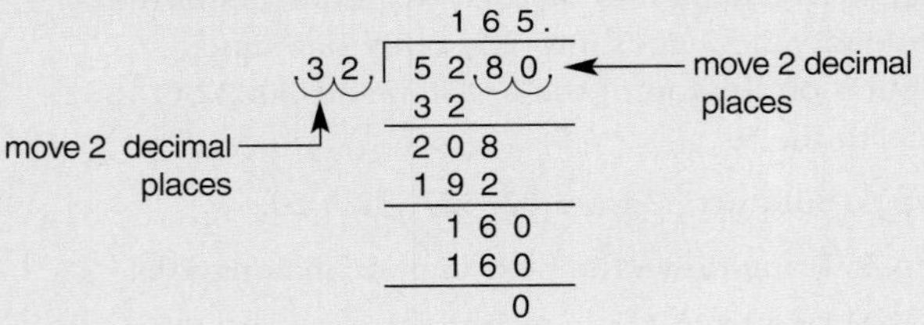

Step 1. Read the problem (i.e., 52.8 divided by 0.32) and identify the divisor and dividend. The divisor is the number after "divided by" and goes outside of the bracket (0.32). The dividend is the number before "divided by" and goes inside the bracket (52.8).

Step 2. Now, move the decimal point to the right in the divisor until it becomes a whole number. In this example, you would move the decimal two places.

Step 3. Now, move the decimal point in the dividend the same number you moved the divisor.

Step 4. Divide as you normally would.

Final answer: 165

Review of Fractions

A **fraction**, like a decimal, indicates part of a whole number, for example: 1/2, 5/6, or 12/100. The top number of a fraction is called the **numerator**; the bottom number is called the **denominator**. An **improper fraction** indicates that the numerator is larger than the denominator, for example: 12/8 or 141/13. A **mixed fraction** includes both a whole number and a fraction, for example: 3-1/2, 24-3/8. When solving a problem with a mixed fraction, begin by converting the whole number into an improper fraction, using the formula: ([whole number × denominator] + numerator)/denominator

EXAMPLE

Convert 5-2/3 to an improper fraction.

Step 1. Identify the numbers to plug into the equation. The whole number is 5; the denominator is 3; the numerator is 2.

Step 2. Plug the numbers into the preceding formula and calculate: (5 × 3) + 2 = 17.

Step 3. Add the denominator, which is 3.

Final answer: 17/3.

TABLE 52–5 Working with Fractions

Adding or Subtracting Fractions	
$\frac{1}{4} + \frac{2}{3}$ (12 is lowest common denominator) $\frac{1(\times 3)}{4(\times 3)} + \frac{2(\times 4)}{3(\times 4)}$ $\frac{3}{12} + \frac{8}{12} = \frac{11}{12}$	**Step 1.** Change any mixed fractions to improper fractions. **Step 2.** The denominator must be the same for each fraction before adding or subtracting. Find the lower common denominator that all denominators divide into evenly. **Step 3.** Convert each fraction into an equivalent fraction with the lowest common denominator. **Step 4.** Add the numerators. **Final Answer: 11/12**
Multiplying Fractions	
$\frac{3}{4} \times \frac{2}{3} =$ $\frac{(3 \times 2)}{(4 \times 3)} =$ $\frac{6}{12} =$ $\frac{1}{2}$	**Step 1.** Change any mixed fractions to improper fractions. **Step 2.** Multiply the numerators straight across. **Step 3.** Multiply the denominators straight across. **Step 4.** Reduce to lowest terms, that is, the lowest equivalent fraction. **Final Answer: 1/2**
Dividing Fractions	
$\frac{2}{3} \div \frac{1}{2}$ $\frac{2}{3} \times \frac{2}{1} = \frac{4}{3} = 1\frac{1}{3}$	**Step 1.** Change any mixed fractions to improper fractions. **Step 2.** Reverse the numerator and denominator of the *second fraction*. **Step 3.** Multiply the numerators straight across. **Step 4.** Multiply the denominators straight across. **Step 5.** Reduce to lowest terms, that is, the lowest equivalent fraction. **Final Answer: 1-1/3**

Table 52–5 reviews adding, subtracting, multiplying, and dividing fractions.

MEDIA LINK

You can also review the "Fractions and Decimals" tutorial on the StudyWARE™ Software to help practice the concepts in this section.

Working with Percentages

Percent means "per hundred," and a **percentage** expresses a value that is part of 100. For instance, 75% means 75/100 or 0.75. When the word *of* is used in conjunction with *percent*, it means to multiply. Before calculating percentages, change the percent number to a decimal (by dividing by 100). Then, multiply the numbers together.

EXAMPLE

150% of 200 = 1.50 × 200 = 300
30% of 88 = 0.30 × 88 = 26.4

Ratio

A **ratio** expresses a relationship between two components and is an alternate way to express a fraction. It contains two numbers separated by a colon. The numerator is to the left of the colon, and the denominator is to the right.

EXAMPLE

A ratio is written as 1:20
The same ratio is spoken as "One to twenty."
The same ratio, expressed as a fraction, would be 1/20.
The same ratio, expressed as a decimal, would be 0.2.
The same ratio expressed as a percent would be 20%.

Proportion

A **proportion** expresses the relationship between two ratios. Two ratios are set, side by side, with either an equal sign (=) or a colon (:) between them.

EXAMPLE

1:2 = 6:12
This proportion is spoken aloud as, "One is to two as six is to twelve."

The values within a proportion are called **means** and **extremes**. The means are the numbers directly to the left and right of the equal sign. The extremes are the two outer numbers.

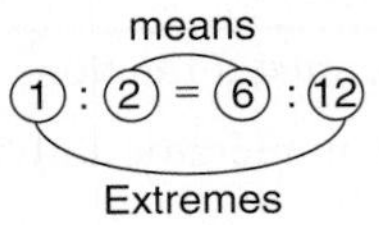

In a true proportion, the product of the means equals the **product** of the extremes. In the example we've been using, 2 × 6 is equal to 1 × 12.

Understanding proportion is important because it allows you to solve for an unknown amount, (x), when the other values are known. This concept is critical to determining dosage calculations.

EXAMPLE

5:15 = x:450

Step 1. Multiply the means (15 × x = 15x)
Step 2. Multiply the extremes (5 × 450 = 2250)
Step 3. Set up an equation, remembering that the means equals extremes (15x = 2250)
Step 4. Divide both sides of the equation by 15 to find the value of x.

$$\frac{\cancel{15}X}{\cancel{15}} = \frac{2250}{15}$$

$$X = 150$$

Step 5. Now, plug 150 back into the original proportion because you have solved the proportion. 5:15 = 150:450 (five is to fifteen as one hundred fifty is to four hundred fifty)

MEDIA LINK

You can also review the "Ratios, Percents, and Equations" tutorial on the StudyWARE™ Software to help practice the concepts in this section.

DOSAGE CALCULATIONS

Basic math skills are necessary for accurately calculating and verifying medication dosages to ensure patient safety before administering any medication. The *wrong dose* of any medication can have profound adverse consequences. Insufficient dosing of an antibiotic does nothing to cure an infection, but an excess dose can cause a toxic reaction. Calculating the *right dose* of medication is a responsibility not to be taken lightly. Familiarity with fractions and equation solving is necessary to convert and calculate drug dosages.

Several methods can be used to calculate dosages; this book will present two methods, the *basic formula* method and the *ratio and proportion* method. The examples for each method will use the same orders and supply numbers, so you can easily compare the methods.

Basic Formula

The basic formula method is:

$$\frac{N}{A} \times V = \text{Dose}$$

The letters in the formula stand for:

$$\frac{\text{Amount Needed}}{\text{Amount Available}} \times \text{Vehicle} = \text{Dose}$$

The amount *Needed* is the dose prescribed, or what the provider has ordered. The amount *Available* is the supply on hand (from the medication label). The *Vehicle* is the form and amount in which the medication comes (capsule, tablet, liquid).

EXAMPLE

Order: Give Baby aspirin 162 mg
Supply: Baby aspirin 81 mg tablets

$$\frac{\text{N (162 mg)}}{\text{A (81 mg)}} \times \text{V(1 Tablet)} =$$

$$\frac{162\ \cancel{\text{mg}}}{81\ \cancel{\text{mg}}} \times 1\ \text{Tablet} =$$

(UNITS CANCEL)

2 Tablets

Final Answer: 2 tablets

EXAMPLE

Order: Give 1000 mg Tylenol elixir
Supply: Tylenol elixir 500 mg per 15 mL

$$\frac{N\ (1000\ \text{mg})}{A\ (500\ \text{mg})} = V(15\ \text{mL}) =$$

$$\frac{1000\ \cancel{\text{mg}}}{500\ \cancel{\text{mg}}} \times 15\ \text{mL} =$$

$$2 \times 15\ \text{mL} =$$

$$30\ \text{mL}$$

Final Answer: 30 mL

Ratio and Proportion Formula

The second method of calculating dosages uses a ratio and proportion formula, which is:

Dosage on hand: Amount on hand = Dosage desired: x (Amount desired)

With this formula, you can follow a three-step process: convert, construct, and calculate.

Step 1. Convert: Ensure that all measurements are in the same system of measurement and the same unit of measurement. Review the next section, "Converting between Units of Measurement."

Step 2. Construct: Use the ratio and proportion formula to construct your equation. The amount desired is the unknown value, x.

Dosage on hand: Amount on hand = Dosage desired: x (Amount desired)

Step 3. Calculate: Solve for x. Insert the answer back into the proportion to identify the units.

CLINICAL PEARL

When calculating dosages for tablets, break tablets in half only when whole tablets in the correct dose are not available.

Converting between Units of Measurement

Medication dosages are ordered by units of measurement. The units tell you how much of the medication to give. The dosage might or might not be the same as the supply of medication on hand.

EXAMPLE

Order: 100 mg of a medication
Supply: The medication is available in 50 mg tablets.

In this example, the units of measurement are the same for both the order and the medication supply; you just need to figure out how many tablets to give. If one tablet equals 50 mg, then two tablets equal 100 mg. The dose for this patient is two tablets.

Frequently, the conversions are more difficult than this. Sometimes a medication is ordered in one unit of measurement but is supplied in another. One way to convert between units of measurement is to set up a proportion of two ratios. To use this method, follow these steps:

- Identify the equivalent.
- Set up a proportion of two equivalent ratios. Remember to label the units in each ratio. The proportion must be set up so the units in the numerators match, and the units in the denominators match.
- Solve for x. Recall that to do this, you multiply the means and extremes and set up the equation to solve for the unknown quantity. Once solved, insert the answer into the original proportion to determine the units.

EXAMPLE

Convert 650 milligrams to grams.
Identify the equivalent. (1 g = 1,000 mg)
Set up the proportion. (1,000 mg:1 g = 650 mg : x g)
Solve for x. Insert the answer back into the proportion to identify the units.

$$(1 \times 650) = (1000 \times X)$$

$$\frac{650}{1000} = \frac{\cancel{1000}X}{\cancel{1000}}$$

$$0.65 = X$$

Final Answer: 0.65 g

EXAMPLE

Convert 12 ounces to mL.
Identify the equivalent. (8 ounces = 240 mL)
Set up the proportion. (8 oz:240 mL = 12 oz:x mL)
Solve for x. Insert the answer back into the proportion to identify the units. (8 oz:240 mL = 12 oz:360 mL)

$$(240 \times 12) = (8 \times X)$$

$$\frac{2880}{8} = \frac{\cancel{8}X}{\cancel{8}}$$

$$360 = X$$

Final Answer: 360 mL

MEDIA LINK

You can also review the "Conversions" tutorial on the StudyWARE™ Software to help practice the concepts in this section.

Practicing the Ratio and Proportion Method

Note that the examples in this section use the same values as the basic formula, so you can compare the two methods easily.

EXAMPLE

Order: Give Baby aspirin 162 mg
Supply: Baby aspirin 81 mg

Step 1. Convert. All measurements are in the same unit of measurement (mg), so no conversion is needed.
Step 2. Construct the proportion.

Dosage on hand: Amount on hand = Dosage desired:*x* (Amount desired)

81 mg:1 tablet = 162 mg:*x* tablets.
Step 3. Calculate, solving for *x*. Insert the answer back into the proportion to identify the units.

$$(1 \times 162) = 81 \times X$$

$$\frac{162}{81} = \frac{\cancel{81}X}{\cancel{81}}$$

$$2 = X$$

Final Answer: 2 tablets

MEDIA LINK

You can also review the "Oral Dosages" and "Parenteral Dosages" tutorials on the StudyWARE™ Software to help practice the concepts in this section.

Ratio and Proportion Method and Calculating Dosages for Liquid Medications

To calculate the dose for medications in liquid form, you must determine how much liquid contains the amount of medication you need to give. The label indicates the amount of drug in a certain volume, for example: 100 mg per 5 mL. Be careful: Sometimes the same medication will come in different concentrations.

EXAMPLE

Order: Give 1000 mg Tylenol elixir
Supply: Tylenol elixir 500 mg per 15 mL

Step 1. Convert. No conversion is necessary because the order and the supply dosage are the same units.
Step 2. Construct your equation.

Dosage on hand:Amount on hand = Dosage desired:Amount desired

500 mg:15 mL = 1000 mg:*x* mL

$$(15 \times 1000) = (500 \times X)$$

$$\frac{15000}{500} = \frac{\cancel{500}X}{\cancel{500}}$$

$$30 = X$$

Step 3. Calculate, solving for *x*. Insert the answer back into the proportion to identify the units.

Final Answer: 30 mL

Calculating Dosages by Weight

Some medications are ordered based on the patient's weight, which usually requires a conversion from pounds to kilograms. To calculate the patient's weight in kilograms (kg), use a conversion factor of 2.2 (1 kg = 2.2 lb).

EXAMPLE

Order: Give Tylenol 30 mg/kg PO now
The child weighs 24 pounds.

Step 1. Convert 24 pounds to kilograms.
- See computations 2.2 lb = 1 kg

$$2.2 \text{ lb:1 kg} + 24 \text{ lb/} \times \text{ kg}$$
$$2.2 \times = 24$$
$$\times = 10.9$$

- Conversion Final Answer: 10.9 kg

Step 2. Set up a proportion by using the number of kilograms and medication order.
- 30 mg:1 kg = *x* mg:10.9 kg

Step 3. Solve for *x*. Insert the answer back into the proportion to identify the units.

$$(1 \times X) = (30 \times 10.9)$$

$$\frac{\cancel{1}X}{\cancel{1}} = \frac{327}{1}$$

$$X = 327$$

Final Answer: 327 mg

CHAPTER SUMMARY

- The metric system is the most commonly used system of measurement in health care; it's based on multiples of ten.
- The three basic units in the metric system are the gram (g), the liter (L), and the meter (m).
- Prefixes in the metric system include: micro-, milli-, centi-, deci-, deka-, hecto-, and kilo-.
- Other systems of measurement include the household measurements and apothecary systems.
- Fractions and decimals indicate part of a whole number, an improper fraction indicates that the numerator is larger than the denominator, and a mixed fraction includes both a whole number and fraction.
- A ratio expresses a relationship between two components and is an alternate way to express a fraction.
- A proportion expresses the relationship between two ratios. Setting up equivalent ratios allows you to solve for an unknown amount (x) when the other values are known.
- Medication dosages are ordered in units of measurement. Sometimes a medication is ordered using one unit of measurement but is supplied in another. One way to convert between units of measurement is to set up a proportion of two ratios.
- Some medications are ordered based on the patient's weight in kilograms; the conversion factor for this is 1 kilogram = 2.2 pounds.
- Calculating dosages follows a three-step process: convert, construct, and calculate.

STUDY TOOLS

Workbook	Activities for Chapter 52
Premium Website	
MEDIA LINK	View these **Media Links** for Chapter 52: • Fractions and Decimals tutorial • Ratios, Percents, and Equations tutorial • Systems of Measurement tutorial • Conversions tutorial • Oral Dosages tutorial • Parenteral Dosages tutorial
StudyWARE	Activities and Quizzes on the **StudyWARE™ Software** for Chapter 52
	Audio Library of medical terms
	Online access to **Critical Thinking Challenge 2.0**
CourseMate	Activities and Quizzes for Chapter 52
WebTutor	Activities and Quizzes for Chapter 52

CHECK YOUR KNOWLEDGE

1. Which system of measurement is most commonly used in health care?
   1. Apothecary
   2. Metric
   3. Standard
   4. Household
2. Drop, cup, and pint are measurements in which system?
   1. Apothecary
   2. Metric
   3. Standard
   4. Household
3. The prefix centi- means what?
   1. 1/10 of a unit
   2. 1/100 of a unit
   3. 10 units
   4. 100 units
4. In the basic formula method, the prescribed amount would be inserted into what place in the formula?
   1. Needed
   2. Available
   3. Vehicle
   4. Dose

5. What are the three steps used in finding the correct amount of medication in the ratio and proportion method?
   1. Calculate, convert, confirm
   2. Convert, calculate, confirm
   3. Convert, construct, calculate
   4. Construct, calculate, convert

6. What is the conversion factor for converting pounds into kilograms?
   1. 1 lb = 2 kg
   2. 1 lb = 2.2 kg
   3. 2 lb = 1 kg
   4. 2.2 lb = 1 kg

Chapter 53 Administering Oral and Non-Injectable Medications

OBJECTIVES

In this chapter, you will learn the following:

KB KNOWLEDGE BASE

1. Spell and define, using the glossary in the back of the text, all the Words to Know in this chapter.
2. Describe the necessary elements that constitute a complete and accurate prescription.
3. List and describe the routes of medication administration.
4. Understand legal aspects of writing prescriptions, including federal and state laws.
5. List the required information and explain the purpose of a medication order.
6. List and explain the Seven Rights of medication administration.
7. Discuss how to avoid and handle a medication error.
8. List and discuss the information required for a complete and accurate medication entry into the patient's record.
9. Recognize and be able to write out correctly the abbreviations used in recording medications.
10. Describe and discuss appropriate measures regarding documentation of medication and immunization side effects and adverse effects.

S SKILLS

1. Prepare a prescription according to the provider's direction.
2. Demonstrate calling in a complete and accurate prescription to a pharmacist.
3. Demonstrate how to record a medication entry accurately in the patient's chart.
4. Measure and administer the ordered dose of oral medication.
5. Administer eye drops.
6. Instill drops into the ears.
7. Administer a rectal medication.
8. Administer a vaginal medication.

B BEHAVIORS

1. Verify ordered dosages before administering medication.
2. Prepare and administer medication following the Seven Rights.
3. Use language and verbal skills that enable patients' understanding.
4. Work within the medical assistant's legal scope of practice.

WORDS TO KNOW

buccal	medication order	prescription	sublingual
dispense as written (DAW)	narcotic	right documentation	suppository
enemas	ointment	salve	topical
Joint Commission	parenteral	Seven Rights	transdermal

ROUTES OF ADMINISTRATION

Drugs may be administered by many routes, depending on the rate of absorption desired, distribution, biotransformation (how the body converts the drug into a form it can use), and elimination. The following list of administration routes is provided as an introduction to the terminology used in orders and prescriptions.

Additional information regarding the proper mechanics of each route the medical assistant is responsible for and authorized to perform are covered later in this chapter and in Chapter 54.

Note: *The medical assistant is not authorized to deliver every route listed, but additional routes have been included for these reasons:*

- *To familiarize you with the terminology to enable you to identify an erroneous or inappropriate order or a typographical error.*
- *To give you a broader understanding of different routes of medication administration and the effects of each.*
- *To enhance your understanding of medication terminology to become a better prepared member of the health care team.*
- *To assist in the preparation or administration of different types of medications to be given by a provider licensed to do so.*
- *To be prepared to provide specific directions to patients for taking medications.*

Different routes of administration include:

- *Oral:* by mouth; medication may be swallowed in solid or liquid form.
- *Buccal:* placed between the cheek and gum for absorption through the mucous membranes in the mouth; medication is a solution, gel, or dissolvable tablet.
- *Sublingual:* placed under the tongue for fast absorption; medication is a dissolvable tablet or gel.
- *Drops:* liquid solution applied directly to eyes, ears, nose, or in the mouth for infants and small children.
- *Inhalation:* breathed in through nose or mouth; delivered by spray or by metered aerosol device.
- *Intradermal:* given by shallow angle injection just under the dermis of the skin.
- *Intramuscular:* injected into muscular tissue for delayed absorption.
- *Intranasal:* given through the nares.
- *Intraosseous:* used in emergencies to deliver drugs directly into the bone marrow; not a commonly used route but used in emergencies when other routes are unavailable.
- *Intrathecal:* delivered into the spinal canal by injection or infusion.
- *Intravenous:* delivered into a vein by injection or infusion.
- *Ophthalmic:* applied directly into the eyelid or lacrimal opening in the corner of the eye; medication in the form of ointment or drops.
- *Otic:* delivered into the ear canal.
- *Rectal:* inserted directly into the rectum; usually in the form of an ointment or dissolvable tablet.
- *Subcutaneous:* injection just below cutaneous layer of the skin.
- *Topical:* applied directly to the skin.
- *Transdermal:* applied directly to the skin; an adhesive patch placed on the skin, containing time-released medication.
- *Vaginal:* delivered directly by manual insertion or applicator into the vaginal vault in the form of ointment or dissolvable tablet.

PRESCRIPTIONS

A **prescription** is a written order prepared by a licensed provider or practitioner authorizing a medication or treatment to be dispensed to the patient for self-administration. The prescription must include the following information, as shown in Figure 53–1.

- Practitioner's name and address
- Date of issue
- Patient's name and address
- Drug name
- Dosage form
- Quantity prescribed
- Directions for use
- Number of refills if any are authorized and are permitted under the law
- Line or check box indicating whether it should be dispensed as written or substitutions are permitted by the prescriber
- Manual signature of prescriber

The medical assistant should *always* return an incomplete prescription or medication order for revision to the prescriber if any required information is missing and should never fill in missing information independently. This standard information is required for the pharmacist to fill the prescription accurately. Prefilled and prepackaged medications now make the pharmacist's job easier, but there is still the occasional need for certain medications to be compounded, or prepared, by a licensed pharmacist from the directions on the prescription.

Prescriptions often contain a box or line with **DAW**, which stands for **dispense as written**, by which the

Parts of a Prescription

1. The physician's name, address, telephone and fax numbers, and DEA registration number.
2. The patient's name, date of birth, address, and the date on which the prescription is written.
3. The *superscription* that includes the symbol Rx ("take thou").
4. The *inscription* that states the names and quantities of ingredients to be included in the medication.
5. The *subscription* that gives directions to the pharmacist for filling the prescription.
6. The *signature* (Sig) that gives the directions for the patient.
7. The physician's signature blanks. Where signed, indicates if a generic substitute is allowed or if the medication is to be dispensed as written.
8. REFILL 0 1 2 3 p.r.n. This is where the physician indicates whether the prescription can be refilled.

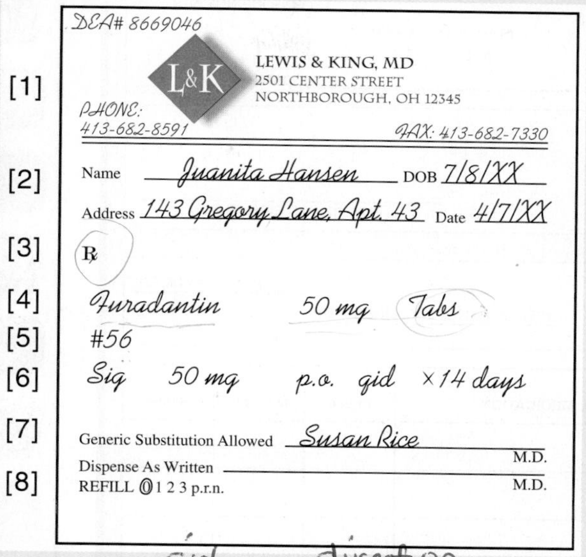

[1]
[2]
[3]
[4]
[5]
[6]
[7]
[8]
DEA# 8669046
L&K
LEWIS & KING, MD
2501 CENTER STREET
NORTHBOROUGH, OH 12345
PHONE:
413-682-8591
FAX: 413-682-7330
Name Juanita Hansen DOB 7/8/XX
Address 143 Gregory Lane, Apt. 43 Date 4/7/XX
℞
Furadantin 50 mg Tabs
#56
Sig 50 mg p.o. qid ×14 days
Generic Substitution Allowed Susan Rice M.D.
Dispense As Written M.D.
REFILL 0 1 2 3 p.r.n.

Figure 53–1: Parts of a prescription. *Delmar/Cengage Learning.*

prescriber may indicate permission for a medication to be substituted with a trade or generic form as appropriate. For example, the prescribed generic might be temporarily unavailable or recommended in place of a trade name drug to save the patient money. Many insurance providers require a generic to be dispensed by formulary unless a condition exists in which the prescriber feels the generic is potentially harmful or ineffective for the patient. The prescriber will indicate whether the medication may or may not be substituted. If not, it should be *dispensed* exactly *as written*.

Preparing Prescriptions

In the past, prescriptions have been predominantly handwritten by the provider, especially those for **narcotics**, but with the advent of electronic medical records, it has become more prevalent for many prescribers to transmit prescriptions directly to the pharmacist. Some handwritten or even electronically prepared prescriptions may be faxed to a pharmacist, providing they are not for certain schedules of narcotics. The practice of telephoning in a prescription to the pharmacy has declined quite a bit in recent years to avoid medication errors made with verbal communication. A copy of the actual prescription should be entered in the patient's chart. In addition to this, a running log of prescriptions with all pertinent information should be included in the medical record for ease of tracking. This is one of many very useful tools included in most electronic medical record software packages.

In offices without electronic medical records, preparing the handwritten prescription may be delegated to the medical assistant except for the final review and signature. Because the prescription is a legal document, the provider is obligated to verify that the information is accurate before signing the prescription. Figure 53–2 shows an example of a prescription blank.

When only one medication is prescribed, the single medication prescription pad is used. These may be printed in many variations, including provider letterhead information at the top in a preprinted pad or an electronic record, and so on, as long as all the legally required information is included. The multiple medication prescription format is useful for patients whose conditions require multiple medications to be prescribed at a time, eliminating the need to write in the patient's information on multiple single prescriptions and the doctor to sign many single prescriptions. In many states, prescriptions for controlled substances may contain only the controlled substance and no other drugs on the same document. The quantity must appear in both numerical and written form.

When patients have their prescriptions filled by a pharmacist, the container often has a supplementary label(s) on it. Pharmacists frequently use one or more of these brightly colored labels to alert the patient of special instructions or warnings regarding a particular medication ordered by the doctor. Bright colors attract attention to important information (Figure 53–3). The medical assistant should encourage patients to read and comply with the warning labels.

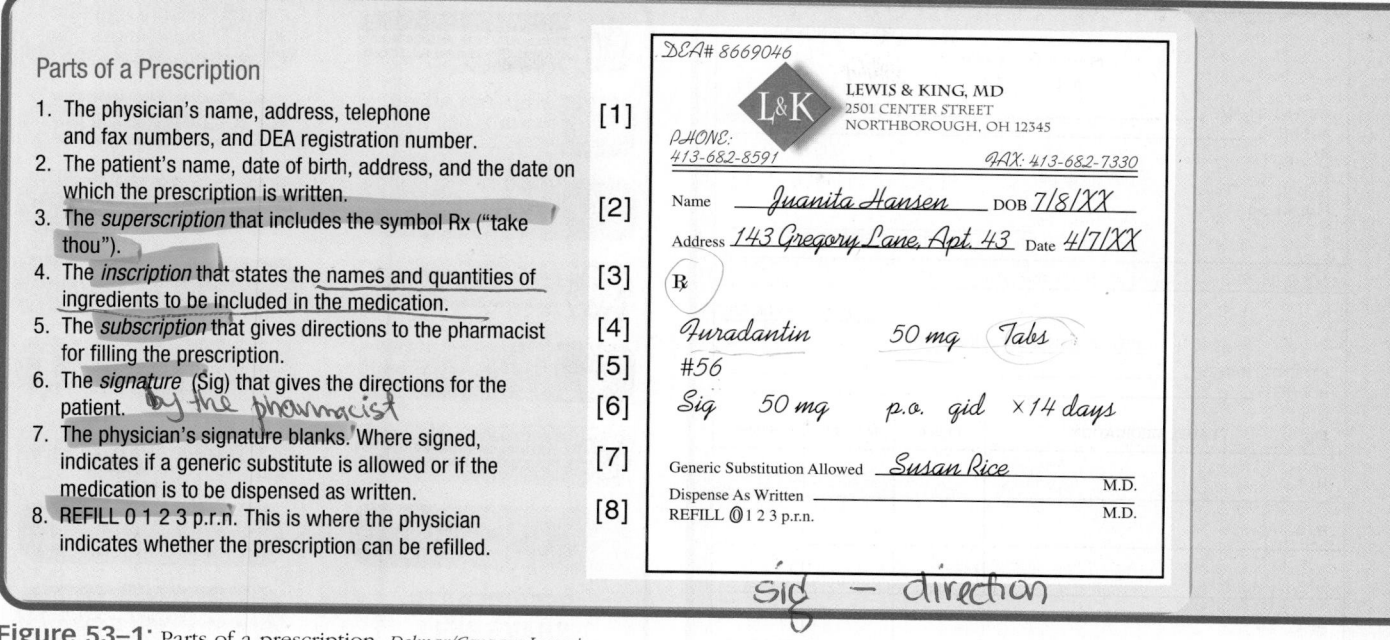

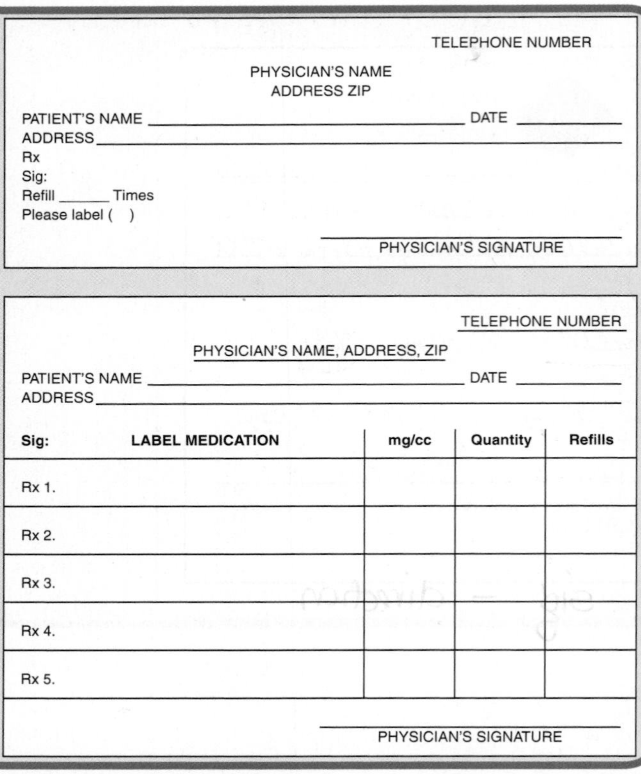

TELEPHONE NUMBER

PHYSICIAN'S NAME
ADDRESS ZIP

PATIENT'S NAME ________________ DATE ________
ADDRESS ________________
Rx
Sig:
Refill ______ Times
Please label ( )

________________ PHYSICIAN'S SIGNATURE

TELEPHONE NUMBER

PHYSICIAN'S NAME, ADDRESS, ZIP

PATIENT'S NAME ________________ DATE ________
ADDRESS ________________

Sig: LABEL MEDICATION	mg/cc	Quantity	Refills
Rx 1.			
Rx 2.			
Rx 3.			
Rx 4.			
Rx 5.			

________________ PHYSICIAN'S SIGNATURE

Figure 53–2: Sample prescription blanks for single medication and multiple medications. *Delmar/Cengage Learning.*

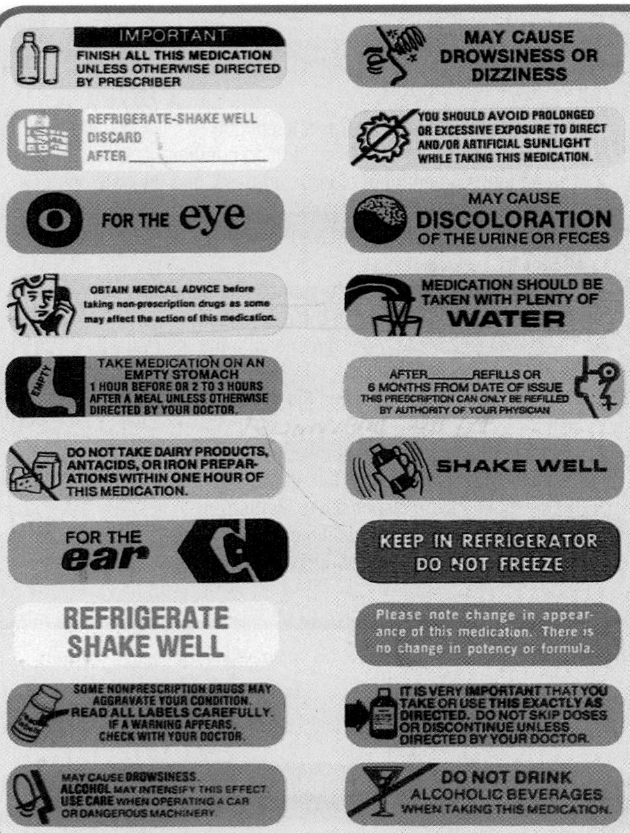

Figure 53–3: Examples of instruction and warning labels for prescription medications. *Delmar/Cengage Learning.*

PROCEDURE 53–1 Prepare a Prescription

MEDIA LINK: View the video, "Prepare a Prescription per Provider's Orders," for this chapter on the Premium Website.

PURPOSE: To ensure patient safety by providing a complete and accurate prescription

EQUIPMENT: Chart, prescription pad, or electronic prescription

S **SKILL:** Prepare a prescription according to the provider's or nurse practitioner's direction.

Procedure Steps	Detailed Instructions and/or *Rationales*
1. Obtain the order from the chart.	Verify that the prescription to be written is exactly what is being prescribed. *Avoids incorrect prescription.*
B 2. ***Compare patient identifiers.***	Check the chart information for the ***right*** patient and compare to the order sheet or note to be sure they match. *Prescribes medication to the **right patient**.*

Procedure Steps	Detailed Instructions and/or *Rationales*
3. Fill in prescription fields.	Enter information in prescription: ***right*** drug, ***right*** amount, ***right*** frequency, ***right*** route, and any special instructions. *Follows the* **Seven Rights.**
B 4. ***Compare the completed prescription to the order.***	Match each item to the order. *Verifies that the prescription is being written accurately.*
5. Obtain prescriber's signature.	Present to prescriber for legal authorization. *Ensures compliance with prescribing laws.*
B 6. ***Compare the completed prescription to the order—again.***	Verify that all fields are completed correctly, including prescription line, DAW, and refills. *Avoids incomplete or incorrect prescriptions.*
7. Present the completed prescription to the patient.	Provide applicable patient teaching and offer opportunity for patient to ask questions. *Ensures patient safety and promotes compliance with prescribed regimen.*
8. Document correctly in the patient's chart.	***Right*** documentation should be included in the chart, including all the elements of the prescription and any patient teaching provided. *Complies with Seven Rights of medications and includes pertinent information in patient's chart for future reference.* Review the following Charting Example and Figure 53–4.

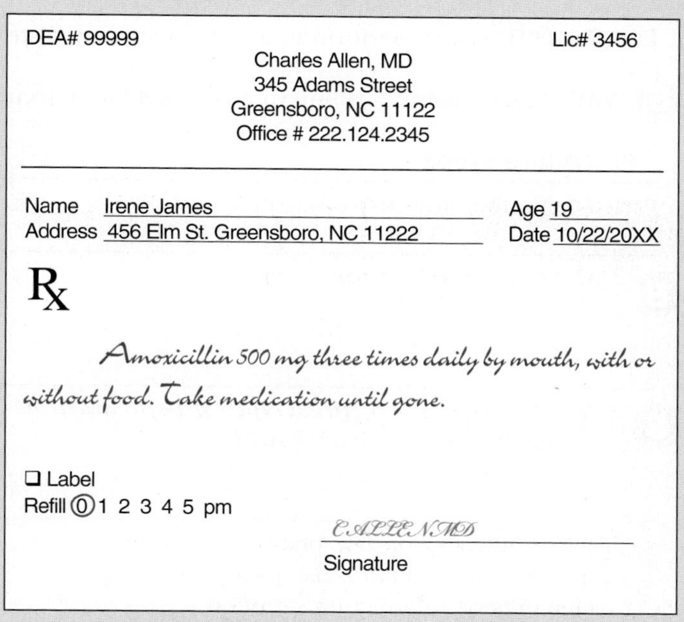
DEA# 99999 Lic# 3456

Charles Allen, MD
345 Adams Street
Greensboro, NC 11122
Office # 222.124.2345

Name Irene James Age 19
Address 456 Elm St. Greensboro, NC 11222 Date 10/22/20XX

℞

Amoxicillin 500 mg three times daily by mouth, with or without food. Take medication until gone.

☐ Label
Refill ⓪ 1 2 3 4 5 pm

C ALLEN MD
Signature

Figure 53–4: Example of a completed prescription. Notice that the handwriting of the prescription and the author belongs to two persons. *Delmar/Cengage Learning.*

Charting Example

10/22/20XX, 9:22 am	Prepared prescription for amoxicillin to be given to Ms. James. Reviewed and signed by Dr. Allen. Patient will take to ABC pharmacy on Green St. Amy Sanderson, RMA (AMT) ————

Calling in a Prescription to a Pharmacy

When telephoning in prescriptions, the medical assistant must provide the pharmacist with ALL the information contained in the prescription. To ensure accuracy, the pharmacist should repeat back this information to avoid dangerous misunderstandings. This practice of repeating back prescription or medication order information is recommended by the **Joint Commission** in all areas of medical practice.

In addition to encouraging the patient to read all warning labels, the medical assistant should ask patients whether they have any questions about the medications and are able to read the instructions completely. If the patient is not literate enough to read the label completely or has a visual impairment that prevents reading small print, the medical assistant may ask the pharmacist to print a second label in the patient's native language, in addition to English, or in larger type.

CLINICAL PEARL

Many patients, not just the elderly, might have arthritis or other fine-motor problems that make it difficult for them to open childproof caps. If this is the case, the medical assistant may request the prescription to be dispensed in a non-childproof bottle. The pharmacist will likely add an additional warning of the importance of keeping an unprotected bottle out of the reach of children.

PROCEDURE 53–2 Call in a Complete and Accurate Prescription to the Pharmacy

PURPOSE: To convey and confirm that a complete and accurate prescription has been transmitted and received

EQIUPMENT: Chart; perform in an area with few distractions

S SKILL: Demonstrate calling in a complete and accurate prescription to a pharmacist.

Procedure Steps	Detailed Instructions and/or *Rationales*
1. Obtain the order from the chart.	Verify that the prescription to be written is exactly what is being prescribed. *Ensures accurate prescription.*
B 2. ***Compare patient identifiers.***	Check the chart information for the ***right*** patient and compare to the order sheet or note to be sure they match. *Ensures that you are prescribing medication to the* ***right*** *patient.*
B 3. ***Verify accuracy of prescription information (demonstrate critical thinking skills).***	Compare all elements of prescription with order, including patient name, address, date of birth, time, date, and provider's signature. *Ensures that the accurate prescription is being provided to pharmacist.*
4. Determine appropriate pharmacy. Call in information to pharmacist, providing all the elements of a correct prescription.	
B 5. ***Have the pharmacist read back the prescription.***	*Verify accuracy by evaluating whether information was received correctly.*
6. Document in patient's chart.	***Right*** documentation should be included in the chart, including all the elements of the prescription. Also include the person and his or her credentials to whom you called in the prescription. Date and time your entry. *Maintain complete documentation in patient's chart for future reference.*

Charting Example

1/31/20XX, 11:53 am	Called in order for "Flexeril 10 mg po every 6 hours as needed for muscle spasms" for Mary L. Anderson to EFG Pharmacy on Elm St. per Ms. Anderson's request, authorized by Dr. Green, see prescription/order in medication section of chart. Joseph, pharmacy tech, took prescription and read back with correct information, including patient name and date of birth verified. Insurance information was on file. Entered prescription in medication flow sheet. Called Ms. Anderson to advise it will be ready by 3 pm today. Elizabeth Parsons, RMA (AMT)

E-Prescribing

With the advancement in health information software, prescriptions may be printed by selecting a particular drug from a drop-down menu in the electronic medical record application with the appropriate strength, dosage, and the quantity to be supplied or days' supply, as ordered. The prescription is printed on special prescription paper with tamper-proof watermark. Computer-generated prescriptions reduce the possibility of forgery through decreasing availability of the prescription document through password controls and tracking of users authorized to print the prescriptions. The most significant benefit of electronic prescriptions is most likely in the elimination of errors that result from illegible handwriting.

CLINICAL PEARL

You might notice different medications prescribed for the same disease process in patients of different color, race, or gender. The clinical decision behind this practice is based on evidence that suggests different medications have varying effectiveness and differing side effects in blacks versus whites and males versus females and is not just a random choice.

CLINICAL PEARL

Providers or nurse practitioners occasionally prescribe a medication for a particular disease or symptom that is considered off-label use. This does not mean that the drug should not be used in this manner or that it is necessarily an improper prescribing practice. It simply refers to the fact that controlled clinical trials have not been done to determine whether the drug is safe. Different weight charts are available, and one been done to determine whether the drug is safe or effective for the indication for which the medication is being prescribed.

MEDICATION ORDERS

Medication orders are direct and complete instructions composed by the provider or other licensed practitioner for administering medications to a patient while he or she is in the facility or office. The medication order is generally written either in the chart or on a separate order sheet that should be included as a permanent part of the patient's chart. If the order is illegible, incomplete, or unclear, the order must not be carried out until it is rewritten or clarified. Many offices are now using electronic medical records, which helps eliminate medication errors and illegible orders. Figure 53–5 compares an example of a handwritten, illegible medication order to a computer-generated order.

Elements of a correct and complete medication order include:

- *Full name of the patient:* There can be patients in a given practice or facility who have similar names,

PRIMARY CARE ASSOCIATES
456 Oak Street * Everywhere, USA 98765 * 444-555-1111

Name: Johnny Jones Date: 2/10/2010

Address: 777 Elm St. Date of birth: 10/1/1985

Anywhere, KS 22200

℞ Lamiclal 25 mg daily for 2 weeks then increase to 50 mg daily.

K Johnson, FNP
Dispense as Written Substitution Permitted

Refills: 0

PRIMARY CARE ASSOCIATES
456 Oak Street * Everywhere, USA 98765 * 444-555-1111

Name: Johnny Jones Date: 2/10/2010

Address: 777 Elm St. Date of birth: 10/1/1985

Anywhere, KS 22200

℞ Lamiclal 25 mg daily for 2 weeks then increase to 50 mg daily.

K Johnson, FNP
Dispense as Written Substitution Permitted

Refills: 0 Disp. # 70/ (4 weeks supply)

Figure 53–5: Compare the readability of the (A) handwritten order to (B) the computer-generated order. *Delmar/Cengage Learning.*

e.g., John Smith, Jane Williams, and so on. Writing the full name of the patient, including any middle names or initials and Jr. or Sr. at the end of the name provides additional information that helps ensure that the order is for the correct patient.

- *Name of the medication:* It is important always to check, check, and check again the name of the medication in the order against the label on the medication to be given. When possible, maintain consistency within a practice by using either a generic or a trade name for a particular medication to avoid errors.
- *Dosage:* Verify that the dosage of a medication being ordered is not only being measured accurately but that it is also an appropriate dosage for that medication. If in doubt, always double-check against drug references.
- *Route of administration:* The wrong route of the medication can be ineffective and even dangerous. Always double-check what is written with what is appropriate for the medication ordered.
- *Frequency, or how often, the medication is ordered:* In the office setting, a medication will likely ordered as a single dose, but the MA should make sure that

the patient understands when the next dose is due to ensure accurate therapeutic levels and avoid any toxic side effects from taking doses too close together.

- *Date and time the order is written:* It is very important to record accurately both the date and time ordered, particularly when other medications are being taken or ordered, and to avoid any duplicated medications.
- *Specific instructions:* Certain medications should be given with food to avoid stomach upset or enhance absorption, whereas others must be taken on an empty stomach for more rapid absorption. Many medications have interactions with foods, supplements, or other medications. For instance, Valium and several cholesterol-lowering drugs should not be taken with grapefruit juice. Coumadin has multiple medication and food interactions and considerations. Osteoporosis medications, such as Boniva®, require the patient to remain upright for at least one hour following administration.
- *Signature of the prescriber:* Although it is the responsibility of the prescriber to sign the order, the person administering the order is responsible for making sure the order is complete and accurate before giving any medication. Even when a verbal or telephone order is taken and signed off on by an authorized health care provider, the order still requires a signature within a given period of time, which varies from state to state and by the type of institution, to be legal.

PROCEDURE 53–3 Prepare a Medication Order

PURPOSE: To write instructions for a medication order accurately and completely.

EQUIPMENT: Chart; direct supervision of the licensed prescribing practitioner.

S **SKILL:** Demonstrate preparing a complete medication order.

Procedure Steps	Detailed Instructions and *Rationales*
1. Obtain the chart for the correct patient.	Verify the ***right*** chart for the ***right*** patient. *Avoids providing medication to wrong patient.*
2. Receive and write order from prescribing practitioner on the patient's permanent medication order sheet.	*Prepares a legal record of the medication order.* To avoid duplicated medication administration, make the entry immediately and prior to any medication being given.
B 3. ***Read back the order to the prescriber if received verbally.***	*Verifies the accuracy of the order. Prevents errors of the Seven Rights: patient, medication, dosage, route, time, technique, and documentation.*
4. Obtain signature of prescriber.	*Not only is this a legal requirement, but it also gives the prescriber yet another opportunity to verify that the information is accurate.*
5. Document in patient's chart.	

Charting Example

11/13/20XX 11:17 am	Janet Yeager, MD, examined patient and reviewed lab work. Verbal order for Coumadin 5 mg po received. Noted order, read back with correct information, verified patient by name and street address correctly provided by patient. Coumadin 5 mg po given with water. Entered in medication flow sheet. Amber Clinton, CMA (AAMA)

THE SEVEN RIGHTS OF MEDICATION ADMINISTRATION

The medical assistant is expected to read and record many types of medications. Accurately recording all medications administered to patients is absolutely necessary. When following the provider's orders in giving medications to patients, always prepare, administer, and record the medication as soon as possible before beginning any other new tasks. When the provider is present and gives the order verbally (verbal orders are discouraged per Joint Commission recommendations), always double-check the specific medicine, the dose, the expiration date, and any other necessary details with the provider *again* just prior to administration.

Medical assistants, as well as other health care personnel, should not prepare medications for someone else to administer nor should they give medications that have been prepared by someone else. One of the few exceptions to this rule is in the case of public health scenarios during which mass immunizations, e.g., flu shots, are given.

Prior to administering *any* medication to *any* patient, the MA should follow a standard format checklist of the **Seven Rights** of medication administration:

1. Right Patient
2. Right Medication
3. Right Dose/amount
4. Right Route/method
5. Right Technique
6. Right Time/schedule
7. Right Documentation

To confirm that the medication is being administered to the ***Right Patient***, ask the patient to cite his or her full name as well as one other identifier from the chart such as birth date, age, address, and so on. *Do not* ask these questions in a way that prompts a "yes" or "no" response from the patient.

To ensure the ***Right Medication***, check the medication order and verify the medication at least four times prior to administration:

1. When preparing the medication
2. Upon bringing the medication to administer to the patient
3. Prior to administering
4. Following administration

Carefully reading the medication order provides instruction on the ***Right Dose*** as well as the ***Right Route*** by which the provider wants the medication to be administered (e.g., topically, transdermally, orally, or by injection). These methods of administration are very different.

The ***Right Technique*** refers to how the medication is administered (e.g., the skill in giving different types of injections, the manner in which you apply a topical preparation, or the way in which you administer an inhalation treatment to a patient).

Attention must be given to the ***Right Time*** and schedule in administering medicines. The time a medication is administered is also important to the well-being of the patient. For instance, some medicines should not be taken when the stomach is full, and some should not be taken when the stomach is empty. Determining the time the patient has eaten last is important. Checking the time also should remind you to check the expiration date of the medication to be sure of its quality strength.

Other considerations for route of administration can include:

- Age of the patient
- General physical condition: whether athletic or debilitated
- Body size or mass
- Gender
- Other medical problems, e.g., kidney or liver disease
- Other medications being taken, e.g., blood thinners

Once the medication has been administered, the medical assistant might be required to observe the patient for a period of time for any signs of adverse events.

All the information regarding the preceding rights described should be documented in complete detail in the patient's record (***Right Documentation***) along with any adverse events and instructions provided to the patient regarding being alert for reactions and what steps to take if a reaction occurs.

Medication Errors

The consequences of medication errors can be serious, and the prevention of these errors cannot be stressed enough. Great care must be taken to identify correctly the patient for whom the medication is intended before it is administered. Offices and clinics care for many patients in the course of the daily schedule. As the number of patients being seen increases, so do the opportunities for errors.

If an error is made, NEVER try to cover it up, even if the intent is to protect the practice. Notify the prescriber or supervising practitioner at once to determine what steps need to be taken. Many errors require only monitoring, but some errors might require emergency intervention; the plan of care is determined only by the ordering provider or advanced practitioner.

A medication error involves one or more of the following:

- Correct drug given to *wrong* ***patient***
- *Wrong* ***drug*** given to the correct patient
- *Wrong* ***dose*** administered

- *Wrong* ***documentation*** placed in the patient's chart: can be either wrong chart or incorrect information
- Drug given by the *wrong* ***route***
- Drug given at the *wrong* ***time***

MEDICATION DOCUMENTATION

Right documentation is the last but very important step that *always* follows the administration of medications. The person who administered the medication verifies AGAIN that all Seven Rights were followed to ensure that no medication error was made. At the end of the order, leaving no lines or spaces, the person administering the order signs his or her name with credential, followed by the date and time the order was given. NEVER document a medication for anyone else or have anyone else record a medication you administer. In some situations, the medical assistant may write down the information regarding a medication administered by the provider in the provider's stead, but the provider should sign, date, and time the entry personally.

Many factors must be included in recording medication information on the patient's chart. The following is a list of the details that should be included in recording medications:

Who—*Who ordered* the medication and *who should take it*. Include the provider's printed name and be sure the patient's name is correctly spelled in the chart.

What—What medication was administered. The medication name should be recorded accurately and legibly; *how much*, meaning the strength and dose of the substance, should also be recorded.

When—The date and time the medication is administered should be recorded. Be sure to check the expiration date of the medication before administering it.

Where—Refers to the route of administration of the medication: oral, sublingual, topical, or parenteral, including site and appearance of the site following injection.

Why—Offer information regarding the reason the medication is being given to the patient verbally and provide printed patient information as necessary. Provide an opportunity for the patient to ask questions before and after the medication has been given. The provider is required by the National Childhood Vaccine Injury Act of 1986 (NCVIA) to provide written information regarding information to the patient or parent of a minor patient prior to immunizations.

Medication records may be kept differently based on types of practice settings or the employer's preference. Private office practices and clinics often keep a running log of medications prescribed and a separate running log for those given in the practice setting. Long-term care facilities may keep a separate medication record of all medications given on a daily basis. Whatever the format used, it is important to become familiar with that setting's practice and maintain consistency when making medication entries, using the desired format.

Appropriate documentation includes:

- Patient's name
- Date of birth
- Medication name; amount, site, and route of administration; time administered; and any reactions observed (This might or might not be necessary, depending on medication administered and patient's history of previous adverse events to other medications or immunizations.)
- Patient education provided
- Ordered by (provider, nurse practitioner, or other legal prescriber)
- For immunizations, also include manufacturer, lot number, serial number if applicable, and expiration date

If any conditions were not met or any variances made, this should also be noted. When a separate medication sheet is maintained, as in a long-term care facility for example, the variance is noted there. If the medication order sheet is the only record, as might be the case in a clinic setting, the notation should go on the order. For example, if a patient was unavailable at the time the medication was ordered, it would be noted that it was administered late and the specific reason it was given late. Other reasons for variances can include withholding the medication for medical judgment (patient vomiting), patient refusal to take the medication, or learning of a potential interaction or contraindication for giving the medication. If this occurs, secure the medication and notify the ordering prescriber at once for further instructions.

After the medication has been administered as ordered, enter next to the order the *date* and *time* and that it was given as ordered, followed by a legible *signature* complete with credential. Follow the last letter of the entry with a line to the edge of the page to signify that nothing follows, preventing unauthorized additions to this chart note.

EXAMPLE

"... given at 1:10 PM, 2/2/2010, by
J. Smith, RMA (AMT) ______________________"

Figure 53–6 shows an example of correct documentation.

10-10-xx
John Smith, dob 1/1/1990, identity verified by Jane Johnson, MA. ADACEL™
8:15 AM
1.0 mL to right deltoid IM, no swelling or bruising at site following injection. Sanofi Plasteur, Lot#12345, expires 12/31/2010. Patient observed for 30 minutes after injection, no adverse events noted. J. Johnson, CMA(AAMA).

Figure 53–6: Example of a correct entry in the patient's chart. *Delmar/Cengage Learning.*

TABLE 53–1 Abbreviations Commonly Used in Administering Medications

Abbreviation	Meaning	Abbreviation	Meaning
ac	before meals	LB, lb	pound
ad lib	as needed or desired	mcg	microgram
am	morning	mL	milliliter
ā	before	noc	night
BID, bid	twice daily	NPO, npo	nothing by mouth
BSA	body surface area	oz	ounce
c̄	with	p	after
CAPS	caps	pc	after meals
comp	compound	po	by mouth
contra	against	PRN, prn	as needed
DAW	dispense as written	pt	patient
DC, DISC, disc, d/c	discontinue	QAM	every morning
EENT	eye, ear, nose, throat	Q or q followed by a number (2, 3, etc.)	every 2,3,etc. hours
elix	elixir	qh	every hour
emul	emulsion	QID, qid	4 times daily
ext	extract	qns	quantity not sufficient
Fe^{++}	iron	qs	quantity sufficient
fl	fluid	Rx	prescription, treatment
garg	gargle	s̄	without
G, Gm, g, gm	gram	sat	saturated
gtt, gtts	drop, drops	Sig, sig	directions, dispense number . . .
GI	gastrointestinal	sol	solution
GU	genitourinary	STAT, stat	immediately
hr	hour	suppos, supp.	suppository
IM	intramuscular	TAB	tablet
inj	injection, injectable	TBSP, tbsp	tablespoon
IV	intravenous	TID, tid	three times daily
K^{+}	potassium	tinc	tincture
kg	kilogram	TSP, tsp	teaspoon
L	liter	w/o	without

Abbreviations Used in Documenting Medications

Table 53–1 presents some of the commonly used abbreviations and symbols in medication administration. Although a number of abbreviations are used in different specialties and types of health care environments, there is no comprehensive list of "approved" abbreviations. The word should always be spelled out if the person making the entry is unsure of the appropriate abbreviation to use or if it could create any confusion about what is being written.

Several organizations have prepared lists of abbreviations that most commonly lead to medication errors. Figure 53–7 shows a list from the Institute of Safe Medication Practices (ISMP). Additionally, the Joint Commission, the accrediting agency for hospitals, has prepared a "Do Not Use" list of abbreviations and recommends that each practice, facility, or system use standardized procedures for documenting medications. However, they do not dictate which abbreviations should be included or excluded other than those indicated in the "Do Not Use" list. To download the "Do Not Use" list, navigate to www.jointcommission.org and search for "Do Not Use List." The CDC also posts a vaccine acronym and abbreviation list on its Website that can be printed and kept where vaccinations are stored as a quick reference for charting. (Navigate to www.cdc.gov and search for "Vaccine Acronyms and Abbreviations.")

Documenting Medication and Immunization Side Effects and Adverse Events

A reaction to any medication that is given at a medical facility or elsewhere, whether observed by a health care professional or reported by the patient, should be documented in the patient's chart. Any corrective actions taken should also be recorded. Proper documentation includes (but may not be limited to):

- Date
- Time
- Type of reaction
- Medication administered to reverse the reaction or restore function
- Airway support, when applicable
- Level of care, that is, office interventions, transfer to emergency department, hospital admission, etc.
- Outcome of interventions
- Instructions provided to the patient and family member for further observation

In addition to these documentation items, immunizations require even further documentation. (Immunizations are discussed in more depth in Chapter 54.) For immunizations, record the name of the medication as well as the following information:

- Name of the manufacturing pharmaceutical company
- Lot number
- Serial number (if applicable)
- Container's expiration date

Companies that produce immunizations are required to assign lot numbers to each batch of the product. These lot numbers are used to track and report any adverse events experienced by one or more patients to the manufacturer. The manufacturer can then conduct an evaluation to find the cause of the patient's problem. Depending on the circumstances and whether there are a significant number of reports, the manufacturer might need to file a report with the Food and Drug Administration (FDA). The expiration date is also a very important piece of information because the manufacturer guarantees the effectiveness and safety of medication only until the expiration date printed on the container. Finally, the provider's name and complete address must be written on the chart and the form the patient provides for legal documentation.

The Immunization Action Coalition (IAC), working in concert with the Centers for Disease Control and Prevention (CDC), offers sample vaccine administration records for both children and adults that may be downloaded and printed or ordered. Figure 53–8 shows the first page of the Adult Form. You can download these forms at www.immunize.org. (Search for "Vaccine Administration Record for Adults" and "Vaccine Administration Record for Children and Teens.") Although use of these particular forms is not required, the information contained in the form should be recorded in the patient's chart.

In addition to forms, the CDC also recommends that each practice participate in a vaccination registry. The CDC cites the benefits of an immunization registry as preventing both under- and over-immunization of children and ensuring that new immunizations are provided as they become available. According to the Healthy People 2010 initiative, sponsored by the U.S. Department of Health and Human Services, immunization registries are to become the "cornerstone of the nation's immunization system by 2010." Most states have developed regional immunization systems, but many do not yet have legal agreements that allow for information sharing between states.

Under the NCVIA, health care providers are required to report certain adverse events that occur following vaccination to the Vaccine Adverse Event Reporting System (VAERS). VAERS is a reporting and vaccination safety surveillance program cosponsored by the FDA and the CDC. Its purpose is to detect new or unusual adverse events, monitor increases in adverse events,

Institute for Safe Medication Practices

ISMP's List of *Error-Prone Abbreviations, Symbols,* and *Dose Designations*

The abbreviations, symbols, and dose designations found in this table have been reported to the Institute for Safe Medication Practices (ISMP) through the ISMP Medication Errors Reporting Program (MERP) as being frequently misinterpreted and involved in harmful medication errors. They should NEVER be used when communicating medical information. This includes internal communications, telephone/verbal prescriptions, computer-generated labels, labels for drug storage bins, medication administration records, as well as pharmacy and prescriber computer order entry screens.

The Joint Commission (TJC) has established a National Patient Safety Goal that specifies that certain abbreviations must appear on an accredited organization's do-not-use list; we have highlighted these items with a double asterisk (**). However, we hope that you will consider others beyond the minimum TJC requirements. By using and promoting safe practices and by educating one another about hazards, we can better protect our patients.

Abbreviations	Intended Meaning	Misinterpretation	Correction
µg	Microgram	Mistaken as "mg"	Use "mcg"
AD, AS, AU	Right ear, left ear, each ear	Mistaken as OD, OS, OU (right eye, left eye, each eye)	Use "right ear," "left ear," or "each ear"
OD, OS, OU	Right eye, left eye, each eye	Mistaken as AD, AS, AU (right ear, left ear, each ear)	Use "right eye," "left eye," or "each eye"
BT	Bedtime	Mistaken as "BID" (twice daily)	Use "bedtime"
cc	Cubic centimeters	Mistaken as "u" (units)	Use "mL"
D/C	Discharge or discontinue	Premature discontinuation of medications if D/C (intended to mean "discharge") has been misinterpreted as "discontinued" when followed by a list of discharge medications	Use "discharge" and "discontinue"
IJ	Injection	Mistaken as "IV" or "intrajugular"	Use "injection"
IN	Intranasal	Mistaken as "IM" or "IV"	Use "intranasal" or "NAS"
HS	Half-strength	Mistaken as bedtime	Use "half-strength" or "bedtime"
hs	At bedtime, hours of sleep	Mistaken as half-strength	
IU**	International unit	Mistaken as IV (intravenous) or 10 (ten)	Use "units"
o.d. or OD	Once daily	Mistaken as "right eye" (OD-oculus dexter), leading to oral liquid medications administered in the eye	Use "daily"
OJ	Orange juice	Mistaken as OD or OS (right or left eye); drugs meant to be diluted in orange juice may be given in the eye	Use "orange juice"
Per os	By mouth, orally	The "os" can be mistaken as "left eye" (OS-oculus sinister)	Use "PO," "by mouth," or "orally"
q.d. or QD**	Every day	Mistaken as q.i.d., especially if the period after the "q" or the tail of the "q" is misunderstood as an "i"	Use "daily"
qhs	Nightly at bedtime	Mistaken as "qhr" or every hour	Use "nightly"
qn	Nightly or at bedtime	Mistaken as "qh" (every hour)	Use "nightly" or "at bedtime"
q.o.d. or QOD**	Every other day	Mistaken as "q.d." (daily) or "q.i.d." (four times daily) if the "o" is poorly written	Use "every other day"
q1d	Daily	Mistaken as q.i.d. (four times daily)	Use "daily"
q6PM, etc.	Every evening at 6 PM	Mistaken as every 6 hours	Use "6 PM nightly" or "6 PM daily"
SC, SQ, sub q	Subcutaneous	SC mistaken as SL (sublingual); SQ mistaken as "5 every;" the "q" in "sub q" has been mistaken as "every" (e.g., a heparin dose ordered "sub q 2 hours before surgery" misunderstood as every 2 hours before surgery)	Use "subcut" or "subcutaneously"
ss	Sliding scale (insulin) or ½ (apothecary)	Mistaken as "55"	Spell out "sliding scale;" use "one-half" or "½"
SSRI	Sliding scale regular insulin	Mistaken as selective serotonin reuptake inhibitor	Spell out "sliding scale (insulin)"
SSI	Sliding scale insulin	Mistaken as Strong Solution of Iodine (Lugol's)	
i/d	One daily	Mistaken as "tid"	Use "1 daily"
TIW or tiw	3 times a week	Mistaken as "3 times a day" or "twice in a week"	Use "3 times weekly"
U or u**	Unit	Mistaken as the number 0 or 4, causing a tenfold overdose or greater (e.g., 4U seen as "40" or 4u seen as "44"); mistaken as "cc" so dose given in volume instead of units (e.g., 4u seen as 4cc)	Use "unit"
Dose Designations and Other Information	**Intended Meaning**	**Misinterpretation**	**Correction**
Trailing zero after decimal point (e.g., 1.0 mg)**	1 mg	Mistaken as 10 mg if the decimal point is not seen	Do not use trailing zeros for doses expressed in whole numbers"
"Naked" decimal point (e.g., .5 mg)**	0.5 mg	Mistaken as 5 mg if the decimal point is not seen	Use zero before a decimal point when the dose is less than a whole unit

Figure 53–7: ISMP's list of error-prone abbreviations, symbols, and dose designations. *ISMP 2008.*
Delmar/Cengage Learning.

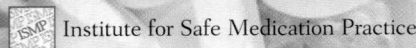

Institute for Safe Medication Practices

ISMP's List of *Error-Prone Abbreviations, Symbols,* and *Dose Designations* (continued)

Dose Designations and Other Information	Intended Meaning	Misinterpretation	Correction
Drug name and dose run together (especially problematic for drug names that end in "l" such as Inderal40 mg; Tegretol300 mg)	Inderal 40 mg Tegretol 300 mg	Mistaken as Inderal 140 mg Mistaken as Tegretol 1300 mg	Place adequate space between the drug name, dose, and unit of measure
Numerical dose and unit of measure run together (e.g., 10mg, 100mL)	10 mg 100 mL	The "m" is sometimes mistaken as a zero or two zeros, risking a 10- to 100-fold overdose	Place adequate space between the dose and unit of measure
Abbreviations such as mg. or mL. with a period following the abbreviation	mg mL	The period is unnecessary and could be mistaken as the number 1 if written poorly	Use mg, mL, etc. without a terminal period
Large doses without properly placed commas (e.g., 100000 units; 1000000 units)	100,000 units 1,000,000 units	100000 has been mistaken as 10,000 or 1,000,000; 1000000 has been mistaken as 100,000	Use commas for dosing units at or above 1,000, or use words such as 100 "thousand" or 1 "million" to improve readability
Drug Name Abbreviations	**Intended Meaning**	**Misinterpretation**	**Correction**
ARA A	vidarabine	Mistaken as cytarabine (ARA C)	Use complete drug name
AZT	zidovudine (Retrovir)	Mistaken as azathioprine or aztreonam	Use complete drug name
CPZ	Compazine (prochlorperazine)	Mistaken as chlorpromazine	Use complete drug name
DPT	Demerol-Phenergan-Thorazine	Mistaken as diphtheria-pertussis-tetanus (vaccine)	Use complete drug name
DTO	Diluted tincture of opium, or deodorized tincture of opium (Paregoric)	Mistaken as tincture of opium	Use complete drug name
HCl	hydrochloric acid or hydrochloride	Mistaken as potassium chloride (The "H" is misinterpreted as "K")	Use complete drug name unless expressed as a salt of a drug
HCT	hydrocortisone	Mistaken as hydrochlorothiazide	Use complete drug name
HCTZ	hydrochlorothiazide	Mistaken as hydrocortisone (seen as HCT250 mg)	Use complete drug name
MgSO4**	magnesium sulfate	Mistaken as morphine sulfate	Use complete drug name
MS, MSO4**	morphine sulfate	Mistaken as magnesium sulfate	Use complete drug name
MTX	methotrexate	Mistaken as mitoxantrone	Use complete drug name
PCA	procainamide	Mistaken as patient controlled analgesia	Use complete drug name
PTU	propylthiouracil	Mistaken as mercaptopurine	Use complete drug name
T3	Tylenol with codeine No. 3	Mistaken as liothyronine	Use complete drug name
TAC	triamcinolone	Mistaken as tetracaine, Adrenalin, cocaine	Use complete drug name
TNK	TNKase	Mistaken as "TPA"	Use complete drug name
ZnSO4	zinc sulfate	Mistaken as morphine sulfate	Use complete drug name
Stemmed Drug Names	**Intended Meaning**	**Misinterpretation**	**Correction**
"Nitro" drip	nitroglycerin infusion	Mistaken as sodium nitroprusside infusion	Use complete drug name
"Norflox"	norfloxacin	Mistaken as Norflex	Use complete drug name
"IV Vanc"	intravenous vancomycin	Mistaken as Invanz	Use complete drug name
Symbols	**Intended Meaning**	**Misinterpretation**	**Correction**
ʒ ♍	Dram Minim	Symbol for dram mistaken as "3" Symbol for minim mistaken as "mL"	Use the metric system
x3d	For three days	Mistaken as "3 doses"	Use "for three days"
> and <	Greater than and less than	Mistaken as opposite of intended; mistakenly use incorrect symbol; "< 10" mistaken as "40"	Use "greater than" or "less than"
/ (slash mark)	Separates two doses or indicates "per"	Mistaken as the number 1 (e.g., "25 units/10 units" misread as "25 units and 110" units)	Use "per" rather than a slash mark to separate doses
@	At	Mistaken as "2"	Use "at"
&	And	Mistaken as "2"	Use "and"
+	Plus or and	Mistaken as "4"	Use "and"
°	Hour	Mistaken as a zero (e.g., q2° seen as q 20)	Use "hr," "h," or "hour"

**These abbreviations are included on TJC's "minimum list" of dangerous abbreviations, acronyms, and symbols that must be included on an organization's "Do Not Use" list, effective January 1, 2004. Visit www.jointcommission.org for more information about this TJC requirement.

Institute for Safe Medication Practices
www.ismp.org

Figure 53–7: *(continued)*

Vaccine Administration Record for Adults

Patient name: ________________

Birthdate: ________________

Chart number: ________________

Before administering any vaccines, give the patient copies of all pertinent Vaccine Information Statements (VISs) and make sure he/she understands the risks and benefits of the vaccine(s). Always provide or update the patient's personal record card.

Vaccine	Type of Vaccine[1]	Date given (mo/day/yr)	Funding source (F,S,P)[2]	Site[3]	Vaccine		Vaccine Information Statement (VIS)		Vaccinator[5] (signature or initials & title)
					Lot #	Mfr.	Date on VIS[4]	Date given[4]	
Tetanus, Diphtheria, Pertussis (e.g., Td, Tdap) Give IM.[6]									
Hepatitis A[7] (e.g., HepA, HepA-HepB) Give IM.[6]									
Hepatitis B[7] (e.g., HepB, HepA-HepB) Give IM.[6]									
Human papillomavirus (HPV2, HPV4) Give IM.[6]									
Measles, Mumps, Rubella (MMR) Give SC.[6]									
Varicella (VAR) Give SC.[6]									
Pneumococcal polysaccharide (PPSV23) Give SC or IM.[6]									
Meningococcal (e.g., MCV4, conjugate; MPSV4, polysaccharide) Give MCV4 IM.[6] Give MPSV4 SC.[6]									

See page 2 to record influenza, zoster, and other vaccines (e.g., travel vaccines).

Figure 53–8: Vaccine Administration Record for Adults. *Acquired from www.immunize.org/catg.d/p2023.pdf on 1/3/2010; We thank the Immunization Action Coalition.*
Delmar/Cengage Learning.

identify potential risk factors, identify an increase in events associated with certain lot numbers, and track the safety of new vaccines. The medical assistant may complete a written VAERS form or enter the information online at http://vaers.hhs.gov/index. Although health care providers are required to report certain events, anyone may submit a report to VAERS. VAERS does not determine the causality between a vaccination and an adverse event but collects information for further investigation to detect unknown side effects of vaccines.

Another useful Website for keeping up to date on the latest information regarding immunizations and vaccinations is the National Network for Immunization Information (NNii) Website, www.immunizationinfo.org.

PROCEDURE 53–4 Record a Medication Entry in the Patient's Chart

MEDIA LINK: View the video, "The Right Documentation," for this chapter on the Premium Website.

PURPOSE: To document a medication entry

EQUIPMENT: Chart; without interruption

S SKILL: Demonstrate how to record a medication entry accurately in the patient's chart.

Procedure Steps	Detailed Instructions and/or *Rationales*
1. Obtain the completed medication order and the medication record if separate documents.	Verify the patient's identity, using at least two identifiers: name, date of birth, last four digits of social security number, spouse's name, street address, etc. Do not ask "yes" or "no" questions. *Confirms that the medication is being given to the **right** patient.*
B 2. ***Prepare and administer medication, following the Seven Rights.***	
3. Record the information in the medication record.	Enter the name of the medication as it appears on the container, date, time, amount (whether it was two 50 mg tablets or one 100 mg capsule), signature of person administering, and any problems or variances. *To keep an accurate medical and legal record of what has been administered.*
4. Sign off the order on the medication order sheet or chart.	Sign off the entry immediately after the medication has been administered. *Prevents a second health care worker from duplicating the order.*

Charting Example

Order:	Dilantin 250 mg po now. K. Jones, MD
Signed off:	Dilantin 250 mg po now. K. Jones, MD. Noted order, patient identified, given at 11:20 am S. Adams, RMA (AMT)

ADMINISTERING ORAL AND NON-INJECTABLE MEDICATIONS

As you've read, there are many methods of medicating patients, and even though the medical assistant is not permitted to administer all routes, you should become familiar with references to each route of administration and be prepared to assist in the preparation of different types of medications. The route of administration of a given drug is chosen based on the rate of absorption desired, distribution, biotransformation, and elimination. The medical assistant is permitted to administer medications by the following routes unless otherwise designated by state laws: oral, inhaled, **topical**, rectal, vaginal, urethral, and injectable. When working in an acute care or extended care facility, it may also be necessary for the medical assistant to administer medications by these routes as well. Additionally, it is important to be prepared to provide patient education regarding medications that are often self-administered vaginally, urethrally, and rectally in the outpatient setting.

Oral medications are intended for absorption through the alimentary canal or digestive system; other methods are said to be **parenteral**, or intended for absorption outside the digestive system.

PATIENT EDUCATION

Patients can be anxious about receiving a new medication, whether it is a medication taken by mouth, given by injection, or given by any other route of administration. Careful and understandable explanations of the disease being treated and the reason the medication is being provided helps reassure the patient. It is essential for the patient to understand not only the benefits of the medication but also any potential unpleasant or harmful side effects to look for, many of which can be avoided or alleviated by proper timing. For example, stomach upset is avoided by taking some medications with meals, and sleeplessness can be reduced by taking other medications in the morning, where appropriate.

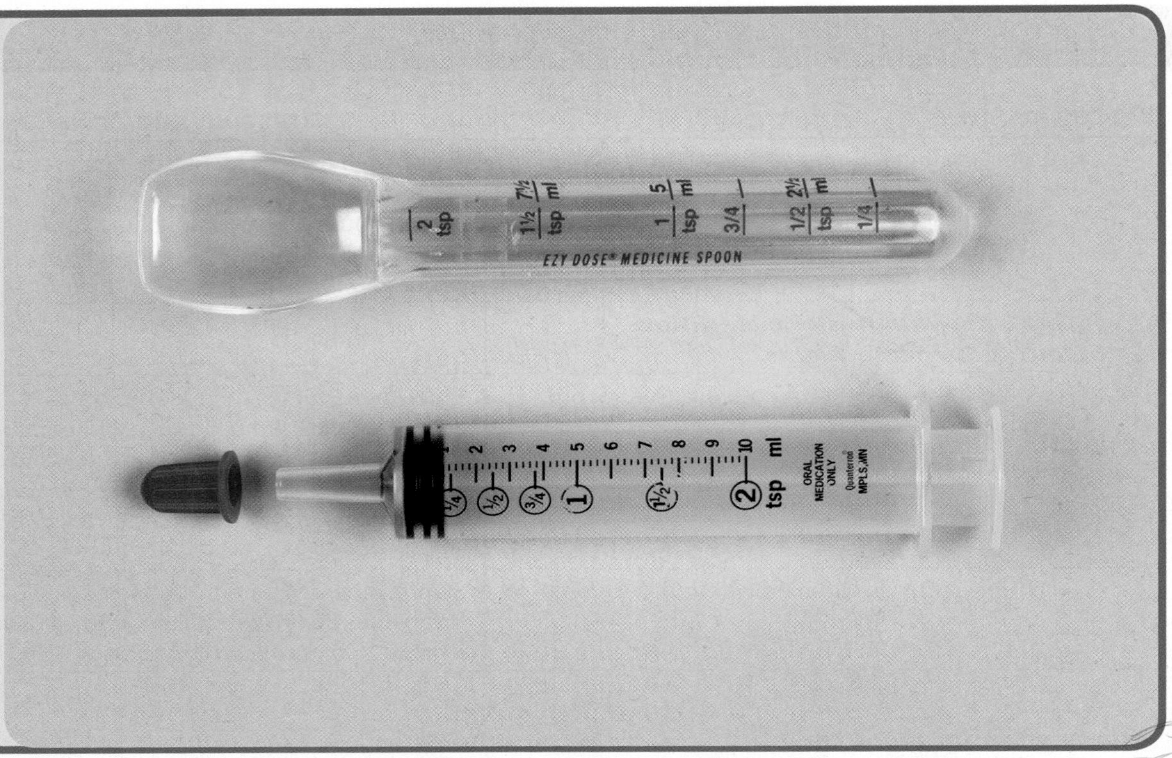

Figure 53–9: Calibrated medication spoon and syringe. *Delmar/Cengage Learning.*

Oral Administration

The most common method of administering medications is orally, or by mouth. Medicines to be swallowed come in the forms of pills, tablets, capsules, caplets, lozenges, syrups, sprays, and other liquids. Prescriptions are most often provided for oral medications but are also administered to patients in the office environment. For example, a patient may be given an analgesic while in the office for more immediate relief of pain and then provided with a prescription for the same or similar medication to be filled at the pharmacy.

Oral medications have many advantages. The most obvious advantage is convenience. If a patient exhibits an intolerance or an adverse reaction to an oral medication, the remedy might be simply to discontinue the medicine. Oral medications are also easily stored, usually requiring only a room temperature or ambient environment, although some require refrigeration. They are generally more economical for the medical practice and for the patient.

Oral medication administration requires care but is generally associated with lower risk and less expense than medication given by injection. An added advantage is that it is easy for a patient or family member to self-administer the medication at home.

If the medication to be given orally is a liquid, one of several devices are available for proper measurement of the dosage: medicine cups, calibrated medicine spoons, oral syringes (Figure 53–9), or calibrated medicine droppers (Figure 53–10).

Procedure 53–5 provides steps for administering oral medication to a patient.

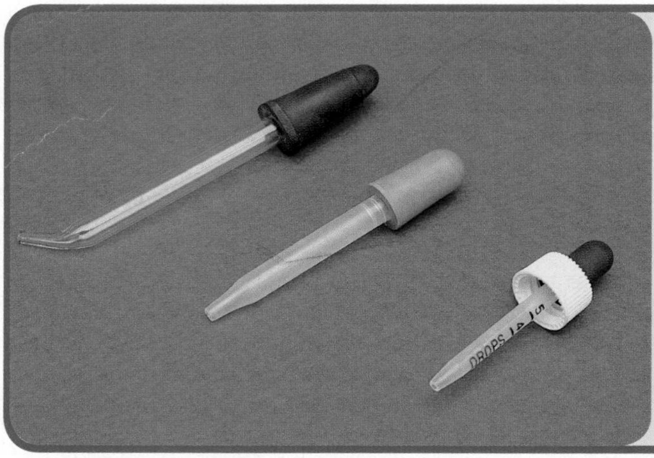

Figure 53–10: Calibrated medicine droppers. *Delmar/Cengage Learning.*

PROCEDURE 53–5 Prepare and Administer Oral Medication

PURPOSE: To demonstrate the steps required to obtain and administer oral medications

EQUIPMENT: Medication order, medicine cup (disposable), disposable paper cup filled with water, medicine tray

S SKILL: Measure and administer the ordered dose of oral medication.

Procedure Steps	Detailed Instructions and/or *Rationales*
B 1. Obtain the medication from the storage area. Read the label carefully, ***comparing it with the order.***	
2. Calculate the dosage, if necessary, and wash hands.	
3. Prepare the medication: a. Take the bottle cap off and place it inside-up on counter. b. If in pill or capsule form, pour the desired amount into the cap. Then pour the medication into a medicine cup. c. If in liquid form, pour it directly into a measuring device to the calibrated line of the ordered amount. Syrup or liquid medications may also be given in disposable plastic measuring spoons or droppers.	*The countertop is considered contaminated and must not come into contact with the inside of the cap. Touching the inside of the bottle or cap likely will result in contamination.* Hold the measuring device at eye level with your thumbnail placed at the desired amount (Figure 53–11). Liquids should be poured from the opposite side of the bottle's label to prevent the contents from dripping and discoloring the label. 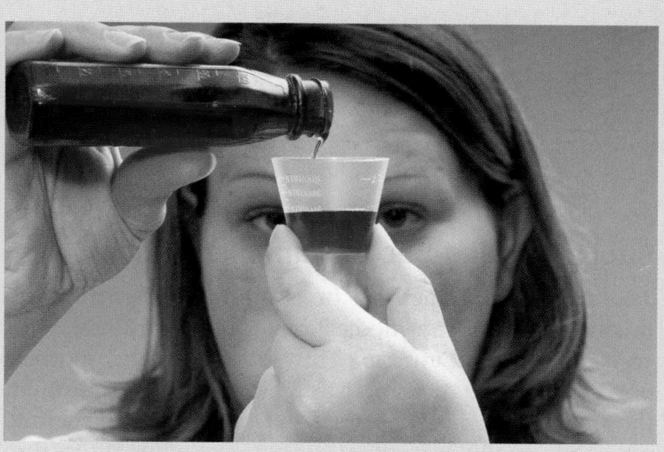 **Figure 53–11:** Hold the medicine cup at eye level when pouring, for accurate measurement. *Delmar/Cengage Learning.*
B 4. Place the medication container on a tray and the ordered dose in a medicine cup. Place a cup of water on the tray for the patient to drink with the medicine, if allowed. ***Read the label a second time and compare with the order.***	*Some liquid medications, such as a cough suppressant, should not be taken with water. Water can wash away the coating created by swallowing the liquid medication.*
5. Take the medication tray to the patient and confirm the patient's identity. Read the label a third time and compare prior to administering.	Verify the patient's identity by using at least two identifiers: name, date of birth, last four digits of social security number, spouse's name, street address, etc. Do not ask "yes" or "no" questions. *Confirms that the medication is being given to the **right** patient.*

(continues)

(continued)

Procedure Steps	Detailed Instructions and/or *Rationales*
B 6. Explain the procedure, ***using language the patient can understand. Make the patient feel comfortable about the procedure and answer any questions***.	
B 7. Give the patient the medication and offer the cup of water, if allowed. ***Observe the patient taking the medication and report any reaction or problem to the provider.***	
B 8. Discard any disposables and return the medication container and tray to the proper storage area. ***Read the label a fourth time***.	
9. Record the information in the medication record. Sign off the order on the medication order sheet or chart.	Enter the name of the medication as it appears on the container, date, time, amount, signature of person administering, and any problems or variances. Sign off the entry immediately after the medication has been administered.

Charting Example

3-19-20XX 2:35 PM	Robitussin 2 teaspoons given orally for nasal congestion and cough; instructed patient per doctor's instructions to take 2 teaspoons every 4 hours. S. Davis, RMA(AMT)

Sublingual and Buccal Administration

The **sublingual** method of administering medication involves placing the medication, usually tiny tablets or spray, under the tongue. This introduces the medication quickly into the bloodstream by absorption through the mucous membranes. One example is nitroglycerine, which is usually prescribed for patients who suffer from angina. Tiny tablets or spray are also administered by the **buccal** method, that is, placed or sprayed in the mouth between the gum and the cheek. The medication is also absorbed through the mucous membranes.

PATIENT EDUCATION

Patients should avoid eating, drinking, or chewing while the medication is in place. Patients should be instructed on how to use these medications properly. These medications should not be swallowed whole because that can cause the intended action to be delayed or rendered ineffective.

Parenteral — Non-injectable

A number of medications are given parenterally (by routes other than through the alimentary canal) but are not injectables. These routes include inhalation, nasal, ointment, otic, rectal, topical, **transdermal,** urethral, and vaginal. (Refer to Chapter 51 for complete descriptions of these routes.) Medications given by these routes may be applied directly to the affected body part or inhaled into the lungs.

PATIENT EDUCATION

Specific instructions are provided for each route as well as for the particular medication being given by that route. For ointments, the skin may require cleansing for one preparation or mild rubbing to enhance absorption for a different medication.

Nasal, Ophthalmic, and Otic Administration

Usually, drops, ointments, or salves are applied directly into the nose, eyes, or ears for immediate relief or direct absorption by the target tissues (see Figures 53–12 and 53–13. Proper technique and aftercare instructions are very important to achieve the maximal benefit from these routes. Refer to Procedures 53–6 and 53–7.

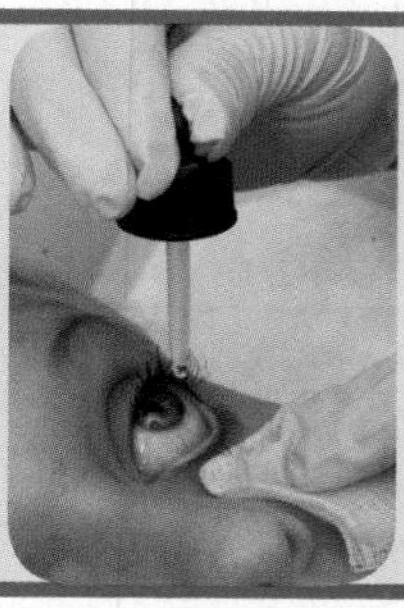

Figure 53–12: Administering eyedrops. *Delmar/Cengage Learning.*

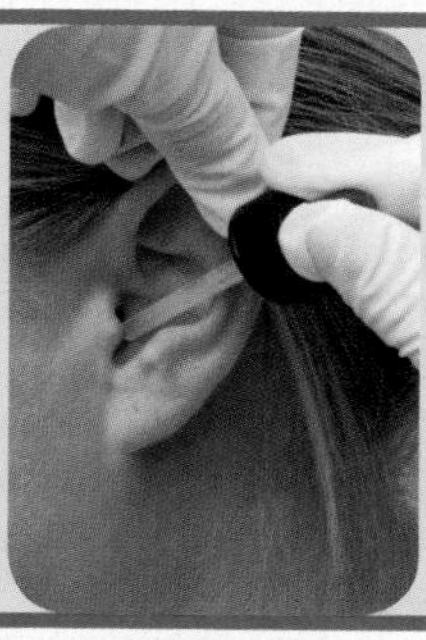

Figure 53–13: Instilling ear drops. *Delmar/Cengage Learning.*

PROCEDURE 53–6 Administer Eyedrops

PURPOSE: To instill medication into the eye without introducing pathogens

EQUIPMENT: Clean gloves, medication with dropper, tissue

S **SKILL:** Demonstrate accurate administration of eyedrops while maintaining aseptic technique.

Procedure Steps	Detailed Instructions and/or *Rationales*
1. Wash hands; don clean gloves.	*Maintain aseptic technique to avoid infection.*
B 2. Explain procedure to patient, ***using language the patient can understand. Make the patient feel comfortable about the procedure and answer any questions***.	*This reassures the patient.*
3. Ask the patient whether he or she is allergic to any medications.	Always check again just prior to administration.
4. Have the patient sit, leaning back slightly in the chair, or lie supine on exam table.	*Position to allow for effective introduction of medication.*
5. Tilt head slightly toward the side drops will be placed. Place gentle traction on the skin slightly below the lower eye lid and place prescribed number of drops, one at a time, in the inner canthus of the eye followed by gentle pressure. Repeat for each drop administered. Do not allow patient to rub, only dab, drops with a clean tissue that run onto the skin.	*Ensures absorption of medication; gentle pressure to the canthus prevents drops from going into the tear duct instead of remaining in the eye.*
6. Document medication, time, date, and patient response to medication in the chart.	*Maintain permanent record of medication and patient response.*

Charting Example

7/2/2010 9:32 am	Zymar 0.3% ordered. Two drops to left eye as ordered. Most of medication remained in eye as administered. Clean tissue provided, advised patient not to rub eyes but only dab excess that escaped onto skin. Instructed patient in proper use. Kelly Smith, NCMA.

PROCEDURE 53–7 Instill Drops in the Ears

PURPOSE: To introduce appropriate medications into the ear canal

EQUIPMENT: Clean gloves, medication with dropper, tissue for dabbing external leakage of excess.

S **SKILL:** Administer medication into the ear while maintaining aseptic technique.

Procedure Steps	Detailed Instructions and/or *Rationales*
1. Wash hands; don clean gloves.	*Maintain aseptic technique to avoid infection.*
B 2. Explain procedure to patient, ***using language the patient can understand. Make the patient feel comfortable about the procedure and answer any questions***.	*This reassures the patient.*
3. Ask the patient whether he or she is allergic to any medications.	Always check again just prior to administration.
4. Have the patient sit, leaning back slightly in the chair, or on the opposite side comfortably positioned on the exam table.	*Position to allow for effective introduction of medication.*
5. Have the patient turn the head so that the affected ear is facing upward. Place gently upward traction on the earlobe to straighten the external canal.	*Ensures that medication enters the ear canal.*
6. Drop prescribed number of drops into ear canal.	Deliver prescribed dose.
7. Have patient remain in position for a few minutes or as indicated by prescriber.	*Allows complete absorption of medication.*
8. Document medication, time, date, and patient response to medication in the chart.	*Maintains permanent record of medication and patient response.*

Charting Example

10/2/2010, 11:33 am	Child positioned on mother's lap with left ear up. Murine ear drops, 5 gtts placed in left ear. Instructed mother to help child lie still for 1 minute following administration to allow for complete absorption. Clean tissue provided to absorb excess after child sits up. Child tolerated procedure well. James Allen, CMA (AAMA)

Inhalation Administration

Medications given to patients by the inhalation method are in the form of gases, sprays, fluids, or powders. These are then mixed with liquid to be used with equipment that will produce a medication-containing mist or vapor that can be breathed into the respiratory tract. The patient often self-administers the medication at home, through either a metered inhaler or a nebulizer machine. Proper instruction should be provided and reinforced until the patient or parent feels comfortable in doing so alone. Manufacturers prepare instruction material on the proper use and care of their equipment. Keeping a file of various manufacturers' instructions for the most commonly prescribed inhalation medications used in the practice would be a valuable resource for helping patients when they call with questions or have trouble locating their own.

A form of inhalation medication that should be kept in every medical practice is oxygen. Although it is not given often in most practices, it should be available for emergency use. The tanks should be checked on a daily basis and maintained as recommended by the manufacturer or providing company. Manufacturers also offer various home oxygen treatment programs for patients who need this treatment daily. The provider or prescribing practitioner will determine the method of delivery (nasal cannula or mask) and the rate of delivery, prescribed in liters of oxygen per minute (LPM). Figures 53–14A and B illustrate the nasal cannula and the simple face mask.

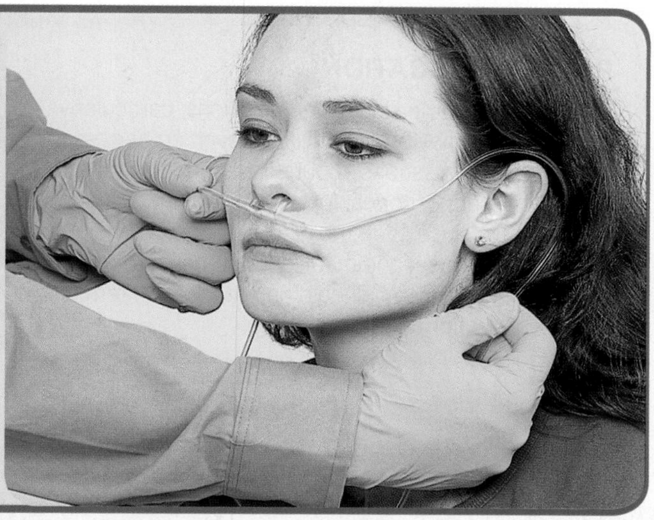

Figure 53–14A: Nasal cannula. *Delmar/Cengage Learning.*

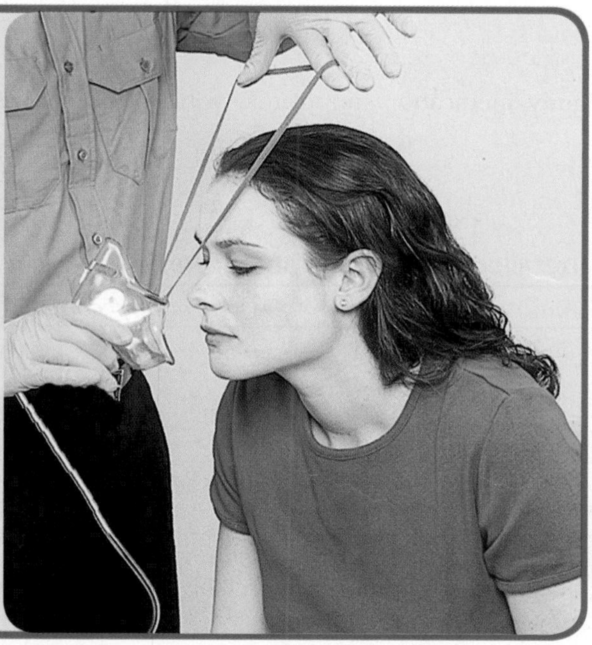

Figure 53–14B: Oxygen mask. *Delmar/Cengage Learning.*

Topical Administration

Topical medications are used in treating diseases or disorders of the skin or mucous membranes. They come in sprays, lotions, creams, **ointments**, paints, **salves**, wet dressings, and transdermal patches.

Topical medications must be applied as prescribed to achieve the desired effect. For example, a patient should apply a medication to reduce itching with gentle single strokes. If the medication is rubbed into the skin vigorously, the itching will increase from the heat produced by the friction of rubbing. Nitroglycerin ointment should be removed at the time scheduled and the area cleaned before applying the next dose in a new area. This prevents an unsafe of excess medication being available for absorption.

The transdermal patch is a convenient method of choice for medicating patients for many medical conditions (Figure 53–15). It is painless and ensures patient compliance. The patch is placed on the skin according to the accompanying manufacturer's directions. The patient receives time-released treatment in a sustained dose over several days or weeks rather than having to remember more frequent dosing schedules.

Several commonly prescribed medications are available as transdermal systems. Examples of medications contained in transdermal patches include nicotine for smoking cessation, nitroglycerin for angina, estrogen for birth control, Fentanyl for chronic pain, Exelon for Alzheimer's disease, and Daytrana for ADHD in children. There are many others, but this illustrates that there are many types of medication for patients of all ages and types of conditions.

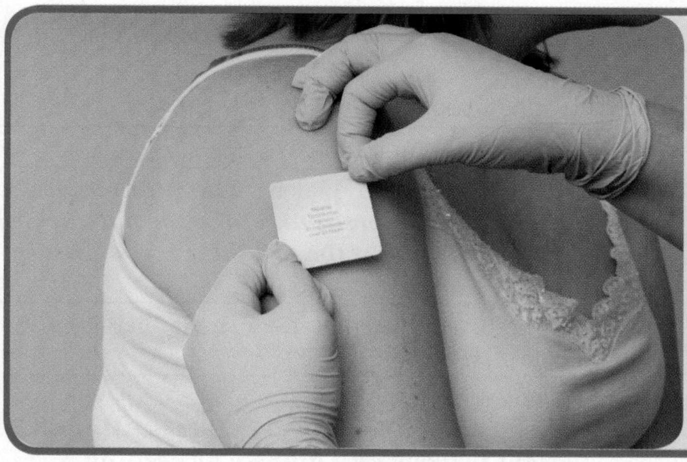

Figure 53–15: Placing a transdermal patch on a patient. *Delmar/Cengage Learning.*

O_2 LPM – liters per minute

PATIENT EDUCATION

Patients should be properly instructed in applying the transdermal patch themselves. In the case of a child or a forgetful patient, the caregiver is instructed in applying it where it cannot be removed by the patient before the next patch is due to be placed. Disposable gloves should be worn when applying a transdermal patch to avoid accidental absorption of the medication by the person applying the patch. A priming dose of medication is in the adhesive edge of the patch. Instruct a caregiver to wash his or her hands with soap and water immediately after application of a patch if any touches his or her skin. The effects of inadvertent transfer could range from undesirable to dangerous to the one person applying it, depending on the medication contained in the patch.

Rectal Administration

Suppositories and enemas are the most prevalent means of delivering medication by the rectal route. A suppository is a conical or ovoid-shaped, solid, compressed amount of medication that is designed to melt at body temperature when inserted into the vagina or rectum. **Enemas** are liquids, either fluid or medication, delivered directly into the rectum by using a flexible tube. This route can be desirable for any of several reasons, including an inability to swallow medication due to disease (esophageal cancer or active ulcer); an inability to ingest medications orally due to temporary symptoms such as nausea and vomiting; the need to introduce imaging material, such as barium, to visualize the lower intestinal tract; or to treat local symptoms such as hemorrhoids. See Procedure 53–8.

PATIENT EDUCATION

Do not overlook the simplest instructions, particularly since patients may be unfamiliar or even embarrassed and fail to ask questions about proper administration. Rectal suppositories, for example, often come in foil wrappers since even the warmth of normal hand temperature causes the medication to begin to melt. Patients (or caregivers) should be reminded to remove the wrapper prior to administering.

PROCEDURE 53–8 Administer Rectal Medication

PURPOSE: To deliver medication suppository rectally

EQUIPMENT: Clean gloves, sheet for protecting patient dignity, medication suppository with or without applicator as appropriate

S **SKILL:** Administer a rectal medication.

Procedure Steps	Detailed Instructions and/or *Rationales*
1. Wash hands; don clean gloves.	*Maintains aseptic technique to avoid infection.*
B 2. Explain procedure to patient, ***using language the patient can understand. Make the patient feel comfortable about the procedure and answer any questions***.	*Reassures patient.*
3. Ask the patient whether he or she is allergic to any medications.	Always check again just prior to administration.
B 4. Position patient on left side, as tolerated, with knees drawn comfortably toward chest. ***Maintain patient privacy and dignity by keeping the room closed and the patient draped appropriately***.	*Positions to allow for effective introduction of medication; maintains respect for patient.*

Procedure Steps	Detailed Instructions and/or *Rationales*
5. Remove foil wrapper on medication and insert into rectum just past the anal sphincter, holding gentle manual pressure against the suppository for a few seconds to avoid involuntary expulsion from the rectum. If medication is supplied as a cream with applicator, follow specific package directions for use, withdrawing accurate amount of medication into applicator for delivery. Advise patient to remain in the same position for a few minutes following administration.	*Ensures absorption of medication.*
6. Document medication, time, date, and patient response to medication in the chart.	*Maintains permanent record of medication and patient response.*

Charting Example

9/3/2010 2:45 PM	Procedure explained to patient, curtain pulled and sheet provided for modesty. Patient disrobed self waist down; assisted patient into position on left side with knees flexed. Wrapper removed, Compazine 5 mg suppository inserted PR with gentle pressure just beyond sphincter. Patient covered and advised to remain in position for a few minutes to allow for absorption. A. James, RMA (AMT)

Vaginal Administration

Vaginal medications can be applied in the form of creams, suppositories, tablets, douches, foams, ointments, tampons, sprays, and salves (Figure 53–16). The patient should be educated in the proper method of self-administration of vaginal medications. Some women might be uncomfortable or embarrassed about asking for clarification of instructions. A woman might not know that, for example, vaginal medications should be used during the menstrual flow because this is an ideal time for growth of microorganisms. Vaginal medications can also seem undesirable because they tend to be messy. Most vaginal medications are ordered for use at bedtime to encourage patient compliance. The medical assistant may advise patients to use disposable panty liners to avoid medication leaking and staining undergarments or clothes.

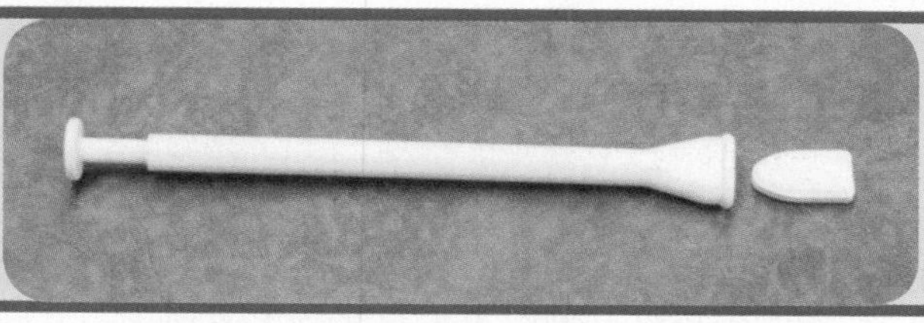

Figure 53–16: Vaginal medication and applicator.
Delmar/Cengage Learning.

PATIENT EDUCATION

Be sure to stress the importance of completing the prescribed treatment plan because it is just as important for the patient to finish medications taken vaginally as medications taken by any other route. Patients too often stop using a medication after a few doses or a few days because the symptoms seem to clear up. Unless all the prescribed medication is used, the condition or problem could return. While using vaginal medications, patients should always be advised to avoid using tampons unless specifically directed by a provider to do so. Many women self-medicate minor symptoms with over-the-counter (OTC) gynecological preparations and should be encouraged to consult with their providers if their complaints do not improve or worsen with a regular course of any OTC products they use.

PROCEDURE 53–9 Administer Vaginal Medication

PURPOSE: To deliver vaginal medication

EQUIPMENT: Clean gloves, suppository or medication with supplied applicator, clean sheet to protect patient privacy and dignity

S **SKILL:** Administer vaginal medication.

Procedure Steps	Detailed Instructions and/or *Rationales*
1. Wash hands before preparing medication; don clean gloves.	*Maintains aseptic technique to avoid introducing microorganisms.*
B 2. Explain procedure to patient, ***using language the patient can understand. Make the patient feel comfortable about the procedure and answer any questions***.	*Reassures patient.*
3. Advise patient to empty bladder.	*Avoids the need to void after medication has been introduced.*
4. Have patient wash or rinse external genitalia with water.	*Prevents contamination of medication as it is introduced.*
5. Have patient lie on her back or side with knees bent.	*Position allows for introduction and retention of medication following insertion.*
6. Apply a small amount of water-soluble lubricant, if needed, to applicator or to suppository and insert medication into vaginal vault toward the posterior wall approximately 2–4 inches toward the spine. If applicator has a plunger, gently push the plunger to release the medication while angling slightly upward. (If suppository, remind patient to remove outer plastic or foil wrapper prior to application.)	*Optimizes effectiveness by delivering into canal.*
7. Encourage patient to remain in a reclining position for 10 minutes following administration.	*Ensures adequate absorption of medication.*
8. Advise patient to use a sanitary napkin or panty liner while using medication.	*To prevent staining of clothes from leaked medication.*
9. If applicable, wash applicator with warm, soapy water, allow to air dry, and store in container with the remainder of the medication.	*Keeps medication and delivery system available for next use and free of microorganisms.*
10. Offer to answer any questions and advise patient to report any adverse reactions immediately.	*Ensures patient safety and encourages compliance with adequate patient education.*

Charting Example

8/21/2009 10:15 am	Patient with contractures, here from nursing home for evaluation. First dose of Metronidazole 750 mg to be administered in office. Medication withdrawn into vaginal applicator. Explained procedure to patient. Gently assisted patient to side lying position with knees flexed, covered with sheet. Inserted applicator into vaginal vault, medication completely dispensed from applicator. Reminded patient to lie still for 10 minutes following administration to allow for absorption. Ensured patient safety with side rails in place. Order for additional doses included in chart to return to nursing home with patient. B. Jones, RMA (AMT)

CHAPTER SUMMARY

- Drugs may be administered by many routes, depending on the rate of absorption desired, distribution, biotransformation (how the body converts the drug into a form it can use), and elimination.
- A prescription is a written order prepared by a licensed provider or practitioner authorizing a medication or treatment to be dispensed to the patient for *self-administration*.
- Medication orders differ from prescriptions in that they are direct and complete instructions composed by the provider or other licensed practitioner for *administering* medications to a patient while he or she is in the facility or office.
- Although they make record keeping more expedient, abbreviations should be used carefully. A number of abbreviations are used in different specialties and types of health care environments, and there is no comprehensive list of "approved" abbreviations. When there is any question of the correct abbreviation, the word should be spelled out instead to avoid any confusion about what is being written.
- The Seven Rights of medication administration should always be followed to avoid medication errors.
- Documentation of immunizations requires additional information beyond what is required for medications, including name of the manufacturing pharmaceutical company, lot number, serial number (if applicable), and container's expiration date.
- Non-injectable medications include those delivered by the following routes: oral, inhaled, topical, rectal, vaginal, and urethral.

STUDY TOOLS

Workbook	Activities for Chapter 53
Premium Website	
MEDIA LINK	View these **Media Links** for Chapter 53. • Prepare a Prescription per the Provider's Orders • The Right Documentation
StudyWARE	Activities and Quizzes on the **StudyWARE™ Software** for Chapter 53
	Audio Library of medical terms
	Online access to the **Critical Thinking Challenge 2.0**
CourseMate	Activities and Quizzes for Chapter 53
WebTutor	Activities and Quizzes for Chapter 53

CHECK YOUR KNOWLEDGE

1. A prescription is best described as:
   a. Instructions for administering medications in the office.
   b. Labeling of a drug container.
   c. Whether a generic medication may be substituted for the trade name.
   d. A written order that authorizes the dispensing of a medication to a patient.
2. The prescription abbreviation "DAW" stands for:
   a. Do As you Wish.
   b. Don't Authorize When (followed by date).
   c. Dispense as Written.
   d. none of the above.
3. If the prescribing practitioner leaves out a minor part of the prescription, the MA's most appropriate action should be to:
   a. Fill in the information if it is minor.
   b. Ask another person in the office what should be included.
   c. Return the prescription to the prescriber to be completed.
   d. Nothing; the pharmacist will know what to put there.

PRIO, T, T, D, M.

4. Which of the following is NOT an advantage of e-prescriptions?
   a. Reduces the possibility of forgery
   b. Helps maintain a running record of patient medications
   c. Prevents handwriting errors
   d. All of the above
5. A medication order should contain the following elements EXCEPT:
   a. Patient name.
   b. Signature of prescriber.
   c. Site where the medication should be given.
   d. Amount of medication to be given.
6. Which of the following list best describes the Seven Rights?
   a. Checklist of criteria to help prevent medication errors
   b. The MA's entitlements while working for a provider
   c. Patient's entitlements under HIPAA
   d. None of the above
7. Which of the following criteria is NOT required in documenting immunizations?
   a. Pharmaceutical company name
   b. Color of contents
   c. Expiration date
   d. Serial number of container

WEB LINKS

Information regarding immunization registries, from the Every Child By Two foundation: www.ecbt.org/registries

Model Interstate Immunization Information Sharing Statute, from the Every Child By Two foundation: www.ecbt.org/registries/modelinterstate.cfm

Additional information on NCVIA and VAERS: www.cdc.gov/vaccinesafety/Vaccine_Monitoring/history.html

Vaccination and immunization requirements for school entry in each state, from the NNii: www.immunizationinfo.org/vaccines/state-requirements

Vaccine information from the CDC: www.cdc.gov/vaccines/about/terms/vacc-abbrev.htm

Chapter 54 Administering Injections and Immunizations

OBJECTIVES

In this chapter, you will learn the following:

KB KNOWLEDGE BASE

1. Spell and define, using the glossary at the back of the text, all the Words to Know in this chapter.
2. List and describe three common parenteral routes by injection that medical assistants perform.
3. Correctly identify the parts of a syringe and needle.
4. Explain how to handle and dispose of needles safely.
5. Identify the proper angles of injection and injection sites for intradermal, intramuscular, intramuscular Z-track, and subcutaneous injections.
6. Describe the proper way to prepare, verify, and administer correct doses of medications for intradermal, intramuscular, intramuscular Z-track, and subcutaneous injections.
7. Discuss the importance of patient education and documentation regarding medications and immunizations.

S SKILLS

1. Accurately draw up the correct amount of medication from an ampule or vial into various types of syringes.
2. Reconstitute a powder medication, correctly preparing it for administration.
3. Prepare, verify, and administer proper doses of medications for intradermal, intramuscular, intramuscular Z-track, and subcutaneous injections.
4. Demonstrate appropriate aseptic technique as it applies to medication administration.
5. Demonstrate proper disposal of used syringes and needles.
6. Maintain medication and immunization records.

B BEHAVIORS

1. Use language and verbal skills that enable patients' understanding of procedures being performed.
2. Show awareness of patients' concerns regarding their perceptions of the procedure being performed.
3. Verify ordered doses and dosages prior to medication administration.

WORDS TO KNOW

anaphylactic
ampule
catarrhal stage
decline stage
diphtheria
epiglottitis
epinephrine
gauge
hepatitis A
hepatitis B
immunization
incubation period
influenza
intradermal (ID)
intramuscular (IM)
intravenous (IV)

meningitis	photosensitivity	sensitivity	varicella zoster
needlesticks	pneumonia	series	vial
paroxysmal stage	rubella	subcutaneous	wheal
pertussis	rubeola	vaccine	Z-track IM

PARENTERAL INJECTABLE MEDICATIONS

Special considerations are required when giving injections and immunizations to patients. The previous chapter introduced the different routes of administration and the Seven Rights of administering medications. Parenteral routes other than those mentioned in Chapter 53 involve injecting medications through the skin or directly into a vein or artery. Some instances when these routes are chosen can include:

- when the patient is unable to tolerate medications by mouth.
- when other routes of administration do not provide the desired effect quickly or predictably enough.
- when medication given by mouth would be destroyed by the gastrointestinal tract.
- when continuous delivery is required to achieve the desired outcome.

Parenteral routes by injection involve increased cost as well as increased risk. Increased cost is related to the requirement of special equipment or personnel to administer the medications correctly. With respect to increased risk, injectables should be handled carefully to avoid infection in the patient but also to avoid inadvertent infection to the health care worker by accidental needlesticks due to unsafe handling or disposal.

The majority of injections administered by medical assistants are given by the following routes:

- **Intradermal (ID)** injections are given by shallow-angle injection just under the dermis of the skin. Placing a small amount of a known antigen between layers of skin by shallow-angle injection is used to test for an allergic response without allowing the antigen to circulate within the bloodstream. Tuberculin skin tests and allergy testing is done in this manner.
- **Subcutaneous** injections insert liquid medication just below the cutaneous skin layer. Insulins are the most commonly used subcutaneous medications. This route of administration involves placing the tip of the needle just below the skin and into the layer of fat underlying the skin for a longer period of absorption. This type of injection can be self-administered as well as by a health care provider.
- **Intramuscular (IM)** injections insert medication into muscular tissue for delayed absorption. Delivering medication deep into the muscle tissue allows for an immediate effect with an additional, predictable absorption of medication over the next several hours. Narcotic pain medications and loading doses of antibiotics are examples of how this method of medication delivery is used.

There are additional injectable routes of administration, including intraarterial, intraosseous, intrathecal, and intravenous (refer to their descriptions in Chapter 53), *but medical assistants are not permitted to administer medications through these routes.* There are serious legal implications for both a medical assistant *as well as* his or her employer for acting beyond the scope of practice. These include fines, certification suspension or revocation, and even criminal charges, depending on the circumstances. Be sure to understand your own state requirements and the limitations the employer can impose beyond state regulations.

CLINICAL PEARL

Intravenous Medications

Injecting medications directly into a vein is a common, effective, and efficient means of delivering multiple types of medications. Medical assistants **are not** permitted to provide direct **intravenous (IV)** injections or to initiate an IV access; but, may see a patient in the office or clinic setting from time to time who has an IV access port or a running IV from a nursing facility. It is important to recognize a problem and report it to the provider immediately. Redness or swelling at the site and who was notified of the problem should be noted in the patient's chart. Any IV fluids that are infusing should also be recorded and the bag maintained above the site to allow for gravity, especially if a volumetric pump is not in use. Medical assistants are not permitted to change the bag whether it contains only fluids or medications. (That task falls under the licensure of either the transporting team or licensed providers or nurses who work in the office.) Do not risk your credentials by doing so, even if it seems to be a simple task.

PREPARING TO ADMINISTER INJECTIONS

To administer injections properly, you must become familiar with and proficient in handling needles and syringes. Figures 54–1 and 54–2 show needles and syringes with labeled parts. Needles come in different sizes, both in length (how long they are) and **gauge** (the diameter of the needle). Different syringes are calibrated in different measurements, as shown in Figure 54–2.

Syringes commonly used in the medical office to administer medication include:

- 3 mL syringe, calibrated in milliliters (Figure 54–3A). Each small line represents one-tenth mL (0.1, 0.2, 0.3, etc.), and the longer lines represent 0.5, 1.0, 1.5, 2.0, 2.5, and 3.0 mL.
- Tuberculin syringe, calibrated in tenths of a milliliter (Figure 54–3B). This syringe has only a 1.0 mL capacity. Each small line represents one-tenth of a milliliter.
- Insulin syringe, calibrated in units (Figure 54–3C). Capacity is 100 units.

When giving injections and immunizations, you must be careful to choose the correct syringe and to draw up the correct dosage according to the medication order. For example, you may never use a tuberculin syringe to give insulin nor use an insulin syringe to give any other medication because either could result in a medication error.

To read the amount of medication in the syringe properly, hold the syringe at eye level and note the innermost line of the black plunger. When medication is pulled into the syringe and all air bubbles have been expelled, the

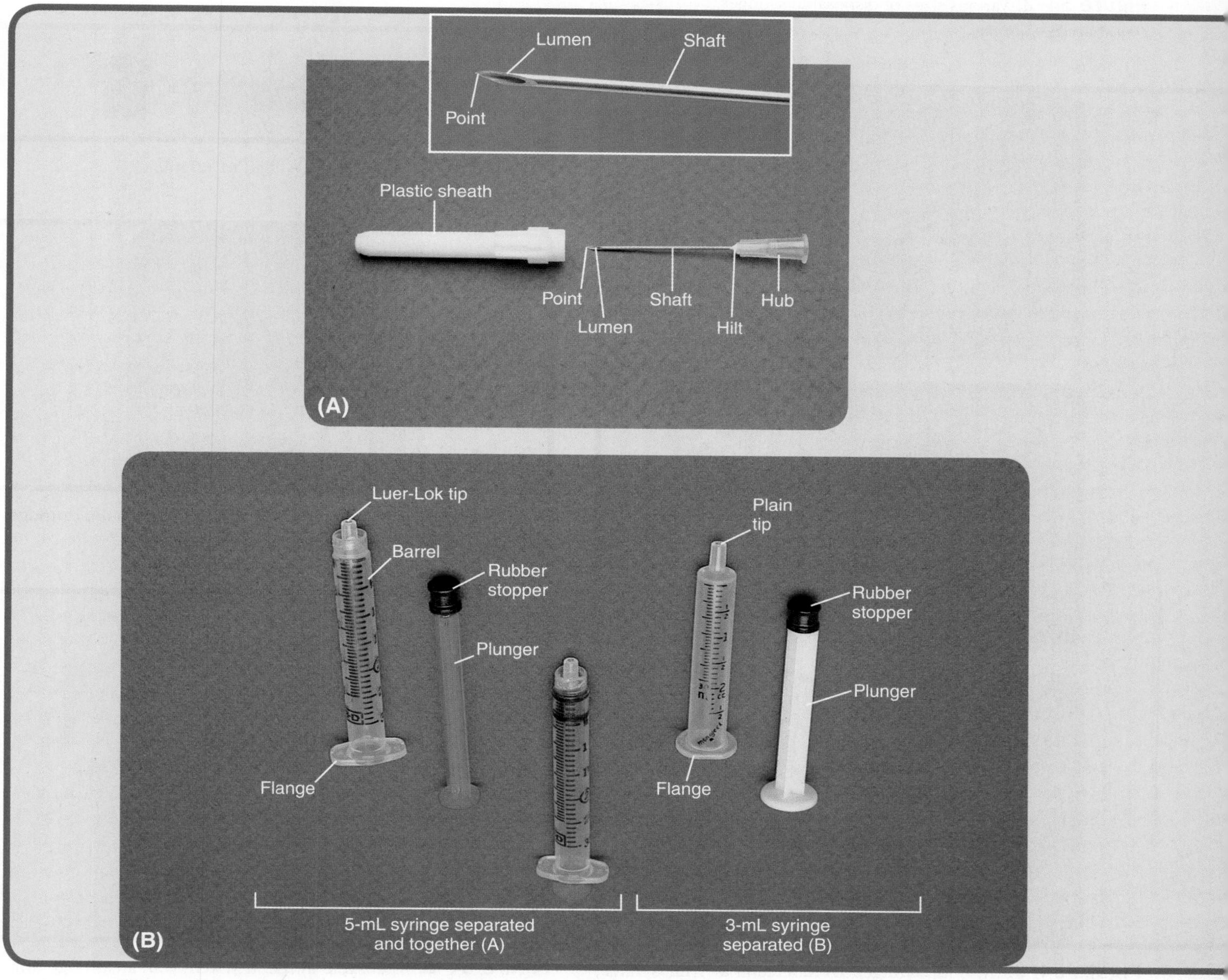

Figure 54–1: (A) Parts of a needle; (B) Parts of a syringe. *Delmar/Cengage Learning.*

amount of medication in the syringe is shown at the end of the black rubber plunger (Figure 54–4). To gain confidence in handling the different types of syringes and needles, practice filling the syringe with varying amounts of sterile water from a **vial** and **ampule**, as instructed in Procedures 54–1 and 54–2.

Injectable medications may be provided in ampules, multi-dose or single-dose vials, prefilled, disposable sterile syringes and cartridges (Figure 54–5). Prefilled, single-dose syringes guarantee an accurate dosage and are convenient and time-saving. Single-dose units are assembled by inserting the cartridge into a reusable injector (Figures 54–6).

Some injectable medications come in powdered form and must be reconstituted before administration. Procedure 54–3 lists the steps necessary to reconstitute a powdered medication in a vial.

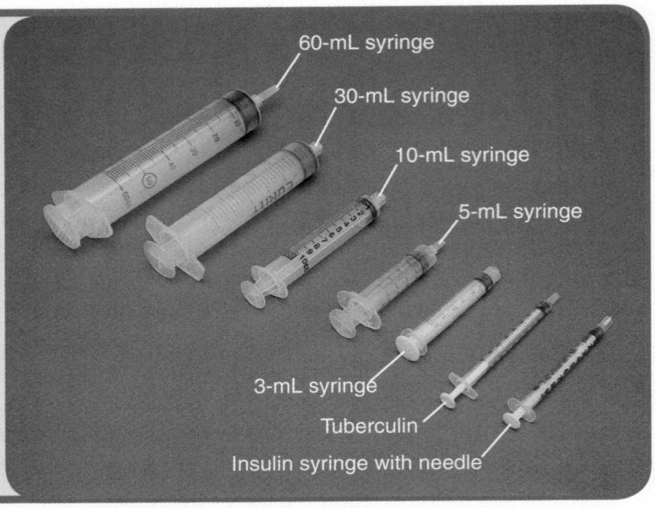

Figure 54–2: Various sizes of disposable syringes. *Delmar/Cengage Learning.*

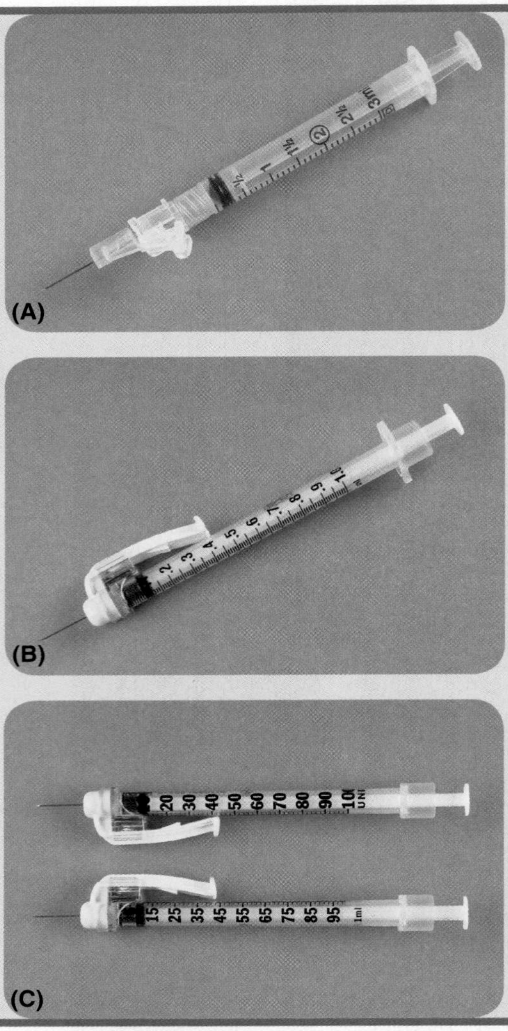

Figure 54–3: (A) 3 mL syringe; (B) tuberculin or 1 mL syringe; (C) insulin syringe. *Delmar/Cengage Learning.*

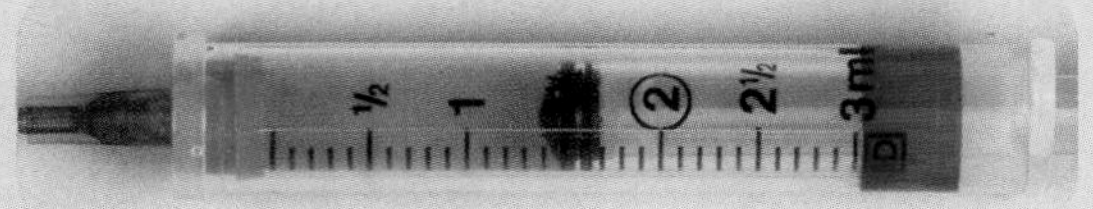

Figure 54–4: A 3 mL syringe filled to 1.5 mL. *Delmar/Cengage Learning.*

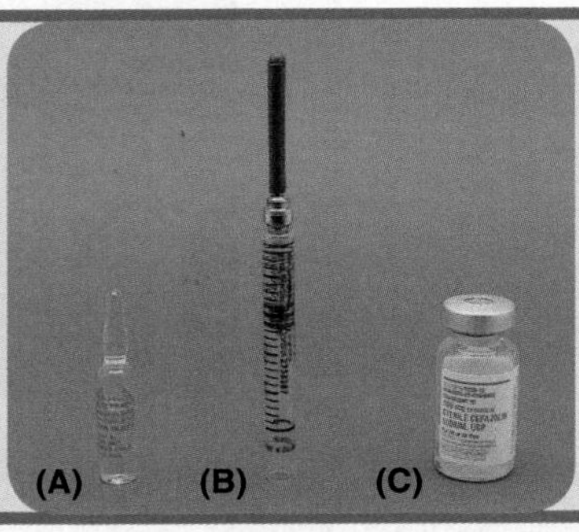

Figure 54–5: Various medication containers: ampule, cartridge unit, and vial. *Delmar/Cengage Learning.*

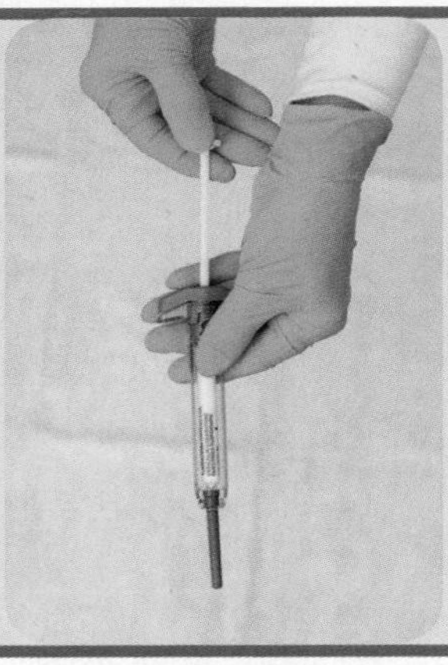

Figure 54–6: A reusable injection system with a cartridge unit; secure the needle by twisting clockwise. *Delmar/Cengage Learning.*

PROCEDURE 54–1 Withdraw Medication from an Ampule

PURPOSE: To demonstrate steps required to prepare medication for injection from an ampule

EQUIPMENT: Medication ampule, medication tray, sterile gauze 2 × 2 dressing, sterile safety needle and syringe, filter needle, disposable gloves

S **SKILL:** Accurately draw up the correct amount of medication from an ampule or vial into various types of syringes.

Procedure Steps	Detailed Instructions and/or *Rationales*
B 1. ***Compare the label of the ampule with all the elements of the ordered medication in the chart.*** Calculate desired dose to be given, if applicable. Wash hands and don clean gloves.	
2. Clean the neck of the ampule with an alcohol swab (54–7A).	
3. Tap the ampule to release any medication into the main part of the ampule; using sterile gauze or alcohol foil, snap the tip of the ampule off and discard in a sharps container (Figure 54–7B).	• Gently tap the top of the ampule to release any medication into the main part of the ampule. • Use a sterile gauze square or alcohol foil to cover the ampule top, including the neck. • Gently, but firmly, "pop" the neck of the ampule away from you by pulling the top toward you.
4. Use a syringe fitted with a filter needle to withdraw the entire contents of the ampule into the syringe, keeping the tip of the needle below the fluid line (Figure 54–7C).	*Keeping the tip of the needle below the fluid line reduces bubbles. This may be done with the ampule directly upright or tilted slightly to the side.*
5. Close the top of the filter needle and remove (Figure 54–7D); discard in sharps container.	
6. Attach a clean needle of appropriate guage for the injection (Figure 54-7E). Expel any air bubbles and then adjust the amount of medication in the syringe to that of the ordered dose.	Holding the syringe with the needle pointing up, gently tap the barrel to encourage air bubbles to travel to the top of the plunger and expel any air bubbles.
7. Discard the ampule in a sharps container.	

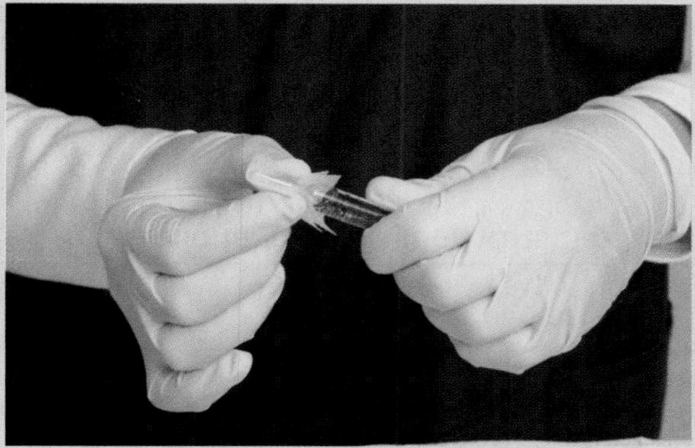

Figure 54–7A: Clean the top of the ampule with an alcohol swab. *Delmar/Cengage Learning.*

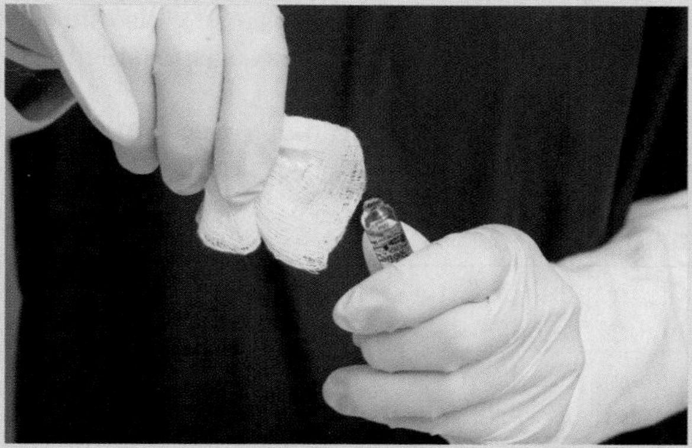

Figure 54–7B: Remove top from ampule. Snap away from you by pulling top toward you. *Delmar/Cengage Learning.*

(continues)

(continued)

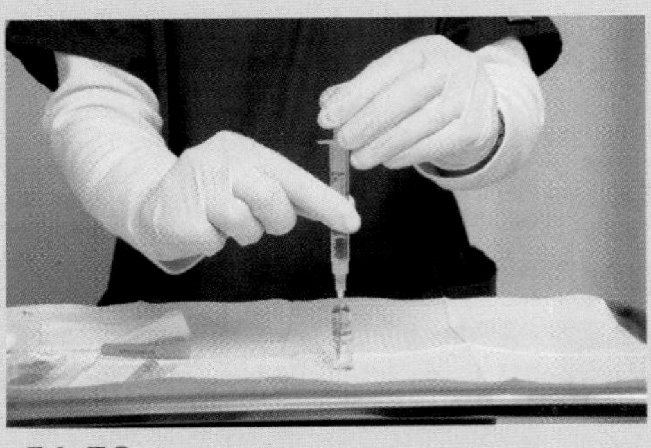

Figure 54–7C: Draw the required dose into the syringe, keeping the tip of the needle below the fluid line. *Delmar/Cengage Learning.*

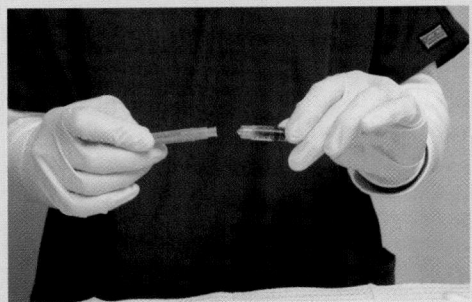

Figure 54–7D: Close the top of the filter needle and remove. *Delmar/Cengage Learning.*

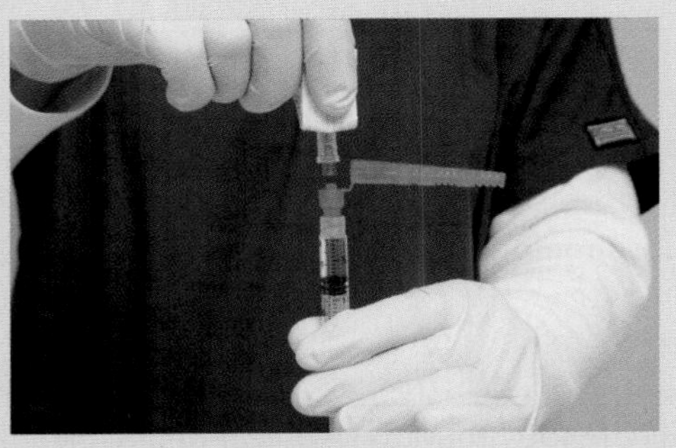

Figure 54–7E: Prepare the syringe with a new needle (and safety device). *Delmar/Cengage Learning.*

PROCEDURE 54–2 Prepare Medication from a Multi- or Single-Dose Vial

PURPOSE: To demonstrate steps required to prepare medication for injection from a multi- or single-dose vial

EQUIPMENT: Multiple- and single-dose vials (sterile water for injection), alcohol-saturated cotton balls, sterile needle and syringe, medication tray, disposable gloves, sharps container

S SKILL: Accurately draw up the correct amount of medication from an ampule or vial into various types of syringes.

Procedure Steps	Detailed Instructions and/or *Rationales*
1. Clean the top of the vial with alcohol swab (Figure 54–8A).	
2. Attach a needle to the syringe. Holding the syringe pointed upward, pull back on the plunger and take in a volume of air into the syringe equal to the order of medication.	Usually a 20- or 18-gauge needle is used.
3. Insert the needle into the vial stopper. Invert the vial and needle and syringe unit.	*This allows the fluid level to be seen clearly.*

Procedure Steps	Detailed Instructions and/or *Rationales*
4. Gently inject the air into the vial above the fluid level (Figure 54–8C).	Injecting the air above the fluid level avoids creating bubbles. This will prevent a vacuum from forming that will prevent the withdrawal of medication.
5. Withdraw the desired amount of medication into the syringe, keeping the needle below the fluid line (Figure 54–8D).	
6. Gently tap the barrel of the syringe to allow air bubbles to travel to the top of the syringe, and push them back in the vial (Figure 54–8E).	
7. Close the safety cover on the needle (Figure 54–8F) and remove. Discard in sharps container.	
8. Using aseptic technique, replace a new needle of the appropriate gauge onto the tip of the syringe. Discard gloves and vial in regular trash.	
9. Label the syringe or place a card with medication information on the medication tray.	

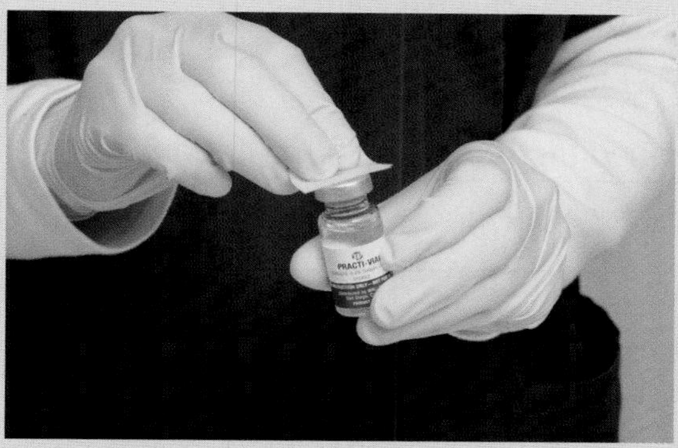

Figure 54–8A: Cleanse the rubber stopper with an alcohol swab. *Delmar/Cengage Learning.*

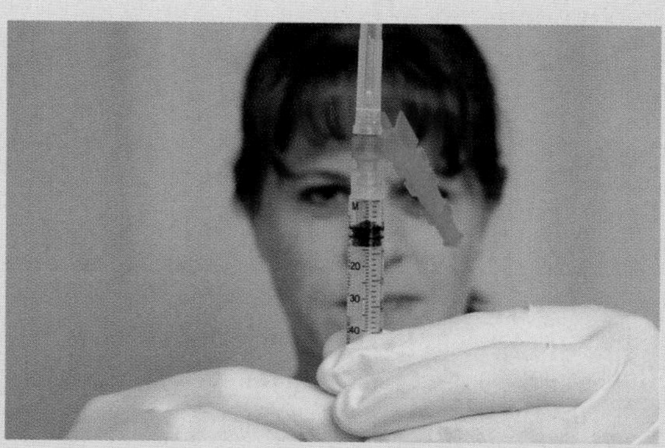

Figure 54–8B: Inject air into the vial, equal to the amount of medication that is ordered. *Delmar/Cengage Learning.*

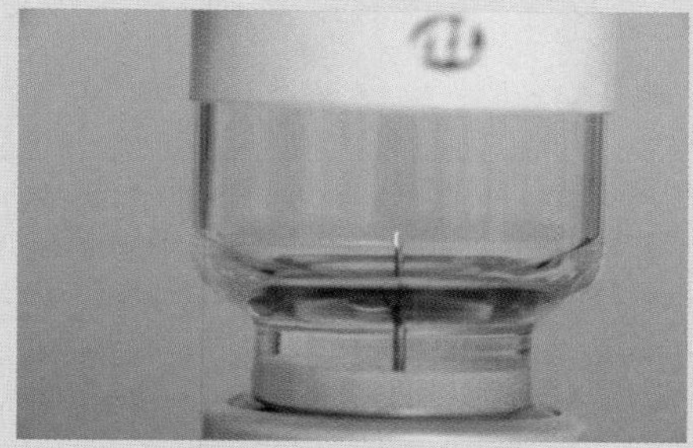

Figure 54–8C: Keeping the needle above the fluid level, inject air into the air space of the vial. *Delmar/Cengage Learning.*

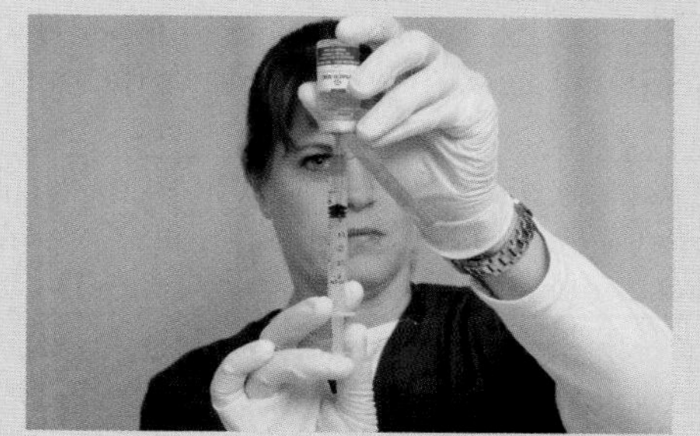

Figure 54–8D: Pull back on the plunger to withdraw the ordered dose of medication. *Delmar/Cengage Learning.*

(continues)

(continued)

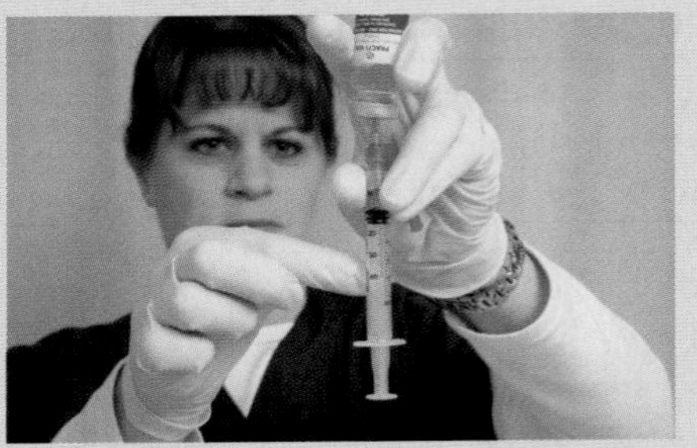

Figure 54–8E: Tap the side of the syringe to remove air bubbles. *Delmar/Cengage Learning.*

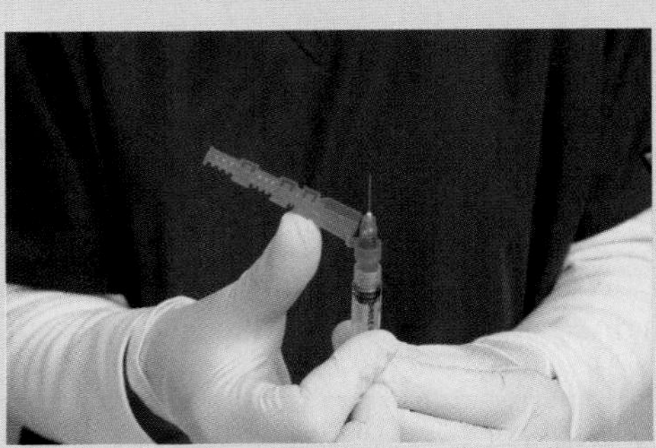

Figure 54–8F: Activate the safety device on the needle, remove, and discard in a sharps container. *Delmar/Cengage Learning.*

PROCEDURE 54–3 Reconstitute a Powder Medication

PURPOSE: To add a diluent to a powdered medication in a vial, preparing it for administration

EQUIPMENT: Powdered medication, diluent, two sterile needles and syringes, alcohol wipes, disposable gloves, sharps container

S SKILL: Reconstitute a powder medication, correctly preparing it for administration.

Procedure Steps	Detailed Instructions and/or *Rationales*
1. Assemble the needle and syringe units; wash hands and don gloves.	
2. Remove the tops from the diluent and powder medication vials and clean with alcohol swabs (Figure 54–9A).	
3. Insert the needle through the rubber stopper of the vial of diluent. The syringe should have an amount of air in it equal to the amount of diluent to be withdrawn. Invert the vial and needle and syringe unit, and withdraw the appropriate amount of diluent to be added to the powdered medication. (Figure 54–9B).	
4. Insert the needle into the rubber stopper of the powdered medication and inject the diluent (Figure 54–9C).	
5. Withdraw the needle from the top of the vial, activate the safety device, and remove it from the syringe. Discard it in a sharps container (Figure 54–9D).	
6. Gently roll the vial of medication between your hands to mix it thoroughly (Figure 54–9E).	*Roll, rather than shake, to prevent excess bubbles and foaming, making it difficult to measure medication accurately.*
7. Label the vial of prepared medication (Figure 54–9F).	The label must include the following information: strength, date and time of preparation, your initials, the expiration date of the medication.

Procedure Steps	Detailed Instructions and/or *Rationales*
8. Prepare the syringe with a second sterile needle, and properly withdraw the medication for administration. Label the syringe or place a card with medication information on the medication tray.	*Avoid using a damaged or dulled needle to minimize pain during injection and risk of infection.*
9. Discard gloves and wash hands.	

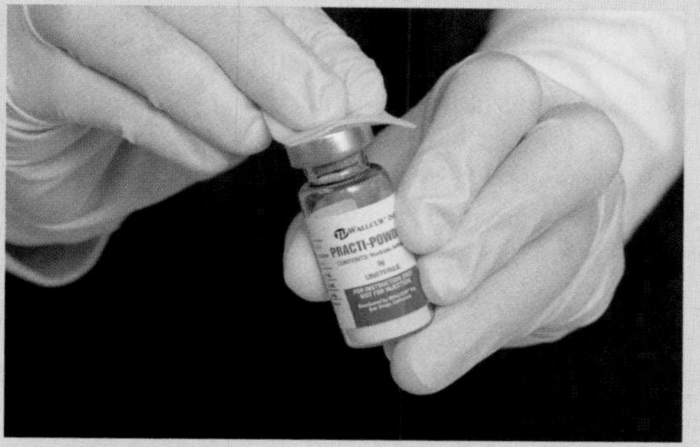

Figure 54–9A: Wipe the tops of the diluent and powdered medication with alcohol swabs. *Delmar/Cengage Learning.*

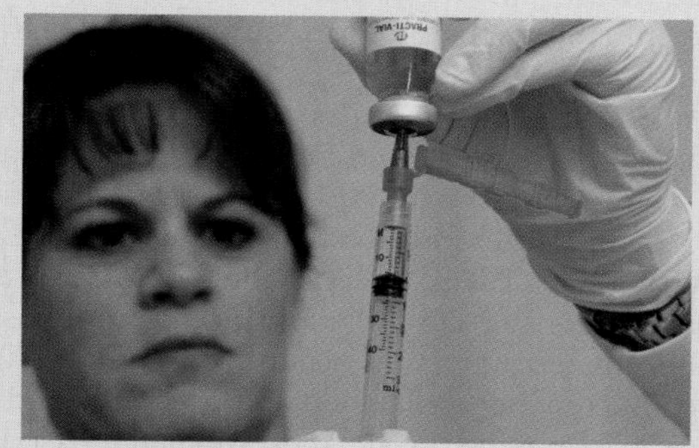

Figure 54–9B: Withdraw the appropriate amount of diluent to be added to the powdered medication. *Delmar/Cengage Learning.*

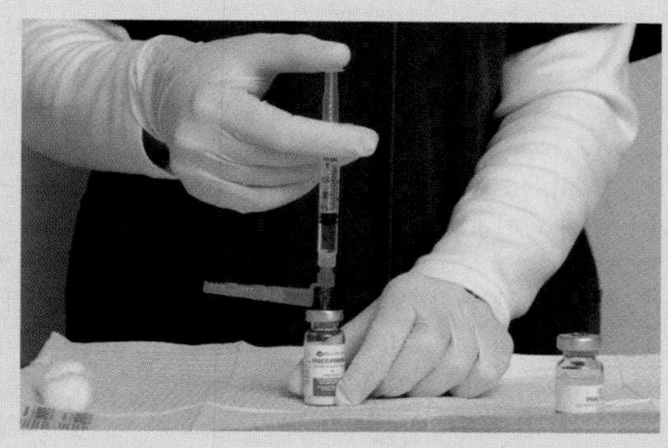

Figure 54–9C: Reconstituting medication with a diluent. *Delmar/Cengage Learning.*

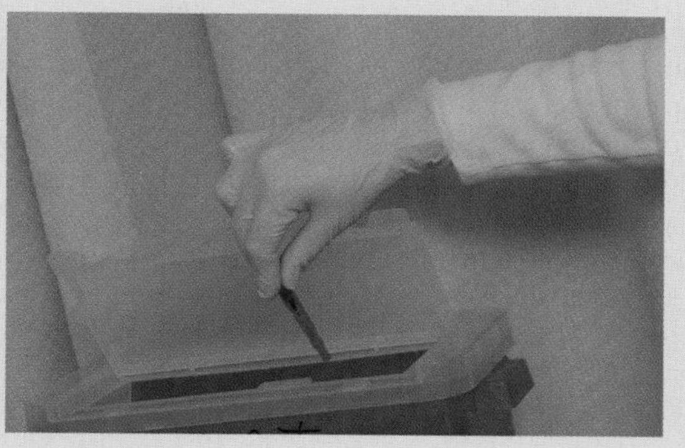

Figure 54–9D: Once diluent is added to the powdered medication, remove the needle, activate the safety, and discard in a sharps container. *Delmar/Cengage Learning.*

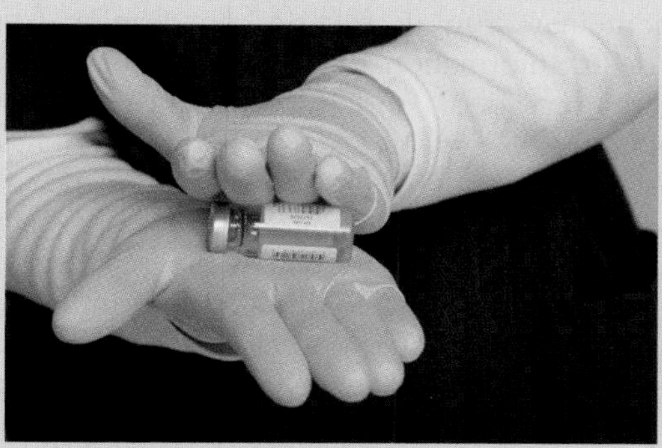

Figure 54–9E: Roll the vial between your hands to mix well. *Delmar/Cengage Learning.*

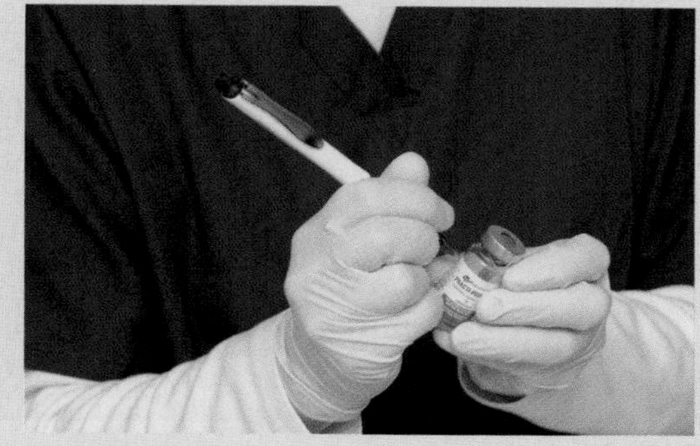

Figure 54–9F: Label the medication vial. *Delmar/Cengage Learning.*

Handling Needles Safely

While handling the syringe and needle, use caution to avoid dangerous **needlesticks**. The needle guard remains on the needle until just before the injection is administered. Needles should NEVER be recapped after use. All used needles and syringes should be discarded, intact, into a biohazard, hard-sided, and appropriately labeled sharps container (Figure 54–10). The container should never be overfilled and always locked appropriately before sending to be destroyed. Proper disposal of used needles and syringes is absolutely necessary to prevent accidental needlesticks and disease transmission to the medical and custodial staff of the facility.

If a needlestick occurs *before* the injection is given, the needle and syringe should be discarded and a new dose of medication prepared. This prevents the patient from becoming infected from a contaminated needle. In the event of a needlestick to either the medical assistant or the patient, consult the provider or other supervising practitioner immediately. The occurrence must be carefully documented on an incident report form, and all actions taken to address the situation should be based on the facility's procedures manual. Careful washing of the needlestick site can help prevent infection and additional resorption of the medication contained in the needle. Testing might be ordered to determine whether there has been an accidental infectious exposure. Antibiotics or other prophylactic medication can be required, but the appropriate steps to be taken require the evaluation of the provider or practitioner. It is also critical to adhere to any reporting requirements mandated by the state in which you work.

Some needle and syringe units have a shield that locks into place over used needles to prevent injury to the user. There are also safety devices that activate by the touch of a finger to click a shield over the used needle or retract the needle into a sleeve on the syringe.

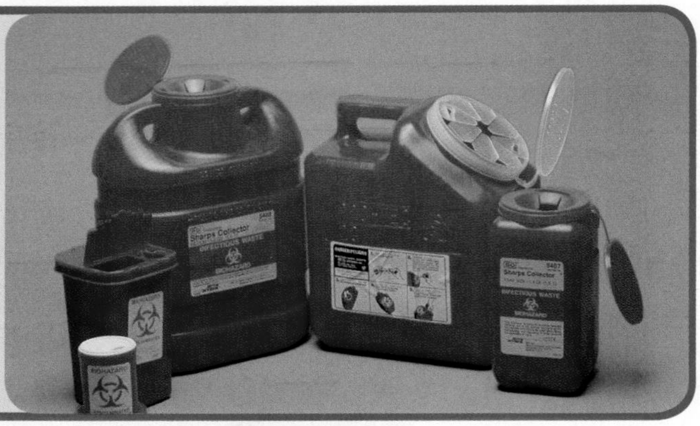

Figure 54–10: Sharps container. *Delmar/Cengage Learning.*

Another safety device to protect users from contaminated needlesticks is a sheath cover that clicks into place to cover the used needle completely. Table 54–1 illustrates these safety devices.

PATIENT EDUCATION

All patients who self-administer injections should receive proper instruction in the safe storage, use, and disposal of used syringes and needles. Remind patients not to remove the needle from the barrel of the syringe after use and to procure a sharps container. When necessary, assist the patient in locating a telephone number for a local disposal company or waste management office or, if the practice or clinic offers the service, advise the patient to return the container to the medical facility to be disposed of properly. Stress that all materials should be kept safely out of the reach of children to avoid accidents.

Other Safety Considerations

Because injections introduce a substance directly into tissues, where it quickly enters the patient's bloodstream, extreme caution must be practiced. Proper technique must be learned under supervision. Latex or vinyl gloves should be worn to administer an injection.

Medication should be given only to patients when a provider is available nearby in case the patient exhibits any adverse reaction; there is always the possibility of an **anaphylactic** reaction. (Refer to Chapter 55 for symptoms of anaphylactic reactions.) If this situation occurs, notify the provider immediately. The provider may choose to administer an injection of **epinephrine**. Continue taking the patient's vital signs until the patient is stable or until the patient's care is transferred to an emergency team.

Even if the patient has no past history of **sensitivity** to a particular drug, a reaction can develop from any given dose. Information regarding an allergic reaction, the care provided, and the patient's response to treatment must always be recorded on the patient's chart. If transferred, a copy of all documentation pertinent to the event should be sent along with the emergency team or faxed to the facility to which the patient is being transported. A brightly colored sticker indicating the medication allergy should be placed on the outside and on the inside of the patient's chart. Advise the patient to wear an identification bracelet containing information about the medication allergy.

TABLE 54–1 Needle Safety Devices

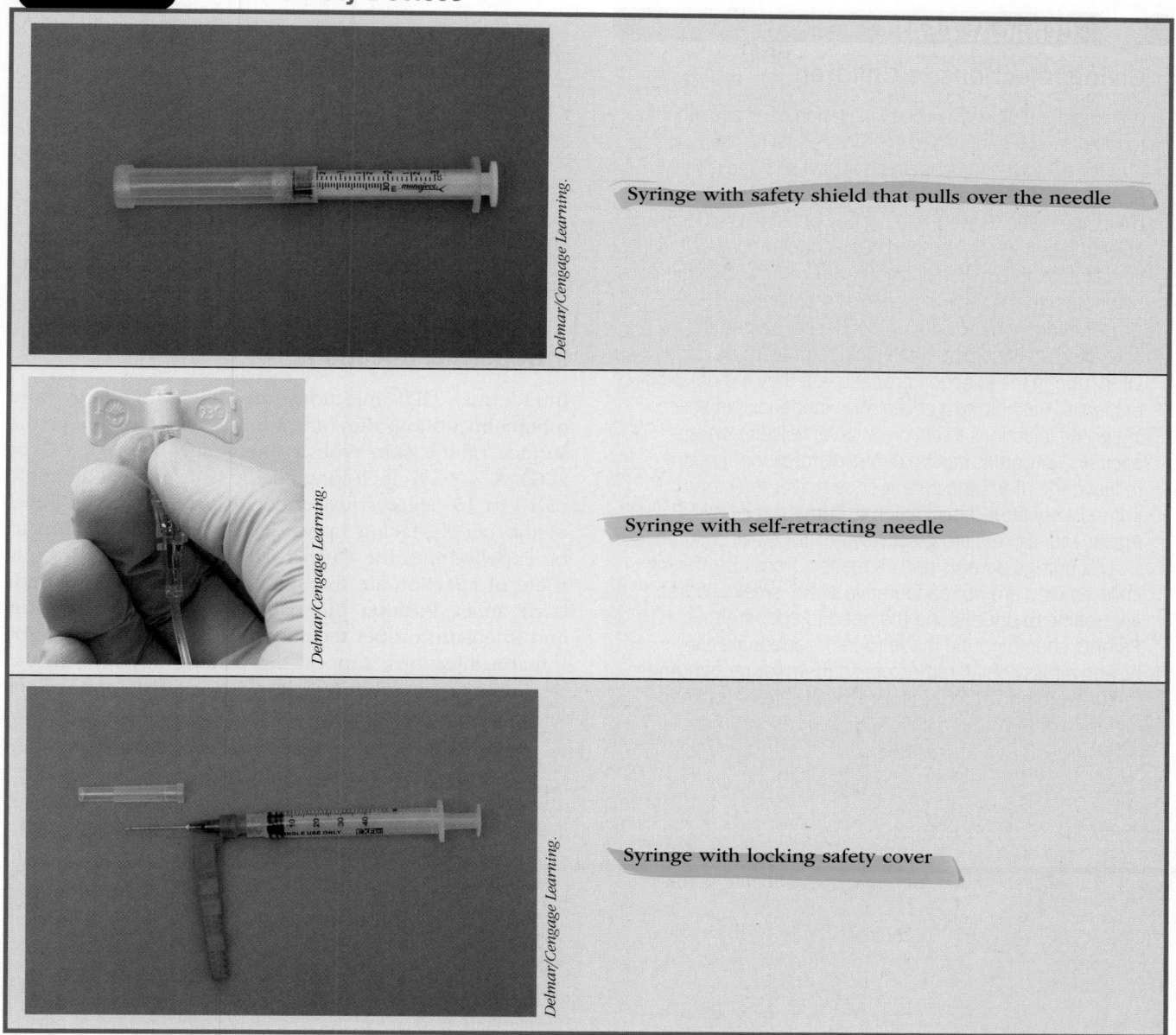

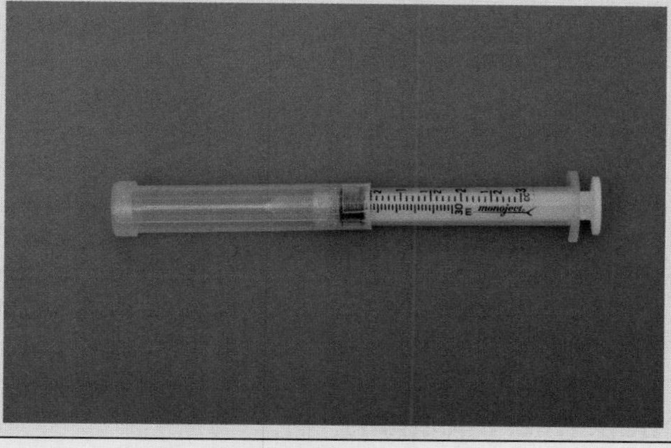 Delmar/Cengage Learning.	Syringe with safety shield that pulls over the needle
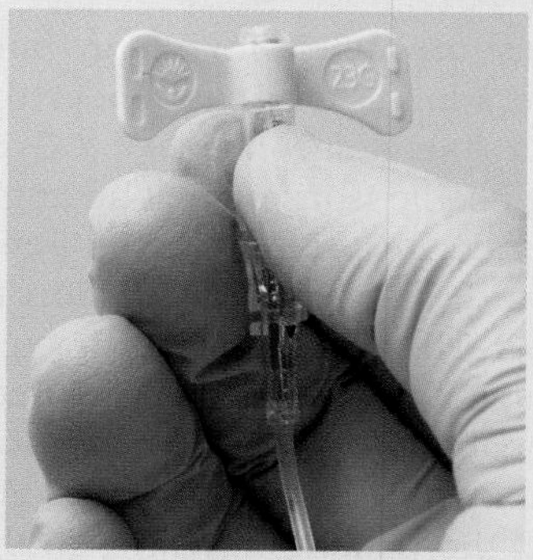 Delmar/Cengage Learning.	Syringe with self-retracting needle
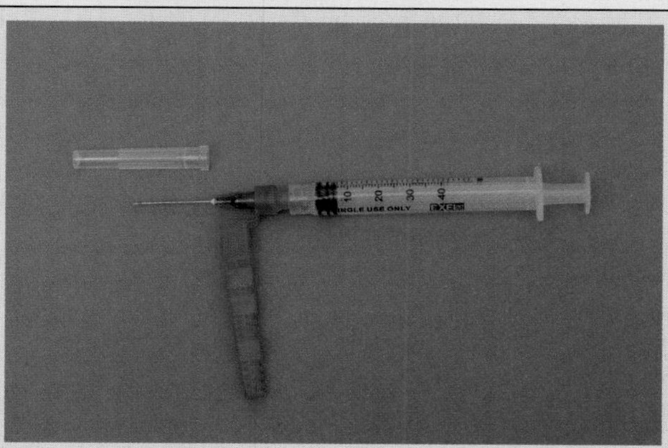 Delmar/Cengage Learning.	Syringe with locking safety cover

Preparing the Patient

Explaining the procedure can relieve the patient's anxiety. Being honest with patients is very important. The site to be injected should be free from restrictive clothing. Patients should be asked to remove these items of clothing while the medication is being prepared. Proper preparation of the skin at the site of injection is necessary before and after injecting the medication because microorganisms can enter the body through a break in the skin. Alcohol is the usual antiseptic because it is least irritating to the skin.

If administering an immunization, ensure that all appropriate authorization forms are in order. Allow sufficient time for parents (or those responsible for a child patient) to read the information regarding the vaccine and have all questions answered before obtaining the authorization signature. This form must be filed in the patient's chart. More information about immunizations is discussed later in this chapter.

CLINICAL PEARL

Giving Injections to Children

Children should be given an explanation of what is about to take place. It can help to emphasize that it might hurt for a few seconds but the pain will be gone quickly. Engage the child as a partner in the procedure, for example, being made to feel like a big boy or big girl by being given the option of helping through cooperation. A simplified explanation of "keeping you from getting sick" might be enough to gain an older child's compliance.

Depending on provider and office policy, parents or caregivers may help hold the child to prevent an undue injury during the injection procedure. If they are not present, enlist the help of a coworker experienced in assisting giving injections to children. Quiet voices, songs, pacifiers, or bottles can be useful distractions. If opting to leave the room, the parent or caregiver may return immediately after the injection to comfort the child. Praise and stickers are great rewards for small children.

Discourage parents and caregivers from threatening children who are not cooperative. Many small children are unable to understand the need to cooperate. Parents should not be made to feel inadequate for having a fussy child; rather, praise them for recognizing the need to bring them in for medical care or for keeping up to date with the child's immunization schedule.

ADMINISTERING INJECTIONS

The administration techniques for injecting medications are extremely important. Improper injection techniques can result in infection as well as damage to nerves, blood vessels, and tissues and can lead to legal action. When proper technique is used, however, giving medications by injection can be a minimally painful experience for the patient.

Each type of injection must be given at a specific angle for the medication to be absorbed properly. Figure 54–11 illustrates the proper angles for the different types of injections.

Intradermal Injections

Intradermal (ID) injections are used in allergy and tuberculin testing; they are administered just under the surface of the skin with a fine-gauge needle (26G or 27G). A ⅜- to ⅝- inch-long needle is inserted at an angle of 10 to 15 degrees just under the skin with the bevel of the needle facing upward, allowing the solution to be expelled into the dermis. The preferred sites for this route of injection are the anterior forearm and the mid-back areas. Position the patient to allow for comfort and to ensure proper technique for accurate results. For forearm injections, support the patient's forearm on the treatment table and, for back injections, have the patient lie down on the treatment table.

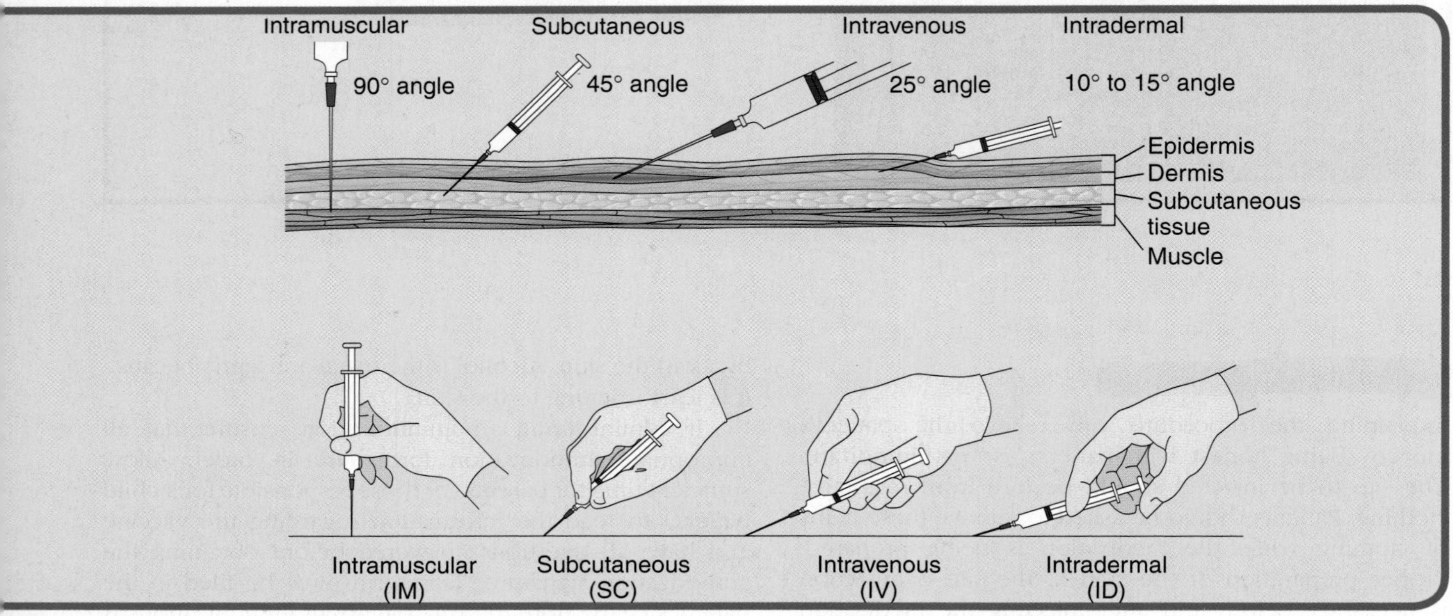

Figure 54–11: Angles of injection with appropriate needles for types of injections. *Delmar/Cengage Learning.*

A small **wheal**, or lump, should develop at the site of the injection to give evidence that the medication is in the dermal layer of the skin (Figure 54–12). Only small amounts of medication, from 0.01 to 0.05 mL, are administered intradermally. The speed of the reaction and the size of the wheal should be recorded and the patient observed carefully for any reaction for at least 20 minutes and sometimes longer. Allergy testing is most often performed under the direct supervision of the provider. In the event of a hypersensitive reaction, be prepared to assist with emergency administration of epinephrine by the provider. Refer to Procedure 54–4 for administering intradermal injections.

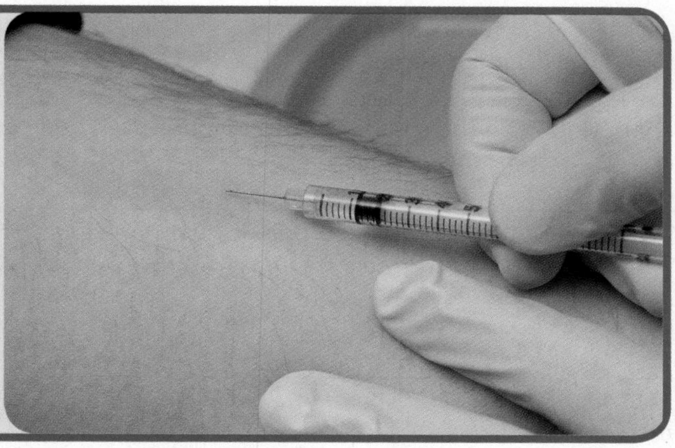

Figure 54–12A: When giving an intradermal injection, hold the patient's skin taut between your thumb and fingers and insert the needle at a 10–15 degree angle. *Delmar/Cengage Learning.*

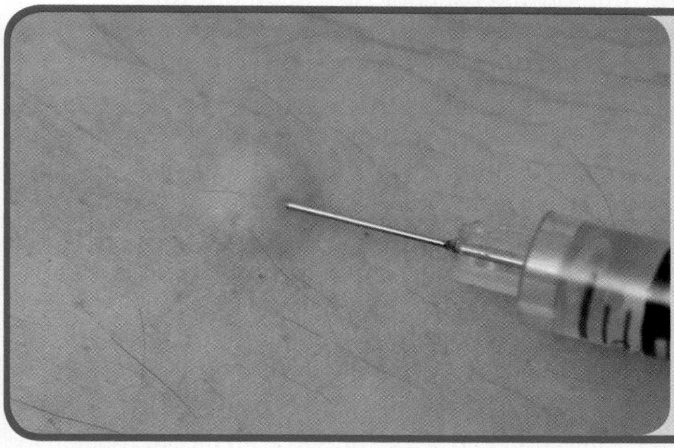

Figure 54–12B: Slowly inject the medication by depressing the plunger. A small wheal should develop at the site of the injection. *Delmar/Cengage Learning.*

PROCEDURE 54–4 Administer an Intradermal Injection

PURPOSE: To inject liquid solutions of 0.01 mL and 0.05 mL into the dermal layer of tissue for allergy and immunity testing of patients

EQUIPMENT: Medication (sterile water for injection in vial or ampule), cotton balls, adhesive bandage or hypoallergenic tape, sterile needle (usually ⅜ to ⅝ inch, 25G to 27G) and syringe, medication tray, alcohol prep, patient's chart, pen, gloves

S **SKILL:** Prepare, verify, and administer proper doses of medications for intradermal injections.

S **SKILL:** Demonstrate appropriate aseptic technique as it applies to medication administration.

S **SKILL:** Demonstrate proper disposal of used syringes and needles.

Procedure Steps	Detailed Instructions and/or *Rationales*
1. Wash and glove hands.	
B 2. Prepare the syringe with the ordered amount of medication, ***verifying the ordered doses or dosages prior to patient administration.***	Read the label of the medication and compare it with the order.

(continues)

(continued)

Procedure Steps	Detailed Instructions and/or *Rationales*
B 3. Identify the patient and explain the procedure, ***using language the patient understands***. Compare the medication order (again) with the patient's chart.	Identify the patient by using two identifiers.
B 4. Allow the patient to ask questions ***and show awareness of any patient concerns regarding the procedure.*** Respond to the patient as appropriate.	
5. Select and prepare the injection site with an alcohol prep. Allow the alcohol to air dry.	Do not blow on the area to dry the alcohol. *The area can be contaminated by microorganisms in the exhaled air.*
6. Holding the patient's skin taut between your thumb and fingers, insert the needle at a 10- to 15-degree angle of insertion and slowly expel the medication from the syringe by depressing the plunger.	The bevel of the needle should be up; *this allows the material to produce a wheal by infiltrating the dermal layer of the skin.*
7. Remove the needle quickly by the same angle of injection and wipe the site with a cotton ball. Do not massage the injection site.	*Massaging distributes the material throughout the tissues.*
8. Observe the patient and time the reaction. Give the patient instructions as ordered and answer any questions.	
9. Apply a bandage.	Determine whether patient is allergic to adhesive before applying the bandage; if so, use hypoallergenic tape.
10. Discard disposable items and gloves into a biohazard waste bag. Place the entire syringe and needle into the biohazard sharps container. Return the medication and tray to the proper storage area.	
11. Document the procedure in the patient's chart or medication log.	

Charting Example

7/21/20XX 8:35 am	Mumps Skin Test Antigen 0.1 mL ID placed left anterior forearm. Patient advised to return to clinic to have site evaluated in 48–72 hours. Instructions provided not to rub or put creams on site of injection and to avoid taking antihistamines. Susan Davis, RMA(AMT)

Subcutaneous Injections

Subcutaneous injections are used to administer small doses of medication, usually not more than 2 mL. The injection is most often given in the upper, outer part of the arm, abdominal area, or upper thigh (Figure 54–13). The length of the needle ranges from ½ to ⅝ inch and the gauge from 25G to 27G. Subcutaneous injections are administered at a 45-degree angle of insertion. Many medications, including allergy injections, insulin, and immunizations, are administered by the subcutaneous method. Refer to Chapter 45 for specific details about giving allergy injections. The patient should be asked to sit or lie on the treatment table for safety. Refer to Procedure 54–5 for administering subcutaneous injections.

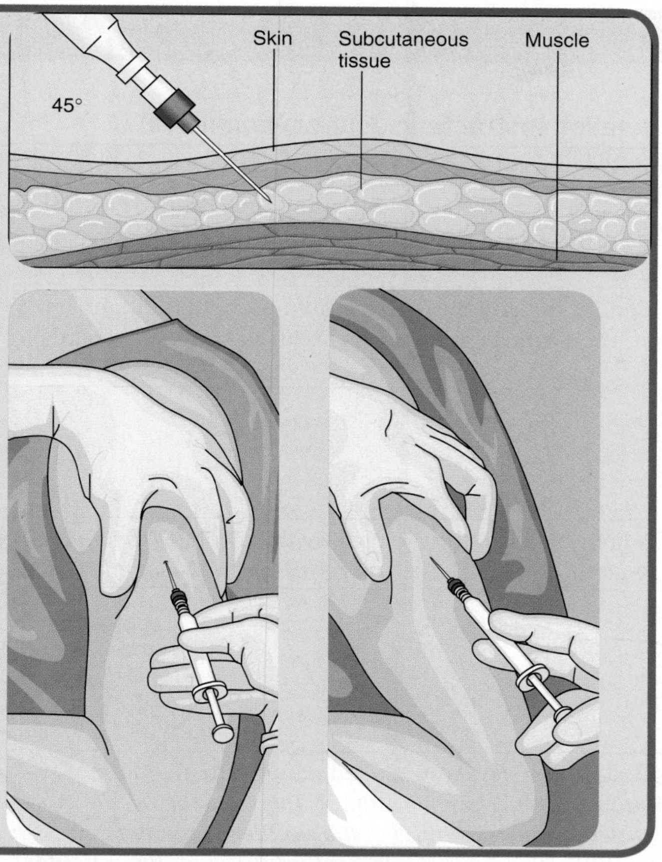

Figure 54–13: Subcutaneous injection. *Delmar/Cengage Learning.*

Intramuscular Injections

As the name suggests, intramuscular (IM) injections are placed into muscle tissue. The most common sites for this method of injection are the deltoid (upper, outer arm), gluteus medius (upper, outer portion of the hip), ventrogluteal (lateral outside portion of the hip), and vastus lateralis (mid-portion of the thigh) (Figure 54–14).

Proper positioning of patients is important. For injections in the deltoid area, the patient should be sitting. If the site is the gluteus muscle, ask the patient to lie in prone position on the treatment table with the toes pointed inward or to lean over the treatment table and stand on the non-injection-site leg to relax the muscle, making the injection less uncomfortable. For injection of the vastus lateralis site, the patient may be sitting or lying in the horizontal recumbent position. Record the site and rotate injection sites to reduce tissue scarring.

When administering IM injections, the needle is 1 to 3 inches in length or longer to penetrate many layers of tissue. The angle of injection is 90 degrees. IM injections are indicated when large doses of medication or oil-based, non–water based, or thicker medications must be given. Dosage can vary from 0.5 to 3.0 mL. Medications given by the IM method are absorbed over several hours by the rich blood supply of the muscle tissue.

The gauge of the needle ranges between 18G and 23G to accommodate the density of the substance. In giving injections intramuscularly to pediatric patients, the gauge and length of the needle are, of course,

PROCEDURE 54–5 Administer a Subcutaneous Injection

MEDIA LINK: View the animation, "Subcutaneous Injection Animation," on the Premium Website for this chapter.

PURPOSE: To inject aqueous solutions of 0.5 to 2.0 mL into the subcutaneous tissue.

EQUIPMENT: Medication (sterile water for injection in vial or ampule), alcohol prep, adhesive bandage or hypoallergenic tape, sterile needle (usually ½ to ⅝ inch, 25G) and syringe, gloves

S **SKILL:** Prepare, verify, and administer proper doses of medications for subcutaneous injections.

S **SKILL:** Demonstrate appropriate aseptic technique as it applies to medication administration.

S **SKILL:** Demonstrate proper disposal of used syringes and needles.

(continues)

(continued)

Procedure Steps	Detailed Instructions and/or *Rationales*
1. Wash and glove hands.	
B 2. Prepare the syringe with the ordered amount of medication, ***verifying all ordered doses or dosages prior to administration.***	Read the label of the medication and compare it with the order.
B 3. Identify the patient and explain the procedure, ***using language the patient understands.*** Ask patient to remove clothes, if necessary.	Identify the patient by using two identifiers. Compare the medication order (again) with the patient's chart.
B 4. Allow the patient to ask questions ***and show awareness of any patient concerns regarding the procedure.*** Respond to the patient as appropriate.	
5. Select and prepare the injection site with an alcohol prep. Allow the alcohol to air dry.	Do not blow on the area to dry the alcohol. *The area can be contaminated by microorganisms in the exhaled air.*
6. Bunch the patient's skin between the thumb and finger of one hand and, with the other hand, hold the syringe securely. Insert the needle at a 45-degree angle with a steady penetration. Let go of the skin.	
7. With one hand, hold the barrel of the syringe while pulling back on the plunger slightly with the other hand to make sure a blood vessel has not been penetrated. If no blood appears in the syringe, proceed by slowly pushing down on the plunger to expel medication into the tissues.	If blood appears in the syringe, pull the needle out carefully at the angle of entry. *Blood in the needle indicates the possibility of the needle placement being within a blood vessel. Medication injected directly into the bloodstream causes rapid absorption and can cause undesirable as well as dangerous results.* Discard the medication, syringe, and needle. Replace with a new syringe and medication.
8. Remove the needle quickly by the same angle of injection and wipe the site with a cotton ball. Gently massage the area.	*Massaging helps distribute the material throughout the tissues.*
9. Observe the patient and time the reaction. Give the patient instructions as ordered and answer any questions.	Report to the provider if a reaction occurs.
10. Apply a bandage.	Determine whether patient is allergic to adhesive before applying the bandage; if so, use hypoallergenic tape.
11. Discard disposable items and gloves into a biohazard waste bag. Place the entire syringe and needle into the biohazard sharps container. Return the medication and tray to the proper storage area.	
12. Document the procedure in the patient's chart or medication log.	

Charting Example

7/28/20XX 9:54 am	Allergy serum from vial # 2345, expires 12/31/2012, 0.6 mL subq Rt arm. Patient will wait for 20 min to observe for allergic reaction prior to leaving clinic. Patient advised not to rub injection site. Susan Davis, RMA(AMT)

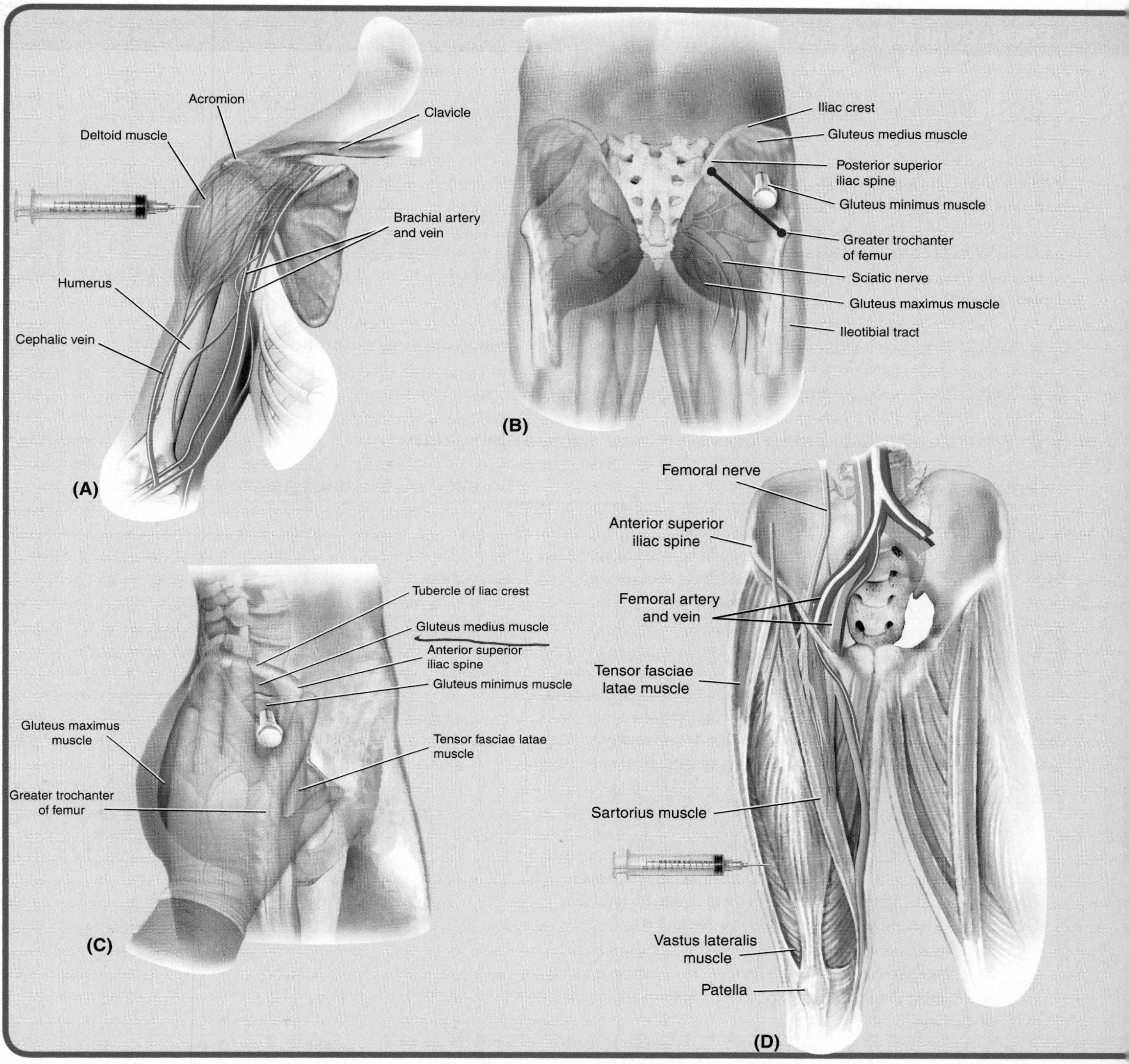

Figure 54–14A–D: (A) Deltoid site; (B) Dorsogluteal site; (C) Ventrogluteal site; (D) Vastus lateralis site, adult patient.
Delmar/Cengage Learning.

smaller than those generally used for adults. Refer to Procedure 54–6 for administering intramuscular injections.

For injecting substances that can be irritating or cause discoloration of the subcutaneous tissues, the **Z-track IM** method is used. Muscle tissue is displaced by holding it to the side of the injection site. Following injection of the medication, the tissue is moved back over the site, blocking any residual substance. Using this technique prevents the medication from following the path of the needle and leaking out into the tissues. After Z-track IM administration, the injection site should *not* be massaged, because this action would encourage the irritating substance to circulate into the subcutaneous tissues. Refer to Procedure 54–7 for administering Z-track intramuscular injections.

PROCEDURE 54–6 Administer an Intramuscular Injection

MEDIA LINK: View the animation, "Intramuscular Injection Animation," on the Premium Website for this chapter

PURPOSE: To inject large amounts of medication, 0.5 mL to 3.0 mL, and oil-based substances or irritating solutions that are more easily tolerated in the muscle tissue

EQUIPMENT: Medication (sterile water for injection in vial or ampule), cotton balls, alcohol prep, adhesive bandage or hypoallergenic tape, sterile needle (usually 1 to 3 inches, 18G to 23G), medication tray, patient's chart, pen, gloves

S **SKILL:** Prepare, verify, and administer proper doses of medications for intramuscular injections.

S **SKILL:** Demonstrate appropriate aseptic technique as it applies to medication administration.

S **SKILL:** Demonstrate proper disposal of used syringes and needles.

Procedure Steps	Detailed Instructions and/or *Rationales*
1. Wash and glove hands.	
B 2. Prepare the syringe with the ordered amount of medication, ***verifying all ordered doses or dosages prior to administration.***	Read the label of the medication and compare it with the order.
B 3. Identify the patient and explain the procedure, ***using language the patient understands.*** Ask patient to remove clothes, if necessary.	Identify the patient by using two identifiers. Compare the medication order (again) with the patient's chart.
B 4. Allow the patient to ask questions ***and show awareness of any patient concerns regarding the procedure.*** Respond to the patient as appropriate.	
5. Select and prepare the injection site with an alcohol prep. Allow the alcohol to air dry.	Do not blow on the area to dry the alcohol. *The area may be contaminated by microorganisms in the exhaled air.*
6. Secure a large area of skin (to accommodate the large amount of medication) between the thumb and finger of one hand and, with the other hand, hold the syringe securely. Insert the needle at a 90-degree angle with a steady penetration. Let go of the skin.	
7. With one hand, hold the barrel of the syringe while pulling back on the plunger slightly with the other hand to make sure a blood vessel has not been penetrated. If no blood appears in the syringe, proceed by slowly pushing down on the plunger to expel medication into the muscle.	If blood appears in the syringe, pull the needle out carefully at the angle of entry. *Blood in the needle indicates the possibility of the needle placement being within a blood vessel. Medication injected directly into the bloodstream causes rapid absorption and can cause undesirable as well as dangerous results.* Discard the medication, syringe, and needle. Replace with a new syringe and medication.
8. Remove the needle quickly by the same angle of injection and wipe the site with a cotton ball. Gently massage the area.	*Massaging helps distribute the material throughout the tissues.*

Procedure Steps	Detailed Instructions and/or *Rationales*
9. Observe the patient and time the reaction. Give the patient instructions as ordered and answer any questions.	Report to the provider if a reaction occurs.
10. Apply a bandage.	Determine whether patient is allergic to adhesive before applying the bandage; if so, use hypoallergenic tape.
11. Discard disposable items and gloves into a biohazard waste bag. Place the entire syringe and needle into the biohazard sharps container. Return the medication and tray to the proper storage area.	
12. Document the procedure in the patient's chart or medication log.	

Charting Example

12/4/20XX 4:15 PM	Ivanz 150 mg [15 mg/kg, child's weight 10 kg] IM Rt hip. Second MA assisted with injection to ensure patient safety. Parent returned to comfort child following injection. Parent will wait with child for 20 min in the waiting room to watch for signs of reaction prior leaving clinic. Bandage lightly placed across injection site. Jorge Watkins, CMA (AAMA)

PROCEDURE 54–7 Administer an Intramuscular Injection by Z-Track Method

MEDIA LINK: View the animation, "Z-Track Injection Animation," on the Premium Website for this chapter

PURPOSE: To inject substances, 0.5 mL to 3.0 mL, which can be irritating or discoloring to the tissues, deep into the muscle layer of tissue

EQUIPMENT: Medication (sterile water for injection in vial or ampule), cotton balls, alcohol prep, adhesive bandage or hypoallergenic tape, sterile gauze square, sterile needle (usually 1 to 3 inches, 18G to 23G), medication tray, patient's chart, pen, gloves

S **SKILL:** Prepare, verify, and administer proper doses of medications for intramuscular Z-track injections.

S **SKILL:** Demonstrate appropriate aseptic technique as it applies to medication administration.

S **SKILL:** Demonstrate proper disposal of used syringes and needles.

Procedure Steps	Detailed Instructions and/or *Rationales*
1. Wash and glove hands.	
B 2. Prepare the syringe with the ordered amount of medication, ***verifying all ordered doses or dosages prior to administration.***	Read the label of the medication and compare it with the order.

(continues)

(continued)

Procedure Steps	Detailed Instructions and/or *Rationales*
B 3. Identify the patient and explain the procedure, ***using language the patient understands.*** Ask patient to remove clothes, if necessary.	Identify the patient by using two identifiers. Compare the medication order (again) with the patient's chart.
B 4. Allow the patient to ask questions ***and show awareness of any patient concerns regarding the procedure.*** Respond to the patient as appropriate.	
5. Select and prepare the injection site with an alcohol prep. Allow the alcohol to air dry.	Do not blow on the area to dry the alcohol. *The area can be contaminated by microorganisms in the exhaled air.*
6. Use a gauze square to hold the patient's skin securely at the injection site to one side to displace skin and tissues until the injection is completed. Insert the needle at a 90-degree angle with a steady penetration.	
7. The first and second fingers may be used to aspirate while the thumb and ring finger hold the syringe near the needle end. If no blood appears in the syringe, proceed by slowly pushing down on the plunger to expel medication into the muscle. Wait a few seconds before removing the needle.	If blood appears in the syringe, pull the needle out carefully at the angle of entry. *Blood in the needle indicates the possibility of the needle placement being within a blood vessel. Medication injected directly into the bloodstream causes rapid absorption and can cause undesirable as well as dangerous results.* Discard the medication, syringe, and needle. Replace with a new syringe and medication.
8. Remove the needle quickly by the same angle of injection and let go of the skin quickly so that displaced tissue will cover the needle track and prevent it from leaking into the surrounding tissues. Cover the site with a cotton ball. Do not massage the area.	*Massaging helps distribute the material throughout the tissues.*
9. Observe the patient and time the reaction. Give the patient instructions as ordered and answer any questions.	Report to the provider if a reaction occurs.
10. Apply a bandage.	Determine whether patient is allergic to adhesive before applying the bandage; if so, use hypoallergenic tape.
11. Discard disposable items and gloves into a biohazard waste bag. Place the entire syringe and needle into the biohazard sharps container. Return the medication and tray to the proper storage area.	
12. Document the procedure in the patient's chart or medication log.	

Charting Example

1/26/20XX 3:15 PM	Rocephin 2 g admixed with 0.5 cc lidocaine, divided into 2 doses of 3 mL injections, injected deep IM to bilateral gluteus maximus. Patient positioned on exam table with toes inverted to relax muscle. Patient tolerated injections well, will remain in waiting room for 20 minutes prior to leaving. Sarah Rodriguez, RMA (AMT)———

Administering Injections to Infants and Small Children

Injections that are given to infants and small children need special attention. The size of the child's arm or leg will help decide the size of the underlying muscle, which determines the needle length appropriate for the muscle thickness. The gauge of the needle is determined by the viscosity of the medication. The vastus lateralis is the preferred injection site for infants and young children (Figure 54–15). Gently aspirate between 5 and 10 seconds (tiny blood vessels take time to flow) before injecting the medication to prevent entering a blood vessel, which would be critical in a child. If a blood vessel is entered while aspirating, withdraw the needle and start over. For injecting the left vastus lateralis, grasp and stabilize the muscle. Lightly prepare the tissue with an alcohol prep and proceed with assistance in holding the child during the procedure. Administer the injection carefully in the center of the muscle while holding the tissue taut.

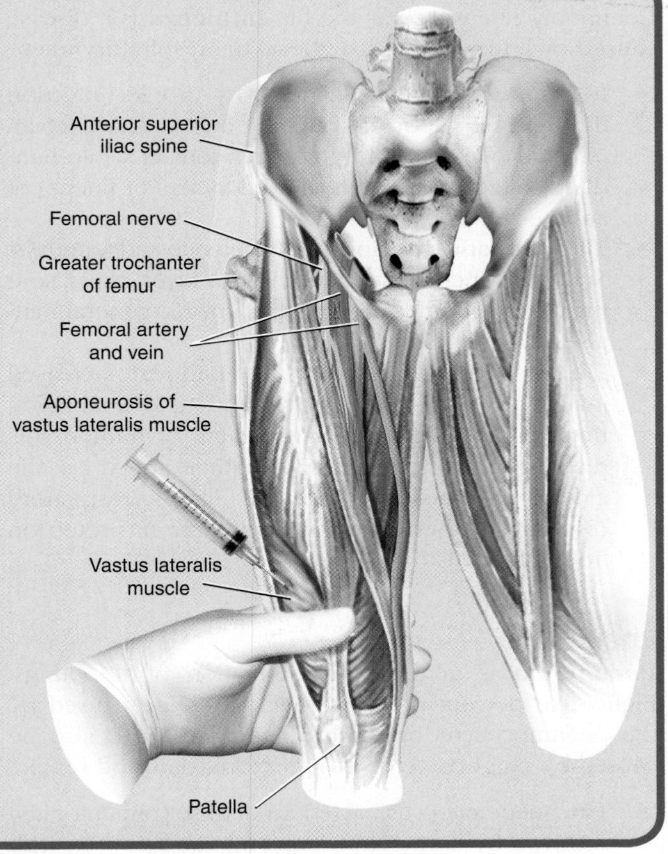

Figure 54–15: Injection technique for vastus lateralis site, pediatric patients. *Delmar/Cengage Learning.*

Assisting with Intravenous Injections

The intravenous, or IV, method of injection is used by the provider or nurse, usually in an institutional setting or emergency situation. The medical assistant is not qualified or licensed to administer medications by this method. Intravenous medications act immediately because they are introduced directly into the bloodstream. Intravenous preparations vary in amount from a few milliliters, given directly into the vein, to much larger doses, given by continuous infusion through a volume-controlled pump.

The medical assistant may be asked to draw up IV medication for the provider or other licensed provider to administer in an emergency. After filling the syringe, be sure to close the safety cap and replace with a new needle. The person giving the medication is responsible for verifying its accuracy so make sure to keep the package with the prepared medication. Label the syringe or tape the vial or ampule to the syringe. Stay with the patient while waiting for the emergency squad or ambulance to transport the patient to the hospital and observe for signs of distress or reactions to the administered medication. Notify the provider immediately of any complications and record all information on the patient's chart. All medication administered is signed off by the person who gave it.

ADMINISTERING IMMUNIZATIONS

Immunity was discussed in detail in Chapter 31. Recall that after recovery from exposure to certain illnesses, antibodies are generated to protect the body from developing the same disease again through a process known as *natural immunity*. *Artificial immunity* is produced by administering **immunizations** or **vaccines** (terms generally used interchangeably) made from dead or weakened infectious agents that trigger an immune response in the body, which in turn stimulates the production of antibodies against that particular disease-causing agent.

Types of Vaccines

Vaccines are categorized according to the type of immune stimulation that occurs:

- *Live attenuated (changed) pathogens:* The pathogen itself is altered or weakened by the manufacturer and then injected into the body, which stimulates the body to produce antibodies. Examples of this type of vaccine include varicella and measles.
- *Pathogenic toxin:* Some pathogenic organisms produce a poisonous substance (toxin), which stimulates antibody production. Examples of this type of vaccine include diphtheria and tetanus.
- *Killed pathogen:* The pathogenic organism is rendered inactive and then injected into the body, which stimulates antibody production. This type of vaccine can require several doses to ensure lasting immunity.

Examples of this type of vaccine include pertussis (whooping cough), rabies, and poliomyelitis.

When more than one dose of a vaccine is necessary to reach adequate immunization against a particular disease, such as the DTaP injections, it is referred to as a primary **series**. Each of these should be given according to the most up-to-date schedule available from the CDC.

Immunization Schedules

The Centers for Disease Control and Prevention (CDC) publish an annual recommended childhood and adolescent immunization schedule for the United States; this can be found at www.cdc.gov/vaccines, the CDC's Vaccines and Immunizations page. Immunization schedules can vary in other countries for infants, children, and adults. Figure 54–16 shows the 2012 adult schedule, but be sure to consult the CDC Website for the most current schedule. Refer to Chapter 42 for the childhood and adolescent schedule.

Immunizations other than those that appear on the CDC immunization schedules are not recommended on a routine basis in most Western countries but might be needed for foreign travel. Travel to some countries requires immunizations against particular diseases before entry is permitted. To acquire up-to-date immunization information by country, visit the Travelers' Health page of the CDC Website at wwwnc.cdc.gov/travel.

Patient Preparation and Documentation

In years past, diseases that people are now immunized against were potentially fatal illnesses that affected children and adults, often resulting in death. Patients need to protect themselves and their families against these diseases for their own well-being but also to prevent the return of epidemics. Cholera and typhoid, for example, can wipe out entire populations. Be patient and attempt to answer patients' questions about immunizations when they ask why they or their children need the prescribed vaccine.

Every patient or parent of a minor patient must be made aware of the benefits and risks of all vaccines, and a signed copy of the VIS, or vaccine information statement, should be made part of the patient's permanent record. Authorization forms should be in order before immunizations are administered. Sufficient time should be allowed for patients and parents (or those responsible for the child) to read the information regarding the vaccine and have all questions answered before obtaining the authorized signature. This form must be filed in the patient's chart. VIS forms can be found on the CDC's Website at www.cdc.gov/vaccines/pubs/vis/default.htm. Sufficient time should be given to the responsible person to read printed material after a verbal explanation is given regarding the vaccine(s). An opportunity must be provided for any questions of the parent or patient to be answered by the doctor before administration of immunization(s).

Concerns that should be addressed prior to administering any immunization include assessing for active illness or fever as well as verifying the patient's health and medical history for a history of convulsions or allergies, especially to any components of the vaccination intended to be given. The provider should be advised of any patient's concerns prior to administering the vaccine. The Immunization Action Coalition (IAC) publishes many resources for vaccine administration, including a sample Vaccine Screening Form (Figure 54–17), on their Website at www.immunize.org.

Provide the patient with a card or booklet to record each immunization accurately and the month, day, and year for each. Record each administered vaccine on the patient's chart. Any reaction to the vaccine, no matter how slight, must also be recorded on the patient's chart. Remind patients to make appointments and carry the immunization record (or a copy) with them at all times.

Common Illnesses Reduced by Immunizations

Influenza

Commonly referred to as the flu, **influenza** is a disease caused by a myxovirus that affects the respiratory tract.

- It is *spread* by direct contact, by droplet infection through the vapor of coughing and sneezing of an infected person, and by indirect contact while handling soiled items (such as used tissues or linens) of an infected patient.
- The **incubation period** is between one and four days.
- *Symptoms* include sudden onset of fever, chills, sore throat, cough, muscle aches and pains, general malaise, and weakness.
- *Treatment* for the flu consists of bed rest, increased intake of fluids, antipyretics, and mild analgesics. Immunization against some strains of influenza is recommended for high-risk patients such as the elderly and those with chronic illness, respiratory distress, or other conditions that warrant protection from infectious disease.

Pneumonia

Pneumonia is an acute inflammation of the lungs. Eighty-five percent of pneumonia cases are caused by the pneumococcus bacterium. Pneumonia can also be caused by other bacteria, a virus, rickettsiae, and fungi.

- The pneumococcus bacterium disease (pneumonitis) is *spread* by droplet infection and direct contact with an infected person.

Recommended Adult Immunization Schedule

UNITED STATES · 2011

Note: These recommendations must be read with the footnotes that follow containing number of doses, intervals between doses, and other important information.

Recommended adult immunization schedule, by vaccine and age group

<table>
<tr><th>VACCINE ▼ AGE GROUP ▶</th><th>19–26 years</th><th>27–49 years</th><th>50–59 years</th><th>60–64 years</th><th>≥65 years</th></tr>
<tr><td>Influenza[1,*]</td><td colspan="5">1 dose annually</td></tr>
<tr><td>Tetanus, diphtheria, pertussis (Td/Tdap)[2,*]</td><td colspan="4">Substitute 1-time dose of Tdap for Td booster; then boost with Td every 10 yrs</td><td>Td booster every 10 yrs</td></tr>
<tr><td>Varicella[3,*]</td><td colspan="5">2 doses</td></tr>
<tr><td>Human papillomavirus (HPV)[4,*]</td><td>3 doses (females)</td><td></td><td></td><td></td><td></td></tr>
<tr><td>Zoster[5]</td><td></td><td></td><td></td><td colspan="2">1 dose</td></tr>
<tr><td>Measles, mumps, rubella (MMR)[6,*]</td><td colspan="2">1 or 2 doses</td><td colspan="3">1 dose</td></tr>
<tr><td>Pneumococcal (polysaccharide)[7,8]</td><td colspan="4">1 or 2 doses</td><td>1 dose</td></tr>
<tr><td>Meningococcal[9,*]</td><td colspan="5">1 or more doses</td></tr>
<tr><td>Hepatitis A[10,*]</td><td colspan="5">2 doses</td></tr>
<tr><td>Hepatitis B[11,*]</td><td colspan="5">3 doses</td></tr>
</table>

*Covered by the Vaccine Injury Compensation Program.

For all persons in this category who meet the age requirements and who lack evidence of immunity (e.g., lack documentation of vaccination or have no evidence of previous infection)

Recommended if some other risk factor is present (e.g., based on medical, occupational, lifestyle, or other indications)

No recommendation

Report all clinically significant postvaccination reactions to the Vaccine Adverse Event Reporting System (VAERS). Reporting forms and instructions on filing a VAERS report are available at http://www.vaers.hhs.gov or by telephone, 800-822-7967.

Information on how to file a Vaccine Injury Compensation Program claim is available at http://www.hrsa.gov/vaccinecompensation or by telephone, 800-338-2382. Information about filing a claim for vaccine injury is available through the U.S. Court of Federal Claims, 717 Madison Place, N.W., Washington, D.C. 20005; telephone, 202-357-6400.

Additional information about the vaccines in this schedule, extent of available data, and contraindications for vaccination also is available at http://www.cdc.gov/vaccines or from the CDC-INFO Contact Center at 800-CDC-INFO (800-232-4636) in English and Spanish, 24 hours a day, 7 days a week.

Use of trade names and commercial sources is for identification only and does not imply endorsement by the U.S. Department of Health and Human Services.

The recommendations in this schedule were approved by:

Centers for Disease Control and Prevention's (CDC) Advisory Committee on Immunization Practices (ACIP)

American Academy of Family Physicians (AAFP)

American College of Obstetricians and Gynecologists (ACOG)

American College of Physicians (ACP).

Vaccines that might be indicated for adults based on medical and other indications

<table>
<tr><th rowspan="2">INDICATION ▶
VACCINE ▼</th><th rowspan="2">Pregnancy</th><th rowspan="2">Immuno-compromising conditions (excluding human immunodeficiency virus [HIV])3,5,6,13</th><th colspan="2">HIV infection3,6,12,13
CD4⁺ T lymphocyte count</th><th rowspan="2">Diabetes, heart disease, chronic lung disease, chronic alcoholism</th><th rowspan="2">Asplenia12 (including elective splenectomy) and persistent complement component deficiencies</th><th rowspan="2">Chronic liver disease</th><th rowspan="2">Kidney failure, end-stage renal disease, receipt of hemodialysis</th><th rowspan="2">Healthcare personnel</th></tr>
<tr><th><200 cells/μL</th><th>>200 cells/μL</th></tr>
<tr><td>Influenza[1,*]</td><td colspan="8">1 dose TIV annually</td><td>1 dose TIV or LAIV annually</td></tr>
<tr><td>Tetanus, diphtheria, pertussis (Td/Tdap)[2,*]</td><td>Td</td><td colspan="8">Substitute 1-time dose of Tdap for Td booster; then boost with Td every 10 yrs</td></tr>
<tr><td>Varicella[3,*]</td><td colspan="3">Contraindicated</td><td colspan="6">2 doses</td></tr>
<tr><td>Human papillomavirus (HPV)[4,*]</td><td></td><td colspan="7">3 doses through age 26 yrs</td><td></td></tr>
<tr><td>Zoster[5]</td><td colspan="3">Contraindicated</td><td></td><td colspan="5">1 dose</td></tr>
<tr><td>Measles, mumps, rubella (MMR)[6,*]</td><td colspan="3">Contraindicated</td><td colspan="6">1 or 2 doses</td></tr>
<tr><td>Pneumococcal (polysaccharide)[7,8]</td><td></td><td colspan="7">1 or 2 doses</td><td></td></tr>
<tr><td>Meningococcal[9,*]</td><td colspan="5">1 or more doses</td><td></td><td colspan="3"></td></tr>
<tr><td>Hepatitis A[10,*]</td><td colspan="6">2 doses</td><td></td><td colspan="2"></td></tr>
<tr><td>Hepatitis B[11,*]</td><td colspan="2"></td><td colspan="2"></td><td colspan="2">3 doses</td><td colspan="3"></td></tr>
</table>

*Covered by the Vaccine Injury Compensation Program.

For all persons in this category who meet the age requirements and who lack evidence of immunity (e.g., lack documentation of vaccination or have no evidence of previous infection)

Recommended if some other risk factor is present (e.g., based on medical, occupational, lifestyle, or other indications)

No recommendation

These schedules indicate the recommended age groups and medical indications for which administration of currently licensed vaccines is commonly indicated for adults ages 19 years and older, as of January 1, 2011. For all vaccines being recommended on the adult immunization schedule, a vaccine series does not need to be restarted, regardless of the time that has elapsed between doses. Licensed combination vaccines may be used

contraindicated. For detailed recommendations on all vaccines, including those used primarily for travelers or that are issued during the year, consult the manufacturers' package inserts and the complete statements from the Advisory Committee on Immunization Practices ((http:// www.cdc.gov/vaccines/pubs/acip-list.htm).

U.S. DEPARTMENT OF HEALTH AND HUMAN SERVICES
CENTERS FOR DISEASE CONTROL AND PREVENTION

Figure 54–16: Recommended adult immunization schedule—United States, 2012. *National Immunization Program, Centers for Disease Control and Prevention.*

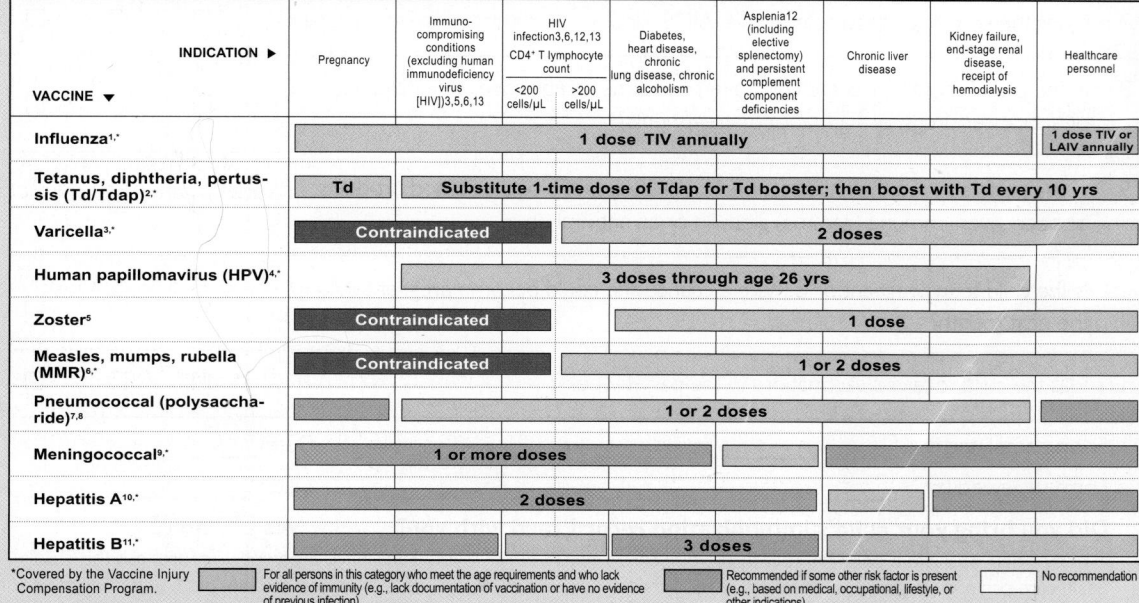

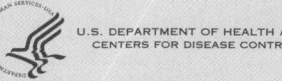

Patient name: ______________________ Date of birth: ____/____/____
(mo.) (day) (yr.)

Screening Questionnaire for Child and Teen Immunization

For parents/guardians: The following questions will help us determine which vaccines your child may be given today. If you answer "yes" to any question, it does not necessarily mean your child should not be vaccinated. It just means additional questions must be asked. If a question is not clear, please ask your health care provider to explain it.

	Yes	No	Don't Know
1. Is the child sick today?	☐	☐	☐
2. Does the child have allergies to latex, medications, food, or any vaccine?	☐	☐	☐
3. Has the child had a serious reaction to a vaccine in the past?	☐	☐	☐
4. Has the child had a health problem with lung, heart, kidney or metabolic disease (e.g., diabetes), asthma, or a blood disorder? Is he/she on long-term aspirin therapy?	☐	☐	☐
5. If the child to be vaccinated is between the ages of 2 and 4 years, has a health care provider told you that the child had wheezing or asthma in the past 12 months?	☐	☐	☐
6. Has the child, a sibling, or a parent had a seizure? Has the child had brain or other nervous system problems?	☐	☐	☐
7. Does the child have cancer, leukemia, AIDS, or any other immune system problem?	☐	☐	☐
8. In the past 3 months, has the child taken cortisone, prednisone, other steroids, or anticancer drugs, or had radiation treatments?	☐	☐	☐
9. In the past year, has the child received a transfusion of blood or blood products, or been given immune (gamma) globulin or an antiviral drug?	☐	☐	☐
10. Is the child/teen pregnant or is there a chance she could become pregnant during the next month?	☐	☐	☐
11. Has the child received vaccinations in the past 4 weeks?	☐	☐	☐

Form completed by: ______________________ Date: __________

Form reviewed by: ______________________ Date: __________

Did you bring your child's immunization record card with you? **yes** ☐ **no** ☐

It is important to have a personal record of your child's vaccinations. If you don't have a personal record, ask the child's healthcare provider to give you one with all your child's vaccinations on it. Keep this record in a safe place and bring it with you every time you seek medical care for your child. Your child will need this important document for the rest of his or her life to enter day care or school, for employment, or for international travel.

Technical content reviewed by the Centers for Disease Control and Prevention, June 2010 www.immunize.org/catg.d/p4060.pdf • Item #P4060 (6/10)

Immunization Action Coalition • 1573 Selby Ave. • St. Paul, MN 55104 • (651) 647-9009 • www.immunize.org • www.vaccineinformation.org

Figure 54–17: Child and Teen Immunization screening questionnaire. *Acquired from www.immunize.org on 8/4/2010; We thank the Immunization Action Coalition.*

- The *incubation* period is only a few hours after exposure to the bacteria.
- The *symptoms* are abrupt in onset and include severe chills, high fever, headache, chest pain, dyspnea, rapid pulse, cyanosis, and cough with blood-stained sputum.
- *Treatment* includes bed rest; increased fluid intake; analgesics; antipyretics; and, in many cases, oxygen for successful treatment of the patient. Pneumovax is a vaccine to protect high-risk patients from contracting the disease generally. Only one immunization is required for life protection, although boosters may be considered after 10 years. Patients age 65 and older are encouraged to get this vaccine.

Haemophilus Influenza Type B

Haemophilus (or Hemophilus), also known as Hib and HIB, is a disease caused by a small, gram-negative, nonmotile parasitic bacterium that leads to severe destructive inflammation of the larynx, trachea, and bronchi.

- The disease is *spread* by droplet airborne infection. Incubation is from one to three days.
- The *symptoms* are sudden onset of fever, sore throat, cough, muscle aches, weakness, and general malaise.
- *Treatment* includes bed rest, increased fluid intake, antipyretics, antibiotics, and analgesics as necessary. Because this particular disease affects infants and small children, immunization is recommended for these age groups. Every year, HIB attacks 1 in every 200 infants in the United States; the most at-risk age group is between 6 months and 5 years. With the rise in popularity of day care centers, immunization against the HIB bacterium is the most sensible way to prevent this often antibiotic-resistant disease from spreading through the very young population in the United States.
- *Complications* of this childhood disease include **meningitis**, which could result in damage to the nervous system or in mental retardation; **epiglottitis**, which could cause a child to choke to death if immediate treatment is not given; joint infections; and forms of crippling arthritis. The HIB vaccine is administered in a series of three subcutaneous or intramuscular injections at 2, 4, and 6 months. A booster is given at 18 months.

Measles, Mumps, and Rubella (MMR)

The MMR vaccine protects children from all three childhood diseases.

Measles, medically termed **rubeola**, is also referred to as "old-fashioned" and "10-day measles."

- It is *spread* by direct contact, droplet infection, and indirect contact from infected items of a patient. It has a 10- to 21-day *incubation* period.
- In the prodromal (earliest) stage, *symptoms* include fever, malaise, runny nose, cough, and sometimes conjunctivitis; it progresses with loss of appetite, **photosensitivity**, sore throat, and, eventually, Koplik's spots (the red skin rash). The cause is the rubeola virus, which is an acute and highly contagious viral disease involving the respiratory tract.
- *Complications* of measles can result in deafness, brain damage, and pneumonia. Treatment for measles is bed rest, increased fluid intake, antipyretics, antibiotics, cough medicine, and calamine lotion.

PATIENT EDUCATION

The patient should be kept in isolation to prevent transmission to others. Quiet activity is suggested for the patient during recovery time, usually a few days.

Mumps is an acute, contagious febrile disease that causes inflammation of the parotid and salivary glands. Parotitis is transmitted by droplet infection or direct contact with an infected person.

- The usual *incubation* period is from 14 to 28 days.
- *Symptoms* include chills and fever, headache, and pain below and in front of the ear(s) for five to seven days' duration. Another symptom is pain between the ear and the angle of the jaw with drinking or eating acidic substances.
- *Treatment* includes bed rest, and a soft diet, including increased fluid intake, is recommended.

Rubella, also called German measles or three-day measles, is an acute, contagious viral disease characterized by an upper respiratory infection.

- Rubella is *transmitted* by droplet infection and by direct contact.
- The *incubation* period is from 12 to 23 days.
- *Symptoms* include slight fever; sore throat; drowsiness; malaise; swollen glands and lymph nodes; arthralgia; and a diffuse, fine, red rash.
- *Treatment* is bed rest, liquids, antipyretics, and sponge baths.
- *Complications* of rubella can result in blindness, deafness, brain damage, heart defects, enlarged liver, and bone malformation.

PATIENT EDUCATION

Fetal abnormalities can result if the mother acquires rubella during her first trimester of pregnancy. Female patients of childbearing age should be advised of this concern. It would be advisable to test a woman planning to become pregnant for a rubella antibody titer so she can be vaccinated before becoming pregnant if indicated. ***Females should not be vaccinated during pregnancy.*** Be sure to determine pregnancy status before administering the vaccine.

Diphtheria

This acute infectious disease is caused by *Corynebacterium diphtheriae*, which is a gram-positive, nonmotile, non-spore-forming, club-shaped bacillus. **Diphtheria** diagnosis is confirmed by throat culture.

- *Transmission* is by direct and indirect contact.
- The *incubation* period is between two and five days.
- *Symptoms* include headache, malaise, fever, and sore throat with a yellowish white or gray membrane.
- *Treatment* consists of adequate liquids and a soft diet; antibiotics; bed rest; and, in cases of severe respiratory compromise, a tracheostomy for extended ventilatory support.

Pertussis

Whooping cough, or **pertussis**, is an acute, infectious disease characterized by respiratory drainage; then a peculiar paroxysmal cough; and, finally, a whooping inspiration (sounds like a shrill trumpeting cry; the name comes from the whooping crane that makes this sound). This disease is most common in children younger than 4 years, although it can affect children of all ages if they have not received immunizations. Pertussis is caused by the small, nonmotile, gram-negative bacillus, *Bordetella pertussis*.

- It is *transmitted* by direct and indirect contact.
- The *incubation* period is from 7 to 14 days.
- *Symptoms* of whooping cough in the **catarrhal stage** (period when it is highly communicable) include an increase in leukocyte count marked by lymphocytosis, respiratory drainage, sneezing, slight fever, dry cough, irritability, and loss of appetite; in the **paroxysmal stage** (when symptoms tend to be at their worst), symptoms include a violent cough with whooping inspiration sounds and forceful vomiting that can evoke hemorrhaging from various portions of the body as a result of straining; and, in the **decline stage**, symptoms a decrease in coughing and return of appetite. A trace cough can last from several months to two years.

Rabies

Rabies is a viral disease found in unvaccinated animals such as dogs, cats, bats, foxes, raccoons, and skunks in the wild.

- Rabies is *spread* through the saliva of infected animals (unvaccinated animals such as dogs, cats, bats, foxes, raccoons, and skunks in the wild) and through airborne transmission, which is possible in heavily infested bat caves.
- Human *symptoms* of the disease can include fever, pain, aggressive behavior, hallucinations, extreme weakness, and thirst.
- *Treatment* involves a series of five injections of a vaccine that is very effective in combating the disease and has been shown to have few if any side effects. The disease is fatal when treatment is delayed until after symptoms appear.

> **PATIENT EDUCATION**
>
> The rabies vaccine for animals is still the best means of prevention. Pets should always be vaccinated and not allowed to roam unsupervised; both are legal requirements for pet owners in most of the United States. Children should not be allowed to approach wild animals for any reason. Patients planning to travel to rural areas of foreign countries might wish to consult with their provider regarding immunization injections against rabies in addition to the established list of required immunizations.

Tetanus

This acute, potentially fatal, infectious disease affects the central nervous system and has commonly been referred to as lockjaw. It is caused by the *Clostridium tetani* bacillus, the toxin of which is one of the most lethal poisons known. The bacillus is found in superficial layers of the soil. It is a normal inhabitant of the intestinal tracts of horses and cows. Tetanus affects only wounds that contain dead tissue, transmitted commonly in puncture wounds, abrasions, lacerations, and burns.

- Immediate cleansing and debridement of the wound are required in *initial treatment*.
- There is a short incubation period of 3 to 21 days and a longer period of four to five weeks. The *symptoms* of tetanus are stiffness of the jaw, esophageal muscles, and sometimes neck muscles. Progressing rigidity follows soon with fixed jaw (thus lockjaw), altered voice, fever, painful spasms of all skeletal muscles, irritability, and headache. Airway maintenance and antitoxin administration are primary concerns.
- *Treatments* can also involve sedation, pharmacologic control of muscle spasms, maintenance of fluid balance, possible tracheostomy, and penicillin G and oxygen administration. A quiet environment is necessary to prevent triggering muscle spasms.

Rotavirus

Rotavirus affects 500,000 children under the age of 3 years in the United States each year. Nausea and vomiting require hospitalization for dehydration in approximately 50,000 patients, and approximately 20 children die annually.

- *Transmission* is through contact with an infected person.
- *Treatment* is mostly supportive and should be provided at once, focusing on maintaining adequate hydration. Infants and children with rotavirus are especially susceptible to dehydration, which can be life-threatening.
- Often, children have no *symptoms* for a couple of days before they begin the diarrhea, and, for several days after the diarrhea stops, the child seems to be better. Even during these times when the child or infant does not seem to be sick, the virus can be passed on to other children. Child day care center workers should strive to prevent this virus by frequent hand washing of the children and of themselves. The rotavirus vaccine can be given to infants along with other immunizations at 2, 4, and 6 months of age, although it has not yet been added to the recommended childhood immunization schedule. If an infant has not had the vaccine by the age of 7 months, it is likely unnecessary.

Varicella Zoster

Better known as "chickenpox," **varicella zoster** is a highly contagious virus that primarily affects young children. A member of the herpes virus family, it is often called herpes zoster.

- It is *transmitted* by direct contact and droplets from the respiratory tract in the *prodromal* or early stages of the rash. The rash develops into vesicular fluid eruptions that are infectious until dry scabs form. Incubation is between two and three weeks.
- *Symptoms* include highly pruritic rash, fever, headache, loss of appetite, and general malaise, which last from a few days to two weeks.
- *Treatment* can include bed rest, liquids, antipyretics, and oral or topical antihistamines or a paste made of baking soda for control of itching. The Varivax vaccine is given by injection to children between 12 and 18 months old, with an additional dose given between 11 and 12 years. The most common complication of chickenpox is secondary infections.

Hepatitis A

Hepatitis A is a liver disease that results from infection with the Hepatitis A virus. It can range in severity from a mild illness lasting a few weeks to a severe illness lasting several months. The hepatitis A virus causes inflammation that affects your liver's ability to function. Mild cases of hepatitis may not require treatment, and most people who are infected recover completely with no permanent liver damage. Practicing good hygiene by washing your hands often is one way to protect against hepatitis A, although the best way to prevent Hepatitis A is by getting vaccinated.

- Transmission occurs usually when a person ingests fecal matter (even in microscopic amounts), from contaminated food or water (when someone with the virus handles the food you eat without first carefully washing his or her hands after using the toilet), or from close contact with someone who's already infected (even if that person has no signs or symptoms). It has also been known to be transmitted from eating raw shellfish from water polluted with sewage or by having sex with someone who has the virus.
- The symptoms normally don't appear until you've had the virus for a few weeks. They include: fatigue, nausea and vomiting, abdominal pain or discomfort, especially in the area of your liver on your right side beneath your lower ribs, loss of appetite, low-grade fever, dark urine, muscle pain, yellowing of the skin and eyes (jaundice). Symptoms usually last less than two months, but can last as long as six months. Not everyone with hepatitis A develops signs or symptoms.
- The hepatitis A vaccine can prevent infection with the virus. The hepatitis A vaccine is typically given in two doses—initial vaccination followed by a booster shot six months later.

Hepatitis B

Hepatitis B is a highly contagious liver disease that results from infection with the Hepatitis B virus (HBV). It can range in severity from a mild illness lasting a few weeks to a serious, lifelong illness.

- Hepatitis B is usually spread when blood, semen, or another body fluid from a person infected with the Hepatitis B virus enters the body of someone who is not infected. This can happen through sexual contact with an infected person or sharing needles, syringes, or other drug-injection equipment. Hepatitis B can also be passed from an infected mother to her baby at birth. It has an incubation period of 60 to 150 days. The symptoms are slow at onset with fever, malaise, loss of appetite, nausea, and vomiting, progressing to include jaundice, weakness, dark urine, and light-colored stool.
- Recommended treatment includes bed rest and fluids with elimination of alcohol and fats from the patient's diet. The hepatitis B vaccine is urged for all who might be at risk, especially all health care workers. It is thought to be in widespread proportions everywhere, and immunization is strongly urged to protect the country's population and to prevent a massive epidemic. The hepatitis B virus vaccine, is given to neonates, whose mothers have not had the disease, before leaving the hospital. The second dose is given between 1 and 2 months of age, and the third dose between 6 and 18 months. A booster dose is recommended for children between 11 and 12 years.

Human Papillomavirus

Human papillomavirus, or HPV, is the most common sexually transmitted infection. There are more than 40 HPV types that affect both males and females, not just in the genital areas but also in the mouth and throat. HPV, which currently affects 20 million Americans, can be present but silent for many years and passed unknowingly to sexual partners. HPV causes genital warts and cervical, vaginal, penile, and anal cancers. Some head and neck cancers are also associated with HPV. Cervarix and Gardasil are two available vaccines. Vaccination is recommended for women under 26 years of age and is encouraged as a series of three shots to be given to girls at age 11 to 12. Boys may also receive the vaccination.

Meningitis (Bacterial)

In the 1990s, there was an increase in the number of cases of bacterial meningitis among young adults between the ages of 15 and 24 years. Bacterial meningitis is a highly contagious disease that can cause serious and long-lasting effects on the nervous system and can be fatal within 24 to 48 hours after contracting the disease. A vaccine is available. Persons who have an altered immune system or a serious health condition, and pregnant women, should not receive this vaccine. Viral meningitis is not as serious as bacterial meningitis, and there is currently no vaccine.

Polio

Polio is caused by poliovirus, which affects only humans. The virus begins to multiply in the back of the throat of the infected person. Incubation can be from 4 to 35 days.

- *Transmission* most often occurs through contact with feces of an infected person.
- *Symptoms* are categorized by three groups: minor or abortive, aseptic meningitis, and paralytic poliomyelitis. Minor symptoms occur in 4 percent to 8 percent of people affected and include fever, sore throat, nausea or vomiting, abdominal pain, constipation, and flu-like symptoms. These can progress to symptoms of meningitis (high fever, stiff neck, and headache), muscle aches, loss of reflexes, or other minor illness symptoms. Paralysis affecting limbs or urinary control is usually permanent if lasting more than six months.
- The current injectable polio vaccine is called IPV (inactivated polio vaccine) and is more potent than the previous oral polio vaccine. It may be given by intramuscular or subcutaneous injection. It is recommended for children to receive IPV at 2 and 4 months with additional doses given from 12 to 18 months of age. If four doses are given prior to age 4 years, a fifth dose should be given after the child's fourth birthday and at least six months after the previous injection. IPV is recommended for those who have a low resistance to serious infections, for those in close daily contact with them, or for adults who have never been vaccinated.

CHAPTER SUMMARY

- Some parenteral routes of medication administration involve injecting medications through the skin or directly into a vein or artery.
- Instances when parenteral routes are desirable include when the patient is unable to tolerate medications by mouth, when other routes of administration do not provide the desired effect quickly or predictably enough, when medication given by mouth would be destroyed by the gastrointestinal tract, or when continuous delivery is required to achieve the desired outcome.
- Select the appropriate needle and syringe size for the type of medication to be administered. Tuberculin and insulin syringes are NEVER interchangeable.
- Not all medications may be injected by different routes. Always verify that the medication ordered is appropriate for the type of injection ordered. Follow the Seven Rights of medication administration at all times.
- Good sterile and aseptic technique should be used when delivering any injectable medication.
- Use additional care and caution when giving injections to children. Due to smaller size and mass, inadvertent entry of medication into a blood vessel will have magnified effects.
- Vaccines are categorized into three types: live attenuated (changed) pathogens, pathogenic toxins, and killed pathogens.
- Immunization schedules are updated periodically and should be continually reviewed for the latest recommendations. Always maintain up-to-date immunization records in the patient's chart.
- Immunizations require additional documentation beyond what is necessary for other medications.
- The MA should understand the different immunizations and effects of the diseases observed in unimmunized patients to be better prepared to educate the patient.

STUDY TOOLS

Workbook	Activities for Chapter 54
Premium Website	
MEDIA LINK	View these **Media Links** for Chapter 54: • Subcutaneous Injection Animation • Intramuscular Injection Animation • Z-Track Injection Animation
StudyWARE	Activities and Quizzes on the **StudyWARE™ Software** for Chapter 54
	Complete the following **Competency Challenge 2.0** activity: • Wednesday, 4 PM: Administer Medications
	Audio Library of medical terms
	Online access to the **Critical Thinking Challenge 2.0**
learninglab	Module 22: Medication Administration Procedures
CourseMate	Activities and Quizzes for Chapter 54
WebTutor	Activities and Quizzes for Chapter 54

CHECK YOUR KNOWLEDGE

1. What is an *anaphylactic* reaction?
   a. The patient faints as a result of the medication administration.
   b. The patient has an allergic reaction as a result of the medication administration.
   c. The patient has a needlestick injury.
   d. The patient develops a wheal.
2. When is the intradermal route of injection used?
   a. To administer medication directly into a vein.
   b. To give immunizations.
   c. To administer small doses of medication.
   d. For allergy testing.
3. All the following are reasons parenteral routes are indicated instead of oral routes except for which?
   a. The patient is unable to tolerate medications by mouth.
   b. The medication would be destroyed by the GI tract.
   c. There is less risk involved with parenteral routes than with oral routes.
   d. The medication needs to be effective more quickly.
4. Which document should always be signed before an immunization is given?
   a. VIS
   b. HIB
   c. MMR
   d. CDC
5. Which of these sites is not used for intramuscular injections?
   a. Anterior forearm
   b. Gluteus medius
   c. Deltoid
   d. Vastus lateralis
6. In the ____________ category of vaccine, the pathogenic organism is rendered inactive and then injected into the body, which stimulates antibody production.
   a. pathogenic toxin
   b. live attenuated pathogen
   c. killed pathogen
   d. passive toxin
7. What do the initials MMR represent?
   a. Mumps, meningitis, rotavirus
   b. Measles, meningitis, rabies
   c. Measles, mumps, rubeola
   d. Measles, mumps, rubella

WEB LINKS

CDC: www.cdc.gov/vaccine

Immunization Action Coalition: www.immunize.org

Unit

18

First Aid and Responding to Emergencies

Individuals working in health care can expect to be confronted with emergency or accident situations. Patients might be brought into the provider's office, you might be witness to an incident in your community or neighborhood, and, almost certainly, you will be responding to phone calls concerning injuries or sudden illness. It is important for you to acquire first aid skills and have a working knowledge of appropriate actions to take in common accident, emergency, or illness situations. It also is your responsibility to maintain current certification to provide the basic life support measures involving obstructed airway, resuscitation, or CPR.

This unit deals with emergency and first aid care in cases of acute illness, accident, or injury, both within the provider's office and outside the health care setting. This information will be valuable not only in your professional life but also in your personal life. When anything happens within your family or immediate neighborhood, your relatives and neighbors might look to you for assistance due to your medical background as a medical assistant.

Certification Connection

	Ch. 55	Ch. 56
CMA (AAMA)		
Telephone techniques: Emergency calls	X	
Principles of infection control	X	X
Emergencies	X	X
First Aid	X	X
RMA (AMT)		
Perform appropriate telephone techniques	X	X
Develop emergency procedures and policies	X	X
Blood-borne pathogens and universal precautions	X	X
Medical asepsis	X	X
First aid and emergency response	X	X
CMAS (AMT)		
Asepsis in the medical office	X	X
Medical office emergencies	X	X

Chapter

55 Emergencies in the Medical Office

OBJECTIVES

In this chapter, you will learn the following:

KB KNOWLEDGE BASE

1. Spell and define, using the glossary at the back of the text, all the Words to Know in this chapter.
2. Define a medical emergency.
3. List items that might be found in a crash cart or emergency kit.
4. Explain the purpose of the universal emergency medical identification symbol.
5. State principles and steps of professional and provider CPR.
6. Discuss the importance of safety when administering CPR.
7. Explain the purpose of an AED and its capabilities.
8. Identify seven descriptive terms that describe the severity or onset of a disease or disorder.
9. List examples of emergency situations.
10. Compare and contrast symptoms of hyperglycemia and hypoglycemia.
11. Identify symptoms of a heart attack.
12. Differentiate the symptoms of heat stroke and heat exhaustion.
13. Name symptoms that might indicate damaged tissue due to cold exposure.
14. Identify the distinguishing characteristics of capillary, vein, and arterial bleeding.
15. List symptoms of internal bleeding.
16. List, in order of occurrence, the chain of events that might happen with a seizure.
17. Discuss instances when obstructed airway can occur.
18. List symptoms of shock.
19. Identify signs of possible stroke.

S SKILLS

1. Perform an abdominal thrust on an adult victim with an obstructed airway.

WORDS TO KNOW

acute
airway
ammonia
aspiration
cardiopulmonary resuscitation (CPR)
coma
cessation
chronic
compressions
consciousness
coroner
diabetic ketoacidosis
diaphoresis
emergency
emergency medical services (EMS)
exhaustion
flushed
frostbite
heat cramps
heat exhaustion
heatstroke
hyperglycemia
hypoglycemia
hypothermia
ingested
insulin shock

intubation
life-threatening
medical emergency
myocardial infarction
obstructed
poison
post mortem
prophylactic
seizure
severe
subtle
sudden
syncope
trauma
universal emergency medical identification
urgent

HANDLING EMERGENCIES IN THE MEDICAL OFFICE

A provider's office must always be ready to react to an **emergency** situation. A **medical emergency** is any situation in which an individual suddenly becomes ill or injured or in circumstances calling for decided action. This can involve a patient already in the office or one brought in already experiencing problems, for example:

- A patient receives a medication or injection and has a severe reaction.
- Someone is injured just outside the office and comes in for immediate treatment.
- A patient brings in a very ill or injured family member.

Knowing how to respond and how to assist the provider in treating the individual is very important. Swift and appropriate action can affect the outcome of the situation. As a medical assistant, it is important to remember that you are not to perform at the level of **trauma** or trained medical emergency personnel, only to provide a standard of care equal to that of any person with like training and experience and within your scope of practice.

Office Policy Manual and Documentation

Every office must identify who is responsible for recording the detailed information of an emergency situation and its handling. The office policy manual should have guidelines to follow when dealing with emergencies. An emergency plan with assigned responsibilities should be developed and made known to each employee (such as who should call 911). All staff members should be capable of administering first aid and **cardiopulmonary resuscitation (CPR)** and hold current certification in CPR. The goal for emergency care in an office is to stabilize patients to release them to their family or send them to a hospital for further treatment.

Emergencies, sudden illness, and accidents can also occur among personnel while they are working in the medical office. It is equally important to document the circumstances surrounding this type of incident. Persons experiencing at-work injuries might be eligible for benefits under workers' compensation if the injury occurred while performing job responsibilities. Employee forms can be placed in the employee's personal file and in the office personnel file. (Refer to Chapter 36 for complete instructions on filling out an OSHA 301 incident report form.)

Emergency Supplies and Equipment

As part of the preparation for emergency care, medical offices should have the necessary supplies and equipment to handle medical emergencies that might arise. These items should be collected and set aside in a special place where they are always ready for use. This could be in the form of a small suitcase or a cart referred to as an emergency kit (Figure 55–1 A) or crash cart. Figure 55–1 B shows a crash cart in the form of a mobile cart with drawers for equipment as well as a shelf on top

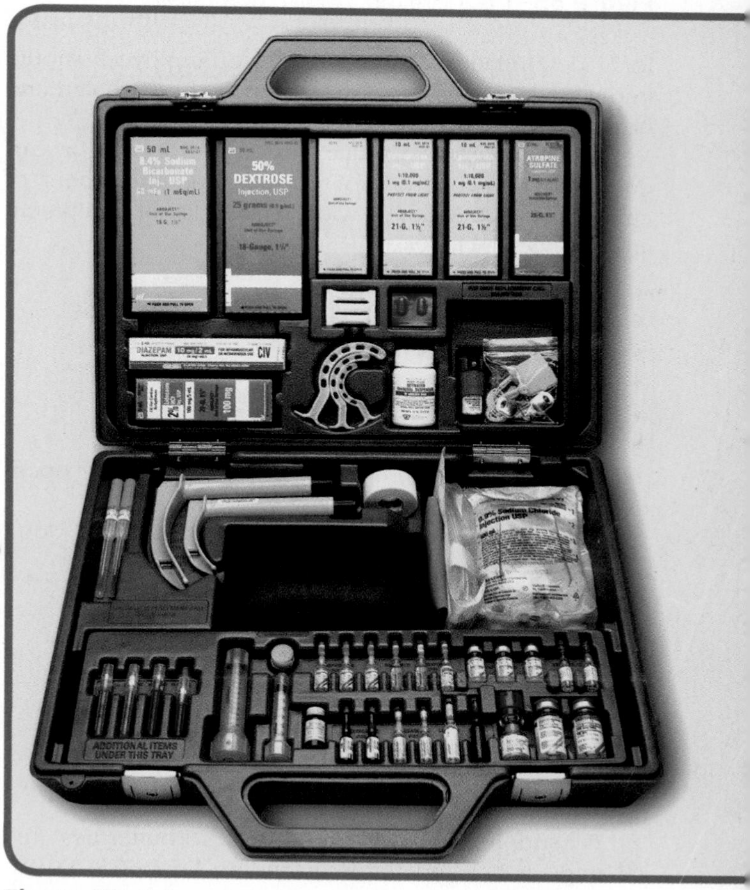

Figure 55–1 A: Medical emergency equipment (prepared kit). *Courtesy of Banyan International Corporation.*

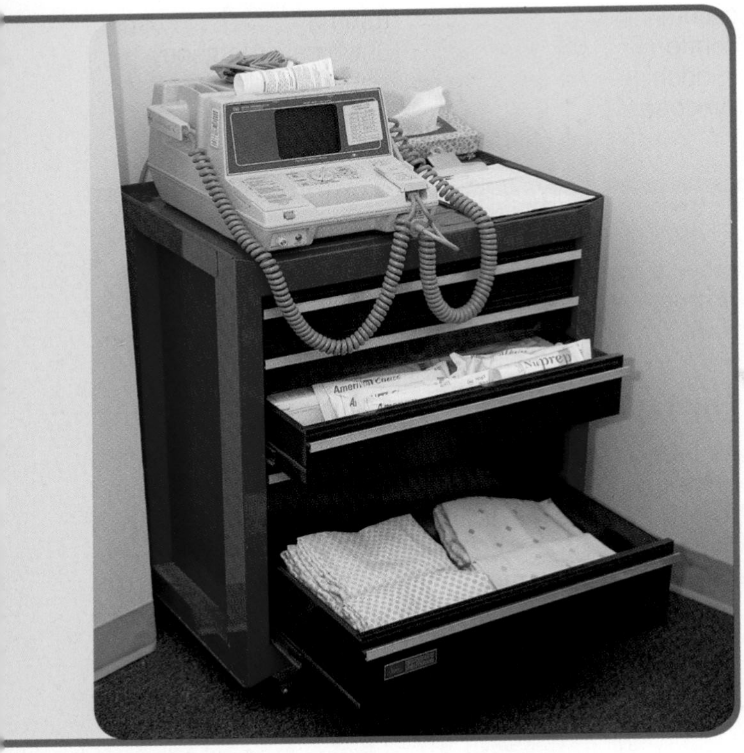

Figure 55–1 B: Crash cart. *Delmar/Cengage Learning.*

for a defibrillation device. All office employees should know the location of the emergency kit or crash cart and how to use the materials.

Although each practice customizes its kit or cart depending on the type of practice and the extent of emergency care it can provide, a basic list of equipment and supplies includes:

- Gloves
- Alcohol wipes
- Stethoscope
- Blood pressure cuff
- Penlight
- Aromatic spirits of **ammonia**
- Oxygen tank with flow meter and wrench for opening the tank
- Tubing, nasal cannula, and pediatric and adult masks
- Ambu bag
- Resuscitation masks in a variety of sizes
- Airways of differing sizes (nasal and oral)
- Bandage material (sterile dressings)
- Adhesive tape
- Bandage scissors
- Disposable syringes
- Tourniquets
- IV supplies: tubing and needles (butterflies and angiocaths) and fluids, including D5W, NS, D10W, and lactated Ringer's
- Medications for emergency use

TABLE 55–1 Medications Commonly Stocked on Crash Cart

Emergency Medications	
• Activated charcoal	• Lidocaine
• Atropine	• Local anesthetics
• Diphenhydramine	• Nitroglycerine
• Epinephrine	• Phenobarbital and diazepam
• Furosemide	• Sodium bicarbonate
• Instant glucose	• Solu-Cortef™
• Insulin	• Verapamil

Table 55–1 includes some of the common medications that can be stocked on the cart.

The kit or cart should be checked regularly to be certain that all items are present and no dated material is past its expiration date. A chart attached to the cart should provide an inventory of the materials and check-off date for inspection to ensure that nothing is overlooked.

In addition, offices should be equipped with a defibrillation unit for responding to cardiac emergencies. A common type of defibrillator is the automated external defibrillator (AED), which is used in addition to CPR if the heart is in fibrillation or arrest. (These arrhythmias were explained in more detail in Chapter 47.) An AED, as well as the oxygen tank and Ambu bag (a mask with an attached inflation bag to assist breathing), should be readily accessible if needed. AED and CPR procedures are discussed later in this chapter.

RECOGNIZING AN EMERGENCY

When severe injury or sudden critical illness occurs, a patient should have the advantages of trauma and critical care facilities as soon as possible. Often, the first hour is so important that it directly correlates with prognosis and the possibility of recovery. Being able to recognize that a situation is an emergency is the first step to providing assistance and medical attention.

Several emergency situations demand immediate medical intervention because of their severity and life-threatening consequences. Lack of breathing or heart action is fatal within a matter of minutes. The following are examples of life-threatening conditions:

- Cardiac arrest
- Respiratory arrest or great difficulty breathing
- Uncontrolled severe bleeding
- Head injury
- Poisoning
- Open chest or abdominal wound

- Shock
- Significant burns

Often the victim's actions will alert you that something is happening. The victim might yell or call out for help, moan from discomfort, be unresponsive, or present abnormal behavior. When you are an eyewitness, you can visually assess the situation and arrive at a decision.

Responding to an Emergency

In any emergency, as a medical assistant, you will be expected to assess the situation and deliver appropriate care as directed. When emergencies occur in the office, as discussed earlier, you might follow an emergency plan developed by the office. The training you receive in procedures such as CPR, AED, obstructed airway, bandaging and splinting, stopping a bleed, and immobilizations can be the treatment you render. The first step in an emergency is to survey the scene to determine whether it is safe for you to encounter without causing harm to yourself. You will also determine the severity of the emergency and determine who needs to be treated first if more than one person is involved. This is determined by assessing the airway, breathing, and circulation of those involved, also known as conducting a primary survey. Those with the more severe injuries or ailments should be treated first.

If you should encounter an emergency situation or if you happen to come upon an unknown person who has become ill or lost **consciousness**, check for a **universal emergency medical identification** symbol (Figure 55–2). This symbol was designed by the American Medical Association (AMA) as a means for individuals with certain medical conditions to alert health care workers of their conditions when they are unable to. The tag is worn around the neck, wrist, or ankle. Some might identify the particular problem the person has; others might not. If a tag is found, the person should have an information card on his or her person, usually inside a wallet, that identifies the condition and provides some directions to follow. All patients who have conditions that could cause emergency episodes, such as heart conditions, diabetes, epilepsy, allergies, or a laryngectomy, should be encouraged to wear a universal emergency medical identification tag.

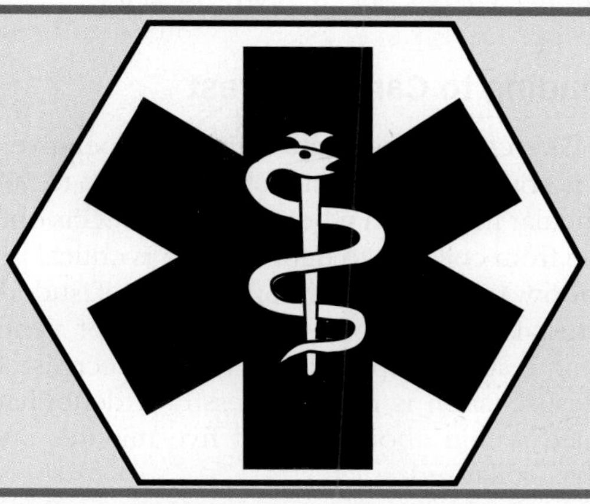

Figure 55–2: Universal emergency identification symbol. *Delmar/Cengage Learning.*

Activating EMS

Activating the emergency medical services (EMS) system by telephoning 911 might also be necessary in a true emergency. Trained personnel usually provided by the police or fire departments (referred to as first responders) are generally the first to arrive on the scene. Depending on the area, emergency coverage can be provided by private ambulance services that employ trained personnel, volunteer firefighters, local law enforcement officers, or the state police.

You should know how to summon assistance in your area. If not, you may check with the office policy manual or manager to identify the appropriate service and determine what help is available and the quickest way to obtain emergency assistance. A list of all emergency numbers should be posted by every phone in the provider's office. All office staff should be aware of this information.

CLINICAL PEARL

Keeping a listing of emergency numbers by the phone is helpful at home as well. When an actual emergency occurs, individuals might experience difficulty finding numbers in a phone directory. Posted information saves critical time.

Some offices might place a card containing this information within the emergency kit or crash cart as well. In a situation when the provider and the medical assistant are both involved in administering first aid and there are no other office personnel present, the card could be handed to a family member to summon help.

Documenting Emergencies

As with any medical procedure, documentation of the emergency is essential. Documenting the who, what, when, and where of the emergency is the protocol generally followed. In addition, the treatment rendered, patient education, and any follow-up for additional care will be addressed in the documentation.

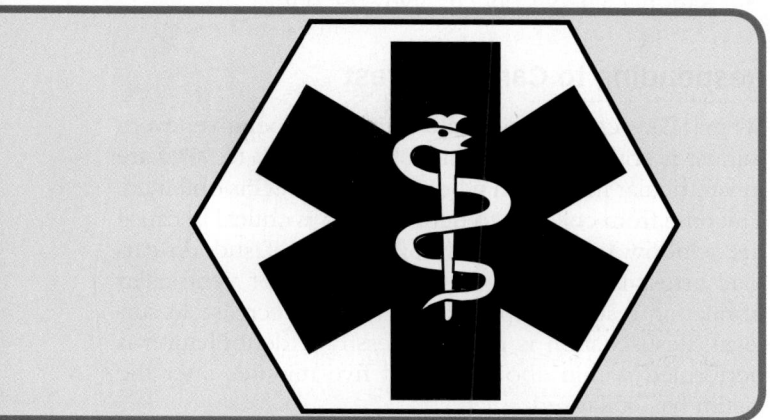

Unfortunately, not all life-saving procedures are effective and occasionally the patient might expire in the office. If that happens, the local law enforcement agency that is generally on the scene will notify the **coroner** to pick up the body for **post mortem** examination. Regulations differ and are determined by local statutes. Normally, if the patient has not been examined by a provider within a fairly recent time frame, an autopsy is required to establish the cause of death to be recorded on the death certificate. If the individual was a patient, you must be certain the specifics regarding the death are recorded on the chart and notations made on additional relevant records so that no inappropriate correspondence is sent to the residence.

Telephone Screening in an Emergency

When a patient calls the office with an emergency situation, you must listen to the caller, ask questions, and follow office policy. You might need to give the call to licensed personnel or a provider who is able to triage the situation. When a caller states there is an emergency, do not put the caller on hold. If it is a true life-threatening emergency, even a minute lost is critical. Obtain the following information:

- The victim's name
- The caller's name and phone number in case the connection is lost
- When did the problem start?
- Is the victim conscious and breathing; does the victim have a pulse?

Some situations require immediate activation of emergency medical services (EMS), for example, if the victim is not breathing or has no pulse. Check with office policy on the correct procedure to follow. Some offices instruct the caller to hang up and call 911 or the local emergency number or keep the caller on the line and have another person in the office call EMS. Either way, you must get immediate information to relay to EMS, including:

- The nature of the situation
- The location of the victim

Then continue to speak with the caller and provide any immediate assistance as appropriate:

- Reassure the caller that EMS is on the way.
- Give appropriate specific instructions in relation to the situation, such as:
  (a) If the victim has a body part pierced by an object, do not remove it.
  (b) If the victim is bleeding severely, apply pressure directly to the area.
  (c) Don't move a patient with a possible spinal injury.
- Try to stay calm and support the caller until EMS arrives and you are assured the victim is being cared for.
- Document in the patient's medical record or EHR all the information obtained and discussed.

CPR AND AED PROCEDURES

Sudden cardiac arrest (SCA) is the total, abrupt, and unexpected loss of heart function and is a leading cause of death in the United States. According to the American Heart Association (AHA), 92% of SCA victims die before reaching the hospital; if more people knew how to perform cardiopulmonary resuscitation (CPR), more lives could be saved. Immediate CPR can double, or even triple, a victim's chance of survival (CPR Statistics, CPR & Sudden Cardiac Arrest Fact Sheet).

All medical assistants should take an approved CPR and a standard first aid course and participate in refresher courses periodically. Several organizations provide CPR training, including the AHA, American Red Cross, American Safety and Health Institute, and the National Safety Council.

Procedures are constantly being refined by these organizations, and the procedure you learn might be altered in the future, which is why it is critical to take periodic refresher courses to maintain CPR certification. In this chapter, the 2010 updates and changes to CPR and ECC (Emergency Cardiovascular Care) are discussed, but step-by-step procedures are not covered because CPR certification must be provided by one of these organizations. During your CPR training, the most up-to-date requirements will be provided along with a training manual. Adult CPR certification consists of both a written examination and a performance test-out on a mannequin similar to the one pictured in Figure 55–3. More information can be found at the organizations' Websites:

- AHA: www.heart.org
- American Red Cross: www.redcross.org
- American Safety & Health Institute: www.ahsi.org
- National Safety Council: www.nsc.org

Responding to Cardiac Arrest

When SCA occurs, immediate action is imperative; every minute is critical. The majority of adults (80% to 90%) are in ventricular fibrillation when the initial ECG is obtained. The time from collapse to defibrillation is critical because the window of opportunity for survival of sudden cardiac arrest is very narrow. Each minute of ventricular fibrillation results in approximately 10% decrease in survival. Resuscitation is most successful if defibrillation is performed within about the first five minutes after the victim has collapsed.

Current guidelines from the AHA and Red Cross advocate immediate defibrillation of the victim using an

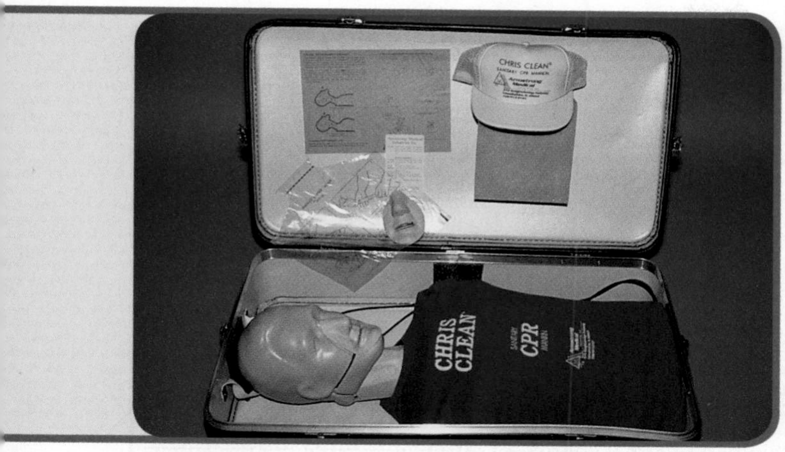

Figure 55–3: Chris Clean CPR training mannequin with disposable parts. *Delmar/Cengage Learning.*

AED, which provides electric stimulation to the chest. CPR should be given until an AED is available. CPR is also necessary immediately after an AED shock because most victims experience a period of no pulse after the shock. CPR and AEDs are beneficial in restoring effective heart rhythm. The chain of survival involves the following sequence of events occurring as quickly as possible:

1. Recognition of early warning signs
2. Activation of the EMS system
3. Basic CPR
4. Early defibrillation with AED
5. Intubation
6. Intravenous administration of medications

Principles of CPR

CPR is a life-saving procedure performed when a person's breathing or heartbeat has stopped. CPR involves two elements: chest compressions and artificial respiration (mouth-to-mouth rescue breathing). The purpose is to keep oxygen flowing to the lungs and blood flowing to the brain and other vital organs until normal heart rhythm can be restored. The CPR procedure was easily remembered by applying the A-B-Cs (airway, breathing, and circulation):

- Clear the **airway**.
- Initiate rescue breathing to provide oxygen to the victim's lungs. A variety of devices are available, from the simple CPR mouth barriers and pocket masks to CPR ventilating masks and Ambu bag and masks.
- Begin chest **compressions** to restore blood circulation. Brain damage or death can occur if blood circulation stops.

However, the 2010 American Heart Association (AHA) guidelines have recommended a change in the basic life support (BLS) sequence to C-A-B (chest compressions, airway, breathing) for adults, children, and infants (excluding newborns). For information on newborns, refer to the neonatal section of the AHA guidelines. The reasoning behind this change is that the majority of cardiac arrests occur in adults, and the highest survival rates are reported when chest compressions are initiated very early on. The old sequence of A-B-C delayed the initiation of compressions while rescuers attempted to open the airway and search for a proper barrier device or ventilation equipment. This change in process should now be minimal (only the time required to deliver the first cycle of 30 chest compressions) for one-person CPR and even less when two rescuers are present. Guidelines for cardiac arrest, respiratory arrest, and obstructed airway are similar but vary according to the age of the patient. Table 55–2 includes the adult, child, and infant CPR skills.

> **CLINICAL PEARL**
>
> For the latest and up-to-date recommendations and procedures, visit the AHA Website, www.heart.org, or American Red Cross Website, www.redcross.org.

AED Procedure

The AED is used in connection with CPR to restore cardiac function. AEDs are easily operated and can be used in the office even in the absence of the provider. They are also being installed for use by the public in many places such as shopping malls, bus stations, and airports. In a provider's office, designated personnel should be trained to operate the equipment to be prepared to respond to life-threatening emergencies. Accurate recording of time, actions, and the use of the defibrillator is very important to document emergency response and provide for risk management. Equally important is the scheduled equipment check to ensure that the battery is charged, the cables are intact, and the dated electrode package remains sealed and has not expired.

The AED can:

- Analyze the heart rhythm of a person in fibrillation or arrest.
- Recognize a shockable rhythm.
- Advise the operator through lights, text, and voice prompts if shock is indicated.
- With built-in diagnostic capability, permit life-saving intervention without the operator needing to evaluate the situation or interpret an ECG.

The AED consists of two large electrodes (pads that are placed on the patient's chest) and cables that connect to the machine. A battery package is the source of power so that the equipment can operate in any location;

TABLE 55–2 Summary of Key BLS Components for Adults, Children, and Infants

Component	Recommendations: Adults	Children	Infants
Recognition	Unresponsive (for all ages)		
	No breathing or no normal breathing (only gasping)	No breathing or only gasping	
	No pulse palpated within 10 seconds for all ages (HCP only)		
CPR sequence	C-A-B		
Compression rate	At least 100/min		
Compression depth	At least 2 inches (5 cm)	At least ⅓ AP diameter about 2 inches (5 cm)	At least ⅓ AP diameter about 1 ½ inches (4 cm)
Chest wall recoil	Allow complete recoil between compressions HCPs rotate compressions every 2 minutes		
Compression interruptions	Minimize interruptions in chest compressions Attempt to limit interruptions to <10 seconds		
Airway	Head tilt—chin lift (HCP suspected trauma: jaw thrust)		
Compression-to-ventilation ratio (until advanced airway placed)	30:2 1 or 2 rescuers	30:2 Single rescuer 15:2 2 HCP rescuers	
Ventilations: when rescuer untrained or trained and not proficient	Compressions only		
Ventilations with advanced airway (HCP)		1 breath every 6–8 seconds (8–10 breaths/min) Asynchronous with chest compressions About 1 second per breath Visible chest rise	
Defibrillation	Attach and use AED as soon as available. Minimize interruptions in chest compressions before and after shock; resume CPR beginning with compressions immediately after each shock.		

Source: 2010 American Heart Association Guidelines for CPR and ECC.

some units have a self-contained battery. The AED is indicated when the victim is unresponsive, is not breathing, and has no pulse. Although AEDs are manufactured by various companies, and some differences exist between the different machines, there are universal steps to follow.

- Turn on the power.
- Attach the electrode pads of the AED to the victim's chest (must be against dry bare skin and might require cutting or shaving of hair. Usually, a disposable razor is with the equipment). Adult pads may be used on victims over 8 years old.
- Analyze the heart rhythm. Some machines respond automatically; others require a button to be pushed. Stop CPR. It is critical for no one to touch the victim while the rhythm is being analyzed.
- Charge the AED if so advised by the AED message; some charge automatically.
- Advise everyone to stay clear and then push the shock button if the AED so indicates. Some AED systems have been designed to deliver both adult and child shock doses. You must follow the AED instructions to select the lower (child) shock doses for children ages 1–8.
- If the victim responds, leave the electrodes in place in case of re-arrest. If no response, repeat the analysis and shock sequence.

- Continue efforts until emergency medical services arrive.

Caution is needed with the use of AED equipment in certain situations:

- For children 1 to 8 years of age, be sure to change the child key or switch and use the child pads. If this is not available, you may use the adult pads and dose.
- For infants under the age of 1, there is not enough evidence to recommend for or against the use of an AED.
- The victim must not be in water; drag the victim from the area before using.
- If the victim has an implanted pacemaker or defibrillator, place the electrode at least one inch to the side.
- Remove and wipe dry any area covered with a transdermal patch that interferes with electrode placement.

nitroglycerine - transdermal patch

Documenting CPR and AED Procedures

If defibrillation or CPR is performed by the provider or an employee within the office, it must be recorded on a chart. If the victim is not a patient, a new chart must be established and the incident recorded. As soon as care is provided, a doctor–patient relationship is established, and there are legal responsibilities.

CPR for Children and Infants

CPR procedures for children and infants vary somewhat from those for adults. Children are considered to be from age 1 to puberty or about 12 to 14 years old. Infants are considered to be from newborn discharge from hospital to 1 year old.

If a rescuer is treating a child *found* in cardiac arrest, the rescuer should initially provide five cycles of CPR before attaching an AED. If the collapse is *witnessed*, the AED should be used as soon as it is available. Recall that the AED device should be dose-attenuated for children under the age of 8, and there is no recommendation for infants at this time.

With infants and children, the prime concern is usually respiratory because arrest from asphyxia is more common than cardiac arrest. Opening the airway might need to be attempted a couple of times before ventilation is successful. A single rescuer in this situation is advised first to give appropriate CPR for five cycles and then to break to summon the EMS system. The provision of CPR first is indicated because arrest from asphyxia is more common than cardiac arrest in children, and the child is much more likely to benefit from initial CPR.

CPR for children and infants also must be taught and the student evaluated for competence by an approved instructor. Providing CPR for infants uses a slightly different technique than for children. A few of the differences are mentioned here:

- When assessing the infant's consciousness, flick the bottom of the foot.
- Using a resuscitation mouthpiece, cover the infant's mouth and nose.
- Observe the infant's chest for evidence of effective breaths.
- Use the brachial artery in the arm to check for a return of the pulse (Figure 55–4).

CPR Safety

It is realistic to believe that any emergency situation involves exposure to certain body fluids and has the potential for disease transmission. These can be minimized by using a face shield or face mask barrier device. They might provide a degree of protection. Masks without one-way valves, including the S-shaped devices, offer little if any protection and should not be considered for routine use. Obviously, **intubation** and bag compression by trained medical emergency personnel is more effective and highly desirable because it does not require personal contact.

The perceived risk of disease transmission during CPR has reduced the willingness of laypersons to provide mouth-to-mouth in unknown cardiac arrest victims. If a lone rescuer refuses to initiate mouth-to-mouth ventilation, he should at least access the EMS system, open the airway, and perform chest compressions until a rescuer

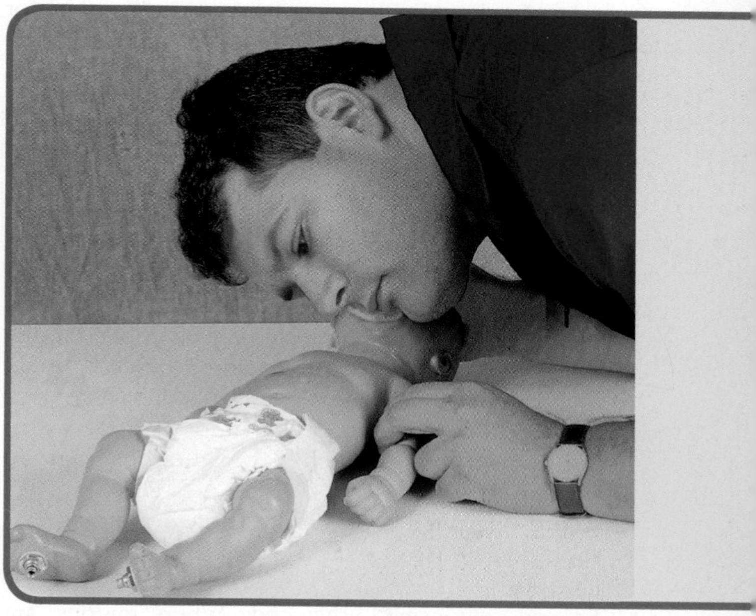

Figure 55–4: Check for a pulse in the brachial artery while observing for breaths. *Delmar/Cengage Learning.*

arrives who is willing to provide ventilation or until EMT or paramedics can use the necessary barrier devices.

The probability that a rescuer will become infected with HBV or HIV as a result of performing CPR is minimal. Although some incidents have been documented from blood exchange or penetration of the skin, infection during mouth-to-mouth has not been documented. HBV-positive saliva has not been shown to be infectious even to oral mucous membranes. Saliva has not been implicated in the transmission of HIV even after bites, percutaneous inoculation, or contamination of cuts and open wounds with HIV-infected saliva. The theoretical risk of infection is greater for salivary transmission of herpes simplex and airborne diseases such as tuberculosis and other respiratory infections. Rare instances of herpes simplex transmission during CPR have been reported. Rescuers with impaired immune systems might be particularly at risk of acquiring tuberculosis and should be tested initially and about 12 weeks after a known exposure. Performance of mouth-to-mouth when blood is apt to be exchanged, such as in trauma cases, does pose a theoretical risk of HBV or HIV transmission.

Public safety and health care personnel should follow the guidelines established by the CDC and OSHA. These involve the use of latex or vinyl gloves and mechanical ventilation equipment. Rescuers who themselves are ill should not perform the procedures if other methods of ventilation are available.

COMMON EMERGENCIES IN THE MEDICAL OFFICE

Several terms describe the severity and length of time for onset of disease or illness. Some of the more common terms are:

- **Chronic**—long, drawn out, not acute. Some diseases have a slow chronic phase but can quickly change into an acute episode.
- **Subtle**—hidden, not apparent, treacherous. Often, disease conditions have a slow, hidden beginning and then quickly develop symptoms.
- **Urgent**—a situation requiring intervention as soon as can be arranged. This term may be applied to the need for care when experiencing a blocked ureter by a kidney stone.
- **Sudden**—occurring quickly and without warning. Onset of headaches or allergies can be sudden.
- **Acute**—having a rapid onset, severe symptoms, and short course. Heart attacks are an example of acute illnesses.
- **Severe**—extensive, advanced. When injuries are severe, it usually implies multiple sites and requires considerable medical attention. The term is also applied to an illness that requires aggressive action and is potentially irreversible.
- **Life threatening**—can cause death. Extensive trauma and massive circulatory or respiratory involvement that might be beyond medical intervention are deemed life threatening.

Almost any injury or illness could be manifest in most of the preceding classifications. Consider a cut that is bleeding: It could be oozing, a slow flow, a pulsating flow, or a hemorrhage that is life threatening. The following conditions are examples of disorders, diseases, or situations that can present emergency events if in an acute phase.

Hyperglycemia and Hypoglycemia

Diabetic patients can present emergency situations by going into **diabetic ketoacidosis** (DKA) or insulin shock. Diabetic ketoacidosis is caused by a lack of insulin, along with an increased amount of sugar in the blood and can lead to diabetic **coma** or death. Patients with uncontrolled **hyperglycemia** are at risk for going into diabetic ketoacidosis. This can be caused by consuming excess carbohydrates, an infection, fever, emotional stress, or failing to take adequate insulin

Insulin shock or **hypoglycemia** can occur from an excess amount of insulin in the body. This can happen if food is not eaten regularly in measured amounts, if the patient vomits after taking insulin, after engaging in excessive exercise, or if too much insulin is taken. The patient might have muscle weakness, anxiety, mental confusion, a pounding heartbeat, hunger, and **diaphoresis**. The skin will be cold, pale, and moist. The patient might lapse into unconsciousness and have seizures. He or she should be given some form of sugar. Sweetened orange juice, sublingual sugar, or tubes of glucose are often used. The sugar should end the shock; if not, the patient must be transported at once to a hospital.

You must be alert to the possibility of diabetic ketoacidosis or insulin shock in a diabetic patient with these symptoms. If the patient can talk, ask if insulin or food has been taken. This will give you a better idea of the need for treatment of diabetic ketoacidosis or insulin shock. If the condition cannot be determined, the provider might suggest giving the patient a little sugar because insulin shock can cause irreversible brain damage. Recent studies indicate that a very small amount of sugar placed under the tongue of an unconscious person will be absorbed rapidly into the bloodstream and return the patient to consciousness.

TABLE 55–3 Causes, Symptoms and First Aid of Diabetic Ketoacidosis and Insulin Shock

	Diabetic Ketoacidosis (DKA)	Insulin Shock
Causes	Too little insulin	Too much insulin
	Illness	Too little food or delayed meal
	Stress	Too much exercise
		Alcohol consumption on empty stomach
Symptoms	Thirst or very dry mouth	Moist and pale, diaphoresis
	Frequent urination	Nervous, anxious, irritable
	Dry or flushed skin	Shaky
	Nausea, vomiting, or abdominal pain	Lightheaded
	Fruity odor on breath	Hungry
	Feeling constantly tired	Fast heartbeat, palpitations
	Difficult time breathing	Blurred vision
	Confusion or difficulty paying attention	Headache
	High blood glucose levels	Confusion
	High levels of ketones in the urine	Seizures
First aid	Keep patient warm	If conscious, give patient food or drink containing 15–20 grams of carbohydrate (sugar, honey, corn syrup, candy, orange juice, soft drink, or glucose tablets)
	Obtain medical help immediately	If unconscious, obtain medical help immediately

Fainting

The medical term for fainting is **syncope**, explained as a brief episode of unconsciousness. Fainting itself is not a disease but rather a symptom of an underlying condition or disease. A patient who feels faint should lower his or her head between the legs or lie down with his or her feet elevated to improve the blood circulation to the brain (Figure 55–5). The patient who is about to faint might be pale; perspiring; have cold, clammy skin; and complain of dizziness or nausea. An emesis basin should be handy in case the patient vomits. Each examination room should be supplied with aromatic spirits of ammonia capsules, which can be easily broken and used to arouse the patient. These should not be held directly under the nose but passed back and forth about six inches under the nose. The patient should be kept in a reclining position until fully recovered and then be gradually allowed to sit up. The patient should regain consciousness within a minute or two from a simple fainting episode; any time longer than that might require EMS activation. The provider should be alerted to examine the patient, and vital signs must be monitored to determine whether they are stabilized before allowing the patient to leave your facility. Realize that in this situation, the patient might need emotional support and reassurance.

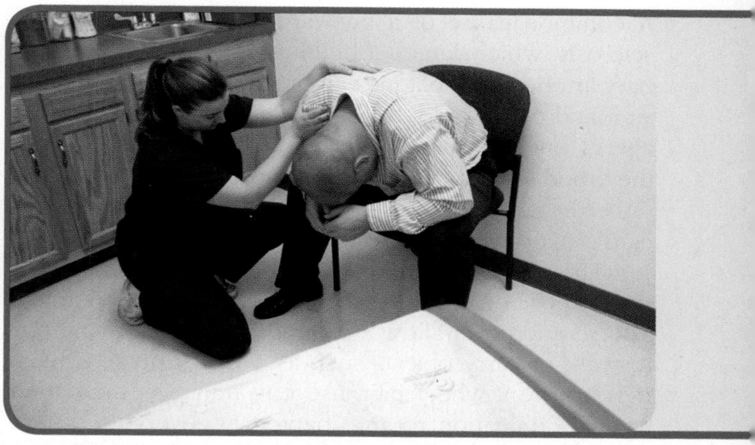

Figure 55–5: Assist the patient to lower the head between the legs when feeling faint. *Delmar/Cengage Learning.*

Heart Attack

Patients might arrive at the office complaining of severe chest pain or pressure. It is extremely important for the provider to be alerted immediately to rule out whether the patient is suffering from a heart attack, otherwise known as a **myocardial infarction**, the leading cause of death for both men and women. The patient might also complain of pain radiating down one or both arms and a tightness of the chest or pain radiating into the left shoulder and jaw (mandible). The pulse is usually rapid and weak. The patient might be perspiring profusely; have cyanotic lips and fingernails; and be nauseated, anxious, and agitated and might be in denial that anything serious is occurring.

These classic symptoms were identified primarily from observation of adult males who were the subjects of research studies. However, findings now indicate that heart disease is also very prominent among women. In fact, statistics indicate that heart disease kills more women than all forms of cancer combined. In recent studies, it has been noted that women can experience symptoms somewhat differently than men. Because of this, women might not recognize they are having a coronary event and do not seek medical attention. In fact, more than 60 percent of women who suffered sudden cardiac death had no known symptoms of heart disease.

Women do experience chest pain and pressure, but they are more likely to have other symptoms as well, such as:

- Shortness of breath
- Burning sensation in the chest (often dismissed as heartburn)
- Nausea and vomiting and other flulike symptoms
- Unexplained fatigue or weakness
- Pain in the jaw, neck, shoulder, back, or ear
- Overwhelming sense of doom

A common cause of a myocardial infarction is atherosclerosis, which causes a buildup of plaque in the coronary arteries. This plaque can break away from the artery wall and cause a clot to form, which can create a blockage of one or more of the coronary arteries, restricting the blood flow to the heart and causing the heart to stop. Other heart conditions such as various arrhythmias and cardiomyopathy can also be the cause.

The first intervention is to help the patient into a sitting position and elevate his or her feet if possible. You should never allow a patient with cardiac symptoms to walk or carry objects such as a heavy purse or coat. If you have a wheelchair, use it to transport the patient to an examination room. Chapter 40 covers the procedures for safely assisting a patient from a wheelchair to an exam table and vice versa. Most cardiac patients prefer to have their head elevated, so once seated, adjust the table as needed.

The provider might want you to administer oxygen or prepare an injection for the patient. Always have the crash cart with IV equipment and emergency medications ready for the provider. If the patient has previously been diagnosed with angina and has a medication such as nitroglycerine, it should be given immediately. Many providers also recommend taking one regular-size aspirin to help dissolve any blood clot that might be present.

If oxygen administration is ordered to assist the patient to breathe more easily, a nasal cannula connected by tubing to a portable oxygen tank will be used. The tank valve is opened and the flow meter set at the amount prescribed by the provider, usually 3 to 4 liters. Feel the area adjacent to the nasal tips to ensure that oxygen is flowing. The woman in Figure 55–6 A is receiving oxygen through a nasal cannula fitted over her face with a nasal tip in each nostril. The cannula is then draped behind each ear and brought forward under the chin. An adjustable slide on the cannula can be moved toward the chin to maintain its position. Figure 55–6 B shows the tips of the cannula, which must be inserted into the nostrils. Monitor the patient's level of anxiety and effects of the oxygen. Be sure to document the use of oxygen on the patient's chart, indicating the method, amount of

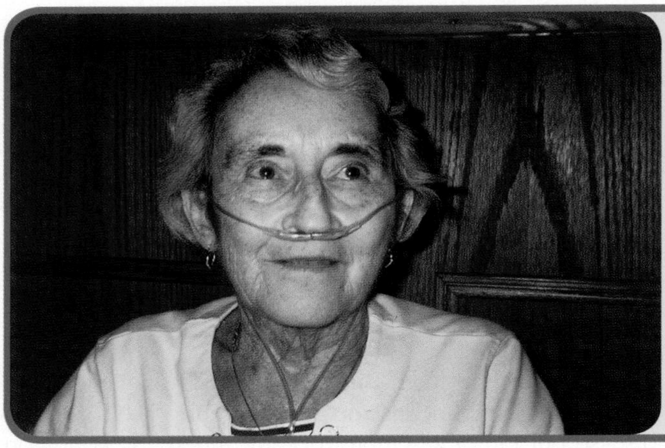

Figure 55–6 A: Administer oxygen by nasal cannula.
Delmar/Cengage Learning.

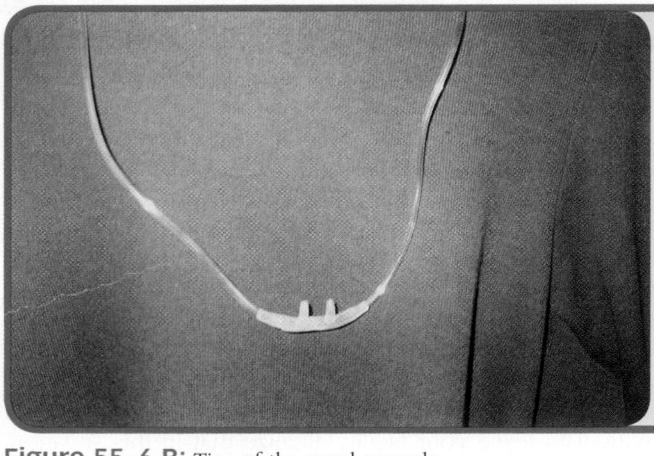

Figure 55–6 B: Tips of the nasal cannula.
Delmar/Cengage Learning.

flow, time begun, and patient's response. The provider might also order an electrocardiogram to be done immediately. Refer to Chapter 47 for the procedure of obtaining an ECG if you need to be refreshed. The emergency medical service should be summoned per the provider's request. If the provider is out of the office, summon EMS immediately on your own so the victim can be stabilized and transported to the hospital as quickly as possible. If the patient stops breathing, start rescue breathing and, if there is no pulse, start chest compressions (CPR). Time is critical in the event of a myocardial infarction. Prompt, appropriate treatment within the first hour of an attack can save lives and reduce damage.

Heat Exposure

The patient who is exposed to high temperatures for a long period in industry or at home can suffer from **heat cramps**. These patients might have diaphoresis (excessive sweating) and should drink large amounts of water because they lose a large amount of body salt. The patient will complain of severe muscle cramps of the abdomen, arms, and legs and might also complain of faintness, dizziness, and exhaustion. First aid to replace salt is provided by giving the patient a balanced electrolyte drink such as Gatorade. The patient should lie down in a cool place. If muscle spasms are severe, IV normal saline may be given. It is important to differentiate between **heatstroke** and **heat exhaustion**.

In heat exhaustion, the skin is pale, cool, and moist and the body temperature is normal. The patient becomes overheated with profuse perspiration, usually after some form of vigorous exercise. He or she might have headaches, muscle cramps, nausea, dizziness, and fatigue. The pulse is weak and rapid, and the respirations are quiet and shallow. The patient should stop all activity, move to a cooler place, and consume cool water or sports drink. If the patient's signs and symptoms worsen or don't resolve within an hour, medical care should be sought. If the body temperature reaches 40°C/104°F, immediate medical treatment is necessary because heatstroke is probably occurring.

Heatstroke is the most severe of the heat-related problems. The patient suffering from heatstroke will have a red, dry face. The skin will be hot and dry, and the body temperature can be above 40°C/104°F. The pulse will be rapid and then gradually slow and weaken. Respirations will be rapid and shallow. The pupils of the eyes will be dilated but equal. Headache, shortness of breath, nausea or vomiting, dizziness, weakness, and dry mouth are common symptoms. Treatment is to get the individual out of the heat immediately and cool the body with cool water or wet cloths. Have the patient drink cool water or other nonalcoholic, caffeine-free beverages. EMS should be activated because this is a potentially life-threatening condition.

Cold Exposure

Hypothermia occurs when your body loses heat faster than it can produce it, resulting in a dangerously low body temperature. This occurs when the body temperature drops lower than 35°C/95°F. If left untreated, respiratory and heart failure can occur and eventually lead to death. Exposure to cold weather and submersion in cold water are the usual causes of hypothermia. Common signs and symptoms include shivering, slurred speech or mumbling, confusion, weak pulse, and shallow breathing. Treatment includes bringing the patient's temperature back up to normal by bringing him or her inside, removing any wet clothing, and covering him or her with layers of blankets. EMS should be activated because this can be a life-threatening condition.

Exposure to freezing temperatures will often result in **frostbite**. The body parts most often damaged by cold are the hands, feet, ears, and nose. Symptoms that might indicate damaged tissue are a tingling sensation with numbness followed by pain and redness of the skin. If exposure is continued, the patient might complain of burning and itching. Sensation might be completely lost. The skin can be white or grayish-yellow and waxy in appearance. Severe frostbite can cause blistering and hardening of the skin. The first aid required is to warm the affected part slowly by placing it in water with a temperature of 40°C/104° to 41.7°C/107°F. This helps reduce tissue damage. Never rub frostbite; you will cause tissue damage. Hot tea or coffee will act as a stimulus and dilate blood vessels to increase circulation. The patient should *not* be allowed to smoke because of the constriction effect on the blood vessels. After warming, wrap the area loosely with sterile dressing. If feet are frostbitten, the patient must avoid the pressure of standing or walking because this causes additional damage to the tissue. If the skin turns red and has a tingling sensation as it warms, circulation is returning. If the skin remains numb or blisters, seek medical care.

Hemorrhage

It is important to understand the different sources of bleeding and determine the seriousness of the hemorrhage. Bleeding can be of three types: arterial, venous, and capillary. The term *hemorrhage* refers to excessive, uncontrolled bleeding. Arterial bleeding produces bright red blood in spurts. If the ruptured artery is a large branch, death can occur in three minutes or less. Bleeding from a vein produces a steady flow of dark red blood. It is important to control bleeding quickly. This is best accomplished by covering the wound with a clean cloth or pad of gauze squares, if available, and exerting pressure directly on the bleeding area (Figure 55–7). The area might also require elevation to stop the bleeding. Sometimes, especially with arterial bleeding, this is not

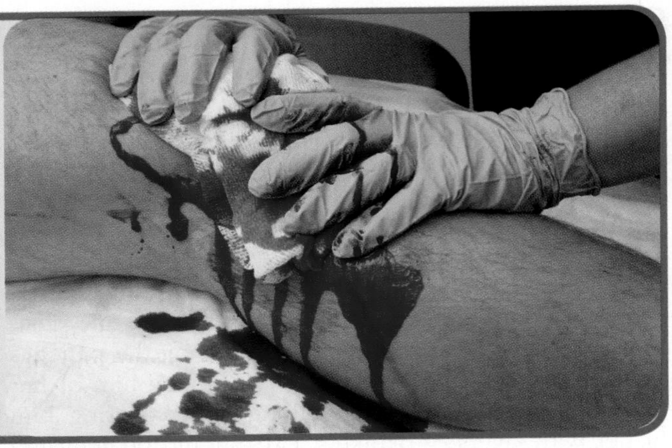

Figure 55–7: Applying direct pressure. *Delmar/Cengage Learning.*

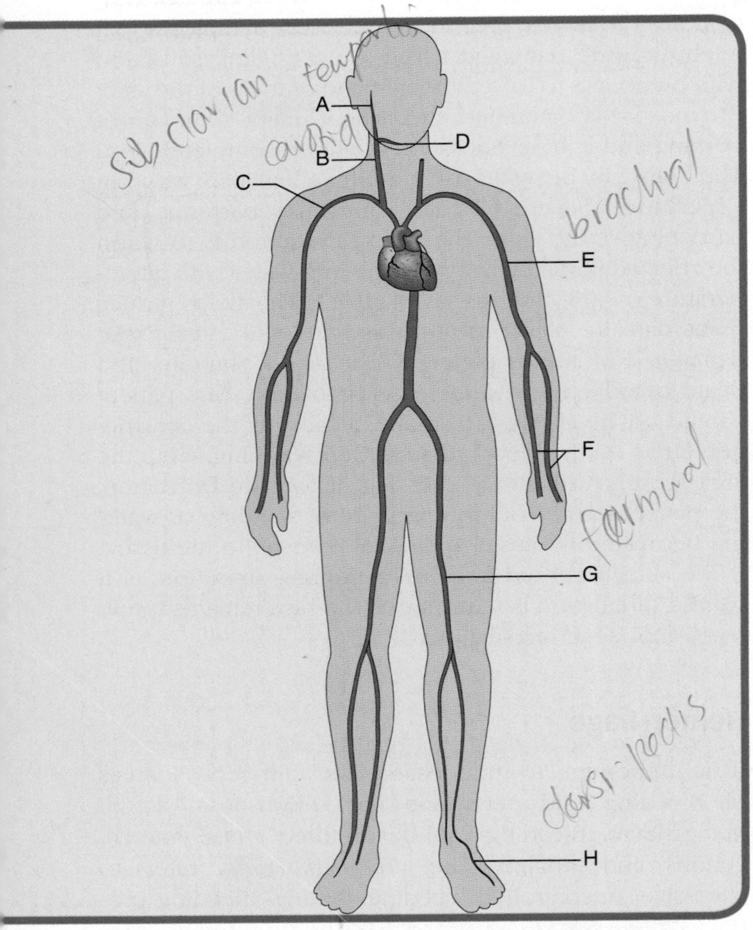

Figure 55–8: Pressure points. *Delmar/Cengage Learning.*

sufficient, and pressure must be exerted at the pressure point proximal to the wound to stop the flow of blood to the area (Figure 55–8). Any bleeding from capillary damage produces a steady ooze from the wound area. This type of bleeding often clots without first aid measures (Figure 55-8; see areas A-H).

Internal bleeding causes symptoms similar to those of shock. The patient can have a rapid, weak pulse; shallow breathing; cold, clammy skin; dilated pupils; dizziness; faintness; thirst; restlessness; and a feeling of anxiety. Internal hemorrhage might need to be controlled by surgery. The patient must be kept in a recumbent position with strictly limited movement until the surgery can be performed.

Internal bleeding can be difficult to detect unless it produces symptoms or external signs. For example, the patient who coughs up bright red blood might have a lung hemorrhage, or vomiting bright red blood might indicate an ulcer has started bleeding. If the patient is vomiting what looks like coffee grounds, it could indicate chronic slow bleeding of the stomach. If the patient notices coal-black stools, a loss of blood in the intestines is probable and, if the patient has bright red rectal bleeding, it is likely to be from a lesion in the rectum or lower colon. A patient with severe abdominal pain from trauma might have internal bleeding from a ruptured organ such as a kidney, liver, or spleen. Internal bleeding that causes symptoms of shock and produces pain probably requires surgical intervention to correct. Slow bleeding, when the cause has been determined, can be treated with medication and, if intestinal, by altering the diet to allow the area to heal. In addition, a hemorrhage that occurs with the rupture of various types of aneurysms is discussed in Chapter 30.

Epistaxis (nosebleed) can be the result of excessively dry air over a prolonged period, hypertension, injury, or simply blowing the nose too hard (see Chapter 25). First aid for epistaxis is to elevate the head and pinch the nostrils closed for at least six minutes. Keep the patient in a sitting position with the head tilted forward so that the blood will not trickle down the throat unseen. The use of a cold compress over the nasal area or on the back of the neck can be helpful. A piece of gauze can be placed between the lips and gums with pressure against this area for several minutes. Specially treated gauze is best for nasal packing because it is less difficult to remove. A provider should be consulted if bleeding is not easily controlled. Sometimes, the addition of humidity to the air will relieve the patient who has recurrent epistaxis.

Another common bleeding condition that can present to the office is that of a pregnant patient experiencing vaginal bleeding. It is necessary to determine the kind of flow. If bleeding is heavy, the patient should lie down immediately with feet elevated, and emergency medical services should be called. If there has been a discharge of clots or tissue substance, this should be collected and sent along with the patient to the hospital for possible analysis. Your employer will let you know the protocol on how to handle these types of emergencies.

Poisoning

Poison can be **ingested**, absorbed, inhaled, injected, or acquired from bites and stings. Poisoning can occur from a medication overdose. It can be accidental or intentional. If someone calls regarding a possible ingestion of **poison**, always obtain the patient's name, age, sex, and weight and ask what was taken, how much was taken, and the time it was taken. Learn the location and the telephone number of the local poison control center, which is staffed with registered nurses, pharmacists, and providers 24 hours a day, seven days a week, so that you can direct callers to the best source of help. The poison control center will determine what the treatment should be.

Children are often the victims of ingested poisonings. They will swallow pills, detergent, household cleaners, painting supplies, and drain cleaners and eat plants. Usually, the evidence is nearby, such as opened pill bottles, pills on the floor or loose in a purse, spilled liquids on clothing and the floor, opened containers, and pieces of plant material. If the poisoning is not discovered quickly, symptoms such as nausea, stomach cramps, shallow breathing, drowsiness, skin color change, and even unconsciousness can occur. Remember, the poison control center is your prime source of information. Follow its instructions to provide the appropriate care. If the provider or treatment center advises examining the patient, instruct the caller to bring in the material ingested and a sample of anything vomited, if possible, so an analysis can be made to verify what was swallowed.

Poisoning by inhalation can be caused by cleaning fluids and sprays used in a poorly ventilated area. Carbon monoxide poisoning can be caused by a faulty exhaust system in an automobile or home heating system. Poisoning by injection is usually the result of drug abuse. The patient might exhibit symptoms ranging from confusion to excitement to hallucinations to convulsions. These poisonings usually require the EMS system to be activated.

Seizures (Convulsions)

A **seizure** is a severe, involuntary contraction of muscles that first causes the patient to become rigid and then to have uncontrollable movements. Seizures can occur when the patient has high body temperature, head injuries, brain disease, or a brain disorder such as epilepsy. The patient becomes unconscious and can be injured during the seizure. The face and lips can become cyanotic, and the patient might stop breathing. He or she might also lose bladder and bowel control and bite the tongue. When the seizure has stopped, the patient might be confused and complain of headache and **exhaustion**.

During the convulsive phase, your main goal is to prevent injury to the patient. If the patient is in the upright position when the seizure occurs, ease him or her to the floor. Do not restrain movement and move any objects out of the way that might cause injury. Do not force any object between the patient's teeth, or it could cause vomiting, **aspiration**, or spasm of the larynx. If mucus or saliva is present, turn the head to the side to prevent choking. If the victim is not breathing, open the airway with the head-tilt or jaw-thrust maneuver. Allow the patient to rest or sleep after the seizure is over. Document the length of the seizure and any other pertinent information. Provide emotional support as the patient regains composure because this situation can cause the person to feel embarrassed. If the seizure is due to the condition of status epilepticus (continuous seizure), EMS must be activated because this is a life-threatening condition. Administration of oxygen and antiseizure medication might be necessary; therefore, alert the provider immediately.

Obstructed Airway

One of the most common medical emergencies is an **obstructed** airway. The most usual cause in adults is food aspirated while eating. This occurs when partially chewed food is sucked into the trachea when talking, laughing, or coughing while eating. Children, on the other hand, can get toys, toy parts, buttons, candy, or a variety of other objects caught in their throat and obstruct their airway. Pieces of food are also a problem for children; the most dangerous food is the hot dog, because if fed in a small sliced portion, it's just the right shape to cause choking.

CLINICAL PEARL

Most people are familiar with the dangers of plastic wrapping and bags because of all the warning labels, but one of the most common airway obstructers is the latex balloon. Safety authorities believe no young child should have a balloon unless it is made of Mylar. Children ages 4 to 8 require supervision if playing with or trying to inflate latex balloons.

The obstruction, if complete, must be cleared away immediately because brain damage can result in about four minutes from lack of oxygen. A person who is choking usually places his or her hand at the throat, which is the universal distress signal (Figure 55–9). This is called conscious choking. The individual might not be able to cough or speak and will simply fall from the chair if

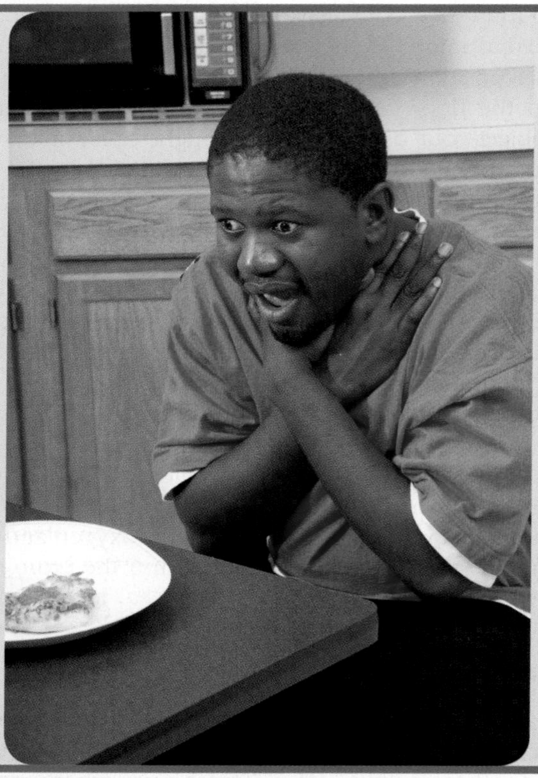

Figure 55–9: Universal distress signal. *Delmar/Cengage Learning.*

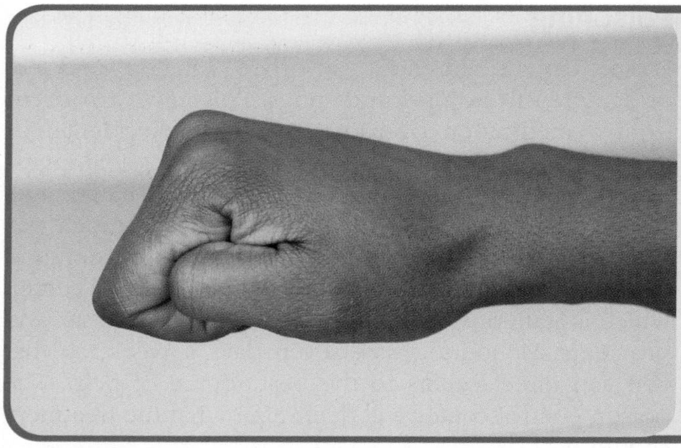

Figure 55–10 A: Fist with thumb flexed. *Delmar/Cengage Learning.*

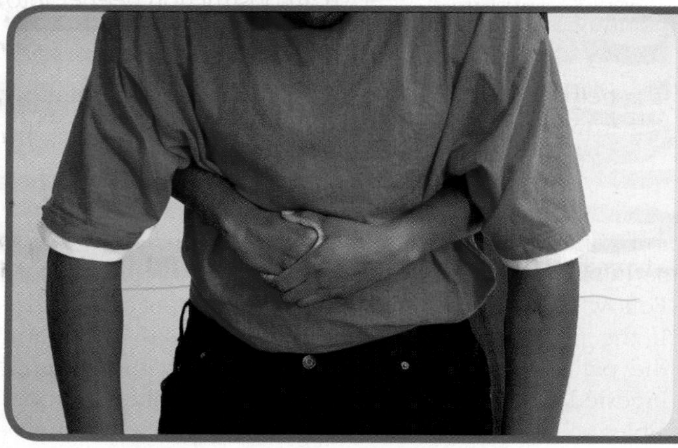

Figure 55–10 B: Hand placement for abdominal thrust. *Delmar/Cengage Learning.*

nothing is done. You should always ask the patient, "Are you choking?" and watch for a response such as the universal distress signal before attempting any intervention.

Chest thrusts, back blows or slaps, or abdominal thrusts are effective for relieving an obstructed airway in conscious adults and children older than 1 year of age, although injuries have been reported with the abdominal thrust. There is insufficient evidence to determine which should be used first. These techniques should be applied in rapid sequence until the obstruction is relieved; more than one technique might be needed. Unconscious victims should receive CPR. The finger sweep should be used in the unconscious patient with an obstructed airway only if solid material is visible in the airway. There is insufficient evidence for a treatment recommendation for an obese or pregnant patient with an obstructed airway. For the abdominal thrust method, while standing behind the victim, reach around the waist. Clench one hand to make a fist, and grasp your fist with the other hand. Place the thumb side of the fist against the midline of the victim's abdomen between the waist and the rib cage (Figure 55–10 A and B). Thrust your fist inward and upward in quick, firm movements to move air out of the lungs with enough force to dislodge the obstruction.

A choking victim who is alone can use the abdominal thrust with his or her own fist or thrust against a chair back or any hard object of appropriate height (Figure 55–11).

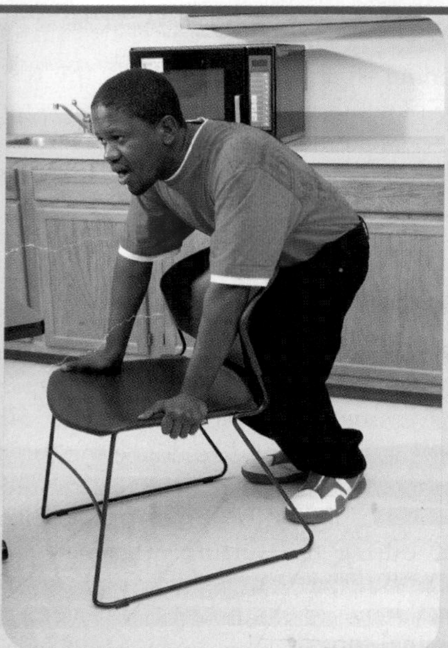

Figure 55–11: Self-administered abdominal thrust. *Delmar/Cengage Learning.*

If a patient is in an advanced stage of pregnancy or is very obese, abdominal thrusting is not possible. A chest thrust can be used to dislodge the material. If the patient is standing, from the back, place your arms around the victim directly under the axillae. Using the abdominal clenched-fist technique, place your thumb over the sternum; place your other hand over the fist, and give firm thrusts, pulling straight back toward yourself.

If the thrusts have dislodged the obstruction but have not expelled it from the victim's mouth, then a finger sweep is performed. Open the victim's mouth by tilting the head back with one hand and moving the jaw forward to lift the tongue away from the back of the throat. Insert an index finger along the inside of the cheek and sweep deeply into the mouth in a hooking action. Be careful not to push an obstruction deeper into the throat. If it is possible to dislodge an obstruction, be sure to remove it from the mouth. If dentures are worn, it is helpful to remove them. If the patient has vomited, it is extremely important to turn the patient on his or her side to keep an open airway and prevent aspiration of material into the lungs.

CLINICAL PEARL

Important

- *Do not* try to remove an object that is stuck in the victim's throat; you might push it farther into the airway. Only if it is lying within the mouth should it be removed.
- If the heart stops, *do not* begin CPR chest compressions until the airway is open.

Follow the steps in Procedure 55–1 to perform an abdominal thrust on an adult victim with an obstructed airway. The procedure is written for an office setting, but obstructed airway incidents usually occur in restaurants, at parties, and other places where food is being eaten.

PROCEDURE 55–1 Perform an Abdominal Thrust on an Adult Victim with an Obstructed Airway

MEDIA LINK: View the video, "Abdominal Thrusts," for this chapter on the Premium Website.

PURPOSE: To dislodge an object obstructing the airway and restore breathing

EQUIPMENT: Disposable gloves and resuscitation mouthpiece

SKILL: Perform an abdominal thrust on a adult victim with an obstructed airway.

Procedure Steps	Detailed Instructions and/or *Rationales*
1. Observe the victim using the universal distress signal.	
2. Ask, "Are you choking?" If yes, ask, "Can you speak?"	A weak cough, a wheezing breath sound, and inability to speak are signs of obstruction.
3. Get into position behind the victim.	*The victim can become worse and go into unconsciousness at any time; this position allows you to perform the maneuver as well as lower the patient to the floor.*
4. Extend your arms around the victim's abdomen and locate his or her umbilicus with the index finger of one hand. With the other hand, make a fist with your thumb bent outward. Place the thumb against the abdomen just above the umbilicus.	
5. Place your other hand over the fist.	
6. Keep your thrusts in the soft high abdominal area to avoid injury to the rib cage and sternum. Give an abdominal thrust by forcefully pulling up and back quickly.	*Force pushes the abdominal organs up against the diaphragm to force out air and the obstruction. Note:* If the patient is pregnant or obese, perform chest thrusts instead of abdominal thrusts.

(continues)

(continued)

Procedure Steps	Detailed Instructions and/or *Rationales*
7. If this is unsuccessful, repeat thrusts until the obstruction is expelled or the victim loses consciousness.	
8. If the victim becomes unresponsive and falls to the floor, position him or her on his or her back and activate the emergency response system by calling 911, open the airway, remove the object if you see it, and begin CPR.	*The victim can go into respiratory and cardiac arrest if the obstruction remains.*
9. Every time you open the airway to give breaths, open the victim's mouth wide and look for the object. If you see it, remove it; if not, continue CPR.	
10. After the victim has resumed breathing and the heart is beating or EMS services have taken over the rescue, remove your gloves and the mouthpiece and dispose of them in the biohazard waste container.	
11. Document the procedure.	

Charting Example

6/24/XX 1:25 PM	Pt. sitting in reception room began choking on piece of candy. Complete airway obstruction. Notified Dr. Green, EMS called. Given multiple abdominal thrusts; candy was expelled. Breathing and heart rate restored. Patient evaluated by Dr. Green to ensure that no complications resulted from abdominal thrusts. G. Jenks, CMA(AAMA)

Special Considerations for Infants

An infant or toddler experiencing a blocked airway will have difficulty breathing, coughing, and crying and might display cyanosis. The recommended AHA and Red Cross course of action is:

1. Place the baby face-down on your forearm, which is extended on your thigh (Figure 55–12). You might also kneel or sit with the infant on your lap to do this.
2. The head should be lower than the body and supported by your hand.
3. With the heel of your other hand, deliver five backslaps, forcefully, in the middle of the back between the infant's shoulder blades.
4. If this is unsuccessful, turn the infant face up; support the head and neck. Keep the head lower than the trunk.
5. Place two fingers on the midsternal area just below the nipple line.
6. Give five quick downward chest thrusts; deliver chest thrusts at a rate of about one per second (Figure 55–13).
7. Continue with five back blows and five chest thrusts until the object is dislodged or the infant becomes unconscious.
8. If unsuccessful, call out for help to notify EMS.
9. If no help arrives, give the infant CPR for one minute and then call 911 yourself.
10. Continue CPR until assistance arrives.

Some additional information:

- Even if the procedure is successful and infant seems fine, check with the provider for further instructions.
- If you can *see* the object, try to remove it with your finger.
- *Do not* try to grasp the object and pull it out if the infant is conscious.
- *Do not* perform the procedure on an infant who stops breathing for other reasons, such as asthma, swelling in the throat, head injury, or an infectious process.

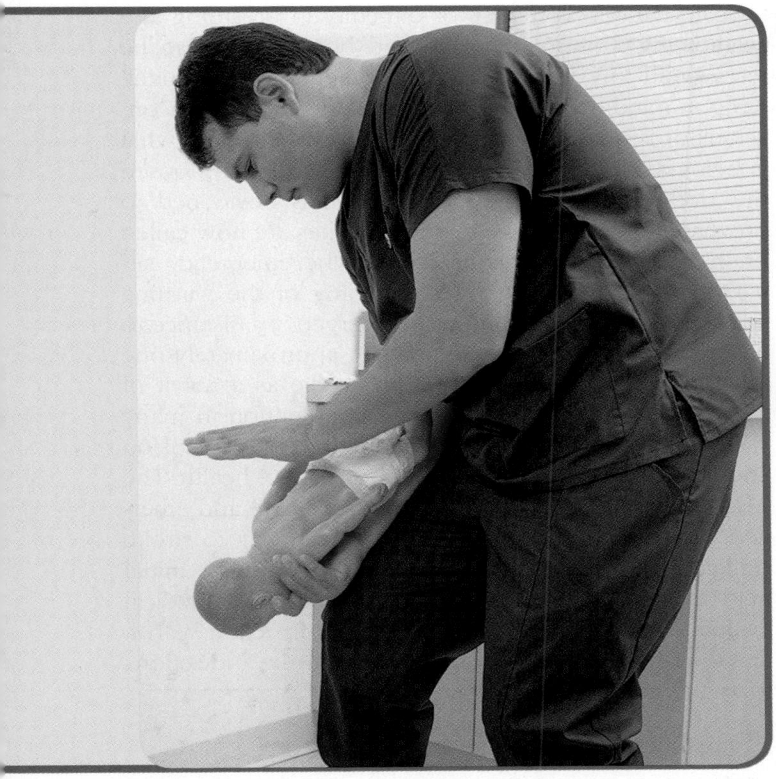

Figure 55–12: Back blows on an infant. *Delmar/Cengage Learning.*

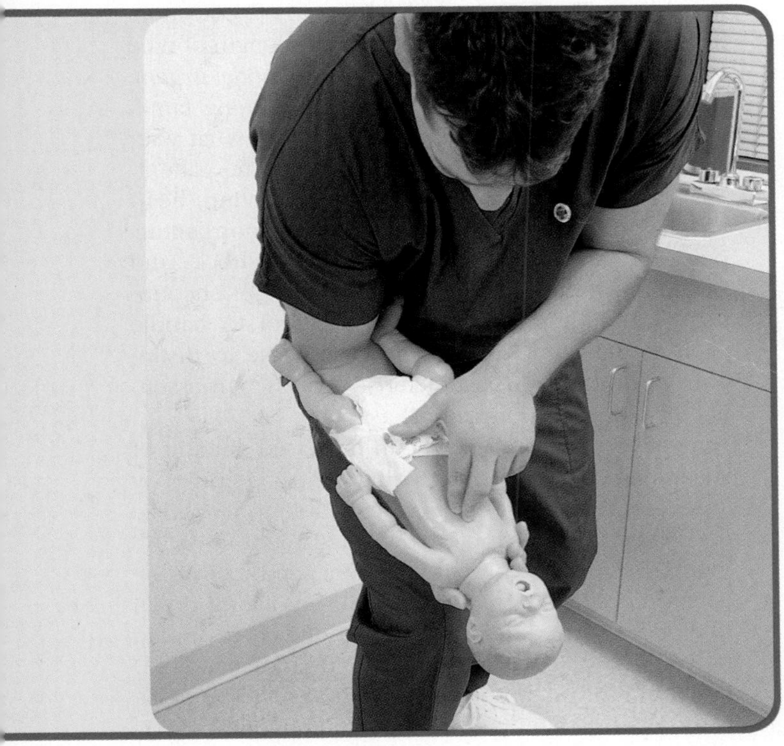

Figure 55–13: Infant chest thrusts. *Delmar/Cengage Learning.*

Accidental, Allergic, and Drug-Induced Distress

Respiratory problems can also arise from other conditions such as:

- A patient suffering from severe edema of the vocal cords as a result of an allergic reaction to food or stings of bees or wasps must be hospitalized as quickly as possible.
- The victim of a drowning must receive rescue breathing immediately. This can be given before the patient is taken from the water if there is help to support the patient while resuscitation is given. A person surviving drowning needs to be hospitalized for follow-up observation.
- Poisoning by toxic gases, such as carbon monoxide, or suffocation can also require immediate rescue breathing.
- A person having an asthma attack might have great difficulty breathing. The provider must determine the treatment needed, but you can be helpful by attempting to calm the patient. Emotional upset often starts an asthma attack.
- Some medications can cause a slowing or **cessation** of breathing.
- Electric shock can cause respiratory paralysis. The victim must be moved away from the source of the electricity by indirect means (never touch the victim) and then be given rescue breathing and CPR if necessary.

Shock

Shock can be associated with many kinds of injuries and is a serious depressor of vital body functions. Symptoms include a rapid, thready, weak pulse; shallow, rapid respirations; dilated pupils; ashen color; and cool, clammy skin. All of these result from decreased blood volume because of diminished cardiac output causing a drop in blood pressure. It is possible for shock to cause death even when the injury causing the shock is not life threatening. First aid measures include placing the patient in a recumbent position with feet elevated unless there is a head injury, in which case the patient is kept flat. If the patient has difficulty breathing or has a chest injury, the head and shoulders should be elevated. It is best to place a blanket under and over the patient to maintain body warmth but not to overheat.

Shock can be caused by various circumstances. It can be associated with a heart attack or respiratory collapse. It frequently follows trauma or physical injury. Extensive burns, electrical shock, hemorrhage, near drowning, and severe infection can all result in shock. Another type, an anaphylactic shock, is an acute allergic reaction to a foreign substance, which can include certain foods, beestings, or injections of therapeutic or **prophylactic** substances. The patient might have dyspnea, cyanosis, and seizures. Epinephrine and oxygen should be immediately available for use by the provider or by the medical assistant under the direction of the provider. No patient should be given an allergy injection and then be allowed to leave the office immediately because anaphylactic shock can result from these injections. Patients can also have severe reactions to penicillin, aspirin, serums, vaccines, local anesthetics, salicylates, and X-ray contrast media.

Stroke

The common term for a cerebrovascular accident (CVA) is stroke. A CVA is the result of a ruptured blood vessel in the brain or an occlusion of a blood vessel. The patient might have a light stroke with very little damage or a more extensive one with immediate paralysis in the form of sagging muscles on one side of the face or the inability to use an arm or leg. One entire side of the body might be paralyzed. The patient might complain of numbness. The pupils of the eyes might be unequal in size. The patient might have mental confusion, slurred speech, nausea, vomiting, or difficulty in breathing and swallowing. Control of urine and bowels can also be lost. Avoid any unnecessary movement of the patient. Keep in mind that the patient who appears to be unconscious or is unable to speak might be able to hear what is being said. If a patient is experiencing a CVA, loosen the clothing and be sure the patient is positioned to prevent choking on excess saliva. Strokes are now called brain attacks and are considered to be emergency situations. The patient who exhibits any of the warning signs of stroke needs immediate emergency assistance to ensure optimal recovery. Remember, approximately one third of patients with a major stroke die as a result of the condition. Quick, appropriate intervention in many cases limits damage caused by blood vessel occlusion and helps restore patients to the prior state of health. The AHA has adapted a series of actions for EMS and emergency personnel to take to evaluate and react to stroke similar to those for cardiac response. It involves initial field evaluation criteria, rapid transportation, medical evaluation, CT scan interpretation, and injection with a clot-dissolving drug if it is an ischemic stroke and actions for acute hemorrhage if not.

CHAPTER SUMMARY

- It is critical for medical office personnel to be ready to react to an emergency situation. A medical emergency is any situation in which an individual suddenly becomes ill or has an injury or circumstances calling for decided action.
- As part of your preparation for emergency care, the office should have the necessary supplies and equipment to handle any emergency that might come under your care. These items should be collected and set aside in an emergency kit or crash cart, where they will always be ready for use.
- A universal emergency medical identification symbol was designed by the AMA as a means for individuals with certain medical conditions to alert health care workers of their conditions when they are unable to.
- CPR is a life-saving procedure performed when a person's breathing or heartbeat has stopped. CPR involves two elements: chest compressions and artificial respiration (mouth-to-mouth rescue breathing).
- AED units are used in addition to CPR if the heart is in fibrillation or arrest and permits life-saving intervention without the operator needing to evaluate the situation or interpret an ECG. The AED unit is computerized and can analyze the heart rhythm of a person in fibrillation or arrest; recognize a shockable rhythm; and advise the operator through lights and voice prompts if shock is indicated.
- It is realistic to believe that any emergency situation involves exposure to certain body fluids and has the potential for disease transmission. These can be minimized by using a face shield or face mask barrier device. They can provide a degree of protection.
- Several terms describe the severity and length of time for onset of disease or illness: *chronic*, *subtle*, *urgent*, *sudden*, *acute*, *severe*, *life threatening*. Being familiar with the terms will help you establish what your steps will be for preparing and directing the patient.
- Diabetic ketoacidosis, insulin shock, fainting, heart attack, heat and cold exposures, hemorrhaging, poisoning, seizures, obstructed airway, shock, and stroke are common emergencies you might encounter. Understanding the proper protocol to handle each of these conditions, and being able to distinguish symptoms and characteristics of each, is essential in your role as a medical assistant.
- Hyperglycemia is caused by an increased amount of sugar in the body, whereas hypoglycemia is caused by an excess amount of insulin. Being able to recognize the differences in symptoms will assist you in notifying the provider so proper treatment can be given.
- Severe chest pain or pressure, pain radiating down one or both arms, and a tightness of the chest or pain radiating into the left shoulder and jaw (mandible) might indicate symptoms of a heart attack. The pulse is usually rapid and weak. The patient might be perspiring profusely; have cyanotic lips and fingernails; be nauseated, anxious, and agitated; and in denial that anything serious is occurring.

- In heat exhaustion, symptoms such as cool, pale, moist skin with a normal body temperature occur usually after some form of vigorous exercise. The patient becomes overheated with profuse perspiration and might have headaches, muscle cramps, nausea, dizziness, fatigue with a pulse that is weak and rapid, and respirations that are quiet and shallow.
- Heatstroke symptoms include a red, dry face with hot and dry skin. The body temperature can be above 40°C/104°F, and the pulse will be rapid but then gradually slow and weaken. Respirations will be rapid and hollow. The pupils of the eyes will be dilated but equal. Headache, shortness of breath, nausea or vomiting, dizziness, weakness, and dry mouth are common symptoms.
- Symptoms that might indicate damaged tissue (frostbite) are a tingling sensation with numbness followed by pain and redness of the skin. If exposure is continued, the patient might complain of burning and itching. Sensation can be completely lost. The skin might be white or grayish-yellow and waxy in appearance.
- Arterial bleeding produces bright red blood in spurts. Bleeding from a vein produces a steady flow of dark red blood. Any bleeding from capillary damage produces a steady ooze from the wound area.
- Internal bleeding causes symptoms similar to those of shock. The patient can have a rapid, weak pulse; shallow breathing; cold, clammy skin; dilated pupils; dizziness; faintness; thirst, restlessness; and a feeling of anxiety. External signs can include coughing or vomiting up bright red blood or vomiting what looks like coffee grounds. In addition, coal-black stools, bright red rectal bleeding, and severe abdominal pain are other symptoms.
- A seizure is a severe involuntary contraction of muscles that first causes the patient to become rigid and then to have uncontrollable movements. The patient becomes unconscious and can be injured during the seizure. The face and lips can become cyanotic, and the patient might stop breathing. He or she might also lose bladder and bowel control and bite the tongue. When the seizure has stopped, the patient might be confused and complain of headache and exhaustion.
- Obstructed airway most often occurs in adults when food is aspirated while eating. This occurs when partially chewed food is sucked into the trachea when talking, laughing, or coughing while eating. Children, on the other hand, can get toys, toy parts, buttons, candy, or a variety of other objects, in addition to food, caught in their throat and obstruct their airway.
- Shock symptoms include a rapid, thready, weak pulse; shallow, rapid respirations; dilated pupils; ashen color; and cool, clammy skin.
- Signs of a possible stroke can include immediate paralysis in the form of sagging muscles on one side of the face or the inability to use an arm or leg. One entire side of the body might be paralyzed. The patient might complain of numbness. The pupils of the eyes might be unequal in size, and the patient might present mental confusion, slurred speech, nausea, vomiting, or difficulty in breathing and swallowing. Control of urine and bowels can also be lost.

STUDY TOOLS

Workbook	Activities for Chapter 55
Premium Website	
MEDIA LINK	View this **Media Link** for Chapter 55: • Abdominal Thrusts
StudyWARE	Activities and Quizzes on the **StudyWARE™ Software** for Chapter 55
	Complete the following **Competency Challenge 2.0** activity: • Thursday, 11 AM: Prepare for Emergencies
	Audio Library of medical terms
	Online access to the **Critical Thinking Challenge 2.0**
CourseMate	Activities and Quizzes for Chapter 55
WebTutor	Activities and Quizzes for Chapter 55

CHECK YOUR KNOWLEDGE

1. This unit is computerized and can analyze the heart rhythm of a person in fibrillation or arrest, recognize a shockable rhythm, and advise the operator through lights and voice prompts if a shock is indicated.
   a. ECG
   b. AED
   c. EMS
   d. Ambu bag
2. The most immediate information you need to relay to EMS includes:
   a. the nature of the situation and the address of the victim's location.
   b. the victim's name.
   c. the caller's name and phone number in case the connection is lost.
   d. when the problem started.
3. When distinguishing the severity and length of time for onset of disease or illness, which of the following common terms describes having rapid onset, severe symptoms, and a short course?
   a. Chronic
   b. Subtle
   c. Acute
   d. Life threatening
4. In which of the following emergency situations should the patient be given some form of sugar to help alleviate the situation?
   a. Diabetic ketoacidosis
   b. Hyperglycemia
   c. Diaphoresis
   d. Hypoglycemia
5. The signs of a patient having heat exhaustion would be:
   a. pale, cool, and moist skin and normal body temperature.
   b. hot and dry skin and body temperature possibly above 40°C/104°F.
   c. a weak pulse and shallow breathing, body temperature dropping lower than 35°C/95°F.
   d. white or grayish-yellow skin waxy in appearance.
6. Symptoms that might include shortness of breath; a burning sensation in the chest; nausea and vomiting; unexplained fatigue or weakness; and/or pain in the jaw, neck, shoulder, back, or ear could indicate:
   a. heart attack.
   b. stroke.
   c. shock.
   d. seizure.
7. If an obstructed airway is complete, the object must be removed immediately, within ________, to prevent brain damage from lack of oxygen.
   a. 30 seconds
   b. 2 minutes
   c. 4 minutes
   d. 6 minutes
8. Vomiting up what appears to be coffee grounds can indicate:
   a. lung hemorrhage.
   b. a chronic slow bleed of the stomach.
   c. epistaxis.
   d. an ulcer has started bleeding.

WEB LINKS

American Academy of Emergency Medicine: www.aaem.org

American Heart Association: www.heart.org

Mayo Clinic: www.mayoclinic.com

National Institutes of Health: www.nih.gov

U.S. National Library of Medicine: www.nlm.nih.gov

American Red Cross: www.redcross.org

National Center for Emergency Medicine Informatics: www.ncemi.org

RESOURCES

Beebe, R., and Funk, D. (2010). *Fundamentals of Emergency Care* (3rd ed.). Clifton Park, NY: Delmar Cengage Learning.

BLS for Healthcare Providers: Guidelines for CPR and ECC (2005). (2006). Dallas, TX: American Heart Association.

CPR & Sudden Cardiac Arrest (SCA) Fact Sheet. "CPR Statistics." www.heart.org/HEARTORG/CPRAndECC/WhatisCPR/CPRFactsandStats/CPR-Statistics_UCM_307542_Article.jsp. (Retrieved 10/12/2010)

Estes, M. E. Z. (2010). *Health Assessment & Physical Examination* (3rd ed.). Clifton Park, NY: Delmar Cengage Learning.

Heller, M., and Veach, L. (2009). *Clinical Medical Assisting: A Professional, Field Smart Approach to the Workplace*. Clifton Park, NY: Delmar Cengage Learning.

Lindh, W., Pooler, M., Tamparo, C., and Dahl, B. (2010). *Delmar's Comprehensive Medical Assisting Administrative and Clinical Competencies* (4th ed.). Clifton Park, NY: Delmar Cengage Learning.

Simmers, L. (2009). *Diversified Health Occupations* (7th ed.). Clifton Park, NY: Delmar Cengage Learning.

Wellness Letter. (2000). *Is It a Heart Attack? If You're a Woman, Will You Know?* Berkeley: University of California.

Chapter 56 First Aid for Accidents and Injuries

OBJECTIVES

In this chapter, you will learn the following:

KB KNOWLEDGE BASE

1. Spell and define, using the glossary at the back of the text, all the Words to Know in this chapter.
2. Identify four pieces of information that can help you evaluate the severity of an illness or injury when screening a patient over the phone.
3. Describe how to remove foreign bodies from the eyes and ears.
4. Compare and contrast the various types of fractures.
5. Discuss the treatment for animal and human bites.
6. Describe the symptoms of an allergy to stings.
7. Name the three types of burns and give examples of each.
8. Explain the classifications of burns and the treatment for each.
9. Explain the effects of cold and heat applications.
10. Identify and describe the various types of wounds.
11. Explain to the patient the proper care of bandages.

S SKILLS

1. Demonstrate the proper method of cleaning a wound.
2. Demonstrate application of a tube gauze bandage.
3. Demonstrate application of a spiral bandage.
4. Demonstrate application of a figure-eight bandage.
5. Demonstrate application of a cravat bandage to the head.

B BEHAVIORS

1. Apply critical thinking skills in performing patient assessment and care.
2. Use language and verbal skills that enable patients' understanding of the procedure being performed.
3. Concepts of effective communication.

WORDS TO KNOW

abrasion
anaphylactic
avulsion
chemical
cravat
electrical
foreign body
friction
immobilize
incision
laceration
molten
puncture
rabies
shock
splinter
superficial
thermal
wound

ACCIDENTS AND INJURIES

Knowing what to do when an accident or injury occurs is very helpful not only in your professional life but also in your personal life. When you have a basic understanding of first aid, you can respond quickly and efficiently to sudden incidents without becoming overly anxious or upset. As you come in contact with injury incidents, you will learn when they can be handled with simple first aid and when they require the assistance of a provider or advanced emergency medical services. Recall that many illnesses and injuries can occur in varying degrees of severity. As an example, consider a burn. A burn confined just to the skin surface may be managed without medical assistance unless it covers extensive body surface, whereas, a relatively small area of burn can require medical attention if it extends into underlying tissue. If you are ever unsure of the severity of an injury, it is always better to seek medical assistance or advanced emergency services than to underestimate the severity and care needed.

Keep in mind what you learned in Chapter 55 about recognizing and responding to an emergency. When screening patients over the phone, you need specific information before you can determine whether the situation warrants emergency medical care, an office visit, or management at home. Ask the caller to give you a brief history of the victim's situation, the nature of the initial injury or accident, the time the accident occurred or the illness began, and a description of the victim's current condition. Unlike cardiac or respiratory arrest, which always requires emergency response, the sudden accidents and injuries discussed in this chapter might or might not require the same level of response. The decision to seek emergency response depends on the extent and severity of the condition and the reaction or response of the individual. After obtaining the facts, you can respond appropriately as directed.

COMMON INJURIES

There are common injuries you might encounter for which your facility must provide treatment. In some cases, the initial care might be delivered and the patient might then need to be sent to the hospital or specialist for further treatment. Common injuries you might see include foreign bodies within various body areas, dislocations and fractures, strains and sprains, and a variety of wounds that need treatment. Many of these injuries tend not to be life-threatening; however, always be prepared for the occasional injury that needs to be treated as an emergency.

Foreign Bodies

Foreign bodies are substances or objects that become lodged in any part of the human body. Common foreign bodies are dirt, metal shavings, and eyelashes to the eyes; small objects such as beads placed by children in the ears and nose; items accidentally swallowed; and splinters and fishhooks in the skin. Foreign bodies require immediate attention by the provider to prevent further damage.

It is fairly common for a speck of dirt, soot from a fire, or an eyelash to lodge in the eye, for example. Always wash your hands before touching the eyes. A foreign body under the lower lid can usually be seen easily and can be removed with a bit of cotton or a fold of tissue moistened with water. If a foreign body is under the upper lid, it might be possible to remove it by pulling the upper lid down over the lower lid. If this procedure is not successful, it might be necessary to grasp the eyelashes and carefully turn back the upper lid over a cotton swab (Figure 56–1).

An object located under the upper lid may also be removed with a folded piece of moistened sterile gauze. If the material cannot be removed easily or is on the cornea, try flushing with large amounts of water to dislodge it (see Chapter 40). Any object imbedded on the cornea must be removed by the provider. Until the object can be removed, the object must be stabilized by covering both eyes with a sterile compress to help keep the injured eye from moving, which will cause discomfort and additional irritation. The eyes move together, so covering only the injured eye could do more harm than good. If the object is protruding, try covering the eyes with Styrofoam or plastic cups and hold in place with a gauze wrap. This will prevent the object from being pushed deeper into the eye. In addition, warn the patient not to rub the affected eye, which would only embed the object deeper into the cornea. When chemicals, either liquid or powder, get in the eyes, use a sterile eye irrigation solution to dilute and neutralize the chemical.

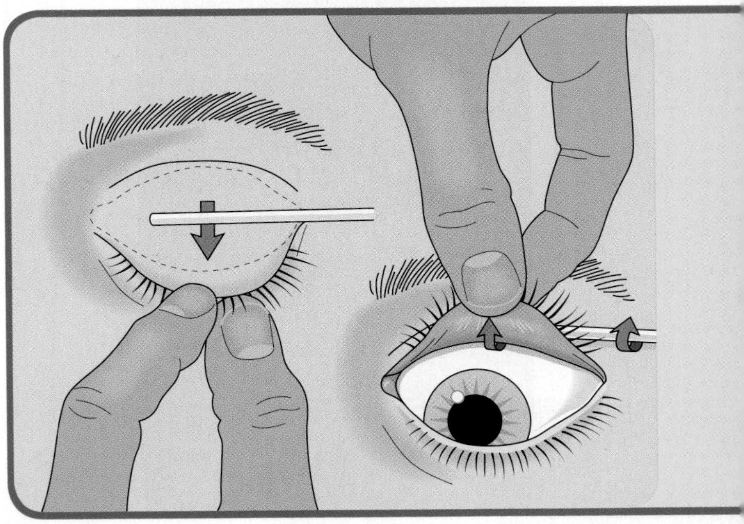

Figure 56–1: Remove a foreign body from upper eyelid by turning the eyelid back over a cotton-tipped swab or the stem of a wooden kitchen match. *Delmar/Cengage Learning.*

This solution should be continuously dripped into the eye for 20 minutes. Pre-packed solutions should be kept in the provider's office for emergency use. If a sterile solution is not available, use any clean tap or bottled water to flush the eye. Eye injuries should be evaluated by a provider as soon as possible.

First aid for an object lodged in the ear consists of placing several drops of warm olive oil, mineral oil, or baby oil into the ear and pulling back on the earlobe to straighten the external canal while the head is tilted toward the unaffected side (Figure 56–2). Then let the oil run out and see whether the object comes out with it. Never try to dig an object out of the ear; damage can be done to the external canal or tympanic membrane. If first aid measures are not successful, a provider should examine the patient.

Children are notorious for putting things, such as beans, pebbles, buttons, or marbles, in their ears or up their noses. Instilling oil in the ear when there are large, smooth objects to be removed might make them more difficult to grasp and retrieve. Often, these can be removed from the nose with forceps or irrigated out of an ear by directing water against the wall of the external canal. (Refer to Chapter 40 on ear irrigation.) However, water should never be used with any object, such as beans or peas that would swell, thereby causing pain and making removal much more difficult.

You might get a call from a parent who is frightened because a child has swallowed a small object. It is best for the provider to perform an X-ray examination such as a fluoroscopic exam to see whether the object is actually in the stomach. If the object is not sharp, it might pass through the intestinal tract and be eliminated in the stool.

Splinters can generally be removed with a sterile needle and splinter forceps in the office. The skin should be washed with soap and water. Lift the end of the exposed splinter with the sterile needle and it remove it by grasping with a pair of sterile splinter forceps. If a splinter or thorn is under a fingernail, it is best to have a provider remove it. After the splinter or thorn is removed, the area should again be washed with soap and water; apply antibiotic ointment and cover with an adhesive bandage.

Another common injury involving a foreign body is that of an embedded fish hook. One of the hazards of fishing, or of being around individuals who are casting for fish, is that hooks can become embedded in fingers, backs, scalps, or any part of the anatomy that is exposed. It is best for a provider to use a local anesthetic for such removal. When the area is numb, the provider can push the barb on through the flesh and then cut if off with a pair of nipper pliers (Figure 56–3). After this is done, you can back out the remainder of the hook. Another possibility is to cut off the shank of the hook and pull out the barbed end. After the hook is removed, the area should be carefully cleaned with an antimicrobial soap or solution; apply antibiotic ointment and a dry dressing. As with any injury, a tetanus toxoid booster might be needed if it has been longer than five years since the last booster. The provider might also prescribe an antibiotic.

Strains and Sprains

Strains are the result of overuse of a muscle or group of muscles or when a muscle or tendon is overextended by stretching. They can be caused by improper lifting or

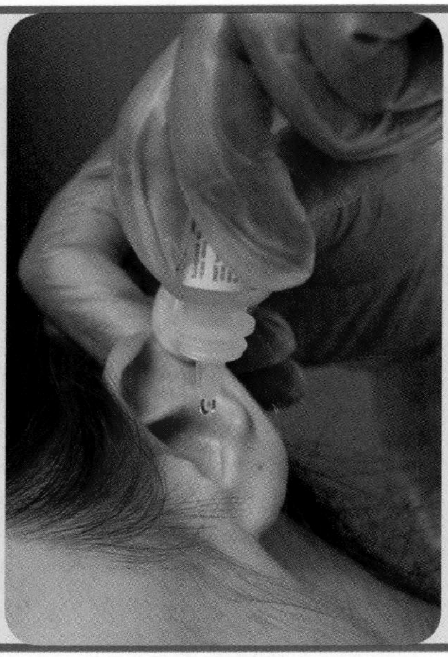

Figure 56–2: After the patient's head is tilted to the side, pull back on the ear to straighten the external canal and instill ear drops. *Delmar/Cengage Learning.*

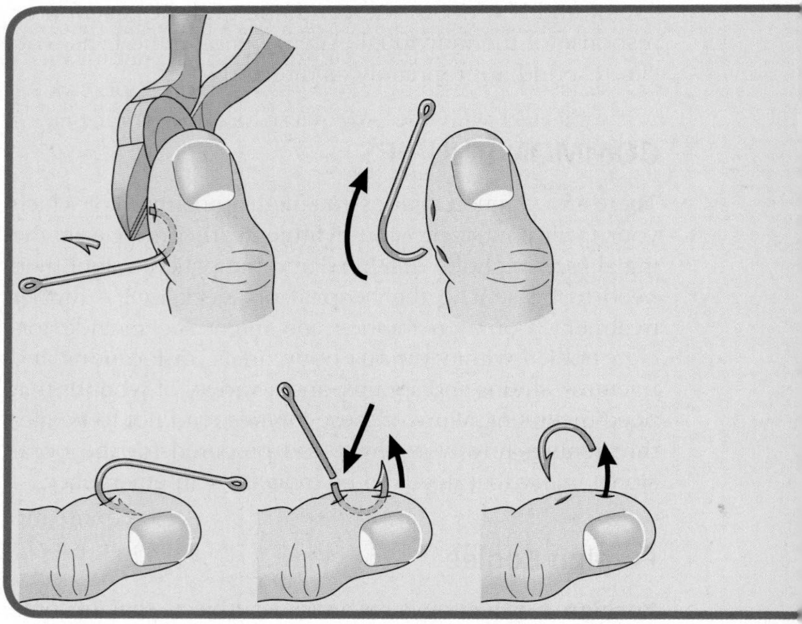

Figure 56–3: Fish hook removal by (A) cutting the barb or (B) cutting the shank. *Delmar/Cengage Learning.*

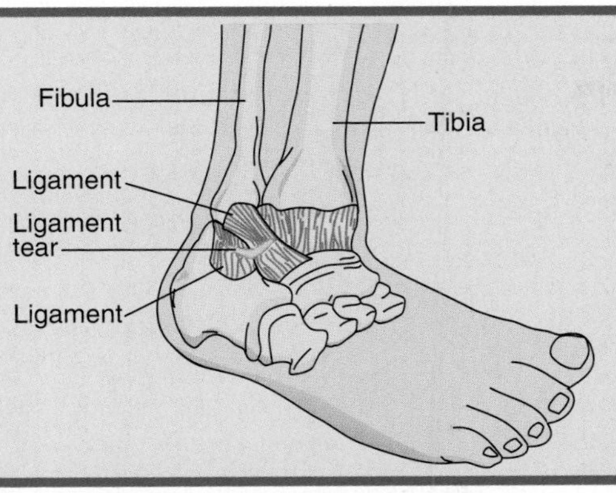

Figure 56–4: In an ankle sprain, one or more of the ligaments can be torn or stretched. *Delmar/Cengage Learning.*

by slipping while moving a heavy object. Muscle strain is common after engaging in any strenuous activity that you are not accustomed to doing (Figure 56–4).

Sprains occur when muscles, tendons, or ligaments surrounding a joint are torn. They are usually the result of overuse or trauma from twisting the joint and are sometimes so severe that a fracture can also occur. A common site is the ankle.

First aid for both sprains and strains is to rest the injured muscles in a comfortable position and use what is known as RICE (rest, ice, compression, elevation) or a newer term, PRINCE (protection, rest, ice, NSAIDS or acetaminophen, compression, and elevation) method. Protect the injury by using some form of support mechanism such as an ACE bandage or ankle stirrup if an ankle is involved. Rest the involved area. If a lower extremity is involved, the patient might want to use crutches until the area is pain free. Ice the area for the first 48 to 72 hours or until the swelling is reduced. Non-steroidal medications (NSAIDS) such as ibuprofen or acetaminophen can be used for pain and swelling. Compression can be accomplished with the ACE wrap or ankle brace if an ankle injury (refer to Procedure 56–4 on applying an elastic bandage); be sure the supportive device is not too loose or tight. Elevate the injured area for approximately two to three days, making sure to elevate the involved area higher than the heart.

Dislocations

At least half of all dislocations involve the shoulder, but dislocations are possible at any freely moving joint. When a bone end slips out of the socket or when the capsule surrounding a joint is stretched or torn, a dislocation is likely to occur. There is usually severe pain and obvious deformity of the joint area and possible loss of function of the affected limb. There is also noticeable swelling. Dislocations are best treated by a provider. The only first aid measure is to **immobilize** the dislocation during the trip to the medical office or hospital. Treat all sprains, strains, and dislocations as if they are a fracture. The injured extremity should be carefully supported in the position in which it was found to avoid additional injury. This involves splinting from the joint above to the joint below the injury. With a shoulder involvement, this probably involves immobilizing the affected arm by wrapping it to the body for support. (Refer to Chapter 57 for applying an arm sling.)

Fractures

Fractures are breaks in a bone caused by trauma or bone disease. There are several types of fractures; however, they are all classified as either open or closed (Figure 56–5). In a *closed* or *simple fracture*, there is no open wound. In an *open* or *compound fracture*, there is an open wound. First aid for an open fracture is to control bleeding and to splint without moving the bone ends. The patient might also need to be treated for **shock**. Check the pulse and motor and sensory reflexes (PMS). Capillary refill of the distal area to all fracture sites on an injured limb will be impaired. To ensure good perfusion and unimpaired neurological function, treatment must be administered as soon as possible. A fracture can be accurately diagnosed only by an X-ray unless bone ends can be seen in an open wound or a severe deformity is present. A provider is the only person who should attempt to straighten, or reduce, a fracture. Refer to Table 56–1 for a description of the various types of fractures.

BITES AND STINGS

Bites and stings are common occurrences that seem more likely in the summertime.

Bites can occur from animals (both pets and strays) and humans. They can be **superficial** or can break the skin, causing a **puncture** or **laceration**. Stings come from, bees, wasps, hornets, and other insects and can present very minimal symptoms such as swelling, redness, and itching or be life threatening.

Animal Bites

An animal bite can tear skin and cause a bruise. The bite is dangerous because of the possibility of infection or **rabies**. The **wound** should be thoroughly cleansed with an antiseptic soap and rinsed well with water. The area should be bandaged and immobilized, and the patient should be examined by a provider as soon as possible. The bite must be reported to the police or local health authorities, who will examine the animal for rabies. Generally, the animal should be held for observation for at least 15 days to see whether it is rabid. The decision must be made regarding the use of anti-rabies serum, depending on what is known about the animal and what type of animal it is. If the skin is broken and

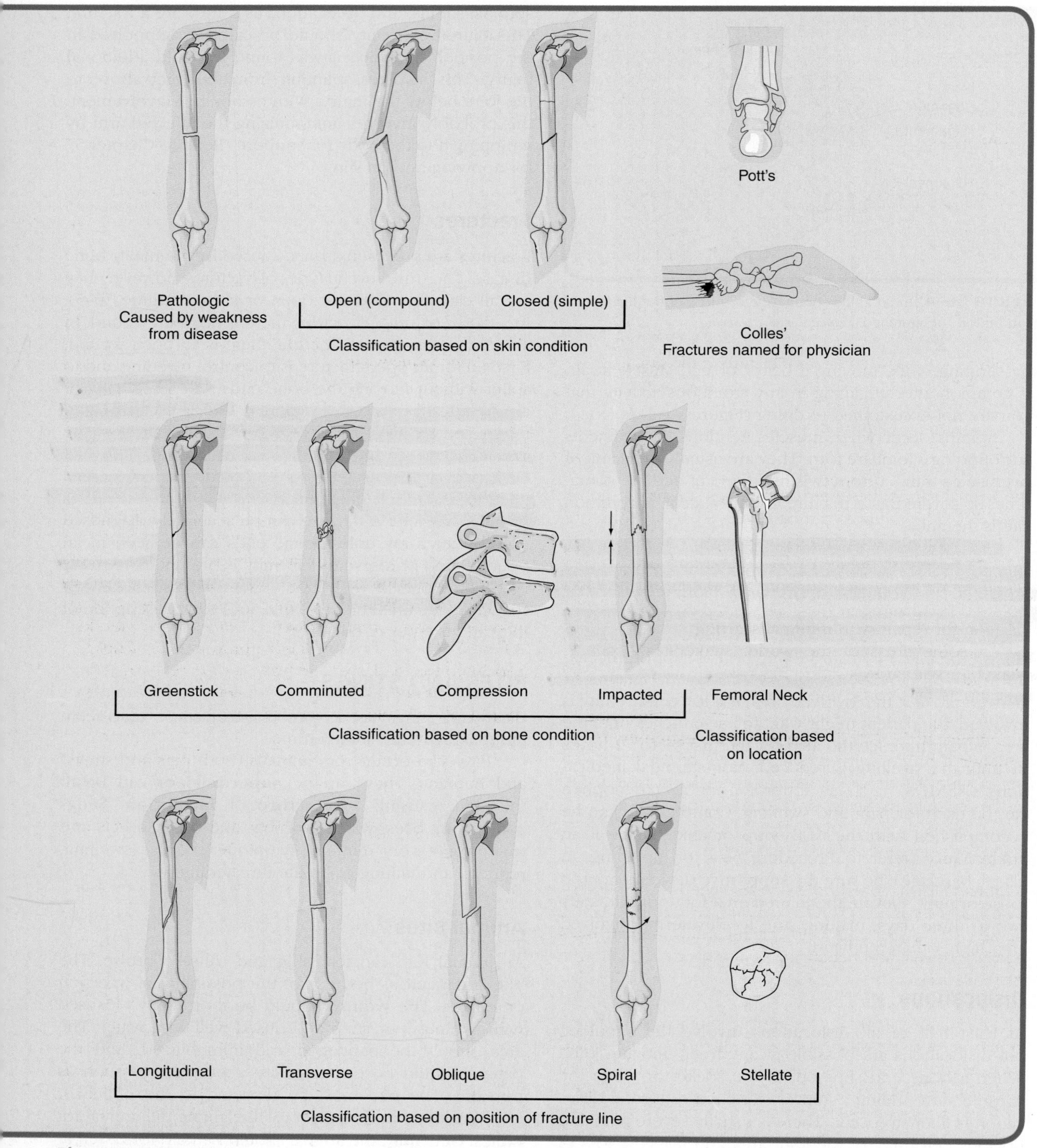

Figure 56–5: Types of fractures. *Delmar/Cengage Learning.*

TABLE 56–1 Types of Fractures

Name	Description
Greenstick (incomplete)	Bone partially bent and partially broken; often occurs in children
Closed (simple, complete)	Skin intact over the fracture; bone is completely broken into two or more pieces.
Transverse	Fracture crosses the bone at a 90° angle to the bone's axis
Oblique	A diagonal fracture of a bone
Open (compound)	Open wound over the ends of the fractured bones; often an end of the bone is visible
Impacted	One bone fragment is wedged into the other bone fragment
Comminuted	Crushing or splintering of the bone
Spiral	Fracture spirals around a long bone; occurs as the result of the bone twisting
Depressed	Fragments or portions of the bone pressed down into the skull; can be into the brain and surrounding tissue
Colles	Fracture of the distal end of the radius bone in the wrist
Potts	Fracture of the lower part of the fibula with serious injury of the lower tibial articulation, usually a chipping off of a portion of the medial malleolus or rupture of the medial ligament

the animal cannot be tested, anti-rabies serum should be used. When the animal can be observed and is found to be free of rabies, no serum is necessary.

Bites can also result in a laceration and need suture repair. Generally, when children are bitten on the face, arms, or hands, the provider will refer them to a plastic surgeon for repair with minimal scarring.

In some areas of the world, snakebites occur. A snakebite will show a two-fang wound. Recommended first aid is to cleanse the area to remove any surface venom with antibacterial soap and water and immobilize the victim. If the bite is located on an extremity, try to maintain the extremity *below* the level of the heart. Do not cut into the wound or attempt to suck out venom. Do not apply cold packs or ice or apply a tourniquet.

Human Bites

A human bite that breaks the skin also needs to be cleaned with antibacterial soap and water, and the patient should be seen by a provider. Concern regarding human bites because of HIV and hepatitis B is also an issue. Although the transmission of HIV is not likely (the only way HIV could be transmitted in this manner is if the bite breaks the skin and the person doing the biting has bleeding gums), it is a possibility. Patients who have sustained such a bite from another person should be advised to have injections to be immunized against hepatitis B. With all bites, a tetanus injection must be administered to the patient if he or she has not received one within five years.

Stings

Bees, wasps, and hornets cause deaths every year. If the victim is not sensitive to the sting, the result can be only a painful swelling with redness and itching. When several stings are received at one time, the victim can become quite ill and might develop severe hives or generalized edema. When a patient is severely allergic to stings, the sting can cause acute illness. The patient can become restless, complain of headache, have shortness of breath, or have mottled blueness of the skin. When shortness of breath is not apparent, the victim can appear to be in shock and have severe nausea, vomiting, and bloody diarrhea. The severely allergic patient should always have a special emergency kit known as an EpiPen, which is a self-administered epinephrine injection, close at hand when a sting is possible (Figure 56–6). If anaphylactic shock is evident, epinephrine should be given as a lifesaving measure. (Refer to Chapter 55 for a discussion about **anaphylactic** shock and stings.)

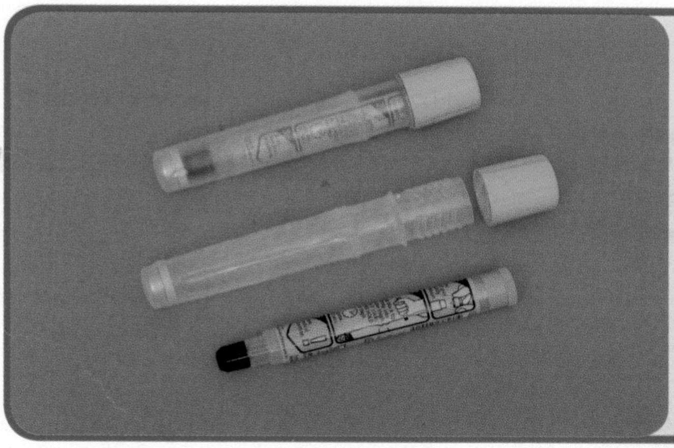

Figure 56–6: EpiPens. *Delmar/Cengage Learning.*

A honeybee leaves the stinger in the skin, and it should be immediately removed by scraping it out carefully with a credit card or other rigid object. This is usually the only treatment needed. You can make a paste of baking soda and water to be applied to the area or apply an anti-itch cream, lotion, or gel such as Benadryl. Never grasp the stinger with your fingers or a tweezers because that would inject more of the venom. Wasps, hornets, and yellow jackets retain their stingers and can unfortunately sting repeatedly; therefore, no stinger can be removed.

BURNS

According to the American Burn Association, there are one million burn injuries in the United States and an estimated 45,000 hospitalizations per year. Extensive burns require painful treatment and a long period of rehabilitation. They often result in permanent disfigurement and physical and emotional problems.

Types of Burns

Burns are basically of three types: **thermal**, **chemical**, and **electrical**, with thermal being the most common.

- *Thermal*—Caused by residential fires; automobile accidents; playing with matches; accidents with gasoline, space heaters, or firecrackers; scalding water from the stove or tub; and coming in contact with curling irons, stoves, or clothing irons. Some childhood burns, such as from cigarettes, can be traced to deliberate abuse. Sunburn occurs from overexposure to the sun.
- *Chemical*—From contact with, ingestion, inhalation, or injection of acids or alkalines.
- *Electrical*—Occur after contact with faulty electrical wiring, a child chewing on an electrical cord, or from downed high-voltage power lines. Although rare, an electrical burn can also come from a lightning strike.

Classification of Burns

Burns are classified by three methods. One is by the percentage of body surface area (BSA) involved in the burn. The Rule of Nines illustrated in Figure 56–7A and the Lund and Browder chart in Figure 56–7B are methods to estimate the size of the burn. These methods establish a standard by which all injuries can be estimated. The Lund and Browder chart is more specific and has a way to estimate areas for different age groups because body proportions are quite different for infants and small children as compared with adults.

A familiar classification reflects the extent of burn as a relationship to the layer of skin involved and is estimated from one to four degrees (Figure 56–8). A first-degree burn (also called a superficial burn) involves an injury primarily to the epidermis, resulting in reddening of the skin and moderately severe pain. A sunburn or contact with boiling water or steam can cause this type of burn (Figure 56–9A). A second-degree burn (also called a partial-thickness burn) involves the epidermis and part of the dermis. The leakage of plasma and electrolytes from the capillaries damaged by the burn into the surrounding tissues raises the epidermis to form blisters and results in mild to moderate edema and pain (Figure 56–9B). Third- or fourth-degree burns (also called full thickness burns) involve the epidermis, dermis, and subcutaneous skin layers, including fat and muscle tissue (Figure 56–9 C). No blisters appear, but white, leathery tissue and thrombosed vessels are visible. Although most providers have combined the third- and fourth-degree burns into the same category and consider them third-degree burns, some use the term *fourth-degree burn* for burns involving all layers of the skin, muscle, and bone. This can result from an industrial injury such as contact with **molten** metal.

Another classification of burns measures the severity of a burn by a combination of two methods. It correlates the burn's depth with its size (BSA) to determine its severity, which is then classified as a minor, moderate, or major burn.

- A *minor* burn has less than 2% of BSA at the third-degree level and burns on less than 15% for adults and 10% for children at the second-degree level.
- A *moderate* burn is when third-degree burns cover 2% to 10% of BSA; second-degree burns cover from 15% to 25% on adults or over 10% on children.
- A *major* burn is when a third-degree burn covers more than 10% of BSA or second-degree burns cover more than 25% in adults or 20% in children; burns of the hands, feet, or genitalia are also major burns; burns that are complicated by fractures, affect poor-risk patients, or are electrical are also major burns.

The classification of burns is at the discretion of the provider or the treatment facility involved.

Treatment of Burns

The treatment of burns depends on the classification of the burn, although the first priority is to stop the burning process. Treat first-degree burns with cold water and a dressing to protect the area. Applying cold water

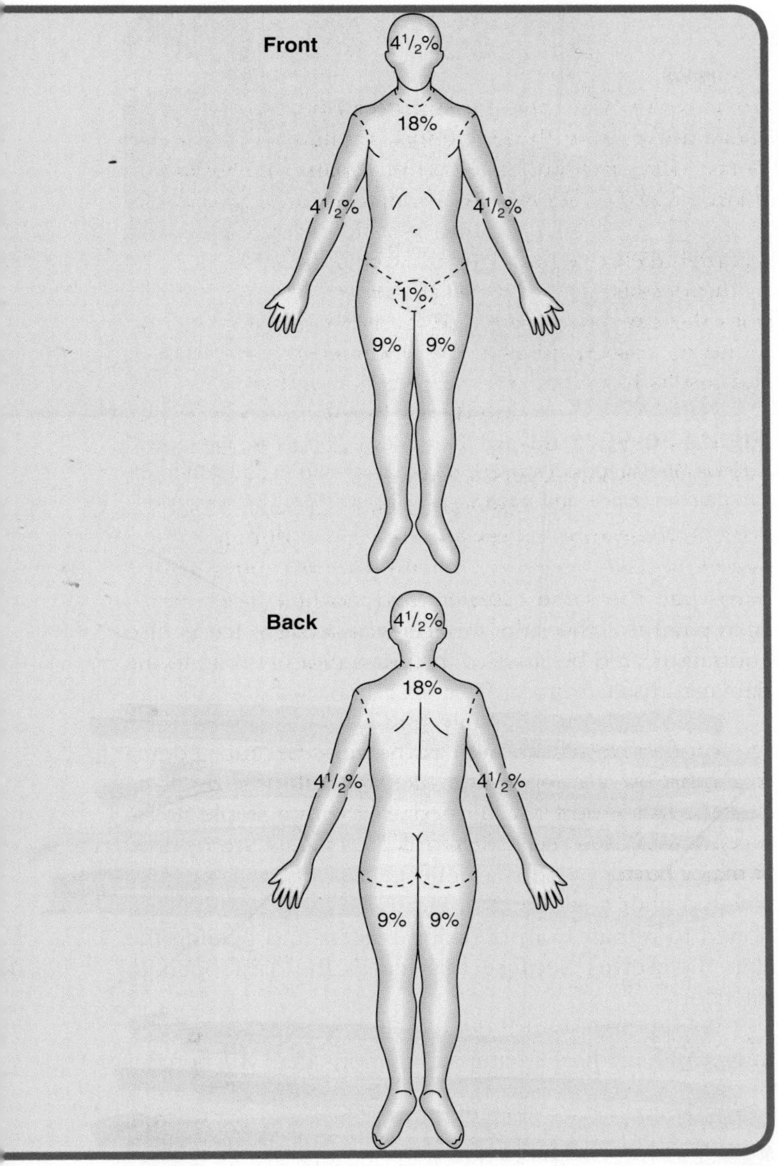

Figure 56–7A: Diagram for use in calculating the extent of burns or other injuries for an adult. *Delmar/Cengage Learning.*

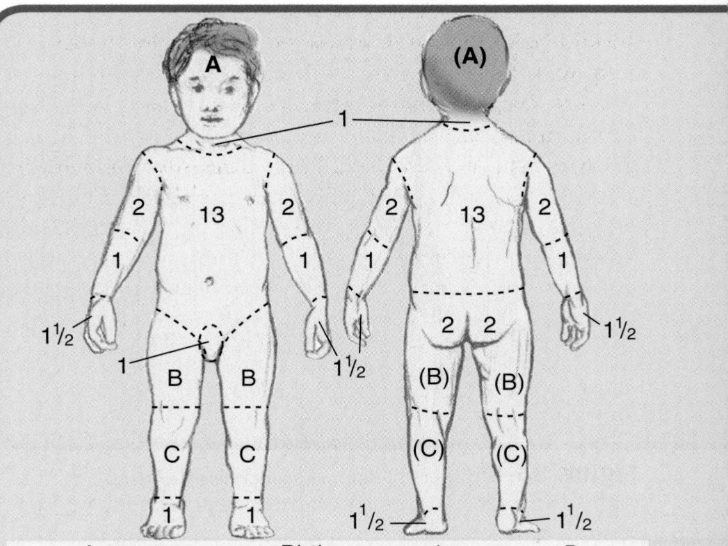

Area	Birth	1 yr	5 yr
A (head)	19	17	14
B (one thigh)	6½	7½	9
C (one leg)	6	6	6

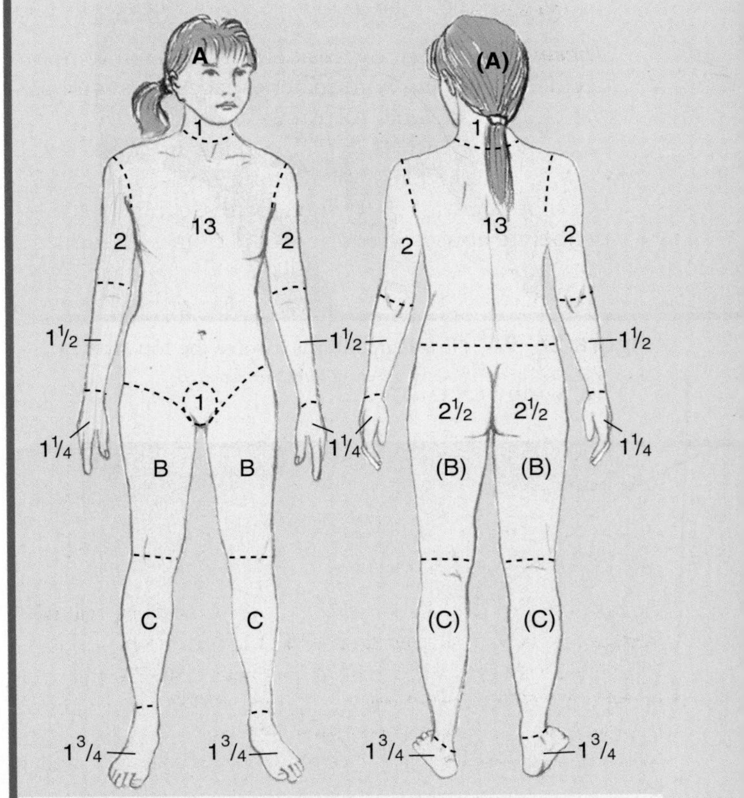

Area	10 yr	15 yr	Adult
A (head)	11	9	8
B (one thigh)	8½	9	9
C (one leg)	6	6½	7

Figure 56–7B: Lund and Browder chart. *Delmar/Cengage Learning.*

to the area should stop the pain and might even keep the burn from progressing into deeper tissue layers. Encourage a victim of severe sunburn to soak in a tub of cool water and drink large amounts of fluids. Patients who are on photosensitive drugs need to be warned about their increased danger from exposure to the sun and the need to wear protective sunscreen and clothing. Pharmacists generally place a warning label on the prescription bottles containing these drugs. The application of butter or ointments is contraindicated for two reasons: it will hold in the burn and cause more pain, and it will be painful to remove when the burn is evaluated and treated. In addition, butter contains salt, which would be

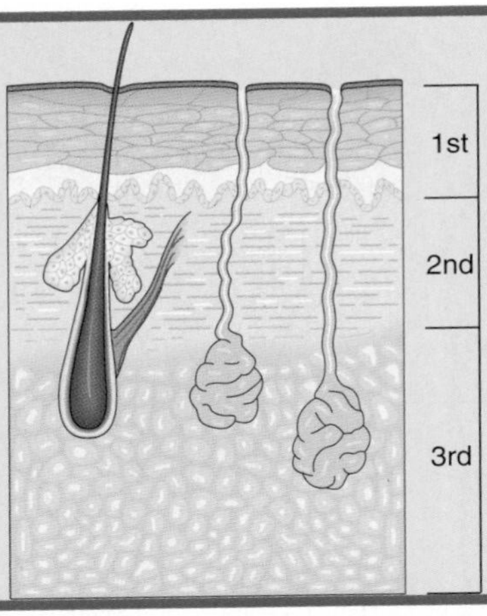

Figure 56–8: Layers of skin. *Delmar/Cengage Learning.*

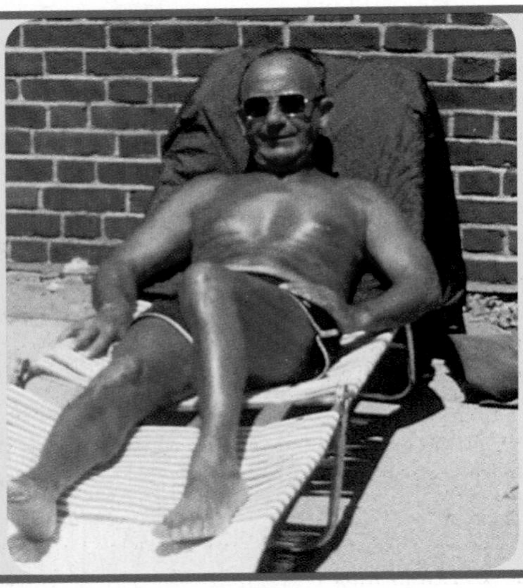

Figure 56–9A: First-degree burns involve the top layer of skin. *Courtesy of the Phoenix Society of Burn Survivors, Inc.*

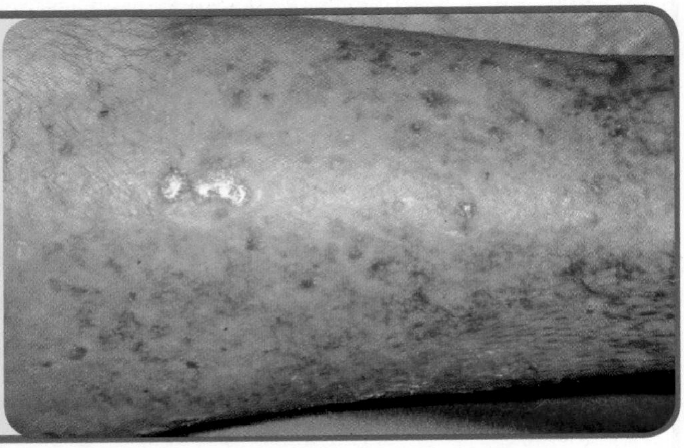

Figure 56–9B: Second-degree, or partial-thickness burns affect the top layers of skin. The healing process is slower, and scarring can occur. *Courtesy of the Phoenix Society of Burn Survivors, Inc.*

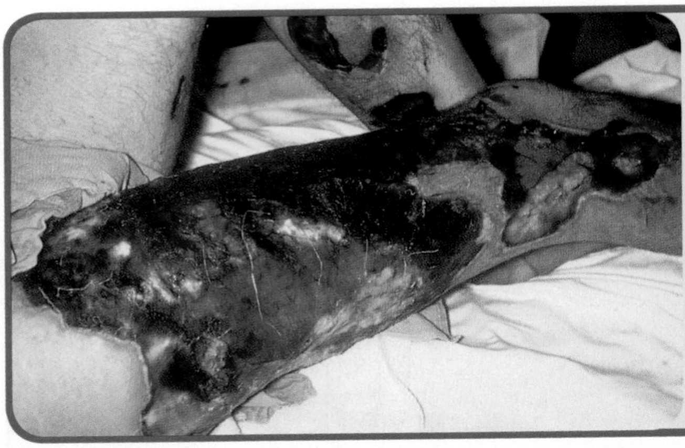

Figure 56–9C: Third- and fourth-degree burns are the most serious, affecting or destroying all layers of skin in addition to the fat, muscle, bones, and nerves. *Courtesy of the Phoenix Society of Burn Survivors, Inc.*

very painful if the skin surface was broken. Ice is also contraindicated because of the chance of frostbite to the damaged tissue.

In second-degree burns, first aid can include treatment for shock, removal of any jewelry because edema might be severe, providing ample amounts of liquid to drink, and covering the burned area with a sterile dressing. Healing can be facilitated if the blisters are opened by the provider under aseptic conditions and the area covered with a sterile dressing. Patients should be cautioned to refrain from breaking blisters and peeling the skin themselves because this leaves the area open to infection.

Third- and fourth-degree burns should receive immediate medical treatment. If more than 10 percent of the BSA is involved, it is considered a major burn and requires surgical intervention, IV fluids for fluid replacement, medication for pain, and probably tetanus antitoxin or a toxoid booster shot if it has been longer than five years since the patient has received one. The only first aid that is appropriate is to cover the burned area with sterile dressings and treat the patient for shock. Remember to avoid applying a dressing to second- and third-degree burns with any material that could adhere to the area because it will cause pain and tissue damage when it has to be removed. No attempt should be made to remove clothing that is in contact with the burn. The patient will need surgical care to remove the burned fabric, clean the area, and dress the wound.

Treating Electrical and Chemical Burns

When burns are caused by electricity or chemicals, other factors must be considered before first aid can be given. An electrical burn results from contact with electrical wiring, power lines, or lightning. The first concern is to remove the victim from the source of electricity—but only *after* the electrical source has been turned off. This situation requires evaluation. If the electrical source is from the wiring within a home, the main electrical supply coming into the house can be shut off at the electrical box, thereby making rescue safe. If the electrical source is power lines, the electric company must be summoned. If the person and the electrical source are in a wet area, keep in mind that electricity conducts well through water. If you come in contact with the water, you could receive a severe shock or be electrocuted. EMS personnel have been electrocuted trying to rescue people from situations involving downed wires and water. Because of this potential for a lethal accident, policy states that they must summon the electric company or the fire department to deal with the electrical source prior to any rescue attempt.

If the voltage is of a sufficient amount, it is possible for the victim to suffer circulatory and respiratory arrest, which necessitates administering CPR and obtaining advanced medical care. The everyday electrical burn is treated like any other burn; however, the extent of the damage might not be readily observable. Electrical burns can cause extensive internal damage along the conduction pathway, which can take a few days to manifest itself. Persons struck by lightning need CPR and immediate emergency treatment. They might have the hallmark ferning markings on their body, which are characteristic of lightning burns. They might, too, have extensive internal damage and, if they were standing when struck, have extensive burns to the soles of the feet where the lightning exits the body.

Chemical burns are treated by removing any clothing from the burn area and then immediately flooding the area with water for at least 15 minutes. A dry chemical should first be brushed off carefully before flushing the patient's skin because some chemicals, such as lime, are activated by water. Following the flooding of water, chemical burns, like all other burns, should be covered with a sterile dressing. A chemical burn of the eye should be flooded with water continuously for at least 20 minutes. A provider should always examine eye burns immediately.

APPLYING HEAT AND COLD TREATMENTS

In the treatment of injuries, providers often order the application of a heat or cold pack. The provider will give specific instructions concerning the length of time and where to apply the treatment.

Many offices and clinics today use disposable heat and cold packs because of their convenience (Figure 56–10).

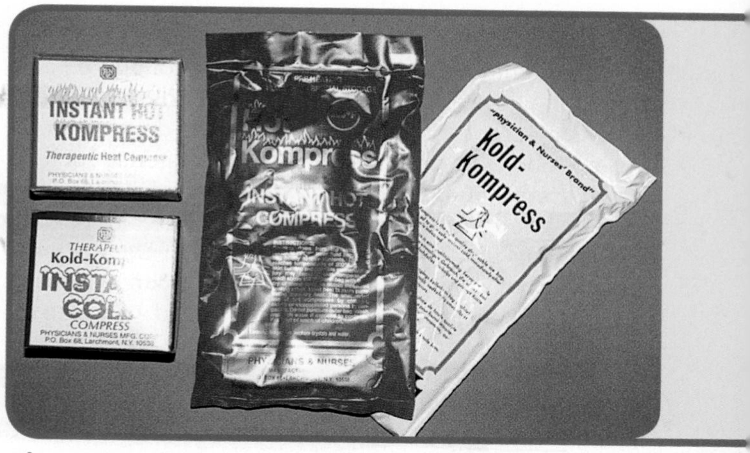

Figure 56–10: Hot and cold packs. *Delmar/Cengage Learning.*

These plastic packs contain chemicals that are activated by either squeezing the bag or mixing the contents to produce cold or by bending a metal disc to initiate heat. Many of these disposable packs are reusable by boiling or freezing them, which is of further convenience to the patient. When using these packs, it is recommended for them to be placed in a cloth covering or a disposable towel to protect the skin. If the provider requests moist heat or cold treatment, you should use a clean, moist cloth towel between the plastic pack and the skin. Moisture facilitates conduction to tissues. Moist heat is less likely to cause burns of the skin, and it provides deeper penetration to tissues. Unless otherwise ordered by the provider, the pack should be left in place for 20 minutes at a time. Generally, the standard instruction is on for 20 minutes and off for 10. This may be repeated to increase circulation, but constant hot or cold is never advised.

The application of cold decreases bacterial growth, body temperature, and local circulation temporarily. It also is a temporary anesthetic, relieves inflammation, helps control bleeding, and reduces swelling. The average temperature is between 10°C and 26.7°C (50°F and 80°F). Cold applications are used in burns, sprains, strains, and bruises and in the initial treatment of injuries to the eye.

Heat applications are used to increase tissue temperature, circulation, and rate of healing. When heat is applied to an injured area, pain decreases. The average temperature is between 40.6°C and 49°C (105°F and 120°F). Heat treatments relieve congestion in deep muscle layers and visceral organs and muscle spasms. The heat dilates blood vessels, which helps increase circulation and reduce localized swelling *after* the initial 48 to 72 hours of cold treatment following the injury.

WOUNDS

It is important to know the characteristics of and be able to identify and treat many types of wounds. **Abrasions** involve a scrape of the epidermis with dots of blood and possibly the presence of foreign material such as dirt or gravel (56–11). First aid is to clean the area carefully with soap and water, apply an antiseptic solution or ointment, and cover with a dressing. If the abrasion resulted from contact with rusty metal or an unusually dirty object, an injection of tetanus toxoid or antitoxin might be required.

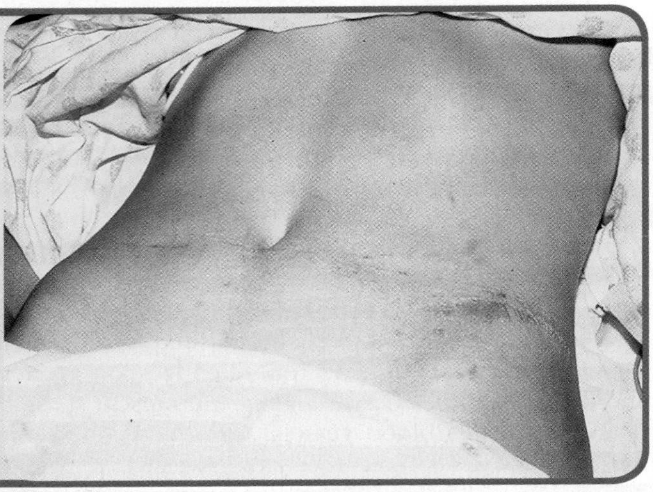

Figure 56–11: Abrasion. *Delmar/Cengage Learning.*

An **avulsion** is when the skin is torn off and the wound is bleeding profusely. Avulsions generally occur on limbs and appendages such as fingers, toes, hands, arms, and legs. Often, they occur during a motor vehicle accident or when a body part gets caught in machinery. Clean the wound with soap and water and replace the skin flap in its original position. Apply pressure to control the bleeding. When the bleeding has stopped, apply a pressure bandage.

A wound caused by a sharp object that leaves a clean cut is called an **incision** and can need sutures to close (Figure 56–12). Some people prefer to use tape Steri-Strips for closure rather than sutures if the wound is not too long and not in an area that bends. The area must be carefully cleaned with soap and water, and an antiseptic can be applied before covering with a sterile dressing.

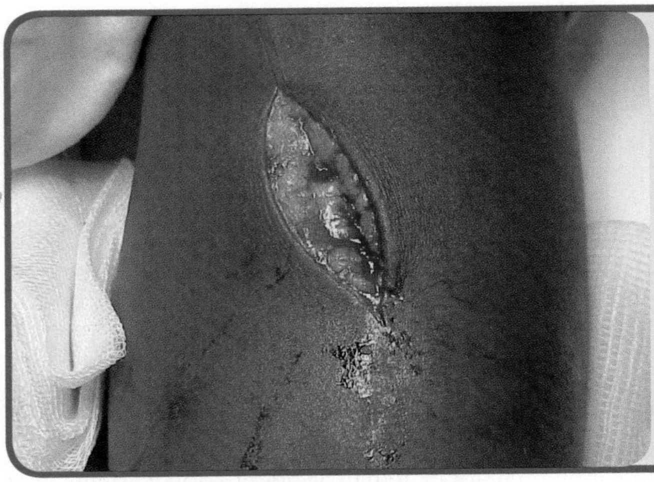

Figure 56–12: Incision. *Delmar/Cengage Learning.*

A laceration is a tearing of body tissue and is more difficult to clean and suture properly (Figure 56–13). Special care must be taken to avoid infection. In the first aid care of an incision or laceration, the first concern must be control of bleeding. Apply direct pressure to the wound area and elevate the extremity. If direct pressure is not effective, apply indirect pressure on the appropriate pressure point.

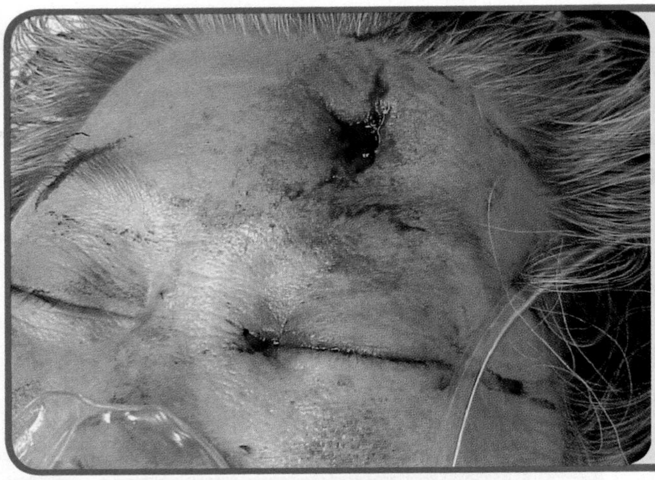

Figure 56–13: Laceration. *Delmar/Cengage Learning.*

A puncture wound is one made with a pointed object, such as an ice pick, knife, or nail (Figure 56–14). First aid is to clean the wound area and, if necessary, enlarge the hole with a probe to allow for irrigation with antiseptic solutions. A puncture wound can also be the result of an animal or human bite, as mentioned earlier. It is usually possible to identify the type of bite by looking at the shape of the wound. A human bite is identified by the shape of the denture and needs to be cleaned carefully.

Cleaning Wounds

Human skin cannot be sterilized, but the microorganisms that might be harmful can be washed off the skin's surface

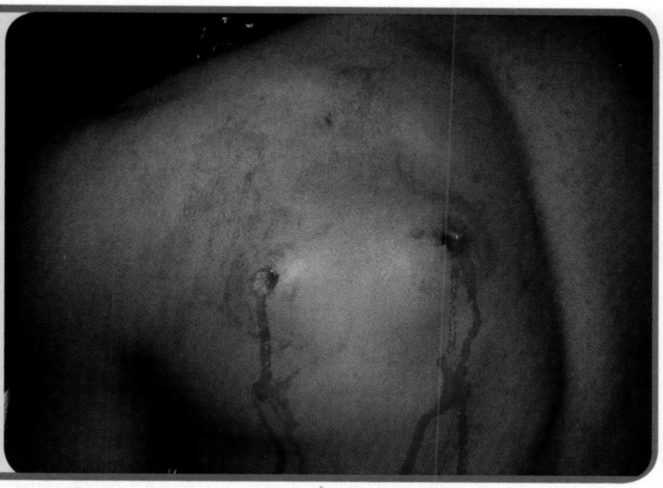

Figure 56–14: Puncture. *Delmar/Cengage Learning.*

with Betadine or other antimicrobial solution, water, and **friction**. Applying an antiseptic following the washing makes the skin essentially germ free. The procedure of cleaning a wound is usually the responsibility of the medical assistant and is presented in Procedure 56–1.

When the wound does not bleed excessively and does not involve tissues below the skin, the area can be thoroughly cleaned. If a wound is superficial and will heal well with simple cleaning and protection from contamination, sutures are unnecessary. Soaking the wound area in an antiseptic solution might be necessary if debris is ground in. This helps loosen the debris and make the cleaning process easier. Some clean cuts can be closed with adhesive Steri-Strips or butterfly closures, depending on the length, depth, and severity of the wound.

PROCEDURE 56–1 Clean Wound Areas

MEDIA LINK: View the video, "Clean Wound Areas," for this chapter on the Premium Website.

PURPOSE: To remove blood, debris, and surface microorganisms from the area of injury

EQUIPMENT: Basin, antibacterial solution (Betadine), warm water, sterile gauze sponges, sterile sponge forceps, gloves, sterile water, irrigation syringe, biohazard and regular waste receptacle, bandage and tape, patient chart or EHR, pen

S **SKILL:** Demonstrate the proper method of cleaning a wound.

Procedure Steps	Detailed Instructions and/or *Rationales*
1. Assemble the equipment and materials, wash hands, and put on gloves.	
B 2. Introduce yourself, identify the patient, and ***explain the procedure, using language the patient can understand.***	*Ensures that you are performing the procedure on the correct patient. Giving patients an explanation helps allay any fears about the procedure.*
3. Grasp several gauze sponges with sponge forceps.	
4. Dip the sponges into warm detergent water.	Make certain the water is at a comfortable temperature.
5. Wash the wound and wound area to remove microorganisms and any foreign matter.	Be careful not to injure the patient further with the instrument. Clean the wound area with sponges only, working from the inside to 2 or 3 inches around the wound as you would for a surgical prep. If there is a lot of debris on the wound, you might soak the wound in an antibacterial solution first. *This prevents bringing microorganisms from the surrounding skin into an open wound.*
6. Discard the sponges in proper waste receptacle.	Unless the sponges are soaked or dripping with blood or body fluids, a regular receptacle is used.

(continues)

(continued)

Procedure Steps	Detailed Instructions and/or *Rationales*
7. Irrigate the wound thoroughly with sterile water.	
8. Blot the wound dry with sterile gauze and dispose of the gauze in the proper waste receptacle.	
B 9. ***Call the provider to inspect the wound and assist as needed with treatment.***	
10. Apply a sterile dressing and bandage it in place (Figure 56–15).	The provider might order an antibiotic ointment to be applied; this not only helps prevent infection but keeps the wound from sticking to the bandage.
B 11. ***Instruct patient in how to care for the bandage and to watch for signs of circulation impairment and infection.***	The patient should be told to watch for redness, swelling, and sensation of pain or fever. Typed instructions should be given to the patient for follow-up care.
12. Clean up the work area.	Place all used materials and gloves in the proper waste receptacle for safe disposal.
13. Wash hands.	
14. Document.	

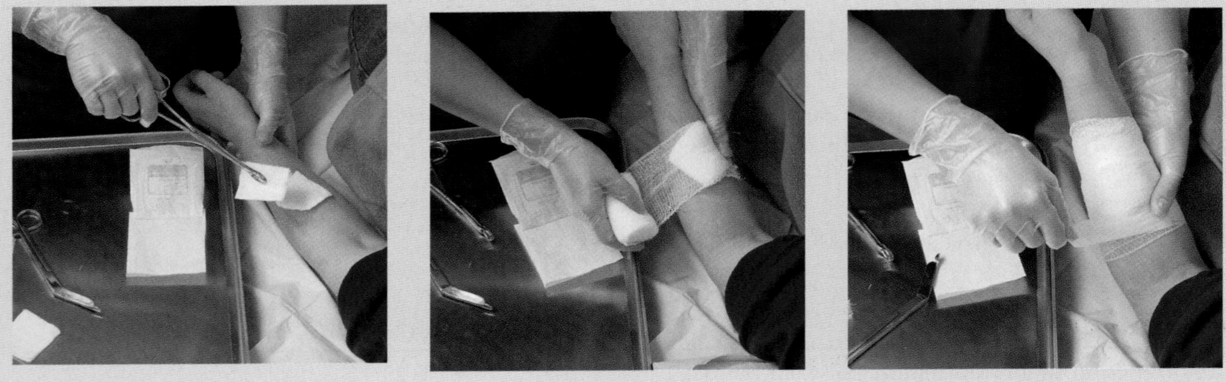

Figure 56–15: Apply sterile gauze and bandage in to place. *Delmar/Cengage Learning.*

Charting Example

65-3-XX 1:25 PM	Extensive wound over knee and lateral surface of right leg from fall off bicycle onto gravel area by road. Also jagged 10 cm laceration from broken glass fragment. Wound cleansed thoroughly with antibacterial solution and water. Two glass fragments removed and wound closed with four sutures by provider. Sterile dressing, antibiotic ointment, and bandage applied. Patient given follow-up instructions and patient education provided. Patient tolerated procedure well. S. Davis, RMA(AMT)

When bleeding has been severe, no attempt should be made to clean the area because it can restart the bleeding. Because the patient will need additional medical care, it can be cleaned then. A pressure bandage should be applied securely and the patient taken for emergency medical care immediately. (A pressure bandage usually consists of multiple layers of gauze squares or pads tightly fastened to the skin with tape or bound with a roller bandage or ACE bandage. If such a patient comes to your office, wait for instructions from the provider before removing the pressure dressing. You will be responsible for having a suture set up for use when the provider is ready. You might question the patient or a relative to find out what caused the wound and how large and deep it is. You should also inquire about the most recent tetanus immunization booster and record the information on the patient's chart. The general rule is for the patient to have a tetanus injection every 10 years; however, for an injury, the requirement changes to every five years. The provider will write the orders for the necessary immunizations. You should not proceed with any medication or injection until the order has been written by the provider.

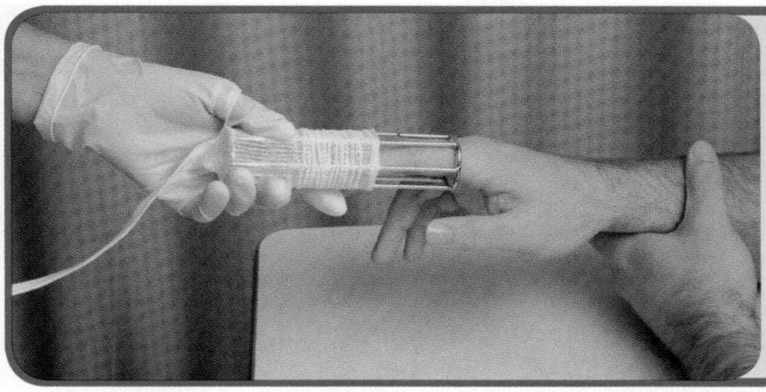

Figure 56–16A: The cylindrical applicator is placed over the finger. *Delmar/Cengage Learning.*

Bandaging Wounds

After the provider has treated the wound, it might become your responsibility to apply the dressing. You must also educate the patient to keep the bandage clean and dry and to watch for signs of infection such as redness, pain, and drainage. He or she should be advised to contact the provider if any of these signs occur. The following illustrations and procedures are guidelines to care for the patient satisfactorily.

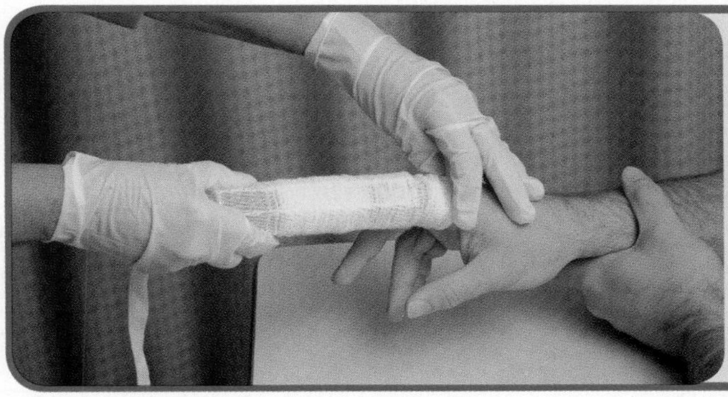

Figure 56–16B: Gauze is stretched over the finger. *Delmar/Cengage Learning.*

Tube Gauze Bandage

The easiest and probably quickest way to bandage arms, legs, fingers, and toes is with a tubular gauze bandage. Use an appropriately sized cylindrical cage applicator. The amount of tube gauze you expect to use is stretched over the applicator and placed over the extremity. By manipulating the cylinder around the extremity, grasping the tube gauze, withdrawing the cylinder, twisting the gauze, and repeating the sequence, a snug gauze bandage can be placed over the dressing (Figures 56–16A–C). Refer to Procedure 56–2 for applying a tube gauze bandage.

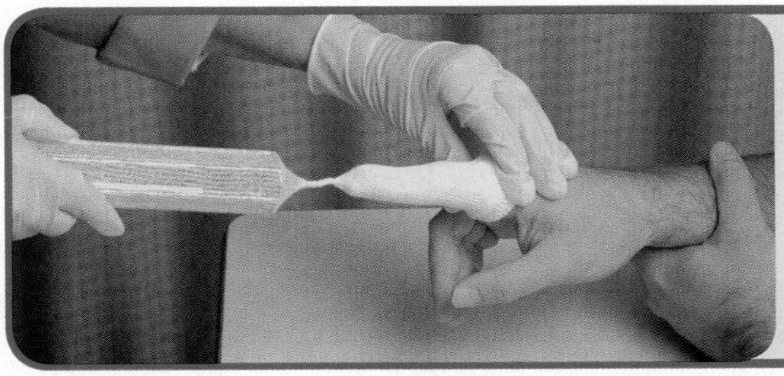

Figure 56–16C: The applicator is pulled off, leaving the bandage. *Delmar/Cengage Learning.*

Spiral Bandage

An injury on the arms or legs requires the dressing to be held in place with a spiral bandage. Refer to Procedure 56–3 for applying a spiral bandage.

reverse spiral

PROCEDURE 56–2 Apply a Tube Gauze Bandage

PURPOSE: To cover a wound or hold a bandage in place on an appendage such as a finger, toe, arm, or leg

EQUIPMENT: Scissors, dressing, adhesive tape, tube gauze bandage, applicator, gloves, a waste container, patient chart or EHR, pen

S SKILL: Demonstrate application of a tube gauze bandage.

Procedure Steps	Detailed Instructions and/or *Rationales*
1. Assemble the equipment and materials, wash hands, and put on gloves.	
B 2. Introduce yourself, identify the patient, and ***explain the procedure, using language the patient can understand.***	*Ensures that you are performing the procedure on the correct patient. Giving patients an explanation helps allay any fears about the procedure.*
3. Choose an applicator that is larger than the appendage to be bandaged.	
4. Cut an appropriate amount of tubular bandage to be applied and slide onto the applicator.	A general rule is to cut three times the applicator size.
5. Slide the applicator over the appendage. (*Apply first layer.*)	Start at the proximal end of the appendage, hold the bandage in place, and then directly pull the applicator approximately 1 inch past the distal end.
6. Turn the bandage gauze one complete turn.	
7. Next, slide the applicator toward the proximal end of the appendage.	
8. Repeat application process until area is completely covered.	
9. Anchor bandage at the proximal end and secure with tape.	Some providers might want you to secure the bandage by tying off the gauze at the wrist. Do this by: a. Cut the excess bandage from the finger and take the end of the bandage diagonally across the back of the hand to the wrist. b. Circle the wrist once or twice. c. Tie off or tape it at the wrist or tape it in place.
B 10. ***Instruct patient in how to care for the bandage and to watch for signs of circulation impairment and infection.***	The patient should be told to watch for redness, swelling, and sensation of pain or fever. Typed instructions should be given to the patient for follow-up care.
11. Clean up area and dispose of used supplies.	
12. Wash hands.	
13. Document.	

Charting Example

1-12-XX 1:25 PM	A tubular gauze bandage and antibiotic ointment applied to the right index finger. Patient education provided on how to keep the bandage clean and dry and to watch for signs of infection. Follow-up appointment scheduled for dressing change and wound recheck in 48 hours. J. Finelli, RMA(AMT)

PROCEDURE 56–3 Apply a Spiral Bandage

MEDIA LINK: View the video, "Spiral Bandage," for this chapter on the Premium Website.

PURPOSE: To apply a spiral bandage *NOTE*: This procedure describes how to apply a dressing to a wound and then cover it with a bandage.*

EQUIPMENT: Bandage, adhesive tape, scissors, sterile dressing, a waste container, patient chart or EHR, pen

S SKILL: Demonstrate application of a spiral bandage.

Procedure Steps	Detailed Instructions and/or *Rationales*
1. Assemble the equipment and materials, wash hands, and put on gloves.	
B 2. Introduce yourself, identify the patient, and ***explain the procedure, using language the patient can understand.***	*Ensures that you are performing the procedure on the correct patient. Giving patients an explanation helps allay any fears about the procedure.*
3. Carefully open a dressing, without contaminating it, and place it over the wound area.	(*Omit step 3 to eliminate dressing application.)
4. Anchor the bandage by placing the end of the bandage on a bias at the starting point (see Figure 56–17A).	
5. Encircle the part, allowing the corner of the bandage end to protrude (see Figure 56–17B).	CAUTION: Take care not to wrap extremities straight around because it impedes circulation to the distal part of the extremity.
6. Turn down the protruding tip of the bandage (see Figure 56–17C).	
7. Encircle the part again (see Figure 56–17D).	
8. Continue to encircle the area to be covered with spiral turns spaced so that they do not overlap (see Figure 56–17E).	
9. If a closed spiral bandage is desired, overlap spiral turns until the dressing is completely covered (see Figure 56–17F).	
10. Complete the bandage by taping it in place (see Figure 56–17G).	
B 11. ***Instruct patient in how to care for the bandage and to watch for signs of circulation impairment and infection.***	The patient should be told to watch for redness, swelling, and sensation of pain or fever. Typed instructions should be given to the patient for follow-up care.
12. Clean the area and discard contaminated materials and gloves in a proper waste receptacle.	
13. Wash hands.	
14. Document.	

(continues)

(continued)

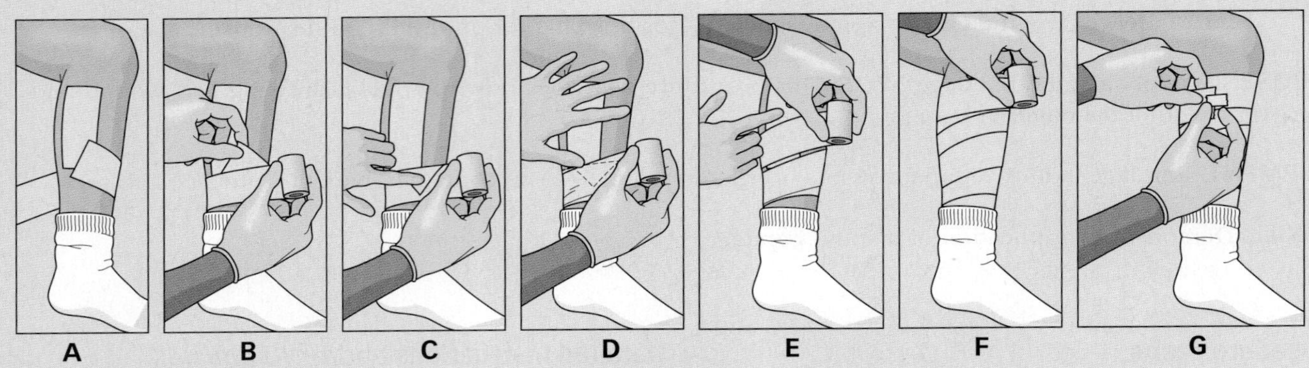

Figure 56–17A–G: Application of a spiral bandage. *Delmar/Cengage Learning.*

Charting Example

4-18-XX 1:25 PM	Open spiral bandage applied over dressing on left lower leg. Patient education provided on how to keep the bandage clean and dry and to watch for signs of infection. Follow-up appointment scheduled for dressing change and wound recheck in 48 hours. C. Spatz, CMA(AAMA)

Figure-Eight Bandage

A wound on the palm or back of the hand may be protected with a dressing and a figure-eight bandage (Figure 56–18). Refer to Procedure 56–4 for applying a figure-eight bandage.

Cravat Bandage

When applying a dressing to the forehead, ears, or eyes, a **cravat** can hold the dressing in place (Figure 56–19). Refer to Procedure 56–5 for applying a cravat bandage.

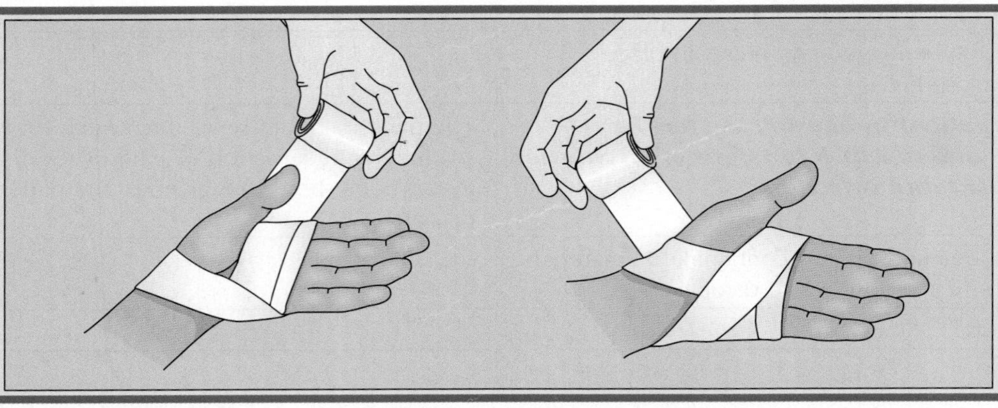

Figure 56–18: Figure-eight bandage to hand and wrist. *Delmar/Cengage Learning.*

PROCEDURE 56–4 Apply a Figure-Eight Bandage

MEDIA LINK: View the video, "Figure-Eight Bandage," for this chapter on the Premium Website.

PURPOSE: To apply a figure-eight bandage *NOTE*: This procedure describes how to apply a dressing to a wound and then cover it with a bandage.*

EQUIPMENT: Sterile dressing, bandage, gloves, scissors, tape, a proper waste receptacle, patient chart or EHR, pen

S SKILL: Demonstrate application of a figure-eight bandage.

Procedure Steps	Detailed Instructions and/or *Rationales*
1. Assemble the equipment and materials, wash hands, and put on gloves.	
B 2. Introduce yourself, identify the patient, and ***explain the procedure, using language the patient can understand.***	*Ensures that you are performing the procedure on the correct patient. Giving patients an explanation helps allay any fears about the procedure.*
3. Apply a dressing over the wound.	(*Omit step 3 to eliminate dressing application.)
4. Anchor the bandage with one or two turns around the palm of the hand.	
5. Roll the gauze diagonally across the front of the wrist and in a figure-eight pattern around the hand.	
6. Cut the gauze and tape at the wrist.	Caution: Do not impair circulation.
B 7. ***Instruct patient in how to care for the bandage and to watch for signs of circulation impairment and infection.***	The patient should be told to watch for redness, swelling, and sensation of pain or fever. Typed instructions should be given to the patient for follow-up care.
8. Discard contaminated materials and gloves in a proper waste receptacle.	
9. Wash hands.	
10. Document.	

Charting Example

6-14-XX 1:25 PM	Figure-eight bandage applied to right hand. Patient education provided on how to keep the bandage clean and dry and to watch for signs of infection. C. Spatz, CCMA

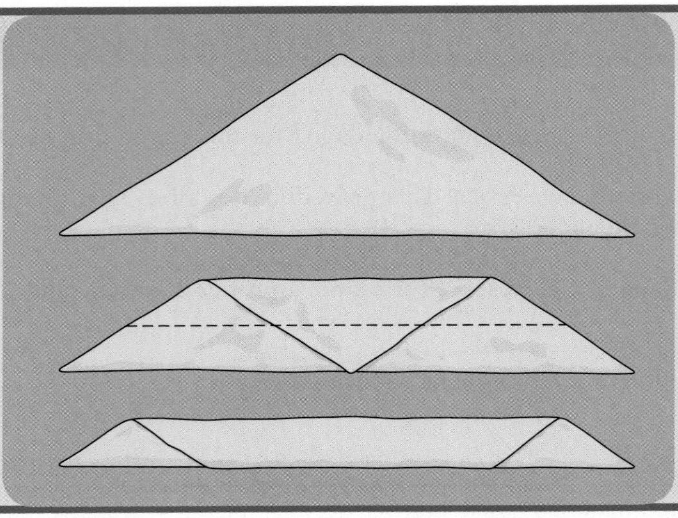

Figure 56–19: Folding a triangular bandage to make a cravat bandage. *Delmar/Cengage Learning.*

PROCEDURE 56–5 Apply a Cravat Bandage to Forehead, Ear, or Eyes

PURPOSE: To apply a cravat bandage to the head *NOTE*: This procedure explains how to apply a dressing to a wound and then cover it with a cravat bandage.*

EQUIPMENT: Sterile dressing, cravat bandage, gloves, a proper waste receptacle, patient chart or EHR, pen

S **SKILL:** Demonstrate application of a cravat bandage to the head.

Procedure Steps	Detailed Instructions and/or *Rationales*
1. Assemble the equipment and materials, wash hands, and put on gloves.	
B 2. Introduce yourself, identify the patient, and ***explain the procedure, using language the patient can understand.***	*Ensures that you are performing the procedure on the correct patient. Giving patients an explanation helps allay any fears about the procedure.*
3. Apply a dressing over the wound.	(*Omit step 3 to eliminate dressing application.)
4. Place the center of the cravat over the dressing.	
5. Take the ends around to the opposite side of the head and cross them. Do not tie.	
6. Bring the ends back to the starting point and tie them (Figure 56–20).	
B 7. ***Instruct patient in how to care for the bandage and to watch for signs of circulation impairment and infection.***	The patient should be told to watch for redness, swelling, and sensation of pain or fever. Typed instructions should be given to the patient for follow-up care.
8. Discard the contaminated materials and gloves in a proper waste receptacle.	
9. Wash hands.	
10. Document.	

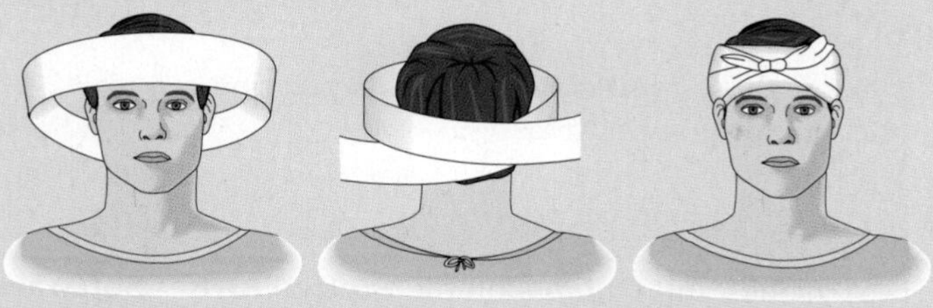

Figure 56–20: Applying a cravat bandage to the head. *Delmar/Cengage Learning.*

Charting Example

8-28-XX 1:25 PM	Cravat bandage applied over dressing on head. Patient education provided on how to keep the bandage clean and dry and to watch for signs of infection. C. Spatz, CCMA

CHAPTER SUMMARY

- When deciding whether the situation warrants emergency medical care, an office visit, or management at home, ask the caller to give you a brief history of the victim's situation, the nature of the initial injury or accident, the time the accident occurred or the illness began, and a description of the victim's current condition.
- Remove a foreign body under the lower eyelid with a bit of cotton or a fold of tissue moistened with water. If a foreign body is under the upper lid, remove it by pulling the upper lid down over the lower lid. If this procedure is not successful, it might be necessary to grasp the eyelashes and carefully turn back the upper lid over a cotton swab.
- Placing several drops of warm olive oil, mineral oil, or baby oil into the ear and pulling back on the earlobe to straighten the external canal, letting the oil run out to see whether the object will come out with it is first aid for an object lodged in the ear.
- Being able to compare and contrast fractures and having knowledge of the various types will help you assist the provider and the patient.
- With animal and human bites, the wounds must be thoroughly cleansed with an antiseptic soap and rinsed well with water. The area should be bandaged and immobilized, and the patient should be examined by a provider as soon as possible to determine further treatment.
- Acute illness can occur in patients that are severely allergic to stings. The patient might become restless, complain of headache, have shortness of breath, or have mottled blueness of the skin. When shortness of breath is not apparent, the victim might appear to be in shock and have severe nausea, vomiting, and bloody diarrhea.
- Burns are classified by three methods: the percentage of body surface area (BSA) involved in the burn, the Rule of Nines, and the Lund and Browder chart. These methods establish a standard by which all injuries can be estimated.
- Hot and cold pack applications are often used in the treatment of injuries. The provider will give specific instructions concerning the length of time and where to apply the treatment.
- Wounds can be caused by trauma or surgical procedures. Open wounds are abrasions, avulsions, incisions, lacerations, and punctures, and closed wounds are contusions. You should be able to identify the wound type and provide patient teaching to identify infection of a wound.

STUDY TOOLS

Workbook	Activities for Chapter 56
Premium Website	
MEDIA LINK	View these **Media Links** for Chapter 56: • Clean Wound Areas • Spiral Bandaging • Figure-Eight Bandaging
StudyWARE	Activities and Quizzes on the **StudyWARE™ Software** for Chapter 56
	Complete the following **Competency Challenge 2.0** activity: • Thursday, 11 AM: Emergency Procedures
	Audio Library of medical terms
	Online access to the **Critical Thinking Challenge 2.0**
learninglab	Module 23: First Aid and Responding to Emergencies
CourseMate	Activities and Quizzes for Chapter 56
WebTutor	Activities and Quizzes for Chapter 56

CHECK YOUR KNOWLEDGE

1. With all human bites, a tetanus injection must be administered to the patient if he or she has not received one within:
   a. one year.
   b. five years.
   c. seven years.
   d. 10 years.
2. At least half of all dislocations involve which of the following body parts?
   a. Shoulder
   b. Wrist
   c. Ankle
   d. Knee
3. A _________ leaves the stinger in the skin, and it should be removed immediately by scraping it out carefully with a credit card or other rigid object.
   a. wasp
   b. hornet
   c. yellow jacket
   d. honeybee
4. Partial-thickness burns are also referred to as:
   a. first-degree burns.
   b. second-degree burns.
   c. third-degree burns.
   d. fourth-degree burns.
5. When using the PRINCE method on a strain or sprain, the injury should be treated with a cold pack for the first __________hours.
   a. 12–24
   b. 24–36
   c. 24–48
   d. 48–72
6. Which of the following types of wounds involves the skin being torn off and the wound bleeding profusely?
   a. Laceration
   b. Avulsion
   c. Abrasion
   d. Puncture
7. This type of fracture involves an open wound.
   a. Simple
   b. Closed
   c. Compound open
   d. Both a and b are correct

WEB LINKS

American Academy of Emergency Medicine: www.aaem.org

American Red Cross: www.redcross.org

National Center for Emergency Medicine Informatics: www.ncemi.org

National Institutes of Health: www.nih.gov

U.S. National Library of Medicine: www.nlm.nih.gov

WebMD: www.webMD.com

RESOURCES

Beebe, R., and Funk, D. (2010). *Fundamentals of Emergency Care* (3rd ed.). Clifton Park, NY: Delmar Cengage Learning.

Estes, M. E. Z. (2010). *Health Assessment & Physical Examination* (3rd ed.). Clifton Park, NY: Delmar Cengage Learning.

Heller, M., and Veach, L. (2009). *Clinical Medical Assisting: A Professional, Field Smart Approach to the Workplace*. Clifton Park, NY: Delmar Cengage Learning.

Lindh, W., Pooler, M., Tamparo, C., and Dahl, B. (2010). *Delmar's Comprehensive Medical Assisting Administrative and Clinical Competencies* (4th ed.). Clifton Park, NY: Delmar Cengage Learning.

Unit

19

Rehabilitation and Healthy Living

As you've learned, one of your roles as a medical assistant is to assist the provider with a variety of treatment modalities and present educational opportunities with patients. The provider prescribes a treatment plan for the patient to follow and typically discusses it with the patient. Your responsibility might be to reinforce the provider's instructions and provide additional teaching on a variety of topics. This unit covers several rehabilitation methods, such as body mechanics, mobility devices, and range of motion exercises, as well as healthy living techniques that include nutritional guidelines and the significance of diet, exercise, weight control, sleep, and the way personal behaviors influence health. These are commonly discussed and conducted in the office on a daily basis. This unit provides you with the knowledge to adopt behaviors that positively influence your own and your patient's health. Hopefully, it also enables you to recognize and provide assistance to individuals who need to change their behavior before their health is compromised. You must have a complete understanding of the tasks at hand and be a positive role model for the patients with whom you will be working.

Certification Connection

	Ch. 57	Ch. 58
CMA (AAMA)		
Adapting communication according to an individual's needs	X	X
Recognizing and responding to verbal and nonverbal communication	X	X
Patient education	X	X
Nutrition		X
RMA (AMT)		
Understand and properly apply communication methods	X	X
Patient education	X	X
Therapeutic modalities	X	X

Chapter

57 Rehabilitation

OBJECTIVES

In this chapter, you will learn the following:

KB KNOWLEDGE BASE

1. Spell and define, using the glossary at the back of the text, all the Words to Know in this chapter.
2. Identify principles of body mechanics and ergonomics.
3. Explain the importance of using good body mechanics.
4. Describe how to make the home safer for people using mobility aids.
5. Identify situations when the use of mobility equipment is indicated.
6. Describe different mobility equipment.
7. Identify the terms related to range-of-motion exercises.

S SKILLS

1. Use proper body mechanics.
2. Demonstrate application of an arm sling.
3. Demonstrate fitting and instruction in use of a cane.
4. Demonstrate fitting and instruction in use of crutches.
5. Demonstrate instruction in use of a walker.

B BEHAVIOR

1. Use language/verbal skills that enable patients' understanding.
2. Apply critical thinking skills in performing patient assessment and care.
3. Adapt to individualized needs.

WORDS TO KNOW

ambulate
angle
axilla
body mechanics
crutches
flexibility
gait
mobility
quad-base
range of motion (ROM)
sling
stabilize
support
walker
wheelchair

sitz bath
— after rectal surgery (hemoroids)
after episiotomy

warm soaks
→ 110°F (44°C)

BODY MECHANICS

Body mechanics is the practice of using certain key muscle groups together with good body alignment and proper body positioning to reduce the risk for injury to both patient and caregiver.

When caring for patients or moving and lifting equipment and supplies, you must always be conscious of using proper body mechanics. This should not be practiced just on the job but in everything that requires moving, lifting, pushing, or pulling heavy or awkward objects.

Practicing good body mechanics starts with good posture. Regularly check your posture by reminding yourself to keep your chin and chest up, shoulders back, pelvis tilted slightly inward. In addition, you want to keep your feet straight at approximately a shoulder width apart and weight evenly distributed to both legs with a slight bend in your knees (Figures 57–1A–B).

When lifting patients or moving or lifting heavy objects, certain techniques should be used to prevent back injury. Refer to Procedure 57–1 for a step-by-step process on using proper body mechanics.

Ergonomics

Ergonomics describes pairing workplace conditions and job demands with the capabilities of the worker. When the conditions are a good fit with the employees, high productivity, prevention of illness and injury risks, and increased satisfaction among the workforce occur. Ergonomics covers a large scope and is often discussed in the front office with employees who are working with computers or spending a lot of time sitting at a desk. In this chapter, it relates to assessing those work-related factors that can pose a risk of musculoskeletal disorders. Examples of ergonomic risk factors are found in jobs requiring repetitive, forceful, or prolonged exertions of the hands; frequent or heavy lifting, pushing, pulling, or carrying heavy objects; and prolonged awkward postures. Jobs or working conditions presenting multiple risk factors will have a higher probability of causing a musculoskeletal problem. Following the proper use of body mechanics can help alleviate the risks. See Chapter 21 for more discussion about ergonomics.

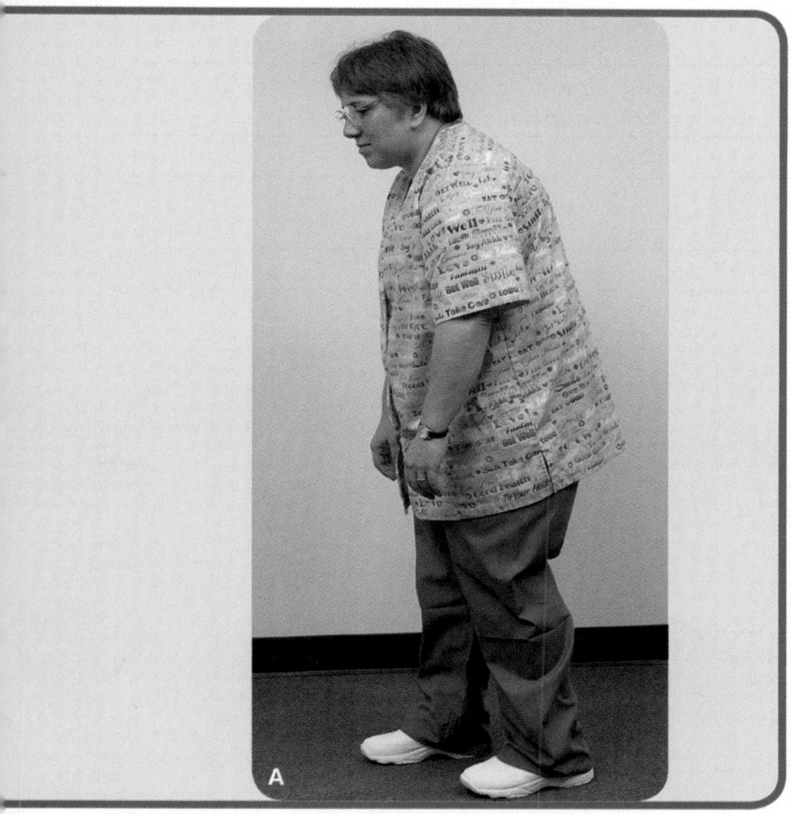

Figure 57–1A: Medical assistant with poor posture. *Delmar/ Cengage Learning.*

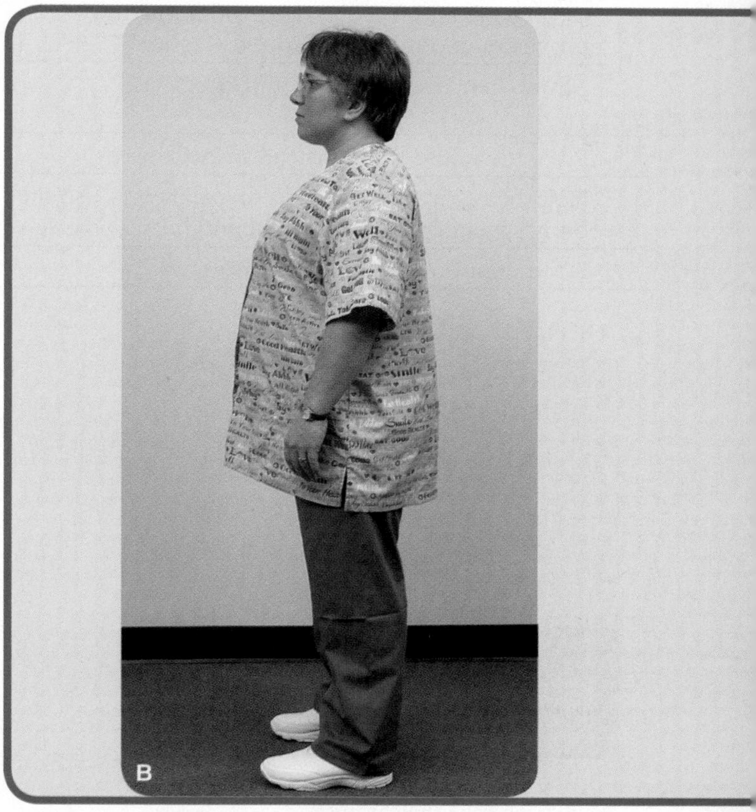

Figure 57–1B: Medical assistant with good posture. *Delmar/ Cengage Learning.*

Active resistance – using resistance band

PROCEDURE 57–1 Use Proper Body Mechanics

MEDIA LINK: View the video, "Use Proper Body Mechanics," for this chapter on the Premium Website.

PURPOSE: To use techniques when lifting or moving objects to prevent back injury

EQUIPMENT: Will vary based on object or person selected

S **SKILL:** Demonstrate using proper body mechanics.

Procedure Steps	Detailed Instructions and/or *Rationales*
B 1. If a patient is involved, introduce yourself and identify the patient. ***Explain the procedure and what you are going to do, using language the patient can understand.***	*Ensures that you are performing the procedure for the correct patient.*
B 2. ***Before lifting anything or anyone, determine whether it is possible for one person to do***; if a patient or object is too heavy, obtain help.	
3. Make sure the path is clear, the floor is clean and dry, and the area is ready to receive the patient or object before lifting or moving.	
4. Face the patient or object; keep the back as straight as possible and feet shoulder-width apart to provide a good base of support (Figure 57–2).	
5. Always bend from the hips and knees.	This allows the largest muscles of the legs to do the hard work, but *never* bend from the waist.
6. Pivot the entire body instead of twisting it.	
7. Hold heavy objects close to the body and use the body's weight to push or pull any heavy object.	
8. Document procedure (if appropriate).	

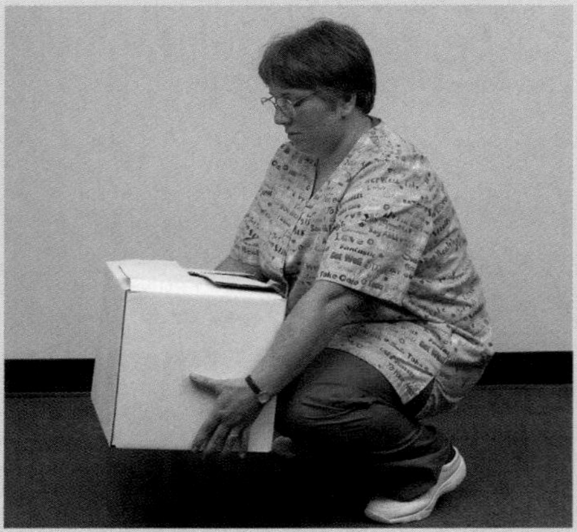

Figure 57–2: Provide a good base of support by keeping the back straight. *Delmar/Cengage Learning.*

Transferring Patients

It might be necessary to transfer patients if they cannot walk or lift themselves. This will be necessary if the patient is in a wheelchair as discussed in Chapter 40. Procedures 39–2 and 39–3 provide step-by-step instructions for transferring a patient from the wheelchair to an exam table and back again; however, it is important to go over a few reminders here. Before beginning any transfer, observe certain precautions:

- Lock the brakes of a wheelchair and make sure the exam table or other surface will not move during the transfer.
- Take small shuffling steps and avoid crossing the feet.
- It is best if the transfer surfaces being used are close to the same height. If possible, lower the exam table or bed to the height of the wheelchair.
- If the patient is stronger on one side, make sure that is the side on which the transfer will take place.
- Always use a gait belt when transferring a patient. Lift the patient by grasping the belt from underneath and lifting up. Never lift a patient by the arms or under the armpits.
- Take advantage of any assistance the patient can provide in lifting and moving.
- Never have patients put their arms around your neck or your shoulders.
- Make sure both you and the patient are wearing footwear that will not slip.
- Thoroughly explain to the patient what you intend to do and make sure the patient understands what to expect during the transfer.

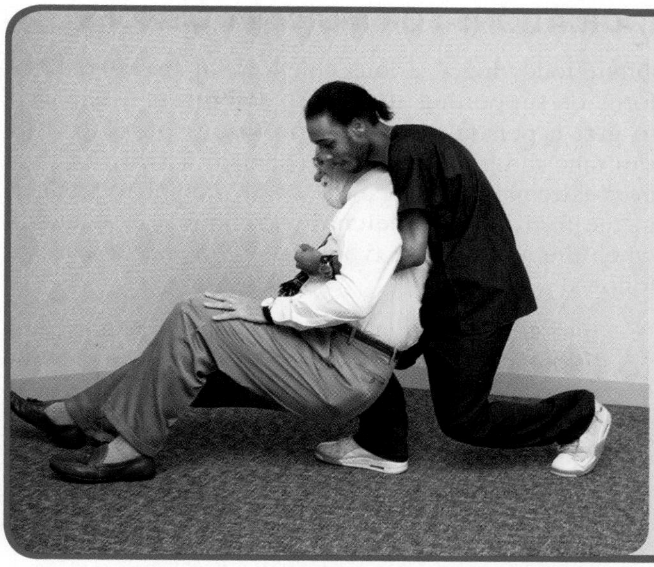

Figure 57–3A: Easing a falling patient safely to the floor from behind the patient. *Delmar/Cengage Learning.*

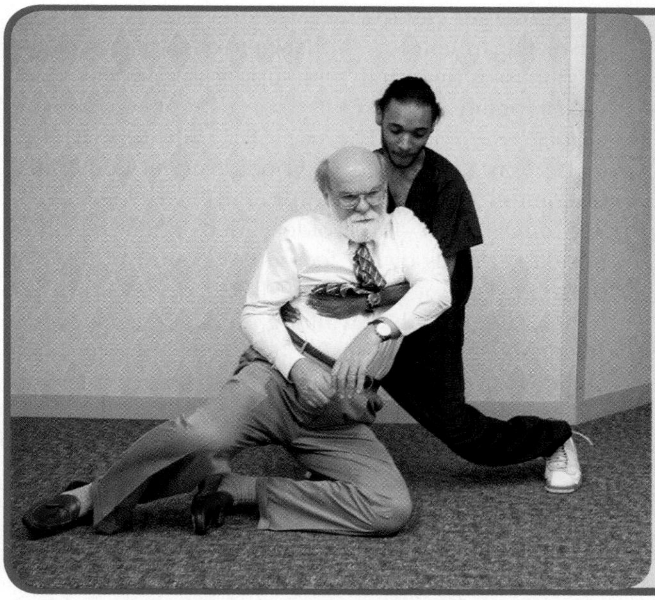

Figure 57–3B: Easing a falling patient safely to the floor from beside the patient. *Delmar/Cengage Learning.*

Assisting Falling Patients

Even being as careful as possible when assisting patients to walk or move about the office, you still might have one who becomes faint, slips, or suddenly becomes weak. Usually, a single person cannot hold up someone who becomes dead weight. The best option in this case is to ease the patient to the floor to prevent injury. If you are supporting the patient from behind and he or she begins to fall backward, grasp him or her under the arms, put one leg back with the foot at a right angle, slide the other leg forward under the patient, and ease him or her to slide down your leg onto the floor (Figure 57–3A). If you are walking beside the patient and he or she begins to fall forward, grasp him or her around the waist, extend your leg farthest from the patient forward, bend at the knees, and slowly lower the patient to the floor (Figure 57–3B). You must be careful to avoid injuring your own back by trying to support too much weight. Keep your back as straight as possible, bend from the knees, and use your large thigh muscles to handle the weight. Whenever a patient falls, have the provider examine him or her as soon as possible and be sure to document the incident carefully on the chart and on an accident or incident form if indicated by your office policy.

INDICATIONS FOR MOBILITY DEVICES

Often, following a serious illness or an accident, some form of supporting device or equipment is needed to give a person as much **mobility** as possible. This can take the form of only a splint or a **sling** to support extremities, or it can be nearly complete reliance in the form of a **wheelchair**. Examples of situations when the use of some type of device is needed are as follows:

- *After an accident or injury*—Sprains, fractures, and dislocations require temporary **support** and abstinence from use to permit healing.
- *Following a stroke*—If there has been a loss of use of the extremities or if the person has become somewhat unsteady on his or her feet, something might be needed to help him or her maintain balance.
- *After surgery*—When joints are replaced, supportive devices are necessary until muscles are strengthened around the new implant and the person is allowed to bear his or her own weight when he or she **ambulates**.
- *With a severe medical condition*—Patients with congestive heart failure, emphysema, or similar debilitating illnesses frequently use supportive devices to aid their mobility.
- *Arthritis sufferers*—The use of a cane or **crutches** to support a portion of the body weight reduces the discomfort in the knees, hips, and lower back.
- *The older adult*—The older adult often becomes unsteady on his or her feet and, because of the fear of falling, use a cane or walker to help **stabilize** him- or herself while walking.
- *Physically challenged*—Persons with physical disabilities often require supportive devices to assist them with mobility.

TYPES OF MOBILTY DEVICES

Many caregivers such as providers, physical therapists, therapy aids, and medical supply representatives are trained to fit and instruct people in how to use various pieces of equipment. When it is known that a disability will occur, as with planned surgery, this should be done prior to the procedure so that the patient is prepared to function as soon as possible after it is performed. This chapter discusses the various devices that might be indicated in the process of recovering and gaining mobility and provides procedures covering the most common ones. Not only should you learn to instruct others in the proper use or application of the various pieces of equipment, but you could also participate in the patient's experience by practicing being the patient so that you can appreciate the patient's dependence and understand the constraints involved. Few people realize the amount of strength and energy required to walk a long hallway or climb a flight of stairs using crutches or the dependence that can be taken away by the use of other devices. Spending a few hours in a wheelchair can also prove to be a very enlightening experience.

PATIENT EDUCATION

Help patients and their families identify techniques to maintain a safe home environment for persons using ambulatory aids. Care must be taken to keep floors free of spills and clutter. It is especially important to remove all loose throw rugs or damaged floor coverings that might cause the patient to fall. Any bare floor-care product, such as floor wax, that might cause the floor to be slippery must be avoided. It is also important to ensure that appropriate footwear is worn. It should be well-fitting and have a nonslip walking surface.

Arm Sling

A sling is often used to support an arm after a fracture or injury to the shoulder or arm (Figure 57–4). This aids the patient by supporting and protecting the injured extremity so that most activities can be continued until it is healed. Arm slings come in a variety of adult and child sizes, and some providers like to use a print material for children. The standard adult sling is about 55 inches

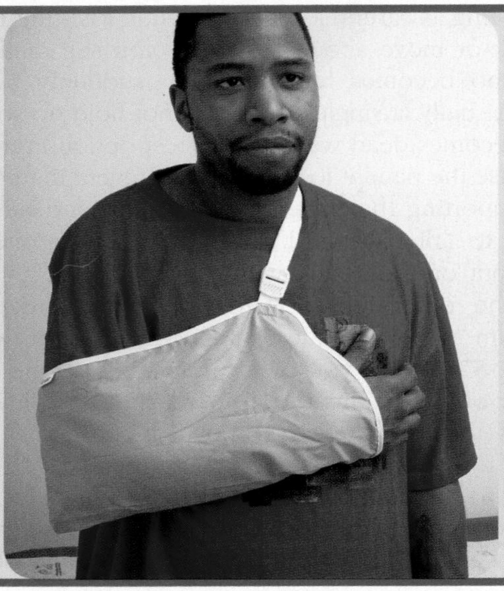

Figure 57–4: Arm sling. *Delmar/Cengage Learning.*

across the base and 36 to 40 inches along the sides. It is important to learn the correct way to apply a sling with the patient standing, sitting, or lying down. Care must be taken to elevate the hand properly to assist the return of circulation and avoid swelling. You must also be sure that the sling is applied properly so the patient gets the best therapeutic treatment from its use. (See Procedure 57–2.)

Canes

The patient who needs only a cane for support should have one that is the proper length to fit comfortably in the hand with the arm hanging naturally at the side and the elbow flexed at about a 25- to 30-degree **angle**. The handle should be just below hip level. Many canes are adjustable; if not, they must be fitted to the correct length. Canes come in a variety of materials and types (Figure 57–5). An older adult patient usually has less trouble with a **quad-base** cane because its four feet provide a stable base that gives better support. The patient should carry the cane on the strong or uninjured side. The cane should swing forward with the injured extremity. Part of the weight is carried by the cane being firmly placed on the floor simultaneously with the injured extremity. Refer to Procedure 57–3.

PROCEDURE 57–2 Apply an Arm Sling

PURPOSE: To apply an arm sling to provide support for an injured arm or shoulder

EQUIPMENT: Commercial, buckle-type arm sling, patient's chart or EHR, and pen

S **SKILL:** Demonstrate application of an arm sling

Procedure Steps	Detailed Instructions and/or *Rationales*
B 1. Introduce yourself, identify the patient, and ***explain the procedure, using language the patient can understand.***	*Ensures that you are performing the procedure for the correct patient.*
2. Wash hands.	
3. Select the proper size arm sling.	You want to make sure the arm sits comfortably at an angle with the elbow in the corner of the pouch and the fingers peeking out the other side.
B 4. ***For patient safety, support the injured arm above and below the injury site.***	
5. Position the arm into a 90° angle and slide it into the pouch-like opening of the sling.	Be sure the ends of the fingers extend slightly beyond the edge of the sling. *It is necessary to be able to observe the fingers for signs of impaired circulation such as swelling or discoloration.*
6. Bring the adjustable strap around the back of the neck on the side of the uninjured arm and slide into the ring attached to end of the sling, fasten, and tighten strap.	The arm should be elevated so the hand is 4 to 5 inches above the elbow and arm snug to the chest. *Elevation aids in the return of circulation, which reduces swelling and discomfort.*
B 7. ***Check arm for circulation impairment.***	Observe for numbness, tingling, and blueness in color.
8. Document procedure in patient's chart.	

Charting Example

6-23-XX 1:25 pm	Commercial arm sling applied to left arm for support following fall. Fingers elevated and extended from sling. No swelling observed, color normal. P. Blair, NC RMA

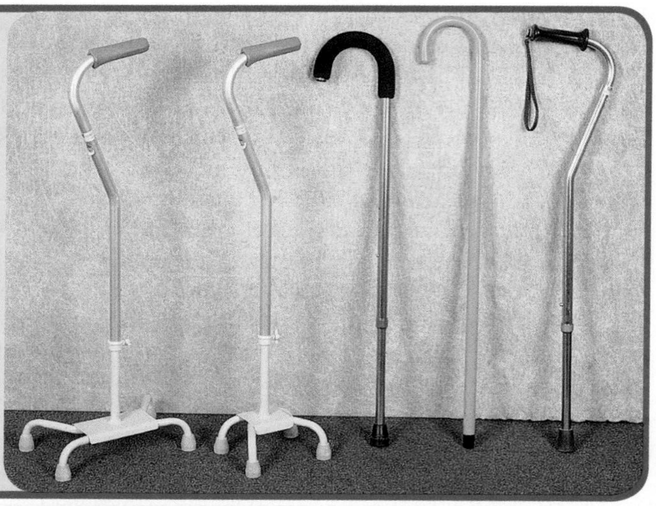

Figure 57–5: Types of standard canes: quad canes and single-tip canes. *Delmar/Cengage Learning.*

Crutches

It is often necessary for a patient to walk with crutches to give a foot, ankle, knee, or leg injury or surgery an opportunity to heal. It is important for the crutches to be adjusted to the correct height (Figure 57–6A). This is accomplished by holding the crutches up to the side of the patient and adjusting them so that the underarm pad is two to three fingers or 2 inches below the **axilla**. The handhold should be adjusted so that the hands fit comfortably with the arms extended. The axillary piece and the handhold should be foam padded for comfort. The patient should be instructed to stand on the uninjured foot while swinging the injured leg forward as the crutches are moved forward (Figure 57–6B). The weight of the body should be on the hands and never on the axillary area because, over time, prolonged pressure on the axillary nerves can cause nerve damage.

PROCEDURE 57–3 Use a Cane

PURPOSE: To adjust a cane for proper height and teach a patient its correct and safe use

EQUIPMENT AND SUPPLIES: Cane, patient's chart or EHR, and pen

S **SKILL:** Demonstrate fitting and instruction in use of a cane.

Procedure Steps	Detailed Instructions and/or *Rationales*
B 1. Introduce yourself, identify the patient, and ***explain the procedure, using language the patient can understand.***	*Ensures that you are performing the procedure for the correct patient.* The patient must be wearing nonskid shoes or foot coverings.
2. Wash hands and assemble the equipment. Check the cane for an intact rubber tip.	*This helps prevent slipping or falling.*
3. Adjust the height of the cane so that the patient's elbow is flexed comfortably at approximately a 25- to 30-degree angle and check that the handle of the cane is positioned just below the hip level of the uninjured or strong side.	
4. Demonstrate for the patient the gait ordered for safe ambulation.	
5. Move the cane and injured extremity forward simultaneously.	
6. Then, move the strong or uninjured extremity forward.	
7. Allow the patient to practice the procedure.	Observe the patient and be alert to assist the patient and rescue him or her in case of a fall.
8. Demonstrate going up stairs. Move the uninjured extremity up first and then move the injured extremity up.	Remind the patient to use the cane for support and have the patient practice. Answer any questions the patient might have and give emotional support.

Cane to be place opposite of injured foot

Procedure Steps	Detailed Instructions and/or *Rationales*
9. Demonstrate going down stairs. Move uninjured extremity down first. Then move the injured extremity down.	
10. Instruct the patient to take small, slow steps.	*This aids in maintaining balance.*
11. Ensure that the cane height is correct and that the patient is using the cane correctly.	
12. Document procedure on the patient's chart.	

Charting Example

7-23-XX 1:25 PM	Cane adjusted for proper height. Rubber tip securely in place. Proper use of cane demonstrated. Patient correctly returned the demonstration. Practiced on level floor and short flight of stairs. Advised patient regarding selection of appropriate shoes to prevent slipping or falling. B. COX, CMA (AAMA)

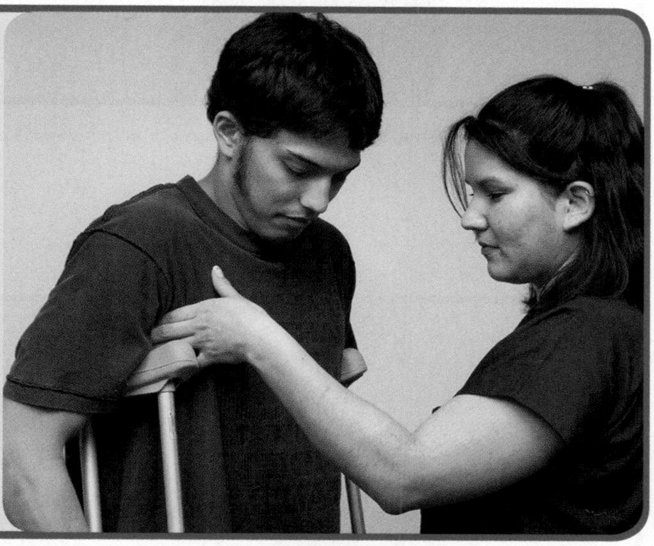

Figure 57–6A: Measuring for axillary crutches: The top of the crutch should be about 2 to 3 inches below the patient's axilla. *Delmar/Cengage Learning.*

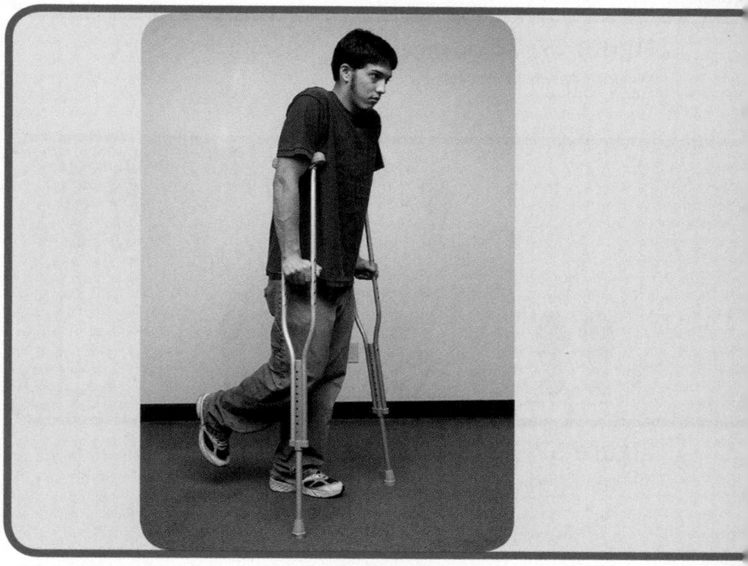

Figure 57–6B: A patient using axillary crutches. *Delmar/Cengage Learning.*

Crutches can be used in different **gait** or step patterns. (Refer to Procedure 57–4.) Five gait walks are commonly used. Practice all five gaits until you are certain you could instruct a patient in the safe use of crutches.

- Two-point gait (Figure 57–7A): Matches the crutch to the opposite foot, moving them together.

To use crutches, pat should have strong upper extremities

- Three-point gait (Figure 57–7B): Positions both crutches and the left foot forward and then brings up the right foot. (The foot moved with the crutches depends upon which extremity is injured.)
- Four-point gait (Figure 57–7C): Shows the right crutch being positioned first, followed by moving the left foot. Then, the left crutch is moved forward, followed by the right foot. This makes for good stability but requires practice to coordinate the movements.

left crutch move and Right leg move. for stability

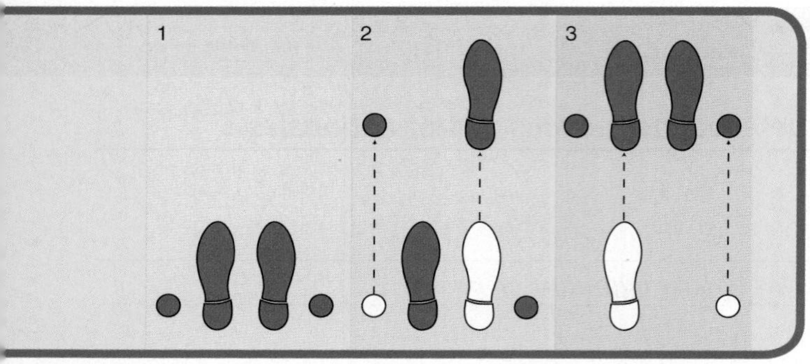

Figure 57–7A: Examples of crutch gaits: two-point. *Delmar/Cengage Learning.*

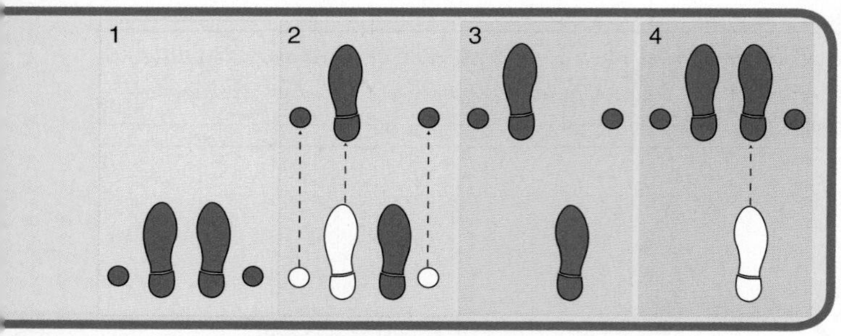

Figure 57–7B: Examples of crutch gaits: three-point. *Delmar/Cengage Learning.*

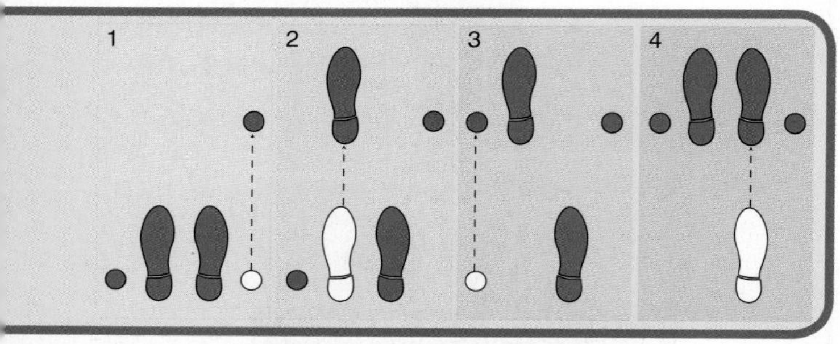

Figure 57–7C: Examples of crutch gaits: four-point. *Delmar/Cengage Learning.*

- Swing-to gait: Crutches are moved forward simultaneously and the weight is transferred forward. Then swing both feet together up to the crutches.
- Swing-through gait: Crutches are moved forward, weight is transferred, and both feet swing through the crutches, stopping slightly in front.

Other varieties of crutches are designed for special situations. The Lofstrand/Canadian crutch, more commonly referred to as forearm crutches (Figure 57–8A), eliminate axillary pressure and, with the forearm cuff, is more stable. This type would be used for long-term rehabilitation. The platform crutch (Figure 57–8B) is used when a patient's hand or forearm is not able to bear the patient's body weight.

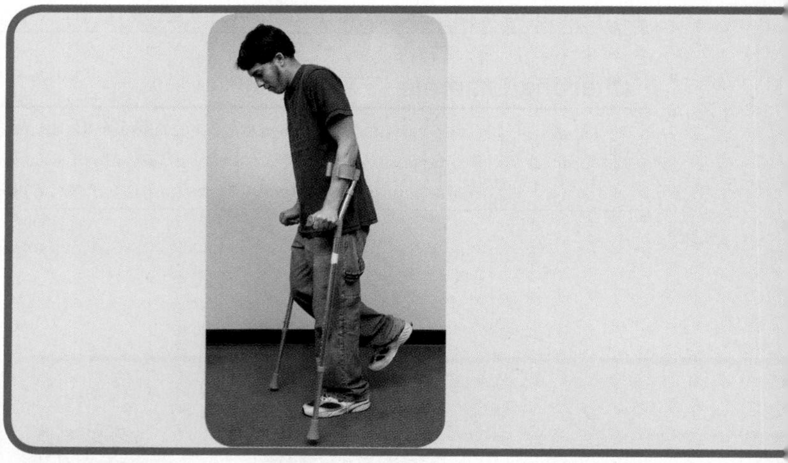

Figure 57–8A: Lofstrand/Canadian or forearm crutches. *Delmar/Cengage Learning.*

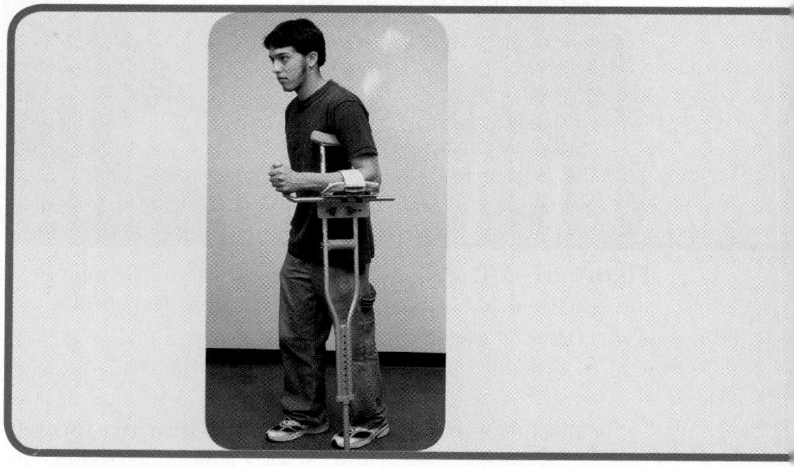

Figure 57–8B: Platform crutch. *Delmar/Cengage Learning.*

PROCEDURE 57–4 Use Crutches

MEDIA LINK: View the video, "Assist a Patient to Use Crutches," for this chapter on the Premium Website.

PURPOSE: To adjust crutches' length and teach a patient to use crutches correctly and safely.

EQUIPMENT: Crutches, hand pads, rubber tips, patient's chart or EHR, and pen.

S SKILL: Demonstrate fitting and instruction in use of crutches.

Procedure Steps	Detailed Instructions and/or *Rationales*
B 1. Introduce yourself, identify the patient, and ***explain the procedure, using language the patient can understand.***	*Ensures that you are performing the procedure for the correct patient.* The patient must be wearing nonskid shoes or foot coverings.
2. Wash hands and assemble the equipment.	Make sure the crutches are intact (hand pads and rubber tips) and stable.
B 3. ***For patient safety, stabilize the patient upright near a wall or chair for support. Apply a gait belt to the patient.***	
4. Adjust the length of the crutches for the patient so that the handles are comfortable, with a 30-degree angle bend of the elbows and 2 inches between the axilla and the top of the crutches.	
5. Explain to the patient to support his or her weight at the handles and not under the arm. Tell the patient to take small steps slowly to avoid losing balance and possibly falling.	*Pressure in the axilla from upper body weight can damage nerves.*
6. Instruct the patient to stand on his or her uninjured foot while swinging the injured leg forward with crutches.	Crutches should be placed approximately 4 to 5 inches in front and 4 to 5 inches to the side of the patient's heels. Use Figure 57–7 to show the ordered gait for walking safely with crutches.
7. Demonstrate the proper use of crutches.	
8. Allow the patient to practice the procedure to ensure correct use.	
9. Document the procedure on the patient's chart.	

Charting Example

2-16-XX 1:25 pm	Measured and adjusted crutches for proper height. Hand pads and tips firmly attached. Demonstrated three-point gait and had patient return demonstration. Instructed not to bear weight on axillary area. Advised to select appropriate shoes to help prevent slipping or falling. J. FINELLI, RMA (AMT)

Walker

A **walker** is useful for patients who, because of age or physical condition, cannot safely use crutches. The walker may be adjusted to proper height for the patient. The patient must be cautioned not to step too far into the walker because this makes it difficult to maintain balance. The patient should move the walker forward and then step into the walker while leaning slightly forward (Figure 57–9 and Procedure 57–5).

Some walkers come with wheels so that patients can push them along as they walk and therefore can move a little quicker. This type of walker is less stable and can cause some patients to fall if it rolls away from them. Some more expensive wheeled walkers come with hand brakes that the patient can use to control the rolling, but this depends upon the response action and hand strength of the patient for control and safety. Some walkers even have a seating area so the patient can stop and rest while walking. Many retirement and nursing home patients use walkers they will bring to the provider's office. Become familiar with their use and be able to instruct or correct a patient's usage.

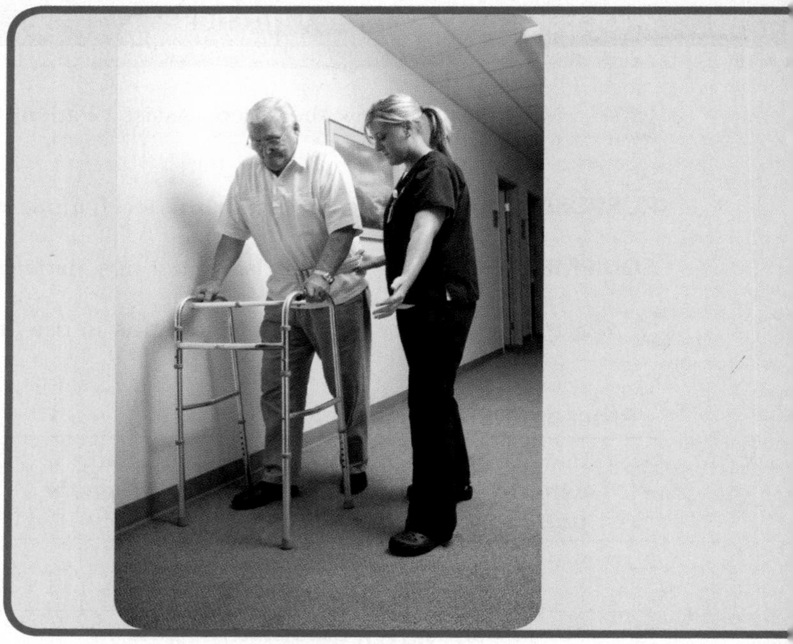

Figure 57–9: Patient using a walker. *Delmar/Cengage Learning.*

PROCEDURE 57–5 Use a Walker

MEDIA LINK: View the video, "Assist a Patient to Use a Walker," for this chapter on the Premium Website.

PURPOSE: To adjust the walker's height and teach a patient the proper and safe use of a walker

EQUIPMENT: Walker, handles, rubber tips, patient's chart or EHR, and pen

S SKILL: Demonstrate instruction in use of a walker.

Procedure Steps	Detailed Instructions and/or *Rationales*
B 1. Introduce yourself, identify the patient, and explain the procedure, ***using language the patient can understand.***	*Ensures that you are performing the procedure for the correct patient.* The patient must be wearing nonskid shoes or foot coverings.
2. Wash hands and assemble the equipment.	Check the walker for rubber tips, pads at the handles, and stability.
B 3. ***For patient safety, stabilize the patient upright near a wall or chair for support. Apply a gait belt to the patient.***	
4. The height of the walker should be adjusted so that the handles are at the patient's hip level and the bend of the patient's elbows is at a comfortable 25- to 30-degree angle.	

Procedure Steps	Detailed Instructions and/or *Rationales*
5. Position the walker around the patient (see Figure 57–9).	
6. Instruct the patient to pick up the walker, move it slightly forward, and walk into it. Instruct the patient to keep all four feet of the walker on the floor. Explain to the patient not to slide the walker. Instruct the patient not to step too close to walker.	*If the patient slides the walker, it can slip or catch and cause a fall. If the patient steps too close to the walker, it can be difficult to maintain balance.*
7. Demonstrate the correct use of a walker.	
8. Have the patient practice the procedure.	
B 9. ***Observe the patient and be ready to assist in case of a fall.***	
10. Document the procedure on the patient's chart.	

Charting Example

1-29-XX 1:25 PM	Walker adjusted to appropriate height and hand grips and rubber tips examined. Demonstrated safe use of the walker and reminded patient to wear nonskid shoes or slippers when walking. We also discussed being aware of floor coverings and possible hazards. Patient returned the demonstration and talked about the presence of hazards at his residence. J. Finelli, RMA (AMT)

Wheelchair

Wheelchairs enable a person to get around who otherwise would be immobile. As discussed in Chapter 39, patients might need to be assisted on and off the exam table and into and out of the wheelchair. Refer to that chapter for specific details on those procedures. Patients who are residents of retirement or nursing facilities are often seen in the office. Many of them arrive by wheelchair and might be accompanied by a nursing aide. You should be familiar with the different types of wheelchairs and their standard features for operation (Figures 57–10A–B).

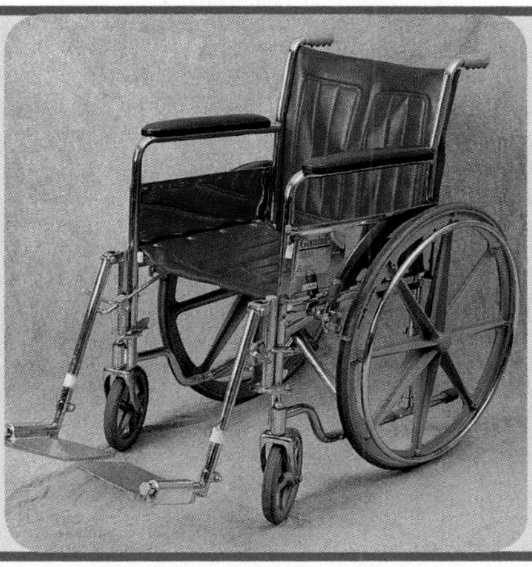

Figures 57–10A: Two types of wheelchairs: manual. *Delmar/Cengage Learning.*

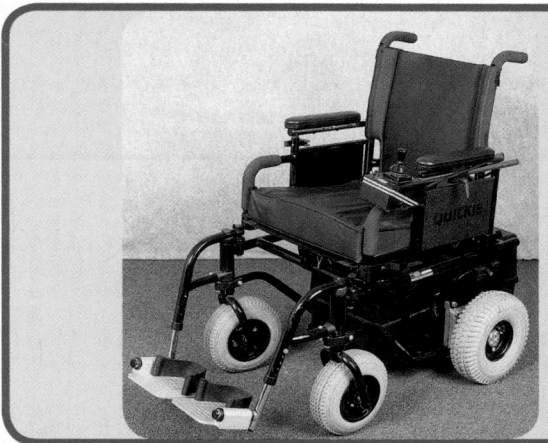

Figures 57–10B: Two types of wheelchairs: motorized. *Delmar/Cengage Learning.*

RANGE-OF-MOTION EXERCISES

In addition to the use of mobility devices, patients can benefit greatly by improving their strength and **flexibility**. This can be accomplished with participation in a regular program of exercise. Regular exercise improves circulation and muscle tone and relieves tension. People who have followed an exercise routine regularly report that they experience a better outlook on life, have more energy, and feel healthier. The degree of exertion in any exercise routine varies with individuals, and the provider's advice should be taken.

For patients who cannot engage in strenuous exercise, walking and **range-of-motion (ROM)** exercises are suggested to improve circulation and flexibility and promote muscle tone. A ROM exercise is defined as any body action involving muscles, joints, and natural directional movements such as abduction, adduction, extension, flexion, pronation, and rotation. Such exercises are usually applied actively or passively in the treatment of orthopedic deformities, assessment of injuries and deformities, and athletic conditioning. These movements help move each joint through its full range. These exercises can help patients who have arthritis, bursitis, and other disabilities. Refer to Table 57–1 for descriptions of the common terms used in ROM exercises.

Study the illustrations in Figure 57–11, and perform the motions yourself. Patients are frequently sent to a physical therapist for treatment and instruction, but the medical assistant can be responsible for reinforcing the therapist's instruction about how to perform the exercises.

TABLE 57–1 ROM Exercise Descriptions

Movement	Description
Abduction	A motion that pulls a structure or part *away* from the midline of the body (or, in the case of fingers and toes, spreading the digits apart)
Adduction	A motion that pulls a structure or part *toward* the midline of the body or toward the midline of a limb
Dorsiflexion	Extension of the entire foot superiorly, as if taking one's foot off an automobile pedal
Extension	The opposite of flexion; a straightening movement that *increases* the angle between body parts
Flexion	Bending movement that *decreases* the angle between two parts. Bending the elbow or clenching a hand into a fist are examples of flexion
Hyperextension	A position of maximum extension or extending a body part beyond its normal limits
Inversion	The movement of the sole toward the median plane (same as when an ankle is twisted)
Plantar Flexion	Flexion of the entire foot inferiorly as if pressing an automobile pedal
Pronation	A rotation of the forearm that moves the palm from an anterior-facing position to a posterior-facing position or palm facing down
Rotation	A motion that turns a part on its axis (the head rotates on the neck)
Supination	The opposite of pronation; the rotation of the forearm so that the palm is anterior facing or palm facing up

circumdance
Passive - assisted motion
Active - voluntary ROM
Goniometry -

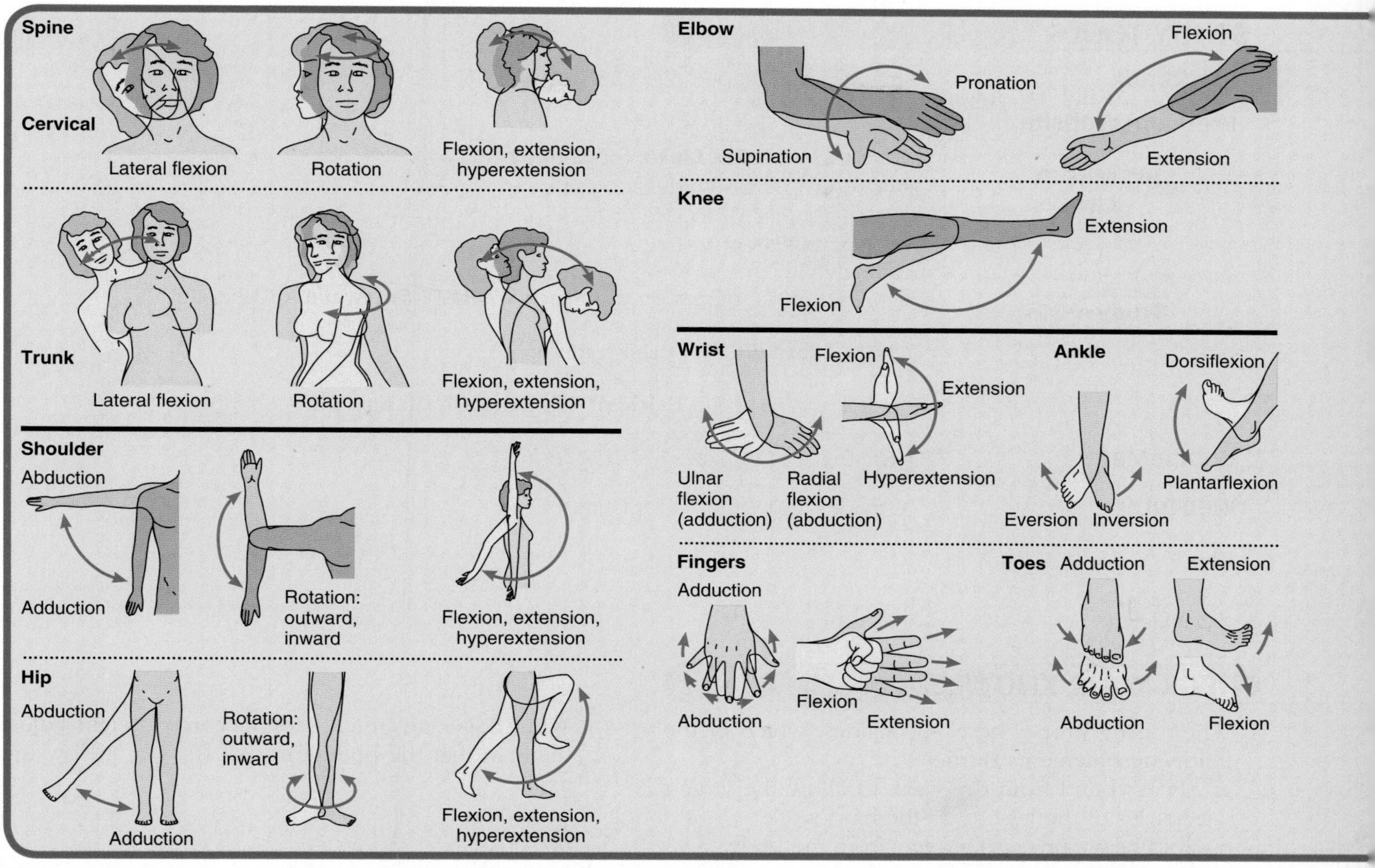

Figure 57–11: ROM exercises. *Delmar/Cengage Learning.*

CHAPTER SUMMARY

- Body mechanics is the practice of using certain key muscle groups together with good body alignment and proper body positioning to reduce the risk for injury to both patient and caregiver. When caring for patients or moving and lifting equipment and supplies, you must always be conscious of using proper body mechanics for safety to yourself and the patients.
- Patients and their families must be informed of the importance of maintaining a safe home environment for persons using ambulatory aids.
- Many times, following a serious illness or an accident, some form of supporting device or equipment is needed to allow a person as much mobility as possible.
- Not only should you learn to instruct others in the proper use or application of the various pieces of equipment, but you could also participate in the patient's experience by practicing being the patient so that you can appreciate the patient's dependence and understand the constraints involved.
- Various devices that might be indicated in the process of recovering and gaining mobility include slings, canes, crutches, and walkers. Understanding how each of these devices operates and being able to educate the patient is essential.
- ROM is defined as any body action involving muscles, joints, and natural directional movements such as abduction, adduction, extension, flexion, pronation, and rotation. Such exercises are usually applied actively or passively in the treatment of orthopedic deformities, assessment of injuries and deformities, and athletic conditioning.

STUDY TOOLS

Workbook	Activities for Chapter 57
Premium Website	
MEDIA LINK	View these **Media Links** for Chapter 57: • Use Proper Body Mechanics • Assist a Patient to Use Crutches • Assist a Patient to Use a Walker
StudyWARE	Activities and Quizzes on the **StudyWARE™ Software** for Chapter 57
	Audio Library of medical terms
	Online access to the **Critical Thinking Challenge 2.0**
CourseMate	Activities and Quizzes for Chapter 57
WebTutor	Activities and Quizzes for Chapter 57

CHECK YOUR KNOWLEDGE

1. When using proper body mechanics, which of the following statements is true?
   a. Always bend from the waist to allow the largest muscles of the legs to do the hard work.
   b. Hold heavy objects far away from the body.
   c. Check your posture by reminding yourself to keep your chin and chest up.
   d. Check your posture by keeping shoulders forward and pelvis tilted slightly inward.
2. An example of a situation when the use of a mobility device would be needed includes:
   a. arthritis sufferers.
   b. after a stroke.
   c. physically challenged.
   d. all of the above.
3. When using a cane for support, the arm should hang naturally at the side with the elbow flexed at about a ______-degree angle.
   a. 10–15
   b. 20–25
   c. 25–30
   d. 30–45
4. When adjusting crutches for the correct height, adjust them so that the underarm pad is _____ below the axilla.
   a. 1 inch
   b. 2 inches
   c. 4 inches
   d. 6 inches
5. Which of the following crutch gaits positions both crutches and the left foot forward and then brings up the right foot?
   a. Three-point
   b. Four-point
   c. Two-point
   d. Swing-through

WEB LINKS

Proper Lifting Techniques, from the Mayo Clinic:
www.mayoclinic.com/health/back-pain/LB00004_D

National Center for Biotechnology Information:
www.ncbi.nlm.nih.gov

Occupational Safety & Health Administration:
www.osha.gov

RESOURCES

Estes, M. E. Z. (2010). *Health Assessment & Physical Examination* (3rd ed.). Clifton Park, NY: Delmar Cengage Learning.

Hegner, B. R., Acello, B., and Caldwell, E., (2008). *Nursing Assistant: A Nursing Process Approach* (10th ed.). Clifton Park, NY: Delmar Cengage Learning.

Heller, M., and Veach, L. (2009). *Clinical Medical Assisting: A Professional, Field Smart Approach to the Workplace*. Clifton Park, NY: Delmar, Cengage Learning.

Lindh, W., Pooler, M., Tamparo, C., and Dahl, B. (2010). *Delmar's Comprehensive Medical Assisting Administrative and Clinical Competencies* (4th ed.). Clifton Park, NY: Delmar Cengage Learning.

Simmers, L. (2009). *Diversified Health Occupations* (7th ed.). Clifton Park, NY: Delmar Cengage Learning.

Venes, D. (ed.). (2009). *Taber's Cyclopedic Medical Dictionary* (21st ed.). Philadelphia: F.A. Davis.

Chapter

58 Nutrition, Exercise, and Healthy Living

OBJECTIVES

In this chapter, you will learn the following:

KB KNOWLEDGE BASE

1. Spell and define, using the glossary at the back of the text, all the Words to Know in this chapter.
2. Discuss the dos and don'ts listed in the Guidelines for Good Health table.
3. Define nutrition.
4. Name the fat- and water-soluble vitamins.
5. Discuss what minerals are and why they are essential.
6. Discuss the MyPyramid Food Guidance System.
7. Discuss some of the ways and foods that promote good general health.
8. Describe the parts of a food label and how to interpret the amounts.
9. Describe and discuss dietary and health concerns of adolescents.
10. Provide instruction to patients for performing stretching exercises.
11. Explain the importance of sleep and a positive outlook toward health.

WORDS TO KNOW

additive
amenorrhea
anorexia nervosa
anorexic
beriberi
binge
bulimia nervosa
calorie
carbohydrate
deprivation
dietician
emaciation
health
infirmity
malnutrition
NREM (non-rapid eye movement)
nutrition
obesity
protein
purge
REM (rapid eye movement)
rickets
scurvy
sleep apnea
tactile

GUIDELINES FOR GOOD HEALTH

Health is defined by the World Health Organization as a state of complete physical, mental, and social well-being. Health is not merely the absence of disease or **infirmity**. All things conducive to good health are referred to as healthful. Healthful living habits are essential for one to maintain good physical condition or to stay physically fit. There are simple guidelines that can keep us in good health, increase vitality, and possibly even increase life expectancy. Table 58–1 outlines the suggestions advised for the general population. Those who are in the health care professions are urged to set a good example to the patients we teach.

With today's attention to physical fitness, the medical assistant must be well informed to answer the inquiries patients make concerning diet and exercise programs. The provider will decide what is best for each patient after all data from the medical history, examination, laboratory findings, and other pertinent information have been evaluated. You can reinforce the provider's orders and help patients adapt those orders to their particular lifestyles.

In some instances, the provider will refer the patient to a registered **dietician** to teach dietary basics and plan for the patient's specific needs. If this is the case, you still might be asked about something that gives you the opportunity to reinforce what the dietician has said and helps the patient understand.

NUTRITION

Nutrition is defined in *Taber's Cyclopedic Medical Dictionary* as "all the processes involved in the taking in and utilization of food substances by which growth, repair, and maintenance of activities in the body as a whole or in any of its parts are accomplished." This includes ingestion, digestion, absorption, and metabolism (assimilation) and means that what you put into your body is all your body has available to use to keep you healthy. If you fail to give it the proper nutrients (ingredients), it can't keep you functioning at the optimum level. Patient education in proper nutrition is one of your many responsibilities.

Nutrients

You are probably familiar with the basic nutrients. The body gets energy from **carbohydrate**, fat, and **protein** nutrients. Other elements such as water, electrolytes, fiber, minerals, and vitamins are nutrients that are essential to the process of metabolism. The body is able to function best with adequate amounts of these essential nutrients, along with exercise and restful sleep. Poor diet and sedentary lifestyle leads to:

- Cardiovascular disease
- Hypertension
- Dyslipedemia
- Type 2 diabetes
- Diverticular disease
- Osteoporosis
- Overweight and **obesity**
- Iron deficiency
- **Malnutrition**
- Certain cancers

Being able to discuss the essential nutrients and other elements for healthy living with patients is a valuable skill. Table 58–2 shows a sample of widely diverse nutrient values and calories in various foods.

Calories

The energy nutrients of carbohydrates, proteins, and fats have calorie values. A **calorie** is a unit of heat. Technically, a calorie is defined as the amount of heat needed to raise the temperature of a kilogram of water one degree centigrade, from 14.5°C to 15.5°C. All of the body's processes burn calories to provide energy and sustain life. Foods are a combination of nutrients and, therefore, calories, but not all nutrients have the same caloric value. For example, a gram of carbohydrate or

TABLE 58–1 Guidelines for Good Health

Do	Don't
Eat a sensible, well-balanced diet including high-fiber, low-fat cereal and grain foods	Overeat or gain too much weight
Practice health and safety rules at home and work	Use drugs or medications unless prescribed for a specific purpose
Exercise regularly	Smoke or use tobacco (including chew and snuff)
Use sunscreen with SPF 15+ as needed	Expose skin to sun for prolonged periods
Get adequate rest and recreation	Drink alcohol in excess
Nurture your spirit daily	Expose yourself to unnecessary X-rays

TABLE 58–2 Examples of Nutrients and Calories in Common Foods

Food	Portion	Total Grams	Calories	Carbohydrates	Protein	Fats
Green beans	1 cup	125	45	10	2	trace
Baked fish	3 oz.	85	80	trace	17	1
Butter	1 tablespoon	14	100	trace	trace	11
Apple	1 large	212	125	32	trace	1
Cheeseburger with bun	4 oz.	194	525	40	30	31
Pecan pie	1/8 pie	138	575	71	7	32

Adapted from Taber's Cyclopedic Medical Dictionary.

CLINICAL PEARL

It is interesting to compare food calories in relation to their amount. For example, reviewing Table 58–2, for 100 calories you could have 1 tablespoon of butter or more than 2 cups of green beans. Which will satisfy your hunger better? Small, inexpensive paperback booklets are available at grocery and bookstores that list the most common food values in calories, carbohydrates, proteins, and fats. Patient education materials can be offered to patients in the reception area also.

protein will have *approximately* 4 calories, whereas a gram of fat has *approximately* 9 calories.

The ideal balance would be to eat an amount of nutrients equal to the amount of energy we use, but that is not easily done. The basic amount of calories required to maintain an average-sized adult expending a low level of energy is 1,500 to 1,800 per day or about 70 calories per hour. This refers to the amount of energy it takes just for normal body functions. Another part of good health, which is discussed in more detail later in the chapter, concerns the amount of exercise we get. Exercise burns calories and keeps us more flexible, strong, and healthy. Table 58–3 lists how many calories you would burn from engaging in one hour of various activities.

Vitamins and Minerals

Vitamins are organic substances found in foods that are essential to good health and growth. Vitamins are called micronutrients. As the name implies, only a trace quantity is required for enzymatic reaction in the body. If the body does not receive adequate vitamins or does not absorb them sufficiently, deficiency diseases can result. (The major ones are **rickets**, **scurvy**, and **beriberi**. Rickets is the result of a deficiency of vitamin D; scurvy, of vitamin C or ascorbic acid; and beriberi, of vitamin B or thiamine.)

Vitamins A, D, E, and K are fat-soluble vitamins. Vitamin C and the B-complex vitamins are water-soluble. With a well-balanced diet, there is little likelihood of vitamin-deficiency diseases. Vitamins are added to many foods because of their loss in the food's preparation. Patients will be advised by the provider if a vitamin or mineral supplement is necessary.

TABLE 58–3 Calories Burned in One Hour of Activity or Exercise by an Average 160-Pound Person

Activity or Exercise	Calories Burned per Hour (approx.)
Sitting, reading	80
Playing golf, not walking or carrying bag	200
Moderate speed walking or bicycling, housework	250
Swimming, tennis doubles, ballet exercises	350
Fast walking, singles tennis, water skiing	400
Running, climbing stairs, heavy manual work	660
Soccer, handball	700

Adapted from Taber's Cyclopedic Medical Dictionary.

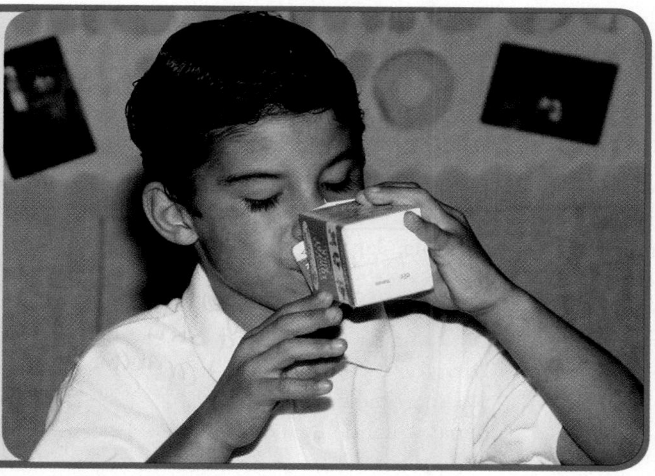

Figure 58–1: Milk is an important source of calcium and phosphorus. *Delmar/Cengage Learning.*

Minerals are naturally occurring, inorganic, homogeneous, solid substances. Thirteen are said to be essential to good health and are supplied by a variety of meats and vegetables (Figure 58–1). Minerals found to be lacking most often from the diet are calcium, iron, and iodine. Insufficient amounts of zinc, copper, magnesium, and potassium can cause metabolic disturbances.

The principal vitamins, minerals, and micronutrients are listed in Table 58–4, and Table 58–5 shows a basic calorie chart. Careful study of these charts will give you an understanding of the food sources, the function of each in the body's growth and repair, the effects of deficiency and toxicity, and the dosages recommended for daily intake.

Table 58–5 lists single servings of some common foods with their total calorie content; carbohydrate, protein, and fat grams; and total calories from fats, proteins, and carbohydrates. This can be used as a guide in meal planning. Prepared foods and many of the fast foods we eat usually have more fat, sugar, and salt than the foods we cook for ourselves. Advise patients that eating fast foods should be the exception and not a regular meal habit.

PATIENT EDUCATION

Several servings of fiber-rich foods (fruits, vegetables, peas and beans, whole grain cereals) should be included in the daily diet to promote a healthy digestive tract and prevent constipation. Encourage patients to modify cooking techniques by using less fat, oil, and sugar and by baking, broiling, boiling, roasting, grilling, poaching, or steaming meats and other foods instead of frying them. These modified cooking practices can also reduce the amount of calories, cholesterol, sodium, sugar, and saturated and total fat from the diet.

HEALTHY EATING

The United States Department of Agriculture (USDA), in cooperation with the Department of Health and Human Services (HHS), is charged to develop and release Dietary Guidelines for Americans (DGA) at five-year intervals, based on the most current and scientific nutritional advice available. The most current guidelines can be found at www.dietaryguidelines.gov.

According to the 2010 report, the following summarizes four major priority action steps for Americans:

1. *Reduce overweight and obesity* of the U.S. population by *reducing overall calorie intake* and *increasing physical activity.*
2. Shift food intake patterns to a *more plant-based diet* that emphasizes vegetables, cooked dry beans and peas, fruits, whole grains, nuts, and seeds. In addition, *increase the intake of seafood* and *fat-free and low-fat milk and milk products* and consume *only moderate amounts of lean meats, poultry, and eggs.*
3. *Significantly reduce intake of foods containing added sugars and solid fats* because these dietary components contribute excess calories and few, if any, nutrients. *Reduce sodium.* Eat *fewer refined grains,* especially those in foods with added sugar, solid fat, and sodium.
4. Meet the *2008 Physical Activity Guidelines for Americans.* (Report of the Dietary Guidelines Advisory Committee on the Dietary Guidelines for Americans, 2010)

The DGA serve as a base for all government programs related to nutrition, such as the National School Lunch Program and the WIC program (Supplemental Nutrition Program for Women, Infants, and Children). They also are the basis for the USDA's MyPlate Food Guidance System (Figure 58–2). The MyPlate program is no longer one-size-fits-all and offers personalized eating

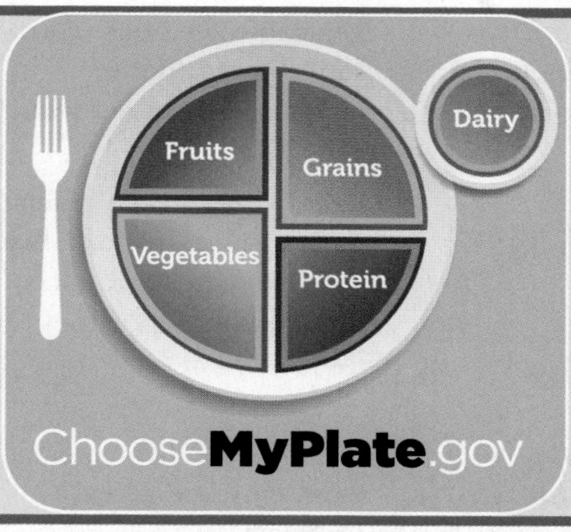

Figure 58–2: MyPlate is the "new generation" food icon to prompt consumers to think differently about their food choices. *Courtesy of the U.S. Department of Agriculture.*

TABLE 58–4 Principal Micronutrients

Micronutrient	Principal Source	Functions	Effects of Deficiency and Toxicity	Usual Therapeutic Dosage
Vitamin A	Fish liver oils, liver, egg yolk, butter, cream, vitamin A–fortified margarine, green leafy or yellow vegetables	Photoreceptor mechanism of retina, integrity of epithelia, lysosome stability, glycoprotein synthesis	*Deficiency:* Night blindness, perifollicular hyperkeratosis, xerophthalmia, keratomalacia *Toxicity:* Headache, peeling of skin, hepatosplenomegaly, bone thickening	10,000–20,000 mcg (30,000–60,000 units/day)
Vitamin D	Fortified milk is main dietary source, fish liver oils, butter, egg yolk, liver, ultraviolet irradiation	Calcium and phosphorus absorption, resorption, mineralization, and collagen maturation of bone; tubular reabsorption of phosphorus	*Deficiency:* Rickets (tetany sometimes associated), osteomalacia *Toxicity:* Anorexia, renal failure, metastatic calcification	*Primary Deficiency* 10–40 mcg (1,400–1,600 units)/day) *Metabolic Deficiency* 1–2 mcg/day $1.25\text{–}(OH)_2D_3$ or $1\alpha\text{–}(OH)D_3$
Vitamin E group	Vegetable oil, wheat germ, leafy vegetables, egg yolk, margarine, legumes	Intracellular antioxidant, stability of biologic membranes	*Deficiency:* RBC hemolysis, creatinuria, ceroid deposition in muscle	30–100 mg/day
Vitamin K (activity) Vitamin K_1 (phytonadione) Vitamin K_2 (menaquinone)	Leafy vegetables, pork, liver, vegetable oils, intestinal flora after newborn period	Prothrombin formation, normal blood coagulation	*Deficiency:* Hemorrhage from deficient prothrombin *Toxicity:* Kernicterus	In situations conducive to neonatal hemorrhage, 2–5 mg during labor or daily for 1 wk prior; or 1–2 mg to newborn
Essential fatty acids (linoleic, arachidonic acids)	Vegetable seed oils (corn, sunflower, safflower); margarines blended with vegetable oils	Synthesis of prostaglandins, membrane structure	Growth cessation, dermatosis	Up to 10 g/day
Thiamine (vitamin B_1)	Dried yeast, whole grains, meat (especially pork, liver), enriched cereal products, nuts, legumes, potatoes	Carbohydrate metabolism, central and peripheral nerve cell function, myocardial function	Beriberi, infantile and adult (peripheral neuropathy, cardiac failure, Wernicke-Korsakoff syndrome)	30–100 mg/day
Riboflavin (vitamin B_2)	Milk, cheese, liver, meat, eggs, enriched cereal products	Many aspects of energy and protein metabolism integrity of mucous membranes	Cheilosis, angular stomatitis, corneal vascularization, amblyopia, sebaceous dermatosis	10–30 mg/day

Micronutrient	Principal Source	Functions	Effects of Deficiency and Toxicity	Usual Therapeutic Dosage
Niacin (nicotinic acid, niacinamide)	Dried yeast, liver, meat, fish, legumes, whole-grain enriched cereal products	Oxidation-reduction reactions, carbohydrate metabolism	Pellagra (dermatosis, glossitis, GI and CNS dysfunction)	Niacinamide 100–1,000 mg/day
Vitamin B_6 group (pyridoxine)	Dried yeast, liver, organ meats, whole-grain cereals, fish, legumes	Many aspects of nitrogen metabolism (e.g., transaminations, porphyrin and heme synthesis, tryptophan conversion to niacin), linoleic acid metabolism	Convulsions in infancy, anemias, neuropathy, seborrhea-like skin lesions Dependency states	25–100 mg/day
Folic acid	Fresh green leafy vegetables, fruit, organ meats, liver, dried yeast	Maturation of RBCs, synthesis of purines and pyrimidines	Pancytopenia, megaloblastosis (especially pregnancy, infancy, malabsorption)	1 mg/day
Vitamin B_{12} (cobalamins)	Liver, meats (especially beef, pork, organ meats), eggs, milk and milk products	Maturation of RBCs; neural function; DNA synthesis, related to folate coenzymes; methionine and acetate synthesis	Pernicious anemia, fish tapeworm and vegan anemias, some psychiatric syndromes, nutritional amblyopia Dependency states	In pernicious anemia 50 mcg/day IM first 2 wk, 100 mcg twice/wk next 2 mo, thereafter 100 mcg/mo
Vitamin C (ascorbic acid)	Citrus fruits, tomatoes, potatoes, cabbage, green peppers	Essential to osteoid tissue, collagen formation, vascular function, tissue respiration and wound healing	Scurvy (hemorrhages, loose teeth, gingivitis)	100–1,000 mg/day
Sodium	Wide distribution—beef, pork, sardines, cheese, green olives, cornbread, potato chips, sauerkraut	Acid–base balance, osmotic pressure, pH of blood, muscle contractility, nerve transmission, sodium pumps	*Deficiency:* Hyponatremia *Toxicity:* Hypernatremia, confusion, coma	
Potassium	Wide distribution—whole and skim milk, bananas, prunes, raisins	Muscle activity, nerve transmission, intracellular acid–base balance and water retention	*Deficiency:* Hypokalemia, paralysis, cardiac disturbances *Toxicity:* Hyperkalemia, paralysis, cardiac disturbances	

(continues)

TABLE 58–4 *(Continued)*

Micronutrient	Principal Source	Functions	Effects of Deficiency and Toxicity	Usual Therapeutic Dosage
Calcium	Milk and milk products, meat, fish, eggs, cereal products, beans, fruits, vegetables	Bone and tooth formation, blood coagulation, neuromuscular irritability, muscle contractility, myocardial conduction	*Deficiency:* Hypocalcemia and tetany, neuromuscular hyperexcitability *Toxicity:* Hypercalcemia, GI atony, renal failure, psychosis	10–30 ml 10% calcium gluconate soln IV in 24 h
Phosphorus	Milk, cheese, meat, poultry, fish, cereals, nuts, legumes	Bone and tooth formation, acid–base balance, component of nucleic acids, energy production	*Deficiency:* Irritability, weakness, blood cell disorders, GI tract and renal dysfunction *Toxicity:* Hyperphosphatemia in renal failure	Potassium acid and di-basic phosphate parenteral 600 mg (18.8 mEq)/day
Magnesium	Green leaves, nuts, cereal grains, seafoods	Bone and tooth formation, nerve conduction, muscle contraction, enzyme activation	*Deficiency:* Hypomagnesemia, neuromuscular irritability *Toxicity:* Hypermagnesemia, hypotension, respiratory failure, cardiac disturbances	2–4 ml 50% magnesium sulfate soln/day IM
Iron	Wide distribution (except dairy products)—soybean flour, beef, kidney, liver, beans, clams, peaches Much unavailable (<20% absorbed)	Hemoglobin, myoglobin formation, enzymes	*Deficiency:* Anemia, dysphagia, koilonychia, enteropathy *Toxicity:* Hemochromatosis, cirrhosis, diabetes mellitus, skin pigmentation	Ferrous sulfate or gluconate 300 mg orally three times a day
Iodine	Seafoods, iodized salt, dairy products Water variable	Thyroxine (T_4) and triiodothyronine (T_3) formation and energy control mechanisms	*Deficiency:* Simple (colloid, endemic) goiter, cretinism, deaf-mutism *Toxicity:* Occasional myxedema	150 mcg iodine/day as potassium iodide added to salt 1:10–40,000 ppm
Fluorine	Wide distribution—tea, coffee Fluoridation of water supplies with sodium fluoride 1.0–2.0 ppm	Bone and tooth formation	*Deficiency:* Predisposition to dental caries, osteoporosis *Toxicity:* Fluorosis, mottling, pitting of permanent teeth, exostoses of spine	Sodium fluoride 1.1–2.2 mg/day orally

Micronutrient	Principal Source	Functions	Effects of Deficiency and Toxicity	Usual Therapeutic Dosage
Zinc	Wide distribution—vegetable sources Much unavailable	Component of enzymes and insulin, wound healing, growth	*Deficiency:* Growth retardation, hypogonadism, hypogeusia; cirrhosis, acrodermatitis enteropathica	30–150 mg zinc sulfate/day orally
Copper	Wide distribution—organ meat, oysters, nuts, dried legumes, whole-grain cereals	Enzyme component	*Deficiency:* Anemia in malnourished children; Menkes kinky hair syndrome *Toxicity:* Hepatolenticular degeneration, some biliary cirrhosis	0.3 mg/kg/day copper sulfate orally
Cobalt	Green leafy vegetables	Part of vitamin B_{12} molecule	*Deficiency:* Anemia in children *Toxicity:* Beer-drinker's cardiomyopathy	20–30 mg/day cobaltous chloride orally
Chromium	Wide distribution—brewer's yeast	Part of glucose tolerance factor (GTF)	*Deficiency:* Impaired glucose tolerance in malnourished children, some diabetics	

Lack of Zinc → hypogonadism – Less function of ovary & testis.

plans and interactive tools to help individuals make healthy food choices. There are daily food plans for various age groups and different lifestyles and nutritional needs. The Website www.ChooseMyPlate.gov allows you to enter your age, gender, height, weight, and level of exercise. In return, you receive a calorie pattern (number of calories) estimated for your needs and your own personal modified pyramid (Figure 58–3A–B). Also available on the site are useful interactive tools (MyFoodapedia, Food Tracker, and Food Planner), sample menus, and recipes.

It is hoped the ChooseMyPlate program will encourage Americans to make healthier food choices and be active every day. Look at the place setting in Figure 58-2, and note the following:

- *The green section refers to vegetables.* Vegetables are naturally low in fat and calories, and are sources of many essential nutrients. Beans and peas are unique in that they may be considered both a vegetable and a protein, because of their high nutrient content.
- *The red section refers to fruits.* Fruits supply nutrients such as Vitamin C, potassium, dietary fiber, and folic acid. They are naturally low in fat, sodium, and calories.
- *The orange section refers to grains.* Grains are divided into two groups: whole grains and refined grains. Make at least half of your grains whole grains. Refined grains have been removed of nutrients and dietary fiber.
- *The purple section refers to protein.* Proteins supply nutrients such as Vitamin E, B vitamins, iron, zinc, magnesium, and omega-3 fatty acids. Meat, poultry, seafood, beans and peas, eggs, processed soy products, nuts, and seeds are considered proteins.
- *The blue section refers to dairy.* Dairy supplies nutrients such as calcium, Vitamin D, potassium, and protein. Milk, calcium-fortified soymilk, yogurt, cheese, and milk-based desserts are part of the dairy group; lactose-free versions of these items are also included. Foods made from milk that have little or no calcium (butter, cream cheese) are not considered dairy. Choose fat-free or low-fat products in this group.

TABLE 58–5 Nutritional Content in a Single Serving of Common Foods

Food	Total Calories	Fat Grams	Calories from Fat	Carbohydrate Grams	Calories from Carbohydrate	Protein Grams	Calories from Protein
Breads and Cereals							
Whole wheat bread							
(1 slice)	65	1	9	11	44	3	12
Biscuit (2-inch diameter)	103	4.8	43.2	12.8	51.2	2	8
Spaghetti (1 cup)	190	1	9	39	156	7	28
Shredded wheat (2/3 cup)	100	0.5	4.5	23	92	3	12
Bran flakes (1 cup)	106	0.6	5.4	28.2	112.8	4	16
Granola (1/3 cup)	125	5	45	19	76	3	12
Dairy Products							
Milk (1 cup)							
Whole	159	8.2	73.8	11.4	45.6	8	32
2% low-fat	121	4.7	42.3	11.7	46.8	8	32
Skim (nonfat)	86	0.44	4	11.8	47.2	8	32
Yogurt (1 cup), plain low-fat	144	3.5	31.5	16	64	12	48
Cottage cheese (1 cup)							
Regular	217	9.4	84.6	5.6	22.4	27	108
Low-fat (2%)	203	4.4	39.6	8.2	32.8	31	124
Cheddar cheese (1 oz)	112	9.4	84.6	0.36	1.4	7	28
Swiss cheese (1 oz)	107	7.8	70.2	0.96	3.8	8	32
Egg (1 large, raw)	82	6.5	58.5	0.5	2	6	24
Fruits and Vegetables							
Apple (1 medium)	96	1	9	24	96	Trace	0
Avocado (1 medium)	334	32.8	295.2	12.6	50.4	5	20
Banana (1 medium)	127	0.3	2.7	33	120	1	4
Broccoli (1 stalk, raw)	40	1	9	8	32	4	16
Carrot (1 large, raw)	30	0.2	1.8	7	28	1	4
Orange (1 medium)	64	0.3	2.7	16	64	1	4

Potato (1 large, baked, no skin)	145	0.2	1.8	32.8	131.2	3	12
Tomato (1 medium, raw)	25	Trace	0	5	20	1	4
Meat, Poultry, Fish, and Legumes							
Beef							
Ground, lean (3 oz)	230	16	144	0	0	21	84
Roast, chuck (3 oz)	226	13	117	0	0	25	100
Lamb, chop (3 oz)	220	15	135	0	0	20	80
Pork, chop (3 oz, pan fried)	335	27	243	0	0	21	84
Chicken, breast (¼ lb, roasted)	140	3	27	0	0	27	108
Turkey, light meat (3 oz)	135	3	27	0	0	25	100
Flounder (3 oz)	80	1	9	0	0	17	68
Shrimp, fresh (¼ lb)	103	0.9	8.1	6.8	27	17	68
Kidney beans (1 cup cooked)	218	0.9	8.1	39.6	158.4	15	60
Lentils (1 cup cooked)	212	0	0	38.6	154.4	16	64
Split peas (1 cup cooked)	230	0.3	2.7	41.6	166.4	16	64
Miscellaneous							
Butter (1 tablespoon)	102	11.3	102	0	0	Trace	0
Margarine (1 tablespoon)	102	11.3	102	0	0	Trace	0
Mayonnaise (1 tablespoon)	102	11.3	102	0	0	Trace	0

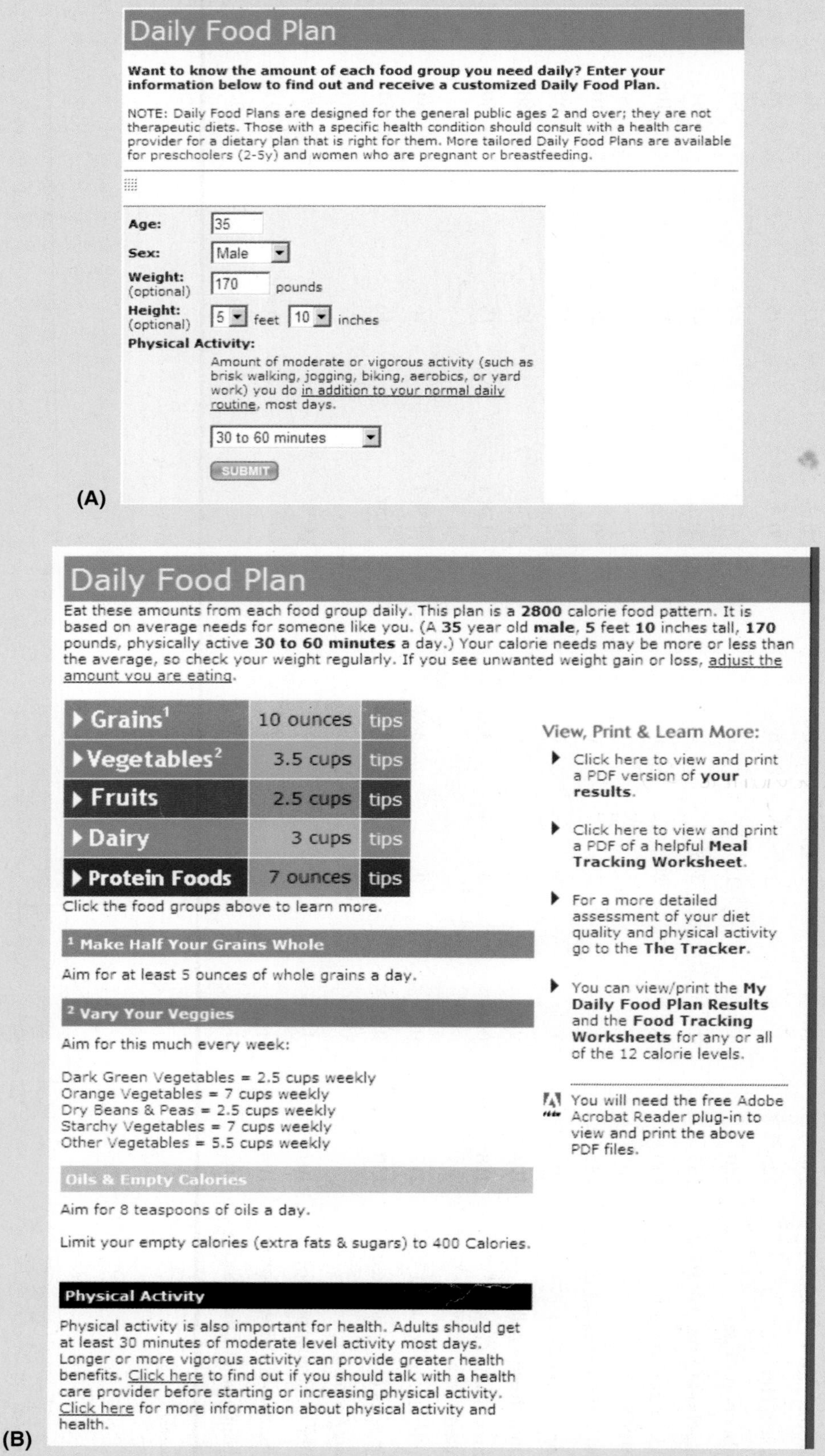
Daily Food Plan
Want to know the amount of each food group you need daily? Enter your information below to find out and receive a customized Daily Food Plan.
NOTE: Daily Food Plans are designed for the general public ages 2 and over; they are not therapeutic diets. Those with a specific health condition should consult with a health care provider for a dietary plan that is right for them. More tailored Daily Food Plans are available for preschoolers (2-5y) and women who are pregnant or breastfeeding.
Age: 35
Sex: Male
Weight: (optional) 170 pounds
Height: (optional) 5 feet 10 inches
Physical Activity:
Amount of moderate or vigorous activity (such as brisk walking, jogging, biking, aerobics, or yard work) you do in addition to your normal daily routine, most days.
30 to 60 minutes
SUBMIT
(A)
Daily Food Plan
Eat these amounts from each food group daily. This plan is a 2800 calorie food pattern. It is based on average needs for someone like you. (A 35 year old male, 5 feet 10 inches tall, 170 pounds, physically active 30 to 60 minutes a day.) Your calorie needs may be more or less than the average, so check your weight regularly. If you see unwanted weight gain or loss, adjust the amount you are eating.
Grains[1] 10 ounces tips
Vegetables[2] 3.5 cups tips
Fruits 2.5 cups tips
Dairy 3 cups tips
Protein Foods 7 ounces tips
Click the food groups above to learn more.
1 Make Half Your Grains Whole
Aim for at least 5 ounces of whole grains a day.
2 Vary Your Veggies
Aim for this much every week:
Dark Green Vegetables = 2.5 cups weekly
Orange Vegetables = 7 cups weekly
Dry Beans & Peas = 2.5 cups weekly
Starchy Vegetables = 7 cups weekly
Other Vegetables = 5.5 cups weekly
Oils & Empty Calories
Aim for 8 teaspoons of oils a day.
Limit your empty calories (extra fats & sugars) to 400 Calories.
Physical Activity
Physical activity is also important for health. Adults should get at least 30 minutes of moderate level activity most days. Longer or more vigorous activity can provide greater health benefits. Click here to find out if you should talk with a health care provider before starting or increasing physical activity. Click here for more information about physical activity and health.
View, Print & Learn More:
Click here to view and print a PDF version of your results.
Click here to view and print a PDF of a helpful Meal Tracking Worksheet.
For a more detailed assessment of your diet quality and physical activity go to the The Tracker.
You can view/print the My Daily Food Plan Results and the Food Tracking Worksheets for any or all of the 12 calorie levels.
You will need the free Adobe Acrobat Reader plug-in to view and print the above PDF files.
(B)

Figure 58–3: Daily food plan screens on www.ChooseMyPlate.gov: (A) You can enter your individual information. (B) The results of your information input. *Courtesy of the U.S. Department of Agriculture.*

Helping patients select materials that can benefit them is a way to keep them motivated to follow a diet plan. Give patients support by letting them know that you are pleased that they are making progress in healthy choices in their diets.

Reading Nutrition Facts Labels

The federal Nutritional Labeling and Education Act requires manufacturers to put Nutrition Facts labels on all their food so consumers can know what they are eating. The labels contain a wealth of information about the food item (Figure 58–4). Note that all labels have the same format:

- *Serving Size:* This indicates how much of the product the figures relate to; it is followed by the weight in total grams.
- *Servings per Container:* This indicates how many servings of the serving size are in the box or package.
- *Amount per Serving:* This indicates the number of calories per serving as well as how many of those calories are from fat. Remember, the number of servings eaten determines the number of calories actually consumed.
- *Listing of the food nutrients with their respective gram amounts:* The nutrients listed first (Total Fat, Cholesterol, and Sodium) are the ones Americans generally eat in adequate amounts or even too much.
- *Percentage (%) of Daily Value amounts:* These percentages represent how much is in the serving of the total daily amount of the item that a person on a 2,000-calorie diet should consume.
- *The Total Fat section:* This is broken down into several types, including saturated fats and trans-fats. As of January 2005, manufacturers were required to list the amount of trans-fat in their product because it has been shown to have a direct relationship with elevated LDL cholesterol and heart disease.
- *The Total Cholesterol section:* This is also broken down into types, including dietary fiber and sugars. A diet high in dietary fiber promotes healthy bowel

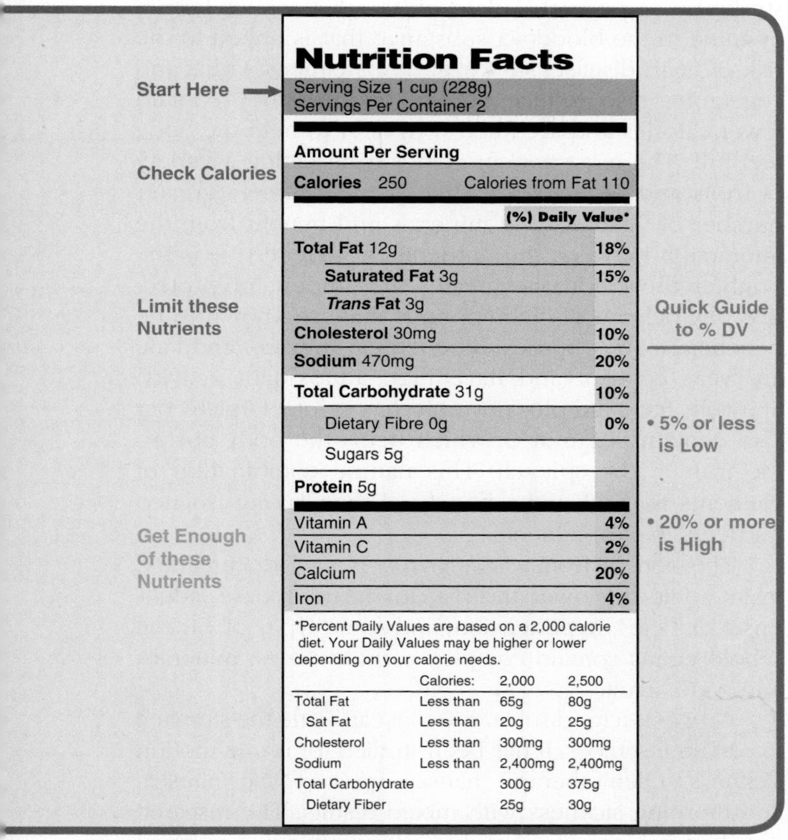

Figure 58–4: Reading a Nutrition Facts label. *Adapted from the U.S. Food and Drug Administration.*

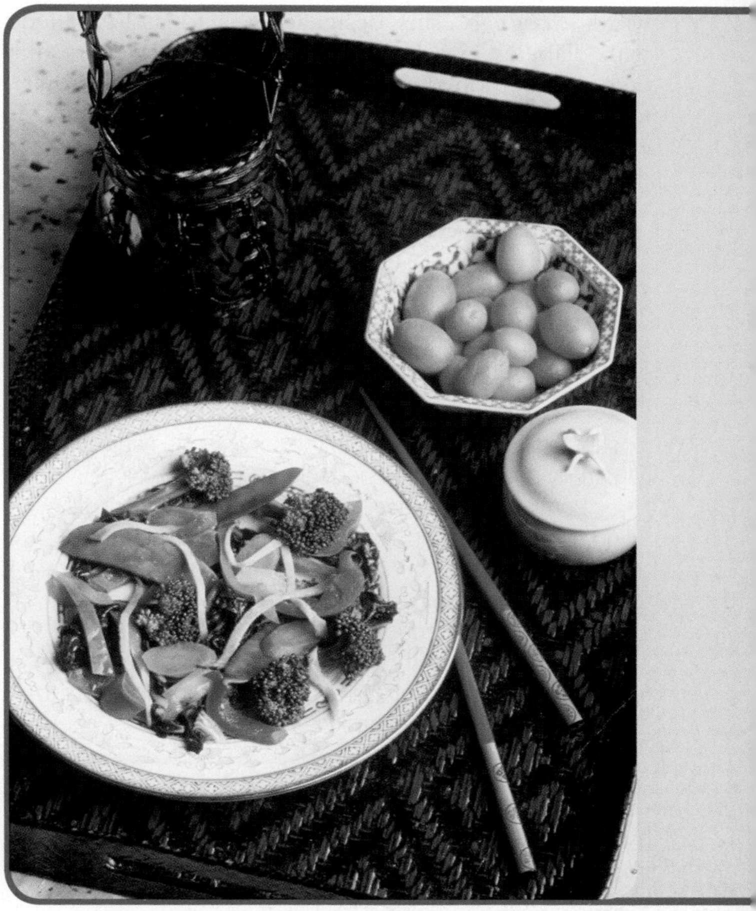

Figure 58–5: Traditional Chinese foods. *Delmar/Cengage Learning.*

function. Sugars include both naturally occurring sugars (such as those in fruit) and added sugars.
- *A list of vitamins and minerals in the serving:* Two of these samples have hardly any listed, but the box of cereal, label (A), lists a large amount. According to the FDA, most Americans don't get enough vitamin A, vitamin C, calcium, and iron in their diets.

A list of ingredients follows the nutritional information and should include everything in the product. You will note many chemical **additives**: Some enhance taste or color, whereas others prolong the shelf life of the product. It is important to understand how the ingredients are listed. The ingredient with the highest content in the product is listed first. The last ingredient listed is the one with the least amount contained in the product.

At the end of the list of ingredients on each label, some of the ingredients are listed again. This identifies quickly the items that might cause allergic reactions in sensitive people. Some of the most common food allergies are peanuts, wheat, milk, fish, and shellfish. A peanut allergy is so serious that it can be life threatening, and even traces of peanuts can be a problem to a person with a severe peanut allergy.

Another feature you will find on some labels is the word *exchange*. This designation is to assist patients with diabetes in selecting food within a category; this time, it is carbohydrates to maintain their carbohydrate-fat-protein balance. Their dietary amounts are stated in exchanges, and they can select any foods up to their daily limit within that food category.

PATIENT EDUCATION

Encourage patients to read food labels at the grocery store before they buy any food. As patients are planning their daily menu, advise them to read food labels again and note the percentage of each of the nutrients. They should also pay attention to the serving size (which is usually not the amount normally consumed).

Remind patients about attractive wording, such as no "cholesterol" and "low fat." Some food labels claim to be low in fat or salt or to contain no (zero) cholesterol, but then they are generally high in sugar and calorie content. Reduced-calorie food items can also have a high salt or sodium content. Manufacturers add increased amounts of salt and other flavor enhancers to make the lower-calorie food item taste better.

Explaining to patients how to count calories, carbohydrates, fat grams, and so on will help them realize the importance of planning meals that are well balanced and sensible. For those who are interested in eating a healthier diet, labels help eliminate the guesswork. Having the contents listed on packages also makes it easier for those who are on special diets and those watching their caloric intake, fat grams, cholesterol content, and so on. Food labels can also make menu planning a more pleasant and interesting project. Remind patients to read *all* labels carefully.

Foods That Promote Health

Volumes are written about the claims of certain foods. Interesting information regarding many unusual treatments can be found on the Internet, but always be cautious and evaluate the content and source. Some reliable sites are operated by the National Institutes of Health (NIH), the U.S. Department of Agriculture, and the U.S. Department of Health and Human Safety. URLs to these sites are listed in the Web Links section at the end of this chapter.

A strong body of evidence shows that *fruits and vegetables* promote good general health. Some fruits and vegetables might even protect against heart disease and certain cancers. Eating a diet with nine servings of fruits and vegetables a day lowers the risk of ischemic stroke by 31 percent. Folates in the diet reduce homocysteine in the blood—a substance that is linked to the risk of heart disease, stroke, and Alzheimer's. Fruits and vegetables also reduce obesity because they contain fewer calories and are filled with fiber to help the body feel full. The most benefit comes from eating a variety of fruits and vegetables so that you consume a greater number of vitamins and minerals and benefit from the interaction between the nutrients. A general rule is the brighter the color, the greater the amount of protective phytochemicals (compounds that are known to be beneficial). Strawberries, blueberries, spinach, and kale are very colorful and have high antioxidant activity. Spinach, for example, not only has a lot of folate but also contains vitamin C, which helps the body absorb the iron in the spinach. This natural combination of elements is much more beneficial than taking isolated nutrients in supplements.

The benefit from *whole grains* is well documented in its ability to lower the risk for heart disease, adult-onset diabetes, hypertension, and some types of cancer. Whole grains contain complex carbohydrates, minerals, and antioxidants.

Ginger is a food substance that can settle the stomach in certain instances. It has been studied for use in motion sickness, chemotherapy nausea, postsurgical nausea, and morning sickness with mixed results. The research did show taking a 1-gram dose 30 minutes before travel could be recommended. *Garlic* is another food item that has been promoted as healthful. It does seem to have some ability to lower cholesterol and blood pressure, thereby preventing heart disease. It has been used for centuries to treat many conditions from tuberculosis to hemorrhoids. Laboratory studies have suggested that garlic might help fight cancer, but human studies have not determined it lowers cancer risk. However, dietary histories of 564 Chinese people with stomach cancer were compared with 1,131 individuals without the disease. It was concluded the risk of developing stomach cancer was 60 percent lower among people who ate the most alliums (garlic, onions, leeks, and shallots), which seems to infer some protective benefit. Its cousin, the onion, was used for a poultice (a hot mashed mass inside a cloth) to treat chest congestion in the past.

Walnuts and other nuts in general have been identified as being able to reduce the risk of heart disease. Even though they are loaded with calories and fat, researchers believe that because they are rich in monounsaturated and polyunsaturated fats, they lower the LDL and raise the HDL cholesterol levels. However, this is possible only when these types of fat *replace* the saturated fats in meats and dairy products.

Meal Supplements

When patients suffer from loss or lack of appetite or they cannot tolerate a normal diet, it might be necessary for the provider to prescribe a protein-vitamin-mineral food supplement. Patients who might need this type of treatment include the older adult and the chronically ill, postoperative, underweight, anemic, and **anorexic** patients. This treatment should be conducted only under the supervision of a provider. Remind patients to take these supplements regularly as directed. The supplements generally come in at least vanilla and chocolate flavors and can be purchased in drug, health, and grocery stores. They are available in individual, ready-to-drink cans or in powder form to be mixed with liquid. They can be ordered as a meal substitute or as between-meal nourishment. They can be beneficial for patients receiving chemotherapy to supply extra nourishment in an easy-to-use liquid format when eating regular food is not appealing.

Herbal Products and Dietary Supplements

According to a national survey conducted in 2007, an estimated 17.7 percent of American adults had used dietary supplements other than vitamins and minerals. The Office of Dietary Supplements (ODS) within the NIH was created by the Dietary Supplement Health and Education Act of 1994. The mission of the ODS is to investigate the safety and effectiveness of dietary supplements, support research and disseminate results of that research, and educate the public. The most important thing to understand about dietary supplements is the big difference between these products and conventional over-the-counter (OTC) drugs, even though they might be displayed on the same shelves in drug and grocery stores. The Food and Drug Administration (FDA) regulates dietary supplements; however, *the regulations are not the same as those for prescription or OTC drugs*. Substances passing OTC regulations require clinical trials, designated dosage establishment, documentation of side effects, and characteristics of people who had adverse reactions. Manufacturers are also required to show the product is at least as good as any previously approved product for the same purpose. These reports are published in scientific journals for professional and public review. One study estimated that the whole process requires 7.5 years from lab testing to consumer market and can cost over $800 million per item. The regulations for dietary supplements are much less strict:

- Manufacturers are expected follow "good marketing practices" to ensure that their products meet quality standards, but a manufacturer does not have to prove the safety and efficacy of a dietary supplement prior to bringing it to the consumer market.
- Manufacturers may make claims about a supplement if there is research to support it; however, it must include a disclaimer stating, "This statement has not been evaluated by the U.S. Food and Drug Administration (FDA). This product is not intended to diagnose, treat, cure, or prevent any disease."
- After it is on the market, the FDA monitors the safety of the dietary supplement. If the FDA finds a product unsafe, it can take action against the manufacturer or distributor, ranging from a warning to requiring the removal of the product from the market.

Labels on dietary supplements should contain a list of ingredients and their strength, a suggested dosage, and any warning about its use. A few of the most common dietary supplements are:

- *St. John's wort*—Widely used for herbal treatment for depression, anxiety, and sleep disorders. According to the National Center for Complementary and Alternative Medicine (NCCAM), there is scientific evidence that it can be useful for short-term treatment of mild to moderate depression. Although some studies have reported benefits for more severe depression, others have not; for example, a large study sponsored by NCCAM found that the herb was no more effective than placebo in treating major depression of moderate severity. No standards for dosage, its

PATIENT EDUCATION

Research has also shown that St. John's wort negatively interacts with many medications, including:

- Antidepressants
- Birth control pills
- Digoxin
- Seizure-controlling drugs
- Warfarin and related coagulants

Herbal and other supplements can negatively interfere with medications; thus it is critical to ask patients about any herbal or other dietary supplements they might be taking.

preparation, or its long-term safety have been developed. Even though classified as a supplement, it has drug-like actions.

- *Black cohosh*—A large woodland plant found in eastern North America, used for menopause relief as an alternative to traditional hormone therapy, to control hot flashes, night sweats, headaches, heart palpitations, and mood changes. Its effect seems to suggest that it contains a natural estrogen-like substance and the known salicylates found in aspirin. The NCCAM is currently funding studies to measure the effects of black cohosh; studies done to date are mixed on whether it actually relieves menopausal symptoms. It appears that side effects are mild when taken in moderate amounts, but it can include vomiting, dizziness, and headaches in larger doses. Because it is not standardized, each manufacturer indicates the dosage. It is recommended to take black cohosh no longer than six months because no long-term studies have been done on its safety.
- *Melatonin*—A hormone produced naturally in the pineal gland within the brain. It plays a part in regulating sleep patterns. As a supplement, it regulates sleep and prevents jet lag. It has also been promoted as an anti-aging agent. Evidence does seem to support its effect on sleep, and laboratory studies indicate that it has antioxidant properties at much larger concentrations than in the body. No evidence exists that it slows the aging process or reduces the risk of developing cancer. A potential risk from melatonin is the resulting drowsiness that impairs function and might cause morning-after headaches. It has also been reported to interfere with conception.
- *Willow bark*—Has been used to relieve pain for more than 2,400 years. Hippocrates prescribed chewing on willow leaves to relieve childbirth pain. In the second century, it was used to reduce fever and inflammation. In 1897, a Bayer chemist determined that acetylsalicylic acid (aspirin) could be extracted from a willow bark–related compound. Now, willow bark is being sold as a natural pain relief medication. Double-blind trials of 210 people with chronic low back pain determined willow bark extract to be a useful and safe treatment, at least for low back pain. Again, remember, it is not controlled or standardized. The recommended maximum daily dose is 240 mg, but it should not be used by people who have problems tolerating aspirin.
- *Echinacea*—An herb reported to stimulate the immune system to help prevent developing a cold or the flu. It has been used for centuries by Native Americans to treat everything from coughs to burns and snakebites. Study results have been mixed about its effectiveness in preventing or treating upper respiratory infections; two NCCAM-funded studies did not find a benefit from echinacea, but other studies have shown that it might be beneficial in treating upper respiratory infections. Echinacea grows in three forms, each with a different concentration of ingredients. Benefits can also depend on which part of the plant is used: the leaf, roots, or flowers. Potential side effects include severe allergic reactions, which indicates that all people with asthma or allergic rhinitis should avoid usage; gastrointestinal system upset; and rash. In addition, some medications are changed and broken down by the liver; echinacea might decrease how quickly the liver breaks down some medications, which might be problematic. It has also been known to increase the effects and side effects of some medications. Before taking echinacea, patients must be instructed to discuss with their provider whether to take it if they are taking any medications that are changed by the liver.
- *Saw palmetto*—A plant that produces berries containing phytosterol compounds that scientists think might slow down the production of male testosterone, which stimulates prostate growth. The compound is used to treat symptoms of benign prostate hypertrophy (BPH). Several traditional medications are available but are sometimes not effective and might cause erectile dysfunction or a decline in sexual desire. Smaller studies have suggested that saw palmetto might be safe and effective for treating BPH, but larger studies and research between 2006 and 2009 indicate that it has not been shown to be more effective than a placebo. Saw palmetto might interact with other medications, including birth control pills, estrogens, and anticoagulant or antiplatelet drugs, but there are no known interactions with food or other herbs and supplements. It is again noted that, without regulation, there is no guarantee of the purity or content of the product.

- *Glucosamine sulfate*—A chemical naturally produced in the human body as well as in nature. It is promoted as a product to relieve the pain of osteoarthritis. It reportedly promotes healthy cartilage formation to maintain or replace that which is worn away by age and use. New data from a long-term study of the glucosamine and chondroitin dietary supplements for knee osteoarthritis pain revealed that patients who took supplements had outcomes similar to those patients who took placebo pills.
- *Ginseng*—The root of a shrub native to China and Korea that has been used medicinally in many cultures for centuries. Ginseng has been used to support overall health and boost the immune system. In addition, it has been used to treat erectile dysfunction, hepatitis C, and menopausal symptoms; to lower blood glucose; and to control blood pressure. Studies and research have been inconclusive, but scientific investigation has failed to support its claims as an aphrodisiac. There is evidence that it improves circulation and elevates mood.
- *Gingko biloba*—A product from the leaves of the ginkgo tree and promoted as an agent to improve memory and mental function by increasing blood flow to the brain. European studies suggest that it might slow the progress of or even prevent Alzheimer's disease. It also appears to be an antioxidant and might help prevent atherosclerotic plaque. Side effects of nausea, vomiting, and diarrhea occur at extremely high doses.

This discussion of common herbs and supplements only scratches the surface of products available in grocery and health food stores. Here are several resources for additional information on these and other herbs and supplements:

- National Center for Complimentary and Alternative Medicine (NCCAM, a division of the National Institutes of Health [NIH]): www.nccam.nih.gov
- NIH Office of Dietary Supplements: www.ods.od.nih.gov
- NIH National Library of Medicine's MedlinePlus: www.nlm.nih.gov/medlineplus

CLINICAL PEARL

The use of supplements requires reading and careful consideration. Discuss all dietary supplement use with a provider. Look for quality of evidence in reports, how many people are using the product, and their experiences. Choose a brand tested in published studies if possible. Learn as much as you can to make the wisest selection.

WEIGHT CONTROL

Providers want their patients to lose weight if they are either on the threshold of obesity or have already been diagnosed as obese. Weighing more than 30 percent above your ideal body weight (obese), can put you at risk for developing serious health problems such as heart disease, stroke, diabetes, cancer, and **sleep apnea**. A good weight-control program should contain foods from the food pyramid to be nutritionally sound. Eating should be an enjoyable, relaxing experience. However, in our fast-food society, people tend to eat more food, with more calories, more often. As discussed earlier, a calorie is a unit of heat, and all food substances have caloric value (see Table 58–5). All the body's processes burn calories to provide energy and sustain life. If you overeat regularly, the unused calories are not wasted but stored as fat. If you reduce calorie intake, the body uses the stored fat for energy, and you will begin to shed the extra weight. Make patients aware that they should eat their meals slowly because it takes approximately 20 minutes for the brain to realize that the stomach is full. Those who follow this practice in a relaxed atmosphere eat *less* and digest their food better. It is now recommended that eating several (five to six) small meals daily not only allows for better use of nutrients by the body for more energy, but it is much easier on the digestive tract. This practice also helps in weight control.

A variety of magazines, books, and businesses offer weight-control plans that promise success for each individual. Over-the-counter drugs promise miraculous weight loss in a matter of weeks. You can be influential in helping patients avoid possible health hazards by warning them of the danger in these quick-weight-loss programs. Many people do lose weight in a short time, but they gain it right back as soon as the program ends. Others do permanent damage to their health.

Most people who reach their weight-loss goals and have maintained a satisfactory weight have learned how to change their eating habits. Positive reinforcement is one of the keys to their success. Encourage patients who are trying to follow a diet by showing a genuine interest as they work to reach their goals.

There is no quick fix or one particular diet to follow for everyone who needs to lose weight. A list of foods with their calorie content or a basic diet as a guide can be helpful to those who wish or need to reduce their weight.

Therapeutic Diets

Therapeutic diets are used in the treatment of patients with a specific disease or disorder. Standard printed diet sheets, pamphlets, booklets, and other patient education topics can be displayed on a wall-mounted rack for convenience to patients and you. Post information about nutrition, heart-healthy cooking classes, and other topics on the bulletin board to involve patients in their health care. Patients who have a medical condition with dietary needs beyond the printed materials in your facility should be referred to a registered dietitian (RD). Reinforce the need for this referral and how important it is to give their full cooperation. A patient's background and lifestyle will be considered and adjustments made as necessary. A dietician will work closely with other health care team members in individual therapeutic diet planning.

The number of special diets is far too numerous to list in this book. A few therapeutic diets that might be helpful to you in providing education to patients are briefly discussed here. These are general guidelines to follow. You should follow the patient education policy established by the providers in your medical facility when advising patients either by phone or in person. If you are uncertain or have any questions regarding what to tell patients about their treatment plan, ask the provider. Providers usually have printed dietary information about the most common types of diets to which you can refer and provide to patients.

- *Clear liquid diet:* Pedialyte for infants and children, Gatorade for adults, clear gelatin, decaffeinated coffee and tea, clear broth, no-caffeine sodas, artificially flavored drink mix, flavored frozen juice bars and treats, clear juice, and water as directed by provider—offered to patients at least every two hours the first 24 hours for patients with diarrhea.
- *BRAT diet:* **B**ananas, **r**ice, **a**pplesauce, **t**oast, and clear liquids or water (Pedialyte for infants) for 24 hours as tolerated by patients after diarrhea stops, or as directed by the provider.
- *Soft diet:* Creamed hot cereals, gelatin, pudding, ice cream, sherbet, mashed or baked potatoes, puréed vegetables, creamed soups, baked turkey/chicken/fish, meatloaf, milk, poached egg, macaroni and cheese, yogurt, applesauce, and graham crackers. These are suggestions for foods that might be more easily tolerated for patients who have gastrointestinal disorders such as a duodenal ulcer or gastritis. This diet is also for those who are just getting over an intestinal virus.
- *Low-calorie diet:* Counting calories and adding up the total will help those who wish to shed a few pounds, especially if cardiovascular exercise is included at least three times a week for a minimum of 30 minutes. Eating no more than a total of 30 percent of calories from fat each day is recommended for a healthy heart, especially if there is a family history of heart disease.
- There are low-fat, no-sugar, high-fiber, low- or no-salt, and low-residue diets, and the list continues with specialized therapeutic diet plans for individual needs.

Popular Diets

Many popular or fad diets over the years have promised rapid weight loss over a short period of time. Most of these diets appear to work initially, usually because of reduced caloric intake, but the only proven long-term and safe method is to take fewer calories in and get more exercise. Some of these diets include the grapefruit diet, in which you consume primarily grapefruit; the cabbage soup diet, in which you eat a mixture of cabbage and other vegetables for a short period of time; and low-carbohydrate diets such as Atkins and South Beach, which actually resulted in the manufacture of special low-carbohydrate foods and meals. More recent popular diets include the master cleanse (also called the maple syrup diet), the zone diet, and the caveman power diet.

Cultural Influence on Diet

Various cultures have a long history of dietary preferences and practices. Because so many cultures have come to the United States, you will surely come in contact with many of them. It is interesting to learn about ethnic and religious practices that differ from your own; it can make your life experiences exciting. Some dietary practices of different cultural or religious groups will be familiar to you. To introduce you to the diversity, a brief listing follows.

- *Asian:* The main foods are rice, vegetables, fruits, and curries. Meat, fish, and chicken are used in small amounts. Most foods are prepared by sautéing in a wok.
- *Catholic:* Abstain from eating meat on Ash Wednesday and Fridays during Lent. Older Catholics might still adhere to the former restriction of no meat on any Fridays. They often choose something, such as a favorite food, to abstain from throughout the total Lenten season.
- *Chinese:* Rice is the main staple, along with soybean products. Pork, eggs, and vegetables are also favorites (Figure 58–5). Tea is the beverage of choice.
- *Hindu:* Followers believe life is sacred and animals are the dwelling places of ancestors' souls. Therefore, they eat primarily vegetables.
- *Islamic:* Followers have dietary laws governing the method of killing animals for food. Eating pork or drinking alcohol is prohibited. During the daylight hours in the month of Ramadan, Muslims do not eat

food or drink water but spend the day in reflection, intense worship, reading the Quran, and developing self-control.

- *Italian:* Pasta with various tomato sauces and cheese are popular foods. Southern Italy natives enjoy fish and highly seasoned food, whereas northern Italy natives eat more meat and root vegetables.
- *Japanese:* Rice, soybean paste, vegetables, fruits, and fish. Food is frequently fried and topped with soy sauce. Sushi is rice combined with fish, eel, or squid, rolled in sheets of dry seaweed, and cut into small wheels. It is very popular in the United States.
- *Jewish:* Orthodox Jews have strict dietary laws, many dating to Biblical times. Foods prepared by these laws are called kosher (Figure 58–6). Meat and poultry must be killed and treated in a specific manner. Meat and milk products must not share the same preparation dishes and must be eaten six hours apart. The laws also forbid eating hindquarters of meat. Shellfish, pork, and many other items are on the forbidden list. No cooking is permitted on the Sabbath (Friday sundown to Saturday sundown), so foods must be made ahead of time.
- *Mexican:* The favorite foods are rice, beans, chili peppers, tomatoes, and cornmeal. The meat is usually cooked with vegetables in a thick, soup-like chili. Tortillas and tamales are flat breads made from cornmeal and are filled with meat and vegetable mixtures and then wrapped in cornhusks and steamed.
- *Seventh-Day Adventist:* Observe Saturday as the day of worship. Members abstain from coffee, tea, and alcohol, which they consider harmful. The diet consists of milk, eggs, and vegetables and no meat, fish, or poultry. Meat substitute from soybeans provides protein.

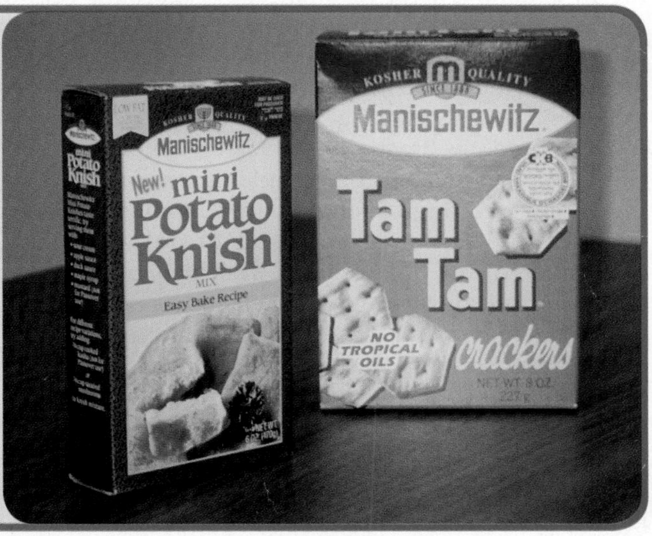

Figure 58–6: Kosher foods. *Delmar/Cengage Learning.*

After this brief introduction to various dietary differences, it is easy to see how some cultural and religious practices could cause challenges to diet modifications that might be needed due to the lack of some nutrients in the diet.

Health Concerns in Adolescents

Special focus should be directed to a predominantly adolescent condition called **anorexia nervosa**. Anorexia nervosa is a psychoneurotic disorder in which the patient—usually but not exclusively a female—refuses to eat over a period of time. Often, vigorous exercise is part of the daily routine to help burn calories. Many problems can stem from the ongoing weight loss, including **emaciation** and **amenorrhea**. This disorder can be the result of emotional stress or conflict. The patient has a poor self-image and is obsessed with a fear of becoming obese. Signs of this disorder are a change in personality, irritability, refusal to eat, and weight loss.

A similar disorder, also seen mainly in adolescent females, is **bulimia nervosa**. Unlike the patient with anorexia, the patient with bulimia eats a very large quantity of food at one time (as much as 5,000 calories) but uses **purging** (vomiting, laxatives, and diuretics) to rid the body of the calories. Usually, the patient eats normal meals with others to conceal the disorder. This is one of the reasons this disorder is sometimes difficult to diagnose. The bulimic's **binge** eating and purge behaviors also originate from poor self-image and feelings of inadequacy. Symptoms of bulimia are dark circles under the eyes, muscle wasting, dental cavities, and damage to tooth enamel caused by stomach acid from frequent vomiting. Problems with gastrointestinal and cardiovascular systems are a potential danger in this disorder.

Referral for psychiatric therapy and nutritional counseling as soon as possible are necessary to arrest these potentially fatal disorders. Make a sincere effort to give positive reinforcement to patients in an area of their personal interest (e.g., hobby, school project, or activity). Your patience and understanding is extremely important in helping these patients feel accepted and supported.

The adolescent in general needs a little extra attention in the promotion of or, possibly, in the initial establishment of good health habits. Give this patient a chance to ask questions and discuss problems in private. Often, fears arise about many timely issues such as sexual behavior, STDs and HIV, pregnancy and birth control, substance abuse (drugs and alcohol), depression and suicide, domestic issues and abuse (emotional, physical, and sexual), peer pressure, and a wealth of other topics the patient might feel he or she cannot talk to anyone else about because of embarrassment or intimidation. You might be the only one who will treat him or her as an individual and listen objectively to his or her problems. Sometimes just getting a chance to let it out is helpful. Offer your listening ear and support and refer the patient to the provider or to an appropriate service agency as necessary (e.g., mental health center, teen pregnancy free clinic). Some teenagers are reluctant to speak to the school nurse or other authoritative figure because of the possibility of having a parent called.

Being a teenager is a very stressful time. Many pressures begin to surface, creating many demands that pile up rapidly on an already confused and mood-swinging adolescent. One very common problem you might be influential in curbing is the cigarette habit. Giving adolescents the facts about smoking and health can make all the difference in their decision to resist this temptation. Health care professionals have a responsibility to give this age group of patients their careful attention whenever the opportunity occurs, simply because they do not appear very often for health care services.

EXERCISE

In addition to a well-balanced diet, adequate exercise and sufficient rest are essential to good health. Exercise is defined as physical exertion for improvement of health or correction of physical deformity. Regular exercise improves circulation and muscle tone and relieves tension. People who have followed an exercise routine regularly report that they experience a better outlook on life, have more energy, and feel healthier. The degree of exertion in any exercise routine varies with individuals, and the provider's advice should be taken.

Many exercise programs are available that people can choose according to their individual needs and goals. A combination of proper diet and proper exercise brings satisfying results in overall good health. Special diet and exercise programs must be approved for individuals by the provider, who will determine the patient's needs and tolerance from careful examination and medical history. This safeguards the patient from overexertion and stress.

It is important also to prepare your muscles for exercise to avoid discomfort and limited motion. This is especially true when you begin an exercise program. If you get sore, aching muscles, you will not be able to participate in exercise and can become discouraged. People who exercise regularly or participate in vigorous activity will go through simple exercises to warm up gently and stretch muscles. Even before walking, proper stretching is recommended to keep from straining muscles and help prevent other injuries. Table 58–6 illustrates the 10 basic stretching exercises to help prepare for exercise.

Repeat the pre-exercise stretches following exercise as a cool-down period. This allows muscles to adjust to a non-exercise state and helps eliminate soreness. Read the instructions and practice the different exercises. Even if you are not preparing to exercise, these will help you relax tense muscles from daily stress or long periods of sitting.

PATIENT EDUCATION

The safest form of exercise, and one almost everyone can participate in, is walking. Often, patients are reluctant to walk if they have to walk alone because they fear for their safety. You can suggest seeking a walking partner and trying to go in daylight hours. The purchase of a treadmill is a good investment (for those who can afford it) because it is available at any time and in any weather. You might suggest inquiring at a local enclosed shopping mall about walking clubs that meet before the mall opens. This way, the patients have a safe and comfortable environment in the company of others with the same interest. This idea could be quite helpful in motivating them to stick to a routine for their better health.

HEALTHY SPIRIT

All the behaviors that influence health are governed by one's mental (or social) health and vice versa. A positive outlook is most helpful in coping with life in general. (Refer to Chapter 8.) Learning coping and problem-solving skills can help us deal with the everyday stress and occasional crisis of routine living. Many providers recognize the power of a patient's belief system. Nurturing the spirit (the soul) has overall benefits. Practicing a chosen religious belief can help the feelings of completeness and belonging. Many meaningful religious ceremonies give us a sense of direction and remind us of purpose. Being a member of an organization in which others offer their support and caring can help boost one's sense of worth and fulfill basic self-esteem needs. Self-esteem needs can also be met with activities that reinforce our significance and our independence of one another. Meditation and other relaxation exercises, including reflection, have a calming effect. These are excellent ways to unwind, relieve stress, and help one get a good night's rest.

TABLE 58–6 Ten Basic Stretching Exercises

Illustration	Area of the body	Description
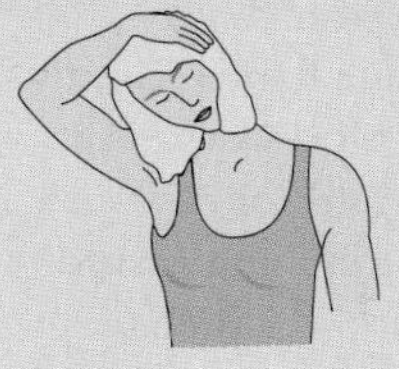	Neck muscles	Keep shoulders down while you tilt your head to the right. Place your right hand on the left side of your head, and pull gently toward your right shoulder for about 15–25 seconds. Repeat for the left side.
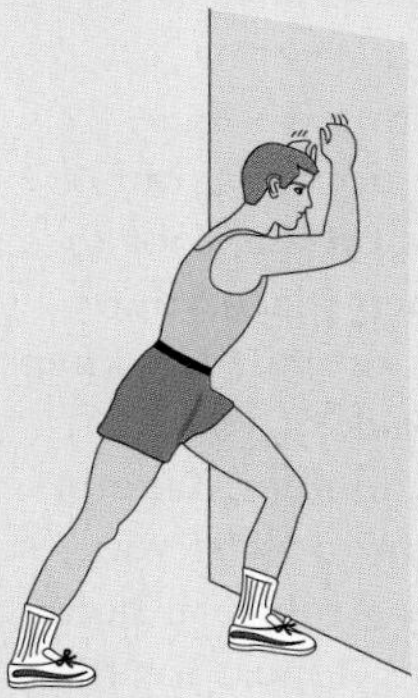	Calf muscles	Place feet flat on the floor, 2–3 feet away from a wall. Lean your forearms flat against the wall, then step toward the wall with the left foot, bending the knee while keeping the heel of the right foot flat on the floor for about 15–25 seconds. Repeat with the right leg.
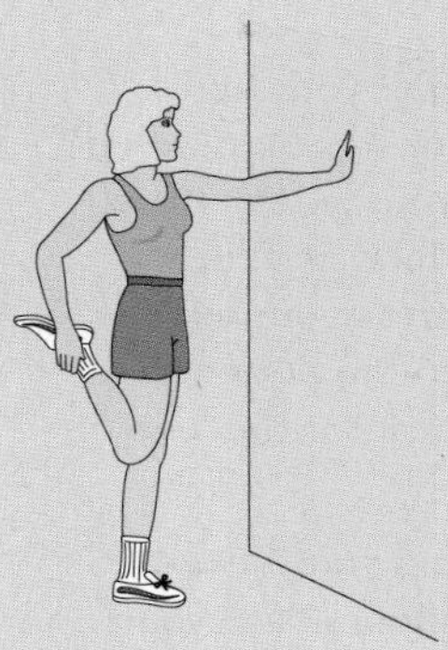	Thigh muscles (quadriceps)	Lean into the wall with your left hand, and pull your right ankle up gently with your right hand for 15–25 seconds. Repeat for the left ankle.
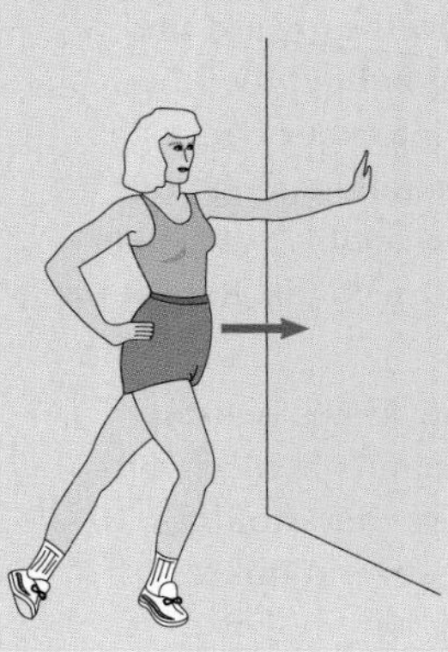	Outer thigh muscles	Stand next to and press your left hand against the wall as you place your right hand on your right hip. Bend the right knee slightly, rest the left foot on its side, and hold for 15–25 seconds. Repeat for the left leg.
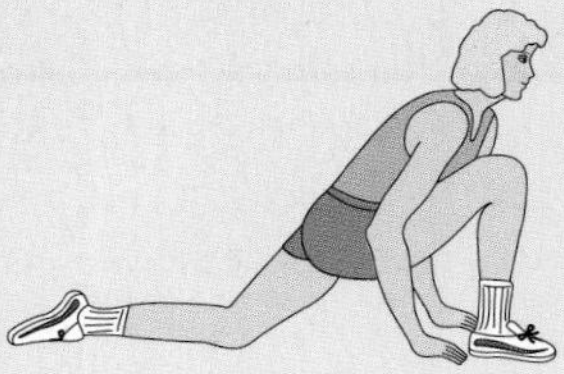	Hip muscles (hip flexor)	Get into a kneeling position with your right foot flat on the floor and bend the right knee up to touch your chest. Keep your left leg on the floor behind you (arms at your sides) and stretch and hold for 15–25 seconds. Repeat; bring the left knee to your chest; keep your right leg on the floor behind you.

(continues)

TABLE 58–6 *(Continued)*

Illustration	Area of the body	Description
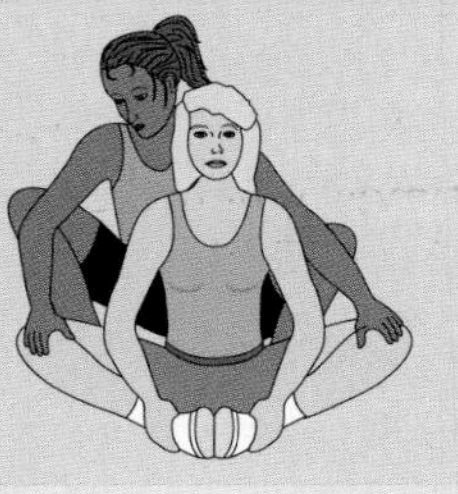	Groin muscles	While sitting on the floor, bring your heels together, and hold them with your hands. Gently push your legs down with your elbows (or ask someone to do it for you), and hold for 5–10 seconds; use resistance to feel stretching (avoid straining) and then relax. Repeat 5–10 times. This is often called the butterfly stretch.
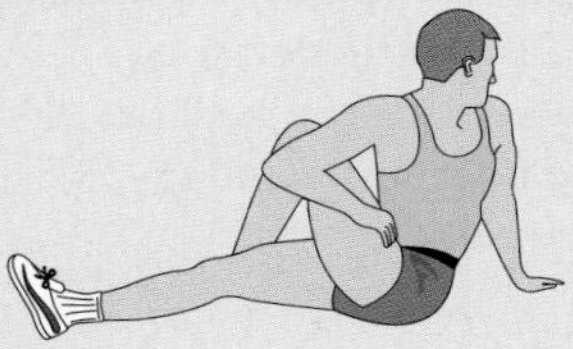	Back and side muscles	Sit up straight on the floor with both legs straight out. Bring the left leg up with your knee bent and place your foot on the floor to the right of the right knee. Then place your right elbow on the upper part of your left knee. Your left hand should be in back of you to help you look over your left shoulder. Take in a deep breath before you begin to twist your upper body and exhale slowly while you hold this posture for 10–25 seconds. Repeat for the right leg.
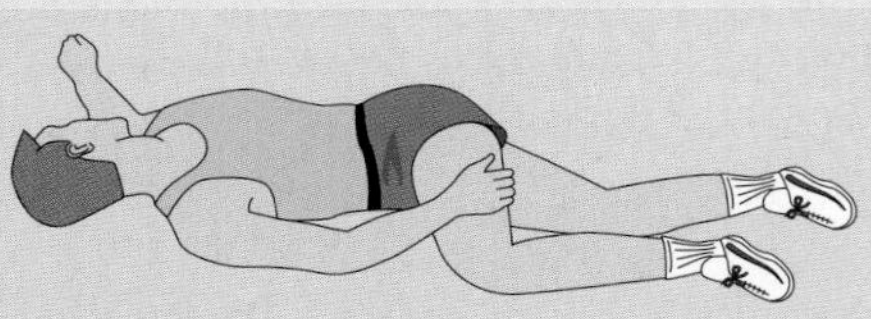	Lower back	Lie flat on your back and bring your left knee up. Cross it over to your right hip (keep your arms stretched out to your sides). Keep your shoulders against the floor, and turn your head to the left, then press your left thigh with your right hand to the floor and hold for 10–25 seconds. Repeat for the right leg.
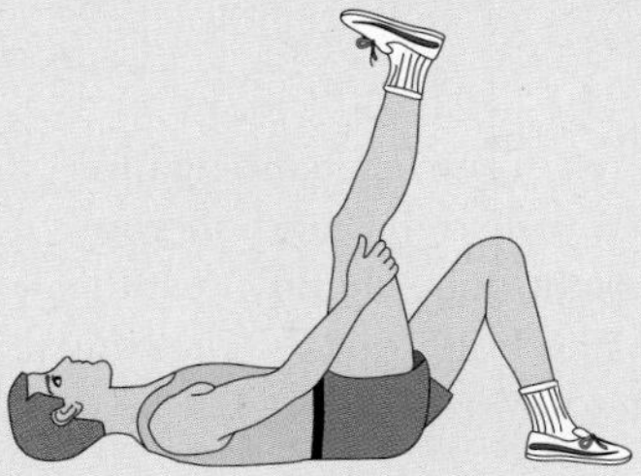	Hamstrings	Lie flat on your back and bend your knees, placing both feet flat on the floor. Raise your right leg up so that your heel is toward the ceiling. Hold your right leg behind the knee with both hands and pull into your chest. Relax your foot and keep straightening your leg until it becomes uncomfortable, and then hold the position for 10–20 seconds. Repeat for the left leg.
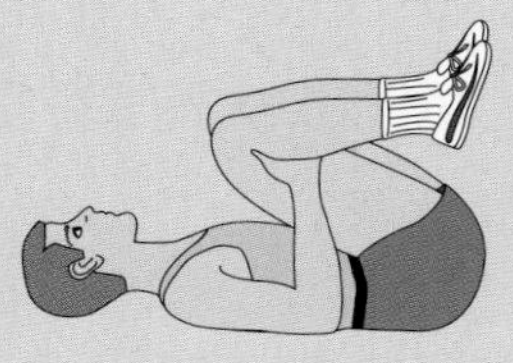	Lumbar muscles (lower back)	Lie on your back with your knees bent up to your chest. Place your hands behind your knees, press into your chest, and hold for 10–25 seconds; relax and repeat several times.

SLEEP

Getting sufficient rest is necessary for good health. Rest is usually thought of as another word for sleep and is defined as a time away from activity. Most people use the words *rest* and *sleep* interchangeably. Sleep is the natural way the body restores itself. Adequate rest or sleep equips us with strength to handle various daily activities. Winding down from strenuous or hectic activity is usually essential before one is able to rest and relax enough to go to sleep. Even though the number of hours of sleep needed varies from person to person, quality sleep should not be interrupted. The average amount of sleep needed is between six and nine hours in a 24-hour period for most adults. However, sleep patterns can change as we age. Each of us has a pattern of sleep and sleep needs specific to us.

When a patient tells you he has not been getting any sleep at night, you must ask how long the patient *does* sleep and *when* the patient sleeps. Often, sleep is sufficient but not all at once at night. If the person is obviously not getting sufficient sleep, the provider needs to be alerted when the patient first mentions it. Often, the patient does not consider it a problem worth telling you because initially it is just an annoyance. *Insomnia* describes not being able to sleep. A serious physical or emotional (psychological) problem can be the reason for the insomnia. Generally, the provider will ask the patient to keep track of when and how long at a time he or she sleeps. Establishing a record of sleep dysfunction helps the provider make a decision about diagnostic and treatment plans. Being comfortable and ready to go to sleep should be stressed to patients who have trouble sleeping. Patients who awaken once in a while, whether the reason is apparent or not, should not be alarmed. Those who wake up several times each night on a regular basis are at risk for health problems if sleep interruption continues. Sleep **deprivation** is a term that means lack of sleep. Many people experience times when sleep is not sufficient but manage to function. Within a day or so of getting sufficient rest and sleep, they are back to a normal sleep pattern.

Those who suffer from sleep deprivation on a long-term basis exhibit irritability, fatigue, poor concentration and remembering ability, clumsiness, and sometimes visual or **tactile** hallucinations. Research studies have shown that a person needs both **REM (rapid eye movement)** and **NREM (non-rapid eye movement)** stages of sleep. The NREM stage begins approximately 90 minutes after a person goes to sleep. Those who can sleep for at least six uninterrupted hours feel better and more rested because they have benefited from the effects of the proper sequence of sleep. Explain to patients that their sleep schedule might need to be altered. Patients often get stuck in a pattern because they think they have to sleep at a certain time. It is possible that some try to change their biological clock. Most people know that is not easy to do. Sometimes, all a patient needs to do is talk to someone about his or her concerns. Just listening and a suggestion from you to read or play soft music or engage in a quiet activity can be helpful. One needs to realize that sleep is not a luxury; it is necessary for the body to function well.

CHAPTER SUMMARY

- Being knowledgeable in the dos and don'ts of guidelines for good health included in the chapter is essential in providing patient education and practicing a healthy lifestyle for yourself.
- Nutrition is defined in *Taber's Cyclopedic Medical Dictionary* as "all the processes involved in the taking in and utilization of food substances by which growth, repair, and maintenance of activities in the body as a whole or in any of its parts are accomplished." This includes ingestion, digestion, absorption, and metabolism (assimilation).
- The MyPyramid Food Guidance System offers personalized eating plans and interactive tools, each geared to different lifestyles and nutritional needs. It is hoped this new design will guide people to healthy eating. You can access the food pyramid information by going to www.mypyramid.gov on the Internet. Vitamins A, D, E, and K are fat-soluble vitamins. Vitamin C and the B-complex vitamins are water-soluble.
- Minerals are naturally occurring, inorganic, homogeneous, solid substances. Thirteen are said to be essential to good health and are supplied by a variety of meats and vegetables. Minerals found to be lacking most often from the diet are calcium, iron, and iodine. Metabolic disturbances can be caused by insufficient amounts of zinc, copper, magnesium, and potassium.
- There is a strong body of evidence showing that *fruits and vegetables* promote good general health. Some foods might even protect against heart disease and certain cancers. Eating a diet with nine servings of fruits and vegetables a day lowers the risk of ischemic stroke by 31%. Folates in the diet reduce homocysteine in the blood—a substance that is linked to the risk of heart disease, stroke, and Alzheimer's. Fruits and vegetables also reduce obesity because they contain fewer calories and are filled with fiber to help the body feel full.
- The federal Nutritional Labeling and Education Act requires manufacturers to put Nutrition Facts labels on all their food so that consumers can know what they are eating. The labels contain a wealth of information about the food item such as serving size, vitamins and nutrients, serving size, serving size per container, and much more information.
- The adolescent in general needs a little extra attention in the promotion of or in the establishment of good health habits. Issues you might need to discuss include dietary issues, alcohol and drugs, and sexual encounters.
- It is very important to prepare your muscles for exercise to avoid discomfort and limited motion. This is especially true when you begin an exercise program. If you get sore aching muscles, you will not be able to participate in exercise and might become discouraged. People who exercise regularly or participate in vigorous activity will go through simple exercises to warm up gently and stretch muscles.
- Getting sufficient rest is necessary for good health. Rest is usually thought of as another word for sleep and is defined as a time away from activity. Most people use the words *rest* and *sleep* interchangeably. Sleep is the natural way for the body to restore itself. Adequate rest or sleep equips us with strength to handle various daily activities. Winding down from strenuous or hectic activity is usually essential before one is able to rest and relax enough to go to sleep.

STUDY TOOLS

Workbook	Activities for Chapter 58
Premium Website	
StudyWARE	Activities and Quizzes on the **StudyWARE™ Software** for Chapter 58
	Audio Library of medical terms
	Online access to the **Critical Thinking Challenge 2.0**
learning**lab**	Module 24: Rehabilitation and Healthy Living
CourseMate	Activities and Quizzes for Chapter 58
WebTutor	Activities and Quizzes for Chapter 58

CHECK YOUR KNOWLEDGE

1. The body gets energy from:
   a. fats.
   b. water.
   c. electrolytes.
   d. vitamins.
2. A gram of fat has *approximately* ________ calories.
   a. four
   b. five
   c. seven
   d. nine
3. The basic number of calories required to maintain an average-sized adult expending a low level of energy is __________ per day.
   a. 1200–1500
   b. 1500–1800
   c. 70
   d. 150
4. Which of the following is a water-soluble vitamin?
   a. Vitamin C
   b. Vitamin D
   c. Vitamin K
   d. Vitamin E
5. Which of the following disorders is characterized by bingeing and purging?
   a. Anorexia
   b. Gluttony
   c. Bulimia
   d. Obesity
6. Which of the following is considered a vitamin C deficiency disease?
   a. Rickets
   b. Scurvy
   c. Beriberi
   d. Spongy bones
7. Which of the following are protective elements found in fruits and vegetables?
   a. Hydro-proteins
   b. Phytochemicals
   c. Amino acids
   d. Tryptophan
8. This dietary supplement is a hormone produced naturally in the pineal gland within the brain. It plays a part in regulating sleep patterns.
   a. St. John's wort
   b. Echinacea
   c. Melatonin
   d. Ginseng
9. Regular exercise is known to:
   a. improve circulation.
   b. improve muscle tone.
   c. relieve tension.
   d. all of the above.
10. Which of the following cultural or religious groups has dietary laws that prohibit eating pork and drinking alcohol?
    a. Hindu
    b. Islamic
    c. Jewish
    d. Catholic

WEB LINKS

American Yoga Association: www.americanyogaassociation.org

American Dietetic Association: www.eatright.org

Department of Health and Human Services Office of Disease Prevention and Health Promotion: www.health.gov/dietaryguidelines

National Institute of Diabetes & Digestive & Kidney Diseases: www.niddk.nih.gov

National Institutes of Health—Center for Complementary and Alternative Medicine: www.nccam.nih.gov

National Library of Medicine: www.nlm.nih.gov

U.S. Department of Agriculture MyPyramid Program: www.mypyramid.gov

RESOURCES

Estes, M. E. Z. (2010). *Health Assessment & Physical Examination* (3rd ed.). Clifton Park, NY: Delmar Cengage Learning.

Heller, M., and Veach, L. (2009). *Clinical Medical Assisting: A Professional, Field Smart Approach to the Workplace*. Clifton Park, NY: Delmar, Cengage Learning.

Lindh, W., Pooler, M., Tamparo, C., and Dahl, B. (2010). *Delmar's Comprehensive Medical Assisting Administrative and Clinical Competencies* (4th ed.). Clifton Park, NY: Delmar Cengage Learning.

U.S. Department of Agriculture and Health and Human Services. (2010). *Dietary Guidelines for Americans, 2010*. Dietary Guidelines Advisory Committee Report. www.health.gov/dietaryguidelines. (Retrieved January 15, 2011)

U.S. Department of Agriculture. www.mypyramid.gov. (Retrieved January 15, 2011)

Venes, D. (ed.). (2009). *Taber's Cyclopedic Medical Dictionary* (21st ed.). Philadelphia: F.A. Davis.

Section

5

Preparing for Employment

Unit

20

Workplace Readiness

Employment as a medical assistant requires administrative or clinical skills or a combination of both. In seeking employment, think about the different opportunities and decide which area of medical assisting you would prefer. Some medical assistants prefer general or family practice because of its variety and challenge; others enjoy the specialty fields with their new developments and rapid change.

Participating in a practicum not only helps you become more competent in medical assisting skills but also helps you decide which area of practice you enjoy the most. The practicum also helps you develop good work habits in preparation for full-time employment. The job search begins with the desire to work. A medical assistant with skills in communication, medical office procedures, and clinical skills should discover excellent opportunities for employment. After employment is obtained, your success and satisfaction depends upon the effort you make to be part of the team.

Certification Connection

	Ch. 59
CMA (AAMA)	
Professionalism	X
RMA (AMT)	
Interpersonal relations	X
CMAS (AMT)	
Professionalism	X

Chapter

59 Practicum and the Job Search

CHAPTER OBJECTIVES

In this chapter, you will learn the following:

KB KNOWLEDGE BASE

1. Spell and define, using the glossary at the back of the text, all the Words to Know in this chapter.
2. Explain the purpose of a practicum and how it differs from an employed position.
3. List the qualities employers regard as most important in an employee.
4. Identify the goal of a résumé and describe the purpose of each style of résumé.
5. Explain the purpose of a cover letter to accompany a résumé.
6. List six places to assist you in your job search.
7. Describe appropriate professional attire and appearance for an interview.
8. Describe the dos and don'ts in preparing for an interview or applying for a job.
9. Explain why you should send a follow-up note after an interview.
10. Describe why continuing education is important.

S SKILLS

1. Prepare a résumé.
2. Compose a professional letter (cover letter, interview follow-up letter).
3. Complete an application form.

WORDS TO KNOW

career laddering
chronological
externship
functional
performance objectives
practicum
résumé
targeted
transcript

THE PRACTICUM EXPERIENCE

A **practicum**, or **externship**, is a period of time when a student is placed in an actual health care setting, under the supervision of a practicing health care provider, to apply the skills learned in the classroom. The practicum must be understood to be a learning, not a working, experience. The student does not replace any employee or assume anyone's job responsibilities. No financial benefits are to be paid.

The experience is an important part of a student's total training and is an opportunity to perform various clinical and administrative procedures learned in the classroom. Practicum sites can be in a physician's offices, internal medicine, OB/GYN, general surgery, or accredited hospital or clinic. The student's performance during the practicum is evaluated and becomes part of the student's record. A minimum of 160 practicum hours is a required component of the curriculum for medical assisting programs that are accredited by the Accrediting Bureau of Health Education Schools (ABHES) or the Commission on Accreditation of Allied Health Education Programs (CAAHEP).

PRACTICUM OBJECTIVES

For your practicum experience to achieve its purpose, a list of **performance objectives** will be compiled by your school coordinator; they will specify a list of administrative, clinical, and general competencies that should be experienced during the practicum. Figure 59–1 displays a partial list of competencies with checks to indicate those

SAMPLE PRACTICUM TRAINING RECORD

Student ______________________________ Facility ______________________________

Coordinator ______________________________ Supervisor ______________________________

Competency	school	Externship	Date
Answer office phone	✓	LK	1/10
Receive phone messages	✓	LK	1/10
Obtain/record messages	✓		
Schedule appointments	✓		
Obtain patient information	✓		
Initiate charge slip	✓		
Calculate charge slip	✓		
Process payment	✓		
File alphabetically	✓		
File numerically	✓		
Pull numerical file	✓		
Operate transcriber	✓		
Prepare letter from machine	✓		
Make corrections	✓		
Compose correspondence	✓	LK	1/15
Total charges	✓		
Use copy machine	✓	LK	1/25
Operate office computer		LK	1/27
Prepare ledger card	✓	N/A	
Record charges	✓		
Collection letter	✓		
Write check	✓		
Deposit slip	✓		
Balance bank statement	✓		
ETC.			

Competency	school	Externship	Date
Handwashing	✓		
Measure infant length	✓		
Weigh infant	✓		
Head circumference	✓		
Snellen chart	✓		
Ishihara method	✓		
Oral temperature	✓		
Rectal temperature	✓		
Axillary temperature	✓		
Electronic thermometer		LK	2/6
Radial pulse	✓	LK	2/6
Apical pulse	✓		
Respirations	✓	LK	2/6
Blood pressure	✓	LK	2/6
Irrigate eye	✓		
Irrigate ear	✓		
Horizontal recumbent	✓		
Prone position	✓		
Sims' position	✓		
Knee-chest position	✓		
Semi-Fowler's	✓		
Lithotomy	✓		
Use microscope	✓		
ETC.			

Figure 59–1: Competency documentation in a practicum training record. *Delmar/Cengage Learning.*

SAMPLE PRACTICUM EVALUATION

(Student)	(Facility)

Please enter your observations that best describe the knowledge and performance of the above named student in the spaces below.

Appearance (personal grooming, uniform, etc.)

Attitude (interested, courteous, confident, cooperative)

Maturity (accepts supervision, adapts to situation, accepts assignments)

Dependability (punctual, completes tasks, accepts responsibility)

Initiative (seeks new learning opportunities, performs extra duties)

Administrative Tasks (performs receptionist, secretarial, and managerial tasks)

Clinical Tasks (completes database, performs lab and diagnostic skills)

Interpersonal (cooperates with co-workers, supervisor, physician)

Evaluated By ______________________ (On-Site Supervisor)

Please complete by ______________________ (Date)

Date ______________________

Thank you, ______________________ (Coordinator)

Figure 59–2: Sample practicum evaluation form. *Delmar/Cengage Learning.*

deemed competent during the school program. The form contains a column for the on-site supervisor to initial when the competency is observed and deemed competent during the practicum. The goal is to gain experience in as many of the areas as possible. To facilitate this goal, the plan might indicate specific periods of time, rotating through various areas of practice, for example, two weeks in clinical, one week in billing, one week filing insurance claims, one week as a receptionist, one week with the manager, and so on. You and your on-site supervisor must be aware of these goals, and both of you should work to achieve them.

PRACTICUM POLICIES AND EVALUATIONS

The school will draft a statement of policy regarding the practicum, which indicates how the practicum should be established. It will include such things as:

- Philosophy and goals of the practicum experience.
- The role of the school.
- The role of the health facility.
- The on-site supervisor's role.
- The student's obligation.

Figure 59–2 shows a sample practicum evaluation form, listing the areas in which a student may be evaluated.

SELF-ASSESSMENT AND CAREER ENTRY

Preparing yourself for employment in your chosen career is an exciting time. A personal review of your strengths and weaknesses will help you uncover some of your best qualities and remind you of what might need extra attention. Ask family and friends to help you sort out ideas. Often, good advice can come from those who know you well. It might be helpful for you to think about your personal characteristics. Think about the regular things in your life. For example:

- Are you outgoing and friendly; do you like having people around or are you more reserved; do you have just a few good friends; or do you enjoy being alone?
- Are you usually on time or a little early or just in time and sometimes a little late?
- Can you work with very little direction or do you like to have things spelled out clearly so you feel you won't make a mistake?
- In your spare time, do you want to engage in some group activity or sport or would you rather attend a cultural event or read?

Everyone has personal characteristics that affect his or her way of doing things. When evaluating yours, you might want to make two lists, one for what you feel are your strong points and another for your weaker ones. Later, when a prospective employer asks you a question about what you think are your strong and weak areas, you will have already thought it through and can answer with responses that have a positive impact. Even negative traits can be expressed in a positive way. For example, if you have an employer reference or school notation about frequent tardiness, you might respond by saying you are taking steps to change your behavior. You are getting up 15 minutes earlier and are rewarding yourself with dinner out on Friday nights for being on time all week.

Another way in which to gain insight into your qualifications is to review the evaluations you had during your school program and, especially, during your practicum. These should indicate your strong and weak areas specific to medical assisting. Again, this helps you realize what you have to offer as a prospective employee in addition to your educational background and any past employment experiences. Getting a good idea about who you are will help you write your résumé and cover letter and prepare you for your in-person interview.

WHAT EMPLOYERS WANT MOST IN EMPLOYEES

The personal investment you have made in your education and skills training, along with the effort you put forth in producing a résumé and interviewing for employment, does not stop with being hired. Even after securing a position, you must continually strive to do your best. Your employer expects you to perform with increasing expertise in your position as you continue to gain experience.

Employers want their employees to possess certain important skills as well as valuable personal qualities or traits, presented in Table 59–1.

MEDIA LINK

View the video, "Employers and Professionalism," for this chapter on the Premium Website.

AT WORK AND ON TIME

Attendance is most important because schedules must be changed and reassignments made when an employee is absent, especially when it is unexpected. An absent employee affects everyone because work must be divided among the other team members. If you must be absent from work due to illness, it is important to follow office policies for notifying your supervisor in a timely manner. If it is necessary to get another member of the health care team to replace you, the team will need enough notice to get ready.

It is equally important to be on time daily. If you are scheduled to be at work at 8:00 AM., you should be at the work site and ready to begin at 8:00 AM. and not just coming in the door at that time. Arriving a few minutes early is a wise practice because it allows time to put your personal belongings away and begin your day without

Table 59–1 Desirable Skills and Personal Qualities in an Employee

Skills	Qualities
Communication skills (listening, verbal, written)	Positive attitude
Computer proficiency	Strong work ethic (hard-working)
Critical thinking and analytical thinking	Dependability (reliable, responsible)
Teamwork and interpersonal skills	Honesty and integrity
Time management	Punctuality
	Flexibility
	Motivated (takes initiative)

being rushed. Being prompt is a valuable personal quality appreciated by both employers and patients.

Leaving early is not advised unless absolutely necessary and with permission of the supervisor in advance. When one leaves before the scheduled time, it puts an added burden on other team members to finish your job. With each member of the health care team doing what is expected, the work is shared, and the group's efficiency will be noticed by your employer. This promotes a harmonious working relationship among employees.

TAKING CARE OF YOURSELF

You have studied throughout this text about various patient education materials and guidelines for better health. You must have realized by now that you should be practicing what you are expected to teach patients. This can only help you feel better about yourself, which will be evident to others with whom you come in contact. In good health, you are more productive and more energetic and display better coping skills. All the qualities important to employers should also be important to you.

PREPARING YOUR RÉSUMÉ

Now that you have assessed yourself and learned about desired characteristics that employers look for in employees, you should develop a personal **résumé**, an outlined summary of your abilities and experiences.

The goal of a résumé is to make a favorable impression so you will obtain an interview for a position. It should be complete, accurate, and neatly organized. The résumé describes to prospective employers your employment objectives, educational background, previous work experience, professional affiliations, community service, personal interests, honors, and whatever else you feel is important for them to know. Basic elements of a résumé are presented in Table 59–2. It need not contain personal information about your marital status, race, religion, or age. Your résumé should demonstrate to the prospective employer how qualified you are for the position for which you are applying. Refer to Procedure 59–1 for steps in creating a résumé.

A résumé that is basic but complete and properly arranged will attract an employer's attention. One that is flashy, too lengthy, or too wordy may well be discarded. A one-page résumé is a preferred length. It must be well organized and grammatically correct. You should always have someone proofread your résumé because, often, our own mistakes go unnoticed. Spelling must be accurate. There is no need to be elaborate in style. A résumé that is printed on a soft ivory or light gray, high-quality paper will stand out and is easily retrieved in a pile of others.

Because many employers accept or require résumés submitted electronically by email or uploaded through a website, think about converting your résumé into PDF (protected document format) if it is possible. This will maintain the format and layout and ensure that the electronic version of your résumé matches the printed version.

CLINICAL PEARL

It is not necessary to include a "references are available upon request" statement on your résumé Employers already expect that references, **transcripts**, and professional certificates will be provided to them. Prepare a list of references, separate from your résumé, that includes three to four nonfamily persons who know you well and can recommend you to an employer. Be sure to ask these individuals whether you may use them for a reference before you put them on your list.

RÉSUMÉ STYLES

Four major styles of résumés are most frequently used, each with a particular focus: the **functional** style, the skills style, the **targeted** style, and the **chronological** style. You can tailor your qualifications and experiences to the most appropriate style to present yourself best for the position specifications.

Chronological Style Résumé

The *chronological style* résumé is the most common and the more traditional format. It lists education achievements followed by work experience, starting with the present or most recent job and progressing back in time. This style is most appropriate for people who have employment experiences that are closely related to their desired position. It works best when there are no long periods of unemployment between jobs, which can become obvious with this style. This format is probably the easiest to prepare and works well for most job applicants. If you have extensive work experience or have worked for several employers, it is appropriate to focus on the last 10 to 15 years of employment. Figure 59–3 is an example of a chronological style format.

Table 59–2 Résumé Elements

Element	Description
Basic Résumé Entries	
Contact Information	• Include your name, address, phone number, and email address. This information can be aligned left, centered, or across the page. • Emphasize this information by bolding or enlarging the print and, perhaps, drawing a line across the page to set it apart.
Objective	• An objective is a one-sentence statement that describes the type of work you want to do, the skills you want to apply to the work, or a combination of both. • It is best to keep this brief and simple.
Education	• List your education, beginning with the most recent experience. • If you have completed several educational programs, perhaps earning a degree, it probably is not appropriate to list your high school. • If listing the dates of completion might be a disadvantage age-wise, the dates can be omitted.
Experience	• Identify your job titles, responsibilities, and specific skills performed with each position. Use phrases rather than complete sentences. • The employment experience format will depend upon which résumé style is most appropriate for the position for which you are applying. Again, dates could be an item to consider if you have long gaps in employment, changed jobs frequently, or lack recent work experience.
Other Résumé Entries	
Certifications	• List certifications relevant to the job position such as training in CPR or successful completion of a medical assisting certification exam.
Professional Affiliations	• List your membership in a professional organization and identify any leadership position you have held. This shows your involvement in your profession and willingness to assume responsibility for its operation. • List these entries alphabetically, in order of importance, or in chronologic order.
Professional Achievements and Awards	• List your certification status to indicate your commitment to a recognized professional credential. • List any awards, scholarships, or recognitions you have been given; these show you have outstanding abilities.
Community Service	• Willingness to give of one's time and energy in community service is an admirable trait and should be listed on the résumé.

Functional Style Résumé

A *functional style* résumé works well for people who have had practicum or cooperative work experience. The style highlights previous work experience that provided you with experience for the job for which you are applying. When listing experience, you enter the job title first, showing the prospective employer your progress at work. If you have experience with a prestigious company, it can be to your advantage to list the company name first and then your job title. Either way is acceptable; however, be consistent and list all experiences in the same format. You can skip any positions that do not apply to the desired position, and they do not have to be listed in chronological order. It is most impressive if the listing is from most important to least, regardless of the dates of employment. As an example, if your work experience is limited prior to a medical assistant program, you might list your practicum as the most applicable, followed by nurse assistant employment and self-employed child care. You may choose to eliminate, for example, fast-food restaurant and housekeeping jobs. Figure 59–4 is an example of the functional résumé of a recent medical assistant graduate.

SANDY LYNN BEACH, CMA(AAMA)
4030 Newbank Road
Wheelersburg, OH 45794
(623) 223-0988
sandy_lynn_beach@email.com

EDUCATION

Present	*Evening courses in Nursing* Southern Ohio Technical College, Lucasville, OH
2007	*Certificate, Medical Assisting* Ohio Valley Training Academy, Wellston, OH
2005	*Diploma, General Business* Portsmouth East High School

WORK EXPERIENCE

2009-Present	**Administrative Medical Assistant** Wilbur Roth, M.D., Rolling Hills, OH
2006–2009	**Admissions Clerk** Green Meadows Community Hospital, Green Meadows, OH
2004–2005	**Cashier** Garden Inn Restaurant, Hilldale, OH

ACHIEVEMENTS

Certified Medical Assistant (CMA) through the American Association of Medical Assistants (AAMA), 2010

PROFESSIONAL ASSOCIATIONS

American Association of Medical Assistants
Ohio Society of Medical Assistants
Scioto County Chapter of Medical Assistants

COMMUNITY SERVICE

Red Cross Volunteer
Big Sisters Association Volunteer

Figure 59–3: Chronological style résumé. *Delmar/Cengage Learning.*

Targeted Style Résumé

The *targeted style* résumé arranges information to focus on a specific job opportunity by highlighting the work experience and job skills that are requested by the employer. For example, if an opening indicated the position was for an administrative assistant with possible opportunity for office management, your résumé should reflect that opportunity. Usually, this style has a position statement such as Targeted Position, Professional Goal, or Career Objective. In this case, it is followed by a statement, for example, Career Objective: Administrative medical assistant position with the opportunity to advance to office manager. The work experiences listed should stress administrative competencies and any areas that could be considered management skills. Remember that positions you hold with organizations could be applicable, such as a treasurer or a committee chairperson. Additional educational accomplishments such as computer training, an insurance seminar, or a time management workshop would be very desirable. Figure 59–5 is an example of a résumé targeted for a clinical position.

Skills Style Résumé

The *skills style* résumé is best for highlighting experiences in a number of unrelated jobs and courses. It might also work well for individuals making a significant

SARAH MILLER
510 State Street
Silverton, MO 63131
(123) 456-7890
Sarah.Miller@email.com

EDUCATION

2011	*AS, Medical Assisting* Silverton Community College, Silverton, MO
January 2012	*CPR for the Professional* Northern University

RELATED EXPERIENCE

2010-2011	**MEDICAL ASSISTING PRACTICUM** (160 Hours) Primary Care Physicians, Silverton, MO • Prepared patients for examination, took vital signs, charted chief complaint • Performed diagnostic tests, including throat cultures, rapid strep test, ECGs • Performed clerical duties, including answering telephones, filing, writing referrals, scheduling appointments • Performed data entry of patient information and insurance payments
2008-Present	**HEALTH CARE AIDE** Manor Care Center, Silverton, MO • Performed personal care, took vital signs, range-of-motion exercises
2005-2008	**SELF-EMPLOYED CHILD CARE PROVIDER** • Responsible for child's care and safety

SPECIAL SKILLS

Keyboarding, 60 wpm
Computer applications: Microsoft Word, Medical Manager (Practice Management Software), Ingenix CareTracker (Electronic Health Records software)

OTHER EXPERIENCE

2003-2005	**CASHIER** Allen's Supermarket, Silverton, MO • Head cashier

Figure 59–4: Functional style résumé. *Delmar/Cengage Learning.*

career field change. It emphasizes what you can do, not where you have been employed. You can list any applicable skills acquired through jobs, education, volunteer activities, and life experiences. For example, your summer receptionist job with an insurance company, a classifieds sales position at a small newspaper, and a volunteer position arranging Meals on Wheels deliveries seem quite diverse, but the common elements of telephone skills and scheduling experience would be your areas of experience. The key is to categorize your experiences to match the skills required for the position. These skills would make you a good candidate for a receptionist in a medical facility.

KEEPING YOUR RÉSUMÉ CURRENT

Remember that as you gain work experience and acquire educational credentials, it will be necessary to update your résumé. Employment dates will change, and, it is hoped, job responsibilities will show growth. Items of less importance should be deleted as more impressive accomplishments are achieved. Always try to maintain your résumé on a single page, using a 12-point font size if at all possible; however, don't reduce the font size below 10 or reduce the margins beyond ¾ inch trying to make it fit. If you do have enough quality items to list that you need to use the second page, be certain the most important information is on the first page.

RAMON WILLIAMS, RMA(AMT)
4270 Hilldale Drive
Fern Ridge, CA 92079
(882) 809-1324
rwilliams@email.com

JOB TARGET

Clinical medical assistant in a family practice

CLINICAL SKILLS

- Assist with patient examinations
- CPR and first aid
- Phlebotomy
- Basic clinical laboratory skills
- Electrocardiography

ACHIEVEMENTS

- Registered Medical Assistant through the American Medical Technologists
- Bachelor's degree in Nutrition
- CPR certification

EMPLOYMENT EXPERIENCE

2010-Present	**Fern Ridge Family Health Center** Clinical Medical Assistant
2005-2010	**Brownville General Hospital** Phlebotomist/ECG Technician
2005-2008	**Ronald L. Botkin, D.O., General Practice** Administrative and Clinical Medical Assistant

PROFESSIONAL AFFILIATIONS

Member, American Medical Technologists

EDUCATION

Baldwin Community College, Baldwin, CA
Brownsville University, San Fernando, CA

Figure 59–5: Targeted style résumé. *Delmar/Cengage Learning.*

PROCEDURE 59–1 Prepare a Résumé

PURPOSE: To prepare a résumé, documenting information concerning education, experience, and abilities for employment consideration

EQUIPMENT: High-quality paper, dictionary, thesaurus, telephone book, computer, and a quality printer

S SKILL: Prepare a résumé.

Procedure Steps	Detailed Instructions and/or *Rationales*
1. Determine the résumé style appropriate for your needs.	Refer to Figures 59–3, 59–4, and 59–5 as example templates.

Procedure Steps	Detailed Instructions and/or *Rationales*
2. Write your complete legal name, address, phone number, and email address. This information may be arranged flush left or centered at the top of the page.	
3. List your educational background, beginning with the most recent or present date.	
4. List all pertinent employment experience, beginning with the most recent or present date, or enter information in an alternative résumé style.	*Listing only the pertinent employment experience allows you to provide necessary information and keep your résumé to the desired one-page limit.*
5. List other information that might be relevant: memberships and affiliations in professional organizations; community service, including volunteer programs; and activities as might be appropriate.	
6. Print the completed résumé and proofread it for errors. Make any necessary edits.	Do not rely on spell check to correct typos or grammatical mistakes. In addition, you can ask a reliable person to proofread your résumé.
7. Prepare the résumé for distribution: a. Print copies of the résumé on quality paper. b. If possible, convert the résumé into PDF format for electronic distribution.	*Converting the résumé into PDF format ensures that formatting remains consistent with the printed version of your résumé.*

PREPARING YOUR COVER LETTER

After you have perfected your résumé, compose a cover letter to send with it. The letter must state *why* you should be hired for the desired position. Discuss the skills and characteristics you would bring to the position. The cover letter should be addressed to the person who decides who is interviewed and hired. Finding out the name of the office manager or supervisor can be done by making a simple phone call and asking (be sure to get the correct spelling). Personalizing the letter will gain more attention than will the standard form letter. Let the employer know that your skills and qualifications will be an asset. Make the letter simple and direct to convey what makes you the person for the job. Be sure to request an interview and make it clear when and how you can be reached. Figure 59–6 provides sample cover letters.

Remember that your résumé should provide a general overall description of your assets and qualifications. The cover letter should be specific and targeted toward a particular person or department. It should be sent in answer to an ad, in request for an interview, or at an individual's request. If an employer requests an email to be sent, type your cover letter in the body of the email and send your résumé as an attachment to that email.

Both cover letter and résumé must be error free. Employers eliminate numerous résumés by pitching those with spelling or grammatical errors, tears, or smudges, or those that are too wordy or unorganized.

Date

Karla Baker, CMA (AAMA)
Office Manager
Hilldale Medical Center
Hilldale, Ohio 45102

Dear Ms. Baker:

I have completed training in medical assisting at Ohio Valley Training Academy. It has provided me with skills in both administrative and clinical areas. I am very interested in securing a position in your health care facility as a medical assistant. I am a Certified Medical Assistant through the American Association of Medical Assistants.

Please let me know if I may schedule an appointment for an interview. I can be reached at home on Tuesday and Thursday afternoons and every evening at 555-8131.

Thank you for your consideration.

Sincerely,

Sandy Lynn Beach, CMA(AAMA)

(A)

4270 Hilldale Drive
Fernridge, CA 95061
(406) 555-1122

Date

Ms. Doreen Castle
Office Manager
Hopkin's Medical Clinic
739 Mountainview Way
Great Valley, CA 95068

Dear Ms. Castle:

I read your ad in the local paper regarding the opening for a full-time clinical medical assistant at Hopkin's Medical Clinic. I feel that my training and experience makes me a worthy candidate for this position. I am a Registered Medical Assistant and have a bachelor's degree in Nutrition.

My experience in patient education regarding therapeutic diets has helped me to sharpen my communication skills. I also have excellent clinical skills and am currently enrolled in a CPR certification class.

At your earliest convenience, I would like to meet with you for an interview to discuss matching my qualifications to your needs. Please call me at the number listed above to schedule an appointment. I can be reached at home every evening and on Wednesday afternoons.

Yours truly,

Ramon Williams, RMA(AMT)

(B)

Figure 59–6A and B: Two cover letter examples. *Delmar/Cengage Learning.*

PROCEDURE 59–2 Prepare a Cover Letter

PURPOSE: To write an error-free cover letter as an indication of interest in being interviewed for a desired position

EQUIPMENT: Computer, printer, high-quality paper, addressee's name and address, dictionary, thesaurus

S SKILL: Compose a professional letter.

Procedure Steps	Detailed Instructions and/or *Rationales*
1. Assemble the needed information and equipment.	
2. Enter your name and address in a letterhead format.	
3. Enter the date.	
4. Enter the addressee information and salutation.	
5. Write the first paragraph, expressing your skills and qualifications that make you an asset to the position desired.	

Procedure Steps	Detailed Instructions and/or *Rationales*
6. Write the second paragraph, making it clear when and how you can be reached.	
7. Enter the closing and then your typed name four spaces below.	
8. Print the cover letter and proofread it for errors. Make any necessary edits.	Do not rely on spell check to correct typos or grammatical mistakes. In addition, you can ask a reliable person to proofread your cover letter.
9. Save, print, and sign the letter and make a copy. Send in answer to an ad or at the request of an individual.	Request may be to send by mail or email.

STARTING YOUR JOB SEARCH

The health care team is made up of many members who are delegated to perform specific functions. Each member should have a job description—a detailed outline of the duties required in their employment position. An example of a simple job description is shown in Figure 59–7. The job description should contain the following information:

- Title of the position
- Person(s) to whom responsible
- Summary of the position
- Primary duties of the job
- Expectations of the person in the job (regarding job performance)
- Requirements of the position (education, certification, and so on)
- Qualifications for the job
- Additional criteria per facility

SAMPLE JOB DESCRIPTION

Position:	Clinical medical assistant
Job Summary:	Prepare patients for exams, assist physician with examinations and treatments, provide patient education
Job Requirements:	Responsibilities: • Follow standard precautions, CLIA/OSHA regulations • Perform patient education regarding exam preparation, treatments, and follow-up care • Assist physician(s) with patient exams and treatments • Document patient information accurately • Assist as needed at the request of office manager • Cleaning and stocking patient rooms as necessary
Responsible to:	Physician(s) and Clinical Supervisor

Job Qualifications: Current CPR certification

Employee's signature ____________ Date ____________

Office Manager's signature ____________ Date ____________

Figure 59–7: An example of a job description.
Delmar/Cengage Learning.

THE INTERNET

You can check out many job opportunities online. Online information about jobs in every field is listed and updated regularly on many sites, including USAJOBS.gov, CareerBuilder.com, Monster.com, or even Craigslist. Performing a job search is quick and easy. You can find opportunities without traveling miles and spending lots of time and money in the process. Taking advantage of one or all the ways to find employment should ensure you of a position in an area of your liking. Some sites allow you to upload a résumé directly onto the site or ask you to email the résumé to a certain contact within the company.

APPT—Appointment	MGR—Manager
ASST—Assistant	MOS—Months
BGN or BEG—Beginning	NEC—Necessary
COL—College	NEG—Negotiable
DEPT—Department	OFC—Office
EDUC—Education	PD—Paid
EOE—Equal Opportunity Employer	POS—Position(s)
EXP—Experience	PT—Part Time
FB—Fringe Benefits	REF—References
FT—Full Time	REQ—Required
GRAD—Graduate	SAL—Salary
H—Handicapped	SEC—Secretary
HS—High School	T—Temporary
HR—Hour	TRANSP—Transportation
HRS—Hours	WPM—Words Per Minute
IMMED—Immediate	WK—Week
INT—Interview	WKENDS—Weekends
LIC—License	W/—With
MED—Medical	Yrs—Years

Figure 59–8: Abbreviations used in classified ads. *Delmar/Cengage Learning.*

NEWSPAPERS AND CLASSIFIED ADS

A classified advertisement (ad) is a request for qualified applicants to send information about themselves to a prospective employer. The employer may then request an interview with those who meet the requirements for the position instead of interviewing all persons who apply. Figure 59–8 shows abbreviations commonly used in classified advertisements.

In responding to a classified ad, it is customary to write a cover letter to accompany your résumé. Begin the letter by stating that you read the ad in the paper so the recipient knows how you learned about the position.

PUBLIC EMPLOYMENT SERVICES

All states offer assistance in locating jobs through a state employment service. Local offices of this agency have job openings on file, possibly including the one you are looking for. You simply walk in, fill out the general forms, wait your turn, and then have a conference with an employment counselor. If there are listings that call for your type of experience and training, you have immediate leads to begin contacting. If no appropriate listings are currently on file, the employment counselor will place your name on file and notify you when listings do materialize. Because this agency is supported by tax dollars, there is no fee for the service.

PRIVATE EMPLOYEMENT AGENCIES

Private employment agencies offer similar services. A cover letter and résumé should be sent to the agency, explaining your area of expertise and desired employment. Many agencies specialize in the medical field and can give efficient service in locating openings in medical assisting. Many potential jobs are fee paid, meaning that the employer pays the agency's fees. In general, you should avoid positions that require you to pay the fee. Fees for finding employment positions are generally based on a percentage of the first year's wages of an employee. Often, arrangements may be made for the fee to be paid in installments. The decision is obviously yours. You might be definitely interested in a particular position for which you have to pay a fee; carefully weighing the advantages and disadvantages will help you decide whether the cost is worth it to you.

OTHER CONTACTS

A résumé with a cover letter requesting an interview may be sent to many medical offices or health care facilities even if there is no position available. If you wish to be employed in a particular facility, making it known may spark an interest in you as a prospective employee if there is an opening. Introducing yourself through correspondence and specifying your interest in employment if a position becomes available can be very productive. Employers may keep your letter and résumé on file for as long as a year and respond as the need arises.

Additional information about job opportunities may be obtained at the public library. Many services, periodicals, and books deal with occupational information, and library personnel can be very helpful.

Membership in professional associations is also quite helpful in the job search. Not only can an association's publications include classified ads, but personal contact with other members at meetings can provide invaluable information about job openings. Participation in community service groups can put you in touch with yet another network of persons who might have information about job openings.

Watch for industry-sponsored job fairs where employers will have a table or booth to meet prospective employees. This type of recruitment is usually reserved for large organizations, but many hospitals, clinics, and care facilities cooperate in health fairs. Finally, you should not overlook your friends and acquaintances; the job one of them happens to mention in conversation could turn out to be just the one you have been waiting for.

COMPLETING AN APPLICATION FORM

Filling out an application for employment might be your next step. These forms can range from the simple to the complex. Figure 59–9 shows an example of an application form that asks for a minimal amount of information.

Application for Employment

Please Print

Position(s) applied for ______ Date of application __/__/__

Name ______ Last First Middle Social Security # ___-__-____

Address ______ Street City State Zip Code

Telephone # ( ) ______ Mobile/Beeper/Other # ( ) ______ E-mail Address ______

Referral Source (How did you hear about us?) ______

If you are under 18, and it is required, can you furnish a work permit? ☐ Yes ☐ No

If **no**, please explain ______

Have you ever been employed here before? If *yes*, give the dates and position ______ ☐ Yes ☐ No

Are you legally eligible for employment in this country? ☐ Yes ☐ No

Date available for work __/__/__ What is your desired salary range? $ ______

Type of employment desired ☐ Full-Time ☐ Part-Time ☐ Temporary ☐ Seasonal ☐ Educational Co-Op

Driver's licence number if driving may be required in position for which you are applying ______ State ______

Answering "yes" to the following question does not constitute an automatic bar to employment. Factors such as date of the offense, seriousness and nature of the violation, rehabilitation and position applied for will be taken into account.

Have you ever pled "guilty" or "no contest" to, or been convicted of a crime? ☐ Yes ☐ No

If **yes**, please provide date(s) and details ______

Employment History

Starting with your most recent employer, provide the following information.

Employer | Telephone # ( )
Street address | City | State
Starting job title/final job title
Immediate supervisor and title (for most recent position held) | May we contact for reference? ☐ Yes ☐ No ☐ Later
Why did you leave?
Dates employed: Month / Year To Month / Year
Compensation (Starting): ☐ Hourly ☐ Salary $ per
Commission/Bonus/Other Compensation $
Compensation (Final): ☐ Hourly ☐ Salary $ per
Commission/Bonus/Other Compensation $
Summarize the type of work performed and job responsibilities.
What did you like the most about your position?
What were the things you liked least about the position?

Employer | Telephone # ( )
Street address | City | State
Starting job title/final job title
Immediate supervisor and title (for most recent position held) | May we contact for reference? ☐ Yes ☐ No ☐ Later
Why did you leave?
Dates employed: Month / Year To Month / Year
Compensation (Starting): ☐ Hourly ☐ Salary $ per
Commission/Bonus/Other Compensation $
Compensation (Final): ☐ Hourly ☐ Salary $ per
Commission/Bonus/Other Compensation $
Summarize the type of work performed and job responsibilities.
What did you like the most about your position?
What were the things you liked least about the position?

Employer | Telephone # ( )
Street address | City | State
Starting job title/final job title
Immediate supervisor and title (for most recent position held) | May we contact for reference? ☐ Yes ☐ No ☐ Later
Why did you leave?
Dates employed: Month / Year To Month / Year
Compensation (Starting): ☐ Hourly ☐ Salary $ per
Commission/Bonus/Other Compensation $
Compensation (Final): ☐ Hourly ☐ Salary $ per
Commission/Bonus/Other Compensation $
Summarize the type of work performed and job responsibilities.
What did you like the most about your position?
What were the things you liked least about the position?

Figure 59–9: An example of a job application form. *Delmar/Cengage Learning.* *(continues)*

Skills and Qualifications

Summarize any special training, skills licenses and/or certification that may assist you in performing the position for which you are applying.

____

Computer Skills (check appropriate boxes. Include software titles and years of experience.)

☐ Word Processing ____________ Years: ______ ☐ E-mail ____________ Years: ______

☐ Spreadsheet ____________ Years: ______ ☐ Internet ____________ Years: ______

☐ Presentation ____________ Years: ______ ☐ Other ____________ Years: ______

Educational Background

Starting with your most recent school attended, provide the following information.

School (include City & State)	Years Completed	Completed	GPA Class Rank	Major/Minor
		☐ Diploma ☐ GED ☐ Degree ______ ☐ Certification ______ ☐ Other ______		
		☐ Diploma ☐ GED ☐ Degree ______ ☐ Certification ______ ☐ Other ______		
		☐ Diploma ☐ GED ☐ Degree ______ ☐ Certification ______ ☐ Other ______		

References

List name and telephone number of three buiness/work references who are *not* related to you and are *not* previous supervisors.
If not applicable, list three school or personal references who are *not* related to you.

Name	Title	Relationship to You	Telephone	Number of Years Known
			( )	
			( )	
			( )	

Figure 59–9: *(continued).*

CLINICAL PEARL

To help you complete application forms, have a *master application* prepared and with you as you complete specific employers' application forms. A master application is one that you have completed beforehand and contains all of your previous education, employers, and references, along with all appropriate dates and contact information. Being prepared with dates, names, addresses, phone numbers, and other detailed information will expedite completion of the form. Some applications are extremely lengthy (several pages).

Be sure to transcribe dates and all other information correctly, completely, and accurately. When you are nervous or if you are hurried, you can make mistakes such as transposing numbers, leaving a space blank, or even placing the wrong information in a space. Take adequate time to complete whatever forms are necessary in a neat and attractive manner. It is not considered proper to ask for a phone directory or any other reference when completing an application because this demonstrates that you are ill-prepared. In filling out an application for employment, you must be accurate and honest.

Because the job application will probably reach the personnel manager's office before you do, it must speak well for you; it must make a good impression on the person who reads it. Applications must be complete, neat, and legible, or they will be discarded promptly. Reading and following the instructions on the form is of utmost importance. Take time to read the instructions and follow them precisely when completing an employment application form. If the printed instructions on the form say to print all information in black ink, you should do just that and not use cursive style or another color of ink. One of the functions served in having candidates complete the application form is to find out how well they follow directions. The application form will provide the employer not only with factual information about you but with many other insights as well. Refer to Procedure 59–3 to practice completing an application.

If you take sufficient time and interest in completing the application, you will be more likely to be given a personal interview. Additionally, because of the Immigration Reform Act of 1986, employers are required by federal law to ask you for documents that show both your identity and eligibility to work in the United States. Employers will make copies of your documents and return them to you. Further, the Employment Eligibility Verification Form I-9 must be completed and filed in the employee's record along with other important documents. Employers must verify that you are legally entitled to work in the United States. All applicants and employers must comply with this law.

CLINICAL PEARL

Because of the professional setting (medical field) for which you are seeking employment, many employers require the background of prospective employees to be checked. Among the areas of concern are the person's credit rating, police record, and drug use or abuse. You might be asked to produce documents or give authorization for the employer to find out about your personal records before you can be considered for hiring. When completing a job application, be honest about your background, references, and skills because a background check will confirm your history. Background checks can go as far back as 7 to 10 years.

PROCEDURE 59–3 Complete a Job Application

PURPOSE: To complete a job application, following all directions and entering all information neatly and without error

EQUIPMENT: Job application; pen; copy of résumé; list of necessary names, addresses, and phone numbers; and copies of educational achievements

S SKILL: Complete a job application.

Procedure Steps	Detailed Instructions and/or *Rationales*
1. Assemble all necessary equipment and supporting documents.	
2. Read the application, noting the instructions for completion.	
3. Neatly enter your personal information.	
4. Enter your educational information, including names, addresses, and phone numbers.	Make sure to refer to diplomas, certificates, and transcripts for accurate dates.
5. Enter work experience information, including employers' names, addresses, and phone numbers.	Begin with current or last position worked and proceed backward. Refer to prepared lists for accurate addresses.
6. Enter any other information requested.	Note that applications vary in information requested.
7. List the names and phone numbers of personal references.	List only those from whom you have received approval.
8. Review the application, checking for missed or incorrectly entered information. Check for accuracy of spelling and general appearance. Make any necessary edits.	
9. Present or mail the application to the prospective employer.	

INTERVIEWING FOR THE JOB

An interview is a face-to-face meeting between you and your prospective employer. As soon as you know the date of the interview, make plans to allocate your time so that you can be stress free to get ready, travel to the site, interview, and return without rushing. Table 59–3 presents dos and don'ts of interviewing and applying for a job. An interview is an investment in yourself and your career. It is worth giving sufficient time and effort for a successful outcome.

PERSONAL APPEARANCE

When applying for a job, your appearance is extremely important. Even if you are merely picking up an application to take home to complete or returning it after you have completed it, your appearance, including your attitude, will certainly be noticed. You should dress for success any time a prospective employer might see you (Figure 59–10). Other employees will surely notice you and relay the information to the employer, especially if a negative impression is given. Appearance is an outward indication of who you are. Remember what you learned about nonverbal communication. If you are a sincere, competent, and dedicated person, then by all means attend to your appearance accordingly. Nonverbal messages, though silent, can speak loudly.

Most employers expect appropriate attire, and some require adherence to a very specific policy concerning type of dress and general appearance. Unprofessional attire and grooming (including facial piercings, unusual hair colors, and long nails) give a negative impression to employers.

If you are interviewing for a clinical position, ask beforehand about what type of clothing to wear. Your inquiry will most likely be taken as showing genuine interest. Women who prefer to wear business attire should dress conservatively in a black, navy, gray, tan, or brown tailored suit or pantsuit. Bright colors, jewelry, miniskirts, and frilly outfits are not considered professional attire. Men should also follow this advice and dress conservatively, avoiding outrageous ties, jewelry, and fad clothes or extreme haircuts. Remember that you want to make a positive impression with the interviewer about

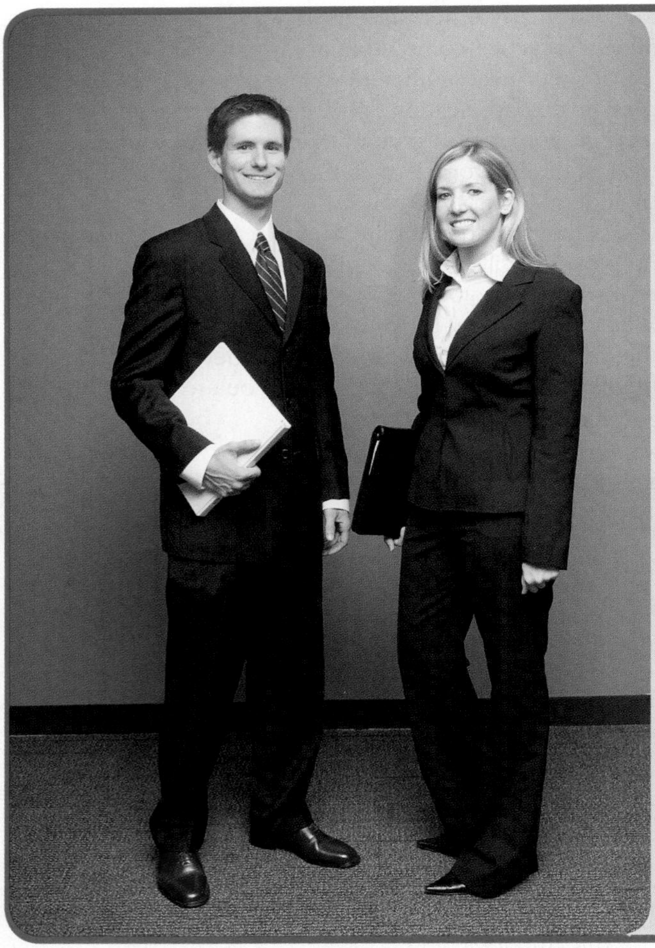

Figure 59–10: Two prospective job candidates dressed for an interview and prepared with portfolios. *Delmar/Cengage Learning.*

TABLE 59–3 Dos and Don'ts When Interviewing or Applying for a Job

Do	Don't
Allow sufficient time to get ready	Be late!
Arrive on time (10–15 minutes early)	Make excuses
Show interest and enthusiasm	Talk about personal problems
Be immaculate about personal appearance and dress appropriately in business attire	Chew gum or smoke (or smell of cigarettes)
Display a positive attitude	Bring your children
Use courtesy and respect	Act overconfident
Maintain good posture (sit still and straight) and positive body language	Drum fingers, swing legs, tap feet

yourself and your qualifications, not about your taste in fashions and accessories. A medical assistant who is more interested in meeting the requirements of the job than in being up with the latest fad is more appealing to a personnel manager.

CLINICAL PEARL

All matters concerning personal cleanliness are vital. The following characteristics are sure to interfere with or negate the possibility of employment: bad breath, dirty or untrimmed fingernails, chipped nail polish, dirty or unkempt hair, overpowering aftershave or perfume, unclean teeth, unpleasant or offensive body odor, or untended complexion problems. The point is this: No matter how well qualified or eager you are, you might not find anyone willing to employ you if you fail in matters of personal hygiene, grooming, and appearance. Take nothing for granted.

PREPARING FOR THE INTERVIEW

Rushing usually detracts from your appearance and demeanor. If the address of the facility is not familiar to you, get directions and plan your time beforehand. (It is a good idea to go to the facility a day or two before the scheduled interview to check out the area to determine the approximate travel time, exact location, parking, bus route, and so on to avoid getting lost or being delayed.) You should arrive about 10 to 15 minutes before the appointment. (You may be instructed to arrive up to an hour or more before the interview to complete an application form or to take required preemployment tests.) Arriving too early makes you appear insecure. Being late for almost any reason makes you appear irresponsible and a poor candidate for the position. If you happen to find yourself in a situation beyond your control, a telephone call explaining the delay and a sincere apology are in order. Being on time is a sign of reliability, dependability, and conscientiousness.

MEDIA LINK

View the video, "What Employers Look for in Job Interviews," for this chapter on the Premium Website.

DURING THE INTERVIEW

It is important to remember your body language when going into an interview. Some key things to be aware of are your handshake, posture, eye contact, and fidgeting:

- Your handshake should be firm and dry (Figure 59–11).
- Your manner should tell the interviewer you are happy to be there.
- Be aware of your posture. Do not slouch. Sit up straight and lean in a little toward your interviewer.
- Try to maintain eye contact with the person interviewing you.
- Avoid fidgeting and talking with your hands. This can distract the person interviewing you. Try to keep your hands in your lap or at your sides.

The interview ought to allow sufficient time for each of you to inquire about the other and to discuss the requirements of the position. You want to leave the interview knowing everything about that position so you can make an honest decision when they call you back to offer you the job.

Be prepared to answer questions concerning your career goals and objectives, how you feel about changes, why you decided on this career, and so on. Look at the questions commonly asked by interviewers in Figure 59–12. Review these and draft answers for yourself. It is good to have thought-out answers before going in for the interview. Your answers should be brief, concise, and honest.

Remember to be prepared with the list of references and verification of your educational achievements and any certifications you hold. You should take the originals with you, but having a copy of each document to give to the interviewer will show your attention to details.

In terms of perspective and dimension, the section of the résumé that lists community services is an appealing area to many prospective employers. It is an indicator of your concern for others, your involvement, and your energy level and time management skills. Some employers might ask what prompted your interest in a particular service area. Be prepared to respond honestly.

Federal laws are designed to deal with arbitrary discrimination in hiring practices. Toward this end, you should not be asked questions concerning your age, cultural or ethnic background, marital status, or parenthood. Nevertheless, these issues can come up in the course of your interview. You are not required to provide this information if you choose not to. The purpose of the

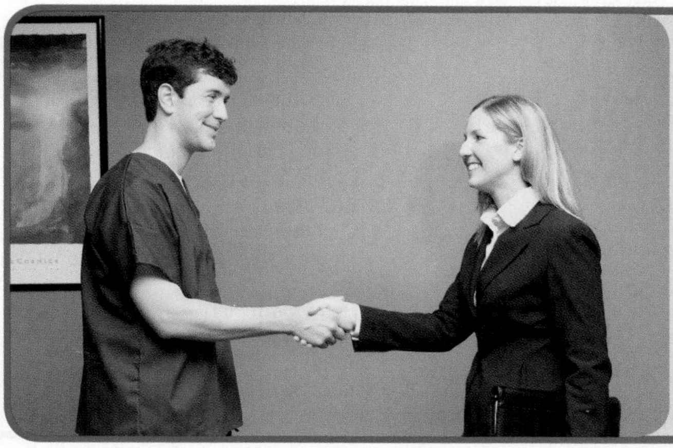

Figure 59–11: A firm handshake and warm smile are positive nonverbal messages. *Delmar/Cengage Learning.*

1. What are your qualifications for employment in our facility?
2. What were your favorite subjects in school and why?
3. Why are you seeking employment with us?
4. What made you decide to enter the medical assisting field?
5. What is your most rewarding experience in life thus far?
6. What are your long-range career goals?
7. What motivates you to do your best?
8. What is the most difficult problem you ever had to deal with? And how did you handle it?
9. What does success mean to you?
10. What relationship should exist between supervisors and those under their supervision?
11. How would you describe yourself?
12. Do you work well under pressure?
13. What are your strengths and weaknesses?
14. What two things are most important to you in a job?

Figure 59–12: A list of commonly asked questions during employment interviews.
Delmar/Cengage Learning.

interview is to ascertain the relevance of your experience and character to the position. If any of these unrelated issues come up, be careful to analyze the context in which they arose (it could be from something you said). In any case, if you are honestly convinced that you have been denied a job because of discrimination, be advised that this is illegal, and you have legal recourse.

At some point during the interview, the interviewer might give you a written job description of the position for which you are applying. You will probably be given time to look it over and then be asked whether you would feel confident about performing the job described. An honest answer is the best. Avoid hedging or bluffing about issues because an experienced interviewer will pick up on your insecurities. Remember that body language tells the rest of the story. If there are one or two duties you have never performed before or one or two pieces of equipment that you know little about, say so but add that you are eager to learn. The employer will appreciate the initiative in your answer. If the job description sounds totally unfamiliar or if you feel it would be an impossible task, it is best to say so. The interviewer will appreciate your openness.

Some positions might have no job description, and the duties involved will be discussed during the interview. Knowing that there are probably as many duties not mentioned as mentioned will give you an idea of the amount of work the job requires.

By the time all these matters have been dealt with, the interview will be starting to wind down. The interviewer beginning to reach closure will ask you whether you have any further questions (Figure 59–13). If issues of salary, benefits, raises, and advancement have not been dealt with previously, this is an appropriate time to mention them. This is also the logical point for you to ask about any other matters you are uncertain about. However, do not drag out this time. Let the interview end smoothly. When it is over, rise and thank the interviewer for his time. Firmly shake hands if the interviewer extends a hand. Remember to smile and be pleasant and polite as you exit with confidence.

1. To see a job description
2. About hours—work day schedule
3. Rate of pay (if not discussed by the close of the interview)
4. Chances for advancement or promotion
5. About continuing education—in-service programs (are expenses paid?)
6. Fringe benefits:
   a. Health insurance plan
   b. Dental insurance plan
   c. Eye care
   d. Vacation/time off
   e. Membership dues in professional organizations
   f. Profit sharing
   g. Retirement plan
   h. Tuition reimbursement
   i. Other
7. Frequency of job performance evaluations

Figure 59–13: A list of questions you, the applicant, might ask during the interview.
Delmar/Cengage Learning.

The interviewer may be interviewing a number of people about a specific job opening in the office. To help the interviewer remember specific facts and traits about each individual, a form such as the one shown in Figure 59–14 can be filled out.

INTERVIEW FOLLOW-UP

You might be one of many candidates interviewing for a particular job. Therefore, any decision can take some time. Out of courtesy and to enhance your image with the interviewer, take the time to compose a follow-up letter shortly after the interview has taken place. A typed thank you letter or a neatly handwritten note reiterates your interest in the position and demonstrates your persistence and follow-through ability. Figure 59–15 offers a sample letter. Refer to Procedure 59–4 to write an interview follow-up letter.

INTERVIEW EVALUATION

Subject	Excellent	Good	Satisfactory	Needs Improvement	Poor
Appearance					
Attitude					
Eye contact					
Self-control					
Voice					
Grammar					
Responses					
Manners					
Resumé					
Comments					
Date					
Employer			Title		
Address			Phone		
Applicant					

Figure 59–14: Employers might use a form such as this after an interview to record information about an applicant. *Delmar/Cengage Learning.*

Sandy Lynn Beach
4030 Newbank Road
Wheelersburg, OH 45794

Date

Karla Baker, CMA(AAMA)
Office Manager
Hilldale Medical Center
Hilldale, OH 45102

Dear Ms. Baker:

Thank you very much for granting me an interview for the clinical medical assistant's position on your staff. The interview was both challenging and stimulating; I found it to be an enjoyable and rewarding experience.

You outlined the duties and responsibilities that come with the position very specifically. This is the type of position for which I have been trained; I feel confident that if I am offered the position, I can handle the responsibilities and become an asset to your staff.

Again, thank you for considering me for this position. I look forward to hearing from you soon.

Sincerely,

Sandy Lynn Beach, CMA(AAMA)

Figure 59–15: A sample follow-up letter. *Delmar/Cengage Learning.*

PROCEDURE 59–4 Write an Interview Follow-Up Letter

PURPOSE: To write an error-free interview follow-up letter or thank you note as an indication of interest and appreciation following an employment interview

EQUIPMENT: Computer, printer, high-quality paper, addressee's name and address, dictionary, and thesaurus

S SKILL: Compose a professional letter.

Procedure Steps	Detailed Instructions and/or *Rationales*
1. Assemble the needed information and equipment.	
2. Enter your name and address in a letterhead format.	
3. Enter the date.	

(continues)

(continued)

Procedure Steps	Detailed Instructions and/or *Rationales*
4. Enter the addressee information and salutation.	
5. Write the first paragraph, expressing appreciation for the interview.	
6. Write the second paragraph, restating your preparation for and confidence in your ability to perform in the position.	
7. Write a closing paragraph, again expressing appreciation and requesting notification of the decision.	You can express willingness to reinterview for further evaluation.
8. Enter the closing and then your typed name four spaces below.	
9. Print the cover letter and proofread it for errors. Make any necessary edits.	Do not rely on spell check to correct typos or grammatical mistakes. Additionally, you can ask a reliable person to proofread your letter.
10. Sign the letter, make a copy, and place the original in an addressed envelope to be mailed.	

AFTER YOU ARE EMPLOYEED

When you obtain employment, you must dedicate yourself to keeping the job. This is when your work history begins, and it will follow you throughout your working life. If the health care field remains your chosen career area and if medical assisting is your point of entry, you must be determined to become the very best medical assistant you can. Ultimately, your eventual advancement into a more responsible position and higher pay will depend largely upon your demonstrated capabilities in performing your administrative and clinical tasks.

Progressing in employment is up to you. The desire to advance in your field of choice is the first step to consider. Job satisfaction is also a major issue. If you enjoy your work and find your duties challenging and rewarding, you might want to stay in that position. If your salary meets your needs and you like what you do, staying with that job can be quite fulfilling. However, a motivating factor in moving up into a higher position or even changing jobs is most often for an increase in pay. *Note*: Cost-of-living raises (given to keep up with the economy) do not reflect one's job performance, but merit raises do. A merit raise is given to those employees who deserve recognition and praise for a job well done.

Chances of advancement in your job depend on several factors. Employees who are offered better-paying positions and positions with more responsibility are the ones who show the greatest interest. Interest can be displayed in several ways. Primarily, the person who shows initiative, is the most dependable, seeks continuing education, acquires new skills, exhibits efficiency in a pleasant manner, and communicates well with others will be the first to be considered for a promotion. To move forward to a higher position in your place of employment means that you have been recognized by your employer or supervisor for your efforts, and you are being rewarded with a raise in pay, a promotion, or both.

CONTINUING EDUCATION

Because the medical field in general is always changing and improving in health care technology, it is your responsibility to keep up with these changes. This is necessary if you want to reach peak performance at your job. To do this, you must take advantage of continuing education. This can be done in a variety of ways. Of course, the primary means of obtaining current information is to read. Providers usually subscribe to several medical news publications that you can read on breaks or at lunchtime. Keeping up with the latest in managed health care, new medications, and other newsworthy items is admirable and will be noticed by your employer.

It will also help you perform your duties and provide the best possible patient care.

Professional organizations such as the American Association of Medical Assistants (AAMA) and American Medical Technologists (AMT), as well as others, specifically address the needs of the medical assistant by offering continuing education programs at national, state, and local levels. These organizations also offer opportunities for certification examinations and credentialing for medical assistants. Continuing education units (CEUs) offered by these organizations is a way to keep your certification status current.

Another way to better yourself and attain further education is to attend courses related to your area of interest in the medical field at a local college. Many night and weekend classes are offered for convenience to those who work during the day. You might take a refresher course in medical terminology or anatomy, for instance. Some find a favorite niche, such as medical records, transcription, or laboratory procedures, and realize that to advance in a particular area, additional education and credentials are necessary. Discussing your goals with your supervisor is certainly advised so that reorganizing your work schedule to allow adequate time for classes can be arranged.

In addition, local hospitals offer educational seminars on a variety of topics for health care professionals. They welcome the attendance of those interested in learning more about patient care. You can ask to be put on the mailing list to keep you informed of future program offerings.

Employers are very receptive to and impressed by employees who take the initiative in self-improvement and involve themselves in professional organizations that offer continuing education to members. This conveys to the employer that you are interested in advancement and are willing to put forth the additional effort to move forward in your profession. Your involvement in leadership roles within the organization also gives the employer further insight into your appreciation of your career and its importance.

Career Laddering

You might be completely satisfied as a medical assistant and find great pleasure in your work. (This is very admirable—you are providing a valuable service!) But perhaps, after a period of time, you decide you would like to pursue another occupation for personal reasons, achievement needs, or financial gain. The term **career laddering** refers to a pathway of job positions in which you may progress based upon your interest, training, and experience.

A "ladder" can be lateral or vertical. Lateral laddering (Figure 59–16A) are moves that generally do not require additional education other than training from the facility that hires you. These positions require skills that you would already possess from education in medical assisting programs. Forward or upward laddering (Figure 59–16B) are other job opportunities that might be possible with additional education. These are good matches for medical assistants because they entail some skills that you have already acquired as well as some courses that you already have taken as a medical assistant (such as medical terminology, anatomy and physiology, and so on). In addition to the advancement to a medical office manager is hospital-based employment that medical assistants can fulfill.

CLINICAL PEARL

Refer to Table 2–3 in Chapter 2 for descriptions of the professions medical assistants may progress to. Additional information is available from the websites of state and federal governments, educational organizations, and professional associations.

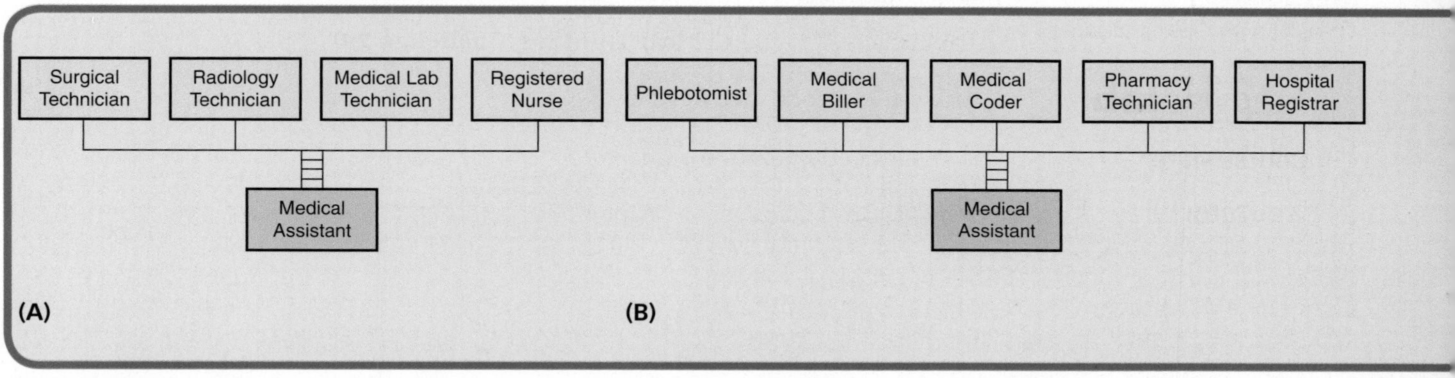

Figure 59–16: Career laddering for medical assistants. (A) Upward laddering. (B) Lateral laddering. *Delmar/Cengage Learning.*

CHAPTER SUMMARY

- The purpose of a practicum is to apply skills learned in the classroom to an actual work environment, although it is not a work experience. The individual does not replace any employee and does not receive a paycheck.
- Employers look for these skills when considering a potential employee: communication skills, computer skills, critical thinking skills, teamwork skills, and time management skills.
- Employers also look for the following desirable qualities in a potential employee: positive attitude, strong work ethic, dependability, honesty and integrity, punctuality, flexibility and adaptability, and motivation.
- The four styles of résumés are functional style (includes relevant work experience), skills style (highlights experiences and skills in unrelated jobs), targeted style (arranges information to focus on a specific job opportunity), and chronological style (lists education and work experience in reverse chronologic order). The chronologic style is the most common and traditional format for résumés.
- A cover letter accompanies a résumé and is a narrative that discusses the skills and characteristics you possess that make you the right fit for the position available.
- When starting your job search, many resources are available to help you locate open positions, including the Internet, newspapers, public and private employment services, professional organizations, job fairs, library resources, and personal networking.
- Preparing for an interview is critical. Make sure to arrive early, in appropriate attire and appearance, and bring copies of your résumé, master application form, and any other documents you might need to reference or pass out. During the interview, try to appear relaxed and professional when speaking and in body language. Be ready to answer common interview questions and to ask the interviewer questions about employment at the facility.
- Sending a follow-up note after the interview is considered courteous and shows your interest in the job along with positive qualities such as follow-though and persistence.
- The health care field is always changing and improving in technology, and it is important to keep up with these changes to provide the best patient care as well as to advance in employment. Continuing education, credentialing, seminars and workshops, and additional classes are all ways to demonstrate your commitment to your employer and profession.

STUDY TOOLS

Premium Website	
MEDIA LINK	View these **Media Links** for Chapter 59: • Employers and Professionalism • Job Interviews and Professionalism
StudyWARE	Activities and Quizzes on the **StudyWARE™ Software** for Chapter 59
	Complete the following **Competency Challenge 2.0** activity: • Friday: Capstone
	Online access to the **Critical Thinking Challenge 2.0**
learninglab	Module 25: Workplace Readiness
CourseMate	Activities and Quizzes for Chapter 59
WebTutor	Activities and Quizzes for Chapter 59

CHECK YOUR KNOWLEDGE

1. A practicum should be treated:
   a. as a work experience.
   b. as a learning experience.
   c. as a possible job lead.
   d. as a regular school day.
2. What is the goal of a résumé?
   a. To present a personal profile
   b. To get a job
   c. To show off your achievements
   d. To receive an interview
3. All of the following are personal qualities except:
   a. critical thinking skills.
   b. initiative.
   c. dependability.
   d. positive attitude.
4. A résumé style that highlights your previous work experiences related to the position you are seeking is which type of résumé?
   a. Skills
   b. Chronological
   c. Targeted
   d. Functional
5. When should you arrive at an interview?
   a. Right on time
   b. 5 minutes early
   c. 10 minutes early
   d. 20 minutes early
6. All of the following are background checks may be performed on an applicant except:
   a. credit rating.
   b. criminal record.
   c. drug screen.
   d. marital status.

WEB LINKS

CareerBuilder.com: www.careerbuilder.com

Job Interview Helper: jobinterviewhelper.com

REFERENCES

Career Services at Virginia Tech. (n.d.) *Contents and Sections of Your Resume.* www.career.vt.edu/ResumeGuide/ContentSections.html (Retrieved 11/15/2010)

USAJobs.gov. Info Center. *Tips on Applying for a Federal Job.* www.usajobs.gov/ei/resumeandapplicationtips.asp (Retrieved 11/15/2010)

Purdue University, Online Writing Lab. (n.d.) *Workplace Writers.* http://owl.english.purdue.edu/owl/resource/681/01/ (Retrieved 11/15/2010)

University of Minnesota, Office of Human Resources. (n.d.). *Resume Tutor!* www1.umn.edu/ohr/careerdev/resources/resume (Retrieved 11/15/2010)

Appendix A
AAMA 2007–2008 Occupational Analysis of the CMA(AAMA)*

In furtherance of its leadership role in the profession, the American Association of Medical Assistants (AAMA) has completed the following *2007–2008 Occupational Analysis of the CMA(AAMA)*. In previous years, this document was titled *AAMA Role Delineation Study: Occupational Analysis of the Medical Assisting Profession*.

A NECESSARY DISTINCTION

A professional's skills are largely determined by professional education. The CMA(AAMA) is the only credential that requires candidates to be graduates of a programmatically accredited medical assisting program. Therefore, it is appropriate and necessary that the qualifying language "of the CMA(AAMA)" be incorporated into this document's title.

ABOUT THE SURVEY

A survey was sent to a random sample of CMAs (AAMA)—AAMA members and nonmembers. The CMA (AAMA) represents a medical assistant who has been certified by the Certifying Board of the AAMA. Of the 15,500 surveys distributed, 3,658 were collected and analyzed, resulting in a 95 percent confidence level. The results obtained from the sample are within ±1.6 percent of the results if all 15,500 individuals had responded.

ANALYSIS HIGHLIGHTS

Today's CMA(AAMA) is expected not only to master the body of knowledge of the profession, but also to apply this knowledge in the complex and fast-paced world of ambulatory health care. Thus, critical thinking is emphasized in this *Occupational Analysis*.

Another dimension in the *Occupational Analysis* reflects the growing awareness that the CMA(AAMA) is uniquely qualified to "speak the patient's language" and serve as a "communication liaison" between the busy physician and patients. The roles of the CMA(AAMA) as "patient advocate" and "health coach," as well as "communication liaison," are given appropriate prominence in this document.

All health professionals have been expected to refine their knowledge and skills in responding to natural and manmade emergencies, and the vital roles of CMAs(AAMA) have come into increasing focus in recent years. In keeping with this priority, the *Occupational Analysis* includes emergency-related functions under Communication, Instruction, and Patient Care.

USES OF THE STUDY

This document provides valuable data to the Certifying Board (CB) and the Continuing Education Board (CEB) of the AAMA, as well as to the Medical Assistant Education Review Board (MAERB). However, the *Occupational*

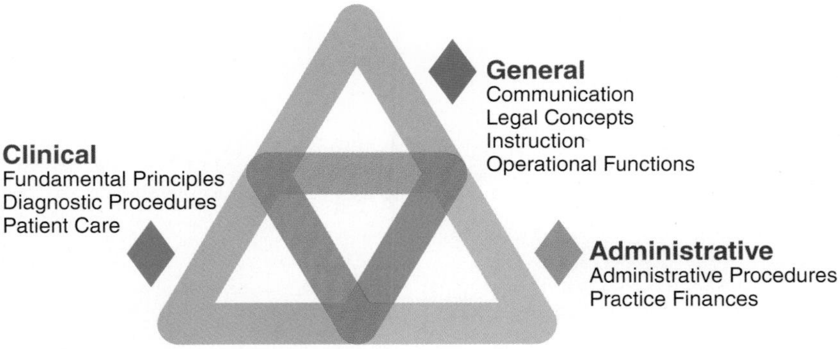
General
Communication
Legal Concepts
Instruction
Operational Functions
Clinical
Fundamental Principles
Diagnostic Procedures
Patient Care
Administrative
Administrative Procedures
Practice Finances

*Permission is granted from the American Association of Medical Assistants.

Analysis should not be confused with the following documents:

- *Content Outline of the CMA(AAMA) Certification/Recertification Examination,* published by the CB
- *Advanced Practice of Medical Assisting,* published by the CEB
- *Standards and Guidelines for Medical Assisting Educational Programs,* published by CAAHEP
- *Curriculum Content and Competencies,* published by the CRB

Legal Scope of Practice

This *Occupational Analysis* does not delineate the legal scope of medical assisting practice. Legally delegable responsibilities vary from state to state. Scope of practice questions should be directed to AAMA Executive Director and Legal Counsel Donald A. Balasa, JD, MBA, at dbalasa@aama-ntl.org.

Occupational Analysis Committee

Chair: Charlene Couch, CMA(AAMA)

Karen Minchella, CMA(AAMA), PhD

Rebecca Walker, CMA(AAMA), CP

Nina Watson, CMA(AAMA), CPC, COS

Ex officio

Linda Brown, CMA(AAMA), 2007-2008 President

Kathryn Panagiotacos, CMA (AAMA), 2007-2008 Vice President

Donald A. Balasa, JD, MBA, Executive Director

AMERICAN ASSOCIATION OF MEDICAL ASSISTANTS®
20 N. WACKER DR., STE. 1575
CHICAGO, ILLINOIS 60606
website: www.aama-ntl.org 800/228-2262

General, Clinical, and Administrative Skills* of the CMA (AAMA)

General Skills

Communication

- Recognize and respect cultural diversity
- Adapt communications to individual's understanding
- Employ professional telephone and interpersonal techniques
- Recognize and respond effectively to verbal, nonverbal, and written communications
- Utilize and apply medical terminology appropriately
- Receive, organize, prioritize, store, and maintain transmittable information utilizing electronic technology
- Serve as "communication liaison" between the physician and patient
- Serve as patient advocate professional and health coach in a team approach in health care
- Identify basics of office emergency preparedness

Legal Concepts

- Perform within legal (including federal and state statutes, regulations, opinions, and rulings) and ethical boundaries
- Document patient communication and clinical treatments accurately and appropriately
- Maintain medical records
- Follow employer's established policies dealing with the health care contract
- Comply with established risk management and safety procedures
- Recognize professional credentialing criteria
- Identify and respond to issues of confidentiality

Instruction

- Function as a health care advocate to meet individual's needs
- Educate individuals in office policies and procedures
- Educate the patient within the scope of practice and as directed by supervising physician in health maintenance, disease prevention, and compliance with patient's treatment plan
- Identify community resources for health maintenance and disease prevention to meet individual patient needs
- Maintain current list of community resources, including those for emergency preparedness and other patient care needs
- Collaborate with local community resources for emergency preparedness
- Educate patients in their responsibilities relating to third-party reimbursements

Operational Functions

- Perform inventory of supplies and equipment
- Perform routine maintenance of administrative and clinical equipment
- Apply computer and other electronic equipment techniques to support office operations
- Perform methods of quality control

Clinical Skills

Fundamental Principles

- Identify the roles and responsibilities of the medical assistant in the clinical setting
- Identify the roles and responsibilities of other team members in the medical office
- Apply principles of aseptic technique and infection control
- Practice Standard Precautions, including handwashing and disposal of biohazardous materials
- Perform sterilization techniques
- Comply with quality assurance practices

Diagnostic Procedures

- Collect and process specimens
- Perform CLIA-waived tests
- Perform electrocardiography and respiratory testing
- Perform phlebotomy, including venipuncture and capillary puncture
- Utilize knowledge of principles of radiology

Patient Care

- Perform initial-response screening following protocols approved by supervising physician
- Obtain, evaluate, and record patient history employing critical thinking skills
- Obtain vital signs
- Prepare and maintain examination and treatment areas
- Prepare patient for examinations, procedures and treatments
- Assist with examinations, procedures, and treatments
- Maintain examination/treatment rooms, including inventory of supplies and equipment
- Prepare and administer oral and parenteral (excluding IV) medications and immunizations *(as directed by supervising physician and as permitted by state law)*
- Utilize knowledge of principles of IV therapy
- Maintain medication and immunization records
- Screen and follow up test results
- Recognize and respond to emergencies

Administrative Skills

Administrative Procedures

- Schedule, coordinate, and monitor appointments
- Schedule inpatient/outpatient admissions and procedures
- Apply third-party and managed care policies, procedures, and guidelines
- Establish, organize, and maintain patient medical record
- File medical records appropriately

Practice Finances

- Perform procedural and diagnostic coding for reimbursement
- Perform billing and collection procedures
- Perform administrative functions, including book-keeping and financial procedures
- Prepare submittable ("clean") insurance forms

All skills require decision making based on critical thinking concepts.

Appendix B
Medical Assisting Task List

The various tasks that medical assistants perform include, but are not necessarily limited to, those on the following list.

The tasks presented in this inventory are considered by American Medical Technologists to be representative of the medical assisting job role. This document should be considered dynamic, to reflect the medical assistant's evolving role with respect to contemporary health care. Therefore, tasks may be added, removed, or modified on an on-going basis.

Medical Assistants that meet AMT's qualifications and pass a certification examination are certified as a Registered Medical Assistant (RMA).

I. GENERAL MEDICAL ASSISTING KNOWLEDGE

A. Anatomy and Physiology

1. Body systems
2. Disorders and diseases of the body

B. Medical Terminology

1. Word parts
2. Medical terms
3. Common abbreviations and symbols
4. Spelling

C. Medical Law

1. Medical law
2. Licensure, certification, and registration

D. Medical Ethics

1. Principles of medical ethics
2. Ethical conduct
3. Professional development

E. Human Relations

1. Patient relations
2. Interpersonal skills
3. Cultural diversity

F. Patient Education

1. Identify and apply proper communication methods in patient instruction
2. Develop, assemble, and maintain patient resource materials

II. ADMINISTRATIVE MEDICAL ASSISTING

A. Insurance

1. Medical insurance terminology
2. Various insurance plans
3. Claim forms
4. Electronic insurance claims
5. ICD-9CM/CPT Coding applications
6. HIPAA mandated coding systems
7. Financial applications of medical insurance

B. Financial Bookkeeping

1. Medical finance terminology
2. Patient billing procedures
3. Collection procedures
4. Fundamental medical office accounting procedures
5. Office banking procedures
6. Employee payroll
7. Financial calculations and accounting procedures

C. Medical Secretarial—Receptionist

1. Medical terminology associated with receptionist duties
2. General reception of patients and visitors
3. Appointment scheduling systems
4. Oral and written communications
5. Medical records management
6. Charting guidelines and regulations
7. Protect, store, and retain medical records according to HIPAA regulations
8. Release of protected health information adhering to HIPAA regulations
9. Transcription of dictation
10. Supplies and equipment management

AMT American Medical Technologists
Allied Health Professionals

11. Medical office computer applications
12. Compliance with OSHA guidelines and regulations of office safety

III. CLINICAL MEDICAL ASSISTING

A. Asepsis

1. Medical terminology
2. State/Federal universal bloodborne pathogen/body fluid precautions
3. Medical/surgical asepsis procedure

B. Sterilization

1. Medical terminology associated with sterilization
2. Sanitization, disinfection, and sterilization procedures
3. Record keeping procedures

C. Instruments

1. Specialty instruments and parts
2. Usage of common instruments
3. Care and handling of disposable and reusable instruments

D. Vital Signs/Mensurations

1. Blood pressure, pulse, respiration measurements
2. Height, weight, circumference measurements
3. Various temperature measurements
4. Recognize normal and abnormal measurement results

E. Physical Examinations

1. Patient history information
2. Proper charting procedures
3. Patient positions for examinations
4. Methods of examinations
5. Specialty examinations
6. Visual acuity/Ishihara (color blindness) measurements
7. Allergy testing procedures
8. Normal/abnormal results

F. Clinical Pharmacology

1. Medical terminology associated with pharmacology
2. Commonly used drugs and their categories
3. Various routes of medication administration
4. Parenteral administration of medications (subcutaneous, intramuscular, intradermal, ZTract)
5. Classes or drug schedules and legal prescriptions requirements for each
6. Drug Enforcement Agency regulations for ordering, dispensing, storage, and documentation of medication use
7. Drug Reference books (PDR, Pharmacopeia, Facts and Comparisons, Nurses Handbook)

G. Minor Surgery

1. Surgical supplies and instruments
2. Asepsis in surgical procedures
3. Surgical tray preparation and sterile field respect
4. Prevention of pathogen transmission
5. Patient surgical preparation procedures
6. Assisting physician with minor surgery including set-up
7. Dressing and bandaging techniques
8. Suture and staple removal
9. Biohazard waste disposal procedures
10. Instruct patient in pre- and postsurgical care

H. Therapeutic Modalities

1. Various standard therapeutic modalities
2. Alternative/complementary therapies
3. Instruct patient in assistive devices, body mechanics, and home care

I. Laboratory Procedures

1. Medical laboratory terminology
2. OSHA safety guidelines
3. Quality control and assessment regulations
4. Operate and maintain laboratory equipment
5. CLIA waived laboratory testing procedures
6. Capillary, dermal, and venipuncture procedures
7. Office specimen collection such as: urine, throat, vaginal, wound cultures – stool, sputum, etc
8. Specimen handling and preparation
9. Laboratory recording according to state and federal guidelines
10. Adhere to the MA Scope of Practice in the laboratory

J. Electrocardiography

1. Standard, 12 lead ECG testing
2. Mounting techniques for permanent record
3. Rhythm strip ECG monitoring on lead II

K. First Aid

1. Emergencies and first aid procedures
2. Emergency crash cart supplies
3. Legal responsibilities as a first responder

American Medical Technologists
10700 W. Higgins Road
Rosemont, Illinois 60018
Phone: (847) 823-5169 – Fax: (847) 823-0458
Website: www.amt1.com

Appendix C
Measurements and Abbreviations

CONVERTING MEASUREMENTS

LENGTH	Centimeters	Inches	Feet
1 centimeter	1.000	0.394	0.0328
1 inch	2.54	1.000	0.0833
1 foot	30.48	12.000	1.000
1 yard	91.4	36.00	3.00
1 meter	100.00	39.40	3.28

VOLUMES	Cubic Centimeters	Fluid Drams	Fluid Ounces	Quarts	Liters
1 cubic centimeter	1.00	0.270	0.033	0.0010	0.0010
1 fluid dram	3.70	1.00	0.125	0.0039	0.0037
1 cubic inch	16.39	4.43	0.554	0.0173	0.0163
1 fluid ounce	29.6	8.00	1.000	0.0312	0.0296
1 quart	946.0	255.0	32.00	1.000	0.946
1 liter	1000.0	270.0	33.80	1.056	1.000

WEIGHTS	Grains	Grams	Apothecary Ounces	Pounds
1 grain (gr)	1.000	0.064	0.002	0.0001
1 gram (gm)	15.43	1.000	0.032	0.0022
1 apothecary ounce	480.00	31.1	1.000	0.0685
1 pound	7000.00	454.0	14.58	1.000
1 kilogram	15432.0	1000.00	32.15	2.205

RULES FOR CONVERTING ONE SYSTEM TO ANOTHER

Volumes

Grains to grams—divide by 15
Drams to cubic centimeters—multiply by 4
Ounces to cubic centimeters—multiply by 30
Minims to cubic millimeters—multiply by 63
Minims to cubic centimeters—multiply by 0.06
Cubic millimeters to minims—divide by 63
Cubic centimeters to minims—multiply by 16
Cubic centimeters to fluid ounces—divide by 30
Liters to pints—divide by 2.1

Weights

Milligrams to grains—multiply by 0.0154
Grams to grains—multiply by 15
Grams to drams—multiply by 0.257
Grams to ounces—multiply by 0.0311

Temperature

Multiply centigrade (Celsius) degrees by $\frac{9}{5}$ and add 32 to convert Fahrenheit to Celsius.
Subtract 32 from the Fahrenheit degrees and multiply by $\frac{5}{9}$ to convert Celsius to Fahrenheit.

COMMON HOUSEHOLD MEASURES AND WEIGHTS

1 teaspoon	= 4–5 mL or 1 dram
3 teaspoons	= 1 tablespoon
1 dessert spoon	= 8 mL or 2 drams
1 tablespoon	= 15 mL or 3 drams
4 tablespoons	= 1 wine glass or ½ gill
16 tablespoons (liq)	= 1 cup
12 tablespoons (dry)	= 1 cup
1 cup	= 8 fluid ounces or ½ pint
1 tumbler or glass	= 8 fluid ounces or 240 mL
1 wine glass	= 2 fluid ounces, 60 mL
16 fluid ounces	= 1 pound
4 gills	= 1 pound
1 pint	= 1 pound

MEDICAL SYMBOLS

O	pint	′	foot, minute
#	pound, number	″	inch, second
℞	recipe, prescription	°	degree
♂	male	%	percent
♀	female	×	multiply
$\bar{s}$	without	÷	divide
$\bar{c}$	with	=	equals
–	minus, negative, alkaline reaction	∞	infinity
$\overline{aa}$	equal parts	↑	increase
		↓	decrease

ABBREVIATIONS

a, aa	of each
abd	abdomen
a.c.	before meals
ad lib	as desired
A & P	anterior and posterior
aq	aqueous, water
b.i.d., BID	twice a day
bm, BM	bowel movement
BP, B/P	blood pressure
BUN	blood urea nitrogen
$\bar{c}$	with
C	Celsius, centigrade
Ca	calcium
cap	capsule
CBC	complete blood count
CC	chief complaint
CCU	coronary care unit
CHF	congestive heart failure
CNS	central nervous system
c/o	complains of
CO_2	carbon dioxide
comp	compound
COPD	chronic obstructive pulmonary disease
CPR	cardiopulmonary resuscitation
CSF	cerebrospinal fluid
CVA	cerebrovascular accident
cysto	cystoscopy
D & C	dilatation and curettage
Dil, dil	dilute
DOA	dead on arrival
DOB	date of birth
DPT	diphtheria, pertussis, tetanus
dx, Dx	diagnosis
ECG	electrocardiogram
EEG	electroencephalogram
EENT	eye, ear, nose, throat
EKG	electrocardiogram
elix	elixir
ER	emergency room
ext.	extract
F	fahrenheit
F	female
FBS	fasting blood sugar
FH	family history
fl	fluid
fl. oz.	fluid ounce
Fx	fracture
GB	gallbladder
GI	gastrointestinal
gm	gram
GP	general practitioner
gtt, Gtt, gtts	drop, drops
GU	genitourinary
GYN	gynecology
H, h	hour
HCL	hydrochloric acid
Hgb	hemoglobin

HPI	history present illness
Hx	history
ICU	intensive care unit
I & D	incision and drainage
IM	intramuscular
inj	injection
I & O	intake and output
IPPB	intermittent positive pressure breathing
IT	inhalation therapy
IUD	intrauterine device
IV	intravenous
IVP	intravenous pyelogram
k	potassium
KUB	kidney, ureter, and bladder
lat	lateral
lb	pound
liq	liquid
LLQ	left lower quadrant
LMP	last menstrual period
LUQ	left upper quadrant
M	male
mm	millimeter
MS	multiple sclerosis
NB	newborn
neg	negative
NKA	no known allergies
no.	number
noct	at night
NPO	nothing by mouth
N & V	nausea and vomiting
OB	obstetrics
OD	overdose
OP	outpatient
OR	operating room
os	mouth
oz	ounce
Path	pathology
PBI	protein bound iodine
p.c.	after meals
Peds	pediatrics
per	through, by
PID	pelvic inflammatory disease
PKU	phenylketonuria
PO, p.o.	by mouth
prn	as desired, needed
pro time	prothrombin time

Psych	psychiatry
pt	patient
pulv	powder
Px	physical examination
q	every
q (2, 3, 4) h	every (2, 3, 4) hours
qh	every hour
q.i.d., QID	four times a day
qns	quantity not sufficient
qs	quantity sufficient
qt	quart
R	right
Ra	radium
RBC	red blood cells
REM	rapid eye movement
rep	let it be repeated
R/O	rule out
ROM	range of motion
ROS	review of systems
Rx	prescription, take
$\bar{s}$	without
sig	instructions, directions
SOB	shortness of breath
sol	solution
solv	solvent
s.o.s.	distress signal
sp. gr.	specific gravity
stat	immediately
syr.	syrup
T	temperature
T & A	tonsillectomy and adenoidectomy
tab	tablet
TIA	transient ischemic attack
t.i.d.	three times a day
tinct.	tincture
TPR	temperature, pulse, respiration
TUR	transurethral resection
UA	urinalysis
ung.	ointment
URI	upper respiratory infection
UTI	urinary tract infection
VD	venereal disease
VS	vital signs
WBC	white blood cells
WNL	within normal limits
wt., Wt.	weight

Glossary

ABHES Accrediting Bureau of Health Education Schools.
abandonment to desert, to give up entirely.
abbess a mother superior; a woman who is the head of an abbey of nuns.
abbreviations shortened form.
abdomen the cavity in the body between the diaphragm and the pelvis.
abdominal pertaining to the abdomen.
abdominopelvic pertaining to the anterior body cavity below the diaphragm.
abduction to move away from the midline.
ablation a surgical procedure using a resectoscope inserted into the uterus through the cervix.
abortion the termination of pregnancy; spontaneous or induced.
abrasion an injury caused by rubbing or scraping off the skin.
abrupt sudden; blunt, curt.
absolute free as to condition, unlimited in power.
absorb to suck or swallow up, to drink in.
abstinent refraining from use; being away from.
absurd contrary to sense or reason.
abuse to maltreat; to use wrongly.
accelerator increasing action or function.
acceptance agreeing verbally or in writing to the terms of a contract, which is one of the requirements of an enforceable contract.
accept assignment Provider agrees to accept the insurer's payment as payment in full for the service provided.
accommodation the process of the lens changing shape to permit close vision.
account record of all transactions made on an individual's financial record that lists debits, credits, and balance
account history the past financial record.
accountant one who keeps, audits, and inspects the financial records of individuals or businesses.
accounting formula The formula which is considered the basis for all financial accounting, which is assets minus liabilities equals net worth.
accounts payable (A/P) The total amounts owed by the practice to suppliers and other service providers for regular business operating expenses, such as medical office supplies and equipment, office rental space, utilities (gas and electric, water, telephone and/or internet services), and office staff salaries.
accounts receivable (A/R) money owed to the practice by patients.
accounts receivable (A/R) ratio The total dollar amount of the outstanding payments or claims due to the office from patients and customers.
accreditation a process in which an educational institution or program establishes credibility or legitimacy by complying with predetermined standards.
accreditation the assignment of credentials; approval given for meeting established standards.
accredited certified as being of a specified quality; accepted as valid.
Accrediting Bureau of Health Education Schools (ABHES) An accrediting body that provides programmatic accreditation for medical assisting and other healthcare programs.
accumulated to pile up; collect; gather.
accuracy correctness, exactness.
accurate correct, exact, without error.
accurate and precise testing (APT) refers to a standard for performing laboratory procedures to ensure reliability of results.
acetylcholine a hormone released at the parasympathetic and skeletal nerve endings.
Achilles' tendon a tendon attaching the gastrocnemius muscle of the leg to the heel.
achromatic a condition of total color blindness.
acidosis a disturbance of the acid–base balance of the body.
acne valgaris a skin condition characterized by inflammation of sebaceous glands and producing pimples.
acquaintance the state of knowing a person or subject.
acquire to gain by one's own efforts or actions; to get.
acquired immunodeficiency syndrome (AIDS) a viral disease that renders the immune system ineffective.
acquisition acquired by one's own efforts.
acromegaly a chronic condition characterized by enlargement of bones of the extremities and some bones of the head; thickening of facial soft tissues.
acronym a word formed from the initial letters of each major word in a term.
action potential the temporary electrical charge within a cell.
activate to make active or more active.
active listening participation in the conversation with another by paraphrasing words and phrases or giving approving or disapproving nods.
acuity refers to the sharpness or clearness of vision or hearing.
Acupuncture A procedure used to treat pain by inserting extremely thin, sterilized needles, sometimes electrified with low-voltage, along the network of 12 body meridians (channels) to connect the different levels from the organs to the skin.
acupuncture involves the insertion of needles at various points in the body to treat disease or relieve pain.
acute sharp, severe; having a rapid onset, severe symptoms, and a short course; not chronic.
acute glomerulonephritis the rapid onset of inflammation of the glomerulus of the kidney.
acute phase a period of increased symptoms and severity of the disease.
acute renal failure the sudden cessation of kidney function.
adapt the act of or the result of adjusting to a new circumstance or change.
addiction the state of being governed or controlled by a habit, as with alcohol or drugs.
additive a substance deliberately added to a material to fulfill some specific purpose such as enhancing taste or color or prolonging shelf life.
additive effect The combined actions of two or more drugs are the same as the sum of each action individually.
adduction to draw together toward the midline.
adenitis inflammation of lymph nodes or a gland.
adequate equal to the requirement or occasion, sufficient.
adhere to stick fast, become firmly attached; to be devoted to.
adjective a word added to (modifying) a noun to quantify or limit it.
adjustment credit entry made on an account to decrease a balance owed to the medical office; may be due to insurance, professional discounts, write-offs, or to correct bookkeeping errors
adjustments changes to fit or bring into harmony.

administer to manage; to conduct, as in business.
administrative duties that manage or direct activities; in medical assisting, refers to tasks other than clinical in nature; front office duties.
Administrative Simplification Compliance Act (ASCA) identifies limited situations where paper claim forms may be submitted for payment (rather than electronic submission); signed into law on December 27, 2001 as Public Law 107-105.
administrative skills skills that help to manage the business affairs of a medical practice and includes two categories—administrative procedures and practice finances.
admissions clerk a person who processes information and forms for a patient who will be entering the health facility.
adrenal pertaining to the adrenal glands, which sit atop each kidney.
adrenaline an internal secretion derived from the adrenal glands; can be commercially prepared from animal glands; acts as a stimulant.
adrenocorticotropic hormone (ACTH) a hormone secreted by the anterior lobe of the pituitary gland.
advance beneficiary notice (ABN) Document used to notify a Medicare beneficiary that it is either unlikely that Medicare will pay or certain that Medicare will not pay for the service they are going to be provided. Beneficiaries are required to sign this document if they wish to have the service with the understanding that they will be responsible for payment.
advance directives a living will; a document, written in advance, that states the patient's wishes regarding end-of-life care.
advantageous beneficial, profitable.
adverb a word added to (modifying) a verb, an adjective, or another adverb.
adverse opposed to; unfavorable.
advocacy Defending or supporting the rights or interests of another. In healthcare, specifically referring to those rights or interests of a patient or other vulnerable party.
advocate one who pleads for or defends a cause or a person.
advocate Someone who speaks for another person.
aerobe a microorganism that can live and grow only in the presence of oxygen.
afebrile without fever.
affiliate to unite, to join, or become connected.
agar a dried mucilaginous substance, or gelatin, extracted from algae, used as a culture medium.
agent one that acts or has the power or authority to act for another.
aggression pushiness, assuming the offensive without cause; forcefulness.
aging of accounts dividing accounts into categories according to the amount of time since the first billing date.
agonist A drug that binds to a receptor in order to produce or trigger a response.
airborne transported or carried through the air.
Al-Anon a support group for family members of alcoholics.
alateen a support for teenagers with an alcoholic parent.
albino a person who lacks pigment in the skin, hair, and eyes, either partial or total; a person with albinoism.
alcohol a liquid generated by the fermentation of sugar and other carbohydrates.
alcoholic an individual who uses alcohol to excess.
Alcoholics Anonymous an organization formed to assist alcoholics to refrain from the use of alcohol.
alcoholism a chronic, progressive, and potentially fatal disease characterized by tolerance and physical dependency on the ingestion of alcohol.
aldosterone a mineralocorticoid hormone secreted by the adrenal cortex.
alignment being in proper position.
alimentary canal the intestinal tract, from the esophagus to the rectum, and accessory organs.
allege to state positively but not under oath and without proof; to affirm.
allergens any substance which causes an allergic reaction.
allergic rhinitis inflammation of the nose caused by an allergy.
allergist a physician specializing in the care of patients with allergies.
allergy an altered or acquired state of sensitivity; abnormal reaction of the body to substances normally harmless.
allosteric protein a protein found in erythrocytes that transports oxygen in the blood; hemoglobin.
alopecia the loss of hair; baldness.
Alpha-Fetoprotein Screening (AFP) a blood test during pregnancy to detect birth defects.
alpha search look by alphabetical order.
alternative different from the usual or conventional.
alternative therapy a therapy that is used in place of conventional therapy—often this therapy is experimental or has not been approved as a credible therapy.
altrusim unselfish concern for the welfare of others.
alveoli microscopic air sacs in the lung.
amber orange/yellowish color.
amblyopia lazy eye; a condition characterized by the inward turning of the affected eye.
ambulate to walk, not be confined to bed.
ambulatory refers to walking, being mobile.
amenity pleasantness, pleasant ways, civilities.
amenorrhea absence of menses; without menstruation.
American Academy of Professional Coders (AAPC) An organization that promotes professionalism and encourage and support education, networking, and certification in the medical billing and coding areas.
American Association of Medical Assistants (AAMA) A professional organization for medical assistants that certifies medical assistants and provides continuing education opportunities.
American Medical Technologists (AMT) A professional organization that provides credentialing opportunities for medical assistants and continuing education opportunities.
ammonia strong-smelling inhalants used to revive a person who has fainted; also known as ammonia inhalants or spirits of ammonia.
amnesia loss of memory.
amniocentesis the use of a needle to withdraw amniotic fluid from the amniotic sac.
amniotic pertaining to the amniotic fluid within the amniotic membrane surrounding the fetus.
amphetamine a central nervous system stimulant, often referred to as an upper.
amplifier a device on an electrocardiograph that enlarges the ECG impulses.
ampule a small glass container that can be sealed and its contents sterilized.
amputate to cut off, remove a part.
anaerobe a microorganism having the ability to live without oxygen.
anal pertaining to the anus or outer rectal opening.
analysis the examination of anything to determine its makeup; a description of the process or the examination, point by point.
analytical characterized by a method of analysis, a statement of point-by-point examination.
anaphylactic a severe and rapid multi-system allergic reaction.
anaphylaxis a hypersensitive reaction of the body to a foreign protein or a drug; the term implies symptoms severe enough to produce serious shock, even death.
anatomic pertaining to the anatomy or structure of an organism.
anatomical the position with the human body upright, facing forward, with the palms facing toward the front of the body.
anatomical position the position with the human body upright, facing forward, with the palms facing toward the front of the body.
anatomy the study of the physical structure of the body and its organs.
anchor the attachment of a skeletal muscle; the wrapping at the start of a gauze or elastic bandage.

anemia a deficiency of red blood cells, hemoglobin, or both.
aneroid operating without a fluid; when used in reference to a sphygmomanometer, measuring by a dial instead of a mercury column.
anesthesia without sensation, with or without loss of consciousness.
anesthesiologist one who studies anesthiology.
anesthesiology the study of anesthesia.
anesthetic an agent that produces insensibility to pain or touch, either generally or locally.
anesthetize to cause a loss of sensation, loss of consciousness.
aneurysm a widening, external dilation caused by the pressure of blood on weakened arterial walls.
angina pain and oppression radiating from the heart to the shoulder and left arm; a feeling of suffocation.
angiography a radiologic study of an artery using a radiopaque medium.
angioplasty an invasive procedure to alter the interior of a blood vessel.
angle the inclination of two straight lines that meet in a point.
annotate to provide with explanatory notes.
annotating to provide critical or explanatory notes.
annuity a sum of money to be received yearly, either in a lump sum or by installments.
anorexia (nervosa) loss of appetite; with anorexia nervosa, loss of appetite for food not explainable by disease, which may be a part of psychosis.
anorexic one suffering from anorexia.
antagonist A drug that blocks the actions of a receptor or its intended ligand.
antagonize to annoy; to arouse opposition.
antecubital the inner surface of the arm at the elbow.
anteflexed abnormal bending forward.
anterior before or in front of.
anteverted a forward placement.
antibody a protein substance carried by cells to counteract the effect of an antigen.
antibody-mediated humoral immunity; when antibodies and complement work together to destroy antigens.
anticipate to predict, based on experience and training, situations or events that may be likely to occur, that may or may not require intervention.
anticipation expect, forsee.
anticoagulant a substance that prohibits the coagulation of blood.
antigen any immunizing agent that, when introduced into the body, may produce antibodies.
antihistamine a class of drugs used to counteract allergic reactions or cold symptoms.
antiseptic an agent that will prevent the growth or arrest the development of microorganisms.
antitoxin a protein that defends the body against toxins.
anuria the absence of urine.
anus the external opening of the anal canal.
anxiety a condition of mental uneasiness arising from fear or apprehension.
aorta the main trunk of the arterial system of the body.
apex the point, tip, or summit of anything; in reference to the heart, the point of maximum impulse of the heart against the chest wall.
Apgar refers to a method for assessing the condition of newborns.
apical referring to the apex.
apnea the absence of breathing.
aponeurosis extension of connective tissue beyond a muscle in round or flattened tendons; a means of insertion or origin of a flat muscle.
apostrophe a punctuation mark showing the absence of a letter or letters or possession.
apothecaries An early term for pharacist.
apothocary one who dispenses drugs and medicines.
appearance outward or visible persona that a person gives to other individuals.
appearance outward show.
appendectomy the excision of the appendix.
appendicitis inflammation of the appendix.
appendicular pertaining to the limbs or things that append (attach) to other parts.
appointment an engagement; a meeting at a particular time.
apprehension anticipation of something feared, dread; a mental conception.
apprenticeship a training or learning period; study under the guidance of a skilled, experienced worker.
apprenticeship a period of time when one is bound by agreement to learn some trade or craft.
apprise to inform.
appropriate correct, suitable.
aqueous humor a watery, transparent liquid that circulates between the anterior and posterior chambers of the eye.
arachnoid a delicate, lacelike membrane covering the central nervous system.
arbitrary depending on will or whim, self-willed; depending on choice or discretion.
ardently eagerly, passionately, intensely.
areola a ringlike coloration about the nipple of the breast.
aromatherapy the use of essential oils from plants for a therapeutic effect.
arrhythmia without rhythm; irregularity.
arteriography a radiologic study of an artery using a radiopaque medium.
arterioles small blood vessels connecting arteries with capillaries.
arteriosclerosis a degeneration and hardening of the walls of arteries.
artery a blood vessel carrying blood away from the heart, usually filled with oxygenated blood.
arthritis inflammation of a joint.
articulate to join together, as in a joint.
artifact something extraneous to what is being looked for, activity that causes interference on ECG's.
artificial insemination the mechanical placement of semen containing viable sperm into the vagina.
ascending referring to that portion of the colon that ascends from the lower right quadrant to the upper right quadrant of the abdomen.
ascertain to make certain.
ascites an abnormal accumulation of fluid in the abdomen.
ASCLS American Society for Clinical Laboratory Science.
asepsis a condition free of organisms.
aseptic technique means of performing tasks without contamination by organisms.
aseptic technique The process of maintaining sterility throughout a surgical procedure.
asphyxiation suffocation, loss of consciousness as the result of too little oxygen and too much carbon dioxide.
aspiration removal by suction.
assault physical harm; a violent attack.
assertive Confident, persistent manner of communicating one's thoughts and ideas, in a positive manner.
assess to determine, to appraise the condition or state.
assets anything owned that has exchange value, all the entries on a balance sheet that show the property or resources of a person or business.
associate's degree a degree granted by a junior college at the end of a two-year course.
asthma an allergic reaction to a substance resulting in wheezing, shortness of breath, and difficulty in breathing.
astigmatism blurring of the vision caused by an abnormal curvature of the cornea.
asymmetry lack of same size, shape, and position of parts or organs on opposite sides.
atelectasis lack of air in the lungs caused by the collapse of the alveoli of the lungs.
atherosclerosis fatty degeneration of the walls of the arteries.
atmosphere any surrounding influence.
atria the upper chambers of the heart.
atrial depolarization the excitement and contraction caused by the SA node at the beginning of the cardiac cycle.
atrioventricular see **AV node.**

atrium cardiac auricle; the upper chamber of the heart.
atrophy wasting away of a muscle.
attachment the point at which something attaches or originates.
attenuated diluted; to reduce virulence of a pathogenic organism.
at the time of service (ATOS) when service is rendered; real time.
attitude state of thought or feeling.
attribute quality or characteristic; to give credit for.
atypical deviated from normal.
audible loud enough to be heard.
audiometer a device to measure the degree of hearing ability.
audiometry testing of the hearing sense.
audit inspection.
audit trail a record of transaction that identifies which what person or persons and at what time and day an electronic record was accessed in order to maintain accountability for the security of the information as it is accessed.
auditory pertaining to the sense of hearing; the external canal of the ear.
augmented refers to leads 4, 5, and 6 of the standard 12-lead ECG tracing; these leads are of different voltage.
aural the ear; temperature measurement using tympanic infrared scanner.
auscultate to listen for sounds produced by the body.
auscultation the process of listening for sounds within the body.
authorization the giving of authority.
authorize to give permission.
autoclave a pressurized device designed to heat aqueous solutions above their boiling point to achieve sterilization. It was invented by Charles Chamberland in 1879.
autoimmune a condition wherein the person's antibodies react against their own normal tissues.
autologous given by oneself.
automated teller machine (ATM) a banking machine operated by inserting a credit or bank card and entering a personal identification number (PIN) code. Deposits, transfers, withdrawals, and other banking functions can be performed at the ATM location 24 hours a day, seven days a week.
automation behavior in an automatic or mechanical fashion.
autonomic spontaneous; the part of the nervous system concerned with reflex control of bodily functions.
autonomous self-governing.
autonomy independence or freedom of an individual's will; the right to choose
autotrophs microorganisms that feed on inorganic matter.
auxiliary to provide aid.
AV node atrioventricular node; the beginning of the bundle of his in the right atrium; nerve fibers responsible for the contraction of the ventricles.
avulsion an injury in which a body structure is forcibly detached
axial pertaining to the spinal column, skull, and rib cage of the skeleton.
axilla the underarm area, armpit.
axillary referring to the underarm area.
axon an extension from a nerve cell.
ayurvedic the traditional healing system of India that may be the oldest formal medical system in the world.
ayuredic medicine traditional healing system of India that addresses mental and spiritual well-being and physical health. ayurveda identifies three types of energies that are present in all things: vata, pitta, and kapha and believe that imbalances in any of these areas can cause disease.

bacteria unicellular microorganism concerned with the fermentation and putrefaction of matter; disease-causing agent.
balance to bring into or keep in equilibrium; to have equal weight and power.
balance sheet Also known as a "statement of financial position" that reveals a company's assets, liabilities and owner's equity (net worth).
bandage a piece of cloth used to hold a dressing in place, to support a body part; provide compression, or to protect from external contamination.
bankruptcy the state of being bankrupt, being legally declared unable to pay debts.
barbiturate a sedative or hypnotic drug, also known as a downer.
barrier to prevent access; bar passage.
barter to give one thing in exchange for another.
bartholin's glands two small mucous glands, situated one on each side of the vaginal opening at the base of the labia minora.
baseline the initial information on which additional data is based.
basophil a granulated white blood cell.
battery any illegal beating of another person.
behaviors a term used to describe professional characteristics or attitudes that are expected in particular professions.
beneficence the doing of good for another; the act of caring
benefits anything that promotes or enhances well-being.
benign nonmalignant; not cancerous.
benign hypertrophy nonmalignant enlargement.
bereavement sadness as a result of death of a loved one.
bereavement time time that an employee can take off when a family member or very close friend dies.
beriberi a disease resulting from lack of vitamin B, thiamine.
Beyond a reasonable doubt being sure of a criminal defendant's guilt to a moral certainty.
Biases A person's slant toward a particular belief.
biceps the muscle of the upper arm that flexes the forearm.
biconvex the curving out on both sides.
bicuspid heart valve between the left atrium and left ventricle, also known as the mitral valve.
biennially happening once in 2 years.
bile a secretion of the liver; a greenish-yellow fluid with a bitter taste.
bilirubin a yellow breakdown product of normal heme catabolism. its levels are elevated in certain diseases, and it is responsible for the yellow color of bruises and the brown color of feces.
bimanual two-handed; with both hands.
bimonthly occurring once in 2 months.
binge a spree; to overindulge, such as with alcohol or food.
binocular pertaining to the use of both eyes; possessing two eyepieces as with a microscope.
biochemistry a science concerned with the chemistry of plants and animals.
biofeedback a method, usually with the help of electronic equipment, that enables a person to learn to control otherwise involuntary bodily functions.
biofeedback a method that enables a person, usually with the help of electronic equipment, to learn to control otherwise involuntary bodily functions.
biohazard organism, or substance derived from an organism, that poses a threat to (primarily) human health.
biohazardous any material that has been in contact with body fluid and is potentially capable of transmitting disease.
biopsy excision of a small piece of tissue for microscopic examination.
birthday rule a means to identify primary responsibility in insurance coverage.
bizarre odd, unusual, strikingly out of the ordinary.
bladder a membranous sac or receptacle for a secretion; the gallbladder, urinary bladder.
bleb an elevation of the epidermis; a blister; in the lungs refers to a bubble-like structure from destroyed alveoli.
bloodborne capable of being transported in blood.
blood pressure the amount of force exerted by the heart on the blood as it pumps the blood through the arteries.
body mass index (BMI) a measure of body fat that is the ratio of the weight of the body in kilograms to the square of its height in meters.
body mechanics the use of appropriate body positioning when moving and lifting objects to avoid injury.
body surface area (BSA) refers to the total surface of the human body.
bolus a mass of masticated food ready to be swallowed.

bonding the attachment of two persons; the relationship between a parent and a baby.
bookkeeper one who records the accounts and transactions of a business.
booster a subsequent injection of immunizing substance to increase or renew immunity.
bowel refers to intestines.
bowman's capsule part of the renal corpuscle; surrounds the glomerulus of the nephron.
brachial refers to the brachial artery in the arm; the artery used in measuring blood pressure.
brachytherapy a type of radiation therapy that places radioactive isotopes in or near the tumor.
bradycardia slow heart rate.
braille printing for the blind, using a system of raised dots.
brain scan a diagnostic test using a scanner to measure radioisotopes within the brain.
breach violation of a law, contract, or other agreement.
brochure a small pamphlet or booklet of information.
bronchi the primary divisions of the trachea.
bronchiole small terminal branches of the bronchi that lack cartilage.
bronchitis inflammation of the mucous membranes of the bronchial tree.
bruit an adventitious sound of venous or arterial origin heard on auscultation; usually refers to the sound produced by the mixing of arterial and venous blood at dialysis shunts.
BSA see **body surface area.**
buccal the mouth; oral cavity.
bulbourethral glands two small glands, one on each side of the prostate gland, terminating in the urethra by way of a duct.
bulimia nervosa a condition characterized by alternating periods of overeating followed by forced vomiting and the use of laxatives to remove food from the body.
bundle a number of things bound together.
bunion a bursa with a callus formation.
bursa a sac or pouch in connective tissue chiefly around joints.
business associate agreement (BAA) an agreement with a company that ensures the company understands the person's expectations as to what the company will do with the privileged information they will have access to and the consequences of an inappropriate disclosure.

CAAHEP Commission on Accreditation of Allied Health Education Programs.
caduceus the wand of hermes or mercury; used as a symbol of the medical profession.
caduceus a medical symbol depicted by a staff with a serpent coiled around its shaft
calculate to compute.
calculator an electronic or mechanical device for the performance of mathematical computations.
calculi commonly called stones; usually composed of mineral salts.
calibration a set of graduated markings to indicate values.
callus in fractures, refers to the formation of new osseous material around the fracture site.
calorie a unit for measuring the heat value of food.
calyces two or more calyx.
calyx the cuplike division of the kidney pelvis.
cancellation to strike out by crossing with lines; marking a postage stamp or check or to delete an appointment or event.
cancellous a latticework structure, as the spongy tissue of bone.
cancer a malignant tumor or growth; specifically the hyperplasia of cells with infiltration and destruction of tissue.
cancerous refers to a malignant growth.
cannula a tube or sheath enclosing a trocar (triangular bore needle); after insertion, the trocar is removed.
capacity having the mental competency to make health care decisions, or execute a will at the time the will was signed and witnessed. The decision-maker must understand the nature of the decision and be aware of the potential risks.
capillary a microscopic blood vessel connecting arterioles and venules.
capitation a structure of payment based on the number served.
caption heading, title, or subtitle.
carbohydrate an organic combination of carbon, hydrogen, and oxygen as a sugar, a starch, or cellulose.
carbon dioxide a gas found in the air, exhaled by all animals; the chemical formula is CO_2.
carbon monoxide a colorless, odorless, poisonous gas caused by the incomplete combustion of carbon.
carboxyhemoglobin combined carbon monoxide and hemoglobin in red blood cells.
carbuncle a staphylococcal infection following furunculosis, characterized by a deep abscess of several follicles with multiple draining points.
carcinoembryonic antigen a tumor marker that can be detected in the blood when tested.
carcinogen cancer-causing agent.
carcinoma a malignant tumor from epithelial tissue.
cardiac pertaining to the heart.
cardiac sphincter the muscle that encircles the esophagus where it enters the stomach.
cardinal signs principal signs: temperature, pulse, respiration, and blood pressure.
cardiologist a physician specializing in the care of patients with diseases of the heart.
cardiology the study of the heart and its diseases.
cardiopulmonary resuscitation (CPR) a combination of rescue breathing and chest compressions delivered to victims thought to be in cardiac arrest
cardiovascular pertaining to the heart and blood vessels.
caregiver the person responsible for another's care and well-being.
carotid pertaining to the carotid artery.
carpal bone of the wrist.
carpal tunnel syndrome (CTS) the symptoms associated with the entrapment of the median nerve within the carpal bones and the transverse ligament at the wrist.
carrel a small, partitioned space.
carrier one who carries, transports; with insurance, it's the company who provides the policy.
cartilage a strong, tough, elastic tissue forming part of the skeletal system; precalcified bone in infants and young children.
CAT scan see **computerized transaxial tomography.**
cataract an opacity of the lens of the eye resulting in blindness.
catarrhal pertaining to inflammation of mucous membranes; causing severe spells of coughing with little or no expectoration.
catarrhal stage inflammation of the mucous membranes.
catastrophic of great consequence; disastrous.
categorize to arrange by class or kind; to place like things together.
catheterization to insert a catheter into a cavity (for example, urinary bladder to remove urine) to remove body fluid.
caudal pertaining to any taillike structure.
caustic capable of burning; an agent that will destroy living tissue.
cauterize to burn with an electrical cautery or chemical substance.
cautery an iron or caustic used to burn tissue.
cavities a hollow space, such as within the body or organs.
cecum the beginning of the ascending portion of the large intestine that forms a blind pouch at the junction with the small intestine.
celiac disease dilation of the small and large intestines.
cell structural and functional unit of all living organisms; sometimes called the building block of life.
cell-mediated direct cellular response to antigens.

cell membrane the structure that surrounds and encloses a cell.
central situated at or related to a center.
centrifuge a machine for the separation of heavier materials from lighter ones through the use of centrifugal force.
centriole an organelle within the cell.
cerebellum lower or back brain below the posterior portion of the cerebrum.
cerebral pertaining to the cerebrum of the brain.
cerebrospinal referring to the brain and spinal cord.
cerebrospinal fluid the liquid that circulates within the meninges of the spinal cord and ventricles and meninges of the brain.
cerebrovascular accident a stroke; hemorrhage in the brain.
cerebrum the largest part of the brain. It is divided into two hemispheres with four lobes in each hemisphere.
certificate a written declaration of some fact.
certificate of completion a document awarded upon fulfillment of a program's criteria.
certificate of waiver refers to a list of basic laboratory tests that may be performed in the physician's office by nonlaboratory personnel.
certification written declaration.
certified holding a certificate; being certificated; guaranteed in writing.
Certified Clinical Medical Assistant (CCMA) credential given by the National Healthcare Association(NHA) after eligible candidates pass the certification exam.
Certified Medical Administrative Assistant (CMAA) credential given by the National Healthcare Association(NHA) after eligible candidates pass the certification exam.
Certified Medical Assistant, CMA (AAMA) the credential given by the American Association of Medical Assistants (AAMA) to eligible candidates that pass the CMA(AAMA) examination.
certified ophthalmic technician (COT) a person trained and certified in diagnostic testing procedures and limited examination of the eye.
cerumen waxlike brown secretion found in the external auditory canal.
cervical pertaining to the neck portion of the spinal column; also to the entrance into the uterus.
cervicitis an inflammation of the cervix of the uterus.
cervix the entrance into the uterus.
cesarean surgical removal of an infant from the uterus.
cessation ceasing or discontinuing.
chaos a state of complete confusion; disorder.
charge slip see encounter form.
charting the recording of observations, subjective and objective findings, diagnostic procedures, treatments, and other pertinent data in the patient file.
chemical a simple or compound substance used in chemical processes.
chemotherapy the use of chemical agents in the treatment of disease, usually associated with cancer therapy.
cheyne-stokes a breathing pattern characterized by alternating periods of apnea and hyperventilation.
chief complaint the main reason for seeking medical care.
Chief complaint, History, Examination, Details, Drugs/Dosages, Assessment, and Return visit (CHEDDAR) Acronym that provides a structured charting method for data acquired during a routine healthcare visit; it encourages more detailed of the information obtained during the patient interview and examination.
chiropractic a system of healing based upon the theory that disease results from a lack of normal nerve function; treatment by scientific manipulation and specific adjustment of body structures, such as the spinal column.
chiropractor a health care provider who uses chiropractic methods to treat patients.
chlamydia a sexually transmitted disease caused by a bacteria that lives as an intracellular parasite.
chloroform a liquid compound that yields a gas that dulls pain and causes unconsciousness.
cholecystectomy surgical removal of the gallbladder.
cholecystolithiasis an abnormal presence of stones in the gallbladder.
cholelithiasis stones in the gallbladder.
cholenergic nerve fibers capable of secreting acetylcholine.
cholera an acute, specific, infectious disease characterized by diarrhea, painful cramps of muscles, and a tendency to collapse.
cholesterol a sterol present in the tissues which contributes to heart disease when elevated; transported in the blood plasma of all animals.
chorionic gonadotropin a hormone detectable in the urine of a pregnant female soon after conception.
choroid the vascular coat of the eye between the sclera and the retina.
chromosome structures within the cell's nucleus that store hereditary information.
chronic continuing a long time, returning; not acute.
chronic glomerulonephritis the slow, progressive destruction of the glomerulus of the kidney.
chronic leukemia a form of leukemia characterized by insidious onset and slower progress.
chronic obstructive pulmonary disease (COPD) a syndrome characterized by chronic bronchitis, asthma, and emphysema, or any combination of these conditions, resulting in dyspnea, frequent respiratory infections, and thoracic deformities from attempting to breathe.
chronic renal failure the end result of the progressive loss of kidney function.
chronologic the arrangement of events, dates, etc., in order of occurrence.
chyme the mixture of partially digested food and digestive secretions found in the stomach and small intestines during digestion of a meal.
cilia hairlike projections from epithelial cells, as in the bronchi.
circulatory refers to the circulatory system; the process of blood flowing through the vessels to all the cells of the body.
circumcision surgical removal of the foreskin of the penis.
circumference the distance around a circle; with mensurations, the measurement of the head.
circumversion rotation of an extremity in a circular motion.
cirrhosis an interstitial inflammation with hardening of the tissues of an organ, especially the liver.
civil law pertaining to the rights of private individuals; legal proceedings concerning rights that are not criminal.
clarity clearness, absence of cloudiness.
classified arranged in a group or classification according to some system.
clause part of a sentence with a subject and a predicate.
claustrophobia an abnormal fear of being in enclosed or confined places.
clavicle the collar bone, articulating with the sternum and scapula.
clearinghouse a private or public company that often serves as the middleman between physicians and billing groups, payers and other health care partners for the transmission and translation of electronic claims information into the specific format required by payers
CLIA see **Clinical Laboratory Improvement Amendments.**
clinical based on observation; in medical assisting, pertains to duties considered "back office"; not administrative in nature.
clinical diagnosis identification of a disease by history, laboratory findings, and symptoms.
Clinical Laboratory Improvement Amendments (CLIA) legislation dealing with the operation of a clinical laboratory.
clinical skills these are skills that are an extension of the provider's responsibilities and can be divided into fundamental practices, diagnostic procedures and patient care.
clitoris an erectile organ located at the anterior junction of the labia minora.

clonal the duplicated copy; with immunity it is the cells produced to attack antigens.
clone an exact copy.
CMS-1500 form the standard claim form designed by the centers for medicare and medicaid services to submit physician services for third-party (insurance companies) payment
coagulation lessening of the fluidity of a liquid substance; clotting or curdling.
coccyx the tailbone; the last four bones of the spine.
cochlea the snail-shaped portion of the inner ear.
coercion to force or compel; to restrain or constrain by force.
coinsurance a percentage that a patient is responsible for paying for each service after the deductible has been met.
coitus sexual intercourse between a man and a woman.
colitis inflammation of the colon.
collaborate to work together.
collateral subordinate, secondary; property deposited as security for a loan.
colleague an associate at work, usually one of similar status.
collections ratio a formula that determines how efficiently and timely an office is collecting payments for services rendered by the physicians.
colon the large intestine.
colorimeter an instrument used for measuring the amount of pigments and determining the amount of hemoglobin in the blood.
colostomy incision of the colon for the purpose of making a more or less permanent opening.
colposcopy a diagnostic examination to visualize the cervix through a colposcope.
coma an abnormal deep stupor from which a person cannot be aroused by external stimuli.
coma scale refers to the Glascow Coma Scale used to determine level of consciousness.
combining forms in medical terminology, the word root with a combining form vowel (usually an "o") that aids in making the word pronounceable, particularly when adding a suffix that begins with a consonant.
comminuted a crushed bone fracture with many fragments.
commiserate to feel or express sympathy or pity for.
Commission on Accreditation of Allied Health Education Programs (CAAHEP) an accrediting body that provides programmatic accreditation for medical assisting and other healthcare programs.
common bile duct a duct carrying bile from the hepatic and cystic ducts to the duodenum.
Common law the traditional unwritten law of england, based on custom and usage, which began to develop over a thousand years before the founding of the united states. today, almost all common law has been enacted into statutes with modern variations by all the states except louisiana, which is still influenced by the napoleonic code. in some states, the principles of common law are so basic they are applied without reference to statute.
commonality people in general; a body corporate or its membership.
communicable capable of being transmitted from one person or species to another, also known as contagious.
communication the act of communicating; information given; a means of giving information.
comorbidity a condition that exists along with the primary diagnosis of a patient.
compatible able to be mixed or taken together without destructive changes (as in blood typing and cross-matching); matching; not opposed to.
compensate to make amends; be equivalent to.
compensation anything given as an equivalent or to make amends; pay.
compensatory damages damages recovered in payment for actual injury or economic loss, which does not include punitive damages (as added damages due to malicious or grossly negligent action).
competency demonstrated capability, being able; a task to achieve.
competent fit, able, capable.
complement a group of about 20 inactive enzyme proteins present in the blood.
complementary something that will add to or make another thing complete or whole.
complete blood count a test requested by a doctor or other medical professional that gives information about the cells in a patient's blood; also known as a CBC; amongst the most commonly performed blood tests in medicine.
complexity the state of being complicated.
compliance consent; conformity to formal or official requirements.
complicated not simple, involved; having many parts; not easy to solve.
complimentary express appreciation; given without charge.
complimentary therapy therapy used in addition to traditional therapies.
compose to form by putting together, creating.
compound not simple, composed of two or more parts; with fractures, refers to bone fragments piercing the skin externally.
comprehensive covering all areas; inclusive.
compression to exert force against, press.
Computed Transaxial Tomography (CAT) computed axial tomography, a medical imaging method employing tomography in which digital geometry processing is used to generate a three-dimensional image of the internals of an object from a large series of two-dimensional x-ray images taken around a single axis of rotation.
computer a mechanical, electric, or electronic device that stores numerical or other information and provides logical answers at high speed to questions bearing on that information.
computerized to store in a computer; to put in a form a computer can use; to bring computers into use to control an operation.
Computerized Axial Tomography (CAT) a series of x-ray views of the body used to construct a three-dimensional picture.
conceal to hide, to keep secret, to withhold, as information.
conceive to become pregnant; the uniting of the sperm and ovum.
conception the union of the sperm of a male and the egg of a female; fertilization.
conceptualize to form a concept, thought, notion, or understanding.
concise condensed, short.
condenser part of a microscope substage that regulates the amount of light directed on a specimen.
confidential revealed in confidence; secret information.
confidential being prudent and conscious—especially in regards to speech.
Confidential Communication Preference (CCP) form a form a patient signs which authorizes other individuals to receive information regarding the patient's care. Individuals not listed will not be permitted to receive or ask for such information.
confidentiality to be held in confidence; a secret.
confinement restriction within certain limits.
confirmation making firm or sure; convincing proof.
confirmed verified or ratified.
confirmed Verification of authenticity
conflict a clash of opinions or interests; a fight or struggle; an inner moral struggle; to come into opposition.
confrontation to stand face to face with.
congenital existing at birth.
congestive heart failure a complex condition of inadequate heart action with retention of tissue fluids; may be either right- or left-side failure, or both.
congratulations to express pleasure; a recognition of accomplishment.
conjunction meeting; a word that connects.

conjunctiva a mucous membrane that lines the eyelids and covers the anterior sclera of the eyeball.
connective that which connects or binds together; one of the five main tissues of the body.
connotations something implied or suggested.
consciousness awareness, full knowledge of what is in one's own mind.
consecutive following in order, successive.
consecutively a series of things that follow each other.
conserve to keep from damage or loss; to maintain.
consideration a vital element in the law of contracts, consideration is a benefit which must be bargained for between the parties, and is the essential reason for a party entering into a contract. consideration must be of value and is exchanged for the performance or promise of performance by the other party.
constipation a sluggish action of the bowel; usually refers to an excessively firm, hard stool that is difficult to expel or lack of a bowel movement over a time.
constrict to narrow; to become smaller because of contraction of a sphincter muscle.
contact dermatitis inflammation and irritation of the skin caused by contact with an irritating substance.
contagious catching; able to be transmitted by contact.
contaminate to place in contact with microorganisms.
contemporary happening or existing at the same time; a person living at the same time as another.
content the matter dealt with in a field of study; matter contained.
context the part of a written or spoken statement that surrounds a particular word or passage and can clarify its meaning.
continuity of care the delivery of services provided to a person that proceeds without a lapse or interruption, with the intended purpose of maintaining a level of health and treatment
contraception against conception.
contract to draw together, reduce in size, or shorten.
contraction the muscle action of the uterus during labor; in spelling and punctuation, the shortening of a word by the omission of one or more letters, which are replaced with an apostrophe.
contracture permanent shortening or contraction of a muscle.
contradiction to deny; to assert to the contrary of.
contrast to show difference; in radiology, refers to a radiopaque medium used to outline body organs.
contrast media a substance used to enhance the visibility of structures or fluids within the body for medical imaging
contributory giving a share; helping toward a result.
contributory factors Additional components that can be considered when selecting an evaluation and management code: time, nature of presenting problem, counseling and coordination of care.
Control testing of machines and testing kits in the laboratory to detect any deficiencies prior to testing patient specimens.
controversial open to dispute; relating to discussion of opposing views.
conventional growing out of custom; not spontaneous.
convey to impart, as an idea; to transfer.
convulsion attack of involuntary muscular contractions often accompanied by unconsciousness.
cooperate to work together.
coordination a state of harmonious adjustment or function.
coordination of benefits when both spouses have health care insurance, the policy provision that limits benefits to 100% of the cost; also known as dual coverage.
coordinator a person who works for harmonious functioning of parts or agents toward the production of a desired result.
COPD see **chronic obstructive pulmonary disease.**
cornea the transparent extension of the sclera that lies in front of the pupil of the eye.
coronal the plane dividing the body into front and back portions.
coronal (plane) a line drawn through the side of the body from head to toe, making a front and back section.
coronary referring to the arteries surrounding the heart muscle; also refers to a "heart attack," which involves the coronary arteries.
coroner an official who investigates a sudden, suspicious, or violent death to determine the cause. In some communities this position has been replaced by the medical examiner.
corpus luteum the yellow body that develops in the ruptured graafian follicle after the ovum has been discharged.
correspondence communication by the exchange of letters.
cortex the outer portion of the kidney.
corticosteroids hormones used to treat inflammation.
cost ratio a formula that demonstrates a cost of a specific procedure or service.
cost-benefit analysis an analysis which allows for program evaluation by demonstrating whether the benefits received will outweigh its costs.
COT see **certified ophthalmic technician.**
countershock (in cardiology) a high-intensity, short-duration, electric shock applied to the area of the heart, resulting in total cardiac depolarization.
courteous polite, considerate, and respectful in manner and action.
CPT see **Current Procedural Terminology.**
cramp a spasmodic, painful contraction of a muscle or muscles.
cranial pertaining to the cranium or skull.
cranium the skull; the eight bones of the head enclosing the brain; generally applied to the 28 bones of the head and face.
cravat a triangular bandage, folded lengthwise; it may be used as a circular, figure-eight, or spiral bandage to control bleeding or to tie splints in place
credit balance occurs when the amount paid is greater than was due or the account is being paid in advance of service provided.
crenated notched or scalloped, as the crenated condition of blood corpuscles.
cretinism a congenital condition caused by the lack of the hormone thyroxin.
criminal law of, involving, or having the nature of a crime.
crisis the turning point of a disease; a very critical period; an emergency situation.
criterion a standard of criticism or judgment (plural: criteria).
critical thinking using deductive reasoning to examine a problem or issue from a variety of different angles in order to arrive at the most appropriate conclusion and using that information in order to guide behaviors.
critique a critical examination of a thing or situation, to determine its nature, worth, or conformity to standards.
crohn's disease an inflammation of the GI tract with debilitating symptoms.
cross-match a blood test used to ensure compatibility of the donor to the recipient when transfusing blood.
crutches staffs with a cross-piece at the top to place under the arms of a lame person.
cryosurgery the use of a substance at subfreezing temperature to destroy or remove tissue.
cryptorchidism failure of the testicles to descend into the scrotum.
CTD see **cumulative trauma disorder.**
CTS see **carpal tunnel syndrome.**
cultivate to form and refine; to improve.
culture a method of growing a microbial organism to determine what it is, its abundance in the sample being tested, or both. It is one of the primary diagnostic methods of microbiology.
cumulative trauma disorder (CTD) an injury resulting from repetitive movement of a body part.
curette an instrument to scrape material from a cavity.

currency any form of money.
current happening now; of the present time; the latest information.
Current Procedural Terminology (CPT) a numerical listing of procedures performed in medical practice; a standardized identification of procedures. Published by the american medical association.
curriculum a course of study at a school or university.
cushing's syndrome a disorder resulting from the hypersecretion of glucocorticoids from the adrenal cortex.
cusp a sharp point or apex.
customarily by custom, the usual course of action under similar circumstances.
cyanosis a bluish discoloration of the skin caused by lack of oxygen.
cyst a bladder; any sac containing fluid.
cystic pertaining to a cyst; of disease, refers to a condition with multiple cysts.
cystic fibrosis a disease condition of fibrous tumors that have undergone cystic degeneration, accumulating fluid in the interspaces; also known as fibrocystic disease.
cystitis inflammation of the urinary bladder.
cystoscope an instrument for examining the interior of the urinary bladder.
cystoscopy a diagnostic procedure performed with a cystoscope that allows a provider to look at the inside of the bladder and urethra, collect urine samples, and examine the prostate gland; it also enables biopsies to be taken or small stones to be removed by way of a hollow channel in the cystoscope.
cytokine a nonantibody protein of the immune system that regulates immune response.
cytologist one who studies cells and interprets slides.
cytology the study of cell life and cell formation.
cytoplasm cellular matter, not including the nucleus of a cell.
cytotechnologist a laboratory specialist who prepares and examines tissue cells to study cell formation.
cytotoxic capable of destroying cells.

DACUM an acronym for "design a curriculum."
daltonism the inability to distinguish between red and green.
data facts from which conclusions can be inferred.
date of birth (DOB) the date a person is born, including the month, day, and year.
date of service (DOS) the calendar date a service begins or is provided.
Daysheet Form used for recording all daily financial transactions of charges made and payments received; also called a daily journal
D & C see **dilatation and curettage.**
DEA see **Drug Enforcement Administration.**
debilitated weakened; impaired the strength of.
debit to deduct, to charge.
debit balance Occurs when the amount paid is less than the total due
débridement to clean up or remove, as is done with damaged tissue around a wound.
decibel a unit of measure to express the degree of loudness of sound.
decimal numbers that are expressed as a fraction of a part using 10 as its base number; it also refers to the period used to separate a whole number from a fraction, as in 10.2, otherwise read as "ten and two-tenths."
decline stage becoming less intense, subsiding; a period of time when the symptoms of disease start to disappear.
dedicated committed to; set apart for a special use.
deductible an amount to be paid before insurance will pay.
deductions to deduct or subtract; remove, take away.
defamation to slander, or to attack the reputation of an individual or group.
defecate to pass stool or move bowels.
defendant the party sued in a civil lawsuit or the party charged with a crime in a criminal prosecution.
defibrillation to cause fibrillation to end; restore to normal action.
defibrillator a device designed to deliver an electric shock to a patient, in an effort to stop pulseless ventricular fibrillation or ventricular tachycardia.
dehydration withdrawal of water from the tissues naturally or artificially.
delegation a person or group of persons officially elected or appointed to represent another or others; to entrust power
delete to remove, erase.
delirium tremens a psychic disorder involving hallucinations, both visual and auditory, found in habitual users of alcohol.
deltoid the muscle of the shoulder.
demeanor behavior; bearing.
demography the study of population statistics concerning births, marriage, death, disease, and many other indicators.
dendrite an extension from a nerve cell.
denial a refusal to believe or accept; disowning.
denomination a category or classification of currency.
denominator The bottom number of a fraction.
denote to indicate, to mean.
dental assistant a health care worker employed by a dentist to perform management and clinical functions and provide chairside assistance.
dental hygienist a licensed health care provider who is trained to x-ray and perform prophylactic treatments on teeth.
dentist (DDS) a licensed health provider who cares for the teeth, repairing and replacing as needed.
deoxyribonucleic acid (DNA) material within the chromosome that carries the genetic information.
dependable that which may be relied upon.
dependence that on which one depends; reliance.
dependent person covered under a subscriber's insurance policy.
dependent children (please remove from key terms list)
depict to represent by a picture; portray.
depleted consumed, emptied, exhausted.
deposit to entrust money to a bank or other institution.
deposit record a record of a financial deposit that is given by the bank to the customer at the time of the deposit.
deposit slip a slip accompanying a bank deposit and containing an itemized list of checks or cash deposited, the date, and the depositer's signature.
deposition testimony given under oath.
depressant a drug that causes a slowing down of bodily function or nerve activity.
depressed a state of depression, a period of low spirits; referring to a fracture, usually a fracture of the skull where bone fragments are driven (depressed) inward.
deprivation to be deprived; without; having to do without or unable to use.
dermatitis an inflammation of the skin, often the result of an irritant.
dermatologist a physician who specializes in the diseases and disorders of the skin.
dermatology the study of the skin and its diseases.
dermis true skin.
descending refers to the portion of the large intestine from the splenic flexure to the sigmoid.
description a word picture.
desensitization the process of making an individual less susceptible to allergens.
desensitizing a process of exposing a patient to small levels of an allergen to gradually build up a nonallergic reaction.
design working plan; layout; sketch.
designate to point out; indicate; appoint.
detection find out or discover.
detrimental harmful, injurious.
deuteranopia the difficulty in differentiating between the shades of green and bluish reds and some neutral shades.
devastate to lay waste, plunder, destroy.
development the advancement of abilities and knowledge.

dextrose a simple sugar, also known as glucose.
diabetes mellitus a metabolic disease caused by the body's inability to use carbohydrates.
diabetic one afflicted with the condition diabetes.
diabetic coma a diabetic emergency that can be fatal if not treated promptly and properly.
diabetic ketoacidosis a complication of diabetes that occurs when the body cannot use sugar (glucose) as a fuel source because the body has no insulin or not enough insulin, and fat is used instead. Byproducts of fat breakdown, called ketones, build up in the body
diagnostic referring to measures that assist in the recognition of diseases and disorders of the body.
diagnostic-related group (DRG) method of determining reimbursement from medical insurance according to diagnosis on a prospective basis.
dialysis removal of the products of urine from the blood by passage of the solutes through a membrane.
diaphanography a type of transillumination used to examine the breast, using selected wavelengths of light and special imaging equipment.
diaphoresis profuse sweating.
diaphragm the muscle of breathing that separates the thorax from the abdomen.
diarrhea frequent bowel movements, usually liquid or semisolid.
diarthrosis a movable joint; another word for synovial.
diastole the relaxation phase of the heartbeat; the period of least pressure.
dictation spoken words; recorded voice communication.
dietician one who is trained in dietetics, which includes nutrition, and in charge of the diet of an institution.
differential refers to determining the number of each type of leukocyte in a cubic millimeter of blood.
diffuse to scatter or spread.
diffusion a process whereby gas, liquid, or solid molecules distribute themselves evenly through a medium.
digestion the process by which food is broken down, mechanically and chemically, in the gastrointestinal tract and converted into absorbable forms.
digestive pertaining to digestion.
digitally pertaining to or resembling a finger or toe, as an examination using a finger or fingers.
digital rectal exam (DRE) examination performed by the provider to check for abnormalities of organs or other structures in the pelvis and lower abdomen.
dilate to enlarge, expand in size; to increase the size of an opening.
dilation and curettage (D & C) dilation of the cervix and scraping of the interior lining of the uterus.
dimpling a condition characterized by indentations in the skin.
diphtheria an acute infectious disease characterized by the formation of a false membrane on any mucous surface, usually in the air passages, interfering with breathing.
diplomate an advanced status of medical practice.
direct payment payment made directly to the physician by the insurance company.
disability a legal incapacity.
disaster an occurrence inflicting widespread destruction and distress.
disciplinary designed to correct or punish breaches of conduct.
discipline self-control, conduct, system of rules.
disclose to uncover, reveal.
discoid a type of lupus that is confined to the skin; also called cutaneous.
discreet wisely cautious, prudent.
discrepancy inconsistencies; variances.
discretion the use of judgment, prudence.
disease sickness, illness, ailment.
disinfection the process of applying antimicrobial agents to non-living objects to destroy microorganisms.
dislocation the displacement of a part; usually refers to a bone temporarily out of its normal position in a joint.
dispense to distribute; to deal out in portions.
dispense as written (DAW) Phrase indicating that substitutions for generics or similar medications are not allowed by the prescriber
displacement the transfer of emotions about one person or situation to another person or situation.
disposition the act or manner of putting in a particular order; arrange.
dissect to cut into parts for examination; to separate.
distal farthest from the center, from the medial line, or from the trunk.
distend to become inflated, to stretch out.
distinctive unmistakable, different from anything else.
distort to misrepresent; to twist out of usual shape.
distributive justice the act of assigning or allotting
diversion the act of diverting or turning aside.
diverticulitis inflammation of the diverticula.
diverticulum a sac or pouch in the walls of a canal or organ, particularly the colon.
dividend The result of dividing one number by another.
divisor The number used to divide into another number.
divulge to make public; to make known; reveal.
DNA see **deoxyribonucleic acid.**
doctorate a postgraduate degree conferred following extensive course work, an individual research project, and the writing of a dissertation; a PhD.
Doctor of Medicine (MD) an individual who has met all the requirements in the state to become licensed as a medical doctor.
Doctor of Osteopathic Medicine (DO) a doctor licensed by the state to practice medicine. These practitioners place special emphasis on the body's musculoskeletal and nervous systems, preventive medicine, and holistic patient care, and patient education.
Doctorate Persons that hold doctoral degrees have attained advanced knowledge through higher education in disciplines such as nursing, mathematics, education, chemistry, philosophy, and so on and have the right to be addressed as doctor.
doctrine the principles of any branch of knowledge; a belief held or taught.
documentary presenting facts without inserting fictional matter.
documentation refers to both the act of preparing, or the evidence created when a healthcare professional records, information regarding a patient during the course of assessment and treatment; can be handwritten or electronically.
domestic not foreign; private.
dominant strongest; prevailing, the prime or main.
dominant gene the prevailing gene.
dorsal pertaining to the back.
dorsal recumbent body position in which the patient is on his or her back, face up, legs separated, knees flexed with feet flat.
dorsalis pedis a pulse point palpable on the instep of the foot.
dosimeter a device which measures exposure to ionizing radiation, such as x-rays, alpha rays, beta rays, and gamma rays.
double-entry bookkeeping system an accounting method in which each financial transaction is recorded in two accounts; equal debits and credits are recorded for each transaction
douche an irrigation of the vagina.
dowel a round piece of wood.
downcoding A practice of third-party payers in which the benefits code has been changed to a less complex or lower cost procedure than was reported.
downtime refers to being offline; computer failure; time when nothing is scheduled.
dribbling uncontrolled leakage of urine from the bladder.

drill disciplined repetitious exercises as a means of perfecting a skill or procedure.
droplet a very small drop.
droplet infection a disease that results from contamination with water-based microorganisms.
Drug Enforcement Administration (DEA) a division of the federal government responsible for the enforcement of laws regulating the distribution and sale of drugs.
dual referring to two; having two parts.
duodenum the first segment of the small intestine.
dura mater the outer membrane covering the brain and spinal cord.
duration the amount of time a thing continues.
dwarfism a condition caused by inadequate growth hormone during childhood.
dysmenorrhea painful menstruation.
dysplasia precancerous cells; with cervix are precursors to cervical cancer.
dyspnea difficult or labored breathing.
dyspneic difficulty in breathing.
dystrophy progressive atrophy or weakening of a part, such as the muscles.
dysuria painful urination; difficulty in urination.

ECG or EKG see **electrocardiogram.**
echocardiography ultrahigh-frequency sound waves directed toward the heart to evaluate function and structure of the organ.
echoes reflections of sound.
ectopic in an abnormal position; in pregnancy refers to the embryo or fetus being outside the uterus.
eczema a noncontagious skin disease characterized by dry, red, itchy, and scaly skin.
edema a condition of body tissues containing abnormal amounts of fluid, usually intercellular; may be local or general.
effacement the thinning out of the cervix during labor.
efficiency the ratio of energy expended to results produced.
ejaculation the expulsion of seminal fluid from the male urethra.
ejaculatory duct the duct from the seminal vesicle to the urethra.
elaborate to improve by successive operations; to work out in detail.
elasticity ability to return to shape after being stretched.
electrical charged with electricity; run by electricity.
electrocardiogram (EKG, ECG) a graphic record of the electric currents generated by the heart; a tracing of the heart action.
electrocardiogram technician (ECG tech) a person trained in obtaining electrocardiograms, a record of cardiac impulses.
electrocardiograph a machine for obtaining a graphic recording of the electrical activity of the heart.
electrocautery an apparatus used to cauterize tissue with heat from a current of electricity.
electrocoagulation coagulation of tissue by means of a high-frequency electric current.
electrode an instrument with a point or a surface that transmits current to the patient's body; also known as a sensor used to conduct electricity from the body to the electrocardiograph.
electroencephalography (EEG) recording of the electric currents generated by the brain; a tracing of brain waves.
electrolyte a substance that, in solution, conducts an electric current.
electromagnet a soft iron core that temporarily becomes a magnet when an electric current flows through a coil surrounding it.
electromagnetic a specialized field of radiology that involves the use of both electrical and magnetic fields for diagnosis of disease processes.
electromagnetic radiation rays produced by the collision of a beam of electrons with a metal target in an x-ray tube.
electromyography the insertion of needles into selected skeletal muscles for the purpose of recording nerve conduction time in relation to muscle contraction.
electron a minute particle of matter charged with the smallest known amount of negative electricity; opposite of proton.
electronic operated by the use of electrons.
Electronic Claims Tracking (ECT) computer software designed for monitoring insurance claims
Electronic Data Interchange (EDI) Refers to the exchange of routine business transactions from one computer to another in a standard format, using standard communications protocols
Electronic health record (EHR) aggregate electronic record of health-related information on an individual that is created and gathered cumulatively across more than one health care organization and is managed and consulted by licensed clinicians and staff involved in the individual's health and care.
Electronic Media Claims (EMC) A flat file format used to transmit or transport claims
Electronic medical record (EMR) the electronic record of health-related information for an individual that is created, gathered, managed, and consulted by licensed clinicians and staff that is maintained through a single organization involved in the individual's health and care.
elements substances in their simplest form; the basic building blocks of all matter.
elicit to draw out, to derive by logical process.
elimination to remove, get rid of, exclude; also to pass urine from the bladder or stool from the bowel.
elite choice, superior, select.
ellipses a mark or series of marks used in writing or printing to indicate an omission, especially of letters or words.
emaciation to become abnormally thin; the loss of too much weight.
emancipated minor no longer under the care, custody, or supervision of a parent or guardian.
embolism the presence of an obstruction in a blood vessel.
embolus a circulating mass in a blood vessel; foreign material that obstructs a blood vessel.
embryo the first 8 weeks of development after fertilization.
emergency an unexpected occurrence or situation demanding immediate action.
Emergency Medical Services (EMS) A group that provides out-of-hospital acute medical care and/or transport to definitive care to patients experiencing a medical emergency
emergency medical technician (EMT) an individual trained to respond in emergency situations and provide appropriate initial medical treatment.
emergency preparedness Preparing for the first and immediate response to any type of hazard or emergency event.
Emergent Arising suddenly and unexpectedly.
emesis to vomit.
emetic medication that induces vomiting.
Empathetic Putting yourself in another person's shoes
empathy sympathetically trying to identify one's feelings with those of another.
emphysema a chronic lung disease characterized by overdistention of the alveolar sacs and inability to exchange oxygen and carbon dioxide.
empirically based on observations or experiment.
empyema exudate (pus) within the pleural space of the chest cavity.
enact to make into law.
Encoder software application that allows searching or browsing within CPT, HCPCS, ICD-9-CM code sets, and Medicare coding guidelines.
encompass to surround, enclose.
encounter to meet, unexpectedly or by chance.
Encounter form a record of information obtained during a health care visit, usually a preprinted document, that designates what services and/or procedures are performed and at what level of acuity those services should be billed. Also called a charge slip.

encounter form Document used to record the services provided to a patient; also known as a superbill.
encounter form Form listing the procedures that are performed in that medical office, with their respective codes; also called superbill or charge slip
endocardium the serous membrane lining of the heart.
endocervical the lining of the canal of the cervix.
endocrine a gland that secretes directly into the blood stream.
endocrinologist a physician specializing in the diseases and disorders of the endocrine system.
endocrinology the study of the endocrine or ductless glands of internal secretion.
endocytosis a cellular process to bring large molecules of material into the cytoplasm of the cell.
endometrium the mucous membrane lining of the uterus.
endoplasmic reticulum an organelle within the cytoplasm of a cell.
endorse to approve, recommend, or sponsor.
endorsement the act of endorsing; approving.
Endorsement when a physician gains licensure in a particular state as a result of passing the national board examination.
endoscope an instrument consisting of a tube and optical system for observing the inside of an organ or cavity.
enema the instillation of fluid into the rectum and colon.
engorge to fill with blood to the point of congestion; to devour or engulf.
enhance to intensify, improve.
enthusiasm intense interest; zeal; passion.
entity a thing having reality.
enucleation surgical excision of the eyeball.
enumerate to count separately, name one by one.
enunciate to speak or pronounce clearly.
envelope to enclose completely with a cover; a paper container for a letter.
environment surroundings.
enzyme a complex chemical substance produced by the body, found primarily in the digestive juices, that acts upon food substances to break them down for absorption.
eosinophil a white blood cell or cellular structure that stains readily with the acid stain eosin; specifically an eosinophilic leukocyte.
epidemic affecting many persons at one time.
Epidemic a disease affecting large numbers of individuals in a population
epidermis the outer layer of the skin; literally *over the true skin*.
epididymis a convoluted tube resting on the surface of the testicle that carries sperm from the testicle to the vas deferens.
epigastric pertaining to the area of the abdomen over the stomach.
epiglottis a cartilagenous lid that closes over the larynx when swallowing.
epilepsy a chronic disease of the nervous system characterized by convulsions and often unconsciousness.
epinephrine a hormone produced by the adrenal medulla.
epiphysis a portion of bone not yet ossified; the cartilagenous ends of the long bones that allow for growth.
episiotomy an incision in the perineum to avoid tearing during childbirth.
epistaxis nosebleed; hemorrhage from the nose.
epithelial pertaining to a type of cell or tissue that forms the skin and mucous membranes of the body.
equity the value of property beyond the total amount owed on it.
equivalent equal to in value, size, or effect.
erectile refers to tissue that is capable of erection, usually caused by vasocongestion.
ergonomics the applied science of being concerned with the nature and characteristics of people as they relate to design and activities with the intention of producing more effective results and greater safety.
erythema diffuse redness over the skin because of capillary congestion and dilation of the superficial capillaries.
erythrocyte a red blood cell (RBC).
erythropoiesis the formation of red blood corpuscles.
eschar slough, especially after a cauterization.
esophagus a collapsible tube from the pharynx to the stomach, through which pass the food and water the body ingests.
essential necessary; when referring to blood pressure, indicates an elevation without apparent cause.
e-statement An electronic bank statement sent via email from the bank to the customer's email address; a paperless bank statement.
esthetic relating to the principles of beauty and taste.
estrogen a female hormone produced by the ovaries.
ether a colorless liquid used to produce unconsciousness and insensibility to pain.
ethical right, according to the principles of ethics.
ethics standards of conduct and moral judgement.
ethics a system of moral principles; the rules of conduct in respect to a particular class of actions
ethnicity Demographic term that indicates with what societal group a patient identifies himself/herself.
etiology the study of the cause of disease.
etiquette conventional rules for correct behavior.
euphoria a feeling of well-being, elation.
eustachian tube refers to the tube of the middle ear that connects to the pharynx.
evacuants a medication that promotes emptying of the bowels.
evacuate to empty, especially the bowels.
evacuated Withdrawal; to remove; to make empty.
evacuation withdrawal, to remove, to make empty.
evaluation assessment; judgment concerning the worth, quality, significance, or value of a situation, person, or product.
eversion the movement of the sole of the foot away from the median plane.
evoke to call forth or up; summon; elicit.
excretion the process of expelling material from the body.
exemplify to show by example.
exempt excluded; not liable; freedom from duty or service; privileged.
exemption freed from or not liable for something to which others are subject.
exfoliate to scale off dead tissue.
exhale to breathe out.
exhaustion extreme fatigue.
exocrine a gland that secretes substances through a duct into the body.
exocytosis a cellular process that moves materials within the cell to the outside.
exogenous originating outside an organ or part.
exophthalmia abnormal protrusion of the eyeball.
Exophthalmos (NOTE: Exophthalmus is already in the glossary as exophthalmia. It can be spelled exophthalmos, exophthalmus or exophthamia).
exorcism the act of expelling an evil spirit.
expectorate to spit, to expel mucus or phlegm from the throat or lungs.
expedient suitable means for achieving or attaining a purpose or end; of immediate advantage, convenient.
expedite to hasten.
expended spent or used, as with money or energy.
expenditure Actual payment of cash or cash-equivalent for goods or services, or a charge against available funds in settlement of an obligation as evidenced by an invoice, receipt, voucher, or other such document.
experience observation or practice resulting in knowledge; knowledge gained by seeing and doing.
expertise special knowledge or skill.
expiration the expulsion of air from the lungs in breathing.
explicit clearly and definitely expressed; unambiguous; leaving no room for questions.

express to utter; to make known in words or by action.
expressed said in words or by action.
extend movement of a joint to increase the angle of that joint.
extensive having a wide range.
extensor the muscle of a muscle team that extends a part, allowing the joint to straighten.
external the outermost part of the body.
externship a supervised employment experience in a qualified health care facility as part of the educational curriculum.
extinguish to put out; put an end to.
extinguisher a device for putting out fire.
extracellular outside the cell.
extract a substance distilled or drawn out of another substance.
extremes The highest or lowest level of a math function on an interval.
extremities the terminal parts of the body—the arms, legs.
extrinsic originating from outside one's self; motivation coming from factors outside of an individual
exudate pus; the collection of purulent material in a cavity.
exudative pertaining to any fluid that filters from the circulatory system into lesions or areas of inflammation.
eyewash a device using water to remove foreign material from the eyes, usually in emergency situations.

facility a building; in medical situations, a building for the care and treatment of patients.
facsimile an exact copy.
facultative able to live under conditions of temperature or oxygen supply that vary; having the capability to adapt to more than one condition, as a facultative anerobe.
failure to thrive (FTT) A description applied to infants and children whose current weight or rate of weight gain is significantly below that of other children of similar age and sex.
faith belief in the doctrines of religion; a firm belief in something for which there is no proof.
fallopian tube the ovaduct; the passageway for the ova from the ovary to the uterus.
familial pertaining to the same family.
family practice one which cares for patients of all ages and all conditions not requiring specialization.
fascia a fibrous membrane covering, supporting, and separating muscles; may also unite the skin with underlying tissue.
fast to abstain from food; without food or water.
fatal causing death.
fax a message that is transmitted over phone lines and printed by the recipient's equipment.
feasible possible; practicable.
febrile pertaining to a fever.
fecal pertaining to feces.
feces stool, bowel movement.
Federal law legislation enacted by Congress and signed by the President.
fee-for-service Payment for each service that is provided.
fee schedule listing of allowable charge.
Felonies crimes sufficiently serious to be punishable by death or a term in state or federal prison.
femoral pertaining to the artery that lies adjacent to the femur.
femoral point the pressure point on the femoral artery.
femur the thigh bone of the leg.
fenestrated having a window or opening.
fertilization impregnation of the ovum by the sperm; conception.
fetal pertaining to a fetus, pregnancy beyond the third month.
fetal alcohol syndrome a group of birth defects in infants born to mothers who persisted to consume alcohol during gestation.
fetal monitor a device to access fetal heart beat.
fetus an embryo after 8 weeks of gestation.
fibrillation the quivering of muscle fibers; ineffective, rapid but weak heart action.
fibroid a tumor made up of fibrous and muscular tissue.
fibrosis abnormal formation of fibrous tissue.
fibula a long bone in the leg from the knee to the ankle.
filtration the movement of solutes and water across a semipermeable membrane as a result of a force, such as gravity or blood pressure.
financial records Records that reflect the financial status of the medical office or business.
fiscal of or pertaining to finances in general.
fissure an ulcer, split, crack, or tear in the tissue.
fistula an abnormal tubelike passage from a normal cavity or an abscess to a free surface.
flatulence the existence of flatus or intestinal gas.
flatus intestinal gas.
flex time refers to the practice of permitting work hours within a range of time.
flexed bent, as at a joint.
flexibility easily bent, compliant, yielding to persuasion.
flexible the ability to adapt to circumstances; ability to flex and bend; nonrigid.
flexible sigmoidoscope A scope used for a flexible sigmoidoscopy exam to evaluate the lower part of the large intestine (colon).
flexible spending account (FSA) Pretax funds set aside for use in payment of medical services and supplies not covered by insurance.
flexor the muscle of a muscle team that bends a part.
flora plant life as distinguished from animal life; plant life occurring or adapted for living in a specific environment, as flora in the intestines.
flu an abbreviation for the word influenza; a respiratory or intestinal infection.
fluoroscope a device consisting of a fluorescent screen in conjunction with an x-ray tube to make visible shadows of objects interposed between the screen and the tube.
flushed sudden reddish coloration of the skin.
follicle a small excretory duct or sac or tubular gland; a hair follicle.
folliculitis a staphylococcal infection of a hair follicle.
Fomite An object (such as clothing, towels, or utensils) that may harbor a disease agent, and is also capable of transmitting it.
Food and Drug Administration (FDA) The government agency responsible for regulating the approval of medications, foods, cosmetics and certain supplements.
forceps an instrument used to grasp tissue and to clamp blood vessels.
foreign (body) anything that is not normally found in the location; usually refers to dirt, splinters, etc.
foreskin loose skin covering the end of the penis.
forge to imitate, especially to counterfeit, as a signature.
formaldehyde a colorless, pungent gas used in its liquid form to harden tissue for pathologic study, or as a germicide, disinfectant, or preservative, according to the strength of the solution.
formalin wood alcohol containing 40% formaldehyde.
fortitude courageous endurance.
fovea centralis a depression in the posterior surface of the retina that is the place of sharpest vision.
Fowler's a full or partial sitting examination position.
fraction A numerical expression of the number of portions of a whole by using the number of portion over the designated whole number, as in 1/8 or "one-eighth."
fracture the sudden breaking of a bone.
fraudulent characterized by cheating and deceit; obtained by dishonest means.
frequency the need to void urine often, though usually only a small amount at one time.
friction resistance of one surface to the motion of another surface rubbing over it.
fringe (benefits) benefits included in or added to the salary paid, such as health insurance, retirement fund, etc.

frontal anterior; the forehead bone; refers to the plane drawn through the side of the body from the head to the foot.
frostbite A condition where localized damage is caused to skin and other tissues due to extreme cold
functional practical, working, useful.
fundus that portion of an organ most remote from its opening; with uterus, the body of the uterus above the openings of the fallopian tubes.
Funduscopy Examination of the fundus of the eye.
fungus a vegetable, cellular organism that subsists on organic matter, such as bacteria or mold; a disease condition that causes growth of fungal lesions on the surface of the skin.
furuncle the medical term for a boil.

gait manner of walking.
gallbladder a small sac suspended beneath the liver that concentrates and stores bile.
galley proofs printed matter in preliminary form, to be corrected.
galvanometer an instrument that measures current by electromagnetic action.
gamete a germ cell; any reproductive body.
ganglion a mass of nerve tissue that receives and sends out nerve impulses.
gangrene a form of necrosis; the putrefaction of soft tissue.
gastric pertaining to the stomach.
gastrocnemius the large muscle in the calf of the leg.
gastroenterologist a physician specializing in the care of patients with diseases and disorders of the gastrointestinal tract.
gastroenterology the study of the stomach and intestines and their diseases.
gastrointestinal (GI) pertaining to the stomach and intestines.
gastrointestinal (GI) system also called the digestive tract, alimentary canal, or gut, the system of organs within multicellular animals that takes in food, digests it to extract energy and nutrients, and expels the remaining waste.
gastroscopy examination of the stomach with a gastroscope.
gatekeeper one who regulates access to someone or something; in insurance, a primary care physician who coordinates the patient's referral to specialists and hospital admissions.
gauge the size of a needle bore; the smaller the number the larger the needle bore.
gene a substance within the chromosome that dictates heredity.
general equivalence mappings (GEMs) provide forward and backward mapping between the ICD-9 and ICD-10 coding systems.
General Skills The skills that are necessary regardless whether working in a clinical or administrative capacity. They include legal functions, communication skills, the ability to deliver education and operational functions.
Generalist Medical assistants work as a generalists when they perform both clinical and administrative duties in addition to general responsibilities.
generate to produce, as heat, ideas, power.
generic general; characteristic of a genus or group.
genetic pertaining to the genes.
genital herpes fluid-filled lesions on the external genitalia, which are contagious upon direct contact.
genitalia the external sexual organs.
genogram a graph of family health history.
genucubital pertaining to the elbows and knees; the knee-elbow position.
genupectoral pertaining to the knees and chest; the knee-chest position.
geriatrics the study and treatment of the diseases of old age.
gerontologist a physician specializing in the care of the aged.
gestation period of intrauterine fetal development.
gestational diabetes form of diabetes found in pregnant women.
gigantism a condition resulting from the overproduction of growth hormone during childhood.
glance a quick look or view.
glaucoma a disease of the eye characterized by increased intraocular pressure.
glomerulonephritis inflammation of the glomerulus of the nephron of the kidney.
glomerulus the microscopic cluster of capillaries within the Bowman's capsule of the nephron.
glucohemoglobin sugar in the blood.
glucose a colorless or yellow, thick, syrupy liquid obtained by the incomplete hydrolysis of starch; a simple sugar.
gluteus maximus the large muscle of the buttocks.
glycohemoglobin test that indicates the average blood sugar over the past 2 months.
glycosuria sugar in the urine.
glycosylation the process of adding sugars to proteins or lipids.
goiter an enlargement of the thyroid gland.
Golgi apparatus an organelle within the cytoplasm of a cell.
gonadotropic related to stimulation of the gonads.
gonads the sex glands, the ovaries in the female and the testicles in the male.
gonorrhea a venereal disease of the reproductive organs, which is highly contagious upon direct contact.
gooseneck lamp a light fixture with a flexible portion that allows adjustment.
graafian follicle the vesicle in which ova are matured and which releases them when ripened.
graft a constructed part.
Gram negative bacteria that take on a pink color with Gram staining process.
Gram positive bacteria that take on a purple color with Gram staining process.
greenstick an incomplete fracture, occurring in children.
grillwork a bar-like device, usually constructed of heavy metal; an open grating for a door or window.
groin the depression between the thigh and the trunk of the body; the inguinal region.
gross exclusive of deductions; total; entire.
gross anatomy refers to the study of those features that can be observed with the naked eye by inspection and dissection.
Gross negligence carelessness which is in reckless disregard for the safety or lives of others, and is so great it appears to be a conscious violation of other people's rights to safety; more than simple negligence or mistake; less than intentionally evil.
guaiac a solution used to test for the presence of occult blood in the stool.
guaiac test paper a screening agent to test for hidden blood.
guarantee assurance that something will be done as specified; a pledge.
guarantor a person who makes or gives a guarantee or pledge, often to pay another's debt or obligation in the event of default.
Guardian a person who has been appointed by a judge to take care of a minor child or incompetent adult personally and/or manage that person's affairs.
guilds associations of persons engaged in the same trade or calling for mutual protection.
Guilds an association of persons engaged in a common trade or calling for mutual advantage and protection. Medicine was divided into three guilds during the seventeen hundreds; Surgeons, barbers and apothecaries.
GYN see **gynecology.**
gynecologist a physician specializing in the care of diseases and disorders of women, particularly the genital organs.
gynecology (GYN) the study of diseases of the female, particularly of the organs of reproduction.

haemophilus bacterial strains that grow best in hemoglobin.
hallucinogen a substance that causes hallucinations.
hamstring a group of muscles of the posterior thigh.

handicap to hinder; those who are physically disabled or mentally retarded.
hangover the malaise that follows ingestion of a considerable amount of alcohol.
harassment continual annoyance; persecution.
harbor place of protection; in health care, surfaces that allow microorganisms to hide and grow.
hard copy information printed on a solid surface, such as paper, instead of displayed on a CRT screen or stored on a disk.
hardware the visible parts of a computer system (keyboard, disk drive, monitor, and printers).
harmonious having parts combined in a proportionate, orderly, or pleasing arrangement; being peaceable or friendly.
hazard danger; risk.
HCFA Health Care Financing Administration.
health a state of complete physical and mental or social well-being.
health maintenance organization (HMO) a type of managed care operation that is typically set up as a for-profit corporation with salaried employees.
health reimbursement arrangement (HRA) an account with employer contributions used to pay for medical expenses.
health savings account (HSA) a tax-sheltered savings account, with contributions from the employer and employee, which can be used to pay for medical expenses.
healthcheck a federally mandated Medicaid program for health care of children up to 21 years of age.
heart block a condition in which impulses from the SA node fail to carry over to the AV node, resulting in a slow heart rate and a different rate of contraction between the upper and lower heart chambers.
heart murmur a sound produced by the leakage of blood through a heart valve.
heartburn a burning sensation beneath the breastbone, usually associated with indigestion.
heat cramps Painful, brief muscle cramps that occur during exercise or work in a hot environment; muscles may spasm or jerk involuntarily
heat exhaustion A condition whose symptoms may include heavy sweating and a rapid pulse, as a result of the body overheating
heat stroke A severe condition caused by impairment of the body's temperature-regulating abilities, resulting from prolonged exposure to excessive heat and characterized by cessation of sweating, severe headache, high fever, hot dry skin, and in serious cases collapse and coma
height the vertical length of an object or person.
hematocrit an expression of the volume of red blood cells per unit of circulating blood.
hematologist a physician specializing in the care of patients with disorders and diseases of the blood and blood-forming organs.
hematology the study of the blood and its diseases.
hematoma a tumor or swelling that contains blood.
hematuria blood in the urine.
hemodialysis a process whereby blood is passed through a thin membrane and exposed to a dialysate solution to remove waste products.
hemoglobin the combination of a protein and iron pigment in the red blood cells that attracts and carries oxygen in the body.
hemolysis dissolution; the breaking down of red blood cells.
hemophilia hereditary condition, transmitted through sex-linked chromosomes of female carriers; affects males only, causing inability to clot blood.
hemorrhage abnormal discharge of blood either internally or externally from venous, arterial, or capillary vessels.
hemorrhoidectomy surgical excision of hemorrhoidal tissue.
hemorrhoids varicose veins of the anal canal.
hemostat a type of forceps.
hemothorax blood within the pleural space of the chest cavity.
heparin a substance formed in the liver that inhibits the coagulation of blood.
hepatic pertaining to the liver.
hepatitis inflammation of the liver.
hepatitis A An acute infectious disease of the liver caused by a virus that is transmitted by contaminated food or water or by direct person-to-person contact
hepatitis B acute infection of the liver transmitted through blood or body fluids.
herbal pertaining to plants, particularly to their medicinal qualities.
hernia a projection of a part from its normal location.
herniorrhaphy the surgical repair of a hernia.
herpes simplex the medical term for fever blister, an acute viral infection of the face, mouth, or nose.
herpes zoster the medical term for shingles, an acute viral infection of the dorsal root ganglia.
hesitancy difficulty in starting a urine stream.
heterosexual sexual attraction toward the opposite sex.
heterotrophs microorganisms that feed on organic matter.
HHS U.S. Department of Health and Human Services.
hiatus pertains to a herniation of the stomach through an opening or hiatus.
HIB/hib *Hemophilus influenzae* type B.
hiccough (also hiccup) a result of the spasmodic closing of the epiglottis and spasm of the diaphragm.
hiccup see **hiccough.**
high-power field (hpf) refers to microscope lens.
hilum the recessed area of the kidney where the ureter and blood vessels enter.
hinge a type of joint.
Hippocratic oath refers to the oath taken by a doctor bonding him to observe the code of medical ethics contained in the oath by Hippocrates in the 4th century.
Hippocratic Oath A code of behavior that doctors are to follow.
histamine a substance normally present in the body.
histologist (histotechnologist) a person engaged in the study of the microscopic structure of tissue.
histology the study of cells.
histoplasmosis a fungal infection caused by an organism found in bird and bat droppings.
histotechnologist a laboratory specialist who prepares tissues for microscopic examination and diagnosis.
HL7 protocol Health Level Seven protocol, the standard for exchanging information between medical applications.
holistic considering the whole or entire scope of a situation.
Holter monitor a device that attaches electrodes to a patient's chest for the purpose of obtaining a 24-hour ECG tracing in an accessory tape recorder.
homeopathy a system of medical practice that treats a disease by the administration of minute doses of a remedy that would in healthy persons produce symptoms similar to those of the disease.
Homeopathy a 200-year-old system of medicine based on the Law of Similars. This means that if a dose of a substance can cause a symptom, that same substance in minuscule amounts can cure the symptom.
homeostasis maintenance of a constant or static condition of internal environment.
homosexual sexual attraction toward the same sex as oneself.
honesty the state of being truthful, trustworthy; genuine.
horizontal not vertical; flat and even; level; parallel to the plane of the horizon.
hormone a chemical substance secreted by an organ or gland.
hospice movement an organization dedicated to providing care with dignity people who are terminally ill.
Hospitalist work with patients admitted to the hospital. These individuals work in many different departments and reduce the load of hospital visits for the primary care provider and specialist.

hourly wage amount of wages paid to an employee per hour; a varying amount of income depending on hours worked
hostility unfriendliness, enmity.
human chorionic gonadotropin (hCG) a hormone produced in pregnancy that is made by the embryo soon after conception.
human immunodeficiency virus (HIV) a retrovirus that causes acquired immunodeficiency syndrome (AIDS), a condition in humans in which the immune system begins to fail, leading to life-threatening opportunistic infections.
human organism the collective higher individual resulting from the organization of cells, tissues, organs, and organ systems.
humble modest, unassuming.
humerus the long bone of the upper arm.
humor something that is designed to be amusing or comical.
humoral antibody-mediated immunity.
hyaline membrane disease a condition resulting from incomplete development of the respiratory system in premature infants.
hydrocele the accumulation of fluid in the scrotum.
hydrochloric acid a digestive juice found in the stomach.
hygiene the study of health and observance of health rules.
hygienist one who provides health-related services, such as dental procedures.
hymen a membranous fold partially or completely covering the vaginal opening.
hyperglycemia increase of blood sugar, as in diabetes.
hyperopia a defect of vision so that objects can only be seen when they are far away; farsightedness.
hypersensitive oversensitive; abnormally sensitive to a stimulus of any kind.
hypertension elevated blood pressure.
hyperthermia higher than normal temperature.
hyperthyroidism a condition caused by excessive secretion of the thyroid glands.
hypertonic having a higher concentration of salt than found in a red blood cell.
hyperventilation excessive deep and frequent breathing.
hyphen a punctuation mark used to divide or create compound words.
hypnosis a state that resembles sleep but is induced by suggestion.
hypoallergenic unlikely to cause an allergic reaction.
hypochondriac pertaining to the upper outer regions of the abdomen below the thorax; also someone with a morbid fear of disease, resulting in abnormal concern about one's health.
hypogastric referring to an abdominal area in the middle lower third of the abdomen.
hypoglycemia deficiency of sugar in the blood.
hypotension abnormally low blood pressure.
hypothalamus a structure of the brain between the cerebrum and the midbrain; lies below the thalamus.
hypothermia below normal body temperature.
hypothyroidism a condition caused by a marked deficiency of thyroid secretion.
hypotonic having a lower concentration of salt than found in a red blood cell.
hypoxia a lack of oxygen.
hysterectomy surgical removal of the uterus.
hysteroscopy a procedure using the hysteroscope to view the endometrium of the uterus.

ICD see **International Classification of Diseases.**
I & D see **incision and drainage.**
identification anything by which a person or thing can be identified.
idiopathic disease without recognizable cause.
idle uninvolved; doing nothing.
ileocecal the valve between the end of the small intestine and the cecum.
ileostomy a surgical opening from the ileum onto the abdominal wall.
ileum the last section of the small intestine.
iliac the edge or crest of the pelvic bone.
ilium the hip bone.
illegible impossible to read.
illicit improper; unlawful; not sanctioned by custom or law; illegal.
illuminating enlightening; throwing light on.
imaging a representation or visual impression produced by a lens, mirror, etc.
immobilize to keep out of action or circulation; stationary.
immune protected or exempt from a disease.
immunization becoming immune or the process of rendering a patient immune.
immunoassays a biochemical test that measures the level of a substance in a biologic liquid, typically serum or urine, using the reaction of an antibody or antibodies to its antigen.
immunodeficiency lacking the components necessary to mount an immune response.
immunoglobulin a large protein molecule that assists in the immune response.
immunologic pertaining to immunology.
immunology a broad branch of biomedical science that covers the study of all aspects of the immune system in all organisms.
immunosuppressed a condition wherein the immune system has been overpowered and cannot function adequately.
impacted refers to a fracture where the broken ends are jammed together.
impaction a collection of hardened feces in the rectum that cannot be expelled.
impending to be at hand or about to happen.
implant something implanted into tissue; a graft; artificial part.
implement a tool or instrument for doing something; to put into effect.
implementation put into effect.
implication involvement, bringing into connection.
implied hinted, suggested.
impotence inability of a male to obtain or maintain an erection.
impulse a charge transmitted through certain tissues, especially nerve fibers and muscles, resulting in physiologic activity.
inappropriate not appropriate, out of place.
incident report a report giving detailed information about an emergency situation and how it was handled.
incineration burn, setting afire.
incision cut.
incision and drainage (I & D) cutting into for the purpose of providing an exit for material, usually a collection of pus.
inclined leaning or tending toward.
income statement A statement that demonstrates the profit and expenses for a given month and also includes year-to-date information for a given year.
incompetent not capable; not legally qualified; deficient.
incomprehensible beyond belief, not to be grasped by the mind.
incongruous lacking harmony or agreement.
incontinent unable to control the bladder or bowel.
increments becoming greater; amount of increase; gain.
incubation the interval between exposure to infection and the appearance of the first symptom.
incus the anvil, the middle bone of the three in the middle ear.
indemnity to compensate for damage done or loss caused.
independent practice association (IPA) An association of independent physicians, or other organization that contracts with independent physicians, and provides services to managed care organizations on a negotiated per capita rate, flat retainer fee, or negotiated fee-for-service basis.
indexing A system of cross-referencing information contained in office files so that the data may be searched using different characteristics as the query term.
Indication The intended purpose or reason for using a particular medication.

indigent needy, poor, destitute.
indigestion difficulty in digesting food.
induction the process of causing or producing; to bring on.
inevitable unavoidable, destined to occur.
infarction infiltration of foreign particles; material in a vessel causing coagulation and interference with circulation.
infectious capable of producing infection; denoting a disease in the body caused by the presence of germs; tending to spread to others.
infectious mononucleosis a disease seen most commonly in adolescents and young adults, characterized by fever, sore throat, leg and muscle soreness and fatigue (symptoms of a common cold or allergies). Mononucleosis is caused by the Epstein-Barr virus (EBV).
inferior below, under.
inferior vena cava the large vein that carries deoxygenated blood from the lower half of the body into the heart.
infertility inability to achieve conception.
infirmity illness, disease.
inflict to strike, to cause punishment.
influenza an acute illness characterized by fever, pain, coughing, and general upper respiratory symptoms.
informed consent agreement to do something or to allow something to happen only after all the relevant facts are known.
infrared pertaining to those invisible rays just beyond the red end of the visible spectrum that have a penetrating heating effect.
infusion to instill; introduction of a substance into a vein.
ingested to eat.
inguinal referring to the region where the thigh joins the trunk of the body; the groin.
inguinal canal a passageway in the groin for the spermatic cord in the male.
inguinal hernia the presence of small intestine in the inguinal canal.
inhale to breathe in.
initial the first; beginning; the first letter of each of a person's names.
initiate to get something started, begin.
initiative the action of taking the first step; ability to originate new ideas.
innate inborn; inherent.
innate characteristics that are inherent or natural, while others must be learned.
inoculating loop a laboratory instrument used to transfer organisms from one source to another.
inorganic not living; occurring in nature independently of living things.
inseminate to impregnate with semen.
insertion the place where a muscle is attached to the bone that it moves.
insidious hidden, not apparent.
insignificant unimportant; petty; of little or no value.
insomnia abnormal inability to sleep.
inspect to examine closely.
inspection the first part of a physical examination; close observation.
inspiration to breathe in, inhale.
instill to slowly drop liquid onto a surface or into a cavity.
institute to originate as a custom.
insufficient not as much as needed.
insulin a hormone secreted by the islets of langerhans in the pancreas.
insulin shock a condition of excess insulin or lack of blood sugar.
insurance a contract to guarantee compensation for a specified situation.
intact unbroken, undamaged.
intangible that which cannot be touched, easily defined, or grasped.
integrity soundness of character; honesty in particular.
integumentary the skin; a covering.
integumentary system the largest organ system by surface area, comprising skin, hair, nails, and sweat glands and their products (sweat and mucus). It distinguishes, separates, and protects. the name derives from the latin *integumentum*, which means "a covering."
intellectualization to employ reasoning to avoid confrontations or stressful situations.
intelligence the ability to learn or understand.
interaction to act upon one another.
intercede to mediate, plead on behalf of another.
intercostal between the ribs.
interference confusion of desired signals caused by undesired signals, as in artifacts on an ECG.
interferon a lymphokine that helps regulate the activities of macrophages and natural killer cells.
interjection a part of speech; an exclamation.
interleukin a substance that is a messenger between leukocytes.
intermediate in the middle.
intermittent stopping and starting again at intervals.
intermuscular within the muscle.
internal the innermost part(s) of the body.
internal revenue service the division of federal government charged with implementing tax laws and collecting taxes.
International Classification of Diseases (ICD) a comprehensive listing of diseases and disorders of the human body.
interneurons neurons connecting sensory to motor neurons.
internist a physician specializing in the care of patients with internal diseases.
internship a time following graduation wherein practice of the profession is performed.
interpersonal between persons.
interpret to explain, translate; to determine the meaning.
interpretive computerized analysis of ECG tracings.
interval time between events; space. On an ECG, the period that includes one segment and one or more waves ie: P-R interval.
intervention taking action to modify, hinder, or change an effect.
interventional hysterosalpingography a diagnostic examination to evaluate the fallopian tubes.
intervertebral between the vertebrae.
interview a meeting between two people where one asks questions of the other.
intestine the alimentary canal extending from the pylorus of the stomach to the anus.
intimidate to make afraid, to frighten.
intimidation to make afraid; to deter with threats.
intolerance an adverse effect of a medication that is not related to an immune response.
intoxicated a condition caused by the overindulgence in alcoholic beverages.
intracellular within the cell.
intracellular leukemia should not be a key term (only *leukemia* should be a key term)
intradermal within the skin.
intramuscular (IM) type of injection administered into a muscle.
intraocular within the eyeball.
intrauterine device (IUD) an object inserted into the uterus to prevent pregnancy.
intravenous to insert into the vein.
intravenous pyelography (IVP) the insertion of a radio-paque material into the vein for the purpose of x-raying the kidneys and ureters.
intricate complicated, complex, elaborately interwoven.
intrinsic belonging to one's self inherently; motivation coming from within an individual
intubation insertion of a tube into the larynx for entrance of air.
intuition the immediate knowing or learning of something without the conscious use of reasoning.
inunction the process of administering drugs through the skin.
invasive (procedure) diagnostic methods involving entry into living tissue.
inventory an itemized list of goods in stock.
inversion the movement of the sole of the foot toward the median plane.
in vivo that which takes place inside an organism.
invoice a document that includes itemization of goods and purchases or services provided together with the charges and terms of the agreement.
involuntary independent of or even contrary to will or choice.

iodine a nonmetallic element belonging to the halogen group.
ipecac an emetic; causes vomiting.
iris the colored, contractible tissue surrounding the pupil of the eye.
irrational lacking the power to reason; senseless.
irreconcilable cannot be brought into agreement.
irrelevant not pertinent, not to the point.
irreparable damaged beyond possibility of repair.
irrigate to wash out with a liquid.
ischemia temporary and localized anemia caused by obstruction of the circulation to a part.
ischium posterior and inferior portion of the hip bone.
ishihara refers to an eye test to determine color vision.
islets of langerhans clusters of cells in the pancreas.
isotonic having the same concentration of salt as found in a red blood cell.
issue to send forth; to put into circulation.
IVP see **intravenous pyelography.**

Jaeger a system for measuring near vision acuity.
Jaeger chart an eye chart is used for reading up close and for determining near vision.
jaundice a yellowish discoloration of the sclera and skin due to the presence of bile pigments in the blood.
jejunum the middle segment of the small intestine, which measures approximately 8 feet in length.
jeopardize to put at risk.
job description a combination of skills and behaviors expected of an employee; effectively fulfill the responsibilities in a designated work position.
joint commission refers to the agency that has oversight for hospitals adhering to regulations that allow them to bill for medicare reimbursement for medical services provided
journal a record of happenings; a diary.
journalizing entries on the daily log.
judgment a decision; ability to make the right decisions.
jurisdiction the authority given by law to a court to try cases and rule on legal matters within a particular geographic area and/or over certain types of legal cases.

keloid an overgrowth of new skin tissue; a scar.
ketone (acetone) products of metabolism generated from carbohydrates, fatty acids, and amino acids in humans.
key components the major factors to be considered when selecting an evaluation and management code: history, exam, medical decision making.
keying pressing a lever or button, as on a typewriter, with the finger to operate the machine.
kidney a bean-shaped organ that excretes urine and is located retroperitoneally, high in the back of the abdominal cavity.
knee-chest body position in which the patient kneels on the exam table with buttocks elevated, back straight, and chest resting on the table
knowledge base a term used to describe the theoretical portion of an educational program.
KUB kidneys, ureters, and bladder; refers to a radiologic study.
kyphosis a convex curvature of the spine; humpback.

L & A light and accommodation.
labia majora the two large folds of adipose tissue lying on each side of the vulva of the female; external genitalia.
labia minora the two mucocutaneous folds of membrane within the labia majora.
laboratory technician a health care worker who performs specialized chemical, microscopic, and bacteriologic tests of blood, tissue, and body fluids.
laboratory a room or building in which scientific tests or experiments are conducted.
laceration a cut or tear.
lacrimal pertaining to tears; the glands and ducts that secrete and convey tears.
Lamaze a program or method of managing labor during birth.
laminectomy the removal of a portion of the vertebral posterior arch.
lancet a sharp, pointed instrument used to pierce the skin to obtain a capillary blood sample.
laryngeal pertaining to the larynx.
laryngectomy surgical removal of the larynx or voice box.
laryngitis inflammation of the vocal cords.
larynx the voice box.
lateral pertaining to the side.
latissimus dorsi the large muscle of the back.
lavage the washing out of a cavity.
laxative a substance that induces the bowels to empty.
ledgers the principal account books of a business establishment, containing the credits and debits.
legible easy to read, readable.
legislating the act of exercising the power and function of making laws that have the force of authority by virtue of their origin by a state legislature or US Congress.
legionnaires' disease an acute bronchopneumonia.
leisure spare or free time, away from the pressure and responsibilities of work.
lens a part of the eye that bends or refracts images onto the retina.
lesion an injury or wound; a circumscribed area of pathologically altered tissue.
lethal deadly; capable of causing death.
lethargic sluggishness, apathy.
leukemia a disease characterized by a great excess of white blood cells; it exists in a lymphatic and myelogenous form; it is often fatal, especially in adults.
leukocyte a white blood cell.
leukocyte esterase a urine test for the presence of white blood cells and other abnormalities associated with infection.
liability anything to which a person is liable, responsible, legally bound.
liaison intercommunication between two entities.
license a legal permit to engage in an activity.
licensed practical nurse (LPN) an individual trained in basic nursing techniques, to provide direct patient care under the supervision of an RN or physician.
life-threatening used to describe diseases or conditions where the likelihood of death is high
ligament fibrous tissue that connects bone to bone.
ligation to tie off; the process of binding or tying.
limbs refers to the arms and legs.
limited to restrict; to hold within fixed bounds.
limited check a check that will be marked void if written for more than a certain amount. This type of check is often used for payroll or insurance payments.
listlessness lack of desire, interest.
liter a unit of measure; 1,000 mL or approximately 1 quart.
lithotomy an examination position wherein the patient lies upon the back with thighs flexed upon the abdomen and legs flexed upon the thighs.
lithotripsy destruction of stone; stonecrusher.
liver the largest gland in the body, located in the upper right quadrant of the abdomen beneath the diaphragm.
living will advance directive; a document, written in advance, that states the patient's wishes regarding end-of-life care.
LMP last menstrual period.
longevity a long duration of life; lasting a long time.
longitudinal fissure the deep cleft between the two hemispheres of the cerebrum.
lordosis abnormal anterior curvature of the lumbar spine.
low-power field (lpf) refers to microscope lens.
lubb dupp sounds made by the heart.
lumbar pertaining to the back, specifically to the five vertebrae above the sacrum.

lumbar puncture the insertion of a needle between the vertebrae in the lumbar area for the purpose of withdrawing spinal fluid.
lumen the space within an artery, vein, or capillary; the space within a tube.
lung the organ of respiration, located within the thoracic cavity.
lupus erythematosus a chronic autoimmune disease that causes changes in the immune system.
luteinizing a hormone effect that causes ovulation and progesterone in the female and sperm production and testosterone in the male.
lyme disease a disease caused by a spirochete that is carried by the deer tick.
lymph a body fluid formed within the tissue spaces and circulated throughout the body.
lymphatic system a network of transparent vessels carrying lymph fluid throughout the body.
lymphedema excess lymph fluid in the tissues.
lymphocyte a type of white blood cell.
lymphokine a cytokine produced by a T-cell.
lymphokine leukemia should not be a key term (only *leukemia* should be a key term)
lymphoma a tumor of the lymphatic tissue. NOTE: This is a new word to be inserted into the Words to Know and added to the glossary.
lysosomes an organelle within the cytoplasm of the cell.

macrophage a phagocytic cell that destroys antigens.
macule a discolored spot or patch on the skin neither elevated nor depressed.
magnet therapy a therapy which involves placing small magnets close to the skin in order to correct an imbalance.
magnetic having the properties of a magnet, able to attract.
magnetic resonance imaging (MRI) a diagnostic test using magnetic waves to visualize internal body structures.
magnify to make something look larger than it really is.
mailable a standard for judging written correspondence as satisfactory for sending.
maintenance to preserve; the act or work of keeping something in proper condition.
malaise a feeling of discomfort or uneasiness.
malignant a cancerous growth; tumor.
malinger to pretend illness to escape dealing with a situation or obligation.
malleus the largest of the three bones of the middle ear, also called the hammer.
malnutrition lack of necessary or proper food substances in the body.
mammary glands the breasts.
mammogram an x-ray of the breast.
mammography the process of using low-dose x-rays to examine the human breast. It is used to look for different types of tumors and cysts.
management the act, manner, or practice of managing, handling, or controlling something.
managerial accounting the study and analysis of financial data as it applies to operational issues within a company. also known as cost accounting.
mandate an order of authorative command; instruction.
manifestation act of disclosing; revelation; display.
manipulation the passive movement of a joint to determine the range of flexion and extension.
manipulation therapy any treatment or procedure involving the use of the hands; additional manual skills used by osteopathic physicians.
marginal close to the lower limit of acceptability.
marrow the soft tissue in the hollow of long bones.
massage manipulation of tissues for therapeutic purposes by rubbing, kneading, or tapping with the hands.
masses a multitude; a large number of people.
mastectomy surgical removal of a breast.
master refers to a reference document used to compare other similar documents or values to, as in a master patient list, or an original document saved to a file which can be copied or modified as needed.
materials safety data sheet (MSDS) printed materials that come with hazardous chemicals that provide basic information to the safety and health of the user.
matrix a format for establishing a time schedule for appointments.
maturation index (MI) a measurement of cellular maturity.
maturation refers to a stage of cellular development.
maturity a state of full development.
meaningful use with reference to healthcare records, this term is used by government agencies to refer to the way in which medical record information is employed in order to provide a means for improving patient care and patient outcomes through evaluating treatment patterns and verifying necessity of medical procedures performed.
means the average which is derived by adding up all the values of a given series and dividing by the number of values.
measles a highly contagious disease characterized by the presence of maculopustular eruptions.
mechanical pertaining to machinery.
medial pertaining to the middle or midline.
medicaid a government health care program.
medical assistant an integral member of the health care delivery team, qualified by education and experience to work in the administrative office, the examining room and the physician office laboratory.
medical emergency an injury or illness that is acute and poses an immediate risk to a person's life or long-term health
medical malpractice an act or continuing conduct of a physician or hospital that does not meet the standard of professional competence and results in provable damages to the patient.
medical necessity services or supplies that are needed for the diagnosis or treatment of your medical condition and meet accepted standards of medical practice.
medication order instructions written by a licensed provider for administration of a medication to a patient
medicare a federal health program for paying certain medical expenses of the aged.
medigap refers to situations not covered by medicare insurance.
medulla the inner section of the kidney.
medulla oblongata enlarged portion of the spinal cord; the lower portion of the brainstem.
melanin a pigment that gives color to the skin, hair, and eyes.
melanocytes cells that produce the pigment of the skin, melanin.
membrane a thin, soft, pliable layer of tissue that lines a tube or cavity or covers an organ or structure.
menarche the first menstrual period.
meniere's disease a disorder of the ear characterized by nausea, vomiting, tinnitus, and hearing loss.
meninges the membranes covering the brain and spinal cord.
meningitis inflammation of the meninges of the brain and/or spinal cord.
meniscus a concave level of fluid in a tube or cylinder.
menopause the permanent cessation of menstruation.
menorrhagia excessive menstrual flow, hemorrhage.
menstruation periodic discharge of bloody fluid from the uterus.
mensuration the process of measuring.
mercury a liquid metal used in measurement devices such as thermometers and sphygmomanometers; chemical symbol, Hg.
merit to deserve reward or praise; excellence.
mesentery a peritoneal fold connecting the intestine to the posterior abdominal wall.

metabolism the successive transformations to which a substance is subjected from the time it enters the body to the time it or its decomposition products are excreted, and by which nutrition is accomplished and energy and living substance are provided.
metabolized the successive transformation of a substance from the time it enters the body to the time it or its decomposition products are excreted, and by which nutrition is accomplished and energy and living substance are provided.
metacarpal pertaining to the five bones of the hand between the wrist and the phalanges.
metastasis movement of cancer cells from one part of the body to another.
metastasize the process whereby malignant cells leave the primary lesion and migrate to another location.
metatarsal the five bones of the feet between the instep and the phalanges.
methodical systematic, following a plan or method.
metric system a system of measurements that uses the base function of ten.
MI see **myocardial infarction.**
microbes organisms that are microscopic (too small to be visible to the human eye).
microbial related to microbes.
microfiche a sheet of microfilm capable of accommodating and preserving a considerable number of book pages in reduced form.
microfilming using a machine to put copies of written data such as a patient file into a smaller, storable format.
microhematocrit packed cell volume (PCV) that measures the proportion of blood volume that is occupied by red blood cells.
microorganism a microscopic living body not perceivable by the naked eye.
microscopic visible only with a microscope.
microscopic anatomy an area of study that deals with features that can be seen only with a microscope.
micturtion the passing of urine.
midbrain that portion of the brain connecting the pons and the cerebellum.
midlevel practitioner healthcare providers such as a nurse practitioner or physician's assistant. they are able to examine patients, order diagnostic tests and prescribe certain types of medications. activities for midlevel practitioners are usually directed and/or dictated by a supervising physician.
midline the middle.
midsagittal an imaginary vertical plane made by dividing the body down the middle, creating equal right and left sides; also known as the midline.
migraine a severe headache with characteristic symptoms.
mineralocorticoid a biologic principle of the adrenal cortex involved in regulating body fluid and electrolytes.
minute a measurement of time equal to 60 seconds; very small, tiny.
misalignment out of alignment; not straight.
misdemeanor a lesser crime than a felony, punishable by a fine and/or county jail time for up to one year.
misspelled to spell incorrectly.
mitochondria an organelle within the cytoplasm of the cell.
mitosis the division of a cell.
mitral the valve in the heart between the chambers of the left side, also known as the bicuspid.
mobile banking a banking method that allows the bank customer to perform banking actions on his or her cell phone or other mobile device.
mobility quality of being mobile; easy to move.
modifier changes; limits the meaning.
modifies changes the form or quality of; alters slightly.
molten melted.
monilia a family of parasitic fungi or molds.
moniliasis an infection of the mucous membranes by yeastlike fungi.
monitor to oversee or observe.
monoclonal a laboratory-produced hybrid cell that produces antibodies.
monocular possessing a single eyepiece, as with a microscope.
monocyte single nucleated cells that leave the blood and enter into tissues to become macrophages.
monogamous an exclusive relationship between two people.
monokine a cytokine produced by macrophages or monocytes.
monotone a single, unvaried tone; having the same pitch; a tiresome sameness.
mons pubis a pad of fatty tissue and coarse skin overlying the symphysis pubis in the female.
moral a principle of right and wrong in conduct.
moral pertaining to distinction of "right" and "wrong"
morality right living; virtue.
mores folkways that, through general observance, develop the force of a law.
morphology a branch of biology dealing with the form and structure of organisms.
motor refers to the nerves that permit the body to respond to stimuli.
mouth the oral cavity; can also refer to the opening to organs.
MRI see **magnetic resonance imaging.**
mucosa pertaining to mucous membrane.
MUGA see **multiple-gated acquisition scan.**
multi-provider clinic group practices, which consists of three or more physicians who share a facility for the purpose of practicing medicine.
multi-skilled having more than one skill area for employment.
multichannel refers to the capability of ECG equipment of processing impulses from multiple leads.
multiple-gated acquisition scan (MUGA) a diagnostic test to evaluate the condition of the myocardium of the heart.
mumps an acute contagious disease characterized by inflammation of the parotid gland and other salivary glands.
murmur a soft blowing or rasping sound heard on auscultation of the heart.
muscle team a pair of skeletal muscles, one that flexes and one that extends the joint.
muscle tone a state of muscle contraction in which a portion of the fibers are contracted while others are at rest.
muscle a type of tissue composed of contractile cells or fibers that effect movement of the body.
muscular pertaining to muscles.
musculoskeletal pertaining to the muscular and skeletal systems.
mutation a change in an inheritable characteristic; cellular change caused by an influence.
myelin a fatlike substance forming the principal component of the myelin sheath of nerve fibers.
myelography an x-ray examination of the spinal cord following an injection of a radiopaque material.
myocardial infarction (MI) blockage of a coronary artery that interrupts the flow of blood to the heart muscle.
myocardium the muscle layer of the heart.
myometrium the muscular structure of the uterus.
myopia a defect in vision so that objects can only be seen when very near; nearsightedness.
myxedema a condition resulting from the hypofunction of the thyroid gland.

nagel's rule a method of predicting the anticipated date of delivery when pregnant.
narcolepsy overwhelming attacks of sleep that the victim cannot inhibit; sleeping sickness.
narcotic a drug capable of producing sleep and relieving pain or inducing unconsciousness and even death, depending upon the dosage.
nasal pertaining to the nose.
nasal speculum an instrument permitting visualization of the inside of the nasal cavity.

national center for competency testing a national certifying organization which certifies medical assistants and other healthcare professionals after successful completion of a certification exam.
National Certified Medical Assistant (NCMA) the credential given by the National Center for Competency testing to successful candidates that pass the NCMA exam.
National Certified Medical Office Assistant (NCMOA) the credential given by the National Center for Competency testing to successful candidates that pass the NCMOA exam.
National Healthcare Association NHA provides products and services to health care professionals, including continuing education, program development, career and networking services, as well as 10 certification exams for several allied health care area, including Certified Clinical Medical Assistant (CCMA) (and Certified Medical Administrative Assistant (CMAA).
National Provider Identifier (NPI) the name of the standard unique health identifier for health care providers
naturopathy a multidisciplinary approach to health care based on the belief that the body has the power to heal itself.
naturopathy a multidisciplinary approach to health care based on the belief that the body has power to heal itself. Treatment is based on assessment of the correct diet, rest, relaxation, exercise, fresh air, clean water, and sunlight the patient is receiving.
nausea an inclination to vomit.
needle holder instrument used to hold a suture needle during the suturing process.
needlesticks unintentional injury that occurs in the course of handling injection materials used for medication administration
negate to deny the existence or truth of.
neglect to ignore or pay no attention to; to leave uncared for.
negligent guilty of neglect; lacking in due care or concern; act of carelessness.
negotiable capable of being discussed and terms arranged.
neoadjuvant new attachment process; giving chemotherapy prior to surgery to shrink the tumor before removal.
neonate a newborn infant.
neoplasm a new growth.
neoplastic new abnormal tissue formation; cancer-related.
nephrologist a physician specializing in the diseases and disorders of the kidney.
nephrology the study of the kidney and its diseases.
nephron the structural and functional unit of the kidney.
nephrotic syndrome term applied to renal disease of whatever cause characterized by massive edema, proteinuria, and usually elevation of serum cholesterol and lipids.
nerve a group of nervous tissues bound together for the purpose of conducting nervous impulses.
nervosa loss of appetite for food not connected with a disease; part of a psychosis.
net remaining after all deductions have been made; to clear as profit.
net worth assets minus liabilities, that demonstrates the value of a business.
neurilemma a thin membranous sheath enveloping a nerve fiber.
neurologist a physician specializing in the diseases and disorders of the nervous system.
neurology the study of the nervous system and its diseases.
neuron a nerve cell.
neurosurgery surgical procedures performed on the nervous system.
neutrophil a granulated white blood cell.
nicotine a poisonous alkaloid extracted from tobacco leaves.
nit the egg of a louse or other parasitic insect.
nitrite a urine test that is positive in urinary tract infections from the presence of bacteria reducing nitrates to nitrite.
nocturia having to void at night.
node a knot, knob, protuberance, or swelling.
nomenclature a system of technical or scientific names.
nominal too small to be considered, or a very small amount.
nomogram representation by graphs, diagrams, or charts of the relationship between numerical variables.
non compos mentis general legal term for all forms of mental illness.
nonchalant unconcerned, indifferent.
noninvasive procedurer a diagnostic method not requiring entry into body tissue.
nonpathogen an organism that does not produce a disease.
nonspecific urethritis inflammation of the urethra in males and vaginitis or cervicitis in females caused by bacteria or an allergy to substances used by a sexual partner.
norepinephrine a hormone secreted by adrenal medulla in response to sympathetic stimulation.
normal saline a solution with the same salt content as that found within a red blood cell.
no show term used to describe a visit in which a patient fails to present for examination without giving the provider advance notice.
noun the name of anything, such as a person, place, object, occurrence, or state.
NREM (non-rapid eye movement) a stage of sleep in which the sleeper does not experience rapid eye movement. In a healthy young adult, NREM sleep usually accounts for 75%–90% of sleep time.
nuclear pertaining to the nucleus of an atom.
nuclear medicine the branch of medicine that uses radionuclides in the diagnosis and treatment of disease.
nuclear medicine technologist an individual trained in the specialized field of operating cameras that detect and map the radioactive drug in a patient's body to create diagnostic images.
nucleolus a structure found within the nucleus of the cell.
nucleus the vital body in the protoplasm of a cell.
numerator the top number of a fraction.
numeric denoting a number or system of numbers.
nurse anesthetist is an RN that is certified to administer anesthesia.
nurse assistant (NA) a person trained to assist nurses and attend to patients.
nurse midwife a nurse trained in the delivery of babies.
nurse midwife a professional RN who has had extensive training and experience in labor and delivery.
nurse practitioner a midlevel practitioner that is able to examine patients, order diagnostic tests and prescribe certain types of medications. Usually supervised by a physician but may work independently in some states.
nurse practitioner an RN with advanced clinical experience and education in a special branch of practice.
nurture to care for, train, or educate.
nutrition refers to edible material, food, things that nourish.
nutritionist a member of the health care team who studies and applies the principles and science of nutrition.

obese weighing more than 30% of ideal body weight.
objective the end toward which action is directed; of a disease symptom, perceptible to persons other than the one affected; on a microscope, a lens or series of lenses.
obligate to bind legally or morally.
obligation responsibility; a moral, social, or legal tie.
obliterate to blot out; leave no trace; destroy.
observant quick to notice, watchful.
obsolete out of use, discarded, no longer useful.
obstetrician a physician who specializes in the care and treatment of women during pregnancy and childbirth.

obstetrics the branch of medicine dealing with women during pregnancy, childbirth, and postpartum.
obstructed blocked.
obturator anything that obstructs or closes a cavity or opening; refers to that internal portion of an examining instrument that facilitates the introduction of the instrument into the body and is then withdrawn, permitting visualization of the internal area.
occipital pertaining to the back part of the head, the posterior lobe of the cerebrum.
occlude to close up, obstruct.
occluder a device to block viewing when conducting an eye examination.
occult obscure; hidden.
occulta obscure; hidden.
occupational medicine diagnosing and treating disease or conditions arising from occupational circumstances.
Occupational Safety and Health Administration (OSHA) an agency of the United States Department of Labor. It was created by Congress under the Occupational Safety and Health Act, signed by President Richard M. Nixon, on December 29, 1970. Its mission is to prevent work-related injuries, illnesses, and deaths by issuing and enforcing rules (called standards) for workplace safety and health.
occupational therapist (OT) a health care worker involved in the use of purposeful activity with individuals who are limited by physical injury or illness, psychosocial dysfunction, developmental or learning diabilities, poverty and cultural differences, or the aging process to maximize independence, prevent disability, and maintain health.
occupational therapy assistant (OTA) a person trained to assist an occupational therapist.
Ocular (1) eyepiece of a microscope; (2) Pertaining to the eye
O.D. oculus dexter, or right eye.
Offer a specific proposal to enter into an agreement with another; an offer is an essential component of an enforceable contract.
office manager (business office manager) an individual responsible for the overall operation of the medical office.
ointment a salve; a fatty, soft substance having antiseptic or healing properties.
olfactory pertaining to the sense of smell.
oliguria scanty production of urine.
oncogenes a gene in a tumor cell.
oncologist a doctor who has been specially trained in the study of tumors and cancer.
oncology the branch of medicine dealing with tumors, usually malignant.
online banking The practice of making bank transactions or paying bills electronically via the Internet.
on-site at the location.
operating information the information that is needed on a day-to-day basis in order for a company to conduct business.
ophthalmic pertaining to the eye.
ophthalmic technician (OT) an individual trained for assisting ophthalmologists with patients as well as procedures associated with the eyes.
ophthalmologist a physician specializing in the diseases and disorders of the eye.
ophthalmology the study of the eye and its diseases.
opportunistic seizing the opportunity; taking advantage of the situation.
opposition action against, resistance.
optic pertaining to the eye or sight.
optic disc the blind spot where the optic nerve exits from the retina of the eye.
optometrist a person who measures the eye's refractive power and prescribes correction of visual defects when needed.
oral pertaining to the mouth.
orbital refers to the cavity within the skull where the eye is located.
organ a part of the body constructed of many types of tissue to perform a function.
organ of Corti terminal acoustic apparatus in the cochlea of the inner ear.
organelles functional structures within the cytoplasm of a cell.
organic pertaining to or derived from animal or vegetable forms of life.
organizational ethics the standards by which an organization will hold itself accountable to proper conduct
origin the beginning or source of anything; of muscles, the anchor.
orthopedics the branch of medicine dealing with the structure and function of bones and muscles.
orthopedist a physician who corrects deformities and treats diseases and disorders of the bones, joints, and spine.
orthopnea respiratory condition in which breathing is possible only in an erect sitting or standing position.
orthostatic standing; concerning an erect position.
O.S. oculus sinister, or left eye.
os pertains to a mouth or opening.
oscilloscope an instrument that displays a visual representation of electric variations on the fluorescent screen of a cathode ray tube.
OSHA U.S. Occupational Safety and Health Administration.
osmosis the process of diffusion of water or another solvent through a selected permeable membrane.
osseous bonelike, concerning bones.
osteopathy any bone disease; also refers to a school of medicine based on the belief that the bony fragment of the body largely determines the structural relations of its tissues.
osteoporosis a condition resulting from a decrease in the amount of calcium stored in the bone.
OTA see **occupational therapy assistant.**
OTC see **over the counter.**
otic pertaining to the ear.
otitis inflammation of the ear; can be referenced to the external, middle, or internal ear.
otorhinolaryngologist a physician specializing in diseases and disorders of the ear, nose, and throat.
otorhinolaryngology the study of the ear, nose, and larynx and their diseases.
otosclerosis condition characterized by progressive deafness caused by the fixation of the stapes of the middle ear.
outsourcing an arrangement by which a task, operation, or job that could be performed by employees within a company is instead contracted to another company.
O.U. oculus uterque, or each eye.
ovary the female gonad, which produces hormones causing the secondary sex characteristics to develop and be maintained.
over-the-counter (OTC) referring to accessible, nonprescription drugs.
overdraft an amount beyond what is currently in the account.
ovulation the periodic ripening and rupture of a mature graafian follicle and the discharge of the ovum.
ovum an egg, the female gamete or reproductive cell.
oxalate a salt of oxalic acid.
oxygen a colorless, odorless, tasteless gas found in the air; chemical symbol, O_2.
oxygenate combine or supply with oxygen.

pacemaker the SA node of the heart; also refers to an artificial device that initiates heartbeat.
pallor lack of color, paleness.
palpate to feel; to examine by touch.
palpation the technique of examination using the fingers or hands.
pancreas an organ that secretes insulin and pancreatic digestive juice.
pancreatitis inflammation of the pancreas.
pandemic epidemic over a large region; epidemic in many regions.
panic value an important indicator on a lab test that indicates immediate notification of the health care provider.
pantomime motions or gestures used for expressive communication.
papanicolaou (Pap) smear a test to detect cancer cells in the mucus of an organ.
papillae small protuberances or elevations, such as the taste buds of the tongue.
papillary muscles muscular attachments to the undersides of the heart valves from the walls of the ventricles, which open the valves during the relaxation phase of the heartbeat.

papule red, elevated area on the skin.
parabasal beside, near, an accessory to the base or lower part.
paralytic ileus paralysis of the intestinal wall with symptoms of acute obstruction.
paramedic health care providers who provide emergency and supportive medical care; have additional training beyond EMT status.
parameter quantity to which an arbitrary value may be given as a convenience in expressing performance or for use in calculations.
parasite an organism that lives in or on another organism without rendering it any service in return.
parasympathetic a division of the autonomic nervous system.
parathyroid small endocrine glands located close to the thyroid gland.
parenteral other than by mouth.
parietal a central portion of the cerebrum located on each side of the brain.
paroxysmal a sudden attack of a disease; fit of acute pain, passion, coughing, or laughter.
paroxysmal stage occurring repeatedly; recurrent symptoms.
partnership two or more physicians that have a legal agreement to share in the total business operation of the practice.
patella the kneecap.
pathogen any microorganism or substance capable of producing a disease.
pathologic a condition caused by a disease.
pathologist a physician specializing in the interpretation and diagnosis of changes caused by disease in tissues and body fluids.
pathology the study of the nature and cause of disease.
pathophysiology the study of mechanisms by which disease occurs, the responses of the body to the disease process, and the effects of both on normal function.
patience calm in waiting, endurance without complaint.
patient care technician (PCT) a health care worker who uses both nursing and medical assisting skills to provide patient care in a hospital setting.
patient centered medical homes a team-based model of care led by a personal physician who provides continuous and coordinated care throughout a patient's lifetime to maximize health outcomes.
patient education Information, instructions and cautions provided to a patient intended to ensure and advance his or her safety, health and/or recovery from injury or illness.
patient portal a component of an Electronic Health Records (EHR) system that allows patients to communicate with their medical office electronically, to request lab results, referrals, appointments, and in some instances communicate with doctors via email.
Patient Protection and Affordability Act a bill passed in 2010 intended to expand access to health insurance, provide additional consumer protections and reduce costs of health care.
patronize to treat condescendingly.
payee a person to whom money is paid.
PCT see **patient care technician**.
PDR *Physician's Desk Reference*.
peak flow the maximum rate of air flow out of the lungs during forced expiration; used especially for monitoring lung capacity of individuals with asthma.
pectoralis major the principal muscle of the chest wall.
pediatric the branch of medicine dealing with the care of children and their diseases.
pediatrician a physician specializing in the diseases and disorders of children.
pediatrics the branch of medicine dealing with the care of children and their diseases.
pediculosis the scientific name for lice.
peer equal; usually refers to someone of similar standing or status.
peer review assessment by other physicians or scientists in the same field.
pelvic pertaining to the pelvis.
penis the male external sex organ.
peptic pertaining to digestion; can also refer to an ulcer of the upper digestive tract.
per capita for each person.
perceive to become aware of through the senses; to understand.
percentage rate or proportion of each hundred.
percentage rate or proportion of each hundred.
percentile any value in a series dividing the distribution of its members into 100 groups of equal frequency.
perception awareness through the senses; the receipt of impressions; consciousness.
percussion tapping the body lightly but sharply to determine the position, size, and consistency of an underlying structure.
percussion hammer a hard, rubber-surfaced instrument used to test tendon reflex action.
performance to execute an undertaking; an action; success in working.
performance objectives statements on a resume which identify a person's specific knowledge, skills, or behaviors
perfusion passing of a fluid through spaces; the act of pouring over or through.
pericarditis inflammation of the pericardium, the covering of the heart.
pericardium the membranous sac that covers the heart.
perineum the region between the vagina and anus of the female and the scrotum and anus of the male.
periodic occurring, appearing, or done again and again, at regular intervals.
periodical appearing at regular intervals of time.
periosteum the fibrous membrane covering the bone except at the articulating surfaces.
peripheral pertaining to a portion of the nervous system; an item attached to a computer system.
peristalsis a progressive, wavelike muscular movement that occurs involuntarily in the urinary and digestive system.
peritoneal pertaining to the peritoneum.
peritoneum the membrane that lines the abdominal cavity and covers the abdominal organs.
permeable capable of being penetrated; allowing entrance.
pernicious anemia a severe anemia characterized by progressive decrease in the production of red blood cells.
perplexing troubling with doubt, puzzling.
PERRLA an acronym meaning pupils equal, regular, react to light and accommodation.
persecute treat badly; do harm to again and again; pursue to injure.
perserverance the act of continuing steadfastly, especially in the face of discouragement.
personal protective equipment (PPE) protective clothing, goggles, or gloves designed to protect the wearer's body or clothing from contamination by blood or other potentially infectious materials for job-related occupational safety and health purposes.
personality the personal or individual qualities that make one person different from another.
perspective a view of things, or facts, in which they are in the right relations.
pertinent having to do with what is being considered; relevant or to the point.
pertussis an acute infectious disease characterized by a paroxysmal cough, ending in a whooping inspiration.
petechiae small, purplish, hemorrhagic spots on the skin.
petition a written plea in which specific court action is sought.
petty small, having little value, mean, narrow-minded.
petty cash a small amount of cash available for small business expenses used for postage stamps, inexpensive office supplies, and small charitable donations, usually maintained in a locked container.
pH a measure of acidity or alkalinity.
phagocyte a white blood cell that engulfs and destroys antigens.

phagocytosis ingestion and digestion of bacteria and particles by phagocytes.
phalanges bones of the fingers and toes.
phalanx any one of the bones of the fingers or toes.
phantom limb an illusion following amputation of a limb that the limb still exists.
pharmaceutical concerning drugs or pharmacy.
pharmacist (RPH) a licensed health care provider who prepares and dispenses drugs.
pharmacology the study and practice of compounding and dispensing medical preparations.
pharmacy technician (PT) an assistant to a pharmacist who prepares and in some situations administers medication.
pharynx the throat; that portion of the alimentary canal between the mouth and the esophagus.
phenylalanine an amino acid of a protein.
phenylketonuria (PKU) a genetic disorder resulting from the body's failure to oxidize an amino acid, perhaps because of a defective enzyme.
phimosis a narrowing of the opening of the foreskin of the penis.
phlebitis inflammation of a vein.
phlebotomist a health care worker who specializes in obtaining blood samples.
photocopy a photographic reproduction of written matter made by a special device.
photophobia sensitive to light; avoiding light.
photosensitivity inability to tolerate light due to medication effects or illness
physical pertaining to the body; also used for the examination of the body.
physical medicine the branch of medicine dealing with the treatment of disorders and diseases with mechanical devices, as in physical therapy.
physical therapist (PT) one who is licensed to assist in the examination, testing, and treatment of physically disabled or handicapped people through the use of special exercise, application of heat or cold, use of sonar, and other techniques.
physician a medical doctor; one skilled in the practice of medicine.
physician's assistant (PA) a person trained in certain aspects of the practice of medicine to provide assistance to the physician.
physician assistant a midlevel practitioner that is able to examine patients, order diagnostic tests and prescribe certain types of medications. Usually supervised by a physician.
Physicians' Desk Reference (PDR) one of the reference books that lists information about medications.
physician's office laboratory (POL) a designated room in the physician's office where laboratory procedures and tests are performed by qualified persons.
physiology the study of the function of the cells, tissues, and organs of the body.
pia mater innermost of the three meninges of the brain and spinal cord.
pigment any coloring matter.
pineal body a small endocrine gland attached to the posterior part of the third ventricle of the brain.
pinocytosis the process whereby a cell engulfs large amounts of liquid.
pitch the frequency of vibrations of sound that enable one to classify sound on a scale from high to low.
pitfall trap or hidden danger.
pituitary a small endocrine gland attached to the base of the brain; the "master" gland.
PKU see **phenylketonuria.**
placebo an inactive substance that is given as a medicine for its suggestive effect.
placebo effect refers to the fact that some people respond favorably to a known ineffective treatment because they believe it is working.
placenta the structure through which the fetus obtains nourishment during pregnancy; the afterbirth.
plague a deadly epidemic or pestilence.
Plague potentially infectious life-threatening diseases, usually transmitted by bites of rodent fleas to humans
Plaintiff the party who initiates a lawsuit by filing a complaint with the clerk of the court against the defendant(s) demanding damages, performance and/or court determination of rights.
planes a flat or relatively smooth surface; points of reference by which positions or parts of the body are indicated.
plasma the liquid part of the lymph and blood.
platelet a type of cell found in the blood that is required for clotting.
pleura a serous membrane that covers the lungs and lines the thoracic cavity.
pleurisy inflammation of the pleura.
plexuses a network of nerves.
plight unfavorable situation or distressed condition.
plural the form of a term that indicates more than one.
pneumoencephalography an x-ray examination of ventricles and subarachnoid spaces of brain following withdrawal of cerebrospinal fluid and injection of air or gas via a lumbar puncture.
pneumonia inflammation of the lung caused primarily by microbes, chemical irritants, vegetable dust, or allergy.
pneumonitis an inflammation of the lungs, also known as pneumonia.
pneumonoconiosis a respiratory condition caused by inhalation of dust particles from mining or stone cutting.
pneumothorax a collection of air or gas in the pleural cavity that displaces lung tissue.
podiatrist (chiropodist) a person trained to diagnose and treat diseases and disorders of the feet.
podiatry the branch of medicine dealing with disorders of the feet.
poison a substance that, if taken internally or applied externally, is a threat to life.
POL see **physician's office laboratory.**
policy a high-level overall plan; general principles of an organization.
polio (poliomyelitis) an acute, infectious, systemic disease that causes inflammation of the gray matter of the spinal cord.
polling pertains to obtaining an unauthorized FAX transmission.
polycystic kidney disease a condition of multiple cysts in the kidney.
polycythemia an excess of red blood cells.
polyneuralgia pain in many nerves.
polyp a tumor with a pedicle, especially on mucous membranes, such as in the nose, rectum, or intestines.
polyuria excessive secretion and discharge of urine.
pons a portion of the brainstem connecting the medulla oblongata and cerebellum with upper portions of the brain.
popliteal pertains to the area in back of the knee.
portal pertaining to the portal circulation of blood from impaired internal organs to the liver for processing before entering the inferior vena cava.
positive strongly affirmative.
positron emission tomography (PET scan) a form of imaging permitting visualizing the physiologic function of the body.
post mortem pertaining to or occurring during the period after death; common term for autopsy.
posted to transfer charges from the day sheet to patient account records.
posterior toward the rear or back or toward the caudal end.
postmark a dated cancellation of a stamp by the post office that also identifies the place of posting.
postoperative (post-op) after or following a surgical procedure.
postpartum the period following delivery of a baby.
postscript (PS) an addition to a letter written after the writer's name has been signed.
posture the position and carriage of the body as a whole.
potential possible; ability to develop into actuality.

power of attorney a legal document authorizing a person to act as another's attorney, legal representative, or agent.
PPM see **provider-performed microscopy.**
practice management system (PMS) computer system used to keep and generate the records and reports of the practice.
Practice Management Software (PMS) a type of medical office software that provides the medical office the electronic component to deal with day-to-day financial operations of a medical practice, and frequently includes the ability for appointment scheduling, patient registration, charge and payment posting, and insurance and billing.
practicum a supervised employment experience in a qualified health care facility as part of the educational curriculum; also known as an externship.
practitioner one who practices the profession of medicine.
preauthorization prior approval of insurance coverage and necessity of procedure.
precancerous a state just prior to the development of cancer.
precautions care beforehand; a preventive measure.
precise exact; definite; very accurate.
precision exactness, accuracy.
precordial pertaining to that area of the chest wall over the heart for the placement of ECG chest leads.
preferred provider organization (PPO) an organization of physicians who network together to offer discounts to purchasers of health care insurance.
prefix a word component added to the beginning of a word root or combining form that typically modifies the remaining part of the term.
pregnancy the condition of being with child.
preliminary coming before, leading up to.
premium the amount paid or payable (for example, an insurance policy premium).
prenatal the period before birth.
preoperative (preop) the preparatory period preceding surgery.
Preponderance of the evidence the greater weight of the evidence required in a civil (non-criminal) lawsuit for the trier of fact (jury or judge without a jury) to decide in favor of one side or the other. this preponderance is based on the more convincing evidence and its probable truth or accuracy, and not on the amount of evidence.
preposition a word that shows the relationship of an object to some other word in the sentence.
presbycusis impairment of acute hearing in old age.
presbyopia a defect of vision in advancing age involving loss of accommodation.
prescribe to lay down as a rule or direction; to order or advise the use of.
prescription a written direction for the preparation of a medicine.
prevention the act of keeping something from coming to pass; to hinder.
preventive tending to prevent or hinder; something used to prevent disease.
primary occurring first in time, development, or sequence; earliest.
primary diagnosis the main reason a patient is seen or cared for during an encounter.
prioritize to arrange in order of importance.
priority preference; state of being first in time, place or mark.
privacy officer the person designated by a healthcare organization, whether hospital system or private practice, who handles and oversees the maintenance of protected health information.
pro tem acting as (a temporary position); for the time being.
Problem-Oriented Medical Record (POMR) A system of recordkeeping used to collect specific pieces of information regarding a patient during a healthcare visit, such as patient profile, chief complaint, review of systems, physical examination, laboratory reports, chronic problems, medication and preventive care lists, and patient education.
process to treat or prepare by some method.
processor performing a whole sequence of actions or operations.
proclivity an inclination or predisposition toward something.
procrastination intentionally delaying action of something that should be done; to postpone.
procrastinator one who intentionally delays or postpones action.
proctological body position that requires the use of a proctologic examination table; the patient kneels on knee board of the table, bends at the hips and rests the chest on the table. the head is supported by a headboard.
proctology the study of the rectum and anus and their diseases.
proctoscope an instrument for the inspection of the rectum.
proctoscopy instrumental inspection of the rectum.
procure to get or obtain.
procurement to obtain; acquire.
product the result of multiplying two numbers together.
productivity the amount of work accomplished in a period of time.
professional conforming to the technical or ethical standards of a profession.
professional ethics a framework of evaluating conduct applicable to members of a given profession
professionalism professional status, methods, character, or standards.
proficiency testing (PT) the measurement of acquired knowledge and skills; a means of assessing the competency of someone or of something.
proficient well advanced in an art, occupation, skill, or branch of knowledge; unusually knowledgeable.
profit sharing a system by which employees receive a share of the profits of a business enterprise.
progesterone a hormone secreted by the graafian follicle following the expulsion of the ovum.
programmed arranged; planned; a sequence of actions performed by a computer.
progress notes record of the continuing progress and treatment of a patient.
progress report an upgrading of current findings.
project to produce and send forth with clarity and distinctness.
projection a defense mechanism of trying to blame another for one's own inadequacies.
prolapse dropping of an internal part of the body; usually refers to uterus or rectum.
prominent conspicuous, outstanding.
promissory containing a pledge to pay.
prompt to urge to action, to inspire.
prone a position, lying horizontal with the face down.
pronoun a word used instead of a noun, to indicate without naming.
proofread reading of printed proofs to discover and correct errors.
property right the entitlement to anything that is owned by a person or entity. Property is divided into two types: "real property," which is any interest in land, real estate, growing plants or the improvements on it, and "personal property," which is everything else.
prophylactic preventing disease.
proportion another way of saying fraction.
proprietary privately owned and managed and run as a profit-making organization.
proprietorship the amount by which assets exceed liabilities.
prosecution in criminal law, the government attorney charging and trying the case against a person accused of a crime, or a common term for the government's side in a criminal case.
prostaglandins a group of chemical substances secreted by mast cells or basophils that constricts smooth muscles in some organs.

prostate a gland of the male reproductive system that surrounds the proximal portion of the urethra.
prostatectomy excision of part or all of the prostate gland.
prosthesis an artificial replacement of a missing body part.
protanopia a problem in which the perception of reds and sometimes yellow and green become confusing.
protected health information (PHI) confidential health information that is protected under Health Insurance Portability and Accountability Act (HIPAA).
protein (albumin) a normal substance found in serum but when found in urine means the presence of an excess of serum proteins excreted in the urine rather than reabsorbed by the renal tubules; a nutrient found in foods such as eggs, meat, fish, legumes, and soy products that provides energy to the body.
prothrombin chemical substance existing in circulating blood which aids in the clotting process.
protocol a plan of treatment, usually experimental, used to determine effectiveness of new treatments or medications.
protozoan a single-cell animal.
Provider is an individual licensed to examine, diagnose and prescribe treatment to patients seeking assistance.
Provider the person that oversees the patient's healthcare. Often a physician, physician's assistant or nurse practitioner.
provider-performed microscopy (PPM) refers to microscopic procedures done in the physician's office laboratory.
provisions the act of providing; something provided for the future; a stipulation.
proximal nearest the point of attachment.
proxy one who has authority to vote or act for another; a certificate of authorization to vote.
prudent careful; wise in practical affairs.
pruritic pertaining to an itching sensation.
pruritus severe itching.
pruritus ani itching around the anus.
PS see **postscript.**
psoriasis a chronic inflammatory disease characterized by scaly patches.
psychedelics hallucinogenic drugs.
psychiatrist a physician specializing in the diseases and disorders of the mind, including neuroses and psychoses.
psychiatry the branch of medicine dealing with the diagnosis, treatment, and prevention of mental illness.
psychological of the mind; mental.
psychologist a person specializing in the study of the structure and function of the brain and related mental processes.
psychology the study of mental processes, both normal and abnormal, and their effects upon behavior.
psychoneuroimmunology a science studying the connection between the brain, behavior, and immunity.
psychopathic concerning or characterized by a mental disorder.
psychosis mental disturbance of such magnitude that there is personality disintegration and loss of contact with reality.
psychosomatic pertaining to interrelationships between the mind or emotions and body.
psychotherapy the treatment of disease by hypnosis, psychoanalysis, and similar means.
PT see **pharmacy technician** or **proficiency testing**.
ptosis a drooping or dropping of an organ or part, for example the eyelid or the kidney.
puberty the period of life at which one becomes functionally capable of reproduction.
pubic pertaining to the middle section of the lower third of the abdomen, also referred to as the hypogastric.
pulmonary concerning or involving the lungs.
pulmonary edema the presence of interstitial fluid in the lung tissue.
pulmonary embolis a blockage in the pulmonary artery or one of its branches.
pulse deficit the difference between the pulse rate measured radially and apically.
pulse oximetry measuring the oxygen saturation of arterial blood in a subject by utilizing a sensor attached typically to a finger, toe, or ear to determine the percentage of oxyhemoglobin in blood pulsating through a network of capillaries and that typically sounds an alarm if the blood saturation becomes less than optimal.
pulse pressure difference between the systolic and diastolic measurements.
pulse throbbing caused by the regular alternating contraction and expansion of an artery.
punctual prompt; being on time.
punctuality a desirable trait of being on time for appointments, work, etc.
punctuation standardized marks in written matter to clarify meaning.
puncture a hole made by something pointed.
Punitive damages damages awarded in a lawsuit as a punishment and example to others for malicious, evil or fraudulent acts.
pupil the contractible opening in the center of the iris for the transmission of light.
purge to empty; to cleanse of impurities; clear.
Purkinje network of fibers found in the cardiac muscle that carries the electrical impulses resulting in the contraction of the ventricles.
pustular pertaining to a collection of pus that has accumulated in a cavity formed by the tissue on the basis of an infectious process.
pustule small elevation of the skin filled with lymph or pus.
pyelonephritis inflammation of the kidney, pelvis, and nephrons.
pyloric pertaining to the opening between the stomach and the duodenum.
pyrogen capable of producing fever.

QNS quantity not sufficient.
quackery the pretense to knowledge or skill in medicine.
quad-base refers to a cane with four "feet."
quadrant one of four regions, as of the abdomen, divided for identification purposes.
quadriceps femoris a large muscle on the anterior surface of the thigh that is composed of four separate muscles.
qualifications a quality or attainment that fits a person for a place or position.
quality assurance (QA) inclusive policies, procedures, and practices as standards for reliable laboratory results that includes documentation, calibration, and maintenance of all equipment, quality control, proficiency testing, and training.
quality control (QC) inclusive laboratory procedures as standards to provide reliable performance of equipment, including test control samples, documentation, and analyzing statistics for diagnostic tests.

Rabies an acute viral disease of the nervous system of warm-blooded animals; usually transmitted by the bite of a rabid animal
radial referring to the radial artery or pulse taken in the radial artery.
radiation the emission and diffusion of rays; a product of x-ray and radium.
radioactive capable of emitting radiant energy.
radioactive agents agents used to diagnose certain medical problems or treat certain diseases.
radiograph a record produced on a photographic plate, film, or paper by the action of x-ray or radium.
radiologist one who diagnoses and treats disease by the use of radiant energy.
radiology the study of radiation and its uses.
radiology technician an individual trained in the administration of x-rays.
radionuclides a type of atom used in nuclear medicine for the diagnosis and treatment of disease.
radiopaque impenetrable to the x-ray or other forms of radiation.
radius a long bone of the forearm.
rales an unusual sound heard in the bronchi on examination of respirations.

ramification a subdivision or consequence.
random by chance; without plan.
range of motion (ROM) refers to the degree of movement of the body's joints and extremities.
rapport relationship characterized by harmony and cooperation.
ratchet locking mechanism of an instrument
rational based on reasoning, sensible.
rationalization to explain on rational grounds, to devise plausible explanations for one's acts.
RAST short for radioallergosorbent test, a blood test used to determine what a person is allergic to. This is different from a skin allergy test, which determines allergy by the reaction of a person's skin to different substances.
Raynaud's phenomenon a symptom of lupus characterized by fingers that turn white or blue in the cold.
reactivity rate of nuclear disintegration in a reactor.
reagent a substance involved in a chemical reaction.
realm kingdom or empire, as used in text.
reason rule refers to the purpose or reason for doing a test or procedure, an insurance company criteria for reimbursement.
receipt a written acknowledgement that something has been received.
reception the fact or manner of being received; a social gathering.
receptionist one employed to greet telephone callers, visitors, patients, or clients.
receptor peripheral nerve ending of a sensory nerve that responds to stimuli.
recessive gene apparently suppressed in crossbred offspring in preference for a characteristic from the other parent.
recipient one who receives.
reciprocity mutual exchange, especially the exchange of special privilege.
Reciprocity a physician who has been licensed in one state and wishes to move to another state may be granted a license by reciprocity if it is determined that the original licensure requirements are equal to or more stringent to the requirements of the new state.
reconcile process to bring checkbook and bank statement into agreement.
rectal referring to the rectum.
rectocele the protrusion of the posterior vaginal wall and anterior wall of the rectum through the vagina.
rectum the lower part of the large intestine between the sigmoid and the anal canal.
recumbent lying down.
recurrent returning at intervals.
reduce to restore the ends of a fractured bone to their usual relationship.
redundant extra, not needed, repetitive.
reference a source of information or authority.
reference points in communication, the sum total of values, culture, education, and experiences that an individual holds that affect the way that a message is received.
referral sending a patient to a provider of a different specialty for treatment beyond the scope of practice for the initial practitioner
reflective communication an interactive communication process in which the receiver uses verbal "mirroring" to restate what the sender has said for optimal clarification by all parties.
reflex an involuntary response to a stimulus.
reflexology massaging of the hands or feet based on the belief that pressure applied to specific points on these extremities benefits other parts of the body.
reflux a return or backward flow.
refractive the degree to which a transparent body deflects a ray of light from a straight path.
regimen regulation of diet, sleep, exercise, and manner of living to improve or maintain health.
register a formal or official recording of items, names, or actions; a record of money that has been spent.
registered legally certified or authenticated.
Registered Medical Assistant, RMA (AMT) the credential the American Medical Technologists (AMT) issues to eligible candidates, which successfully pass the RMA examination.
registered nurse (RN) an individual trained through formal training in the field of nursing.
registry a list of persons qualified in a particular area of expertise.
regression a defense mechanism of retreating to the thoughts and actions of an earlier, "safer," age.
regulate control or direction.
regulations in the POL standards set for quality assurance and quality control in the physician's office laboratory to ensure reliable diagnostic tests.
regulatory to control according to a rule; to adjust so as to make work accurately.
rehabilitate to put back in good condition; to restore.
rehabilitation centers facilities that assist in developing appropriate socialization skills, family and community reintegration, and increased independence.
rehabilitative therapy treatment that offers the highest level of patient care and programs that will enhance the physical, psychological, and emotional health of the population served in most of these facilities.
reimbursement to pay back or compensate for money spent, or losses or damages incurred.
reiterate to say or do again.
rejuvenate to make young again; to give youthful qualities to.
relapse recurrence of a disease or symptoms; returning to a previous condition.
reliable dependable, can be relied upon.
reluctant marked by unwillingness.
rely to depend on, to trust.
REM (rapid eye movement) a stage of sleep in which the sleeper experiences rapid eye movement. In a healthy young adult, REM sleep accounts for 10%–25% of sleep time.
remedy anything that relieves or cures a disease.
remission a period that is disease- and symptom-free.
remote from a distance; far removed in time and place; indirect.
renal pertaining to the kidney.
renal failure loss of function of the kidneys' nephrons.
renal threshold the concentration at which a substance in the blood normally not excreted by the kidney begins to appear in the urine.
render to present or to deliver, as a service or statement.
renovate restore; to make new again.
repolarization reestablishment of a polarized state in a muscle or nerve fiber following contraction or conduction of a nerve impulse. On a ECG, the time of recovery before another contraction.
repression to force painful ideas or impulses into the subconscious.
reproductive concerning reproduction.
reputable having a good reputation; well thought of.
res ipsa loquitur the thing speaks for itself.
residency physician training period in a specialty field of medicine.
residual barium barium remaining in the intestinal tract following evacuation at the completion of x-ray studies.
residual pertaining to that which is left as a residue.
resistance opposition, ability to oppose.
resonance quality of the sound heard on percussion of the chest; the intensification and prolongation of a sound by reflection or by vibration of a nearby object.
resource a source of support or supply.
respectful showing respect; honoring; treat with consideration.
respiration the taking in of oxygen and its use in the tissues and the giving off of carbon dioxide.
respiratory therapy technician a person trained to perform procedures of treatment that maintain or improve the ventilatory function of the respiratory tract.
respiratory pertaining to respiration.

respite a temporary cessation of something that is painful or tiring; to delay, postpone.
respondeat superior let the master answer.
restricted limited; only for a certain group.
resumé a summary, especially of work experiences.
resuscitation an emergency first aid procedure for a victim of cardiac arrest. It is part of the chain of survival, which includes early access (to emergency medical services), early CPR, early defibrillation, and early advanced care. It is also performed as part of the choking protocol if all else has failed; revival from apparent or possible death.
retardation slowing, delay, lag; slow in development, mental or physical.
retention inability to void urine that is present in the bladder.
reticuloendothelial pertaining to that group of cells that appear to aid in the making of new blood cells and the disintegration of old ones.
retina the innermost layer of the eye that receives the image formed by the lens.
retinopathy a degeneration of the retina caused by a decrease in blood supply.
retraction a shortening; the act of drawing backward or state of being drawn back.
retractor instrument used to hold back tissue, making the operative site easier to visualize.
retroflexed refers to the body of the uterus being bent backward.
retrograde refers to an x-ray procedure in which a radiopaque material is instilled by catheter into the bladder, ureters, and kidneys.
retrograde pyelogram a urologic procedure in which the physician injects contrast into the ureters in order to visualize the ureters and kidney.
retroperitoneal behind the peritoneum; posterior to the peritoneal lining of the abdominal cavity.
retroverted refers to the entire uterus being tilted backward.
retrovirus one with RNA (ribonucleic acid) genetic material.
revalidation the renewing or reconfirmation of credentials.
revocation temporary of permanent suspension of a license.
revoke to cancel, withdraw, take back.
Rh factor an antigenic substance in human blood similar to the A and B factors that determine blood groups; apparently present only in red blood cells.
rhinitis inflammation of the nasal mucosa.
rhinoplasty plastic surgery of the nose.
rhythm a measured time or movement; regularity of occurrence.
ribosome an organelle within the cytoplasm of the cell.
rickets a disease of the bones primarily due to the deficiency of vitamin D.
Rickettsiae Any of a family of rod-shaped, coccoid, or diplococcus-shaped, often pleomorphic gram-negative, bacteria that are intracellular parasites of arthropods (such as lice or ticks) and when transmitted to humans cause various diseases (such as typhus).
risk chance; hazard; chance of loss or injury; degree of probability of loss.
R/O rule out.
roentgen refers to x-rays.
role delineation study occupational analysis study conducted by AAMA and the National Board of Medical Examination in 1997 that identifies the most up-to-date entry-level areas of competence of the medical assisting profession.
ROM see **range of motion.**
rotate to move around; to turn on an axis.
rubella (German measles) a mild contagious viral disease that may cause severe damage to an unborn child.
rubeola (measles) an acute, highly contagious disease marked by a typical cutaneous eruption.

SA node see **sinoatrial node.**
sacrilege the crime of misappropriating what is consecrated to God or religion.
sacrum five fused vertebrae that lie between the coccyx and the lumbar vertebrae of the spinal column.
safety freedom from danger or loss.
sagittal refers to a plane that is made by dividing the body down the center, creating a right and left side.
salary a fixed amount of wages paid to an employee on a regular basis for a prescribed period of time, i.e., weekly or monthly
saliva a digestive secretion of the salivary glands that empties into the stomach.
salivary glands three pairs of glands that secrete the saliva that begins the digestion of food, primarily the breakdown of starch or complex carbohydrates.
salpingectomy surgical removal of the fallopian tube or tubes.
salpingo-oophorectomy surgical excision of the ovary and fallopian tube.
salve an ointment.
sanitization the process of applying antimicrobial agents to nonliving objects to destroy microorganisms.
sarcoma malignant tumors of the connective, muscle, or bone tissue.
sartorius a long narrow muscle of the thigh; the longest muscle of the body.
scan to look over quickly but thoroughly.
scapula the shoulder blade.
schedule to arrange a timetable; to place in a list of things to be done.
sciatica inflammation and pain along the sciatic nerve felt at the back of the thigh running down the inside of the leg.
scientific based upon or using the principles and methods of science; systematic; exact.
sclera the white or sclerotic outer coat of the eye.
scoliosis lateral curvature of the spine.
screening a preliminary or indicating procedure.
Scribe A person who documents by hand as a profession and helps providers keep track of records.
script manuscript; type designed to look like handwriting.
scrotum the double pouch containing the testes and part of the spermatic cord.
scrub specific and thorough hand washing procedure performed for 6 minutes before taking part in any sterile surgical procedure.
scrupulously with great attention to detail; with great care.
scurvy a disease caused by lack of fresh fruits, vegetables, and vitamin C in the diet.
sebaceous an oily, fatty matter; glands secreting such matter.
sebum oily secretion of the sebaceous glands of the skin.
secondary one step removed from the first; not primary.
Secondary insurance exists when a patient is covered under more than one insurance plan; charges are first submitted to the primary carrier and any charges not covered are then submitted to the secondary carrier.
secretary one employed to conduct correspondence; a person responsible for records and correspondence.
secretion separation of certain materials from the blood by the activity of a gland.
sector a section or division.
security freedom from fear or anxiety.
sedate to produce a state of calmness; process of allaying nervous excitement; using an agent to produce a tranquilizing effect.
sedentary pertaining to sitting; inactivity.
sedimentation formation or depositing of sediment; of blood, refers to the speed at which erythrocytes settle when an anticoagulant is added to blood.
segment a part or section of an organ or a body. The Portion of ECG between two waves.
seizures a sudden attack of pain, disease, or certain symptoms.
self-control control of ones emotions, desires.
semen the mixture of secretions from the various glands and organs of the reproductive system of the male, which is expelled at orgasm.
semicircular canals structures located in the inner ear.

semilunar the valves of the heart located between the ventricles and the pulmonary artery and aorta.
senility feebleness of body or mind caused by old age.
sensitivity abnormal susceptibility to a substance.
sensorineural refers to a sensory nerve.
sensorineural deafness a loss of hearing caused by transmission failure of the nerves within the inner ear or the auditory nerve.
sensory refers to the nerves that receive and transmit stimuli from the sense organs.
septum a membranous wall dividing two cavities, as within the heart or the nose.
sequence order of succession.
sequentially arranged in sequence; in an order.
series a group; a set of things in the same class coming one after another.
serrated notched, toothed.
serrations etchings located on the blades of an instrument to keep it from slipping.
serum blood plasma in which clotting factors (such as fibrin) have been removed naturally by allowing the blood to clot prior to isolating the liquid component
service charge a fee charged for a service, often in addition to a basic fee.
Seven Rights Refers to seven elements that must be considered when administering medication, which are: right patient, right medication, right dose (amount), right route (method), right technique, right time (schedule), and right documentation
sharps any object that can cut, prick, stab, or scrape the skin.
sheath a covering structure of connective tissue, such as the membrane covering a muscle.
shelf life that length of time that sterile items are given before they are considered unsuitable as maintaining sterility.
shiatsu a massage with the fingers applied to those specific areas of the body used in acupuncture.
shock a condition in which the pulse becomes rapid and weak, the blood pressure drops, and the patient is pale and clammy.
sickle cell anemia a blood disorder in which the red blood cells are shaped like sickles.
side effect unintended or adverse effects of a medication, ranging from mild to intolerable
sigmoid an S-shaped section of the large intestine between the descending colon and the rectum.
sigmoidoscopy an inspection of the sigmoid with an instrument.
signature a signing of one's own name.
simple referring to a bone fracture, one without involvement of the skin surface.
Sims' an examination position with the patient lying on the left side.
simultaneous occurring at the same time.
Single-booking a method of scheduling in which only one patient is assigned to one block of time in a visit schedule.
single-entry bookkeeping system an accounting method in which each financial transaction is recorded only once in account books.
singular the form of a term that indicates the presence of only one.
sinoatrial (SA) node the source of the nerve impulse that initiates the heartbeat; the pacemaker.
sinusitis inflammation of the sinuses.
site review visit, examination, or inspection to the medical office by an outside agency (such as, insurance companies, OSHA, CLIA, etc).
skeletal pertaining to the skeleton or bony structure; also to the muscles attached to the skeleton to permit movement.
skills a term used to describe procedures that are taught in an educational program or work setting.
skip a person who owes money but cannot be located.
skull x-ray a radiologic examination of the skull.
sleep apnea brief episodes of the cessation of breathing during sleep.
sling a hanging support for an injured arm.
slough to cast off, as dead tissue.
smooth a type of involuntary muscle tissue found in internal organs.
snap locks metal locking devices.
snellen chart the chart of alphabetic letters used to evaluate distant vision.
Social Security number (SSN) unique nine-digit number assigned by the U.S. government.
software computer programs necessary for directing the computer hardware to perform specific functions.
solace an easing of grief, to comfort.
sole only.
solicit to ask for.
Solo Practice When an individual provider/physician makes all the decisions for the practice.
somatic Pertaining to the body as distinguished from the mind; physical. Pertaining to the structures of body wall such as the skeletal muscles.
sonar a device that transmits high-frequency sound waves in water and registers the vibrations reflected back from an object.
sonogram record obtained by ultrasound.
sophisticated not simple or natural; very refined; highly complex or developed in form, technique, etc.
sound that which is or can be heard; free from damage, safe, secure.
spasm an involuntary sudden movement or convulsive muscular contraction.
spastic colon spasmodic contractions of the large intestine.
specific gravity the ratio of dissolved substances in a solvent as compared with the ratio of dissolved substances in distilled water, most commonly comparing the ratio of dissolved substances in a urine specimen when compared with distilled water.
specifications any point or particular specified; mention in detail.
specificity something specially suited for a given use or purpose; a remedy regarded as a certain cure for a particular disease.
specified named particularly; mentioned in detail.
specimen a sample; a representative piece of the whole.
speculum an instrument that permits viewing inside a body cavity.
sperm the male gamete or sex cell.
spermatozoan a sperm cell.
sphincter a circular muscle constricting an opening.
sphygmomanometer a device that measures blood pressure; also called manometer.
spina bifida occulta a disorder characterized by a defect in the spinal vertebrae with or without protrusion of the spinal cord and meninges.
spinal pertaining to the spinal column, canal, or cord.
spinal fusion the surgical implanting of a bone fragment between the processes of two or more spinal vertebrae to render them immobile.
spiral having a circular fashion.
spirometer an apparatus that measures the volume of inhaled and exhaled air.
spleen an oval, vascular, ductless gland below the diaphragm in the upper left quadrant of the abdomen.
splinter a thin sharp piece of wood.
spontaneous involuntary; produced by itself; unforced.
spores hard capsules formed by certain bacteria that allow them to resist prolonged exposure to heat.
sports medicine the branch of medicine dealing with the care of athletes to prevent and treat sports-related injuries.
sprain the forcible twisting of a joint with partial rupture or other injury of its attachments.
sputum substance ejected from the mouth containing saliva and mucus; usually refers to material coughed up from the bronchi.
stability the ability of a reagent to remain constant after being opened.
stabilize to make steady; firmly fixed; constant.
staging a method for determining the extent of the disease process with cancer.

standard conforming to a custom or law.
Standard of care the watchfulness, attention, caution and prudence that a reasonable person in the circumstances would exercise.
Standard of proof the burden that the plaintiff or prosecution must meet in presenting their case; the measure by which evidence is judged to show a "preponderance of evidence" in a civil action and "beyond a reasonable doubt" in a criminal case.
standard precautions guidelines for the prevention of infectious diseases and nosocomial infections established by the centers for disease control and prevention.
standardization process of bringing into conformity with a standard; pertaining to ECG, a mark made at the beginning of each lead to establish a standard of reference.
stapes one of the three bones of the middle ear.
stasis ulcer an open lesion caused by stagnant or inade quate blood supply to an area.
STAT (statim) immediately.
state law legislation enacted by the state legislature and signed by the governor.
stationery writing materials, especially paper and envelopes.
stature height.
Statute / statutory law a federal or state written law enacted by the Congress or state legislature respectively.
statutory legally enacted; deriving authority from law.
stem cells Cells with the ability to divide for indefinite periods in culture and to give rise to specialized cells.
stenosis narrowing or constriction of a passage or opening.
sterile without any organisms.
sterile gauze square a piece of dressing for a wound.
sterilization the elimination of all transmissible agents (such as bacteria and viruses) from a surface, a piece of equipment, food, or biologic culture medium, including spores.
sternocleidomastoid a muscle of the chest arising from the sternum and inner part of the clavicle.
sternum the breastbone.
stethoscope an instrument used in auscultation to convey to the ear the sounds produced by the body.
stimulant a substance that temporarily increases activity.
stipulations terms of an agreement.
stomach a dilated, saclike, distensible portion of the alimentary canal below the esophagus and before the small intestine.
stool bowel movement, feces.
strabismus an eye disorder caused by imbalance of the ocular muscles.
strain injury to muscles from tension caused by overuse or misuse.
stratagem a trick or deception.
stress to put pressure on; emphasize; urgency; tension, strained exertion. Topical; causing strain or injury to the skin.
striated a type of muscle tissue marked with stripes or striae.
stricture the narrowing of an opening, tube, or canal, such as the urethra or esophagus.
strikethrough condition in which fluid is able to penetrate through a drape
stylus a pen; the ECG writer.
subarachnoid the space between the pia mater and the arachnoid containing cerebrospinal fluid.
subcutaneous beneath the skin.
subdural beneath the dural mater; the space between the arachnoid and the dura mater.
subjective relating to the person who is thinking, saying, or doing something; personal; of a disease symptom, felt by the individual but not perceptible to others.
Subjective Objective Assessment Plan (SOAP) one of the most widely used methods of charting, to collect patient visit information; appropriate for most types of patient encounters.
sublimation to express certain impulses, especially sexual, in constructive, socially acceptable forms.
sublingual under the tongue.
subpoena duces tecum court process initiated by a party in litigation, compelling production of specific documents and other items, and material in relevance to facts in issue in appending judicial proceedings.
subsequent coming after, following.
substantial considerable, large.
subtle so slight as to be difficult to detect or describe; elusive
suction withdrawal by pressure; a sucking action.
sudden happening without warning or in a short space of time
sudden infant death syndrome (SIDS) the sudden, unexplainable death of an infant.
suffix an addition to the end of a term that changes the grammatical function of the term.
superficial on the surface.
superior vena cava large but short vein that carries deoxygenated blood from the upper half of the body to the heart's right atrium.
superior above or higher than.
supernatant floating on the surface.
supervisor one who oversees; has control; in charge.
supine lying horizontally on the back.
supplement something added; an additional or extra section.
support to hold up; to bear part of the weight of.
suppository a medicated conical- or cylindrical-shaped material that is inserted into the rectum or vagina.
suppression the shutdown of kidney function; the absence of urine excretion; in psychology, it is the deliberate exclusion of an idea, desire, or feeling from consciousness.
suppressor one that holds back or stops an action.
suprapubic above the pubic arch.
Supremacy Clause article VI, section 2 of the U.S. Constitution, which allows a Supreme Court ruling to be binding on state courts if involving a constitutional issue. The Clause reads: "This Constitution, and the Laws of the United States which shall be made in pursuance thereof; and all treaties made, or which shall be made, under the authority of the United States, shall be the supreme law of the land; and the judges in every state shall be bound thereby, anything in the Constitution or laws of any state to the contrary notwithstanding."
surfactant a fatty molecule on the respiratory membranes.
surgeon a physician with advanced training in operative procedures.
surgery the branch of medicine dealing with manual and operative procedures for correction of deformities and defects and repair of injuries.
surgical asepsis techniques used to destroy all pathogenic organisms before they can enter the body.
surrogate a substitute; in place of another.
surveillance the process of watching or observing.
susceptible having little resistance to a disease or foreign protein.
suspicion mistrust, not believing statements.
suture to unite parts by stitching them together.
symmetry the state in which one part exactly corresponds to another in size, shape, and position.
sympathetic a portion of the autonomic nervous system.
symphysis pubis the junction of the pubic bones on the midline in front.
symptom any perceptible change in the body or its functions that indicates disease or the phase of a disease.
synapse the minute space between the axon of one neuron and the dendrite of another.
syncope fainting; a transient form of unconsciousness.
syndrome the combination of symptoms with a disease or disorder.
synergism something stimulating the action of another so that the effect of both is greater than the sum of the individual effects.

synergistic describes the action of a medication that augments or enhances the actions of another medication.
synovial a movable joint; also called diarthroses.
synthetic not real or natural.
syphilis a communicable venereal disease spread by sexual contact.
system a group of organs working together to perform a function of the body.
systematically by a system or plan.
systemic pertaining to a whole system.
systole the contraction phase of the heart; the greatest amount of blood pressure.

tachycardia abnormal rapidity of heart action.
tact delicate perception of the right things to say and do without offending.
Tachypenia Increased rate of respiration.
tactful being able to perceive a situation and know the right thing to say or do. Tact is especially difficult and important when dealing with ill people.
tactile relating to the sense of touch.
tar a sticky, brown or black carcinogenic substance.
targeted marked, the object of desire; aimed for.
tarry a stool that has the appearance of tar.
tarsal pertaining to the seven bones of the instep of the foot.
taut tightly drawn; tense.
technical relating to some particular art, science, or trade; also, requiring special skill or technique.
technologist one skilled in technology; able to apply the technical methods in a particular field of industry or art.
technology the practice of any or all of the applied sciences that have practical value and/or industrial use.
teleconference a meeting held over phone lines incorporating video equipment.
teletherapy radiation therapy administered by a machine that is positioned at some distance from the patient.
temperature degree of heat of a living body; degree of hotness or coldness of a substance; usually refers to an elevation of body heat.
template an electronic file (or preprinted document) with a pre-designed, customized, format. Examples include fax cover sheets or patient information letters, ready to be filled in.
temporal relating to the temporal bone on the skull.
tendon fibrous connective tissue serving to attach muscles to bones.
tendonitis inflammation of the tendon.
tentative experimental, provisional, temporary.
terminal final, end; a terminal illness, refers to a condition that cannot be reversed.
termination ending.
testes the male gonads of the scrotum that produce sperm.
testosterone a male hormone secreted by the testes that causes and maintains male secondary sex characteristics.
tetanus an acute infectious disease caused by the toxins of the bacillus tetani.
tetany intermittent tonic spasms resulting from inadequate parathyroid hormone.
thalamus a portion of the brain lying between the cerebrum and the midbrain.
theories beliefs not yet tested in practice; the general principles on which a science is based.
therapeutic having medicinal or healing properties; pertaining to results obtained from treatment.
therapist one who practices the curative and preventive treatment of disease or an abnormal condition.
thermal characterized by heat; heat activated.
thermally pertaining to heat activation.
thermography a technique for sensing and recording on film hot and cold areas of the body by means of an infrared detector that reacts to blood flow.
thermometer an instrument used to measure temperature.
thesaurus a treasury of words, quotations, knowledge; a collection of words with their synonyms and antonyms.
thinprep a method for preparing cytology specimens.
third-party someone other than the two principals in a transaction; when referring to checks, a type of check made out to the patient by another unknown person
third-party a check made out to someone from an unknown party.
third-party reimbursement payment made by a party other than the one providing or receiving the service, such as a physician or patient. Examples of whom you would receive third-party reimbursement from are an insurance company or an attorney.
thoracic pertaining to the thorax or chest.
thorax the chest; the body cavity enclosed by the ribs and containing the heart and lungs.
thready term used to describe a weak pulse that may feel like a thread under the skin surface.
threshold a minimum amount of supplies to be maintained; also known as par level
thrive vigorous growth.
thrombophlebitis inflammation of a vein associated with the formation of a blood clot.
thrombosis the formation of a blood clot or thrombus.
thymus an unpaired organ located in the mediastinal cavity anterior to and above the heart.
thyroid an endocrine gland located anteriorly at the base of the neck.
thyroidectomy the surgical removal of the thyroid gland.
tibia a long bone in the leg from the knee to the ankle.
tibialis anterior a muscle of the leg.
Time Management an assortment of skills, tools, and practices used to manage time during daily activities and when accomplishing specific projects.
tinnitus a ringing or tinkling sound in the ear that is heard only by the person affected.
tissue a collection of similar cells and fibers forming a structure in the body.
tolerance the difference between the maximum and minimum; the amount of variation allowed from a standard.
tongue the muscular organ of the mouth that assists in the production of speech, contains the taste buds, and provides the ability to swallow.
tongue depressor a flat wooden stick used to depress the tongue.
tonometer instrument for measuring intraocular tension or pressure.
tonometry measuring tension or pressure and especially intraocular pressure.
topical pertaining to a specific area; local.
tort any wrongful act, damage, or injury done willfully, negligently.
torticollis stiff neck caused by spasmotic contraction of neck muscles drawing the head to one side with the chin pointing to the other; can be congenital or acquired.
total quality management (TQM) refers to a management style that uses QA and QC to maintain quality of performance throughout the total process, not just to ensure the end result is satisfactory or corrected.
tourniquet any constrictor used on an extremity to produce pressure on an artery and control bleeding; also used to distend veins for the withdrawal of blood or the insertion of a needle to instill intravenous injections.
toxin poisonous substance or compound of vegetable, animal, or bacterial origin.
toxoid a toxin treated so as to destroy its toxicity, but it is still capable of inducing formation of antibodies on injection.
TQM see **total quality management.**
trace the production of a sketch by means of a stylus passing over the paper, as in electrocardiography.
trachea a cartilaginous tube between the larynx and the main bronchus of the respiratory tree.
tracheotomy a surgically made opening in the trachea through which a person will breathe.

traction the process of pulling; with fractures, traction is applied in a straight line to stretch the contracted muscles and permit realignment of the bone fragments.
trade name The name a manufacturer assigns to a given medication compound for marketing purposes or to simplify referencing the medication.
trait a feature; a distinguishing feature of character or mind.
transaction dealing accomplished.
transcript a copy made directly from an original record, especially an official copy of a student's educational record.
transcription writing over from one book or medium into another; typing in full in ordinary letters.
transdermal through the skin.
transducer a device that transforms power from one system to another in the same or different form.
transfusion injection of the blood of one person into the blood vessels of another.
transient ischemic attack (TIA) temporary interruption of blood flow in the brain caused by small clots closing off blood vessels.
transillumination inspection of a cavity or organ by passing a light through its walls.
transition passing from one condition, place, or activity to another.
transmission the process of sending from one place to another.
transmitted sent from one person, thing, or place to another.
transpose putting one in place of another, the accidental misplacing of words or letters.
transurethral literally means through the urethra; refers to the removal of the prostate by going through the urethral wall.
transverse lying across; the segment of large intestine that lies across the abdomen; a line drawn horizontally across the body or a structure.
trapezius the large muscle of the back and neck.
trauma any injury, physical or mental.
traumatic caused by or relating to an injury.
traumatize to cause trauma or injury.
treadmill an apparatus with a movable platform that permits walking or running in place.
tremulousness the process of involuntary shaking or trembling.
Trendelenburg a position with the head lower than the feet.
trephining cutting out a circular section.
triage a system of sorting and identifying the severity of injuries.
trial balance bookkeeping strategy to confirm accuracy in debits and credits in ledger.
triangular having three angles and three sides.
triangular bandages bandages having three angles and three sides.
triceps the posterior muscles of the arm that work as a team with the biceps; the triceps straighten the elbow.
trichomoniasis infestation with parasitic protozoa; usually refers to vaginal involvement.
tricuspid a valve in the right side of the heart, between the chambers; literally means three cusps or leaflets.
triglycerides a combination of glycerol and fatty acids in the blood.
trimester divided into three sections; the third segment or period.
tritanopia the inability to distinguish the color blue.
trivial of little value, insignificant.
truncated to cut the top or end off; to lop; with insurance.
Truth in Lending Act (TILA) federal law designed to protect consumers in credit transactions; it specifies that when there is an agreement between the physician and a patient to accept payment in more than four installments, the physician is required to provide disclosure of finance charges
tuberculosis an infectious disease caused by the tubercle bacillus; pulmonary tuberculosis is a specific inflammatory disease of the lungs that destroys lung tissue.
tumor a swelling or enlargement; a neoplasm; often used to indicate a malignant growth.
tuning fork an instrument used to determine the sensation of hearing.
turbidity flaky or granular particles suspended in a clear liquid giving it a cloudy appearance; usually refers to cloudy urine.
turgor normal tension; with the skin means the resistance to being deformed and the length of time to return to normal.
tympanic membrane the eardrum.
typhoid an acute infectious disease acquired by ingesting contaminated food or water.
tzanck smear examination of tissue from the lower surface of a lesion in vesicular disease to determine the cell type.

ulcer an open lesion on the skin or mucous membrane of the body characterized by loss of tissue and the formation of a secretion.
ulceration suppuration of the skin or mucous membrane; an open lesion.
ulna a long bone in the forearm from the elbow to the wrist.
ultimately in the end, finally.
ultrasonic scanning a process of scanning the body with sound waves to produce a picture on a screen of underlying internal structures.
ultrasound technologist also known as diagnostic medical sonographers, these individuals are specially trained to use ultrasound equipment to direct high-frequency sound waves into specific areas of a patient's body to produce images of the shape, position, or movement of organs, fluid accumulations, masses, or fetuses.
umbilical pertaining to the umbilicus or navel of the abdomen.
unbundled reporting multiple codes for a service when there is one code that will report the entire service.
unemployment the state of being without work; also, a limited federal program to provide some income for those who are without work.
unique one of a kind, unmatched.
unit clerk a secretarial position on the health care team of a patient care facility.
universal relating to the universe; general or common to all.
universal emergency medical identification worn by patients who have conditions that could have emergency episodes, such as heart conditions, diabetes, epilepsy, allergies, or a laryngectomy, to alert health workers of the patients' conditions when they cannot do so on their own.
universal precautions steps taken by health care workers to prevent exposure to communicable diseases.
unobtrusive not forced upon others; not thrusted forward or pushed out.
unproductive not productive; no accomplishment.
unstructured without specific arrangement.
unwittingly not knowing, unaware; unintentional.
upcoding reporting a higher level code than is appropriate for the service that was rendered resulting in higher reimbursement.
upper respiratory infection (URI) inflammatory process involving the nose and throat, may include the sinuses; refers to symptoms associated with the common cold.
uremia a condition in which products normally found in the urine are found in the blood.
ureter a tube carrying urine from the kidney to the urinary bladder.
urethra a membranous canal for the external discharge of urine from the bladder.
urgency the sudden need to expel urine or stool.
urgent requiring immediate attention.
urgent care center ambulatory care centers that take care of patients with acute illness or injury and those with minor emergencies. Used quite often when patients can get into to see their own provider.
URI see **upper respiratory infection.**

urinalysis an analysis of the urine; a test performed on urine to determine its characteristics.
urinary pertaining to secreting and containing urine: the kidneys, ureters, bladder and urethra.
urinary meatus the opening through which urine passes from the body.
urinary tract infection (UTI) infection occurring within the kidneys, ureters, and/or urinary bladder.
urination the act of urinating or voiding of urine.
urine fluid secreted from the blood by the kidneys, stored in the bladder, and discharged from the body by voiding.
urobilinogen the colorless product of bilirubin reduction formed in the intestines by bacterial action.
urologist a doctor who has been specially trained in studies of the urinary system.
urology the study of the urine and diseases of the urinogenital organs.
urticaria an inflammatory condition characterized by the eruption of wheals that are associated with severe itching; commonly called hives.
uterus a muscular, hollow, pear-shaped organ of the female reproductive tract in which a fertilized ovum develops into a baby.
UTI see **urinary tract infection.**
utilization to put to profitable use.
utilize to use or make use of.

vaccination inoculation with modified harmless viruses or other microorganisms to produce immunity, a preventive against diseases.
Vaccination Information Statement (VIS) information sheets produced by the Centers for Disease Control and Prevention that explain to vaccine recipients by the benefits and risks of a particular vaccine.
vaccine any substance for prevention of a disease.
vagina a musculomembranous tube that forms the passageway from the uterus to the exterior.
vaginal pertaining to the tissues of the vagina.
vaginitis inflammation of the vagina.
vagus the 10th cranial nerve that has both motor and sensory function, affecting the heart, stomach, and other organs.
values beliefs which are important to a person or organization, which influence attitudes or behavior
valve any one of various structures for temporarily closing an opening or passageway or for allowing movement of fluid in one direction only.
varicella The virus responsible for causing chicken pox
varices enlarged, twisted veins.
varicose pertaining to varices; distended, swollen veins, most commonly found in the legs.
vas deferens the excretory duct of the testes.
vasectomy the cutting out of a portion of the vas deferens.
vector an organism (such as an insect) that transmits a pathogen.
vein a blood vessel carrying blood toward the heart after receiving it from a venule.
vena cava one of two large veins that empty into the right atrium of the heart.
venereal pertaining to or transmitted by sexual contact.
venipuncture the puncture of a vein; the insertion of a needle into a vein for the purpose of obtaining a blood sample or instilling a substance.
venom any of a variety of toxins used by several groups of animal species.
venous pertaining to a vein.
ventilation admission and circulation of fresh air; with the lungs, refers to a diagnostic test to determine air exchange and presence of an embolism.
ventilatory that which ventilates, lets in fresh air.
ventral pertaining to the anterior or front side of the body.
ventricle one of the two lower chambers of the heart; also used in reference to cavities within the brain.
venule a minute vein; a blood vessel that connects a capillary with a vein.
verb the part of speech that expresses an action.
verify to prove to be true; to support by facts.
veritable actual, genuine.
vermiform appendix the appendix; a small tube attached to the cecum.
verrucae warts; small, circumscribed elevations of the skin formed by hypertrophy of the papillae.
vertebrae the bones in the spinal column.
vertex the top of the head, the crown.
vesicle a small sac or bladder containing fluid; a small, blisterlike elevation on the skin containing serous fluid.
vested settled; complete; absolute; continuous.
Viability capable of normal growth and development
viable capable of living.
vial a small glass tube or bottle containing medication or a chemical.
Vicariously liable attachment of responsibility to a person for harm or damages caused by another person in either a negligence lawsuit or criminal prosecution.
video display terminal the computer monitor.
vigilance the act of watching for something to happen or watching for danger.
vigilant alertly watchful, especially to avoid danger or harm.
villi tiny projections from a surface; the villi of the small intestine that absorb nutrients during the process of digestion.
villous adenoma a type of polyp that is invasive and malignant.
viral shedding that time when a virus is the most active and most contagious.
Virulence Disease-evoking power of a pathogen.
virulent full of poison; deadly; malignant.
virus a very simple, frequently pathogenic, microorganism capable of replicating within living cells.
viscera internal organs.
visceral pertaining to viscera, the internal organs, especially the abdomen.
visualization the formation of mental visual images.
vital capacity the total volume of air exchanged from forced inspiration and forced expiration.
vital essential; pertaining to the preservation of life (the vital signs).
vital signs Signs of life; specifically, the pulse rate, respiratory rate, body temperature, and often blood pressure of a person.
vitreous humor the substance that fills the vitreous body of the eye behind the lens.
void to pass urine from the urinary bladder; to make ineffective or invalid.
volatile easily changed into a gas or tending to change into a vapor; usually considered potentially dangerous.
voltage a measure of electromotive force.
volume the amount of space occupied by an object as measured in cubic units.
voluntary under one's control; done by one's own choice.
vomit to expel the contents of the stomach through the mouth.
voucher a document that serves as proof that terms of a transaction have been met.
vulnerable liable to injury or hurt; capable of being wounded.
vulva the female external genitalia, including the clitoris, the labia minora, and the labia majora.

waived laboratory testing that is simple in nature and nonthreatening to the patient if performed or interpreted incorrectly.
waiver to give up; forgo; waiving of a right or claim.
walker a type of mobility device, useful for patients who cannot safely use crutches or a cane.
warrant to justify, to give definite assurance as to the value of; to authorize.
warranted justification for some act, belief.
wart see **verrucae.**
watermark a mark imprinted on paper that is visible when it is held to the light, usually a sign of quality.

WBC differential a white blood cell count in which each type of white blood cell is classified and counted.
weight the amount of heaviness.
wheals more or less round and evanescent elevations of the skin, white in center with a pale red edge, accompanied by itching.
wheelchair a chair fitted with wheels by which a person can propel oneself.
whorl a type of fingerprint in which the central papillary ridges turn through at least one complete circle.
wick a small piece of cotton to absorb or provide moisture or medication.
withdrawal a removal of something that has been deposited.
womb nonmedical name for the uterus.
word processor a system or machine that produces typewritten documents.
word root a component of a medical term that does not have a combining form vowel attached.
work-in to make time or space for.
wound an injury to living tissue, especially an injury involving a cut or break in the skin
write-offs a reduction in the value of an asset or earnings by the amount of an expense or loss, usually deemed uncollectible by any business.
writer the person who writes; the author.
wrongful death the death of a human being as the result of a wrongful act of another person. Examples include negligence (such as a misdiagnosis), assault and/or battery, vehicular manslaughter, manslaughter or murder.
xiphoid a process that forms the tip of the sternum.
x-linked connected to the cell's sex chromosome; a characteristic of the sex chromosome.
x-ray technician a person with specialized training in the techniques to prepare x-ray films to visualize the tissues and organs of the body.

year to date (YTD) begins with the 1st date of the calendar year to present.
yoga a system of exercises for attaining bodily or mental control and well-being.

Z-track (IM) a method of injecting medication intramuscularly.
zygote a cell produced by the union of an ovum and a sperm.

Glosario

abadesa madre superiora; una mujer que es la cabeza de una abadía de monjas.
abandono desertar, dejar por completo.
abdomen la cavidad en el cuerpo entre el diafragma y la pelvis.
abdominal perteneciente al abdomen.
abdominopélvico perteneciente a la cavidad anterior del cuerpo bajo el diafragma.
ABHES por sus siglas en inglés, Oficina de Acreditación de las Escuelas de Educación en las Ciencias de la Salud.
ablación procedimiento quirúrgico en que se usa un resectoscopio insertado en el útero por la cervix.
abogado uno que alega o defiende una causa o a una persona.
aborto la terminación del embarazo antes de la etapa de viabilidad; espontáneo o inducido.
abrasión una lesión causada por el frote o raspadura de la piel.
abreviación forma corta.
abrupto súbito; brusco, seco.
absoluto libre de condición, ilimitado en su poder.
absorber chupar o tragar, tomar.
abstinente Persona que renuncia a algo.
abstracto resumen de las partes principales de una obra extensa.
absurdo contrario al sentido o a la razón.
abusar maltratar, lastimar una y otra vez.
accesible capaz de ser alcanzado.
accidente cerebrovascular embolia cerebral; hemorragia en el cerebro.
acción potencial la carga eléctrica temporal en una célula.
acelerador aumento de la acción o de la función.
acetilcolino hormona liberada en las terminaciones nerviosas parasimpatéticas y las terminaciones nerviosas esqueléticas.
acidez sensación de quemazón bajo el hueso del esternón, usualmente asociada con indigestión.
ácido clorhídrico jugo digestivo encontrado en el estómago.
ácido desoxirribonucleico (ADN) el material dentro del cromosoma que porta la información genética.
acidosis disturbio del balance ácido-base del cuerpo.
acné una condición de la piel caracterizada por la inflamación de las glándulas sebáceas y que produce barros.
acomodación proceso por el cual el lente cambia de forma para permitir la visión cercana.
acoso molestia continuada; persecución.
acreditación la asignación de credenciales; aprobación otorgada por reunir los estándares establecidos.
acreditado certificado; que cumple los estándares establecidos; aceptado como válido.
acromegalia condición crónica caracterizada por el agrandamiento de los huesos de las extremidades y de algunos huesos de la cabeza; engrosamiento de los tejitos suaves faciales.
acrónimo una palabra formada de las letras iniciales de cada palabra principal de un término.
actitud estado de pensamiento o de sentimiento.
activar hacer activo o más activo.
actual que sucede ahora; del tiempo presente; la última información.
acumulado amontonar; recoger; juntar.
acupuntura involucra la inserción de agujas en varios puntos del cuerpo para tratar una enfermedad o aliviar el dolor.
adaptabilidad el acto o el resultado de ajustarse a nuevas circunstancias o cambios.
adecuado igual a lo requerido o a la ocasión, suficiente.
adenitis inflamación de los ganglios linfáticos o de una glándula.
adherir pegarse rápido, unirse de manera firme; ser devoto a.
adicción el estado de estar gobernado o controlado por un hábito, como por alcohol o drogas.
adjetivo una palabra añadida a (que modifica) un sustantivo para cuantificarlo o limitarlo.
administración acción o práctica para manejar o controlar una situación.
administrador de consultorio persona responsable por el funcionamiento del consultorio médico.
administrar manejar; conducir-dirigir, como un negocio.
administrativo deberes que manejan o dirigen actividades; en asistencia médica, se refiere a los deberes diferentes de aquellos por naturaleza clínica; deberes de oficina de recepción.
ADN ver ácido desoxirribonucleico.
adquirir obtener por esfuerzos o acciones propias; contraer.
adquisición obtenido por esfuerzo personal.
adrenalina una secreción interna derivada de las glándulas adrenales; se puede preparar comercialmente de glándulas animales; actúa como estimulante.
adrenal relacionado con las glándulas adrenales que se sientan encima de cada riñon.
aducción alejarse del eje del cuerpo.
aductar acercar al eje del cuerpo.
adverbio una palabra añadida (que modifica) un verbo, un adjetivo, u otro verbo.
adverso opuesto, desfavorable.
aerobio un microorganismo que sólo puede vivir y crecer en la presencia de oxígeno.
afebril sin fiebre.
afiliarse unirse, adherirse o conectarse.
agar sustancia seca mucilaginosa, o gelatina, extraída de alga, usada como medio de cultivo.
agente uno que actúa o tiene el poder o la autoridad de actuar por otro.
agotado consumido, vacío, exhausto.
agravio cualquier acto malintencionado, daño o lesión causada en forma intencional o por negligencia.
agresión cualquier paliza ilegal a otra persona.
agresivo insistente, que asume la ofensiva sin causa, vigoroso.
agudo cortante, severo; tiene un comienzo rápido, síntomas severos y un curso corto; no crónico.
ajustes cambios para que se acomode o poner en armonía.
Al-Anon grupo de apoyo para familiares de alcohólicos.
Al-Ateen apoyo para adolescentes de un padre o madre alcohólico.
albino persona que carece de pigmentación en la piel, cabello u ojos, total o parcialmente; una persona con albinismo.
alcohol líquido generado por la fermentación de azúcar y de otros carbohidratos.
alcohólico individuo que usa alcohol en exceso.
Alcohólicos Anónimos una organización formada para ayudar a que los alcohólicos se abstengan de usar alcohol.
aldosterona hormona mineralocorticoide secretada por la corteza adrenal.
aleatorio al azar; sin plan.
alegar afirmar pero no bajo juramente y sin prueba; aducir.

alergia estado alterado o adquirido de sensibilidad; reacción anormal del cuerpo a sustancias normalmente inofensivas.
alergista médico especializado en el cuidado de pacientes con alergias.
alineamiento estar en la posición adecuada.
alopecia pérdida del cabello; calvicie.
alostérico una proteína que se encuentra en los eritrocitos que transporta oxígeno en la sangre; hemoglobina.
alquitrán sustancia carcinógena pegajosa, de color café o negro.
alquitranado feces que tienen la apariencia del alquitrán.
alucinógeno una sustancia que causa alucinaciones.
alvéolos sacos microscópicos de aire en el pulmón.
ámbar color anaranjado/amarilloso.
ambiente lo que nos rodea.
ambliopía ojo perezoso; condición del ojo caracterizada porque el ojo afectado se voltea hacia adentro.
amenidad agradabilidad, amabilidades, cortesías.
amenorrea ausencia de períodos menstruales; sin menstruación.
aminiocentesis el uso de una aguja para extraer el fluido amniótico del saco amniótico.
amniótico relacionado con el fluido amniótico adentro de la membrana amniótica que rodea al feto.
amplificador un dispositivo en un electrocardiograma que amplía los impulsos del ECG.
ámpula un pequeño contenedor de vidrio que puede ser cerrado y su contenido esterilizado.
amputar cortar, remover una parte.
anaerobio un microorganismo que tiene la habilidad de vivir sin oxígeno.
anafilaxis una reacción hipersensitiva del cuerpo a una proteína o droga extraña; el término implica síntomas lo suficientemente severos para producir un shock serio, o aun la muerte.
análisis el examen de cualquier cosa para determinar su composición; descripción del proceso o del examen, paso por paso.
analítico caracterizado por un método de análisis, una declaración del examen paso por paso.
anal relacionado con el ano o la apertura exterior del recto.
anatomía general se refiere al estudio de aquellas características que pueden ser observadas a simple vista por inspección y disección.
anatomía microscópica area que estudia las características que sólo son visibles a través del microscopio.
anatomía el estudio de la estructura física del cuerpo y de sus órganos.
anatómico relacionado con la anatomía o la estructura de un organismo.
ancla la atadura de un músculo esquelético; la envoltura al principio de una gasa o de un vendaje elástico.
anemia drepanocítica trastorno de la sangre en el cual los glóbulos rojos presentan la forma de la hoz.
anemia perniciosa anemia severa caracterizada por la reducción progresiva en la producción de glóbulos rojos.
anemia una deficiencia de células rojas de la sangre, hemoglobina, o de ambas.
aneroide operando sin fluido; cuando se usa en referencia a un esfigmomanómetro, se mide por el marcador en vez de por la columna de mercurio.
anestesia sin sensación, con o sin consciencia.
anestésico un agente que produce insensibilidad al dolor o al toque, ya sea general o local.
anestesiología el estudio de la anestesia.
aneurisma ensanchamiento, dilación externa causada por la presión de la sangre en las paredes arteriales débilitadas.
anfetamina estimulante del sistema nervioso central.
angina dolor u opresión que irradia del corazón al hombro y al brazo izquierdo; sensación de asfixia.
angiografía un estudio radiológico de una arteria usando un medio radiopaco.
ángulo la inclinación de dos líneas derechas que se encuentran en un punto.
ano la apertura externa del canal anal.
anorexia pérdida de apetito; con anorexia nerviosa, pérdida del apetito por comida sin explicación por enfermedad, que puede ser parte de una psicosis.
anormalidad persona, cosa o condición que no es normal.
anotación entradas en un diario.
anotaciones del progreso relación escrita del tratamiento y progreso de un paciente.
anotando proveer notas críticas o de explicación.
anotar proveer notas explicatorias.
ansiedad la condición mental de desasosiego que surge del miedo o de la aprensión.
antagonizar molestar; crear oposición.
antecubital la superficie interior del brazo o del codo.
anteflexión doblarse hacia delante de manera anormal.
anterior antes o enfrente de.
anticipación esperar, prever.
anticoagulante una sustancia que prohibe la coagulación de la sangre.
anticonceptivo contra la concepción.
anticuerpo una sustancia proteínica cargada por las células para contrarrestar el efecto del antígeno.
antígeno carcinoembriónico un marcador de tumor que puede ser detectado en la sangre cuando es examinada.
antígeno cualquier agente inmunizante que cuando es introducido en el cuerpo, puede producir anticuerpos.
antihistamínico una clase de drogas usada para contrarrestar reacciones alérgicas o síntomas del resfriado.
antiséptico agente que va a prevenir el crecimiento o impedir el desarrollo de microorganismos.
antitoxina una proteína que defiende al cuerpo de toxinas.
antógeno dado por uno mismo.
anualidad una suma de dinero que se recibe anualmente, ya sea en una sola suma o por cuotas.
anuria la ausencia de orina.
aorta el tronco principal del sistema arterial del cuerpo.
aparato de Golgi un organelo dentro del citoplasma de una célula.
apariencia representación exterior.
apendectomía la extirpación del apéndice.
apéndice vermiforme apéndice; tubo pequeño adherido al ceco.
apendicitis la inflamación del apéndice.
apendicular perteneciente a las extremidades o cosas que son apéndices (adheridas) a otras partes.
apical en referencia al ápice.
ápice el punto, la punta o la cumbre de cualquier cosa; en referencia al corazón, el punto de impulso máximo del corazón contra la pared del pecho.
aplicable capaz de ser aplicado, adecuado.
apnea la ausencia de respiración.
apoderado persona que tiene la autoridad de votar o actuar por otra persona.
aponeurosis extensión del tejido conectivo más allá del músculo en tendones redondos o aplanados; medio de inserción u origen de un músculo plano.
apóstrofe un signo de puntuación que muestra la ausencia de una letra o letras; posesión.
aprehensión anticipación de algo temido, tener miedo; una concepción mental.
apremio situación desfavorable o condición desesperada.
aprendizaje un entrenamiento o período de aprendizaje; estudio bajo la guía de un trabajador calificado o con experiencia.
apropiado correcto, adecuado.
aracnoides una membrana delicada como encaje que cubre el sistema nervioso central.
arbitrario dependiente de un deseo o capricho, obstinado; que depende de elección o discreción.
ardientemente ansiosamente, apasionadamente, intensamente.
área de superficie corporal (ASC) se refiere a la superficie total del cuerpo humano.

aréola coloración como anillo alrededor del pezón del seno.
armonioso que tiene sus partes combinadas en un arreglo proporcionado, ordenado o placentero; el ser pacífico o amistoso.
arritmia sin ritmo; irregularidad.
artefacto algo ajeno a aquello que se está buscando. Actividad que causa interferencia en los ECG.
arteria un vaso sanguíneo que lleva la sangre desde el corazón, usualmente lleno de sangre oxígenada.
arterioesclerosis una degeneración y endurecimiento de las paredes de las arterias.
arteriolas pequeños vasos sanguíneos que conectan las arterias con los capilares.
articular unir, como en una articulación.
artritis inflamación de una articulación.
artrografía estudio radiológico de una arteria usando un medio radiopaco.
asalto daño físico; un ataque violento.
ASC área de superficie corporal.
ascendiente se refiere a la porción del colon que asciende del cuadrante inferior derecho al cuadrante superior derecho del abdomen.
ASCLS siglas que en inglés significan American Society for Clinical Laboratory Science, en español corresponden a la Sociedad Americana de la Ciencia del Laboratorio Clínico.
asepsis una condición libre de organismos.
asfixia sofocación, pérdida de conocimiento como resultado de poco oxígeno o de mucho dióxido de carbono.
asimetría ausencia del mismo tamaño, forma y posición de partes u órganos en lados opuestos.
asistente del terapeuta ocupacional (OTA por sus siglas en inglés) persona entrenada para asistir al terapeuta ocupacional.
asistente dental trabajador de la salud empleado por un dentista para llevar a cabo funciones administrativas y clínicas y darle asistencia.
asma reacción alérgica a una sustancia que produce respiración sibilante, falta de respiración y dificultad para respirar.
asociado conectar en pensamiento; unirse como amigo o como socio; un grado otorgado por una universidad al finalizar un programa de dos años.
aspirar remover por succión.
astigmatismo visión borrosa causa da por una curvatura anormal de la córnea.
astilla pedazo de madera delgado y puntiagudo.
ataque repentina ocurrencia de dolor, enfermedad o de ciertos síntomas.
atelectasis falta de aire en los pulmones causada por el colapso de los alvéolos de los pulmones.
atenuado diluido; reducir la virulencia de un organismo patógeno.
ateroesclerosis degeneración adiposa de las paredes de las arterias.
atípico desviado de lo normal.
atmósfera cualquier influencia alrededor.
atributo cualidad o característica; dar crédito.
atrio aurícula cardíaca; cámara superior del corazón.
atrofia mengua de un músculo.
audible lo suficientemente alto para ser escuchado.
audiometría prueba del sentido de audición.
auditorio perteneciente al sentido de audición; canal externo del oído.
aumentado se refiere a los conductores 4, 5 y 6 de los 12 conductores estándar del trazo del ECG; estos conductores son de diferente voltaje.
auricular del oído; medida de temperatura usando un escáner timpánico infrarrojo.
auriculoventricular ver AV.
auscultar escuchar los sonidos producidos por el cuerpo.
autocontrol dominio de los deseos y las emociones.
autoinmune la condición por la cual los anticuerpos de una persona reaccionan en contra de sus propios tejidos normales.
automatización comportamiento de modo automático o mecánico.
autónomo autogobernado; espontáneo; parte del sistema nervioso relacionado con el control reflejo de las funciones corporales.
autorización la concesión de autoridad.
autótrofo microorganismos capaces de elaborar su propia materia orgánica a partir de materia inorgánica.
axial perteneciente a la columna vertebral, cráneo, y la pared torácica.
axila área debajo del brazo, sobaco.
axilar referente al área debajo del brazo.
axón una extensión de la célula nerviosa.
ayuno abstenerse de comida; sin comida o agua.

bacteria microorganismo unicelular relacionado con la fermentación y putrefacción de la materia; agente causante de enfermedades.
balance poner o mantener en equilibrio; tener igual peso y poder.
bancarrota el estado de estar quebrado, haber sido declarado legalmente incapaz de pagar deudas.
barbitúrico un sedativo o droga hipnótica, también llamado tranquilizante.
bario residual bario remanente en el tracto intestinal después de la evacuación al final de una sesión de exámenes de rayos X.
barrera prevenir el acceso; prohibir el paso.
basófilo célula blanca granulada de la sangre, que se tiñe fácilmente.
bazo glándula ovalada, vascular y sin conductos localizada debajo del diafragma en el cuadrante posterior izquierdo del abdomen.
beneficio cualquier cosa que promueve o aumenta el bienestar.
beneficios adicionales beneficios incluidos en o agregados al salario pagado, como seguro de salud, pensión de retiro, etc.
benigno no maligno; no canceroso.
beriberi enfermedad como resultado de falta de vitamina B, tiamina.
bíceps el músculo de la parte alta del brazo que flexiona el antebrazo.
biconvexo la curvatura en ambos lados.
bicúspide válvula del corazón entre el atrio izquierdo y el ventrículo izquierdo, también llamada válvula mitral.
bienal que sucede una vez en 2 años.
bien cualquier cosa que tiene valor de cambio, todas las entradas en una hoja de balance que muestran las posesiones o recursos de una persona o de un negocio.
bilis una secreción del hígado; fluido verdoso-amarillento que tiene un sabor amargo.
bimanual a dos manos; con las dos manos.
bimensual que ocurre una vez en 2 meses.
binocular perteneciente al uso de los dos ojos; que posee dos piezas para el ojo como en un microscopio.
biopsia extracción de un pequeño pedazo de tejido para ser examinado bajo microscopio.
bioquímica la ciencia relacionada con la química de las plantas y de los animales.
bisagra un tipo de articulación.
bizarro extraño, inusual, llamativamente fuera de lo ordinario.
bloqueo del corazón una condición en la cual los impulsos del nódulo sinoatrial no traspasan al nódulo atrioventricular, causando un ritmo cardíaco lento y una rata diferente de contracción entre las cámaras alta y baja del corazón.
boca cavidad bucal; también, relativo a la apertura de los organismos.
bolo masa de comida masticada lista para ser tragada.
borradura el adelgazamiento del cervix durante el parto.
borrar remover, suprimir.
boticario persona que dispensa drogas y medicinas.
bradicardia ritmo cardíaco lento.
braille impresión para los ciegos, usando un sistema de puntos en relieve.
braquial se refiere a la arteria braquial del brazo; la arteria que se usa para medir la presión sanguínea.
broche de cerradura mecanismo de metal para cerrar.
bronquíolo pequeñas ramas terminales de los bronquios que carecen de cartílago.

bronquios las divisiones primarias de la tráquea.
bronquitis inflamación de las membranas mucosas del árbol bronquial.
bucal de la boca; cavidad oral.
bulimia una condición caracterizada por períodos alternos de comer en exceso seguidos de vómito forzado y del uso de laxativos para eliminar comida del cuerpo.
bulto número de cosas ligadas.
bursa saco o bolsillo con tejido conectivo principalmente alrededor de las coyunturas.
búsqueda alfa buscar por orden alfabético.
búster inyección subsecuente de sustancia inmunizante para aumentar o renovar la inmunidad.

CAAHEP por sus siglas en inglés, Comisión de Acreditación de Programas de Educación en las Ciencias de la Salud.
cabestrillo venda sujeta al hombro para sostener la mano o el brazo lastimado.
caduceo la vara de Hermes o Mercurio; usada como símbolo de la profesión médica.
calambre una contracción espásmica y dolorosa de un músculo o músculos.
calcitonina hormona producida por la glándula tiroides esencial en el metabolismo del calcio en los huesos.
calcular computar.
cálculos comúnmente llamados piedras; compuestos usualmente de sales minerales.
calibraciones juego de marcas graduadas para indicar valores.
calibre el tamaño del ojo de la aguja; mientras más pequeño el número, más grande el ojo de la aguja.
cálices dos o más cáliz.
calificaciones cualidades o talentos de los que dispone una persona para ocupar ciertos cargos o ejecutar ciertas acciones.
cáliz la división que se parece a una tasa de la pelvis del riñon.
callos en las fracturas se refiere a la formación de nuevo material óseo alrededor del sitio de la fractura.
caloría unidad para medir el valor calórico de la comida.
campo de baja potencia (LPF, low-power field, por sus siglas en inglés) relativo al lente del microscopio.
canal alimenticio el tracto intestinal, del esófago al recto y órganos accesorios.
canal inguinal un pasaje en la ingle para el cordón espermático en el macho.
canales semicirculares estructuras localizadas en el oído interno.
cancelación tachar cruzando con líneas; marcar una estampilla o un cheque para borrar una cita o un evento.
cáncer un tumor o crecimiento maligno; específicamente la hiperplasia de las células con infiltración y destrucción de tejido.
cánula un tubo o envoltura que rodea un trocar (aguja triangular de perforación); después de la inserción, se remueve el trocar.
caos estado de confusión completa: desorden.
capa Estructura que recubre un tejido conectivo, como la membrana que cubre el músculo.
capacidad vital Volumen total de aire intercambiado entre la inspiración forzada y la expiración forzada.
capción encabezamiento, título o subtítulo.
capilar un vaso sanguíneo microscópico que conecta las arteriolas y las vénulas.
capitación una estructura de pago basado en el número servido.
cápsula de Bowman parte del corpúsculo renal; rodea el glomérulo de la nefrona.
carbohidrato una organización orgánica de carbón, hidrógeno y de oxígeno como en azúcar, un almidón o celulosa.
carboxihemoglobina la combinación de monóxido de carbón y hemoglobina en las células rojas de la sangre.
carbúnculo una infección de estafilococo que sigue a la forunculosis, caracterizada por abcesos profundos de varios folículos con múltiples puntos de drenaje.
carcinogenesis la transformación maligna de una célula.
carcinogénico agente causante de cáncer.
carcinoma un tumor maligno de tejido epitelial.
cardíaco perteneciente al corazón.
cardiología el estudio del corazón y sus enfermedades.
cardiólogo médico especializado en el cuidado de los pacientes con enfermedades del corazón.
cardiovascular perteneciente al corazón y a los vasos sanguíneos.
carótida perteneciente a la arteria carótida.
carpales huesos de la muñeca.
cartílago un tejido fuerte, duro, elástico, que forma parte del sistema esquelético; hueso precalcificado en bebés y niños pequeños.
CAT scan ver tomografia axial computarizada.
catarata una opacidad del lente del ojo que resulta en ceguera.
catarral perteneciente a la inflamación de las membranas mucosas; causando ataques severos de tos con poca o ninguna expectoración.
catastrófico de gran consecuencia; desastroso.
categorizar organizar por clase o naturaleza; poner juntas las cosas que son similares.
cateterizar insertar un catéter en una cavidad (por ejemplo, en la vejiga para remover orina) y para remover fluidos corporales.
caudal perteneciente a caulquier estructura como la cola.
caústico capaz de quemarse; un agente que destruirá tejido vivo.
cauterio una plancha o un caústico usado para quemar tejido.
cauterizar quemar con un cauterio eléctrico o con una sustancia química.
cavidades espacio hueco como dentro del cuerpo o de los órganos.
central situado o relacionado a un centro.
centrífuga una máquina para la separación de materiales pesados de los más livianos a través del uso de la fuerza centrífuga.
centríolo organelo dentro de la célula.
cerciorarse asegurarse.
cerebelo parte baja o trasera del cerebro bajo la parte posterior del encéfalo.
cerebral que pertenece al encéfalo del cerebro.
cerebro medio Porción del cerebro que conecta el pons y la corteza cerebral.
cerebroespinal que se refiere al cerebro y a la columna vertebral.
certificación una declaración escrita.
certificado de renuncia se refiere a una lista de exámenes básicos de laboratorio que pueden ser realizados en la oficina de un médico por personal que no pertenece a un laboratorio.
certificado en posesión de un certificado; estar certificado; una garantía por escrito; una declaración escrita de un hecho.
cerumen la secreción café y serosa que se encuentra en el canal auditivo externo.
cervical perteneciente a la porción del cuello de la columna vertebral; también a la entrada del útero.
cervix la entrada al útero.
cesación cesar o descontinuar.
cesárea extracción quirúrgica de un bebé del útero.
Cheyne-Stokes un patrón de respiración caracterizado por períodos alternos de apnea e hiperventilación
cianosis una decoloración azulosa de la piel causada por falta de oxígeno.
ciática Inflamación y dolor a lo largo del nervio ciático que corre desde la parte posterior del muslo hacia abajo por el interior de la pierna.
ciego el comienzo de la porción ascendente del intestino grueso que forma una bolsa ciega en la unión con el intestino delgado.
científico Basado en, o que utiliza los principios y métodos de la ciencia; sistemático, exacto.
CIE ver Clasificación Internacional de las Enfermedades.
cifosis Curvatura convexa de la espina; joroba.
cigoto Célula producida por la unión de un óvulo y de una esperma.
cilia proyecciones como cabellos de las células epiteliales como en los bronquios.

circulación portal Relativo a la circulación de la sangre desde órganos internos hasta el hígado para procesamiento antes de entrar la vena cava inferior.
circulatorio se refiere al sistema circulatorio; el proceso de fluido de la sangre a través de los vasos a todas las células del cuerpo.
circundar rodear, cerrar.
circunscición extirpación quirúrgica del prepucio del pene.
circunvolutivo Tipo de huella dactilar en la cual los surcos centrales dan por lo menos una vuelta completa.
cirrosis una inflamación intersticial con endurecimiento de los tejidos de un órgano, especialmente del hígado.
cirugía Rama de la medicina que estudia los procedimientos manuales y operativos para la corrección de deformidades y defectos, y para reparar lesiones.
cirujano Médico con entrenamiento avanzado en operaciones para la corrección de deformidades y defectos, y para reparar lesiones.
cistitis inflamación de la vejiga urinaria.
cistoscopio instrumento para examinar el interior de la vejiga urinaria.
cita un compromiso; una reunión a una hora en particular.
citología el estudio de la vida celular y de la formación celular.
citoplasma materia celular sin incluir el núcleo de una célula.
citotecnólogo un especialista de laboratorio quien prepara y examina el tejido de las células para estudiar su formación.
citotóxico capaz de destruir células.
civil perteneciente a los derechos de los individuos privados; procedimientos legales que conciernen derechos que no son criminales.
clamidia bacteria que vive como un parásito intracelular y causa una enfermedad de transmisión sexual.
claridad claro, ausencia de opacidad.
Clasificación Internacional de Enfermedades (CIE) listado comprensivo de enfermedades y desórdenes del cuerpo humano.
clasificado arreglado en un grupo o clasificación de acuerdo a algún sistema.
claustrofobia temor anormal de estar en espacios cerrados o confinados.
cláusula parte de una frase con sujeto y predicado.
clavícula el hueso del cuello, que se articula con el esternón y la escápula.
CLIA ver Enmienda al Mejoramiento del Labotarorio Clínico.
clínico basado en observación; en asistencia médica, pertenece a los deberes considerados tras bambalinas; de naturaleza no administrativa.
clítoris órgano eréctil localizado en la unión anterior de la labia menor.
clon copia exacta.
cloroformo un compuesto líquido que produce un gas que mitiga el dolor y causa inconsciencia.
coagular disminuir la fluidez de una sustancia líquida; coágular o agrumar.
cocle porción en forma de concha del oído interno.
coerción forzar, imponer; restringir o constreñir a la fuerza.
coito relación sexual entre hombre y mujer.
colaborar trabajar juntos.
colateral subordinado, secundario; propiedad depositada como garantía por un préstamo.
colecistomía la extirpación quirúrgica de la vejiga.
colega un asociado en el trabajo, usualmente uno de estatus similar.
colelitiasis piedras en la vejiga.
cólera una enfermedad aguda, específica e infecciosa caracterizada por diarrea, calambres dolorosos de los músculos y tendencia al colapso.
colinérgicas fibras nerviosas capaces de secretar acetilcolina.
colirio un objeto que usa agua para remover material extraño de los ojos, usualmente en situaciones de emergencia.
colitis inflamación del colon.
colon intestino grueso.
colon espástico contracciones espasmódicas del intestino grueso.
colonoscopia un examen diagnóstico para visualizar el colon por medio de un colonoscopio.
colorímetro instrumento usado para medir la cantidad de pigmentos y determinar la cantidad de hemoglobina en la sangre.
colostomía incisión en el colón con el propósito de hacer una apertura más o menos permanente.
coma un letargo profundo y anormal del que una persona no puede ser despertada por un estímulo externo.
compatibilidad relación caracterizada por la armonía y la cooperación.
compatible capaz de ser mezclado o tomado en conjunto sin cambios destructivos (como en tipo de sangre y pruebas sanguíneas cruzadas); asemejar; no opuesto a.
compensación cualquier cosa dada como un equivalente o para hacer enmiendas; pagar.
compensar hacer enmiendas; ser equivalente.
competencia habilidad demostrada.
competente persona con los conocimientos necesarios y aptitudes avanzadas para la realización de una actividad artística o un trabajo determinado.
competente apto, hábil, capaz.
complejidad el estado de ser complicado.
complementario expresar aprecio; dar sin cobrar.
complemento un grupo de cerca de 20 proteínas enzimáticas inactivas presentes en la sangre.
complicado no simple, involucrado; tener muchas partes; no fácil de resolver.
componer formar juntando, creando.
comprensivo que cubre todas las áreas; inclusivo.
compresión ejercer fuerza contra, presionar.
compuesto no simple, formado por dos o más partes; con fracturas, se refiere a los fragmentos de hueso que perforan la piel externamente.
computador un aparato mecánico, eléctrico o electrónico que guarda información numérica o de otra clase y provee respuestas lógicas a alta velocidad a preguntas basadas en esa información.
computarizado guardar en un computador; poner de forma que el computador pueda usar; poner los computadores en uso para controlar una operación.
comunal gente en general; un cuerpo corporativo y su membresía.
comunicación el acto de comunicar; información dada; forma de dar información.
concebir quedar embarazada; la unión del esperma y del óvulo.
concepción la unión del esperma del macho y del huevo de la hembra; fertilización.
conciso condensado, corto.
condensador parte debajo de la platina del microscopio que regula la cantidad de luz dirigida a un espécimen.
conducta comportamiento, presencia.
conducto biliar común un conducto que lleva la bilis de los conductos hepáticos y cístico al duodeno.
conducto eyaculatorio el ducto de la vesícula seminal a la uretra.
conectivo que conecta o une; uno de los cinco tejidos principales del cuerpo.
confiabilidad seriedad, fiabilidad.
confiable fiable, seguro.
confiable sobre lo cual se puede contar.
confiar fiar, tener fe en algo o alguien.
confidencialidad ser tenido en confidencia; secreto.
confidencial revelado en confidencia; información secreta.
confinamiento restricción dentro de ciertos límites.
confirmación hacer firme o seguro; prueba convincente.
confirmar verificar o ratificar.
conflicto colisión de opiniones e intereses; una pelea o lucha; una lucha interna moral; estar en oposición.
confrontar encarar.
conjunción reunión; una palabra que conecta.

conjuntiva membrana mucosa que cubre los párpados y cubre la esclerótica anterior de la bola del ojo.
conminuto una fractura del hueso con muchos fragmentos.
conmiseración sentir o expresar simpatía o lástima.
connotación algo implicado o sugerido.
conocido el estado de conocer a una persona o sujeto.
consciencia pleno conocimiento de lo que está en la propia mente.
consecutivamente una serie de cosas que se siguen una a la otra.
consecutivo que sigue en orden, sucesivo.
conservar evitar daño o pérdida, mantener.
constipación una acción indolente del intestino; usualmente se refiere a una deposición excesivamente firme y dura que es difícil de expeler o a la falta de movimiento del intestino por un período de tiempo.
constreñir angostar; volverse más pequeño por contracción de un músculo del esfínter.
consuetudinario por costumbre, la conducta habitual bajo circunstancias similares.
contable persona que registra las cuentas y transacciones de un negocio.
contador aquel que mantiene, verifica e inspecciona los registros financieros de individuos o negocios.
contagioso pegadizo; capaz de ser transmitido por contacto.
contaminar poner en contacto con microorganismos.
contemporáneo que sucede o existe al mismo tiempo; una persona que vive al mismo tiempo que otra.
contenido la materia que hace parte de un campo de estudio; materia contenida.
contexto la parte de una declaración escrita o hablada que rodea una palabra o un pasaje en particular y que puede clarificar su significado.
contracciones la acción del músculo uterino durante la labor del parto.
contrachoque (en cardiología) un choque eléctrico y de corta duración, aplicado al área del corazón y que resulta en una despolarización total cardíaca.
contractura acortamiento permanente o contracción de un músculo.
contradicción el acto de contradecir; negar; afirmar lo contrario de.
contraer juntar, reducir en tamaño o acortar.
contraste mostrar diferencia; en radiología, se refiere al medio radiopaco que se usa para resaltar los órganos del cuerpo.
contributivo dar una parte; ayudar hacia un resultado.
controvertido abierto a la disputa; relativo a la discusión de puntos de vista opuestos.
convencional dejar de estar de moda; no espontáneo.
convulsión ataque de contracciones musculares involuntarias a menudo acompañadas de inconsciencia.
cooperar trabajar juntos.
coordinación un estado de ajuste o función armoniosa.
coordinador persona que se encarga del funcionamiento armónico de las personas o agentes involucrados en una tarea o proyecto con el fin de obtener los resultados esperados.
copia dura información impresa en una superficie sólida, como papel, en lugar de estar exhibida en una pantalla o guardada en un disco.
córnea la extensión transparente de la esclerótica que yace enfrente de la pupila del ojo.
coroide la envoltura vascular del ojo entre la esclerótica y la retina.
coronario se refiere a las arterias que rodean el músculo del corazón; también se refiere a un "ataque al corazón", que involucra las arterias coronarias.
corregir pruebas leer pruebas impresas con el objeto de corregir errores.
cortés educado, considerado y respetuoso en manera y acciones.
cortex la porción externa del riñón.
corticoesteroides hormonas usadas para tratar la inflamación.
coto un agrandamiento de la glándula tiroides.
coxis el hueso de la cola; los últimos cuatro huesos de la columna vertebral.
craneal perteneciente al cráneo o a la calavera.
cráneo la calavera; los ocho huesos de la cabeza que contienen el cerebro; generalmente se aplica a los 28 huesos de la cabeza y la cara.
creación de imágenes una representación o impresión visual producida por un lente, espejo, etc.
crenado dentado u ondulado, como la condición dentada de los corpúsculos sanguíneos.
cretinismo una condición congénita causada por la falta de la hormona tiroxina.
criminal involucrar o tener la naturaleza de un crimen.
criocirugía el uso de una sustancia a temperaturas bajo cero para destruir y/o extirpar tejido.
criptorquidismo incapacidad de los testículos de descender al escroto.
crisis el momento crucial de una enfermedad; un período muy crítico; una situación de emergencia.
criterio un estándar de crítica o juicio.
crítica un examen crítico de una cosa o situación, para determinar su naturaleza, valor o conformidad a estándares.
cromosoma estructuras dentro del núcleo de la célula que almacenan la información hereditaria.
crónico que continúa por un largo tiempo, que retorna; no agudo.
cronológico la organización de eventos, fechas, etc., en orden de ocurrencia.
cuadrante cuarta una de las cuatro partes del círculo. Este término se utiliza para identificar regiones en partes del cuerpo, como en el abdomen, por ejemplo.
cubículo un espacio dividido, pequeño.
cubierta cerrar completamente con algo que cubre; el contenedor de papel de una carta.
cúbito hueso largo del antebrazo que se encuentra entre el codo y la muñeca.
cuerpo lúteo el cuerpo amarillo que se desarrolla en la ruptura del folículo de De Graaf después de que el óvulo ha sido soltado.
cuerpo pineal glándula endocrina pequeña adjunta a la parte posterior del tercer ventrículo del cerebro.
cultivar formar y refinar; mejorar.
cumplimiento consentimiento; conformidad con requerimientos formales u oficiales.
curandero persona que pretende practicar medicina, pero que realmente no tiene mucho entrenamiento y usa métodos muy cuestionables.
cureta un instrumento para raspar material de una cavidad.
currículo un programa de estudio en un colegio o universidad.

D & C ver dilatación y curetaje.
DACUM un acrónimo en inglés que en español significa "diseño de currículo".
dar parte informar
datos hechos a partir de los cuales se infieren conclusiones.
deambular caminar, no estar confinado a una cama.
DEA ver Drug Enforcement Administration.
debilitado endeble; menoscabar la fortaleza de.
débito deducir, cobrar.
débridement limpiar o remover, como se hace con el tejido dañado alrededor de una herida.
dedicado comprometido a; apartar para uso especial.
deducciones deducir o restar; remover, quitar.
deducible una cantidad que debe pagarse antes de que el seguro pague.
deducir inferir, derivar por proceso lógico.
defecar expeler los excrementos o mover los intestinos.
defibrilación causar la terminación de la fibrilación; restaurar la acción normal.

deficiencia renal pérdida de función de los nefrones en el riñón.
déficit de pulso diferencia entre el pulso radial y el pulso apical.
delegación una persona o grupo de personas oficialmente elegidas o nombradas para representar a otro u otros; para empoderar.
delirium tremens un desorden síquico que involucra alucinaciones, tanto visuales como auditivas, encontrado en usuarios habituales del alcohol.
deltoide el músculo del hombro.
demografía el estudio de las estadísticas de población que conciernen nacimientos, matrimonios, muertes, enfermedades y otros indicadores.
dendrita una extensión de una célula nerviosa.
denominación una categoría o una clasificación de dinero.
denotar indicar, significar.
dentista un proveedor de salud licenciado que se ocupa de los dientes, de repararlos y reemplazarlos en la medida de lo necesario.
deposición testimonio dado bajo juramento.
depositar confiar dinero en un banco o en otra institución.
deprimido un estado de depresión, un período de desanimo; refiriéndose a una fractura, usualmente una fractura del cráneo donde los fragmentos de hueso son empujados (deprimidos) hacia dentro.
deprivación estar deprivado; sin; tener que arreglárselas sin algo o incapaz de usar.
dermatitis por contacto inflamación e irritación de la piel causada por contacto con una sustancia irritante.
dermatitis una inflamación de la piel, a menudo el resultado de un irritante.
dermatología el estudio de la piel y sus enfermedades.
dermatólogo un médico que se especializa en las enfermedades y los desórdenes de la piel.
dermis piel de verdad.
desalineamiento no alineado, no derecho.
desastre una ocurrencia que inflije destrucción y aflicción extendidas.
descendente se refiere a una porción del intestino grueso del pliegue esplénico al sigmoide.
desconcertante sorprendente, extraño, misterioso.
describir representar con un dibujo; retratar.
descripción un dibujo con palabras.
desempleado estado de no tener trabajo.
desensibilización el proceso de hacer a un individuo menos susceptible a los alérgenos.
deshidratación privación de agua de los tejidos natural o artificialmente.
designar senalar; indicar; nombrar.
desorden traumático acumulativo (DTA) lesión como resultado de movimientos repetitivos de una parte del cuerpo.
desplazamiento la transferencia de emociones acerca de una persona o situación a otra persona o situación.
despolarización atrial la excitación y contracción causada por el SA node al principio del ciclo cardíaco.
detección encontrar o descubrir.
detrimento dañino, lesionante.
devastar desperdiciar, saquear, destruir.
dextrosa un azúcar simple, también conocida como glucosa.
diabetes mellitus una enfermedad metabólica causada por la inhabilidad del cuerpo de usar carbohidratos.
diabético alguien afectado con la condición de diabetes.
diafanografía un tipo de transiluminación usado para examinar el seno, usando diferentes longitudes de onda luz y equipo especializado de creación de imágenes.
diaforesis sudor profuso.
diafragma el músculo de la respiración que separa al tórax del abdomen.
diagnóstico se refiere a las medidas que asisten en el reconocimiento de las enfermedades y los desórdenes del cuerpo.
diálisis remoción de los productos de la orina de la sangre por el paso de solutos a través de una membrana.
diario un registro de acontecimientos; periódico.
diarrea movimientos frecuentes de los intestinos, usualmente líquidos o semisólidos.
diartrosis una articulación movible; otra palabra para sinovial.
diástole la fase de relajación del latido cardíaco; el período de menor presión.
dictado palabras habladas; comunicación de voz grabada.
dietista el que es entrenado en dietética, que incluye nutrición, y a cargo de la dieta de una institución.
difamación calumniar o atacar la reputación de un individuo o grupo.
diferencial se refiere a la determinación del número de cada tipo de leucocitos en un milímetro cúbico de sangre.
difteria una enfermedad aguda e infecciosa caracterizada por la formación de una falsa membrana en cualquier superficie mucosa, generalmente en los pasajes del aire, interfiriendo con la respiración.
difusión un proceso por el cual gas, líquido o moléculas sólidas se distribuyen en forma uniforme a través de un medio.
difuso regado o esparcido.
digestión el proceso por el cual la comida es descompuesta mecánica y químicamente, en el tracto gastrointestinal y convertida en formas absorbibles.
digestivo perteneciente a la digestión.
digital perteneciente a o pareciéndose a un dedo de la mano o del pie, como a un examen usando uno o varios dedos.
dilatación y curetaje (D & C) dilatación de la cervix y raspado del forro interior del útero.
dilatar agrandar, expandir en tamaño; aumentar el tamaño de una apertura.
dióxido de carbón un gas encontrado en el aire, exhalado por todos los animales; la fórmula química es CO2.
diplomado estatus avanzado de práctica médica.
directiva plan general a alto nivel; principios de una organización.
disciplina autocontrol, conducta, sistema de reglas.
disciplinario diseñado para corregir o castigar faltas de conducta.
disco óptico punto ciego donde el nervio óptico sale de la retina.
discoide un tipo de lupus confinado a la piel; también llamado cutáneo.
discreción el uso de juicio, prudencia.
discrepancia inconsistencias; variaciones.
discreto poco llamativo, que no molesta.
discreto sabiamente cuidadoso, prudente.
disectar cortar en partes para examinar; separar.
diseño un plan de trabajo; esquema; trazado.
dislocar el desplazamiento de una parte; usualmente se refiere a un hueso temporalmente fuera de su posición normal en una articulación.
dismenorrea menstruación dolorosa.
disnea respiración difícil o trabajosa.
dispensa renuncia.
dispensar distribuir; repartir en porciones.
disposición el acto o la manera de poner en un orden particular; arreglar.
dispositivo intrauterino (DIU) un objeto insertado en el útero para impedir embarazos.
distal lo más alejado del centro, de la línea media o del tronco.
distender inflarse, estrecharse.
distintivo inconfundible, diferente de cualquier otra cosa.
distorsionar tergiversar; cambiar de su forma usual.
distribución de ganancias sistema a través del cual los empleados reciben una parte de las ganancias de la empresa.
distrofia atrofia progresiva o debilitamiento de una parte, como de los músculos.
disuria dolor al orinar; dificultad para orinar.
diversión el acto de divertir o poner a un lado.
diverticulitis inflamación de los divertículos.
divertículo un saco o vejiga en las paredes o un canal u órgano, particularmente el colon.

divulgar descubrir, revelar; hacer público; hacer conocido; revelar.
doctorado un grado de posgrado conferido después de completar extensos cursos, un proyecto individual de investigación y escribir una disertación; un Ph.D.
doctrina los principios de cualquiera rama del conocimiento; una creencia que se tiene o se enseña.
documental la presentación de hechos sin incluir aspectos de ficción.
doméstico no extranjero; privado.
dominante el más fuerte; el que prevalece, el primero o principal.
dorsalis pedis un punto de pulso palpable en el empeine del pie.
dorsal perteneciente a la espalda.
Drug Enforcement Administration (DEA por sus siglas en inglés) en español equivale a la Administración para el Cumplimiento de las Leyes Antidrogas; una división del gobierno federal responsable del cumplimiento de las leyes que regulan la distribución y venta de drogas.
DTA ver desorden traumático acumulativo.
ducha irrigación de la vagina.
duelo tristeza como resultado de la muerte de una persona querida.
duodeno el primer segmento del intestino delgado.
duración la cantidad de tiempo por la que algo continúa.
duramadre la membrana exterior que cubre el cerebro y la médula espinal.

ECG/EKG ver electrocardiograma.
ecocardiografía ondas de sonido de frecuencia ultra-alta dirigidas hacia el corazón para evaluar la función y la estructura del órgano.
ecos reflejo de sonido.
ectópico en posición anormal; en embarazo se refiere a cuando el embrión o feto está fuera del útero.
eczema enfermedad no contagiosa de la piel caracterizada por piel seca, roja, con picazón y escamosa.
edema pulmonar presencia de fluido intersticial en el tejido pulmonar.
edema una condición de los tejidos del cuerpo que contienen cantidades anormales de fluido, usualmente intercelular; puede ser local o general.
eficiencia la rata de energía utilizada para producir resultados.
ejemplificar mostrar con ejemplo.
elasticidad la habilidad de volver a la forma original después de haber sido estirado.
eléctrico cargado con electricidad; que funciona con electricidad.
electrocardiógrafo una máquina para obtener un registro gráfico de la actividad eléctrica del corazón.
electrocardiograma (ECG, EKG) un registro gráfico de las corrientes eléctricas generadas por el corazón; un trazado de la actividad del corazón.
electrocauterio un aparato usado para cauterizar el tejido con calor de una corriente de electricidad.
electrocoagulación coagulación de tejido por medio de una corriente eléctrica de alta frecuencia.
electrodo un instrumento con una punta o una superficie que transmite corriente al cuerpo del paciente.
electroencefalograma registro gráfico de las corrientes eléctricas generadas por el cerebro; un trazado de las ondas cerebrales.
electroimán un núcleo de hierro suave que se convierte en imán de manera temporal cuando una corriente eléctrica fluye a través de un alambre que lo rodea.
electrolito una sustancia que, en solución, conduce una corriente eléctrica.
electromiografía la inserción de agujas en músculos esqueléticos selectos con el propósito de registrar el tiempo de conducción de los nervios en relación con la contracción muscular.
electrónico operado por el uso de electrones.
electrón una partícula diminuuta de materia cargada con la cantidad más pequeña conocida de electricidad negativa; lo opuesto al protón.
elementos sustancias en su forma más simple; los bloques básicos de construcción de toda materia.
eliminar remover, descartar, excluir; también el paso de la orina desde la vejiga o las heces desde el intestino.
elipsis una marca o serie de marcas usadas en la escritura o en la impresión para indicar una omisión, especialmente de letras o palabras.
elite escogencia, superior, selecto.
emaciado convertirse en delgado anormalmente; la pérdida de demasiado peso.
embarazo período desde el momento de la concepción hasta el parto.
embolia pulmonar obstrucción en la arteria pulmonar o en una de sus ramas.
émbolo una masa que circula en un vaso sanguíneo; material extraño que obstruye un vaso sanguíneo.
embrión las primeras 8 semanas de desarrollo después de la fertilización.
emergencia un evento o situación inesperados que demandan acción inmediata.
emesis vomitar.
emético medicina que induce el vómito.
empatía tratar de identificar los sentimientos propios con los de otra persona.
empiema un exudado (pus) dentro del espacio pleural de la cavidad torácica.
enanismo una condición causada por el crecimiento hormonal inadecuado durante la niñez.
encéfalo la parte más grande del cerebro. Se divide en dos hemisferios con cuatro lóbulos en cada hemisferio.
encuentro encontrarse, inesperadamente o por suerte.
endocardio la membrana serosa que reviste el corazón.
endocervical el revestimiento del canal del cervix.
endocitosis un proceso celular para traer grandes moléculas de material al citoplasma de la célula.
endocrinología el estudio de las glándulas endocrinas o sin ductos de secreción interna.
endocrinólogo un médico que se especializa en las enfermedades y desórdenes del sistema endocrino.
endocrino una glándula que secreta directamente en el torrente sanguíneo.
endometrio la membrana mucosa que recubre el útero.
endosar aprobar, recomendar, patrocinar.
endoscopio un instrumento que consiste de un tubo y un sistema óptico para observar el interior de un órgano o cavidad.
endoso el acto de endosar; aprobar.
enema la instalación de fluido en el recto y colon.
enfermedad celíaca dilatación de los intestinos grueso y delgado.
enfermedad de Crohn una inflamación del tracto gastrointestinal con síntomas debilitantes.
enfermedad de Lyme enfermedad que se transmite a través de la picadura de una garrapata que se encuentra en los venados.
enfermedad de membrana hialina una condición que resulta del desarrollo incompleto del sistema respiratorio en bebés prematuros.
enfermedad del Legionario bronconeumonía aguda.
enfermedad policística condición caracterizada por muchos quistes.
enfermedad pulmonar crónica obstructiva (EPCO) un síndrome caracterizado por bronquitis crónica, asma y enfisema, o cualquier combinación de estas condiciones, que resulta en disnea, infecciones respiratorias frecuentes y deformaciones torácicas como resultado de dificultad para respirar.
enfermedad dolencia, achaque, indisposición.
enfermedad dolencia, afección.
enfermera practicante enfermera registrada (RN por sus siglas en inglés) con experiencia clínica avanzada y educación especializada en una rama particular de la medicina.
enfermera practicante licenciada (LPN por sus siglas en inglés) persona entrenada en técnicas básicas de enfermería, con el objeto de proporcionar cuidado directo al paciente bajo la

supervisión de una enfermera registrada (RN por sus siglas en inglés) o de un médico.
enfisema una enfermedad crónica del pulmón caracterizada por la sobredistención de los sacos alveolares y la inhabilidad para el intercambio de oxígeno y dióxido de carbono.
engullir llenar con sangre hasta el punto de congestión; devorar o absorber.
Enmienda al Mejoramiento del Labotarorio Clínico (EMLC) legislación relacionada con la operación de un laboratorio clínico.
enrejado un artefacto como barra, usualmente construído de metal pesado; una rejilla abierta para una puerta o ventana.
entidad una cosa que tiene realidad.
entusiasmo interés intenso; celo; pasión.
enucleación la extracción quirúrgica del ojo.
enumerar contar separadamente, uno por uno.
enunciar hablar o pronunciar claramente.
enzima una sustancia química compleja producida por el cuerpo, que se encuentra principalmente en los jugos digestivos, que actúa sobre las sustancias alimenticias para descomponerlas para ser absorbidas.
eosinófilo una célula blanca sanguínea o estructura celular que se mancha fácilmente con el ácido eosino; específicamente un leucocito eosinofílico.
EPCO ver enfermedad pulmonar crónica obstructiva.
epidemia que afecta a muchas personas al mismo tiempo.
epidermis la capa superior de la piel; literalmente sobre *la verdadera piel*.
epidídimo tubo enroscado que descansa en la superficie del testículo que lleva la esperma del testículo al vas deferens.
epífisis una porción del hueso que todavía no se ha osificado; las terminaciones cartilaginosas de los huesos largos que permiten el crecimiento.
epigástrico perteneciente al área del abdomen sobre el estómago.
epiglotis tapa cartilaginosa que se cierra sobre la laringe al tragar.
epilepsia una enfermedad crónica del sistema nervioso caracterizada por convulsiones y a menudo inconsciencia.
epinefrina una hormona producida por la médula adrenal.
episiotomía una incisión en el perineo para evitar rasgaduras durante el parto.
epistaxis sangrado nasal; hemorragia de la nariz.
epitelial perteneciente a un tipo de célula o tejido que forma la piel y las membranas mucosas del cuerpo.
equidad el valor de la propiedad más allá de la suma total que se debe.
equipo muscular par de músculos, uno flexiona mientras el otro extiende.
equivalente igual a en valor, tamaño o efecto.
eréctil se refiere al tejido que es capaz de erección, usualmente causado por vasocongestión.
ergonomía la ciencia aplicada que se preocupa por la naturaleza y las características de la gente en cuanto se relaciona con el diseño y actividades, con la intención de producir resultados efectivos y mayor seguridad.
eritema enrojecimiento disperso sobre la piel causado por una congestión capilar y por la dilatación de capilares superficiales.
eritrocito una célula roja de la sangre (CRS)
eritropoyesis la formación de corpúsculos de glóbulos rojos.
escanear observar rápida pero cuidadosamente.
escáner del cerebro prueba de diagnóstico en que se usa un escáner para medir los radioisótopos dentro del cerebro.
escaner ultrasónico procedimiento de inspección del cuerpo a través de ondas sonoras que producen una imagen de las estructuras internas del cuerpo en una pantalla.
escápula omóplato, paletilla.
escara costra, especialmente después de una cauterización.
esclera membrana de color blanco nacarado, gruesa, resistente y fibrosa, que constituye la capa externa del globo ocular.
escoliosis curvatura lateral de la columna vertebral.
esconder mantener secreto, retener, como información.
escorbuto enfermedad causada por la falta de frutas frescas, vegetales y vitamina C en la dieta.
escroto bolsa de piel que cubre los testículos y parte del tubo espermático.
esencial necesario; cuando se refiere a presión arterial, indica una elevación sin causa aparente.
esfigmomanómetro aparato que mide la presión sanguínea; también llamado manómetro.
esfínter cardíaco el músculo que rodea el esófago donde entra al estómago.
esfínter músculo circular que encoge una apertura.
esguince torcedura contundente de una articulación con ruptura parcial, o lesión de sus ligamentos.
esófago un tubo plegable de la faringe al estómago a través del cual pasa la comida y el agua que ingiere el cuerpo.
espasmo movimiento repentino involuntario o contracción muscular convulsiva.
especificado declarado en particular; mencionado en detalle.
específico dícese de algo idóneo para un propósito o fin particular; medicamento que obra especialmente en una enfermedad.
espécimen muestra; pedazo representativo del todo.
esperma gameto masculino o célula sexual masculina.
espermatozoon célula de la esperma.
espina bífida trastorno caracterizado por un defecto en la espina vertebral con o sin protrusión de la columna vertebral y de las meninges.
espinal relativo a la columna vertebral, al canal vertebral o a la espina dorsal.
espiral curva abierta que se aleja cada vez más de su centro.
espirómetro aparato que mide el volumen de aire inhalado y exhalado.
esponjoso estructura enrejada, como el tejido esponjoso del hueso.
espontáneo de propio movimiento; natural; no forzado.
espora cápsula dura formada por ciertas bacterias que le permiten resistir una exposición prolongada al calor.
esputo sustancia expectorada que contiene saliva y moco; usualmente se refiere al material que se escupe proveniente de los bronquios.
esqueletal relativo al esqueleto o a la estructura ósea; relativo también a los músculos adjuntos al esqueleto para permitir el movimiento.
estabilizar devolver a un estado constante; firme, seguro.
establecimiento un edificio; en situaciones médicas, un edificio para el cuidado y tratamiento de pacientes.
estandarización proceso a través del cual se logra la conformidad con unas normas establecidas; en un electrocardiograma, la marca de referencia establecida al comienzo de una curva.
estatura altura de una persona medida desde los pies hasta la cabeza.
estatutorio legalmente representado; promulgado.
estenosis estrechamiento o restricción de un conducto o apertura.
estéril sin organismos; que no produce.
esternocleidomastoideo músculo del pecho que surge del esternón y la parte interior de la clavícula.
esternón hueso plano del pecho con el cual se articulan las costillas.
estético relativo a los principios de belleza y gusto.
estetoscopio instrumento utilizado en auscultación para transmitir al oído los sonidos producidos por el cuerpo.
estilógrafo instrumento de tinta para escribir; instrumento que escribe en el electrocardiograma.
estimulante sustancia que aumenta la actividad en forma temporal.
estipulaciones términos de un acuerdo.

estómago órgano en forma de saco, dilatado y distensible, que forma parte del canal alimenticio y está localizado bajo el esófago y antes del intestino delgado.
estrabismo trastorno del ojo causado por un desequilibrio de los músculos oculares.
estratagema ardid, treta, engaño.
estresar ejercer presión; enfatizar; tensionar; agotamiento. Tópico: causar lesión en la piel.
estriado tipo de tejido muscular marcado por rayas o estrías.
estribo uno de los tres huesos del oído medio.
estrictura estrechamiento de una apertura, tubo o canal, como la uretra o el esófago.
estrógeno hormona femenina producida por los ovarios.
etapa de declinación volverse menos intenso, subsidir; período de tiempo en que los síntomas de la enfermedad empiezan a desaparecer.
éter un líquido incoloro utilizado para producir inconsciencia e insensibilidad al dolor.
ética estándares de conducta y juicio moral.
ético correcto, de acuerdo a los principios de la ética.
etiología el estudio de la causa de las enfermedades.
etiqueta reglas convencionales para un comportamiento correcto.
euforia sensación de bienestar, exaltación.
evacuación separación, remover, vaciar.
evacuar pasar orina desde la vejiga; vaciar, especialmente los intestinos.
evaluación estimación; juicio concerniendo la importancia, calidad, significado, o valor de una situación, persona o producto.
evocar provocar o llamar; invitar; sacar.
examen de conocimientos prácticos medida de los conocimientos y las aptitudes de una persona para la realización de un trabajo determinado. Medida de evaluación de la competencia de alguien.
examen de Tzanck inspección de tejido proveniente de la superficie inferior de una lesión para determinar el tipo de célula.
exceso gasto extraordinario; demasiada indulgencia, como con el alcohol o la comida.
excreción el proceso de expeler material del cuerpo.
exención librado o no responsable por algo a que otros están sometidos.
exento excluido, no responsable; exoneración del servicio o deber; privilegiado.
exfoliación viral período durante el cual un virus presenta mayor actividad y es más contagioso.
exfoliar desescamar tejido muerto.
exhalar expirar.
exocitosis un proceso celular que mueve materiales desde el interior de la célula hacia fuera.
exocrino una glándula que secreta sustancias a través de un ducto al cuerpo.
exoftalmia protrusión anormal del ojo.
exógeno que se origina fuera de un órgano o parte.
exorcismo el acto de expeler un espíritu maligno.
expectorar escupir, expeler moco o flema de la garganta o pulmones.
expediente una forma adecuada para lograr u obtener un propósito o un fin; de ventaja inmediata, conveniente.
expedir apurar.
expedir enviar; poner en circulación.
experiencia conocimiento que resulta de la observación y la práctica.
expiración la expulsión del aire de los pulmones al respirar.
explícito claramente y definidamente expresado; no ambiguo; sin espacio para preguntas.
exploración investigación preliminar o indicación de un procedimiento.
expresado dicho en palabras o por acción.
expresar decir; dar a saber por palabras o por acción.
extenso que tiene una amplia gama.
extensor el músculo de un grupo de músculos que extiende una parte, permitiendo que la articulación se enderezca.
externado una experiencia de empleo supervisada en un establecimiento de salud calificado como parte del currículo educativo.
extinguidor aparato para extinguir fuego.
extinguir apagar; terminar.
extracelular fuera de la célula.
extraer una sustancia destilada u obtenida de otra sustancia.
extraño cualquier cosa que no se encuentre normalmente en el sitio; usualmente se refiere a sucio, astillas, etc.
extremidad fantasma ilusión de que la extremidad aún existe, después de ser amputada.
extremidad se refiere a las partes terminales del cuerpo—los brazos, las piernas.
exudar pus; la recolección de material purulento en una cavidad.
eyaculación la expulsión de líquido seminal de la uretra masculina.

facsímil una copia idéntica.
factible posible; practicable.
factor Rh sustancia antígena en la sangre similar a los factores A y B que determinan el grupo sanguíneo; aparentemente, el factor Rh sólo está presente en los glóbulos rojos.
facultativo capaz de vivir bajo condiciones de temperatura o suministro de oxígeno variable; tener la capacidad de adaptarse a más de una condición, como una anerobia facultativa.
fagocito glóbulo blanco que absorbe y destruye antígenos.
fagocitosis ingestión y digestión de bacterias y otras partículas por parte de fagocitos.
falanges huesos de las manos y los pies.
falsificar imitar, especialmente falsear, como una firma.
familiar perteneciente a la misma familia.
faringe garganta; porción del canal alimentario entre la boca y el esófago.
farmaceuta profesional licenciado que prepara y dispensa medicinas.
farmacéutico relativo a las medicinas.
farmacología el estudio y la práctica de preparar y dispensar medicinas.
fascia una membrana fibrosa que cubre, sostiene y separa músculos; también puede unir la piel por debajo con tejido.
fatal que causa muerte.
febril perteneciente a una fiebre.
fecal perteneciente a heces.
feces desecho de los intestinos.
felicitaciones expresar placer; reconocimiento de un logro.
femoral pertenece a la arteria que yace adyacente al fémur.
fémur el hueso del muslo de la pierna.
fenestrado que tiene una ventana o apertura.
fenilalanina aminoácido de una proteína.
fenilcetonuria (PKU por sus siglas en inglés) trastorno genético que afecta el modo en que el cuerpo procesa las proteínas, probablemente debido al déficit de una encima. Se manifiesta por una deficiencia intelectual grave y trastornos neurológicos.
fenómeno de Raynaud síntoma del lupus caracterizado por dedos que se vuelven azules o blancos a causa del frío.
fertilización la impregnación del óvulo por el esperma; concepción.
fetal perteneciente a un feto, embarazo después del tercer mes.
feto un embrión después de la octava semana de gestación.
fibrilación la vibración de fibras musculares; inefectiva, acción rápida pero débil del corazón.
fibroide un tumor hecho de tejido fibroso y muscular.
fibrosis quística una condición de una enfermedad de tumores fibrosos que ha sufrido degeneración quística, acumulando fluido en los intersticios; también conocida como enfermedad fibroquística.
fibrosis formación anormal de tejido fibroso.
fiebre tifoidea enfermedad infecciosa aguda adquirida tras la ingestión de comida o agua contaminada.

filigrana marca transparente en el papel y los billetes de banco que sólo es visible cuando se ve en contraluz.
filo cualquier objeto afilado que puede cortar, pinchar, punzar, apuñalar o rasguñar la piel.
filtración el movimiento de solutes y agua a través de una membrana semipermeable como resultado de una fuerza, como la gravedad o la presión arterial.
fimosis estrechez de la "boca" del prepucio, piel que recubre el glande.
firma nombre de una persona en un papel.
fiscal de o perteneciente a las finanzas en general.
fisiatría rama de la medicina que estudia los trastornos y enfermedades de la mecánica del cuerpo, y sus formas de tratamiento. También conocida como Medicina Física y Rehabilitación.
físico relativo al cuerpo.
fisiología estudio de la función de las células, tejidos y órganos del cuerpo.
fisioterapista persona licenciada para examinar y ofrecer tratamiento a pacientes con deficiencias fisiológicas o anatómicas a través de ejercicios especiales, aplicación de terapias de frío o calor, utilización del sonar y otras técnicas.
fístula un pasaje anormal en forma de tubo de una cavidad normal o un absceso a una superficie libre.
fisura una úlcera, división, apertura o rasgadura en el tejido.
fisura longitudinal incisura profunda que divide los dos hemisferios del cerebro.
flato gas intestinal.
flatulencia la existencia de flato o gas intestinal.
flebitis inflamación de una vena.
flebotomista trabajador en el área de la salud con formación especial en la práctica de abrir venas para extraer muestra de sangre para ser analizadas en el laboratorio.
flexibilidad fácilmente doblado, que acata, cediendo a la persuasión.
flexionado doblado, como en una articulación.
flexor el músculo de un grupo de músculos que dobla una parte.
flora la vida de la planta en cuanto se distingue de la vida animal; la vida de las plantas que ocurre o se adapta para vivir en un entorno específico, como la flora de los intestinos.
fluido cerebroespinal el líquido que circula dentro de las meninges de la columna vertebral y ventrículos y meninges del cerebro.
fluoroscopio un aparato que consiste de una pantalla fluorescente junto con un tubo de rayos X que hace visibles las sombras de los objetos interpuestos entre la pantalla y el tubo.
foliculitis una infección de estafilococo del folículo piloso.
folículo grafiano el vesículo en el cual los huevos son madurados y que los libera cuando están maduro.
folículo un pequeño conducto o saco excretor o glándula tubular; un folículo piloso.
folleto un pequeño panfleto u opúsculo de información.
fondo la porción de un órgano más remota de su apertura; en el útero, la porción del útero que se encuentra arriba de las aperturas de las trompas de falopio.
formaldehído un gas incoloro y punzante, usado en su forma líquida para endurecer tejidos para estudios patológicos, o como germicida, desinfectante o preservativo, de acuerdo a la fortaleza de la solución.
formalina alcohol de madera que contiene 40% de formaldehído.
fortaleza resistencia valerosa.
forúnculo el término médico para un nacido.
fotocopia reproducción fotográfica de material escrito.
fotofobia sensitividad hacia la luz.
fovea centralis una depresión en la superficie posterior de la retina que es el lugar de la visión más aguda.
fractura la ruptura repentina de un hueso.
fraudulento caracterizado por hacer trampa y engaño; obtenido por medios deshonestos.
frecuencia la necesidad de vaciar orina a menudo, aunque usualmente sólo en una pequeña cantidad cada vez.
fricción la resistencia de una superficie al movimiento de otra superficie que frota sobre ella.
frontal anterior; el hueso de la frente; se refiere al plano dibujado por el lado del cuerpo de la cabeza a los pies.
fuera de línea se refiere a no estar en línea; falla de computador; tiempo en el que nada ha sido programado.
funcional práctico; que funciona; útil.
fundido derretido por el calor.
fusión espinal implantación quirúrgica de un fragmento óseo entre los espacios de dos o tres vértebras espinales para inmovilizarlas.

galvanómetro un instrumento que mide corriente por acción electromagnética.
gameto una célula germen; cualquier cuerpo reproductivo.
ganglión una masa de tejido nervioso que recibe y envía impulsos nerviosos.
gangrena una forma de necrosis; la putrefacción de tejidos suaves.
garante una persona que hace o da una garantía o promesa, a menudo pagar la deuda o la obligación del otro en el evento de incumplimiento.
garantía seguridad de que algo será hecho como está especificado; una promesa.
garantizar justificar; dar certeza definitiva del valor de algo; autorizar.
gastar disponer o usar, como de dinero o energía.
gástrico perteneciente al estómago.
gastrocnemio el músculo grande en la pantorrilla.
gastroenterología el estudio del estómago e intestinos y sus enfermedades.
gastroenterólogo un médico especializado en el cuidado de pacientes con enfermedades y desórdenes del tracto gastrointestinal.
gastrointestinal (GI) perteneciente al estómago y a los intestinos.
gastroscopia examen del estómago con un gastroscopio.
generar producir, como calor, ideas, poder.
genérico general; características de un género o grupo.
genético perteneciente a los genes.
genitales órganos sexuales externos.
genograma registro de la historia de la salud de la familia.
genucubital perteneciente a los codos y rodillas; la posición rodilla-codo.
gen una sustancia dentro del cromosoma que dicta la herencia.
genupectoral perteneciente a las rodillas y al pecho; la posición rodilla-pecho.
geriatría el estudio y tratamiento de las enfermedades de la vejez.
gerontólogo un médico especializado en el cuidado de los ancianos.
gestación período de desarrollo fetal intrauterino.
gigantismo una condición que resulta de la sobreproducción de la hormona de crecimiento durante la niñez.
ginecología (GIN) el estudio de las enfermedades de las mujeres, particularmente de los órganos de reproducción.
ginecólogo un médico especializado en el cuidado de las enfermedades y desórdenes de las mujeres, particularmente de los órganos genitales.
GIN ver ginecología.
glándula bulbouretral dos pequeñas glándulas, una en cada lado de la glándula de la próstata, que terminan en la uretra por medio de un ducto.
glándulas de Bartholin dos pequeñas glándulas mucosas, situadas una a cada lado de la apertura vaginal en la base de la labia minora.
glándulas mamarias senos.
glándulas salivares tres pares de glándulas que secretan la saliva, la cual inicia la digestión de la comida, y se encarga primordialmente de la descomposición de los almidones y los carbohidratos complejos.
glándulas sebáceas órganos de la piel que secretan sebo.
glaucoma una enfermedad del ojo caracterizada por aumento de presión intraocular.

glicosuria azúcar en la orina.
glomerulonefritis inflamación de los glomérulos del nefrón del riñón.
glomérulo un racimo microscópico de capilares dentro de la cápsula de Bowman del nefrón.
glucohemoglobina azúcar en la sangre.
glucosa un líquido incoloro o amarillo, espeso y almibarado obtenido de la hidrólisis incompleta del almidón; un azúcar simple.
glúteo máximo el músculo grande de los glúteos.
gónadas las cláusulas del sexo, los ovarios en la hembra y los testículos en el macho.
gonadotrópico relacionado con el estímulo de las gónadas.
gonadotropina coriónica una hormona que se encuentra en la orina de una mujer embarazada poco después de la concepción.
gonorrea una enfermedad venérea de los órganos reproductivos, que es altamente contagiosa por contacto directo.
goteo filtración incontrolada de orina de la vejiga.
gotica una gota muy pequeña.
graficar registro de observaciones, hallazgos subjetivos y objetivos, procedimientos diagnósticos, tratamientos y otros datos pertinentes en la carpeta del paciente.
gram-negativo bacteria que se tiñe de rosado con el proceso de teñido de Gram.
gram-positivo bacteria que se tiñe de morado con el proceso de teñido de Gram.
gremios asociaciones de personas interesadas en el mismo oficio o reunidas para protección mutua.
gripe influenza; una infección respiratoria o intestinal.
guayaco una solución usada para probar la presencia de sangre oculta en las heces.
guión manuscrito.

HCFA siglas en inglés para Health Care Financing Administration que en español significan Administración para la Financiación del Cuidado de la Salud.
heces materia fecal, movimientos intestinales.
hematocrito una expresión del volumen de las células rojas por unidad de sangre circulante.
hematología el estudio de la sangre y de sus enfermedades.
hematólogo un médico especializado en el cuidado de los pacientes con desórdenes y enfermedades de la sangre y de los órganos que la forman.
hematoma un tumor o hinchazón que contiene sangre.
hematuria sangre en la orina.
hemodiálisis un proceso en el cual la sangre es pasada a través de una membrana delgada y expuesta a una solución dializada para remover productos de desecho.
hemofilia condición hereditaria, trasmitida a través de cromosomas ligados al sexo de portadores femeninos; afecta a los hombres únicamente, causando inhabilidad de coagular la sangre.
hemófilo cepa bacterial que crece mejor en la hemoglobina.
hemoglobina la combinación de una proteína y un pigmento de hierro en los glóbulos rojos que atrae y lleva oxígeno en el cuerpo.
hemorragia descarga anormal de sangre tanto interna como externamente de vasos venosos, arteriales o capilares.
hemorroidectomía extirpación quirúrgica de tejido hemorroidal.
hemorroides venas varicosas del canal anal.
hemotórax sangre dentro del espacio pleural de la cavidad del pecho.
heparina una sustancia formada en el hígado que inhibe la coagulación de la sangre.
hepático perteneciente al hígado.
hepatitis inflamación del hígado.
hernia inguinal la presencia del intestino delgado en el canal inguinal.
hernia una proyección de una parte de su localización normal.
herniografía la reparación quirúrgica de una hernia.
herpes genital lesiones llenas de fluido en los genitales externos, que son contagiosos al contacto directo.
herpes simple el término médico para ampollas de fiebre, una aguda infección viral en la cara, la boca o la nariz.
herpes zóster un término médico para culebrilla, una infección viral aguda de los ganglios dorsales.
heterosexual atracción sexual hacia el sexo opuesto.
heterótrofo microorganismos que se alimentan de materia orgánica.
HHS siglas en inglés para Health and Human Services que en español significan Servicios Humanos y de Salud.
hiato pertenece a la herniación del estómago a través de una apertura o hiato.
hidrocele acumulación de fluido en el escroto.
hígado la glándula más grande del cuerpo, localizada en el cuadrante superior derecho del abdomen debajo del diafragma.
higiene el estudio de la salud y de la observancia de las reglas de la salud.
higienista el que provee servicios relacionados con la salud, tales como procedimientos dentales.
higienista dental proveedor de salud licenciado que está entrenado para tomar rayos X y efectuar tratamientos profilácticos en los dientes.
hilio el área retirada del riñón donde entran la uretra y los vasos sanguíneos.
himen un pliegue membranoso que cubre parcial o completamente la apertura vaginal.
hiperglicemia un aumento del azúcar en la sangre, como en diabetes.
hiperopia un defecto de la visión que hace que los objetos sólo puedan ser vistos cuando están muy lejos; hipermetropía.
hipersensitivo muy sensible; anormalmente sensible a un estímulo de cualquier clase.
hipertensión elevada presión arterial.
hipertermia temperatura más alta de lo normal.
hipertiroidismo una condición causada por excesiva secreción de las glándulas tiroides.
hipertónico que tiene una concentración más alta de sal que las encontradas en los glóbulos rojos.
hipertrofia benigna agrandamiento no maligno.
hiperventilación respiración excesivamente profunda y frecuente.
hipo el resultado del cierre espástico de la epiglotis y espasmo del diafragma.
hipoalergénico poco probable que cause una reacción alérgica.
hipocondríaco perteneciente a las regiones superiores y exteriores del abdomen bajo el tórax, también alguien con temor mórbido a la enfermedad, resultando en una preocupación anormal acerca de la propia salud.
hipocrático se refiere al juramento tomado por un doctor que lo obliga a observar el código de ética médica contenido en el juramento hecho por Hipócrates en el siglo IV.
hipogástrico se refiere a un área abdominal en el tercio medio bajo del abdomen.
hipoglicemia deficiencia de azúcar en la sangre.
hipotálamo una estructura del cerebro entre el cerebelo y el cerebro medio; yace bajo el tálamo.
hipotensión presión arterial anormalmente baja.
hipotermia temperatura corporal más baja de lo normal.
hipotiroidismo una condición causada por una marcada deficiencia de secreción tiroidea.
hipotónico que tiene una menor concentración de sal que la encontrada en un glóbulo rojo.
hipoxia falta de oxígeno.
histamina una sustancia presente normalmente en el cuerpo.
histerectomía extirpación quirúrgica del útero.
histeroscopia un procedimiento que usa el histeroscopio para ver el endometrio del útero.
histólogo (histotecnólogo) una persona comprometida al estudio de las estructuras microscópicas de los tejidos.

histoplasmosis una infección de hongos causada por un organismo que se encuentra en las heces de pájaros y murciélagos.
historia financiera los registros financieros pasados.
hoja de vida sumario de experiencia laboral.
holístico considera la totalidad o el alcance completo de una situación.
homeostasis el mantenimiento de una condición constante o estática de un entorno interno.
homólisis disolución; descomposición de los glóbulos rojos.
homosexual atracción sexual hacia el mismo sexo de uno mismo.
honestidad el estado de ser verdadero, confiable; genuino.
hongo un organismo vegetal y celular, que subsiste en materia orgánica, como bacteria o moho; la condición de una enfermedad que causa el crecimiento de lesiones de hongos en la superficie de la piel.
honrado de buena reputación.
horizontal no vertical; plano y parejo; nivelado; paralelo a la línea del horizonte.
hormona adrenocorticotrópica (HACT) una hormona secretada por el lóbulo anterior de la glándula pituitaria.
hormona una sustancia química secretada por un órgano o glándula.
hostilidad animadversión, enemistad.
hoyuelos una condición caracterizada por las hendiduras en la piel.
hpf siglas en inglés que significan high-power field; en español significa campo de alto poder; se refiere al lente del microscopio.
húmero el hueso largo del brazo.
humilde modesto, no pretensioso.
humor acuoso líquido aguado y transparente que circula entre la cámara anterior y posterior del ojo.
humor vítreo sustancia que ocupa el cuerpo vítreo del ojo detrás del lente.
humoral inmunidad mediada por anticuerpos.

I & D ver incisión y drenaje.
ictericia una descoloración amarillenta de la esclerótica y de la piel debida a la presencia de pigmento de bilis en la sangre.
identificación cualquier cosa por la cual una persona o una cosa puede ser identificada.
idiopático una enfermedad sin causa reconocible.
IHB/ihb influenza hemófila tipo B.
ilegible imposible de leer.
Íleo paralítico parálisis de la pared intestinal con síntomas de obstrucción aguda.
ileocecal la válvula entre el final del intestino delgado y el ciego.
íleon la última sección del intestino delgado.
ileostomía una apertura quirúrgica del íleon encima de la pared abdominal.
ilíaco el borde o la cresta del hueso pélvico.
ilícito impropio, ilegal; no permitido por la costumbre o la ley; fuera de la ley.
ilion el hueso de la cadera.
iluminar aclarar, esclarecer.
impacción una colección de heces endurecidas en el recto que no puede ser expulsada.
impactado se refiere a una fractura cuando los extremos rotos están apretujados.
impedimento obstaculizar; aquellos que están físicamente incapacitados o mentalmente retardados.
implante algo implantado en un tejido; un injerto; parte artificial.
implementación poner en práctica.
implemento una herramienta o instrumento para hacer algo; poner en práctica.
implicación envolvimiento, poner en contacto.
implicado insinuado, sugerido.
impotencia inhabilidad de un macho para obtener o mantener una erección.
improductivo que no logra resultados.
impulso una carga transmitida a través de ciertos tejidos, especialmente fibras nerviosas y músculos, que resultan en actividad fisiológica.
inapropiado no apropiado, fuera de lugar.
incapacidad una inhabilidad legal.
incas el yunque, el hueso de la mitad de los tres en el oído medio.
incinerar quemar, poner fuego.
incisión y drenaje (I & D) cortar con el propósito de proveer una salida para un material, usualmente una colección de pus.
incisión corte.
inclinado recostado o propender a.
incompetente no capaz; no calificado legalmente; deficiente.
incomprensible increíble, sin que pueda ser entendido por la mente.
incongruo falta de armonía o acuerdo.
inconscientemente involuntariamente, sin tener conocimiento, sin intención.
incontinente incapaz de controlar la vejiga o el intestino.
incrementos agrandar; cantidad de aumento; ganancia.
incubación el intervalo entre la exposición a la infección y la aparición del primer síntoma.
indemnización compensar por daño hecho o pérdida causada.
indigente necesitado, pobre, destituto.
indigestión dificultad en digerir comida.
inducción acción de causar o producir; generar.
inevitable ineludible, destinado a ocurrir.
infarto infiltración de partículas extrañas; en un vaso el material que causa coagulación e interferencia con la circulación.
infarto del miocardio (MI por sus siglas en inglés) obstrucción de la arteria coronaria que interrumpe el flujo de sangre hacia el músculo del corazón.
infeccioso capaz de producir infección; denota una enfermedad en el cuerpo causada por la presencia de gérmenes; tendencia a extenderse a otros.
inferior abajo, debajo.
infertilidad inhabilidad de lograr concepción.
infligir asestar, causar castigo.
influenza una enfermedad aguda caracterizada por fiebre, dolor, tos y síntomas generales del aparato respiratorio superior.
infrarojo perteneciente a esos rayos invisibles que se encuentran más allá del final rojo del espectro visible que tienen el penetrante efecto de calentar.
infusión infundir; introducción de una sustancia en una vena.
ingenio inteligencia; facultad para discurrir o inventar.
ingerir comer.
ingle la depresión entre la cadera y el tronco del cuerpo; la región inguinal.
inguinal se refiere a la región donde el muslo se une con el tronco del cuerpo; la ingle.
inhalar respirar hacia adentro.
inicial el primero; comienzo; la primera letra del nombre de cada persona.
iniciar comenzar algo; empezar.
iniciativa la acción de dar el primer paso; la habilidad de originar nuevas ideas.
injerto una parte construída.
inminente estar a la mano o a punto de suceder.
inmovilizar mantener fuera de acción o circulación; estacionario.
inmune protegido o exento de una enfermedad.
inmunización volverse inmune o el proceso de hacer a un paciente inmune.
inmunodeficiencia falta de los componentes necesarios para crear una respuesta inmune.
inmunoglobulina una molécula de proteína grande que ayuda a la respuesta inmune.
inmunológico perteneciente a la inmunología.
inmunosuprimido una condición en la cual el sistema inmune ha sido vencido y no puede funcionar adecuadamente.
innato congénito; inherente.
inorgánico no viviente; ocurre en la naturaleza de forma independiente de las cosas vivas.
inseminar impregnar con semen.
inserción el lugar donde un músculo se une al hueso que mueve.
insidioso oculto, no aparente.
insignificante pequeño, de poco valor; mezquino.
insignificante no importante; mezquino; de poco o ningún valor.

insomnio incapacidad anormal de dormir.
inspeccionar examinar de cerca.
inspección la primera parte de un examen físico; observación cercana.
inspiración respirar hacia adentro, inhalar.
instituir originar como una costumbre.
insuficiencia cardíaca congestiva una condición compleja de una acción cardíaca inadecuada con retención de líquidos de tejidos; puede ser una falla del lado derecho, izquierdo, o de ambos.
insuficiente no tanto como se necesita.
insulina una hormona secretada por las isletas de Langerhans en el páncreas.
intacto no roto, no dañado.
intangible lo que no puede ser tocado, fácilmente definido o captado.
integridad solidez de carácter; honestidad en particular.
integumentario la piel; una cubierta.
intelectualización el empleo del racionamiento para evitar confrontaciones o situaciones de estrés.
inteligencia la habilidad de aprender o entender.
interacción actuar el uno con el otro.
interceder mediar, rogar por otro.
intercostal entre las costillas.
interferencia confusión de las señales deseadas causada por señales indeseadas, como en artefactos en un ECG.
interferón una lymphokina que ayuda a regular las actividades de los macrófagos y células destructoras naturales.
interjección parte del habla; una exclamación.
interleukina una sustancia mensajera entre leucocitos.
intermedio en el medio.
intermitente que para y arranca de nuevo a intervalos.
internado etapa después de la graduación en que se practica la profesión.
internista un médico especializado en el cuidado de pacientes con enfermedades internas.
interpersonal entre personas.
interpretar explicar, traducir; determinar el significado.
intervalo tiempo entre eventos; espacio.
intervención tomar acción para modificar, impedir o cambiar un efecto.
intervertebral entre las vértebras.
intestinal se refiere a los intestinos.
intestino el canal alimentario que se extiende desde el píloro del estómago al ano.
intimidación producir miedo; impedir con amenazas.
intimidar producir miedo, asustar.
intoxicación condición causada por la exageración en el consumo de bebidas alcohólicas.
intracelular dentro de la célula.
intradermal dentro de la piel.
intramuscular dentro del músculo.
intraocular dentro del ojo.
intravenoso insertar en la vena.
intrincado complicado, complejo, entretejido elaboradamente.
intubación la inserción de un tubo en la laringe para la entrada de aire.
intuición el conocimiento o aprendizaje inmediato de algo sin el uso consciente del razonamiento.
inunción el proceso de administrar drogas a través de la piel.
invasivo método de diagnóstico que involucra la entrada en el tejido vivo.
inventario una lista pormenorizada de productos en existencia.
involuntario independiente o aun en contra de la voluntad o escogencia.
iris el tejido coloreado, contráctil que rodea la pupila del ojo.
irracional sin el poder de la razón; sin sentido.
irreconciliable situación en la que no se puede llegar a un acuerdo.
irrelevante no pertinente.
irreparable dañado más allá de la posibilidad de ser reparado.
ishahara se refiere a una prueba del ojo para determinar visión de color.
isletas de Langerhans ramos de células en el páncreas.
isotónico que tiene la misma concentración de sal que se encuentra en un glóbulo rojo.
isquemia anemia temporal y localizada causada por la obstrucción de la circulación de una parte.
isquión porción posterior e inferior del hueso de la cadera.

Jaeger un sistema para medir la agudeza de la visión cercana.
juanete una bursa con formación callosa.
juicio una decisión; la habilidad de tomar las decisiones correctas.

KUB (por sus siglas en inglés) riñones, uréteres y vejiga. Relativo a un estudio radiológico.

L&A luz y acomodación.
labia mayor los dos pliegues grandes de tejido adiposo que se encuentran a cada lado de la vulva; genitales externos.
labia menor los dos pliegues mucocutáneos de membrana dentro de la labia mayor.
laboratorio espacio o edificio en el cual se conducen análisis o experimentos científicos.
laceración cortadura o herida.
lagrimal (o lacrimal) relativo a las lágrimas; las glándulas y ductos que secretan las lágrimas.
Lamaze programa o método que prepara a la mujer embarazada para el momento del parto.
laminectomía extirpación de una porción del arco posterior vertebral.
lanceta instrumento afilado y punteado utilizado para perforar la piel con el objeto de obtener una muestra de sangre a nivel capilar.
laringe caja vocal. Parte superior de la tráquea cuyos cartílagos sostienen las cuerdas vocales.
laríngeo relativo a la laringe.
lateral relativo al lado o costado.
lattissimus dorsi el músculo grande de la espalda.
laxativo sustancia que induce la evacuación de los intestinos.
legible fácil de leer.
lengua órgano muscular de la boca que ayuda en la producción de palabras, contiene las papilas gustativas y asiste en la acción de tragar.
lente parte del ojo que refracta las imágenes en la retina.
lesión herida; área circunscrita de tejido patológicamente alterado.
letal mortal; capaz de causar la muerte.
letra script fuente diseñada para parecer escrita a mano.
leucemia enfermedad caracterizada por un exceso de glóbulos blancos; existe en forma linfática y mielógena; es a menudo fatal, especialmente en adultos.
leucocito glóbulo blanco.
liaison término francés que significa intercomunicación entre dos entidades.
libro de contabilidad documento que contiene el registro de los créditos y débitos de una empresa.
licencia permiso legal para ejecutar una actividad determinada.
liendre huevo del piojo o de otro insecto parasítico.
ligado al cromosoma X conectado al cromosoma sexual de la célula; una característica del cromosoma sexual.
ligadura proceso a través del cual se amarra o se aprieta.
ligamento tejido fibroso que conecta los huesos entre sí.
limitar restringir, confinar, circunscribir.
línea de base la información inicial en la que se basan datos adicionales.
linfa fluido que se forma al interior de los espacios entre los tejidos y que circula a través del cuerpo.
linfocito tipo de glóbulo blanco.
lisosoma organelo que se encuentra al interior del citoplasma en la célula.
lista de honorarios listado de cobros permitidos.
litotomía posición para examinar al paciente en la cual el paciente se acuesta de espaldas con los muslos flexionados sobre el abdomen y las piernas flexionadas sobre los muslos.
litotripsia destrucción de cálculos renales.
litro medida de capacidad equivalente a 1,000 ml o aproximadamente un cuarto.
longevidad larga duración de vida.

lordosis curvatura anterior anormal de la espina lumbar.
lubb dupp sonidos cardiacos normales.
lumbar relativo a la espalda, específicamente a las cinco vértebras sobre el sacro.
lumen espacio al interior de una arteria, una vena o un vaso capilar; espacio al interior de un tubo.
lupus eritomatoso enfermedad autoinmune crónica que causa cambios en el sistema inmunológico.
luteinización efecto hormonal que causa ovulación y progesterona en la mujer, y producción de esperma y testosterona en el hombre.

macrófago célula fagocítica que destruye antígenos.
mácula parche en la piel descolorado pero sin elevaciones o depresiones.
maduración relativo a las fases de desarrollo celular.
madurez fase de mayor desarrollo.
magnético que tiene las propiedades de atracción del imán.
magnificar hacer aparecer algo más grande de lo que es realmente.
malestar sensación de incomodidad.
maligno bulto o tumor canceroso.
malinger fingir enfermedad para escapar una situación u obligación.
malleus el más grande de los tres huesos del oído medio, también llamado "martillo".
mamografía rayos X de los senos.
mandato orden de mando; instrucción.
manifestación acción de revelar o de exponer.
mantenimiento actividad de preservar; acciones para conservar algo en condición apropiada.
marcapasos nodo sinoatrial del corazón; también, aparato eléctrico que provoca en forma artificial la contracción del corazón cuando ésta no puede efectuarse normalmente.
marginal cercano al límite más bajo de aceptación.
masa multitud; grupo grande de personas.
mastectomía operación quirúrgica para extirpar un seno.
matasellos cancelación fechada de una estampilla por la oficina de correos; también identifica la dirección de la oficina de correos.
matriz formato para establecer horarios para citas.
meato urinario apertura a través de la cual la orina es evacuada del cuerpo.
mecánica corporal el uso de posicionamiento adecuado del cuerpo cuando se mueve o cuando se levantan objetos para evitar lesiones.
mecánico relativo a maquinaria.
mediado por anticuerpos inmunidad humoral; cuando los anticuerpos y complementos trabajan juntos para destruir los antígenos.
medial relativo al medio o a la línea central.
Medicaid programa de salud del gobierno.
Medicaire programa de salud a nivel federal destinado a pagar ciertos tratamientos de salud para pacientes de edad avanzada.
medicina deportiva rama de la medicina que estudia la manera de prevenir y tratar lesiones causadas por la práctica del deporte.
medicina nuclear rama de la medicina que utiliza radionúclidos en el diagnóstico y tratamiento de enfermedades.
medicina ocupacional rama de la medicina que estudia el diagnóstico y tratamiento de enfermedades ocurridas en el trabajo.
médico doctor entrenado en la práctica de la Medicina.
médico asistente persona entrenada en ciertos aspectos de la práctica de la medicina con el objeto de proporcionar ayuda al médico.
médico de familia el que cuida los pacientes de todas las edades y todas las condiciones que no requieren especialización.
Medigap relativo a situaciones no cubiertas por Medicare.
médula tejido suave que se encuentra en el hueco de los huesos largos.
médula renal sección interna del riñón.
medulla oblongata porción alargada de la médula espinal; la porción más baja del tronco encefálico.
melanina pigmento que da color a la piel, cabello y ojos.
melanocito células que producen el pigmento de la piel, melanina.
membrana capa de tejido muy delgada, suave y doblable que cubre un tubo, cavidad, órgano o estructura.
membrana celular estructura que rodea y encierra la célula.
membrana timpánica tímpano.
menarquía primer período menstrual.
meninges membranas que cubren el cerebro y la médula espinal.
meningitis inflamación de las meninges.
menisco concavidad que forma la superficie de un líquido contenido dentro de un tubo o cilindro.
menopausia cesación permanente de la menstruación.
menor emancipado que ya no está bajo el cuidado, la custodia o supervisión de un padre o guardián.
menorragia flujo menstrual excesivo; hemorragia.
menstruar descargar fluido sanguíneo del útero en forma periódica.
mensura medida, medición.
mercurio metal líquido utilizado en aparatos de medida tales como termómetros y esfigmomanómetros. Su símbolo químico es el Hg.
mérito lo que hace digna de elogio o recompensa a una persona; excelencia.
mesenterio doblez peritoneal que conecta al intestino con la pared abdominal posterior.
metabolismo transformaciones sucesivas a las que se somete una sustancia desde el momento en que entra en el cuerpo hasta que dicha sustancia o sus desechos son excretados, y a través de las cuales el cuerpo se nutre y adquiere la energía para su subsistencia.
metacarpos los cinco huesos de la mano que se encuentran entre la muñeca y las falanges.
metástasis movimiento de células cancerosas de una parte del cuerpo a otra.
metatarsos los cinco huesos de los pies que se encuentran entre el empeine y las falanges.
metódico sistemático, que sigue un plan o método.
MI—Índice de maduración (por sus siglas en inglés) medida de maduración celular.
MI infarto del miocardio (por sus siglas en inglés).
microbiano relativo a los microbios.
microficha hoja de microfilme con la capacidad de almacenar una cantidad considerable de información en forma reducida.
microorganismo cuerpo viviente microscópico que no se puede percibir a simple vista.
microscópico visible sólo a través de un microscopio.
micturación acción de orinar.
mielina sustancia grasosa que envuelva las fibras nerviosas.
mielografía examen de la médula espinal a través de rayos X con inyección de un material radio-opaco.
miembros relativo a los brazos y/o las piernas.
migraña dolor de cabeza severo con síntomas característicos.
mineralocorticoide hormona de la corteza adrenal que influye en el metabolismo del sodio y del potasio y regula el fluido del cuerpo y los electrolitos.
minuto medida de tiempo equivalente a 60 segundos.
miocardio capa muscular del corazón.
miometrio estructura muscular del útero.
miopía defecto de la vista que sólo permite ver los objetos próximos al ojo.
mitocondria organelo que se encuentra en el citoplasma de la célula.
mitosis división celular.
mitral válvula en el corazón localizada entre las cámaras del lado izquierdo.
mixedema condición que resulta de la hipofunción de la glándula tiroidea.

modificador que cambia; que limita el significado.
modificar cambiar la forma o cualidad de alguna cosa; alterar ligeramente.
moneda cualquiera forma de dinero.
monilia familia de hongos parásitos o mohos.
monitor fetal un dispositivo para tener acceso al latido del corazón fetal.
monitor Holter un aparato que adhiere electrodos al pecho de un paciente con el propósito de obtener el trazado de un electrocardiograma de 24 horas en una grabadora portátil.
monitorear observar.
monocitos células mononucleares que abandonan el sistema sanguíneo y entran en los tejidos para convertirse en macrófagos.
monoclonal célula híbrida producida en laboratorio capaz de producir anticuerpos.
monocular que posee un solo ojo, como el microscopio.
monograma registro obtenido por ultrasonido.
monótono tono único; invariable, aburrido, rutinario.
monóxido de carbón un gas venenoso incoloro, inodoro, causado por la combustión incompleta del carbón.
mons pubis relleno de tejido graso y piel gruesa que recubre el symphisis pubis en la mujer.
moralidad virtud.
mores acciones que, a través del acatamiento general, adquieren la fuerza de la ley.
morfología rama de la biología que estudia la forma y estructura de los organismos.
motor relativo a los nervios que permiten que el cuerpo responda a estímulos.
motricidad cualidad del movimiento; de fácil movimiento.
MRI resonancia magnética (por sus siglas en inglés). Examen de diagnóstico que utiliza ondas magnéticas para visualizar las estructuras internas del cuerpo.
mucosa perteneciente a la membrana mucosa.
mudar dejar una cosa como, por ejemplo, tejido muerto.
MUGA (multiple-gated acquisition scan) por sus siglas en inglés, examen de diagnóstico para evaluar la condición del miocardio del corazón.
muleta un bastón con una pieza atravesada en la parte superior para ponerlo bajo el brazo de la persona lisiada.
multicanal relativo a la capacidad del equipo de ECG de procesar impulsos provenientes de múltiples procedencias.
murmuro soplo suave o sonido áspero que se escucha durante la auscultación del corazón.
muscular relativo a los músculos.
músculo tipo de tejido compuesto de células contráctiles o fibras que generan el movimiento del cuerpo.
musculoesqueletal relativo a los sistemas muscular y esqueletal.
músculos papilares grupos de músculos que van agarrados desde las paredes de los ventrículos del corazón hasta la parte inferior de las válvulas del corazón y cuya función es abrir las válvulas durante la fase de relajación del latido.
mutación cambio en una característica heredada; cambio celular causado por una influencia.

narcolepsia deseo irresistible e incontrolable de dormir a cualquier hora.
narcótico droga capaz de producir el sueño y la relajación muscular, o capaz de inducir inconsciencia e incluso la muerte, dependiendo de la dosis.
nasal relativo a la nariz.
náusea ganas de vomitar.
nefrología el estudio del riñón y de sus enfermedades.
nefrólogo médico especializado en las enfermedades y los trastornos del riñón.
nefrón unidad estructural y funcional del riñón.
negación el rechazo a creer o a aceptar; desconocer.
negar no admitir la existencia o veracidad de algo.
negligente descuidado; que no pone todo el cuidado y aplicación que debiera.
negociable asunto capaz de ser discutido y sus términos acordados.
neonato infante recién nacido.
neoplástico nueva formación de tejido anormal (cancerosa).
nervio grupo de tejidos nerviosos que conducen la sensibilidad y el movimiento.
nervosa pérdida de apetito sin conexión con una enfermedad; parte de una psicosis.
neto valor restante después de deducir los gastos y descuentos; beneficios y ganancias; excluyente de deducciones; total; entero.
neumoconiosis condición respiratoria causada por la inhalación de partículas de polvo provenientes de labores como la minería o el trabajo con piedra.
neumoencefalografía examen por rayos X de los ventrículos y espacios subaracnoides del cerebro después de extraer fluido cerebroespinal e inyectar aire o gas a través de una puntura lumbar.
neumonía inflamación del pulmón causada primordialmente por microbios, irritantes químicos, polvo vegetal o alergias.
neumotórax colección de aire o gas en la cavidad pleural que desplaza el tejido pulmonar.
neurilema capa membranosa delgada que recubre la fibra nerviosa.
neurocirugía procedimientos quirúrgicos efectuados en el sistema nervioso.
neurología estudio del sistema nervioso y de sus enfermedades.
neurólogo médico especializado en las enfermedades y los trastornos del sistema nervioso.
neurona internuncial neuronas que conectan las neuronas sensoriales a las motoras.
neurona célula nerviosa.
neutrófilo glóbulo blanco granulado.
nicotina alcaloide venenoso extraído de las hojas de tabaco.
nicturia necesidad de evacuar durante la noche.
no estructurado sin orden.
no invasivo método de diagnóstico que no requiere penetrar el tejido corporal.
no patógeno organismo que no produce enfermedad.
nodo nudo, protuberancia o inflamación.
nódulo AV nódulo auriculoventricular; principio del nodo de His en la aurícula derecha/atrio; fibras nerviosas responsables de la contracción de los ventrículos.
nomenclatura sistema de nombres científicos o técnicos.
nominal demasiado pequeño para ser considerado, o cantidad muy pequeña.
nomograma representación—a través de gráficos, diagramas, cuadros o tablas—de las relaciones entre variables numéricas.
non compos mentis término legal general para todas las formas de enfermedad mental.
nonchalant término francés que alude a una persona indiferente o despreocupada.
norepinefrina hormona secretada por la médula adrenal en respuesta a una estimulación simpática.
norma de cumpleaños manera de identificar la responsabilidad primaria en caso de cobertura de seguros.
nuclear relativo al núcleo de un átomo.
núcleo cuerpo vital en el protoplasma de la célula.
nucleolo estructura que se encuentra en el interior del núcleo de la célula.
numérico denota un número o sistema de números.
nutrición relativo al material comestible, comida, cosas que nutren.
nutricionista miembro del equipo de profesionales de la salud que estudia y aplica los principios de la ciencia de la nutrición.
nutrir alimentar, cuidar.

O. D. por sus siglas en latín (oculus dexter), u ojo derecho.
O. S. por sus siglas en latín (oculus sinister), u ojo izquierdo; también, boca o apertura.
O. U. por sus siglas en latín (oculus uterque), o cada ojo.

objetivo fin hacia el cual se dirige la acción; del síntoma de una enfermedad, perceptible por personas diferentes de la afectada; en un microscopio, lente o serie de lentes.
obligar atar legal o moralmente.
obliterar borrar, no dejar trazo alguno; destruir.
observante quien percibe rápidamente; agudo observador.
obsoleto anticuado; caído en desuso.
obstetra médico especializado en el cuidado y tratamiento de mujeres durante el embarazo y parto.
obstetricia rama de la medicina que se encarga del cuidado y tratamiento de mujeres durante el embarazo y parto.
obturador cualquier cosa que obstruye o cierra una cavidad o apertura; relativo a la porción interna de un instrumento de examen que facilita la introducción del instrumento dentro del cuerpo y es después retirada, permitiendo la visualización del área interna.
occipital perteneciente a la parte posterior de la cabeza, el lóbulo posterior del cerebro.
ocluir cerrar, obstruir.
oculto oscuro, escondido.
oficinista de admisiones una persona que procesa la información y los formularios para un paciente que va a ingresar al establecimiento de salud.
oftalmología el estudio del ojo y de sus enfermedades y trastornos.
oftalmólogo médico especializado en las enfermedades y trastornos del ojo.
ojeada una mirada o visión rápida.
olfativo perteneciente al sentido del olfato.
oliguria producción escasa de orina.
oncogén gene en la célula de un tumor.
oncología rama de la medicina que estudia tumores, usualmente malignos.
oportunista persona que aprovecha la oportunidad o toma ventaja de una situación.
oposición actividad en contra de algo, resistencia.
óptico relativo al ojo o a la visión.
optómetra técnico que mide el poder refractivo del ojo y, de ser necesario, prescribe una fórmula correctiva de cualquier defecto visual.
oral relativo a la boca.
orbital relativo a la cavidad del cráneo donde está ubicado el ojo.
organelo estructura funcional al interior del citoplasma de la célula.
orgánico perteneciente a o derivado de formas de vida animal o vegetal.
órgano parte del cuerpo construida a partir de diferentes tipos de tejidos para desempeñar una función necesaria para la vida.
órgano de Corti aparato acústico terminal en la cóclea del oído interno.
origen principio o procedencia de algo.
orina fluido secretado de la sangre por los riñones, depositado en la vejiga, y evacuado del cuerpo a través de la orinación.
orinación acto de orinar.
ortopedia rama de la medicina que estudia la estructura y función de huesos y músculos.
ortopedista médico que corrige las deformidades y trata enfermedades y trastornos de los huesos, las articulaciones y la columna vertebral.
ortopnea condición respiratoria en la cual el paciente sólo puede respirar cuando está sentado o parado.
ortostático relativo a la posición erecta; parado.
osciloscopio instrumento de medida electrónico para la representación gráfica de variaciones eléctricas.
óseo relativo a los huesos.
OSHA (Occupational Safety and Health Administration) organización gubernamental encargada de la seguridad y la salud ocupacional.
osmosis proceso de difusión de agua o de otro solvente a través de una membrana permeable.
osteopatía cualquier enfermedad de los huesos; relativo a la escuela de medicina basada en la creencia según la cual el fragmento óseo del cuerpo determina en gran medida las relaciones estructurales de sus tejidos.
osteoporosis condición causado por la reducción del calcio en los huesos.
OTC por sus siglas en inglés "over the counter" se refiere a los medicamentos que se pueden adquirir sin prescripción médica.
otitis inflamación del oído; puede referirse al oído externo, medio o interno.
otorrinolaringología rama de la medicina que estudia las enfermedades y trastornos del oído, la nariz y la laringe.
otorrinolaringólogo médico especializado en las enfermedades y trastornos del oído, la nariz y la garganta.
otosclerosis condición caracterizada por la pérdida progresiva de la audición. El hueso esponjoso que rodea el laberinto del oído y los huesillos de éste van perdiendo progresivamente la facultad de conducir el sonido.
ovario gónada femenina encargada de producir las hormonas que desarrollan y mantienen las características sexuales de la mujer.
"over the counter" (OTC, por sus siglas en inglés) se refiere a los medicamentos que se pueden adquirir sin prescripción médica.
ovulación proceso de formación y de su maduración de un folículo ovárico que culmina en la emisión de un óvulo.
ovum huevo, el gameto o célula reproductora femenina.
oxalato sal de ácido oxálico.
oxigenar combinar con oxígeno o proveer oxígeno.
oxígeno gas incoloro, inodoro y sin sabor que se encuentra en el aire. Su símbolo químico es O2.

paciencia esperar con tranquilidad, soportar con resignación.
pagaré que contiene la promesa de pagar.
palidez falta de color.
palpar sentir, examinar con el tacto.
páncreas órgano que secreta insulina y jugos digestivos.
pancreatitis inflamación del páncreas.
pandémico relativo a la extensión de una enfermedad contagiosa a muchas regiones o a una región extensa.
pantomima expresarse por medio de gestos y movimientos.
Papanicolau (Pap por sus siglas en inglés) examen que detecta células cancerosas en la mucosa de un órgano.
papelería materiales para escribir, especialmente papel y sobres.
paperas enfermedad contagiosa caracterizada por la inflamación de la glándula parótida y otras glándulas salivares.
papila pequeñas protuberancias o elevaciones de la piel o de las membranas mucosas, tales como las papilas gustativas que se encuentran en la lengua.
pápula área roja y elevada en la piel; elevación evanescente de la piel, más o menos redonda, blanca en el centro con un borde rojo pálido, acompañada de comezón.
par igual. Usualmente se refiere a alguien con un status o una posición similar.
parabasal al lado a cerca de la base o a la parte inferior.
paramédico profesional de la salud que proporciona cuidado médico de emergencia y cuidado de apoyo.
parámetro cantidad que se determina en forma arbitraria con el objeto de establecer comparaciones.
parasimpático división del sistema nervioso autónomo.
parásito organismo que vive en o sobre otro organismo, a expensas de ese otro organismo.
paratiroides glándulas endocrinas situadas cerca de la glándula tiroides.
parenteral que no se administra a través de la boca.
parietal porción central de la corteza cerebral localizada a cada lado del cerebro.
paroxístico ataque repentino de una enfermedad; ataque de dolor agudo, ataque de tos, ataque de risa, ataque de pasión.
paso manera de caminar.
patela rótula.
patofisiología estudio de los mecanismos mediante los cuales ocurre una enfermedad, las respuestas del cuerpo al proceso de la enfermedad, y los efectos de ambos en una función normal.

patógeno cualquier microorganismo o sustancia capaz de producir una enfermedad.
patología estudio de la naturaleza y la causa de las enfermedades.
patológico condición causada por una enfermedad.
patólogo médico especializado en la interpretación y diagnóstico de cambios generados por una enfermedad determinada en tejidos y fluidos corporales.
pectoral mayor el músculo principal de la pared del pecho.
pediatra médico especializado en las enfermedades y los trastornos de la infancia.
pediatría rama de la medicina que proporciona cuidad y tratamiento a los niños que sufren enfermedades.
pediculosis enfermedad de la piel producida por el rascamiento motivado por la infestación de piojos.
peligro biológico cualquier material que ha estado en contacto con un fluido corporal y que es potencialmente capaz de transmitir una enfermedad.
peligroso arriesgado, de cuidado.
pélvico relativo a la pelvis.
pene órgano sexual externo masculino.
péptico relativo a la digestión; también se refiere a una úlcera en el tracto digestivo superior.
per cápita expresión latina que significa por cabeza. Se aplica a lo que corresponde por persona.
percentil cualquier valor en una serie que divide la distribución de sus miembros en 100 grupos de igual frecuencia.
percepción adquisición de consciencia o de conocimiento a través de los sentidos; recepción de impresiones.
percibir adquirir consciencia de una sensación; comprender.
percusión acción de golpear el cuerpo suave pero puntualmente para determinar la posición, el tamaño y la consistencia de una estructura subyacente.
perfusión acción de verter o hacer correr un líquido.
pericardio saco membranoso que recubre el corazón.
pericarditis inflamación del pericardio, la cubierta del corazón.
pericia un conocimiento especial o una habilidad.
periférico relativo a una porción del sistema nervioso; aparato conectado a un computador.
perineo región entre la vagina y el ano en la mujer, o la región entre el escroto y el ano en el hombre.
periódico relativo a una acción que ocurre una y otra vez, a intervalos regulares.
periostio membrana fibrosa que recubre la superficie del hueso excepto las las articulaciones que están cubiertas por cartílago.
peristalsis serie de contracciones musculares normales, coordinadas y rítmicas que ocurren automáticamente para hacer pasar los alimentos a través del tracto digestivo, y para hacer pasar los líquidos por el sistema urinario.
peritoneal relativo al peritoneo.
peritoneo membrana serosa que forma la envoltura de la cavidad abdominal, y que rodea la mayor parte de los órganos abdominales.
permeable capaz de ser penetrado; que permite la entrada.
peroné un hueso largo en la pierna de la rodilla al tobillo.
perseverancia cualidad de quien persiste sin flaquear.
personalidad cualidades individuales que hacen a cada individuo diferente de los demás.
perspectiva visión de cosas o hechos desde un punto deter-minado.
pertinente perteneciente a una cosa. Relevante, relacionado con lo que está siendo considerado; que viene a propósito.
petechiae manchas hemorrágicas pequeñas en la piel.
petición súplica que se expresa por escrito a una autoridad con el fin de demandar acción legal.
pH medida de acidez o alcalinidad.
piamadre de las tres meninges del cerebro y la columna vertebral, es la que se encuentra más hacia el interior.
pielografía intravenosa (PIV) la inserción de un material radiopaco en la vena con el propósito de tomarle radiografías a los riñones y uréteres.
pielonefritis inflamación del riñón, pelvis y nefrones.
pigmento todo material que genera color.
pilórico relativo a la apertura entre el estómago y el duodeno.
pinocitosis proceso a través del cual una célula absorbe grandes cantidades de líquido.
pirógeno capaz de producir fiebre.
pituitaria glándula endocrina adjunta a la base del cerebro; la glándula "maestra".
PIV ver pielografía intravenosa.
placenta estructura a través de la cual el feto se alimenta durante el embarazo.
plaga epidemia o pestilencia que puede llegar a ser fatal.
plano coronal una línea trazada de la cabeza a los pies, creando una sección delantera y trasera.
plano superficie lisa; también, punto de referencia.
plasma componente líquido de la linfa y la sangre.
plateleta células de la sangre que evitan y detienen el sangrado.
pleura membrana serosa que cubre los pulmones y reviste la cavidad torácica.
pleuresía inflamación de la pleura.
plexo red de filamentos nerviosos o vasculares.
poder documento legal por el cual se autoriza a una persona a actuar en representación de otra.
podiatra médico entrenado para diagnosticar y tratar enfermedades y trastornos de los pies.
podiatría rama de la medicina que estudia las enfermedades y trastornos de los pies.
POL laboratorio en consultorio médico (por sus siglas en inglés). Algunos consultorios han designado un espacio para establecer su propio laboratorio en el cual personas calificadas efectúan análisis y otros procedimientos de laboratorio comunes.
policitemia trastorno en el cual hay un exceso de glóbulos rojos en la sangre.
polio (poliomielitis) enfermedad sistémica aguda e infecciosa que causa inflamación de la materia gris de la espina dorsal.
pólipo tumores o crecimientos exagerados de tejido que pueden estar adheridos por un pedículo. Generalmente, se encuentran en membranas mucosas como el útero, los intestinos, el recto y la nariz.
poliuria secreción excesiva de orina.
"polling" término inglés que significa obtener una transmisión de fax no autorizada.
pons porción de la corteza cerebral que conecta la médula oblongada y el cerebelo con las porciones superiores del cerebro.
popliteo perteneciente al área posterior de la rodilla.
porcentaje tasa o proporción por cada cien.
posdata lo que se añade a una carta después de la firma.
posparto período siguiente al parto.
posterior la parte de atrás.
postoperatorio etapa siguiente a una operación quirúrgica.
postura posición y manejo del cuerpo en su totalidad.
potencial que tiene la posibilidad de suceder o existir.
PPMP (por sus siglas en inglés) análisis microscópicos realizados en el laboratorio del consultorio médico.
práctica ejercicios disciplinados y repetitivos como medio para perfeccionar una destreza o un procedimiento.
preautorización decisión por parte de la compañía de seguros de establecer la necesidad de un procedimiento médico antes de efectuarse, y de cubrir los gastos por dicho procedimiento.
precanceroso grado previo al desarrollo del cáncer.
precaución cuidado previo; medida preventiva.
precisión exactitud, certeza.
precisión corrección, exactitud.

preciso exacto, definido, certero, correcto.
precordial perteneciente al área del pecho sobre el corazón donde se ubican los electrodos para realizar el electrocardiograma.
preliminar antes de; que precede.
prenatal período antes del nacimiento.
preoperatorio período preparatorio que precede a la cirugía.
prepucio la piel suelta que cubre el final del pene.
presbicusis pérdida de la audición relacionada con la edad.
presbiopía defecto de la visión que consiste en la dificultad para enfocar objetos que están cerca.
prescribir señalar, determinar, dar dirección. Ordenar o aconsejar el uso de.
prescripción orden escrita para la preparación y administración de una medicina.
presentar pronunciar una declaración u ofrecer un servicio.
presión de pulso diferencia entre la medida sistólica y la medida diastólica.
presión sanguínea la cantidad de fuerza que ejerce el corazón en la sangre cuando bombea la sangre por las arterias.
prevención acción de evitar que algo suceda; disposición que se toma para evitar algún peligro.
preventivo que impide que algo suceda. Acción tomada para evitar una enfermedad.
prima cantidad pagada o pagable (por ejemplo, la prima de una póliza de seguros).
primario primero en orden o grado.
prioridad preferencia; el primero.
priorizar dar preferencia; ordenar en orden de importancia.
pro tem posición temporal; por el momento.
procesador ejecutar una secuencia de acciones u operaciones.
procesar tratar o preparar información por medio de un método.
proclividad inclinación o predisposición hacia algo.
procrastinación diferir o aplazar una acción.
proctología estudio del recto y el ano y de sus enfermedades.
proctoscopia inspección instrumental del recto.
proctoscopio instrumento para la inspección del recto.
procurar hacer esfuerzos por conseguir una cosa. Ocasionar, originar.
productividad cantidad de trabajo efectuado en un período de tiempo.
profesional persona que se ciñe a las técnicas y normas de su trabajo.
profesionalismo óptima realización de un trabajo.
progesterona hormona secretada por el folículo graafiano después de la expulsión del óvulo.
programado planeado, planificado. Secuencia de acciones ejecutadas por un computador.
programar establecer un calendario; ingresar en la lista de actividades por realizar.
prolapsis caída de una parte interna del cuerpo; usualmente se refiere al recto o al útero.
prominente eminente, destacado, preponderante.
prono acostado contra el vientre.
pronombre palabra que hace las veces del nombre y toma el género y número de éste.
propiedad dominio que se tiene sobre lo que se posee.
propietario persona que posee un inmueble o finca raíz y que lo administra en forma privada con ánimo de lucro.
prostaglandinas grupo de sustancias químicas secretadas por mastocitos o basófilos. Estas sustancias químicas encogen los músculos lisos en algunos órganos.
próstata glándula del sistema reproductivo masculino que rodea la porción proximal de la uretra.
prostatectomía intervención quirúrgica para extraer la totalidad o parte de la glándula prostática (próstata).
prótesis extensión artificial que reemplaza una parte del cuerpo que falta.
protocolo plan de tratamiento, a menudo experimental, utilizado para determinar la efectividad de nuevos tratamientos o medicinas.
protozoario animal unicelular.
protrombina sustancia química existente en la sangre que ayuda a la coagulación.
provechoso beneficioso, lucrativo.
provisiones conjunto de cosas necesarias; estipulación.
provocar mover a alguien a hacer algo; inspirar.
proximal punto más cercano al centro (tronco del cuerpo) o al punto de unión al cuerpo.
proyectar disponer, preparar con intención y claridad.
prudente cauteloso. Que actúa con juicio.
prueba de galera material impreso en forma preeliminar, para ser corregido.
prueba precisa y cierta (PPC) se refiere a un estándar para realizar procedimientos de laboratorio para asegurar la veracidad de los resultados.
pruebas sanguíneas cruzadas prueba de sangre usada para asegurar la compatibilidad del donante con el receptor cuando hay transfusión de sangre.
prurito picazón severo.
pruritus ani picazón alrededor del ano.
psicodélicos drogas alucinógenas.
psicología estudio de los procesos mentales, tanto normales como anormales, y sus efectos sobre el comportamiento.
psicológico relativo a la mente.
psicólogo persona especializada en el estudio de la estructura y función del cerebro y sus procesos mentales.
psiconeuroinmunología ciencia que estudia la conexión entre el cerebro, el comportamiento y la inmunología.
psicopático relativo a un trastorno mental.
psicosis disturbio mental de tal magnitud que se presenta una desintegración de la identidad y una pérdida del contacto con la realidad.
psicosomático relativo a la interrelación entre las emociones y el cuerpo.
psicoterapia tratamiento de enfermedades mentales a través de hipnosis, psicoanálisis y otras técnicas.
psiquiatra médico especializado en las enfermedades y los trastornos de la mente, incluyendo neurosis y psicosis.
psiquiatría rama de la medicina que se encarga del diagnóstico, tratamiento y prevención de las enfermedades mentales.
psoriasis enfermedad inflamatoria crónica caracterizada por parches escamosos en la piel.
ptosis caída de un órgano o parte, por ejemplo el párpado superior o el riñón.
pubertad época de la vida en que se manifiesta la aptitud para la reproducción.
púbico perteneciente a la sección media del tercio bajo del abdomen, también llamado hipogastro.
pulmón órgano de la respiración localizado al interior de la cavidad torácica.
pulmonar relativo a los pulmones.
pulso palpitación causada por el proceso intermitente de contracción y expansión de una arteria.
punción perforación realizada por un instrumento puntudo.
puntuación conjunto de signos ortográficos que se emplean para puntuar y aclarar el significado de una frase.
puntual pronto, diligente, exacto; a tiempo.
puntura lumbar inserción de una aguja entre las vértebras en el área lumbar con el objeto de extraer fluido de la espina.
pupila apertura del iris para la transmisión de luz.
purgar evacuar, purificar.
Purkinje red de fibras en el músculo cardiaco que transportan los impulsos eléctricos resultantes en la contracción de los ventrículos.
pústula elevación pequeña de la piel llena de linfa o pus.

QA certificación de calidad (por sus siglas en inglés). Conjunto de reglas, procedimientos y prácticas que se utilizan como estándares para obtener resultados de laboratorio confiables. La certificación de calidad se aplica a los diferentes procesos que incluyen la calibración y el mantenimiento del equipo, el control de

calidad, los exámenes de competencia y entrenamiento para los técnicos del laboratorio.
QC control de calidad (por sus siglas en inglés). El control de calidad determina estándares confiables para garantizar el óptimo desempeño del equipo de laboratorio.
QNS cantidad no suficiente (por sus siglas en inglés).
quadriceps femoris músculo grande en la superficie anterior del muslo que está compuesto de cuatro músculos.
queloide engrosamiento de nuevo tejido de piel; una cicatriz.
químico una sustancia simple o compuesta usada en procesos químicos.
quimo la mezcla de comida parcialmente digerida y las secreciones digestivas que se encuentran en el estómago y el intestino delgado durante la digestión de una comida.
quimoterapia el uso de agentes químicos en el tratamiento de la enfermedad, asociado usualmente con terapia de cáncer.
quiropráctica un sistema de sanación basado en la teoría de que la enfermedad resulta de la falta de función normal de los nervios; el tratamiento por la manipulación científica ajuste específico de las estructuras del cuerpo, como la columna vertebral.
quiropráctico proveedor de salud que usa los métodos quiroprácticos para tratar pacientes.
quiste una vejiga; cualquier saco que contiene fluido.
quístico perteneciente a un quiste; en enfermedad, se refiere a una condición con múltiples quistes.

R/O descartar (por sus siglas en inglés).
racional basado en la razón.
racionalización explicar con la razón; concebir explicaciones plausibles por actos determinados.
radiación electromagnética rayos producidos por la colisión de haz de electrones con un objetivo de metal en un tubo de rayos X.
radiación emisión y difusión de rayos; producto de los rayos X y del radio.
radial relativo a la arteria radial o al pulso que se ha tomado en la arteria radial.
radio hueso largo del antebrazo.
radioactivo capaz de emitir energía radiante.
radiografía fotografía por rayos X o por efecto del radio que visualiza los tejidos y órganos del cuerpo.
radiología estudio de la radiación y de sus usos y beneficios en el diagnóstico y tratamiento de enfermedades.
radiólogo médico que diagnostica y trata enfermedades a partir del uso de energía radiante.
radionúclidos tipo de átomo utilizado en medicina nuclear para el diagnóstico y tratamiento de enfermedades.
radio-opaco impenetrable por los rayos X y otras formas de radiación.
rales sonido inusual escuchado en los bronquios durante el examen de la respiración.
ramificación subdivisión o consecuencia.
raquitismo enfermedad de los huesos debida primordialmente a una deficiencia de vitamina D.
rasgo característica.
RDS examen de certificación (por sus siglas en inglés). RDS (Role Delineation Study) es un estudio de análisis ocupacional realizado en 1997 por la AAMA (Asociación Americana de Asistentes Médicos) y por NBME (Junta Nacional de Exámenes para Médicos) con el fin de identificar los conocimientos y aptitudes básicas necesarias para los profesionales de la salud entrenados en asistencia médica.
reactividad tasa de desintegración nuclear de un reactor.
reagente sustancia involucrada en una reacción química.
realzar intensificar, mejorar.
reason rule se refiere al propósito o razón para ejecutar un examen o procedimiento; criterio utilizado por una compañía de seguros para determinar la cobertura.
recepción acción o efecto de recibir; reunión social.
recepcionista persona encargada de recibir a los visitantes, pacientes o clientes, y de contestar llamadas.
receptor terminación nerviosa periférica de un nervio sensorial que responde a estímulos.
recesivo que tiende a la recesión; característica aparentemente suprimida durante la concepción para dar prioridad a una característica dominante; organismo que posee una o más características recesivas.
recibo constancia escrita de que algo ha sido recibido.
recipiente aquel que recibe.
reciprocidad intercambio mutuo, especialmente el intercambio de privilegios especiales.
reconciliar proceso a través del cual se comparan las cuentas llevadas en el talonario de cheques con el extracto de cuenta.
recreo tiempo libre, alejado de las tensiones y responsabilidades del trabajo.
rectal relativo al recto.
recto parte inferior del intestino grueso entre el sigmoide y el canal anal.
rectocel protrusión de la pared vaginal y de la pared anterior del recto a través de la vagina.
recurrente que vuelve a suceder.
recurso fuente de apoyo o de provisiones y suministros.
reducir restaurar las terminaciones de un hueso fracturado a su relación normal.
redundante repetitivo; reiterativo; superfluo.
reembolsar pagar o recompensar por dinero que ya se ha gastado, o por pérdidas o daños en los que se ha incurrido.
referencia fuente de información o autoridad.
reflejo responsa involuntaria a un estímulo.
refracción modificación en la dirección y velocidad de una onda al cambiar el medio en que se propaga. Se produce refracción de la luz cuando ésta pasa del medio aéreo al líquido.
refractivo que produce refracción.
régimen regulación de dieta, hábitos de sueño, ejercicio y estilo de vida para mantener una buena salud y/o mejorarla.
registrado legalmente certificado o autenticado.
registro documentación formal u oficial de ítems, nombres o acciones; relación de dinero que se ha gastado; listado de personas calificadas en un área particular.
regla de Nagel método para predecir la fecha de nacimiento.
regulaciones en el POL estándares establecidos para certificación de calidad (QA por sus siglas en inglés) y control de calidad (QC por sus siglas en inglés) en el laboratorio de un consultorio médico (POL por sus siglas en inglés) con el fin de garantizar resultados confiables.
regular establecer control o dirección.
regulatorio control basado en reglas establecidas; acción de adaptarse a ciertas reglas con el fin de alcanzar la mayor eficiencia y resultados precisos y confiables.
rehabilitar devolver a su condición de funcionamiento normal; restaurar.
reincidencia recurrencia de una enfermedad o de unos síntomas; vuelta a una condición previa.
reino dominio, esfera.
reiterar decir o hacer más de una vez.
rejuvenecer renovar, otorgar cualidades juveniles.
reluctante reacio, contrario a algo.
remedio cualquier cosa que alivie o cure una enfermedad.
remisión período durante el cual el paciente está libre de síntomas o de la enfermedad que lo aquejó.
remoto a distancia; que sucedió hace mucho tiempo o en un lugar lejano.
renal relativo al riñón.
renovar restaurar, dar la apariencia de nuevo.
Rentas Internas Internal Revenue en inglés; la división del gobierno federal encargada de implementar las leyes de impuestos y de la recolección de impuestos.
repolarización reestablecimiento de un estado polarizado en una fibra nerviosa o muscular después de la contracción o conducción de un impulso nervioso.

represión acción de contener o forzar ideas o impulsos dolorosos en el inconsciente.
reproductivo relativo a la reproducción.
res ipsa loquitur expresión latina que significa que la cosa habla por sí misma.
resaca malestar que sigue a la ingestión de una cantidad considerable de alcohol.
residencia período durante el cual el médico recibe entrenamiento y especialización en la rama de la medicina de su escogencia.
residual relativo a lo que queda como residuo o remanente.
resistencia oposición.
resonancia cualidad del sonido escuchada en la percusión del pecho; intensificación y prolongación del sonido por reflexión o por la vibración de un objeto cercano.
respetuoso considerado, honorable.
respiración acción de tomar oxígeno para el funcionamiento del cuerpo y de soltar dióxido de carbono.
respiratorio relativo a la respiración.
respiro tregua, aplazamiento de algo que es doloroso o agotador.
respondeat superior expresión latina que significa "dejar que el maestro responda".
responsabilidad deber, obligación.
responsabilidad legal cualquier cosa por la que una persona es responsable o por la que está legalmente atada u obligada.
restringido limitado; exclusivo para cierto grupo.
retención incapacidad de evacuar la orina que está en la vejiga.
retículo endoplásmico un organelo dentro del citoplasma de una célula.
reticuloendotelial relativo al grupo de células que parecen ayudar en la producción de glóbulos rojos y en la desintegración de los que ya han cumplido su función.
retina capa más profunda del ojo que reciba la imagen formada por el lente.
retinopatía degeneración de la retina causada por una reducción del suministro de sangre.
retiro remoción de algo que ha sido depositado.
retracción reducción o disminución en el volumen de los tejidos; acción de echarse para atrás.
retraso acción de ir despacio, de llegar tarde o de posponer. Desarrollo físico o mental lento.
retroflexionado relativo al útero cuando éste se voltea hacia atrás.
retrógrado relativo a un procedimiento con rayos X para el cual un material radioopaco se instila a través de un catéter en la vejiga, uréteres y riñones.
retroperitoneal detrás del peritoneo; posterior a la cubierta peritoneal de la cavidad abdominal.
retrovertido relativo al útero cuando el órgano se voltea hacia atrás en su totalidad.
retrovirus partículas infecciosas que contienen sólo el material genético RNA.
revalidación renovación o confirmación de credenciales.
revocar cancelar, retirar, retractar.
ribosoma organelo al interior del citoplasma de la célula.
riesgo peligro. Probabilidad de pérdida, daño o lesión.
rinitis inflamación de la mucosa nasal.
rinitis alérgica inflamación de la nariz causada por una alergia.
riñon un órgano en forma de frijol que excreta orina y está localizado retroperitonealmente, alto en la parte de atrás de la cavidad abdominal.
rinoplastia cirugía plástica de la nariz.
ritmo espacio de tiempo o movimiento medido; que ocurre en forma regular.
roentgen relativo a los rayos X. Unidad de cantidad de radiación.
ROM rango de movimiento (por sus siglas en inglés). Se refiere al grado de movimiento de articulaciones y extremidades.
rotar mover(se) alrededor de un eje.
rubéola enfermedad viral contagiosa leve pero que puede causar graves daños en el feto de la mujer embarazada que desarrolla la enfermedad.
rubor repentina coloración rojiza de la piel.
ruptura violación de la ley, de un contrato o de otro acuerdo.

sacrilegio profanación de una cosa sagrada. Atentado contra una persona digna de veneración.
sacro cinco vértebras fusionadas que se encuentran entre el cóccix y la vértebra lumbar de la columna vertebral.
sagital relativo al plano resultante de la división del cuerpo por la mitad creando un lado derecho y un lado izquierdo.
saliva secreción digestiva de las glándulas salivares.
salpingectomía remoción quirúrgica de una o de las dos trompas de Falopio.
salpingo-ooforectomía extirpación quirúrgica de uno o ambos ovarios y de una o las dos trompas de Falopio.
salud estado de completo bienestar físico y mental o social.
sancionar convertir en ley.
sarampión enfermedad aguda altamente contagiosa caracterizada por la presencia de erupciones maculopustulares.
sarcoma tumor maligno de los tejidos conectivos, músculos o huesos.
sartorio músculo largo y delgado del muslo; el músculo más largo del cuerpo.
sebo secreción grasa de la piel.
secreción separación de ciertos materiales por actividad glandular.
secretaria persona encargada de la correspondencia.
sector sección y división.
secuencia orden o sucesión.
secuencialmente organizado en secuencia, en orden.
secundario que viene en segundo lugar.
sedar producir un estado de calma; utilizar un fármaco u otro agente para producir un efecto tranquilizante.
sedentario que permanece sentado demasiado tiempo; inactividad.
sedimentación formación o depósito de sedimento. En la sangre, se refiere a la velocidad en la que los eritrocitos se asientan cuando se agrega un anticoagulante a la sangre.
segmento parte o sección de un órgano o del cuerpo.
seguridad ausencia de miedo o ansiedad; ausencia de peligro o pérdida.
seguro a salvo, libre de daño; un contrato que garantiza una compensación por una situación específica.
semen mezcla de secreciones de varias glándulas y órganos del sistema reproductivo masculino, que se expele durante el orgasmo.
semilunar válvulas del corazón localizadas entre los ventrículos y la arteria pulmonar y la aorta.
senilidad debilidad del cuerpo y de la mente debida a la vejez.
sensibilidad susceptibilidad anormal a una sustancia.
sensorial relativo a los nervios que reciben y transmiten estímulos desde los órganos de los sentidos.
septo pared membranosa que divide dos cavidades, como en el corazón o la nariz.
serie grupo de cosas de la misma clase ordenadas una después de otra.
serrado que tiene dientes como un serrucho.
SIDS por sus siglas en inglés, fallecimiento repentino e inexplicable de un infante menor de un año.
sífilis enfermedad venérea comunicable que se propaga por contacto sexual.
sigmoide sección del intestino largo en forma de S localizada entre el colon descendiente y el recto.
sigmoidoscopia inspección del sigmoide con un instrumento.
signos cardíacos principales signos: temperatura, pulso, respiración y presión arterial.
simetría estado en el cual una parte corresponde exactamente a la otra en tamaño, forma y posición.
simpático porción del sistema nervioso autónomo.
simple relativo a una fractura ósea sin implicación de la superficie de la piel.
simultáneo que ocurre al mismo tiempo.
sinapsis el espacio diminuto entre el axón de una neurona y la dendrita de otra.

síncope colapso. Condición en la cual el pulso se vuelve rápido pero débil, la presión sanguínea disminuye, y el paciente se ve pálido y sudoroso.
síncope desvanecimiento, desmayo; forma transciende de inconsciencia.
síndrome combinación de síntomas con una enfermedad o trastorno.
síndrome de alcoholismo fetal grupo de defectos en infantes nacidos de madres que consumieron alcohol durante el embarazo.
síndrome de Cushing un desorden que resulta de la hipersecreción de los glucocorticoides de la corteza adrenal.
síndrome del tunel carpal (STC) los síntomas asociados con el atrapamiento del nervio intermedio en los huesos carpales y en el ligamento transverso de la muñeca.
síndrome nefrótico término aplicado a la enfermedad renal de cualquier causa caracterizada por edema masivo, proteinuria, y a menudo elevación de los niveles de colesterol y de lípidos.
sinergismo una cosa que estimula la acción de otra que hace que el efecto de las dos es más grande que la suma de los efectos individuales.
sinovial articulación móvil, también llamada diartrosis.
síntoma cualquier cambio perceptible del cuerpo o de sus funciones que indica una enfermedad o la fase de una enfermedad.
sinusitis inflamación de los senos nasales.
sistema grupo de órganos que trabajan juntos con el fin de ejecutar una función del cuerpo.
sistema linfático red de vasos transparentes que transportan el fluido linfático a través del cuerpo.
sistemático que sigue un sistema o plan.
sístole la fase de contracción del corazón; la cantidad de presión sanguínea máxima.
SN nodo sinoatrial (por sus siglas en inglés). Fuente del impulso nervioso que origina el latido del corazón; marcapasos.
sobregiro cantidad que excede de los créditos o fondos disponibles en una cuenta.
Sociedad Americana para la Ciencia del Laboratorio Clínico American Society for Clinical Laboratory Science (ASCLS por sus siglas en inglés).
sofisticado opuesto a lo simple o natural; muy refinado; altamente complejo o avanzado en forma, estilo, técnica, etc.
solaz descanso, placer. Consuelo de una pena.
solicitar pedir.
sólo solamente.
solución normal salina solución con el mismo contenido salino al que se encuentra en el interior de una célula sanguínea.
somático físico. Relativo al cuerpo, a diferencia de la mente.
sonar aparato que transmite ondas sonoras de alta frecuencia en agua y registra las vibraciones reflejadas desde un objeto.
sonido lo que se puede oír.
soplo sonido adventicio de origen venoso o arterial que se escucha en la auscultación; usualmente se refiere al sonido producido por la mezcla de la sangre arterial y venosa at dyalisis shunts.
soportar sostener; aguantar parte del peso.
sordera sensorineural pérdida de audición causada por una falla en la transmisión de los nervios al interior del oído interno del nervio auditivo.
STC ver síndrome de tunel carpal.
suave tipo de tejido muscular involuntario que se encuentra en órganos internos.
subaracnoide espacio entre la piamadre y el aracnoide que contiene fluido cerebroespinal.
subcutáneo debajo de la piel.
subdural debajo de la dura-madre; espacio entre el aracnoide y la dura-madre.
subjetivo relativo a la persona que está pensando, diciendo o haciendo algo; personal; relativo al síntoma de una enfermedad, sentido por el paciente pero no percibido por otros.
sublimación expresión de ciertos impulsos, especialmente sexuales, en formas constructivas y socialmente aceptables.
sublingual bajo la lengua.
subpoena duces tecum expresión latina que se refiere a un proceso en la corte iniciado por una parte en litigio, producción contundente de documentos específicos y otros ítems, y material relevante a los hechos en cuestión en procedimientos judiciales adjuntos.
subsecuente siguiente, que viene después.
substancial considerable, importante, grande.
succión aspiración por presión; acción de chupar o sorber.
superficial en la superficie.
superior sobre o más alto.
supernatante que flota en la superficie.
supervisor persona a cargo; que se asegura de que se cumplan las reglas y los procedimientos para lograr los resultados esperados.
supino acostado boca arriba.
suplemento algo agregado; sección adicional o extra.
supositorio material medicado en forma de cono o de cilindro para insertar en el recto o vagina.
suprapúbico sobre el arco púbico.
supresión cesación del funcionamiento del riñón, ausencia de secreción de orina; en psicología, se refiere a la exclusión deliberada de una idea, deseo o sentimiento de la consciencia.
supresor persona que calla o impide una acción.
surfactante molécula grasa en las membranas respiratorias.
susceptible que tiene poca resistencia a una enfermedad o a una proteína foránea.
sustituto persona que reemplaza a otra persona.
sutura costura de los bordes de una llaga o herida.
symphisis pubis conexión de los huesos púbicos en la media línea al frente.

tabla de Snellen tabla de letras del alfabeto utilizada para evaluar la visión a distancia.
tacto sentimiento delicado de las conveniencias; destreza en la manera de decir las cosas sin ofender.
tálamo porción del cerebro que descansa entre el cerebro y el mesencéfalo o cerebro medio.
tallo verde una fractura incompleta que le ocurre a los niños.
taquicardia rapidez anormal de la acción cardiaca.
tarsos los siete huesos del empeine.
TCO ver técnico certificado de oftalmología.
teclear presionar una palanca o tecla, como en una máquina de escribir, operar la máquina con el dedo.
técnica aséptica forma de realizar tareas sin contaminación de organismos.
técnico certificado de oftalmología una persona entrenada y certificada en procedimientos de exámenes de diagnóstico y en el examen limitado del ojo.
técnico de emergencia médica (TEM) un individuo entrenado para responder en situaciones de emergencia y proveer tratamiento médico inicial adecuado.
técnico de laboratorio profesional especializado en el área de la salud que lleva a cabo análisis químicos, microscópicos y bacteriológicos en sangre, tejidos y fluidos corporales.
técnico en radiología persona entrenada en las técnicas para preparar el filme y tomar la radiografía.
técnico farmaceuta (PT por sus siglas en inglés) trabajador de la salud entrenado para asistir al farmaceuta en la preparación y la dispensación de medicinas.
técnico para el cuidado de pacientes (PCT por sus siglas en inglés) trabajador de la salud entrenado tanto en enfermería como en asistencia médica para proporcionar ayuda a pacientes durante su permanencia en el hospital.
técnico relativo a un arte, ciencia u oficio particular; que requiere un talento especial.
tecnología la práctica de una ciencia o de todas las ciencias aplicadas que tienen un valor práctico o un uso industrial.

tecnólogo persona entrenada en una tecnología particular; capaz de aplicar los métodos de la técnica necesaria en un área o arte particular.
tejido colección de células similares y fibras que forman la estructura del cuerpo.
teleconferencia reunión sostenida a través de líneas telefónicas con la incorporación de equipos de video.
temblor movimiento involuntario.
temperatura grado de calor de un cuerpo viviente; grado de calor o frío de una sustancia; usualmente se refiere a la elevación del calor corporal.
temporal relativo al hueso temporal del cráneo.
tendinitis inflamación de un tendón.
tendón de Aquiles un tendón que une el músculo gastrocnemio de la pierna al talón.
tendón de la corva un grupo de músculos del muslo posterior.
tendón tejido conectivo fibroso cuya función es unir los músculos a los huesos.
tentativo experimental; provisional, temporal.
teoría creencia no comprobada en la práctica; principio general en el que se basa una ciencia.
terapeuta de la respiración persona entrenada para efectuar procedimientos con el fin de mantener o mejorar la función ventilatoria del tracto respiratorio.
terapeuta ocupacional trabajador de la salud encargado de diseñar y llevar a cabo actividades con pacientes que están limitados por enfermedad o lesión física, disfunción psicológica, retraso mental o problemas de aprendizaje, pobreza o diferencias culturales, o vejez, con el objeto de maximizar la independencia de estos pacientes, prevenir su invalidez y mejorar su salud.
terapeuta persona que practica los tratamientos curativos y preventivos de una aenfermedad o de una condición anormal.
terapéutico que tiene propiedades medicinales o curativas; relativo a los resultados obtenidos después de un tratamiento.
terapia de manipulación tratamiento o procedimiento que implica el uso de las manos; movimiento de una coyuntura para determinar su rango de extensión y de flexión; técnicas manuales utilizadas por osteópatas.
tercera parte en la industria de los seguros médicos, persona que no es el paciente, esposo o pariente responsable de pagar una porción o la totalidad de los costos médicos incurridos por el paciente.
térmico relativo al calor; activado por el calor.
terminación finalización.
terminal final; enfermedad terminal, se refiere a una condición que no se puede revertir.
terminología procedimental actual (TPA) listado numérico de procedimientos efectuados en una práctica médica; identificación estandarizada de procedimientos. Publicado por la Asociación Médica Americana.
termografía técnica para detectar y registrar en filme áreas frías y áreas calientes del cuerpo por medio de un detector infrarrojo que reacciona al flujo sanguíneo.
termómetro instrumento utilizado para medir la temperatura.
testículos gónadas masculinas del escroto que producen la esperma.
testosterona hormona masculina secretada por los testículos que causa y mantiene las características masculinas secundarias.
tetania espasmos tónicos intermitentes causados por una inadecuada cantidad de hormona paratiroides.
tétano enfermedad infecciosa aguda causada por las toxinas del bacilo tetani.
thesaurus diccionario de sinónimos y antónimos.
thin prep método para preparar especimenes para citología.
TIA ataque isquémico transiente, por sus siglas en inglés. Interrupción temporal del flujo sanguíneo en el cerebro causado por pequeñas coagulaciones que obstruyen los vasos sanguíneos.
tibia hueso largo de la pierna que se encuentra entre la rodilla y el tobillo.
tibialis anterior músculo de la pierna.
tiempo flexible se refiere a la práctica de permitir horas de trabajo dentro de un rango de tiempo.
timo órgano localizado en la cavidad mediastinal anterior y sobre el corazón.
tinnitus zumbido o tintineo en el oído que sólo lo oye la persona afectada.
tirante tenso, ajustado.
tiroidectomía extracción quirúrgica de la tiroides.
tiroides glándula endocrina localizada en la base anterior del cuello.
tolerancia diferencia entre lo máximo y lo mínimo; cantidad de variación permitida por un estándar.
tomografía axial computarizada (TAC) una serie de imágenes de rayos X del cuerpo usadas para construir una imagen tridimensional.
tono muscular estado de contracción muscular en el cual una porción de lasa fibras se contraen mientras las otras están en estado de relajación.
tono frecuencia de vibraciones de sonido que permite clasificar el sonido en una escala de alto a bajo.
tonómetro instrumento para medir la tensión o presión intraocular.
tópico relativo a un área específica; local.
torácico relativo al tórax o al pecho.
tórax pecho; cavidad encerrada por las costillas y que contiene el corazón y los pulmones
torcedura lesión de un músculo debido a la tensión causada por el uso incorrecto o el abuso.
torniquete cualquier método utilizado para apretar una extremidad para producir presión en una arteria y controlar el sangrado; también se utiliza para dilatar una vena para la extracción de sangre o para la inserción de una aguja con el fin de instilar inyecciones intravenosas.
tortícolis rigidez del cuello causada por la contracción de los músculos del cuello. Dichos músculos tiran la cabeza hacia un lado mientras tiran la barbilla hacia el otro lado. Este trastorno puede ser congénito o adquirido.
tosferina enfermedad infecciosa aguda que afecta la parte superior de las vías respiratorias. Se caracteriza por vigorosos y repetidos ataques de tos. Típicamente, la persona tose de 5 a 10 veces sin poder tomar aliento. Cuando la tos finaliza, el aire es inhalado con tanta fuerza que suena al entrar en la tráquea.
toxina sustancia venenosa o compuesto de vegetal, animal o bacterial.
toxoide toxina tratada con el fin de destruir su toxicidad, pero sigue siendo capaz de inducir la formación de anticuerpos mediante su inyección.
TPA ver terminología procedimental actual.
TQM gestión de calidad total, por sus siglas en inglés. Se refiere a un estilo de gestión que utiliza QA (certificación de calidad) y QC (control de calidad) para mantener la más alta calidad de ejecución a través de la totalidad del proceso, y no sólo para asegurar que los resultados sean correctos o satisfactorios.
tracción acción de tirar; en el caso de fracturas, se aplica tracción en línea recta para estirar los músculos contraídos y permitir el reajuste de los fragmentos óseos.
trampa peligro escondido para engañar a alguien.
tranquilizante droga que causa el retraso de la función corporal o de la actividad nerviosa.
transacción acuerdo entre persona s o empresas.
transcribir escribir en un libro o documento lo que está escrito en otro libro o documento.
transcripción copia realizada directamente de un registro original, especialmente de una copia oficial de los registros educativos de un estudiante.
transdermal que atraviesa la piel.
transductor dispositivo que recibe la potencia de un sistema mecánico, electromagnético o acústico y la transmite a otro, generalmente en forma distinta.

transfusión inyección de la sangre de una persona en las venas de otra persona.
transición acción de pasar de una condición, lugar o actividad a otra.
transiluminación colocación de una luz a través de una cavidad u órgano del cuerpo para inspeccionarlo.
transmitido enviado de una persona, lugar o cosa a otra.
transmitir impartir, como una idea; transferir.
transponer poner una cosa en lugar de otra; trastocar letras o palabras.
transportador el que carga, transporta: en seguros, es la compañía que provee la póliza.
transuretral a través de la uretra; se refiere a la extirpación de la próstata a través de la pared uretral.
transverso acostado a través; segmento del intestino grueso que reposa de un lado al otro del abdomen; línea horizontal dibujada de un lado al otro del cuerpo o de cualquier estructura.
trapecio músculo grande de la espalda y cuello.
tráquea tubo cartilaginoso entre la laringe y el bronquio principal del árbol respiratorio.
traqueotomía apertura en la tráquea realizada quirúrgicamente para lograr que el paciente pueda respirar.
trastorno condición patológica de la mente o del cuerpo.
traumático causado por o relacionado con una lesión.
traumatizar causar trauma o lesión.
trazo en electrocardiografía, dibujo básico producido por el estilógrafo en una hoja de papel.
"treadmill", trotadora o cinta rodante aparato con una plataforma móvil que permite caminar o correr en un mismo sitio.
trendelenburg posición con la cabeza ubicada más abajo que los pies.
trepanar cortar una sección circular.
trial balance balance de comprobación, balance de sumas y saldos. Listado de los saldos de toda cuenta del libro mayor que se prepara al cierre del período contable. Incluye la sumatoria de todos los débitos y créditos en forma separada, debiendo ser iguales ambas columnas. Garantiza que el pase del libro diario al libro mayor ha sido realizado correctamente. Sirve de base para la preparación del balance general.
triangular figura que tiene tres ángulos y tres lados.
tríceps músculos posteriores del brazo que trabajan en conjunto con el bíceps; los tríceps enderezan el codo.
tricomoniasis infestación de parásitos protozoarios; usualmente sucede en la vagina.
tricúspide válvula al lado derecho del corazón, entre las cámaras. Literalmente significa tres cúspides.
trimestral dividido en tres secciones; el tercer segmento o período.
trivial insignificante, de poco valor.
trocar dar una cosa a cambio de otra.
tromboflebitis inflamación de una vena asociada con la formación de un coágulo sanguíneo.
trombosis formación de un trombo o coágulo sanguíneo.
truncar mutilar, disminuir.
tuberculosis enfermedad infecciosa causada por el bacilo tubercle; la tuberculosis pulmonar es una enfermedad inflamatoria específica de los pulmones que destruye los tejidos pulmonares.
tubo de eustaquio se refiere al tubo del oído medio que conecta con la faringe.
tubo de falopio el ovaducto; el pasaje del ovario al útero.
tumor inflamación o agrandamiento; neoplasma; a menudo se utiliza este término para indicar un crecimiento maligno.
turbidez partículas escamosas o granulares suspendidas en un líquido transparente que le dan una apariencia turbia o nublada; este término se utiliza en referencia a la orina.

úlcera lesión abierta en la piel o en las membranas mucosas del cuerpo, caracterizada por pérdida de tejido y la formación de una secreción.
úlcera stasis lesión abierta causada por estagnación o por un inadecuado suministro de sangre a un área.
umbilical relativo al ombligo.
umbral renal concentración en la cual una sustancia en la sangre no excretada normalmente por el riñón empieza a aparecer en la orina.
ungüento medicamento externo compuesto de resina y diversos cuerpos grasos; sustancia grasosa y suave con propiedades antisépticas o curativas.
único que no tiene igual. Sólo hay uno en la especie.
universal relativo al universo; general o común a todos.
UPM ultimo período menstrual (LMP por sus siglas en inglés).
uremia condición en la cual productos que normalmente sólo se encuentran en la orina se encuentran también en la sangre.
uréter tubo que lleva la orina del riñón a la vejiga.
uretra canal membranoso para la descarga externa de la orina desde la vejiga.
uretritis no específica inflamación de la uretra en hombres, y vaginitis o cervicitis en mujeres, causada por bacteria o por una alergia a una sustancia utilizada por el compañero sexual.
urgencia necesidad repentina de evacuar orina o feces.
URI infección de las vías respiratorias superiores, por sus siglas en inglés. Proceso inflamatorio que involucra la nariz y la garganta, y puede incluir los senos nasales; se refiere a los síntomas asociados con la gripa común.
urianálisis análisis de la orina para determinar sus características.
urología rama de la medicina que estudia las enfermedades y trastornos de los órganos genitourinarios.
urticaria condición inflamatoria caracterizada por la erupción de pápulas acompañadas de comezón severa.
útero órgano muscular hueco en forma de pera que pertenece al sistema reproductivo femenino al interior del cual un óvulo fertilizado se desarrolla hasta convertirse en un bebé.
UTI infección del tracto urinario, por sus siglas en inglés. Infección que ocurre al interior de los riñones, uréteres o vejiga.
utilizar usar para algún beneficio.

vacilación dificultad en comenzar un torrente de orina.
vacuna sustancia que ayuda a prevenir una enfermedad.
vacunación inoculación con virus inofensivos modificados o con otros microorganismos con el fin de producir inmunidad y prevenir enfermedades.
vagina tubo musculomembranoso que forma el conducto que va desde el útero hasta el exterior del cuerpo de la mujer.
vaginitis inflamación de la vagina.
vago el décimo nervio craneal que tiene una función motora y una función sensorial y que afecta el corazón, el estómago y otros órganos.
vale documento que sirve como prueba de que los términos de una transacción se han cumplido.
valorar determinar, evaluar la condición o el estado.
válvula una de las varias estructuras que cierran temporalmente una apertura o conducto, o que permiten el movimiento de fluido en una sola dirección.
várices venas agrandadas y retorcidas.
varicoso relativo a las várices; venas hinchadas y dilatadas, a menudo de las piernas.
vas deferens tubo excretorio de los testículos.
vasectomía corte de una porción del vas deferens.
vejiga un saco membranoso o recipiente para una secreción; la vesícula biliar, la vejiga urinaria.
vena vaso sanguíneo que conduce la sangre hacia el corazón después de recibirla de una vénula.

vena cava una de las dos venas grandes que llevan la sangre al atrio derecho del corazón.
venipuntura puntura de una vena; inserción de una aguja con el propósito de obtener una muestra de sangre o de instilar una sustancia.
venoso relativo a la vena.
ventilatorio que permite la circulación de aire fresco.
ventral relativo a la parte anterior o frontal del cuerpo.
ventrículo una de las dos cámaras inferiores del corazón; también se refiere a las cavidades al interior del cerebro.
vénula vena diminuta; vaso sanguíneo que conecta un capilar con una vena.
veraz genuino, real.
verbo parte de la frase que expresa una acción.
verificar comprobar la veracidad; certificar con hechos.
verruga elevación pequeña de la piel formada por la hipertrofia de una papila.
vértebra huesos en la espina dorsal.
vértice corona, tope de la cabeza.
vértigo de Meniere trastorno del oído caracterizado por náuseas, vomito, tinnitus y pérdida auditiva.
vesícula vejiga o pequeño saco que contiene fluido; elevación de la piel parecida a una ampolla, que contiene fluido seroso.
vesícula biliar un pequeño saco suspendido debajo del hígado que concentra y guarda la bilis.
viable con posibilidad de vida.
vial botella o tubo pequeño de vidrio en el que se guarda medicina o un químico.
vientre nombre no médico del útero.
villi vellosidades. Proyecciones pequeñas de una superficie; las vellosidades del intestino delgado absorben nutrientes durante el proceso de la digestión.
virulento venenoso, letal, maligno.
virus microorganismo simple, con frecuencia patógeno, capaz de reproducirse al interior de las células.
visceral relativo a las vísceras, los órganos internos, especialmente el abdomen.
vital esencial; relativo a la preservación de la vida.
volátil sustancia que se convierte fácilmente en gas o en vapor; esta cualidad es a menudo altamente peligrosa.
voltaje medida de fuerza electromotora.
volumen cantidad de espacio ocupado por un objeto. Se mide en unidades cúbicas.
voluntario bajo control propio.
vomitar expeler los contenidos del estómago a través de la boca.
vulnerable propenso a sufrir lesiones o accidentes.
vulva genitales externos femenino, incluidos el clítoris, la labia menor y la labia mayor.

xifoide proceso que forma la punta del esternón.

yacente acostado.
yeyuno el segmento medio del intestino delgado, que mide aproximadamente 8 pies de longitud.
yodo un elemento no metálico que pertenece al grupo alógeno.

z-tract método a través del cual se inyecta una medicina en forma intramuscular.

Index

A

B

C

D

F

J

K

L

M

N

O

P

Q

R

U